Nancy Caroline's
Emergency
Care in the Streets

Volume 2

Trauma
Shock and Resuscitation
Special Patient Populations
Operations

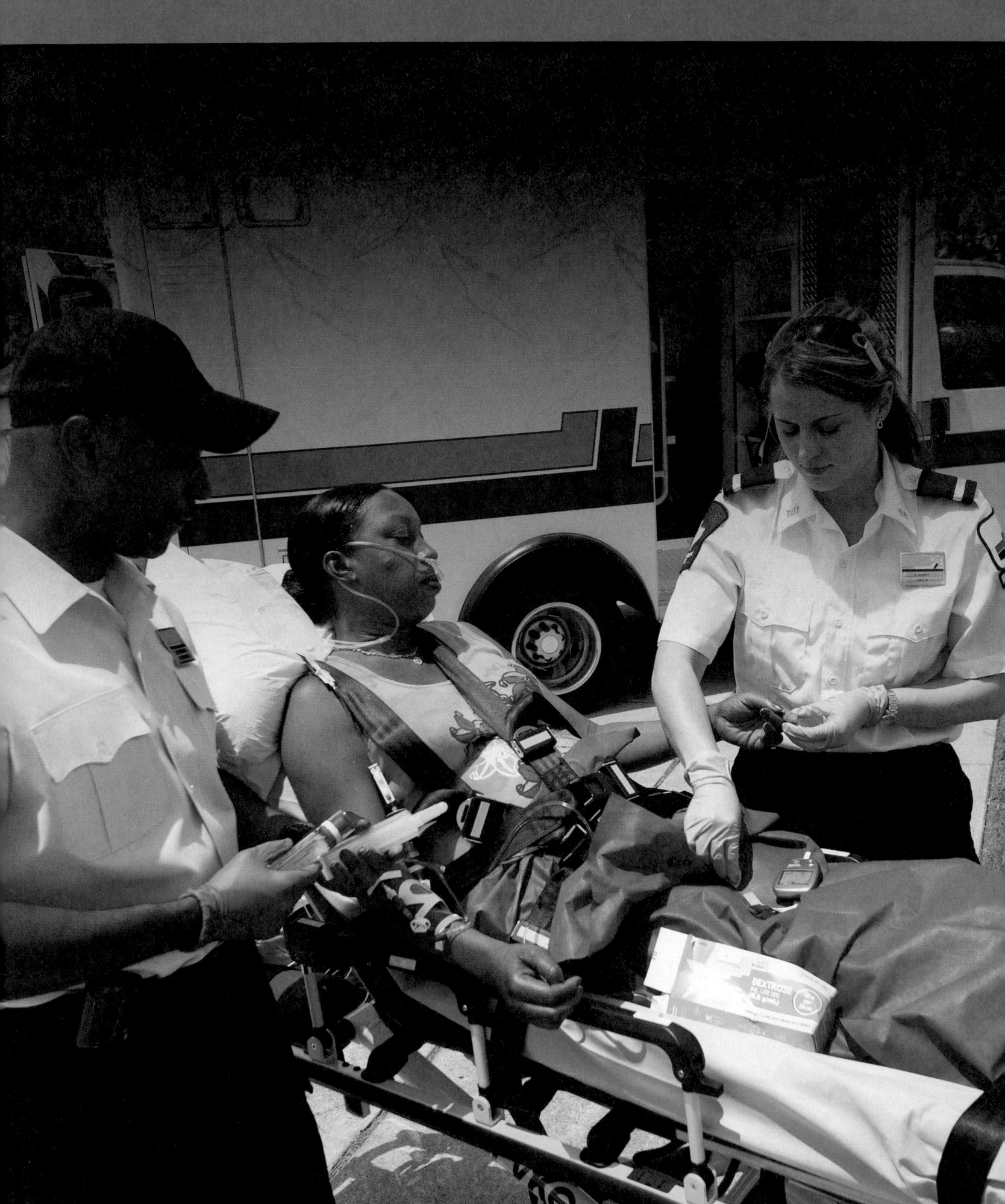

Nancy Caroline's
Emergency
Care in the Streets

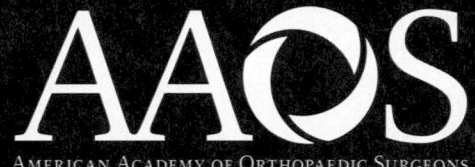

AMERICAN ACADEMY OF ORTHOPAEDIC SURGEONS

Series Editor:

Andrew N. Pollak, MD, FAAOS

Lead Editors:

Bob Elling, MPA, EMT-P
Mike Smith, BS, MICP

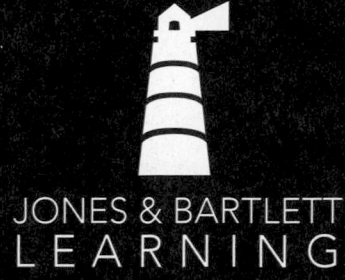

JONES & BARTLETT
LEARNING

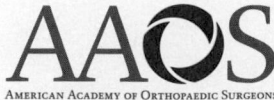

World Headquarters
Jones & Bartlett Learning
5 Wall Street
Burlington, MA 01803
978-443-5000
info@jblearning.com
www.jblearning.com

Jones & Bartlett Learning books and products are available through most bookstores and online booksellers. To contact Jones & Bartlett Learning directly, call 800-832-0034, fax 978-443-8000, or visit our website, www.jblearning.com.

Substantial discounts on bulk quantities of Jones & Bartlett Learning publications are available to corporations, professional associations, and other qualified organizations. For details and specific discount information, contact the special sales department at Jones & Bartlett Learning via the above contact information or send an email to specialsales@jblearning.com.

Editorial Credits
Chief Education Officer: Constance M. Filling
Director, Department of Publications: Marilyn L. Fox, PhD
Managing Editor: Barbara A. Scotese
Associate Senior Editor: Gayle Murray

Production Credits:

Chief Executive Officer: Ty Field
President: James Homer
SVP, Editor-in-Chief: Michael Johnson
SVP, Chief Marketing Officer: Alison M. Pendergast
Executive Publisher: Kimberly Brophy
Vice President of Sales, Public Safety Group: Matthew Maniscalco
Director of Sales, Public Safety Group: Patricia Einstein
Executive Acquisitions Editor—EMS: Christine Emerton
Managing Editor: Carol B. Guerrero
Managing Editor: Amanda J. Mitchell
Senior Editorial Assistant: Carly Lavoie

Editorial Assistant: Marisa Hines
Production Manager: Jenny L. Corriveau
Production Editor: Marcia Murray
Director of Marketing: Alisha Weisman
VP, Manufacturing and Inventory Control: Therese Connell
Composition: diacriTech
Cover Design: Kristin E. Parker
Rights & Photo Research Assistant: Gina Licata
Cover Image: © Glen E. Ellman
Printing and Binding: Courier Companies
Cover Printing: Courier Companies

To order this product, use ISBN: 978-1-4496-4586-1

Library of Congress Cataloging-in-Publication Data
Caroline, Nancy L.
  Nancy Caroline's emergency care in the streets. — 7th ed. / American Academy of Orthopaedic Surgeons.
     p. ; cm.
  Emergency care in the streets
  Includes index.
  ISBN-13: 978-1-4496-0922-1 (hardcover)
  ISBN-10: 1-4496-0922-8 (hardcover)
1. Medical emergencies. 2. Emergency medical technicians. I. American Academy of Orthopaedic Surgeons. II. Title. III. Title: Emergency care in the streets.
  [DNLM: 1. Emergency Treatment. 2. Emergency Medical Services. 3. Emergency Medical Technicians. WB 105]
  RC86.7.C38 2012
  616.02'5—dc23
                          2011017160
6048
Printed in the United States of America
16 15 14 13 12   10 9 8 7 6 5 4 3 2 1

Brief Contents

Contents

Skill Drills

Resources

Instructor Resources

Instructor's ToolKit DVD

ISBN: 978-1-4496-3609-8

The DVD includes:

- PowerPoint presentations
- Lecture outlines
- Teaching tips, enhancements, support materials, and preparation guidance
- Student activities and assignments
- Image and table bank
- Skill sheets
- Answers to end-of-chapter student questions

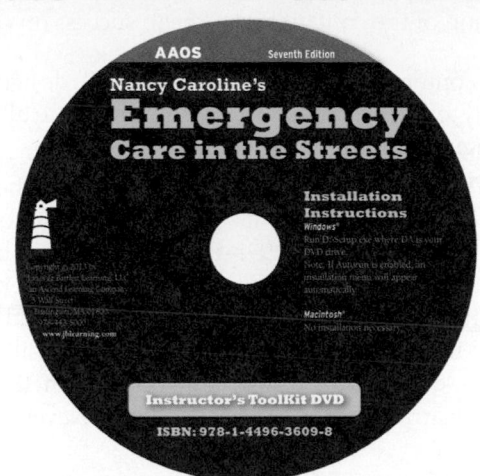

Instructor's TestBank CD

ISBN: 978-1-4496-3688-3

This powerful evaluation tool allows educators to gauge student competency through both general knowledge and critical-thinking questions. Each scenario-based, multiple-choice question is page-referenced to *Nancy Caroline's Emergency Care in the Streets, Seventh Edition*. Educators can originate tailor-made tests quickly and easily by selecting, editing, and printing a test along with an answer key.

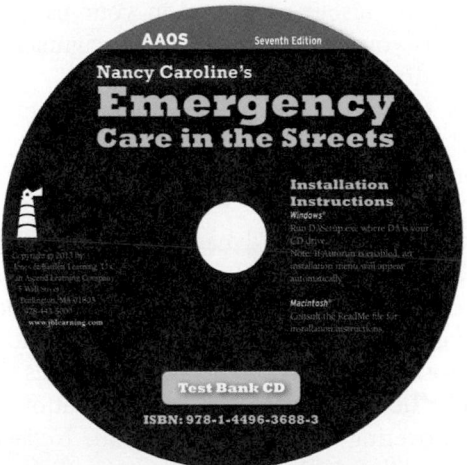

Student Resources

Student Workbook

ISBN: 978-1-4496-0924-5

This resource is designed to encourage critical-thinking and aid comprehension of the course material through a variety of activities:

- Realistic and engaging case studies
- ECG interpretation exercises
- "What would you do?" scenarios
- Skill drill activities
- Anatomy labeling exercises
- Medical vocabulary building exercises
- Complete the Patient Care Report

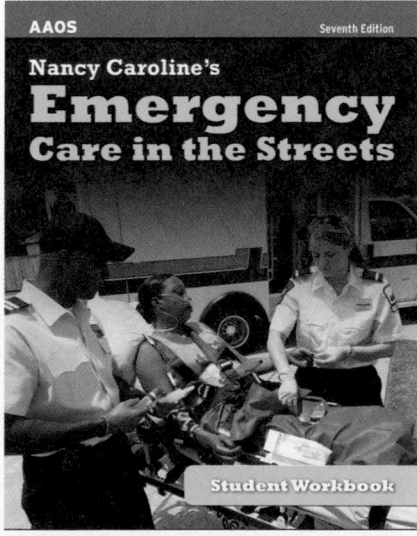

Digital Curriculum Solution Packages

Digital Curriculum Solution Packages allow educators to offer their students cutting-edge digital resources based on world-class medical content. The innovative, multifaceted online tools facilitate absolute understanding—how the human body works, how to apply the patient assessment process, how to be a confident, effective paramedic. This total comprehension and command of the content is the key to success on certification exams and in the field.

Gold standard content joins sound instructional design in a user-friendly online interface to give students a truly interactive, engaging learning experience with:

- **eBook/eWorkbook**: With the content of the *Seventh Edition* at the students' fingertips, students can take notes, listen to 9-1-1 calls, and watch animations and skill videos. Students can then reinforce their general knowledge, hone their critical-thinking skills, and perfect their psychomotor skills in the eWorkbook. The results are recorded in the integrated learning management system, *Navigate Course Manager*.
- **Navigate Course Manager**: Navigate is your complete online classroom environment. In addition to unlocking the resources offered in your package of choice, it is your tool for managing assignments, automatic grading, and classroom discussion.
- **Web Tools**: Unlock additional interactive and mobile educational resources such as a complete audio book, chapter pretests, interactive skill drills, and skill evaluation sheets.
- **Navigate TestPrep**: This dynamic tool is designed to help prepare students for state or national certification examinations by providing practice examinations and simulated certification examinations using case-based questions and detailed rationales.
- **Interactive Lectures**: Take the lectures out of the classroom! Covering the entire scope of the *National EMS Education Standards*, these interactive lectures provide anytime, anywhere access for students to an innovative educational environment.

Available packages include:

Advantage Package Print Edition:
ISBN: 978-1-4496-3817-1

- Printed Textbook
- Printed Student Workbook
- Navigate Course Manager
- Web Tools, including an Audio Book

Advantage Package Digital Edition:
ISBN: 978-1-4496-3818-4

- eBook/eWorkbook
- Navigate Course Manager
- Web Tools, including an Audio Book

Preferred Package:
ISBN: 978-1-4496-3821-4

- Printed Textbook
- Printed Student Workbook (optional)
- eBook/eWorkbook
- Navigate Course Manager
- Web Tools, including an Audio Book
- Navigate TestPrep

Premier Package:
ISBN: 978-1-4496-3822-1

- Printed Textbook
- Printed Student Workbook (optional)
- eBook/eWorkbook
- Navigate Course Manager
- Web Tools, including an Audio Book
- Navigate TestPrep
- Interactive Lectures

www.Paramedic.EMSzone.com

ISBN: 978-1-4496-3778-1

www.Paramedic.EMSzone.com is specifically designed to complement *Nancy Caroline's Emergency Care in the Streets, Seventh Edition*.

This engaging companion website provides a wealth of resources that are free and available to all, including:

- Anatomy Review
- Flashcards
- Glossary
- Ready for Review

The code printed on the front inside cover of Volume 1 provides students with special user privileges to:

- Audio Book
- Case Studies

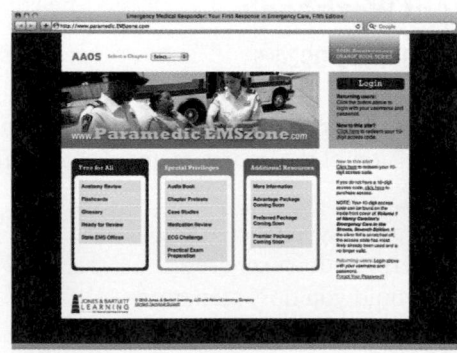

- Chapter Pretests
- Practical Exam Preparation
- Much More

Acknowledgments

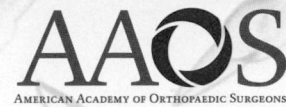

The American Academy of Orthopaedic Surgeons would like to acknowledge the editors, authors, and reviewers of Volume 2 of *Nancy Caroline's Emergency Care in the Streets, Seventh Edition*.

Series Editor

Andrew N. Pollak, MD, FAAOS
Professor of Orthopaedics, Head, Division of Orthopaedic Traumatology, University of Maryland School of Medicine
Associate Director of Trauma, R Adams Cowley Shock Trauma Center, University of Maryland Medical Center
Medical Director, Baltimore County Fire Department
Baltimore, Maryland

Lead Editors

Bob Elling, MPA, EMT-P
Albany Medical Center—Clinical Instructor
Colonie EMS Department
Times Union Center EMS
Whiteface Mountain Medical Services
Colonie, New York

Mike Smith, BS, MICP
Program Chair, Emergency Medical and Health Services
Tacoma Community College
Tacoma, Washington

Authors

Chapter 29: Bruce Butterfras, MS Ed, LP
Assistant Professor, Director of Bachelor Degree Program
Department of Emergency Health Sciences
The University of Texas Health Science Center at San Antonio
San Antonio, Texas

Chapter 30: Barry Jensen, NREMT-P, NCEE
David Geffen School of Medicine at UCLA
Center for Prehospital Care
Los Angeles, California

Chapter 31: Chad E. Brocato, DHSc, REMT-P
Adjunct Faculty
Kaplan University

Chapter 32: Charles D. Bortle, EdD, RRT, NREMT-P
Director, Center for Clinical Competency
Albert Einstein Medical Center
Philadelphia, Pennsylvania

Chapter 33: Bryan Hess, NREMT-P
EMS Chief, Department and Education Director
Gunnison Valley Health EMS
Gunnison, Colorado

Chapter 34: Bryan Hess, NREMT-P
EMS Chief, Department and Education Director
Gunnison Valley Health EMS
Gunnison, Colorado

Chapter 35: Edward "Ted" Lee, AAS, BS, MEd, NREMT-P, CCEMT-P
EMT Paramedic Program Coordinator
Trident Technical College
Charleston, South Carolina

Chapter 36: Edward "Ted" Lee, AAS, BS, MEd, NREMT-P, CCEMT-P
EMT Paramedic Program Coordinator
Trident Technical College
Charleston, South Carolina

Chapter 36: Astra Paro, NREMT-P, CCEMT-P
Meducare Ambulance
Medical University of South Carolina
Charleston, South Carolina

■ Authors continued

Chapter 37: David Ellis, BS, CCEMT-P, FP-C, CMTE
Program Manager
EagleMed, LLC
Greenville, South Carolina

Chapter 37: Daniel Doherty, AS, NREMT-P, CIC
Captain, Albany Fire Dept. (ret.)
Lead Instructor
SUNY, Cobleskill Paramedic Program
Cobleskill, New York

Chapter 38*: Frederick "Fritz" Fuller, BS, PA-C, REMT-P, MPH&TM
Former Firefighter/Paramedic West Thurston (WA) Fire and Rescue
Foreign Service Health Practitioner, United States Department of State
US Embassy Lao PDR
*The content herein represents the views of the authors and not the Department of Defense or Department of State.

Chapter 38: Bridgett Sinnott, MD
Department of Emergency Medicine
Madigan Army Medical Center
Tacoma, Washington

Chapter 38: COl Ian Wedmore, MD, FACEP, FAWM, DiMM
Austere and Wilderness Medicine Fellowship
Department of Emergency Medicine
Madigan Army Medical Center
Tacoma, Washington

Chapter 39: Bob Elling, MPA, EMT-P
Albany Medical Center—Clinical Instructor
Colonie EMS Department
Times Union Center EMS
Whiteface Mountain Medical Services
Colonie, New York

Chapter 40: Bob Elling, MPA, EMT-P
Albany Medical Center—Clinical Instructor
Colonie EMS Department
Times Union Center EMS
Whiteface Mountain Medical Services
Colonie, New York

Chapter 41: Carol Gupton, BS, NREMT-P
Emergency Provider Instruction
Omaha, Nebraska

Chapter 42: Patricia R. Chess, MD
Associate Professor of Pediatrics (Neonatology) and Biomedical Engineering
Director, Neonatal-Perinatal Medicine Fellowship Program
University of Rochester Medical Center
Golisano Children's Hospital at Strong
Rochester, New York

Chapter 42: Yogangi Malhotra, MD
Assistant Professor of Pediatrics
Division of Neonatology
Regional Perinatal Center QA Coordinator
Maria Fareri Children's Hospital at Westchester Medical Center
Valhalla, New York

Chapter 42: Nirupama Laroia, MD
Associate Professor, Department of Pediatrics/Neonatology
Medical Director, Special Care Nursery, Rochester General Hospital
Golisano Children's Hospital at Strong
University of Rochester Medical Center
Rochester, New York

Chapter 43: Stephen John Cico, MD, MEd
Assistant Professor, Pediatrics
University of Washington School of Medicine
Seattle, Washington
Associate Fellowship Director, Pediatric Emergency Medicine
Attending Physician, Emergency Medicine
Seattle Children's Hospital
Seattle, Washington

Chapter 43: Derya Caglar, MD
Assistant Professor, Pediatrics
University of Washington School of Medicine
Seattle, Washington
Attending Physician, Emergency Medicine
Seattle Children's Hospital
Seattle, Washington

■ Authors continued

Chapter 43: Kimberly P. Stone, MD, MS, MA
Assistant Professor, Pediatrics
University of Washington School of Medicine
Seattle, Washington
Co-Director, Pediatric Emergency Simulation
Attending Physician, Emergency Medicine
Seattle Children's Hospital
Seattle, Washington

Chapter 44: Keith Widmeier, NREMT-P, CCEMT-P, EMSI, BA
Wayne County EMS
Monticello, Kentucky

Chapter 45: Andrew Bartkus, RN, MSN, JD, CEN, CCRN, CFRN, NREMT-P, FP-C
Lifeguard Air Emergency Services
Albuquerque, New Mexico

Chapter 46: Anne Austin, NREMT-P, AAS
H.E.R.O. Training Company
Thomaston, Georgia

Chapter 47: Anne Austin, NREMT-P, AAS
H.E.R.O. Training Company
Thomaston, Georgia

Chapter 48: James W. Call
Fire Captain / Paramedic
Alameda County Fire Department
San Leandro, California

Chapter 49: Rob Schnepp
Division Chief, Special Operations
Alameda County Fire Department
San Leandro, California

Chapter 50: Donnell Harvin, MPH, MPA
Deputy Director, Special Operations
New York City
Office of Chief Medical Examiner
New York, New York
Adjunct Instructor, Protection Management Department, John Jay College
Executive Committee, Regenhard Center for Emergency Response Studies (RaCERS)
New York, New York

Chapter 50: Daniel Doherty, AS, NREMT-P, CIC
Captain, Albany Fire Dept. (ret.)
Lead Instructor
SUNY, Cobleskill Paramedic Program
Cobleskill, New York

Chapter 51: Daniel Doherty, AS, NREMT-P, CIC
Captain, Albany Fire Dept. (ret.)
Lead Instructor
SUNY, Cobleskill Paramedic Program
Cobleskill, New York

Chapter 52: Donnell Harvin, MPH, MPA
Deputy Director, Special Operations
New York City
Office of Chief Medical Examiner
Adjunct Instructor, Protection Management Department, John Jay College
Executive Committee, Regenhard Center for Emergency Response Studies (RaCERS)
New York, New York

Contributors

Rhonda J. Beck, NREMT-P
EMT/Paramedic Instructor
Darton College
Albany, Georgia
Crisp County EMS-Paramedic
Cordele, Georgia

Julie Chase, MSEd, FAWM, FP-C
Program Director, Immersion EMS Academy
Berryville, Virginia

Gail C. Larkin, BS, EMT-P
Medical Administrator, Medcor, Inc.
MTA East Side Access Tunnel Construction Project
Long Island City, Queens, New York

Patty Maher, MPA, EMTP
Professor/Assistant Chair—EMS
Daytona State College
Daytona Beach, Florida

Dean C. Meenach, RN, BSN, CEN, CCRN, CPEN, EMT-P
Director of EMS Education
Assistant Professor
Mineral Area College
Park Hills, Missouri

Jeanine Newton-Riner, EdD (c), MHSA, RRT, CICP, EMT-P
Operations Manager
CoastalEMS
Savannah, Georgia

Brittany Ann Williams, MHSc, BSRT, NREMT-P
Associate Professor EMS
Santa Fe College
Gainesville, Florida

Reviewers

Sean M. Ahlers, MS, NREMT-P
Emergency Training Associates
Fargo, North Dakota

Chip Anderson, EMT-P
BFC Emergency Preparedness
Training Center
Randolph, Alabama

Linda Bell, MSN, ARNP, EMT-P
Consultant Services Educational
Company
Middleburg, Florida

Tim Bobbitt, EMT-P
St. Charles County Ambulance
District
Florissant, Missouri

Kathy Boyle, MEd, MS, RRT-NPS, NREMT-P
Southeast Arkansas College
Pine Bluff, Arizona

Joyce S. Bradley, NREMT-P I/C AAS, BHCS
Program Director
Dona Ana Community College
Las Cruces, New Mexico

Serena L. Brafford, BS, NREMT-P, CCT-P
Mathias-Baker EMS
Baker, West Virginia

Scott A. Brandenburg, BS, CCEMT-P, EMS I/C
Southwestern Michigan College
Dowagiac, Michigan

Terry Brandt, NREMT-P
Montana State University – Great
Falls
South Great Falls, Montana

Max Todd Bridges, NREMTP, MBA
Upstate EMS Council
Greenville, South Carolina

Rick Brown, RN, BSN, CEN
Kaweah Delta Medical Center
Visalia, California

Shirley Bonnie Burtman, RN, NREMT-P, CIC, FMCC
Johnstown, New York

Anthony M. Caliguire, AS, REMT-P
Lieutenant
Scotia Fire Department
Scotia, New York
Paramedic Instructor Coordinator
Hudson Valley Community College
Paramedic Program
Troy, New York

Amy K. Cantwell, FP-C, NREMT-P
Stafford, Virginia

Tiffany L. Cattey, NREMT-P, ACLS-F, PALS-F, BLS-I
Campion Ambulance Service, Inc.
Waterbury, Connecticut

Ted Chialtas
Fire Captain/Paramedic
San Diego Fire-Rescue Department
Clinical Coordinator
EMSTA College
Santee, California

Russ Christiansen, NREMT-P, CCEMTP
Casper College
Casper, Wyoming

Reviewers continued

Jen Collins-Brown, MS, EMT-P
Topsfield Fire Department
Essex County Fire Chiefs Association
Topsfield, Massachusetts

Darby L. Copeland, EdD, RN, NREMT-P
Parkway West Career & Technology Center
Oakdale, Pennsylvania

Sharon Ann Cotter, APRN, FNP, MSN, NREMT-P
Foster Ambulance Corps
Foster, Rhode Island

Christopher Crabtree, MPA, CHEP, NREMT-P
Healthcare Association of Hawaii
Emergency Services
Aiea, Hawaii

Michael Crabtree, EMT-P
McLean County Area EMS System
Bloomington, Illinois

Rocky E. Cramer
Paramedic, I/C
Flint Hills Technical College
Emporia, Kansas

Jeanne Curry, RN, BSN, TNS
Paramedic, EMS Lead Instructor
Passavant Area Hospital
Jacksonville, Illinois

Jeffery D. Denney
Paramedic, Level II Instructor
Med Ed
Newnan, Georgia

Annie Dorchak, BA, NREMTP
Evergreen Fire/Rescue
Evergreen, Colorado

Rommie L. Duckworth
New England Center for Rescue and Emergency Medicine
Sherman, Connecticut

William Faust, MPA, NREMT-P
Gaston College
Dallas, North Carolina

Ronald L. Feller Sr, NRP, BS Ed
Oklahoma City Community College
Moore, Oklahoma

Melvin Dennis Fortney III, NREMTP, MS
Battalion Chief
Frederick County Division of Fire and Rescue Services
Frederick, Maryland

Scott R. Frasard, PhD, EMT-P
Cardinal Health
Albuquerque, New Mexico

Brian Fullgraf, NREMT-P, FP-C
UPMC Prehospital Services
Canonsburg, Pennsylvania

Glenn Goodman, NREMT-P
Health Education Design Solutions Inc.
Ft. Meade, South Dakota

Lt. Kathleen D. Grote, NREMTP
Anne Arundel County Fire Department
Millersville, Maryland

Chris Hainsworth, MS, NREMTP
Delaware Technical Community College
Dover, Delaware

Wendy Steel Hastings, EMT-P
LTS EMS Council
Eagles Mere, Pennsylvania

Lynn Henley, NREMT-P I/C
Director of Education & QA
AAA Ambulance Service
AHA TC Coordinator
Hattiesburg, Mississippi

Glenn R. Henry, MA, EMT-P
Athens Technical College
Athens, Georgia

David Hiltbrunn, NRP, CCTP
EMT Institute, St. Mary Corwin Pore-Hospital Care Services
Pueblo, Colorado

Catie Holstein, CCEMTP, SEI
Clinical Manager
Rural/Metro Ambulance of Greater Seattle, Inc.
Everett, Washington

James B. Huettenmueller, BS
EMS Clinical Coordinator/Instructor
Tulsa Tech
Tulsa, Oklahoma

Brian E. Johns, CCEMT-P, I/C
Lifestar EMS/Tri-State EMS Educators
West Ossipee, New Hampshire

Stacy Johnson, BS, EMT-P, I/C
EMS Program Director
Motlow State Community College
Fayetteville, Tennessee

Joe H. Jones, NREMT-P
Affiliate Faculty
Mississippi Gulf Coast Community College
Gulfport, Mississippi

Sue A. Kartman, CCEMT-P, BS
Wisconsin Indianhead Technical School
Rice Lake, Wisconsin
Madison Area Technical College
Reedsburg, Wisconsin
Northcentral Technical College
Wausau, Wisconsin

Kimberly Kidd, BS, EMT-P
Cape Fear Community College
Wilmington, North Carolina

Joshua L. Kingsmore, NRP
Spartanburg Community College
Inman, South Carolina

Tom Lateulere
Chief of Education and Training
Suffolk County Division of EMS
Hauppauge, New York

Kristina A. Long, NREMT-P, BAS
Flathead Valley Community College
Paramedicine Program
Kalispell, Montana

Reviewers continued

Eric T. Mayhew, AAS, NREMT-P
EMS Program Coordinator
Carteret Community College
Morehead City, North Carolina

Stephen E. McClure
Director
Jackson County EMS
Cottageville, West Virginia

Roger L. McDiffett, MBA, NREMT-P
Director of Community Health Services
Maniilaq EMS
Kotzebue, Alaska

Rich Meadows, EMT-P, RN, CCRN, BA, NCEE, CCT-RN
Kanawha County Emergency Ambulance Authority
Charleston, West Virginia

Travis A. Myklebust
Lewiston Fire Department
Lewiston, Idaho

Tamera Nailen, AAS, NREMT-P
Hinds Community College
Pearl, Mississippi

Thomas R. Neal
Indianapolis Fire Department
Battalion Chief of US&R Training
IN-TF1
FEMA US&R Haz Mat/WMD Work Group Chair
Indianapolis, Indiana

Melissa Osborne, BS, EMS-I, CCEMTP, NREMT-P
Ambulance Service of Manchester
Manchester, Connecticut

Elizabeth H. Owen, BS, RN, CCEMT-P
Colorado Mountain College
Edwards, Colorado

Erica Marie Paredes, EMT, MBA
EMS Clinical Specialist
Snowy River EMS Productions, LLC
Phoenix, Arizona

Vincent J. Parker, MS, NREMT-P
Faulkner State Community College
Gulf Shores, Alabama

Corey S. Pittman, NREMT-P, CCEMT-P, AASc-EMS, I/C
Mayland Community College
Spruce Pine, North Carolina

Stephen Post, NREMT-P, CIC, RF
SUNY Rockland Community College
Middletown, New York

Scott Reasor, Paramedic
EMT & Fire Training, Inc.
Priest Lake, Idaho

Lori Reeves, BA, EMT-P
Indian Hills Community College
Ottumwa, Iowa

Joseph J. Rubino
Paramedic, Instructor /Coordinator
Denton Township EMS Education
Prudenville, Michigan

Robert Russell, CCEMT-P, NREMT-P
North East Mobile Health Services
Scarborough, Maine

Todd Schanze, EMT-P
Moses Lake, Washington

Jason G. Scheiderer, BA, NREMT-P, PI
Wishard Health Service/UPUI/Indianapolis EMS
Indianapolis, Indiana

Lieutenant Jared Schreher, EMT-LP
Collin College
McKinney, Texas

Robert W. Seltzer, BS, EFO
Chief of Department
Central Coventry Fire District
Adjunct Faculty
Community College of Rhode Island
Coventry, Rhode Island

Elizabeth A. Sheils, MPH, NRP, CCEMT-P, EMS-I
Capitol Community College
Hartford, Connecticut

Brock Snedeker, MEd, NREMT
Parkway West Career and Technology Center
Oakdale, Pennsylvania

Pamela N. Taylor, EMT-P, PI
Division Chief of EMS
Westfield Fire Department
Westfield, Indiana

Eric Victorin, MBA, EMT (I), NREMTP
The Valley Hospital Emergency Medical Services
Ridgewood, New Jersey

Dawn K. Vogt, MICP, NREMTP, CCEMTP
EMS Programs Director
Denali Medical Education
Wasilla, Arkansas

Carl Voskamp, LicP
The Victoria College
Victoria, Texas

Walter B.A. Webel, BSHS, AS, NREMT-P
Savannah Technical College
Savannah, Georgia

Brittany Ann Williams, MHSc, BSRT-NPS, NREMT-P
Santa Fe College
Gainesville, Florida

David A. Young, BS, NREMT-P
Western Piedmont Community College
Morganton, North Carolina

Thomas Andrew Young Jr
Fayetteville High School Criminal Justice
Fayetteville, Tennessee

■ Photoshoot Acknowledgments

We would like to thank the following people and institutions for their collaboration on the photoshoots for this project. Their assistance was greatly appreciated.

Medical Advisor: Anthony M. Caliguire, AS, REMT-P
Lieutenant
Scotia Fire Department
Scotia, New York
Paramedic Instructor Coordinator
Hudson Valley Community College
Paramedic Program
Troy, New York

Barry Bashkoff
Cromwell Emergency Vehicles Inc.
Clifton Park, New York

Erica D'Errico
Schenectady, New York

Glen E. Ellman
Fort Worth Fire Department
Fort Worth, Texas

Paul Felts
Ballston Lake, New York

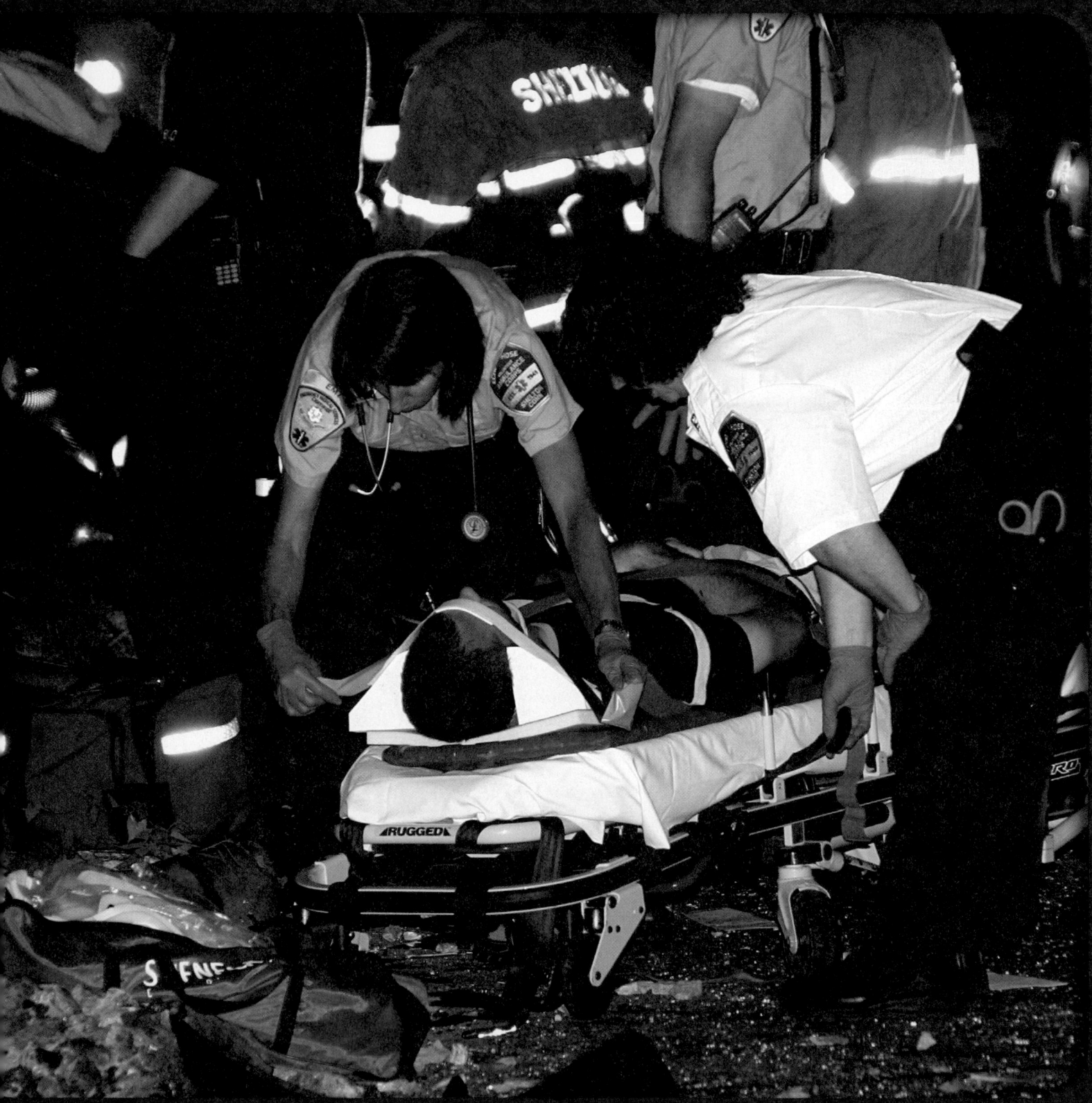

Trauma Systems and Mechanism of Injury

National EMS Education Standard Competencies

Trauma

Integrates assessment findings with principles of epidemiology and pathophysiology to formulate a field impression to implement a comprehensive treatment/disposition plan for an acutely injured patient.

Trauma Overview

Pathophysiology, assessment, and management of the trauma patient

- Trauma scoring (p 1503)
- Rapid transport and destination issues (pp 1507-1508)
- Transport mode (pp 1508-1511)

Multisystem Trauma

Recognition, pathophysiology, assessment, and management of

- Multisystem trauma (pp 1503-1511)

Pathophysiology, assessment, and management of

- Blast injuries (pp 1499-1503)

Knowledge Objectives

1. Define the term trauma and explain its relationship to energy, kinetics, and biomechanics. (pp 1483-1486)
2. Describe some of the factors that affect types of injury. (p 1484)
3. Define the terms mechanism of injury and index of suspicion and explain their relationship to the paramedic's assessment of trauma. (p 1484)
4. Define the term blunt trauma and provide an example of the mechanism of injury that would cause it to occur. (pp 1486-1497)
5. Describe how impact patterns can help the paramedic to determine or predict types of injury following motor vehicle crashes. (pp 1488-1493)
6. Describe the five types of motor vehicle crashes and the injury patterns associated with each one. (pp 1488-1493)
7. Describe the benefits of seat belt restraints during a motor vehicle crash. (p 1493)
8. Describe the four types of motorcycle crashes. (pp 1494-1495)
9. Describe the three predominant mechanisms of injury during a pedestrian versus automobile collision. (pp 1495-1496)
10. Discuss five specific factors to consider during assessment of a patient who has been injured in a fall. (pp 1496-1497)
11. Define the term penetrating trauma and provide examples of the mechanisms of injury that would cause low-, medium-, and high-velocity injuries to occur. (pp 1497-1499)
12. Describe the factors to consider during the assessment of a patient who has sustained a gunshot wound. (pp 1498-1499)
13. Discuss primary, secondary, tertiary, quaternary (miscellaneous), and quinary blast injuries, and describe the anticipated damage each one will cause to the body. (pp 1499-1503)
14. Describe the components of a blast shock wave. (p 1501)
15. Discuss considerations in the assessment and management of a patient with a blast injury. (pp 1502-1503)
16. Describe multisystem trauma and the special considerations that are required for patients who fit this category. (p 1503)
17. Outline the major components of trauma patient assessment, including considerations related to multisystem trauma. (pp 1503-1506)
18. Provide a general overview of trauma management, including considerations related to multisystem trauma. (pp 1507-1511)
19. Summarize the American College of Surgeons Committee on Trauma and Centers for Disease Control and Prevention triage decision scheme for referral to a trauma center. (p 1507-1509)
20. Describe the American College of Surgeons Committee on Trauma classification of trauma centers and how it relates to making an appropriate destination selection for a trauma patient. (pp 1507-1509)
21. Describe trauma patient management in relation to scene time and transport selection, and list the Association of Air Medical Services criteria for the appropriate use of emergency air medical services. (pp 1508-1511)

Skills Objectives

There are no skills objectives for this chapter.

Introduction

According to the Centers for Disease Control and Prevention, trauma has emerged as the primary cause of death and disability in people between ages 1 and 44 years. With improvements in health care and management of chronic diseases, death rates due to conditions such as heart disease, neoplasms, cerebrovascular events, and respiratory illnesses have decreased significantly in younger age groups.

Basic concepts of the mechanics and biomechanics of trauma will help you analyze and manage your patient's injuries. Analyzing a trauma scene is a vital skill because at the scene you are the eyes and ears of the emergency department physicians. Your paramedic-written patient history is the *only* source for physicians and surgeons to understand the events and mechanisms that led to your trauma patient's chief complaint. Your information is critical as a foundation to visualize and search for injuries that may not be apparent on physical examination.

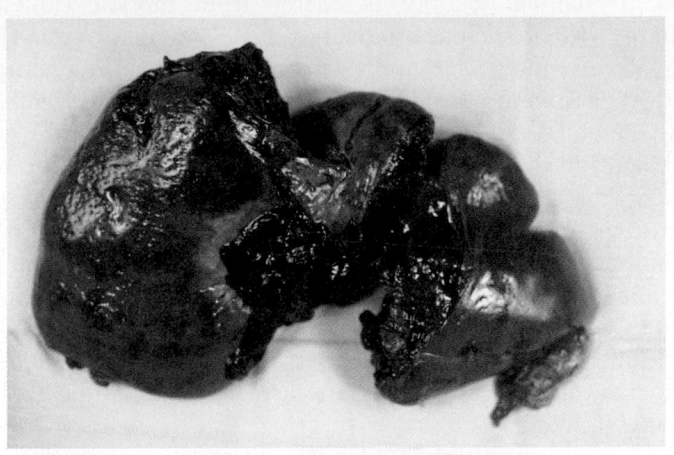
Figure 1 Traumatic injury occurs when the body's tissues are exposed to energy levels beyond their tolerance. Some traumatic injuries may not be visible. This photo shows a ruptured spleen.

Trauma, Energy, and Kinetics

<u>Trauma</u> is the acute physiologic and structural change (injury) that occurs in a patient's body when an external source of energy affects the body beyond its ability to sustain and dissipate it **Figure 1**.

Words of Wisdom

> The top five causes of trauma death are motor vehicle crashes, falls, poisonings, burns, and drownings.

If a body—your patient's body—is in an automobile that smashes into a wall, the energy delivered by an external source—the moving automobile—is released when the car is stopped by the wall. Your patient's body is moving at the same speed as the automobile, and his or her body does not have bumpers to absorb the energy from stopping. If the energy is not absorbed in other ways, the patient's body absorbs it, often resulting in bones that break and internal organs that rupture—what you see as traumatic injuries.

Different forms of energy produce different kinds of trauma. These external energy sources can be mechanical, chemical, thermal, electrical, and barometric.

YOU *are the Medic*   PART 1

You and your partner are enjoying the warm evening breeze, watching people stroll to the nearby mall and amusement park. You see someone running out of a crowd toward the ambulance, waving frantically, just as the dispatcher reports an injury in the amusement park.

The person running toward you shouts, "Someone fell! I don't know what happened—in the park—please hurry!"

You hear the dispatcher's voice, over the shouts of the people, "Report of a fall from the ferris wheel at Sixth Avenue Amusements. Park first aid employees on the scene requesting a rush."

As you arrive at the entrance, a man with a radio is waving you into the gate. He runs ahead, clearing people off of the narrow pathway. There is loud music and a large crowd. As you approach, you see a female teenager, supine, contorted, and unmoving, on the ground beneath the ferris wheel.

1. Looking up at the ferris wheel, what possible mechanisms of injury (MOIs) should you consider?

2. In addition to trauma sustained in the fall, what other information might you want to elicit from witnesses and friends of the patient?

<u>Mechanical energy</u> is energy from motion (<u>kinetic energy (KE)</u>—such as a moving vehicle) or energy stored in an object (<u>potential energy</u>—a brick sitting on a building ledge). KE would be found in two moving vehicles colliding. Potential energy would be present in an object sitting at a height. In that case, gravity would be the *potential* source of energy that converts to KE if the object falls. <u>Chemical energy</u> is the energy released as a result of a chemical reaction and can be found in an explosive or an acid or even from a reaction to an ingested or medically delivered agent or drug. <u>Electrical energy</u> comes in the form of high-voltage electrocution or a lightning strike. <u>Barometric energy</u> can result from sudden and radical changes in pressure, as can occur during scuba diving or flying.

<u>Biomechanics</u> is the study of the physiology and mechanics of a living organism using the tools of mechanical engineering. Biomechanics provides a way of analyzing the mechanisms and results of trauma sustained by the human body. <u>Kinetics</u> studies the relationships among speed, mass, direction of the force, and, for paramedics, the physical injury caused by speed, mass, and force. Knowledge of kinetics can help you predict injury patterns found in a patient.

Factors Affecting Types of Injury

The kind of injury resulting after trauma is sustained will be determined by the ability of the patient's body to disperse the energy delivered by the traumatic event. Some patients' bodies can stretch and bend adequately to absorb the energy of the traumatic event, while other patients' bone and tissue cannot absorb the energy. A healthy football player can absorb a "hit" on the playing field better than an older person with diminished bone and muscle mass.

External factors that determine types of injury include the amount of *force* and *energy* delivered. The amount of injury your patient sustains varies with the size (or mass) of the objects delivering the force, with the velocity (how fast the object is traveling), with acceleration or deceleration (how fast the object speeds up or slows down), and with the body area affected by the application of the force. The primary reasons for the extent of trauma your patients sustain are the amount of energy in the object and the mechanism by which the object is delivered to the body. The body would experience more widespread trauma from a cannon ball (more surface area and mass) than it would from a bullet (traveling the same speed), although both would likely be lethal.

Duration and direction of the force of application are also important. In vehicle crashes, paramedics learn to recognize the directional patterns in injuries from frontal or head-on impacts, side or lateral impacts, and rear-end impacts. The larger the area of force dissipation, the more the pressure is reduced to a specific spot on the body, often without breaking the skin. Injury from a bullet is less severe if the energy of the bullet is dissipated over the ceramic plate inside a bulletproof vest than if all the force of the bullet is applied at a small location on the skin.

In trauma medicine, this spreading of impact without breaking the skin is defined as <u>blunt trauma</u>. EMS providers at all levels quickly learn in the field that blunt trauma is difficult to diagnose because there is often little external damage. Paramedics study kinetics to help recognize this lethal, but almost invisible, trauma.

Words of Wisdom

Suspect a spinal injury when you see a cracked windshield, steering wheel or dashboard damage, intrusion into a vehicle, or an open ankle fracture after a fall. It will make a difference in how you approach the ABCs.

The *duration of force application* affects trauma because rapidly applied amounts of energy are less tolerated than an identical amount of energy delivered over a longer period of time. Rapidly delivered energy causes broken wrists, whereas longer term energy delivery might show up as repetitive stress injuries—even though the total amount of energy ultimately might be exactly the same.

The position of the trauma victim—how he or she is positioned—at the time of the event is an external factor. Seat belt use has done a great deal to affect the reduction in lethal injuries by keeping occupants in positions less likely to cause fatal injuries.

Internal injuries sustained when the break point of an organ is exceeded are easier to diagnose. In the skin, they include contusions, abrasions, lacerations, punctures, and degloving injuries. Bones will fracture or splinter. The viscera covering structures of internal organs will have ruptures, or disruptions.

The *impact resistance of body parts* will also have a bearing on types of tissue disruption. Impact resistance is often determined by what is inside your patient's organs: gas, liquid, or solid.

Biomechanical engineers would measure the densities of tissues that are traumatized. Paramedics need to know that organs that have gas inside, such as in the lungs and intestinal tract, will scatter energy more than liquid or solid boundaries. This means that the organ around the gas will be easily compressed, so look for lung and intestinal trauma first. Liquid-containing organs include the vascular system, the liver, the spleen, and muscle. Liquid-containing tissues are less compressible than tissues containing gases. Solid density interfaces occur mostly in bones such as in the cranium, spine, and long bones.

Because many injuries are not obvious on first presentation, understanding the effects of forces and energy transfer patterns will help in the assessment of the <u>mechanism of injury (MOI)</u>, which in turn can help predict the most likely type of injuries you will see when you are in the field **Figure 2**. Paramedic students need to learn to have a high <u>index of suspicion</u> for injuries that otherwise might be undetected for several hours. Anticipate the possibility of specific types of injury: you will help your patient and the trauma team who will need your assessment of the scene. You will find you need to be aggressive with your primary assessment and interventions to prevent further problems for your patient.

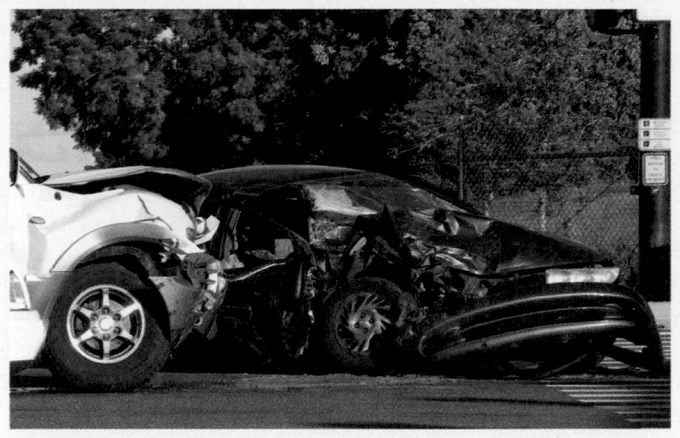

Figure 2 The appearance of the car can provide you with critical information about the severity of the crash and the possible injuries to the occupants.

Kinetics

Although drivers of motor vehicles might not obey the community's traffic laws, they must—whether they want to or not—obey the laws of physics that govern all objects on our planet. A little familiarity with these laws will help you understand more about the mechanisms of trauma.

Velocity (V) is the distance an object travels per unit time. The difference between velocity and speed is that velocity is also defined by moving in a specific direction. **Acceleration (a)** of an object is the rate of change of velocity that an object is subjected to, whether speeding up or slowing down. **Gravity (g)** is the downward acceleration that is imparted to any object moving toward the earth caused by the effect of the earth's mass. During each second of a fall, the velocity or speed of the falling object increases by 9.8 m/sec^2 (approximately 32 ft/sec^2).

Controversies

Some situations may have contraindications or relative contraindications for aeromedical transport. These situations include traumatic cardiac arrest, inclement weather conditions, extremely combative patients, morbidly obese patients, patients with barotrauma (diving injuries may necessitate lower flying altitudes), and situations in which ground transport and appropriate level of care are available and would permit quicker care.

As mentioned previously, the KE of an object is the energy associated with that object in motion. It reflects the relationship between the weight (mass) of the object and the velocity at which it is traveling and is expressed mathematically as:

$$\text{Kinetic energy} = \frac{\text{Mass}}{2} \times \text{Velocity}^2$$

$$\text{or } KE = \frac{m}{2} \times V^2$$

Thus, velocity has a much greater effect on KE than weight because it is squared **Figure 3** .

In other words, an object increases its KE more by increasing its velocity than by increasing its mass. The KE of an object involved in a crash must be dissipated as the object comes to rest. The KE of a car in motion that stops suddenly must be transformed or applied to another object **Figure 4** . In a car, KE can be dissipated by braking, transforming it into heat (another form of energy). If all the energy is not transformed into heat, however, the KE is applied to deform the metal of the car, which results in damage to the car and potentially to its occupants. The mechanics of dissipation can easily result in injury. For example, a car traveling at 35 mph hits a wall, which stops the

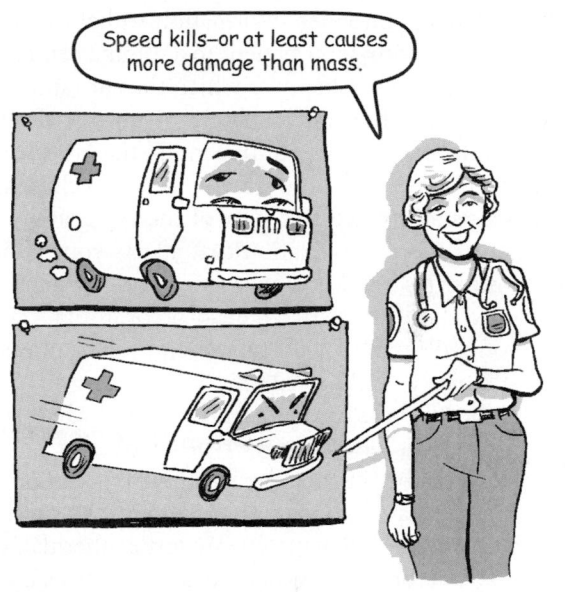

Figure 3 Velocity has a greater effect on KE than Mass.

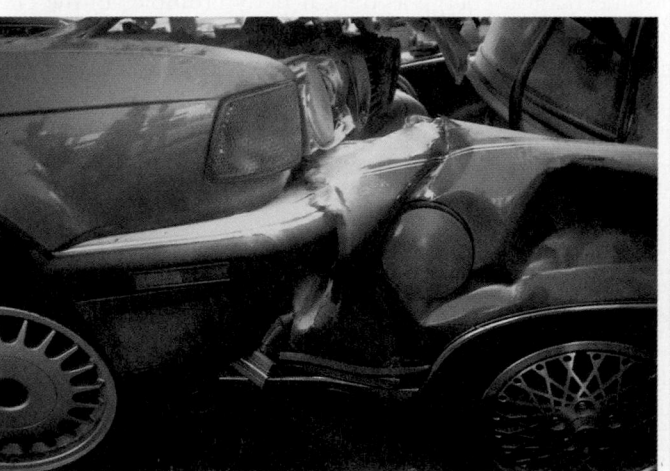

Figure 4 The kinetic energy of a speeding car is converted into the work of stopping the car, usually by crushing the car's exterior.

car, but the driver is still traveling at 35 mph until stopped by the seat belt or the air bag, or, if not wearing a seat belt, the steering wheel, dashboard, or windshield.

Speed affects energy exponentially: look what happens when velocity increases 10 mph versus when the person weighs in at 10 lb heavier **Table 1**.

Note that when weight increases by 10 lb but velocity remains the same, there is not much change in the KE. However, when the velocity increases from 40 to 50 mph (a difference of only 10 mph), for the 160-lb person, the KE increases by 72,000 KE units!

Modern cars are designed to have crumple zones to maximize the amount of energy absorbed by deformation before the passenger compartment is involved. Because the automobile damage so often shows just how fast the car was going, the amount of damage provides information to help in your decision about transferring your patient to a trauma center.

In addition to the velocity at which the car (and its passengers) are traveling, the vehicle's **angle of impact** (front impact versus side impact, or how your patient hit the inside of an automobile), the differences in the sizes of the two vehicles, and the restraint status and protective gear of the occupants will affect the amount of energy dissipation that affects your patients in a crash. Consider that if two vehicles are involved, each one contributes KE to the crash so that a head-on or frontal crash of two vehicles going 60 mph would be the equivalent of one vehicle hitting a stationary object at 120 mph.

Remember the laws of physics that no driver can break? Here's a quick review. The **law of conservation of energy** states that energy can be neither created nor destroyed; it can only change form. Energy generated from a sudden stop or start must be transformed to one of the following energy forms: thermal, electrical, chemical, radiant, or mechanical (as discussed earlier).

Energy dissipation is the process by which KE is transformed into one of these forms of mechanical energy. When a car stops slowly, its KE is converted to thermal energy—heat—by friction of the braking action. If the car crashes, KE is also converted into mechanical energy as the car body crumples in the crash. Mechanical energy is further dissipated in the form of injury as the occupants sustain fractures or other bodily harm.

Protective devices such as seat belts, air bags, and helmets are designed to manipulate the way in which energy is dissipated into injury. For example, a seat belt converts KE of the occupants into a seat belt-to-body pressure force rather than into a steering wheel deformation against the torso or a windshield shattering against the head.

Newton's first law of motion states that a body at rest will remain at rest unless acted on by an outside force. Similarly, a body in motion tends to remain in motion at a constant velocity, traveling in a straight line, unless acted on by an outside force. Most bodies in motion (without the assistance of a motor or other propulsion device) tend to eventually stop due to the action of forces of friction, wind resistance, or other force resulting in deceleration.

Newton's second law of motion states that the force that an object can exert is the product of its mass times its acceleration:

Force = Mass (Weight) × Acceleration (or Deceleration)

The higher an object's mass and acceleration, the higher the force that needs to be applied to make a change of course or stop the object. Force equals mass × acceleration or deceleration. **Deceleration** is slowing down or slowing to a stop. Rapid deceleration, as may occur in a crash, dissipates tremendous forces and, therefore, creates the potential for major injuries. Deceleration and acceleration can also be measured in numbers of g forces. One g force is the normal acceleration due to gravity. A two-or three-g acceleration or deceleration force is, logically enough, two or three times the force associated with the acceleration of gravity. A two-g deceleration force would make you feel like you are twice as heavy as you are at rest. Three-g acceleration force would make you feel three times heavier. High-speed crashes can generate decelerations in hundreds of g's. The human limit to deceleration is about 30 g.

In a head-on crash with two vehicles traveling in opposite directions along a straight line, transferred energy is represented in part as the sum of both their speeds. If a car strikes an immovable object, forces generated come only from the speed of the moving object. In a rear impact of two vehicles traveling along the same line, the energy potential is lessened because it is the difference in speed between them, also known as the closing speed.

It is important to have an understanding of these laws of physics because they help define the types and patterns of trauma you will see in the field. You are the most important witness the hospital trauma team has. The information you learn from physics will affect the outcome of your patient's life.

Table 1 Effects of Velocity and Weight		
Miles per hour (mph)	150 lb patient	160 lb patient
10	7,500 KE units	8,000 KE units
20	30,000 KE units	32,000 KE units
30	67,500 KE units	72,000 KE units
40	120,000 KE units	128,000 KE units
50	187,500 KE units	200,000 KE units

Blunt Trauma

Injuries are generally described as the consequence of blunt or penetrating trauma. Blunt trauma refers to injuries in which the tissues are not penetrated by an external object **Figure 5**. Blunt trauma commonly occurs in motor vehicle crashes, in pedestrians hit by a vehicle, in motorcycle crashes, in falls from heights, in serious sports injuries, and in blasts when no shrapnel is involved and the pressure wave is the primary cause of the injuries.

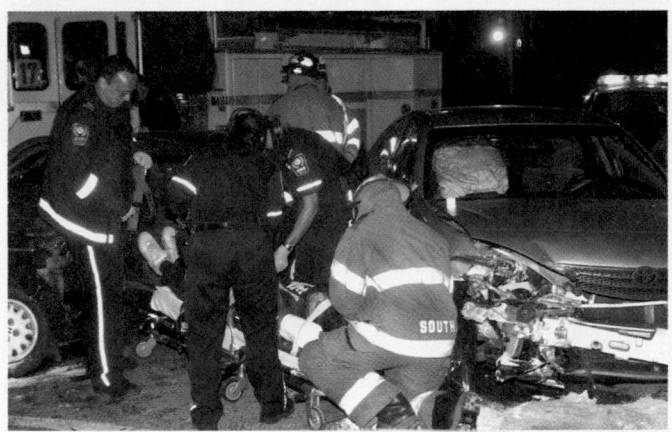

Figure 5 Blunt trauma typically occurs in motor vehicle crashes like this, head-on collision.

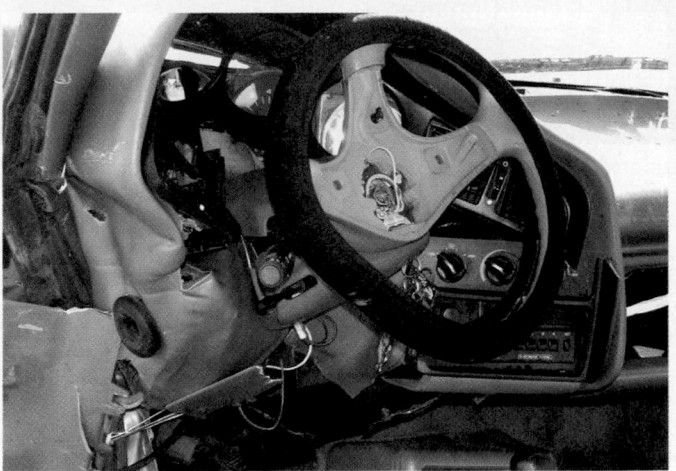

Figure 6 Deceleration of the occupant starts during sudden braking and continues during the impact of the crash. The appearance of the interior of the car can provide you with information about the severity of the patient's injuries.

Motor Vehicle Crashes

According to the National Highway Traffic Safety Administration, in 2009, 33,808 people were killed in an estimated 5,505,000 police-reported motor vehicle traffic crashes; 2,217,000 people were injured; and 3,957,000 crashes involved property damage only. That year, an average of 93 people died each day in motor vehicle crashes.

When a motor vehicle collides with another object, trauma in the crash is composed of five phases tied to the effects of progressive deceleration. The first phase, *deceleration of the vehicle*, occurs when the vehicle strikes another object and is brought to an abrupt stop. The forward motion of the car continues until its KE is dissipated in the form of mechanical deformation and damage to the vehicle and occupant or until the restraining force of the object is removed (for example, sheared-off pole, or the yielding of a guard rail) and the vehicle motion continues until its KE is gently dissipated by drag or continued braking. The second phase is *deceleration of the occupant*, which starts during sudden braking and continues during the impact of the crash. This results in deceleration, compression, and shear trauma to the occupants **Figure 6**. The effects on vehicle occupants will vary depending on the mass of each occupant, protective mechanisms in the vehicle such as restraints and air bags, body parts involved, and points of impact. The third phase, *deceleration of internal organs*, involves the body's supporting structures (skull, sternum, ribs, spine, and pelvis) and movable organs (brain, heart, liver, spleen, and intestine) that continue their forward momentum until stopped by anatomic restraints **Figure 7**. Energy is dissipated by internal organs as they are injured. Movement of fixed and suspended organs may result in tears and shearing injuries. The fourth phase is the result of *secondary collisions*, which occur when a vehicle occupant is hit by objects moving within the auto such as loose objects, packages, animals, or other passengers. These objects may continue to travel at the auto's initial speed and then hit a passenger who has come to rest. These types of collisions have been known to cause severe spine and head trauma. The final phase is the result of *additional impacts* that the vehicle may receive, such as when it is hit by a

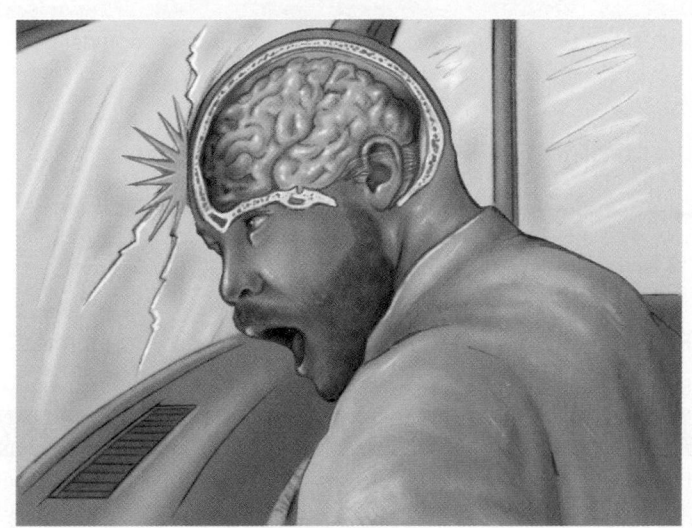

Figure 7 Deceleration of internal organs involves the body's supporting structures and movable organs that continue their forward momentum until stopped by anatomic restraints. In this illustration, the brain continues its forward motion and strikes the inside of the skull, resulting in a compression injury to the anterior portion of the brain and stretching of the posterior portion.

second vehicle, or is deflected into another vehicle, tree, or other object. This may increase the severity of the original injuries or cause further injury. For example, a frontal impact may cause a posterior hip dislocation and an acetabular fracture via a dashboard mechanism, and a subsequent side impact from another vehicle may add a lateral compression pelvic ring injury, resulting in complex pelvic and acetabular trauma. **Table 2** shows the structural clues, body clues, and resulting injuries for different types of crashes.

Table 2 Mechanism of Injury: Motor Vehicle Crash

Structural Clues	Body Clues	Look for These Injuries
Head-on or frontal impact		
Deformed front end Cracked windshield	Bruised or lacerated head or face	■ Brain injury ■ Scalp, facial cuts ■ Cervical spine injury ■ Tracheal injury
Deformed steering column	Bruised neck Bruised chest	■ Sternal or rib fracture ■ Flail chest ■ Myocardial contusion ■ Pericardial tamponade ■ Pneumothorax or hemothorax ■ Exsanguination from aortic tear
Deformed dashboard	Bruised abdomen Bruised knee, misplaced kneecap	■ Ruptured spleen, liver, bowel, diaphragm ■ Fractured patella ■ Dislocated knee ■ Femoral fracture ■ Dislocated hip
Lateral or side impact		
Deformed side of car	Bruised shoulder	■ Clavicular fracture ■ Fractured humerus ■ Multiple rib fractures
Door smashed in	Bruised shoulder or pelvis	■ Fractured hip ■ Fractured iliac wing ■ Fractured clavicle or ribs
"B" pillar deformed	Bruised temple	■ Brain injury ■ Cervical spine fracture
Broken door or window handles	Bruised or deformed arms	■ Contusions
Broken window glass	Dicing lacerations	■ Multiple lacerations
Rear-end impact		
Posterior deformity of the auto	Secondary anterior injuries, especially if the patient was unrestrained	■ "Whiplash" injuries ■ Deceleration injuries of a head-on impact
Headrest not adjusted	None detected	■ Bleeding, bruising, or tearing inside skull

Words of Wisdom

Do not forget that the collision of internal organs striking against the body can result in severe damage, though this may not always be obvious.

Words of Wisdom

When the windshield is cracked or broken, the front seat occupant, whose head struck the windshield, has a cervical spine injury until proven otherwise.

Impact Patterns

Important clues to predict injury types can be obtained by paying attention to the history of the crash and by an examination of the scene. Using your newfound knowledge of the physics of trauma, you can make a good estimate of how injured your patients might be by looking at the amount of damage around the scene. How dented and deformed the vehicle looks is a clear indication of the forces involved and of the degree of deceleration sustained by your patient. Dents and deformities on the inside of the vehicle will show you the point of impact on the patient. Do a quick check for injury types visible on your patient: head injury or seat belt marks show what parts of the body may have been involved in energy absorption. Tire skid marks at the scene indicate whether significant energy was dissipated by braking before the crash. Debris along the course of the crash may indicate multiple collisions and different force vectors acting on the patient along the course of the crash.

There are primarily five types of impact patterns: frontal or head-on impact, lateral or side impact, rear impact, rotational or quarter-panel impact, and rollovers.

Frontal or Head-on Impacts In frontal or head-on impacts, the front end of the car distorts as it dissipates KE and decelerates its forward motion. Passengers decelerate at the same rate as the vehicle. At a 30-mph crash, the front end of an average American car will crush 2 ft at the rough estimate of 1 inch of deformity for each 1 mph. The forces applied to the driver will differ based on car design, materials, and safety features of the vehicle. The interior will also suggest possible injuries by the damage your patient's body has done to the dash, windshield, or steering wheel, for example.

Abrupt deceleration injuries are produced by a sudden stop of a body's forward motion. Whether from a fall, shaking a baby, or a high-speed vehicle crash, decelerating forces can induce **shearing**, **avulsing**, or rupturing of organs and their restraining fascia, vasculature, nerves, and other soft tissues. These injuries are often invisible during examination, so every paramedic needs to understand how such injuries are sustained.

The head is particularly vulnerable to deceleration injuries. The brain is a fairly heavy organ that is suspended in fluid inside the skull. Any trauma that will jerk the patient's head can cause the brain to strike the inside of the skull, potentially causing bleeding, bruising, or tearing injuries. All of these potential injuries are extremely dangerous and will not show up on a physical examination because they occur within the skull. Your index of suspicion should be on high alert for these injuries.

The chest is vulnerable to aortic injury. The aorta, the largest blood vessel in the body, is the most common site of deceleration injury in the chest. The aorta is often torn away from its points of fixation in the body. Shearing of the aorta due to rapid deceleration can result in loss of the total blood volume and immediate death.

Blunt abdominal trauma results as the forward motion of the body stops and internal organs continue their motion, causing tearing at their points of attachment, shearing injuries, and/or tearing of the abdominal walls. Organs that are commonly affected include the liver, kidneys, small intestine, large intestine, pancreas, and spleen.

Kidneys are injured as forward motion produces tears to the organ or to points of attachment with the abdominal aorta or the renal arteries. Also, as motion is restrained by the large bowel, the small bowel can tear and result in spillage of contents into the abdomen. Trauma can also do damage without tearing by reducing the supply of blood to the bowel. The spleen can be torn as well, resulting in left upper quadrant pain and life-threatening internal bleeding.

Crush and compression injuries are the result of forces applied to the body by things external to the body at the time of impact. Crush and compression injuries occur at the time of impact. Crush and compression injuries are often caused by dashboards, windshields, the floor, or heavy objects falling on the body. Crush and compression injuries can also occur when the body or one of its parts gets trapped between two objects such as in a machine or the closing of a door.

Compression head injuries may result in skull fracture, and often are associated with cervical spine injury. Therefore, you need to assume spinal cord injuries and severe injury to the brain when this mechanism is observed. Brain tissue does not compress well; it swells within the enclosed area of the skull when injured. As the brain swells inside the skull, it is compressed, causing a highly lethal condition.

> ### Words of Wisdom
>
> - According to 2010 National Highway Transportation Safety Administration statistics, the overall traffic fatality rate dropped to 1.10 fatalities per 100 million vehicle miles traveled.
> - This still represents a total of 32,885 fatal crashes.

Compression injuries of the chest may produce fractured ribs that can lead to internal injuries of the lungs and heart. One of the signs of lung injury is a flail chest, a condition resulting from multiple consecutive rib fractures (two or more ribs broken in two or more places), in which the chest wall moves paradoxically (opposite of normal) with respirations. Fractured ribs may also cause blood or air to enter the chest cavity, leading to a pneumothorax or hemothorax, which would ultimately require decompression or placement of a chest tube. Blunt cardiac injury can compress the heart between bones in the chest, causing dysrhythmias and direct injury to the heart muscle. If the lungs are compressed, acute respiratory distress syndrome can result, requiring intubation to maintain the patient's breathing.

Almost all abdominal organs can be affected by hitting an external object. Organs often injured include the pancreas, spleen, liver, and, occasionally, kidneys. Compression against the seat belt may result in bowel rupture, bladder rupture, diaphragm tearing, and spinal injuries. The abdomen has two large blood-carrying vessels called the abdominal aorta and the inferior vena cava. Rupture of either of these large blood vessels can lead quickly to exsanguination.

Pelvic fractures also result from external compressive trauma, potentially injuring the bladder, vagina, rectum, lumbar plexus, and pelvic floor and leading to severe bleeding from the iliac arteries.

Position at the precise time of impact is very important in determining an occupant's movements and injuries during a crash. Unrestrained occupants usually follow one of two trajectories, a *down-and-under pathway*, or an *up-and-over pathway* Figure 8.

The down-and-under pathway is traveled by an occupant who slides under the steering column or dash. As the vehicle is decelerating, the occupant continues to travel downward and forward into the dashboard or steering column, led by the knees. The knees hit the dashboard, transmitting the energy of

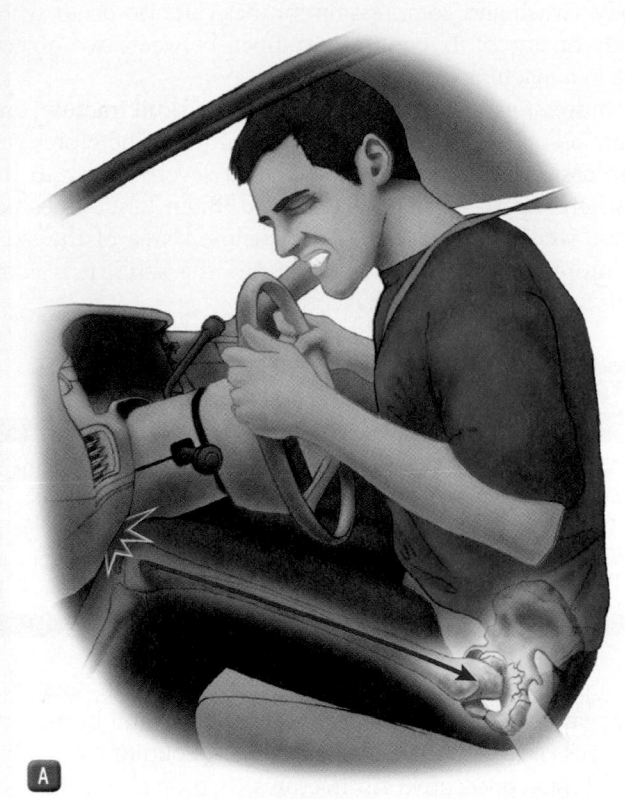

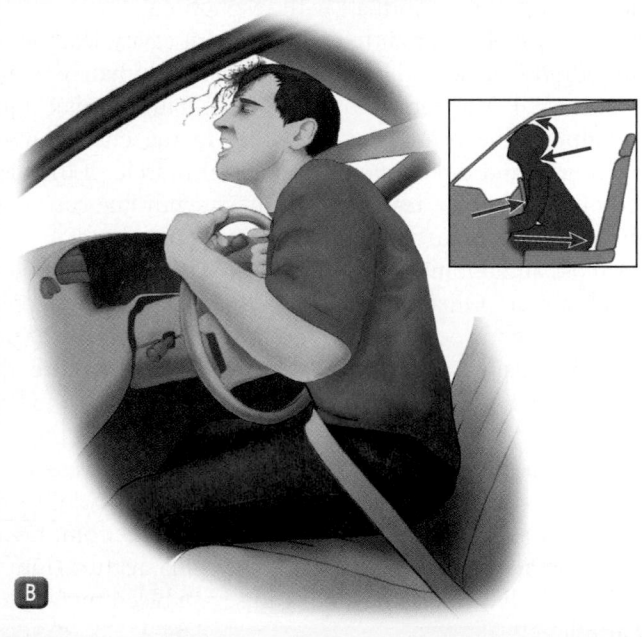

Figure 8 **A.** The down-and-under pathway. **B.** The up-and-over pathway.

the femur will dislocate. If the occupant's knees hit the dashboard, look for a fracture-dislocation of the knee or other related injuries. Look also for hip and pelvic fractures or hip dislocation. Your patient's torso can twist in such a way that his or her head hits the steering column. Always look for spinal injuries.

Words of Wisdom

When there is damage to the steering column, there is critical injury to the driver until proven otherwise. In order to visualize the steering column, you may need to move the inflated airbag.

The upper torso continues forward until it impacts the car—the steering wheel, the dash, or the seat belt and air bag protection system. Look for rib fractures or pulmonary and cardiovascular injuries caused by internal striking and compressing. When your patient is a child, assume that there will be pulmonary or cardiac injuries—children have more flexible ribs but often sustain compression injuries. Remember how gas-containing organs absorb more of the energy of the crash?

In the up-and-over pathway, the lead point is the head. In this sequence, rotation occurs around the ankles with the torso moving in an upward and forward direction. The head takes a higher trajectory, impacting the windshield, roof, mirror, or dashboard, causing compression and deceleration injuries in your patient that can include significant head and cervical spine trauma. The anterior part of the neck may strike the steering wheel, causing laryngeal fracture, serious lacerations, and other soft-tissue injury.

Ejection is possible if the windshield does not stop the body from projecting through it. Ejection leads to second-impact injuries when the body contacts the ground or objects outside of the car. These injuries can be as severe as initial-impact injuries, and they increase the likelihood of great vessel damage and death. The spine absorbs energy as it is compressed between the stationary head and the moving torso, which leads to injury.

A dangerous lung injury may occur if your patient reflexively takes a deep breath just before impact, hyperinflating the lungs and closing the glottis. The impact of the steering wheel can injure the lungs by generating pressures in the lungs beyond the capabilities of the lung tissue, like a "paper bag being exploded" (60% to 70% of pneumothoraces may occur this way) **Figure 9** .

The abdomen, pelvis, or upper thigh contacts the lower aspect of the steering wheel or dash, and lower leg fractures could be present. **Table 3** lists the "ring" of chest injuries that can occur from impact with the steering wheel or the dashboard.

Lateral or Side Impacts Lateral impact, "T"-bone, and side impacts impart energy to the near-side occupant almost directly to the pelvis and chest **Figure 10** . Unrestrained occupants will remain almost motionless, literally having the car pushed out from under them. Seat belts do little to protect these passengers because they are designed to limit forward hinging injuries, not side impacts. As one vehicle makes contact with the side of the other vehicle, the occupant nearest the impact is hit by the door

the deceleration up the femurs to the pelvis. With knees locked in the dash and hips in the seat, force vectors go down the tibia and along the femur. If the feet are not locked by folding floorboards or brake pedals, energy along the tibia will be transferred to the lower leg, with no immediate injury. If the feet are locked in place, femur fracture can occur. In some cases, the head of

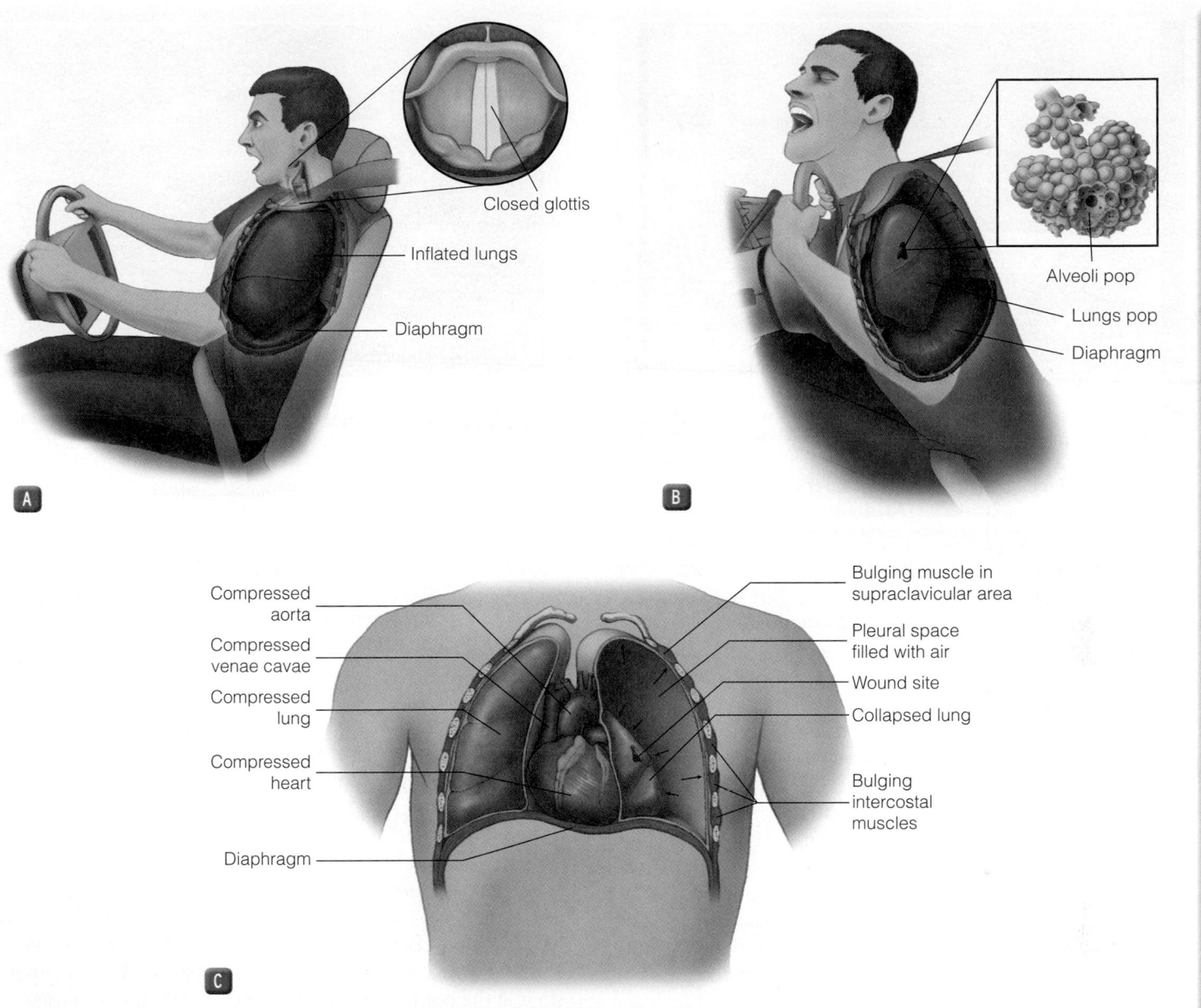

Figure 9 The paper-bag syndrome. **A.** The occupant takes a deep breath just before crashing, closing the glottis and filling the lungs with air. **B.** The occupant's chest hits the steering wheel, popping the alveoli in the lungs. **C.** A pneumothorax results.

Table 3 "Ring" of Chest Injuries from Impact With the Steering Wheel or Dashboard

- Facial injuries
- Soft-tissue neck trauma
- Larynx and tracheal trauma
- Fractured sternum
- Myocardial contusion
- Pericardial tamponade
- Pulmonary contusion
- Hemothorax, rib fractures
- Flail chest
- Ruptured aorta
- Intra-abdominal injuries

of the car as the passenger compartment begins to deform and collapse. As the passenger compartment deforms, the victim's head can strike the impacting vehicle or object. Injury results from direct trauma to the affected side and to tension developed on the far side. Upper extremity trauma depends on the spatial orientation of the arm at impact. The shoulder frequently rotates outward and posteriorly, exposing the chest and ribs to injury. Forces transmitted to the chest cause rib fractures, lateral flail chest, and lung contusions. If the humerus remains between the door and chest, the clavicle may absorb side motion and fracture. As the body of the occupant is pushed in one direction, the head moves toward the impacting object, creating a line of tension along the contralateral side of the spine. This may result in ligamentous disruption and dislocation of the spine on the opposite side of the impact. The far-side occupant, if properly restrained, has the advantage of "riding down" with the car,

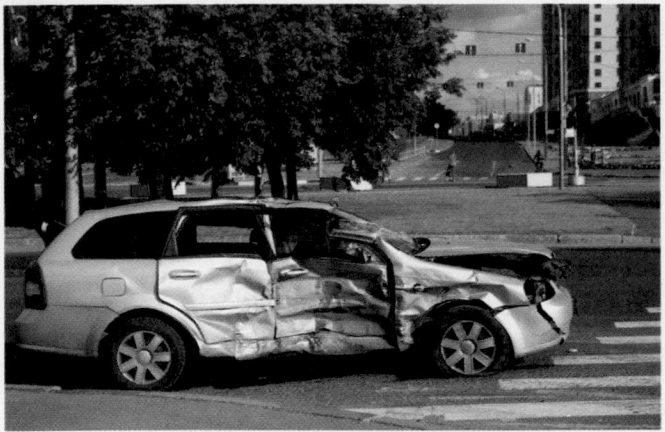

Figure 10 In a lateral impact, the car may be struck above its center of gravity and begin to rock away from the side of impact. This causes a type of lateral whiplash in which the passenger's shoulders and head whip toward the intruding vehicle.

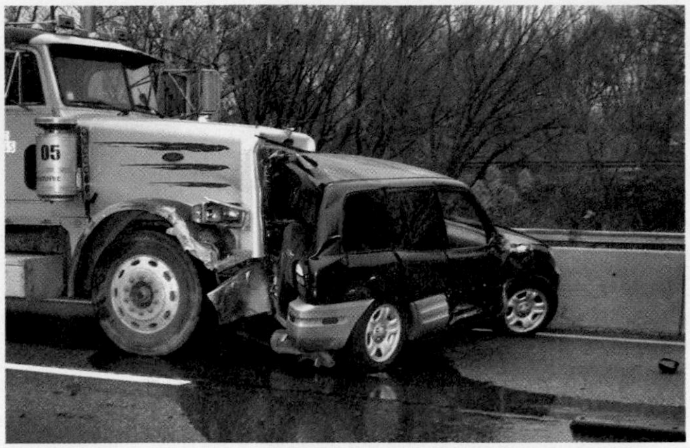

Figure 11 Rear-end impacts often cause whiplash-type injuries, particularly when the head and/or neck is not restrained by a headrest.

thereby receiving considerably less force. If unrestrained, he or she may move in a direction parallel but opposite to the impact. This passenger receives forces similar to any unrestrained occupant. Furthermore, because both passengers travel in a direction parallel to impact but in opposite directions, they collide with each other, causing additional injury.

In a lateral crash, if the greater trochanter of the femur is impacted and transmits forces to the pelvis, sometimes it may be driven through the acetabulum into the pelvis. If the force reaches the ilium, the pelvis may also fracture. The typical pattern of pelvic injury that occurs in this scenario is a lateral compression injury that trauma surgeons call pelvic ring disruption. Lateral compression injuries are less serious than anterior compression injuries. Death in lateral crashes is usually the result of associated torso or head injuries. Remember that the occupants of the other vehicle will most likely be subjected to the forces of a frontal impact.

Rear Impacts Rear impacts or rear-end impacts have the most survivors, if the driver and passengers are properly restrained **Figure 11**. If the vehicle coming from the rear is traveling at excessive speed, however, most bets on survivability are off. Most often in this kind of crash, a stationary (or slower moving) vehicle is struck from behind and the impact energy is transmitted as a sudden forward accelerating force. The neck hyperextends as the body moves forward relative to the head. The head does not move forward with the body unless a headrest is in the proper position; if the headrest is not in proper position, the head is snapped back and then forward. Because most seats have some degree of elasticity after the sudden forward acceleration has ended, the stored potential energy in the seat is converted to an energy of forward motion, which can aggravate the hyperextension trauma to the neck and then follow with some rebound forward flexion of the head on the chest resulting in hyperflexion. A third episode of extension may occur as the chest moves forward. This is the so-called <u>whiplash</u> injury.

In a rear-impact crash, energy is imparted to the front vehicle, which accelerates rapidly, while frontal impact energy to the rear driver is reduced because energy is being transferred to the front car. One concern with rear-impact crashes is the frequency with which seat backs collapse, causing unrestrained occupants to be propelled into the back seat. Head restraints, developed to prevent the head and torso from moving separately, are not always adjusted correctly. Many are placed too low and act as a fulcrum that may actually facilitate the extension injury. They need to be adjusted so they are behind the head and not behind the neck.

Rotational or Quarter-panel Impacts A rotational or quarter-panel impact occurs when a lateral crash is off center. In this case, rotation occurs as part of the car continues to move and part of the car comes to a stop. The vehicle's forward motion stops at the point of impact, but the side continues in rotational motion around the impact point. The point of greatest speed loss of the vehicle is the site where the greatest damage to the occupant will occur. The resultant forces act along a vector oblique to the direction of travel. For example, in a ten o'clock impact with twelve o'clock being frontal, the driver would initially move forward and then diagonally as the auto rotates, striking the A pillar, the support for the windshield. The front seat passenger would strike the rearview mirror area. The point of greatest deceleration becomes the location of the most severely injured patients. Occupants tend to receive a combination of frontal and lateral injuries. Because rigid objects may be in line with vector forces, head injuries may result. Three-point seat belts are effective in preventing injury in angled crashes of up to 45°.

Rollovers Rollover scenarios have the greatest potential to cause lethal injuries. Injuries will be serious even if seat belts are worn. However, if your patients did not wear seat belts, they may be ejected, and/or they will have been struck hard against the interior of the vehicle with each change in direction the car makes during the rollover. Even a restrained occupant's head and neck will change direction with each change in the vehicle's position.

Ejection of the patient from the vehicle increases the chance of death by 25 times **Figure 12**. One of three ejected victims will sustain a cervical spine fracture. A partial ejection can result in an arm or leg injured by being caught between the vehicle and the ground.

Restrained Versus Unrestrained Occupants

Seat belts are highly effective because they stop the motion of any automobile occupant who is traveling at the same speed as the vehicle, until stopped. The seat belt, although capable of delivering some injury at high speeds, will prevent the serious-to-fatal injuries of being unrestrained in the car and being ejected from the car. One of every 13 victims of ejection sustains major and permanent cervical spine damage. Restrained victims "ride down" the deceleration with belt elasticity and crush time of the car, with a nearly 45% reduction in fatalities. Restraints limit the contact of the occupants with the

interior of the vehicle, prevent ejection, distribute deceleration energy over a greater surface, and prevent the occupants from violently contacting each other. As a result, all types of injuries are decreased, including head, facial, spinal, thoracic, intra-abdominal, pelvic, and lower extremity, and ejection is also limited.

All arguments against seat belt use are unfounded. Every unrestrained passenger poses a hazard to themselves and to other occupants in the vehicle, especially for front seat passengers who are at higher risk for injury in a front-end crash if the back seat occupants are unrestrained.

Specific injuries associated with seat belt use include cervical fractures due to flexion stresses and neck sprains due to deceleration and hyperextension. Most serious injuries occur because the patient did not use the seat belt correctly. If the occupant does not use the shoulder strap, severe upper body injuries, including spinal injuries and decapitation, can occur. If the seat belt is placed above the pelvic bone, abdominal injuries and lumbar spine injuries result.

Air bags were another great step up for patient safety. The National Highway Traffic Safety Administration has estimated that air bags have reduced deaths in direct frontal crashes by about 30%. Front air bags will not activate in side impact crashes or impacts to the front quarter panel, and without the use of a seat belt, they are insufficient to prevent ejection. They are self-deflating and function only for a first impact, not a secondary one. The rapidly inflating bag can also result in secondary injuries from direct contact with the air bag or from the chemicals used to inflate it. Common injuries include abrasions to the face, chest, and arms; minor corrosive effects from irritation of the abrasions by the cornstarch used to load the air bag, chemical keratitis, conjunctivitis, or corneal abrasion, and inhalation injuries **Figure 13**.

Small children can be severely injured or killed if air bags inflate while they are in the front seat. That is why all EMS providers are encouraged to participate in teaching parents how to properly place and secure children's car seats.

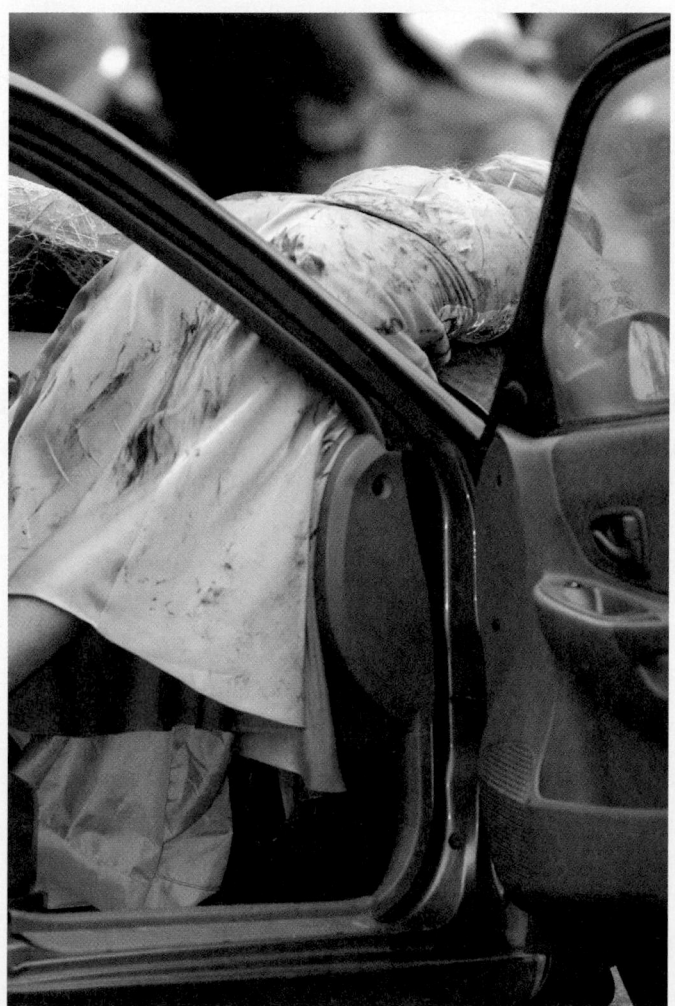

Figure 12 Occupants who have been ejected or partially ejected may have struck the interior of the car many times before ejection.

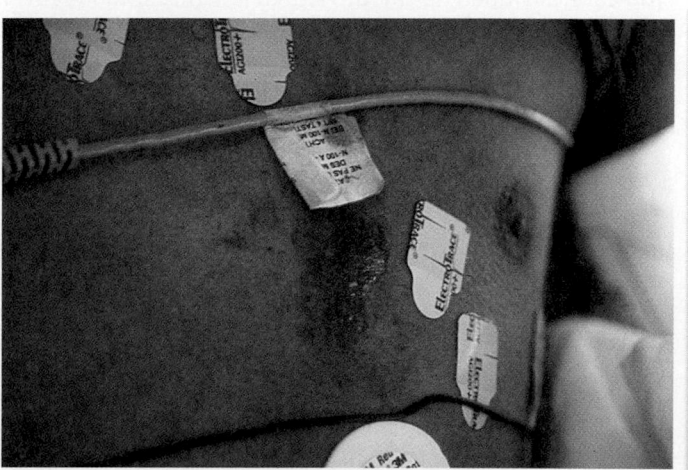

Figure 13 Air bags can cause abrasions to the face, chest, and arms.

Pregnant women in general wear seat belts less frequently than do nonpregnant women owing to discomfort, or the unproven concern that the seat belt may increase damage to the unborn child in the case of a crash. However, no study has reported that seat belts increase fetal mortality. If lap belts are worn alone and too high, they allow enough forward flexion and subsequent compression to rupture the uterus because deceleration forces are transmitted directly to the uterus. Lap belts with shoulder harnesses are essential to provide equal distribution of forces and to prevent forward flexion of the mother. Without the shoulder harness, the protuberant uterus will also receive the impact of the steering wheel or dashboard.

Increased morbidity and mortality, especially chest trauma, is more common in geriatric patients, particularly rib and sternal fractures. Fatalities also increase if child restraint devices are improperly installed or used. Children who have outgrown a car seat but are too small to be restrained by belts designed for adults are at risk for hyperflexion and abdominal injury.

Motorcycle Crashes

In 2009, 4,462 motorcyclists were killed compared with 5,312 motorcycle-related deaths in 2008. Although fatalities declined between 2008 and 2009, from 2000 to 2009, motorcycle fatalities increased by 54%. In 2009, 9,000 motorcyclists were injured in motorcycle crashes. The increase in the number of deaths parallels an increase in engine capacity of production motorcycles.

In a motorcycle crash, any structural protection afforded to the victims is not derived from a steel cage, as is the case in an automobile, but from protective devices worn by the rider—that is, helmet, leather or abrasion-resistant clothing, and boots. While helmets are designed to protect against impact forces to the head, they transmit any impact into the cervical spine, and as such, do not protect against severe cervical spine injury. Leather and synthetic gear worn over the body were initially designed to protect professional riders in competition, where falls tend to be controlled and result in long sliding mechanisms on hard surfaces rather than multiple crashes against road objects and other vehicles. Leather clothing will protect mostly against road abrasion but offers no protection against blunt trauma from secondary impacts. In a street crash, impacts occur usually against other larger vehicles or stationary objects.

When you are assessing the scene of a motorcycle crash, attention should be given to the deformity of the motorcycle, the side of most damage, the distance of skid in the road, the deformity of stationary objects or other vehicles, and the extent and location of deformity in the helmet **Figure 14**. These findings can be helpful in estimating the extent of trauma in a patient.

There are *four types of motorcycle impacts*. In a *head-on impact*, the motorcycle strikes another object and stops its forward motion

YOU are the Medic   PART 2

The scene appears safe and stable. A park employee is kneeling on the grass beside the patient. You instruct her on how to hold and maintain cervical stabilization and call to the patient and try gently squeezing her shoulder. You do not get a response. You ask another employee to find the patient's friends.

You carefully open her mouth with a jaw-thrust manueuver. There is no evidence of blood, broken teeth, or foreign bodies; breathing seems adequate but rapid and shallow. Attempting to insert an oropharyngeal airway (OPA), she gags and the OPA is removed.

Recording Time: 1 Minute	
Appearance	Unmoving, supine, legs bent to sides
Level of consciousness	U (unresponsive to verbal and painful stimuli)
Airway	Clear, does not tolerate an OPA
Breathing	Rapid, shallow
Circulation	Rapid, weak radial pulse

3. The patient is unresponsive with what appears to be adequate breathing. Your partner applies a nonrebreathing mask with 15 L/min of oxygen. What should you do next to continue your primary assessment?

4. The patient's friend comes forward and tearfully explains that her friend, who is a diabetic and was drinking "a few shots of tequila" earlier in the evening, was standing up in the ride's car, yelling and waving to her boyfriend, when the ride suddenly jerked to a stop, sending her tumbling out of the car. What important questions will you ask the friend?

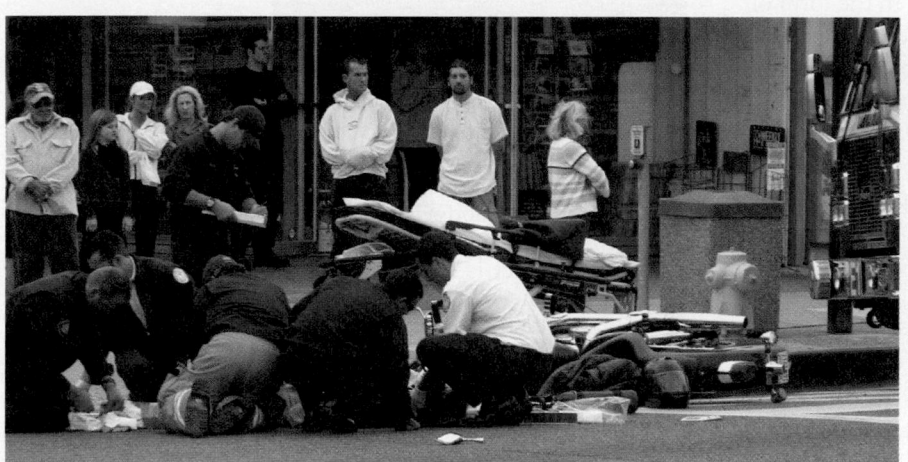

Figure 14 At a motorcycle crash scene, attention should be given to the deformity of the motorcycle, the side of most damage, the distance of skid in the road, the deformity of stationary objects or other vehicles, and the extent and location of deformity in the helmet.

Special Populations

Changes in vision, hearing, posture, and motor ability predispose older people to a greater risk of being struck by a vehicle.

while the rider and parts of the motorcycle that are broken off continue their forward motion until stopped by an outside force, such as contact with the road or another opposing force from a secondary crash. Because the motorcycle's center of gravity is above the front axle, there is a forward and upward motion at the point of the impact, causing the rider to go over the handlebars. If the rider's feet remain on the pegs or pedals, the forward and upward motion of the upper torso is restrained by the femurs and tibias, producing bilateral femur or tibia fractures and severe foot injuries.

For motorcycles with a low riding seat below the level of the gas tank, such as Japanese racing bikes or Italian transalpine style motorcycles, the tank can act as a wedge on the pelvis during the initial phase of the crash. This can result in severe anterior-posterior compression injuries to the pelvis that can cause severe neurovascular compromise. Open pelvic fractures are also common, resulting in severe perineal injuries with loss of the pelvic floor. Mortality associated with open pelvic fractures has been reported to be as high as 50%.

In an *angular impact*, the motorcycle strikes an object or another vehicle at an angle so that the rider sustains direct crushing injuries to the lower extremity between the object and the motorcycle. This usually results in severe open and comminuted lower extremity injuries with severe neurovascular compromise, possibly requiring surgical amputation.

Traumatic amputations are also common high-speed injuries. After the initial crush injury to the lower extremity, mechanisms such as those described in a head-on impact also apply. Often the rider is propelled over the hood of the colliding

vehicle. Because the impact is at an angle, severe thoracoabdominal torsion and lateral bending spine injuries can result, in addition to head injury and pelvic trauma.

An *ejected* rider will travel at high speed until stopped by a stationary object, by another vehicle, or by contact with the road. Severe abrasion injuries (road rash) down to bone can occur. An unpredictable combination of blunt injuries can occur from secondary crashes.

A technique used to separate the rider from the body of the motorcycle and the object to be hit is referred to as *laying the bike down*. It was developed by motorcycle racers and adapted by street bikers as a means of achieving a controlled crash. As a crash approaches, the motorcycle is turned flat and tipped sideways at 90° to the direction of travel so that one leg is dropped to the grass or asphalt. This slows the occupant faster than the motorcycle, allowing for the rider to become separated from the motorcycle. If properly protected with leather or synthetic abrasion-resistant gear, injuries should be limited to those sustained by rolling over the pavement and any secondary crash that may occur. When executed properly, this maneuver prevents the rider from being trapped between the bike and the object. However, a rider unable to clear the bike will continue into the vehicle, often with devastating results.

With any type of crash, the helmet should be removed carefully if airway management techniques cannot be performed with the helmet in place or the helmet does not fit snuggly to the head. Dents and abrasions must be assumed to have caused cervical spine fractures until proven otherwise by a radiograph. Precautions should be taken to remove the helmet, which should be cut if it cannot be removed without introducing further deformation to the neck.

Pedestrian Injuries

In 2009, 4,092 traffic fatalities in the United States involved pedestrians, a 7% decrease from 2008. The largest number of pedestrians killed was in the 45- to 54-year-old age group (19.8%); children younger than 9 years accounted for about 4% of the deaths. The greatest number of deaths (25%) occurred between 6:00 PM and 9:00 PM, and an additional 22% died between 9:00 PM and midnight. Of all deaths, 75% occurred in areas other than intersections, and 25% occurred at intersections. In 2009, 630 deaths were a result of bicycles being hit by a vehicle.

Almost 87% of pedestrians are struck by a vehicle's front end, sustaining a predictable pattern of injuries starting with those caused by direct impact with the bumper. Adult injuries are generally lateral and posterior because adults tend to turn to the side or away from impact, whereas children will face forward into the oncoming vehicle.

There are *three predominant MOIs* during a pedestrian versus automobile crash. The *first impact*, when the auto strikes an adult body with its bumpers, creates lower extremity injuries, particularly to the knee and leg. These injuries are in the form of various patterns of tibia-fibula fractures, often open knee dislocations and tibial plateau fractures. Usually the tibia is fractured on the side of impact; the impact potentially fractures the other leg as well. Knee dislocations are common with severe multiligamentous injury.

In the field, a dislocated knee should be splinted in the position found if the patient has good distal PMS—pulse, and motor and sensory function. It is key to remember that if the knee reduces spontaneously, you must communicate this to the trauma team verbally and in your report. Knee dislocation is an indication of possible vascular injury that can be missed by the trauma team if you do not report that you found the knee in a dislocated position initially.

A *second impact* occurs as the adult is thrown on the hood and/or grille of a vehicle, resulting in head, pelvis, chest, and coup-contrecoup traumatic brain injuries. Lateral compression pelvic fractures are common in this mechanism and can cause open fractures with bony punctures in viscera in this area of the body, or in the vagina in women. A *third impact* occurs when the body strikes the ground or some other object after it has been subjected to a sudden acceleration by the colliding vehicle.

Pediatric patterns of pedestrian injury are different from patterns in adults. Small children are shorter, so the car bumper is more likely to strike them in the pelvis or torso, causing severe injuries from direct impact **Figure 15**. Although they are less likely than adults to fly over the hood of the car, they are more likely to be run over by the vehicle as they are propelled to the ground by the impact. Multiple extremity and pelvic fractures and abdominal and thoracic crush injuries are to be expected. Traumatic brain injury often kills young patients.

The **Waddell triad** refers to the pattern of automobile pedestrian injuries in children and people of short stature: (1) the bumper hits the pelvis and femur instead of the knees and tibias; (2) the chest and abdomen hit the grille or low on the

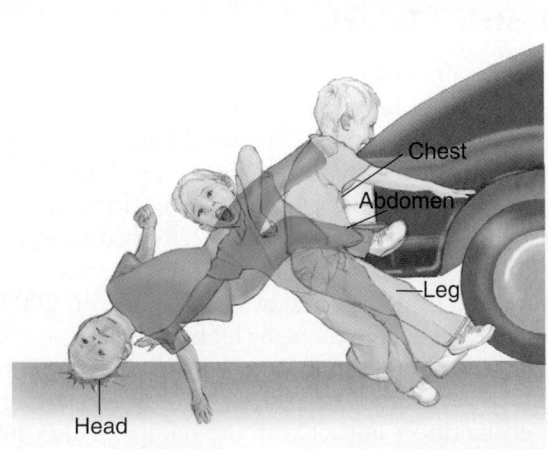

Figure 15 In car versus pedestrian crashes, children frequently sustain multisystem injuries involving the head, chest, abdomen, and long bones. This is called the Waddell triad.

The different mechanisms of injury in children and the unique anatomic features of children together produce predictable patterns of injury. Because penetrating injuries are uncommon and because the head (compared with the rest of the body) is larger in childhood, injured children often have blunt injuries primarily involving the head. If the energy impact is severe and involves the entire body, the child may have a pattern involving the head, chest, abdomen, and long bones.

hood of the car (sternal and rib fractures as well as abdominal injuries are likely); (3) the head strikes the vehicle and then the ground (skull and facial fractures, facial abrasions, and closed head injury).

Falls From Heights

High falls most commonly involve children younger than 5 years of age who are left unsupervised near a high window (more than 10 ft) or on a porch higher than 10 ft with inadequate railings. Adult falls from heights usually occur in the context of criminal activity, attempted suicide, or intoxication such as in alcohol, narcotic, or hallucinogen use, especially PCP.

Remember that a fall produces acceleration downward at 9.8 m/sec². On contact with the floor or ground, an instantaneous stop occurs that decelerates the victim from whatever velocity had been achieved at the end of the fall to zero velocity. If a person falls for 2 seconds, the speed at impact is nearly 20 m/sec.

The severity of injuries you can expect to find in your patient will depend on a number of factors, all of which will be important in your patient assessment:

- **Height.** The height from which the patient has fallen will determine the *velocity* of the fall. A person falling one story (12 ft) onto concrete, for example, will fall at about 28 ft per second (fps) and experience an impact force of about 48 *g*. A person falling from the second story (24 ft) will reach a velocity of 39 fps and experience an impact force of 95 *g* on the same surface. Height plus stopping distance predicts the magnitude of deceleration forces. A fall greater than 15 ft or 2.5 to 3 times the height of the patient will have a greater incidence of morbidity and mortality, although it is usually assumed that a fall from four stories may be survivable. At five stories, survival is questionable; at six stories, survival is unlikely, and a fall from seven stories or higher is rarely survivable.
- **Position.** The position or orientation of the body at the moment of impact will also be a determinant of the type of injuries sustained and their survivability. Children tend to fall headfirst, owing to the relatively greater mass of a child's head, so head injuries are common in children, as are injuries to the wrists and upper extremities when the child attempts to break his or her fall with outstretched

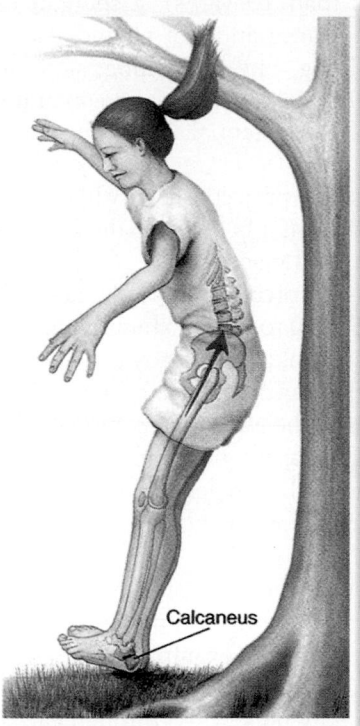

Figure 16 When an adult jumps or falls and lands on his or her feet, the energy is transmitted to the spine, sometimes producing a spinal injury in addition to injuries to the legs and pelvis.

arms. Adults, on the other hand, usually try to land on their feet, thus controlling their fall. However, they often tilt backward, landing on their buttocks and outstretched hands. The group of potential injuries from a vertical fall to a standing position is commonly referred to as the *Don Juan syndrome* or *lover's leap* pattern of injuries **Figure 16**. Injuries include foot and lower extremity fractures, along with hip, acetabular, and pelvic ring and sacral fractures. Lumbar spine axial loading also results in vertebral compression and burst fractures particularly of T12-L1 and L2. Vertical deceleration forces to organs (liver, spleen, and aorta) and fractures of the forearm and wrist (Colles fracture) are also common.

- **Area.** The area over which the impact is distributed—the larger the area of contact at the time of impact, the greater the dissipation of the force and the lesser the peak pressures generated.

- **Surface.** The surface onto which the person has fallen and the degree to which that surface can deform (degree of plasticity) under the force of the falling body can help dissipate the forces of sudden deceleration. Deep snow, for example, has a relatively large capacity to deform, whereas concrete has scarcely any plasticity. Also, contrary to what might be expected, water also has very little plasticity at high-speed impacts. The surface of contact may also present hazards in the form of irregularities or protruding structures; it is far more dangerous to fall onto a wrought-iron picket fence, for example, than onto the grass beside it. If the surface does not conform, the unprotected body will.

- **Physical condition.** The physical condition of the patient in the form of preexisting medical conditions may also influence the injuries sustained. Most notably is the case of older patients with osteoporosis, a condition that predisposes to fractures even with minimal falls. Patients with hematologic conditions resulting in an enlarged spleen may also be more prone to ruptured spleen in a fall. Children younger than 3 years of age have fewer injuries from falls greater than three stories than do

older children and adults, most likely because of the more elastic nature of their tissues and less ossification.

■ Penetrating Trauma

Unlike blunt trauma, which can involve a large surface area, <u>penetrating trauma</u> involves a disruption of the skin and underlying tissues in a small, focused area. Although a variety of objects may cause penetrating injuries in a variety of settings, penetrating trauma is usually interpreted as being more specific to injuries caused by firearms, knives, and other devices used as a means to cause intentional or accidental harm **Figure 17**. Penetrating trauma is classified as low, medium, or high velocity. Low-velocity penetrating trauma, such as a stab wound, is caused by the sharp edges of the object moving through the body. In medium- and high-velocity penetrating trauma, the path of the object (usually a bullet) may not be easy to predict because the bullet may flatten out, tumble, or even ricochet within the body before exiting.

In the United States, the most common sources of penetrating injuries are firearms **Figure 18**. According to US National

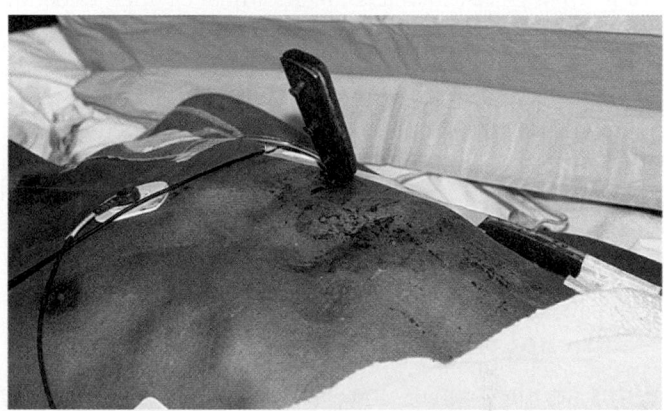

Figure 17 Injuries from low-energy penetrations, such as a stab wound, are caused by the sharp edges of the object moving through the body.

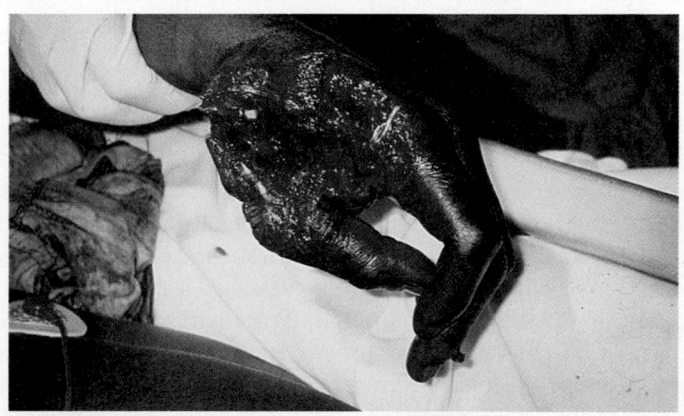

Figure 18 Guns are a common cause of penetrating trauma, as shown in this case.

Vital Statistics Reports, in 2009, 31,285 people died by gunfire in the United States. The number of deaths, while staggering, actually represents a 21% decline in firearm-associated deaths from a peak in 1993. Of the gun-related deaths in 2009, 60% were suicides, 38% were homicides (including justified shootings by law enforcement personnel and gun owners), and 2% were accidental discharge or undetermined.

Stab Wounds

The severity of a stab wound depends on the anatomic area involved, depth of penetration, blade length, and angle of penetration. A stab wound may also involve a cutting- or hacking-type force such as in machete wounds, which not only can result in laceration, but also can cause fractures and blunt injury to underlying soft tissues and bone and potentially amputation.

Neck wounds can involve critical anatomic structures such as the carotid arteries, jugular veins, subclavian vessels, apices of the lung, the upper mediastinum, trachea, esophagus, and thoracic duct. Deep neck wounds of sufficient energy can result in spinal cord involvement and cervical fracture.

Lower chest or upper abdominal wounds have the potential of involving the thoracic and abdominal cavities, depending on the location of the diaphragm at the time of injury—that is, whether the person was taking a breath or exhaling.

The pattern of stab wounds closely relates to the mechanism involved and should be documented in detail because your records may be needed in criminal proceedings. Be sure to record the directions of the stab wounds. Wounds delivered to the back are generally downward, whereas stab wounds from the front are generally upward.

Gunshot Wounds

Firearms are the primary mechanism resulting in penetrating trauma. The amount of damage a firearm can cause will depend on a number of factors, including the type of firearm (rifle, shotgun, or handgun), velocity of the projectile, physical design and size of the projectile, the distance of the victim from the muzzle of the firearm, and the type of tissue that is struck.

There are hundreds if not thousands of firearm models and designs. However, they can be classified *primarily into three types: shotguns, rifles, and handguns.*

Shotguns fire round pellets (referred to as "shot"), from about half a dozen to several dozen at a time, depending on the type of load used. The load denominated 00 or 000 "buckshot" is the larger pellets, and smaller shot such as No. 7 is a common fowl hunting shot or "birdshot." At short range, even the smaller shot can cause devastating injuries. Shotgun shells can also be loaded with a single large and heavy projectile called a sabot, which can cause even worse harm. A shotgun typically has a smooth bore, and its numerous projectiles are not stabilized in flight by spin, as is the single projectile fired from a rifle barrel. The pellets, therefore, leave the barrel and immediately start dispersing so that the shot density (that is, the separation between any two pellets) at the time of impact on a target will be determined by the distance traveled.

At very close range (less than 10 yards), a shotgun can induce destructive injuries. Entrance and exit wounds can be very large, with shotgun wadding, bits of clothing, skin, and hair driven into the wound that can cause massive contamination, leading to increased infection potential should the patient survive the initial trauma.

Rifles are firearms firing a single projectile at very high velocity through a grooved barrel that imparts a spin to the projectile that stabilizes the projectile's flight for accuracy.

Handguns are of two types: revolvers and pistols. Revolvers have a cylinder holding from 6 to 10 rounds of ammunition, and pistols have a separate magazine holding as many as 17 rounds of ammunition in some models. Handguns also have rifled barrels to impart spin to a bullet, but their accuracy is more limited than a rifle's because their barrels (and sight radius) are shorter. The ammunition handguns fire is also, in general, less powerful than ammunition fired from rifles, and handguns fire at lower velocities.

The most important factor for the seriousness of a gunshot wound is the *type of tissue* through which the projectile passes. Tissue of high elasticity like muscle, for example, is better able to tolerate stretch (temporary cavitation) than tissue of low elasticity, like the liver. A high-velocity bullet fired through a fleshy part of the leg may do much less damage than a relatively low-velocity bullet that punctures the aorta or the liver. Many bullet wounds of the extremities that are found to have caused no fracture or neurovascular compromise will be treated by the trauma team with splinting and a single dose of antibiotic without a need for wound exploration or bullet retrieval.

An **entry wound** is characterized by the effects of initial contact and **implosion**. Skin and subcutaneous tissues are pushed in, cut, or abraded externally as missile fragments pass and heat is transferred to the tissues. At close range, tattoo marks from powder burns can occur. At extremely close ranges, burns can occur from muzzle blast. Heavy wound contamination results from negative pressure generated behind the traveling projectile, which sucks surrounding elements such as clothing into the wound, greatly increasing infection potential.

Words of Wisdom

As a general rule, the entrance wound (usually funnel shaped) is always smaller than the exit wound. Assume that cavitation involves internal structures that are not readily visible on your clinical exam.

Deformation and tissue destruction sustained in soft tissues and bone is based on a combination of factors, including density, compressibility, missile velocity, and missile fragmentation. The initial path of tissue destruction is caused by the projectile crushing the tissue during penetration. This creates a **permanent cavity** that may be a straight line or an irregular pathway as the bullet is deflected into a number of angles after initial penetration. **Pathway expansion** refers to the tissue displacement that occurs as the result of low-displacement sonic pressure waves that travel at the speed of sound in tissue (four times the speed of sound in air). These sonic pressure waves push tissues in front of and lateral to the projectile and may not necessarily increase the wound size or cause permanent injury, but they result in **cavitation** (cavity formation). Tissue is compressed and accelerated away, causing injury. The waves of tissue are similar to throwing a rock into a pond. The rock creates a hole in the pond that quickly refills while waves emanate from the penetrating "wound," or hole in the pond.

Bowel, muscle, and the lungs are relatively elastic, resulting in fewer permanent effects of temporary cavitation. The liver, spleen, and brain are relatively inelastic, and the temporary cavity may become a permanent defect. **Missile fragmentation** is a major cause of tissue damage as the projectile sends off fragments that create their own separate paths through tissues. Secondary missiles can also be generated by pieces of bone, teeth, buttons, or other objects encountered in the projectile's path as it enters the body. **Exit wounds** occur when the projectile has sufficient energy that is not entirely dissipated along its trajectory through the body. The projectile then exits the patient and can injure other bystanders as well.

The size of the exit wound depends on the energy dissipated and the degree of cavitation at the point of exit. Exit wounds usually have irregular edges and may be larger than entry wounds Figure 19 . There may be multiple exit wounds in the case of fragmentation. The number of exit wounds and the extent of tissue damage encountered must be assessed and carefully documented.

Words of Wisdom

Don't assume that a bullet followed a straight path between the entrance and exit sites. It may ricochet inside the body, especially off bones, and travel in many different directions.

Shotgun wounds are the result of tissue impacted by numerous projectiles. As described earlier, the greater the distance

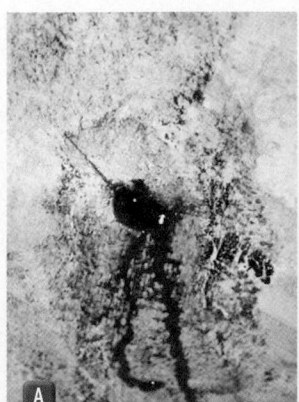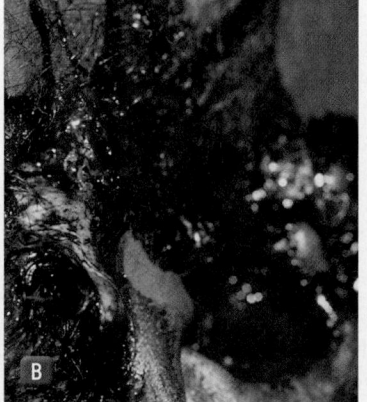

Figure 19 **A.** Entrance wound from a gunshot. **B.** Exit wound from a gunshot.

from the muzzle to the target, the more dispersion the multiple projectiles will have and the more KE that will be lost before impact. Thus, shotguns are most lethal when used as short-range weapons. Also, the velocity of each pellet is less than the velocity of any bullet fired from a rifle.

Wounding potential from an injury sustained from a shotgun depends on the powder charge, the size and number of pellets, and the dispersion of the pellets. Dispersion is in turn determined by the range at which the weapon was fired, the barrel length (shorter barrels have more scatter), and the type of choke at the end of the barrel.

To give the trauma team at the hospital as much information as possible, try to obtain the following information:

- What kind of weapon was used (handgun, rifle, or shotgun; type and caliber, if known)?
- At what range was it fired?
- What kind of bullet was used? (Ideally, see if the police can find an unfired cartridge.)

What to look for:

- Powder residue around the wound
- Entrance and exit wounds (the exit wound is usually larger and more ragged)

In the real world, the assailant is usually gone, along with the weapon, and patient care is the first goal of paramedics, a far more pressing matter than obtaining answers to the previous questions.

■ Blast Injuries

Although most commonly associated with military conflict, blast injuries are also seen in civilian practice in mines, shipyards, and chemical plants, and, increasingly, in association with terrorist activities. People who are injured in explosions may be injured by any of five different mechanisms, often causing multisystem trauma Figure 20 .

■ Primary Blast Injuries

Primary blast injuries are due entirely to the blast itself—that is, damage to the body caused by the pressure wave generated by the explosion. When an explosion occurs, a pressure wave rapidly develops; this tremendous, concentrated pressure results from air displacement and heat originating from the center of the blast. The organs generally affected by primary blast effects are the lungs, eardrums, and other compressible organs. The pressure wave damages air-filled cavities. Burns also may occur.

Close proximity to the origin of the pressure wave carries a high risk of injury or death. Explosions from a bomb start at the center and move outward, so persons closer to the device will be affected to a greater extent. Explosions from fumes or dust involve an entire area, so there is no "safe" region. Underwater blasts have a three times greater range because of the near incompressibility of water. Explosions that occur within a confined space result in more force applied to the body.

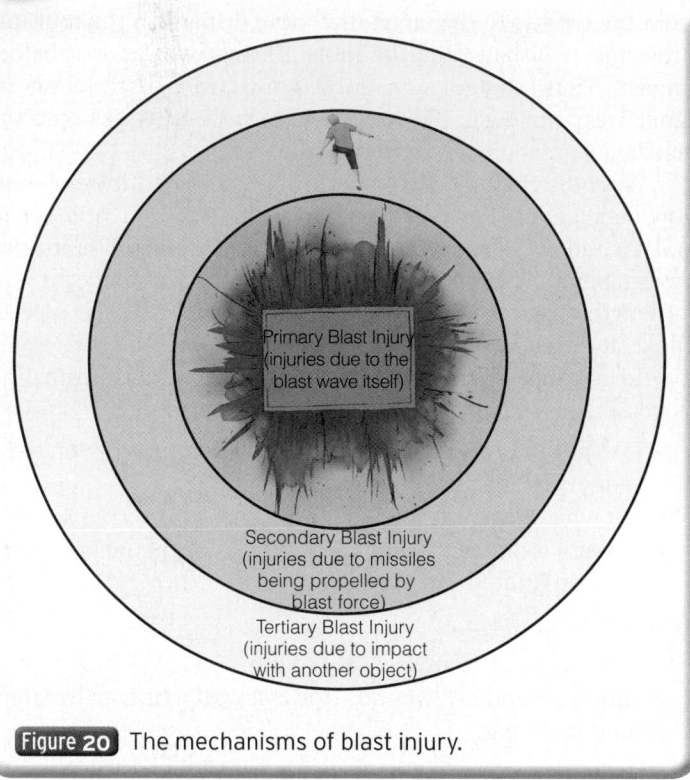

Primary Blast Injury (injuries due to the blast wave itself)

Secondary Blast Injury (injuries due to missiles being propelled by blast force)

Tertiary Blast Injury (injuries due to impact with another object)

Figure 20 The mechanisms of blast injury.

Secondary Blast Injuries

Secondary blast injuries result from being struck by flying debris (such as shrapnel from the device or from glass or splinters) that has been set in motion by the explosion. Objects are propelled by the force of the blast and strike the victim, causing injury. These objects can travel great distances and can be propelled at tremendous speeds, up to nearly 3,000 mph for conventional military explosives.

A blast wind occurs as the shock wave applies force to air molecules. Although less forceful than the pressure wave, the blast wind is longer lasting and can hurt projectiles at high velocities. Projectiles present serious hazards—flying debris may cause blunt and penetrating injuries. With bombs, the casing fragments rip apart with monumental force, spreading in all directions. Structural elements can break apart and travel at high rates of speed. Nails, wood splinters, and glass shards can impale victims located in the area of the blast.

Tertiary Blast Injuries

There may be multiple victims as a result of a tertiary blast. These blast injuries occur when a person is hurled by the force of the explosion (or blast wind) against stationary, rigid objects,

YOU are the Medic   PART 3

The next steps in your primary assessment include an assessment of respiratory status. A quick look at the trachea shows that it is midline and the chest appears to be expanding equally. Breath sounds are present and no crepitus is noted.

A quick look does not reveal any open chest wounds or impaled objects. Using the mnemonic "O I PASS" (or IPASSO) will help you to quickly move through this phase of the primary assessment. The mnemonic stands for Oxygen (high concentration), Inspect, Palpate (quickly for subcutaneous emphysema and crepitus), Auscultate, Seal (open or sucking wounds), and Stabilize (impaled objects). Remember, at this point you are doing just the primary assessment to identify and treat immediate life threats. The radial pulse is present only in her right wrist, but it is very weak and rapid. The left arm is deformed and her hand is cold with no palpable pulse. As you quickly move from head to toe looking for any severe bleeding, your partner reminds you that on-scene time is now approaching 6 minutes. The patient's friend tells you that they were just past the top of the ride and the patient initially fell head first, striking the car below them and then tumbled to the ground.

Recording Time: 5 Minutes	
Respirations	22 breaths/min, unlabored
Pulse	140 beats/min, weak right radial pulse
Skin	Pale, cool, moist
Blood pressure	140/110 mm Hg
Oxygen saturation (Spo$_2$)	97%
Pupils	Left pupil dilated, nonreactive

5. The patient's rapid, weak pulse and cool, moist skin indicate likelihood of inadequate perfusion, yet the blood pressure does not indicate advanced shock. What are some possible reasons for this finding?

6. According to the friend who witnessed the fall, the patient's initial impact was with her head against the metal car below. What is the significance of a smaller surface area of the body absorbing the initial impact as opposed to a larger body surface area?

such as the ground, or walls. Physical displacement of the body is also referred to as ground shock when the body impacts the ground. The injuries that result are numerous and result from both blunt and penetrating mechanisms. A blast wind also causes the patient's body to be hurled or thrown, causing further injury. In some cases, wind injuries can amputate limbs.

Victims may also be injured from displacement away from the blast site. Displacement occurs when a person is in close proximity to the explosion; survival in this circumstance is highly unlikely.

Quaternary (Miscellaneous) Blast Injuries

Injuries result from the miscellaneous events that occur during an explosion. For example, the heat generated during an explosion may cause burns, ranging from superficial flash burns to full-thickness burns involving the entire or large areas of the body. These injuries can include burns from hot gases or fires started by the blast, respiratory injury from inhaling toxic gases, and crush injury from the collapse of buildings. There is also a risk for entrapment that may be prolonged for days.

Quinary Blast Injuries

Quinary blast injuries are caused by biologic, chemical, or radioactive contaminants that have been added to a traditional explosive device. The initial explosion disperses these materials, causing additional long-term damage to victims through biologic, chemical, or radioactive mechanisms. This type of blast injury is associated with "dirty bombs" and is of increased concern due to the threat of its use by terrorist organizations.

The vast majority of patients who survive an explosion will have some combination of the five types of injury mentioned. The discussion here is confined to primary blast injuries because they are the most easily overlooked.

The Physics of an Explosion

When a substance is detonated, a solid or liquid is chemically converted into large volumes of gas under pressure with resultant energy release. Propellants, like gunpowder, are explosives designed to release energy relatively slowly compared with high explosives (for example, trinitrotoluene, or TNT), which are designed to detonate very quickly. Explosives such as composition C4 can create initial pressures of more than 4 million pounds per square inch. This generates a pressure pulse in the shape of a spherical blast wave that expands in all directions from the point of explosion. Flying debris and high winds commonly cause conventional blunt and penetrating trauma.

Components of Blast Shock Wave

The leading edge of an explosion pressure blast wave is called the **blast front**. A **positive wave pulse** refers to the phase of the explosion in which there is a pressure front higher than atmospheric pressure. The peak magnitude of the wave experienced by a patient becomes lessened the farther the person is from the center of the explosion. The increase in pressure from a blast can

be so abrupt that high-explosive blast waves are also referred to as "shock waves." Shock waves possess a characteristic, **brisance**, that describes the shattering effect of the wave and its ability to cause disruption of tissues as well as structures. Tissue damage is dependent on the magnitude of the pressure spike and the duration of force application. The **negative wave pulse** refers to the phase in which pressure is less than atmospheric; it may last 10 times as long as the positive wave pulse. It occurs as air displaced by the positive wave pulse returns to fill the space of the explosion. It can lead to massive movements of air resulting in high-velocity winds.

The speed, duration, and pressure of the shock wave are affected by the following:

- The *size* of the explosive charge. The larger the explosion, the faster the shock waves and the longer they will last.
- The nature of the *surrounding medium*. Pressure waves travel much more rapidly in water, for example, and are effective at greater distances in water than in air.
- The *distance* from the explosion. The farther one is from the explosion, the slower the shock wave velocity and the longer its duration.
- The presence or absence of *reflecting surfaces*. If the pressure wave is reflected off a solid object, its pressure may be multiplied several times. For example, a shock wave that might cause minimal injury in the open can cause devastating trauma if the patient is standing beside a wall or similar solid object.

The changes in pressure produced by the shock wave produce transient *winds*, sometimes of very high velocity, that can accelerate small objects to speeds of hundreds of feet per second. A missile traveling at 50 fps can easily penetrate human skin; at 400 fps, a missile can enter any of the major body cavities and cause serious internal injury. Blast winds can also send the human body flying against larger, more stationary objects, or as mentioned previously, amputate limbs.

In an underwater explosion, a shock wave travels at greater velocity than in open air, thereby making it possible to receive injuries at three times the distance that would normally be required to receive such injuries. This is because positive pressures are higher and there are no negative pressures or high-velocity wind. Blast fragments and gases move shorter distances in water.

An explosion is significantly more damaging in closed spaces because of a limited dissipation environment for the forces involved and for the generation of toxic gases and smoke. The shock wave is magnified when it comes into contact with a solid surface such as a wall, causing persons near a wall to be hit with significantly higher pressure, resulting in increased risk of injury and death.

Remember the discussion of the types of tissue and the effect of trauma on tissues that contain air, water, or hard bone? Blast pressures cause destruction at the interface between tissues of different densities or the interface between tissues and trapped air. When the shock wave passes from a higher to lower density medium, a severe pressure disturbance develops at the interface of the denser medium. The result is fragmentation of the heavier medium, or **spalling**. When the shock wave contacts small gas bubbles, the bubbles are compressed and high local pressures are created, called implosion. The bubbles can then reexpand and cause further damage. Acceleration and deceleration of organs at their fixation points will occur in a manner similar to that in blunt trauma.

Tissues at Risk

Air-containing organs such as the middle ear, heart, lungs, major blood vessels, and the gastrointestinal tract are most susceptible to pressure changes. Junctions between tissues of different densities and exposed tissues such as the head and neck are prone to injury as well. The ear is the organ system most sensitive to blast injuries. The <u>tympanic membrane</u> evolved to detect minor changes in pressure and will rupture at pressures of 5 to 7 pounds per square inch above atmospheric pressure. Thus, the tympanic membranes are a sensitive indicator of the possible presence of other blast injuries. The patient may complain of ringing in the ears, pain in the ears, or some loss of hearing, and blood may be visible in the ear canal. Dislocation of structural components of the ear, such as the ossicles within the inner ear, may occur. Permanent hearing loss is possible.

> ### Words of Wisdom
>
> When hearing is abnormal after an explosion, look for serious injury to the lungs.

Primary <u>pulmonary blast injuries</u> occur as contusions and hemorrhages. When the explosion occurs in an open space, the side toward the explosion is usually injured, but the injury can be bilateral when the victim is located in a confined space. The patient may complain of tightness or pain in the chest and may cough up blood and have tachypnea or other signs of respiratory distress. Subcutaneous emphysema (crackling under the skin) over the chest can be palpated, indicating underlying pneumothorax. Tension pneumothorax may develop and may require emergency decompression in the field for your patient to survive. Pulmonary edema may ensue rapidly. If there is *any* reason to suspect lung injury in a blast victim (even just the presence of a ruptured eardrum), administer oxygen. Avoid giving oxygen under positive pressure. Tension pneumothorax may develop because that may simply increase the damage to the lung. Be cautious as well with intravenous (IV) fluids, which may be poorly tolerated in patients with this lung injury and result in pulmonary edema.

> ### Words of Wisdom
>
> If the victim of a blast injury has any neurologic abnormalities, notify the base physician at once!

One of the most concerning pulmonary blast injuries is <u>arterial air embolism</u>, which occurs on alveolar disruption with subsequent air embolization into the pulmonary vasculature. Even small air bubbles can enter a coronary artery and cause myocardial injury. Air embolisms to the cerebrovascular system

can produce disturbances in vision, changes in behavior, changes in state of consciousness, and a variety of other neurologic signs.

Solid organs are relatively protected from shock wave injury but may be injured by secondary missiles or a hurled body. Hollow organs, however, may be injured by similar mechanisms as for lung tissue. Petechiae, or pinpoint hemorrhages that show up on the skin, to large hematomas are the dominant form of pathology. Perforation or rupture of the bowel and colon is a risk. Underwater explosions result in the most severe abdominal injuries.

Neurologic injuries and head trauma are the most common causes of death from blast injuries. Subarachnoid (beneath the arachnoid layer covering the brain) and subdural (beneath the outermost covering of the brain) hematomas are often seen. Permanent or transient neurologic deficits may be secondary to concussion, intracerebral bleeding, or air embolism. Instant but transient unconsciousness, with or without retrograde amnesia, may be initiated not only by head trauma, but also by cardiovascular problems. Bradycardia and hypotension are common after an intense pressure wave from an explosion. This is a vagal nerve–mediated form of cardiogenic shock without compensatory vasoconstriction (for example, vasovagal syncope).

Extremity injuries, including traumatic amputations, are common. Other injuries are often associated with tertiary blasts. Patients with traumatic amputation by postblast wind are likely to sustain fatal injuries secondary to the blast. In the global war on terror, improved body armor has increased the number of survivors of blast injuries from shrapnel wounds to the torso. The number of severe orthopaedic and extremity injuries, however, has increased. In addition, while body armor may limit or prevent shrapnel from entering the body, it also "catches" more energy from the shock wave, possibly resulting in the victim being thrown backward, thus increasing potential spine and spinal cord injury.

Although blast injuries have usually been the domain of military surgeons, they often occur in industrial settings and are, unfortunately, more common today owing to the increased use of explosives as a tool for urban terrorism and, in the US, from methamphetamine lab explosions. Although civilian blast injuries in an industrial or mining setting were mostly characterized by blast injuries and burns, terrorist bombs often have shrapnel. Modern EMS and trauma services personnel should be fully educated and aware of what to expect in these scenarios.

Assessment and Management of Blast Injuries

When you are at the scene of an explosion, expect significant trauma and multiple victims. The forces generated by the blast have the potential to cover a wide area with devastating effect. If the explosion was intentional, examine the immediate area for a secondary device. When scene safety cannot be ensured, evacuate to a safe distance until qualified personnel advise you that it is safe to approach the patient. Also assess the scene for other hazards that may lead to EMS crew injury, such as exposed electrical wiring, structural instability, and sharp objects.

After standard precautions have been taken and determination of a safe scene has been completed, form a general impression as you approach the patient. Rapidly perform a primary assessment to detect and manage life threats. Immobilize the cervical spine, and assess the airway by performing the jaw-thrust maneuver. Determine whether the airway is patent, and correct airway compromise immediately on discovery. Identify whether breathing is abnormally fast or slow, or deep or shallow, and note the gross respiratory pattern. Assess circulation by checking the carotid and radial pulses. Reassess the patient's mental status while examining the patient for injury.

Pulmonary injuries are common when an explosion occurs and can be life threatening. Assess breath sounds frequently throughout care because the pressure wave generated by an explosion can lead to a pneumothorax. Should the air within the chest cavity continue to collapse the affected lung, a tension pneumothorax can develop. Needle decompression is a lifesaving intervention in such a case.

Noncardiogenic pulmonary edema can develop after an explosion. A massive pulmonary contusion can lead to microhemorrhage within the lungs, further compromising ventilation and respiration. Ask the patient about the ease or difficulty of breathing early in your assessment. Have your team members examine the patient rapidly for the presence of DCAP-BTLS, and manage life threats rapidly. Establish a baseline pulse oximetry value, and reassess this measure frequently. Although pulse oximeter readings are important, administer high-flow supplemental oxygen even in the presence of a high reading. Patient compromise is likely to develop, even if the initial symptoms are not severe.

A patient injured in a blast commonly sustains abdominal trauma that includes ruptured organs and internal hemorrhage. The pressure wave can cause air-filled cavities, such as the small and large bowels, to burst. Although these injuries can be catastrophic, they often take time to emerge. An absence of overt signs of abdominal injury should not lead you to conclude that an injury is not present. Recall the KE forces involved during an explosion, and maintain a high index of suspicion.

Ask the patient about the presence of abdominal pain. If he or she reports discomfort, use the OPQRST mnemonic to guide your history taking. Examine all abdominal quadrants for the presence of DCAP-BTLS, noting tenderness on the patient care report.

During the blast, victims' ears are often adversely affected by the pressure wave. The likelihood of rupture of the tympanic membrane is high. Hearing loss is common when the patient is in proximity to the blast. Because the ears are essential in establishing body position, dizziness can occur when they are affected. Such dizziness can lead to vomiting, which may interfere with airway patency and protection.

Projectiles can produce penetrating wounds during the secondary blast phase. If you discover an impaled object in your patient's body, follow the basic points outlined in the next section regarding management of an impaled object, which is also discussed in the chapter, *Soft-Tissue Trauma*. If an object is impaled in the eye, follow the principles outlined in the chapter, *Diseases of the Eyes, Ears, Nose, and Throat*.

■ Multisystem Trauma

Multisystem trauma describes injuries that involve several body systems. Examples of these injuries include trauma to the head and spine, chest and abdomen, or chest and multiple extremities. The body can compensate fairly well to an isolated injury, but it has a much harder time dealing with multiple injuries that involve several major body areas. In general, multisystem trauma is caused by events that affect the entire body such as a motor vehicle crash or a fall from a height. Often, both blunt and penetrating trauma occurs, with a high level of morbidity and mortality. Be alert for multisystem trauma—assess the patient's entire body if you suspect that multiple body systems are affected by trauma, prioritize the treatment of the injuries, and transport multisystem trauma patients without delay.

■ Trauma Score

Paramedics must have a strong understanding of trauma scoring systems to appropriately classify patients. Use of trauma scoring systems to determine injury severity is a common practice in the health care profession. It was thought that implementing a scoring system would assist health care providers in rapidly identifying the severity of the patient's injuries. There are several different trauma scoring systems. The trauma score is used to determine the likelihood of patient survival, which is calculated on a scale of 1 to 16, with 16 being the best possible score. It takes into account the Glasgow Coma Scale (GCS) score, respiratory rate, respiratory expansion, systolic blood pressure, and capillary refill. The GCS is an evaluation tool used to determine level of consciousness; scores are assigned for eye opening, verbal response, and motor response. The sum of these scores can be used to predict patient outcomes. However, this scoring system does not accurately predict survivability in patients with severe head injuries because motor and verbal deficits make those criteria difficult to assess; in these instances, the Revised Trauma Score is used.

■ Revised Trauma Score

The Revised Trauma Score (RTS) is a physiological scoring system used to assess injury severity in patients with head trauma. This system is heavily weighted to compensate for major head injury without multisystem injury or major physiologic changes.

Objective data used to calculate the RTS include the GCS score, systolic blood pressure, and respiratory rate. In addition to assessing injury severity, the RTS has also demonstrated reliability in predicting survival in patients with severe injuries. The highest RTS a patient can receive is 12; the lowest is 0. An RTS calculation is shown in Table 4.

■ General Assessment of Trauma

Managing a trauma scene involves more consideration of external factors than a typical scene with a medical patient. When a trauma patient arrives at the hospital, the staff there will not have the benefit of the scene information; therefore your observations are critical to them. Trauma patients also tend to have visible injuries and an MOI that is fairly easy to identify. At the same time, very few trauma injuries can be truly stabilized on

Table 4   Revised Trauma Score Calculation

Glasgow Coma Score	Systolic Blood Pressure (mm Hg)	Respiratory Rate (breaths/min)	Value
13 to 15	> 89	> 29	4
9 to 12	76 to 89	10 to 29	3
6 to 8	50 to 75	6 to 9	2
4 to 5	1 to 49	1 to 5	1
3	0	0	0

scene, and in some cases there may be hidden traumatic injuries that will not be identified until the patient reaches surgery. The way you handle the trauma scene can make a huge difference in the outcome of your patient.

◼ Scene Size-up

As with all calls, attention to personal protective equipment is required. Gloves are extremely important because the likelihood of bleeding is much higher in trauma patients than in medical patients. On trauma scenes, it is a good idea to have an extra pair of gloves in your pocket, in case one of your gloves becomes torn and needs to be replaced. In addition to gloves, protective

eyewear is important. Blood and bodily fluids from a traumatically injured patient can easily be splashed into your eyes. Other protective equipment including helmets, heavy coats, and boots may be required based on the MOI.

Anticipate possible scene hazards while en route to the scene. As you identify potential hazards, call for assistance in dealing with them before you move on to patient assessment and care. Fire, rescue, hazardous materials, and police responders require time to travel to the scene; the sooner you call for them, the sooner they will arrive and help you control the scene. Assess your environment carefully.

As you locate and approach your patient(s), also consider whether you will need additional medical resources. Be observant as you locate the patient and work to determine the MOI.

◼ Primary Assessment

Form a General Impression

The general impression formed when you first approach your patient can guide assessment and treatment. Patients who look very ill or present with obvious bleeding injuries often have serious injuries, whereas those who appear to be relatively stable may not be as seriously injured. Obviously, it is wrong to make major patient decisions based strictly on your first impression; however, using the instincts you have developed throughout your career to anticipate what you might need to do is appropriate.

Keeping the MOI in mind as you approach the patient, consider whether spinal stabilization will be necessary and be

YOU are the Medic   PART 4

Your partner places the backboard next to the patient, informing you that it has been almost 9 minutes on the scene. As you cut away her clothing, you see a large contusion on the right lower quadrant and the abdomen appears distended. Her outward-bent legs are gently moved to center and you and your partner, after applying the cervical collar, gently roll the patient and immobilize her on the backboard. You close the buckles over the blanket and load her into the ambulance. As the clock ticks to the 10-minute mark, your partner maneuvers the ambulance out of the park and onto the road to the nearby trauma center.

Recording Time: 9 Minutes	
Respirations	24 breaths/min, irregular
Pulse	88 beats/min, weak right radial pulse
Skin	Pale, cool, moist
Blood pressure	130/116 mm Hg
Oxygen saturation (Spo$_2$)	98%
Pupils	Left pupil dilated, nonreactive

7. What criteria does this patient meet in order to warrant transport to the trauma center?

8. As you continue your examination and observation of your patient en route to the trauma center, you think about the presentation of your patient to the waiting emergency department staff. What MOI will you relate to the staff?

prepared to protect the patient from *movement-induced* spinal injury. As you approach, ask the patient not to move his or her head and have your partner apply manual cervical stabilization. Evaluate the patient's level of consciousness using the AVPU. If the patient is awake, introduce yourself. Check pupil size and reactivity. If the patient does not appear to be awake, see if he or she responds to verbal or light painful stimulus. Make a mental note of this status for later reference.

Airway and Breathing

Continue your evaluation by assessing the patient's airway status. If your patient is unconscious, ask your partner, who is manually stabilizing the cervical spine, to open the airway using the jaw-thrust maneuver. Remember, if there is any possibility of a cervical spine injury, you should avoid using the head tilt–chin lift maneuver. Observe for obvious oral or facial trauma that may contribute to airway obstruction. Be prepared to remove foreign objects and to suction out blood or vomitus to make sure the airway remains clear. If the patient is unconscious, consider the need for an oral or nasopharyngeal airway to maintain the airway once it has been opened. These may be replaced later with an endotracheal tube or a blind insertion airway device if necessary. If you suspect a blockage of the airway due to a foreign object, apply the appropriate manual airway clearing technique and be prepared to use an advanced technique, such as visualization with a laryngoscope or even a needle or surgical cricothyrotomy.

Once the airway is clear, assess the patient's breathing. Absence of breathing will require you to initiate bag-mask ventilation and to consider a more advanced airway adjunct. If the patient is breathing, note the relative rate and quality of the respirations as well as the patient's ability to speak. Dyspnea or difficulty breathing may be caused by many traumatic injuries. Note the skin color, remembering that cyanosis is caused by inadequate oxygenation, and observe the chest wall movement with respirations. If you observe a sucking chest injury, take immediate action to seal the wound to prevent exacerbation of the patient's condition. Assess the thorax and neck for a deviated trachea, tension pneumothorax, neck and chest crepitation, broken ribs, a fractured sternum, or other problems that may inhibit breathing. On the basis of all of the information you find, determine how best to support your patient's breathing. Most trauma patients will benefit from application of oxygen even in the absence of dyspnea. Rapid shallow respirations generally do not provide adequate volumes of air to an injured patient, so you may want to consider assisted ventilation with oxygen using the bag-mask device for these patients.

Circulation

Next, you need to evaluate circulation. Checking both radial and carotid pulses simultaneously will allow you to estimate the patient's blood pressure as well as the pulse. Note the relative rate and quality of the pulse. If there is no pulse, begin CPR immediately. Skin condition (color, temperature, and condition) can also be a good indicator of circulation. Quickly scan the patient for any significant external bleeding. Bleeding that is flowing heavily or spurting should be controlled immediately.

Transport Decision

Once you have identified and treated life threats, and before you continue the assessment, you should be able to make a preliminary transport decision. Patients with altered mental status, airway or breathing problems, multisystem trauma or significantly compromised circulation should be categorized for immediate transport or "load and go." Patients who do not meet these criteria should be categorized as nonurgent (sometimes referred to as "stay and play"). If a patient is considered "load and go," continue your assessment en route to the trauma center, and move as quickly as possible to begin transport. In most patients with multisystem trauma, definitive care requires surgical intervention; therefore, on-scene time should be limited to 10 minutes or less. This is referred to as the "platinum 10 minutes." Spend as little time as possible on scene with patients who have sustained significant trauma. After the first 60 minutes in shock, often termed the "Golden hour," the body has progressively increased difficulty compensating.

History Taking

Gathering patient history includes obtaining a SAMPLE history as well as OPQRST for any symptoms reported. For trauma patients, medical history should be obtained as soon as possible in case the patient's level of consciousness deteriorates. If the patient is unconscious when you arrive, this information should be gathered from bystanders or family members who may be present. Identification of patient symptoms, including where they are feeling the most amount of pain, can be very helpful in the physical exam. Allergies, medications, and past medical history may seem relatively unimportant at this time, but this information will be critical when the patient is treated at the trauma center. The patient's last oral intake is important in case the patient needs to be intubated in preparation for surgery to treat the injuries. Events leading up to the situation may have already been identified, but if not, the last letter of the SAMPLE history should remind you to get more information about what happened.

Secondary Assessment

Trauma patients are classified into two major groups: those with an isolated injury and those with multisystem trauma. From a secondary assessment perspective, the biggest difference between the groups is that an isolated injury allows you to immediately focus on the main problem.

Controversies

After the first 60 minutes, also known as the "Golden hour," the body has increasing difficulty in compensating for shock and traumatic injuries. Because many injured patients require definitive care in less than an hour, this time frame may also be referred to as the "Golden Period." If your patient's condition is nonurgent, continue to monitor him or her during the remainder of your assessment. If your patient's condition deteriorates, you can upgrade the status to urgent and expedite transport at that time.

In contrast, with multisystem trauma, you must first find all (or as many as you can reasonably find) of the various problems (for example, a hematoma on the forehead, a fractured arm, and neck and lower back pain). Then you need to prioritize the injuries by severity and the order in which you plan to address them. During the assessment, you must continually think about how each injury or condition relates to the others. For example, the mortality rate doubles for a patient with a serious traumatic brain injury who has a single episode of hypotension. In such a case, not recognizing and addressing the hypotension and the lack of adequate perfusion pressure has a huge impact—in some cases, a fatal impact. Another important consideration is the high visibility factor of many injuries, which sometimes creates a visual distraction.

Vital Signs

Obtaining a full set of initial or baseline vital signs is critical. The sooner these baselines are established, the better they will serve to help determine whether your patient's condition is improving or deteriorating. The vital signs should include an accurate assessment of pulse and respirations as well as an auscultatory blood pressure. Other measurements that should be considered as part of this assessment include pulse oximetry, blood glucose level, and cardiac monitoring as appropriate. Automatic blood pressure monitoring should be instituted at this time if it is available.

Physical Examinations

Traumatic patients with an isolated injury such as a sprained ankle or a possible isolated fracture may not require a full head to toe exam, but most traumatic injury patients should have a thorough physical exam prior to or during transport. The head to toe exam should be done in a systematic manner.

Head and Neck

Begin by palpating and visualizing the head and neck for injuries. Observe for deformities, contusions, abrasions, penetrations, burns, tenderness, lacerations, and swelling in each body area as you examine it. At the head, be sure to look in the nose, mouth and ears for evidence of bleeding. Bleeding from the nose or ears may indicate a head injury, and bleeding from the mouth may obstruct the airway. At the neck, check for jugular vein distension and tracheal deviation because these can be signs of a serious internal chest injury. The tracheal position can be checked by pressing a finger down in the notch at the top of the sternum. If the trachea is palpated in this position, it is midline (normal). If it is off to one side, it is considered deviated, a fairly reliable sign of an advanced tension pneumothorax. After you complete your assessment of the neck, consider applying a cervical collar to stabilize your patient while you continue with your assessment.

Chest, Abdomen, and Pelvis

As you continue your assessment to the chest, examine and palpate the chest wall carefully. Fractured ribs are common chest injuries and generally result in rapid, shallow respirations. Look for penetrating injuries and assess for bruising,

thoroughly examining the entire chest area. If you have not already done so, use your stethoscope to listen to breath and heart sounds. As you check breath sounds, be sure to auscultate the same area on both sides of the chest so that you can compare the sounds. Unequal breath sounds from right to left may be an indication of a pneumothorax. Be sure to take enough time to evaluate this carefully; overlooking unequal breath sounds can prevent you from providing life-saving treatment to the patient.

After you complete the examination of the chest, proceed to the abdomen and pelvis. Gently palpate the abdomen across the upper and lower quadrants. A rigid and distended abdomen is a serious sign, usually indicating significant internal abdominal bleeding, which may be fatal. Press the iliac crests down and squeeze them inward to determine pelvic stability. Be careful because this will cause significant pain in a conscious patient with a pelvic or lower back injury. Consider palpation of the pubic symphysis and examine the patient for signs of incontinence and/or bleeding from the groin area.

Extremities

Palpate the legs from top to bottom while looking for signs of injury. Palpate each leg separately, and note any difference between the legs. Check for distal pulse, motion, and sensation (PMS), in both feet. Examine the arms in the same manner. Be sure to check for PMS in both hands and wrists.

Back

Prepare to move the patient to a backboard. While the patient is on his or her side, examine the back for injuries. Once the back has been examined, the physical examination is complete.

■ Reassessment

While en route to the hospital, consider performing another head to toe physical examination to identify anything you may have missed and to recognize any patient condition that might have changed. Repeat the primary assessment (ABCs), reevaluate vital signs (every 5 minutes for patients in serious condition), and review the status of the interventions you have performed. Notify the hospital staff as quickly as possible, and give them adequate information to prepare for your arrival. Many trauma patients will be taken to surgery after a quick evaluation in the emergency department, so early notification can help the hospital begin to prepare for this possibility.

Words of Wisdom

Because traumatic injuries are as varied as the mechanisms that cause them, it is almost impossible to prepare for every possible situation. In all situations, you must remain calm, complete an organized assessment, stabilize life-threatening injuries, and do no harm. Avoid tunnel vision; sometimes the obvious injury is not the critical injury.

Management of Trauma

Management of trauma requires a thorough, accurate assessment of the patient and a good working knowledge of the mechanics of injury. During transport, begin any interventions that you consider necessary based on your physical examination of the patient. Specific injuries and their treatment are discussed in later chapters, but most trauma patients will need to be treated for shock, which may include establishing IV access and administering a fluid bolus, and rapid transport. If the patient is being transported by ground, IV access may be delayed until the patient is en route to the hospital. Unresponsive trauma patients will most likely need an advanced airway placed; this should be done before transport, if possible. However, other treatment, including bandaging minor wounds and splinting fractured extremities, should be done en route if the patient is in critical condition.

Blood loss, fluid shifts, and massive vasodilation (widening of the blood vessels) all lead to shock. Shock resuscitation techniques are fairly general; however, you need to find the primary cause to treat the patient properly. Most patients who are in shock should be given oxygen, be kept supine with extremities slightly elevated, if possible, and be transported rapidly to a trauma center. You should also consider fluid resuscitation. If shock is caused by a large fluid shift, which can occur in patients with severe burns, large quantities of fluid may be required. If shock is caused by blood loss, however, too much fluid could dilute the blood and raise blood pressure to the point that clots could be dislodged and bleeding can increase. If shock is caused by vasodilation due to a spinal cord injury, consider administration of medications to constrict the blood vessels instead of adding more fluid through IV boluses. It is important to critically analyze your patient's condition so that you can administer the most appropriate treatment. Consult with medical control.

Traditional shock treatment also includes keeping the patient warm to maintain cardiac output and improve blood clotting. Recent studies involving induced hypothermia used to manage the decrease in blood supply to the brain related to shock may lead to changes in this approach. You should begin fluid resuscitation at volumes that maintain a minimum blood pressure to allow clots to form at sites of bleeding within the body, which will reduce ongoing blood loss. Excessive blood clotting is also a concern in victims with blood loss; clots circulating in blood can be fatal.

Management of specific trauma injuries is covered in other chapters. Several techniques can be used to treat multisystem trauma. Remember that multisystem trauma patients cannot be stabilized in the field. You need to use a team approach to rapidly assess and transport your patient. Work with emergency medical responders, bystanders, and your partner to get the patient assessed and moved to the ambulance as quickly as possible.

Many tasks can be done simultaneously when you use a team approach; for example, you can administer oxygen while your partner maintains cervical spine control, or your partner can prepare the backboard and stretcher while you perform the physical examination. One team member can obtain vital signs while another can question family members or bystanders to gather more information. The team approach requires extra attention on the part of the lead paramedic, but it can be an efficient way to treat the patient.

Critical thinking is important when treating a patient with multisystem trauma. When a person sustains many injuries at once, the body tries to resolve all the injuries, resulting in signs and symptoms that are related to different response mechanisms. For example, in a patient with a closed head injury and internal bleeding elsewhere in the body, the body will try to maintain blood flow to the brain by increasing blood pressure and lowering the pulse. However, the body's response to the shock created by blood loss in other parts of the body can increase the pulse rate and decrease blood pressure. You must analyze the MOI and the patient's signs and symptoms, and anticipate the injuries that need to be managed. Your ability to critically analyze and choose the best treatment will be a major factor in your patient's chance for survival.

Criteria for Referral to a Trauma Center

Paramedics are responsible for determining whether a patient should go to a trauma center—and at what level. Before you even get to the scene, you should know the criteria for referral to a trauma center and what hospital resources are available in your area. It is important to transport your trauma patient to the most appropriate facility based on his or her injuries. The National Study on the Costs and Outcomes of Trauma reported a 25% decrease in mortality for severely injured adult patients who received care at a Level I trauma center compared with those treated at a nontrauma center.

In 2011, the American College of Surgeons Committee on Trauma (ACS-COT) and the Centers for Disease Control and Prevention published an updated field triage decision scheme. Changes to the criteria are outlined below in red font, and the 2011 decision scheme is shown in Figure 21 :

1. Physiologic criteria: If one of the following is present, the patient should be referred to the highest level trauma center:
   - GCS (Glasgow Coma Scale) score of less than or equal to 13
   - SBP (systolic blood pressure) of less than 90 mm Hg
   - RR (respiratory rate) of less than 10 or more than 29 breaths/min (more than 20 breaths/min in infants younger than 1 year old) or need for ventilator support
2. Anatomic criteria: If one of the following is present, transport the patient to the highest level trauma center:
   - All penetrating trauma to the head, neck, torso, and extremities proximal to elbow or knee
   - Chest wall instability or deformity (eg, flail chest)
   - Two or more proximal long bone fractures
   - Crushed, degloved, mangled, or pulseless extremity
   - Amputation proximal to wrist or ankle
   - Pelvic fractures
   - Open or depressed skull fractures
   - Paralysis
3. MOI criteria: Evaluate at this point the MOI and examine the trauma scene for evidence of high-energy trauma. If one of the following is present, and depending on the

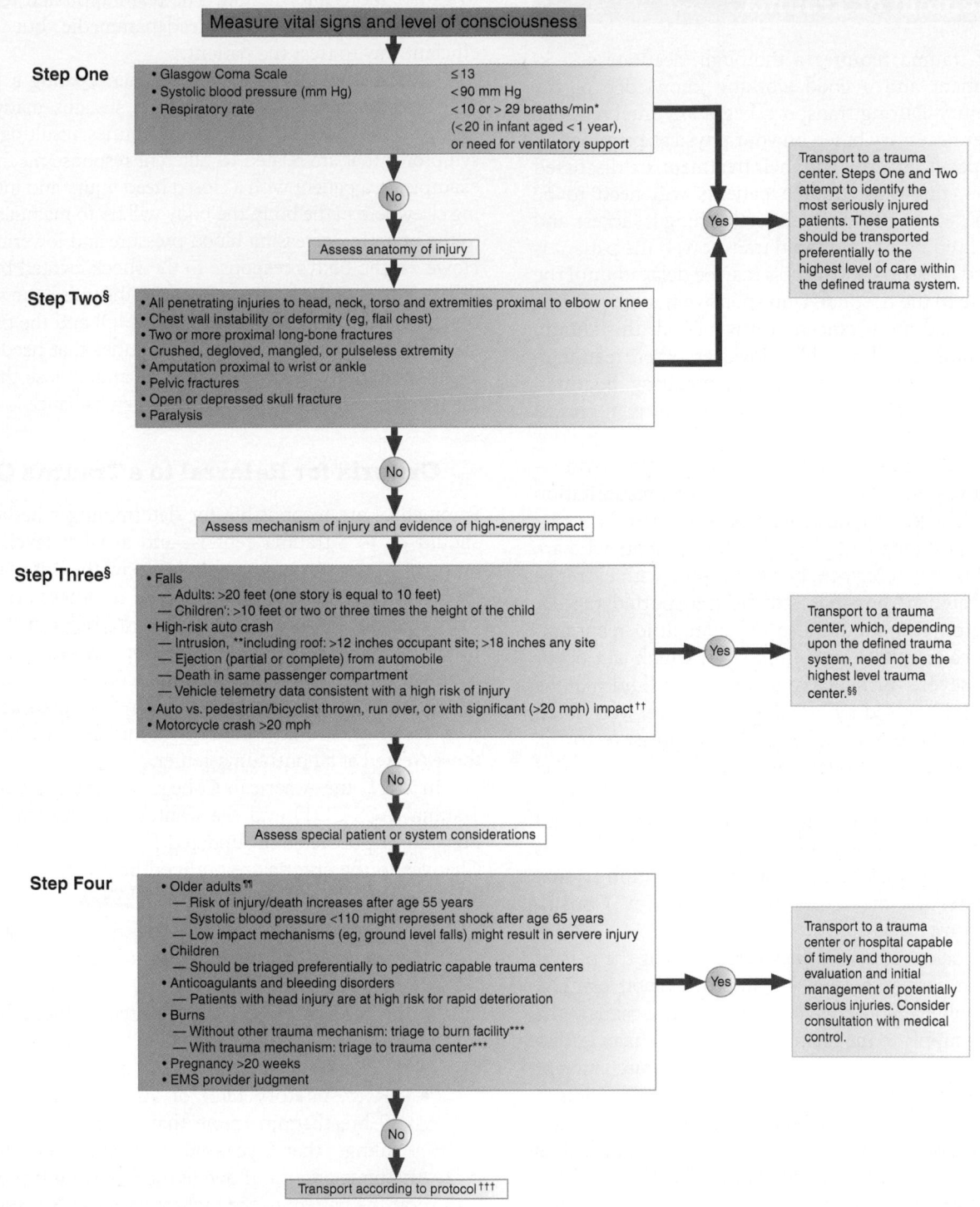

Measure vital signs and level of consciousness

Step One
- Glasgow Coma Scale ≤13
- Systolic blood pressure (mm Hg) <90 mm Hg
- Respiratory rate <10 or >29 breaths/min* (<20 in infant aged <1 year), or need for ventilatory support

No

Assess anatomy of injury

Step Two§
- All penetrating injuries to head, neck, torso and extremities proximal to elbow or knee
- Chest wall instability or deformity (eg, flail chest)
- Two or more proximal long-bone fractures
- Crushed, degloved, mangled, or pulseless extremity
- Amputation proximal to wrist or ankle
- Pelvic fractures
- Open or depressed skull fracture
- Paralysis

Yes → Transport to a trauma center. Steps One and Two attempt to identify the most seriously injured patients. These patients should be transported preferentially to the highest level of care within the defined trauma system.

No

Assess mechanism of injury and evidence of high-energy impact

Step Three§
- Falls
  — Adults: >20 feet (one story is equal to 10 feet)
  — Children¹: >10 feet or two or three times the height of the child
- High-risk auto crash
  — Intrusion, **including roof: >12 inches occupant site; >18 inches any site
  — Ejection (partial or complete) from automobile
  — Death in same passenger compartment
  — Vehicle telemetry data consistent with a high risk of injury
- Auto vs. pedestrian/bicyclist thrown, run over, or with significant (>20 mph) impact††
- Motorcycle crash >20 mph

Yes → Transport to a trauma center, which, depending upon the defined trauma system, need not be the highest level trauma center.§§

No

Assess special patient or system considerations

Step Four
- Older adults¹¹
  — Risk of injury/death increases after age 55 years
  — Systolic blood pressure <110 might represent shock after age 65 years
  — Low impact mechanisms (eg, ground level falls) might result in servere injury
- Children
  — Should be triaged preferentially to pediatric capable trauma centers
- Anticoagulants and bleeding disorders
  — Patients with head injury are at high risk for rapid deterioration
- Burns
  — Without other trauma mechanism: triage to burn facility***
  — With trauma mechanism: triage to trauma center***
- Pregnancy >20 weeks
- EMS provider judgment

Yes → Transport to a trauma center or hospital capable of timely and thorough evaluation and initial management of potentially serious injuries. Consider consultation with medical control.

No

Transport according to protocol†††

When in doubt, transport to a trauma center

Abbreviation: EMS = emergency medical services.
  * The upper limit of respiratory rate in infants is >29 breaths per minute to maintain a higher level of overtriage for infants.
  § Any injury noted in Step Two or mechanism identified in Step Three triggers a "yes" response.
  ¹ Age <15 years.
  ** Intrusion refers to interior compartment intrusion, as opposed to deformation which refers to exterior damage.
  †† Includes pedestrians or bicyclists thrown or run over by a motor vehicle or those with estimated impact >20 mph with a motor vehicle.
  §§ Local or regional protocols should be used to determine the most appropriate level of trauma center within the defined trauma system; need not be the highest-level trauma center.
  ¹¹¹ Age >55 years.
  *** Patients with both burns and concomitant trauma for whom the burn injury poses the greatest risk for morbidity and mortality should be transferred to a burn center. If the nonburn trauma presents a greater immediate risk, the patient may be stabilized in a trauma center and then transferred to a burn center.
  ††† Patients who do not meet any of the triage criteria in Steps One through Four should be transported to the most appropriate medical facility as outlined in local EMS protocols.

Figure 21 2011 decision scheme for field triage of injured patients.

Source: Adapted from Centers for Disease Control and Prevention, Morbidity and Mortality Weekly Report (MMWR), January 13, 2012.

Documentation and Communication

Determining the MOI and getting a complete history of the incident can help you to anticipate as many as 95% of a patient's injuries. After ensuring your personal safety and maintaining the patient's ABCs, the MOI is key information to obtain from the trauma scene (Table 5). You must relay the suspected MOI by radio and by written report to the receiving trauma center. You are the eyes and ears of the emergency department trauma team.

Table 5 Significant Mechanisms of Injury

Age	Mechanisms
Adults	- Multiple body systems injured - Ejection from a vehicle - Death of another person in the same vehicle - Fall > 3 times the patient's height - Vehicle rollover - High-speed (≥ 35 mph) vehicle collision - Vehicle-pedestrian collision - Motorcycle crash - Unresponsiveness or altered mental status following trauma - Penetrating trauma to the head, chest, or abdomen
Children	All mechanisms in the adult list, with the following additions or modifications: - Fall > than 10 ft or two to three times the child's height - Falls of < 10 ft with loss of consciousness - Medium- to high-speed vehicle collision (≥ 25 mph) - Bicycle crash

MOI, transport to the closest appropriate trauma center (may not be the highest level trauma system):

- Adults: falls more than 20 ft
- Children: falls more than 10 ft or two or three times the height of the child
- High-risk auto crash
  - Intrusion, including roof, into passenger compartment (more than 12 inches occupant site or more than 18 inches any other site)
  - Ejection (partial or complete) from automobile
  - Death of another occupant in same passenger compartment
  - Vehicle telemetry data consistent with a high risk of injury
- Pedestrian/bicyclist thrown or run over or auto-pedestrian injury with significant (more than 20 mph) impact
- Motorcycle crash at more than 20 mph

4. Special Considerations: If none of the above criteria are met, then consider transfer to an emergency department or low-level trauma center if:

- Patient's age is more than 55 years
- Systolic blood pressure of less than 110 mm Hg in persons older than 65 years
- Children should be triaged to a pediatric-capable trauma center
- Patient uses anticoagulants or has a bleeding disorder (patients with head injury are at high risk for rapid deterioration)
- Patient is pregnant (more than 20 weeks of gestation)
- Low-impact mechanism in older adults (ground-level falls) may result in severe injury
- Burns with other trauma (without other trauma, triage to burn facility)
- EMS provider judgment

Note: The criteria, "end-stage renal disease requiring dialysis" and "time-sensitive extremity injury" have been removed from the decision scheme.

Words of Wisdom

The criteria for transport to a trauma center may vary from system to system.

The updates are intended to help prehospital care providers recognize injured patients who are likely to benefit from transport to a trauma center compared with transport to an emergency department. It is not intended as a mass-casualty or disaster triage tool; it is intended for individual patients only.

The ACS-COT publishes a list of criteria defining four separate levels of trauma centers (Level I, II, III, and IV). The ACS-COT also provides verification for those institutions seeking to achieve and maintain trauma center capabilities. The verification process includes a site visit by experienced reviewers to ensure that the centers have appropriately designated resources to care for trauma patients. The guidelines in (Table 6) are an overview of the ACS-COT's verification criteria.

In addition, it is important to know which hospitals specialize in neurology, burns, pediatric trauma, cardiac care (centers for heart transplantation, coronary catheter labs), microsurgery (hand and limb reimplantation), or hyperbaric therapy. Your patient should be transported to the most appropriate facility to receive optimal care. It is essential to give the trauma center early notice of the patient's arrival, including: age, sex, MOI, vital signs, GCS, intubation and airway status, SAMPLE history, significant comorbidities, and estimated time of arrival. This way all the right people can be in the ED when you arrive.

Mode of Transport

You must decide which mode of transport will offer the greatest benefit to your patient. Should you call for air transport, or is ground transport sufficient? When making the decision to transport by ground, several factors should be taken into consideration. Can

Table 6 Key Elements for Trauma Centers

Level	Definition	Key Elements
Level I	A comprehensive regional resource that is a tertiary care facility. Capable of providing total care for every aspect of injury—from prevention through rehabilitation.	1. 24-hour in-house coverage by general surgeons 2. Availability of care in specialties such as orthopaedic surgery, neurosurgery, anesthesiology, emergency medicine, radiology, internal medicine, and critical care 3. Should also include cardiac, hand, pediatric, and microvascular surgery and hemodialysis 4. Provides leadership in prevention, public education, and continuing education of trauma team members 5. Committed to continued improvement through a comprehensive quality assessment program and organized research to help direct new innovations in trauma care
Level II	Able to initiate definitive care for all injured patients.	1. 24-hour immediate coverage by general surgeons 2. Availability of care in specialities such as orthopaedic surgery, neurosurgery, anesthesiology, emergency medicine, radiology, and critical care 3. Tertiary care needs such as cardiac surgery, hemodialysis, and microvascular surgery may be referred to a Level I trauma center 4. Committed to trauma prevention and continuing education of trauma team members 5. Provides continued improvement in trauma care through a comprehensive quality assessment program
Level III	Able to provide prompt assessment, resuscitation, and stabilization of injured patients and emergency operations.	1. 24-hour immediate coverage by emergency medicine physicians and prompt availability of general surgeons and anesthesiologists 2. Program dedicated to continued improvement in trauma care through a comprehensive quality assessment program 3. Has developed transfer agreements for patients requiring more comprehensive care at a Level I or Level II trauma center 4. Committed to continuing education of nursing and allied health personnel or the trauma team 5. Must be involved with prevention and have an active outreach program for its referring communities 6. Also dedicated to improving trauma care through a comprehensive quality assessment program
Level IV	Able to provide Advanced Trauma Life Support (ATLS) before transfer of patients to a higher level trauma center.	1. Include basic emergency department facilities to implement ATLS protocols and 24-hour laboratory coverage 2. Transfer to higher level trauma centers follows the guidelines outlined in formal transfer agreements 3. Committed to continued improvement of these trauma care activities through a formal quality assessment program 4. Involved in prevention, outreach, and education within its community

the appropriate facility be reached within a reasonable time frame by ground? Ground transportation EMS units are generally staffed by traditional EMTs, advanced EMTs, and paramedics. What is the extent of injuries? If in a congested area, can the patient be transported to a more accessible landing zone for air medical transport?

Words of Wisdom

The National Trauma Data Standard (formerly known as the National Trauma Registry, or NTR) of the National Trauma Data Bank is a reporting system designed to collect standardized trauma-related data in an effort to improve the quality and cost-effectiveness of care and to aid in outcome research. Your contribution as a paramedic is the record of what you found at the scene.

Air transportation EMS units or critical care transport units are generally staffed by critical care transport professionals such as critical care nurses and critical care paramedics Figure 22. All levels of prehospital providers should recognize the need for and criteria used in making the decision to use aeromedical transport in their service area.

The Association of Air Medical Services and MedEvac Foundation International identify the following criteria for the appropriate use of emergency air medical services for trauma patients in the white paper, *Air Medicine: Accessing the Future of Healthcare*:

- There is an extended period required to access or extricate a remote (eg, injured hiker, snowmobiler, or boater) or trapped patient (eg, in a crashed car) that depletes the time frame to get the patient to the trauma center by ground.
- Distance to the trauma center is greater than 20 to 25 miles.

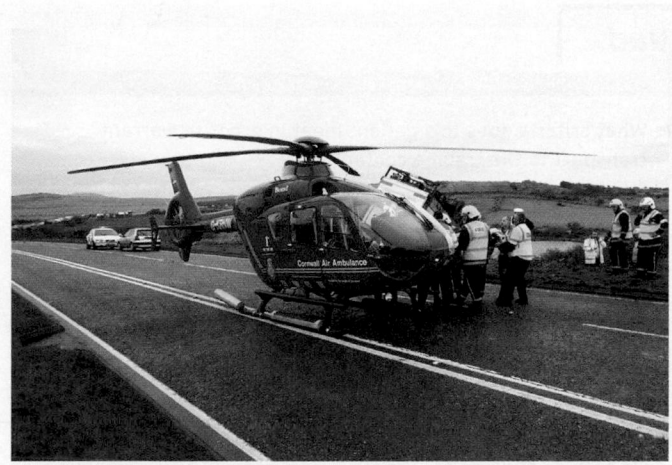

Figure 22 A helicopter may be used to transport patients quickly to a trauma center.

- The patient needs medical care and stabilization at the Advanced Life Support (ALS)-level, and there is no ALS-level ground ambulance service available within a reasonable time frame.
- Traffic conditions or hospital availability make it unlikely that the patient will get to a trauma center via ground ambulance within the ideal time frame for best clinical outcome.

- There are multiple patients who will overwhelm resources at the trauma center(s) reachable by ground within the time frame.
- EMS systems require that the patient be brought to the nearest hospital for initial evaluation and stabilization, rather than bypassing those facilities and going directly to a trauma center. This may add delay to definitive surgical care and necessitate air transport to mitigate the impact of that delay.
- There is a multiple-casualty incident.

These recommendations serve as a guideline for local decision makers to develop comprehensive protocols for the use of air medical transport. You should always follow your local protocols when determining what type of patient transportation is appropriate. If the patient can be transported by ground to definitive care within a reasonable amount of time, there is no need to call for air transport. The time it will take for the aircraft to lift off, travel, and land, just to reach the scene should be considered as well. By weighing the time frame for air transport against transport by ground, you will be able to make an informed decision. Also take into account the terrain. Is there a safe area for landing? If not, how far will the patient need to be transported to reach a secure landing zone? If the distance is great, ground transport may be a more reasonable option. Once the decision is made to call for air medical transport, contact your dispatcher to request a unit, or follow local protocols regarding contacting air support. For more information about establishing landing zones, see the *Transport Operations* chapter.

YOU *are the Medic* | SUMMARY

1. Looking up at the ferris wheel, what possible MOIs should you consider?

First, the most obvious is the height from which the patient fell. Remember that with increased height comes incremental increases in velocity. This in turn helps you to determine the force of impact. In addition, the objects that the body may have struck while falling contribute to the index of suspicion of certain injuries as well. The patient landed on grass. Were there any other objects the patient's body may have struck? Are there rocks protruding? Is the ground wet with some plasticity or dry and hard packed?

2. In addition to trauma sustained in the fall, what other information might you want to elicit from witnesses and friends of the patient?

All of the following information plays a part in helping determine the index of suspicion for possible injury: body position, location on the ride, whether the patient was pushed, fell, or jumped, motion of the ferris wheel, part of the car patient exited (front, side, back).

3. The patient is unresponsive with what appears to be adequate breathing. Your partner applies a nonrebreathing mask with 15 L/min of oxygen. What should you do next to continue your primary assessment?

Remember the steps for the primary assessment—ABCs. Don't allow the stress of a seriously injured patient impair your ability to stay focused and organized. A quick glance shows what appears to be adequate breathing. Your partner is applying oxygen. You need to quickly expose the chest and inspect, palpate, auscultate, seal, and stabilize. Remember, the primary assessment is only for identifying and treating life threats.

4. The patient's friend comes forward and tearfully explains that her friend, who is a diabetic and was drinking "a few shots of tequila" earlier in the evening, was standing up in the ride's car, yelling and waving to her boyfriend, when the ride suddenly jerked to a stop, sending her tumbling out of the car. What important questions will you ask the friend?

Did she take her insulin and/or eat? Was she acting strangely prior to the fall? How much alcohol did she have and at what time? Did the patient ingest any other substances, such as drugs?

YOU *are the Medic*   **SUMMARY,** *continued*

5. **The patient's rapid, weak pulse and cool, moist skin indicate likelihood of inadequate perfusion, yet the blood pressure does not indicate advanced shock. What are some possible reasons for this finding?**

   Mixed or multisystem trauma will often result in injuries whose signs and symptoms may appear contradictory or confusing. The head injury could be causing development of severe and increasing intracranial pressure. This condition often causes fluctuations in vital signs, most notably, increasing blood pressure with narrowing pulse pressure and an eventual drop in pulse rate. The large contusion and possible pelvic fracture and potential for other internal injuries likely have resulted in hypovolemia. The body is responding to both the decrease in blood volume and the increase in intracranial pressure.

6. **According to the friend who witnessed the fall, the patient's initial impact was with her head against the metal car below. What is the significance of a smaller surface area of the body absorbing the initial impact as opposed to a larger body surface area?**

   Remember that the larger the surface area absorbing energy, the more the energy will be spread out. The witness reports seeing her friend hit her head first before hitting the ground; it is possible that the patient's head experienced a significant impact. Your index of suspicion for serious head and cervical spine injury should be very high.

7. **What criteria does this patient meet in order to warrant transport to the trauma center?**

   Upon your arrival, you immediately ascertain that the patient's GCS score is less than 13. This score, due to trauma, is all you need to justify transport to the nearest trauma center. Upon noting this, you ask other officials on scene to call the dispatcher and ask them to notify the trauma center of the impending arrival.

8. **As you continue your examination and observation of your patient en route to the trauma center, you think about the presentation of your patient to the waiting emergency department staff. What MOI will you relate to the staff?**

   First, it is important to relate the patient's medical history and behavior prior to the fall because this will greatly assist the staff in evaluating the patient's mental status and determining the course of treatment. Next, relay the height of the ride, possible trajectory, and points of impact while falling; the materials impacted (steel bars, metal cars); the surface on which the patient landed (soft, wet grass as opposed to hard, packed earth or concrete), and the position of body to the staff.

YOU *are the Medic*   **SUMMARY,** *continued*

EMS Patient Care Report (PCR)

Date: 07-02-11	**Incident No.:** 1056	**Nature of Call:** Injury		**Location:** Sixth Ave Amusement Park	
Dispatched: 1940	**En Route:** 1941	**At Scene:** 1943	**Transport:** 1953	**At Hospital:** 1959	**In Service:** 2018

Patient Information

Age: 18 **Sex:** F **Weight (in kg [lb]):** 55 kg (120 lb)	**Allergies:** Unknown **Medications:** Insulin **Past Medical History:** Type I diabetes **Chief Complaint:** Multisystem trauma

Vital Signs

Time: 1948	**BP:** 140/110	**Pulse:** 140 weak, regular	**Respirations:** 22	**Spo$_2$:** 97%
Time: 1952	**BP:** 130/116	**Pulse:** 88	**Respirations:** 24	**Spo$_2$:** 98%
Time: 1957	**BP:** 120/112	**Pulse:** 60	**Respirations:** 26 irregular	**Spo$_2$:** 96%

EMS Treatment
(circle all that apply)

Oxygen @ __15__ L/min via (circle one): NC (NRM) Bag-mask device	**Assisted Ventilation**	**Airway Adjunct**	**CPR**
Defibrillation	**Bleeding Control**	**Bandaging**	(**Splinting**)	(**Other:** Spinal immobilization)

Narrative

Dispatched by 9-1-1 for an injury at Sixth Avenue Amusement Park. Pt reportedly fell from a car near the top of the 30-ft ferris wheel. Upon arrival, 18-year-old female found supine on wet, grassy area beneath the ferris wheel. Pt unresponsive to verbal and painful stimuli. Witnesses stated that pt fell forward from a standing position and struck her head while tumbling to the ground. Pt was allegedly drinking tequila earlier in the night, has a history of diabetes, and was acting "crazy" according to friends. Cervical stabilization applied immediately upon arrival. Pt airway is open, clear, and maintained. OPA insertion attempted but removed due to patient gag reflex. Breathing was adequate with trachea midline, equal chest rise, no skin breaks, no discoloration, no crepitus noted. Breath sounds present and equal. No severe bleeding noted. Left pupil is dilated and nonreactive. Exposed body shows large hematoma on right lower quadrant extending to pelvic region. Abdominal distention noted. Pt legs both bent outward upon arrival and moved without resistance to midline for immobilization on backboard. Left arm is deformed and cool to the touch. No radial pulse palpable. Immobilized against body and on backboard. No skin breaks or discoloration noted on back. Pt remained unresponsive en route with fluctuating vital signs (see chart). Airway monitored but self-maintained. Blood glucose obtained en route at 1956 hours from right index finger is 73. Trauma center staff notified and waiting for pt arrival—1959 hours. Return to service at 2018 hours. **End of report**

Prep Kit

- Trauma is the primary cause of death and disability in people between ages 1 and 44 years.

- The amount of force and energy delivered are factors in the extent of trauma sustained. Duration and direction of the force of application are also important.

- Understanding the effects of forces and energy will help in developing a high index of suspicion for the mechanism of injury and the likely types of injuries.

- Kinetic energy (KE) of an object is the energy associated with that object in motion. It reflects the relationship between the weight (mass) of the object and the velocity at which it is traveling.

- The law of conservation of energy states that energy can be neither created nor destroyed; it can only change form.

- Blunt trauma refers to injuries in which the tissues are not penetrated by an external object, as commonly occurs in motor vehicle crashes, in pedestrians hit by a vehicle, in motorcycle crashes, in falls from heights, in serious sports injures, and in blasts when no shrapnel is involved.

- In a motor vehicle crash, the angle of impact, mechanical characteristics of the vehicle, and the occupant's position at the time of impact will determine types of injury.

- Trauma in a crash is composed of five phases representing the effects of progressive deceleration: deceleration of the vehicle, deceleration of the occupant, deceleration of internal organs, secondary crashes, and additional impacts.

- There are five primary types of impacts: frontal or head on, lateral or side, rear, rotational, and rollover.

- The front seat occupants of vehicles during a frontal or head-on crash usually follow one of two trajectories, a down-and-under pathway or an up-and-over pathway.

- Protective devices such as seat belts, air bags, and helmets are designed to manipulate the way in which energy is dissipated into injury.

- In a motorcycle crash, any structural protection afforded to the victims is not derived from a steel cage, as is the case in an automobile, but from protective devices worn by the rider such as helmets and leather or abrasion-resistant clothing.

- There are four types of motorcycle impacts: head-on collisions, angular collisions, ejected riders, or laying the bike down.

- Adult pedestrians involved in a crash experience three predominant mechanisms of injury: lower extremity injuries from the initial hit, second impact injuries from being thrown onto the hood or grille, and third impact injuries when the body strikes the ground or another object.

- The severity of injuries from falls from heights depends on the height, position, and orientation of the body at the moment of impact; the area over which the impact is distributed; the surface onto which the person falls; and the physical condition of the patient.

- Penetrating trauma involves a disruption of the skin and underlying tissues in a small, focused area, as commonly occurs with stab wounds and gunshot wounds.

- The severity of a stab wound depends on the anatomic area involved, depth of penetration, blade length, and angle of penetration.

- Firearms are the primary mechanism resulting in penetrating trauma. The magnitude of tissue damage depends on the projectile's velocity, the orientation of the projectile as it entered the body, the distance from which the weapon was fired, the design of the projectile, and the type of tissue through which the projectile passed.

- Blast injuries include primary, secondary, tertiary, quaternary (miscellaneous) injuries.

- A blast wave or shock wave is dependent on many factors including the size of the explosive charge, the nature of the surrounding medium, the distance from the explosion, and the presence or absence of reflecting surfaces.

- Air-containing organs such as the middle ear, heart, lungs, major blood vessels, and gastrointestinal tract are most susceptible to pressure changes and blast injuries.

- Multisystem trauma describes trauma that involves several body systems. Most trauma affects more than one system, often includes both blunt and penetrating trauma, and has a high level of morbidity and mortality.

- Management of trauma patients requires a thorough and accurate assessment of the patient as well as a good working knowledge of the mechanisms of injury. In treating multisystem trauma, remember that if a generalized mechanism is present, you should anticipate multisystem injuries. It is also important to remember that multisystem trauma patients cannot be stabilized in the field.

Prep Kit, continued

- The criteria for transport to a trauma center vary from system to system. However, there are key variables for transport to a trauma center as defined by the Centers for Disease Control and Prevention National Trauma Triage Protocol.

- There are four categories of trauma centers. Your system may include a Level I, which is the highest level trauma center.

- The Association of Air Medical Services and MedEvac Foundation International identify criteria for the appropriate use of emergency air medical services for trauma patients. The criteria include situations in which there is extended transport time by ground, mass-casualty incidents, prolonged extrication times, critically injured patients, or when there is a long distance to an appropriate facility.

Vital Vocabulary

acceleration (a) The rate of change in velocity; speeding up.

angle of impact The angle at which an object hits another; this characterizes the force vectors involved and has a bearing on patterns of energy dissipation.

arterial air embolism Air bubbles in the arterial blood vessels.

avulsing A tearing away or forcible separation.

barometric energy The energy that results from sudden changes in pressure as may occur in a diving accident or sudden decompression in an airplane.

biomechanics The study of the physiology and mechanics of a living organism using the tools of mechanical engineering.

blast front The leading edge of the shock wave.

blunt trauma An impact on the body by objects that cause injury without penetrating soft tissues or internal organs and cavities.

brisance The shattering effect of a shock wave and its ability to cause disruption of tissues and structures.

cavitation Cavity formation; shock waves that push tissues in front of and lateral to the projectile and may not necessarily increase the wound size or cause permanent injury but can result in cavitation.

chemical energy The energy released as a result of a chemical reaction.

deceleration A negative acceleration—that is, slowing down.

electrical energy The energy delivered in the form of high voltage.

entry wound The point at which a penetrating object enters the body.

exit wound The point at which a penetrating object leaves the body, which may or may not be in a straight line from the entry wound.

gravity (g) The acceleration of a body by the attraction of the earth's gravitational force, normally 32.2 ft/sec^2.

implosion A bursting inward.

index of suspicion Anticipating the possibility of specific types of injury.

kinetic energy (KE) The energy associated with bodies in motion, expressed mathematically as half the mass times the square of the velocity.

kinetics The study of the relationship among speed, mass, vector direction, and physical injury.

law of conservation of energy The principle that energy can be neither created nor destroyed; it can only change form.

mechanical energy The energy that results from motion (kinetic energy) or that is stored in an object (potential energy).

mechanism of injury (MOI) The way in which traumatic injuries occur; the forces that act on the body to cause damage.

missile fragmentation A primary mechanism of tissue disruption from certain rifles in which pieces of the projectile break apart, allowing the pieces to create their own separate paths through tissues.

multisystem trauma Trauma caused by generalized mechanisms which affect numerous body systems.

negative wave pulse The phase of an explosion in which pressure from the blast is less than atmospheric pressure.

Newton's first law of motion The principle that a body at rest will remain at rest unless acted on by an outside force.

Newton's second law of motion The principle that the force that an object can exert is the product of its mass times its acceleration.

pathway expansion The tissue displacement that occurs as a result of low-displacement shock waves that travel at the speed of sound in tissue.

penetrating trauma Injury caused by objects that pierce the surface of the body, such as knives and bullets, and damage internal tissues and organs.

permanent cavity The path of crushed tissue produced by a missile traversing part of the body.

positive wave pulse The phase of the explosion in which there is a pressure front with a pressure higher than atmospheric pressure.

potential energy The amount of energy stored in an object, the product of mass, gravity, and height, that is converted into kinetic energy and results in injury, such as from a fall.

pulmonary blast injuries Pulmonary trauma resulting from short-range exposure to the detonation of high explosives.

Revised Trauma Score (RTS) A scoring system used for patients with head trauma.

shearing An applied force or pressure exerted against the surface and layers of the skin as tissues slide in opposite but parallel planes.

spalling Delaminating or breaking off into chips and pieces.

trauma Acute physiologic and structural change that occurs in a victim as a result of the rapid dissipation of energy delivered by an external force.

trauma score A score that relates to the likelihood of patient survival with the exception of a severe head injury. It is calculated on a scale from 1 to 16, with 16 being the best possible score. It takes into account the Glasgow Coma Scale score, respiratory rate, respiratory expansion, systolic blood pressure, and capillary refill.

tympanic membrane The eardrum; a thin, semitransparent membrane in the middle ear that transmits sound vibrations to the internal ear by means of the auditory ossicles.

velocity (V) The distance an object travels per unit time.

Waddell triad A pattern of automobile-pedestrian injuries in children and people of short stature in which (1) the bumper hits pelvis and femur, (2) the chest and abdomen hit the grille or low hood, and (3) the head strikes the ground.

whiplash An injury to the cervical vertebrae or their supporting ligaments and muscles, usually resulting from sudden acceleration or deceleration.

Assessment in Action

You and your partner arrive at the scene of a pedestrian struck by a bicycle. The scene is safe and traffic has been rerouted by police on the scene. As you approach the patient you see a messenger bicycle on its side. A young man is standing next to the bicycle explaining to a police officer, "I didn't see her. I had no time to even slow down. She walked in front of me like I was invisible." An elderly woman is lying supine on the pavement with her left leg rotated outward. A bystander is holding the patient's hand and talking to her.

Your partner is holding cervical stabilization and the patient is responding appropriately to your questions. She is shaking and tells you she feels cold. Her airway appears clear and she is maintaining it on her own. Her chest is expanding equally and her respirations are adequate, although rapid. As you carefully inspect the chest you see some discoloration over the left side. The site is tender to palpation but no crepitus is noted. Lung sounds are equal and clear. She has numerous deep abrasions on her left side, left arm, and left leg, with no severe bleeding. Both radial pulses are present and you notice that her hands are very cold. Covering her with a blanket, you continue with your assessment. Her pupils are constricted and nonreactive. She tells you she was diagnosed with cataracts when she was 75 years old and has been using eye drops for them for about 5 years. She denies any other medical problems.

EMTs arrive and assist with your patient. Baseline vitals are obtained. Her blood pressure is 118/60 mm Hg, pulse is 90 beats/min, and respirations are 22 breaths/min. Pulse oximetry shows an Spo_2 of 96% on high concentration oxygen via nonrebreathing mask.

1. The patient's vital signs seem to indicate that the patient is stable. At this point, you should:
   A. immobilize the patient on a backboard and rapidly transport.
   B. continue with a secondary assessment.
   C. ask the patient to attempt to sit up.
   D. help the patient onto the stretcher.

2. What information contributes significantly to the potential severity of the patient's injuries?
   A. A history of cataracts
   B. The speed and lack of braking of the bicyclist
   C. The weight of the bicyclist
   D. The angle at which the bicycle struck the patient

3. The type of energy with which the patient was initially hit was:
   A. potential energy.
   B. thermal energy.
   C. kinetic energy.
   D. converted energy.

4. Your patient is approximately 80 years old. The significance of age in terms of being able to disperse the energy is:
   A. important because elderly people may not be able to move quickly out of the way.
   B. insignificant.
   C. significant because of reduced bone and muscle mass.
   D. significant due to age-related organ deterioration.

5. During your primary assessment, you found a hand-sized discoloration on the left side of the patient's chest. The patient is telling you that she feels cold but her vital signs seem normal. You would treat her for shock:
   A. only when her vital signs show significant changes.
   B. based on the injuries you observe.
   C. based on the mechanism of injury.
   D. not at all.

6. You and your partner decide that this patient needs to go to the nearest trauma center. Your decision is based on:
   A. her vital signs.
   B. discoloration over the left side of the chest.
   C. the possible fractured hip.
   D. the impact speed at which the bike hit the patient.

Additional Question

7. An elderly patient with multiple injuries presents with a baseline blood pressure of 118/60 mm Hg. You and your partner discuss whether or not this is an important finding. What other information will you need to help determine whether your patient is experiencing shock?

Bleeding

National EMS Education Standard Competencies

Trauma

Integrates assessment findings with principles of epidemiology and pathophysiology to formulate a field impression to implement a comprehensive treatment/disposition plan for an acutely injured patient.

Bleeding

Recognition and management of
- Bleeding (pp 1523–1525, 1526–1527)

Pathophysiology, assessment, and management of
- Bleeding (pp 1523–1525, 1526–1538)

Fluid resuscitation (pp 1535–1538)

Knowledge Objectives

1. Discuss the anatomy and physiology of the cardiovascular system. (pp 1519–1521)
2. Discuss the pathophysiology of external and internal hemorrhage. (pp 1523–1524)
3. Describe the body's physiologic response to hemorrhaging. (pp 1524–1525)
4. Describe the assessment and management of a bleeding patient. (pp 1526–1538)
5. Discuss the pathophysiology of hemorrhagic shock. (p 1526)
6. Describe the types of shock. (pp 1525–1526)
7. Discuss the phases of shock. (p 1526)
8. Discuss the classes of hemorrhage. (pp 1523–1525)
9. Describe the assessment and management of a patient with hemorrhagic shock. (pp 1526–1538)
10. Describe how to assess and manage a patient with external hemorrhage. (pp 1530–1535)
11. Describe how to apply a commercial tourniquet. (pp 1532–1534)
12. Describe how to assess and manage a patient with internal hemorrhage. (pp 1535–1536)
13. Describe how to assess and manage a patient with hemorrhagic shock. (pp 1536–1538)

Skills Objectives

1. Demonstrate the assessment and management of a patient with signs and symptoms of external hemorrhage. (pp 1530–1531, Skill Drill 1)
2. Demonstrate how to apply a commercial tourniquet. (pp 1532–1534, Skill Drill 2)
3. Demonstrate the assessment and management of a patient with signs and symptoms of internal hemorrhage. (pp 1535–1536, Skill Drill 3)
4. Demonstrate the assessment and management of a patient experiencing hemorrhagic shock. (pp 1536–1538, Skill Drill 4)

■ Introduction

After managing the airway, recognizing bleeding (hemorrhage) and understanding how it affects the body are perhaps the most important skills you will learn as a paramedic. Any type of bleeding is potentially dangerous because it may first cause weakness and then lead to shock. Uncontrolled bleeding may eventually lead to serious injury and, ultimately, death. The most common cause of shock after trauma is bleeding.

This chapter begins with a review of the anatomy and physiology of the cardiovascular and respiratory systems and their roles in keeping blood flowing between the lungs and peripheral tissues. The control of external hemorrhaging including the use of tourniquets and the role of hemostatic agents are discussed. Hemorrhagic shock, or shock resulting from bleeding, both internal and external, is also discussed.

■ Anatomy and Physiology

The cardiovascular system is designed to carry out one crucial job: keep blood flowing between the lungs and the peripheral tissues. The right side of the heart pumps blood to the lungs, and the left side of the heart receives blood from the lungs and then pumps it around the body. In order for perfusion to take place, the circulatory system must function efficiently to deliver oxygen to the tissues of the body.

In the lungs, blood unloads the gaseous waste products of metabolism—chiefly carbon dioxide—and picks up life-sustaining oxygen. In the peripheral tissues, the process is reversed: blood unloads oxygen and picks up wastes. If blood flow were to stop or slow significantly, the results would be catastrophic. The cells of the brain, heart, and other organs of the body would have nowhere to eliminate their wastes and would be rapidly engulfed by the toxic by-products of their own metabolism. Oxygen delivery to the tissues also would be disrupted. For a few minutes, the cells could switch to an emergency metabolic system—one that does not require oxygen (anaerobic metabolism), but that form of metabolism produces even more acids and toxic wastes. Within a few minutes of circulatory failure, cells throughout the body would begin to suffocate and die. In an attempt to survive during this state of widespread inadequate perfusion, or shock, the body compensates in an organized manner in order to maintain the systolic blood pressure and perfusion to the brain and heart, at the expense of other areas such as the skin, muscles, liver, and kidneys.

To keep the blood moving continuously through the body, the circulatory system requires three intact components **Figure 1** listed as follows:

- A functioning pump: the heart
- Adequate fluid volume: the blood and body fluids
- An intact system of tubing capable of reflex adjustments (constriction and dilation) in response to changes in pump output and fluid volume: the blood vessels

All three components must interact effectively to maintain life. If any one becomes damaged or is deficient, the whole system is in jeopardy.

Words of Wisdom

Cellular respiration is a series of metabolic processes the body uses to make energy. Cellular respiration has three steps: glycolysis, the citric acid cycle, and the electron transport chain. During glycolysis, glucose is broken down into pyruvic acid and produces 2 adenosine triphosphate (ATP) molecules. In the citric acid cycle a sequence of enzymatic reactions occur to convert pyruvic acid into ATP, water, CO_2, acetyl coenzyme A and high energy electrons. The electron transport chain converts these high-energy electrons into more ATP and releases heat and water as by-products. This is known as the aerobic pathway since oxygen is the final electron donor in this process. A high amount of ATP is produced via this process, which the cells utilize to do the work of life. In the absence of oxygen, only glycolysis and then fermentation occurs and the pathway is known as anaerobic. During fermentation, pyruvic acid is converted into ethanol or lactic acid, and in the process regenerates intermediates for glycolysis. This process only yields a small amount of ATP and cannot sustain life if it is the only pathway available.

YOU *are the Medic*   PART 1

On a quiet Saturday morning the dispatcher receives a call and notifies you that a man is down at a construction site and serious injuries are possible.

On your arrival, a man in a hard hat rushes over to the ambulance. "I'm Dave, the foreman. One of my guys was up there on the scaffold and was hit by a steel beam that was being lowered into place. His harness lanyard didn't hold. He fell and landed on his back. Hurry! He's hurt bad, I think." He is pointing to a scaffold about 15 ft off the ground, on the side of a building under construction.

1. Is there a possibility of more than one mechanism of injury (MOI) in this scenario?
2. This is a high-rise, commercial construction site. What could some of the potential hazards be for you and your partner?

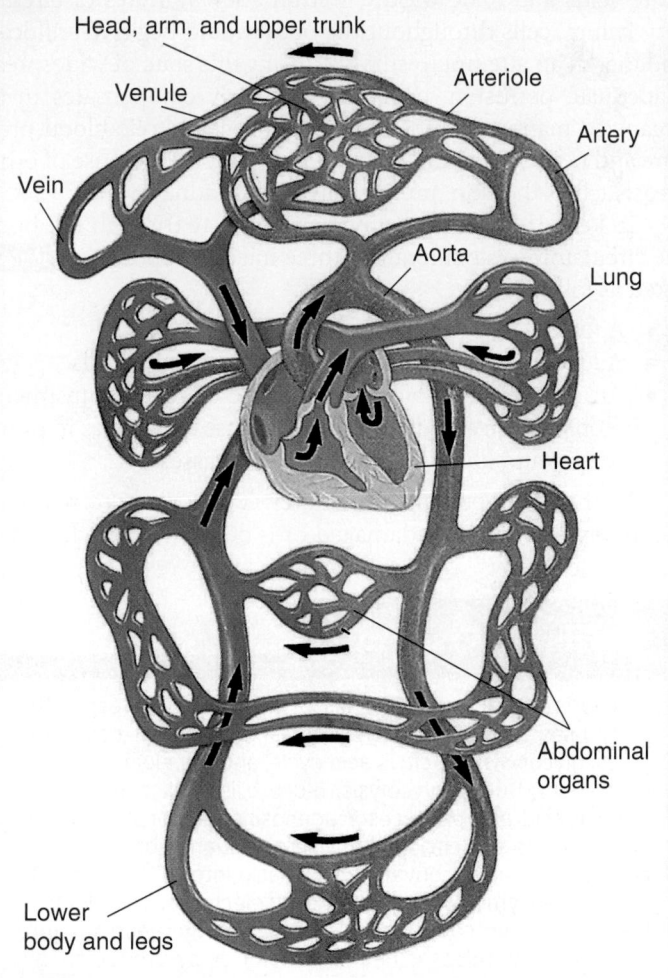

Head, arm, and upper trunk

Venule

Vein

Arteriole

Artery

Aorta

Lung

Heart

Abdominal organs

Lower body and legs

Figure 1 The circulatory system requires continuous operation of its three components: the heart, the blood and body fluids, and the blood vessels.

Structures of the Heart

The heart is a muscular, cone-shaped organ whose function is to pump blood throughout the body. Located behind the sternum, the heart is about the size of a closed fist—roughly 5 inches long, 3 inches wide, and 2.5 inches thick. It weighs 10 to 12 oz in men and 8 to 10 oz in women. Roughly two thirds of the heart lies in the left part of the mediastinum, the area between the lungs that also contains the great vessels.

The human heart consists of four chambers: two atria (upper chambers) and two ventricles (lower chambers). Each atrium receives blood that is returned to the heart from other parts of the body; each ventricle pumps blood out of the heart. The upper and lower portions of the heart are separated by the atrioventricular valves, which prevent backward flow of blood. The semilunar valves, which serve a similar function, are located between the ventricles and the arteries into which they pump blood. Blood enters the right atrium via the superior and inferior venae cavae and the coronary sinus, which consists of veins that collect blood returning from the walls of the heart. Veins often act as blood reservoirs, containing over 60% of the blood volume. Blood from four pulmonary veins enters the left atrium.

Blood Flow Within the Heart and Lungs

Two large veins, the superior vena cava and the inferior vena cava, return deoxygenated blood from the body to the right atrium **Figure 2**. Blood from the upper part of the body returns to the heart through the superior vena cava; blood from the lower part of the body returns through the inferior vena cava (the larger of the two veins). From the right atrium, blood passes through the tricuspid valve into the right ventricle. The right ventricle then pumps the blood through the pulmonic valve into the pulmonary artery and then to the lungs.

In the lungs, oxygen is returned to the blood and carbon dioxide and other waste products are removed from it. The freshly oxygenated blood returns to the left atrium through the pulmonary veins. Blood then flows through the mitral valve into the left ventricle, which pumps the oxygenated blood through the aortic valve, into the aorta (the body's largest artery), and then to the entire body.

The Cardiac Cycle

The cardiac cycle is the repetitive pumping process that begins with the onset of cardiac muscle contraction and ends with the beginning of the next contraction. Myocardial contraction results in pressure changes within the cardiac chambers, causing the blood to move from areas of high pressure to areas of low pressure.

Preload is the amount of blood returned to the heart to be pumped out and directly affects the afterload. The pressure in the aorta or the peripheral vascular resistance, against which the left ventricle must pump blood, is called the **afterload**. The greater the afterload, the harder it is for the ventricle to eject blood into the aorta. A higher afterload, therefore, reduces the **stroke volume (SV)**, or the amount of blood ejected per contraction. To a large degree, afterload is governed by arterial blood pressure.

The amount of blood pumped through the circulatory system in 1 minute is referred to as the **cardiac output (CO)**. CO is expressed in liters per minute (L/min). The CO equals the SV multiplied by the pulse rate:

Cardiac Output = Stroke Volume × Pulse Rate

Factors that influence the SV, the pulse rate, or both will affect CO and, therefore, oxygen delivery (perfusion) to the tissues.

Increased venous return to the heart stretches the ventricles somewhat, resulting in increased cardiac contractility. This relationship, which was first described by the British physiologist Ernest Henry Starling, is known as the Frank-Starling mechanism or Starling law of the heart. Starling noted that if a muscle is stretched slightly before it is stimulated to contract, it would contract with greater force. Thus, if the heart is stretched, the muscle contracts more forcefully.

Although the amount of blood returning to the right atrium varies somewhat from minute to minute, a normal heart continues to pump the same percentage of blood returned, a measure

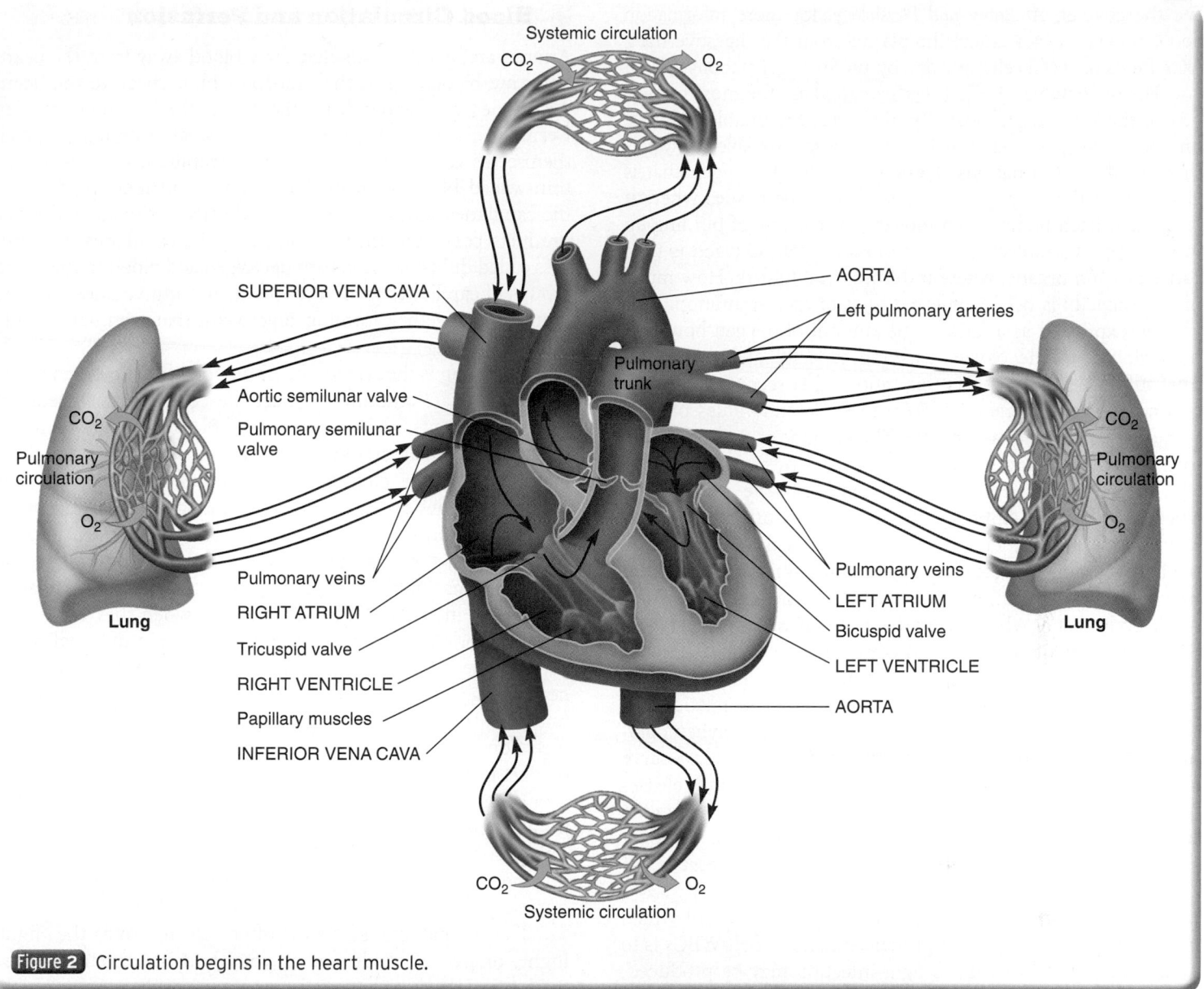

Systemic circulation

CO_2 O_2

AORTA

SUPERIOR VENA CAVA

Left pulmonary arteries

Pulmonary
trunk

CO_2

Pulmonary
circulation

CO_2

Pulmonary
circulation

Aortic semilunar valve

Pulmonary semilunar
valve

O_2

O_2

Pulmonary veins

RIGHT ATRIUM

Lung

Pulmonary veins

LEFT ATRIUM

Bicuspid valve

LEFT VENTRICLE

AORTA

Lung

Tricuspid valve

RIGHT VENTRICLE

Papillary muscles

INFERIOR VENA CAVA

CO_2 O_2

Systemic circulation

Figure 2   Circulation begins in the heart muscle.

called the <u>ejection fraction (EF)</u>. If more blood returns to the heart, the stretched heart pumps harder rather than allowing the blood to back up into the veins. As a result, more blood is pumped with each contraction, yet the ejection fraction remains unchanged: The amount of blood that is pumped increases, but so does the amount of blood returned. This relationship maintains normal cardiac function when a person changes positions, coughs, breathes, or moves.

Blood and Its Components

<u>Blood</u> consists of plasma and formed elements or cells that are suspended in the plasma. These cells include red blood cells (RBCs), white blood cells (WBCs), and platelets. RBCs make up about 45% of blood volume. WBCs and platelets make up less than 1% of blood volume.

The purpose of blood is to carry oxygen and nutrients such as glucose, proteins, fats, and electrolytes to the tissues and

Words of Wisdom

Red blood cells are about one third hemoglobin, a protein that gives them their red color. Hemoglobin is responsible for the ability of the cells to transport oxygen and carbon dioxide. When hemoglobin binds with oxygen, oxyhemoglobin is formed. Oxyhemoglobin is bright red. When oxygen is released, deoxyhemoglobin is formed. Deoxyhemoglobin is darker red, and blood rich in deoxyhemoglobin may appear bluish when seen through blood vessels.

cellular waste products away from the tissues. In addition, the formed elements serve as the mainstay of numerous other body functions, such as fighting infections and controlling bleeding.

<u>Plasma</u> is a watery, straw-colored fluid that accounts for more than half of the total blood volume. It consists of 92% water and 8% dissolved substances such as chemicals, minerals, and nutrients.

See the chapter, *Anatomy and Physiology*, for more information about plasma. Water enters the plasma from the digestive tract, from fluids between cells, and as a by-product of metabolism.

The disk-shaped RBCs (<u>erythrocytes</u>) are the most numerous of the formed elements. Erythrocytes are unable to move on their own; instead, the flowing plasma passively propels them to their destinations. <u>Hemoglobin</u> binds oxygen that is absorbed in the lungs and transports it to the tissues where it is needed. Each hemoglobin molecule is capable of binding up to four gaseous molecules, most often oxygen. Oxygen is then carried to end organs, where it diffuses into tissues. How much of this capacity is used is referred to as oxygen saturation. This is often expressed as a ratio of the amount of oxygen bound to hemoglobin, to the oxygen-carrying capacity of hemoglobin. The pulse oximeter reports this ratio and is recorded as SpO_2. Normal oxygen saturation is 97% to 99%, and values of 95% or more are clinically acceptable. The amount of oxygen bound to the hemoglobin is related to the partial pressure of oxygen (Po_2) to which the hemoglobin is exposed. In the lungs, at the alveolar-capillary membrane, the partial pressure of oxygen is normally high, and therefore oxygen binds easily and rapidly to the hemoglobin. This arterial oxygen saturation is important for proper delivery of oxygen to the tissues. As the blood circulates to the body tissues where the partial pressure of oxygen is lower, the hemoglobin releases the oxygen into the tissues because the hemoglobin cannot maintain its full load of oxygen in the presence of lower oxygen partial pressures. The relationship between the Po_2 and the SpO_2 is represented by the oxyhemoglobin dissociation curve. The oxyhemoglobin dissociation curve is determined by how readily hemoglobin acquires and releases oxygen molecules from its surrounding tissue. This is called the "hemoglobin's affinity for oxygen." Shifts in this affinity for oxygen and the ability for hemoglobin to be released to tissues can occur in certain disease states.

Several types of WBCs (<u>leukocytes</u>) exist, each of which has a different function. The primary function of all WBCs is to fight infection. Antibodies to fight infection may be produced, or leukocytes may directly attack and kill bacterial invaders.

<u>Platelets</u> are small cells in the blood that are essential for clot formation. The blood clotting (coagulation) process is a complex series of events involving platelets, clotting proteins in the plasma (clotting factors), other proteins, and calcium. During coagulation, platelets aggregate in a clump and form much of the foundation of a blood clot. Clotting proteins produced by the liver solidify the remainder of the clot, which eventually includes RBCs and WBCs.

Words of Wisdom

<u>Hematocrit</u> is a blood test that measures the portion of RBCs in whole blood. Normal results vary, but in general are as follows:

- Male (any age): 40.7% to 50.3%
- Female (any age): 36.1% to 44.3%

If a patient's hematocrit value is out of range, disease may be indicated. However, many different diseases or conditions could cause an abnormal value, such as anemia.

Blood Circulation and Perfusion

Arteries are blood vessels that carry blood away from the heart. Veins are blood vessels that transport blood back to the heart. As arteries get farther from the heart, they become smaller. Eventually, they branch into many small arterioles, which themselves divide into even smaller capillaries (microscopic, thin-walled blood vessels). Oxygen and nutrients pass out of the capillaries and into the cells, and carbon dioxide and waste products pass from the cells and into the capillaries in a process called diffusion. To return deoxygenated blood to the heart, groups of capillaries gradually enlarge to form venules. Venules then merge together, forming larger veins that eventually empty into the heart.

<u>Perfusion</u> is the circulation of blood within an organ or tissue in adequate amounts to meet the cells' current needs for oxygen, nutrients, and waste removal. Blood must pass through the cardiovascular system at a speed that is fast enough to maintain adequate circulation throughout the body, yet slow enough to allow each cell time to exchange oxygen and nutrients for carbon dioxide and other waste products. Although some tissues, such as the lungs and kidneys, never rest and require a constant blood supply, most tissues require circulating blood only intermittently, but especially when they are active. Muscles, for example, are at rest and require a minimal blood supply when you sleep. In contrast, during exercise, muscles need a large blood supply. As another example, the gastrointestinal (GI) tract requires a high flow of blood after a meal. After digestion is completed, a small fraction of that flow is adequate to meet its needs.

The autonomic nervous system monitors the body's needs from moment to moment, adjusting the blood flow as required. This system is responsible for maintaining homeostasis and is divided into sympathetic and parasympathetic components that oppose each other and keep vital functions in balance.

The sympathetic system is often referred to as the "fight, flight, or freeze" mode and is your body's normal response to stress. This stressor can be external, such as an immediate danger or it can be internal, such as having a myocardial infarction or experiencing rapid blood loss. Actions of the sympathetic system include faster and stronger heart contractions, faster and deeper respirations along with bronchodilation, shunting of blood to vital areas in the core of the body and away from the skin, and the slowing and cessation of digestive functions.

The parasympathetic nervous system is often referred to as the "rest and digest" mode. The activities of this part of the autonomic nervous system are reparative and restorative. The actions of the parasympathetic system include a slowing of the heart rate, slowing of the breathing rate, and an increase in digestive functions.

The vasomotor center in the medulla oblongata helps to regulate blood pressure. If a drop in blood pressure is detected in the aortic arch or the carotid sinus, such as during blood loss, the baroreceptors (stretch or pressure sensors) send stimuli to the brain via cranial nerves IX and X, which causes an increase in sympathetic stimulation. The opposite is true in cases in which blood pressure is rising.

Another important system that responds to blood pressure changes is the endocrine system. For instance, a fall in blood pressure and the resultant changes in plasma osmolality cause the release of aldosterone from the adrenal glands and antidiuretic hormone (ADH) from the pituitary gland. This causes additional peripheral vasoconstriction as well as a conservation of water in the kidneys.

Thus, the cardiovascular system, working in conjunction with the nervous and endocrine systems, is dynamic and constantly adapting to changing conditions. Sometimes, however, it fails to provide sufficient circulation for every body part to perform its function, resulting in **hypoperfusion** or shock.

The delivery of oxygen to the tissues is dependent on an adequate heart rate, stroke volume, hemoglobin levels, and arterial oxygen saturation. If this is not adequate, tissues will become ischemic.

The brain and spinal cord cannot go for more than 4 to 6 minutes without perfusion, or the nerve cells will be permanently damaged—recall that cells of the central nervous system do not have the capacity to regenerate. The kidneys will be permanently damaged after 45 minutes of inadequate perfusion, which is the same for most other vital organs. Skeletal muscles cannot tolerate more than 2 hours of inadequate perfusion. The GI tract can exist with limited (but not absent) perfusion for several hours. These times are based on a normal body temperature (98.6°F [37.0°C]) and constitute what is known as the "warm ischemic time." An organ or tissue that is considerably colder is better able to resist damage from hypoperfusion because of the slowing of the body's metabolism.

Pathophysiology of Hemorrhage

Hemorrhage means bleeding. Hemorrhage can range from a "nick" to a capillary while shaving, to a severely spurting artery from a deep slash with a knife, to a ruptured spleen from striking the steering column during a car crash. External visible hemorrhage usually can be controlled by using direct pressure or a pressure bandage. Internal hemorrhage is not visible and is usually not controlled until a surgeon locates the source and sutures it closed. Because internal hemorrhage is not as obvious, you must rely on signs and symptoms to determine the extent and severity of the bleeding.

External Hemorrhage

The extent or severity of external hemorrhage is often a function of the type of wound and the types of blood vessels that have been injured. (Wound types are discussed in detail in the *Soft-Tissue Trauma* chapter.) Hemorrhage from a capillary usually oozes, bleeding from a vein flows, and bleeding from an artery spurts.

These descriptions are not infallible. For example, considerable oozing from capillaries is possible when a patient sustains a large abrasion (such as road rash when a cyclist slides along the pavement without protective clothing). Likewise, varicose veins on the leg can produce copious bleeding.

YOU *are the Medic*   PART 2

After grabbing the backboard and trauma kit, you and your partner approach the scene. The foreman assures you that no work is underway and that the site is safe to enter.

As you approach the scene, you see a worker crouched next to the injured man. "I'm an EMT. I work on a volunteer unit back home. I was down here when he fell. I rushed over and told him not to move."

The EMT is maintaining in-line cervical immobilization on the patient who is supine on the hard-packed dirt and rock ground. As you approach, he looks at you and says, "I'm okay. My back hurts, but I think I'm okay. I'm just a little light-headed." As you communicate with the patient you check his radial pulse and notice that his skin is cool and his pulse is very rapid and weak.

Recording Time: 1 Minute	
Appearance	Awake, harness and tool belt attached
Level of consciousness	Alert
Airway	Open and clear, self-maintained
Breathing	Rapid, unlabored
Circulation	Rapid, weak radial pulse

3. The patient is alert, is breathing adequately, and has a rapid but weak radial pulse. His coworker is holding proper manual stabilization of the cervical spine. What is your next priority?

4. You and your partner decide that the MOI indicates that this patient has a high risk of serious injury and you want to move quickly. Do you leave the harness and tool belt in place or remove them before completing your assessment?

Arteries may spurt initially, but as the patient's blood pressure decreases, often the blood simply flows. In addition, an artery that is incised directly across or in a transverse manner will often recoil and attempt to slow its own bleeding. By contrast, if the artery is cut vertically, or along its length, it does not recoil and continues to bleed.

Some injuries that you might expect to be accompanied by considerable external hemorrhage are not severe. For example, a person who falls off the platform at the train station and is run over by a train may have amputations of one or more extremities, yet experience little bleeding because the wound was cauterized by the heat of the train's wheels on the rail. Conversely, a person who is on the shoulder of the road and removing the jack from his car's trunk when another motorist slams into the rear of the car, pinning him between the two vehicles, may have severely crushed legs. In such a case, hemorrhage may be severe, with the only effective means of bleeding control being tourniquets.

Internal Hemorrhage

Internal hemorrhage as a result of trauma may appear in any portion of the body. A fracture of a long bone (such as humerus, ankle, or tibia) produces a somewhat controlled environment in which a relatively small amount of bleeding can occur. By contrast, bleeding in the trunk (that is, thorax, abdomen, or pelvis), because of its much larger space, tends to be severe and uncontrolled. Nontraumatic internal hemorrhage usually occurs in cases of GI bleeding from the upper or lower GI tract, ruptured ectopic pregnancies, ruptured aneurysms, or other conditions.

Any internal hemorrhage must be treated promptly. The signs of internal hemorrhage (such as discoloration, hematoma) do not always develop quickly, so you must rely on other signs and symptoms and an evaluation of the mechanism of injury (MOI) to make this diagnosis. Pay close attention to patient complaints of pain or tenderness, development of tachycardia, and pallor. In addition to evaluating the MOI, be alert for the development of shock when you suspect internal hemorrhage.

Words of Wisdom

Not every person has the same amount of blood, so you must be able to estimate the patient's blood volume before the trauma occurred. Blood volume is relative to weight—it accounts for 6% to 8% of the total body weight. One pint of blood weighs approximately 1 lb.

The Significance of Hemorrhage

Human adult male bodies contain approximately 70 mL of blood per kilogram of body weight, whereas adult female bodies contain approximately 65 mL/kg. For a typical adult weighing 80 kg (176 lb), the total blood volume is approximately 5 L. The body cannot tolerate an acute blood loss of more than 20% of this total blood volume **Figure 3**. Thus, if the typical adult loses more than 1 L (approximately 2 pints) of blood, significant changes in

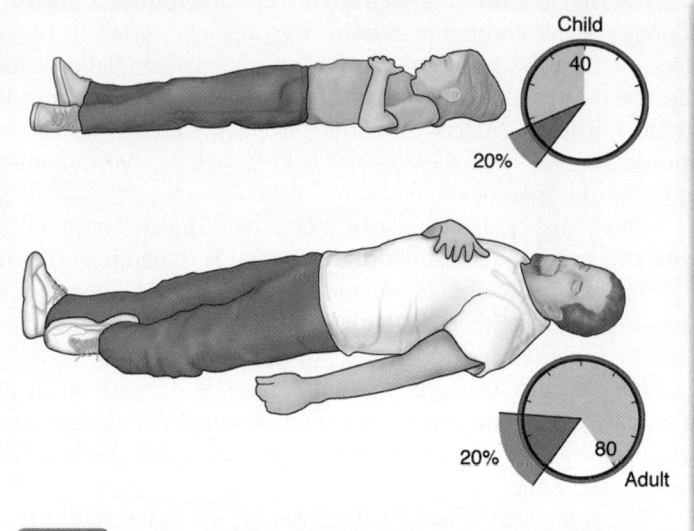

Figure 3 The body will not tolerate an acute blood loss of greater than 20% of blood volume. This equates to approximately 1 L in an adult and proportionally less in a child.

vital signs will occur, including increasing heart and respiratory rates and decreasing blood pressure. An isolated femur fracture, for example, can easily result in the loss of 1 L or more of blood in the soft tissues of the thigh.

Because infants and children have less blood volume than adults, they may experience the same effect with smaller amounts of blood loss. For example, a 1-year-old child has a total blood volume of about 800 mL, so significant symptoms of blood loss may occur after only 100 to 200 mL of blood loss. To put this in perspective, remember that a soft drink can hold roughly 345 mL of liquid.

How well people compensate for blood loss is related to how rapidly they bleed. A healthy adult can comfortably donate one unit (500 mL) of blood in a period of 15 to 20 minutes without having ill effects from this decrease in blood volume. If a similar blood loss occurs in a much shorter period, hemorrhagic shock, may rapidly develop, a condition in which low blood volume results in inadequate perfusion and even death. Consider bleeding to be serious if any of the following conditions are present:

- A significant MOI, especially when the MOI suggests that severe forces affected the abdomen or chest
- Poor general appearance of the patient
- Signs and symptoms of shock (hypoperfusion)
- Significant amount of blood loss
- Rapid blood loss
- Uncontrollable bleeding

Physiologic Response to Hemorrhage

Typically, bleeding from an open artery is bright red (because of the high oxygen content) and spurts in time with the pulse. The pressure that causes the blood to spurt also makes this type of bleeding difficult to control. As the amount of blood circulating in the body drops, so does the patient's blood pressure and, eventually, the arterial spurting diminishes.

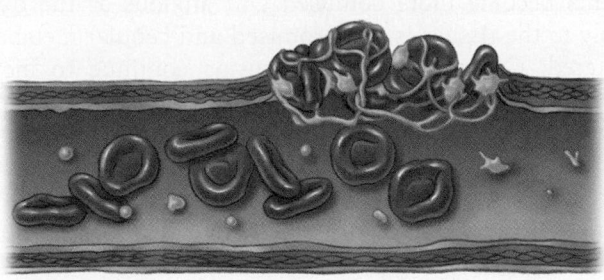

Figure 4 The forming blood clot continues trapping blood components until the bleeding, and eventually the plasma secretions, have stopped.

Table 1 Causes of Shock

Respiratory Failure

- Obstruction—airway or embolism
- Chest wall movement problems—such as flail chest
- Diffusion failure—acute respiratory distress syndrome (ARDS)
- Toxic exposures—such as carbon monoxide and cyanide

Pump Failure

- Cardiogenic shock
- Intrinsic
- Extrinsic
  - Cardiac tamponade
  - Tension pneumothorax

Poor Vessel Function

- Distributive shock
- Septic shock
- Central nervous system loss
  - Neurogenic shock
  - Psychogenic shock
- Anaphylactic shock

Low Fluid Volume

- Hypovolemic shock
  - Hemorrhagic shock such as internal or external bleeding
  - Nonhemorrhagic shock such as dehydration
  - Third space loss such as with some fractures and burns

Blood from an open vein is much darker (low oxygen content) and flows steadily. Because it is under less pressure, most venous blood does not spurt and is easier to manage. Bleeding from damaged capillary vessels is dark red and oozes from a wound steadily but slowly. Venous and capillary bleeding is more likely to clot spontaneously than arterial bleeding.

On its own, bleeding tends to stop rather quickly, within about 10 minutes, in response to internal clotting mechanisms and exposure to air. When vessels are lacerated, blood flows rapidly from the open vessel. The open ends of the vessel then begin to narrow (vasoconstrict), which reduces the amount of bleeding. Platelets aggregate at the site, plugging the hole and sealing the injured portions of the vessel, a process called **hemostasis** **Figure 4** . Bleeding will not stop if a clot does not form, unless the injured vessel is completely cut off from the main blood supply. Direct contact with body tissues and fluids or the external environment commonly triggers the blood's clotting factors.

Despite the efficiency of this system, it may fail in certain situations. A number of medications, including anticoagulants such as aspirin and prescription blood thinners, interfere with normal clotting. Beta blockers can also prevent vasoconstriction, resulting in excessive bleeding. With a severe injury, the damage to the vessel may be so extensive that a clot cannot completely block the hole. Sometimes, only part of the vessel wall is cut, preventing it from constricting. In these cases, bleeding will continue unless it is stopped by external means. In a situation involving acute blood loss, the patient might die before the body's hemostatic defenses of vasoconstriction and clotting can help. In addition, cold will inhibit the enzymes involved in the clotting process; therefore, all bleeding patients must be kept warm.

A small portion of the population lacks one or more of the blood's clotting factors. This condition is called **hemophilia**. There are several forms of hemophilia, most of which are hereditary and some of which are severe. Sometimes, bleeding may occur spontaneously in a person with hemophilia. Because the patient's blood does not clot, all injuries, no matter how trivial, are potentially serious. A patient with hemophilia should be transported immediately.

Shock

Shock can result from many conditions, including bleeding, respiratory failure, acute allergic reactions, and overwhelming infection **Table 1** . In all cases, the damage occurs because of insufficient perfusion of organs and tissues. According to the Centers for Disease Control and Prevention, in 2008, unintentional injury remains the leading cause of death for people ages 1 to 44 years. Your early and rapid actions can help to significantly reduce the morbidity and mortality rates from shock.

When shock comes about because of inadequate blood volume, it is termed **hypovolemic shock** (*hypo* = deficient + *vol* = volume + *emia* = in the blood). There are hemorrhagic and nonhemorrhagic causes of hypovolemic shock. Volume can be lost as blood (internal or external **hemorrhagic shock**), plasma (burns), or electrolyte solution (vomiting, diarrhea, sweating) (nonhemorrhagic shock). When a patient has severe thermal burns, intravascular plasma is lost, leaking from the circulatory system into the burned tissues that lie

Words of Wisdom

You should suspect a hypovolemic component of shock in any patient with unexplained shock, and treat for hypovolemia first.

adjacent to the injury. Likewise, crushing injuries may result in the loss of blood and plasma from damaged vessels into injured tissues.

Hemorrhagic shock is the most common cause of shock and will be discussed in this chapter. See the chapter, *Management and Resuscitation of the Critical Patient*, for information about the other causes of shock, including nonhemorrhagic shock.

Hemorrhagic Shock

The major life threat to most trauma patients is blood loss. Hemorrhage is most prevalent due to blunt or penetrating injuries to vessels or organs, long bone or pelvic fractures, major vascular injuries (as in traumatic amputation), and multisystem injury. The organs and organ systems with a high incidence of exsanguination from penetrating injuries include the heart, thoracic vascular system, abdominal vascular system (such as abdominal aorta, superior mesenteric artery), venous system (such as inferior vena cava or portal vein), and liver.

Hypovolemic shock caused by hemorrhagic trauma has been classified by the American College of Surgeons Committee on Trauma into four classes, each with their own specific characteristics and treatments Table 2 .

Shock occurs in three successive phases (compensated shock [classes I and II], decompensated shock [class III], and irreversible shock [class IV]). Your goal is to recognize the clinical signs and symptoms of shock in its earliest phase and begin immediate treatment before permanent damage occurs Table 3 .

The initial stage of hemorrhagic shock is characterized by low circulating blood volume with minimal signs of hypoperfusion. However, as the body begins to compensate for low venous return, decreased SV, and low CO, patients begin to have tachycardia, hypotension, and signs of poor tissue perfusion, including pallor and delayed capillary refill.

Patients become more confused and anxious as the oxygen supply to the tissues is compromised and cellular metabolism is altered. Compensatory mechanisms continue to increase systemic vascular resistance (SVR) in an attempt to improve hemodynamics. As SVR increases and CO drops, patients have cold, mottled, and pulseless extremities with worsening mental status. Left untreated, the shock will eventually progress to decompensated shock that is refractory to any therapy Table 4 .

Patient Assessment

Scene Size-up

The assessment of any patient begins with a scene size-up. This includes the recognition of hazards and traffic safety, protection of bystanders, and stability of vehicles involved, if applicable. Once the scene is deemed safe to enter, follow standard precautions. Depending on the severity of bleeding and your general impression, this will entail use of gloves, a mask, an eye shield, and, when the patient is bloody or blood is spurting, a gown. Determine the number of patients present.

A high-energy MOI should increase your index of suspicion for the possibility of serious unseen injuries such as internal bleeding Table 5 . Internal bleeding is possible whenever the MOI suggests that severe forces affected the body. These forces include blunt and penetrating trauma. Internal bleeding commonly occurs as a result of falls, blast injuries, and automobile or motorcycle crashes. Also, keep in mind that internal bleeding is not always caused by trauma. Many illnesses such as bleeding ulcers, bleeding from the colon, ruptured ectopic pregnancy, and aneurysms can cause internal bleeding.

Table 2 **Estimated Fluid and Blood Loss for a 70-kg (154 lb) Male**				
	Class I	Class II	Class III	Class IV
Blood loss (mL)	< 750	750-1,500	1,500-2,000	> 2,000
% Blood loss	< 15	15-30	30-40	> 40
Heart rate (beats/min)	< 100	> 100	> 120	> 140
Systolic blood pressure	Within normal limits	Normal	Low	Low
Pulse pressure	Within normal limits	Narrow	Narrow	Very narrow
Capillary refill	Within normal limits	Delayed	Delayed	Absent
Respiratory rate (breaths/min)	14-20	20-30	30-40	> 35
Central nervous system/ mental status	Slightly anxious	Mildly anxious	Anxious and confused	Confused and lethargic
Skin condition	Cool, pink	Cool, pale	Cold, pale, moist	Cold, cyanotic
Urine output (mL/h)	> 30	20-30	5-15	Minimal or none
Fluid replacement	Crystalloid	Crystalloid	Crystalloid and blood	Crystalloid and blood

Table 3 Compensated Versus Decompensated Hypoperfusion

Compensated Hypoperfusion	Decompensated Hypoperfusion
■ Agitation, anxiety, restlessness ■ Sense of impending doom ■ Weak, rapid (thready) pulse ■ Clammy (cool, moist) skin ■ Pallor with cyanotic lips ■ Shortness of breath ■ Nausea, vomiting ■ Delayed capillary refill in infants and children ■ Thirst ■ Normal systolic blood pressure	■ Altered mental status (verbal to unresponsive) ■ Hypotension ■ Labored or irregular breathing ■ Thready or absent peripheral pulses ■ Ashen, mottled, or cyanotic skin ■ Dilated pupils ■ Diminished urine output (oliguria) ■ Impending cardiac arrest

Table 4 Findings in Hemorrhagic Shock

Heart rate	Increased
Blood pressure	Within normal limits in the early stages, then decreases as patient decompensates
Central venous pressure/renal artery pressure	Decreased
Pulmonary capillary wedge pressure	Decreased
Cardiac output/cardiac index	Decreased
Systemic vascular resistance/systemic vascular resistance index	Increased
Systemic vascular oxygen	Decreased
Urinary output	Decreased
Jugular vein distention	Flat
Hematocrit (percentage of whole blood components versus plasma)	Decreased with hemorrhage; increased with dehydration

Words of Wisdom

Regardless of the type of bleeding—whether hidden in the body cavities or visible on the surrounding surfaces—all patients will proceed through the phases of shock if their bleeding is not controlled. In hemorrhagic shock, the specific phase of shock is a function of the percentage of blood volume lost. Because internal bleeding is more likely to be uncontrolled, you should stay alert for the subtle signs of shock and be aggressive in your management of its early phase to help your patient avoid deteriorating toward shock's later phases.

Documentation and Communication

Just as they make for thorough written reporting, taking and recording frequent serial vital signs—and observing perfusion indicators such as skin condition and mental status—will give you a window into the progression of shock. Use your documentation to remind you to suspect shock early and treat it aggressively.

It is often difficult to determine visually the amount of blood lost. You should attempt to determine the amount of external blood loss, but remember that this is not crucial and the presentation and assessment of the patient must direct patient care and treatment.

For patients who have sustained significant MOIs, scene time should not exceed 10 minutes and the most appropriate transportation destination must be considered.

■ Primary Assessment

During the primary assessment, you need to determine the patient's mental status using the AVPU scale (*Alert* to person, place, and day; responsive to *Verbal* stimuli or *Pain*; *Unresponsive*), and locate and manage immediate threats to life involving the airway, breathing, and circulation. Ensure that the patient has a patent airway and there is no structural damage. Check the patient's breathing patterns, chest wall integrity, and

Table 5   Significant Mechanisms of Injury

Multisystem trauma
Ejection from vehicle or vehicle rollover
Fall of more than 20 ft without loss of consciousness
Fall of less than 20 ft with loss of consciousness
High-speed vehicular crash
Vehicle versus pedestrian crash
Motorcycle crash
Significant external blood loss
Penetration of the head, chest, abdomen, or pelvis
Unresponsive or altered mental status with suspected traumatic origin
Death or major injury of another occupant in the same vehicle

pulse rate. Assess for signs of hemorrhagic shock. If you observe bleeding from the mouth or facial areas, keep the suction unit within reach.

Special Populations

In older patients, dizziness, faintness, or weakness may be the first sign of nontraumatic internal bleeding.

If major external hemorrhage is present, manage it immediately, treat the patient for shock, and transport the patient to the emergency department. Continue with the assessment en route to the emergency department.

Most external hemorrhage can be managed with direct pressure and pressure dressings, although arterial bleeding may take 5 or more minutes of direct pressure to form a clot. Previously, pressure points and elevation were the means used to control bleeding in the extremities. However, recent studies have brought into question the effectiveness of using pressure points to control severe external hemorrhage. Military experience in Afghanistan and Iraq has proven that tourniquets can effectively control hemorrhage that does not respond to direct pressure techniques. For this reason, the use of a tourniquet is preferred for external hemorrhage to an extremity that cannot be controlled with direct pressure and a pressure bandage. In addition, there is good evidence to support the use of hemostatic agents for external bleeding. Consult your local protocols for guidance on these agents.

Because most cases of internal hemorrhage are rarely fully controlled in the prehospital setting, a patient with this type of injury needs rapid transport to the emergency department.

Late signs of hypoperfusion suggesting internal hemorrhage include the following:

- Tachycardia
- Weakness, fainting, or dizziness at rest
- Thirst
- Nausea and vomiting
- Cold, moist (clammy) skin
- Shallow, rapid breathing
- Dull eyes

YOU are the Medic   PART 3

The patient's breath sounds are clear and equal with full expansion. The patient tells you that his chest hurts a little bit when he breathes. Your partner applies a nonrebreathing mask, setting the oxygen at 15 L/min and then obtains vital signs as you continue your assessment. As you are cutting away his harness and removing the tool belt, you see a deep laceration on the right flank where one of the tools penetrated the skin. There is no impalement but the wound is bleeding heavily.

Recording Time: 5 Minutes	
Respirations	20 breaths/min, unlabored
Pulse	122 beats/min, very weak radial pulses
Skin	Pale, cool, moist
Blood pressure	108/70 mm Hg
Oxygen saturation (Spo$_2$)	97% on oxygen
Pupils	Equal, reactive to light

5. The patient has unlabored breathing, normal lung sounds, and high concentration oxygen in place. His Spo$_2$ reading seems adequate. Could he still be suffering from poor perfusion?

6. If you measure his end-tidal carbon dioxde (ETCO$_2$), would you expect it to be high, low, or normal range? What are some factors that affect the measured levels of ETCO$_2$?

- Slightly dilated pupils that are slow to respond to light
- Capillary refill of more than 2 seconds in infants and children
- Weak, rapid (thready) pulse
- Decreasing blood pressure
- Altered level of consciousness

Even if their bleeding stops, it could begin again at any moment. Therefore, prompt transport is necessary for these patients.

If you suspect internal hemorrhage, begin management by keeping the patient warm and administering supplemental oxygen by a nonrebreathing mask at 15 L/min en route to the emergency department.

If the patient has minor external hemorrhage, you should make note of it and move on with the assessment process; management of this problem can wait until the patient has been properly assessed and prioritized. Do not get sidetracked by applying dressings and bandages to a patient who may have more serious problems.

Words of Wisdom

When you are managing a bleeding patient, be sure to take necessary precautions to protect yourself from splashing or splattering. Wear appropriate personal protective equipment, including gloves, gown, mask, and eye protection. This is especially essential when arterial bleeding is present. Also remember that frequent, thorough handwashing between patients and after every run is a simple yet important protective measure.

History Taking

As you continue with the assessment, investigate the chief complaint using the OPQRST mnemonic, and obtain a history of the present illness using SAMPLE. Ask the patient if he or she experiences any dizziness or syncope. Ask the patient about current medications that may thin the blood and about any history of clotting insufficiency. For example, patients with a history of a previous myocardial infarction may be taking anticoagulants, in which case a "minor" injury such as an extremity fracture can lead to significant blood loss and shock. Ask about beta blockers, calcium channel blockers, antidysrhythmics, and use of nitroglycerin because these medications will interfere with the body's ability to compensate for shock. Is there any pain, tenderness, bruising, guarding, or swelling? These signs and symptoms may indicate internal bleeding.

Words of Wisdom

Consider any patient exhibiting signs and symptoms of shock without obvious injury to have probable internal bleeding, usually in the abdominal cavity.

Secondary Assessment

When you are performing a secondary assessment, the examination should include a systematic full-body scan. The most common symptom of internal hemorrhage is pain. Significant internal hemorrhage will generally cause swelling in the area of bleeding. Intra-abdominal hemorrhage will often cause pain and distention. A contusion or ecchymosis is a sign of internal hemorrhage. It most commonly occurs in head, extremity, and pelvic injuries and can be a sign of significant trauma. It may not be present initially, and the only sign of severe pelvic or abdominal trauma may be redness, skin abrasions, or pain. Bleeding into the chest may cause dyspnea in addition to tachycardia and hypotension.

Hemorrhage, however slight, from any body opening is serious. It usually indicates internal hemorrhage that is not easy to see or control. Bright red bleeding from the mouth or rectum or blood in the urine (hematuria) may suggest serious internal injury or disease. Nonmenstrual vaginal hemorrhage is always significant. Note the characteristics of the bleeding and try to determine its source. For example, bright red blood from a wound or the mouth, rectum, or other orifice indicates fresh arterial bleeding. Coffee-ground emesis is a sign of upper GI bleeding; this type of blood is old and looks like used coffee grounds.

Other signs and symptoms of internal hemorrhage in both trauma and medical patients include the following:

- **Hematoma**. A mass of blood in the soft tissues beneath the skin; indicates bleeding into soft tissues and may be the result of a minor or a severe injury.
- **Hematemesis**. Vomited blood. It may be bright red or dark red, or, if the blood has been partially digested, it may look like coffee-grounds vomitus; a sign of upper GI bleeding.
- **Hemoptysis**. Coughed-up blood. It is usually bright red.
- **Melena**. Black, foul-smelling, tarry stool that contains digested blood; indicates lower GI bleeding.
- **Hematuria**. Blood in the urine; may suggest serious renal injury or illness.
- **Hematochezia**. The passage of bloody stools. If they contain bright red blood, this may indicate hemorrhage near the external opening of the anus. Hemorrhoids in the lower colon tend to cause hematochezia.
- Pain, tenderness, bruising, guarding, or swelling. These signs and symptoms may mean that a closed fracture is hemorrhaging.
- Broken ribs, bruises over the lower part of the chest, or a rigid, distended abdomen. These signs and symptoms may indicate a lacerated spleen or liver. Patients with an injury to either organ may have referred pain in the right shoulder (liver) or left shoulder (spleen). You should suspect internal abdominal bleeding in a patient with referred pain.

Assess the respiratory system. Specifically assess the airway for patency and determine the rate and quality of respirations. In the neck, look for distended neck veins and a deviated trachea.

In the chest, check for paradoxical movement of the chest wall and bilateral breath sounds.

Assess the cardiovascular system, specifically the rate and quality of pulses. Be careful with the use of a pulse oximeter for patients in shock. When the body uses vasoconstriction to compensate for shock, the pulse oximeter probe, being placed on an extremity, will not be able to give an accurate measurement of the body's oxygen saturation. The ECG should be used to monitor the patient's cardiac rhythm. The presence of pulses is related to perfusion status. As a person's blood pressure begins to drop, the radial pulse will disappear, then the brachial and femoral pulses will disappear, and lastly, the carotid pulse will go absent. Keep in mind that the blood pressure appears normal in the early stages of shock as the body compensates and will not drop until the patient begins to decompensate. Medications may also mask changes in vital signs. For example, beta blockers interfere with the body's normal sympathetic response and will not allow the heart to speed up or pump harder. Calcium channel blockers can interfere with vasoconstriction and not allow for shunting of blood to vital areas. Patients who have recently taken nitroglycerin or are wearing a patch may not be able to achieve vasoconstriction because of the vasodilation effect from the nitroglycerin. Other antidysrhythmics can interfere with the heart's ability to speed up or pump with more force. Normally, in an effort to maintain central perfusion, blood will be shunted away from the periphery and the patient will present with pale, cool, mottled skin and decreased or absent radial pulses with an increased capillary refill time.

Assess the neurologic system to formulate baseline data to guide further decisions. This examination should include level of consciousness, pupil size and reactivity, motor response, and sensory response.

Assess the musculoskeletal system. Perform a detailed full-body examination. Look for DCAP-BTLS to be sure that you have found all of the problems and injuries quickly.

Assess all anatomic regions. When you are examining the head, be alert for raccoon eyes, Battle sign, and/or drainage of blood or fluid from the ears or nose. In the abdomen, feel all four quadrants for tenderness or rigidity. In the extremities, record the pulse and motor and sensory function.

Reassessment

Patient reassessment is an important tool to see how your patient is doing over time. Reassess the patient, especially in the areas that showed abnormal findings during the primary assessment. Be sure to reassess any interventions used to control hemorrhage and ensure they remain adequate. The signs and symptoms of internal hemorrhage are often slow to present because of their covert nature.

Vital signs show how well your patient is doing internally. In all cases of severe hemorrhage, obtain the patient's vital signs every 5 minutes en route to the emergency department. Whenever you suspect significant hemorrhage, either external or internal, provide high-flow oxygen. If significant hemorrhage

Special Populations

Older patients are more likely to be on medications that interfere with normal compensatory mechanisms, such as beta blockers, calcium channel blockers, nitroglycerin, and other antiarrhythmics. The kidneys will atrophy with age and therefore be less responsive to fluid conservation; the blood vessels may be affected by atherosclerosis and less able to shunt blood to vital areas. In addition, other medical problems can be exacerbated during shock states; for instance, ischemia is more likely to interfere with cardiac output in patients with a history of myocardial infarction or angina.

Pediatric patients have underdeveloped kidneys, resulting in an inability to conserve fluid like an adult. This results in a lower tolerance for volume loss. In addition, they will compensate by vasoconstriction better than adults. This will lead to a longer compensatory state and good blood pressure until a point is reached where there is an abrupt collapse of the vital signs and possibly death. An additional complication in small children is their relatively large surface area to weight ratio. Children get cold easier, which results in coagulation difficulties.

Pregnant patients normally will have a faster pulse, greater blood volume, lower blood pressure, and nausea. Therefore, manage these patients aggressively according to the MOI and treat for shock; do not just assume the altered signs are due to the pregnancy.

is visible at any time during the assessment process, begin the steps to control the bleeding, discussed next.

■ Emergency Medical Care of Bleeding and Hemorrhagic Shock

Always follow standard precautions when you are treating bleeding patients and suspect shock if the patient is severely hemorrhaging. As with all patient care, ensure that the patient has an open airway and is breathing adequately. Provide high-flow supplemental oxygen, and assist ventilation if needed, paying special attention to cervical spine control in trauma patients.

■ Managing External Hemorrhage

To control external hemorrhaging in an extremity, follow these steps Skill Drill 1 :

Skill Drill 1

1. Follow standard precautions.
2. Maintain the airway with cervical spine immobilization if the MOI suggests the possibility of spinal injury.
3. Apply direct pressure over the wound with a dry, sterile dressing. Elevate the injury if no fracture is suspected Step 1 .

4. Apply a pressure dressing. Hold the pressure dressing in place using gauze (**Step 2**).

5. If direct pressure with a pressure dressing does not rapidly control bleeding on an extremity injury, apply a tourniquet above the level of the bleeding (**Step 3**).

6. Apply high-flow oxygen as necessary, once hemorrhaging is controlled.

7. Monitor the serial vital signs, and watch diligently for developing shock.

If the patient shows any signs of shock (hypoperfusion), transport rapidly while providing aggressive management en route. Because a patient in shock is usually emotionally upset, you should provide psychological support as well.

Hemorrhaging From the Nose, Ears, and Mouth

Hemorrhaging from the nose (epistaxis) or the ears following a head injury may indicate a skull fracture. In such a case, you should not attempt to stop the blood flow. Applying excessive pressure to the injury may force the blood leaking through the ear or nose to collect within the head, ultimately increasing intracranial pressure and possibly causing permanent damage. If you suspect a skull fracture, cover the bleeding site loosely with a sterile gauze pad to collect the blood and help keep contaminants away from the site—there is always a risk of infection to the brain with a skull fracture. Apply light compression by wrapping the dressing loosely around the head. If blood or drainage contains cerebrospinal fluid (CSF), the dressing will show a characteristic staining of the dressing that resembles a bull's-eye target. Another method that can be used to check for CSF in the blood is the glucometer. Because the CSF has a high glucose content, the glucometer will detect this in the blood of a normoglycemic patient.

For a nosebleed from other conditions, such as trauma directly to the nose or bleeding caused by environmental factors such as dry air, cold compresses can be applied to the bridge of the nose. An alternative is to roll gauze and place it under the upper lip. This will generate pressure on the blood supply to the nose and often works within 5 minutes. Always be sure to check the patient's blood pressure and evaluate for a hypertensive emergency as the cause of epistaxis, especially in older patients.

Hemorrhaging From Other Areas

When there is hemorrhaging from other areas of the body, control it through use of direct pressure. Apply pressure dressings, and consider the use of a tourniquet and hemostatic dressings, per your local protocol. In addition, use splints (or air splints) as necessary, always following your local protocols. Air splints can control venous bleeding but will not apply enough pressure to control arterial bleeding until the patient's blood pressure is extremely low (around 50 mm Hg systolic). Pack large, gaping wounds with sterile dressings.

Once hemorrhaging is controlled and a sterile dressing and pressure bandage have been applied, keep the patient warm and in the appropriate position. Allow the patient's condition to dictate the mode of transport.

Skill Drill 1

Controlling External Hemorrhage

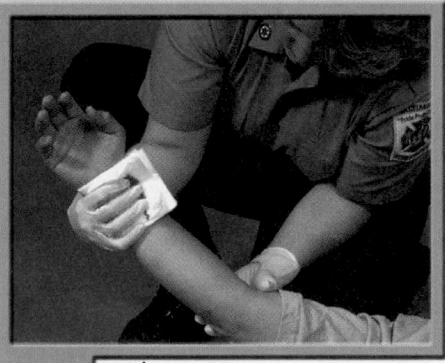
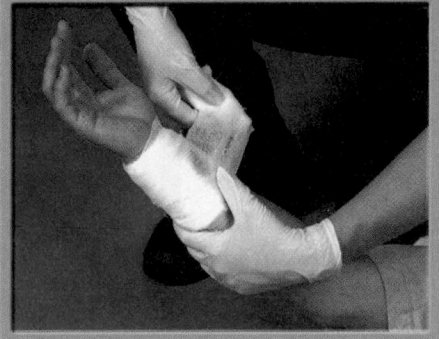
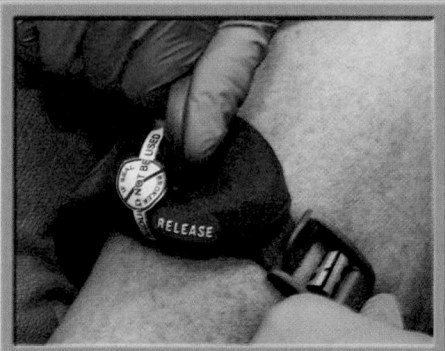

Step 1 Apply direct pressure over the wound with a dry, sterile dressing. Elevate the injury if no fracture is suspected.

Step 2 Apply a pressure dressing.

Step 3 If direct pressure with a pressure dressing does not rapidly control bleeding on an extremity, apply a tourniquet above the level of bleeding.

Special Management Techniques for External Hemorrhage

Tourniquets

The tourniquet is especially useful if a patient is hemorrhaging severely from an extremity injury below the axilla or groin and other methods of control are ineffective. Tourniquets have proven so efficient and easy to use that the military has issued tourniquets to all field personnel **Figure 5** .

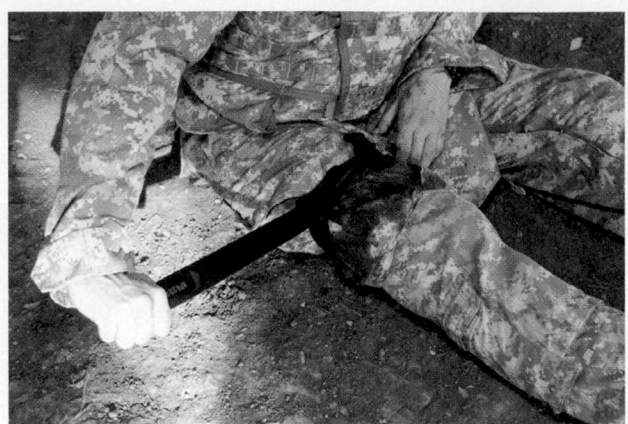

Figure 5 This tourniquet uses a windlass rod to apply pressure to an extremity.

The use of commercial tourniquets generally involves the following steps **Skill Drill 2** :

Skill Drill   2

1. Follow standard precautions.
2. Hold direct pressure over the bleeding site.
3. Place the tourniquet around the extremity proximal to the injury **Step 1** .
4. Click the buckle into place and pull the strap tight.
5. Turn the tightening dial clockwise until pulses are no longer palpable distal to the tourniquet **Step 2** .
6. To release the tourniquet at the hospital, or if otherwise instructed by medical control, push the release button and pull the strap back. Be aware that bleeding may rapidly return upon tourniquet release and that you should be prepared to reapply it immediately if necessary.

If a commercial tourniquet is not available, follow these steps to apply a tourniquet using a triangular bandage and a stick or rod:

1. Fold a triangular bandage until it is 4 inches wide and six to eight layers thick.
2. Wrap the bandage around the extremity twice. Choose an area proximal to the injury to ensure control of the bleeding.
3. Tie one knot in the bandage. Then place a stick or rod on top of the knot, and tie the ends of the bandage over the stick in a square knot.

Words of Wisdom

Historically, if direct pressure and elevation proved ineffective to control bleeding, EMS providers were advised to apply pressure to a proximal arterial pressure point. A pressure point is a spot where a blood vessel lies near a bone. This technique should be considered interesting from a historic perspective only. Because a wound usually draws blood from more than one major artery, proximal compression of a major artery rarely stops bleeding completely. In rare cases, it may help to slow the loss of blood. You would need to be thoroughly familiar with the location of the pressure points for this to work **Figure 6** . Even if you are familiar with the arterial pressure points, there is no real evidence that this is an effective or safe method to control potentially fatal hemorrhage. If the patient has an open fracture of an extremity, bleeding can be substantial. Consider a tourniquet early if bleeding is not easily controlled with direct pressure or if pressure results in excessive pain. The method used to control severe external bleeding may be governed by local protocol; regardless of the method, it must be quick and effective. Remember that uncontrolled bleeding may result in hemorrhagic shock and death. Patients can and do bleed to death from extremity injuries. It is imperative that you use effective techniques to stop bleeding when you encounter it.

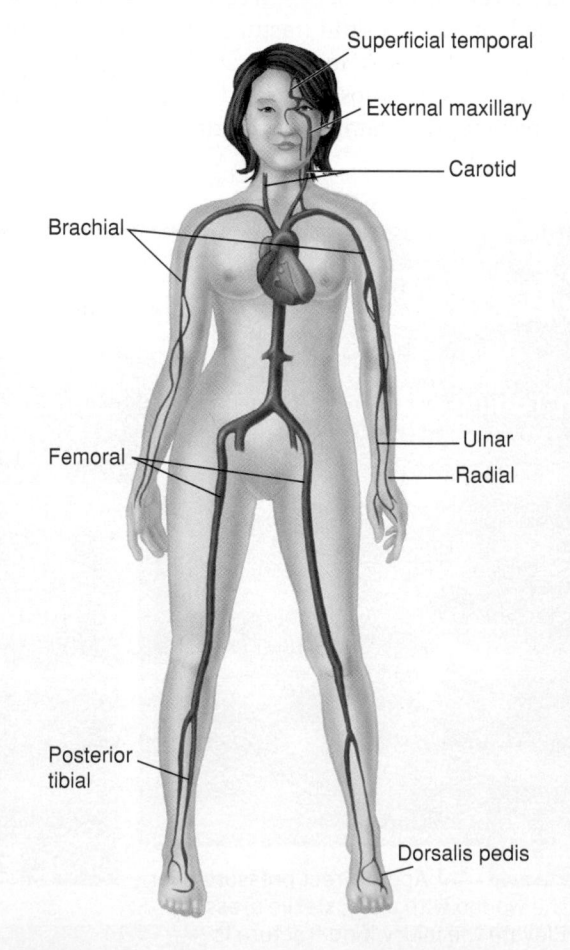

Figure 6 Locations of arterial pressure points.

Skill Drill | 2

Applying a Commercial Tourniquet

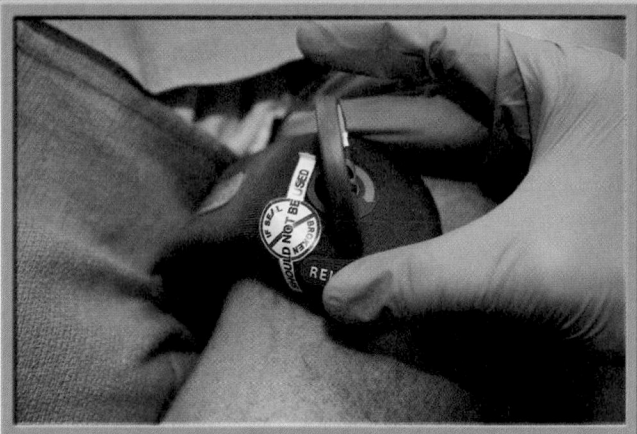

Step **1** Hold direct pressure over the bleeding site and place the tourniquet proximal to the injury.

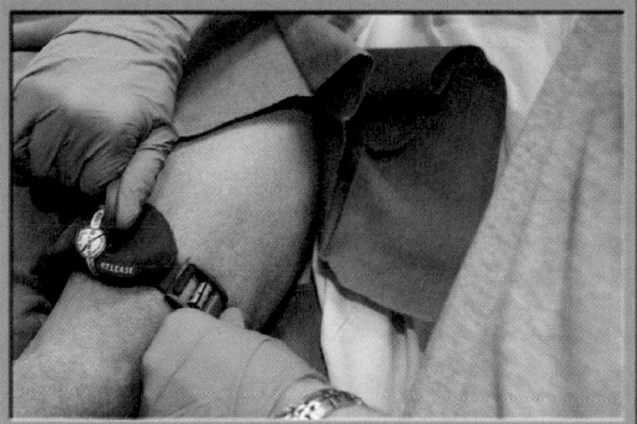

Step **2** Click the buckle into place, pull the strap tight, and turn the tightening dial clockwise until pulses are no longer palpable distal to the tourniquet.

YOU are the Medic | PART 4

With proper PPE already in place, you apply direct pressure to the gaping wound and stop the bleeding. The ground has a small puddle of congealed blood on it and the patient's sweatshirt is soaked with blood. You complete a quick check for any other heavy bleeding but do not find any. Your patient is now complaining of feeling cold and tells you that his vision "feels strange."

Recording Time: 8 Minutes	
Respirations	24 breaths/min, unlabored
Pulse	132 beats/min, very weak radial pulses
Skin	Pale, cool, moist
Blood pressure	92/60 mm Hg
Oxygen saturation (Spo$_2$)	98% on oxygen
Pupils	Equal, reactive to light

7. Despite stopping the flow of heavy bleeding, your patient seems to deteriorate further. What are some of the possible causes of his deteriorating condition?

8. At this point, what is your next priority?

4. Use the stick as a handle, and twist it to tighten the tourniquet until the bleeding has stopped and distal pulses are no longer palpable; then stop twisting **Figure 7** .

5. Secure the stick in place, and make the wrapping neat and smooth.

6. Write "TK" and the exact time (hour and minute) that you applied the tourniquet on a piece of adhesive tape. Use the phrase "time applied." Securely fasten the tape to the patient's forehead. Notify hospital personnel on your arrival that your patient has a tourniquet in place. Record this same information on the patient care report form.

7. As an alternative method, you can use a blood pressure cuff as an effective tourniquet. Position the cuff proximal to the bleeding point, and inflate it enough to eliminate distal pulses and stop the bleeding. Leave the cuff inflated. If you use a blood pressure cuff, monitor the gauge continuously to make sure that the pressure is not gradually dropping. You may have to clamp the tube with a hemostat leading from the cuff to the inflating bulb to prevent loss of pressure.

Whenever you are applying a tourniquet, make sure you observe the following precautions:

- Do not apply a tourniquet directly over any joint. Make sure it is proximal to the zone of injury.
- Use the widest bandage possible. Make sure that it is tightened securely.
- Never use wire, rope, a belt, or any other narrow material as the tourniquet; it could cut into the skin.
- Use wide padding under the tourniquet, if possible, to protect the tissues and help with arterial compression.
- Never cover a tourniquet with a bandage. Leave it open and in full view.
- Inform the hospital in your radio report and verbal report on arrival at the emergency department that a tourniquet has been applied.

- Do not loosen the tourniquet after you have applied it unless directed to do so by hospital personnel or medical control.

Splints

Much of the bleeding associated with broken bones occurs because the sharp ends of the bones lacerate vessels, muscles, and other tissues. As long as a fracture remains unstable, the bone ends will move and continue to damage tissues and vessels. They may also break up clots that have partially formed, resulting in ongoing hemorrhage. For these reasons, immobilizing a fracture is a priority in the prompt control of bleeding. Often, simple splints will quickly control the bleeding associated with a fracture. For example, a fractured pelvis should be stabilized using a pelvic binder or sheets used to bind the pelvis and stabilize the area **Figure 8** .

Air Splints Air splints can control the hemorrhage associated with venous bleeding **Figure 9** . They also stabilize the fracture itself. An air splint acts like a pressure dressing applied to an entire extremity rather than to a small, local area.

Once you have applied an air splint, monitor circulation in the distal extremity. Because an air splint is typically inflated to approximately 50 mm Hg (so you can still dent the splint with your fingertips), it would not be appropriate to use on a patient with arterial hemorrhage because the splint would not actually control the hemorrhage until the patient's systolic blood pressure dropped to the pressure of the splint. Use only approved, clean or disposable valve stems when orally inflating air splints.

Rigid Splints Rigid splints can help stabilize fractures as well as reduce pain and prevent further damage to soft-tissue injuries. Once you have applied a rigid splint, be sure to monitor circulation in the distal extremity.

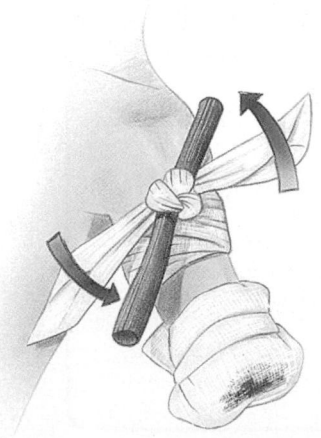

Figure 7 Twist the stick or rod to tighten the tourniquet until the bleeding has stopped and distal pulses are no longer palpable; then stop twisting.

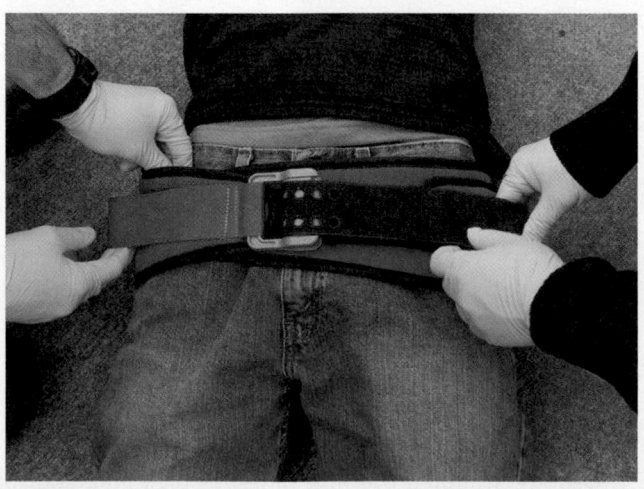

Figure 8 Pelvic binders are meant to provide temporary stabilization and reduce hemorrhage from pelvic bleeding.

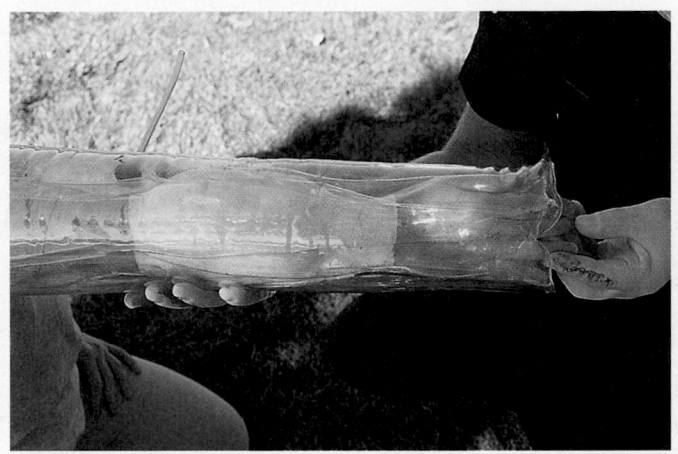

Figure 9 Air splints can control bleeding because they act as a pressure bandage for the entire extremity.

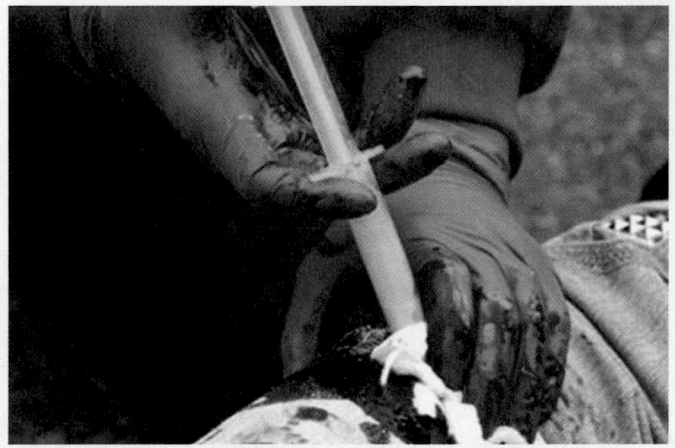

Figure 10 Hemostatic agents are being used in some areas to control profuse bleeding.

Traction Splints Traction splints are designed to stabilize femur fractures. When traction is pulled to the ankle, countertraction is applied to the ischium and groin. This reduces the thigh muscle spasms and prevents one end of the fracture from impacting or overriding the other. Be sure to pad these areas well to prevent applying excessive pressure to the soft tissue of the pelvis. Once you have applied a traction splint, be sure to monitor circulation in the distal extremity.

Hemostatic Agents

The military has successfully used hemostatic agents to control severe hemorrhage, especially to areas where a tourniquet cannot be placed **Figure 10** . These agents work by causing vasoconstriction in the wound site. Hemostatic agents come in powder forms as well as impregnated in dressings. Complications with the use of hemostatic agents in the form of powder include the introduction of emboli through open vasculature as well as the introduction of a foreign substance into the wound (the powder); the use of impregnated bandages instead avoids this complication. Because the evidence supporting the use of hemostatic agents is based on military experience, many physicians are not convinced of their appropriateness in civilian medicine, especially where transport times are short. You will need to consult your local protocols for guidance on the use of hemostatic agents.

Managing Internal Hemorrhage

Management of a patient with internal hemorrhaging focuses on the treatment of shock, minimizing movement of the injured or bleeding part or region, and rapid transport. Eventually, the patient will likely need a surgical procedure to stop the bleeding. In recent years, ultrasound has been used to locate bleeding in the emergency department before moving the patient to the surgical suite for the ultimate resolution of the problem.

Controversies

In the 1980s, researchers began to question whether the military antishock trousers/pneumatic antishock garment (MAST/PASG), and IV fluid infusion, were really effective in the treatment of shock. At the time of this writing, the MAST/PASG is rarely applied in the treatment of hemorrhagic shock. Consult your medical director and regional protocols if you still carry the device.

Follow the steps in **Skill Drill 3** to care for patients with possible internal hemorrhage:

Words of Wisdom

Hemostatic agents such as Celox, HemCon, and QuikClot are primarily used in the military to promote hemostasis or, in other words, to stop profuse bleeding. The agent may be granules poured into a wound or contained in a dressing. The agent absorbs the water component of blood thereby concentrating the clotting factors, activating platelets, and enhancing the coagulation cascade. Some of these agents have an exothermic effect that can damage the surrounding tissue.

Skill Drill   3

1. Follow standard precautions.
2. Maintain the airway with cervical spine immobilization if a MOI suggests the possibility of spinal injury.
3. Administer high-flow supplemental oxygen and assist ventilation if needed **Step 1** .
4. Control all obvious external bleeding.
5. Treat suspected internal bleeding in an extremity by applying a splint. If a pelvic fracture is suspected, use a pelvic binder or sheets to bind the pelvic area **Step 2** .

Skill Drill 3

Controlling Internal Hemorrhage

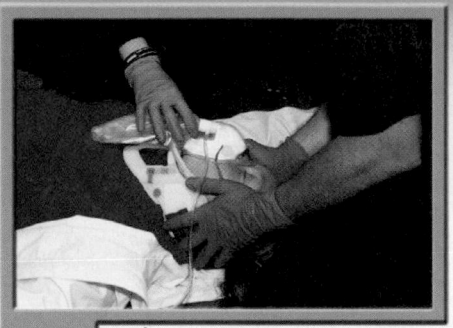

Step 1 Follow standard precautions. Maintain the airway and be alert for cervical spine injury. Administer oxygen and provide ventilation as necessary.

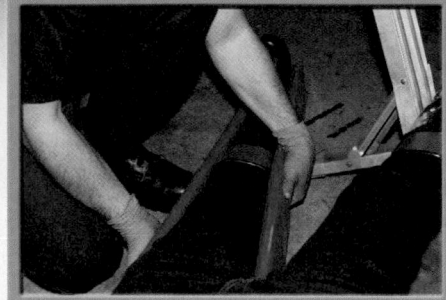

Step 2 Control obvious external bleeding and treat suspected internal extremity bleeding using a splint. If a pelvic fracture is suspected, use a pelvic binder or sheets to bind the pelvic area.

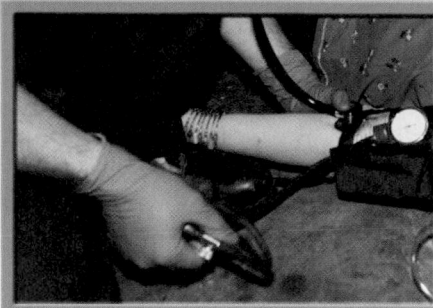

Step 3 Monitor and record vital signs at least every 5 minutes.

6. Monitor and record vital signs at least every 5 minutes (Step 3).

7. Give the patient nothing by mouth.

8. Insert a large-bore (14- or 16-gauge) IV catheter, and administer a fluid bolus of 20 mL/kg of normal saline or lactated Ringer's solution (provided the lungs are clear) en route to the emergency department. Insert an IV line at the scene only if transport is delayed (such as if the patient is pinned). A second large-bore IV line should be obtained if possible. Whenever possible, use warm IV fluids to prevent the patient from becoming hypothermic.

9. Keep the patient warm.

10. Consider giving pain medication if the vital signs are stable and after consultation with medical control.

11. Provide immediate transport. Monitor the serial vital signs, and watch diligently for developing shock en route. If the patient shows any signs of shock (hypoperfusion), transport rapidly while providing aggressive management en route. Because a patient in shock is usually emotionally upset, you should provide psychological support as well.

■ Management of Hemorrhagic Shock

The priorities in treating a patient in hemorrhagic shock are the same as in treating any other patient—namely, the ABCs. Follow the steps in Skill Drill 4:

Skill Drill 4

1. Follow standard precautions. Establish and maintain an open airway. Maintain manual immobilization if necessary. Check the patient's breathing and pulse. Keep suction at hand to clear the mouth and pharynx if the patient should vomit. Comfort, calm, and reassure the patient in the supine position. Never allow the patient to eat or drink anything (Step 1).

2. Control all obvious external bleeding (Step 2).

3. Splint the patient on a backboard. If possible, splint individual extremity fractures during transport (Step 3).

4. Administer supplemental oxygen, assist ventilation as needed and use airway control adjuncts as needed, and continue to monitor the patient's breathing.

5. Keep the patient warm (Step 4).

6. Once you have positioned the patient on the backboard or a stretcher, consider placing the patient in the Trendelenburg position. This technique is easily accomplished by raising the foot of the backboard or stretcher about 6 inches to 12 inches. If the patient is not on a backboard and no lower extremity fractures are suspected, place the patient in the position dictated by local protocol for shock patients. Do not use the Trendelenburg or shock position for patients who have associated chest injury or intra-abdominal injury, which may be aggravated by causing the abdominal contents to push against the diaphragm and further impair breathing.

Skill Drill 4

Managing Hemorrhagic Shock

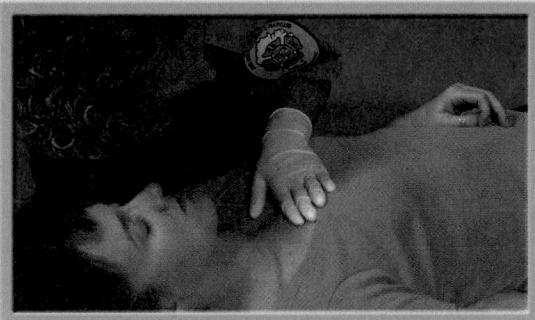

Step 1 Keep the patient supine, open the airway, and check breathing and pulse.

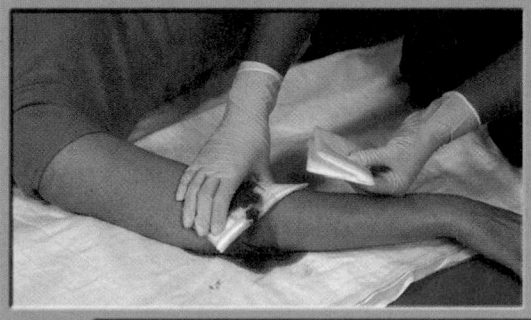

Step 2 Control obvious external bleeding.

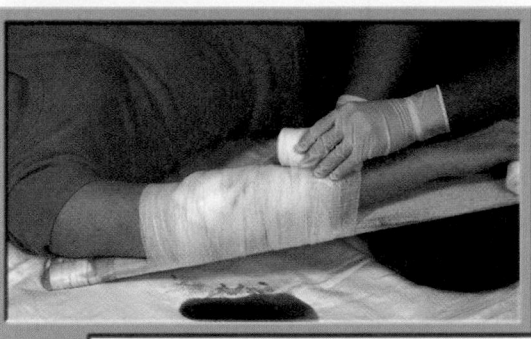

Step 3 Splint the patient on a backboard. Splint any broken bones or joint injuries during transport.

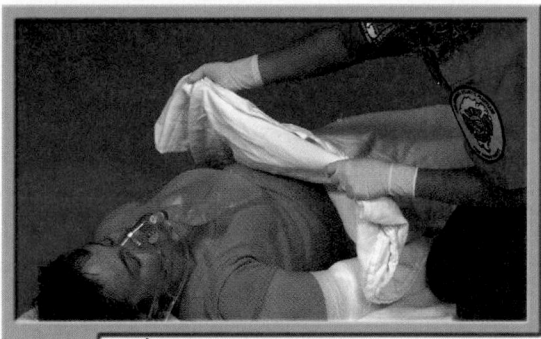

Step 4 Administer high-flow oxygen if you have not already done so, and keep the patient warm.

7. En route to the ED, insert at least one, and preferably two, large-bore peripheral IV lines (14 to 16 gauge), using an over-the-needle catheter. Obtain IV access at the scene only if transport of the patient is delayed.

8. If allowed by protocol, draw blood (two red-top blood collection [Vacutainer] tubes and one purple-top tube) so that hospital personnel may obtain a hematocrit, type- and crossmatch, and other tests immediately on your arrival.

9. Unless local protocol favors a different resuscitation fluid, administer warm isotonic crystalloids of normal saline or lactated Ringer's solution in 250- to 500-mL increments to maintain systolic blood pressure in low normal ranges. Many trauma surgeons prefer lactated Ringer's solution over normal saline because lactated Ringer's may help decrease the acidosis in patients with severe hemorrhagic hypovolemia. However, this belief

remains controversial and either solution will benefit the patient. The use of hypertonic saline, 5 mL/kg of 7.5% sodium chloride, in 250-mL increments may also be effective in treating hemorrhagic shock. Studies have shown that hypertonic solutions may optimize blood pressure, CO, intracranial pressure, and microvascular flow without increasing bleeding or volume overloading patients. However, there has been no change in survival rates compared with standard fluid resuscitation. More research in this area may change the face of fluid therapy, but for now, most disciplines in the United States continue to use isotonic crystalloid therapy. There is some evidence that suggests that titration of blood pressure to 80 to 90 mm Hg systolic is best for hemorrhagic shock. Permitting this low pressure (permissive hypotension) may allow the body to clot better and not dislodge clots already formed.

Blood products should be started early if hemorrhage is suspected. However, blood products will require typing and cross-matching in the emergency department and will take some time to accomplish. The American College of Surgeons recommends starting blood products in class III and IV hemorrhage after an initial 2 L of isotonic solution is administered. Colloids have not shown to be any more benefit than crystalloids in improving patient outcome and, therefore, are not typically recommended. For more information about IV therapy and guidance on IV fluid flow rates, refer to the chapter, *Management and Resuscitation of the Critical Patient.*

Do not give the patient anything by mouth because he or she is likely to vomit. Keep the patient at normal temperature, which usually means covering the patient with a blanket—patients in shock are often unable to conserve body heat effectively and are easily chilled. Monitor the ECG rhythm because any critically ill or injured patient is apt to have dysrhythmias. Also monitor the state of consciousness, pulse, and blood pressure. In a patient with substantial vasoconstriction, the blood pressure sounds may be difficult to hear. If you can feel a pulse over the femoral artery but not over the radial artery, for example, the systolic blood pressure is probably somewhere between 70 and 80 mm Hg. Depending on local protocol, medical control may order sodium bicarbonate to treat acidosis or a vasopressor such as dopamine, metaraminol, or norepinephrine to enhance vasoconstriction.

Words of Wisdom

Remember that a patient's blood pressure may be the last measurable factor to change in shock. The body has several automatic mechanisms to compensate for initial blood loss and to help maintain the blood pressure. Thus, by the time you detect a drop in the blood pressure, shock is well developed. This is particularly true in infants and children, who can maintain their blood pressure until they have lost close to half their blood volume.

YOU *are the Medic*   SUMMARY

1. Is there a possibility of more than one MOI in this scenario?

There can be more than one MOI. The foreman reported that the worker was first struck by a steel beam being lowered into place. Where was the patient struck? What does the path through which he fell look like? Are there outcroppings or other obstacles he may have struck during the fall? What about the failed safety harness? Check to see if there are buckles that may have struck his body when he hit the ground. What is on the ground under or near the injured worker? At this type of scene, like most scenes, you have to play the role of detective in an attempt to reconstruct the incident. Important details, such as being struck by a steel beam or hitting a concrete outcropping or landing on tools are all important in determining the extent of the patient's injuries. Remember that you cannot increase your on-scene time to accomplish this investigation. Multi-task and observe the scene while other tasks are being accomplished.

2. This is a high-rise, commercial construction site. What could some of the potential hazards be for you and your partner?

Most construction sites require anyone on the site to be wearing work boots, a hard hat, a bright reflective vest, and to have specific safety training for that site. Any construction site, especially high-rise commercial sites, have several trades working at the same time. It is important to be sure that all work around the rescue area is stopped and that there is no further risk of falling equipment, moving machines, or other hazards. When you are at a construction site, be sure you are escorted by a supervisor, safety officer, foreman, or another person with the authority to determine whether the scene is safe to enter.

3. The patient is alert, is breathing adequately, and has a rapid but weak radial pulse. His coworker is holding proper manual stabilization of the cervical spine. What is your next priority?

Further assess any life threats. In this case, the patient is maintaining his own airway and does not appear to have any difficulty breathing. Complete your initial primary pulmonary assessment. Some emergency medical personnel like to use the mnemonic: IPASSO. This is to remind you to Inspect, Palpate, Auscultate, Seal, Stabilize, and then apply Oxygen. Next, look for any life-threatening bleeding and bring it under control. Remember, at this point you are identifying and correcting life threats.

4. You and your partner decide that the MOI indicates that this patient has a high risk of serious injury and you want to move quickly. Do you leave the harness and tool belt in place or remove them before completing your assessment?

You should not leave the harness and belt in place. Just as you would do with any trauma patient, you need to inspect the body for any serious injuries. Anything (clothing, harness, tool belt) that gets in the way of a thorough examination needs to be removed. Do not make the mistake of assuming you have

YOU *are the Medic*   SUMMARY, *continued*

corrected all life threats if you have not examined the whole body before you reach the hospital.

5. The patient has unlabored breathing, normal lung sounds, and high concentration oxygen in place. His Spo₂ reading seems adequate. Could he still be suffering from poor perfusion?

Yes. In cases of hypovolemia, a patient's hemoglobin may be saturated with oxygen but because there is so much less hemoglobin, the body's cells cannot be adequately perfused.

6. If you measure his ETCO₂, would you expect it to be high, low, or normal range? What are some factors that affect the measured levels of ETCO₂?

A patient who is hypovolemic may have deceptively low levels of carbon dioxide simply because of poor perfusion and the resultant decrease in metabolism. Decreased lung perfusion can also register as a low carbon dioxide measurement. If he is hyperventilating because of shock, this can also lower his end-tidal carbon dioxide.

7. Despite stopping the flow of heavy bleeding, your patient seems to deteriorate further. What are some of the possible causes of his deteriorating condition?

Although the assessment revealed a large contusion over the flank area, this still may not be the whole picture. The patient fell from a significant height and had heavy tools attached to his belt. This added mass increases the likelihood of injury, especially internal injury due to blunt force trauma of hitting the ground. The MOI in this case dictates a decision for high priority transport, monitoring vital signs, administration of fluids and oxygen, and rapid transfer to a trauma center.

8. At this point, what is your next priority?

Transport! The dropping blood pressure is a late sign of shock. As the blood pressure drops, the body is beginning to fail at its attempts to compensate for the blood loss. Decompensated shock is characterized by dropping blood pressure. This patient needs the definitive emergency treatment available only at a trauma center.

EMS Patient Care Report (PCR)

Date: 10-01-11	Incident No.: 1056	Nature of Call: Man down		Location: 1425 Church Street	
Dispatched: 0930	En Route: 0931	At Scene: 0936	Transport: 0950	At Hospital: 0958	In Service: 1018

Patient Information

Age: 57	Allergies: Denies
Sex: M	Medications: Denies
Weight (in kg [lb]): 90 kg (198 lb)	Past Medical History: High blood pressure, diet controlled
	Chief Complaint: Back and chest pain

Vital Signs

Time: 0941	BP: 108/70	Pulse: 122 weak, regular	Respirations: 20	Spo₂: 97%
Time: 0944	BP: 92/60	Pulse: 132	Respirations: 24	Spo₂: 98%
Time:	BP:	Pulse:	Respirations:	Spo₂:

EMS Treatment
(circle all that apply)

Oxygen @ __15__ L/min via (circle one): NC (NRM) Bag-mask device	Assisted Ventilation	Airway Adjunct	CPR
Defibrillation	(Bleeding Control) (Bandaging)	Splinting	(Other:) Spinal immobilization

Narrative

9-1-1 dispatch for a man down at a construction site with possible serious injuries. Upon arrival, pt, a 57-year-old male supine and alert on the ground. Witnesses report seeing pt fall from scaffold approximately 15 feet from the ground. Ground is hard packed dirt with rocks; pt fall encumbered by tools and tool belt as well as safety harness with large metal buckles. Both still on pt upon arrival. Pt answers all questions appropriately and witnesses deny seeing any loss of consciousness, reporting that pt hardhat stayed on during fall and then bounced off after impact. Coworker/EMT maintained manual cervical spine stabilization within seconds of fall. Pt airway open and clear with no apparent respiratory distress. Trachea midline. Lungs equal and clear with no evidence of limited chest excursion. Radial pulses both palpable but very weak and rapid. Skin pale, cool, and moist.

YOU *are the Medic*   **SUMMARY,** *continued*

High-concentration oxygen administered via nonrebreathing mask. Significant blood flow from a deep laceration in the right flank controlled during primary assessment. Pt apparently landed on tools (hammer, pry bar, large wrench) upon impact. No other external bleeding noted, although subsequent assessment reveals large area of discoloration over right flank, right buttocks, and right forearm. Pt denies any head pain and remained alert and oriented throughout treatment and transport. No visible discoloration, skin breaks, or deformities noted on scalp, face, anterior/posterior neck. Chest movement normal with some complaint of discomfort (pain 5/10) upon palpation of ribs on both sides upon inspiration. No crepitus noted. Abdomen is soft, nontender. Pelvis is painful to palpation and pt complains of weakness in both legs. No incontinence or priapism noted. Pt denies any pain in legs; palpation reveals no deformities or skin breaks. Pt unable to push feet against hands due to stated weakness and pain in pelvic area. Distal (dorsalis pedis) pulses palpated (very weak) with equal strength, capillary nail bed refill slightly more than 2 seconds in both feet.

Pt has large (approx 15-cm) laceration to right flank with bleeding controlled. Some discoloration noted over right buttocks where tools rested as well as across lower back where harness buckle contacted skin upon impact. Large discoloration and abrasions noted on both forearms where patient states that he tried to grab building while falling. Full range of motion noted in both arms with equal but weak radial pulses. Capillary nail bed refill of both hands slightly greater than 2 seconds.

Pt was examined, bleeding controlled with direct pressure and bandaging. Cervical spine immobilization on backboard performed due to MOI and suspected pelvic fracture. High-concentration oxygen maintained throughout transport. 2 large-bore (14-gauge) IV lines started (left and right antecubital) for 2 L of normal saline en route. Upon arrival at hospital, approximately 500 mL of normal saline infused through each IV line. Spo$_2$ monitored and vital signs measured every 5 minutes throughout transport. Pt remained alert and oriented and stated that he was feeling a little bit better upon arrival at emergency department. Hospital ED notified of trauma pt en route. Return to service at 1018 hours. **End of report**

Prep Kit

- The cardiovascular and respiratory systems have distinct roles in keeping blood flowing between the lungs and peripheral tissues.
- Perfusion is the circulation of blood within an organ or tissue in adequate amounts to meet the cells' current needs for oxygen, nutrients, and waste removal.
- Hemorrhage simply means bleeding. Bleeding can range from a "nick" to a capillary while shaving, to a severely spurting artery from a deep slash with a knife, to a ruptured spleen from striking the steering column during a car crash.
- External hemorrhage can usually be easily controlled by using direct pressure or a pressure bandage. For extremities, if these methods are not sufficient, use a tourniquet.
- Internal hemorrhage is often not controlled until a surgeon locates the source and sutures it closed.
- Hemorrhagic shock is the most common cause of shock.
- Hypovolemic shock caused by hemorrhagic trauma has been classified by the American College of Surgeons Committee on Trauma into four classes, each with its own specific characteristics and treatments.
- Shock occurs in three successive phases—compensated shock (classes I and II), decompensated shock (class III), and irreversible shock (class IV).
- Hypoperfusion (shock) occurs when the level of tissue perfusion decreases below normal.
- Early decreased tissue perfusion may result in subtle changes, such as aberrant mental status, long before a patient's vital signs (that is, blood pressure, pulse rate, respiratory rate) appear abnormal.
- As with any patient, airway and ventilatory support take top priority when treating a patient with suspected shock.
- Stabilizing a serious fracture has a high priority in the control of bleeding. Splinting the fracture helps control bleeding, and splinting should occur before other bleeding control.
- Methods for controlling external hemorrhage include direct, even pressure; pressure dressings and/or splints; and tourniquets. Most cases of external hemorrhage can be controlled with direct pressure to the bleeding site.
- If direct pressure fails to immediately stop the hemorrhaging of an extremity, apply a tourniquet above the level of the bleeding. If a commercial tourniquet is not available, a tourniquet can be improvised with a triangular bandage and a stick or rod.
- If bleeding is present at the nose and a skull fracture is suspected, place a gauze pad loosely under the nose.
- Management of a patient with internal hemorrhaging focuses on the treatment of shock, minimizing movement of the injured or bleeding part or region, and rapid transport.
- Patients who have suspected shock, whether compensated or decompensated, can benefit from early surgical intervention and should be transported to a facility with those capabilities.
- Be alert, and search for early signs of shock.

Prep Kit, continued

Vital Vocabulary

afterload The pressure in the aorta against which the left ventricle must pump blood; increasing this can decrease cardiac output.

blood The fluid tissue that is pumped by the heart through the arteries, veins, and capillaries and consists of plasma and formed elements or cells, such as red blood cells, white blood cells, and platelets.

cardiac output (CO) Amount of blood pumped by the heart per minute. Calculated by multiplying the stroke volume by the heart rate per minute.

compensated shock (classes I and II) The early stage of shock, in which the body can still compensate for blood loss. The systolic blood pressure and brain perfusion are maintained.

decompensated shock (class III) The late stage of shock, when blood pressure is falling.

ejection fraction (EF) The percentage of blood that leaves the heart each time it contracts.

erythrocytes Red blood cells.

hematemesis Vomited blood.

hematochezia Passage of stools containing bright red blood.

hematocrit A blood test that measures the portion of red blood cells in whole blood.

hematoma A mass of blood in the soft tissues beneath the skin; indicates bleeding into soft tissues and may be the result of a minor or a severe injury.

hematuria Blood in the urine.

hemoglobin The oxygen-carrying pigment in red blood cells.

hemophilia Lacking one or more of the blood's clotting factors.

hemoptysis Coughed-up blood.

hemorrhage Bleeding.

hemorrhagic shock Volume lost as blood.

hemostasis Stopping hemorrhage.

hypoperfusion A condition that occurs when the level of tissue perfusion decreases below that needed to maintain normal cellular functions.

hypovolemic shock A condition that occurs when the circulating blood volume is inadequate to deliver adequate oxygen and nutrients to the body.

irreversible shock (class IV) The final stage of shock, prior to death.

leukocytes White blood cells.

melena Passage of dark, tarry stools.

perfusion The delivery of oxygen and nutrients to the cells, organs, and tissues of the body.

plasma The fluid portion of the blood from which the cells have been removed.

platelets Small cells in the blood that are essential for clot formation.

preload The precontraction pressure in the heart as the volume of blood builds up.

shock An abnormal state associated with inadequate oxygen and nutrient delivery to the metabolic apparatus of the cell.

stroke volume (SV) The amount of blood that the left ventricle ejects into the aorta per contraction.

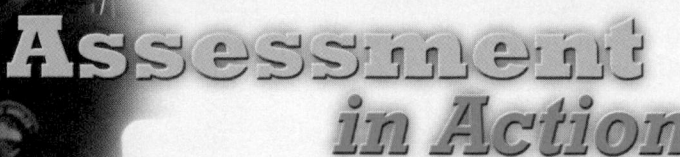

Assessment in Action

You and your partner arrive at the scene of a motorcyclist down. You assess the scene to be safe and, wearing appropriate PPE, you walk toward the police officers waving you over. You walk past a large motorcycle on its side. The front wheel is twisted, pieces of red plastic and chrome are scattered on the surrounding pavement, and a white helmet is nearby. About 30 ft away a man is lying on his back, not moving. A bystander who is kneeling by the man says that the man's name is Jim and he thinks his leg is broken.

A backup crew has just arrived and you instruct one of the crew members to maintain stabilization of the cervical spine. The other crew member administers 15 L/min of oxygen via a nonrebreathing mask.

Your patient looks at you as you call to him. He tells you his name, the day, and what happened. His airway is open and he is maintaining it on his own. No blood or other foreign matter is in his mouth. His radial pulse is barely palpable at 130 beats/min. His skin is pale and cool. Blood is oozing steadily from a tear in the right lower leg of his jeans. As you cut the jeans, you see bone protruding from the anterior lower leg. Bleeding is controlled with direct pressure. His right thigh is swollen and deformed. His right foot is twisted in an unnatural angle and he tells you that he cannot feel his foot. While one of the EMTs brings the backboard and stretcher, you perform a secondary assessment. During this assessment you notice that the radial pulses are no longer palpable. The patient is asking if he can get up and find his bike.

1. The EMTs assist you in packaging the patient for transport. To immobilize the patient's right leg, you should:
   A. apply two splints and attach them to the backboard.
   B. manually support the limb.
   C. use a traction splint.
   D. do nothing except strap the leg to the backboard and provide rapid transport.

2. Baroreceptors in the aortic arch and carotid sinus detect a change in pressure as the patient's blood pressure drops. This would most likely result in:
   A. inhibition of the vasomotor center and antidiuretic hormone release.
   B. stimulation of the vasomotor center and antidiuretic hormone release.
   C. inhibition of the vasomotor center and antidiuretic hormone inhibition.
   D. stimulation of the vasomotor center and antidiuretic hormone inhibition.

3. Initially, your primary assessment of the patient included a finding of rapid but weak peripheral pulses. In this scenario, this is most likely an indication of:
   A. injuries to the arms.
   B. decompensated shock.
   C. compensated shock.
   D. irreversible shock.

4. During your secondary assessment, you once again checked the radial pulses and found them to be absent. In this scenario, you should strongly suspect:
   A. compensated shock.
   B. decompensated shock.

C. irreversible shock.
D. injuries to the arms.

5. During your reassessment of the patient, the best early indicator of a significant change in tissue perfusion is:
   A. a decrease in the blood pressure.
   B. a rise in the pulse rate.
   C. a sudden change in mental status.
   D. the amount of visible blood loss from the leg.

6. As the patient's condition deteriorates, you are quickly packaging him for transport to a trauma center. You should attempt to start at least one, preferably two, large-bore IV lines for rapid infusion of normal saline. This action should be taken:
   A. immediately.
   B. en route.
   C. on arrival at the emergency department.
   D. in the emergency department only.

7. The patient is approximately 150 pounds. He lost 1 L of blood from his femur fracture and another 500 mL from his open tibial fracture. In addition, you suspect that he has other injuries that may be causing blood loss. When fluids are infused, an attempt should be made to:
   A. infuse as much fluid as possible over the shortest time possible.
   B. infuse enough fluid to bring the blood pressure back to normal for that patient.
   C. infuse enough fluid to maintain the systolic pressure at about 80 mm Hg.
   D. infuse enough fluid to maintain the diastolic pressure at about 80 mm Hg.

Soft-Tissue Trauma

National EMS Education Standard Competencies

Trauma

Integrates assessment findings with principles of epidemiology and pathophysiology to formulate a field impression to implement a comprehensive treatment/disposition plan for an acutely injured patient.

Soft-Tissue Trauma

Recognition and management of

- Wounds (pp 1547-1549, pp 1554-1567)
- Burns (see chapter, *Burns*)
  - Electrical (see chapter, *Burns*)
  - Chemical (see chapter, *Burns*)
  - Thermal (see chapter, *Burns*)
- Chemicals in the eye and on the skin (see chapters, *Diseases of the Eyes, Ears, Nose, and Throat* and *Burns*)

Pathophysiology, assessment, and management of

- Wounds
  - Avulsions (p 1562)
  - Bite wounds (pp 1563-1564)
  - Lacerations (p 1560)
  - Puncture wounds (pp 1560-1562)
  - Incisions (p 1560)
- Burns
  - Electrical (see chapter, *Burns*)
  - Chemical (see chapter, *Burns*)
  - Thermal (see chapter, *Burns*)
  - Radiation (see chapter, *Burns*)
- High-pressure injection (pp 1566-1567)
- Crush syndrome (pp 1565-1566)

Knowledge Objectives

1. Discuss the anatomy and physiology of the skin, including the layers of the skin. (pp 1545-1547)
2. Understand the functions of the skin, and its role in the inflammatory process. (pp 1545-1547)
3. Discuss the pathophysiology of soft-tissue injuries, including closed injuries, open injuries, and crush injuries. (pp 1547-1549)
4. Discuss the process of wound healing, including hemostasis, inflammation, epithelialization, neovascularization, and collagen synthesis. (pp 1549-1550)
5. Explain skin tension lines and how they relate to wound healing. (p 1547)
6. Discuss alterations in the wound healing process, including anatomic reasons, high-risk wounds, abnormal scar formation, pressure injuries, and wounds requiring closure. (pp 1549-1550)

7. Discuss the pathophysiology of wound healing, including infection, gangrene, tetanus, and necrotizing fasciitis. (pp 1550-1551)
8. Describe the assessment process for patients with a soft-tissue injury, with a focus on when to perform a physical exam. (pp 1551-1554)
9. Describe the relationship between airway management and the patient with closed and open injuries. (p 1552)
10. Discuss emergency medical care of a patient with a soft-tissue injury. (pp 1554-1560)
11. Discuss the principles for treating a closed wound. (p 1554)
12. Discuss the principles for treating an open wound. (p 1554)
13. List the steps in controlling external bleeding. (pp 1556-1558)
14. List the steps for applying a tourniquet. (pp 1557-1558)
15. Understand the functions and types of sterile dressings and bandages. (pp 1558-1560)
16. Discuss methods and materials for site-specific dressings. (pp 1554-1555)
17. Describe complications of improperly applied dressings. (pp 1555-1556)
18. Discuss the role of pain control when managing patients with soft-tissue injuries. (p 1558)
19. Discuss the pathophysiology, assessment, management of abrasions, lacerations, puncture wounds, impaled objects, avulsions, amputations, animal and human bites, crush syndrome, compartment syndrome, and high-pressure injection. (pp 1560-1567)

Skills Objectives

1. Demonstrate the assessment and management of a patient with signs and symptoms of soft-tissue injury, including:
   a. Contusion (p 1554)
   b. Hematoma (p 1554)
   c. Abrasion (p 1560)
   d. Laceration (p 1560)
   e. Puncture wound (pp 1560-1562)
   f. Impaled object (pp 1560-1562)
   g. Avulsion (p 1562)
   h. Amputation (pp 1562-1563)
   i. Animal and human bites (pp 1563-1564)
   j. Crush syndrome (pp 1565-1566)
   k. Compartment syndrome (p 1566)
   l. Blast injuries (p 1549 and see chapter, *Trauma Systems and Mechanism of Injury*)
   m. High-pressure injection injuries (pp 1566-1567)
2. Describe the method for controlling bleeding from a soft-tissue injury. (pp 1556-1558)
3. Describe the method for applying a tourniquet. (pp 1557-1558)

Introduction

The skin is the largest organ of the human body and serves as the interface between the body and outside world. For that reason, injuries involving the skin are common. Injuries to the skin are often the most immediately obvious of a person's injuries, although not necessarily the most serious. Do not be distracted by dramatic external wounds and neglect to check for higher-priority problems, such as an obstructed airway or significant hypotension. You can avoid making this critical mistake by ensuring that you have a thorough understanding of the anatomy and physiology of the skin.

A wound is any injury to the soft tissues—that is, an injury to the skin with or without involvement of the subcutaneous tissues and muscle. Most soft-tissue wounds are relatively low-priority injuries. Although they may be the most obvious and dramatic injuries, they are seldom the most serious of the patient's problems unless they compromise the airway or are associated with massive bleeding. You should always search systematically and thoroughly for other injuries or life-threatening conditions before tending to soft-tissue trauma. *Do not let dramatic soft-tissue injuries distract you from conducting a thorough primary assessment!*

Incidence, Mortality, and Morbidity

The soft tissues of the body can be injured through a variety of mechanisms. A blunt injury occurs when the energy exchange between the patient and an object is more than the tissues can tolerate, as can happen in an automobile crash that leads to the person striking the steering wheel. A penetrating injury occurs when an object, such as a bullet or knife, breaks through the skin and enters the body, creating an entrance wound and possibly an exit wound. Burns (discussed in the chapter, *Burns*) may also result in soft-tissue injuries.

Soft-tissue trauma is the leading form of injury. Open wounds account for approximately 6.5 million emergency department (ED) visits, and nearly 5 million patients present with contusions. In fact, wound care is one of the most frequently performed procedures in EDs across the United States. Most of these injuries require basic interventions such as wound irrigation, dressing, bandaging, and limited suturing.

Death due to soft-tissue injury is extremely rare. When it occurs, it is typically related to either hemorrhage or infection. Uncontrolled hemorrhage can quickly lead to shock and death. When the skin barrier is breached, invading pathogens—bacteria, fungi, and viruses—can cause local or systemic infection. Infection can be life or limb threatening, especially in people with diabetes. Preventing soft-tissue injuries and their associated complications involves simple protective actions. The use of gloves when working with abrasive materials, for example, can prevent skin injuries. Workplace safety measures to reduce injury include use of safety devices to prevent interaction between machine parts and body parts. Teaching children to avoid using sharp objects also helps prevent injury. Plastic scissors, plastic knives, and plastic drinking cups are all designed in part to reduce the risk of cuts and other skin injuries among children.

Structure and Function of the Skin

The human skin is much more than a wrapping. Rather, skin, or <u>integument</u>, is a complex organ with a crucial role in maintaining the constancy of the internal environment (<u>homeostasis</u>):

- The skin protects the underlying tissue from injury, including that caused by extremes of temperature, ultraviolet radiation, mechanical forces, toxic chemicals, and invading microorganisms.
- The skin aids in temperature regulation, preventing heat loss when the core body temperature starts to fall and facilitating heat loss when core temperature rises.

YOU *are the Medic* **PART 1**

You and your partner are dispatched to a call for a man under a car. You arrive at the address and see a woman waving frantically from the driveway. "I was out shopping. My husband was working on the car—it fell. He's under there. I don't know how badly he's hurt." She runs toward the garage where a man is lying on the ground. Only his head, torso, groin, and arms are visible. He is pale and appears very anxious.

He says, "I—I didn't have my cell phone. I've been yelling—for hours. Nobody—around. I can't—feel my feet."

Police are with you and several neighbors are now running over to the scene. You hear someone shouting, "We can lift the car off him!"

1. As the crowd rushes over, you and your partner begin assessing the scene. After you ascertain that the car is stable and that no other risks are a threat to you and your partner, what other scene precautions must be taken?

2. After you ensure the scene is safe, what are your next actions?

- As a watertight seal, the skin prevents excessive loss of water from the body and drying of tissues, thereby helping maintain the chemical stability of the internal environment.
- The skin serves as a sense organ, keeping the brain informed about the external environment. Changes in temperature, touch, and body position and sensations of pain are mediated through the sense receptors in the skin.

Significant damage to the skin may make the body vulnerable to bacterial invasion, temperature instability, and major disturbances of fluid balance—precisely what happens when an injury results in an opening in the skin.

Epidermis

The skin is composed of two layers: the epidermis and the dermis Figure 1 . The epidermis, or outermost layer, is the body's first line of defense, the principal barrier against water, dust, microorganisms, and mechanical stress. It consists of five layers: an outermost layer (stratum corneum) of hardened, nonliving cells, which are continuously shed through a process called desquamation; and four inner layers of living cells that constantly divide to give rise to the cells of the stratum corneum.

The deeper layers of the epidermis also contain variable numbers of cells bearing melanin granules; these cells are known as melanocytes. The darkness of a person's skin is directly proportional to the amount of melanin present.

Dermis

Underlying the epidermis is a tough, highly elastic layer of connective tissues called the dermis. This complex material is composed chiefly of collagen fibers, elastic fibers, and a mucopolysaccharide gel. Numerous fibroblasts—cells that secrete collagen, elastin, and ground substance—are found within the dermis as well. Collagen, a fibrous protein with a high tensile strength, gives the skin high resistance to breakage under mechanical stress. Elastin, as the name implies, imparts elasticity to the skin, allowing the skin to spring back to its usual contours. Ground substance, which is found in connective tissues in differing amounts, is a transparent mucopolysaccharide gel that gives the skin resistance to compression.

The dermis is subdivided into the papillary dermis and a reticular layer. The vasculature inside the papillary dermis serves two functions: It provides nutrients to the epidermis, and it aids in thermoregulation. Dilation of these vessels increases blood flow to the skin, allowing heat to dissipate. Conversely, blood vessel constriction results in retention of heat. The reticular layer is made of dense, irregular connective tissue, which provides strength and elasticity.

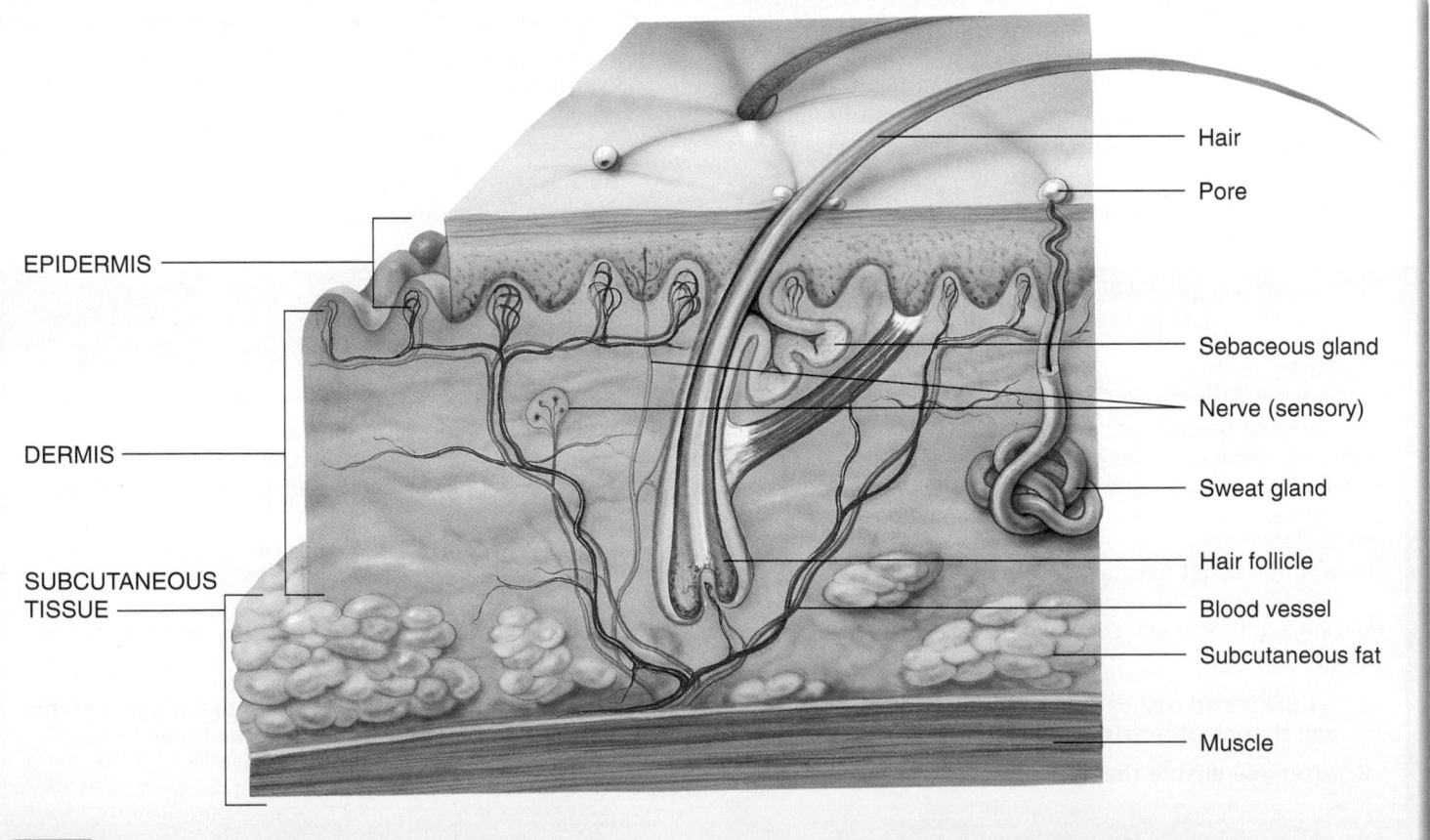

EPIDERMIS

DERMIS

SUBCUTANEOUS TISSUE

Hair

Pore

Sebaceous gland

Nerve (sensory)

Sweat gland

Hair follicle

Blood vessel

Subcutaneous fat

Muscle

Figure 1 The skin is composed of a tough external layer called the epidermis and a vascular inner layer called the dermis.

Macrophages and lymphocytes are also found within the dermal layer. Both are part of the inflammatory process and are responsible for combating microorganisms that breach the epidermal layer. Once a pathogen enters the dermis, macrophages and lymphocytes destroy the invading microorganism and signal other cells to migrate into the area. Physical injury will trigger mast cells to degranulate and synthesize special chemical mediators. The result is increased blood flow to the affected area, manifested as redness and warmth.

Several specialized structures can be identified in the dermis:

- Nerve endings—mediate the senses of touch, temperature, pressure, and pain.
- Blood vessels—carry oxygen and nutrients to the skin and remove carbon dioxide and metabolic waste products.

    Cutaneous blood vessels also have a crucial role in regulating body temperature by regulating the volume of blood that flows from the body's warm core to its cooler surface.
- Sweat glands—produce sweat and discharge it through ducts passing to the surface of the skin. Sweat consists of water and salts, and sweating is regulated through the action of the sympathetic nervous system. The average volume of sweat lost during 24 hours under normal conditions ranges from 500 to 1,000 mL; during strenuous exercise, however, sweat glands may secrete as much as 1,000 mL in an hour. This evaporation of water from the skin surface is one of the body's major mechanisms for shedding excess heat.
- Hair follicles—produce hair and enclose the hair roots. Each follicle contains a single hair. Attached to the hair follicle is a small muscle that, on contraction, causes the follicle to assume a more vertical position. Hairs in each part of the body have definite periods of growth, after which they are shed and replaced; scalp hair, for example, has a life span of 2 to 5 years and grows 1.5 to 3.9 mm per week.
- Sebaceous gland—located at the neck of each hair follicle, is a specialized secretory mechanism that produces an oily substance called sebum. The secretions of the sebaceous glands empty into the hair follicles and from there reach the surface of the skin. The precise function of sebum is not well understood, although it may keep the skin supple so that it does not crack.

Subcutaneous Tissue

The layer of tissue beneath the dermis—that is, the subcutaneous layer (superficial fascia)—consists mainly of adipose tissue (fat). Blood vessels, lymph vessels, and hair follicle roots are also found in this layer. Subcutaneous fat insulates the underlying tissues from extremes of heat and cold. It also provides a cushion for underlying structures and an energy reserve for the body.

Deep Fascia

Below the subcutaneous tissue is a thick, dense layer of fibrous tissue known as the deep fascia. The deep fascia is composed of tough bands of tissue that ensheath muscles and other internal structures. It supports and protects underlying structures from injury. Muscles and bones are found below this layer.

Skin Tension Lines

The skin is arranged over the body structures in a manner that provides tension. This tautness varies by body region but occurs in patterns known as tension lines. Static tension develops over areas that have limited movement, such as the scalp. Lacerations occurring parallel to the skin tension lines may remain closed with little or no intervention. Larger wounds may be pulled open by the normal tension and require closure with sutures, staples, or a biodegradable "glue." Even small lacerations that lie perpendicular to the tension lines result in a wound that remains open. Healing occurs more slowly in an open wound, and abnormal scar formation is more likely.

Dynamic tension is found in areas that lie over muscle. The tension varies according to the contraction of the underlying muscle and subsequent movement of the skin. Open injuries to dynamic tension lines interfere with healing because they disrupt the clotting process and the tissue repair cycle, resulting in slowed healing and a tendency toward abnormal scar formation.

An abnormal scar may prompt the patient to seek scar revision—surgery to improve its appearance. The surgeon takes skin tension into account when determining the best procedure for revision. This factor must also be considered when wound débridement is necessary or when hospital personnel must remove an impaled object.

General Pathophysiology: Closed Versus Open Wounds

Closed Wounds

In a closed wound, soft tissues beneath the skin surface are damaged, but there is no break in the epidermis. A patient with a closed wound can have underlying trauma to organs and other important structures beneath the skin. You should always consider underlying injury when a patient has a closed wound.

The characteristic closed wound is a contusion **Figure 2**. In a contusion (bruise), the skin is intact, but damage has occurred beneath the epidermis. Trauma to the nerve endings produces pain, and leakage of fluid into spaces between the damaged cells produces swelling (edema). If small blood vessels in the dermis are disrupted, a black-and-blue mark (ecchymosis) will cover the injured area; if large blood vessels are torn beneath the contused area, a hematoma—a collection of blood beneath the skin—will be evident as a lump with a bluish discoloration **Figure 3**.

Open Wounds

An open wound is characterized by a disruption in the skin. Types of open wounds include abrasions, lacerations, avulsions, amputations, bites, impaled objects, blast injuries, high-pressure injection injuries, and puncture wounds. Open wounds are potentially much more serious than closed wounds for two

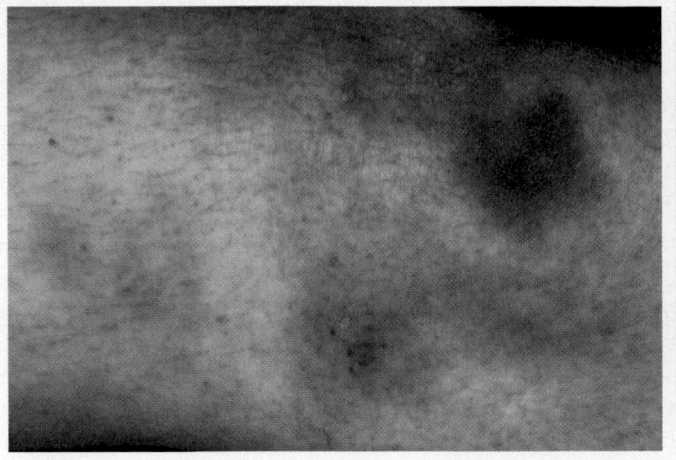

Figure 2 A contusion, or bruise, produces characteristic black-and-blue discoloration (ecchymosis).

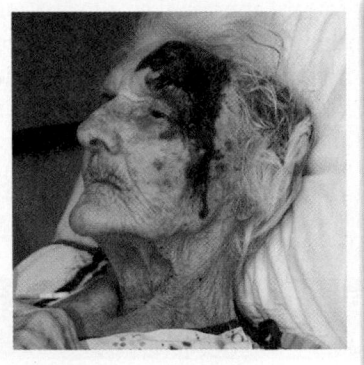

Figure 3 A hematoma.

reasons. First, they are vulnerable to infection. An open wound is contaminated—that is, microorganisms enter it. Whether the contamination produces infection depends in large measure on how the wound is managed. Second, open wounds have a greater potential for serious blood loss. When the skin is unbroken, bleeding from a disrupted blood vessel is limited. Although a significant volume of blood—up to about two units—can be lost into the soft tissues of the leg, eventually the increasing pressure within the leg will prevent further bleeding. In an open wound, the patient's entire blood volume may be lost.

Certain wounds should always be evaluated by a physician. The injuries in Table 1 require transport, even if they appear minor.

Table 1 Conditions That Require Transport

- Compromise of:
  - Nerves
  - Vessels
  - Muscles
  - Tendons or ligaments
- Foreign body or cosmetic complications
- Heavy contamination

Crush Injuries

When a body part is crushed between two solid objects, a **crush injury** may occur to the underlying soft tissues and bones Figure 4 . Such injuries range from a simple finger injury to a life-threatening entrapment of the torso. The latter is likely to be encountered in cases involving structural collapse (such as in collapse of masonry or steel structures, earthquakes, tornadoes, construction accidents, mudslides, motor vehicle crashes, warfare injuries, and industrial accidents). **Compartment syndrome**, discussed later in this chapter, can occur when an unresponsive patient has an upper extremity pinned between the body and the floor. Likewise, compartment syndrome may develop if a pneumatic antishock garment (PASG) is used and is left in place for an excessive period (can vary, but thought to be greater than 2 hours), or a cast or splint is applied too tightly.

The forces involved in a crush injury may be great enough to rupture internal organs. You must rapidly assess the mechanism of injury (MOI) and determine the likelihood for massive internal trauma. Also, note that the longer an injured area remains compressed, the greater the chance for systemic complications.

In a crush injury, the external appearance may not adequately represent the level of internal damage. An upper extremity that merely appears swollen may, in fact, have enough muscle destruction to cause systemic problems, especially if the extremity has been trapped for longer than 4 hours, which is enough time to develop crush syndrome. In other cases, the injured region may be mangled beyond recognition. Remember that grotesque injuries may not necessarily be the primary problem. Always concentrate on threats to life before addressing injured extremities, no matter how bad the initial appearance.

One of the body's first responses to a vessel injury is localized vasoconstriction that reduces the flow of blood. When vessels are crushed and torn, they often lose the ability to constrict, resulting in a free flow of blood from any unnatural opening. Crush injuries tend to result in hemorrhage that cannot easily be controlled by standard methods. Inability to precisely locate bleeding or massive extremity trauma may also lead to difficulty in controlling hemorrhage.

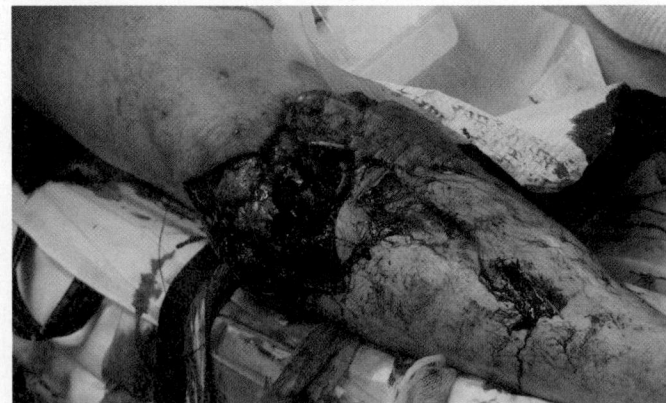

Figure 4 A crush injury is characterized by extensive tissue damage and deformity that is often accompanied by swelling and extreme pain.

Blast Injury

Recall that an explosion is an MOI that can result in many types of injuries, including soft-tissue trauma, abdominal trauma, skeletal trauma, and blast lung, among others. Blast injuries as an MOI are covered in detail in the chapter, *Trauma Systems and Mechanism of Injury*. Always remember to assess the scene for hazards to yourself and your EMS crew, and do not enter the scene until safety can be ensured.

Wound Healing

The Process of Wound Healing

Healing of wounds is a natural process that involves several overlapping stages, all directed toward the larger goal of maintaining homeostasis. Ultimately, the goal is for the body to return to a functional state, although the injured area may not always be restored to the preinjury condition.

Hemostasis

Among the primary concerns in wound healing is the cessation of bleeding. Loss of blood, internal or external, hinders the provision of vital nutrients and oxygen to the affected area. It also impairs the tissue's ability to eliminate wastes. The end result is abnormal or absent function, which interferes with homeostasis. To stop the flow of blood, the vessels, platelets, and clotting cascade must work in unison.

Injury to soft tissue causes chemicals in the vessel wall to be released. These chemicals constrict the blood vessels, resulting in less space through which blood can flow. The muscular layer in the arteries, arterioles, and some veins constricts to reduce the size of the lumen. Skeletal muscles also have a role in the constriction process. Because capillaries lack smooth muscle, bleeding continues, albeit at a slower rate.

Platelets are also activated by the release of these chemicals. Activated platelets adhere to the affected area and to other platelets. This aggregation of platelets forms a platelet plug. Although not the permanent repair, the plug temporarily stops the blood loss and is the beginning of blood clot formation.

Inflammation

In inflammation (the next stage of wound healing), additional cells move into the damaged area to begin repair. White blood cells migrate to the area to combat pathogens that have invaded exposed tissue. Chemicals and proteins known as <u>chemotactic factors</u> are released and signal repairing cells to migrate to the area of injury. <u>Granulocytes</u> and macrophages, among the first restoration cells to arrive, engulf bacteria through phagocytosis, which involves ingestion of damaged cellular parts. Foreign products and bacteria can also be removed from the body by phagocytosis. Similarly, lymphocytes (a type of white blood cell) destroy bacteria and other pathogens.

Mast cells release histamine as part of the body's response in the early stages of inflammation. Histamine causes dilation of blood vessels, increasing blood flow to the injured area and resulting in a reddened, warm area immediately around the site.

Histamine makes capillaries more permeable, and swelling may occur as fluid seeps out of these "leaky" capillaries.

Inflammation ultimately leads to the removal of foreign material, damaged cellular parts, and invading microorganisms from the wound site. Reconstruction of the injured region through epithelialization, neovascularization, and collagen synthesis can then begin.

Epithelialization

In the outer layer of skin, epithelial cells are stacked in layers. To replace the area damaged in a soft-tissue injury, a new layer of epithelial cells must be moved into this region—a process known as <u>epithelialization</u>. Cells from the stratum germinativum quickly multiply and redevelop across the edges of the wound. Except in cases of clean incisions, the appearance of the restructured area seldom returns to the preinjury state. For example, large wounds or injuries that result in significant disruption of the skin will often have incomplete epithelialization. In persons with lightly pigmented skin, a pink line of scar tissue may signal the presence of collagen, a structural protein that has reinforced the damaged tissue. Despite the changed appearance, the function of the area may be restored to near normal.

Neovascularization

In <u>neovascularization</u>, new blood vessels form as the body attempts to bring oxygen and nutrients to the injured tissue. New capillaries bud from intact capillaries that lie adjacent to the damaged skin. These vessels provide a conduit for oxygen and nutrients and serve as a pathway for waste removal. Because they are new and delicate, bleeding might result from a minor injury. It may take weeks to months for the new capillaries to be as stable as preexisting vessels.

Collagen Synthesis

Collagen is a tough, fibrous protein found in scar tissue, hair, bones, and connective tissue. This vital structural repair unit is synthesized by fibroblasts, repair cells that migrate into damaged tissue. In wound healing, collagen provides stability to the damaged tissue and joins wound borders, thereby closing the open tissue. Unfortunately, collagen cannot restore the damaged tissue to its original strength.

Alterations of Wound Healing

Wound healing does not always follow the pattern described previously. Infection or an abnormal scar may develop, excessive bleeding may occur, or healing may be slow. This section discusses altered wound healing and potential complications.

Anatomic Factors

Areas of the body subjected to repeated motion throughout the day, such as the fingers, tend to heal slowly. One strategy used to speed healing in such cases is to splint the affected part, preventing movement. The arrangement of an open wound in relation to skin tension lines also affects how the wound will heal and determines whether an abnormal scar will form.

Some medications can delay healing—namely, corticosteroids, nonsteroidal anti-inflammatory drugs, penicillin, colchicine, anticoagulants, and antineoplastic agents. Likewise, a variety of medical conditions may interfere with normal healing—advanced age, severe alcoholism, acute uremia, diabetes, hypoxia, severe anemia, peripheral vascular disease, malnutrition, advanced cancer, hepatic failure, and cardiovascular disease.

High-Risk Wounds

Wounds that carry a high risk for developing infection include human and animal bites. Because the mouth is warm and constantly moist, it offers a hospitable environment for growth of bacteria. Injection of human saliva into tissue can result in significant infection. In particular, rabies is a serious infection that can develop from the bite of an infected animal (such as wild raccoons, dogs, and cats).

Cases in which a foreign body or organic matter is embedded in an open wound are considered high-risk injuries because of the likelihood that the material involved is impregnated with microorganisms. Once the material breaches the skin barrier, the pathogen has easy entry into the rest of the body. A foreign body that remains in place on evaluation should be left in place because a lacerated blood vessel may not be bleeding freely because of the foreign body's position. *Do not remove an impaled object in the field unless it interferes with the patient's airway*.

Other high-risk wounds include injection wounds, wounds with significant devitalized tissue, crush wounds, wounds in immunocompromised patients, and injuries to patients with poor peripheral circulation.

Abnormal Scar Formation

Excessive collagen formation can occur if the healing process is not balanced between the building up and breaking down phases of healing. A hypertrophic or keloid scar may develop from the excess protein. **Hypertrophic scar** formation occurs in areas subject to high tissue stress, such as the elbow and knee. Such a scar does not extend past the borders of the wound margins and tends to form in people with lightly pigmented skin. In contrast, a **keloid scar** typically develops in people with darkly pigmented skin. It grows over the wound margins and can become larger than the wound area. Keloid scars tend to form on the ears, upper extremities, lower abdomen, and sternum.

Pressure Injuries

Pressure injuries may occur when a patient is bedridden or when pressure is applied for a prolonged period in an unresponsive patient or a patient immobilized on a backboard. The involved tissues are deprived of oxygen, which leads to localized hypoxia and cell deterioration. Prevention involves determining the risk and providing a mechanism to reduce or release the pressure on the skin.

Wounds Requiring Closure

Many open wounds heal without medical intervention, but some require closure with sutures, staples, or medical glue (octyl-2-cyanoacrylate). Closure involves bringing the wound edges together to allow for optimal healing. Open injuries that require closure include those that affect cosmetic areas, such as the lips, face, or eyebrows. Such injuries should be considered for closure because scarring often has psychological implications. Gaping wounds and those occurring over tension lines also require closure. **Degloving** injuries require substantial irrigation and débridement before closing. Closure is also indicated for ring injuries and skin tears.

Open injuries should be closed within 24 hours in most cases, although the scientific evidence to support that recommendation is minimal. Initial hospital management for open wounds involves assessment for foreign material followed by irrigation. The physician can then determine appropriate wound closing options.

Three types of wound closure are performed: primary closure, secondary intention, and delayed primary closure. In primary closure, the wound margins are brought together as primary treatment. Secondary intention entails dressing high-risk wounds and allowing them to heal from inside out. Delayed primary closure, involves delayed closure of wounds initially managed by secondary intention.

Patients who receive sutures need appropriate follow-up care to determine whether healing is normal or abnormal. Serious complications, including localized or systemic infection, can arise. In some cases, sutures may need to be removed early to allow a wound to drain infectious material.

■ Pathophysiology of Wound Healing

Infection

Because the skin serves as an initial barrier against microorganisms, any break in its surface can lead to infection. Larger openings and deeper penetrations result in a higher level of risk for the development of an infection. Not only will there be a delay in healing from the infection, but additional complications or systemic infection can result.

Once pathogens have entered the body tissues, they begin to grow and multiply, although clinical signs of infection may not appear for several days. Visible clues of infection include **erythema**, pus, warmth, edema, and local discomfort. Red streaks adjacent to the wound indicate that the patient has developed **lymphangitis**, an inflammation of the lymph channels. More serious infections can cause systemic signs, such as fever, shaking, chills, joint pain, and hypotension.

Gangrene

Approximately 3,000 cases of **gangrene** occur in the United States each year, of which 60% result from trauma and 25% end in the patient's death. *Clostridium perfringens* is an anaerobic, toxin-producing bacterium that leads to the development of gangrene. Once it enters deeply into tissue, it causes the production of a foul-smelling gas. If the gangrene is not treated, the skin will become necrotic and the infection may lead to sepsis. Prompt recognition and early, aggressive hospital therapy offer the best chance for reducing morbidity and mortality.

Tetanus

Tetanus is caused by infection with an anaerobic bacterium, *Clostridium tetani* (a member of the same family that causes gangrene). This bacterium causes the body to produce a potent toxin, which results in painful muscle contractions that are strong enough to fracture bones. Muscle stiffness may be noted first in the jaw ("lockjaw") and neck, with progression down the remainder of the body. Early recognition is important because conventional therapy does not result in rapid recovery.

Tetanus has become a rare occurrence because of the availability of a vaccine. In the United States, vaccination against tetanus is part of childhood immunization programs. A booster is needed every 10 years, although an inoculation is typically provided to patients who are injured and have not been immunized in the last 5 years. Given the severity of tetanus, you should ask injured patients about the last time they received a tetanus booster.

Necrotizing Fasciitis

Necrotizing fasciitis involves the death of tissue from bacterial infection. This disease is caused by more than one infecting organism—most commonly, *Staphylococcus aureus* and hemolytic streptococci. Although necrotizing fasciitis is rare, the mortality rate can be very high. Antibiotic therapy and surgical débridement are among the available treatments.

Patient Assessment

Although skin trauma is often dramatic, it rarely is immediately life threatening. It is important for you to stay focused on the assessment process used throughout this book to help you first identify threats to you and your crew using the scene size-up and then identify life threats to the patient using the primary assessment.

Scene Size-up

The first aspect to address in any scenario is safety. If you are responding to a vehicle crash, ensure that traffic is controlled and personnel are operating with protective measures in place. When you are responding to a reported explosion, wait for law enforcement personnel to secure the scene and declare it safe before you approach any victims. When a blast seems to be intentional, look for possible secondary devices. Responders have been injured and killed by other explosive devices planted away from the original detonation site.

Once you have determined that the scene is safe, begin evaluating the MOI. Maintain a high index of suspicion whenever a significant MOI is present, even if a patient's external injuries appear minor. Carefully consider the forces involved as you determine the likelihood of internal damage. Remember, the severity of the injury may not be initially apparent, but it will be revealed as you perform a rapid exam or focused assessment.

Next, determine how many patients are involved. Diligently search for patients who may have been ejected during a significant vehicle crash.

As a part of your scene size-up, be aware that skin injuries typically result in a risk of exposure to blood and other bodily fluids. Significant exposures include contact with body fluids through open wounds or mucous membranes. Less worrisome exposures include body fluid contact with intact skin. Be sure to protect yourself and the patient, and review the chapters,

YOU *are the Medic* | PART 2 |

The police and neighbors appear to be making a plan regarding how to best lift the car off the patient. Taking charge of the scene, you explain that the car will not be moved yet. You explain the risks to the officer in charge and have the police officers keep bystanders away from the scene. As with the scene of any illness or injury, you now move on to your general impression and think before taking any immediate action. Your patient is responsive and alert. He has informed you that the car fell on him earlier in the day, at least 3 or 4 hours ago. The patient's wife states that she left to do errands at about 8:30 this morning, while her husband was under the car working. She just arrived home a few minutes after 1:00 PM.

Recording Time: 1 Minute	
Appearance	Supine, legs trapped under car
Level of consciousness	Alert, oriented
Airway	Open, clear, self-maintained
Breathing	Adequate, slightly fast
Circulation	Pale skin, radial pulses equal/strong, rapid

3. Controlling the crowd was an important first step in saving your patient's life. What are the most serious risks of lifting the car off the patient without having performed an examination and without having made preparations?

4. What is the significance of the patient's report of not being able to feel his feet?

Workforce Safety and Wellness and *Infectious Diseases*, regarding infection control procedures.

Primary Assessment

Form a General Impression

When the scene has been secured and standard precautions have been taken, rapidly determine whether any life threats are present. First, form your general impression as you approach the patient. Much information can be obtained from simply looking at the patient and the immediate surroundings. For example, a patient who is lying prone on the ground in a large pool of blood is clearly in worse shape than a patient who meets you at the door with a cut finger.

Many patients have potential injuries to the neck or spine. In such cases, you should assign a crew member to manually immobilize the patient's head and neck. This is an important step because it will determine which maneuvers are used to open the airway.

Evaluation of the patient's initial level of consciousness is also important. Determine whether the patient is alert, responsive to verbal stimuli, responsive to painful stimuli, or completely unresponsive. This assessment may reveal a potential brain injury even when the patient has a seemingly innocuous soft-tissue injury to the head.

Airway and Breathing

Assess the airway as soon as you arrive at the patient's side. Determine whether air is moving from the nose, mouth, or stoma. If blood, vomit, or anything else is present in the airway, provide immediate suctioning. If direct trauma is present, it may severely compromise the airway. Soft-tissue injuries that result in a flow of blood into the airway can also interfere with airway patency. You should immediately correct anything that interferes with airway patency; failure to provide a patent airway can quickly lead to the patient's death.

Assess the patient's breathing. During the primary assessment, it is not important to obtain an exact rate—just determine whether the patient's breathing is abnormally slow or rapid or excessively deep or shallow. Address a significant alteration in breathing by using a nonrebreathing mask with oxygen at 15 L/min or a bag-mask device and supplementary oxygen. An inadequate depth or rate that results in compromised breathing should prompt you to take immediate action.

Circulation

Assessment of circulatory status involves palpating a pulse and checking the skin signs. In an unresponsive adult, assess the carotid pulse; in a responsive patient, assess the radial pulse. If no pulse is present, take resuscitative measures (see the chapter, *Responding to the Field Code*). When you are palpating a pulse, determine whether it is abnormally fast or slow (an exact rate will be calculated later). The goal at this step is for you to determine whether immediate intervention is necessary.

Palpate and inspect the skin (CTC—Color, Temperature, and Condition). Pale or ashen skin points to inadequate perfusion. Cool, moist skin is an early indicator of shock. When present, determine whether the skin is cool and moist only in the extremities or over the entire body.

Ensure that the patient is adequately exposed during the primary assessment. Sometimes, you need to look at only the chest area. On more serious calls, the patient may need to be completely exposed from head to toe. Gunshot wounds and stab wounds, for example, warrant complete removal of the patient's clothing in order to look for entrance and exit wounds **Figure 5** . If severe hemorrhage from a wound is present, control of that hemorrhage with a tourniquet takes precedence over anything else in the primary assessment.

Transport Decision

Once the primary assessment has been completed, you will need to make a priority decision to rapidly package and transport or to stabilize and treat on scene. Patients with significant trauma (significant MOI) should be rapidly transported. Patients with isolated injuries (no significant MOI) are often better managed by carefully treating the injuries on scene.

Patients are stratified into two categories: patients with a significant MOI and patients with no significant MOI. When serious trauma is present, soft-tissue injuries take a lower priority than airway control, breathing inadequacy, and bleeding. *Do not let soft-tissue injuries distract you from life threats that may not be readily apparent.* Patients with less serious injuries will need an exam focused on the specific body part and its function but probably will not need a full-body exam.

Significant MOI

Serious trauma is indicated by an altered level of consciousness, lack of airway protection or lack of patency, inadequate breathing, uncontrolled bleeding, and a significant MOI. If any of these findings are present or your analysis points to a possibility for serious injury, perform a rapid exam. Life threats should have been addressed during the primary assessment; if additional life threats are found now, manage them immediately. For example, if examination of the chest reveals absent breath sounds on one side, the chest may need ventilation, sealing with an occlusive dressing, and decompression if there is a tension

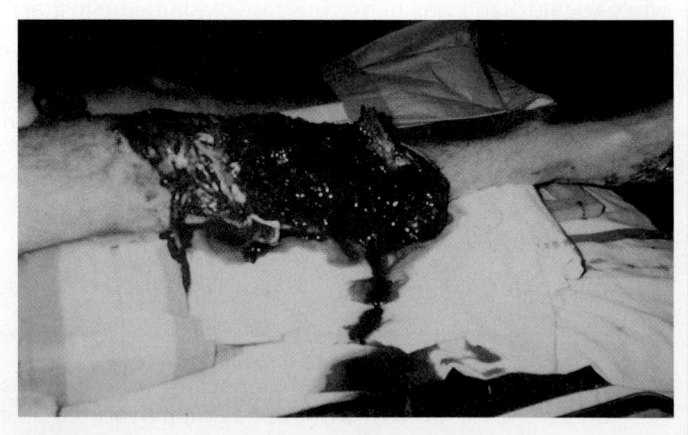

Figure 5 A high-velocity gunshot wound to the leg.

pneumothorax. Interventions can occur simultaneously during the primary assessment of the patient.

A rapid exam involves a full-body exam that focuses on detecting serious injury to major body compartments. Rapidly assess the head, neck, chest, abdomen, pelvis, lower extremities, upper extremities, and posterior. Identify deformities, discolorations, impaled objects, open injuries, and other trauma that demand immediate attention. The mnemonic DCAP-BTLS is a useful reminder of what to look at: Deformities, Contusions, Abrasions, Punctures or penetrations, Burns, Tenderness, Lacerations, and Swelling. Also assess for instability and crepitus. Assess areas with alterations in sensation, uneven temperature, or abnormal muscle tone. Note if any blood appears on your gloves. For example, hair can conceal hemorrhage, but if you find blood on your gloves during your exam of the head, you have identified an injury.

Address airway compromises, breathing inadequacies, and uncontrolled hemorrhage that may have been missed in the primary assessment. Trauma patients are often critically injured, and life threats evolve over time, so reassessments may reveal problems not found in the initial examination. Airway takes priority over breathing issues, and both take precedence over active bleeding. In practice, you will work as a part of a team to manage each issue as it is found rather than addressing each life threat sequentially. For example, the paramedic positioned at the head can manage the airway while another provider performs bleeding control. Prioritize the injuries that need to be addressed first. Remember that optimal on-scene time for seriously injured trauma patients is less than 10 minutes, and any intervention that can be done en route should be delayed until you are in the ambulance.

Once you have assessed the head and neck, you can apply a cervical collar to limit motion and prevent secondary injury. Collars are designed to allow assessment of the front of the neck while in place but do not offer a means to assess the back of the neck without their removal. Completely assess the neck before applying a cervical collar. Once it is in position, a rescuer must continue to stabilize the neck until the patient's torso and head are properly fixed to a long backboard. Be diligent about ensuring that the airway stays open and clear. If the collar is in the way, you may need to resort to manual immobilization of the neck while maintaining an open airway with a jaw-thrust maneuver.

At the conclusion of a rapid exam, you must decide whether to rapidly transport or remain on scene for more detailed care. A full-body exam is typically performed en route to the ED. Completion of a rapid exam should prompt you to reconsider or reconfirm the initial transport priority. A complete set of baseline vital signs and the SAMPLE history should also be obtained on concluding this assessment.

No Significant MOI

A full-body exam is not always warranted. Patients with isolated extremity trauma do not require a full body evaluation. If you are unsure whether a significant MOI exists, conduct a complete rapid exam and then perform a full-body exam en route to the ED. In all other cases, direct your attention to assessing the chief complaint and the area with outward signs of injury.

When local protocols allow, some patients can be treated on scene and released. For example, a patient at a rock concert with a minor laceration; good distal pulses, motor response, and sensation; and recent history of a tetanus shot might be able to be released to an alert and oriented adult. Some systems have established a means for referring the patient for further medical care at a local emergency clinic or other suitable medical facility. Release or referral may be preferred for a patient with relatively minor injuries, such as a simple laceration or abrasion. Providers must still provide basic care, such as dressing and bandaging. You should clearly understand your local protocols prior to "releasing" any patients. Most systems consider this practice to be potentially very dangerous and well beyond the scope of care and training of a paramedic.

History Taking

Gathering information is also an important step in determining how the patient was injured. Ask the patient (if responsive and able to respond) or family members and bystanders about the events leading to injury:

- Was the patient wearing a seat belt?
- How fast was the vehicle traveling?
- How high is the location from which the patient fell?
- Was there a loss of consciousness?
- What type of weapon was used?

When time and patient condition permit, you should determine when the last tetanus booster was given. Record the information on the patient care report, and relay it during patient transfer at the hospital. Ask the patient about prescribed and over-the-counter medications, paying particular attention to those that interfere with hemostasis. A higher priority should be given to patients taking warfarin (Coumadin) or other anticoagulants. Other medications that can lead to continued bleeding include aspirin, ticlopidine (Ticlid), and clopidogrel bisulfate (Plavix). To obtain a complete history, use the mnemonic SAMPLE described in previous chapters.

Secondary Assessment

After obtaining the history and performing the rapid exam, a more thorough examination should generally be conducted en route when there is a significant MOI and adequate time and the patient is in stable condition. This detailed assessment examines every anatomic region, looking for hidden injuries and clinical signs. A full-body exam is an excellent way for you to gather information, but it should never delay transport of a patient in critical condition. As mentioned previously, this assessment can be completed while traveling to the ED.

Reassessment

Frequent reassessment of the patient's conditions should be made en route to the hospital and in conjunction with any necessary interventions. A patient in stable condition should be reassessed every 15 minutes; a more serious condition warrants reexamination every 5 minutes. As part of this assessment, vital signs should be obtained and evaluated, any interventions checked, and the patient monitored.

Written documentation must be completed for every patient contact. When you are filling out the patient care report, include all relevant scene findings, such as a severely damaged vehicle or caliber of weapon used. Also record patient findings, including patency of airway, ventilation, and circulation, and any interventions administered. Describe the patient's presentation on your arrival at the scene, and note the body position on arrival (for example, prone or supine).

Note specific injuries. Describe wounds in terms of size, location, depth, and associated complications. Note your assessment findings for distal neurovascular status, range of motion, and the presence or absence of infection. Obtain patient demographic information, such as age, date of birth, and home address. Include the patient's medical history, medications, and allergies.

If you performed an intervention, record it on the patient care report. Note how the patient responded to the therapy (ie, the same, better, or worse condition). Also document the patient's level of understanding for each intervention. Finally, note which provider attended to the patient en route to the receiving facility.

Documentation and Communication

Most people charged with shooting another person end up in court at some point, and you may be called to testify. In cases of gunshot wounds, it is especially important that you carefully document the circumstances surrounding the scene, the injury, the patient's condition, and the treatment you provided.

■ Emergency Medical Care

Management of soft-tissue trauma varies according to the injury present; however, some basic management principles apply to nearly every scenario. Although attending to clinical issues is important, you must also tend to the patient's feelings about the injury. Be empathetic, because the injury may be perceived very differently in the patient's eyes. From a clinical standpoint, bleeding is controlled using direct pressure, elevation, and if persistent, a tourniquet. Immobilization of an injury site can also be helpful in caring for soft-tissue damage. Once all assessments and interventions are complete and patient care has been transferred, thoroughly document any care provided.

■ Treatment of Closed Wounds

Small contusions do not require any special treatment. When an extensive closed injury is present, however, bleeding beneath the skin may reach significant proportions, and swelling may compromise vital structures. In such cases, take steps to minimize the bleeding and swelling by following the ICES mnemonic:

I Apply *Ice* or cold packs to the injured area. Cold will stimulate blood vessels to constrict, slowing the bleeding.

C Apply firm *Compression* over the injured area to decrease bleeding. Compression may be manual initially, but is most effectively applied with an air splint thereafter.

E *Elevate* the injured part to a level above the heart, to encourage drainage and decrease swelling.

S Apply a *Splint* to an injured extremity. By preventing motion, a splint decreases bleeding. An air splint provides a double benefit—splinting *and* compression, though an air splint will not control arterial bleeding.

Recall that edema in the context of an injury is the body's way of dealing with injury to the soft tissues or connective tissues. Swelling can be due to blood from a developing hematoma, or can simply be the result of fluid. Use of ice as early as possible (20 minutes on and 20 minutes off to cool the injured tissue) may help to decrease the extent of the swelling and in turn speed up the rehabilitation time for the injury.

■ Treatment of Open Wounds: General Principles

Two general principles govern the treatment of all open wounds:

- Control bleeding by whatever method is most effective.
- Keep the wound as clean as possible. Cut away clothing covering the wound. For severely contaminated wounds, wash away loose dirt and debris by pouring sterile water, saline, or tap water over the area. Do *not* try to pick out foreign matter embedded in a wound. Simply irrigate the site copiously, and then cover the wound with a dry, sterile dressing.

Determine the magnitude of the injury and relay the findings to the receiving facility. If bleeding is present, determine the color of the blood, amount lost, and site of origin. Obtaining an accurate history is important when bleeding has stopped before EMS arrival. Ask the patient to describe the bleeding in terms of color and type of flow.

For wounds already in the healing stage, examine the edges to determine whether the wound is closing properly or if the edges are separating. Inspect the area to identify signs of infection, such as redness, swelling, and pain. Discolored pus may also be present. Signs of systemic infection—fever, general malaise, and altered mental status—warrant evaluation in a hospital.

■ Bandaging and Dressing Wounds

Dressing and bandage materials are used to cover the wound, control bleeding, and limit motion. Simple application of a dressing over an open wound will help prevent infection by providing an artificial barrier against microorganisms. Using bleeding control techniques with dressings will stop all but the most serious active blood loss. Correct application of bandage material will limit motion of the affected area, helping the body to recover from the injury.

A variety of materials are used to dress and bandage wounds. A **dressing** directly covers a wound and controls bleeding, whereas a **bandage** keeps the dressing in place. When properly applied, both keep pathogens from entering the open injury. Table 2 reviews specific types of dressings and bandages.

■ Complications of Improperly Applied Dressings

Improper application of dressing and bandage material can result in significant complications. It is important for you to learn how to properly dress a wound in the laboratory, clinical, and field settings to avoid causing harm.

Although it is not always possible to use sterile technique, you should make every effort to avoid further wound

Table 2 Specific Types of Dressings and Bandages	
Type	**Considerations**
Sterile	■ Completely free of microorganisms ■ Used when a high probability of infection is present (eg, large open wounds) ■ Sterility is lost when the package is opened; it is important to use quickly
Nonsterile	■ Used when there is a lower risk of infection ■ First dress the wound with a sterile dressing, then apply multiple nonsterile dressings to increase the ability to absorb blood
Hemostatic dressing	■ Used to control serious hemorrhage when application of a tourniquet is not possible (for example, on the chest or pelvis) ■ Contains a hemostatic agent impregnated into the dressing ■ Unlike with other dressings, it is important to remove all other dressings before applying a hemostatic dressing
Occlusive	■ Used when it is important to keep air from entering the wound ■ When applying to an open wound in the thorax, seal on three sides to allow air to escape (helps prevent development of tension pneumothorax)
Adherent	■ Allows exudate from the wound to mesh with dressing material; facilitates clotting and aid in bleeding control ■ Removal of the dressing is painful and may precipitate additional bleeding
Nonadherent	■ Allows the products of wound repair to pass through the material; does not aid in clot formation ■ Applied after wound closure
Dry	■ Most commonly used in prehospital care
Wet	■ Limited use in the field ■ Used in burn care of superficial burns
Roller bandage	■ Self-adherent; overlapping material adheres to itself to keep the bandage in place ■ Used to wrap extremity injuries
Gauze bandage	■ Similar to roller bandage, but nonadherent ■ Used to secure a dressing ■ Does not stretch much; can result in excess pressure to areas that begin to swell
Absorbent gauze sponges	■ Used to create a thicker, bulkier dressing to control heavy bleeding
Elastic bandage	■ Stretches to allow some pressure to be applied ■ Useful in controlling bleeding ■ Used in musculoskeletal trauma to facilitate healing of damaged tendons and ligaments ■ Avoid applying excessive pressure, which could compromise blood flow
Triangular bandage	■ Ideal for making slings and swathes ■ These do not stretch; are therefore not ideal if pressure must be applied ■ Can be wrapped into a thin strip to be used as a tourniquet
Medical tape	■ Used to secure a dressing ■ Use caution when applying on patients with skin conditions that might lead to damage upon removal of the tape (such as in older patients, who often have thin skin)

contamination. Irrigate open wounds with normal saline to flush out contaminants. If available, apply antibiotic ointment to smaller open wounds to help speed healing and decrease risk of infection. Large open injuries should not have ointment applied but should be dressed. Once the wound is irrigated, apply a dressing over the site. Clean blood around the dressing site, and neatly wrap a bandage over the dressing.

Hemodynamic complications include the possibility for continued bleeding. Once a dressing has been placed, it should not be removed because of the risk of disrupting clot formation. If a wound continues to bleed, additional dressings should be applied in conjunction with bleeding control interventions such as a tourniquet. Frequent reassessments will help prevent unchecked blood loss and hemodynamic complications. Exsanguination is a possibility when a pressure dressing does not stop blood loss; the same is true for an improperly applied tourniquet. If a tourniquet occludes only venous flow, bleeding may actually increase. A properly applied dressing in conjunction with direct pressure is often sufficient to stop blood loss. If not, do not hesitate to apply a tourniquet to achieve bleeding control.

Structural elements—blood vessels, nerves, tendons, muscles, skin, and internal organs—can be damaged, particularly when dressings are excessively tight. Prevention of damage entails assessing and readjusting the dressing and bandage as necessary. Distal pulses, motor, and sensation should be assessed when extremity dressings are in place. Tight dressings may cause pain in a patient who already has an injury.

■ Control of External Bleeding

External bleeding is bleeding that can be seen coming from a wound when the integrity of the skin has been violated. Theoretically, bleeding can be characterized according to the type of blood vessel that has been damaged Figure 6 . Capillary bleeding is characterized by a slow, even flow of bright or dark red blood and is present in minor injuries, such as abrasions or superficial lacerations. Venous bleeding is more likely to be slow and steady, and the color of the blood is darker. Arterial bleeding occurs in spurts, and the blood is usually bright red because of the fully saturated hemoglobin. In reality, most large open wounds show a combination of arterial and venous bleeding.

Four methods are used in the field to control external bleeding: direct pressure, elevation, immobilization, and a tourniquet.

Direct Pressure

Application of pressure over a bleeding wound stops blood from flowing into the damaged vessels, allowing the platelets to seal the vascular walls.

Words of Wisdom

Steady, direct pressure against the bleeding site is the most effective means to control bleeding.

YOU *are the Medic* | PART 3

Your patient has an open, patent airway and does not appear to be in any respiratory distress. He has no discoloration, flail segments, crepitus, or other abnormal findings on chest examination. Lung sounds are equal. No severe bleeding is seen. Your partner has administered high-concentration oxygen via a nonrebreathing mask and the patient's vital signs are measured. You establish two large-bore intravenous (IV) lines in his arms and begin slowly infusing normal saline and sodium bicarbonate under the direction of medical control.

Recording Time: 5 Minutes	
Respirations	22 breaths/min, nonlabored
Pulse	96 beats/min, strong radial pulses
Skin	Pale, warm, dry
Blood pressure	142/96 mm Hg
Oxygen saturation (Spo$_2$)	98%
Pupils	Equal, reactive

5. The patient's blood pressure seems within the normal range, but medical control instructed you to establish two large-bore IV lines. What reasons might justify this order?

6. Assuming the patient has been trapped for several hours, you wish to extricate him and transport him to the hospital as soon as his condition is stable. Medical control does not order any additional medications. What other actions can you take to increase the chances for your patient's survival?

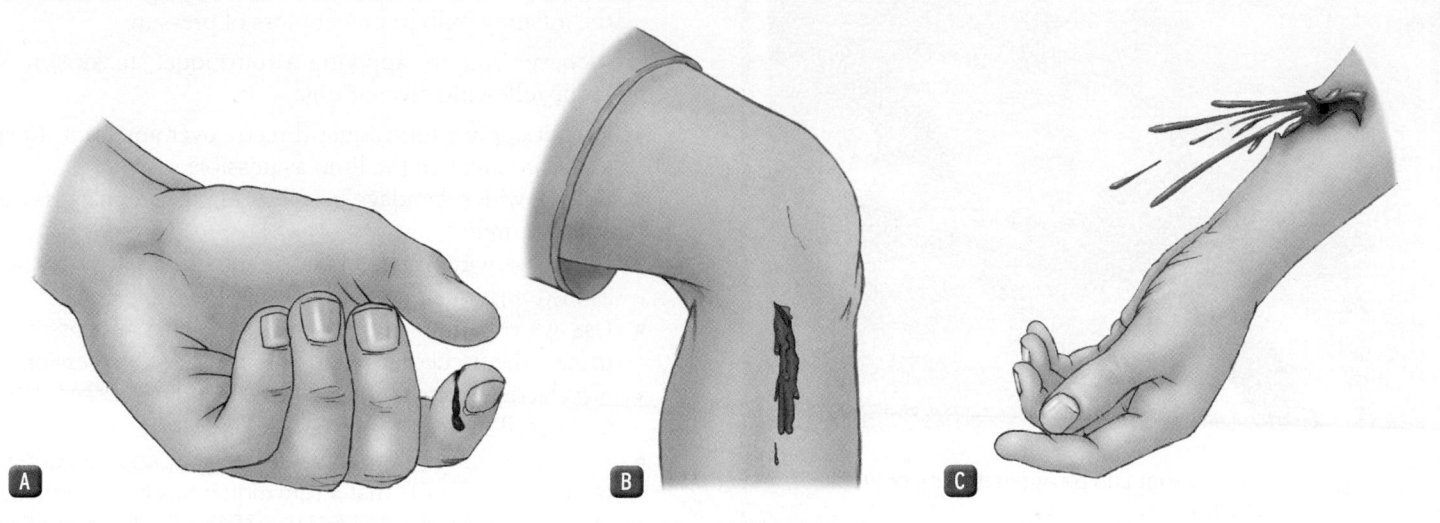

Figure 6 **A.** Capillary bleeding is dark red and oozes from the wound slowly but steadily. **B.** Venous bleeding is darker than arterial bleeding and flows steadily. **C.** Arterial bleeding is characteristically brighter red and spurts in time with the pulse.

If possible, you should use a sterile dressing to exert pressure, and then use your gloved hand to apply pressure over the bleeding site. The steps for controlling bleeding are shown in the chapter, *Bleeding*, and are summarized as follows:

1. Follow standard precautions.
2. Maintain the airway with cervical spine immobilization if the MOI suggests the possibility of spinal injury.
3. Apply direct pressure over the wound with a dry, sterile dressing. Elevate the injury if no fracture is suspected.
4. Apply a pressure dressing. Hold the pressure dressing in place using gauze.
5. If direct pressure with a pressure dressing does not control bleeding on an extremity injury, apply a tourniquet above the level of the bleeding.
6. Apply high-flow oxygen as necessary, once hemorrhaging is controlled.
7. Monitor the serial vital signs, and watch diligently for developing shock. If the patient shows any signs of shock (hypoperfusion), transport rapidly while providing aggressive management en route. Because a patient in shock is usually emotionally upset, you should provide psychological support as well.

Some commercially available pressure dressings allow for simultaneous dressing of the wound and application of pressure. If one of these products is not available, standard dressing material may be used in conjunction with triangular bandages to create localized pressure. This type of dressing will often allow you to focus on other tasks while pressure is applied. Always assess distal circulation before and after you apply a pressure dressing. Adjust the dressing as needed in case of a complication, such as loss of distal pulse, diminished sensation, or change in skin color and temperature distal to the dressing.

Elevation

In patients with venous bleeding from an extremity, the rate of bleeding can be substantially slowed by elevating the extremity above the level of the heart. This measure alone will not control bleeding, but it may be helpful in conjunction with other measures, such as direct pressure.

Immobilization

Any movement of an extremity, even an uninjured extremity, promotes blood flow within that extremity. When the extremity is also injured, motion may disrupt the clotting process and lacerate more blood vessels. Therefore, you should attempt to limit motion of an injured extremity. Advise the patient to make every effort to minimize movement. If that is not possible and conditions warrant, apply a splint to prevent motion.

An air splint or padded board works well to keep an upper or lower extremity immobilized. Use of an air splint provides a double benefit—splinting *and* direct pressure. Remember to assess distal pulses, motor function, and sensation distal to the splint before and after application.

Tourniquet

A tourniquet is especially useful if a patient is bleeding severely from an extremity injury below the axilla or groin and other methods of bleeding control are ineffective.

Some commercial tourniquets can be applied with one arm **Figure 7**, although you may not have access to them. If a tourniquet is required, observe the following application guidelines, shown in the chapter, *Bleeding*:

1. Follow standard precautions.
2. Hold direct pressure over the bleeding site.
3. Place a tourniquet around the extremity above the bleeding site.

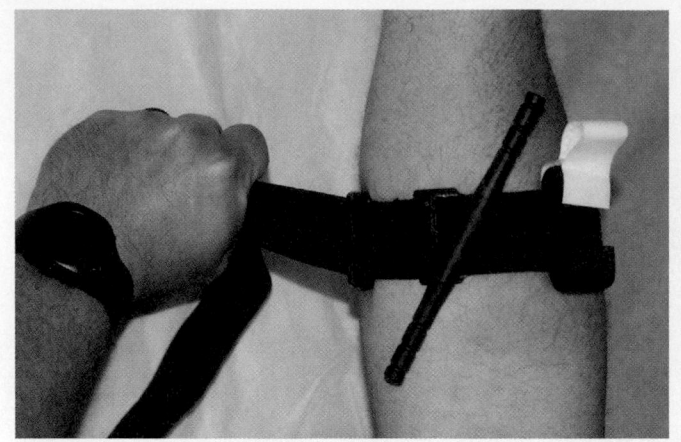

Figure 7 A tourniquet that can be applied using only one arm has been developed.

to clamp the tube with a hemostat leading from the cuff to the inflating bulb to prevent loss of pressure.

Whenever you are applying a tourniquet, make sure you observe the following precautions:

- Do not apply a tourniquet directly over any joint. Keep it as far proximal on the limb as possible.
- Use the widest bandage possible. Make sure that it is tightened securely.
- Never use wire, rope, a belt, or any other narrow material as the tourniquet; it could cut into the skin.
- Use wide padding under the tourniquet, if possible, to protect the tissues and help with arterial compression.
- Never cover a tourniquet with a bandage. Leave it open and in full view.
- Inform the hospital in your radio report and verbal report on arrival at the ED that a tourniquet has been applied.
- Do not loosen the tourniquet after you have applied it unless directed to do so by hospital personnel or medical control.

4. Click the buckle into place and pull the strap tight.
5. Turn the tightening dial clockwise until pulses are no longer palpable distal to the tourniquet and bleeding has been controlled. Then secure the tightening dial.
6. To release the tourniquet at the hospital, or if otherwise instructed by medical control, push the release button and pull the strap back. Be aware that bleeding may rapidly return on tourniquet release and that you should be prepared to reapply it immediately if necessary.

If a commercial tourniquet is not available, follow these steps to apply a tourniquet using a triangular bandage and a stick or rod:

1. Fold a triangular bandage until it is 4 inches wide and six to eight layers thick.
2. Wrap the bandage around the extremity twice. Apply the tourniquet proximal to the bleeding.
3. Tie one knot in the bandage. Then place a stick or rod on top of the knot, and tie the ends of the bandage over the stick in a square knot.
4. Use the stick as a handle, and twist it to tighten the tourniquet until the bleeding has stopped; then stop twisting.
5. Secure the stick in place, and make the wrapping neat and smooth.
6. Write "TK" and the exact time (hour and minute) that you applied the tourniquet on a piece of adhesive tape, preferably in red ink. Use the phrase "time applied." Securely fasten the tape to the patient's forehead. Notify hospital personnel on your arrival that your patient has a tourniquet in place. Record this same information on the ambulance run report form.
7. As an alternative method, you can use a blood pressure cuff as an effective tourniquet. Position the cuff proximal to the bleeding point, and inflate it just enough to stop the bleeding. Leave the cuff inflated. If you use a blood pressure cuff, monitor the gauge continuously to make sure that the pressure is not gradually dropping. You may have

Pain Control

Application of a cold compress will help reduce pain and diminish blood flow to an open wound. Once the dressing is in place, apply the cold pack. Avoid placing the compress directly on the site because excessively cold temperatures may cause further injury. A pressure dressing may alleviate pain and minimize swelling.

If basic life support measures fail to relieve pain, consider administering morphine sulfate or other agents as allowed by protocol. The common dosage for morphine is 0.05 mg/kg IV every 5 minutes to a maximum of 10 mg. As with all medications, carefully assess the patient for allergies, and document pertinent information.

Managing Wound Healing and Infection

In the prehospital setting, management of altered wound healing and infection entails basic measures. Wounds that are not healing properly or show signs of infection should be dressed and bandaged appropriately. In severe cases, pain control measures may be indicated.

Dressing Specific Anatomic Sites

Dressing and bandaging wounds is not the same for every part of the body. This section describes the various factors that need to be considered for a given body region.

Scalp Dressings

Scalp injuries tend to bleed profusely owing to their rich blood supply. When bleeding is present, application of direct pressure is often effective because of the rigid skull that lies under the scalp. Be careful to accurately determine the extent of the injury because significant trauma may lead to skull damage, such as a fracture. In that case, control of bleeding must be balanced against the issue of not causing additional damage. When the skull has been compromised and bleeding must be controlled, apply pressure to the areas around the break. Use a bulky dressing that assists in stopping blood loss and helps prevent excessive direct pressure on the already damaged cranium.

The shape of the skull is a consideration when you are dressing wounds that involve the scalp. Improperly applied dressings can easily slide up or down the scalp, becoming ineffective. In addition, hair may interfere with securing dressings in place.

Facial Dressings

Facial injuries tend to cause significant anxiety for patients and family. While you are tending to the clinical needs, take the time to reassure the patient. Application of direct pressure is an effective means to control bleeding from soft-tissue disruption along the face. If an avulsed piece of tissue is present, attempt to replace the pedicle to its normal anatomic location as closely as possible. Note that bleeding tends to be quite heavy because of the rich blood supply in this area.

Assess the patient for the presence of or potential for airway compromise early in your encounter. Blood pouring into an unprotected airway is a serious concern, so be prepared to suction and position the patient to facilitate drainage. Do not allow a gruesome facial injury to distract you from attending to life threats.

Ear or Mastoid Dressings

Trauma to the ear is commonly external, although internal injury is a possibility. Never place a dressing in the ear canal, but loosely apply it along the entire length of the external ear. Gauze sponges work well to aid in stopping blood loss. If blood is flowing from the ear canal, do not attempt to control it directly. Cerebrospinal fluid may be leaking, and halting the blood flow may increase pressure within the skull. Place a bulky dressing over the external ear, and transport the patient rapidly.

Neck Dressings

Important anatomic structures in the neck include large blood vessels, the airway, and the cervical spine. There is little room for error when trauma is present in this area. A minor neck laceration can lead to an air embolism, a small puncture can penetrate the spinal canal, and an anterior open wound can disrupt the airway **Figure 8**. Pay close attention to the clinical signs that accompany the external trauma.

Open injuries to the neck require use of an occlusive dressing to prevent the drawing of air into the circulatory system. Apply dressings carefully so that they do not interfere with blood flow or movement of air through the trachea.

Shoulder Dressings

The shoulder is relatively easy to dress and bandage. Apply direct pressure to control external hemorrhage in this region. If immobilization is indicated, a sling and swathe will prevent motion of the shoulder girdle.

Truncal Dressings

Injuries to the torso require vigilant assessment for underlying internal trauma. A seemingly innocuous hole may be the only indication that a gunshot wound is present. Cover open wounds with an occlusive dressing that is taped on three sides.

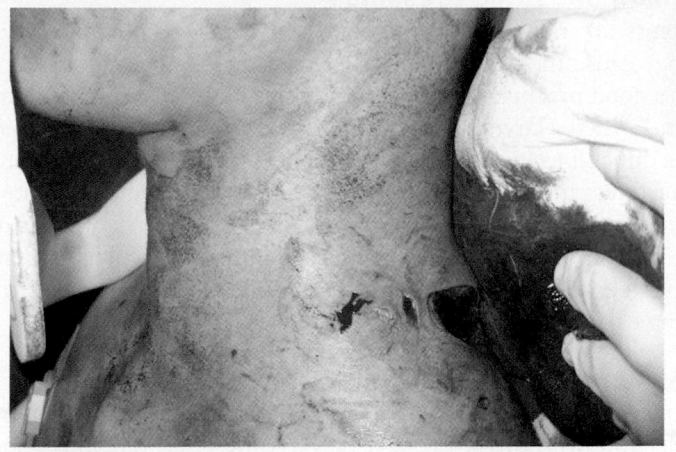

Figure 8 Neck wounds can lead to other serious situations such as air embolism and airway problems. Seal with an occlusive dressing right away.

Assessment of breath sounds becomes a high priority when you find an open chest wound because a pneumothorax or hemothorax may develop from penetrating trauma to the thorax. Continually reassess a patient with thoracic soft-tissue injuries.

The best choice for securing a truncal dressing in place is medical tape. Wrapping the entire torso may interfere with air movement.

Groin and Hip Dressings

Soft-tissue injuries to the groin and hip are typically managed with application of a dressing and bandage in combination with direct pressure to control blood loss in this region. Injuries to the genitalia are best managed by a provider of the same gender, whenever feasible. As always, you should remain professional and protect the patient's privacy while you are providing care. There may be times when a patient is averse to allowing a provider to dress a wound located near his or her genital area. In such cases, provide the patient with a dressing and allow self-directed care, if this is the only way the patient will cooperate.

Hand, Wrist, and Finger Dressings

The hands, wrists, and fingers are among the easiest sites to properly dress and bandage. A dressing is applied over any open wound, and bandage material is wrapped completely around the affected area. When possible, the hand should be placed in the position of function. This is accomplished by placing a roll of gauze in the patient's hand **Figure 9**. If limited motion is necessary, the hand and wrist can be easily splinted. If possible, leave fingers exposed to access circulation.

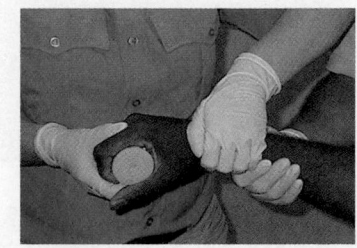

Figure 9 The position of function for the hand.

Elbow and Knee Dressings

Joints are not difficult to dress and bandage, but movement may cause the materials to shift from their original position. It is a good practice to provide immobilization of the elbow or the knee when a larger wound is present. Even smaller wounds may be difficult to manage because of skin tension lines and high tissue stress in these areas. When either of these joints is injured, it is important for you to assess distal neurovascular status. Elbow injuries have a higher risk for neurovascular compromise because of the limited space available for blood vessels and nerves.

Ankle and Foot Dressings

The ankle and foot are simple to dress and bandage. Control bleeding with direct pressure. If bleeding is arterial and cannot be controlled by direct pressure or with a hemostatic dressing, consider applying a tourniquet proximal to the injury. In cases in which bleeding can be readily controlled, application of a bandage must not be so tight that it interferes with circulation or sensation. Always assess distal neurovascular function before and after caring for the wound.

Pathophysiology, Assessment, and Management of Specific Injuries

Abrasions

An abrasion **Figure 10** is a superficial wound that occurs when the skin is rubbed or scraped over a rough surface and part of the epidermis is lost. So-called road rash or mat burns are good examples.

Assessment and Management

Abrasions typically ooze small amounts of blood and may be quite painful. They may also be contaminated with dirt and debris; for example, road rash is caused by sliding on the

pavement in a motorcycle crash. Because the skin has been disrupted, infection is a danger.

Do not attempt to clean an abrasion in the field. Rubbing, brushing, or washing the wound will cause additional bleeding and unnecessary pain. Care should consist of covering the wound lightly with a sterile dressing.

Words of Wisdom

Remember that a soft-tissue wound from an extremity injury can bleed enough to cause shock and death. If you cannot be certain that direct pressure and a pressure dressing have controlled bleeding, do not hesitate to apply a tourniquet to the limb in a position well proximal to the zone of injury.

Lacerations

A laceration **Figure 11** is a cut inflicted by a sharp instrument, such as a knife or razor blade, that produces a clean or jagged incision through the skin surface and underlying structures. Sometimes the word *laceration* is reserved for jagged or irregular cuts, and incision is used to refer to a clean (linear) cut. Incisions tend to heal better than lacerations because of their relatively even wound margins. Lacerations can injure important structures beneath the skin, including tendons, ligaments, organs, body cavities, and bones.

Assessment and Management

The seriousness of a laceration will depend on its depth and the structures that have been damaged. Lacerations may be the source of significant bleeding if they disrupt the wall of a blood vessel, particularly in regions of the body where major arteries lie close to the surface (as in the wrist).

The first priority in treating a laceration is to control bleeding, initially by applying direct manual pressure over the wound. Laceration of a major artery can be fatal due to the severe bleeding that can occur.

Puncture Wounds

A puncture wound **Figure 12** is a stab from a pointed object, such as a nail or a knife. Technically speaking, a bullet wound is a puncture wound. Puncture wounds can result in injury to underlying tissues and organs; the depth of a puncture wound cannot always be easily determined in the field. Many seemingly superficial wounds are later found to involve vital organs. Always suspect further internal injury, as well as potential shock, in patients with puncture wounds.

Assessment and Management

When you are assessing a puncture wound, consider the potential depth of the wound. The type of object and the speed at which

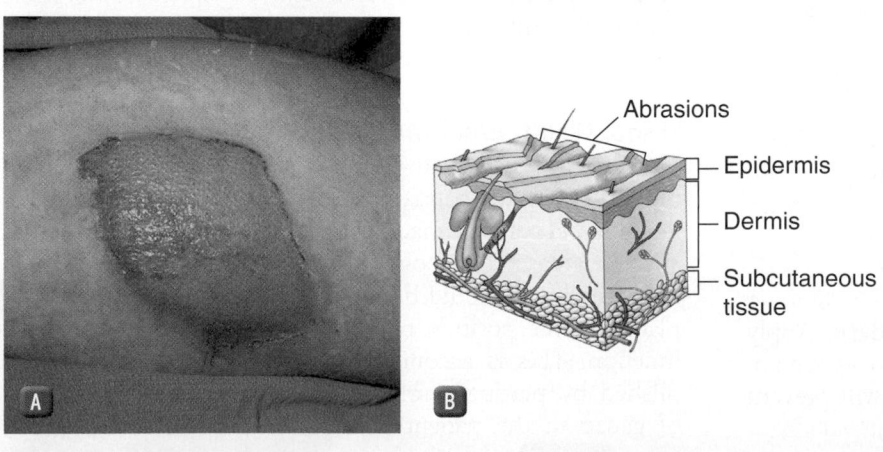

Figure 10 Abrasions usually do not penetrate completely through the dermis, but blood may ooze from the capillaries. These wounds are typically superficial and result from rubbing or scraping across a hard, rough surface. **A.** An abrasion. **B.** Anatomic diagram of an abrasion.

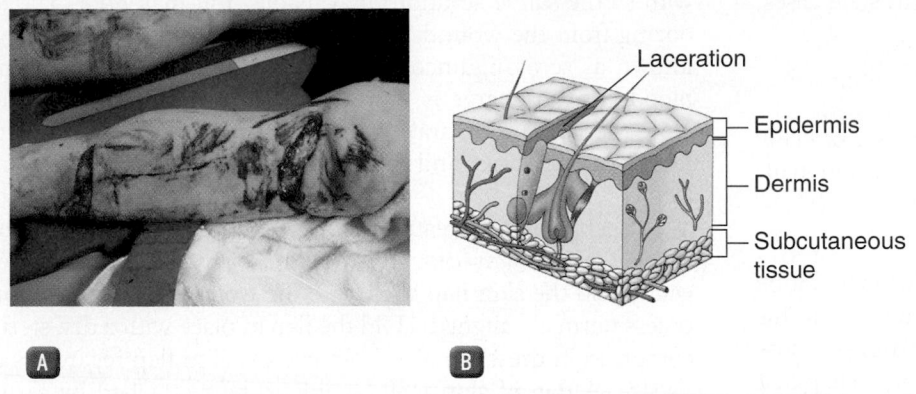

Figure 11 Lacerations can vary in depth and can extend through the skin and subcutaneous tissue to the underlying muscles, nerves, and blood vessels. These wounds can be smooth or jagged as a result of a cut by a sharp object or a blunt force that tears the tissue. **A.** Lacerations. **B.** Anatomic diagram of a laceration.

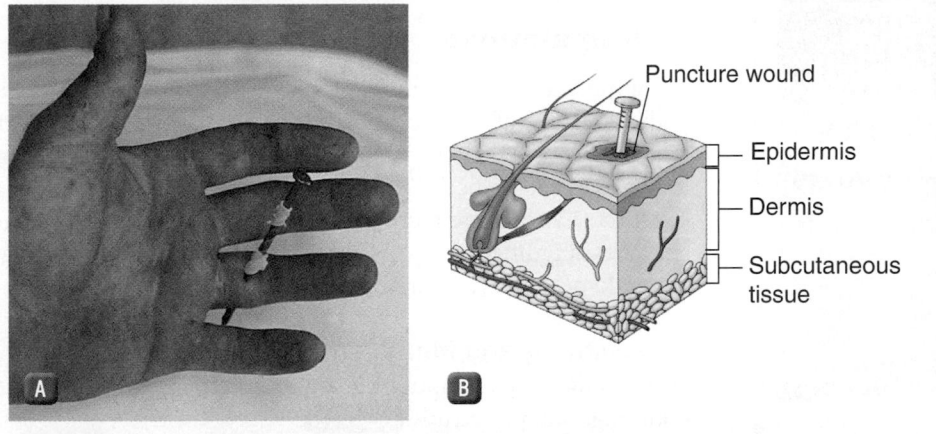

Figure 12 Puncture wounds may cause little external bleeding but can damage structures deep in the body. **A.** Puncture wound. **B.** Anatomic diagram of a puncture wound.

for edema, and be sure to treat swelling with ice.

A special case of the puncture wound is the impaled foreign object **Figure 13**. When the instrument that caused the injury remains embedded in the wound, immobilize the object and transport the patient. Follow the basic points below regarding management of an impaled object.

- Do not try to remove an impaled object. Efforts to do so may precipitate uncontrolled internal hemorrhage, which may lead to exsanguination or further injury to underlying structures.
- Control hemorrhage by direct compression, but do not apply pressure on the impaled object itself or on immediately adjacent tissues.
- Do not try to shorten an impaled object unless it is extremely cumbersome (such as a fence post impaled in the chest); any motion of the object may damage surrounding tissues.
- Stabilize the object in place with a bulky dressing, and immobilize the extremity (if the object is impaled in an extremity) with a splint to prevent motion.

The goal for prehospital care is to limit motion of the impaled object as soon as possible to minimize additional damage. One technique that is effective for thin objects is to use gauze pads cut midway through the center. Stack several pads vertically, and arrange the cut portions so that each stack of pads overlaps. Once it is determined that enough pads are in place for stabilizing the object, tape or bandage them securely. This technique has the dual benefits of providing stabilization and aiding in bleeding control. Larger objects that are impaled in the body can be secured with rolled towels or splinting materials.

Whatever presentation you may encounter, it is important to avoid causing additional harm. Secure the object as best as possible, and be creative in using securing materials. Provide reassurance to the patient and family. Constantly assess the risk for developing threats to life, such as airway compromise, breathing inadequacy, and uncontrolled hemorrhage.

On rare occasions, removal of an impaled object may be the best course of action. If the object directly interferes with airway control and the patient's condition is deteriorating rapidly, medical direction may authorize removal. It may also be necessary to remove an object that interferes with chest compressions in a patient who is in cardiac arrest sond deemed viable. In severe cases, it may be impossible to leave the object in place, such as

it created the wound are factors that relate to the potential depth and severity of the wound. The location of the puncture wound also relates to its severity. Consider whether the wound could involve important internal organs.

Most puncture wounds do not cause significant external bleeding, but they may produce extensive—even fatal—internal bleeding and cause damage to other structures and systems that cannot be seen from the outside of the body. Treatment of puncture wounds is similar to caring for other types of open wounds. Be sure to look for both entrance and exit wounds. Remember to take measures to prevent infection. Also, should a patient with a puncture wound refuse care, it is important to inform him or her of potential infection that could result from not seeking care.

With certain puncture wounds, it is possible for air to be injected under the skin, such as in a wound from a gun at close range, or in a wound from an air-pressurized device. Be alert when the patient is impaled on an immovable object. Establish direct contact with medical control immediately in such cases, and ask for guidance.

Avulsions

An **avulsion** occurs when a flap of skin is torn loose, partially **Figure 14** or completely. The amount of bleeding from an avulsion relates to the depth of injury.

Assessment and Management

Depending on where the avulsion occurs, it may or may not be accompanied by profuse bleeding. The principal danger in this type of injury—besides blood loss and contamination—is loss of the blood supply to the avulsed flap. If the part of the flap that connects it to the body (the **pedicle**) is folded back or kinked, circulation to the flap will be compromised and that piece of skin will die if the circulation is not restored quickly.

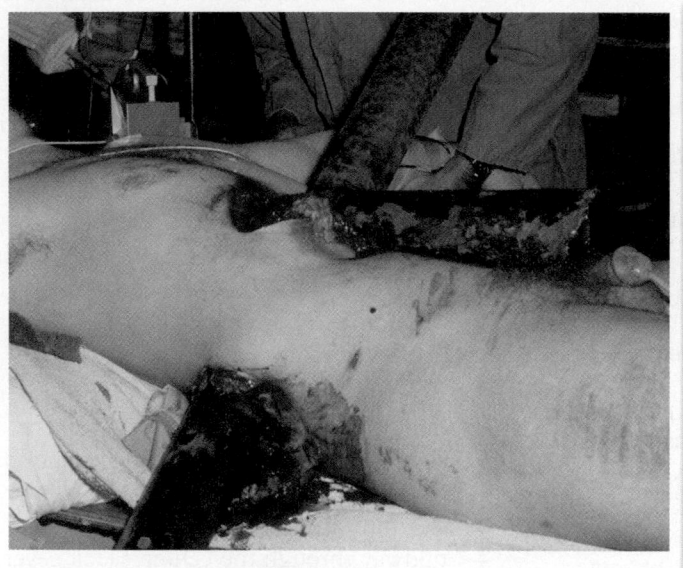

Figure 13 An impaled object remains embedded in the wound.

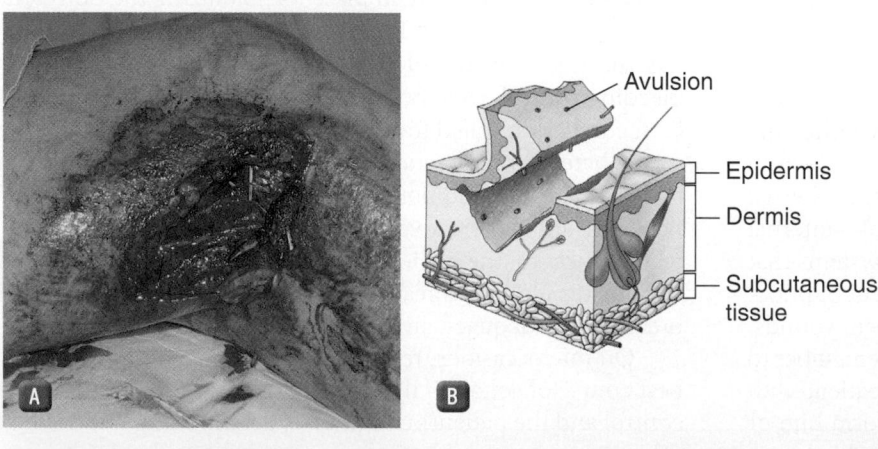

Figure 14 Avulsions are characterized by complete separation of tissue or tissue hanging as a flap. Significant bleeding is common. **A.** An avulsion. **B.** Anatomic diagram of an avulsion.

If the wound is contaminated, provide gentle irrigation with sterile saline solution, if available. You may note exudate oozing from the wound. In some cases, there will be drainage known as serosanguineous, which is a mixture of serum and blood. The discharge is typically thin and has a pinkish hue. Note the amount of drainage seeping from the wound, document your findings, and relay the information to the receiving facility.

When you are treating a partially avulsed piece of skin, quickly irrigate any dirt or debris out of the wound and then gently fold the skin flap back onto the wound so that it is more or less normally aligned. Hold the flap in place with a dry, sterile compression dressing. *Never* remove the skin flap regardless of its size. A flap of skin may be able to be reattached by a surgeon. Care also includes applying ice packs to the surrounding area to decrease pain and swelling. The cooling effect can also increase the length of time that damaged underlying muscle tissue remains viable. In patients who are in any way unstable or potentially unstable, management of these wounds should never be accomplished in a way that prolongs your on-scene time or otherwise delays your transport time. Become accustomed to managing wounds en route to the hospital.

Amputations

An **amputation** is an avulsion involving the complete loss of a body part, typically one or more of the extremities. If the amputation was produced by a sharp object, blood loss is often much less than expected because the blood vessels retain the ability to constrict. In contrast, a crushing or tearing amputation can result in exsanguination (excessive blood loss due to hemorrhage) if you do not intervene rapidly.

Assessment and Management

Wound edges in an amputation are commonly jagged, and sharp bone edges may protrude **Figure 15** .

During wound care, be aware of any sharp bone protrusions that may lead to an exposure. Large, thick dressings should be used to cover the site. In some cases, the body part will be completely detached. In a partial amputation, soft tissues remain attached. A degloving injury is a specific form of amputation that involves unraveling of skin from the hand, much like partial removal of a glove.

When a part of the body is completely avulsed (ie, amputated)—whether a section of skin or an entire limb—it is important for you to try to preserve the amputated part in optimal condition to maximize the chances of successful reimplantation. Once the patient's injuries have been stabilized, turn your attention to the amputated part, which will also require meticulous care. Follow these guidelines:

- Rinse off any debris on the amputated part using cool, sterile saline.
- Wrap the part loosely in saline-moistened sterile gauze.

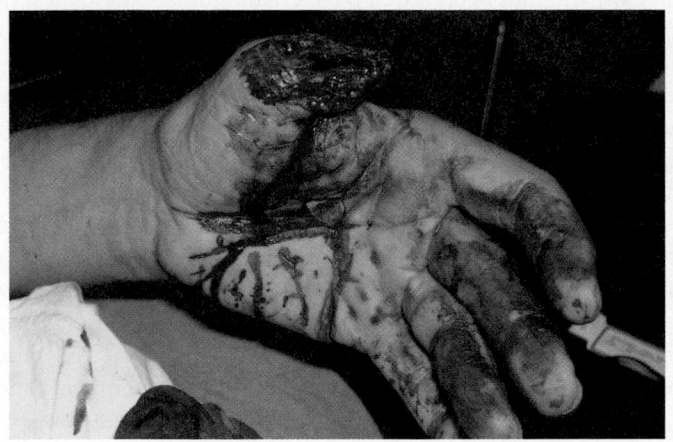

Figure 15 An amputation involving the thumb.

- Seal the amputated part inside a plastic bag, and place it in a cool container (such as a refrigerator or polystyrene foam cooler). Keep it cold, but do not allow it to freeze.
- Never warm an amputated part.
- Never place an amputated part in water.
- Never place an amputated part directly on ice.
- Never use dry ice to cool an amputated part.

Transport the patient and the amputated part as expeditiously as possible. When the amputated part is a limb or part of a limb, notify ED staff in advance of the type of amputation and your estimated time of arrival so that a surgical team can be mobilized while you are en route. Consider whether transport to the nearest reimplantation center is the best option, and whether air medical support is needed.

Words of Wisdom

Never place an amputated part directly on ice because this may cause frostbite and make the part unsalvagable.

■ Bite Wounds

Animal bites and human bites can cause soft-tissue injury. Most people who are bitten by animals do not report the incident to a physician, believing that such bites are not serious; however, in certain instances, they can be very serious, particularly if the animal has certain types of infections. The mouths of dogs and cats are heavily contaminated with virulent bacteria. Cat bites are especially dangerous due to *Pasteurella multocida*, a small gram-negative bacterium that can cause a host of dangerous clinical conditions in humans, including epiglottitis, endocarditis, and brain abscesses. You should consider all such bites as contaminated and potentially infected wounds that may require antibiotics, tetanus prophylaxis, and suturing **Figure 16**. Occasionally, dog bites result in mangled, complex wounds that require surgical repair.

Bites from humans most commonly occur on the hand. The human mouth, more so than even the dog's or cat's mouth,

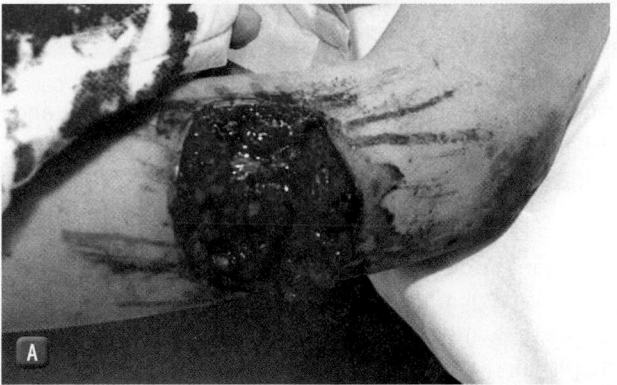

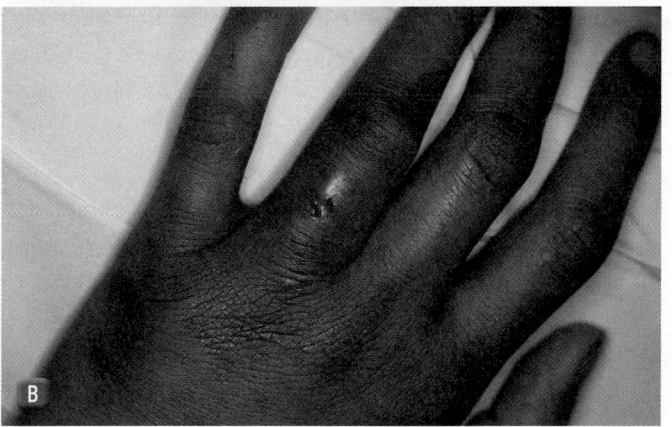

Figure 16 Small animal bite wounds should be examined at the hospital because these wounds are heavily contaminated with virulent bacteria. **A.** Dog bite. **B.** Cat bite.

contains an exceptionally wide range of virulent bacteria and viruses. Infection can be caused by multiple types of bacteria. For this reason, you should regard any human bite that has penetrated the skin as a serious injury. Infection can occur due to a delay in treatment. Similarly, any laceration caused by a human tooth can result in a serious, spreading infection.

Bites can also be caused by spiders and insects. Such bites are discussed in the chapter, *Environmental Emergencies*.

Special Populations

When you are assessing and managing a very young child or older person with an animal or human bite, remember that these patients are more susceptible to infection.

Assessment and Management

In the case of an animal bite, place a dry, sterile dressing over the wound and provide prompt transport to the ED. If there is gross contamination, irrigation of the wound with sterile water may be considered prior to applying a dressing. If an arm or leg is injured, splint that extremity. Often, the patient will be extremely upset and frightened, a situation that calls for calm reassurance on your part.

In addition, find out and document when the bite occurred, and note the type of animal the bite is from. If the bite is from a human, note that, and note what led to the biting incident.

A major concern with dog bites is the spread of *rabies*, an acute, fatal viral infection of the central nervous system that can affect all warm-blooded animals. Although rabies is extremely rare today, particularly with widespread inoculation of pets, it still exists. Once a person shows signs of rabies infection, it is almost always fatal. Stray dogs that have not been inoculated can be carriers of the disease, as can any mammal—squirrels, bats, foxes, skunks, and raccoons. The virus is in the saliva of a <u>rabid</u> or infected animal and is transmitted through biting or through licking an open wound. Infection can be prevented in

a person who has been bitten by such an animal only by a series of special vaccine injections that must be initiated soon after the bite. Because animals that have rabies do not always show it immediately in their behavior, a person's only chance to avoid the vaccine is to find the animal and turn it over to the health department for observation, testing, or both. Refer to your local animal control procedures.

Children, particularly young ones, may be seriously injured or even killed by dogs. The dogs are not always vicious or rabid; sometimes, the child unknowingly provoked the animal. However, you must assume that the dog may turn and attack you as well. Therefore, you should not enter the scene until the animal has been secured by the police or an animal control officer. Then you may carry out the necessary emergency care and transport the child to the ED.

The emergency treatment for human bites consists of the following steps:

1. Promptly control all bleeding, and apply a dry, sterile dressing.
2. Immobilize the area with a splint or bandage.
3. Provide transport to the ED for surgical cleansing of the wound and antibiotic therapy.

Most jurisdictions require health care providers to report all animal bites to the appropriate authority, which is typically the ED physician. Human bites may require notification of the authorities because they are a form of battery. Paramedics should know the local reporting requirements, as failure to report any type of bite can lead to fines or other legal actions against the health care provider.

YOU *are the Medic*   PART 4

Knowing that dangerous levels of metabolic waste have likely accumulated in your patient's lower extremities, you and your partner place tourniquets at the proximal end of each leg. IV lines of normal saline are in place, and nearly 50 mEq of sodium bicarbonate have been infused. Your patient is still receiving oxygen and is alert. Police rescue personnel are in place to use a hydraulic lift to free the patient.

Recording Time: 10 Minutes

Respirations	24 breaths/min, adequate
Pulse	110 beats/min, radial pulses
Skin	Pale, warm, dry
Blood pressure	148/98 mm Hg
Oxygen saturation (Spo$_2$)	98%
Pupils	Equal, reactive

7. What changes might you expect as soon as the car is lifted off the patient?
8. Explain the importance of rapid, immediate transport following extrication.

Crush Syndrome

When an area of the body is trapped for longer than 4 hours and arterial blood flow is compromised, <u>crush syndrome</u> can develop Table 3 . When muscles are crushed beyond repair, tissue necrosis develops and leads to release of harmful products, a process known as <u>rhabdomyolysis</u>. As muscle cells are destroyed, they experience an influx of water, sodium chloride, and calcium from extracellular fluid. In addition, the body develops an efflux of potassium, phosphate, lactic acid, <u>myoglobin</u>, thromboplastin, creatine, and creatine kinase. The oppressing force prevents the return of blood from the injured body part, so the release of these products into the systemic circulation does not occur until *after* the limb is freed from entrapment. For this reason, rescuers must intervene *before* lifting the crushing object off the body.

Crush syndrome has been widely studied in recent years. In January 1995, a massive earthquake occurred in the southern part of Hyogo Prefecture, Japan, producing 41,000 casualties and 5,500 deaths. When researchers evaluated 372 patients who were diagnosed with crush syndrome, they found that most had lower extremity injuries that led to the development of crush syndrome. Upper extremity injuries and trunk entrapment also caused some cases of crush syndrome, albeit to a much lesser extent.

Freeing the limb or other body part from entrapment not only results in release of by-products of metabolism and harmful products of tissue destruction, but also involves the potential for cardiac arrest. In prolonged entrapment, "smiling death" may occur if providers do not take proactive measures. In this situation, the trapped person is alert and conversing with rescuers; however, when the entrapped body part is freed, cardiac arrest is almost instantaneous.

Renal failure is another serious complication that may develop after release of the crushing force. <u>Glomerular filtration</u> can be impaired when the kidneys do not receive enough blood, such as when hypotension develops from bleeding. In addition, the release of large quantities of myoglobin into the central circulation can clog the filtering tubules. The high levels of acids and phosphates can directly damage the kidneys. This problem is compounded by the development of oxygen free radicals. These products travel throughout the affected area, scavenging oxygen molecules and damaging and destroying cells that might otherwise survive the initial injury.

Life-threatening dysrhythmias may also develop from increased blood potassium levels (<u>hyperkalemia</u>). <u>Hyperphos-</u><u>phatemia</u> can lead to calcifications that can interfere with normal blood flow and normal nervous tissue function. Increased levels of uric acid, lactic acid, and potassium may also cause metabolic acidosis.

Assessment and Management

The first issue to consider when you are dealing with crush syndrome is scene safety. Given that most instances of crush syndrome involve building collapse, rescuers face a serious risk. Interaction with technical rescue professionals will often be necessary when you are called to the scene of a collapsed building, irrespective of whether the cause was a natural or human-made disaster. On the scene of an intentional explosion, there is an added danger of a secondary device. You must work closely with law enforcement officials to determine the relative risk to everyone at the scene.

After scene safety has been ensured, the first step is for you to conduct as much of the primary assessment as possible given the nature of the entrapment. If debris can be removed by hand, it should be cleared away on gaining access to the patient. Larger items may require removal by technical rescue teams; removal should be conducted after intervention from caregivers, particularly if the patient has been trapped for longer than 4 hours.

Renal failure—a key complication of crush syndrome—can be prevented with aggressive fluid therapy. In some cases, 8 to 24 L has been provided in the first day to prevent kidney failure. In the field setting, IV access should be obtained before removing the object. Although two large-bore IV lines should be established, the entrapment scenario may rule out typical IV sites. If access to the extremities is not possible, you can establish access at the external jugular veins. When available, a sternal intraosseous needle can be inserted in unresponsive patients.

Once IV access is established, normal saline should be infused. Lactated Ringer's solution contains potassium, so it is not recommended for use in cases of crush syndrome.

Alkalinizing the blood and urine with sodium bicarbonate helps prevent kidney failure, treats hyperkalemia, and reverses metabolic acidosis. High potassium levels released from damaged muscles can be expected on removal of the crushing item. To prevent this complication, sodium bicarbonate may be administered as part of the IV fluid. Mannitol may be used for its diuretic effect. Furosemide is not indicated because it acidifies the urine. If pretreatment with medications is not possible, you should apply a tourniquet above the crush site. The tourniquet will not prevent crush syndrome, but it will reduce some of the reperfusion damage.

Severe hyperkalemia may be treated with 25 mL of $D_{50}W$ followed by 10 units of regular insulin IV. Although caregivers in the field typically do not administer insulin, a medical team may potentially be deployed to the site equipped to provide additional medications. Calcium chloride is not indicated to treat hyperkalemia except in cases of significant dysrhythmia.

Once the patient is freed, rapid transport is indicated. En route to the facility, you should complete a rapid exam and care for injuries not treated on scene. Open injuries can be

---

Table 3 The Progression of Crush Syndrome

1. A body part is trapped for more than 4 hours.
2. Rhabdomyolysis occurs.
3. The trapped body part is freed.
4. By-products of metabolism and harmful products from tissue destruction are released, possibly resulting in cardiac arrest, dysrhythmias, kidney damage, hyperkalemia, and hyperphosphatemia.

handled with dressings and bandaging, and fractures can be splinted, if time permits. Be prepared to administer additional fluids as indicated by patient condition or via online medical direction. Obtain vital signs every 5 minutes at a minimum. Attach an ECG monitor to detect dysrhythmias caused by acidosis, hyperkalemia, hypotension, or other related conditions.

ED care for crush syndrome includes maintaining a urine output of at least 300 mL/h. Additional medications include amiloride, a potassium-sparing diuretic. Allopurinol is a xanthine oxidase inhibitor that will ideally be administered before reperfusion or quickly thereafter. Hemodialysis may help preserve renal function in nonseptic patients. A tetanus toxoid booster may be administered.

Amputation of unsalvageable limbs may occur in the ED. In some cases, a mangled extremity must be amputated on scene to facilitate extrication. When this procedure is performed in the field by a surgeon who has been brought to the scene, there is a higher risk for infection. The benefit must clearly outweigh the risk to warrant this step. Except in the most desperate situations, an on-scene emergency practitioner (physician, osteopath, or authorized physician assistant) should perform the field amputation.

When you transport the patient, consult with medical control regarding the use of a hyperbaric chamber. The physician may opt to have the patient undergo hyperbaric oxygen therapy to aid in tissue recovery and facilitate management of anaerobic bacteria. Hyperbaric therapy, especially when performed early in the course of care, has been shown to decrease muscle necrosis for patients with crush injuries and decrease muscle edema.

Compartment Syndrome

Compartment syndrome develops when edema and swelling result in increased pressure within a closed soft-tissue compartment. Because the tissues can stretch only so far, pressure begins to increase within the compartment, which in turn leads to compromised circulation. Compartment syndrome commonly develops in the extremities and may occur in conjunction with either open or closed injuries. As pressure develops, delivery of nutrients and oxygen is impaired and by-products of normal metabolism accumulate. The longer this situation persists, the greater the chance for tissue necrosis.

Assessment and Management

Compartment syndrome presents with the six Ps: Pain, Paresthesia, Paresis, Pressure, Passive stretch pain, and Pulselessness. Many of these signs may be delayed or nonspecific. Distal perfusion, sensation, and motor function may be intact.

Compartment syndrome that persists for more than 8 hours carries a serious risk for death of local tissues. In such cases, disfiguring débridement. There is also a risk of sepsis. In-hospital intervention includes **fasciotomy**, or incision of the skin and underlying soft tissue with a scalpel. In the upper extremity, this limb-saving procedure can prevent a **Volkmann contracture**—a deformity of the hand, fingers, and wrist resulting from damage to the forearm muscles—and preserve cutaneous sensation.

High-Pressure Injection Injuries

High-pressure injection injuries occur when a foreign material is forcefully injected into soft tissue. The typical scenario involves a tool or machine failure in which liquid or air was compressed and suddenly released from the hose, tool, or other device. Hydraulic tools used to perform patient extrication from entrapment within a crashed vehicle are an example, with some systems using 10,000 psi (pounds per square inch) or greater. Other examples include high-pressure systems used to paint automobiles and to clean surfaces. A force as small as 100 psi can break the skin while 5,100 psi is able to penetrate both clothing and skin.

Injury results directly from the injected material entering the body under great pressure. Acute and chronic inflammation occur following the injection. Damage arises from the direct insult, chemical inflammation, ischemia from compressed blood vessels, and secondary infection. Inflammation tends to be most severe when fuel or paint is injected into the soft tissues. However, it is possible that the patient may experience no pain at all and continue to work. In some cases, the product is able to be absorbed into the body, leading to systemic complications.

Whereas the injuries often appear innocuous, the rate of amputations related to high-pressure injection injuries is approximately 50%. Paint solvent injected into the tissue increases the risk of amputation.

Assessment and Management

The assessment process for this unique form of injury is similar to that performed for any other type of injury—perform a primary assessment, address any life threats, and determine the level of severity. Once the basics are complete and time permits, there are some specific considerations when you are caring for a patient injured by high-pressure machinery or equipment. Question the patient about the nature of the injury. Determine what type of equipment was being used and at what pressure the foreign material was under during the circumstances surrounding the injury. An owner's manual may be of assistance if available. Ask about the type of fluid used for the operation. It is important to pass this information on to the receiving ED physician because certain fluids result in a higher rate of amputation.

Carefully inspect the injury to determine the extent of visibly damaged tissue. Understand that the greatest amount of injury is often under the tissue involved. Seemingly innocuous injuries can lead to amputation, and, thus, you should err on the side of caution and transport the patient for further evaluation. Palpate the affected area for signs of edema and compare the affected area with the uninjured side. Subcutaneous emphysema may be present and it is possible to detect crepitus at the site of injury. Because the hand is the most commonly injured site for high-pressure injection, assess capillary refill, ability to move the fingers, and distal sensation to determine whether there is distal neurovascular compromise.

Treatment for high-pressure injection injuries is typically limited in the prehospital setting. Gently irrigate any open wounds with normal saline. Dress and bandage open injuries as indicated by patient presentation. In some cases, pain management will be indicated. Consult your local protocols to determine the appropriate medication and dosage on the basis of patient presentation. Depending on the type of material injected, the injury may require emergent surgery in an effort to prevent amputation. Gathering adequate information and relaying it to the ED staff can greatly aid the chances for reduced morbidity. Do not underestimate the importance of this aspect of caring for a patient with a high-pressure injection injury.

Pathophysiology, Assessment, and Management of Soft-Tissue Injuries to Specific Anatomic Sites

Soft-tissue injuries that involve the face and neck, thorax, or abdomen deserve special attention. Because the underlying structures in these regions are vital to life, additional concerns arise when they are involved in a traumatic event.

Facial and Neck Injuries

Injuries to the face and neck may involve the airway or large blood vessels. Airway compromise can arise from substantial bleeding or disruption of soft tissue. In such cases, suctioning and patient positioning may become necessary to maintain airway patency. Open injuries involving the jugular or carotid vessels can result in exsanguination if they are not rapidly addressed. These factors, combined with the psychological impact of facial damage, can create challenging scenarios.

Assessment and Management

As always, the airway is the first priority. Immediate assessment of patency, protection, and flow of oxygen with removal of carbon dioxide is paramount.

Suction secretions or blood as indicated by patient presentation. Ensure delivery of high-flow oxygen with a nonrebreathing mask or, if ventilations are compromised, with a bag-mask device. More invasive management may require use of an advanced airway such as an endotracheal tube, a Combitube, or a laryngeal mask airway. When neither ventilation nor intubation is possible, a surgical airway is indicated.

Control of bleeding can be accomplished while airway control is underway. If only one EMS provider is available, bleeding control is addressed only after ensuring an open airway. Manage significant bleeding by applying bulky dressings and direct pressure. Open wounds to the neck require occlusive dressings to prevent air emboli. Realign avulsed skin along the face or neck to its original anatomic position, if possible.

Thoracic Injuries

Thoracic injuries that appear minor may lead you to believe that minimal trauma is present. This is a serious mistake. In reality, gunshot and stab wounds may present as small openings and yet produce internal damage that can quickly lead to death. It is important to determine the MOI while conducting the primary assessment to detect life threats.

Assessment and Management

Assessment includes four steps: inspection, palpation, auscultation, and percussion. Examine the entire chest for signs of visible injury. Listen to breath sounds in at least two sites on each side of the chest. If breath sounds are diminished or absent on one side, suspect a pneumothorax. Palpate the entire chest wall, noting any abnormalities. Subcutaneous emphysema is indicative of a disruption in the tracheobronchial tree. Percussion along the chest wall can help you differentiate between a pneumothorax and a hemothorax—either of which can lead to the patient's death.

Open wounds to the thorax require the application of an occlusive dressing to prevent a pneumothorax or at least stop its progression. Tape the dressing on only three sides to allow air to escape. Failure to provide a small opening for relief of pressure can result in a tension pneumothorax, which can be fatal.

Abdominal Injuries

Abdominal injuries range from minor abrasions to evisceration. Inspect the abdomen for visible signs of injuries. Palpate the area to identify pain, rigidity, and distention. As the diaphragm travels downward during inspiration, the relative sizes of the thoracic and abdominal cavities change. This process increases the risk of drawing air into the pleural space when an open wound is present.

Assessment and Management

Maintain a high index of suspicion when an abdominal injury is readily evident. Soft-tissue injuries in the abdominal area are typically not the primary concern; rather, the focus should be on any injury to underlying organs and blood vessels. Injury to organs and blood vessels could quickly lead to more serious complications, including death. Specific care of abdominal organ injuries is covered in the chapter, *Abdominal and Genitourinary Trauma*.

YOU *are the Medic* | SUMMARY

1. As the crowd rushes over, you and your partner begin assessing the scene. After you ascertain that the car is stable and that no other risks are a threat to you and your partner, what other scene precautions must be taken?

   Crowd control. Care must be taken to keep bystanders away and to prevent anyone from attempting to lift the car off the patient.

2. After you ensure the scene is safe, what are your next actions?

   Continue with patient assessment, as usual. It is important not to allow disturbing scenes or grotesque injuries to distract you from your organized approach to patient assessment.

3. Controlling the crowd was an important first step in saving your patient's life. What are the most serious risks of lifting the car off the patient without having performed an examination and without having made preparations?

   An important part of patient assessment is listening to the patient and determining the most likely mechanism(s) of injury. Your patient, who is alert and oriented, informed you that he was trapped under the car for at least 3 to 4 hours, enough time for crush syndrome to occur. You and your partner need to infuse normal saline, administer sodium bicarbonate to help prevent kidney failure, treat hyperkalemia, and reverse metabolic acidosis that will likely occur as the by-products of metabolism rush back into the circulation. You will likely want to obtain online medical direction prior to proceeding with extrication to ensure that you are maximally prepared to deal with any of the complications of crush syndrome that develop.

4. What is the significance of the patient's report of not being able to feel his feet?

   This is a good indication that circulation is severely impaired. Precautions must be taken to prevent rapid extrication before treatment or the patient's condition will likely deteriorate rapidly, severely, and potentially fatally.

5. The patient's blood pressure seems within the normal range but medical control instructed you to establish two large-bore IV lines. What reasons might justify this order?

   Infusing saline will help prevent kidney failure and will also maintain access for administration of bicarbonate and other medications as ordered.

6. Assuming the patient has been trapped for several hours, you wish to extricate him and transport him to the hospital as soon as his condition is stable. Medical control does not order any additional medications. What other actions can you take to increase the chances for your patient's survival?

   Placing tourniquets proximally on the legs will slow the release of metabolic waste back to the general circulation, perhaps 'buying' your patient enough time to survive the trip to the hospital.

7. What changes might you expect as soon as the car is lifted off the patient?

   Changes such as a drop in the patient's blood pressure or change in level of consciousness. You may also need to address the response of bystanders or family members to seeing the severely injured limbs (have a blanket on hand).

8. Explain the importance of rapid, immediate transport following extrication.

   Infusion of bicarbonate and fluids is only a partial, temporary solution. Crush syndrome is a serious condition requiring aggressive, expert assessment and in-hospital treatment.

YOU *are the Medic* | SUMMARY, *continued*

EMS Patient Care Report (PCR)

Date: 10-15-2011	Incident No.: 1061	Nature of Call: Man trapped		Location: 639 Trevor Lane	
Dispatched: 1310	En Route: 1310	At Scene: 1314	Transport: 1348	At Hospital: 1352	In Service: 1410

Patient Information

Age: 31 Sex: M Weight (in kg [lb]): 90 kg (198 lb)	Allergies: No known drug allergies Medications: Denies Past Medical History: Denies Chief Complaint: Cannot feel feet, trapped underneath car

Vital Signs

Time: 1319	BP: 142/96	Pulse: 96, strong, regular	Respirations: 22	Spo$_2$: 98%
Time: 1324	BP: 148/98	Pulse: 110	Respirations: 24	Spo$_2$: 98%
Time: 1329	BP: 150/96	Pulse: 100	Respirations: 24	Spo$_2$: 98%
Time: 1334	BP: 146/94	Pulse: 96	Respirations: 22	Spo$_2$: 99%
Time: 1339	BP: 120/82	Pulse: 102	Respirations: 26	Spo$_2$: 97%
Time: 1344	BP: 118/78	Pulse: 106	Respirations: 28	Spo$_2$: 97%
Time: 1349	BP: 112/72	Pulse: 108	Respirations: 30	Spo$_2$: 95%

EMS Treatment
(circle all that apply)

Oxygen @ __15__ L/min via (circle one): NC (NRM) Bag-mask device	Assisted Ventilation	Airway Adjunct	CPR
Defibrillation	Bleeding Control	Bandaging	Splinting	Other: Spinal immobilization, IV

Narrative

9-1-1 dispatched to a report of a man trapped under a car. Upon arrival wife states that she left early this morning while her husband was working on car. Husband states that the car collapsed on him shortly after his wife left at least 4 hours earlier. Pt is alert and oriented, supine on asphalt driveway with legs trapped under Ford Explorer from proximal thigh and downward. Pt reports that he is unable to feel his feet and his legs are hurting. Pt denies any other injuries. Physical exam shows a healthy-appearing physically fit male, pale and anxious but alert. No visible injuries initially.

    Treatment included psychological support, administration of high-concentration oxygen via nonrebreathing mask, and vital signs every 5 minutes. Two large-bore IV lines established with infusion of normal saline and 50 mEq sodium bicarbonate at 1319 hours. Tourniquets applied to proximal legs prior to removing pt from under vehicle. Upon lifting vehicle, pt reported light-headedness and became cool, pale, and diaphoretic. Vital signs changed en route with significant blood pressure drop and increase in pulse rate. Pt remained conscious and alert throughout transport. ECG monitor applied en route shows sinus tachycardia with peaked T waves and unifocal PVCs—about 8-10 per minute. Arrived at St. Catherine's Hospital trauma center at 1352. Pt handed off to trauma team in room 10. Return to service at 1410 hours. **End of report**

Prep Kit

- The skin is a complex organ that fulfills several crucial roles, including maintaining homeostasis, protecting tissue from injury, and regulating temperature.

- The main layers of the skin are the epidermis and the dermis. The epidermis, the outer layer, serves as the principal barrier. The dermis, the inner layer, includes collagen, elastin, and ground substance, which contribute to the skin's strength. It also contains nerve endings, blood vessels, sweat glands, hair follicles, and sebaceous glands.

- The subcutaneous layer lies beneath the dermis and contains adipose tissue. Below the subcutaneous layer is the deep fascia, which offers support and protection to underlying structures such as muscle and bone.

- The skin is arranged in patterns of tautness known as tension lines. Wounds that occur parallel to skin tension lines may remain closed. Wounds that run perpendicular to tension lines may remain open.

- Soft-tissue injuries may be dramatic looking but are seldom the most serious injuries. Do not let them distract you from performing a thorough primary assessment!

- In a closed wound, the skin is not broken but soft tissues beneath the skin are damaged. An example is a bruise. A hematoma (collection of blood beneath the skin) can also form.

- In an open wound, the skin is broken. Such an injury can become infected and can result in serious blood loss. Open wounds include abrasions, lacerations, puncture wounds, avulsions, bites, and amputations.

- In a crush injury, a body part is crushed between two solid objects, resulting in damage to soft tissues and bone. The patient's external appearance may not adequately represent the level of internal damage.

- The first stage of wound healing is cessation of bleeding. The body uses several mechanisms to control bleeding, such as constricting the size of vessels and releasing platelets to form a blood clot.

- The second stage of healing is inflammation, in which additional cells enter the damaged area in an effort to repair it. Epithelialization (creation of a new layer of epithelial cells) occurs, followed by neovascularization (formation of new vessels).

- Wound healing is affected by factors such as the amount of movement the part is subjected to, medications, and medical conditions. A wound is more likely to become infected if it is caused by a human or an animal bite or if a foreign body has been impaled. Pressure injuries can develop when a patient is bedridden or remains on a backboard for too long.

- Signs of infection include redness, pus, warmth, edema, and local discomfort. Gangrene, tetanus, and necrotizing fasciitis are serious infection-related conditions that must be recognized early.

- Observe scene safety before assessing patients with soft-tissue injuries; hazards that caused the injury may still be present. Regardless of how dramatic a soft-tissue injury looks, assess the ABCs first.

- When you are obtaining a patient history, ask about the event that caused the injury, such as whether a weapon was used or whether the patient lost consciousness. Find out when the patient last had a tetanus booster. Pay attention to whether the patient is taking any medications that may affect hemostasis.

- Depending on the mechanism of injury, complete your physical exam en route or at the scene, respectively. Direct your attention to the chief complaint and area of injury, and perform frequent reassessments.

- Document scene findings, including vehicle damage or the caliber of weapon used; patient presentation and position; size, location, depth, and complications of injuries; assessment findings; and interventions.

- Be empathetic to patients with soft-tissue injuries.

- Managing soft-tissue injuries includes controlling bleeding. With closed injuries, follow the ICES mnemonic: Ice, Compression, Elevation, and Splinting.

- When you are managing open wounds, control bleeding and keep the wound as clean as possible by irrigating and using sterile dressings. Try to determine the color and type of bleeding and the amount of blood the patient has lost.

- Dressings and bandages are used to cover the wound, control bleeding, and limit motion. Types of dressings include sterile and nonsterile, occlusive and nonocclusive, adherent and nonadherent, and wet and dry. Types of bandages include roller and gauze, absorbent gauze sponges, elastic, and triangular bandages.

- Medical tape may be used to secure a bandage in place, except for patients with thin skin such as older individuals because it can cause damage on removal. Do not apply dressings too tightly.

- Methods of bleeding control include direct pressure, elevation, immobilization, and tourniquets. Cold compresses may help reduce pain. IV medications may be administered if basic measures do not relieve pain.

- Dressing and bandaging techniques vary for different parts of the body. For example, the shape of the skull and the presence of hair make dressing the scalp challenging.

- Management of an avulsion includes irrigation, gently folding the flap back onto the wound, and applying a dry, sterile compression dressing. If the wound is an amputation, preserve the amputated part and transport it with the patient to the ED.

- Do not remove impaled objects in the field. Instead, stabilize the object in place with a bulky dressing. Control bleeding with direct compression, but do not apply pressure on the object or on the immediately adjacent tissues.

- Animal and human bites can lead to serious infection and must be treated by a physician. Dogs and cats can carry rabies, a fatal viral infection present in their saliva. By law, all animal bites must be reported to the appropriate authority.

- Crush syndrome may develop after a body part has been trapped for more than 4 hours. Necrosis occurs in crushed muscles, and harmful products are released in a process called rhabdomyolysis. Freeing the trapped body part can cause these harmful products to be released into the circulation, which can prove fatal. Kidney damage, cardiac arrest, and dysrhythmias can also result.

- Patients who have been trapped for a prolonged period of time must be managed before being freed from the crushing object because this approach improves their chances of survival after experiencing crush syndrome. Aggressive fluid resuscitation can help prevent kidney failure. Normal saline should be infused. Administration of sodium bicarbonate may help prevent an efflux of potassium. Contact online medical control before treatment and rapidly transport the patient once freed.

- Compartment syndrome results when pressure increases inside a closed soft-tissue compartment. Tissue necrosis and sepsis may then develop. Patients present with all or some of the six Ps: Pain, Paresthesia, Paresis, Pressure, Passive stretch pain, and Pulselessness.

- Blasts (explosions) can result in soft-tissue injuries. Blast injuries can include pulmonary damage such as tension pneumothorax and pulmonary contusion, abdominal trauma such as ruptured organs and internal hemorrhage, damage to the ears, and penetrating wounds. Use the DCAP-BTLS guideline to assess the patient rapidly.

- High-pressure injection injuries involve the injection of foreign material into soft tissue. High-pressure injection may cause acute or chronic inflammation, even leading to systemic complications or amputation. Gathering and relaying appropriate information to the receiving facility can potentially reduce mortality.

- Soft-tissue injuries of the face, neck, thorax, and abdomen deserve special attention because these areas contain vital structures. Do not underestimate the seriousness of these injuries, and maintain a high index of suspicion.

■ Vital Vocabulary

abrasion An injury in which a portion of the body is denuded of the epidermis by scraping or rubbing.

adipose Fat tissue.

amputation An injury in which part of the body is completely severed.

avulsion An injury that leaves a piece of skin or other tissue partially or completely torn away from the body.

bandage Material used to secure a dressing in place.

chemotactic factors The factors that cause cells to migrate into an area.

closed wound An injury in which damage occurs beneath the skin or mucous membrane but the surface remains intact.

collagen Protein that gives tensile strength to the connective tissues of the body.

compartment syndrome A condition that develops when edema and swelling result in increased pressure within soft tissues, causing circulation to be compromised, possibly resulting in tissue necrosis.

contusion A bruise; an injury that causes bleeding beneath the skin but does not break the skin.

crush injury An injury in which the body or part of the body is crushed, preventing tissue function and, possibly, resulting in permanent tissue damage.

crush syndrome Significant metabolic derangement that can lead to renal failure and death. It develops when crushed extremities or other body parts remain trapped for prolonged periods.

deep fascia A dense layer of fibrous tissue below the subcutaneous tissue; composed of tough bands of tissue that ensheath muscles and other internal structures.

degloving A traumatic injury that results in the soft tissue of a part of the body being drawn downward like a glove being removed.

degranulate To release granules into the surrounding tissue.

dermis The inner layer of skin, containing hair follicle roots, glands, blood vessels, and nerves.

dressing Material used to directly cover a wound.

ecchymosis Extravasation of blood under the skin to produce a "black-and-blue" mark.

elastin A protein that gives the skin its elasticity.

epidermis The outermost layer of the skin.

epithelialization The formation of fresh epithelial tissue to heal a wound.

erythema Reddening of the skin.

fasciotomy A surgical procedure that cuts away fascia to relieve pressure.

gangrene An infection commonly caused by *Clostridium perfringens*. The result is tissue destruction and gas production that may lead to death.

glomerular filtration The first step in the formation of urine; calculated to determine renal function.

granulocytes Cells that contain granules.

ground substance Material between cells.

hematoma A localized collection of blood in the soft tissues as a result of injury or a broken blood vessel.

high-pressure injection injuries Types of injuries that occurs when a foreign material is forcefully injected into soft tissue.

homeostasis The tendency to constancy or stability in the body's internal environment.

hyperkalemia An increased level of potassium in the blood.

hyperphosphatemia An increased level of phosphate in the blood.

hypertrophic scar An abnormal scar with excess collagen that does not extend over the wound margins.

incision A wound usually made deliberately, as in surgery; a clean cut, as opposed to a laceration.

integument The skin.

keloid scar An abnormal scar commonly found in people with darkly pigmented skin. It extends over the wound margins.

laceration A wound made by tearing or cutting tissues.

lymphangitis Inflammation of a lymph channel.

lymphocytes White blood cells that function to remove invading pathogens.

macrophages Cells that are responsible for protecting the body against infection.

melanin The pigment that gives skin its color.

mucopolysaccharide gel A key component of ground substance that is a polysaccharide that forms complexes with proteins.

myoglobin A protein found in muscle that is released into the circulation after a crush injury or other muscle damage and whose presence in the circulation may produce kidney damage.

necrotizing fasciitis Death of tissue from bacterial infection, caused by more than one infecting organism—most commonly, *Staphylococcus aureus* and hemolytic streptococci; this condition has a high mortality rate.

neovascularization Development of new blood vessels to aid in healing injured soft tissue.

open wound An injury in which there is a break in the surface of the skin or the mucous membrane, exposing deeper tissue to potential contamination.

pedicle A narrow strip of tissue by which an avulsed piece of tissue remains connected to the body.

puncture wound A stab injury from a pointed object, such as a nail or a knife.

rabid Describes an animal that is infected with rabies.

rhabdomyolysis The destruction of muscle tissue leading to a release of potassium and myoglobin.

scar revision A surgical procedure to improve the appearance of a scar, reestablish function, or correct disfigurement from soft-tissue damage, surgical incision, or lesion.

sebaceous gland The gland located in the dermis that secretes sebum.

sebum An oily substance secreted by the sebaceous glands.

subcutaneous Beneath the skin.

tension lines The pattern of tautness of the skin, which is arranged over body structures and affects how well wounds heal.

Volkmann contracture Deformity of the hand, fingers, and wrist resulting from damage to forearm muscles; develops from muscle ischemia and is associated with compartment syndrome.

Assessment in Action

You and your partner are dispatched to a severe injury at a house under renovation. As you pull up to the scene, all appears to be safe and a man is waving you over to the site where a man about 50 years old is sitting on the stairs with a bloody towel wrapped around his lower arm. As he watches you approach, he is shaking his head and pointing to a bag on the ground next to him. He is very pale and diaphoretic but alert as he tells you he was using a table saw. "I took the blade guard off, can't see the cut of the wood with that thing in the way. The blade must have hit a knot and the wood kicked back. Next thing I know, my hand! My hand! It's in the bag, inside the glove."

1. Your patient is alert and has an open, clear airway. He is breathing without difficulty and has equal chest movement. No other injuries are noted and he denies having any significant medical history. Your next action should be to:
   A. keep the arm wrapped and transport, with the severed hand, to the hospital.
   B. retrieve the severed hand and examine and bandage it right away.
   C. unwrap the injured limb, checking first for severe bleeding.
   D. examine the table saw for additional pieces of his hand.

2. Unwrapping his arm, you see a clean severing of his hand just distal to his wrist. You see some bone exposed and you are also surprised to see that most of the bleeding has stopped. This cessation of bleeding is most likely due to:
   A. the pressure he applied to the wound.
   B. the clean cut of the vessels allowing them to retain their ability to contract.
   C. the large amount of blood already lost.
   D. the crushing of the blood vessels.

3. The wound where the hand was severed is barely bleeding. The best way to control the bleeding is by applying:
   A. direct pressure with a dry, sterile dressing.
   B. direct pressure with a moist, sterile dressing.
   C. sterile 4×4s bandaged loosely over the wound.
   D. a tourniquet close to the wound.

4. In addition to a pressure dressing, the patient's arm should be:
   A. immobilized at his side.
   B. splinted and elevated.
   C. left with a pressure bandage only.
   D. compressed at the site of the brachial artery pressure point.

5. Retrieving the patient's gloved hand, you should first:
   A. gently cut away the glove.
   B. leave the severed hand inside the glove.
   C. cut the glove open, leave the hand inside, and place it on ice.
   D. pack sterile dressings inside the glove to minimize blood loss.

6. In preparation for transport, the patient's arm is bandaged and the hand is prepared by:
   A. placing the entire gloved hand inside a plastic bag and placing it on ice.
   B. placing the hand inside moist, sterile dressings and then on ice.
   C. placing the hand inside moist, sterile dressings and then in a sealed plastic bag, and then inside a cooler or loosely wrapped in cool packs.
   D. placing the hand inside dry, sterile dressings and then in a sealed plastic bag, and then inside a cooler or loosely wrapped in cool packs.

Additional Questions

7. After using a stretch gauze to keep sterile dressing in place on a patient's lacerated forearm, he tells you that his hand feels tingly. His hand distal to the bandage is slightly paler than the noninjured hand and cool to the touch. What is your next action?

8. Explain the difference between nonadherent and occlusive dressings. In which types of injuries would each be the best choice?

Burns

National EMS Education Standard Competencies

Trauma

Integrates assessment findings with principles of epidemiology and pathophysiology to formulate a field impression to implement a comprehensive treatment/disposition plan for an acutely injured patient.

Soft-Tissue Trauma

Recognition and management of

- Wounds (see chapter, *Soft-Tissue Trauma*)
- Burns
  - Electrical (pp 1595-1597)
  - Chemical (pp 1590-1595)
  - Thermal (pp 1578-1579; 1590)
- Chemicals in the eye and on the skin (pp 1590-1595)

Pathophysiology, assessment, and management of

- Wounds
  - Avulsions (see chapter, *Soft-Tissue Trauma*)
  - Bite wounds (see chapter, *Soft-Tissue Trauma*)
  - Lacerations (see chapter, *Soft-Tissue Trauma*)
  - Puncture wounds (see chapter, *Soft-Tissue Trauma*)
  - Incisions (see chapter, *Soft-Tissue Trauma*)
- Burns
  - Electrical (pp 1595-1597)
  - Chemical (pp 1590-1595)
  - Thermal (pp 1578-1579; 1590)
  - Radiation (pp 1599-1600)
- High-pressure injection (see chapter, *Soft-Tissue Trauma*)
- Crush syndrome (see chapter, *Soft-Tissue Trauma*)

Knowledge Objectives

1. Describe the anatomy and physiology of the skin, including the layers of the skin. (pp 1575-1577)
2. Describe the anatomy of the surface of the eye. (p 1577)
3. Summarize the general pathophysiology of burn injury. (pp 1577-1581)
4. Describe five types of thermal burns. (pp 1578-1579)
5. Discuss the symptoms of burn shock. (pp 1577-1578)
6. Identify some of the warning signs of intentional burns associated with the potential abuse of children, elders, and people with disabilities. (pp 1578-1579)
7. Define and describe the characteristics of superficial, partial-thickness, and full-thickness burns. (pp 1579-1580)

8. Describe the pathophysiology of inhalation burns. (pp 1580-1581)
9. Summarize the safety concerns that must be addressed during the size-up of a burn scene. (pp 1582-1583)
10. Summarize the primary and secondary assessment processes for a burn patient. (pp 1583-1586)
11. Compare three different methods for determining burn severity. (p 1584)
12. Contrast the burn severity classification for infants and children with that for adults. (pp 1584-1586)
13. List the referral criteria for transporting a patient to a burn unit. (pp 1584-1586)
14. Discuss emergency medical care of a patient with a burn injury, including specific airway management techniques, fluid resuscitation techniques, and pain management. (pp 1586-1589)
15. State the Consensus formula, and discuss its use as it pertains to the prehospital environment, including types of solutions to use and amounts to administer during the prehospital phase. (pp 1588-1589)
16. Describe the management of thermal burns, including the use of sterile dressings. (p 1590)
17. Describe the management of burn shock. (pp 1589-1590)
18. Describe the management of inhalation burns. (p 1590)
19. Describe the pathophysiology, assessment, and management of chemical burns of the skin and eye. (pp 1590-1595)
20. Describe the pathophysiology, assessment, and management of electrical burns. (pp 1595-1597)
21. Describe the pathophysiology, assessment, and management of radiation burns. (pp 1599-1600)
22. Discuss the special considerations involved in the treatment of pediatric and geriatric patients. (p 1600)
23. Summarize some of the long-term consequences of burn injury on the patient's quality of life and on the paramedic's psychological well-being. (p 1601)

Skills Objectives

1. Demonstrate how to care for a burn. (pp 1586-1590)
2. Demonstrate the emergency medical care of a patient with a thermal burn. (p 1590)
3. Demonstrate the emergency medical care of a patient with an inhalation burn. (p 1593)
4. Demonstrate the emergency medical care of a patient with a chemical burn. (pp 1590-1595)
5. Demonstrate the emergency medical care of a patient with an electrical burn. (pp 1595-1597)
6. Demonstrate the emergency medical care of a patient with a radiation burn. (pp 1599-1600)

Introduction

Approximately 80% of all civilian fire-related deaths occur in residential constructions **Figure 1**. The incidence of burn injuries and death in the United States has decreased somewhat with the advent of stricter building codes and widespread use of smoke detectors. Other effective burn prevention techniques include reducing domestic water heater temperatures to 120°F (49°C) to prevent severe scalds and making disposable lighters child-safe. While national trends demonstrate a consistent decrease in fire deaths, more than 3,000 people still die of fire-related causes each year. Children younger than 5 years and elderly people are at particularly high risk of dying in fires.

Just as code enforcement and smoke detectors have decreased fire-related deaths, our ability to treat large burns effectively has steadily improved. Before the medical advances of the 20th century, death was almost inevitable when more than one third of the body was burned. Now, however, better understanding of "burn shock," advances in the use of fluid therapy and antibiotics, improved ability to excise dead tissue,

and the use of biologic dressings to aid early wound closure have vastly improved burn care. The formation of specialized teams to resuscitate patients from burn shock, delay infection, and achieve wound closure has resulted in impressive gains in survival rates.

Deaths and serious injuries also occur from electrical and chemical burns. As a consequence, numerous public safety campaigns have focused on the use of smoke detectors and the dangers that surround the use of flammable liquids, petroleum products, solvents, propane, and fireworks.

Although you probably won't see moderate or severe burns on a daily basis, you will encounter some serious thermal burn injuries during your career, and you might encounter serious electrical, chemical, and radiation injuries as well. Accurate recognition of the severity of burn injuries can dramatically enhance the care of burned patients by allowing you to institute proper emergency care. It is important to understand the treatment for burn shock. In addition, contacting the receiving facility en route will allow burn specialists to provide triage over the phone and will allow them to prepare for the incoming patient.

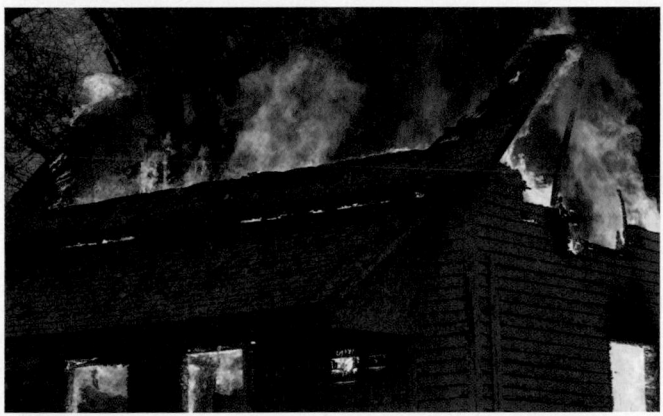

Figure 1 Of all civilian fire fatalities, approximately 80%–the vast majority–occur in the home.

Anatomy and Physiology of the Skin

As discussed in the chapter, *Soft-Tissue Trauma*, the human skin, also known as the **integument**, is the largest and one of the most complex organs in the body. It has a crucial role in maintaining **homeostasis** (balance) within the body. The skin is durable, flexible, and usually able to repair itself. It varies in thickness from almost 1 cm on the heel to 1 mm on the eyelid. The skin has four functions:

- It acts as an all-purpose fortress to protect the underlying tissue from injury and exposure to extremes of temperature, ultraviolet radiation, mechanical forces, toxic chemicals, and invading microorganisms.
- The skin aids in temperature regulation (**thermoregulation**), preventing heat loss when the core body temperature starts to fall and facilitating heat loss when core temperature rises.

YOU *are the Medic*   PART 1

Your patient is standing at the entrance to the office of the gas station. His blistered, reddened arm is stretched out in front of him. His face and neck appear flushed. The gas station owner walks him over to the ambulance as you slow to a stop. "He pulled into the station and before I could say anything, he opened the hood of the car. All of a sudden there was a big burst of steam. I guess a hose blew. It got him pretty good." The scene is safe and both you and your partner have appropriate personal protective equipment (PPE) in place. Your patient is alert and oriented and, grimacing in pain, he tells you in a quiet raspy voice that he can't stand the pain in his arm.

1. **Your next steps should include which actions?**

2. **Based on just the information given so far, would transport of this patient be a low priority ("stay and play") or a high priority ("load and go") at this time?**

- As a watertight seal, the skin prevents excessive loss of water from the body and drying of tissues, thereby helping maintain the chemical stability of the internal environment. Without skin, a person would become water-logged after the first rain and would resemble a prune after the first hot day of summer.
- The skin serves as a sense organ, keeping the brain informed about the external environment. Changes in temperature and sensations of pain are mediated through skin sense receptors.

Significant damage to the skin may make the body vulnerable to bacterial invasion, temperature instability, and major disturbances of fluid balance. People who survive serious burns must live with the ramifications of the damage to large portions of the integument:

- Difficulty with thermoregulation
- Inability to sweat from the scarred portions of the skin
- Impaired vasoconstriction and vasodilation in the areas of severe damage
- Little or no melanin (pigment) in the scar tissue, which makes the skin susceptible to sunburn
- Inability to grow hair on the injured site and little or no sensation in the scarred areas

All of these factors may restrict a person's ability to function even many years after the burn trauma has healed **Figure 2**. Patients who survive serious burns also have a high rate of depression.

Layers of the Skin

To carry out its functions, the skin has a specialized structure **Figure 3**. The skin is composed of two principal layers: the epidermis and the dermis.

The <u>epidermis</u>, or outermost layer, is the body's first line of defense, constituting the major barrier against water, dust, microorganisms, and mechanical stress. The epidermis is itself composed of several layers: an outermost layer of hardened, nonliving cells, which are continuously shed through a process called <u>desquamation</u>, and three inner layers of living cells that constantly divide to give rise to new "dead layer" skin cells. The deeper layers of the epidermis also contain variable numbers of cells bearing <u>melanin</u> granules. The darkness of a person's skin is directly proportional to the amount of melanin present.

Underlying the epidermis is a tough, highly elastic layer of connective tissues called the <u>dermis</u>. The dermis is a complex material composed chiefly of collagen fibers, elastin fibers, and a mucopolysaccharide gel. <u>Collagen</u> is a fibrous protein with a very high tensile strength, so it gives the skin high resistance to breakage under mechanical stress. <u>Elastin</u> imparts elasticity to the skin, allowing it to spring back to its usual contours. The <u>mucopolysaccharide gel</u> gives the skin resistance to compression.

Enclosed within the dermis are several specialized skin structures. Nerve endings mediate the senses of touch, temperature, pressure, and pain, for example. Blood vessels carry oxygen and nutrients to the skin and remove the carbon dioxide and metabolic waste products. <u>Cutaneous</u> blood vessels, which

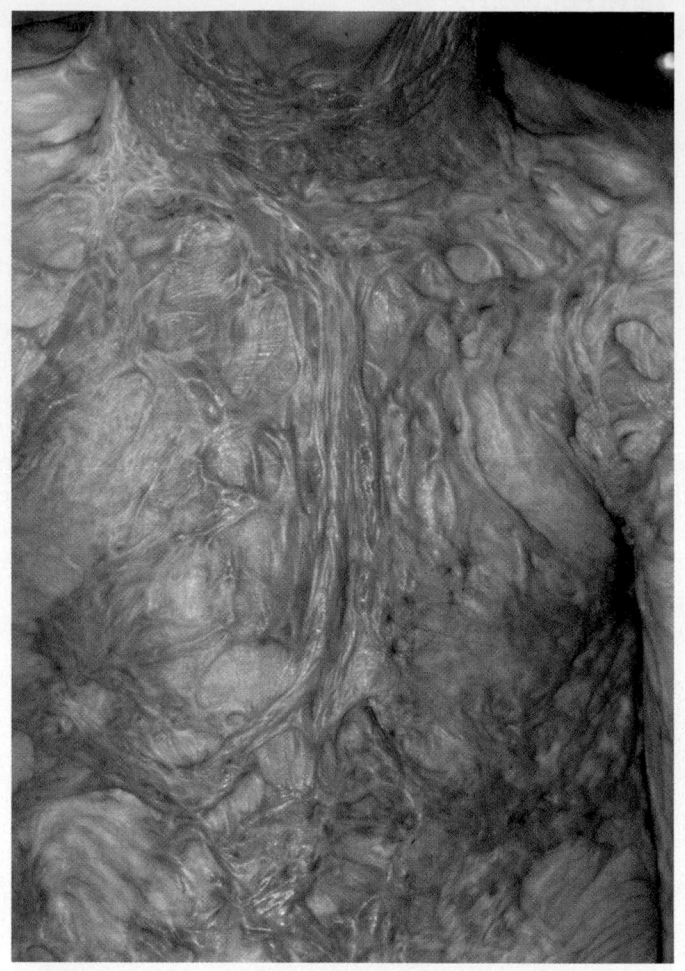

Figure 2 People who survive serious burns must live with the ramifications of their injury.

supply the skin, also serve a crucial role in regulating body temperature by regulating the volume of blood that flows from the body's warm core to its cooler surface.

Also in the dermis, sweat glands produce sweat and discharge it through ducts passing to the surface of the skin in a process regulated by the sympathetic nervous system. Sweat consists of water and salts. The average volume of sweat lost during 24 hours under normal conditions ranges from 500 to 1,000 mL. During strenuous exercise, sweat glands may secrete as much as 1,000 mL in an hour. Evaporation of water from the skin surface is one of the body's major mechanisms for shedding excess heat.

Hair follicles are structures that produce hair and enclose the hair roots. Each follicle contains a single hair. Attached to the hair follicle is a small muscle that, on contraction, causes the follicle to assume a more vertical position. Sensations such as cold and fright stimulate the autonomic nervous system, which in turn brings about contraction of those muscles and results in "gooseflesh." Hairs in each part of the body have definite periods of growth, after which they are shed and replaced; scalp hair, for example, has a life span of 2 to 5 years and grows at an average rate of 1.5 to 3.9 mm per week.

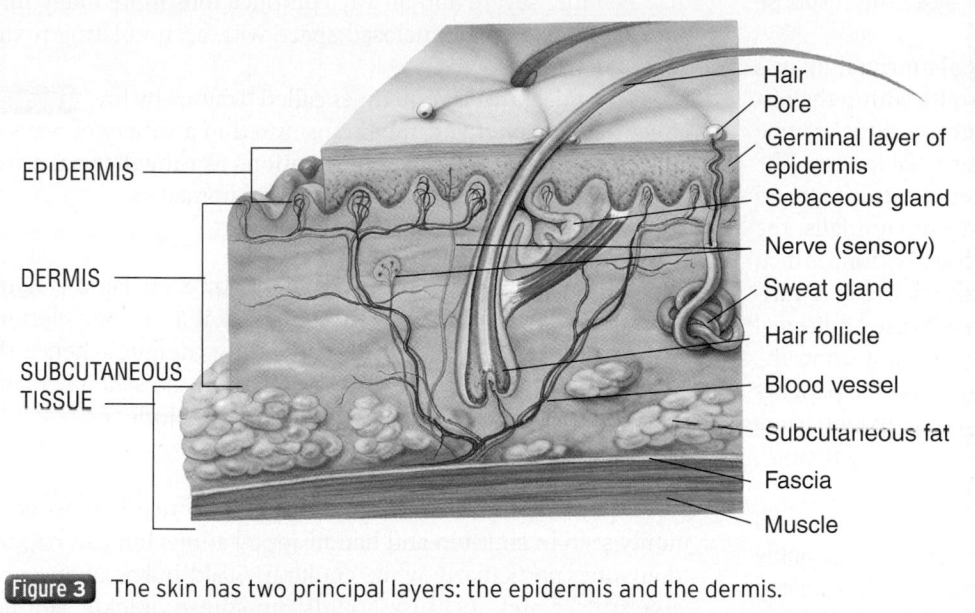

Figure 3 The skin has two principal layers: the epidermis and the dermis.

Labels: EPIDERMIS, DERMIS, SUBCUTANEOUS TISSUE, Hair, Pore, Germinal layer of epidermis, Sebaceous gland, Nerve (sensory), Sweat gland, Hair follicle, Blood vessel, Subcutaneous fat, Fascia, Muscle

Face and Neck Trauma. Clearly, the eyes are sensitive to burn injuries—from a flame, superheated gases, light source (such as a welder's torch), or chemicals. The tear ducts and eyelids combine to constantly lubricate the surface of the eyes **Figure 4** . Unfortunately, intense heat, light, or chemical reactions on the surface of the eye can quickly burn the thin membrane or skin covering the surface of the eye. Ocular damage is a common result of alkali (base) injury: The higher the pH of the substance, the more severe the damage to the eye. When a patient gets a substance like lime in the eyes, the damage is worsened by repeatedly rubbing the eyes as opposed to initiating copious irrigation and essential treatment in the emergency department (ED).

Words of Wisdom

Hair melts when it burns, yet sometimes appears to remain on the patient. When you brush your hand over it, you may find that what you thought was a mustache is now simply a streak of ash. Closely observe nasal hair, eyebrows, and eyelashes in burn patients because damage to them may indicate airway injury. When hair on the arms or legs "falls out" or can be removed without pain, deeper skin structures have been damaged.

◾ Pathophysiology

Burns are diffuse soft-tissue injuries created by destructive energy transfer via radiation, thermal, or electrical energy. The skin serves as a barrier between the environment and the body. When a person is burned, this barrier is destroyed; the victim is now at a high risk for infection, hypothermia, hypovolemia, and shock. Burns to the airway are significant because the loose mucosa in the hypopharynx can swell, leading to complete airway obstruction.

◾ Burn Shock

Burns are not isolated soft-tissue injuries. They can affect the cardiovascular, respiratory, renal, gastrointestinal, hematologic,

At the neck of each hair follicle is a **sebaceous gland** that produces an oily substance called **sebum**. The secretions of the sebaceous glands empty into the hair follicles and ultimately reach the surface of the skin. Sebum is believed to keep the skin supple so it doesn't dry out and crack. When sebaceous glands become obstructed, a hard **comedo** forms, which may serve as the base of an acne pimple.

The tissue beneath the dermis, called the **subcutaneous layer**, consists mainly of **adipose tissue** (fat). Subcutaneous fat insulates the underlying tissues from extremes of heat and cold. It also provides a substantial cushion for underlying structures and serves as an energy reserve for the body.

Finally, beneath the subcutaneous layer are the muscles, tendons, bones, and vital organs. Muscles have thick, fibrous capsules that are prone to hypoxia and anaerobic metabolism in a burn state. Bones are living tissue that can be severely affected by burn injury. Vital organs may also be damaged by thermal, chemical, or electrical energy.

◾ The Eye

The specific anatomy and physiology of the eye is covered in the chapters, *Diseases of the Eyes, Ears, Nose, and Throat* and

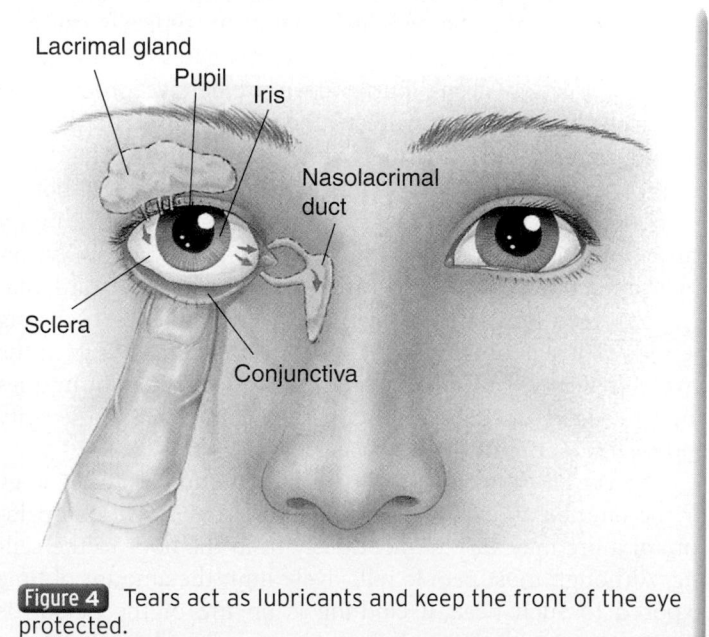

Labels: Lacrimal gland, Pupil, Iris, Nasolacrimal duct, Sclera, Conjunctiva

Figure 4 Tears act as lubricants and keep the front of the eye protected.

and endocrine systems. The most important systemic response to significant burn trauma is burn shock.

Burn shock occurs because of two types of injury: fluid loss across damaged skin and a series of volume shifts within the rest of the body. Capillaries become leaky, so intravascular volume oozes out of the circulation and into the interstitial spaces. The cells of normal tissues then take in increased amounts of salt and water from the fluid around them. As blood pressure falls, the body responds with tachycardia and vasoconstriction, which limits blood flow further and continues the shock cycle. A variety of chemical mediators are released that may cause additional damage and worsen the chain of events. Depending upon the nature of the burn, coagulation disorders may cause the patient's blood to clot more easily, resulting in emboli, or fail to clot, causing excessive bleeding (disseminated intravascular coagulation), as discussed in the chapter, *Hematologic Emergencies*.

Burn shock involves the entire body, not just the area burned. You may have experienced sunburn over a reasonably large surface area, like your back. In addition to the skin-related discomfort from the sunburn, you may have developed chills and nausea and felt sick as a result of the fluid shifts and electrolyte disturbances. This is a mild form of burn shock. Just as in other forms of shock, these changes limit the effective distribution of oxygen and glucose to the tissues and hamper the circulation's ability to remove waste products from healthy and damaged tissues. Adequate fluid resuscitation is essential to avoid the devastating consequences of burn shock.

■ Thermal Burns

Thermal burns can occur when skin is exposed to temperatures higher than 111°F (44°C), or when the heat absorbed exceeds the tissue's capacity to dissipate it. In general, the severity of a thermal injury correlates directly with temperature, concentration, or amount of heat energy possessed by the object or substance, and the duration of exposure. For example, solids generally have higher heat content than gases, so exposure to a hot solid (such as the rack inside an oven) typically causes a more significant burn than exposure to hot gases (such as those coming out of an oven). Burns are a progressive process: the greater the heat energy, the deeper the wound. Superficial burns may injure only the epidermis, while deeper burns extend into or through the dermis, subcutaneous tissue, muscle, and bone.

Exposure time is another important factor. Thermal injury can occur to unresponsive or paralyzed patients from seemingly innocuous heat sources such as heating pads, transcutaneous oxygen sensors, and heat lamps left unattended for long periods. The age of the patient and thickness of the skin in the involved area will affect the burn severity. Concomitant injuries and preexisting medical conditions also complicate the severity and treatment of burn injuries.

It may be difficult to evaluate the amount of heat energy or the amount of exposure time in many cases. The temperature of a fire may vary tremendously from the floor to the ceiling. Although most people reflexively limit the amount of time exposed to such heat, if clothing is on fire or the person is trapped or unresponsive, exposure time will be longer. A burn

may be more severe and airway complications more likely for a patient trapped in an enclosed space with accumulating toxins versus an open space.

A thermal burn is sometimes called "trauma by fire" Figure 5 . However, heat energy can be transmitted in a variety of ways in addition to fire. Many different situations causing thermal burns can pose a safety hazard to responding paramedics.

Flame Burns

Most commonly, thermal burns are caused by open flame. A flame burn is very often a deep burn, especially if a person's clothing catches fire Figure 6 . The fire is fanned by running—hence the adage "stop, drop, and roll" that is taught in the schools. Flame burns may also be associated with inhalation injuries.

Scald Burns

Hot liquids produce scald injuries. A scald burn is most commonly seen in children and handicapped adults but can happen to anyone, particularly while cooking. Scald burns often cover large surface areas because liquids can spread quickly. Hot liquids can soak into clothing and continue to burn until the clothing is removed. Some hot liquids, such as oil and grease, adhere to the skin, causing particularly deep scald injuries.

About 100,000 scald burns result annually from spilled food and beverages. A child may pull a pot or other container of hot liquid off the stove or counter, a toddler may bump into an adult carrying or holding a hot beverage or food, or a toddler may pull the tablecloth, spilling a hot food or beverage off the table.

Contact Burns

Coming in contact with hot objects produces a contact burn. Ordinarily, reflexes protect a person from prolonged exposure to a very hot object; so contact burns are rarely deep unless the patient was prevented from drawing away from the hot object (for example, unresponsive, intoxicated, restrained,

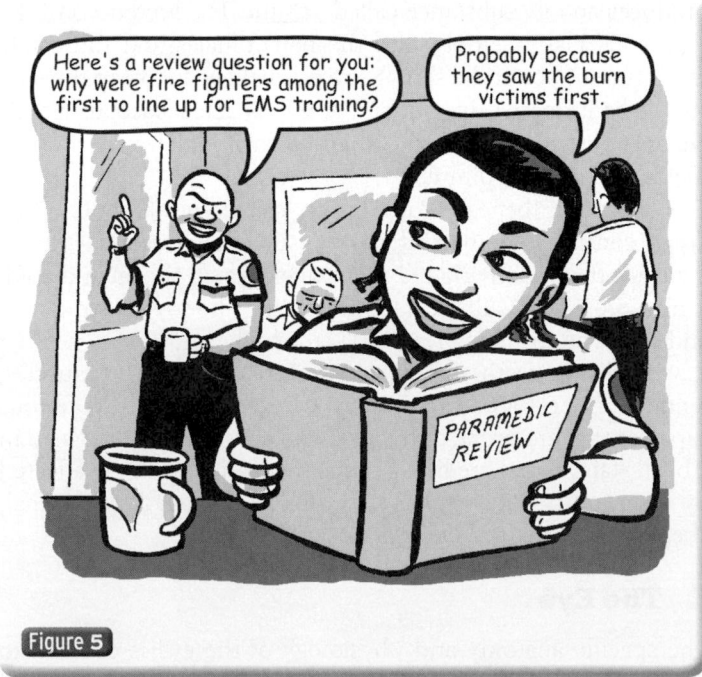

Figure 5

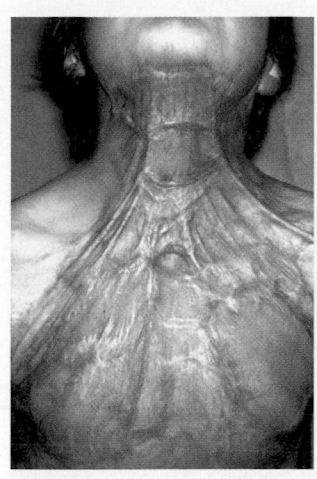

Figure 6 Flame burns are often very deep burns.

or impaired). Prolonged contact with something that is just moderately hot can eventually result in a severe burn, however. A patient who has a stroke and falls against a household radiator, for example, may end up with severe burns.

Scald and contact burns in children, older people, and people with disabilities may be signs of abuse, especially when they include unusual history patterns. Burns with formed shapes or unusual patterns and burns in atypical places such as the genitalia, buttocks, and thighs are often consistent with abuse **Figure 7**.

Steam Burns

A <u>steam burn</u> can produce a topical (scald) burn. Minor steam burns are common when microwaving food covered with plastic wrap. When the plastic is peeled away, hot steam escapes directly onto the hand of the hungry chef. Steam (that is, gaseous water) is also notorious for causing airway burns. Inhalation of other hot gases may cause <u>supraglottic</u> (upper airway) trauma but rarely leads to burns in the lower airway. Steam is unique because the minute particles of hot water can cause significant injury to the lower airway.

Flash Burns

A relatively rare source of thermal burns is the flash produced by an explosion, which may briefly expose a person to very intense heat. Lightning strikes can also cause a <u>flash burn</u>. These injuries are usually minor compared with the potential for trauma from whatever caused the flash **Figure 8**.

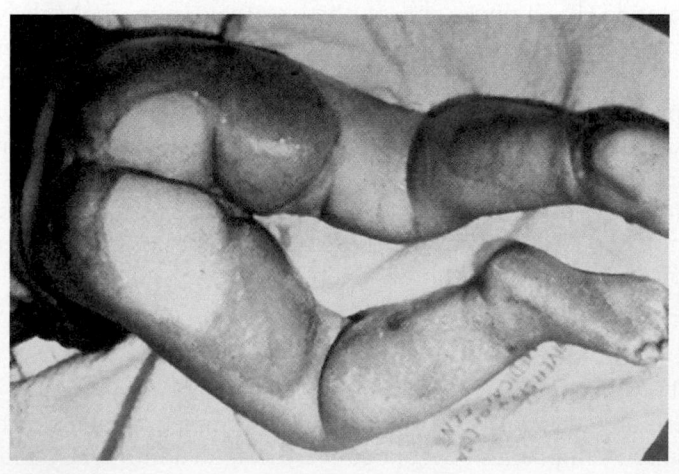

Figure 7 Scalds are sometimes associated with child abuse.

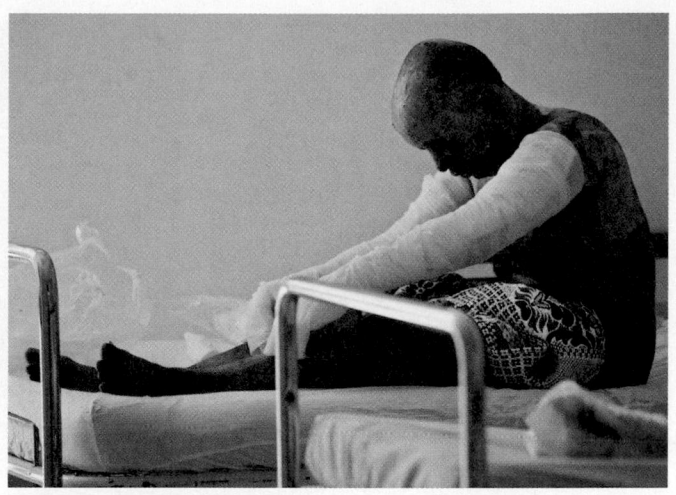

Figure 8 Flash burns may be minor compared with the additional trauma inflicted by an explosion.

Burn Depth

A burn wound is categorized by the degree of injury. Historically, such an injury has been described by three pathologic progressions or zones, which radiate from the central zone of greatest damage. Skin nearest the heat source suffers the most profound cellular changes. The central area of the skin, which suffers the most damage, is called the <u>zone of coagulation</u>. There is little or no blood flow to the injured tissue in this area. The peripheral area surrounding the zone of coagulation has decreased blood flow and inflammation; it is known as the <u>zone of stasis</u>. This area may undergo necrosis within 24 to 48 hours after the injury, particularly if perfusion is compromised by burn shock. Last, the <u>zone of hyperemia</u> is the area least affected by the thermal injury. In this area, cells will typically recover in 7 to 10 days. Similar to a myocardial infarction or stroke, the role of treatment is to salvage as much of the injured tissue as possible by improving perfusion and limiting the secondary changes that turn damaged tissue into dead tissue.

Burn depth is also categorized by severity—first, second, and third degree. Additional categories exist, such as fourth-, fifth-, and sixth-degree burns, for describing deeper destruction into tissue, muscle, and bone. Although these categorizations are still used by burn centers, paramedics should limit their assessment to superficial, partial-thickness, and full-thickness burns to simplify the process and avoid confusion and miscommunication **Figure 9**. Do not spend a significant amount of time categorizing burns in the field; the hospital needs to know the approximate type of burn, and you need to generally categorize the burn in order to properly determine the level of care that the patient requires.

Superficial Burns

A <u>superficial burn</u> involves the epidermis only. The skin is red and swollen and, when touched, the color will blanch and return. Usually blisters are not present. Patients will experience pain because nerve endings are exposed to the air. Such a

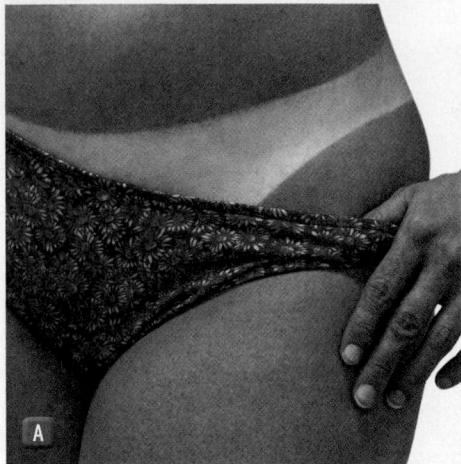 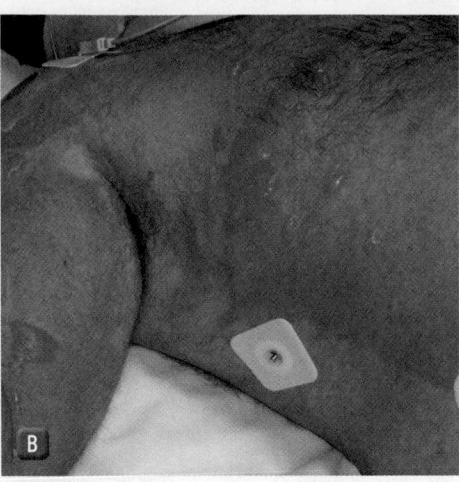 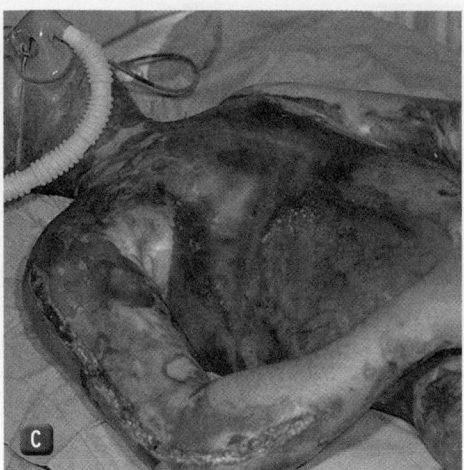

Figure 9 Classification of burns. **A.** Superficial burns involve only the epidermis. **B.** Partial-thickness burns involve some of the dermis but do not destroy the entire thickness of the skin. The skin is mottled, white to red, and often blistered. **C.** Full-thickness burns extend through all layers of the skin and may involve subcutaneous tissue and muscle. The skin is dry, leathery, and often white or charred.

burn will heal spontaneously in 3 to 7 days. The most common example is a sunburn.

Partial-Thickness Burns

A **partial-thickness burn** involves the epidermis and varying degrees of the dermis. In general, the deeper the partial-thickness burn, the more painful it is. The sensation of deep pressure remains intact. This burn category can be subdivided into moderate partial-thickness and deep partial-thickness burns.

With a *moderate partial-thickness burn*, the skin is red; when touched, the color will blanch and return. Usually there are blisters or moisture present, and the patient may experience extreme pain. Hair follicles remain intact. A moderate partial-thickness burn will typically heal spontaneously but may scar or have a changed appearance.

In contrast, a *deep partial-thickness burn* extends into the dermis, damaging the hair follicle and sweat and sebaceous glands. Hot liquids, steam, or grease are often to blame for these injuries. The color of the burn may be deceptive, and the delineation between deep partial thickness and full thickness may be difficult to determine in the field.

Full-Thickness Burns

A **full-thickness burn** involves destruction of both layers of the skin, including the basement membrane of dermis that produces new skin cells; therefore, the skin is incapable of self-regeneration. In such an injury, the skin may appear white and waxy, brown and leathery, or charred. Leathery skin is called eschar, and is dry and hard. No capillary refill occurs with this type of burn because the capillaries have been destroyed. Sensory nerves are destroyed as well, so there may be no pain in the full-thickness section. Because patients usually have mixed depths of burns, they will often experience significant pain in the areas surrounding the full-thickness burns. Treatment of a full-thickness burn will often require skin grafting because the dermis has been destroyed.

Inhalation Burns and Intoxication

Inhalation burns can cause rapid and serious airway compromise. Heat and/or toxic chemicals can be an irritant to the lungs and the airway, causing coughing, wheezing, and swelling of the upper airway tissues, often evidenced by stridor. Infraglottic (vocal cords and larynx) and lower airway damage is more often associated with the inhalation of steam or hot particulate matter. Supraglottic (upper airway) damage is more often associated with the inhalation of superheated gases. In rare cases, you may encounter severe upper airway swelling, requiring intervention immediately after a severe burn, although this problem may not manifest itself until transport.

Smoke Inhalation

According to the National Fire Protection Association, the vast majority of deaths from fires are not from burns, but rather from inhalation of toxic gases, upper airway compromise, or pulmonary injury. When materials such as plastic, polyvinyl chloride (PVC) pipes, and synthetic carpets burn, they release toxic chemicals **Figure 10**. Fire fighters routinely protect themselves from these toxins by wearing self-contained breathing apparatus. Anyone who is exposed to smoke from a fire, however, may experience thermal burns to the airway, hypoxia from lack of oxygen (oxygen is consumed by the burning process), and tissue damage and toxic effects caused by chemicals in the smoke. Such problems are particularly common when a person is caught in a burning building, stands up, and breathes in superheated gases.

Carbon Monoxide Intoxication

The combustion process produces a variety of toxic gases. Carbon monoxide (CO) evolves from incomplete combustion of carbon compounds (just about everything that burns). Cyanide evolves from the combustion of nitrogen-containing polymers (many plastics, polystyrene, PVC). Hydrogen chloride evolves from the combustion of PVC (pipes, insulating materials).

their garages or ambulance bays. Fire fighters who are performing an overhaul after a fire may be exposed to high levels of CO, as may people who are exposed to large amounts of car exhaust (such as toll takers and auto mechanics). Methylene chloride, which is found in some paint removers and bubble lamps and is used as an industrial solvent, is metabolized to CO by the body.

CO can displace oxygen (O_2) from the alveolar air and the blood hemoglobin. Because CO binds to receptor sites on hemoglobin at least 250 times more easily than O_2, the patient's hemoglobin may become saturated with the wrong chemical. Being exposed to relatively small concentrations of CO (such as in cigarette smoke) will result in progressively higher blood levels of CO. Most people have approximately 2% CO attached to their hemoglobin, but these levels may be as high as 4% to 8% in heavy smokers. Levels of 50% or higher may be fatal.

CO intoxication should be considered whenever a group of people in the same place all complain of headache or nausea (a malfunctioning furnace or car exhaust being sucked into the air-handling system can cause CO intoxication in groups of people). Similarly, you should be suspicious when people complain of feeling sick at home but not when they go to work or school.

Traditional wisdom tells us that patients with CO intoxication will appear "cherry red." Most practitioners agree that this cherry red skin is most commonly seen in people who have died, not living people. So, never rule out CO intoxication because the patient's skin is not cherry red.

Patients with severe CO intoxication usually present with an O_2 saturation of normal or better. For this reason, you should never trust a pulse oximeter when dealing with a suspected CO poisoning case **Figure 11** . New devices that can measure CO levels will soon be common in prehospital care; they will allow us to find and treat low-level CO intoxication far more readily than we can today.

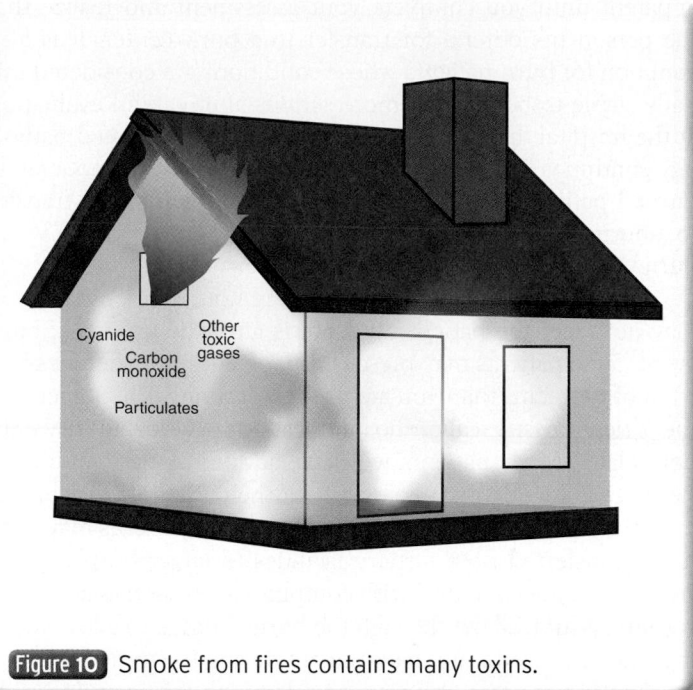

Cyanide
Other toxic gases
Carbon monoxide
Particulates

Figure 10 Smoke from fires contains many toxins.

The less efficient the combustion process, the more toxic the gases—such as carbon monoxide (CO) and carbon dioxide (CO_2)—that may be created. When furnaces, kerosene heaters, and other heating devices are in poor repair, they may emit unsafe levels of these toxic gases. Internal combustion engines may emit many of the same gases and, consequently, should always have their exhaust vented to the outdoors. A common cause of CO exposure is running a small engine in an enclosed space like a garage or basement. For this reason, many ambulance services and fire departments have added CO detectors to

YOU are the Medic PART 2

Your patient is attempting to climb into the ambulance even before you get the equipment. "Please, give me something for the pain. I can't stand it." He sits on the stretcher and as you ask questions to determine what happened, he becomes more agitated. While his airway appears open and maintained, his mouth appears reddened. His voice is raspy and his lips are red. "I can breathe fine, but I'm in a lot of pain. My arm. It hurts so bad." He is breathing rapidly with equal chest expansion. His mouth, neck, and chest are bright red. Lung sounds are present bilaterally. There are no adventitious sounds on inspiration or expiration. Both radial pulses are present, strong, and rapid. There is no severe bleeding and no mechanism indicating cervical spine injury.

Recording Time: 1 Minute	
Appearance	Flushed face and neck, walking
Level of consciousness	Alert (oriented to person, place, and day) and also very agitated
Airway	Open, clear, self-maintained with raspy voice
Breathing	Adequate, slightly fast
Circulation	Radial pulses strong and rapid

3. Your patient is clearly experiencing significant pain. At what point in treatment should this be addressed?

4. How significant is the patient's apparent raspiness as he is speaking to you?

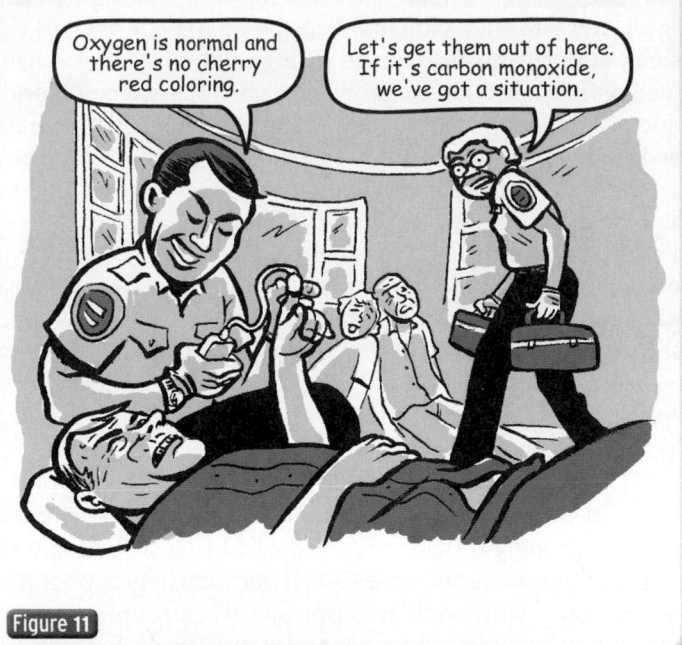

Figure 11

apparent until you complete your assessment and realize that the person fits criteria for transfer to a burn center. It is also common for burn patients whose conditions are considered initially stable to be deemed more serious after careful evaluation at the hospital, because the progression of burn-related pathology continues long after the initial incident. Even a moderately burned patient may ultimately require intubation and transfer to a burn center. Maintain a high index of suspicion even when burn injuries do not initially seem severe.

In other cases, burns may occur in remote locations, and you may not meet the patient until hours after the traumatic burn event. Such patients may present with an entirely different spectrum of problems than you are used to dealing with. Sometimes the patient doesn't realize the ramifications of a burn injury until hours later. Some patients will have additional traumatic injuries from falling debris, explosions, or their attempts to get away from the source of the burn. Seriously burned patients may need to be transferred from tertiary facilities to larger burn centers, and you may need to deal with complex issues such as an <u>escharotomy</u>, a surgical cut through the burned tissue to allow swelling, and advanced fluid management during the transport.

The many types of burns, coupled with the many possible presentations of burn patients, can challenge your assessment skills. As with any trauma patient, it is important to address burned patients in a consistent, efficient, and systematic manner so you do not develop tunnel vision for the major burn trauma and miss other occult injuries that could affect the patient's outcome.

Words of Wisdom

Hyperbaric oxygen has long been recommended for acute carbon monoxide intoxication and a variety of other asphyxiants, but the treatment is logistically difficult because the patient needs to be transported to an appropriate chamber in a reasonable period of time. A meta-analysis of hyperbaric oxygen therapy (HBO) concluded that it is of little value in acute carbon monoxide intoxication, but that it may be beneficial in reducing long-term complications. The availability of HBO in your area and the local medical opinions may result in protocols that differ significantly from place to place.

Words of Wisdom

Signs and symptoms of vascular compromise in a burned extremity that may necessitate an escharotomy include cyanosis, pallor, deep tissue pain, progressive paresthesia, progressive decrease or absence of the pulse, or sensation of a cold extremity.

■ Patient Assessment

Burns can fool paramedics, because we expect critically injured patients to act sick. Most severely injured and dying cardiac and trauma patients are hypotensive, unresponsive, or in obvious distress. In contrast, patients with an isolated severe burn injury may walk up to you at a scene. The chief complaint may be "I'm terribly cold," and the severity of the injuries may not become

■ Scene Size-up

Should you run into a burning building to save a patient? Not if you are not a trained and properly equipped fire fighter. Be wary of entering closed spaces if you see evidence of a recent fire. Toxic gases are often present, even if the fire is out. Never enter a burning building—there is the danger of flashover, when the contents of a room rise in temperature to the point where they all ignite at once. Remember also that plastics contain cyanide, which may be released when they burn.

With modern building construction, be concerned about structural damage to the building. Burning (or recently burned) buildings are notoriously dangerous places; the floors, roofs, beams, and walls may collapse at any time. Electrical wires, gas lines, and plumbing and heating systems can be unstable and dangerous. Look for placards indicating hazardous materials or other signs that hazardous materials may be present. Never enter an area that may contain hazardous materials.

Words of Wisdom

Antidotes for cyanide poisoning are now widely available, but they are expensive. A case can be made that cyanide is a dangerous component in the smoke of residential fires, but it is less clear whether the administration of cyanide antidotes improves survival. Local protocols will dictate whether these agents are available.

Only properly trained and protected personnel should enter such areas.

Safety is a primary concern whenever you are operating near a fire scene. Stage yourself and others in a place where it is safe to provide patient care. This distancing allows you to stay far enough from the scene to keep a global focus. Remember that your role may include treating victims of the fire and providing rehabilitation for fire fighters and other emergency personnel. When EMS providers are too close to the hot zone, it is detrimental to their own safety, the care they provide, and the overall medical response to the situation.

When a recently burned patient comes before you, your initial actions must include extinguishing the flame and cooling the burn. That step may seem obvious, but it is remarkable how many patients arrive by ambulance at hospital EDs with clothes still smoldering. A person whose clothing is on fire should not be permitted to run because running fans the flames; nor should the person remain standing because inhaling flame and igniting hair are more likely in the upright position. Rather, have the patient stop, drop to the ground, and roll. If the patient cannot roll, lower the patient to the ground, cover with a blanket, and pat the fire out.

Remove all smoldering clothing and any articles that may retain heat. Watchbands, zippers, and rings not only can retain enough heat to continue burning the patient, but also can melt through your gloves and burn you as well. Make sure that any jewelry on a patient has been cooled appropriately. If the person's hands are burned, they will swell considerably and rings may become tourniquets if not removed quickly enough. If bits of smoldering cloth adhere to the skin, do not pull them off; instead cut them away. Let burn center or hospital personnel deal with materials that are melted to the flesh.

If possible, determine the mechanism of injury (MOI). As mentioned earlier, patients who have been burned also often have sustained other trauma. Consider and examine other mechanisms associated with the burn: Did the patient jump from a high window to escape flames? Does the patient have musculoskeletal trauma from tetanic spasms after an electrical burn? Was the patient trapped in an enclosed space? Did the patient lose consciousness?

As a part of your scene size-up, do not forget to wear the most appropriate personal protective equipment, perhaps including gloves and a combination mask/eye shield. The burned patient may be "leaking" body fluids and is highly susceptible to infection. Use the most appropriate standard precautions to ensure that you are not exposed and the patient is not exposed to you!

■ Primary Assessment

Form a General Impression

As you approach a burn trauma patient, simple clues may help identify how serious the injuries are and how quickly you need to assess and treat the patient. If the patient greets you with a hoarse voice and a chief complaint of "trouble breathing," your general impression might be that the patient has a potential airway and/or breathing problem. In the absence of hypoxia or

Words of Wisdom

Heat loss is a critical problem for burn patients, particularly children. Take immediate steps to prevent hypothermia, such as heating the ambulance until it is uncomfortable for the crew, covering the patient with warm blankets, and administering fluids.

other trauma, a patient with a severe burn may be responsive and is often able to hold a conversation. Although burns are often painful, the more serious burns may present with little or no pain. Indeed, the chief complaint is often "I'm cold." What may first appear to be tattered clothing could turn out to be sheets of the patient's own skin hanging from his or her burned limbs. Recently burned patients may appear dazed or disconnected from events around them.

Despite what the injuries may look or smell like, you must use compassion when approaching the patient. Burns are obviously traumatic for the patient; if the person survives, he or she may face significant hospitalization and years of rehabilitation. But burns are also traumatic for you, the provider. Focusing on the basic principles of emergency care—the ABCs—can help you perform properly in this chaotic situation.

Patients with a burn injury may demonstrate varied mental status responses. Combative patients should be considered hypoxic until proven otherwise. Because partial-thickness burns are extremely painful, a patient with this type of injury may be awake and in pain. Even patients with excessive burns will often be awake and attempting to communicate. Isolated burns do not cause unresponsiveness (although toxic inhalations can). Unresponsive burn patients must be carefully assessed for the presence of other deadly injuries.

Airway and Breathing

As in any other seriously ill or injured patient, airway management is a priority in a patient with a burn. The airway may be in particular jeopardy because the same heat and flames that caused the external burn may have produced potentially life-threatening damage to the airway. Be prepared to assist ventilations.

The following are signs of airway involvement in a burn patient:

- Hoarseness
- Cough
- Singed nasal or facial hair
- Facial burns
- Carbon in the sputum
- History of burn in an enclosed space

Although rare, laryngeal edema can develop with alarming speed in burn patients, especially in infants and children. Early endotracheal (ET) intubation—before the airway has closed off—could be lifesaving in such cases and should be performed by the most experienced paramedic on your team. To intervene early, however, you need to spot the problem early. Airway management is discussed in greater detail later in this chapter.

Listen to lung sounds, with special attention to stridor, which may be a sign of impending upper airway compromise. Note if signs and symptoms of edema are present.

Note that patients with preexisting lung disease may have bronchospasm after even relatively minor exposure to smoke; they may respond well to inhaled beta-2 agonists.

Anyone suspected of having a burn to the upper airway may benefit from humidified, cool O_2. If you do not carry a high-output humidifier (a bubble humidifier is *not* a high-output humidifier), consider using an aerosol nebulizer to administer nebulized normal saline. This approach will not provide a high concentration of O_2, so you will need to balance the need for a high O_2 concentration against the desire for cool humidity. Keep in mind that the patient's O_2 saturation may be suspect if there is the possibility of CO intoxication.

Circulation

During the first 24 to 48 hours of a patient's burn care, a great deal of emphasis is placed on fluid resuscitation to prevent burn shock. Burn shock is a result of hypovolemia caused by fluid shifts that typically occur 6 to 8 hours after the burn. Severely burned patients will ultimately require large volumes of fluid, but they do not need it during the first minutes of prehospital care unless their burn injury occurred some time ago. Most patients will ultimately require central venous access, and most intravenous (IV) lines placed in the prehospital setting will be removed owing to tissue swelling and infection risk. Do not delay transport by making multiple attempts at vascular access. Of course, if the patient has an obvious peripheral vessel, your early vascular access will be put to good use by hospital or burn center staff for fluid replacement and pain management.

Patients with other trauma may require immediate vascular access just like any other trauma patient. Although it is preferable to avoid starting IV lines through burned tissue, it is not frankly contraindicated. Burn patients may challenge your vascular access skills. Intraosseous access may provide you with more choices than were available to your predecessors.

Assess Burn Severity

Once ABCs are addressed, the severity of the patient's burns should be evaluated to determine which facility the patient should be transported to for the best care. While evaluating the patient's burns, you must approximate the total body surface area (TBSA) burned. Most practitioners advocate counting only the areas of partial- and full-thickness burns (ignoring the areas of superficial burns). The most universal mechanism of calculating the area burned is the **rule of nines**, which is based on dividing the body into 9% segments. The provider adds the

portions of the body to obtain a total of the body area affected by the burn injury. Because our proportions change as we grow, different rules of nines apply to infants, children, and adults **Figure 12**.

Another mechanism of assessing the TBSA is the **rule of palms**, also called the rule of ones. This assessment uses the size of the patient's palm (excluding the fingers) to represent about 1% of the patient's body surface area. This calculation is helpful when the burn covers less than 10% of the body surface area or is irregularly shaped. The **Lund and Browder chart** is an even more specific method used to estimate the burned area by dividing the body into even smaller and more specific regions **Figure 13**.

In the field, providers may disagree on the extent of a given burn; reaching a consensus is not important enough to justify spending time on the discussion. Hospital personnel need a report that includes an estimate of the depth and severity of burns. The American Burn Association has also published burn severity classifications **Table 1**.

Transport Decision

During your primary assessment, your goal is to identify and manage life threats and to determine the level of care the patient requires (eg, burn center, trauma center, local hospital). This means you will need to estimate the burn's size and severity to report to the receiving facility. The nature of the patient's burns will evolve during the next 24 hours, and estimations of their size and severity will inevitably change, so little is to be gained

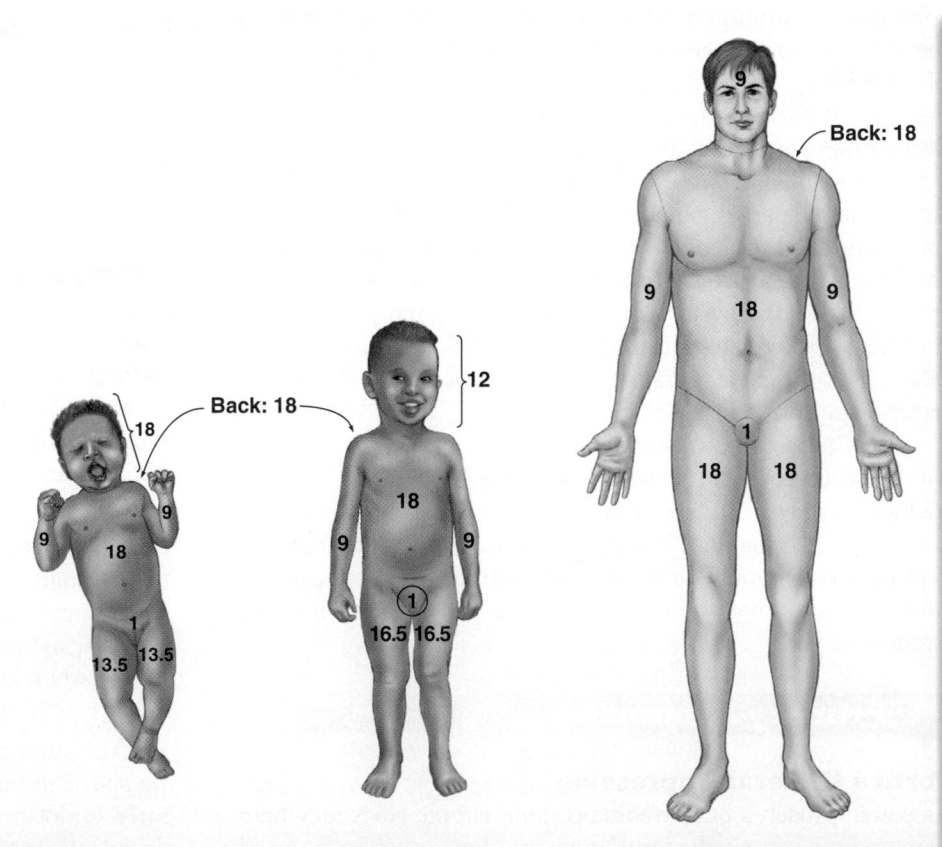

Figure 12 The rule of nines is a quick way to estimate the amount of surface areas that has been burned. It divides the body into sections, each representing approximately 9% of the total body surface area. The proportions differ for infants, children, and adults.

Region	%
Head	
Neck	
Ant. Trunk	
Post. Trunk	
Right arm	
Left arm	
Buttocks	
Genitalia	
Right leg	
Left leg	
Total burn	

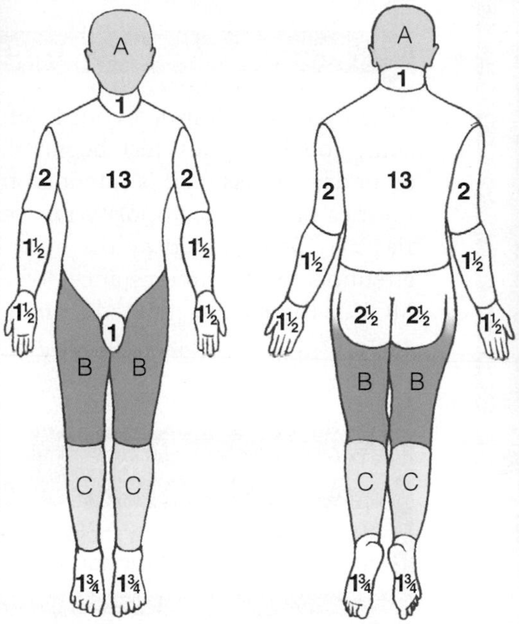

Relative percentages of body surface area affected by growth

Age (years)	A ($\frac{1}{2}$ of head)	B ($\frac{1}{2}$ of one thigh)	C ($\frac{1}{2}$ of one leg)
0	$9\frac{1}{2}$	$2\frac{3}{4}$	$2\frac{1}{2}$
1	$8\frac{1}{2}$	$3\frac{1}{4}$	$2\frac{1}{2}$
5	$6\frac{1}{2}$	4	$2\frac{3}{4}$
10	$5\frac{1}{2}$	$4\frac{1}{4}$	3
15	$4\frac{1}{2}$	$4\frac{1}{2}$	$3\frac{1}{4}$
Adult	$3\frac{1}{2}$	$4\frac{3}{4}$	3

Figure 13 The Lund and Brower chart.

by conducting a comprehensive and time-consuming evaluation of every inch of the patient's body in the field. Nevertheless, a reasonably accurate estimation of the scope of the patient's injuries is helpful for determining both the appropriate destination for the patient and the care to be delivered.

According to the referral criteria identified by the American Burn Association, patients with the following injuries should be transferred to a burn specialty center, also called a burn unit:

- Partial-thickness burns of more than 10% of the body surface area
- Burns that involve the face, hands, feet, genitalia, perineum, or major joints
- Full-thickness burns in any age group
- Electrical burns, including lightning
- Chemical burns
- Inhalation burns

Table 1 Classification of Burns in Adults

Burn Classification	Criteria
Critical (severe) burns	- Full-thickness burns involving hands, feet, face, upper airway, or genitalia or circumferential burns of other areas - Full-thickness burns covering more than 10% of the body's total surface area - Partial-thickness burns covering more than 30% of the body's total surface area - Burns associated with respiratory injury (smoke inhalation or inhalation injury) - Burns complicated by fractures - Burns on patients younger than 5 years or older than 55 years that would be classified as "moderate" in young adults
Moderate burns	- Full-thickness burns involving 2% to 10% of the body's total surface area (excluding hands, feet, face, genitalia, and upper airway) - Partial-thickness burns covering 15% to 30% of the body's total surface area - Superficial burns covering more than 50% of the body's total surface area
Minor burns	- Full-thickness burns covering less than 2% of the body's total surface area - Partial-thickness burns covering less than 15% of the body's total surface area - Superficial burns covering less than 50% of the body's total surface area

Special Populations

Burns to children are generally considered more serious than burns to adults Table 2. This is because infants and children have more surface area relative to total body mass, which means greater fluid and heat loss. In addition, children do not tolerate burns as well as adults do. Children are also more likely to experience shock, hypothermia, and airway problems because of the unique differences of their ages and anatomy.

Some burns in infants and children result from child abuse. The classic burn resulting from deliberate immersion involves the hands and wrists, as well as the feet, lower legs, and buttocks. Similarly, burns around the genitals and multiple cigarette burns should be viewed as possible abuse. You should report all suspected cases of abuse to the proper authorities (see the chapter, *Pediatric Emergencies*).

- Burn injuries in conjunction with preexisting medical conditions that could complicate management, prolong recovery, or affect mortality
- Burns and concomitant trauma in which the burn injury poses the greatest risk of morbidity or mortality
- Burn injury that requires special social, emotional, or long-term rehabilitation

You must balance the need for accuracy against the time required to make an estimate of the TBSA. The prehospital estimation is used to guide the patient to the correct place for treatment. The ED estimation of burned area may be used to initiate fluid therapy. The burn center's estimation of injured area will undoubtedly be more accurate and specific.

History Taking

To the degree possible, get a brief history from the patient. Patients with preexisting diseases, such as chronic obstructive pulmonary disease or acute coronary syndromes, may be triaged as critical even if the burn injury is small. As in any other trauma,

Table 2 Classification of Burns in Infants and Children
Severe Burns
Any full-thickness burn Partial-thickness burns covering more than 20% of the body's total surface area
Moderate Burns
Partial-thickness burns covering 10% to 20% of the body's total surface area
Minor Burns
Partial-thickness burns covering less than 10% of the body's total surface area

allergies, medications, and other pertinent medical history may influence the patient's care plan.

Secondary Assessment

When you have finished your brief inspection of the patient's skin, you have only just begun the head-to-toe exam. The secondary assessment is intended to make sure that no other injuries have higher priority for treatment. Often, such injuries may be obscured by the burn itself, so you need to pay attention to the circumstances of the burn and the possible MOI. If the patient jumped from a second-story window, for example, there may be fractures beneath the obvious burns on the legs.

Words of Wisdom

If a burned patient is in shock in the prehospital phase, look for another injury as the source of shock.

Look for injuries to the eyes, and cover injured eyes with moist, sterile pads. Check the neck, chest, and extremities for **circumferential burns**. Progressive edema beneath a circumferential burn—especially when the burned skin has become leathery and unyielding—may act as a tourniquet. In the neck, a circumferential burn may obstruct the airway; in the chest, it may restrict respiratory excursion; and in an extremity, it may cut off the circulation and put the extremity in jeopardy. Patients with circumferential burns must reach a medical facility quickly because it may be necessary to make an incision into the burned area to decompress it. Check and document the distal pulses in burned extremities often.

Obtaining vital signs may be challenging if the patient has extensive burns on the arms. Nevertheless, you should try to document vital signs accurately because the management of shock, airway compromise, and pain control depends on them to some degree.

Reassessment

If the patient is considered to have a significant MOI, en route to the ED, you should perform a full-body exam and reassessment. Reassessment of vital signs to establish trends is done every 5 minutes for critical patients and every 15 minutes for lower priority patients (in stable condition).

Emergency Medical Care

Definitive burn care can be divided into four phases: initial evaluation and resuscitation, initial wound excision and biologic closure, definitive wound closure, and rehabilitation, reconstruction, and reintegration. Although paramedics will be most heavily involved in the first phase, it is important to appreciate the magnitude of care that a patient with a severe, or even moderate, burn must receive. Early actions of the paramedic may dramatically affect the patient's long-term outcome. Paramedics may also find themselves transporting patients to specialty or rehabilitation facilities at later stages of their care. The four phases of burn care are outlined in **Table 3**.

Table 3 Phases of Definitive Burn Care

Phase	Time Frame	Treatment Objectives
Initial evaluation and resuscitation	First 72 hours	To provide initial resuscitation, secure the airway, achieve accurate fluid resuscitation, and perform a thorough evaluation
Initial wound excision and biologic closure	Days 1 through 7	To identify and remove all full-thickness wounds and obtain biologic closure
Definitive wound closure	Day 7 through week 6	To replace temporary covers with definitive ones and close small, complex wounds
Rehabilitation, reconstruction, and reintegration	Entire hospitalization	To maintain range of motion and reduce edema and to strengthen and prepare the patient for return to the community

Unlike many emergencies you will encounter, burn patient care is measured in weeks, not hours. Burns are devastating multisystem traumatic injuries that dramatically alter a person's life. You should recognize not only the massive physical trauma caused by burns, but also the emotional, psychological, and financial burdens these horrific injuries impose. Once these costs are appreciated, it is easy to understand the importance of teaching injury prevention strategies to the people we serve.

■ General Management

Management of a burned patient begins with the steps taken during the scene size-up and primary assessment to extinguish the fire and ensure adequate ABCs. Only when the ABCs are under control should you turn your attention to the burn itself. It is important to have all resuscitative equipment ready for use when treating a burn patient, including advanced airway equipment and your ECG monitor.

Airway Management

Many burn patients will ultimately require intubation, even though they were talking to you and in no distress in the field. Although it is obviously preferable to have such patients intubated in a controlled environment with a full complement of anesthesia agents, a few patients will absolutely require an emergency advanced airway in the field. Burn patients fall into four general categories for airway management:

1. **The patient with an acutely decompensating airway who requires field intubation.** This group includes burn patients who are in cardiac or respiratory arrest and responsive patients whose airways are swelling before your eyes. In these chaotic and difficult situations, you need to plan

YOU *are the Medic* | **PART 3**

Your partner administers high-concentration oxygen via a nonrebreathing mask and applies cool, moist, sterile dressings to the burns on the patient's arm and neck. Working on his unburned arm, you obtain vital signs and prepare to establish an intravenous (IV) line.

Recording Time: 5 Minutes	
Respirations	22 breaths/min, unlabored
Pulse	120 beats/min, strong radial pulses
Skin	Flushed, warm
Blood pressure	160/110 mm Hg
Oxygen saturation (Spo$_2$)	98%
Pupils	Equal, reactive

5. What is the likely cause of the patient's elevated blood pressure?

6. At what point might you consider aggressive airway management including sedation and intubation?

for the possibility that you cannot intubate. Supraglottic swelling or complete obstruction can occur in some burn scenarios. Surgical airways or rescue devices may be necessary if intubation is not possible and bag-mask ventilation fails.

2. **The patient with a deteriorating airway from burns and toxic inhalations who might require intubation.** It is obviously better for the patient to defer treatment of this airway problem to hospital teams with anesthesia, surgery, specialized equipment, and a fully stocked pharmacy. Patients will often be responsive and may become combative with attempts to place them supine, let alone intubate them. "Awake" techniques, such as nasal intubation, are dramatically more complicated in patients with upper airway burns and should be avoided. Attempt to intubate only if left with no other choice. If the patient's airway continues to swell and intubation will become impossible if you wait for arrival at the hospital, you have little choice but to attempt intubation. Try to consult medical control for advice.

   Intubation of an awake, scared patient in the field is difficult, and considerable damage may be inflicted on the airway if the patient continues to struggle. If intubation becomes necessary under such circumstances, explain carefully to the patient what is to be done, why it is necessary, and how he or she can best cooperate. Have all equipment set up at your side so that intubation, once begun, can proceed rapidly and smoothly. Serious consideration should be made toward performing rapid-sequence intubation if you have been trained in this procedure, carry the appropriate medications, and have medical control authorization. The procedure for rapid-sequence intubation is discussed in the chapter, *Airway Management*. It is also advised that the "most experienced" intubator perform this procedure because the swelling can make for a difficult intubation.

   An airway compromised by advancing edema represents another classic scenario in which administering a neuromuscular blocker to provide respiratory paralysis may be extremely dangerous. It places the paramedic in the dangerous position of having a patient with no gag reflex or ability to breathe and an airway you may be unable to control.

   The choice of ET tube may present another conundrum. It would obviously be beneficial to use the largest tube possible. Sometimes the ET tube will clog with soot from the patient's airway, causing complete occlusion. At the same time, a smaller-than-usual ET tube may be necessary owing to airway edema. Select the largest ET tube that will not cause additional trauma during insertion. Never cut the ET tube down to make it shorter. Edema of the face can actually cause ET tube dislodgment on postburn day 2 or 3.

3. **The patient whose airway is currently patent but who has a history consistent with risk factors for eventual airway compromise.** Cool, humidified O_2 from a high-output nebulizer (not a bubble humidifier) is appropriate. Alternatively, you may use an aerosol nebulizer with saline. The patient will probably *not* require acute interventions in the field, but make sure you report the patient's history to hospital personnel. Many patients will ultimately undergo elective intubation.

4. **The patient with no signs of or risk factors for airway compromise who is in no distress.** While current trends in prehospital care include limiting the aggressive use of O_2, providing supplemental O_2 to burn patients continues to be considered reasonable treatment, even if patients are not in distress. The potential for CO poisoning and the resultant inaccuracy of pulse oximetry and the potential for airway compromise favor the application of O_2.

Fluid Resuscitation

Patients with burns covering more than 20% of the body's total surface area will need fluid resuscitation. Depending upon the patient's age and other medical conditions, too much fluid may be as harmful as too little. If fluid resuscitation is delayed more than 2 hours from the time of the burn in severely burned patients, resuscitation is complicated and mortality increases. The goal is to begin to deliver an appropriate amount of fluid to the burn patient as soon as is reasonable. An IV line may be inserted in the field to administer fluids and/or pain medications. A large-bore IV catheter should be inserted as early as possible in any patient who has been severely burned. Do not delay transport to do so, but try to get a large-bore IV catheter into a large vein, and give lactated Ringer's solution or normal saline. You can use the burned extremity for the IV site if you cannot find another site—an IV line in a burned upper extremity is still preferable to an IV line in a lower extremity. Most seriously burned patients will need central venous access, and IV lines placed in the prehospital setting will most often be lost as peripheral swelling begins.

   Approximate the amount of fluid the burned patient will need by using the __Consensus formula__ (previously known as the Parkland formula) **Table 4**, which states that *during the first 24 hours*, the burned patient will need:

$$4\,\text{mL} \times \text{body weight (in kg)} \times \text{percentage of body surface burned}$$

Half of that amount needs to be given during the first 8 hours, and the other half needs to be given over the subsequent 16 hours. For example, if a 70-kg man has sustained burns to 30% of his body, his fluid needs during the first 24 hours will be:

$$4\,\text{mL} \times 70\,\text{kg} \times 30 = 8{,}400\,\text{mL}$$

Half of the 8,400 mL—that is, 4,200 mL—should be administered during the first 8 hours. The original Parkland formula used normal saline solution, but lactated Ringer's solution has also gained popularity in many burn centers. Consult your local protocol for fluid choice.

Table 4 Consensus Formula Chart

% Burn	10 kg	20 kg	30 kg	40 kg	50 kg	60 kg	70 kg	80 kg	90 kg	100 kg
10	25	50	75	100	125	150	175	200	225	250
20	50	100	150	200	250	300	350	400	450	500
30	75	150	225	300	375	450	525	600	675	750
40	100	200	300	400	500	600	700	800	900	1,000
50	125	250	375	500	625	750	875	1,000	1,125	1,250
60	150	300	450	600	750	900	1,050	1,200	1,350	1,500
70	175	350	525	700	875	1,050	1,225	1,400	1,575	1,750
80	200	400	600	800	1,000	1,200	1,400	1,600	1,800	2,000
90	225	450	675	900	1,125	1,350	1,575	1,800	2,025	2,250
20 mL/kg	200	400	600	800	1,000	1,200	1,400	1,600	1,800	2,000

This table represents the fluid recommended in the *first hour* (1/8 of the initial 8-hour dose) by the Parkland formula. The second dose, administered over the remaining 16 hours, is equal to the amount given in the initial dose. The final row represents the amount of a 20-mL/kg bolus.

Even though this formula implies that burn patients need enormous amounts of fluid, remember that you do not need to attempt to deliver the entire initial amount in the field. The large amounts of fluid suggested by the Consensus formula often lead providers to give more fluid than necessary prior to the patient's arrival at a burn center, a phenomenon known as fluid creep. Interestingly, the Parkland formula was devised to give guidelines to limit fluid overload so burn patients do not develop pulmonary edema and acute respiratory distress syndrome. Ongoing fluid resuscitation at the hospital is based on urine output and vital signs. Even though burn patients will need large amounts of fluid, giving it too early or too fast can lead to rapidly increasing peripheral edema that may compromise airway devices and vascular access and lead to compartment syndrome. It is even more important to monitor geriatric and pediatric patients for fluid overload during this critical period. In short, you have to administer a lot of fluid while simultaneously monitoring the patient to ensure that you are not administering too much.

Words of Wisdom

The adequacy of resuscitation is based on monitoring the patient's vital signs, mentation, and urine output.

Pain Management

With any patient with burns, you should provide aggressive pain management. Assess the patient's pain before administering any analgesia. Reassessment should be completed using the same scale (for example, 1 to 10) every 5 minutes.

Burn patients may require higher doses than usual of pain medications to achieve relief. Their metabolism rates are accelerated, which creates the need for higher doses than normal of analgesics. Consult your protocols or contact medical control for guidance in administering analgesics.

Pain medication is best given via the IV route. Owing to changes in fluid volume and tissue blood flow, absorption of any intramuscular or subcutaneous drug is unpredictable. Accurately measure and assess the patient's pain, and continuously monitor response to pain medication.

Narcotics such as morphine and fentanyl remain the drugs of choice for the extreme pain that often accompanies burns. Dosing is typically considerably heavier than what you might be used to giving for other conditions. This is because the pathophysiology of burns may prevent all of the dose from reaching the intended receptor sites. Doses equivalent to 10 to 20 mg of morphine are not uncommon in previously healthy adults. Administering narcotics to geriatric and pediatric patients, or those with respiratory compromise, requires careful assessment of the patient's response to the medications. As always, titrate multiple doses to the patient's response.

Burn Shock

Burn shock sets in during a 6- to 8-hour period, so you will not typically witness it in the field. Therefore, if an acutely burned patient is in shock in the prehospital phase, look for another injury as the source of shock. People who are caught in fires may fall through floors, jump out of windows, and have debris fall on them. There are ample opportunities for traumatic injuries at fire and explosion scenes, so you must be diligent in your assessment. Although seriously burned patients (greater than 15% to 20% TBSA) will not immediately show evidence of burn shock, mortality increases if fluid resuscitation is delayed longer than 2 hours from the time of the burn. It is therefore helpful to obtain vascular access and begin fluid resuscitation in the field if practical. Consider time from hospital, difficulty of obtaining vascular access, need for analgesia, and possibility of additional pathologies that require vascular access in your decision to begin fluid resuscitation in the field.

Thermal Burns

While assessing a patient's burns, consider the presence or absence of pain, swelling, skin color, capillary refill time, moisture and blisters, the appearance of the wound edges, the presence of foreign bodies, debris and contaminants, bleeding, and circulatory adequacy. Also assess for concomitant soft-tissue injury. Cool small burn areas and any large areas that remain hot. Apply dry, sterile, nonadherent dressings to help prevent infection and provide comfort. (Use a moist dressing if the burn covers less than 10% of the TBSA.) Remember that patients with a large area of the body's surface burned are likely to also have hypovolemia and hypothermia.

Superficial Burns

Although superficial burns can be very painful, they rarely pose a threat to life unless they involve nearly the entire surface of the body. If you reach a patient with superficial burns within the first hour after the injury occurred, immerse the burned area in cool water or apply cold compresses to the burn. Burned hands or feet may be soaked directly in cool water; and towels soaked in cold water may be applied to burns of the face or trunk.

The objectives of this exercise are twofold: stop the burning process and relieve pain. Commercial products that meet both objectives are available Figure 14 . Regardless of the method used to cool the burn, take care not to cool the whole body—don't let the patient become chilled. A dry sheet or blanket applied over the wet dressings will help prevent systemic heat loss.

Do not use salves, ointments, creams, sprays, or any similar materials on any type of burn. They will just have to be scrubbed off in the ED or burn unit, causing the patient further pain. Never apply ice to burns because it can exacerbate the tissue injury.

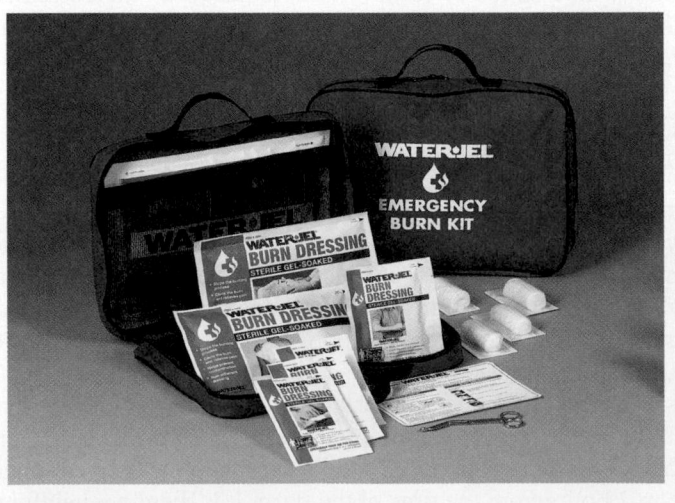

Figure 14 Sample burn dressing (Water-Jel).

No further treatment should be necessary in the field for an uncomplicated, superficial burn. Simply transport the patient in a comfortable position to the hospital.

Partial-Thickness Burns

Treatment of partial-thickness burns in the field is similar to that of superficial burns. Cooling the burned area with water or application of wet or Water-Jel dressings within the first hour can diminish edema and provide significant pain relief. Burned extremities should be elevated to minimize edema formation.

Do not attempt to rupture blisters over the burn; they initially act as a physiologic burn dressing. Establish IV fluids with lactated Ringer's solution or normal saline as dictated by local protocol. Pain in the patient with partial-thickness burns may be severe, so complete a pain assessment and administer pain medication as allowed by your protocols.

Full-Thickness Burns

Although full-thickness burns may not cause pain, most patients will have varying degrees of burns within the affected region of injury. For this reason, a pain assessment should be completed and pain medication should be administered as described earlier. Usually, dry dressings are used after the fire is out. Check with your burn center or medical center on their view on wet dressings or analgesia. Begin fluid resuscitation, if possible, preferably within 2 hours of injury.

Thermal Inhalation Burns

Application of cool mist or aerosol therapy may help reduce some minor edema. Because most ambulances do not carry misters, apply an ice pack to the throat.

More aggressive airway management may be necessary if supraglottic tissue swelling threatens the patient's airway. In addition, heat inhalation may produce laryngospasm and bronchospasm in the lower airway. Patients sometimes experience pulmonary damage from direct thermal injury. Later pulmonary involvement may be from toxic inhalation injury.

Pathophysiology, Assessment, and Management of Specific Burns

Chemical Burns of the Skin

Chemical burns occur when the skin comes in contact with strong acids, alkalis or bases, or other corrosive materials Table 5 . The burn progresses as long as the corrosive substance remains in contact with the skin. The cornerstone of therapy is, therefore, removal of the chemical from contact with the patient's body. Typical management for removal of chemical solutions

Table 5 Chemical Burns

Chemical Type	Examples	Injury
Acids	Battery acid (sulfuric acid), hydrochloric acid, hydrofluoric acid	Causes immediate pain and coagulation necrosis; deeper tissue typically not injured
Bases and alkalis	Potassium hydroxide, sodium hydroxide, lime, drain cleaner, oven cleaner, lye	Causes little pain but extensive damage by liquefaction necrosis: breakdown of protein and collagen, saponification of fats, dehydration of tissues, thrombosis of blood vessels
Oxidizing agents	Hydrogen peroxide, sodium chlorate	Exothermic (heat) reaction in addition to tissue destruction; could cause systemic poisoning
Phosphorus	White phosphorus, tracer ammunition, fireworks	Burns when exposed to air; could cause systemic poisoning
Vesicants	Lewisite, sulfur mustard (mustard gas), phosgene oxime	Blister agents; respiratory compromise if inhaled

is copious flushing with water; while management of powders requires brushing off as much of the substance as possible before washing.

The amount of damage from a chemical burn depends on the nature of the chemical involved, as well as:

- **The concentration and quality of the agent.** Common agents that are not particularly dangerous may be much more reactive in their concentrated or commercial forms. The hydrogen peroxide that you put on cuts is typically a 3% to 6% solution. The hydrogen peroxide being transported in a tanker might be a 70% to 98% solution and is a highly volatile oxidizer.
- **The chemical state or temperature of the agent.** Many gases (nitrogen, oxygen, anhydrous ammonia) are transported in their liquid form, which can cause severe burns because they are so cold. Liquid oxygen systems, which are becoming increasingly popular for home use, can cause severe burns if their contents are inadvertently released (such as during a building collapse or motor vehicle crash).
- **The length of exposure.** Agents that do not cause significant pain sometimes soak into clothing and are held against the skin for long periods of time where they eventually can cause significant injury. Phenol (carbolic acid) causes a painless burn that can result in significant damage before it is identified. Unresponsive patients and patients

with paralyzed limbs sometimes suffer significant burns from contact with simple household items like radiators or cooking grease.

- **The depth of penetration.** One reason that alkaline burns are often worse than acid burns is that acids create a coagulative necrosis that is painful and forms a tough layer of dead tissue that may prevent deeper burning. Bases break down protein and collagen, creating a liquefactive necrosis that burns deeper.

Typically, chemical burns react with the skin and tissues quickly. In some cases, however, the injury may take time to develop, as in a person who is exposed to cement (calcium oxide). Cement tends to penetrate clothing and can react with sweat on the surface of the skin. Hours later, the patient may notice that a burn injury has occurred.

Acid Burns Hydrogen ions formed by an acid are relatively easy to neutralize because they do not form soluble products. Acids cause destruction and coagulation of tissues, resulting in a coagulative necrosis that may actually limit the depth of the burn.

Alkali Burns Hydroxide ions of an alkaline burn form soluble products that sink into the tissue, carrying the burn deeper and making it more difficult to neutralize. This effect is particularly pronounced in chemical burns of the eye. Flushing, including flushing with the patient's own tears, quickly helps to disperse an acid, while alkali burns to the eye are profoundly destructive, often within just a few minutes.

Assessment

Typically, chemical burns are the result of unexpected contact with a caustic substance, so your assessment must begin by ensuring your own safety followed by appropriate decontamination of the patient. Be careful not to get any of the hazardous chemicals on your own clothing or skin. Consider wearing additional protective materials; your nitrile or vinyl gloves may not protect you from many chemicals.

Documentation and Communication

It is difficult to assess the size and depth of chemical burns, but you should certainly relay your impression of the burned area and type of chemical to the emergency department.

It is also important for you to try to determine what agent the patient came into contact with. Secure product labels, Material Safety Data Sheets, or other documentation available for the chemical agent. Be sure to protect yourself from exposure. Consider consulting poison control if you can ascertain the name of the specific chemical involved. Remember that if the burn took place at an industrial site, experts may be available at the scene.

Management

Speed is essential when treating chemical burns. Begin flushing the exposed area of the patient's body immediately with copious quantities of water Figure 15 . If the patient is in or near the home, the shower or a garden hose is ideal. In an industrial setting,

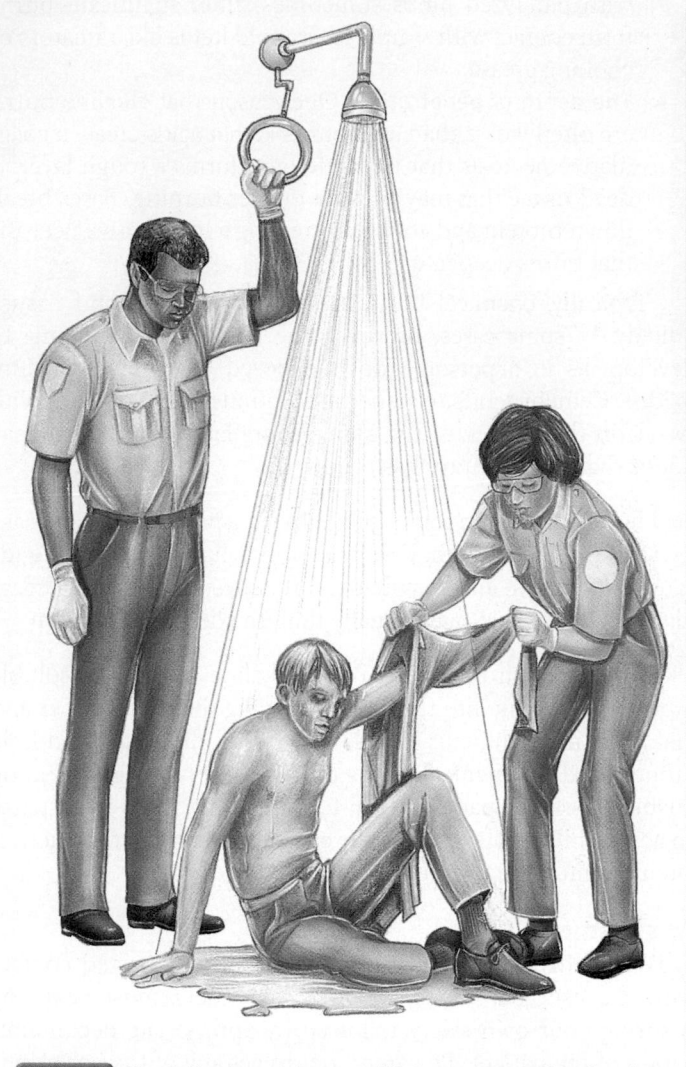

Figure 15 Flush the burned area with large amounts of water.

weigh the realities of flushing on the scene for long periods against the benefits of transport and their ability to continue flushing en route. After flushing, limit hypothermia by keeping the patient covered and warm.

Several types of chemical burns require special management techniques:

- **Dry lime.** In alkali burns caused by dry lime, combination with water will produce a highly corrosive substance. For that reason, when a patient has been in contact with dry lime, *first* remove the patient's clothing and *brush* as much lime as you can from the skin (wear gloves!). *Then* start flushing copiously with a garden hose or shower. Your intention is to completely overwhelm any damaging chemical reaction with a deluge of water.

- **Sodium metals.** Sodium metals produce considerable heat when mixed with water and may explode. Cover this type of burn with oil, which will stop the reaction by preventing the sodium from coming in contact with the atmosphere.

- **Hydrofluoric (HF) acid.** HF acid is used in drain cleaners in the home and for etching glass and plastic in industrial settings. Burns that exceed 3% to 5% of the TBSA can be fatal. The patient will complain bitterly of pain (caused by the HF acid sucking calcium out of the body), and the pain will not improve even with continuous flushing—a sign that the process of tissue destruction is ongoing. Calcium chloride (CaCl) jelly may be available in an industrial setting that uses HF acid; this jelly is placed on small-area HF acid burns (small burns from splashing or pinholes in gloves) to help reduce continued pain and injury. An ampule of CaCl (10 mL of a 10% CaCl solution) can be mixed with a water-based lubricant to make CaCl jelly in an emergency. Medical control may order IV CaCl for HF acid burns.

- **Gasoline or diesel fuel.** Since we come into contact with these almost every day, and they are present at virtually all vehicle crashes, it is easy to forget the multitude of potential problems caused by gasoline, kerosene, and other hydrocarbons. Prolonged contact may produce a chemical injury to the skin. This would be managed like any other chemical irritant and washed off as soon as possible. Most hydrocarbons are more effectively removed with a soap solution than water alone. Hydrocarbons also stimulate gamma-aminobutyric acid receptors and can cause sleepiness and even coma. Many hydrocarbons can also cause a fire or explosion under certain circumstances.

- **Hot tar.** Burns caused by hot tar are, strictly speaking, thermal burns, not chemical burns, although they tend to be

use the decontamination shower or a hose. While flushing, rapidly remove the patient's clothing, especially shoes and socks that may have become contaminated with the offending agent. Removing a patient's clothes typically removes at least 85% of external contamination.

Have the patient bend over when washing the hair and head to avoid having residual chemicals run over the rest of the body. Chemicals can collect in skin folds, where they remain in contact with the tissue and continue to cause more severe damage. Care must be taken to meticulously wash the skin folds at joints and between fingers and toes. Once you think washing is complete, wash the body again. Some chemicals may adhere to the skin, and a mild detergent (dishwashing liquid) will aid in removal. Rinse and wash gently to avoid abrading the skin and exacerbating the injury or absorption of the chemical.

Do not waste time looking for specific antidotes or neutralizing agents; copious flushing with water is more effective and more immediately available. Flushing is preferable for 30 minutes before moving the patient; for chemical burns caused by strong alkalis (such as oven and drain cleaners), 1 to 2 *hours* of flushing has been recommended. Paramedics must

classified with chemical burns. The most important step in the prehospital phase is to immerse the affected area in cold water to dissipate the heat from the tar and speed up the hardening process. Once the tar has cooled, it will not do further damage, and there is no need to try to remove it in the field.

Inhalation Burns From Other Toxic Chemicals

A variety of irritant gases can cause local swelling of the airway or a more systemic response. In many cases, the solubility properties of the gas will determine where it affects the airway Table 6 . Highly water-soluble gases such as ammonia and hydrogen chloride will react with the moist mucous membranes of the upper airway and cause immediate irritation and swelling. Slightly water-soluble gases such as phosgene and nitrogen dioxide will react with tissue over time. Since they are not initially as irritating, they will be breathed deep into the lungs, causing damage at the alveolar level hours or even days after they are inspired. These patients may present with pulmonary edema long after the exposure took place. Some other very common irritant gases can be categorized as moderately water soluble, and their site of action will depend on the concentration breathed. For example, chlorine is a common chemical found in powdered and liquid forms in homes, businesses, and on the highways. When high concentrations are released, such as after a rail car or tanker collision, the evolved gas can be irritating and causes immediate upper airway irritation. The same product in lower concentrations may not be as irritating, resulting in less intense symptoms that do not present until hours or days later.

HF acid is a special case. Fluoride dust can be inhaled in an industrial setting or at the scene of fires or explosions where fluorides are stored. As discussed in the chapter, *Toxicology*, HF acid aggressively binds with calcium ions and may require the administration of IV calcium. Significant inhalation frequently results in death.

Assessment

Your usual airway assessment should always include a high index of suspicion for irritant gas exposure if the patient was involved in a fire, explosion, or contaminated environment situation. The irritant gases that affect the upper airway will also usually cause burning of the eyes. Signs of upper airway swelling, such as stridor, are ominous and may signal the potential for acute upper airway obstruction. Signs of lower airway involvement may include wheezing and desaturation or may present as pulmonary edema, ranging from crackles in the lung bases to the expectoration of pink froth.

Management

Maintaining an acceptable O_2 saturation level and monitoring for signs of continued airway compromise are the mainstays of therapy. Aerosolized beta-agonists are usually helpful. Some authorities aerosolize sodium bicarbonate to help buffer acidic irritant gases, but this treatment is controversial. Be sure to follow your local protocols.

Chemical Burns of the Eye

Chemicals known to cause burning injuries to the eyes include acids (eg, concentrated liquid chlorine), alkalis (eg, cement powder or a strong cleaning agent), dry chemicals (eg, lye or lime), and phenols Figure 16 . Always wear eye protection when working with chemicals!

Assessment and Management

If chemicals have splashed into the patient's eyes, flush the eyes with copious amounts of water. It may be most expeditious to simply support the patient's head under a faucet or at an eyewash station, directing a steady stream of lukewarm tap water

Water Solubility	Examples of Substances	Effects
Highly water soluble	Ammonia Formaldehyde Hydrogen chloride (HCl) Sulfur dioxide	Corrosive local effects upon reacting with water in the upper airways. Effect usually immediate.
Moderately water soluble	Chlorine	Site of action depends on concentration inhaled. Effect may be immediate or delayed.
Slightly water soluble	Phosgene Nitrogen dioxide	Inflammation and pulmonary edema at the alveolar level. Effect may occur hours or days after exposure.

Table 6 Irritant Gases and Their Effects

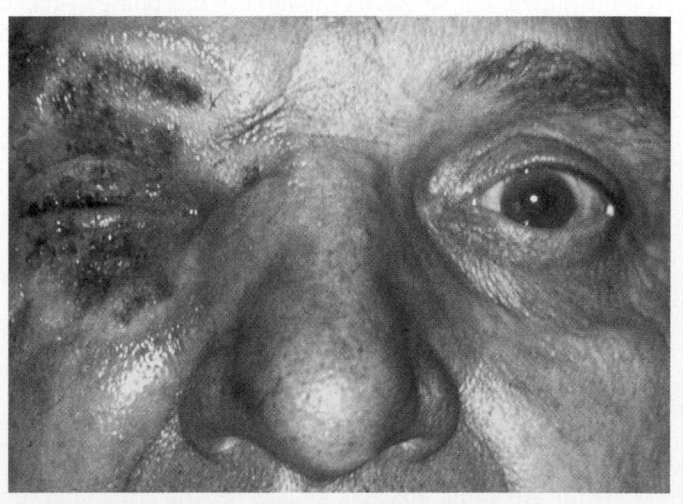

Figure 16 The eyes are particularly vulnerable to chemical burns.

into the affected eye **Figure 17**. If the patient wears contact lenses and the stream of water does not flush them out, pause after a minute or two of irrigation to allow the patient to remove the contact lenses—if they remain in place, they will prevent water from reaching the cornea underneath. Be sure to irrigate well underneath the eyelids.

Never use chemical antidotes (such as vinegar or baking soda) in the eyes; except possibly in the special case of irritation from tear gas or pepper spray. Irrigate with water only. After

irrigating, patch the patient's eyes with lightly applied dressings and begin transport to the hospital for evaluation.

Eye irrigation is extremely important whenever a chemical has gotten into the eye. However, it may be uncomfortable and inefficient to attempt to irrigate an eye by prying it open and rinsing with a standard normal saline IV set. Another option is the Morgan lens, which may make eye irrigation more comfortable, efficient, and effective. It is essentially a plastic contact lens with IV tubing attached to it, which allows IV fluids to flow directly over the surface of the eye **Figure 18**. Ocular anesthetic drops are preferable, but care must be taken when the eye is "numb" to keep the patient from scratching or rubbing it. Some authorities suggest that 100 mg of lidocaine can be placed in a liter of normal saline to produce an analgesic flush solution.

It is important to keep fluid running through the Morgan lens during insertion and removal. Suction can occur between the lens and the eye if the fluid flow is stopped before removal. After flushing, the pH of the eye can be tested with hydrazine paper

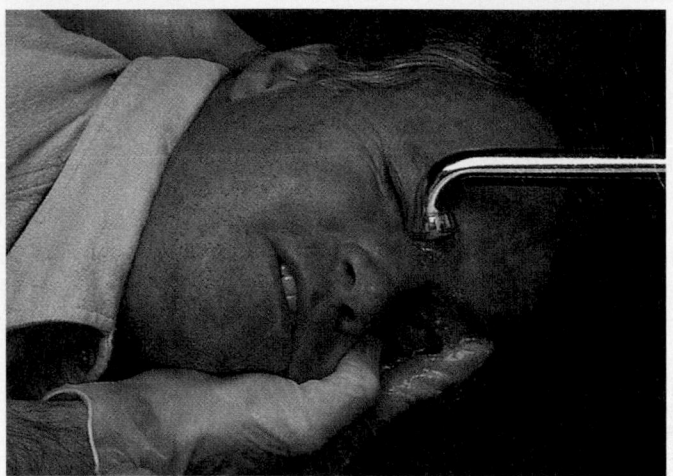

Figure 17 Flood the affected eye with a gentle stream of water. Hold the eyelids open–a challenging task because the patient's reflex is to keep the eye shut. Take care to prevent the chemical from getting into the other eye during the flushing.

YOU *are the Medic*   PART 4

An intravenous line is established and your patient receives 3.5 mg of morphine sulfate for pain. He is quiet during the ride to the hospital and it seems as though the morphine is helping to control the pain. A few minutes from the hospital you notice that the pulse oximetry numbers are dropping and your patient's breathing has become slow and shallow. His color is poor and you take action to correct and control the airway.

Recording Time: 9 Minutes	
Respirations	24 breaths/min, labored
Pulse	120 beats/min, radial pulses
Skin	Flushed, warm
Blood pressure	150/100 mm Hg
Oxygen saturation (Spo$_2$)	92%
Pupils	Equal, reactive

7. What are some possible causes for the change in respiratory status?

8. Explain the steps you would take to identify the cause of a change in respiratory status and explain how you would correct the problem.

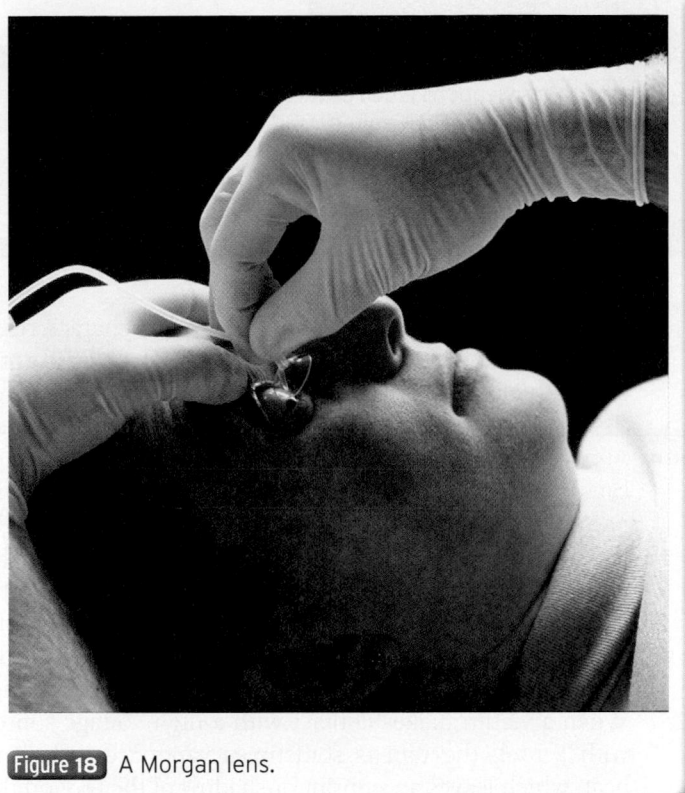

Figure 18 A Morgan lens.

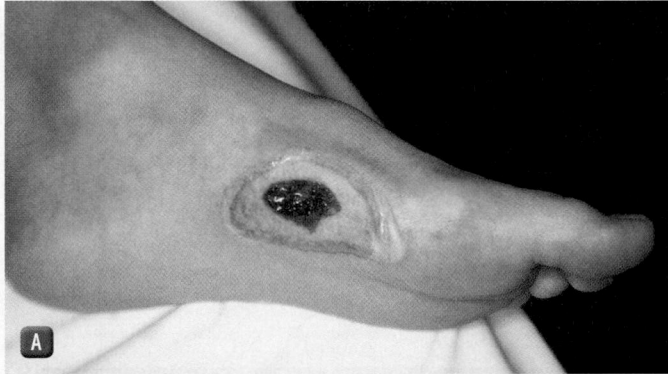

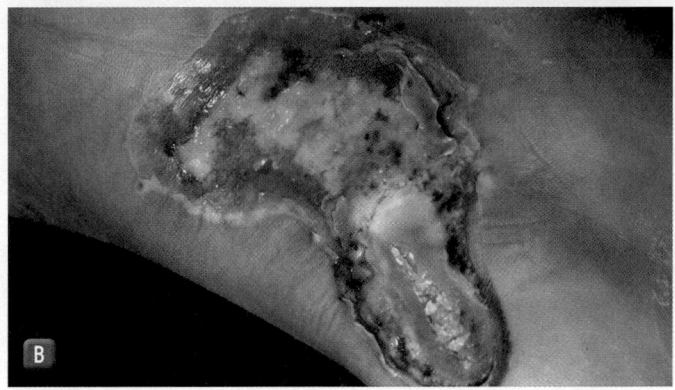

Figure 19 Electrical burns have entrance and exit wounds. **A.** The entrance wound is often quite small. **B.** The exit wound can be extensive and deep.

(pH paper) to determine if all of an acid or base has been removed, but this is typically done at the hospital with topical anesthetic.

Electrical Burns and Associated Injuries

Four percent of burn center admissions are from electrical burns. One of every five construction deaths is caused by electrical contact. Statistics from the National Institute of Occupational Safety and Health indicate that electrocution is the fourth leading cause of death in the workplace, causing more than 250 deaths per year. Children are involved in the majority of electrocutions in the home.

Electrical burns may produce devastating internal injuries with little external evidence. This type of burn may result in two injury sites: one at the point where electricity entered the body (an entrance wound) and another where it exited (an exit wound). The entrance wound may be quite small, but the exit wound can be extensive and deep Figure 19 . The degree of tissue injury is related to the resistance of the body tissues, the intensity of current that passes through the victim, and the duration of exposure.

When a person comes in contact with an electrical source, the amount of current delivered to the inside of the body depends to some extent on the resistance of the skin. Wet, thin, clean skin offers less resistance than dry, thick, dirty skin; thus a moist inner surface of the forearm will have much less resistance than a dry, callused palm.

As electric current travels from the contact site into the body, it is converted to heat, which follows the current flow—usually along blood vessels and nerves—causing extensive damage to the tissues in its path Table 7 . The greater the current flow, the greater the heat generated. When the voltage is low (less than 1,000 volts, as in household sources), current follows the path

of least resistance, generally along blood vessels, nerves, and muscles. When the voltage is high (as from high-tension lines), current takes the shortest path. The initial damage is usually the greatest at the entry and exit points, because this is where the amperage is concentrated (due to resistance from the skin).

Alternating current is considerably more dangerous than direct current because the alternations cause repetitive muscle contractions, which may "freeze" the victim to the conductor until the current source is turned off. Furthermore, alternating current is more likely than direct current to induce ventricular fibrillation.

Special Populations

A common electrical injury occurs when toddlers chew on electrical wires **Figure 20**. Children 1 to 2 years old have a greater propensity to chew or suck on electrical cords. Therefore, they may sustain significant burns to the oral cavity that can result in erosion of the labial and facial arteries, causing life-threatening hemorrhage. The electrolyte-rich saliva completes the circuit between the two wires when they bite the cord. Five percent of these toddlers will manifest dysrhythmias.

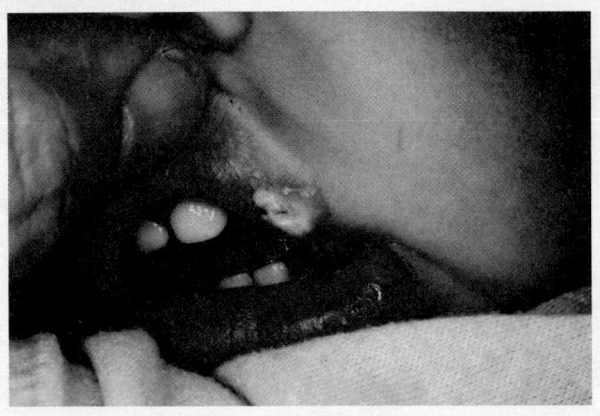

Figure 20 Children often sustain electrical burns.

Table 7 The Effects of Electric Current on the Body

Current (milliamps)	Effect on Body
1-4	Tingling sensation/perception
3-4	"Let go"* current–Children
6-8	"Let go" current–Women
7-9	"Let go" current–Men
16-20	Skeletal muscle tetany
20-50	Respiratory muscle paralysis
50-120	Ventricular fibrillation

*"Let go" current is the average amount of current at which a person is still physically able to let go of the source. Above this level, skeletal muscle contraction prevents the person from being able to release his or her grip.

The direction of current flow is also significant. Current moving from one hand to the other is particularly dangerous because current may then flow across the heart; a current of only 0.1 amp to the heart can provoke ventricular fibrillation.

Electricity can cause three types of burns:

- **True electrical injury.** This is the most common type of electrical burn. Because the current was most intense at

Words of Wisdom

Electroshock weapons (such as the Taser) use a high voltage/low amperage (50,000 volts/0.004 amps) shock to cause neuromuscular incapacitation, demonstrating that even low-amperage electrical shocks can have significant effects on the nervous system.

the entrance and exit sites, you may see a characteristic bull's-eye lesion at these sites, with a central, charred zone of full-thickness burns; a middle zone of cold, gray, dry tissue; and an outer, red zone of coagulation necrosis.

- **Arc-type or flash burn.** This is an electrothermal injury caused by the arcing of electric current. A person who passes close enough to a source of high-voltage current will reach a point where the resistance of the air between the current source and the person is sufficiently low that the current arcs through the air, from the current source to the passerby. This arc has a temperature from 3,000°C to 20,000°C—high enough to produce significant charring. When a victim makes contact with a high-voltage source with a tool, the tool is sometimes vaporized, releasing heat, which leaves an imprint or shadow of the tool on the patient's body.
- **Flame burn.** This kind of thermal injury occurs when electricity ignites a person's clothing or surroundings.

Electrical burns are most often classified as critical burns because there is a strong possibility of severe internal injury between the point of entry and the point of exit from the body. In some cases, the electricity may have flowed across the chest, potentially injuring the cardiac conduction system.

Burns may be only one of the problems experienced by a patient who has come in contact with an electrical source—and not necessarily the most serious. The two most common causes of death from electrical injury are asphyxia and cardiac arrest.

Asphyxia may occur when prolonged contact with alternating current induces tetanic contractions of the respiratory muscle. It may also result from current passing through the respiratory center in the brain and knocking out the impulse to breathe.

Cardiac arrest may occur secondarily, from hypoxia, or as a direct result of the electrical shock. Even currents as small as 0.1 amp can trigger ventricular fibrillation if they pass directly through the heart, as when current travels across the body from hand to hand. When cardiac arrest does not occur, cardiac damage may still be manifest in various rhythm disturbances on the electrocardiogram tracing.

Words of Wisdom

Dysrhythmias commonly seen with electrical injury include atrial fibrillation and atrial flutter.

Electricity can disrupt the nervous system; ask anyone who has been on the receiving end of a Taser. A host of neurologic complications have been reported in connection with electrical injury, including peripheral nerve deficit, seizures, delirium, confusion, coma, and temporary quadriplegia. Damage to the kidneys after electrical injury resembles the syndrome seen after a crush injury, which occurs when the breakdown products of damaged muscle (myoglobin) are liberated into the circulation. Electrical contact may affect muscle coordination and strength. Electricity that contacts the eyes may cause cataracts.

Severe, tetanic muscle spasms may lead to fractures and dislocations, which are often overlooked because of the preoccupation with the electrical injury. Posterior dislocation of the shoulder and fracture of the scapula—otherwise rare injuries—have been reported in several cases of electrocution. And don't forget the cervical spine, especially in a worker who has fallen from a utility pole.

All of the potential injuries that can result from an electrical injury conspire to make the victim of an electrical contact a very complex assessment challenge. Never let obvious injuries distract you from a complete assessment, including the neurologic, respiratory, cardiac, and musculoskeletal systems. In dealing with a patient who has an electrical injury, the usual priorities apply.

Assessment

The first priority at the scene of an electrical injury is to protect yourself and bystanders from becoming the next victims. Do *not* use a rope, wooden pole, or any other object to try to dislodge the patient from the current source. Do *not* try to cut the wire. Do *not* go anywhere near a high-tension line.

Many parts of the electrical grid are protected by automatically resetting breakers. When the wind blows a branch into wires or a rambunctious squirrel bridges the gap between two wires, it is desirable to have the breaker reset after a few moments to avoid power outages. As a consequence, a downed wire that "looks dead" can jump back to life, perhaps several times. There is only one safe way to deal with a downed high-tension wire: Call the electric company. Wait until a qualified person has shut off the power before you approach the patient. This can be a traumatic event for paramedics, who will feel helpless waiting for the power to be shut down while a possibly critical patient lies on the ground nearby. But remember—*rescuers die in these situations.* You can help the greatest number of people by being cautious and safe in this circumstance.

Once the electric hazard has been neutralized, assess the patient. Start CPR as indicated, and attach the monitor to identify ventricular fibrillation. Open the airway using the jaw-thrust maneuver, keeping in mind the possibility of cervical spine injury. If the patient is not in cardiac arrest, dysrhythmias remain a risk, and cardiac monitoring is indicated for 24 hours after the injury. Make careful note of the patient's state of consciousness, and record his or her vital signs.

Try to determine the path the current has taken through the body by looking for entrance and exit wounds and by carefully palpating the skin and soft tissues. When deep tissues have been seriously damaged by heat, the surrounding muscle may swell and become rock-hard. Thus, a rigid abdomen or rigid extremity may indicate a serious internal injury. Be alert for fractures or dislocations, and check the distal pulses in all four extremities.

Words of Wisdom

Many electrical injuries are obvious. Even so, you should always consider the possibility of an "occult" electrical exposure in patients with findings that suggest injury and no obvious mechanism of injury.

Management

Management of an electrical burn injury includes prioritizing care of the patient. If the patient has life-threatening injuries, begin related care and prepare to transport the patient as soon as practical. Generally, aside from the fluid therapy for hypotension, no specific pharmacologic interventions are indicated, other than the normal medications used to manage a cardiac dysrhythmia or extreme pain (if authorized by medical control).

Early O_2 therapy is helpful, as is managing the patient for impending shock. Transport decisions should be made early and take into consideration the regional resources for the care of a patient with a severe (electrical) burn. Contact medical control for advice in making a transport decision or regarding the need to use aeromedical evacuation directly to the burn center. The patients will be very anxious and scared, so be sure to talk with them calmly and explain what you are doing and how you plan to obtain the best care for them.

■ Lightning-Related Injuries

One special case of electrical injury deserves specific mention—the injury sustained from lightning. Over the last 30 years, there have been 55 reported lightning fatalities in the US. Those who do not die from their injuries are left with varying degrees of disability.

Lightning strikes when a massive discharge of electricity occurs between two bodies that have different charges—for example, between a thundercloud and the ground. The stream of current takes the path of least resistance from its origin to its destination. If any object projects above the surface of the earth that is a better conductor of electricity than the air—such as a building, a light pole, an antenna, a flagpole, or a tree—that object will "attract" the lightning bolt.

A person need not sustain a direct hit from lightning to be injured; in fact, most victims are not struck directly. Much more commonly, the victim is splashed by lightning striking a nearby tree or other projecting object, resulting in an arc-type or flash burn that leaves a characteristic "feathering" pattern on the skin **Figure 21**. Ground current produced by lightning striking the ground near the victim can also cause severe injury and accounts for incidents in which there are multiple casualties in an extended area, such as on a golf course or in an open field.

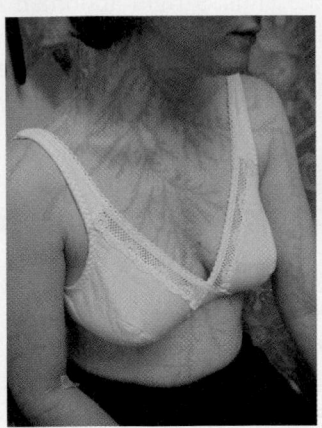

Figure 21 An arc-type burn resulting from a nearby lightning strike may leave a characteristic feathering pattern on the skin.

The best treatment for lightning injuries is prevention, and all health care professionals have a responsibility to educate the public in preventive measures. Clearly, the most effective precaution is to come in out of the rain, but that is not always possible. Bear in mind that a lightning strike may happen before or after the actual storm has passed, and it can strike up to 10 miles away from the storm. Lightning tends to strike the tallest objects that are good conductors. The following rules can help avoid lightning injuries:

- **Rule 1.** *Don't be the tallest object that is a good conductor.* Stay away from the middle of fields, lakes, golf courses, and other large, open areas. If you are stuck in the middle of an open area, try to be as small as you can. Don't hold up an umbrella, golf club, or lightning rod. Don't fly a kite.
- **Rule 2.** *Don't stand under or near the tallest object that is a good conductor.* Although you don't want to be in the middle of the field, you also don't want to be under the tallest tree, radio antenna, or golf umbrella.
- **Rule 3.** *Take shelter in the most substantial structure that you can to remain safe if it is hit by lightning.* A large building with a lightning suppression system is the best choice. An enclosed building is better than an open one (shed, lean-to). Close the shelter as much as possible. If in a car, keep the windows rolled up. Lightning tends to flash over the outside of objects (and people). It can travel substantial distances through conductors, however.
- **Rule 4.** *Avoid touching good conductors during a lightning storm.* Examples of good conductors include plumbing fixtures, fences, and electrical appliances, particularly those connected to wires outside (such as the telephone, TV, and computer).

Lightning carries enormous electrical power—its energy can reach 100 *million* volts, and peak currents can be in the range of 200,000 amps. Unlike other high-voltage electric current, it is *direct*—not alternating—current, and the duration of exposure is measured in milliseconds. Thus, lightning injuries tend to resemble blast injuries more than they do high-voltage injuries, with damage to the tympanic membranes of the ears and air-containing internal organs. Many reports of lightning strikes indicate victims' clothes were "blown off" of their bodies. Muscle damage may occur, and the release of myoglobin from injured muscle may jeopardize the kidneys.

For the cardiovascular system, lightning acts as a cosmic defibrillator, delivering a massive direct-current countershock that depolarizes the entire heart. The heart may resume beating spontaneously shortly after the shock or after 5 cycles (30:2) or approximately 2 minutes of CPR that is started immediately. Because respiratory arrest is apt to persist in patients who have been struck by lightning, continued ventilatory support may be required. The phenomenon of someone regaining a pulse after a lightning strike and having respiratory arrest is known to lead to a secondary cardiac arrest if left untreated. The central nervous system is almost invariably affected by a lightning strike. At least 70% of victims will lose consciousness for some period, and nearly 90% will have some confusion or amnesia (loss of memory). Temporary paralysis of the legs has occurred, and permanent paralysis and quadriplegia have been reported in a few cases.

Despite its unique appearance, the immediate threats to life caused by a lightning strike are the same as those caused by a high-voltage power line injury: airway obstruction, respiratory arrest, and cardiac arrest.

Assessment

When you reach the scene of a lightning strike, all the usual priorities apply, but there are two special considerations to keep in mind.

First, if the electrical storm is still going on, your first priority is to get any patients and rescuers to a safe place, preferably indoors, or at least inside the ambulance. Lightning *can* strike twice in the same place. There is, however, no hazard in touching the victim of a lightning strike—contrary to what your grandmother may have told you, electricity does not remain within the body of a person who has been hit by lightning.

Words of Wisdom

In a lightning strike with multiple victims, priority goes to the victims who are not breathing.

Second, be aware that a lightning strike is apt to injure more than one person. Therefore, the first thing you need to do on arrival at the scene—before you leave the safety of the ambulance—is a rapid size-up of the entire scene to determine the number of patients.

Start CPR when necessary. Carry out the primary assessment as usual. When establishing an airway, bear in mind the possibility of cervical spine injury, and do not hyperextend the neck; use the jaw-thrust maneuver.

Patients with cardiac arrest caused by a lightning strike deserve aggressive, continuing CPR. The chances of a successful resuscitation in such a case are good, even when the patient appears beyond help initially and even when there is a long delay in the return of spontaneous breathing. Minimize the interruption in compressions, and push hard and fast with full chest recoil!

Words of Wisdom

Don't give up quickly on a patient in cardiac arrest due to a lightning strike.

Management

Treatment of lightning injuries is similar to that of injuries sustained from high-voltage lines:

- Make sure the scene is safe. Move the victim to a safer location if necessary.
- Priority for treatment goes to patients who are not breathing.
- Perform CPR as needed. Establish an airway, with cervical spine precautions.
- Administer supplemental oxygen.
- Monitor cardiac rhythm.
- Insert a large-bore IV catheter and run in normal saline solution wide open to keep the kidneys flushed out.
- Cover any surface burns with dry, sterile dressings.
- Splint fractures.
- If the patient has fallen, immobilize the cervical spine.

■ Radiation Burns

Acute radiation exposure has become more than a theoretical issue as use of radioactive materials increases in industry and medicine, and you must understand it to function effectively in the prehospital arena. Between 1944 and 2010 there were more than 400 radiation accidents worldwide involving significant radiation exposure to more than 3,000 people. More recent events in Japan (March 11, 2011) highlight that radiation accidents continue to be a threat. Potential threats include incidents related to the use and transportation of radioactive isotopes and intentionally released radioactivity in terrorist attacks. To be effective, you must first suspect radiation and attempt to determine whether ongoing exposure exists. Increasingly, special response units are equipped with pager-sized radiation detectors, or such detection may be provided by other public safety services.

There are three types of ionizing radiation: alpha, beta, and gamma. Alpha particles have little penetrating energy and are easily stopped by the skin. Beta particles have greater penetrating power and can travel much farther in air than alpha particles. They can penetrate the skin but can be blocked by simple protective clothing designed for this purpose. The threat from gamma radiation is directly proportional to its wavelength. This type of radiation is very penetrating and easily passes through the body and solid materials.

Radiation is measured in units of radiation equivalent in man (rem) or radiation absorbed dose (rad). One hundred rad are equal to 1 gray (Gy). Small amounts of everyday background radiation are measured in rad; the amount of radiation released in a major incident may be measured in Gy. The average human exposure from background radiation is 0.36 rem per year. Mild radiation sickness can be expected with exposures of 1 to 2 Gy (100 to 200 rad), moderate sickness at 2 to 5 Gy, and severe sickness at 4 to 6 Gy. Exposure to more than 8 Gy is immediately fatal.

The vast majority of ionizing radiation accidents involve gamma radiation, or x-rays. People who have suffered a radiation exposure generally pose no risk to the people around them. However, in some types of incidents—particularly those involving explosions—patients may be contaminated with radioactive particulate matter. It is speculated that after a nuclear explosion, most patients will have sustained some type of trauma in addition to the radiation exposure.

Acute Radiation Syndrome <u>Acute radiation syndrome</u> causes hematologic, central nervous system, and gastrointestinal changes. Many of these changes occur over time and so will not be apparent during contact with EMS providers. Patients who are rendered unresponsive by radiation or who manifest vomiting within 10 minutes of exposure will not survive. Those who manifest vomiting in less than an hour have severe exposure and a 30% to 80% survival rate. Many people with moderate exposure will vomit within 1 to 2 hours and have a 95% to 100% survival rate. Clearly, the onset of vomiting soon after exposure is a predictor of poor outcomes. Consider this fact when triaging patients or considering the risks of entering a high-radiation environment to attempt rescue.

Radiation Contact Burns A person who handles a radioactive source briefly may sustain a local soft-tissue injury without a lot of total body irradiation. This scenario might arise, for example, in a collision involving a vehicle transporting radioactive material or after the detonation of a "dirty bomb." The injury could resemble anything from superficial sunburn to a chemical burn. Although chemical burns usually become apparent almost immediately after exposure, radiation burns could appear hours or even days after exposure.

Assessment

First and foremost, the assessment of a patient who may have been exposed to radiation involves a scene size-up to determine if the scene is safe for rescuers to enter. Determine what protective gear you will need to shield yourself from the radiation before entering the scene **Figure 22**. In most cases, it will be appropriate to contact the hazardous materials response team so they may determine the appropriate precautions, including exposure-limiting suits and the most appropriate ED for the patient's treatment. Not all EDs are set up to treat a patient who

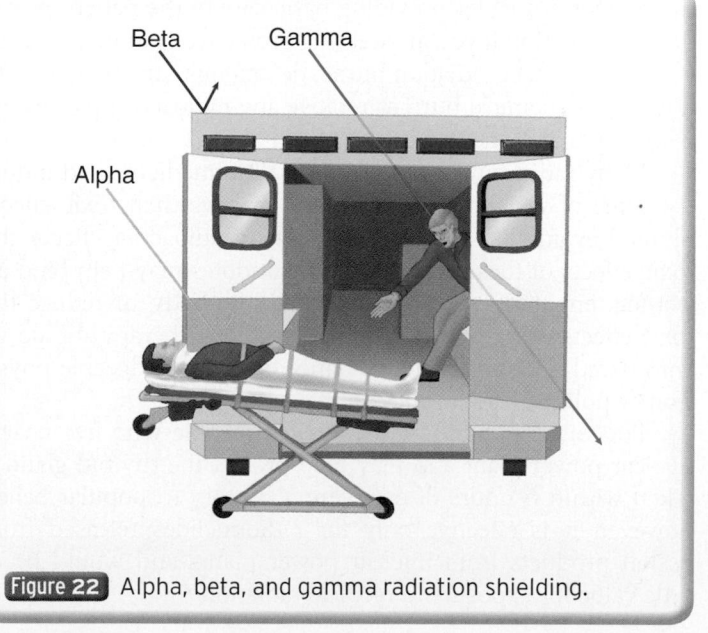

Figure 22 Alpha, beta, and gamma radiation shielding.

has been exposed to radiation, so learn the capabilities of your hospitals before an incident occurs! EMS agencies that operate in an area where there is a nuclear power plant or other research facility typically have additional training offered by the facility and regularly practice responding to radiation-related emergencies.

Clothing will protect from alpha radiation. Simple protective clothing will protect from beta radiation. Gamma radiation will pass through the body and solid materials. Special protective clothing such as lead shielding is necessary to protect from gamma radiation.

Once the scene is deemed safe, you may proceed with your primary assessment of the patient. Assess the patient's mental status and ABCs, and then prioritize the patient's care. Unfortunately, patients who have sustained significant radiation exposure and a major burn are unlikely to survive, even with major resources expended to keep them alive (a burn of greater than 70% of the TBSA is probably fatal by itself; a burn and radiation of greater than 30% of the TBSA are probably fatal). When confronted with large numbers of patients who have been exposed to radiation and simultaneously received thermal burns, keep the 30% rule in mind when triaging and making transport decisions. Of course, you should also consult with medical control in these complicated cases. In the field, it is difficult to determine the extent of the patient's internal injuries.

Management

Patients with radiation burns may be contaminated with radioactive material, so they should be decontaminated before transport. The majority of contaminants can be removed by simply disrobing the patient.

Irrigate open wounds. Washing should be gentle to avoid further damage to the skin, which could result in additional internal radiation absorption. The head and scalp should be irrigated the same way. The ED should be notified as soon as practical if you are transporting a potentially contaminated patient. In contrast with other types of contamination, radioactive particulate matter probably poses a relatively small risk to the rescuer. Consider providing basic care to the patient before decontamination if you are wearing protective clothing.

With contact radiation burns, decontaminate the wound as if it were a chemical burn to remove any radioactive particulate matter. You may then treat it as a burn.

Many radioactive isotopes are used in medicine and industry, some of which can be absorbed or have their toxic effects blunted by another substance. Like their radioactive effects, the toxic effects of these isotopes vary. Antidotes may help bind an isotope, enhance its elimination from the body, or reduce the toxic effects on other organs. Such antidotal therapy should be considered only under the guidance of a knowledgeable physician or public health agency.

Potassium iodide is distributed to people who live near a nuclear power plant and may help protect the thyroid gland if taken within 6 hours of exposure. Contrary to popular belief, however, it is effective only for radionuclides released from fission products from nuclear power plants and would be of little value for exposure to medical radiation.

Radiation injury follows the "inverse square law": Exposure drops exponentially as distance is increased. Increasing your (and your patient's) distance from the source by even a few feet may dramatically decrease your exposure, so it is important to identify the radioactive source and the length of the patient's exposure to it. You must try to limit your duration of exposure, increase your distance from the source, and attempt to place shielding between yourself and sources of gamma radiation.

■ Management of Burns in Pediatric Patients

Escaping from a fire can be difficult for children. More than half of the fire-related deaths and injuries in children involve preschoolers. Research suggests that young children are not as effectively awakened by smoke detectors, and they are often disoriented immediately after waking. The "reliable waking rate" in children younger than 15 years may be as low as 6%. Young children are also more likely to sustain severe scald injuries. Children's thin skin and delicate respiratory structures are more easily damaged by thermal insults than are those of older children and adults.

In children, fluid resuscitation may be more challenging because of their increased body surface/weight ratio. As a consequence, children may require more fluid per kilogram than adults. You may start with the Consensus formula in children, only to find that medical control orders additional fluids for severe burns. Also, because of poor glycogen stores, children may require dextrose-containing solutions earlier than adults. Blood glucose monitoring should be routinely performed in seriously burned children.

Burns may raise the suspicion of child abuse. Pay careful attention to the MOI, and relay this information to the hospital staff.

■ Management of Burns in Geriatric Patients

Approximately 1,200 older adults die of fire-related causes each year, making it the sixth leading cause of death in this population. Some 13% of older adults smoke, and smoking is the leading cause of fires that lead to death of elderly people. Burns from fires caused by smoking while wearing supplementary O_2 are the leading sentinel event in home care. Cooking fires represent another distinct hazard to elderly people, who may be less able to smell a gas leak or a fire in the kitchen. Elderly patients are also particularly sensitive to respiratory insults. Relatively small fires can produce toxic fumes before detection or suppression devices are activated.

Geriatric patients may also have poor glycogen stores, so their blood glucose levels should be checked to assess for hypoglycemia. Cardiac monitoring should, of course, be implemented. Although fluid resuscitation is important, pulmonary edema is more likely to develop in geriatric patients. Routinely assess lung sounds.

Long-Term Consequences of Burns

The Patient

Serious burn injuries are devastating events that leave patients with long-term physical and psychological challenges. People with major injuries average about 1 day of inpatient treatment for each 1% of the TBSA burned. Extensive rehabilitation may also be necessary to regain function. Survivors of serious burns are left with a host of long-term consequences, including problems with thermoregulation, motor function, and sensory function. Although tremendous improvements in the care of critical burn patients have made long-term survival possible for many who would have died of their injuries a decade ago, large surface area burns remain a critical care challenge on par with other forms of severe multisystem trauma.

The Provider

Caring for patients with severe burn emergencies can be one of the most horrifying tasks undertaken by paramedics. Fire scenes are chaotic and dangerous. Patients are often in severe pain. The smell of burned hair and flesh permeates your clothes and equipment. Sheets of tissue may peel off the patient when you perform simple tasks like attempting to take vital signs or moving the patient. Despite the traumatic circumstances, with the proper training and the right mix of confidence and courage, you can make a tremendous impact in the treatment and overall survival of burn patients.

YOU *are the Medic*   SUMMARY

1. Your next steps should include which actions?

Continue with your patient assessment. Painful or gruesome injuries are very distracting to the patient. It's up to you, the paramedic, to stay on track so that significant injuries will not be overlooked.

2. Based on just the information given so far, would transport of this patient be a low priority ("stay and play") or a high priority ("load and go") at this time?

High priority. Airway burns, in this case, inhalation of superheated gases (steam), can cause serious damage both in the upper and lower airways.

3. Your patient is clearly experiencing significant pain. At what point in treatment should this be addressed?

While pain is significant, the primary concern is first to identify and correct life threats. Inhalation burns can cause rapid and serious airway compromise. Although this patient is breathing without difficulty, his reddened face and neck, as well as the raspiness of his voice, indicate the potential for a sudden airway compromise that the paramedic must be ready to aggressively manage with advanced airway techniques and sedation if necessary.

4. How significant is the patient's apparent raspiness as he is speaking to you?

This is a red flag that should alert you and your partner that the airway has been injured. Be alert for other developments such as stridor, wheezes, and a poor Spo_2.

5. What is the likely cause of the patient's elevated blood pressure?

Severe and acute pain leads to increased sympathetic nerve activity and subsequent increased peripheral vascular resistance.

6. At what point might you consider aggressive airway management including sedation and intubation?

Based on the mechanism of injury, you should be prepared to perform rapid intubation at any time. The burns on the patient's face and neck are good indications that a significant airway burn may have occurred. Heat can be an irritant to the lungs, and you need to be alert for development of wheezing, coughing, stridor, and other indicators of swelling of airway structures.

7. What are some possible causes for the change in respiratory status?

Two possibilities should immediately come to mind. First, the patient was just given morphine sulfate to help control pain. Because it acts on the central nervous system, morphine is a respiratory depressant. The other likely possibility is the development of swelling in the airways due to burns.

8. Explain the steps you would take to identify the cause of a change in respiratory status, and explain how you would correct the problem.

The differential diagnosis between respiratory difficulty from a central nervous system depressant and that of airway burns should be fairly clear. First, if adventitious sounds, such as wheezing or stridor were absent, this would make it unlikely that respiratory difficulty is due to burns. To treat such a condition, small doses of naloxone are indicated. On the other hand, difficulty breathing with the absence of sounds may be due to external injury. The patient's burns on the neck may be causing a circumferential swelling that may not involve the inner airway and therefore no abnormal sounds may be heard. Another possibility is that the back of the ambulance is too noisy to hear lung sound changes. In the case in which airway swelling is visible or sounds such as stridor are audible, immediate and aggressive airway management is needed. This patient is most likely experiencing airway compromise due to burns; airway management using a bag-mask device followed by intubation is indicated.

YOU *are the Medic*   **SUMMARY,** *continued*

EMS Patient Care Report (PCR)					
Date: 09-02-11	**Incident No.:** 0930	**Nature of Call:** Man burned		**Location:** 457 Main Blvd. in gas station	
Dispatched: 1530	**En Route:** 1531	**At Scene:** 1534	**Transport:** 1544	**At Hospital:** 1550	**In Service:** 1610

Patient Information

Age: 22 **Sex:** M **Weight (in kg [lb]):** 70 kg (155 lb)	**Allergies:** No known drug allergies **Medications:** Denies **Past Medical History:** Denies **Chief Complaint:** My arm is burned and it hurts

Vital Signs

Time: 1539	BP: 160/110	Pulse: 120, strong, regular	Respirations: 22	Spo$_2$: 98%
Time: 1543	BP: 150/100	Pulse: 120	Respirations: 24, labored	Spo$_2$: 92%
Time: 1547	BP: 130/90	Pulse: 108	Respirations: 12, assisted	Spo$_2$: 99%

EMS Treatment
(circle all that apply)

Oxygen @ __15__ L/min via (circle one): NC (NRM) (Bag-mask device)	(Assisted Ventilation) 12/min	(Airway Adjunct) ET tube	CPR
Defibrillation	**Bleeding Control**	(Bandaging) Sterile dressings	**Splinting**	(Other:) Spinal immobilization, IV with pain medication

Narrative

9-1-1 dispatched to a report of a man burned at a gas station. Upon arrival, 22-year-old man found standing at gas station, alert and oriented and reporting severe pain as indicated by facial grimace and agitation. Gas station owner reports seeing pt drive in to gas station with what appeared to be an overheating car radiator. The pt got out and opened the hood and owner states that he heard him scream and saw large plumes of steam coming from under the opened hood. Pt walked over to ambulance as we arrived and was able to speak comfortably in complete sentences although his voice seemed raspy. Initially, he denied any difficulty breathing and reported only pain in right arm. Slight swelling of lips noted. Pt has first-degree burns over face, lips, and anterior neck. Lung sounds are equal and clear. Right forearm (palmar surface) has blistering and redness. Distal (radial) pulse present and strong. Capillary nailbed refill of injured arm is < 2 seconds.

    Prior to transport, pt given 3.5 mg IV morphine sulfate at 1540 hours. Pt showed relief of pain, reporting an initial pain scale rating of 10/10; after morphine, 4/10 and blood pressure declined significantly. En route, pt developed respiratory difficulty. Respirations were assisted with bag-mask ventilation; pt not intubated due to quick arrival at hospital. ECG monitored en route with sinus tachycardia. Pt delivered to Mercy Hospital and turned over in ED to Dr. Anthony. Return to service at 1610 hours.
End of report

Prep Kit

Ready for Review

- Although you probably will not see moderate or severe burns on a daily basis, you will encounter some serious burn injuries during your career.

- The skin has four functions: to protect the underlying tissue from injury and exposure, to regulate temperature, to prevent excessive loss of water from the body, and to act as a sense organ.

- Burns are diffuse soft-tissue injuries created from destructive energy transferred via thermal, electrical, or radiation energy.

- Significant burn damage to the skin may make the body vulnerable to bacterial invasion, temperature instability, and major disturbances of fluid balance resulting in burn shock.

- Thermal burns include flame, scald, contact, steam, and flash burns.

- Beyond the visible soft-tissue injury, burns can affect the cardiovascular, respiratory, renal, gastrointestinal, hematological, and endocrine systems. The most important systemic response to significant burn trauma is burn shock.

- When burn shock occurs, capillaries leak out of the circulation into the interstitial spaces. Cells take in increased amounts of salt and water from the fluid around them. As with other types of shock, the body's ability to distribute oxygen and glucose is hampered. Adequate fluid resuscitation is essential treatment.

- Burn wounds of the skin may be superficial, partial thickness, or full thickness.

- A superficial burn involves only the epidermis, and skin appears red and swollen.

- A partial-thickness burn involves the epidermis and part of the dermis. Moderate partial-thickness burns usually are blistered, red, and extremely painful. Deep partial-thickness burns damage the hair follicle and sweat and sebaceous glands.

- A full-thickness burn involves destruction of the epidermis, the dermis, and the basement membrane of the dermis. After this type of burn, skin will not regenerate. Such a burn may appear white and waxy, brown and leathery, or charred.

- Inhalation burns may cause rapid airway compromise via heat and/or toxic chemicals entering the airway and lungs. Signs of irritation include coughing, wheezing, and possible stridor, signifying airway swelling. Carbon monoxide intoxication is also a concern.

- Establishing scene safety should be your first priority in responding to a burn call. Significant threats are likely to remain at the scene of a fire, chemical spill, electrical burn incident, lightning strike, or radiation leak.

- The many types of burns, coupled with the many possible presentations of burn patients, can challenge your assessment skills. Address a burned patient in a consistent, efficient, and systematic manner so you do not develop tunnel vision for the major burn trauma and miss other occult injuries that could affect the patient's outcome.

- Once ABCs are addressed, assess the total body surface area (TBSA) burned, using the rule of palms, rule of nines, or Lund and Browder chart. This is an important step because burn severity relates to the need for transport to a burn unit. Most practitioners advocate counting only the areas of partial- and full-thickness burns (ignoring the areas of superficial burns). Remember that when using the rule of nines, different rules apply for infants, children, and the elderly.

- Three cornerstones of the emergency medical care of burns are airway management, with the potential need for field intubation, fluid resuscitation to prevent shock, and pain management. Cooling and sterile bandaging are indicated for certain thermal burns. Chemical burns of the skin or eyes generally require copious flushing with water, with certain exceptions.

- Many burn patients will ultimately require intubation, even if during their initial presentation they were able to talk to you. Patients who are in cardiac or respiratory arrest, or whose airways are rapidly swelling, will need field intubation. A deteriorating airway may or may not require field intubation. A patient whose airway is currently patent but who has a history consistent with risk factors for airway compromise may or may not need field intubation.

- Patients with more than 20% body surface area burns will need fluid resuscitation. It is important to give the correct amount of fluid; too much fluid may be as bad as too little. If fluid resuscitation is delayed more than 2 hours from the time of the burn in severely burned patients, resuscitation is complicated and mortality increases. Deliver an appropriate amount of fluid to the burn patient as soon as is reasonable.

- The Consensus formula is an equation used to determine the amount of fluid a burned patient will need during the first 24 hours. Note that only a small portion of this time will occur in the prehospital environment. Half of the amount must be given during the first 8 hours. The remainder is given over the remaining 16 hours.

- Remember to assess the patient's pain and provide aggressive pain management. Pain medication is best given intravenously. Burn patients may require higher than usual doses of pain medications to achieve relief. Reassess the patient's pain every 5 minutes.

- Chemical burns may affect the skin, eyes, or airway. Alkali burns are especially devastating. Typical management for removal of chemical solutions from the skin is copious flushing with water; management of powders requires brushing off as much of the substance as possible before washing. Management of chemicals from the eye involves flushing the eyes with copious amounts of water, and possibly removing contact lenses. Consider use of a Morgan lens.

- In cases of electrical burn, electric current is converted to heat as it travels through the body, causing extensive damage. Electrical burns generally leave two wounds, an entrance wound and a much larger exit wound. Assessment of electrical injuries first includes scene safety considerations, then beginning CPR if indicated. Management includes treating life-threatening injuries and potential shock.

- Most radiation burns are caused by gamma radiation, or x-rays. Assessment includes scene safety concerns. Management involves decontamination, irrigation, washing, possibly antidote administration, and transport.

- Pediatric patients can be more easily harmed by thermal injuries than other patients, and fluid resuscitation may be more challenging. Children may require dextrose-containing solutions earlier than adults; perform blood glucose monitoring routinely in seriously ill children. Pay careful attention to mechanism of injury; burns may raise the suspicion of child abuse.

- Elderly patients are also particularly sensitive to respiratory insults. They may have poor glycogen stores; check their blood glucose levels for hypoglycemia. Perform cardiac monitoring. Watch for pulmonary edema if performing fluid resuscitation.

Prep Kit, continued

■ Vital Vocabulary

acute radiation syndrome The clinical course that usually begins within hours of exposure to a radiation source. Symptoms include nausea, vomiting, diarrhea, fatigue, fever, and headache. The long-term symptoms are dose-related and are hematopoietic and gastrointestinal.

adipose tissue Fat tissue.

burn shock The shock or hypoperfusion caused by a burn injury and the tremendous loss of fluids; capillaries leak, resulting in intravascular fluid volume oozing out of the circulation and into the interstitial spaces, and cells take in increased amounts of salt and water.

circumferential burns Burns on the neck or chest that may compress the airway or on an extremity that might act like a tourniquet.

collagen A protein that gives tensile strength to the connective tissues of the body.

comedo A noninflammatory acne lesion.

Consensus formula A formula that recommends giving 4 mL of normal saline for each kilogram of body weight, multiplied by the percentage of body surface area burned; sometimes used to calculate fluid needs during lengthy transport times; formerly called the Parkland formula.

contact burn A burn produced by touching a hot object.

cutaneous Pertaining to the skin.

dermis The inner layer of skin containing hair follicle roots, glands, blood vessels, and nerves.

desquamation The continuous shedding of the dead cells on the surface of the skin.

elastin A protein that gives the skin its elasticity.

epidermis The outermost layer of the skin.

escharotomy A surgical cut through the eschar or leathery covering of a burn injury to allow for swelling and minimize the potential for development of compartment syndrome in a circumferentially burned limb or the thorax.

flame burn A thermal burn caused by flames touching the skin.

flash burn An electrothermal injury caused by arcing of electric current.

full-thickness burn A burn that extends through the epidermis and dermis into the subcutaneous tissues beneath; previously called a third-degree burn.

homeostasis A tendency to constancy or stability in the body's internal environment.

integument The skin.

Joule's law A description of the relationship between heat production, current, and resistance.

Lund and Browder chart A detailed version of the rule of nines chart that takes into consideration the changes in body surface area brought on by growth.

melanin The pigment that gives skin its color.

mucopolysaccharide gel One of the complex materials found, along with the collagen fibers and elastin fibers, in the dermis of the skin.

Ohm's law The formula that describes the relationship between voltage and resistance. Current (I) = Voltage (V) divided by Resistance (R).

partial-thickness burn A burn that involves the epidermis and part of the dermis, characterized by pain and blistering; previously called a second-degree burn.

rule of nines A system that assigns percentages to sections of the body, allowing calculation of the amount of skin surface involved in the burn area.

rule of palms A system that estimates total body surface area burned by comparing the affected area with the size of the patient's palm, which is roughly equal to 1% of the patient's total body surface area; also called rule of ones.

scald burn A burn produced by hot liquids.

sebaceous gland A gland located in the dermis that secretes sebum.

sebum An oily substance secreted by sebaceous glands.

steam burn A burn that has been caused by direct exposure to hot steam exhaust, as from a broken pipe.

subcutaneous layer Beneath the skin.

superficial burn A burn involving only the epidermis, producing very red, painful skin; previously called a first-degree burn.

supraglottic Located above the glottic opening, as in the upper airway structures.

thermal burn An injury caused by radiation or direct contact with a heat source on the skin.

thermoregulation The ability of the body to maintain temperature through a combination of heat gain by metabolic processes and muscular movement and heat loss through respiration, evaporation, conduction, convection, and perspiration.

zone of coagulation The reddened area surrounding the leathery and sometimes charred tissue that has sustained a full-thickness burn.

zone of hyperemia In a thermal burn, the area that is least affected by the burn injury. This is an area of increased blood flow where the body is attempting to repair injured but otherwise viable tissue.

zone of stasis The peripheral area surrounding the zone of coagulation that has decreased blood flow and inflammation. This area can undergo necrosis within 24 to 48 hours after the injury, particularly if perfusion is compromised due to burn shock.

Assessment in Action

You and your partner are dispatched to a patient with possible burns at a construction site. Upon arrival, a construction worker rapidly leads a second man with a cloth over his eyes to the ambulance. He is wearing work clothes and heavy boots that appear to be covered in gray mud. The patient is alert and oriented and readily answers all of your questions appropriately. He tells you that he was working with a special type of concrete—"the kind that sets real fast" and some splashed into his eyes. His coworker tells you that the pH of the concrete is "very high—it causes nasty burns." The patient removes the cloth from his eyes as he climbs into the ambulance and you see that his eyes are red, swollen, and tearing with spillover onto his face. He is alert, is breathing adequately with no respiratory compromise, and has no visible skin breaks or bleeding. He denies any other injuries.

1. The coworker tells you that the pH of the substance in the patient's eyes is "somewhere around 13 or so." Immediate treatment should include:
   A. rapid transport to the hospital.
   B. a secondary assessment.
   C. keeping the patient sitting up and flushing his eyes for 30 minutes before transport and while en route.
   D. keeping the patient flat and flushing his eyes for 30 minutes before transport and while en route.

2. Which of the following concurrent situations do you need to take action on right away?
   A. The presence of cataracts
   B. The presence of contact lenses
   C. Blindness in one eye due to an old injury
   D. Recent laser surgery on one of the eyes

3. Your partner hands you a small bottle of eye drops to numb the patient's eyes. You should:
   A. use them primarily to reduce the pain.
   B. not use them since numbness will mask the extent of injury.
   C. use them to help the patient keep his eyes open.
   D. not use them since you will be holding the patient's eyes open.

4. While irrigating his eyes, you notice that the patient has dried concrete specks on his cheeks and forehead. You should:
   A. remove them from the skin while wearing gloves and flush the skin for 30 minutes.
   B. leave them in place but continue to irrigate the skin for 30 minutes.
   C. do nothing, as they are probably harmless.
   D. make a note of this on the patient report and get to it when you can.

5. Following copious irrigation, the patient should first be questioned and examined for:
   A. visual acuity and any vision changes.
   B. redness.
   C. pupillary reaction.
   D. the presence of pain.

6. Following delivery of this patient to the emergency department, you and your partner return to the ambulance. You notice clumps of grey grit and dirt on the floor of the ambulance. The stretcher bar and the overhead rail both have concrete dried on them from the patient's gloved hands. Before going back into service, you should:
   A. sweep the ambulance and wipe away any debris.
   B. clean the ambulance and decontaminate it before returning to service.
   C. wipe the stretcher and overhead bar, not concerning yourself with the floor.
   D. keep the ambulance out of service.

Additional Questions

7. Many construction sites have chemicals unique to the work being performed. When dealing with an injury related to chemical exposure, what are some important considerations?

8. What are some of the similarities between radiation burns and electrical burns?

Face and Neck Trauma

National EMS Education Standard Competencies

Trauma

Integrates assessment findings with principles of epidemiology and pathophysiology to formulate a field impression to implement a comprehensive treatment/disposition plan for an acutely injured patient.

Head, Facial, Neck, and Spine Trauma

Recognition and management of
- Life threats (pp 1617-1618)
- Spine trauma (pp 1634-1635, and see chapter, *Head and Spine Trauma*)

Pathophysiology, assessment, and management of
- Penetrating neck trauma (pp 1631-1634)
- Laryngotracheal injuries (pp 1631-1634)
- Spine trauma
  - Dislocations/subluxations (see chapter, *Head and Spine Trauma*)
  - Fractures (see chapter, *Head and Spine Trauma*)
  - Sprains/strains (see chapter, *Head and Spine Trauma*)
- Facial fractures (pp 1618-1621)
- Skull fractures (see chapter, *Head and Spine Trauma*)
- Foreign bodies in the eyes (pp 1621-1626)
- Dental trauma (p 1630)
- Unstable facial fractures (pp 1618; 1621)
- Orbital fractures (pp 1619; 1623)
- Perforated tympanic membrane (p 1629)
- Mandibular fractures (pp 1618-1619; 1621)

Knowledge Objectives

1. Discuss the anatomy and physiology of the head, face, and neck, including major structures and specific important landmarks. (pp 1609-1615)
2. Describe the factors that may cause the obstruction of the upper airway following a facial injury. (pp 1618-1619)
3. Discuss the general patient assessment process for a patient with a face or neck injury. (pp 1614-1617)
4. Discuss general emergency care of a patient with a face or neck injury, including the importance of airway management. (pp 1617-1618)

5. Discuss different types of facial injuries, including soft-tissue injuries, nasal fractures, mandibular fractures, maxillary fractures, orbital fractures, and zygomatic fractures and patient care considerations related to each one. (pp 1618-1621)
6. Describe the process of providing emergency care to a patient who has sustained face and neck injuries, including assessment of the patient, review of signs and symptoms, and management of care. (pp 1620-1621)
7. List the steps in the emergency medical care of the patient with soft-tissue wounds of the face and neck. (p 1621)
8. Discuss different types of eye injuries, including lacerations, foreign bodies, impaled objects, blunt trauma, and burns, and related patient care considerations. (pp 1621-1625)
9. List the steps in the emergency medical care of the patient with an eye injury, including lacerations, blunt trauma, foreign object, impaled object, and burns. (pp 1625-1629)
10. Discuss different types of ear injuries, including soft-tissue injuries and a ruptured eardrum, and related patient care considerations. (p 1629)
11. List the steps in the emergency medical care of the patient with injuries of the ear, including lacerations and foreign body insertions. (p 1629)
12. Discuss different oral injuries, including soft-tissue injuries and dental injuries, and related patient care considerations. (p 1630)
13. List the steps in the emergency medical care of the patient with dental and cheek injuries, including how to handle an avulsed tooth. (p 1630)
14. Discuss specific injuries to the anterior part of the neck, including soft-tissue injuries, injuries to the larynx, injuries to the trachea, and injuries to the esophagus. (pp 1631-1632)
15. List the steps in the emergency medical care of the patient with a penetrating injury to the neck, including how to control regular and life-threatening bleeding. (pp 1633-1634)
16. Discuss spine trauma that does not involve the spinal cord, including the pathophysiology of sprains and strains, and their assessment and management. (pp 1634-1635)

Skills Objectives

1. Demonstrate the stabilization of a foreign object that has been impaled in a patient's eye. (p 1626)
2. Demonstrate irrigation of a patient's eye using a nasal cannula, bottle, or basin. (p 1627)
3. Demonstrate the care of a patient who has a penetrating eye injury. (p 1626)
4. Demonstrate how to control bleeding from a neck injury. (pp 1633-1634)

Introduction

As a paramedic, you will commonly encounter patients with injuries to the face and neck. For example, approximately 70% of patients who survive motor vehicle collisions experience facial trauma. In addition to motor vehicle collisions, violence is a common cause of facial trauma. Preventive measures such as the use of air bags and the creation of laws related to speed limits, seat belt use, and operating under the influence have helped lead to a decline in facial bone fractures that result from motor vehicle collisions.

Facial trauma ranges in severity from a broken nose to penetration of the great vessels of the neck. As one of the most exposed regions of the body, the face and neck are frequently subjected to traumatic forces ranging from simple falls and assaults to direct blunt forces in a motor vehicle crash. Whereas other regions of the body are often covered with clothing and protective equipment, the face and neck generally do not share this same level of protection. The injuries in this region often are some of the first you see when you arrive at the side of the patient. Additionally these injuries can be some of the most graphic. You should use caution to prevent yourself from focusing solely on these distracting injuries at the risk of missing other life threats.

This chapter provides a detailed review of the anatomy and physiology of the face and neck. It also discusses injuries to the face and neck, including their respective signs and symptoms and appropriate prehospital care. Topics included in this chapter are as follows:

- Soft-tissue injuries to the region
- Maxillofacial injuries
- Injuries to the eye
- Ear injuries
- Oral and dental injuries
- Injuries to the anterior part of the neck including penetrating injuries
- Injuries to the spine, not including spinal cord injuries

The chapter, *Head and Spine Trauma*, will discuss injuries specific to the head and injuries to the spine and spinal cord. These often occur in conjunction with facial trauma. Injuries that will be discussed there include traumatic brain injuries, skull fractures, and spine fractures.

Anatomy and Physiology

The Facial Bones

The frontal and ethmoid bones are part of the cranial vault and the face. The 14 facial bones form the structure of the face, without contributing to the cranial vault. They include the maxillae, vomer, inferior nasal concha, and the zygomatic, palatine, nasal, and lacrimal bones Figure 1 .

The facial bones protect the eyes, nose, and tongue; they also provide attachment points for the muscles that allow chewing. The zygomatic process of the temporal bone and the temporal process of the zygomatic bone form the zygomatic arch Figure 2 , which lends shape to the cheeks.

Two major nerves provide sensory and motor control to the face: the trigeminal nerve (fifth cranial nerve) and the facial nerve (seventh cranial nerve). The trigeminal nerve branches into the ophthalmic nerve, maxillary nerve, and mandibular nerve. The **ophthalmic nerve** (a sensory nerve) supplies the skin of the forehead, upper eyelid, and conjunctiva. The **maxillary nerve** (another sensory nerve) supplies the skin on the posterior part of the side of the nose, lower eyelid, cheek, and upper lip. The **mandibular nerve** (a sensory and motor nerve) supplies the muscles of chewing (mastication) and skin of the lower lip, chin, temporal region, and part of the external ear. The **facial nerve** supplies the muscles of facial expression.

Blood supply to the face is provided primarily through the external carotid artery, which branches into the temporal, mandibular, and maxillary arteries. Because the face is highly vascular, it tends to bleed heavily when injured.

YOU are the Medic   PART 1

Your unit is dispatched as a second unit for a motor vehicle crash. The first unit at the scene advises you they have two critical trauma patients. Your unit will be responsible for a 21-year-old woman with facial injuries. When you arrive at the scene, you are directed to your patient. The other crew informs you that she was riding with some friends in the bed of a pick-up truck when the driver lost control and struck a tree head-on. The patient was not restrained and was thrown forward into the cab face first. First responders have secured spinal precautions prior to your arrival and the patient is supine on the board. The patient has numerous cuts and contusions to her face. She is unresponsive with noisy respirations, and blood is coming from her mouth.

1. What is your primary concern after scene safety is established?

2. What is your first step in controlling the patient's airway?

The Orbits

The <u>orbits</u> are cone-shaped fossae that enclose and protect the eyes. In addition to the eyeball and muscles that move it, the orbit contains blood vessels, nerves, and fat.

A blow to the eye may result in fracture of the orbital floor because the bone is extremely thin and breaks easily. A <u>blowout fracture</u> **Figure 3** results in transmission of forces away from the eyeball itself to the bone. Blood and fat are then free to leak into the maxillary sinus.

The Nose

The nose is one of the two primary entry points for oxygen-rich air to enter the body. The <u>nasal septum</u>—the separation between the nostrils—is located in the midline. Often, it bulges slightly to one side or the other. The external portion of the nose is formed mostly of cartilage.

Several bones associated with the nose contain cavities known as the <u>paranasal sinuses</u> **Figure 4**. These hollowed sections of bone, which are lined with mucous membranes, decrease the weight of the skull and provide resonance for the voice. The contents of the sinuses drain into the nasal cavity.

The Mandible and Temporomandibular Joint

The <u>mandible</u> is the large movable bone forming the lower jaw and containing the lower teeth. Numerous muscles of chewing attach to the mandible and its rami. The posterior condyle of the mandible articulates with the temporal bone at the <u>temporomandibular joint (TMJ)</u>, allowing movement of the mandible **Figure 5**.

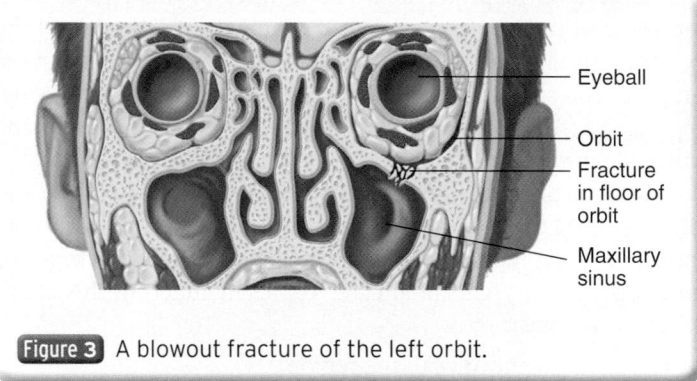

Figure 3 A blowout fracture of the left orbit.

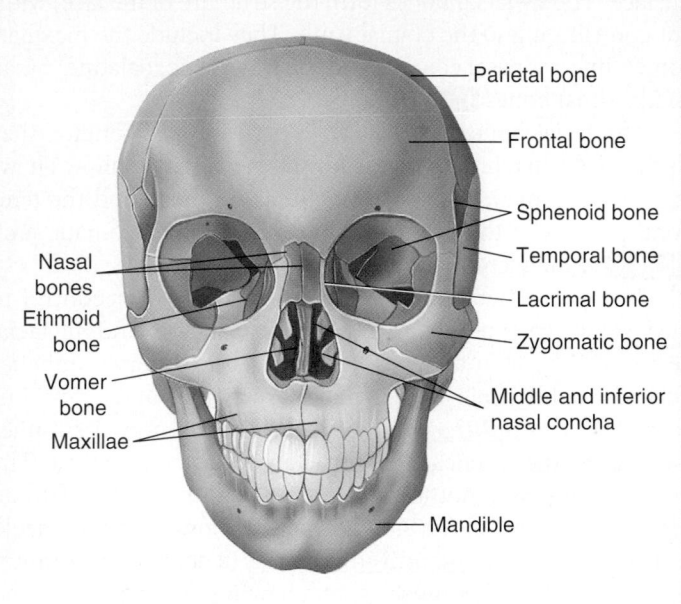

Figure 1 The skull and its components (front view).

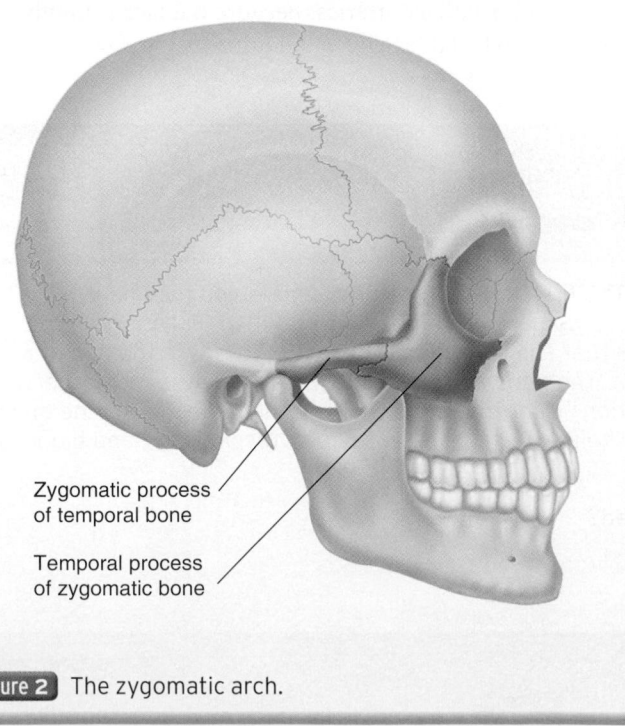

Figure 2 The zygomatic arch.

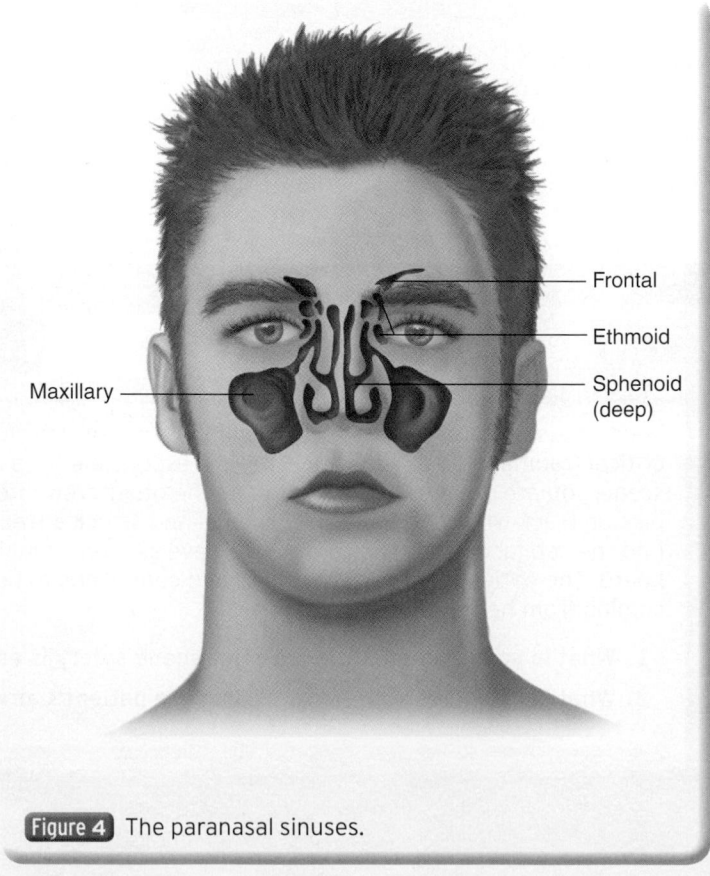

Figure 4 The paranasal sinuses.

The Hyoid Bone

The semicircular <u>hyoid bone</u> "floats" in the superior aspect of the neck just below the mandible. Whereas it is not actually part of the face or skull, it supports and stabilizes the larynx and serves as a point of attachment for many important neck and tongue muscles.

The Eyes, Ears, Teeth, and Mouth

The Eye

The <u>globe</u>, or eyeball, is a spherical structure measuring about 1 inch in diameter that is housed within the orbit, or eye socket. The eyes are held in place by loose connective tissue and several muscles. These muscles also control eye movements. The <u>oculomotor nerve</u> (third cranial nerve) innervates the muscles that cause motion of the eyeballs and upper eyelids. It also carries parasympathetic nerve fibers that cause constriction of the pupil and accommodation of the lens. The <u>optic nerve</u> (second cranial nerve) provides the sense of vision Figure 6 .

The structures of the eye Figure 7 include the following:

- The <u>sclera</u> ("white of the eye") is a tough, fibrous coat that helps maintain the shape of the eye and protect the contents of the eye. In some illnesses, such as hepatitis, the sclera become yellow (icteric) from staining by bile pigments.
- The <u>cornea</u> is the transparent anterior portion of the eye that overlies the iris and pupil. Clouding of the cornea during aging results in a condition known as cataracts.
- The <u>conjunctiva</u> is a delicate mucous membrane that covers the sclera and internal surfaces of the eyelids but not the iris. Cyanosis can be detected in the conjunctiva when it is not easily assessed on the skin of dark-skinned patients.
- The <u>iris</u> is the pigmented part of the eye that surrounds the pupil. It consists of muscles and blood vessels that contract and expand to regulate the size of the pupil.
- The <u>pupil</u> is the circular adjustable opening within the iris through which light passes to the lens. A normal pupil dilates in dim light to permit more light to enter the eye and constricts in bright light to decrease the light entering the eye.
- Behind the pupil and iris is the <u>lens</u>, a transparent structure that can alter its thickness to focus light on the retina at the back of the eye.
- The <u>retina</u>, which lies in the posterior aspect of the interior globe, is a delicate, 10-layered structure of nervous tissue that extends from the optic nerve. It receives light impulses and converts them to nerve signals that are conducted to the brain by the optic nerve and interpreted as vision.

The <u>anterior chamber</u> is the portion of the globe between the lens and the cornea. It is filled with <u>aqueous humor</u>, a clear watery fluid. If aqueous humor is lost through a penetrating injury to the eye, it will gradually be replenished.

The <u>posterior chamber</u> is the portion of the globe between the iris and the lens that is filled with <u>vitreous humor</u>, a jellylike substance that maintains the shape of the globe. If vitreous humor is lost, it cannot be replenished, and blindness may result.

Light rays enter the eyes through the pupil and are focused by the lens. The image formed by the lens is cast on the retina, where sensitive nerve fibers form the optic nerve. The optic nerve transmits the image to the brain, where it is converted into conscious images in the <u>visual cortex</u>.

There are two types of vision: central and peripheral. <u>Central vision</u> facilitates visualization of objects directly in front of you, and is processed by the macula, the central portion of the retina. The remainder of the retina processes <u>peripheral vision</u>, which allows visualization of lateral objects while you are looking forward.

The <u>lacrimal apparatus</u> secretes and drains tears from the eye. Tears produced in the lacrimal gland drain into lacrimal ducts, then into lacrimal sacs that pass into the

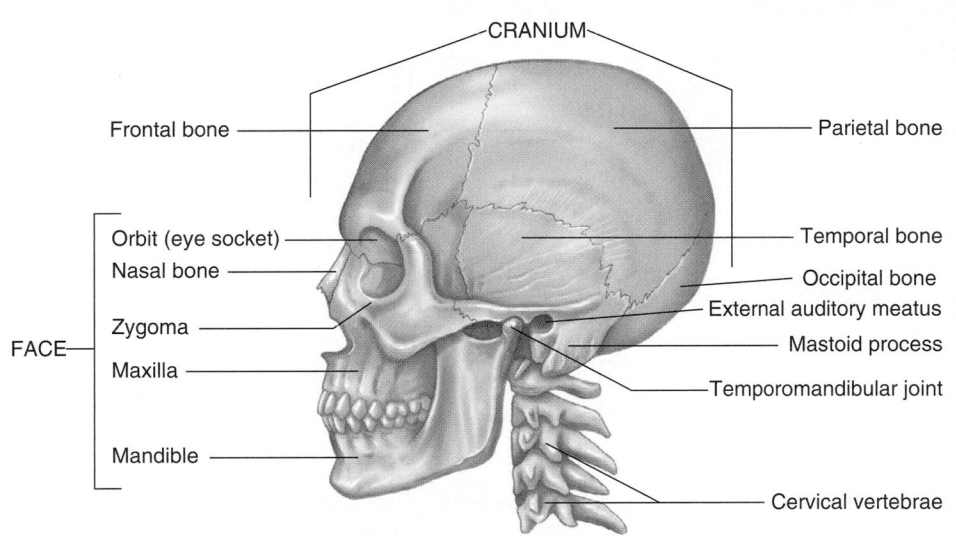

Figure 5 The mastoid air cells are located in the mastoid process. Just anterior to the mastoid is the external auditory meatus, which is associated with the ear canal.

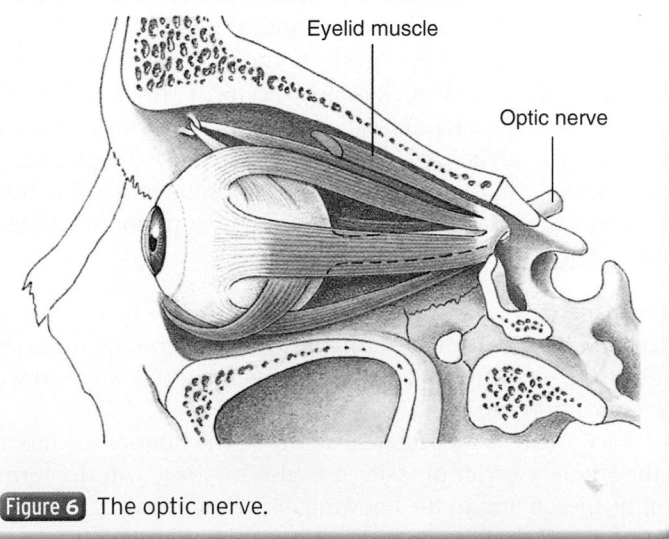

Figure 6 The optic nerve.

nasal cavity via the **nasolacrimal duct**. Tears moisten the conjunctivae **Figure 8** .

The Ear

The ear is divided into three anatomic parts: external, middle, and inner **Figure 9** . The **external ear** consists of the pinna, external auditory canal, and the exterior portion of the tympanic membrane or what is commonly known as the eardrum. The **middle ear** consists of the inner portion of the tympanic membrane and the ossicles. The **inner ear** consists of the cochlea and semicircular canals.

Sound waves enter the ear through the **auricle**, or **pinna**, the large cartilaginous external portion of the ear. They then travel through the **external auditory canal** to the **tympanic membrane**. Vibration of sound waves against the tympanic membrane sets up vibration in the **ossicles**, the three small bones on the inner side of the tympanic membrane. These vibrations are transmitted to the **cochlear duct** at the **oval window**, the opening between the middle ear and the vestibule. Movement of the oval window causes fluid within the **cochlea**, a shell-shaped structure in the inner ear, to vibrate. Within the cochlea at the **organ of Corti**, vibration stimulates hair movements that form nerve impulses that travel to the brain via the auditory nerve. The brain then converts these impulses into sound.

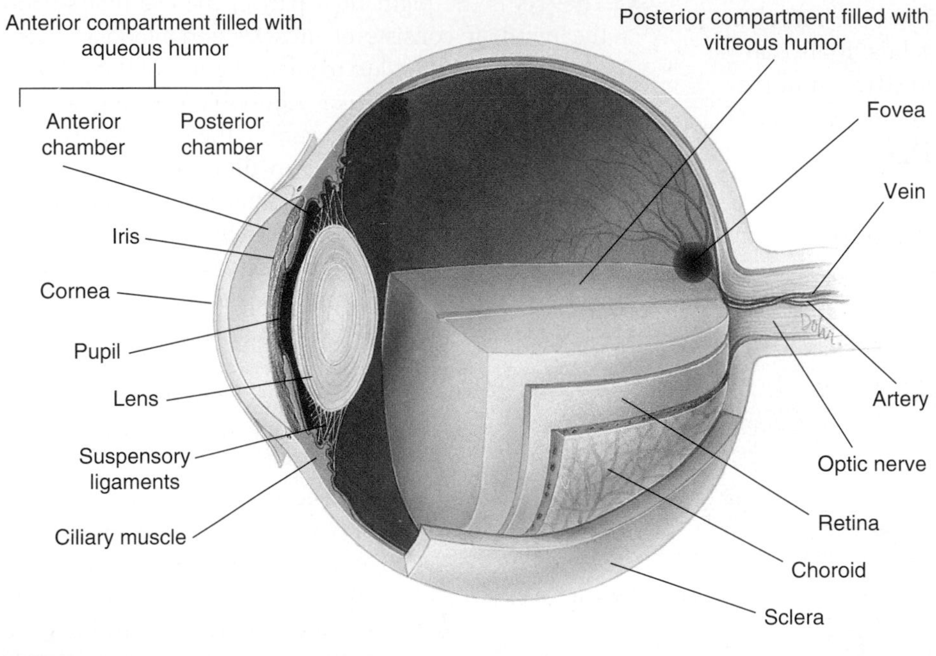

The Teeth

The normal adult mouth contains 32 permanent teeth. The primary or deciduous teeth are lost during childhood. Adult teeth are distributed about the maxillary and mandibular arches. The teeth on each side of the arch are mirror images of each other and form four quadrants: right upper, left upper, right lower, and left lower. Each quadrant contains one central incisor, one lateral incisor, one canine, two premolars, and three molars **Figure 10A** . The third molars, or what are called wisdom teeth, do not appear until late adolescence.

The top portion of the tooth, external to the gum, is the **crown**, containing one or more **cusps**. Below the crown lie the neck and the root. The pulp cavity fills the center of the tooth and contains blood vessels, nerves, and specialized connective tissue, called **pulp**. Dentin and enamel surround the pulp cavity and protect the tooth from damage. **Dentin**, which forms the principal mass of the tooth, is much denser and stronger than bone. The bony sockets for the teeth that reside in the mandible and maxilla are called **alveoli**. The ridges between the teeth, the **alveolar ridges**, are covered by the gingiva, or gums, which are thickened connective tissue and epithelium. Teeth are attached to the alveolar bone by a periodontal membrane **Figure 10B** .

The Mouth

Digestion begins in the mouth with **mastication**, or the chewing of food by the teeth. During mastication, food is mixed with secretions from the salivary glands.

The tongue, a muscular structure in the floor of the mouth, is the primary organ of taste; it is also important in the formation of speech and in the chewing and swallowing of food. The tongue is attached at the mandible and hyoid bone, is covered

Anterior compartment filled with aqueous humor

Anterior chamber

Posterior chamber

Iris

Cornea

Pupil

Lens

Suspensory ligaments

Ciliary muscle

Posterior compartment filled with vitreous humor

Fovea

Vein

Artery

Optic nerve

Retina

Choroid

Sclera

Figure 7 The structures of the eye.

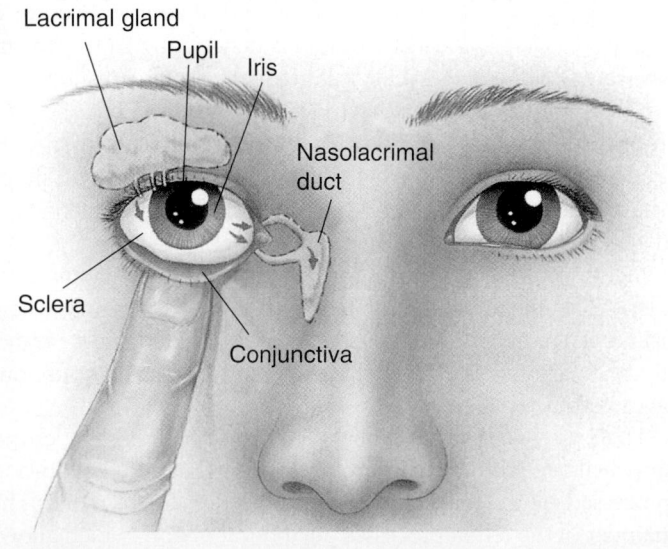

Lacrimal gland

Pupil

Iris

Nasolacrimal duct

Sclera

Conjunctiva

Figure 8 The lacrimal system consists of tear glands and ducts. Tears act as lubricants and keep the anterior part of the eye from drying.

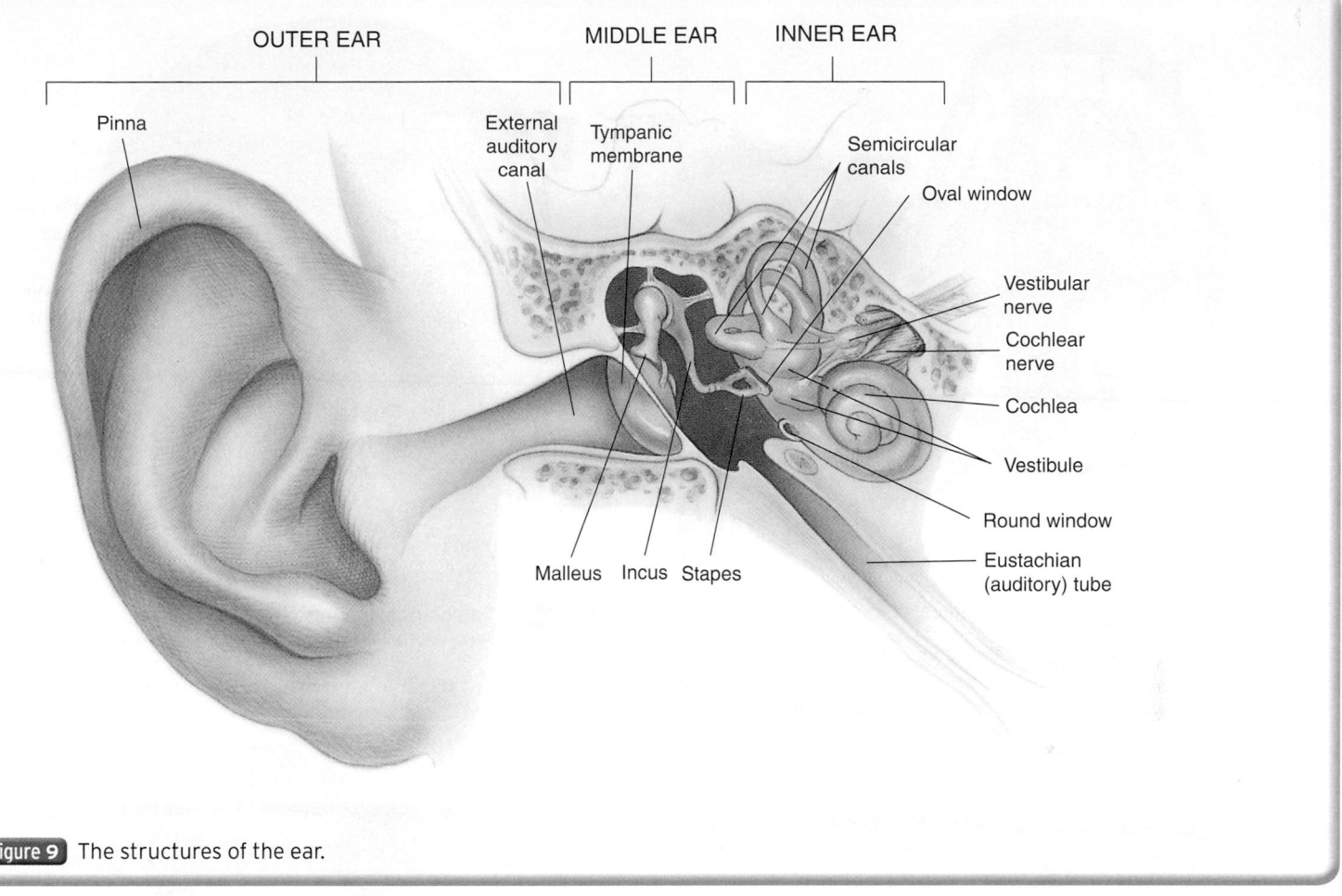

OUTER EAR · MIDDLE EAR · INNER EAR

Pinna

External auditory canal

Tympanic membrane

Semicircular canals

Oval window

Vestibular nerve

Cochlear nerve

Cochlea

Vestibule

Round window

Eustachian (auditory) tube

Malleus Incus Stapes

Figure 9 The structures of the ear.

by a mucous membrane, and extends from the back of the mouth upward and forward to the lips **Figure 11**.

The hypoglossal, glossopharyngeal, trigeminal, and facial nerves supply the mouth and its structures. The **hypoglossal nerve** (12th cranial nerve) provides motor function to the muscles of the tongue. The **glossopharyngeal nerve** (ninth cranial nerve) provides taste sensation to the posterior portions of the tongue and carries parasympathetic fibers to the salivary glands on each side of the face. The mandibular branch of the **trigeminal nerve** (fifth cranial nerve) provides motor innervation to the muscles of mastication. The facial nerve (seventh cranial nerve), in addition to supplying motor activity to all muscles of facial expression, provides the sense of taste to the anterior two thirds of the tongue and cutaneous sensations to the tongue and palate.

The Anterior Region of the Neck

The principal structures of the anterior region of the neck include the thyroid and cricoid cartilage, trachea, and numerous muscles and nerves **Figure 12**. The major blood vessels in this area are the internal and external carotid arteries **Figure 13** and the internal and external jugular veins **Figure 14**. The vertebral arteries run laterally to the cervical vertebrae in the posterior part of the neck.

The major arteries of the neck—the carotid and vertebral arteries—supply oxygenated blood directly to the brain. Therefore, in addition to causing massive bleeding and

hemorrhagic shock, injury to any of these major vessels can produce cerebral hypoxia, infarct, air embolism, and/or permanent neurologic impairment.

Special Populations

Young and old patients are more prone to falling, and therefore have an increased risk of injury. Non-accidental trauma is also a higher risk factor in both the elderly and the pediatric populations.

Other key structures of the anterior part of the neck that may sustain injury from blunt or penetrating mechanisms include the vagus nerves, thoracic duct, esophagus, thyroid and parathyroid glands, lower cranial nerves, brachial plexus (which is responsible for function of the arm and hand), soft tissue and fascia, and various muscles.

Special Populations

The proportionately larger amount of body surface area in the head and scalp of infants and toddlers allows for higher chances of injuries to the face and scalp, and the resultant blood loss in this age group can quickly become significant.

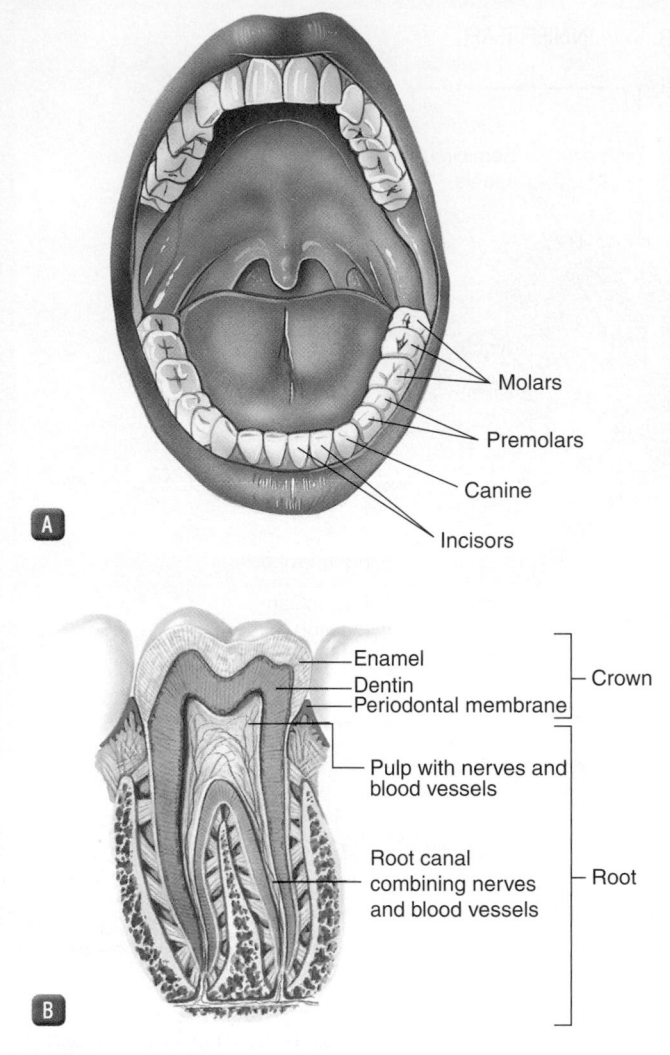

Figure 10 The teeth of the adult mouth. **A.** The incisors are used for biting. Canines are used for tearing food. The premolars and molars are used for grinding and crushing. **B.** Each tooth contains nerves and blood vessels.

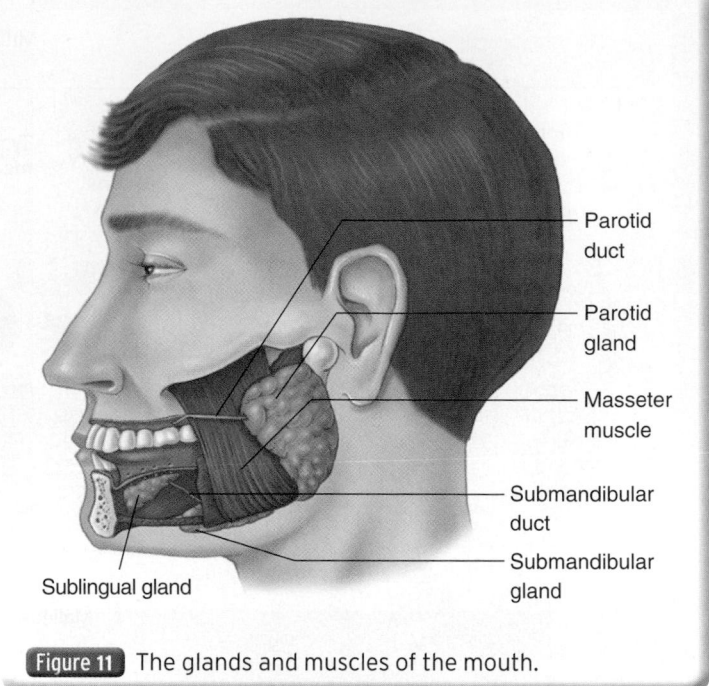

Figure 11 The glands and muscles of the mouth.

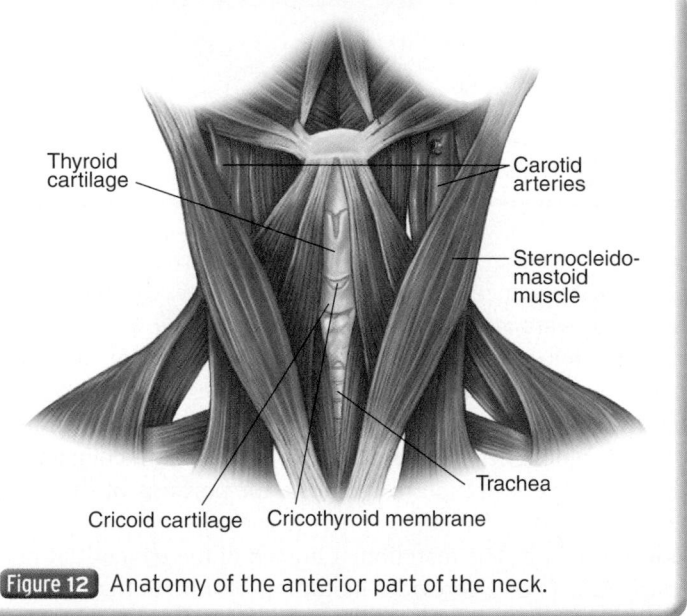

Figure 12 Anatomy of the anterior part of the neck.

Patient Assessment

Scene Size-up

The first aspect for you to address in any scenario is safety. Assess the impact of hazards on patient care, and address the hazards. Also assess for the potential for violence. If you are responding to a vehicle crash, ensure that traffic is controlled and personnel are operating with protective measures in place, including following federal safety vest requirements.

Ensure that you and your crew have taken standard precautions—a minimum of gloves and eye protection. Apply standard precautions before you approach the scene to minimize your direct exposure to body fluids. Because of the color of blood and how well it soaks through clothing, you can often identify patients with an open injury as you approach the scene. Determine the number of patients, and consider whether you need additional or specialized resources on the scene.

Once you have determined that the scene is safe, begin evaluating the mechanism of injury (MOI). Maintain a high index of suspicion whenever a significant MOI is present. Determine how many patients are involved.

Primary Assessment

When serious trauma is present, soft-tissue injuries take a lower priority than airway control, breathing inadequacy, and

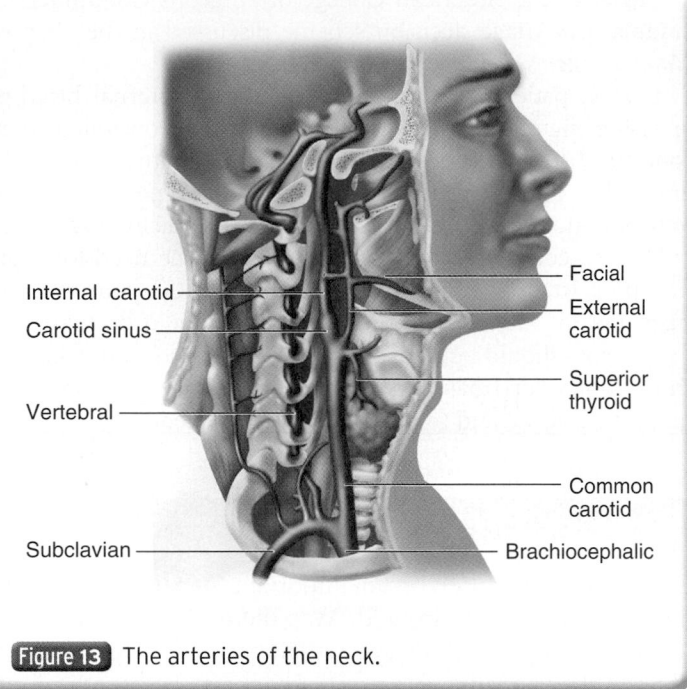

Figure 13 The arteries of the neck.

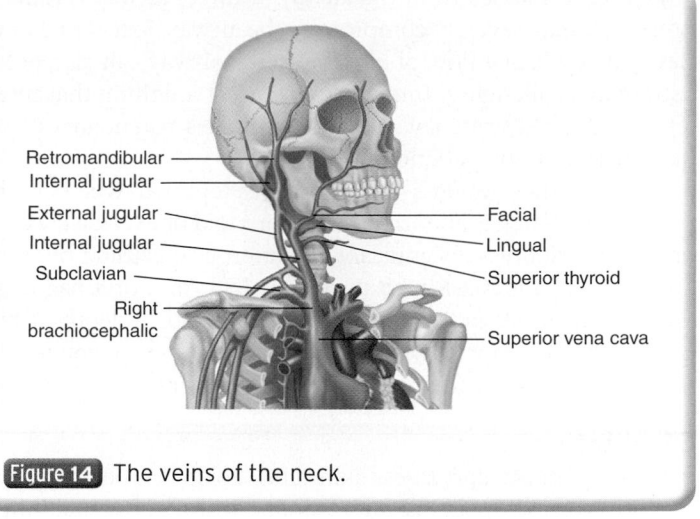

Figure 14 The veins of the neck.

responsiveness even when the patient has a seemingly innocuous soft-tissue injury to the head. Administer high-flow oxygen to all patients whose level of consciousness is altered, and provide immediate transport.

Airway and Breathing

Assess the airway as soon as you arrive at the patient's side. Continue to protect the patient from further spinal injury. If the patient is unresponsive or has a significantly altered level of consciousness, consider inserting an oropharyngeal or nasopharyngeal airway. Remember that nasopharyngeal airways are contraindicated if there is suspicion of a basilar skull or cribriform plate fracture.

Determine whether air is moving from the nose, mouth, or stoma. When present, immediately suction blood, vomit, or

bleeding. *Do not let soft-tissue injuries distract you from life threats that may not be readily apparent.*

Form a General Impression

When the scene has been secured and standard precautions have been taken, rapidly determine whether threats to life are present. Form a general impression as you approach the patient. If the patient has a potential neck or spine injury, assign a crew member to perform manual immobilization. Check for

YOU *are the Medic* | **PART 2** |

Your partner sets up the portable suction. When your partner opens the patient's mouth to insert the suction catheter, she reports that she feels crepitus and it seems the maxilla is moving. Your partner also notices blood and a clear fluid coming from the patient's nose.

Recording Time: 1 Minute	
Appearance	U (unresponsive), facial trauma
Level of consciousness	Unresponsive
Airway	Obstructed with blood
Breathing	Snoring
Circulation	Diminished

3. What type of facial fracture may this patient have?

4. How will this type of fracture affect selection of an appropriate airway method?

any other substance from the airway. If direct airway trauma is present, it may severely compromise the airway. Soft-tissue injuries that result in a flow of blood into the airway can also prove extremely challenging. Immediately correct anything that interferes with airway patency; failure to provide a patent airway can quickly lead to the patient's death.

Assess the patient's breathing. Determine whether the patient's breathing is abnormally slow or rapid or excessively deep or shallow. Address a significant alteration in breathing by using a nonrebreathing mask with oxygen at 15 L/min or a bag-mask device and supplementary oxygen. An inadequate depth or rate that results in compromised breathing should prompt you to take immediate action. Advanced airway management may be needed.

Circulation

Palpate the pulse, and assess skin CTC (color, temperature, and condition). If no pulse is present, take resuscitative measures. When you are palpating a pulse, determine whether it is abnormally fast or slow. Palpate and inspect the skin for color, temperature, and condition. Pale or ashen skin points to inadequate perfusion. Cool, moist skin is an early indicator of shock.

If visible significant bleeding is seen, you must begin the steps necessary to control bleeding. Significant bleeding is an immediate life threat and must be controlled quickly using appropriate methods. After you consider the MOI and form suspicions as to where bleeding may occur, expose that part of the body.

If significant trauma has likely affected multiple systems, expose the patient and perform a rapid exam to ensure that you have found all of the problems and injuries. A rapid 60- to 90-second exam may identify factors that assist you in determining whether a patient requires rapid transport. Begin with the head and neck while manually holding the head in place. When you are done, apply a cervical spine immobilization device if you have not done so already. If you identify conditions that have the potential to become unstable, such as a distended abdomen or femur fracture, the patient requires rapid and immediate transport.

Transport Decision

Patients with significant trauma (significant MOI) should be rapidly transported. Optimal on-scene time is less than 10 minutes (called the "platinum 10"), and any intervention that can be done en route should be delayed until you are in the ambulance. Patients with isolated injuries (no significant MOI) are often better managed by carefully treating the injuries on scene.

Although most patients do not require immediate load-and-go transportation, there are certain conditions for which treatment is limited in the field, and, therefore, immediate transport is the better choice. The following list will help to guide you in determining the findings in patients who need immediate transportation:

- Poor initial general impression
- Altered level of consciousness
- Dyspnea
- Abnormal vital signs
- Shock
- Severe pain

Refer to the American College of Surgeons Committee on Trauma field triage decision scheme discussed in the chapter, *Trauma Systems and Mechanism of Injury*.

When patients have signs of significant internal bleeding or visible significant bleeding that cannot be controlled, their condition may quickly become unstable. Treatment must be directed at quickly addressing life threats and providing rapid transportation. Signs such as tachycardia; tachypnea; weak pulse; and cool, moist, and pale skin imply the need for rapid transport. In any patient with a significant MOI, your index of suspicion for internal injuries and shock should be high, and the patients should be transported early. Do not wait for signs of shock to develop, maintain a high index of suspicion, and reassess your priority and transport decision as needed.

History Taking

Gathering information is an important step in determining how the patient was injured. Was there a precipitating factor? For example, did the patient fall because she got dizzy or because she tripped over the cat? There may be a medical reason that led to the trauma. Ask the patient (if alert and able to respond) or family members and bystanders about the injury, such as:

- Was the patient wearing a seat belt?
- How fast was the vehicle traveling?
- How high is the location from which the patient fell?
- Was there a loss of consciousness?
- What type of weapon was used?

Record the information on the patient care record, and relay it during patient transfer at the hospital.

Make every attempt to obtain a SAMPLE history from your patient. Using OPQRST may provide some background on isolated extremity injuries. You have the opportunity to interview the patient well before the ED physician's examination. Any information you receive will be valuable if the patient loses consciousness.

If your patient is unresponsive and bystanders or family cannot provide information, the scene and any Medic Alert jewelry maybe your only sources of information for a SAMPLE history.

Secondary Assessment

The secondary assessment is a more systematic head-to-toe or focused examination of the patient that is used to reveal injuries that may have been missed during the primary assessment. In some cases, such as with a critically injured patient or a short transport time, you may not have time to conduct a secondary assessment. In other cases, the secondary assessment may occur en route to the ED.

Physical examinations typically will be performed en route to the hospital, and they should result in reconsidering or reconfirming your initial transport decision.

Assessment of the respiratory system should involve looking and listening for signs of airway problems. Look at the patient and ask yourself the following questions:

1. Is the patient in a tripod position?
2. What is the skin's color and condition?
3. Are there any signs of increased respiratory efforts such as retractions, nasal flaring, pursed lip breathing, or use of accessory muscles?

Next, listen for air movement at the patient's mouth and nose. Then listen to breath sounds with a stethoscope. Breath sounds should be clear and equal bilaterally, anteriorly, and posteriorly. Determine the patient's rate and quality of respiration. Finally, assess for asymmetric chest wall movement and feel for crepitus or subcutaneous emphysema.

You must be able to quickly assess pulse rate and quality; determine the skin condition, color, and temperature; and check the capillary refill time.

Assess the neurologic system to gather baseline data on your patient. This examination should include the following:

- Level of consciousness—use AVPU
- Pupil size and reactivity
- Motor response
- Sensory response

Assess the musculoskeletal system by performing a detailed full-body exam. Look for DCAP-BTLS. Assess the chest, abdomen, and extremities for hidden bleeding and injuries. Log roll the patient, and assess the posterior torso for injuries. Once the back has been assessed, the patient can be log rolled back down onto a backboard, followed by complete spinal stabilization. Log rolling and securing the patient to a backboard or other full-body stabilization device should take into consideration injuries found during the primary assessment.

Assess all anatomic regions, looking for the following signs and symptoms:

- Raccoon eyes, Battle sign, and/or drainage of blood or fluid from the ears or nose
- Jugular vein distention and tracheal deviation (Be alert for patients with a stoma or tracheostomy.)
- Pelvic instability (Look at the patient's face while palpating for instability. If a grimace or instability is noted during medial palpation, do not continue with posterior palpation of the iliac crests.)
- Abdominal distention, swelling, guarding, tenderness, or rigidity in any of the four quadrants (If the abdomen is tender, expect internal bleeding.)

In addition to assessing for the preceding signs and symptoms, check the extremities, and record pulse, motor, and sensory function. Note whether any blood appears on your gloves.

It is important to reassess the vital signs to identify whether a patient's condition is becoming unstable. Remember that soft-tissue injuries, even without a significant MOI, can cause shock. The reassessment of your patient's vital signs will give you a good understanding of how well or how poorly your patient is tolerating the injury.

Reassessment

Frequent reassessments of the patient's condition should be made en route to the hospital and in conjunction with any necessary interventions. A patient in stable condition should be reassessed every 15 minutes; a more serious condition warrants reexamination every 5 minutes. As part of this assessment, vital signs should be obtained and evaluated, any interventions checked, and the patient's condition monitored.

Repeat the primary assessment and confirm whether the treatments you provided are still effective. Identify and treat changes in the patient's condition. Reassessing a patient with an open soft-tissue injury is extremely important. Frequently, other emergency care personnel may have dressed and bandaged the wound before your arrival. Therefore, you should regularly reassess the injury; you may need to add additional dressings over the original dressing or bandages.

Special Populations

In the geriatric population, poor skin tone and loss of body fat can produce significant soft-tissue injury in the presence of even a simple MOI. Anticoagulation therapy in older patients can lead to significant blood loss from minor insults. Additionally, normally trivial physical findings such as bruises and minor lacerations can belie severe underlying trauma such as traumatic brain injury.

Your communication and documentation must include a description of the MOI, the position in which you found the patient, the location and description of injuries, and an accurate account of how you treated these injuries. In patients who have open injuries with severe external bleeding, it is important to recognize, estimate, and report the amount of blood loss that has occurred and how rapidly it occurred.

Special Populations

Adolescents who experience facial trauma are likely to fear disfigurement. It is important for you to have a plan to address this with them.

Emergency Medical Care

General emergency care of face and neck injuries must focus on protection of the airway. Airway issues are the most dangerous of the results of injuries to both the face and the neck.

Assess all bandaging frequently. If blood continues to soak through bandages, use additional methods to control bleeding as discussed later in the chapter.

Although most open soft-tissue injuries are not serious, if not appropriately treated, they can lead to substantial blood loss and even shock. By appropriately treating open soft-tissue injuries, you can minimize the common complications such as bleeding, shock, pain, and infection. You should expose all wounds, control bleeding, and be prepared to treat the patient for shock.

Closed soft-tissue injuries can be life threatening if not appropriately treated. Assess and manage all threats to the patient's airway, breathing, and circulation. All patients with major closed soft-tissue injury should receive oxygen via a nonrebreathing mask.

Extremities that are painful, swollen, or deformed should be splinted. When you are splinting these types of injuries, remember to assess the patient's pulses and motor and sensory function before and after applying the splint. Do not forget to document the presence or absence of pulses and any changes.

The next sections cover assessment and treatment of specific injuries, but regardless of the injury type, always constantly manage the airway of any patient with face or neck injuries.

Pathophysiology, Assessment, and Management of Face Injuries

Pathophysiology

Soft-Tissue Injuries

Although open soft-tissue injuries to the face—lacerations, abrasions, and avulsions—by themselves are rarely life threatening, their presence, especially following a significant MOI, suggests the potential for more severe injuries (eg, closed head injury, cervical spine injury). Furthermore, massive soft-tissue injuries to the face, especially if associated with oropharyngeal trauma and bleeding, can compromise the patient's airway and lead to ventilatory inadequacy.

Maintain a high index of suspicion when a patient presents with closed soft-tissue injuries to the face, such as contusions and hematomas **Figure 15** . These indicators of blunt force trauma suggest the potential for more severe underlying injuries.

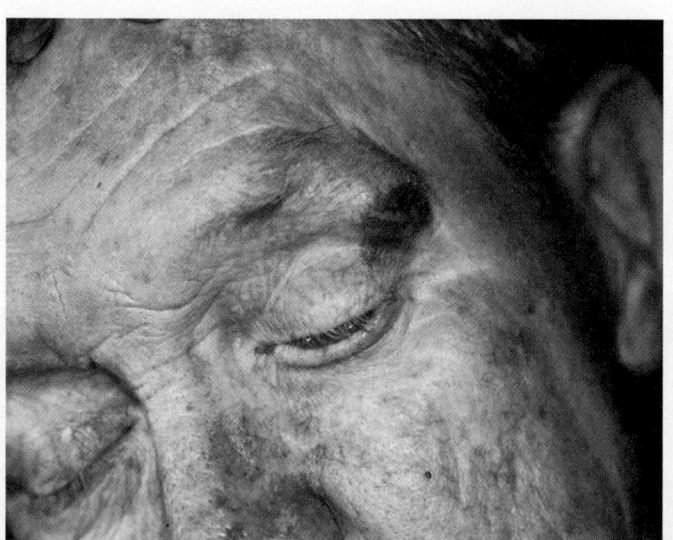

Figure 15 Closed soft-tissue injuries to the face may indicate more severe underlying injuries.

Impaled objects in the soft tissues or bones of the face may occur in association with facial trauma. Although these objects can damage facial nerves, the risk of airway compromise is of far greater consequence. This is especially true when an impaled object penetrates the cheek, because massive oropharyngeal bleeding can result in airway obstruction, aspiration, and ventilatory inadequacy. In addition, blood is a gastric irritant. Swallowing as little as a few tablespoons of blood can make a patient vomit, further increasing the likelihood of aspiration.

> ### Words of Wisdom
>
> Be careful when you are assessing a patient with soft-tissue injuries to the face, especially if he or she has experienced a significant mechanism of injury. Although facial lacerations and avulsions are often the most obvious and dramatic, they are not always the most life-threatening injury the patient has sustained.

Maxillofacial Fractures

Maxillofacial fractures commonly occur when the facial bones absorb the energy of a strong impact. The forces involved may be massive. For example, a force of 150 g (g = acceleration of the body due to gravity) is required to fracture the maxilla; a force of that magnitude is also likely to produce traumatic brain injuries and cervical spine injuries. Therefore, when you are assessing a patient with a suspected maxillofacial fracture, you should protect the cervical spine and monitor the patient's neurologic signs, specifically the patient's level of consciousness.

The first clue to the presence of a maxillofacial fracture is usually ecchymosis; therefore, a black-and-blue mark on the face should alert you to this possibility. A deep facial laceration should likewise increase your index of suspicion that the underlying bone may have been fractured, and pain over a bone tends to support the suspicion of fracture. General signs and symptoms of maxillofacial fractures include ecchymosis, swelling, pain to palpation, crepitus, dental malocclusion, facial deformities or asymmetry, instability of the facial bones, impaired ocular movement, and visual disturbances.

Nasal Fractures Because the nasal bones are not as structurally sound as the other bones of the face, nasal fractures are the most common facial fracture. These fractures are characterized by swelling, tenderness, and crepitus when the nasal bone is palpated. Deformity of the nose, if present, usually appears as lateral displacement of the nasal bone from its normal midline position.

Nasal fractures, like any maxillofacial fracture, are often complicated by the presence of an anterior or a posterior nosebleed (**epistaxis**) that can compromise the patient's airway.

Mandibular Fractures and Dislocations Second only to nasal fractures in frequency, fractures of the mandible typically result from massive blunt force trauma to the lower third of the face; they are particularly common following an assault injury.

Because of the shape of the mandible and the force required to fracture it, this structure may be fractured in more than one place and, therefore, unstable to palpation. The fracture site itself is most commonly located at the angle of the jaw.

Mandibular fractures should be suspected in patients with a history of blunt force trauma to the lower third of the face who present with dental **malocclusion** (misalignment of the teeth), numbness of the chin, and inability to open the mouth. Other findings include swelling and ecchymosis over the fracture site (for example, on the floor of the mouth), and teeth may be partially or completely avulsed. As the patient moves his or her jaw to speak and answer your questions, take note of symptoms of pain, such as decreased normal range of motion. There may be incidences where you might elicit tenderness, for example, by palpating specific locations on the mandible such as near the joints or specific impact points. This so-called "point tenderness" and pain on motion can identify injuries that patients might not have otherwise reported because they may be distracted by other injuries.

Temporomandibular joint (TMJ) dislocations may occur as the result of blunt force trauma to the lower third of the face, but this outcome is rare. These dislocations are most often the result of exaggerated yawning or otherwise widely opening the mouth. The patient commonly feels a "pop" and then cannot close his or her mouth; it is locked in a wide-open position. The jaw muscles eventually go into spasm, causing severe pain.

Maxillary Fractures Maxillary fractures are most commonly associated with mechanisms that produce massive blunt facial trauma, such as motor vehicle crashes, falls, and assaults. They produce massive facial swelling, instability of the midfacial bones, malocclusion, and an elongated appearance of the patient's face. Midfacial structures include the maxilla, zygoma, orbital floor, and nose.

Le Fort fractures **Figure 16** are classified into three categories:

- **Le Fort I fracture.** A horizontal fracture of the maxilla that involves the **hard palate** and inferior maxilla, separating them from the rest of the skull
- **Le Fort II fracture.** A fracture with a pyramidal shape, involving the nasal bone and inferior maxilla
- **Le Fort III fracture** (**craniofacial disjunction**). A fracture of all midfacial bones, separating the entire midface from the cranium.

Le Fort fractures can occur as isolated fractures (Le Fort I) or in combination (Le Fort I and II), depending on the location of impact and the amount of trauma.

Orbital Fractures The patient with an orbital fracture (such as a blowout fracture [Figure 3]) may report double vision (**diplopia**) and lose sensation above the eyebrow or over the cheek secondary to associated nerve damage. The isolated injury is usually caused by application of pressure to the globe of the eye by objects with a radius of curvature of 2 in or less. Typically this would be an object that strikes the region during sporting events, such as a baseball or hockey puck. The injury may cause the patient to have reduced sensation to areas that are innervated by the infraorbital nerve. This area extends from

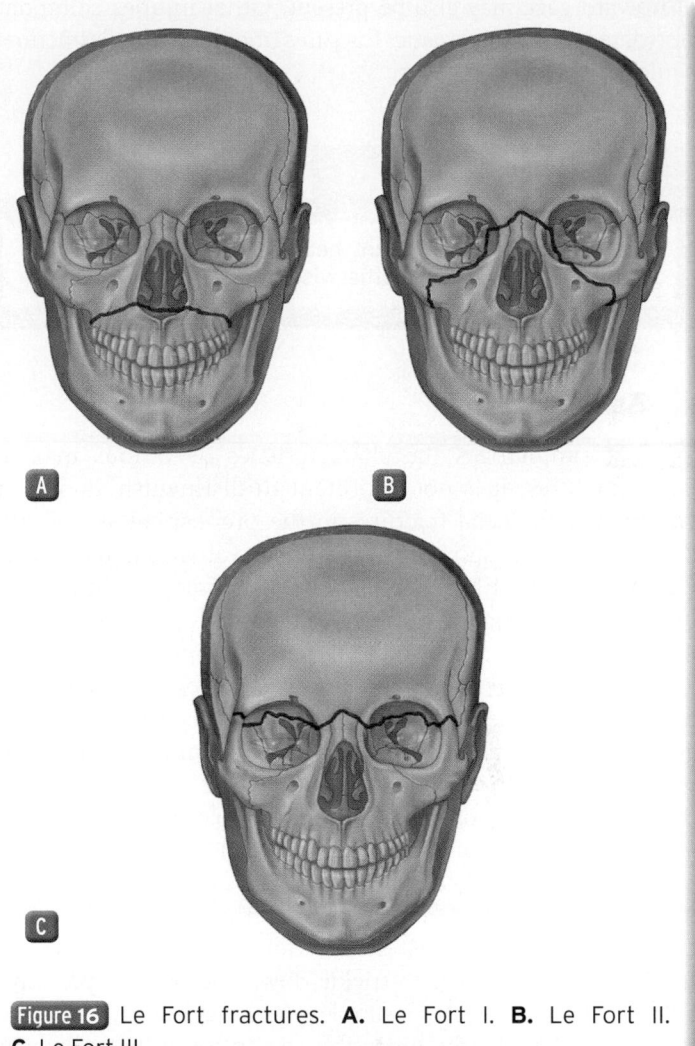

Figure 16 Le Fort fractures. **A.** Le Fort I. **B.** Le Fort II. **C.** Le Fort III.

the tip of the nose, including the nares, and follows the margin of the maxilla, curving up to meet the temple. This symptom is called *infraorbital hypoesthesia*. Also, the eyeball may retract posteriorly into the space created when the cavity is enlarged; this is called *enophthalmos traumaticus*.

Massive nasal discharge may occur, and vision is often impaired. Fractures of the inferior orbit are the most common type and can cause paralysis of upward gaze (the patient's injured eye will not be able to follow your finger above the midline).

Words of Wisdom

Check eye movements in all planes in the patient with possible facial fractures.

Zygomatic Fractures Fractures of the zygomatic bone (cheekbone) commonly result from blunt trauma secondary to motor vehicle crashes and assaults. When the zygomatic bone is fractured, that side of the patient's face appears flattened, and there is loss of sensation over the cheek, nose, and upper lip; paralysis of upward gaze may also be present. Other injuries commonly associated with zygomatic fractures include orbital fractures, ocular injury, and epistaxis.

Words of Wisdom

Any patient with significant head injury also has cervical spine injury until proven otherwise.

Assessment

Table 1 summarizes the characteristics of various maxillofacial fractures. It is not important to distinguish among the various maxillofacial fractures in the prehospital setting; this determination requires radiographic evaluation, usually via CT scan, in the ED. Rapid patient assessment, management of life-threatening conditions, full spinal precautions, and prompt transport are far more important considerations.

Because the region is difficult to assess without radiologic capabilities and because the underlying structures can be damaged easily, your assessment is primarily clinical, meaning that you will use your observation skills of sight and touch in contrast to using diagnostic equipment. Pay particular attention to swelling, deformity, instability, and blood loss. Evaluate the cranial nerve function because subtle signs can help you to determine the extent of the injury. Make certain to visually inspect the oropharynx for signs of posterior epistaxis. This includes frank blood continuing to trickle down the back of the throat after you have controlled a simple anterior epistaxis. A posterior epistaxis can be nearly impossible to control in the prehospital

setting; therefore, alert the ED to this situation so that advanced airway management can be in place on your arrival.

Management

Management of the patient with facial trauma begins by protecting the cervical spine. Because many severe facial injuries are complicated by a spinal injury, you must assume that one exists.

If the patient is unresponsive, open the airway with the jaw-thrust maneuver while simultaneously maintaining manual stabilization of the head in the neutral position unless the patient reports severe pain or discomfort upon movement. Should that occur, the head and neck should be immobilized in the position found. Inspect the mouth for fragments of teeth, dentures, or any other foreign bodies that could obstruct the airway, and remove them immediately. Suction the oropharynx as needed to keep the airway clear of blood and other liquids.

Insert an airway adjunct as needed to maintain airway patency. However, remember that *blind nasotracheal intubation is considered relatively contraindicated in the presence of midface trauma*. This means such a maneuver, or insertion of a nasopharyngeal airway, should not be performed in any patient with suspected nasal fractures or in patients with cerebrospinal fluid (CSF) or blood leakage from the nose or with any evidence of midface trauma, unless it is absolutely necessary. If necessary, such maneuvers must be performed using extreme caution and with medical direction's approval. After establishing and maintaining a patent airway, assess the patient's breathing and intervene appropriately. Apply 100% oxygen via a nonrebreathing mask if the patient is breathing adequately. Patients who are breathing inadequately (ie, fast or slow rate, inadequate tidal volume [shallow breathing], irregular pattern of inhalation and exhalation) should receive bag-mask ventilation with 100% oxygen. Maintain the patient's oxygen saturation at greater than 95%. Airway management can be especially challenging in patients with massive facial injuries **Figure 17**. Oropharyngeal bleeding poses an immediate threat to the airway, and unstable facial bones can hinder your ability to maintain an effective mask-to-face seal for bag-mask ventilation. Therefore,

Table 1	Summary of Maxillofacial Fractures
Injury	**Signs and Symptoms**
Multiple facial bone fractures	■ Massive facial swelling ■ Dental malocclusion ■ Palpable deformities ■ Anterior or posterior epistaxis
Zygomatic and orbital fractures	■ Loss of sensation below the orbit ■ Flattening of the patient's cheek ■ Paralysis of upward gaze
Nasal fractures	■ Crepitus and instability ■ Swelling, tenderness, lateral displacement ■ Anterior or posterior epistaxis
Maxillary (Le Fort) fractures	■ Mobility of the midface ■ Dental malocclusion ■ Facial swelling
Mandibular fractures	■ Dental malocclusion ■ Mandibular instability

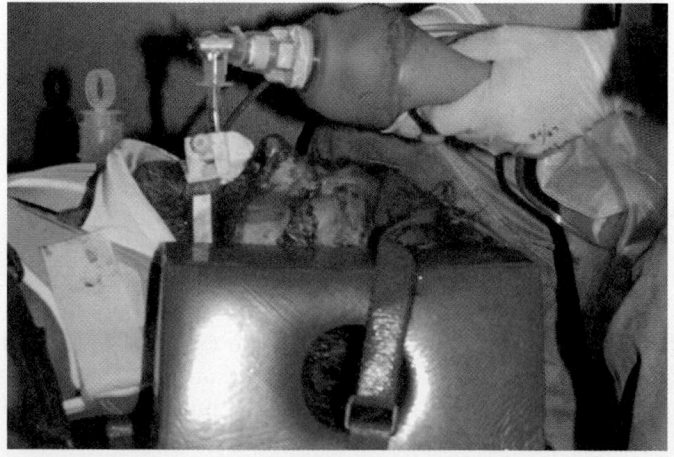

Figure 17 Airway management can be especially challenging in patients with massive facial injuries.

perform endotracheal (ET) intubation of patients with facial trauma, especially those who are unresponsive, to protect their airway from aspiration and to ensure adequate oxygenation and ventilation. Remember that the forces that produce the insult to the victim are often transferred to the spinal column; therefore, it is imperative for you to provide in-line cervical spinal motion restriction while attempting ET intubation. Cricothyrotomy (surgical or needle) may be required for patients with extensive maxillofacial injuries when ET intubation is extremely difficult or impossible to perform (ie, in patients with unstable facial bones, massive swelling, or severe oral bleeding).

Soft-Tissue Injuries

Treat facial lacerations and avulsions as you would any other soft-tissue injury. Control all bleeding with direct pressure, and apply sterile dressings. If you suspect an underlying facial fracture, apply just enough pressure to control the bleeding. Leave impaled objects in the face in place and appropriately stabilize them, unless they pose a threat to the airway (such as an object impaled through the cheek). When you are removing an object from the cheek, carefully remove it, preferably from the same side that it entered. Next, pack the inside of the cheek with sterile gauze and apply counterpressure with a dressing and bandage firmly secured over the outside of the wound. If profuse bleeding continues, position the patient on his or her side—while maintaining stabilization of the cervical spine—to facilitate drainage of secretions from the mouth and suction the airway as needed.

For severe oropharyngeal bleeding in patients with inadequate ventilation, suction the airway for 15 seconds and provide ventilatory assistance for 2 minutes; continue this alternating pattern of suctioning and ventilating until the airway is cleared of blood or secured with an ET tube. Monitoring the pulse oximeter during this process can further serve to keep the patient from becoming hypoxic.

Epistaxis following facial trauma can be severe and is most effectively controlled by applying direct pressure to the nares. If the patient is responsive and spinal injury is not suspected, instruct the patient to sit up and lean forward as you pinch the nares together. Unresponsive patients should be positioned on their side, unless contraindicated by a spinal injury. Proper positioning of the patient with epistaxis is important to prevent blood from draining down the throat and compromising the airway either by occlusion or by vomiting and then aspirating gastric contents. If the responsive patient with severe epistaxis is immobilized on a backboard, you should consider pharmacologically assisted intubation (eg, rapid-sequence intubation [RSI]) to gain definitive control of the airway.

Although facial lacerations and avulsions can contribute to hemorrhagic shock, they are rarely the sole cause of this condition in adults. Severe epistaxis, however, can result in significant blood loss. To counter this problem, you should carefully assess the patient for signs of hemorrhagic shock and administer IV crystalloid fluid boluses as needed to maintain adequate perfusion.

Maxillofacial Fractures

If the facial fracture is associated with swelling and ecchymosis, cold compresses may help minimize further swelling and alleviate pain. Do not apply a compress to the eyeball (globe) if you suspect that it has been injured following an orbital fracture; doing so may increase the intraocular pressure (IOP) and further damage the eye. Other than protecting the airway, there is little you can do to treat instability resulting from facial fractures.

After addressing all life-threatening injuries and conditions, you should ask questions to learn about the events that preceded the injury and determine whether the patient has any significant medical problems. The incident that caused the injury may have been preceded by exacerbation of an underlying medical condition (such as acute hypoglycemia, cardiac dysrhythmia, seizure). For unresponsive patients, medications that the patient is taking may provide information about his or her medical history. Determine the approximate time that the injury occurred, and ask about any drug allergies and the last oral intake during your SAMPLE history.

Special Populations

In contrast to younger, healthy adults, elderly patients are at high risk for severe epistaxis following even minor facial injuries, especially in those patients with a history of hypertension or anticoagulant medication use (such as warfarin [Coumadin]). This bleeding often originates in the posterior nasopharynx and may not be grossly evident unless you look in the patient's mouth.

■ Pathophysiology, Assessment, and Management of Eye Injuries

Approximately 1.5 million eye injuries occur in the United States each year, of which 50,000 result in some degree of visual loss. Because trauma to the eyes is so common and the potential consequences are so serious, you must know how to assess and manage ocular injuries.

Blunt trauma, penetrating trauma, or burns frequently cause eye injuries. Blunt MOI may include motor vehicle crashes, motorcycle crashes, falls, and assaults. Penetrating injuries are often secondary to foreign bodies on the surface of the eye (such as sand) or an object impaled in the globe. Burns to the eye can result from a variety of corrosive chemicals or during industrial accidents (such as welding burns).

■ Pathophysiology

Lacerations, Foreign Bodies, and Impaled Objects

Lacerations of the eyelids require meticulous repair to restore appearance and function. *If there is a laceration to the globe itself, apply no pressure to the eye*; compression can interfere with the blood supply to the back of the eye and result in loss of vision from damage to the retina. Furthermore, pressure may squeeze the vitreous humor, iris, lens, or even the retina out of the eye and cause irreparable damage or blindness **Figure 18**.

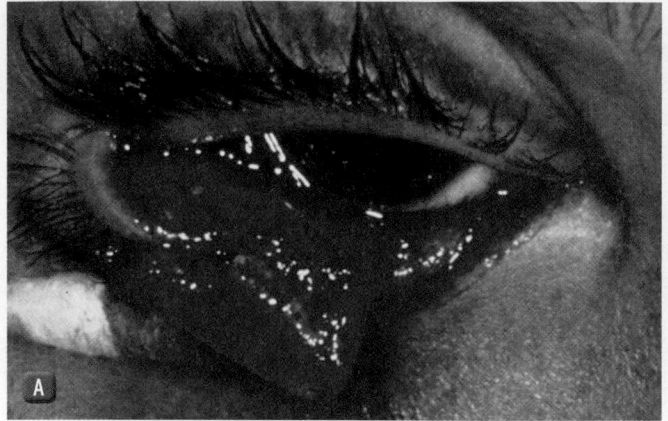

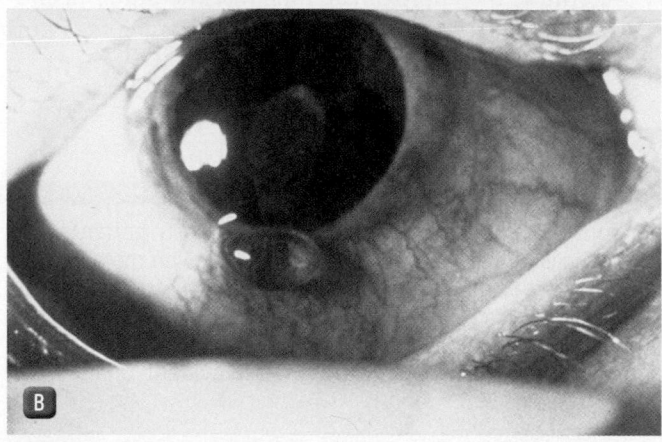

Figure 18 Eye lacerations are serious injuries that require prompt transport. **A.** Although bleeding can be heavy, never exert pressure on the eye. **B.** Pressure may squeeze the vitreous humor, iris, lens, or retina out of the eye.

The protective orbit prevents large objects from penetrating the eye. However, moderately sized and smaller foreign objects can still enter the eye and, when lying on the surface of the eye, produce severe irritation **Figure 19**. The conjunctiva becomes inflamed and red—a condition known as <u>conjunctivitis</u>—almost immediately, and the eye begins to produce tears in an attempt to flush out the object **Figure 20**. Irritation of the cornea or conjunctiva causes intense pain. The patient may have difficulty keeping the eyelids open because the irritation is further aggravated by bright light.

Foreign bodies ranging in size from a pencil to a sliver of metal may be impaled in the eye **Figure 21**. These objects must be removed by a physician.

Words of Wisdom

Large and small foreign bodies, particularly small metal fragments, can become completely embedded in the globe. The patient may not even be aware of the cause of the problem. Suspect such an injury when the history includes metal work (such as hammering, exposure to splinters, grinding, vigorous filing) and when you observe signs of ocular injury (such as redness, irritation, inflammation).

Blunt Eye Injuries

Blunt trauma can cause serious eye injuries, ranging from swelling and ecchymosis **Figure 22** to rupture of the globe. <u>Hyphema</u> is bleeding into the anterior chamber of the eye that obscures vision, partially or completely **Figure 23**. It often follows blunt trauma and may seriously impair vision. Approximately 25% of hyphemas are associated with globe injuries.

YOU are the Medic   PART 3

You set up your equipment in preparation for performing endotracheal intubation on this patient. Your partner is attempting to insert an oral airway that is not properly seating because of the free-floating maxilla injury. You direct one of the first responders to start ventilating the patient using a bag-mask device. Your partner returns to suctioning blood from the airway.

Recording Time: 5 Minutes	
Respirations	8 breaths/min
Pulse	130 beats/min
Skin	Cool, pale, moist
Blood pressure	90/60 mm Hg
Oxygen saturation (Spo$_2$)	92% on room air
Pupils	Equal and slow to react

5. What challenges do facial fractures present during ventilation with a bag-mask device?

6. What precautions will you need to take when you attempt endotracheal intubation?

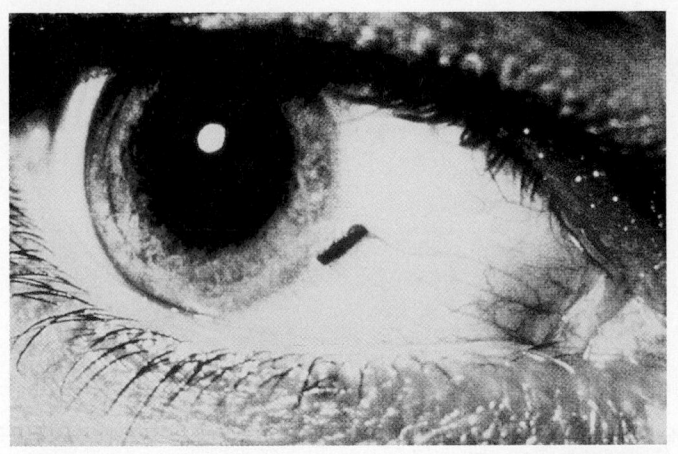

Figure 19 A foreign object on the surface of the eye.

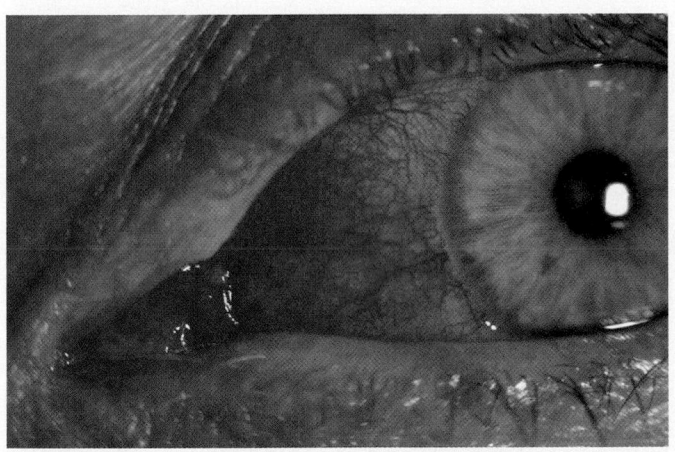

Figure 20 Conjunctivitis is often associated with the presence of a foreign object in the eye.

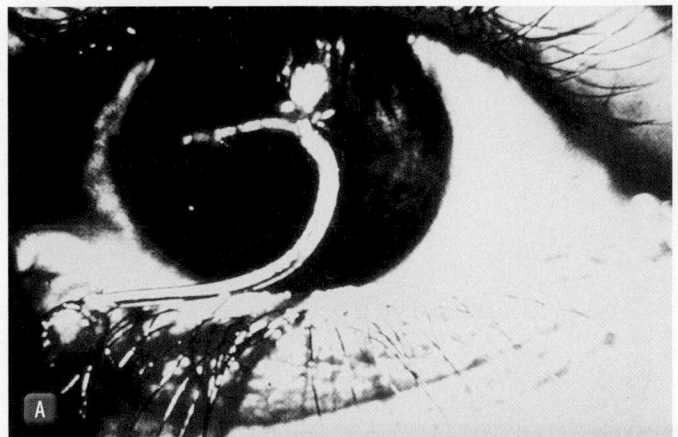

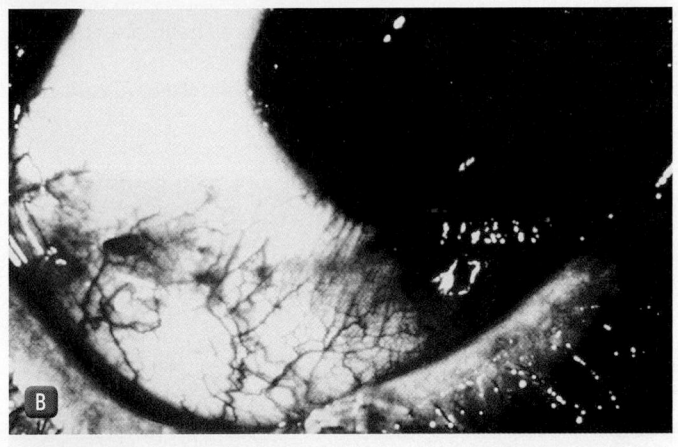

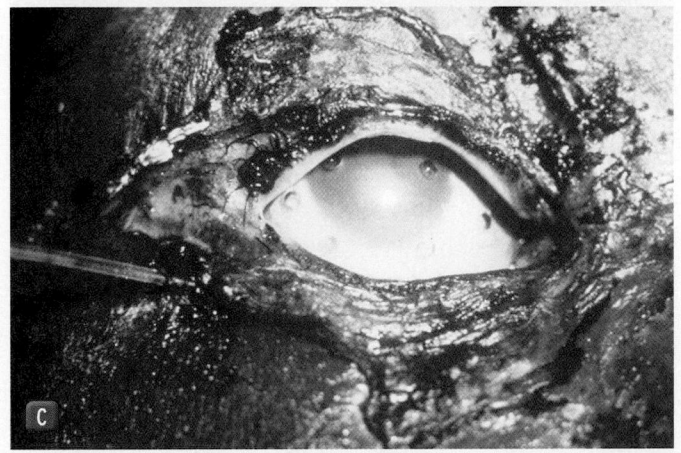

Figure 21 Any number of objects can be impaled in the eye. **A.** Fishhook. **B.** Sharp, metal sliver. **C.** Knife blade.

In orbital blowout fractures, the fragments of fractured bone can entrap some of the muscles that control eye movement, causing double vision (diplopia) **Figure 24**. Any patient who reports pain, double vision, or decreased vision following a blunt injury about the eye should be assumed to have a blowout fracture and should be promptly transported to an appropriate trauma center.

Another potential result of blunt eye trauma is **retinal detachment**, or separation of the inner layers of the retina from the underlying choroid (the vascular membrane that nourishes the retina). Retinal detachment is often seen in sports injuries, especially boxing. This painless condition produces flashing lights, specks, or "floaters" in the field of vision and a cloud or shade over the patient's vision. Because it can cause devastating damage to vision, retinal detachment is an ocular emergency and requires urgent medical attention.

Burns of the Eye

Chemicals, heat, and light rays can all burn the delicate tissues of the eye, often causing permanent damage. Your role is to stop the burning process and prevent further damage.

Chemical burns, which are usually caused by acid or alkali solutions, require immediate emergency care **Figure 25**. Flush the eye with water or a sterile saline solution. If sterile

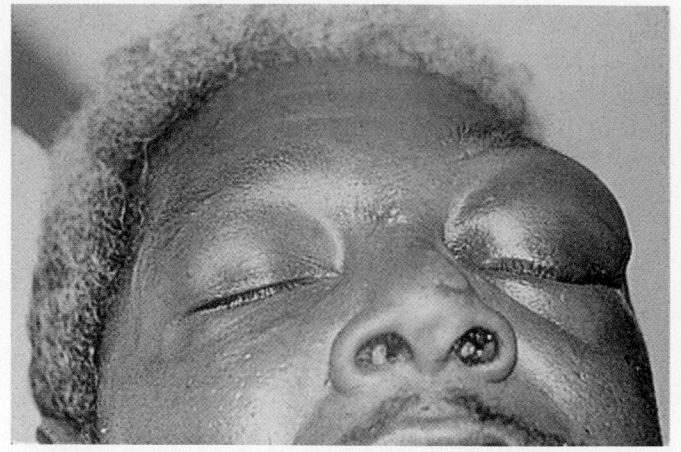

Figure 22 Swelling and ecchymosis are hallmark findings associated with blunt trauma to the eye.

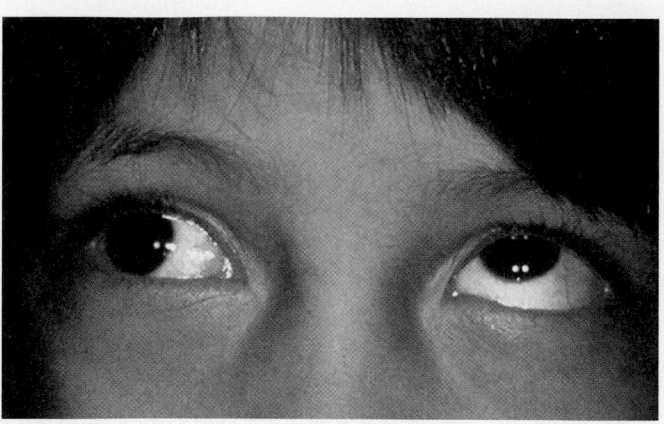

Figure 24 In a patient with a blowout fracture, the eyes may not move together because of muscle entrapment, so the patient sees double images of any object.

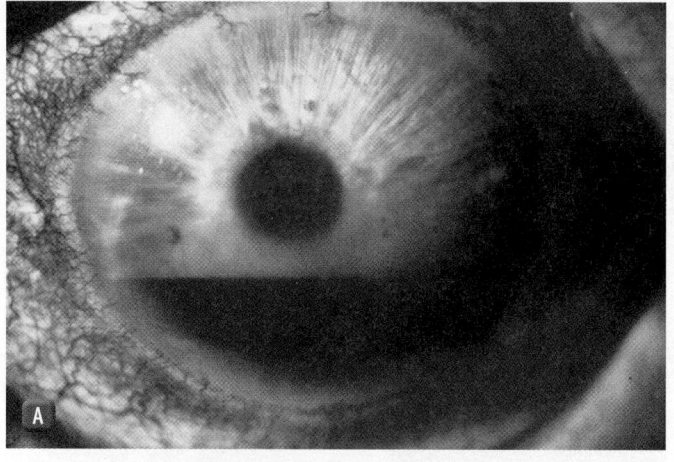

A

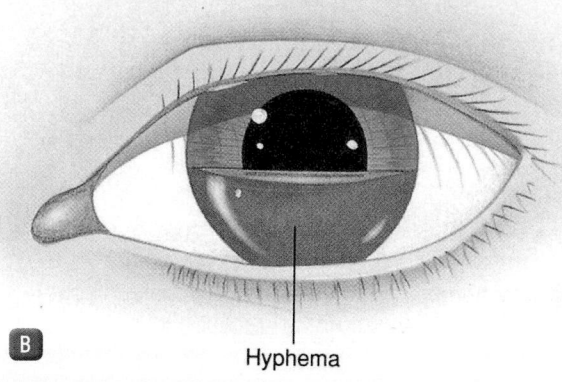

B

Hyphema

Figure 23 A hyphema, characterized by bleeding into the anterior chamber of the eye, can occur following blunt trauma to the eye. This condition should be considered a sight-threatening emergency. **A.** Actual hyphema. **B.** Illustration.

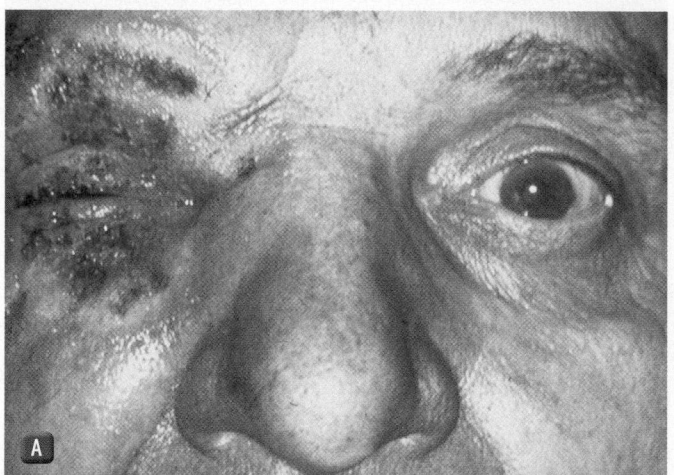

A

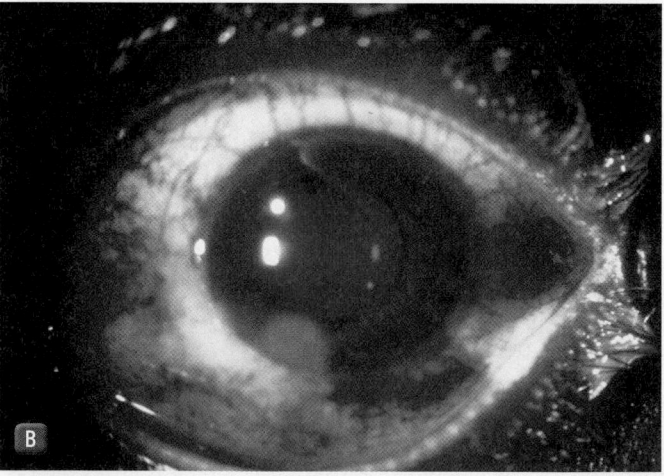

B

Figure 25 **A.** Chemical burns typically occur when an acid or alkali is splashed into the eye. **B.** A chemical burn from lye, an alkaline solution.

saline is not available, you can use any clean water. Specific techniques for irrigating the eyes are discussed later in this section.

Thermal burns occur when a patient is burned in the face during a fire, although the eyes usually close rapidly because of the heat. This reaction is a natural reflex to protect the eyes from further injury. However, the eyelids remain exposed and are frequently burned **Figure 26**.

Infrared rays, eclipse light (if the patient has looked directly at the sun), and laser burns can cause significant damage to the sensory cells of the eye when rays of light become focused on the retina. Retinal injuries that are caused by exposure to extremely bright light are generally not painful but may result in permanent damage to vision.

Superficial burns of the eye can result from ultraviolet rays from an arc welding unit, prolonged exposure to a sunlamp, or reflected light from a bright snow-covered area (snow blindness). This kind of burn may not be painful initially but may become so 3 to 5 hours later, as the damaged cornea responds to the injury. Severe conjunctivitis usually develops, along with redness, swelling, and excessive tear production.

Assessment

The first step when you are assessing a patient with an eye injury is to note the MOI (ie, blunt or penetrating trauma,

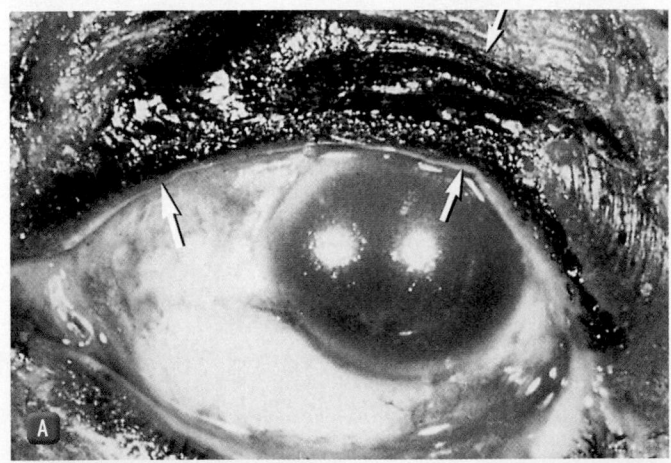

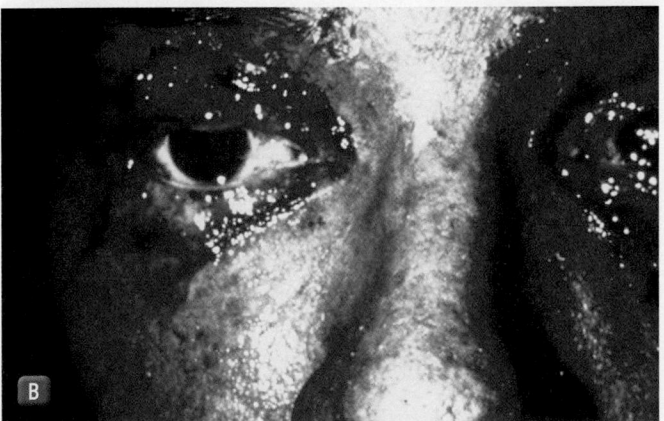

Figure 26 Thermal burns occasionally cause significant damage to the eyelids. **A.** Arrows show some full-thickness burns. **B.** Burns of the eyelids require immediate hospital care.

burn). If it suggests the potential for a spinal injury, use spinal motion restriction precautions. Ensure a patent airway and adequate breathing, and control any external bleeding. If the MOI is significant, or if the patient's clinical status dictates it, perform a rapid exam.

When you are obtaining the history, determine how and when the injury happened, when the symptoms began, and what symptoms the patient is experiencing. Were both eyes affected? Does the patient have any underlying diseases or conditions of the eye (such as glaucoma)? Does the patient take medications for his or her eyes?

A variety of symptoms may indicate serious ocular injury:

- *Visual loss* that does not improve when the patient blinks is the most important symptom of an eye injury. It may indicate damage to the globe or to the optic nerve.
- *Double vision* usually points to trauma involving the extraocular muscles, such as a fracture of the orbit.
- *Severe eye pain* is a symptom of a significant eye injury.
- A *foreign body sensation* usually indicates superficial injury to the cornea or the presence of a foreign object trapped behind the eyelids.

During the physical examination of the eyes, evaluate each of the visible ocular structures and ocular function:

- **Orbital rim:** for ecchymosis, swelling, lacerations, and tenderness
- **Eyelids:** for ecchymosis, swelling, and lacerations
- **Corneas:** for foreign bodies
- **Conjunctivae:** for redness, pus, inflammation, and foreign bodies
- **Globes:** for redness, abnormal pigmentation, and lacerations
- **Pupils:** for size, shape, equality, and reaction to light
- **Eye movements in all directions:** for paralysis of gaze or discoordination between the movements of the two eyes (**dysconjugate gaze**)
- **Visual acuity:** Make a rough assessment by asking the patient to read a newspaper or a hand-held visual acuity chart. Test each eye separately and document the results.

Treatment for specific eye injuries begins with a thorough examination to determine the extent and nature of any damage. Always perform your examination using standard precautions, taking great care to avoid aggravating the injury.

Although isolated eye injuries are usually not life threatening, they should be evaluated by a physician. More severe eye injuries often require evaluation and treatment by an ophthalmologist.

Management

Lacerations and Blunt Trauma

Injuries to the eyelids—lacerations, abrasions, and contusions—require little in the way of prehospital care other than bleeding control and gentle patching of the affected eye. No eyelid injury is trivial, however, so every patient with eyelid trauma should be transported to the hospital. Bleeding from lacerations to the soft tissue of the eye, such as the eyelids, may be heavy, but it usually can be controlled by gentle, manual pressure. Remember not to apply pressure to the globe even when attempting to control bleeding of the soft tissues surrounding it, because this could ultimately result in loss of vision.

Most injuries to the globe—including contusions, lacerations, foreign bodies, and abrasions—are best treated in the ED, where specialized equipment is available. Aluminum eye shields (not gauze patches) applied over *both* eyes are generally all that are necessary in the field. Follow these three important guidelines in treating penetrating injuries of the eye:

1. *Never exert pressure* on or manipulate the injured globe in any way.
2. If part of the globe is exposed, gently apply a moist, sterile dressing to prevent drying.
3. *Cover the injured eye* with a protective metal eye shield, cup, or sterile dressing. Apply soft dressings to both eyes, and provide prompt transport to the hospital.

If hyphema or rupture of the globe is suspected, take spinal motion restriction precautions. Such injuries indicate that a significant amount of force was applied to the face and, thus, may include a spinal injury. Elevate the head of the backboard approximately 40° to decrease intraocular pressure (IOP) and discourage the patient from performing activities that may increase IOP (eg, coughing).

On rare occasions following a serious injury, the globe may be displaced (avulsed) out of its socket **Figure 27**. Do not attempt to manipulate or reposition it in any way! Cover the protruding eye with a moist, sterile dressing and stabilize it along with the uninjured eye to prevent further injury due to **sympathetic eye movement**, the movement of both eyes in unison. Place the patient in a supine position to prevent further loss of fluid from the eye, and provide prompt transport to the hospital.

Foreign Bodies and Impaled Objects

When a foreign body is impaled in the globe, *do not remove it!* Prehospital care involves stabilizing the object and preparing the patient for transport. The greater the length of the foreign object sticking out of the eye, the more important stabilization becomes in avoiding further damage. Cover the eye with

a moist, sterile dressing; place a cup or other protective barrier over the object, and secure it in place with bulky dressing **Figure 28**. Cover the unaffected eye to prevent further damage that could occur from movement as the patient tries to use the uninjured eye to compensate for the loss or limited vision of the injured eye. Promptly transport the patient to the hospital.

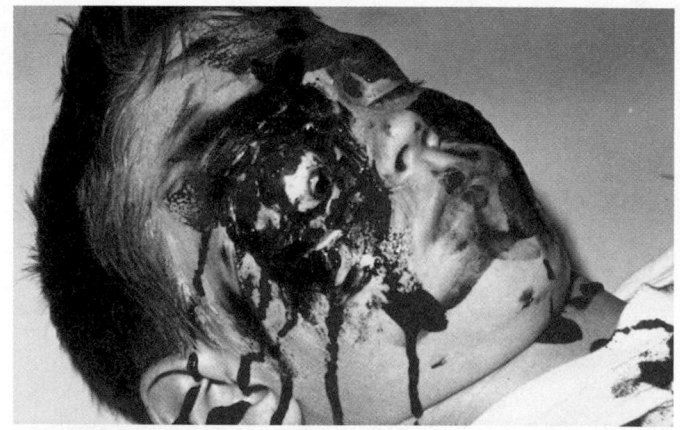

Figure 27 Do not attempt to manipulate or reposition a globe that is displaced (avulsed) out of its socket.

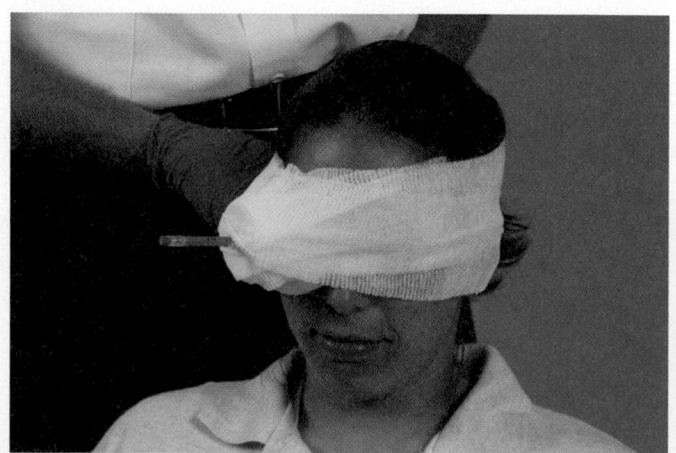

Figure 28 Secure an impaled object in the eye with a protective barrier and bulky dressing.

Burns of the Eye

Burns to the eye that are caused by ultraviolet light are most effectively treated by covering the eye with a sterile, moist pad and an eye shield. The application of cool compresses *lightly* over the eye may afford the patient pain relief if he or she is in extreme distress. Place the patient in a supine position during transport, and protect the patient from further exposure to bright light.

Chemical burns to the eye—acid or alkali—can rapidly lead to total blindness if not immediately treated. The most important prehospital treatment in such cases is to begin immediate irrigation with sterile water or saline solution. *Never use any chemical antidotes (such as vinegar, baking soda) when you are irrigating the patient's eye; use sterile water or saline only.*

The goal when you are irrigating the eye is to direct the greatest amount of solution or water into the eye as gently as possible. Because opening the eye spontaneously may cause the patient pain, you may have to force the lids open to irrigate the eye adequately. Ideally, you should use a bulb or irrigation syringe, a nasal cannula, or some other device that will allow you to control the flow Figure 29 . In some circumstances, you may have to pour water into the eye by holding the patient's head under a gently running faucet. You can have the patient

immerse his or her face in a large pan or basin of water and rapidly blink the affected eyelid. If only one eye is affected, take care to avoid contaminated water getting into the unaffected eye.

Irrigate the eye for at least 5 minutes. If the burn was caused by an alkali or a strong acid, irrigate the eye continuously for 20 minutes because these substances can penetrate deeply. One type of eye injury you may encounter occurs from the use of anhydrous ammonia, which is used during the process of cooking methamphetamine. If the patient's eyes are not irrigated promptly and efficiently, permanent damage is likely. Whenever you have to irrigate the eye(s), continue irrigation en route to the hospital if possible.

Irrigation with a sterile saline solution will frequently flush away loose, small foreign objects lying on the surface of the eye. Always flush from the nose side of the eye toward the outside to avoid flushing material into the other eye. After its removal, a foreign body will often leave a small abrasion on the surface of the conjunctiva, which leads to continued irritation; for this reason, you should transport the patient to the hospital for further assessment and treatment.

Gentle irrigation usually will not wash out foreign bodies that are stuck to the cornea or lying under the upper eyelid.

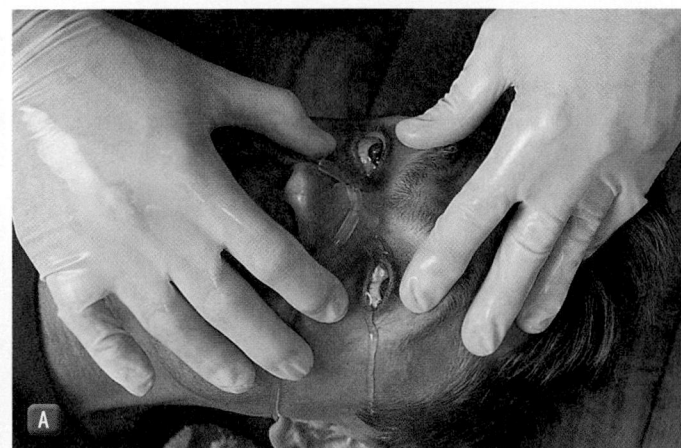
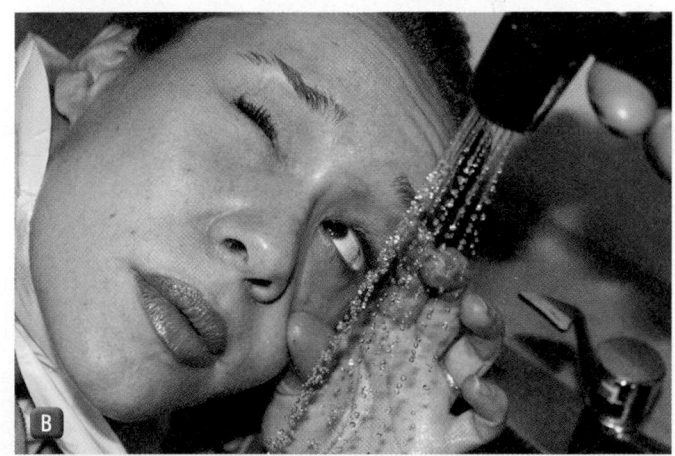
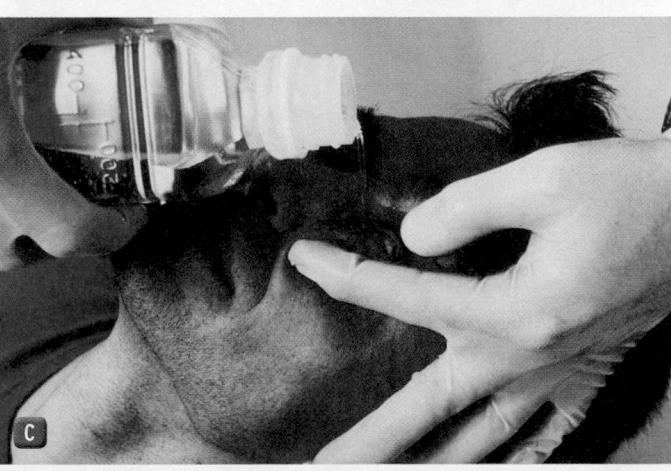
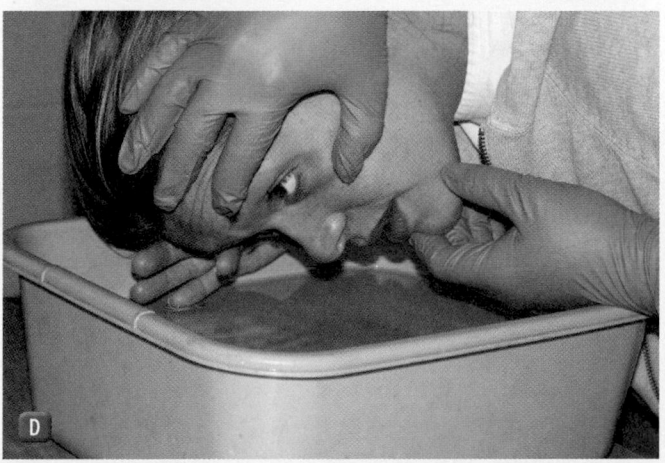

Figure 29 Four ways to effectively irrigate the eye: **A.** Nasal cannula. **B.** Shower. **C.** Bottle. **D.** Basin. Always protect the uninjured eye from the irrigating solution to prevent exposure to the substance.

Words of Wisdom

There are three types of contact lenses: hard, rigid gas-permeable, and soft (hydrophilic). Small, hard contact lenses usually are tinted, making them relatively easy to see. Large, soft contact lenses are clear and can be difficult to see, even more so if they "float" up or down under an eyelid.

In general, you should not attempt to remove contact lenses from a patient with an eye injury because removal could further aggravate the injury. The only indication for removing contact lenses in the prehospital setting is a chemical burn of the eye. In this situation, the lens can trap the offending chemical and make irrigation difficult, thus worsening the injury.

To remove a hard contact lens, use a small suction cup, moistening the end with saline solution **Figure 30A**. To remove soft contact lenses, place one to two drops of saline solution in the eye **Figure 30B**, gently pinch the lens between your gloved thumb and index finger, and lift it off the surface of the eye **Figure 30C**. Place the contact lens in a container with sterile saline solution. Always advise ED staff if a patient is wearing contact lenses.

Occasionally, you may care for a patient who is wearing an eye prosthesis (artificial eye). You should suspect that an eye is artificial when it does not respond to light, move in concert with the opposite eye, or appear quite the same as the opposite eye. If you are unsure as to whether the patient has an eye prosthesis, ask the patient about it. Although no harm will be done if you care for an artificial eye as you would a normal one, you need to clearly understand the patient's eye function.

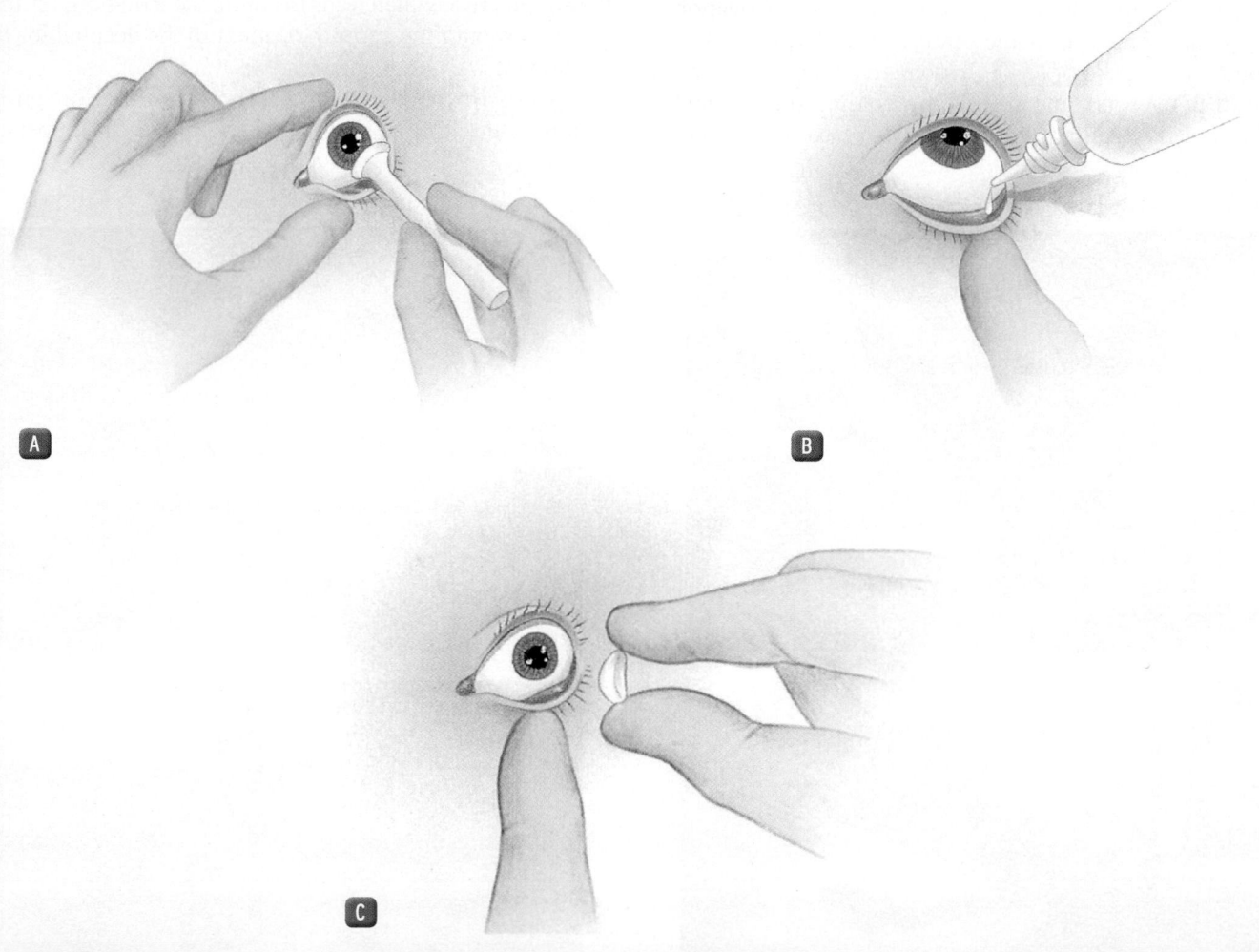

Figure 30 Removing contact lenses should be limited to patients with chemical burns to the eye. **A.** To remove hard contact lenses, use a specialized suction cup moistened with sterile saline solution. **B.** To remove soft contact lenses, place 1 or 2 drops of saline solution in the eye. **C.** Pinch off the lens with your gloved thumb and index finger.

To examine the undersurface of the upper eyelid, pull the lid upward and forward. If you spot a foreign object on the surface of the eyelid, you may be able to remove it with a moist, sterile, cotton-tipped applicator. *Never attempt to remove a foreign body that is stuck or imbedded in the cornea.*

■ Pathophysiology, Assessment, and Management of Ear Injuries

Injuries to the ear may be isolated, or they may occur in conjunction with other injuries to the head or face. Although isolated ear injuries are typically not life threatening, they can result in sensory impairment and permanent disfigurement.

■ Pathophysiology

Soft-Tissue Injuries

Lacerations, avulsions, and contusions to the external ear can occur following blunt or penetrating trauma. The pinna can be contused, lacerated, or partially or completely avulsed. Trauma to the earlobe can result in similar injuries.

The pinna has an inherently poor blood supply, so it tends to heal poorly. Healing of the cartilaginous pinna is often complicated by infection.

Ruptured Eardrum

Perforation of the tympanic membrane (ruptured eardrum) can result from direct blows, foreign bodies in the ear, or pressure-related injuries, such as blast injuries resulting from an explosion, or diving-related injuries that result in barotrauma to the ear. Signs and symptoms of a perforated tympanic membrane include loss of hearing and blood drainage from the ear (hemorrhagic otorrhea). Although the injury is extremely painful for the patient, the tympanic membrane typically heals spontaneously and without complication. Nevertheless, a careful assessment should be performed to detect and treat other injuries, some of which may be life threatening.

■ Assessment and Management

Assessment and management of the patient with an ear injury begin by ensuring airway patency and breathing adequacy. If the MOI suggests a potential for spinal injury, apply full spinal motion restriction precautions.

An adequate assessment of the external ear canal and middle ear cannot be performed in the field. In general, the ears' poor blood supply limits the amount of external bleeding. If manual direct pressure does not control this bleeding, first place a soft, padded dressing between the ear and the scalp because bandaging the ear against the tender scalp can be extremely painful. Then apply a roller bandage to secure the dressing in place **Figure 31**. An ice pack can also help reduce swelling and pain.

If the pinna is partially avulsed, carefully realign the ear into position and gently bandage it with sufficient padding that

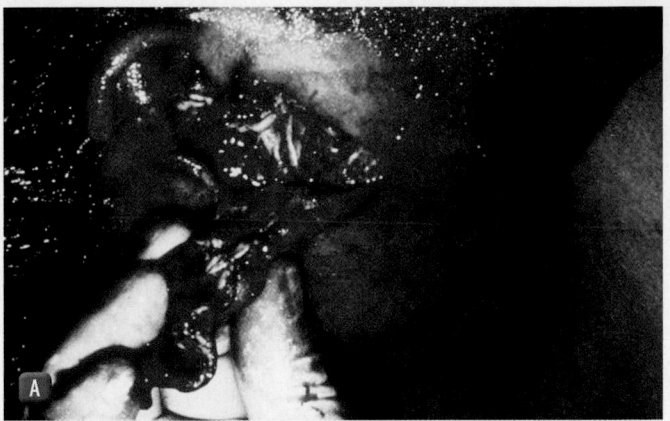
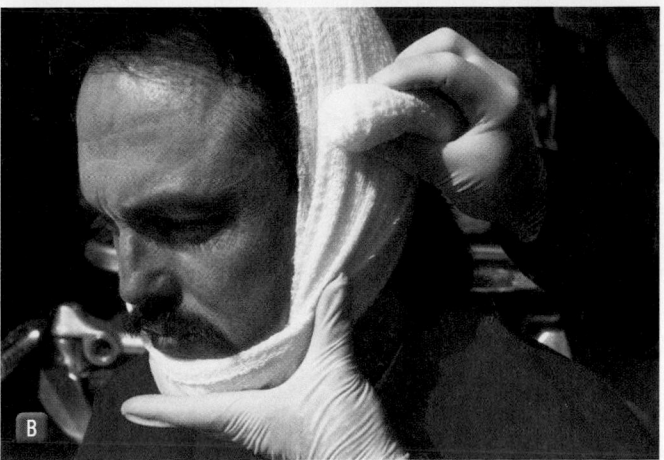

Figure 31 **A.** A major laceration of the ear. **B.** Place a soft, sterile pad behind the ear, between it and the scalp. Then wrap a roller gauze bandage (ie, Kling, Kerlex) around the head to include the entire ear.

has been slightly moistened with normal saline. If the pinna is completely avulsed, attempt to retrieve the avulsed part, if possible, for reimplantation at the hospital. If the detached part of the ear is recovered, treat it as any other amputation; wrap it in saline-moistened gauze, place it in a plastic bag, and place the bag on ice.

If a chemical ice pack is used, it is recommended to shield the avulsed part with several gauze 4 × 4s to diffuse the cold because chemical ice packs are actually colder than ice and inadvertent freezing of the part can occur. If blood or CSF drainage is noted, apply a loose dressing over the ear—taking care *not* to stop the flow—and assess the patient for other signs of a basilar skull fracture.

Do not remove an impaled object from the ear. Instead, stabilize the object and cover the ear to prevent gross movement and minimize the risk of contamination of the inner ear.

Because isolated ear injuries are typically not life threatening, you must perform a careful assessment to detect or rule out potentially more serious injuries. You may then proceed with specific care of the ear, provide emotional support, and transport the patient to an appropriate medical facility.

Pathophysiology, Assessment, and Management of Oral and Dental Injuries

Oral and dental injuries are commonly associated with trauma to the face. Blunt mechanisms are commonly the result of motor vehicle crashes or direct blows to the mouth or chin. Penetrating mechanisms are commonly the result of gunshot wounds, lacerations, and punctures.

The primary risk associated with oral and dental injuries is airway compromise from oropharyngeal bleeding, occlusion by a displaced dental appliance such as a bridge or partial plate, or possibly by the aspiration of avulsed or fractured teeth. Any patient with significant facial trauma should be carefully assessed for injuries to the mouth and teeth.

Pathophysiology

Soft-Tissue Injuries

Lacerations and avulsions in and around the mouth are associated with a risk of intraoral hemorrhage and subsequent airway compromise. Therefore, your assessment of any patient with facial trauma should include a careful examination of the mouth, including the teeth. Fractured or avulsed teeth and lacerations of the tongue may cause profuse bleeding into the upper airway Figure 32 . A responsive patient with severe oral bleeding is often unable to speak unless he or she is leaning forward—this position facilitates drainage of blood from the mouth.

Patients may swallow blood from lacerations inside the mouth, so the bleeding may not be grossly evident. Because blood irritates the gastric lining, the risks of vomiting and aspiration are significant. Objects that are impaled in or through the soft tissues of the mouth (such as the cheek) can also result in profuse bleeding and once again, the threat of vomiting with aspiration.

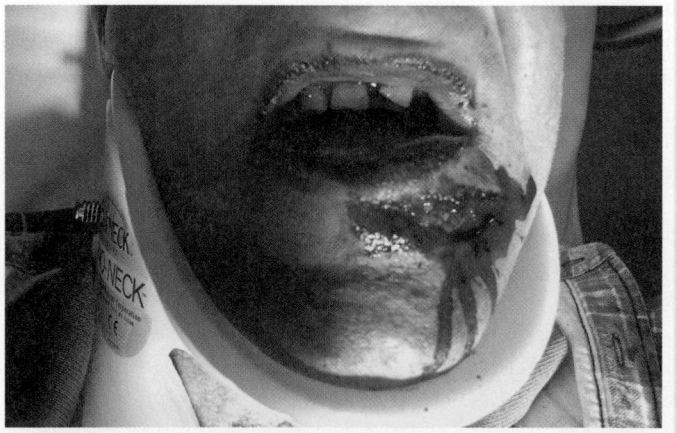

Figure 32 Soft-tissue injuries around the mouth can be associated with profuse oral bleeding and airway compromise.

Dental Injuries

Fractured and avulsed teeth—especially the anterior teeth—are common following facial trauma. Dental injuries may be associated with mechanisms that cause severe maxillofacial trauma (such as motor vehicle crashes), or they may occur in isolation (such as a direct blow to the mouth from an assault).

You should always assess the patient's mouth following a facial injury, especially in cases of fractured or avulsed teeth. Teeth fragments (or even whole teeth) can become an airway obstruction and should be removed from the patient's mouth immediately.

Words of Wisdom

When you are assessing a patient with fractured or avulsed teeth following an assault, you should also assess the person who struck the patient, *if it is safe to do so*. The human mouth is filled with bacteria and other microorganisms, and lacerations to the person's hands or knuckles can easily become infected without proper care. Occasionally, you may encounter fragments of broken teeth impaled in a person's knuckles!

Assessment and Management

Ensuring airway patency and adequate breathing is the priority of care when you are managing patients with oral or dental trauma. Suction the oropharynx as needed, and remove fractured tooth fragments to prevent airway compromise. Apply spinal motion restriction precautions as dictated by the MOI. If profuse oral bleeding is present and the patient cannot spontaneously control his or her own airway (such as with a decreased level of consciousness), pharmacologically assisted intubation (such as RSI) may be necessary.

Impaled objects in the soft tissues of the mouth should be stabilized in place unless they interfere with the patient's breathing or your ability to manage the patient's airway. In those cases, remove the impaled object from the direction that it entered, if possible, and control bleeding with direct pressure.

An avulsed tooth may be successfully reimplanted even if it has been out of the mouth for up to 1 hour. Medical control may sometimes ask you to reimplant the tooth in its original socket. Carefully place the tooth in its socket, and hold it in place with your fingers or have the patient gently bite down. If prehospital reimplantation of a tooth is not possible, follow the guidelines established by the American Association of Endodontists and the American Dental Association Table 2 .

Retrieval and reimplantation or storage of an avulsed tooth is a low priority if the patient is in a clinically unstable condition (such as a compromised airway or shock). In such cases, aggressive airway management, spinal precautions, and rapid transport of the patient are obviously more important, with the dental problem being addressed at a later time.

Table 2 Care for an Avulsed Tooth
Handle the tooth by the crown only. Avoid touching the root surface of the tooth.
Gently rinse the tooth with sterile saline solution or water. Avoid the use of soap or chemicals, and do not scrub the tooth!
Do not allow the tooth to dry. Place it in one of the following: ■ Emergency tooth preservation system (such as EMT Tooth Saver, 3M Save-a-Tooth): a break-resistant storage container with soft inner walls and a pH-balanced solution (such as Hanks Balanced Salt Solution) that nourishes and preserves the tooth ■ Cold whole milk ■ Sterile saline solution (for storage periods of less than 1 hour)
Transport the tooth with the patient, and notify the hospital of the situation.

Pathophysiology, Assessment, and Management of Injuries to the Anterior Part of the Neck

The neck is a vulnerable stretch of anatomy because it houses a critical portion of the airway (ie, larynx, trachea), the major blood vessels to and from the head, and the spinal cord. Other structures contained within the neck that are also vulnerable to injury include portions of the upper gastrointestinal system, such as the esophagus, as well as other muscles, nerves, and glands located in the region. Any injury to the anterior part of the neck—blunt or penetrating—must be considered critical until proved otherwise.

Pathophysiology

Soft-Tissue Injuries

Blunt and penetrating mechanisms can damage the soft tissues of the anterior part of the neck and its associated structures. In both cases, you must be alert for the possibility of cervical spine injury and airway compromise.

Common mechanisms of blunt trauma include motor vehicle crashes, direct trauma to the neck (so-called "clothesline" type injury), and hangings. Such injury often results in swelling and edema; injury to the various structures such as the trachea, larynx, epiglottis, or esophagus; or injury to the cervical spine. Less commonly, blunt injuries may damage the vasculature of the anterior part of the neck. Because blunt trauma to the neck is associated with a high incidence of airway compromise and ventilatory inadequacy, you must carefully assess the patient and be prepared to initiate aggressive management.

Common mechanisms of penetrating trauma include gunshot wounds, stabbings, and impaled objects. The lacerations or puncture wounds produced may be superficial and involve only the fascia or fatty tissues of the neck, or they may be deep and involve injury to the larynx, trachea, esophagus, nerves, or major blood vessels. The primary threats from penetrating neck trauma are massive hemorrhage from major blood vessel disruption and airway compromise secondary to soft-tissue swelling or direct damage to the larynx or trachea.

A special danger associated with open neck injuries is the possibility of a fatal air embolism. If the jugular veins of the neck

YOU are the Medic PART 4

Your partner assists the first responder by gently holding the mask of the bag-mask device in place while the bag is squeezed. When you are ready to intubate, you instruct your partner to gently hold the mandible and sides of the patient's face to provide stability. You gently lift your laryngoscope and visualize the vocal cords. You successfully watch the endotracheal (ET) tube slide through the vocal cords.

Recording Time: 10 Minutes	
Respirations	12 breaths/min, assisted
Pulse	126 beats/min
Skin	Cool, pale, moist
Blood pressure	90/60 mm Hg
Oxygen saturation (Spo$_2$)	95% 15 L/min via bag-mask device
Pupils	Equal and slow to react

7. Describe the steps in determining proper placement of an ET tube.

8. How are you going to secure the ET tube in place with this type of facial fracture?

are exposed to the environment, they may entrain (suck) air into the vessel and occlude the flow of blood to the lungs **Figure 33**. As such, open neck wounds should be sealed with an occlusive dressing immediately. Use caution to avoid constriction of the vessels and structures of the neck and be alert for swelling and expanding hematomas because they can turn the occlusive dressing into a constricting band.

Impaled objects in the neck can present several life-threatening problems for the patient—namely, injury to major blood vessels with massive hemorrhage; damage to the larynx, trachea, or esophagus; or injury to the cervical spine **Figure 34**. Impaled objects should not be removed but rather stabilized in place and protected from movement. The *only* exception is if the object is obstructing the airway or impeding your ability to effectively manage the airway. In some cases, an emergency

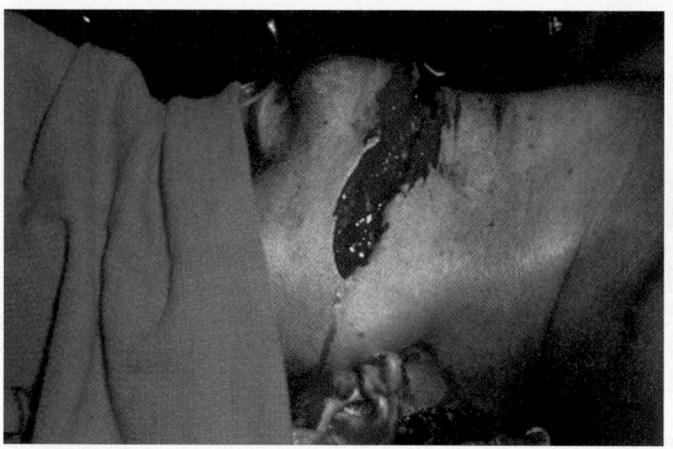

Figure 33 Open injuries to the neck can be dangerous. If veins are exposed to the environment, they can suck in air, resulting in a potentially fatal air embolism.

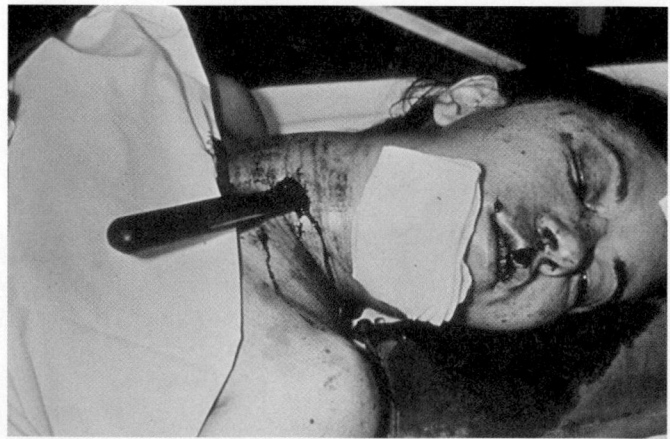

Figure 34 Impaled objects in the neck can cause profuse bleeding, if the major blood vessels are damaged, and direct injury to the larynx, trachea, esophagus, or cervical spine.

cricothyrotomy may be necessary to establish and maintain airway patency.

Injuries to the Larynx, Trachea, and Esophagus

A variety of life-threatening injuries can result if the structures of the anterior part of the neck are crushed against the cervical spine following blunt trauma or if they are penetrated by a knife or similar object. The larynx and its supporting structures (ie, hyoid bone, thyroid cartilage, and cricoid ring) may be fractured, the trachea may be separated from the larynx (<u>tracheal transection</u>), or the esophagus may be perforated. Many injuries to the larynx, trachea, and esophagus are occult; because they are not as obvious and dramatic as penetrating neck injuries, they can be easily overlooked. Therefore, you must maintain a high index of suspicion and perform a careful assessment of *any* patient with blunt trauma to the anterior part of the neck. Significant injuries to the larynx or trachea pose an *immediate* risk of airway compromise due to disruption of the normal passage of air, soft-tissue swelling, or aspiration of blood into the lungs. In addition, esophageal perforation can result in <u>mediastinitis</u>, an inflammation of the mediastinum often due to leakage of gastric contents into the thoracic cavity. Mediastinitis has a very high mortality rate, particularly without rapid surgical treatment. Patients with injuries to the anterior part of the neck may experience concomitant maxillofacial fractures, which can make bag-mask ventilation difficult (usually because of an inadequate mask-to-face seal). Likewise, ET intubation may be extremely challenging, if not impossible, owing to distortion of the normal anatomic structures of the upper airway. If basic and advanced techniques to secure the patient's airway are unsuccessful or impossible, a surgical or needle cricothyrotomy may be your only means of establishing a patent airway and ensuring adequate oxygenation and ventilation. Prior to deciding to perform a surgical airway, use of a lighted stylette or a gum bougie may allow you to get the airway secured in a timely fashion while avoiding more risky procedures.

◼ Assessment

Bruising, redness to the overlying skin, and palpable tenderness are common signs associated with all injuries to the anterior part of the neck. **Table 3** summarizes the signs and symptoms of specific injuries.

Words of Wisdom

Any force that is powerful enough to disrupt the larynx, trachea, or esophagus is powerful enough to injure the cervical spine, so the use of spinal motion restriction precautions is important. Carefully assess the patient for signs of a spinal injury: vertebral deformities (step-offs), paralysis, paresthesia, and signs of neurogenic shock (hypotension, normal or slow pulse rate, lack of diaphoresis). Even a grunt or groan, or withdrawal by the patient during palpation should be assumed to be a positive finding; therefore, spinal motion restriction precautions should be implemented.

Injury	Signs and Symptoms
Laryngeal fracture, tracheal transection	▪ Labored breathing or reduced air movement ▪ Stridor ▪ Hoarseness, voice changes ▪ **Hemoptysis** (coughing up blood) ▪ Subcutaneous emphysema ▪ Swelling, edema ▪ Structural irregularity
Vascular injury	▪ Gross external bleeding ▪ Signs of shock ▪ Hematoma, swelling, edema ▪ Pulse deficits
Esophageal perforation	▪ **Dysphagia** (difficulty swallowing) ▪ Hematemesis ▪ Hemoptysis (suggests aspiration of blood)
Neurologic impairment	▪ Signs of a stroke (suggests air embolism or cerebral infarct) ▪ Paralysis or paresthesia ▪ Cranial nerve deficit ▪ Signs of neurogenic shock

Table 3 Signs and Symptoms of Injuries to the Anterior Part of the Neck

Begin your assessment by noting the MOI and maintaining a high index of suspicion, especially if the patient has experienced blunt or penetrating trauma between the upper part of the chest and head. Fractures of the first rib are associated with close to 50% mortality, not because of the rib fracture, but because the force it takes to fracture such a short, stout bone takes so much force that significant face, head, and neck trauma are often present as well. Remember that obvious and dramatic-appearing soft-tissue injuries may mask occult injuries to the larynx, trachea, or esophagus. Also, the patient may have experienced trauma to multiple body systems, especially following a significant MOI. As you begin your primary assessment, manually stabilize the patient's head in a neutral in-line position and simultaneously open the airway with the jaw-thrust maneuver if the patient is unresponsive. Use suction as needed to clear the airway of blood or other liquids. Assess the patient's breathing—rate, regularity, and depth—and intervene immediately. If the patient is breathing adequately, apply a nonrebreathing mask at 15 L/min. If breathing is inadequate (ie, reduced tidal volume, fast or slow respirations), assist with bag-mask ventilation and 100% oxygen.

Management

Your primary focus when caring for a patient is to always treat the injuries that will be the *most rapidly fatal*. Because death following trauma to the anterior part of the neck is usually the result of airway compromise or massive bleeding, aggressive airway management and external bleeding control are the highest priorities of care. After addressing any life-threatening or other serious problems with the ABCs during the primary assessment, you may perform a rapid exam to detect and treat other injuries. To control bleeding from an open neck wound and prevent an air embolism, immediately cover the wound with an occlusive dressing. In the case of a small wound, or wounds, use of ECG electrodes can be a fast and effective way to seal a small hole or holes. Apply manual direct pressure over the occlusive dressing with a bulky dressing. As a last resort, you can secure a pressure dressing over the wound by wrapping roller gauze loosely around the neck and then firmly through the opposite axilla **Figure 35**. *Do not* circumferentially wrap bandages around the neck to secure the dressing in place. This is contraindicated and could even be fatal because it may impair cerebral perfusion by occluding both carotid arteries or interfere with the patient's breathing. Monitor the patient's pulse for reflex bradycardia, which indicates parasympathetic nervous stimulation due to excessive pressure on the carotid artery.

Whenever injury to the anterior part of the neck (specifically the larynx) is recognized or suspected, it is prudent to advise the patient to refrain from speaking to allow the vocal cords to rest and recuperate. This will require asking questions that can be

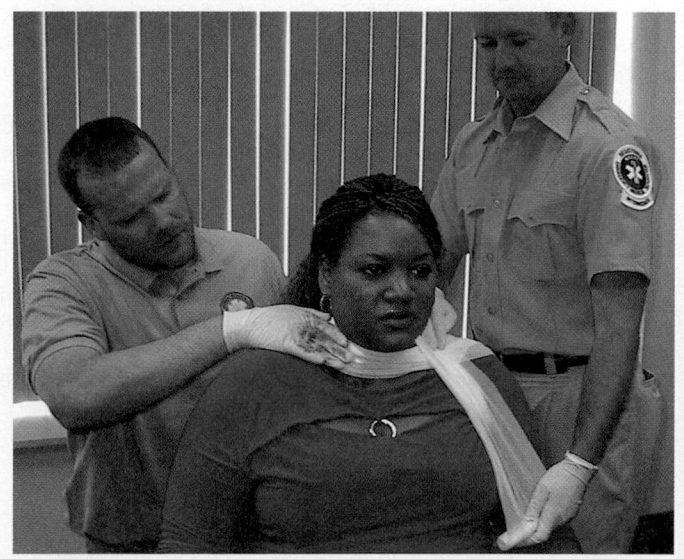

Figure 35 Cover open neck wounds with an occlusive dressing, and apply manual pressure to control bleeding. Do not compress both carotid arteries simultaneously because this may impair cerebral perfusion.

simply answered with yes or no. Alternatively, you may ask the patient to write answers for you. Keep in mind that if the larynx is injured, the incidence of cervical spine involvement is relatively high; therefore, the patient should avoid shaking his or her head when answering.

Words of Wisdom

Never use a flow-restricted, oxygen-powered ventilation device (ie, a manually triggered ventilator) on a patient with trauma to the anterior part of the neck and signs of laryngeal or tracheal injury. The high pressure delivered by such devices can cause barotrauma and potentially exacerbate the patient's injury. If ventilatory support is necessary, use bag-mask ventilation.

If signs of shock are present, keep the patient warm, establish vascular access with at least one large-bore IV en route to the hospital if possible, or on-scene if indicated, and infuse an isotonic crystalloid solution (such as lactated Ringer's or normal saline) as needed to maintain adequate perfusion.

Many patients with serious laryngeal trauma have airway obstruction and may require a surgical or percutaneous airway. Consult your local protocols regarding whether these procedures are performed at the paramedic level in your area. ET intubation may be hazardous in these patients because you cannot see the tip of the ET tube once it passes between the vocal cords; it may pass straight through a defect in the laryngeal or tracheal wall or could result in the complete transection of the trachea. Signs of this complication include increased swelling of the neck and worsening subcutaneous emphysema during assisted ventilation.

If the patient has experienced an open tracheal wound, you may be able to pass a cuffed ET tube directly through the wound to establish a patent airway. However, you must use caution because the trachea may be perforated anteriorly *and* posteriorly, thereby increasing the risk of false passage of the ET tube outside the trachea. It is critical to use *multiple* techniques for confirming correct ET tube placement: Frequently monitor breath sounds, directly measure the expired carbon dioxide (waveform capnography is preferred), assess for adequate chest rise, and assess for vapor mist in the ET tube during exhalation.

■ Pathophysiology, Assessment, and Management of Spine Trauma

■ Pathophysiology

The neck, because of its relative exposure to forces both directly applied and referred, is subject to injury that does not necessarily result in specific bony injury such as fracture or dislocation. Predominately these nonpenetrating injuries are classified as sprains and strains.

Controversies

Performing spinal clearance in the prehospital environment is considered controversial and requires significant training, competency, and oversight. Spinal clearance refers to the act of declaring that, based on your findings, a spinal injury is not present. In the United States, protocols either do not allow spinal clearance in the field, or only allow paramedics to perform spinal clearance on patients who are awake and alert. Such patients may be cleared through history taking and physical examination. All other patients must be cleared by other medical personnel—for example—at the receiving facility with the use of radiologic studies, including plain radiographs, computed tomography, and magnetic resonance imaging.

If a patient does not exhibit any precluding signs or symptoms and if your system and medical direction allow, you can proceed to manual or clinical spinal clearance procedures according to several established criteria. The NEXUS Clinical Criteria uses the following to define a possible spinal injury:

1. Tenderness at the posterior midline of the cervical spine
2. Focal neurologic deficit
3. Decreased level of alertness
4. Evidence of intoxication
5. Clinically apparent pain that might distract the patient from the pain of a cervical spine injury. This might be a fracture of a long bone or a deep laceration or significant burn.

The presence of any one of the above findings is considered to be clinical evidence that a patient is at increased risk for cervical spine injury and requires radiographic evaluation.

Alternatively, the spine can be cleared in the field using the Canadian C-Spine Rule. The patient does not need to be touched when using this rule. It asks three main questions:

1. Is there a high-risk factor? Examples include a patient age of 65 years or older, high-risk MOI, or paresthesias (tingling or sensory change) in the extremities. In such cases, radiography is necessary.
2. Is there a low-risk factor? In such cases, it is safe to assess range of motion. Examples include simple rear-end motor vehicle collision, patient being ambulatory at any time since the injury, delayed onset of neck pain, or absence of midline cervical spine tenderness.
3. Is the patient able to actively rotate the neck 45 degrees to the left and right?

Manual spinal clearance is performed as follows: While your partner is manually providing spinal stabilization, palpate the cervical vertebral spinous processes individually, stopping the evaluation if any pain is encountered. If no pain is encountered, continue to evaluate each of the vertebrae through C7, which is represented by the prominent protrusion at the base of the neck. Then palpate the muscles of the neck individually, again stopping the evaluation if any tenderness or pain is encountered. As one of the final steps of the cervical evaluation, have the patient resist your attempts to cautiously turn the head laterally to both sides individually, and then attempt extension and flexion, again individually. Finally, gently compress the neck by applying pressure to the superior portion of the head.

A <u>sprain</u> is a stretching or tearing of ligaments—the tough bands of fibrous tissue that connect one bone to another. The response to such injuries is for the muscle to contract. The muscles attempt to support the neck. It is believed that this response is the result of injury to the facet joint. This injury can be difficult, if not impossible, to determine in the prehospital setting. As a result, you should maintain a high index of suspicion of cervical involvement and provide cervical spine stabilization.

A <u>strain</u> is a stretching or tearing of muscle or tendon. The most common form of cervical strain is often called <u>whiplash</u> and can be quite difficult to differentiate from injuries that involve the bony structures. It is estimated that over a million cases of whiplash from motor vehicle crashes are reported annually in the United States. That is around 3.8 per 1,000 persons. Most crashes that produce injury are at speeds of greater than 10 mph. Whiplash can be difficult to differentiate from unstable spine fracture or dislocation. If the scope of practice involves clearing the spine after injury, findings of point tenderness and pain on movement often preclude "ruling out" a spinal injury, and cervical precautions should be taken and maintained throughout contact and transport. Whereas mortality is rare from whiplash, morbidity can occasionally develop in the form of persistent and chronic cervical pain, with some patients experiencing prolonged spasms and exacerbation. Fortunately, such cases are rare and often associated with the potential for secondary gain such as insurance or disability payments.

Assessment

Because the evaluation of complaints of neck pain can be difficult, it is recommended that you transport patients to the ED for radiologic studies. Conduct a visual inspection for signs of soft-tissue injury, which may indicate muscular and bony involvement. If the patient is symptomatic with pain (either with or without movement and palpation), maintain spinal stabilization. If the MOI dictates spinal clearance protocol (see Controversies box) and your examination produces any pain or resistance, most protocols require that the provider stop the examination, maintain spinal stabilization, and transport the patient for further evaluation in the ED.

Management

Because of the risk of orthopaedic and central nervous system involvement, most specialists recommend that patients reporting neck pain after injury should be evaluated in the ED. You should address any airway, ventilation, and oxygenation considerations and ensure there is no major circulatory compromise. Prehospital management should focus on preventing further injury with provision of motion restrictions, typically with application of an extrication collar and placement of the patient on a long backboard or vacuum mattress. In critical patients, it may be necessary to perform these tasks simultaneously. If the patient requires advanced airway control, it is acceptable to open the extrication collar while providing in-line stabilization to facilitate the intubation. During application of a long backboard or vacuum mattress, as in all splinting procedures, it is essential for you to check distal circulation, and sensory and motor function before and after the full-body splint (long backboard or vacuum mattress) is applied and document those findings in your patient care report. If your examination and questioning of the patient reveal no obvious MOI, you may consider treatment of the suspected strain as you would for any other muscular strain. This can include rest, ice, and elevation. A soft collar may help to gently support the head and decrease the workload on the strained muscles. An extrication collar can provide limited similar benefit. It is still recommended that patients reporting neck pain be evaluated for occult injuries and prevention of long-term consequences.

Injury Prevention

Because injuries to the face and neck in all of their varying degrees can be life altering and permanent, many improvements and advancements have been made in providing protection to these regions of the anatomy. This is especially true in the area of organized events such as contact sports and wheel-borne sports. Helmets, face shields, mouth guards, and safety glasses help to prevent injury during activities in which the risk of being hit with objects that are in motion is proportionately high. The same holds true for advances in motor vehicle safety. Better occupant safety restraints and air bags help to prevent contact with the interior of the vehicle, and improvements to the headrests, if they are used properly, are reducing the number of neck strains.

YOU are the Medic   SUMMARY

1. **What is your primary concern after scene safety is established?**

   Your immediate concern is the condition of the patient's airway. The patient is unresponsive and has snoring respirations. Without conducting any further assessment, you know the patient has an incomplete airway that needs immediate management.

2. **What is your first step in controlling the patient's airway?**

   You know the patient sustained a significant impact to her face, but you do not know how extensive the damage is at this point. You can suction the patient to remove blood as you begin the assessment of facial structures.

3. **What type of facial fracture may this patient have?**

   The crepitus, the free-floating feel of the maxilla, and clear fluid coming from the nose lead to the suspicion of a Le Fort fracture. Whether it is a type I, II, or III will be determined in the clinical setting. What is important is for you to understand that a Le Fort fracture is an unstable facial fracture. The instability will require extra caution when you are ventilating the patient or using invasive airway techniques.

4. **How will this type of fracture affect selection of an appropriate airway method?**

   As mentioned, Le Fort fractures are unstable and will move with manipulation. Movement will cause further injury, which in turn will cause more damage and swelling. A definitive airway needs to be placed immediately. In this case, endotracheal intubation, if possible, would be best.

5. **What challenges do facial fractures present during ventilation with a bag-mask device?**

   When you think of the method used to perform bag-mask ventilation on a patient with normal facial features, you can imagine how unstable facial fractures will complicate the process.

   If you have an adequate number of care providers, use two people to operate the bag-mask device. The provider responsible for placement of the mask needs to use extreme caution to not press inward to maintain a seal. Care should also be taken to not move the mask laterally.

6. **What precautions will you need to take when you attempt endotracheal intubation?**

   Because blood has already been noted in the patient's upper airway, be ready to perform suctioning when you are inserting the laryngoscope. There may be more blood, tissue, bone, or teeth in the airway on visualization. Have your forceps ready should you need them. Have a second provider gently hold the patient's face for stability while you visualize and insert the airway.

7. **Describe the steps in determining proper placement of an ET tube.**

   Proper placement of the ET tube begins with visualizing the tip of the tube passing through the vocal cords. If you did not see the tube, you cannot be certain where it is. After inflating the cuff (if supplied), auscultate starting with the epigastrium. If you hear air movement, your tube is not in the trachea. If there is no air movement in the stomach, auscultate over both lungs to ensure equal inflation. Repeat the listening process after securing the ET tube in place. Finally, apply capnography and monitor the readings.

8. **How are you going to secure the ET tube in place with this type of facial fracture?**

   As with the bag-mask device, securing the ET tube in place may be challenging because of the injury to the maxilla. Commercially available devices may still work as long as you use caution when tightening the straps. Alternatively, tape may be used.

YOU *are the Medic* | **SUMMARY,** *continued*

EMS Patient Care Report (PCR)

Date: 03-27-11	Incident No.: 23542	Nature of Call: MVC		Location: Hwy 12/River Rd	
Dispatched: 1115	En Route: 1116	At Scene: 1121	Transport: 1135	At Hospital: 1142	In Service: 1200

Patient Information

Age: 21 Sex: F Weight (in kg [lb]): 55 kg (120 lb)	Allergies: Unknown Medications: Unknown Past Medical History: Unknown Chief Complaint: Facial trauma

Vital Signs

Time: 1126	BP: 90/60	Pulse: 130	Respirations: 8	Spo₂: 92% RA
Time: 1131	BP: 90/60	Pulse: 126	Respirations: 12	Spo₂: 95% bag-mask device
Time:	BP:	Pulse:	Respirations:	Spo₂:

EMS Treatment
(circle all that apply)

Oxygen @ __15__ L/min via (circle one): NC NRM ⟨Bag-mask device⟩	⟨Assisted Ventilation⟩	⟨Airway Adjunct⟩	CPR	
Defibrillation	Bleeding Control	Bandaging	Splinting	Other: Spinal immobilization, suction, IV

Narrative

Arrived to find a 21-year-old female who was riding in the bed of a pickup that hit a tree head-on. This pt was unrestrained and was projected forward, striking her face on the cab. Pt was placed in spinal precautions prior to our arrival by Engine 21 crew. Pt is unresponsive with snoring respirations. Attempted oral airway w/o success. Pt has what appears to be a free-floating maxilla with associated blood and clear fluid coming from nose. Suction applied and bag-mask device used with two providers so as to not push in on the maxilla. ET tube 7.5 mm inserted with visualization of the tube passing the cords. No epigastric sounds and positive equal lung sounds noted on ventilation with ET tube. Tube secured using a commercially manufactured device and ET tube placement reassessed. Capnography applied. IV NS established with 12 gauge left AC. Transported emergency without incident to the trauma center and no change in pt condition. Report to Dr. Sterrett on arrival. **End of report**

Prep Kit

- A strong working knowledge of anatomy and physiology of the face, head, and brain is essential to accurately assess and manage patients with injuries to these locations.

- Personal safety is your initial primary concern when you are treating any patient with head or face trauma; never enter an unsafe scene.

- Head and face trauma most often result from direct trauma or rapid deceleration forces.

- Trauma to the face can range from a broken nose to more severe injuries, including massive soft-tissue trauma, maxillofacial fractures, oral or dental trauma, and eye injuries.

- Your primary concerns with assessing and managing a patient with facial trauma are to ensure a patent airway and maintain adequate oxygenation and ventilation. Trauma to the face or neck can compromise the patient's airway. Airway management is crucial in managing these injuries.

- Any patient with head or face trauma should be suspected of having a spinal injury. Apply spinal motion restriction precautions as indicated.

- Blind nasotracheal intubation is relatively contraindicated in the presence of midface fracture; such maneuvers, as well as insertion of a nasopharyngeal airway, should not be performed unless absolutely necessary and with approval of medical control.

- Remove impaled objects in the face or throat only if they impair airway patency or breathing or if they interfere with your ability to effectively manage the airway. Otherwise, stabilize them in place and protect them from further movement.

- Injuries to the eye can be varied, including lacerations, blunt trauma, impaled objects, or burns. Never exert pressure or manipulate an injured globe in any way.

- Never remove impaled objects from the eye; stabilize them in place and put a protective cone (such as a cup) over the object to prevent accidental movement. You should also bandage the unaffected eye to prevent sympathetic movement.

- Chemical burns to the eye should be treated with gentle irrigation using sterile water or saline.

- Ear injuries should be realigned and bandaged. If a part is avulsed, transport with the patient if possible. Stabilize an object that is impaled in the ear.

- The primary threat from oral or dental trauma is oropharyngeal bleeding and aspiration of blood or broken teeth. Keep the airway clear, and ensure adequate oxygenation and ventilation. Endotracheal intubation may be required.

- Aggressively manage injuries involving the anterior neck, ensuring that airway management and external bleeding control remain the top priority. Treat for shock if signs are present, and transport rapidly.

- The spine can sustain trauma that does not produce a spinal cord fracture or dislocation; such trauma is categorized as a sprain or strain. Such patients should be transported for further evaluation at the emergency department.

Vital Vocabulary

alveolar ridges The ridges between the teeth that are covered with thickened connective tissue and epithelium.

alveoli Small pits or cavities, such as the sockets for the teeth.

anisocoria A condition in which the pupils are not of equal size.

anterior chamber The anterior area of the globe between the lens and the cornea that is filled with aqueous humor.

aqueous humor The clear, watery fluid in the anterior chamber of the globe.

auricle The large outside portion of the ear through which sound waves enter the ear; also called the pinna.

blowout fracture A fracture to the floor of the orbit usually caused by a blow to the eye.

central vision The visualization of objects directly in front of you.

cochlea The shell-shaped structure within the inner ear that contains the organ of Corti.

cochlear duct A canal within the cochlea that receives vibrations from the ossicles.

conjunctiva A thin, transparent membrane that covers the sclera and internal surfaces of the eyelids.

conjunctivitis An inflammation of the conjunctivae that usually is caused by bacteria, viruses, allergies, or foreign bodies; should be considered highly contagious if infectious in orgin; also called pink eye.

cornea The transparent anterior portion of the eye that overlies the iris and pupil.

craniofacial disjunction A Le Fort III fracture involves a fracture of all of the midfacial bones, thus separating the entire midface from the cranium.

crown The part of the tooth that is external to the gum.

cusps Points at the top of a tooth.

dentin The principal mass of the tooth that is made up of a material that is much more dense and stronger than bone.

diplopia Double vision.

dysconjugate gaze Paralysis of gaze or lack of coordination between the movements of the two eyes.

dysphagia Difficulty swallowing.

epistaxis Nosebleed.

external auditory canal The area in which sound waves are received from the auricle (pinna) before they travel to the eardrum; also called the ear canal.

external ear One of three anatomic parts of the ear; it contains the pinna, the ear canal, and the external portion of the tympanic membrane.

facial nerve The seventh cranial nerve; supplies motor activity to all muscles of facial expression and anterior two thirds of the tongue; and also relates to the sense of taste and cutaneous sensation to the external ear, tongue, and palate.

globe The eyeball.

glossopharyngeal nerve Ninth cranial nerve; supplies motor fibers to the pharyngeal muscle, providing taste sensation to the posterior portion of the tongue, and carrying parasympathetic fibers to the parotid gland.

hard palate The bony anterior part of the palate that forms the roof of the mouth.

hemoptysis Coughing up blood.

hyoid bone A bone at the base of the tongue that supports the tongue and its muscles.

hyphema Bleeding into the anterior chamber of the eye; results from direct ocular trauma.

hypoglossal nerve Twelfth cranial nerve; provides motor function to the muscles of the tongue and throat.

inner ear One of three anatomic parts of the ear; it consists of the cochlea and semicircular canals.

iris The colored portion of the eye.

lacrimal apparatus The structures in which tears are secreted and drained from the eye.

Le Fort fractures Maxillary fractures that are classified into three categories based on their anatomic location.

lens A transparent body within the globe that focuses light rays.

malocclusion Misalignment of the teeth.

mandible The movable lower jaw bone.

mandibular nerve A sensory and motor nerve that supplies the muscles of chewing and skin of the lower lip, chin, temporal region, and part of the external ear.

mastication The process of chewing with the teeth.

maxillary nerve A sensory nerve; supplies the skin on the posterior part of the side of the nose, lower eyelid, cheek, and upper lip.

mediastinitis Inflammation of the mediastinum, often a result of the gastric contents leaking into the thoracic cavity after esophageal perforation.

middle ear One of three anatomic parts of the ear; it consists of the inner portion of the tympanic membrane and the ossicles.

nasal septum The separation between the right and left nostrils.

nasolacrimal duct The passage through which tears drain from the lacrimal sacs into the nasal cavity.

oculomotor nerve Third cranial nerve; innervates the muscles that cause motion of the eyeballs and upper eyelid.

ophthalmic nerve A sensory nerve that supplies the skin of the forehead, the upper eyelid, and conjunctiva.

optic nerve Either of the second cranial nerves that enter the eyeball posteriorly, through the optic foramen.

orbits Bony cavities in the frontal part of the skull that enclose and protect the eyes.

organ of Corti A structure located in the cochlea that contains hairs that are stimulated by vibrations to form nerve impulses that travel to the brain and are perceived as sound.

ossicles The three small bones in the middle ear that transmit vibrations to the cochlear duct at the oval window.

oval window An oval opening between the middle ear and the vestibule.

paranasal sinuses The sinuses, or hollowed sections of bone in the front of the head, that are lined with mucous membrane and drain into the nasal cavity.

peripheral vision Visualization of lateral objects while looking forward.

pinna The large outside portion of the ear through which sound waves enter the ear; also called the auricle.

posterior chamber The posterior area of the globe between the lens and the iris.

pulp Specialized connective tissue within the cavity of a tooth.

pupil The circular opening in the center of the eye through which light passes to the lens.

retina A delicate 10-layered structure of nervous tissue located in the rear of the interior of the globe that receives light and generates nerve signals that are transmitted to the brain through the optic nerve.

retinal detachment Separation of the inner layers of the retina from the underlying choroid, the vascular membrane that nourishes the retina.

sclera The white part of the eye.

spinal clearance The act of declaring that a spinal injury is not present.

sprain Stretching or tearing of ligaments

strain Stretching or tearing of a muscle or tendon

sympathetic eye movement The movement of both eyes in unison.

temporomandibular joint (TMJ) The joint between the temporal bone and the posterior condyle that allows for movements of the mandible.

tracheal transection Traumatic separation of the trachea from the larynx.

trigeminal nerve Fifth cranial nerve; supplies sensation to the scalp, forehead, face, and lower jaw and innervates the muscles of mastication, the throat, and the inner ear.

tympanic membrane A thin membrane that separates the middle ear from the outer ear and sets up vibrations in the ossicles; also called the eardrum.

visual cortex The area in the brain where signals from the optic nerve are converted into visual images.

vitreous humor A jellylike substance found in the posterior compartment of the eye between the lens and the retina.

whiplash An injury to the neck in which hyperextension occurs as a result of the head moving abruptly forward or backward; can be difficult to differentiate from injuries that involve cervical bony structures and the spine.

Assessment in Action

Your unit is dispatched to a local baseball field for a player hit by a baseball bat. When you arrive on scene you are directed to a man who was hit in the neck by a broken bat. The patient is responsive, alert, and oriented. The patient reports difficulty swallowing and his voice sounds raspy. There is no bleeding noted but a hematoma is developing on the right lateral neck.

1. What cartilage is commonly referred to as the "Adam's apple"?
   A. Cricoid
   B. Thyroid
   C. Hyoid
   D. Laryngeal

2. If you feel a crackling sensation on your fingers when palpating the patient's neck, what condition may be present?
   A. Subcutaneous emphysema
   B. Hemoptysis
   C. Hypoxia
   D. Air embolism

3. The large vein that runs laterally on both sides of the neck is called the:
   A. carotid.
   B. thyroid.
   C. jugular.
   D. esophageal.

4. If the patient had a penetrating injury to the neck, what type of dressing should be applied?
   A. Bulky dressing, lightly bandaged in place
   B. Bulky dressing, tightly bandaged in place
   C. Occlusive dressing, sealed on all sides
   D. Occlusive dressing, sealed on three sides

5. What should also be considered in this patient as a result of the symptoms and mechanism?
   A. Partial airway obstruction
   B. Lower airway swelling
   C. Cervical spine involvement
   D. Patient is a chronic smoker

6. You start to provide spinal motion restriction to the patient using a cervical collar and a long backboard. The patient is unable to tolerate lying supine and reports increased shortness of breath. What is the most suitable alternative treatment?
   A. Provide supplemental oxygen and elevate the head of the backboard to facilitate breathing.
   B. Force the patient to comply with the protocols in place.
   C. Provide stabilization with a short backboard or extrication vest to allow him to sit upright and control his airway.
   D. Provide nasal tracheal intubation to bypass the laryngeal fracture.

7. If the patient had a foreign body impaled in the globe, what type of dressing should be applied?
   A. Bulky dressing, lightly bandaged in place for both eyes
   B. Bulky dressing, tightly bandaged in place for the affected eye
   C. Moist, sterile dressing and protective cup for the affected eye
   D. Moist, sterile dressing; protective cup for affected eye; and bandage unaffected eye

8. What is the medical term for persons with normally unequal pupils?
   A. Dysconjugate
   B. Glaucoma
   C. Anisocoria
   D. Diplopia

9. When should a flow-restricted, oxygen-powered ventilation device be used in neck trauma?
   A. Only if the patient is responsive
   B. Only when ventilating through an endotracheal tube
   C. Only after occlusive dressings have been applied
   D. Never

Additional Question

10. How would you manage an open wound to a carotid artery?

Head and Spine Trauma

National EMS Education Standard Competencies

Trauma

Integrates assessment findings with principles of epidemiology and pathophysiology to formulate a field impression to implement a comprehensive treatment/disposition plan for an acutely injured patient.

Head, Facial, Neck, and Spine Trauma

Recognition and management of

- Life threats (pp 1653-1655)
- Spine trauma (p 1656)

Pathophysiology, assessment, and management of

- Penetrating neck trauma (see chapter, *Face and Neck Trauma*)
- Laryngotracheal injuries (see chapter, *Face and Neck Trauma*)
- Spine trauma
  - Dislocations/subluxations (p 1670)
  - Fractures (p 1671)
  - Sprains/strains (pp 1683-1684)
- Facial fractures (see chapter, *Face and Neck Trauma*)
- Skull fractures (pp 1662-1664)
- Foreign bodies in the eyes (see chapter, *Face and Neck Trauma*)
- Dental trauma (see chapter, *Face and Neck Trauma*)
- Unstable facial fractures (see chapter, *Face and Neck Trauma*)
- Orbital fractures (see chapter, *Face and Neck Trauma*)
- Perforated tympanic membrane (see chapter, *Face and Neck Trauma*)
- Mandibular fractures (see chapter, *Face and Neck Trauma*)

Nervous System Trauma

Pathophysiology, assessment, and management of

- Traumatic brain injury (p 1664)
- Spinal cord injury (pp 1670, 1671-1673)
- Spinal shock (p 1672)
- Cauda equina syndrome (p 1672)
- Nerve root injury (p 1650)
- Peripheral nerve injury (p 1650)

Knowledge Objectives

1. List the major bones of the skull and spinal column and their related structures, and describe their functions as related to the nervous system. (pp 1644-1646, 1648-1650)
2. Describe the regions of the brain, including the cerebrum, diencephalon, brainstem, and the cerebellum, and their functions. (pp 1645-1647)
3. Describe the anatomy and physiology of the spinal cord and spinal nerves. (pp 1648-1650)
4. Describe the steps in the patient assessment process for a person who has a suspected head or spine injury, including specific variations that may be required as related to the type of injury. (pp 1652-1655)
5. Discuss mechanisms of injury (MOIs) that are potential causes of head and spine injuries, and which the paramedic should consider when performing a patient assessment. (pp 1652, 1655-1656)
6. Describe when endotracheal intubation should be performed in a patient with a head injury versus a spinal cord injury. (pp 1653-1654)
7. Discuss specific assessments to perform for a patient with possible spinal cord injury, including a neurologic exam. (pp 1658-1661)
8. Discuss when it would be appropriate to establish intravenous access in a patient with a head or spine injury, including the importance of judicious fluid administration. (p 1655)
9. Discuss general signs and symptoms of a head injury. (p 1668)
10. Discuss types of skull fractures, including linear, depressed, basilar, and open skull fractures. (pp 1662-1664)
11. Define traumatic brain injury and explain the difference between a primary (direct) injury and a secondary (indirect) injury, providing examples of possible MOIs that may cause each one. (p 1664)
12. Discuss the pathophysiology of intracranial pressure and posturing that can occur in the presence of brain injury. (pp 1664-1665)
13. Discuss diffuse brain injuries including cerebral concussion and diffuse axonal injury, and their corresponding signs and symptoms. (pp 1665-1666)
14. Discuss focal brain injuries including cerebral contusion and the various types of intracranial hemorrhage, and signs and symptoms of each. (pp 1666-1668)
15. Describe management of head and brain injuries, including thermal management, treatment of associated injuries, and pharmacologic therapy. (pp 1668-1669)
16. Discuss assessment and management of scalp lacerations. (pp 1669-1670)
17. Discuss MOI that may damage the cervical, thoracic, or lumbar spine, including flexion, rotation with flexion, vertical compression, and hyperextension. (pp 1670-1671)
18. Define primary spinal cord injury versus secondary spinal cord injury, including complete versus incomplete cord injury. (pp 1671-1673)
19. Discuss various cord syndromes and their signs and symptoms, including anterior cord syndrome, central cord syndrome, posterior cord syndrome, cauda equina syndrome, and Brown-Séquard syndrome. (p 1672)
20. Discuss signs and symptoms of neurogenic shock and spinal shock. (pp 1672-1673)
21. Describe the process of providing emergency medical care to a patient with a spinal injury, including the implications of not properly caring for patients with injuries of this nature, and the steps for performing manual in-line stabilization, including immobilizing a supine patient, a seated patient, and a standing patient. (pp 1673-1677, 1679-1680)

22. Discuss when rapid extrication should be performed, and how to perform it. (pp 1677-1679)

23. Discuss how to package and remove a patient who is found in the water with a potential spinal injury. (pp 1680-1681)

24. Explain the different circumstances in which a helmet should be either left on or taken off a patient with a possible head or spinal injury, and then list the steps paramedics must follow to remove a helmet, including the alternate method for removing a football helmet. (pp 1680-1682)

25. Describe prehospital pharmacologic treatment of patients with spinal cord injury. (p 1682)

26. Discuss complications of spinal cord injury, including prehospital management of autonomic dysreflexia. (pp 1682-1683)

27. Discuss nontraumatic spinal conditions, including causes of low back pain and prehospital treatment. (pp 1683-1684)

Skills Objectives

1. Demonstrate how to immobilize a supine patient with a suspected spinal injury to a long backboard. (pp 1674-1676)

2. Demonstrate how to immobilize a patient with a suspected spinal injury who was found in a sitting position. (pp 1676-1677)

3. Demonstrate how to perform rapid extrication. (pp 1677-1679)

4. Demonstrate how to immobilize a patient with a suspected spinal injury who was found in a standing position. (pp 1679-1680)

5. Demonstrate how to immobilize a patient who is found in the water. (pp 1680-1681)

6. Demonstrate how to remove a helmet from a patient with a suspected head or spinal injury. (pp 1680-1682)

Introduction

In this chapter you will learn about injury to the central nervous system. The <u>central nervous system (CNS)</u> consists of the brain and the spinal cord, both of which are encased in and protected by bone. The <u>brain</u>, located within the cranial cavity, is the largest component of the CNS. It contains billions of neurons that serve a variety of vital functions. An understanding of the form and function of spinal anatomy coupled with a high level of suspicion for spinal cord injury (SCI) is required to decipher the often subtle findings associated with a possible SCI.

The two primary divisions of insult are head injuries, most often subdivided into skull fractures and traumatic brain injury, and spinal cord injuries. It is important for you to realize that while these topics will be covered separately, the head and spine are often injured in association with each other. That is not to say that there are not isolated cases of each, but you should remind yourself to be observant for coexisting injury.

Anatomy and Physiology

The Scalp

The brain—the most important organ in the body—requires maximum protection from injury. The human body ensures that the brain receives this protection by housing it within several layers of soft and hard wrappings.

Starting from the outside and proceeding inward toward the brain, the first protective layer is the scalp, which consists of the following layers, given in descending order:

- Skin, with hair
- Subcutaneous tissue that contains major scalp veins that bleed profusely when lacerated
- <u>Galea aponeurotica</u>, a tendon expansion that connects the frontal and occipital muscles of the cranium
- Loose connective tissue (alveolar tissue) that is easily stripped from the layer beneath in "scalping" injuries. The looseness of the alveolar layer also provides room for blood to accumulate between the scalp and skull bone (subgaleal hematoma) after blunt trauma.
- Periosteum, the dense fibrous membrane covering the surface of bones.

The Skull

At the top of the axial skeleton is the <u>skull</u>, which consists of 28 bones in three anatomic groups: the auditory ossicles, the cranium, and the face. The six <u>auditory ossicles</u> function in hearing and are located, three on each side of the head, deep within the cavities of the temporal bone. The remaining 22 bones constitute the cranium and the face Figure 1 .

The <u>cranial vault</u> consists of eight bones that encase and protect the brain: the parietal, temporal, frontal, occipital, sphenoid, and ethmoid bones. The brain connects to the spinal cord through a large opening at the base of the skull called the <u>foramen magnum</u>.

The bones of the skull are connected at special joints known as sutures Figure 2 . The paired parietal bones join together at the <u>sagittal suture</u>. The parietal bones abut the frontal bone at the <u>coronal suture</u>. The occipital bone attaches to the parietal bones at the <u>lambdoid suture</u>. Fibrous tissues called <u>fontanelles</u>, which are soft in infants, link the sutures. The tissues felt through the fontanelles are layers of the scalp and thick membranes overlying the brain. Under normal conditions, the brain may not be felt through the fontanelles. Around the time a child is age 18 months, the sutures should have solidified and the fontanelles closed.

At the base of each temporal bone is a cone-shaped section of bone known as the <u>mastoid process</u>. This area is an important site for attachment of various muscles. In addition, a portion of the mastoid process contains hollow mastoid air cells Figure 3 .

The Floor of the Cranial Vault

Viewed from above, the floor of the cranial vault is divided into three compartments: the anterior fossa, middle fossa, and posterior fossa Figure 4 . The <u>crista galli</u> forms a prominent bony ridge in the center of the anterior fossa and is the point of attachment of the meninges, the three layers of membranes that surround the brain and spinal cord. On the other side of the crista galli is the <u>cribriform plate</u> of the ethmoid bone, a horizontal bone that is perforated with numerous openings (<u>foramina</u>), allowing the passage of the olfactory nerve filaments from the nasal cavity. The <u>olfactory nerves</u>, the cranial nerves for smell, send projections through the foramina in the cribriform plate and into the <u>nasal cavity</u>, the chamber inside the nose that lies between the floor of the cranium and the roof of the mouth.

YOU *are the Medic* | PART 1

It is 1:30 AM when you are dispatched to a public swimming pool. While en route to the scene, dispatch tells you that the police were called after a neighbor heard screams. You arrive to find a teenage boy lying on his back next to the pool. Even with the dim light, you immediately notice that he is having difficulty breathing.

1. Given the updated information, what should you consider doing?

2. What safety concerns do you have?

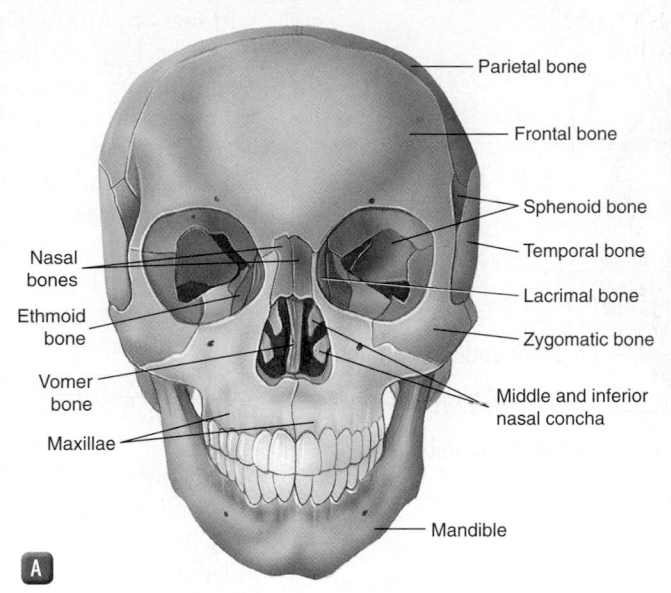

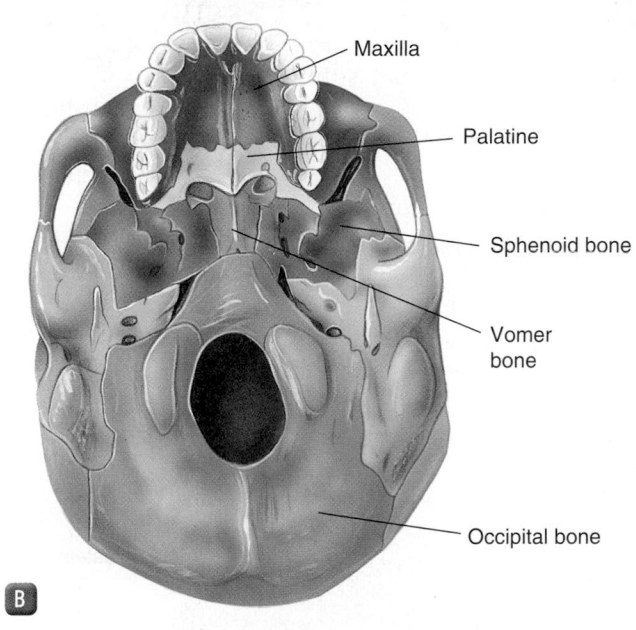

Figure 1 The skull and its components. **A.** Front view. **B.** Bottom view.

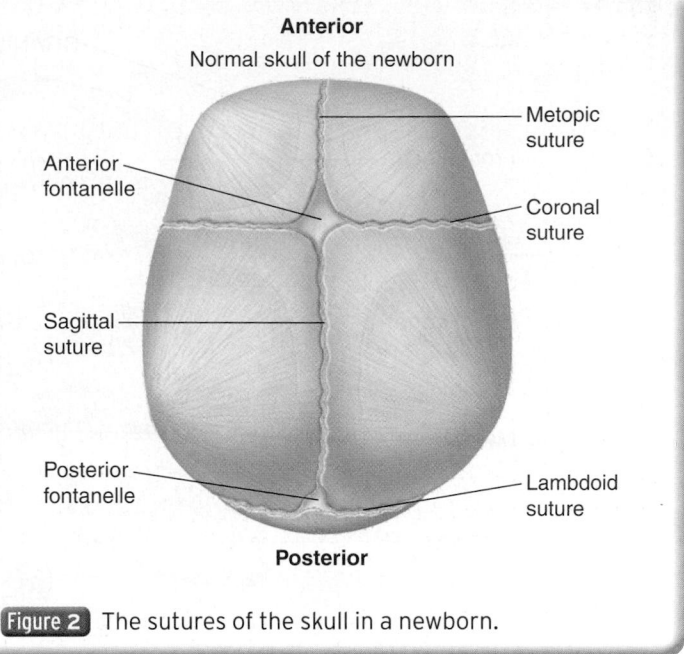

Figure 2 The sutures of the skull in a newborn.

The Base of the Skull

When the mandible is removed, the base of the skull appears amazingly complex, with numerous foramina visible **Figure 5** . The <u>occipital condyles</u> on the occipital bone, which are the points of articulation between the skull and the vertebral column, lie on either side of the foramen magnum. Portions of the maxilla and the <u>palatine bone</u>, the irregularly shaped bone in the posterior nasal cavity, form the <u>hard palate</u>, which is the bony anterior part of the palate, or roof, of the mouth. The <u>zygomatic arch</u> is the bone that extends along the front of the skull below the orbit.

The Brain

The brain, which occupies 80% of the cranial vault, contains billions of neurons (nerve cells) that serve a variety of vital functions **Figure 6** . The major regions of the brain are the cerebrum, diencephalon (thalamus and hypothalamus), brainstem (medulla, pons, midbrain [mesencephalon]), and the cerebellum. The remaining intracranial contents include cerebral blood (12%) and cerebrospinal fluid (8%).

The brain accounts for only 2% of the total body weight, yet it is the most metabolically active and perfusion-sensitive organ in the body. The brain metabolizes 25% of the body's glucose, burning approximately 60 mg/min, and consumes 20% of the total body oxygen (45 to 50 L/min). Because the brain has no storage mechanism for oxygen or glucose, it is totally dependent on a constant source of both fuels via cerebral blood flow provided by the carotid and vertebral arteries. As such, the brain will continually manipulate the physiology as needed to guarantee that a ready supply of oxygen and glucose are available. Also, a loss of blood flow to the brain for 5 to 10 seconds will result in unconsciousness.

The Cerebrum

The largest portion of the brain is the <u>cerebrum</u>, which is responsible for higher functions, such as reasoning. The cerebrum is divided into right and left hemispheres by a longitudinal fissure. The hemispheres of the cerebrum are not entirely equivalent functionally. In a right-handed person, for example, the speech center is usually located in the left cerebral hemisphere, which is then said to be the dominant hemisphere.

The largest portion of the cerebrum is the <u>cerebral cortex</u>, which regulates voluntary skeletal movement and the level of awareness. Injury to the cerebral cortex may result in paresthesia, weakness, and paralysis of the extremities.

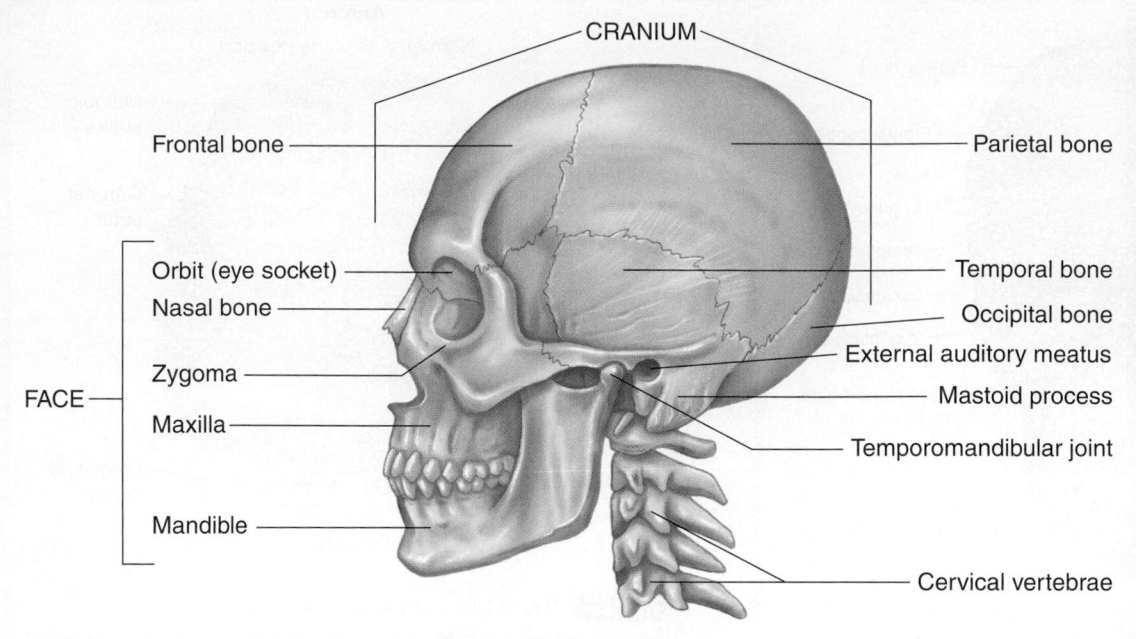

CRANIUM

Frontal bone

Parietal bone

Orbit (eye socket)

Nasal bone

Zygoma

Maxilla

FACE

Mandible

Temporal bone

Occipital bone

External auditory meatus

Mastoid process

Temporomandibular joint

Cervical vertebrae

Figure 3 The mastoid air cells are located in the mastoid process. Just anterior to the mastoid is the external auditory meatus, which is associated with the ear canal.

for processing visual information. After a blow to the back of the head, a person may "see stars," which results when the occipital poles of the brain (the vision centers) bang against the back of the skull.

The speech center is located in the **temporal lobe**. In approximately 85% of the population, the speech center is located on the left side of the temporal lobe. The temporal lobe also controls long-term memory, hearing, taste, and smell. It is separated from the rest of the cerebrum by a lateral fissure.

The Diencephalon

The **diencephalon**, which is located between the brainstem and the cerebrum, includes the thalamus, subthalamus, hypothalamus, and epithalamus **Figure 8**. The **thalamus** processes most sensory input and influences mood and general body movements, especially those associated with fear and rage. The **subthalamus** controls motor functions. The functions of the epithalamus are unclear. The most inferior portion

Each cerebral hemisphere is divided functionally into specialized areas called lobes **Figure 7**. The **frontal lobe** is important for voluntary motor action and personality traits. Injury to the frontal lobe may result in seizures or placid reactions (flat affect). The **parietal lobe** controls the somatic or voluntary sensory and motor functions for the opposite (contralateral) side of the body, as well as memory and emotions; it is separated from the frontal lobe by the central sulcus. Posteriorly, the **occipital lobe**, from which the optic nerve originates, is responsible

Crista galli

Cribriform plate

Sphenoid bone

Optic foramen

Sella turcica

Carotid canal

Jugular foramen

Foramen magnum

Frontal bone

Anterior fossa

Temporal bone

Middle fossa

Occipital bone

Posterior fossa

Figure 4 The floor of the cranial vault and its anatomy.

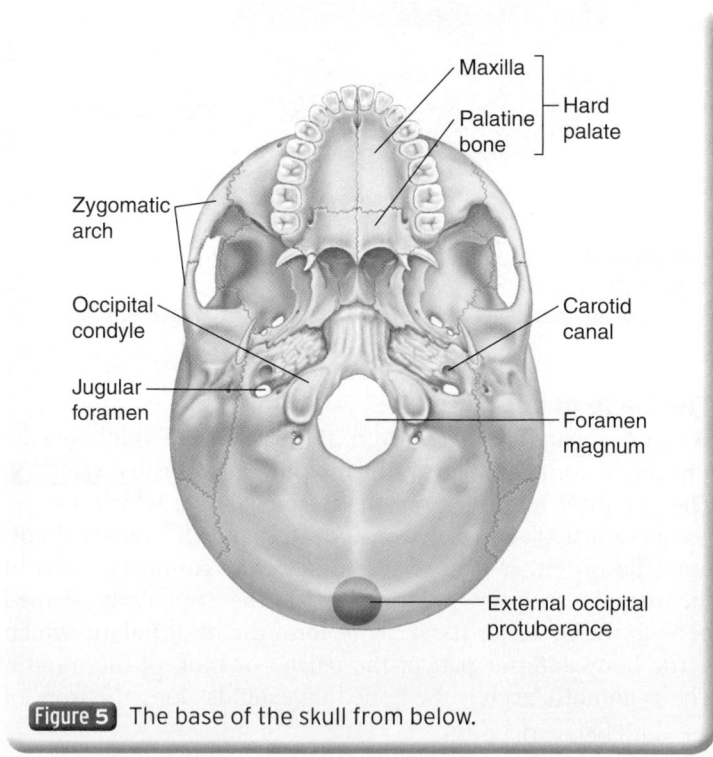

Maxilla

Palatine bone

Hard palate

Zygomatic arch

Occipital condyle

Jugular foramen

Carotid canal

Foramen magnum

External occipital protuberance

Figure 5 The base of the skull from below.

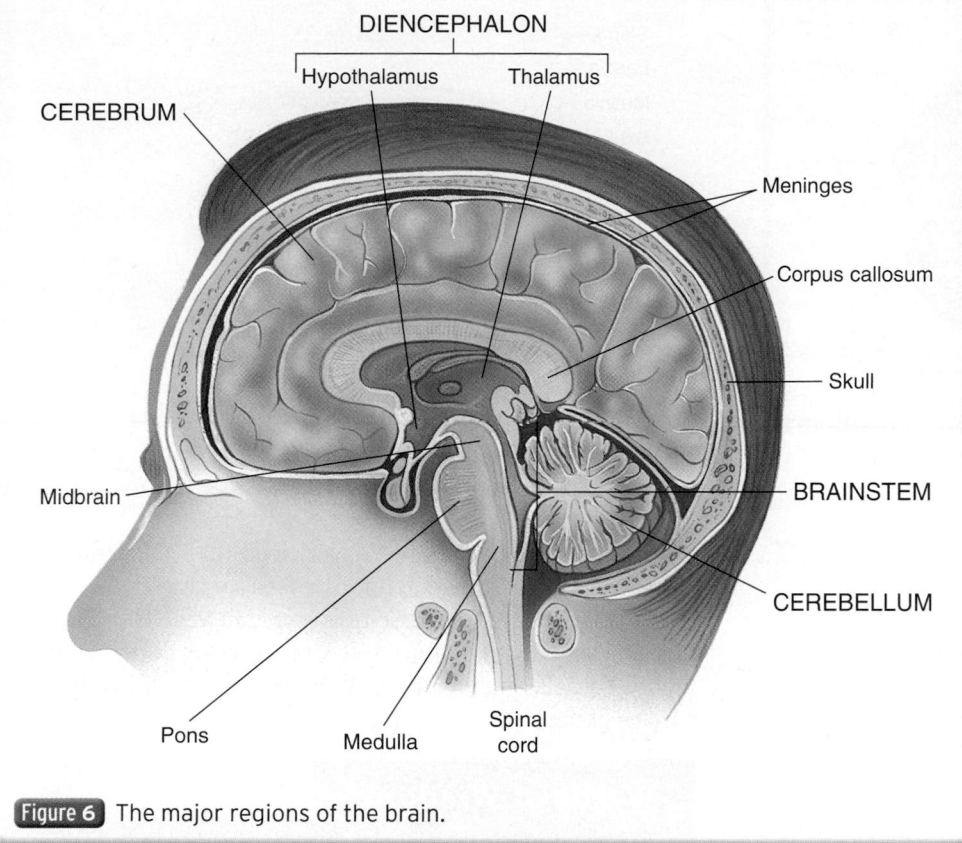

Figure 6 The major regions of the brain.

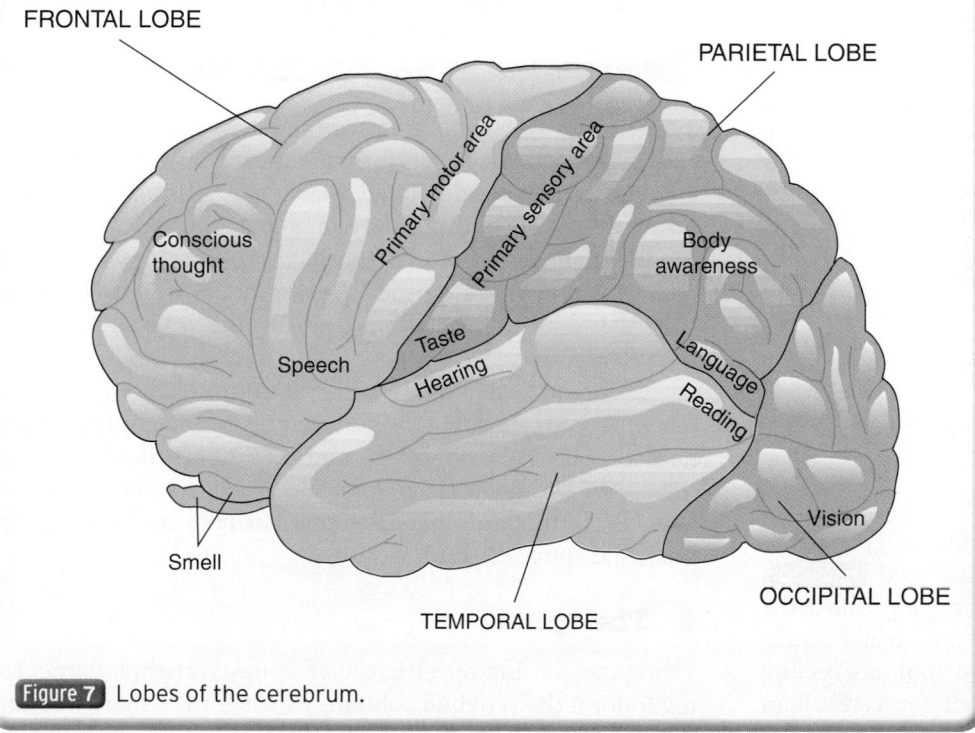

Figure 7 Lobes of the cerebrum.

The Cerebellum

The <u>cerebellum</u> is located beneath the cerebral hemispheres in the inferoposterior part of the brain. It is sometimes called the "athlete's brain" because it is responsible for the maintenance of posture and equilibrium and the coordination of skilled movements.

The Brainstem

The <u>brainstem</u> consists of the midbrain, pons, and the medulla. It is located at the base of the brain and connects the spinal cord to the remainder of the brain. The brainstem houses many structures that are critical to the maintenance of vital functions. High in the brainstem, for example, is the <u>reticular activating system (RAS)</u>, which is responsible for maintenance of consciousness, specifically one's level of arousal. The centers that control basic but critical functions—heart rate, blood pressure, and respiration—are located in the lower part of the brainstem. Damage to this area can easily result in cardiovascular derangement, respiratory arrest, or death.

The midbrain lies immediately below the diencephalon and is the smallest region of the brainstem. Deep within the cerebrum, diencephalon, and midbrain are the <u>basal ganglia</u>, which have an important role in coordination of motor movements and posture. Portions of the cerebrum and diencephalon constitute the <u>limbic system</u>, which influences emotions, motivation, mood, and sensations of pain and pleasure **Figure 9**. The oculomotor nerve (third cranial nerve) originates from the midbrain; it controls pupillary size and reactivity.

The <u>pons</u>, which lies below the midbrain and above the medulla, contains numerous important nerve fibers, including those for sleep, respiration, and the medullary respiratory center.

The inferior portion of the midbrain, the <u>medulla</u>, is continuous inferiorly with the spinal cord (see Figure 6). It serves as a conduction pathway for ascending and descending nerve tracts. It also coordinates heart rate, blood vessel diameter, breathing, swallowing, vomiting, coughing, and sneezing. The vagus nerve (tenth cranial nerve), a bundle of nerves that primarily innervates the parasympathetic nervous system, originates from the medulla.

of the diencephalon, the **hypothalamus**, is vital in the control of many body functions, including heart rate, digestion, sexual development, temperature regulation, emotion, hunger, thirst, vomiting, and regulation of the sleep cycle.

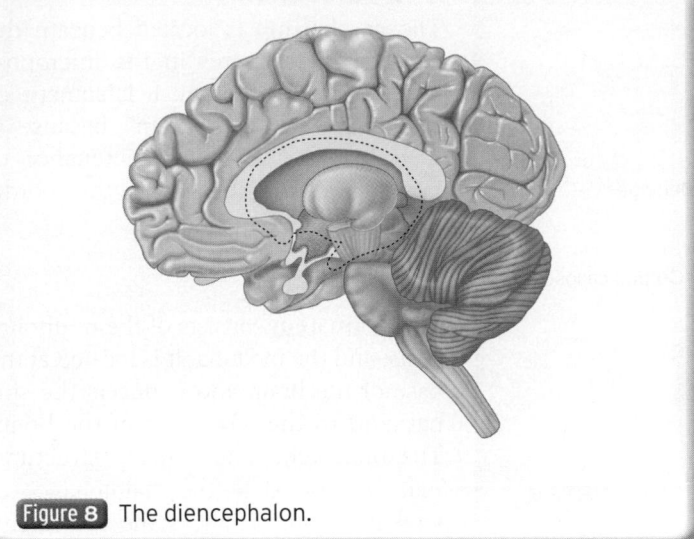

Figure 8 The diencephalon.

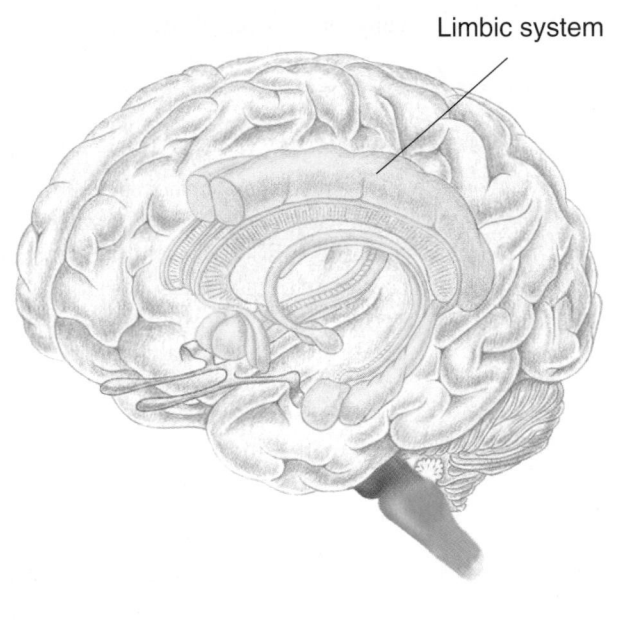

Limbic system

Figure 9 The limbic system is the seat of emotions, instincts, and other functions.

The Meninges

The **meninges** are protective layers that surround and enfold the entire CNS—specifically the brain and spinal cord Figure 10. The outermost layer is a strong, fibrous wrapping called the **dura mater** (meaning "tough mother"). The dura mater covers the entire brain, folding in to form the **tentorium**, a structure that separates the cerebral hemispheres from the cerebellum and brainstem. The dura mater is firmly attached to the internal wall of the skull. Just beneath the suture lines of the skull the dura mater splits into two surfaces and forms venous sinuses. When those venous sinuses are disrupted during a head injury, blood can collect beneath the dura mater to form a subdural hematoma.

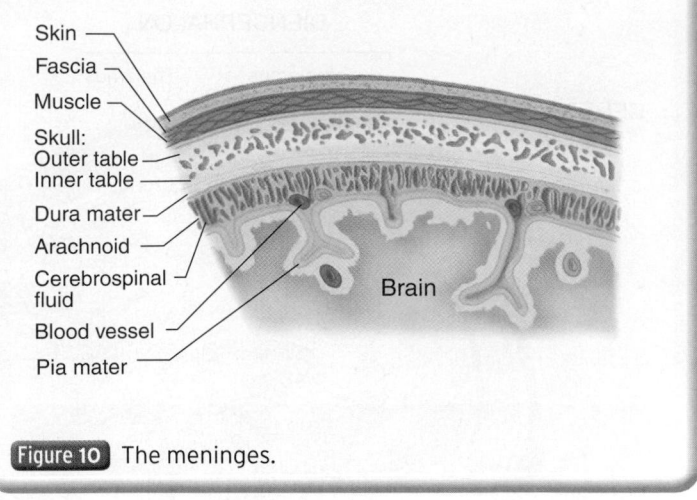

Figure 10 The meninges.

The second meningeal layer is a delicate, transparent membrane called the **arachnoid**. It is so named because the blood vessels it contains resemble a spider web. The third meningeal layer, the **pia mater** ("soft mother"), is a thin, translucent, highly vascular membrane that firmly adheres directly to the surface of the brain.

Words of Wisdom

A tip for remembering the names of the meningeal layers is to think of them as a "PAD" from the inside out. The innermost layer of the pad is the pia (P); the middle layer is the arachnoid (A); and the outer layer is the dura (D).

The meningeal arteries are located between the dura mater and the skull. When one of these arteries (usually the middle meningeal artery) is disrupted, bleeding occurs above the dura mater, resulting in an epidural hematoma.

The meninges float in **cerebrospinal fluid (CSF)**, which is manufactured in the ventricles of the brain. CSF flows in the **subarachnoid space**, located between the pia mater and the arachnoid.

CSF is manufactured by cells within the **choroid plexus** in the **ventricles**, hollow storage areas in the brain. These areas normally are interconnected, and CSF flows freely between them. CSF is similar in composition to plasma. The meninges and CSF form a fluid-filled sac that cushions and protects the brain and spinal cord.

The Spine

The spine consists of 33 irregular bones (vertebrae) articulating to form the vertebral column, which is the major structural component of the axial skeleton Figure 11. These skeletal components are stabilized by both ligaments and muscle. Together these components support and protect neural elements while allowing for fluid movement and erect stature.

Vertebrae are identified according to their location as cervical, thoracic, lumbar, sacral, or coccyx. The **vertebral body**, the

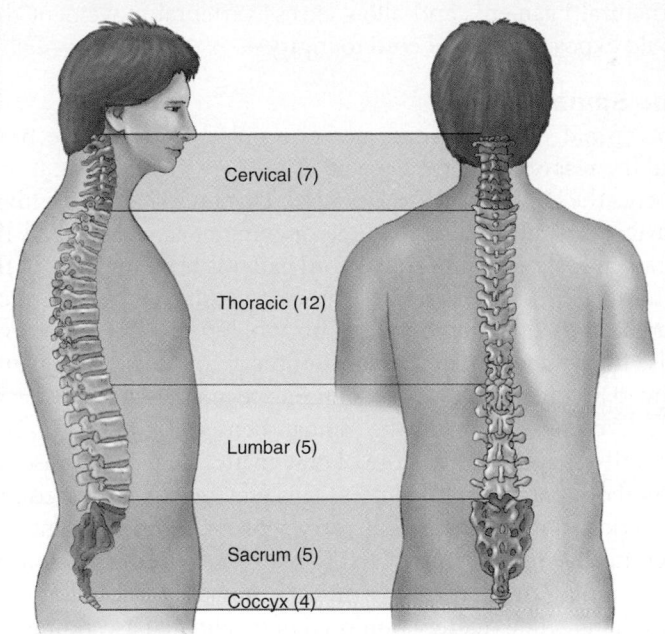

Figure 11 The spinal column consists of 33 bones divided into five sections. Each vertebra is numbered and referred to by a letter corresponding to the section of the spine where it is located plus its number. For example, the fifth thoracic vertebra is referred to as T5.

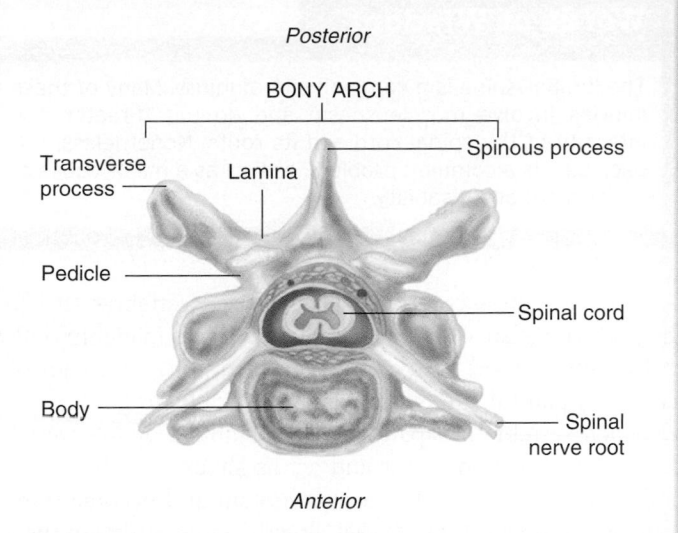

Figure 12 The human vertebra. Vertebrae in different sections of the spinal column vary in shape; this is a general representation. The space through which the spinal cord passes is called the canal, and the space through which a nerve root passes is called a foramen.

anterior weight-bearing structure, is made of bone that provides support and stability. Components of the vertebra include the lamina, pedicles, and spinous processes **Figure 12** . Each vertebra is unique in appearance and, with the exception of the atlas and axis (C1 and C2) **Figure 13** , shares basic structural characteristics.

The inferior border of each pedicle contains a notch forming the intervertebral foramen. This space in the middle of the vertebra allows the exit of a peripheral nerve root and spinal vein as well as the entrance of a spinal artery on both sides at each vertebral junction.

The transverse spinous processes comprise the junction of each pedicle and lamina on each side of a vertebra. They project laterally and posteriorly and form points of attachments for muscles and ligaments. The posterior spinous process is formed by the fusion of the posterior lamina and serves as an attachment site for muscles and ligaments.

The cervical spine includes the first seven bones of the vertebral column and its supporting structures. In addition to protecting the vital cervical spinal cord, the cervical spine supports

the weight of the head and permits a high degree of mobility in multiple planes. The atlas (C1) and axis (C2) are uniquely suited to allow for rotational movement of the skull.

The thoracic spine consists of 12 vertebrae in addition to the supporting muscles and ligaments found in the vertebral column; the thoracic spine is further stabilized by the rib attachments. The spinous processes are slightly larger, reflecting their role as attachment points for muscles that hold the upper body erect and assist with the movement of the thoracic cavity during respiration.

The lumbar spine includes the five largest bones in the vertebral column, and is integral in carrying a large portion of the upper body weight. The lumbar spine is especially susceptible to injury because of this weight-bearing capacity.

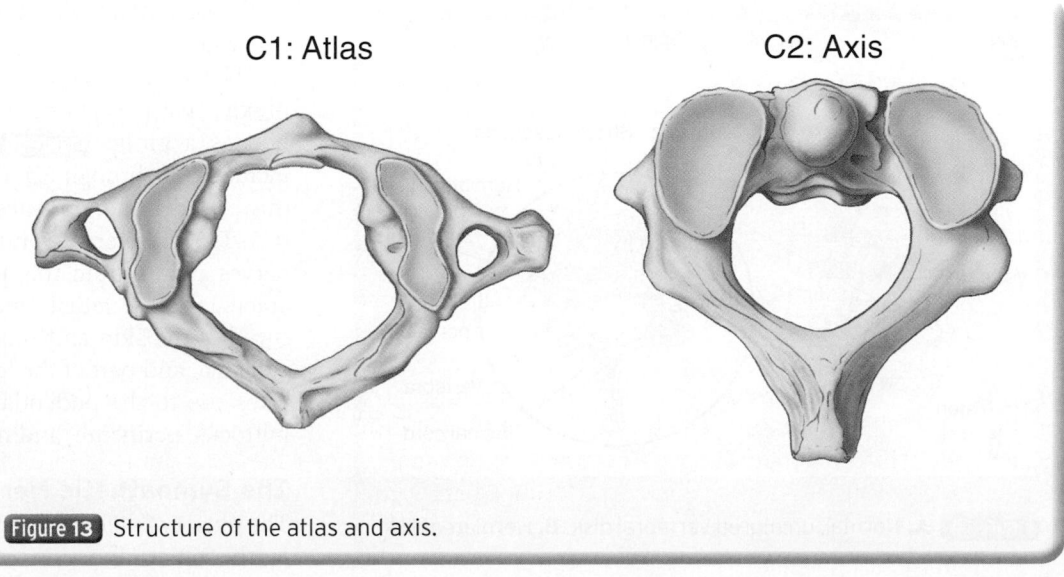

Figure 13 Structure of the atlas and axis.

Words of Wisdom

The lumbar spine is a common site of injury. Many of these injuries involve muscle spasm and do not threaten the integrity of the spinal cord and its roots. Nonetheless, low back pain is a common problem, as well as a major cause of impairment and disability.

The sacrum is composed of five fused vertebrae that form the posterior plate of the pelvis. The coccyx is made up of three to five small fused vertebrae. Coccyx injuries, although often extremely painful, are typically neurologically insignificant.

Each vertebra is separated and cushioned by intervertebral disks that limit bone wear and act as shock absorbers. As the body ages, these disks lose water content and become thinner, causing the height loss associated with aging. Stress on the vertebral column may cause a disk to herniate into the spinal canal, resulting in an injury to the spinal cord or a **nerve root injury** Figure 14. Nerves can also be injured at the peripheral level (anywhere in the body outside of the spinal cord); this is called **peripheral nerve injury**.

The muscles, tendons, and ligaments that connect the vertebrae allow the spinal column a degree of flexion and extension, limited to an extent by the stabilization they must provide to the spinal column. The vertebral column can sustain normal flexion and extension of 60% to 70% without stressing the spinal cord. Flexion or extension beyond those limits may damage structural ligaments and allow excess vertebral movement that could expose the spinal cord to injury.

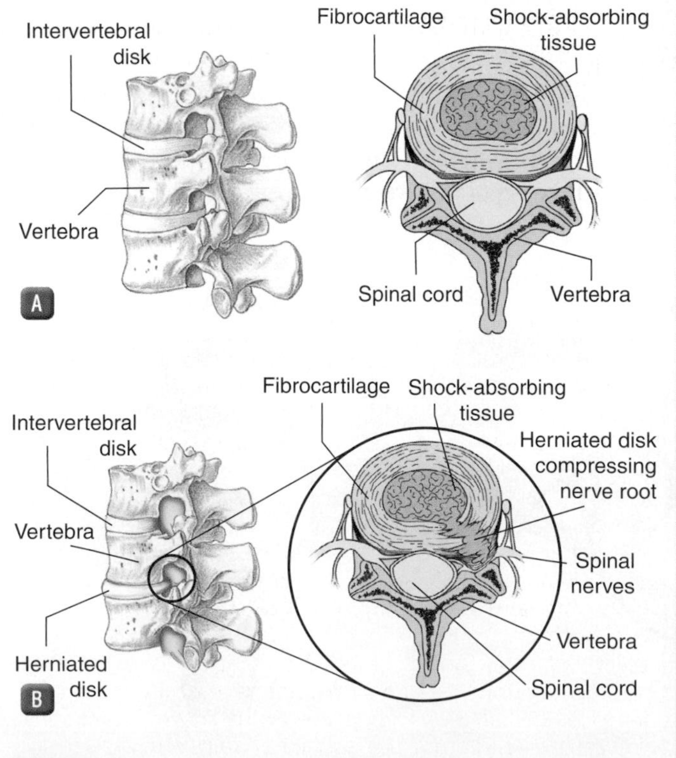

Figure 14 **A.** Normal, uninjured vertebral disk. **B.** Herniated disk.

The Spinal Cord

The **spinal cord** transmits nerve impulses between the brain and the rest of the body. Located at the base of the brain, it represents the continuation of the CNS. This bundle of nerve fibers leaves the skull through a large opening at its base called the foramen magnum. The spinal cord extends from the base of the skull to L2; here it separates into the **cauda equina**, a collection of individual nerve roots. Thirty-one pairs of spinal nerves arise from the different segments of the spinal cord; each pair is named according to its corresponding segment.

A cross-section of the spinal cord Figure 15 reveals a butterfly-shaped central core of gray matter that is composed of neural cell bodies and synapses. This gray matter is divided into posterior (dorsal) horns that carry sensory input, and anterior (ventral) horns that innervate the motor nerve of that segment. Surrounding the gray matter on each side are three columns of peripheral white matter composed of myelinated ascending and descending fiber pathways. Messages are relayed to and from the brain through these spinal tracts.

Specific groups of nerves are named based on their source of origin and point of termination. Ascending tracts carry information to the brain, and descending tracts carry information to the rest of the body Table 1.

Spinal Nerves

The 31 pairs of spinal nerves emerge from each side of the spinal cord and are named for the vertebral region and level from which they arise. The eight cervical roots perform different functions in the scalp, neck, shoulders, and arms. The 12 thoracic nerve roots have varying functions; the upper thoracic nerves supply muscles of the chest that help in breathing and coughing, whereas the lower thoracic nerves provide abdominal muscle control and contain nerves of the sympathetic nervous system. The five lumbar nerve roots supply hip flexors and leg muscles, as well as provide sensation to the anterior legs. The five sacral nerves provide for bowel and bladder control, sexual function, and sensation in the posterior legs and rectum. The coccyx has a single nerve root.

Nerve roots occasionally converge in a cluster called a **plexus** that permits peripheral nerve roots to rejoin and function as a group Figure 16. For example, the cervical plexus includes C1 through C5; the phrenic nerve (C3–C5) arises from this plexus and innervates the diaphragm. The brachial plexus (C5–T1) joins nerves controlling the upper extremities; the main nerves arising from this plexus are the axillary, median, musculocutaneous, radial, and ulnar. The lumbar plexus (L1–L4) supplies the skin and muscles of the abdominal wall, external genitalia, and part of the lower limbs. The sacral plexus (L4–S4) gives rise to the pudendal and sciatic nerves and supplies the buttocks, perineum, and most of the lower limbs.

The Sympathetic Nervous System

The sensory (afferent) and motor (efferent) nerves are responsible for the somatic functions of the spinal cord and often overshadow

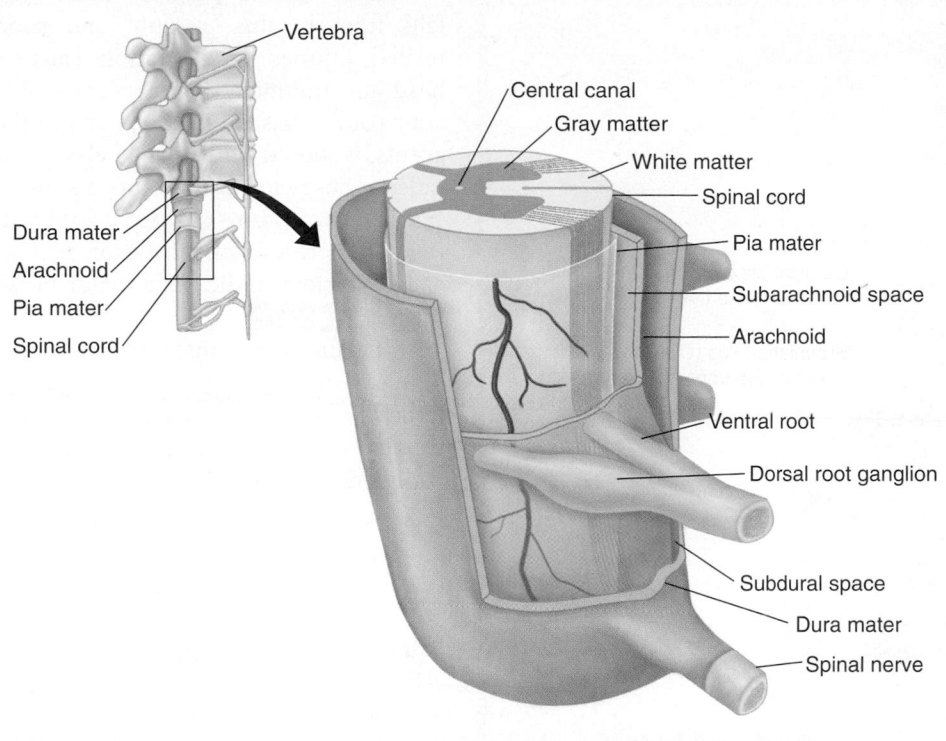

Vertebra

Central canal

Gray matter

White matter

Spinal cord

Pia mater

Subarachnoid space

Arachnoid

Ventral root

Dorsal root ganglion

Subdural space

Dura mater

Spinal nerve

Dura mater
Arachnoid
Pia mater
Spinal cord

Figure 15 The spinal cord and its layers. The meninges enclose the brain and spinal cord.

through the brainstem and the cervical spinal cord and then exits at the thoracic and lumbar levels of the spine to reach target structures. The thoracolumbar system provides sympathetic stimulation to the periphery largely through alpha and beta receptors. Alpha receptor stimulation induces smooth muscle contraction in blood vessels and bronchioles. Beta receptors respond with relaxation of smooth muscles in blood vessels and bronchioles, and have chronotropic and inotropic effects on myocardial cells. The sympathetic nervous system is also responsible for sweating, pupil dilation, and temperature regulation, as well as the shunting of blood from the periphery to the core—the "flight or fight" responses.

SCI at or above the level of T6 may disrupt the flow of sympathetic communication. Loss of sympathetic stimulation can disrupt homeostasis and leave the body poorly equipped to deal with changes in its environment. Stimulation of sympathetic nerves without parasympathetic input can cause sympathetic overdrive, resulting in autonomic dysreflexia; this complication of SCI is discussed later in this chapter.

The Parasympathetic Nervous System

The **parasympathetic nervous system** includes fibers arising from the brainstem and upper spinal cord that carry signals to organs of the abdomen, heart, lungs, and the skin above the waist. The vagus nerve travels from its origins outside of the medulla to the heart via the carotid arteries; thus vagal tone remains intact following a spine injury. When the sympathetic nerves are stimulated and produce autonomic dysreflexia, the parasympathetic nerves attempt to control the rapidly increasing blood pressure by slowing

Table 1 Major Spinal Tracts	
Anterior Spinal Tracts	
Anterior spinothalamic tracts (ascending)	Carry sensation of crude touch and pressure sensation to the brain
Lateral spinothalamic tracts (ascending)	Carry pain and temperature
Spinocerebellar tracts (ascending)	Coordinate impulses necessary for muscular movements by carrying impulses from muscles in the legs and trunk to the cerebellum
Corticospinal tracts (descending)	Voluntary motor commands
Reticulospinal tracts (descending)	Muscle tone and sweat gland activity
Rubrospinal tracts (descending)	Muscle tone
Posterior Spinal Tracts	
Fasciculus gracilis and cuneatus	**Proprioception**, vibration, light touch, deep pressure, two-point discrimination, and stereognosis (recognition of objects by touch)

Special Populations

In elderly patients, SCI can occur even in the presence of seemingly innocuous falls. This is due to the decrease in bone density or osteoporosis, arthritis, and a general weakening of the ligaments and musculature of the neck. For example, a fall down a small flight of stairs may be enough to cause significant injury to the spine.

Similarly, infants and children are more susceptible to direct brain injury due to the incomplete skull formation along the suture lines during development. This flexibility may also mask injuries that may be obvious in the older child and adult patient. A force that compresses an adult skull and readily fractures it will not necessarily cause fracture in a pediatric skull; because of the sutures, that same force could compress the pediatric brain without causing fracture.

the role of the spinal cord in the involuntary autonomic nervous system. The **sympathetic nervous system** is controlled by the brain's hypothalamus. Information from the brain is transmitted

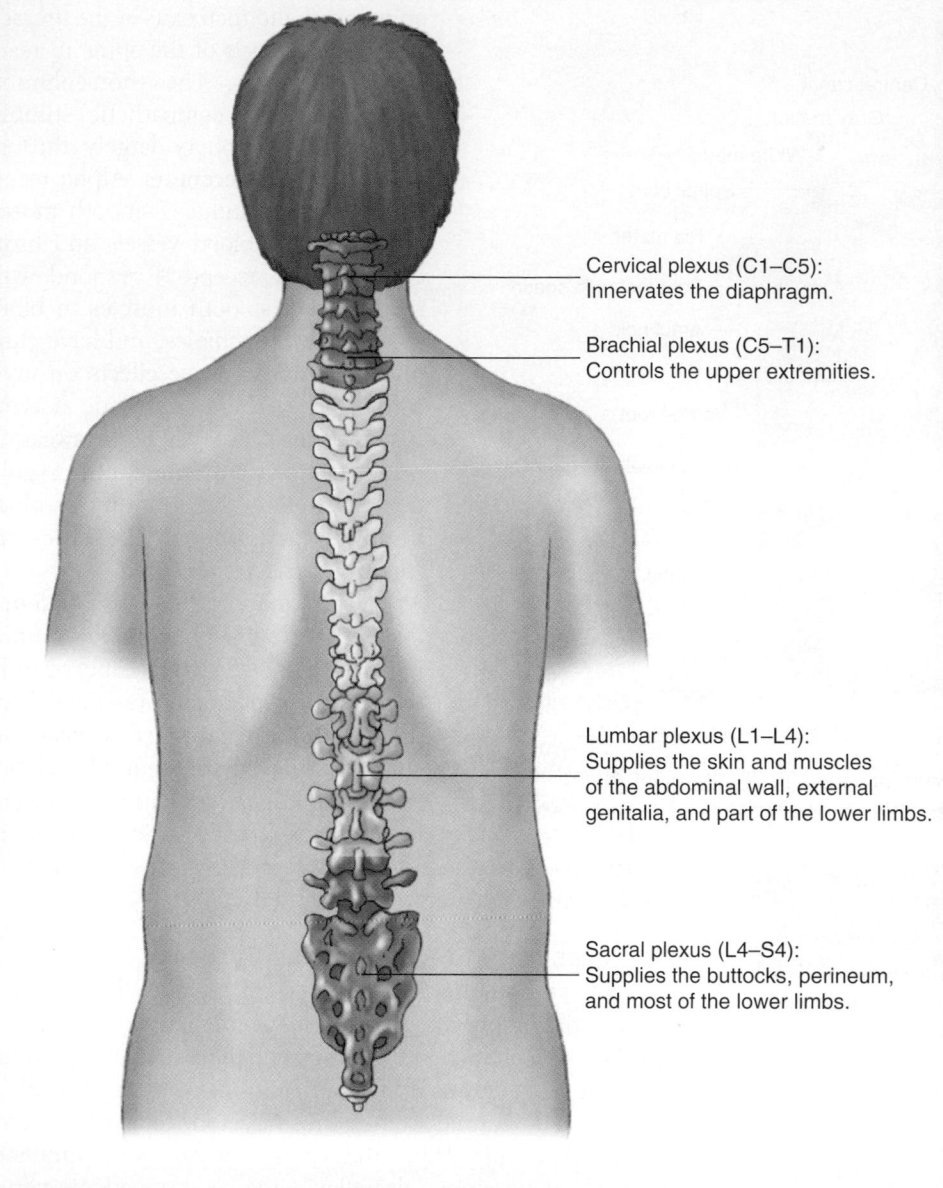

Cervical plexus (C1–C5):
Innervates the diaphragm.

Brachial plexus (C5–T1):
Controls the upper extremities.

Lumbar plexus (L1–L4):
Supplies the skin and muscles
of the abdominal wall, external
genitalia, and part of the lower limbs.

Sacral plexus (L4–S4):
Supplies the buttocks, perineum,
and most of the lower limbs.

Figure 16 Nerve roots originating from groups of vertebrae along the spine converge in plexuses, allowing them to function as a group.

Motor vehicle crashes, direct blows, falls from heights, assault, and sports-related injuries are common causes of head and traumatic brain injuries. When your patient has experienced any of these events, it should immediately elevate your index of suspicion and prompt a search for signs and symptoms of these types of injuries. A deformed windshield or dented or cracked helmet indicates a major blow to the head **Figure 17** .

The following high-risk mechanisms of injury strongly suggest spine injury and indicate that full spinal motion restriction should be applied unless there is a compelling reason not to:

- High-velocity crash (greater than 40 mph) with severe vehicle damage
- Unrestrained occupant of moderate-to high-speed motor vehicle crash
- Vehicular damage with compartmental intrusion (12 inches) into the patient's seating space
- Fall from three times the patient's height
- Penetrating trauma near the spine
- Ejection from a moving vehicle
- Motorcycle crash of greater than 20 mph with separation of the rider from the vehicle
- Diving injury
- Auto-pedestrian or auto-bicycle crash of greater than 5 mph
- Death of occupant in the same passenger compartment
- Rollover crash (unrestrained)

Mechanisms of uncertain risk for spine injury include the following events:

- Moderate- to low-velocity motor vehicle crash (less than 40 mph)
- Patient involved in a motor vehicle crash has an isolated injury without positive assessment findings for SCI
- Isolated minor head injury without positive mechanism for spine injury
- Syncopal event in which the patient was already seated or supine
- Syncopal event in which the patient was assisted to a supine position by a bystander

the heart rate. Parasympathetic nerves that supply the reproductive organs, pelvis, and leg begin at the sacral level (S2–S4). Disruption of the lower parasympathetic nerves in the sacrum results in the loss of bowel/bladder tone and sexual function.

■ Patient Assessment

■ Scene Size-up

After you have taken standard precautions, the initial step of any assessment is to make a determination about scene safety and consider the need for any additional resources. Decide whether the trauma system should be activated (eg, air evacuation of the patient to a Level 1 trauma center).

Words of Wisdom

Any patient with significant head injury also has cervical spine injury until proved otherwise.

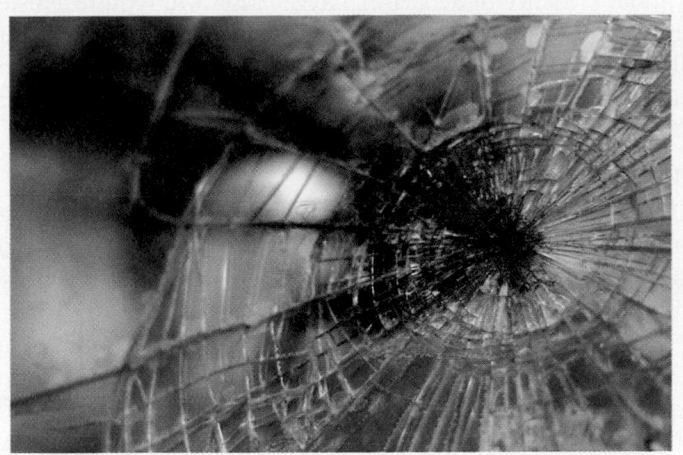

Figure 17 The classic "star" on the windshield after a motor vehicle crash is a significant indicator of injury. Be alert for the signs and symptoms of head and cervical spine injury.

Primary Assessment

Form a General Impression

Note the general age and gender of the patient. Observe the position in which the patient is found and determine whether the patient's condition is life threatening.

Patients with head injuries often have cervical spine injuries as well. Therefore, as you begin your primary assessment of a patient with a head injury, manually stabilize the cervical spine in a neutral, in-line position. While you are maintaining the head and neck in a neutral position through manual stabilization, determine the level of consciousness. A cervical collar may be applied as soon as the assessment of the airway and the anterior and posterior neck is complete. Avoid moving the neck unnecessarily, and continue manual stabilization until full spinal motion restriction precautions have been applied. Sedation or rapid sequence intubation (RSI) procedures, depending on local protocols, may be required for a combative patient to ensure the patient's protection and spine stabilization.

Airway and Breathing

After confirming that the scene is safe and determining the patient's mental status, the next priority is to ensure an open airway. Sonorous respirations usually indicate a positional problem, whereas gurgling respirations often indicate a need for suction. The oropharynx may become occluded by the tongue, secretions, blood, vomitus, foreign bodies, or improperly inserted airways. A retropharyngeal hematoma associated with injury of the upper cervical spine (C2) may also compromise the airway.

While you are maintaining the head and neck in neutral alignment, clear the mouth and carefully but quickly suction if necessary. Patients with a head injury often vomit (especially children). Therefore, after opening the airway, you must be prepared to roll the patient to the side—while maintaining spinal stabilization—to prevent aspiration. If it is safe to do so,

manually remove any large debris from the patient's mouth by sweeping the oropharynx with your gloved finger. Use suction to clear secretions, such as blood or thin secretions from the oropharynx. *Mortality increases significantly if aspiration occurs.*

Open the airway with the jaw-thrust maneuver if the patient is unresponsive or is otherwise unable to maintain his or her own airway spontaneously. If this technique is successful, insert an oropharyngeal airway or a nasopharyngeal airway as appropriate. An intact gag reflex is a contraindication for an oropharyngeal airway because vomiting will increase the likelihood of airway compromise and increase the risk of aspiration. Facial fractures and physical findings or suspicion for a basilar skull fracture are relative contraindications for a nasopharyngeal airway. *If your local protocol allows you to insert a nasal airway, use caution if CSF or bloody rhinorrhea is present or if you suspect a nasal fracture. If resistance is met at any point during insertion, it is advisable to abandon the attempt and establish control using other methods.*

In a patient with a spinal injury, a definitive airway with an advanced airway device should follow the placement of any temporary airway device. If the patient is awake with an impaired airway or has a deteriorating Glasgow Coma Scale (GCS) score (8 or less), consider drug-assisted advanced airway placement with in-line stabilization (ie, RSI). Turn the patient to the side to allow gravity to assist in evacuation of the airway while secured to a long backboard or while you maintain manual in-line stabilization of the head and neck. Follow up with suction to remove the secretions. Local protocols may include sedation or RSI.

Conversely, advanced airway management of a patient with a head injury requires special precautions or it may precipitate dangerous increases in intracranial pressure (ICP). If intubation of the patient is required (eg, unresponsive, unable to effectively perform bag-mask ventilation), observe the following guidelines:

1. Preoxygenate with 100% oxygen for at least 2 to 3 minutes or to a saturation level of 100%.
2. Administer 1 to 1.5 mg/kg of lidocaine IV push. Lidocaine has been shown to blunt an acute increase in ICP that may occur during intubation.
3. Perform intubation with the patient's head in a neutral in-line position. Intubation of a head-injured patient or any patient with significant trauma should be performed by two people: one to maintain manual stabilization of the patient's head and the other to intubate.

If a patient with a head injury requires intubation but will otherwise not tolerate laryngoscopy and endotracheal (ET) tube placement (for example, because of combativeness or clenched teeth [**trismus**]), perform pharmacologically assisted intubation (ie, RSI). This procedure involves using a sedative-hypnotic drug (such as midazolam [Versed]) and a neuromuscular blocking drug (such as vecuronium bromide [Norcuron] or rocuronium bromide [Zemuron]) to facilitate placement of the ET tube. (Refer to the chapter, *Airway Management and Ventilation* for more on pharmacologically assisted intubation.)

After you have cleared the airway, assess the patient's ventilatory status. Evaluate the patient's breathing, noting the rate, depth, and symmetry of each respiration. Closely monitor the patient's oxygen saturation (Spo_2), and maintain it at 95% or higher. Cerebral edema and ICP are aggravated by hypoxia and hypercarbia; therefore, you must constantly ensure adequate oxygenation and ventilation in any patient with a head injury. Administer 100% oxygen via a nonrebreathing mask if the patient is breathing adequately (ie, adequate rate and depth [tidal volume], regular respiratory pattern). An injured brain is even less tolerant of hypoxia than a healthy one, and research has demonstrated that prompt administration of supplemental oxygen can reduce the amount of brain damage and improve neurologic outcome.

If the respiratory center of the brain (pons, medulla) has been injured, the rate, depth, or regularity of breathing may be ineffective. Ventilation may also be impaired by concomitant chest injuries or, if the spinal cord is injured, by paralysis of some or all of the respiratory muscles. Patients with inadequate ventilation, especially if associated with a decreased level of consciousness, should receive bag-mask ventilation and 100% oxygen. Ventilate a brain-injured adult at a rate of 10 breaths/min or as dictated by local protocols. *Avoid routine hyperventilation of brain-injured patients.* Although hyperventilation causes cerebral vasoconstriction, which will shunt blood from the cranium and lower the ICP, this outcome will merely provide additional room for the injured brain to swell or for more blood to accumulate in the skull. Most important, cerebral vasoconstriction shunts oxygen away from the brain, resulting in a drop in cerebral perfusion pressure (CPP) and bringing on cerebral ischemia. The Brain Trauma Foundation (BTF) recommends hyperventilation (20 breaths/min for adults) *only* if signs of cerebral herniation are present **Table 2**. In such brain-injured patients, brief periods of hyperventilation may be beneficial. If available, end-tidal carbon dioxide ($ETco_2$) should be monitored with digital capnometry. Optimally, you should ventilate the patient to maintain the $ETco_2$—an approximation of arterial $Paco_2$—between 30 and 40 mm Hg. Under no circumstances should the $Paco_2$ be allowed to ever drop below 25 mm Hg because the subsequent vasoconstriction will almost assuredly result in brain death due to anoxia.

The diaphragm is innervated by the phrenic nerve (C3–C5). Lesions occurring at or above C3–C4 may consequently lead to diaphragmatic paralysis that is seen clinically as abdominal breathing with use of the accessory muscles of the neck. An injury involving the lower cervical or upper thoracic spinal cord (T2) may result in paralysis of the intercostal muscles, leaving the patient dependent on the diaphragm and accessory muscles of the neck for breathing. Inadequate respirations with or without evidence of decreased oxygenation will require assisted ventilation with a bag-mask device with 12 to 15 L/min of supplementary oxygen flowing at 10 to 12 breaths/min. If a head injury is suspected but you do not suspect brain herniation, use $ETco_2$ monitoring to maintain co_2 levels at 35 to 45 mm Hg.

Circulation

After you have secured the patient's airway and ensured adequate oxygenation and ventilation, you must turn your attention to supporting the patient's circulation. In the absence of a pulse, immediately initiate CPR.

Control major bleeding with direct pressure, taking care not to apply excessive pressure to scalp lacerations in which an underlying fracture is present or suspected. When you are applying direct pressure digitally to injuries that are suspicious for depressed skull fractures, it may be necessary to apply it circumferentially around the suspected fracture site as opposed to on the injury site itself **Figure 18**. Active bleeding will cause or worsen hypoxia, as well as decrease CPP, by reducing the number of oxygen-carrying red blood cells.

To assess perfusion, compare the radial and carotid pulses for their presence, rate, quality, regularity, and equality, and

Words of Wisdom

When you are assessing and managing an adult with a severe head injury, remember the Brain Trauma Foundation's "90-90-9 rule":

- A *single* drop in the patient's oxygen saturation (Spo_2) to less than 90% doubles his or her chance of death.
- A *single* drop in the patient's systolic blood pressure to less than 90 mm Hg doubles his or her chance of death.
- A *single* drop in the patient's GCS score to less than 9 doubles his or her chance of death. A drop in the GCS score of two or more points, at any time, also doubles mortality.

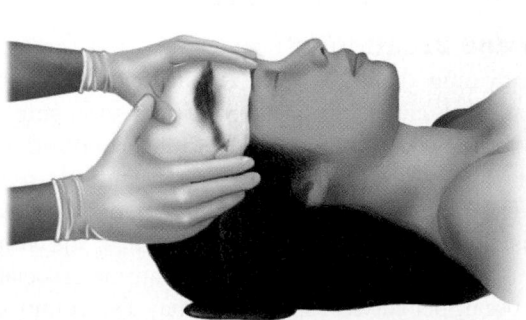

Figure 18 When you suspect a depressed skull fracture, do not apply excessive pressure to the fracture to control bleeding; rather, apply direct pressure circumferentially around the suspected fracture site.

Table 2 Signs of Cerebral Herniation

Unresponsive patient with both of the following:
- Asymmetric (unequal) pupils *or* bilaterally fixed and dilated pupils
- Decerebrate (extensor) posturing *or* no motor response to painful stimuli

examine the patient's skin color, temperature, and moisture. Patients with significant sensory loss from SCI may equilibrate to the surrounding environmental temperature due to the lack of input from the periphery for temperature control. In neurogenic shock, the skin is usually warm, dry, and flushed due to vasodilation and the absence of sweating. These findings should be correlated with the patient's mental status.

Volume resuscitation may be necessary in patients with absent or diminished pulses, especially in the setting of multisystem trauma with hypovolemic shock. An isolated closed head injury will not cause hypovolemic shock in an adult because the skull does not have enough room to accommodate large volumes of blood. If signs of shock are present (ie, persistent hypotension, tachycardia, diaphoresis), carefully assess the patient for occult injuries, such as intra-abdominal or intrathoracic hemorrhage.

Establish at least one large-bore IV line with normal saline or lactated Ringer's solution. Do not administer dextrose-containing solutions (such as 5% dextrose in water [D_5W]) because they may worsen cerebral edema. The *only* indication for administering glucose to a head-injured patient is confirmed hypoglycemia (ie, a glucometer reading of less than 70 mg/dL).

Patients with a severe closed head injury are often hypertensive—a sign of the body's autoregulatory response. Restrict your use of IV fluids for these patients to minimize cerebral edema and ICP, typically at a rate of 25 to 50 mL/h. However, if hypotension develops, infuse fluids as needed—usually 20 mL/kg boluses or as directed by medical control—to maintain a systolic blood pressure of at least 110 to 120 mm Hg in patients with a closed traumatic brain injury (TBI) and a GCS score of less than 9. Hypotension in a brain-injured patient can be lethal because it may decrease the CPP, with resultant cerebral ischemia, permanent brain damage, and death.

Patients with SCI in pure neurogenic shock may not require large amounts of volume resuscitation but may need vagolytic drugs (eg, atropine) and vasopressors (such as dopamine) to reverse the uninhibited vagal stimulation and alpha receptor blockade associated with this type of shock.

Finally, severe head injuries, especially if the lower brainstem is involved, can produce a variety of cardiac rhythm disturbances, so use a cardiac monitor for any critically injured patient. Use of a cardiac monitor also allows you to monitor the patient for acute heart rate changes. If cardiac arrest occurs, follow the ACLS cardiac arrest algorithm.

Transport Decision

Early on in the primary assessment, you must decide whether to obtain the history and perform the secondary assessment on scene, or transport the patient immediately with interventions performed en route. The patient in unstable or potentially unstable condition should be transported as soon as possible to the most appropriate hospital per local trauma guidelines or online medical control instruction.

Prompt transport to a definitive care facility (ie, a trauma center) is crucial to the survival of a brain-injured patient. If available, consider air transport if your transport time will be prolonged. If you are transporting the patient by ground, do so expeditiously, yet cautiously; the use of lights and a siren could precipitate seizures and exacerbate ICP.

Many patients with severe brain injuries and increased ICP require neurosurgical intervention. The extra time it takes to move the patient from one hospital to another could mean the difference between life and death. Therefore, transport the patient *directly* to a trauma center that has neurosurgical capabilities, even if it means bypassing the nearest hospital.

History Taking

An accurate history and physical examination are critical for directing management of patients with potential SCIs.

YOU *are the Medic*   PART 2

As you begin to manage the patient's airway and breathing, your partner asks the bystanders, "What happened?" A young woman tells you they were drinking when they decided to sneak into the pool for a skinny dip. The young man dove into the pool and did not come up. Several of his friends jumped into the water and pulled him out.

Recording Time: 1 Minute	
Appearance	Wet, naked, and lying on his back
Level of consciousness	U (unresponsive)
Airway	Snoring
Breathing	Rapid and shallow
Circulation	Slow, weak radial pulse

3. What injuries do you suspect?

4. What interventions are required?

The history of present illness typically provides most of the information necessary to reach a diagnosis.

A patient's reliability as a historian must always be assessed before performing a secondary assessment. The patient should appear calm, cooperative, and not impaired, and able to perform cognitive functions appropriately. Patients who present with an acute stress reaction, distracting injuries (eg, long bone fractures, rib fractures, pelvic fractures, or clinically significant abdominal pain), or an alteration in mental status due to brain injury or intoxication from drugs and/or alcohol must be considered unreliable in terms of the neurologic exam. These patients should have continuous spine protection until the presence of an injury can be excluded radiographically at the receiving hospital.

You should maintain a high index of suspicion in any patient for whom the mechanism of injury suggests the possibility of SCI. Associated injuries, especially those that reflect involvement of massive forces, may also provide clues of the presence of SCI. Treat all patients who experience multiple trauma or those who are found unresponsive after trauma as if a spine injury exists, because the majority of cervical spine injuries are associated with head injury. Patients with evidence of major trauma above the clavicle should be considered at risk for an associated spine injury.

Obtain a SAMPLE history. Determine as precisely as possible the circumstances of the incident and types of energy imparted to the patient, including the degree of force and the speed and trajectory of impact. Was there blunt or penetrating trauma? Was it a flexion injury, such as the classic diving accident? Was there torsion on the neck? In the case of a fall, estimate the height of the fall and determine whether anything was struck on the way down, how the patient landed, and what the patient landed on. In vehicular crashes, note the use and positioning of restraints, the patient's position in the vehicle, and the degree of damage to the vehicle. Find out the exact time of the initial injury, and record any times and changes in the patient's presentation throughout the prehospital phase.

Controversies

There are several states that have adopted statewide protocols for prehospital spinal clearance. Spinal clearance refers to the act of declaring that, based on your findings, a spinal injury is not present. This practice is controversial, and is discussed in more depth in the chapter, *Face and Neck Trauma*. If there is any doubt, the patient should be immobilized. As always, follow local protocols.

■ Secondary Assessment

The secondary assessment should begin with you obtaining a complete set of baseline vital signs. Modify the physical examination of any patient with suspected SCI based on the patient's level of consciousness, reliability as a historian, and mechanism of injury. In cases of high- or intermediate-risk mechanisms,

whenever possible complete the physical exam with the patient in a neutral position without any movement of the spine. Apply manual stabilization while asking the patient not to move unless specifically asked to do so. The neck and trunk must not be flexed, extended, or rotated.

In case of potential spine injuries, the exam includes rapid inspection and palpation of the head, neck, chest, abdomen, pelvis, extremities, and back for injuries. Use the mnemonic DCAP-BTLS—Deformity, Contusion, Abrasion, Puncture/penetration wounds, Bruising, Tenderness, Laceration, and Swelling—to help you remember specific points. An evaluation of neurovascular integrity should include distal PMS (pulse, motor, and sensory function; also called CMS for circulation, motor, and sensory function) for all four extremities. Any deficits in the neurologic examination must be noted and monitored.

You will need to expose the patient for your examination. Cut away the patient's clothes to minimize motion of the spine during examination or treatment. Directly observe the back to assess for penetrating trauma. Palpate the spine to assess for deformity or displacement (step off) of vertebral bodies. Once the exam is completed, cover the patient with a blanket to maintain normal body temperature. Hypothermia will impair the patient's ability to unbind oxygen from hemoglobin and increase the risk of mortality and morbidity. In colder climates, move the patient to a warmer environment, such as the ambulance, as quickly as possible without compromising the spine further.

Special Populations

The indications for long backboard spinal immobilization of infants and toddlers are unknown. Infants and young children cannot verbally communicate symptoms such as weakness, numbness, or pain, so the threshold for immobilization must be lower than for older children and adults. However, restraining a responsive child on a long backboard will often cause pain and agitation. Reassure nervous children that the immobilization is necessary but only temporary. Try distraction techniques.

Placement on the Backboard

Before you immobilize a patient, be sure you have documented your assessment thus far. It will also be important to document your findings after the patient has been immobilized.

Most patients can be log rolled with visualization for deformity or injury as well as palpation over each posterior spinous process for pain, deformity, or step off. The absence of pain or tenderness along the spine, coupled with a normal neurologic exam and low-risk mechanism of injury, may eliminate the need for manual in-line spinal immobilization. In contrast, paralyzed limbs should always be protected with appropriate backboard and stretcher immobilization.

Patients in severe pain may require an alternative method of transfer to a long backboard. Use of a scoop stretcher often results in less movement of the patient. Once the scoop is in place, another crew member can slide the backboard, air mattress, or vacuum mattress underneath the patient. Although the patient can still be palpated with this method, inability to conduct visual inspection of the area is a disadvantage of this procedure.

Time on a backboard should be kept to a minimum because skin breakdown can be a major complication of SCI **Figure 19**. This problem occurs as a result of excessive pressure over the bones of the buttocks, the scapular ridges, and the base of the occiput. These five areas are the primary points supporting the patient's weight. The initial stages of pressure lesions may occur in a matter of hours; 32% of patients with SCI develop a skin lesion within 24 hours of injury. Blood distribution shifts to the skin and subcutaneous tissues, and decreased muscle tone and sensation predispose the SCI patient to these injuries.

Several devices have been developed to enhance patient comfort. If you have a high suspicion of spinal injury or a long transport time, consider using a vacuum mattress to help prevent pressure ulcers from forming. Use of a vacuum mattress may also be wise if the patient exhibits diaphragmatic breathing, or if you note dermatome changes; in these cases, the patient may remain immobilized longer, until he or she can be seen by a neurosurgeon. The Back Raft is a device that takes pressure off specific areas of the back and fills voids that may otherwise allow patient movement. This low-profile air mattress fits under the patient from the shoulders to the waist **Figure 20**. Slightly flexing the knees with towel rolls or a blanket and slightly separating the legs with a pillow or blanket increases patient comfort and decreases the likelihood of postimmobilization problems, yet still provides adequate immobilization of the patient **Figure 21**. Concave backboards also conform more closely to a patient's anatomy than do flat boards. Three straps should be used to properly immobilize a patient.

A full-body exam for a trauma patient with a significant mechanism of injury should take place while en route to the hospital. Closely examine the head, neck, chest, abdomen, pelvis, extremities, back, and buttocks. A detailed head-to-toe

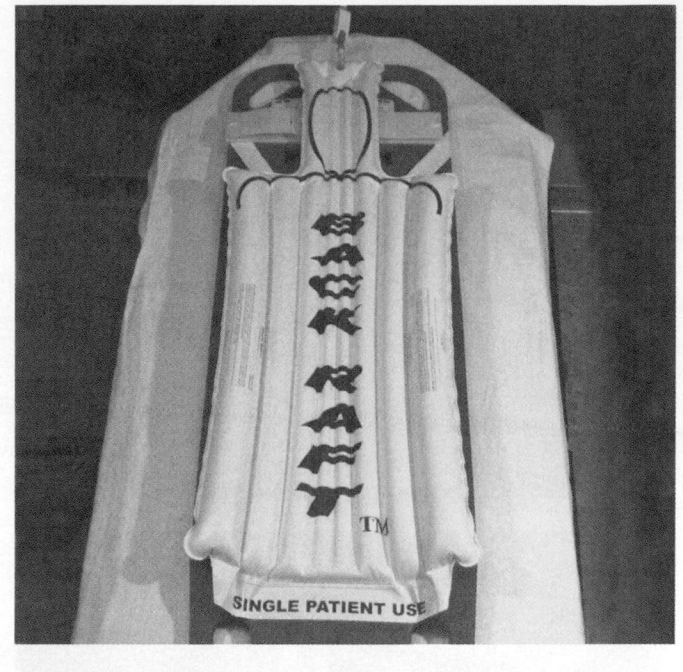

Figure 20 The Back Raft.

Words of Wisdom

Always palpate over the spinous process before concluding that a patient "has no neck tenderness." You must perform a physical exam, not simply ask the patient.

exam can often reveal significant findings, especially in patients with questionable reliability, unclear mechanisms, or multisystem trauma.

Thoroughly assess the head and neck because many SCI patients will have associated head and facial injuries; a complaint of pain is most predictive of a spine injury. Examination of the neck should include gentle palpation of the cervical spine for pain, deformity, or dislocation (step off).

Evaluate the chest and abdomen for both internal and external injuries. Fractures of the ribs, sternum, clavicle, scapula, or pelvis are often associated with SCI in patients with multisystem trauma. Visualization and palpation are the mainstays of this evaluation. Bear in mind that the physical exam in the SCI patient may be skewed due to potentially decreased sensation below the level of the spine injury. Assess the chest wall visually for symmetry of chest wall movement, work of breathing, and use of accessory muscles. Auscultation to assess breath sounds may reveal a shortened inspiratory phase. Inadequate ventilation, accessory muscle use, or paradoxical respirations may indicate diaphragmatic impairment due to SCI.

Continually monitor the cardiovascular system for signs of shock. Neurogenic shock may require pharmacologic management, volume replacement, and/or transcutaneous pacing.

Examination of the gastrointestinal system may be unreliable in the presence of a neurologic deficit. First, inspect the

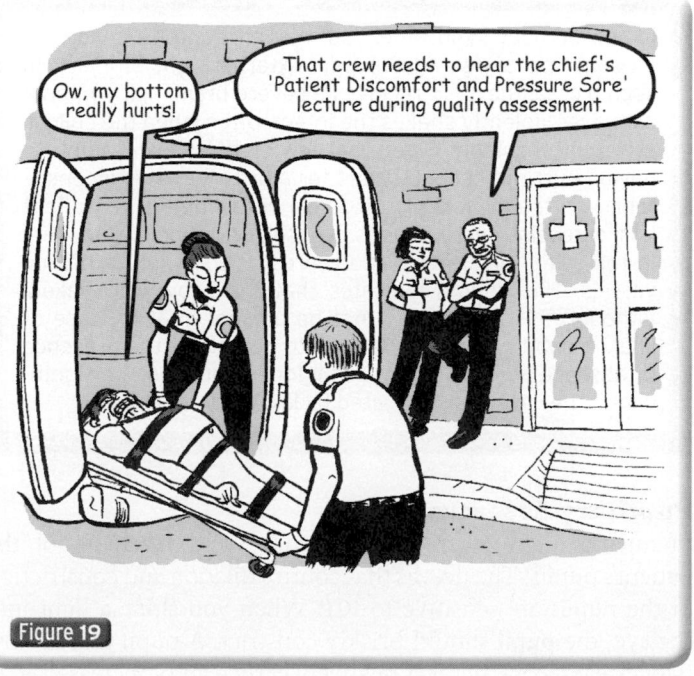

Figure 19

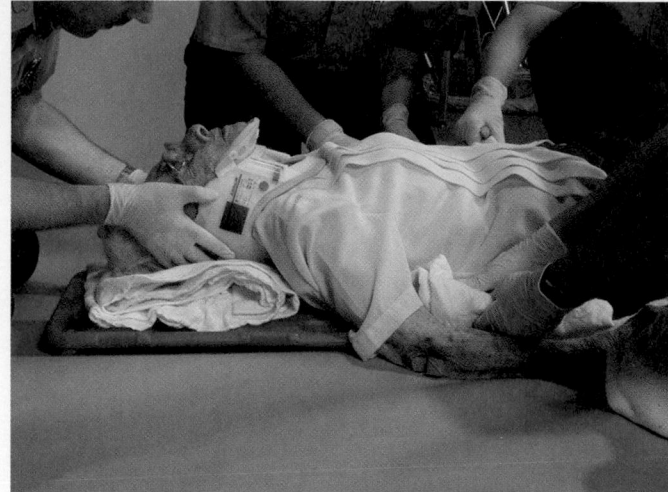

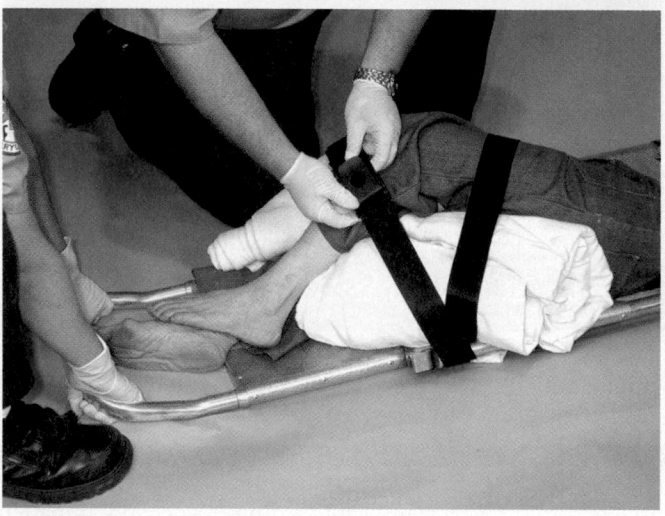

Figure 21 Using towel rolls or blankets to pad the backboard will increase patient comfort and can minimize problems resulting from immobilization of the older patient.

abdomen for evidence of trauma, noting its contour. Severe gastric distention may impair respiration and lead to airway compromise due to vomiting. Palpate all four quadrants for tenderness, guarding, or rigidity, but remember that patients may be insensitive to pain and may not develop a rigid abdomen because of absence of muscle tone. Lower abdominal distention with or without suprapubic tenderness may be due to urinary retention. In men, assess the ureteral meatus for evidence of blood, scrotal swelling, and scrotal ecchymosis, which may be present with pelvic fractures. Assess for priapism as well.

Inspect all extremities for deformity, contusion, abrasions, punctures, lacerations, and edema. Palpate for deformity, tenderness, instability, or crepitus. Look for any abnormal posturing, and assess the patient for potential long bone or other significantly distracting painful injuries that may mask a potential spine or cord injury.

Finally, if possible, obtain a glucose level in patients who show evidence of alterations in sensation.

Level of Consciousness

In addition to evaluating responsiveness with AVPU during your primary assessment, you should also obtain a GCS score because it provides more specific clinical information. A change in the level of consciousness is the single most important observation that you can make when you are assessing the severity of brain injury. The level of consciousness usually indicates the extent of brain dysfunction. Whenever you suspect a head injury, you should perform a baseline neurologic assessment using the AVPU scale (Alert; responsive to Verbal stimuli; responsive to Pain; Unresponsive) and record the time.

Use the more detailed Glasgow Coma Scale (GCS) when you are performing serial neurologic assessments of a head-injured patient Table 3. The GCS—a widely accepted method of assessing level of consciousness—is based on three independent measurements: eye opening, verbal response, and motor response. The GCS score is used to classify the severity of the patient's brain injury. The GCS score is a reliable predictor of the brain-injured patient's outcome. Note that there is an adjusted GCS scoring system for infants and children shown in the chapter, *Pediatric Emergencies.*

Pupillary Assessment

Frequently monitor the size, equality, and reactivity of the patient's pupils. The nerves that control dilation and constriction of the pupils are sensitive to ICP. When you shine a light into the eye, the pupil should briskly constrict. A pupil that is slow (sluggish) to constrict is a relatively early sign of increased ICP;

Table 3 Glasgow Coma Scale

Test	Response	Score
Eye opening	Spontaneous	4
	Voice	3
	Pain stimulation	2
	None	1
Verbal	Oriented conversation	5
	Confused conversation	4
	Inappropriate words	3
	Incomprehensible sounds	2
	None	1
Motor	Obeys commands	6
	Localizes pain	5
	Withdraws from pain	4
	Abnormal flexion (decorticate)	3
	Abnormal flexion (decerebrate)	2
	None	1

Score: 15 indicates no neurologic disabilities.
Score: 13-14 may indicate mild dysfunction.
Score: 9-12 may indicate moderate dysfunction.
Score: 8 or less is indicative of severe dysfunction.

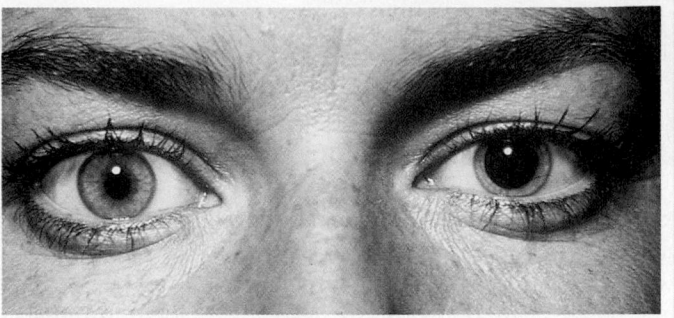

Figure 22 Unequal (shown above) or bilaterally fixed and dilated pupils in a head-injured patient are ominous signs and indicate a significantly increased ICP.

Table 4 Levels of ICP

Mild elevation	■ Increased blood pressure; decreased pulse rate ■ Pupils still reactive ■ **Cheyne-Stokes respirations** (respirations that are fast and then become slow, with intervening periods of apnea) ■ Patient initially attempts to localize and remove painful stimuli; this is followed by withdrawal and extension ■ Vomiting (often without nausea) ■ Headache ■ Altered level of consciousness ■ Seizures ■ Effects are reversible *with prompt treatment*
Moderate elevation (indicates middle brainstem involvement)	■ Widened pulse pressure and bradycardia ■ Pupils are sluggish or nonreactive ■ **Central neurogenic hyperventilation** (deep, rapid respirations; similar to Kussmaul, but without an acetone breath odor) ■ Decerebrate posturing ■ Survival possible but not without permanent neurologic deficit
Marked elevation (indicates involvement of lower portion of brainstem/ medulla)	■ Unilaterally fixed and dilated ("blown") pupil ■ Ataxic respirations (**Biot respirations**; characterized by irregular rate, pattern, and volume of breathing with intermittent periods of apnea) or absent respirations ■ Flaccid paralysis ■ Irregular pulse rate ■ Changes in the QRS complex, ST segment, or T wave ■ Fluctuating blood pressure; hypotension common ■ Most patients do not survive this level of ICP

a sluggish pupil could also indicate cerebral hypoxia. Unequal or bilaterally fixed and dilated ("blown") pupils are later, more ominous signs of increased ICP and in the context of other evidence of severe traumatic brain injury, indicate pressure on one or both oculomotor nerves **Figure 22**.

Assessing ICP

Although ICP cannot be quantified (assigned a numeric value) in the prehospital setting, the severity of increase can be estimated based on the patient's clinical presentation **Table 4**. Critical treatment decisions for brain-injured patients are based on the presence or absence of certain key findings—specifically, posturing, hypotension or hypertension, and abnormal pupil signs. Use serial assessments of the patient's GCS scores and pupillary assessment as indicators of the progression of ICP.

Words of Wisdom

The most important aspect of neurologic assessment is whether the patient's findings are changing and in what direction. Be sure to document in which area the patient's GCS score decreased.

Neurologic Exam

The focused neurologic evaluation in the field is intended to establish a baseline level of the lesion for later comparison—that is, to determine the completeness of the lesion and to identify cord syndromes if the lesion is incomplete. A normal neurologic examination does not rule out the possibility of SCI. Patients who experienced vehicular trauma have been known to walk away from the crash only to become totally paralyzed hours later, when a simple nod of the head squeezed an unstable vertebral column down against the spinal cord. Accordingly, when the mechanism of injury indicates that the patient could have sustained SCI, treat the patient as having a spine injury regardless of the neurologic findings. The neurologic assessment is intended not only to determine whether the patient should be immobilized, but also to furnish data to the hospital about the precise initial presentation of the patient so that personnel there may evaluate any changes in condition and determine whether immediate surgery is necessary.

The initial step of any neurologic assessment is a determination of the level of consciousness. First note the patient's AVPU in the primary assessment, and then address the GCS level during further assessment. When you are assigning the GCS score, do not score the patient as having no motor response if the patient's limbs are paralyzed. Ask the patient to blink or move some facial muscles that would be innervated by a cranial nerve. Remember that an unresponsive patient is always at risk for having a spinal injury.

Motor components of spinal nerves innervate discrete tissues and muscles of the body in regions called **myotomes** Table 5 . The examination of these myotomes should take place in the typical head-to-toe fashion, starting with an assessment of the cranial nerves. Cranial nerve assessment is especially important in circumstances suggestive of a high cervical injury. Observe the patient for drooping of the upper eyelid and a small pupil (Horner syndrome) that would indicate an injury to C3.

Bilaterally assess each major motor group from the top down to identify the lowest spinal segment associated with normal voluntary motor function. Because of the possibility of incomplete spinal cord lesions, it is important to determine the extent of function in segments below this level. Monitor for possible ascending lesions, paying special attention to alterations in respiratory patterns with cervical lesions.

Ask the patient to flex (C5) and extend (C7) both elbows and then both wrists (C6). Have the patient abduct the fingers and keep them open against resistance, and then adduct the fingers and attempt to close them against resistance (T1) Figure 23 . As an alternative maneuver, have the patient curl all four fingers while the examiner applies opposing pull with his or her fingers to determine strength against resistance. This will test the finger flexors (C8).

To evaluate the lower extremities, ask the patient to bend and extend the knees. Next ask the patient to plantar flex the feet and ankles as if pressing down on the gas pedal of a car (S1–S2) and to dorsiflex the toes to gravity and against resistance (L5) Figure 24 .

Assessment of motor integrity in an unresponsive patient is largely based on the patient's response to a painful stimulus. Spine injury with loss of motor function is likely if an unresponsive patient grimaces, vocalizes, or opens his or her eyes to a painful response above the level of the neurologic deficit but does not move the limbs. Pain responses should be tested at several locations before assuming an absence of response. If the motor exam cannot be completed due to local injury, the exam is considered unreliable and spine motion restriction is necessary.

Sensory components of spinal nerves innervate specific and discrete areas of the body surface called **dermatomes** Table 6 Figure 25 . In addition to testing a general loss of sensation, ask the patient about abnormal sensations in these areas such as "pins and needles," electric shock, or hyperacute pain to touch (**hyperesthesia**). As with the motor exam, sensory integrity must be assessed bilaterally but from the feet up. Determine the lowest level of normal sensation and any areas of intact or "spared" sensation below this level. In the responsive patient, a thorough evaluation will include perception of light touch, temperature, and position (proprioception).

Reflexes are usually not assessed in the field but can provide valuable information regarding sensory input, especially in the unresponsive patient. In significant SCIs, reflexes are usually

Table 5 Landmark Myotomes

Nerve Root	Muscle Group	Nerve Root	Muscle Group
C3–C5	Diaphragm	L2	Hip flexors: iliopsoas
C5	Elbow flexors: biceps, brachialis, brachioradialis	L3	Knee extensors: quadriceps
C6	Wrist extensors	L4	Ankle dorsiflexors: tibialis anterior
C7	Elbow extensors: triceps	L5	Long toe extensors: extensor hallucis longus
C8	Finger flexors: flexor digitorum profundus to middle finger	S1	Ankle plantar flexors (gastrocnemius, soleus)
T1	Hand intrinsics: interossei, small finger abductors	S4–S5	Anus, bowel, bladder
T2–T7	Intercostal muscles		

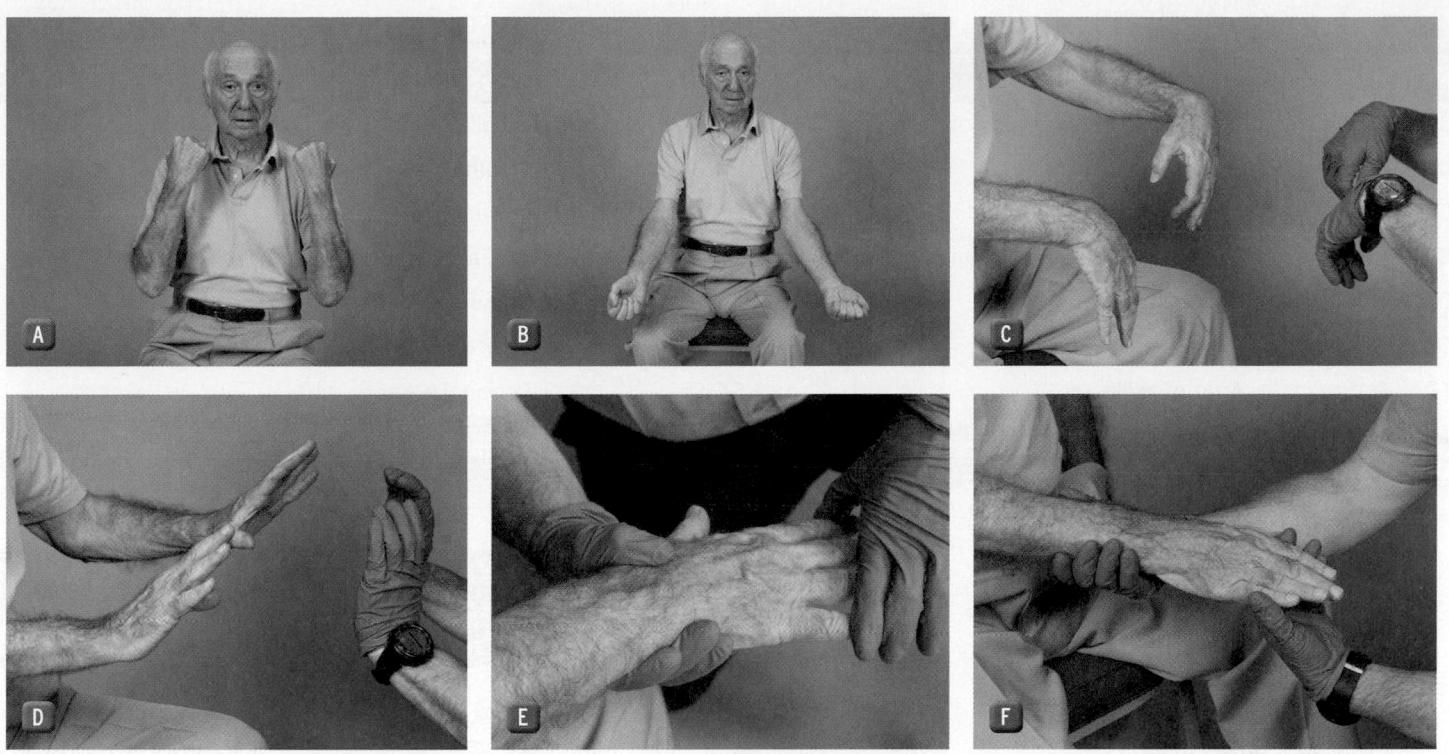

Figure 23 Neurologic evaluation of the upper extremities. Ask the patient to flex (**A**) and then extend (**B**) both elbows. Ask the patient to flex (**C**) and then extend (**D**) both wrists. Have the patient abduct the fingers and keep them open against resistance (**E**). Have the patient try to curl four fingers against resistance (**F**).

absent but return several hours to several weeks after injury. If reflexes are intact, the preservation of motor and sensory activity in the same spinal cord segments is likely. A positive <u>Babinski reflex</u> occurs when the toes move upward in response to stimulation of the sole of the foot. Under normal circumstances, the toes move downward.

■ Reassessment

Frequent reassessments are necessary to help you determine whether the patient is stabilizing, improving, or deteriorating. Vital signs should be monitored every 5 minutes (unstable patients) to 15 minutes (stable patients), with special attention to the patient's cardiovascular status. Be alert for hypotension without other signs of shock. The combination of hypotension with a normal or slow pulse and warm skin is highly suggestive of neurogenic shock. The SCI responsible for neurogenic shock also generally produces a flaccid paralysis and complete loss of sensation below the level of the injury. In contrast to

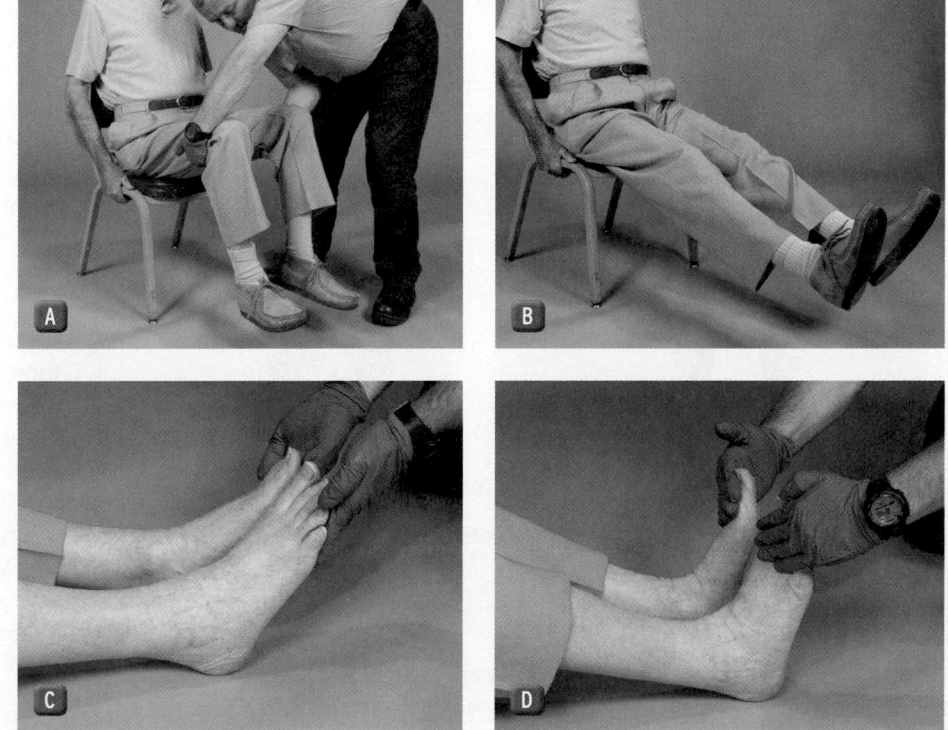

Figure 24 Neurologic evaluation of the lower extremities. Ask the patient to bend (**A**) and extend (**B**) the knees. Ask the patient to flex the feet sand ankles downward (**C**) and flex the toes upward (**D**).

Table 6 Landmark Dermatomes

Nerve Root	Anatomic Location	Nerve Root	Anatomic Location
C2	Occipital protuberance	T10	Umbilicus
C3	Supraclavicular fossa	L1	Inguinal line
C5	Lateral side of antecubital fossa	L2	Mid anterior thigh
C6	Thumb and medial index finger (6-shooter)	L3	Medial aspect of the knee
C7	Middle finger	L5	Dorsum of the foot
C8	Little finger	S1-S3	Back of leg
T2	Apex of axilla	S4-S5	Perianal area
T4	Nipple line		

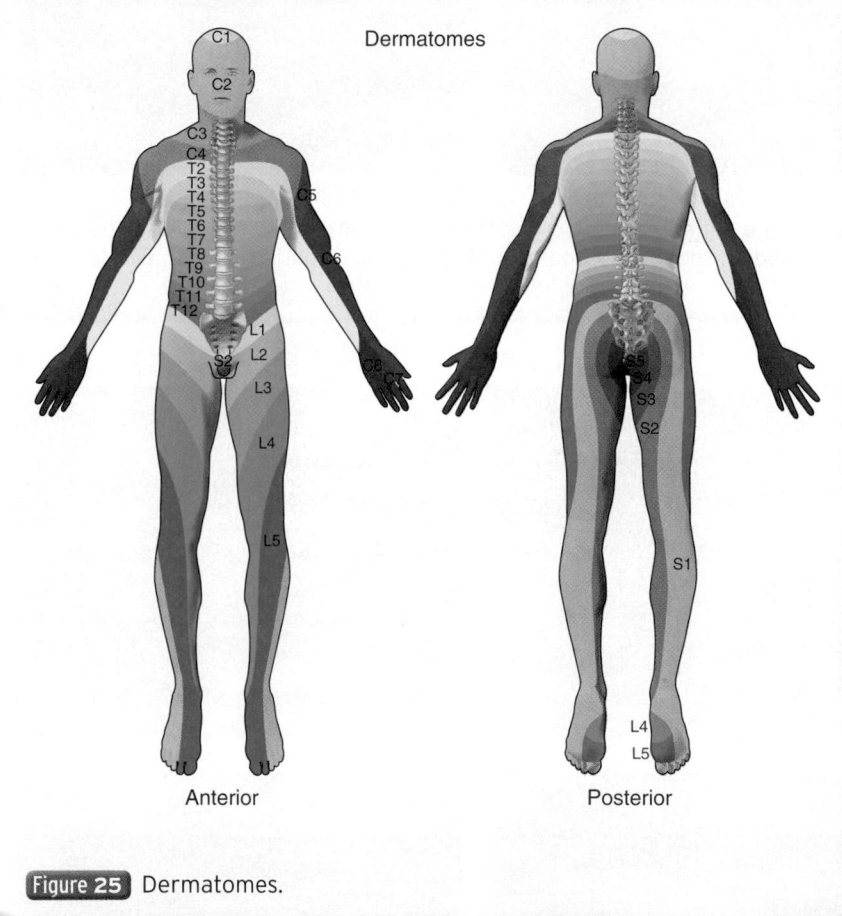

Figure 25 Dermatomes.

neurogenic shock, hypovolemic shock is associated with pale, cold, clammy skin and tachycardia.

Check interventions such as oxygen flow and spinal immobilization to ensure that they are still effective. Some EMS systems may administer an antiemetic or corticosteroid per medical control. Repeat the physical exam and reprioritize the patient as necessary.

Be sure to document suspected spinal cord injury, noting the area involved, sensation, dermatomes, motor function, and areas of weakness.

■ Pathophysiology, Assessment, and Management of Head Injuries

A **head injury** is a traumatic insult to the head that may result in injury to soft tissue, bony structures, or the brain. Approximately 4 million people experience head injuries of varying severity in the United States each year. According to the Brain Trauma Foundation (BTF), 52,000 deaths occur annually as the result of severe head injury. More than 50% of all traumatic deaths result from a head injury. When head injuries are fatal, the cause is invariably associated injury to the brain.

Motor vehicle crashes are the most common mechanism of injury, with more than two thirds of people involved in motor vehicle crashes experiencing a head injury. Head injuries also occur commonly in victims of assault, when elderly people fall, during sports-related incidents, and in a variety of incidents involving children.

There are two general types of head injuries: open and closed. A closed head injury (the most common type) is usually associated with blunt trauma. Although the dura mater remains intact and brain tissue is not exposed to the environment, closed head injuries may result in skull fractures, focal brain injuries, or diffuse brain injuries. Furthermore, these injuries are often complicated by increased ICP.

With an open head injury, the dura mater and cranial contents are penetrated, and brain tissue is open to the environment. Gunshot wounds—the most common penetrating mechanism of injury—have a high mortality rate, and for those who survive there are almost always significant neurologic deficits and a decreased quality of life.

■ Skull Fracture

Four types of skull fractures are distinguished: linear, depressed, basilar, and open **Figure 26**. The significance of a skull fracture

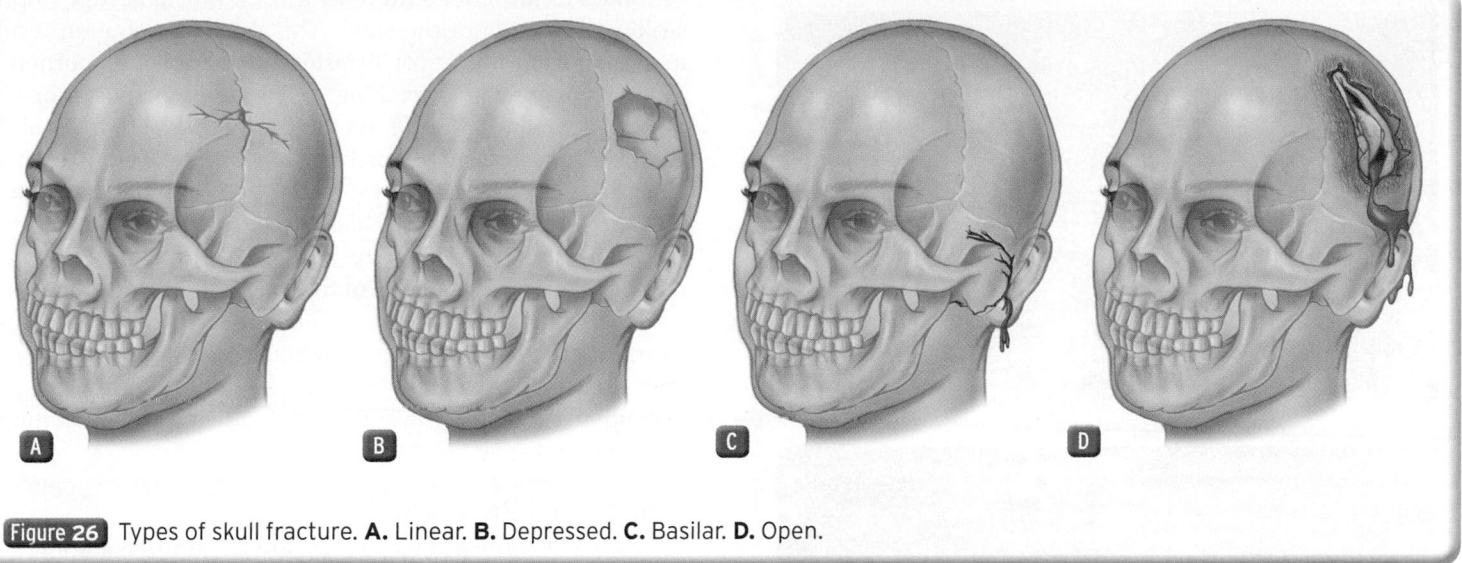

Figure 26 Types of skull fracture. **A.** Linear. **B.** Depressed. **C.** Basilar. **D.** Open.

is directly related to the type of fracture, the amount of force applied, and the area of the head that sustained the blow. Skull fractures are most commonly seen following motor vehicle crashes and significant falls. They may or may not be associated with soft-tissue scalp injuries. Potential complications of any skull fracture include intracranial hemorrhage, cerebral damage, and cranial nerve damage, among others.

Linear Skull Fractures

Linear skull fractures (nondisplaced skull fractures) account for approximately 80% of all fractures to the skull; approximately 50% of linear fractures occur in the temporal-parietal region of the skull (see **Figure 26A**). Radiographic evaluation is required to diagnose a linear skull fracture because there are often no gross physical signs (such as deformity, depression). If the brain is uninjured and the scalp is intact, linear fractures are relatively benign. However, if a scalp laceration occurs in conjunction with a linear fracture—making it an open fracture—there is a risk of infection. In addition, if the fracture occurs over the temporal region of the skull, injury to the middle meningeal artery may result in epidural bleeding.

Depressed Skull Fractures

Depressed skull fractures result from high-energy direct trauma to a small surface area of the head with a blunt object (such as a baseball bat to the head) (see **Figure 26B**). The frontal and parietal regions of the skull are most susceptible to these types of fractures because the bones in these areas, compared with other bones of the skull, are relatively thin. As a consequence, bony fragments may be driven into the brain, resulting in underlying injury. The overlying scalp may or may not be intact. Patients with depressed skull fractures often present with neurologic signs (such as loss of consciousness).

Basilar Skull Fractures

Basilar skull fractures also are associated with high-energy trauma, but they usually occur following diffuse impact to the head (eg, falls, motor vehicle crashes). These injuries generally result

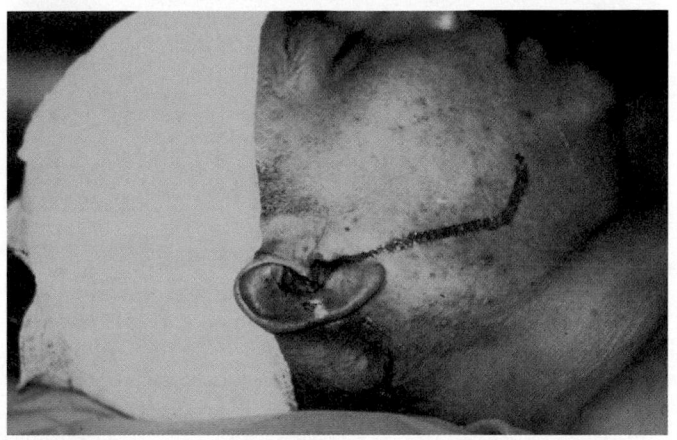

Figure 27 Blood or CSF draining from the ear after a head injury suggests a basilar skull fracture.

from extension of a linear fracture to the base of the skull and can be difficult to diagnose with radiography (x-ray) (see **Figure 26C**).

Signs of a basilar skull fracture include CSF drainage from the ears **Figure 27**, which indicates rupture of the tympanic membrane and freely flowing CSF through the ear. Patients with leaking CSF are at risk for bacterial meningitis.

Other signs of a basilar skull fracture include periorbital ecchymosis that develops under or around the eyes, which is also known as raccoon eyes **Figure 28A**, or ecchymosis behind the ear over the mastoid process known as Battle sign **Figure 28B**. Depending on the extent of the damage, raccoon eyes and Battle sign may appear relatively quickly, but in many cases, they may not appear until up to 24 hours following the injury, so their absence in the prehospital setting does not rule out a basilar skull fracture.

Open Skull Fractures

Open fractures of the cranial vault result when severe forces are applied to the head and are often associated with trauma

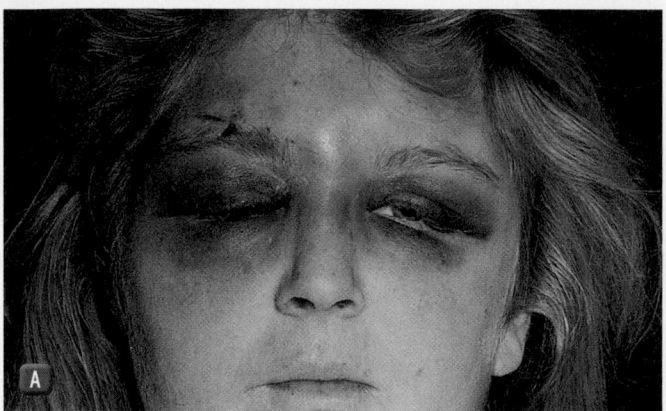

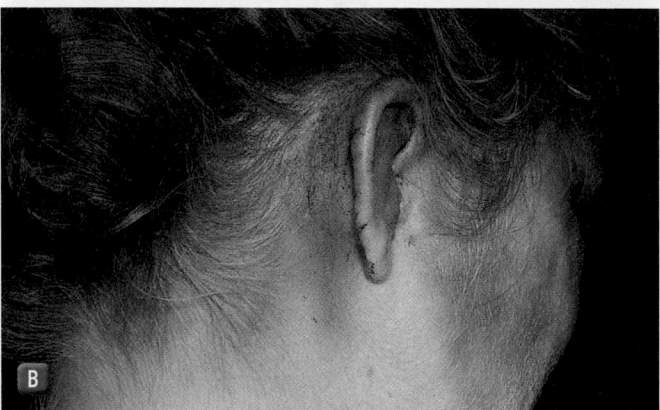

Figure 28 Suspect a basilar skull fracture if a head trauma patient has ecchymosis. **A.** Ecchymosis under or around the eyes (raccoon eyes). **B.** Ecchymosis behind the ear over the mastoid process (Battle sign).

to multiple body systems (see **Figure 26D**). Brain tissue may be exposed to the environment, significantly increasing the risk of a bacterial infection (such as bacterial meningitis). Open cranial vault fractures have a high mortality rate.

■ Traumatic Brain Injury

The National Head Injury Foundation defines a <u>traumatic brain injury (TBI)</u> as "a traumatic insult to the brain capable of producing physical, intellectual, emotional, social, and vocational changes." Traumatic brain injuries are classified into two broad categories: primary (direct) injury and secondary (indirect) injury. <u>Primary brain injury</u> is injury to the brain and its associated structures that results instantaneously from impact to the head. <u>Secondary brain injury</u> refers to the "after effects" of the primary injury; it includes abnormal processes such as cerebral edema, intracranial hemorrhage, increased ICP, cerebral ischemia and hypoxia, and infection. Secondary brain injury can occur anywhere from a few minutes to several days following the initial injury.

The brain can be injured directly by a penetrating object, such as a bullet, knife, or other sharp object. More commonly, such injuries occur indirectly, as a result of external forces exerted on the skull. Consider the most common cause of brain injury, the motor vehicle crash. When the passenger's head hits the windshield on impact with a fixed object, the brain

continues to move forward until it comes to an abrupt stop by striking the inside of the skull. This rapid deceleration results in compression injury (or bruising) to the anterior portion of the brain along with stretching or tearing of the posterior portion of the brain **Figure 29**. As the brain strikes the front of the skull, the body begins its path of moving backward. The head falls back against the headrest and/or seat, and the brain slams into the rear of the skull. This type of front-and-rear injury is known as a <u>coup-contrecoup injury</u>. The same type of injury may occur on opposite sides of the brain in a lateral crash.

The injured brain starts to swell, initially because of cerebral vasodilation. An increase in cerebral water (<u>cerebral edema</u>) then contributes to further brain swelling. Cerebral edema may not develop until several hours following the initial injury, however.

Intracranial Pressure

For adults the skull is a rigid, unyielding globe that allows little, if any, expansion of the intracranial contents. It also provides a hard and somewhat irregular surface against which brain tissue and its blood vessels can be injured when the head sustains trauma.

Accumulations of blood within the skull or swelling of the brain can rapidly lead to an increase in <u>intracranial pressure (ICP)</u>, the pressure within the cranial vault. Increased ICP squeezes the brain against bony prominences within the cranium. Normal ICP in adults ranges from 0 to 15 mm Hg. An increase in ICP (such as from cerebral edema or intracranial hemorrhage) decreases cerebral perfusion pressure and cerebral blood flow. <u>Cerebral perfusion pressure (CPP)</u>, the pressure of blood flow through the brain, is the difference between the <u>mean arterial pressure (MAP)</u>, the average (or mean) pressure against the arterial wall during a cardiac cycle, and ICP (CPP = MAP − ICP). Obviously, decreasing cerebral blood flow is a potential catastrophe because the brain depends on a

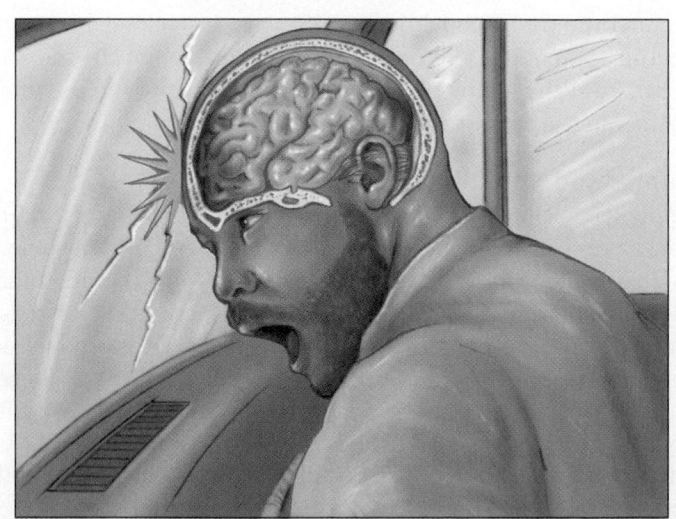

Figure 29 For the unrestrained victim in a motor vehicle crash, the brain continues its forward motion and strikes the inside of the skull, resulting in compression injury to the anterior portion of the brain and stretching of the posterior portion.

constant supply of blood to furnish the oxygen and glucose it needs to survive.

The **critical minimum threshold**, or minimum CPP required to adequately perfuse the brain, is 60 mm Hg in the adult. A CPP of less than 60 mm Hg will lead to cerebral ischemia, potentially resulting in permanent neurologic impairment or even death. In fact, according to the BTF, a *single* drop in CPP below 60 mm Hg *doubles* the brain-injured patient's chance of death!

The body responds to a decrease in CPP by increasing MAP, resulting in cerebral vasodilation and increased cerebral blood flow; this process is called **autoregulation**. However, an increase in cerebral blood flow causes a further increase in ICP. As ICP continues to increase, CSF is forced from the cranium into the spinal cord.

Clearly, the patient with increased ICP is caught in the midst of a vicious cycle. As ICP increases, cerebral blood flow increases secondary to autoregulation, which in turn leads to a potentially fatal increase in ICP. Conversely, if cerebral blood flow decreases, CPP decreases as well, and the brain becomes ischemic.

CPP cannot be calculated in the prehospital setting. Therefore, prehospital treatment must focus on maintaining CPP (and cerebral blood flow), while mitigating ICP as much as possible—a fine balance to maintain.

If increased ICP is not promptly treated in a definitive care setting, cerebral herniation may occur. In **herniation**, the brain is forced from the cranial vault, either through the foramen magnum or over the tentorium. The most common type of brain herniation occurs when a portion of the temporal lobe is displaced (uncal herniation), resulting in compression of cranial nerve III, the midbrain, and the posterior cerebral artery. Uncal herniation typically leads to coma and respiratory arrest. Another type of brain herniation occurs when part of the cerebellum is displaced through the foramen magnum (tonsillar herniation). This compresses the brainstem, resulting in destruction of the respiratory center, apnea, decreased perfusion to the rest of the brain, and death. These patients need immediate surgery to install a drain to remove blood and fluids to alleviate pressure. Other areas of the brain may suffer herniation, although such injuries occur with less frequency than either uncal herniation or foramen magnum herniation.

You must closely monitor the head-injured patient for signs and symptoms of increased ICP. The exact clinical signs encountered depend on the amount of pressure inside the skull and the extent of brainstem involvement. Early signs and symptoms include vomiting (often without nausea), headache, an altered level of consciousness, and seizures. Later, more ominous signs include hypertension (with a widening pulse pressure), bradycardia, and irregular respirations (**Cushing triad**), plus a unilaterally unequal and nonreactive pupil (caused by oculomotor nerve compression), coma, and posturing. **Decorticate (flexor) posturing** is characterized by flexion of the arms and extension of the legs; **decerebrate (extensor) posturing** is characterized by extension of the arms and legs **Figure 30** .

Diffuse Brain Injuries

Brain injuries are broadly classified as diffuse or focal. A **diffuse brain injury** is any injury that affects the entire brain. These injuries include cerebral concussion and diffuse axonal injury.

Cerebral Concussion A **cerebral concussion** occurs when the brain is jarred around in the skull. This kind of mild diffuse brain injury is usually caused by rapid acceleration-deceleration forces (coup-contrecoup), such as those seen following motor vehicle crashes or falls.

A concussion injury results in transient dysfunction of the cerebral cortex; its resolution is usually spontaneous and rapid and is not associated with structural damage or permanent neurologic impairment. Signs of a concussion range from transient confusion and disorientation to confusion that may last for several minutes. Loss of consciousness may or may not occur.

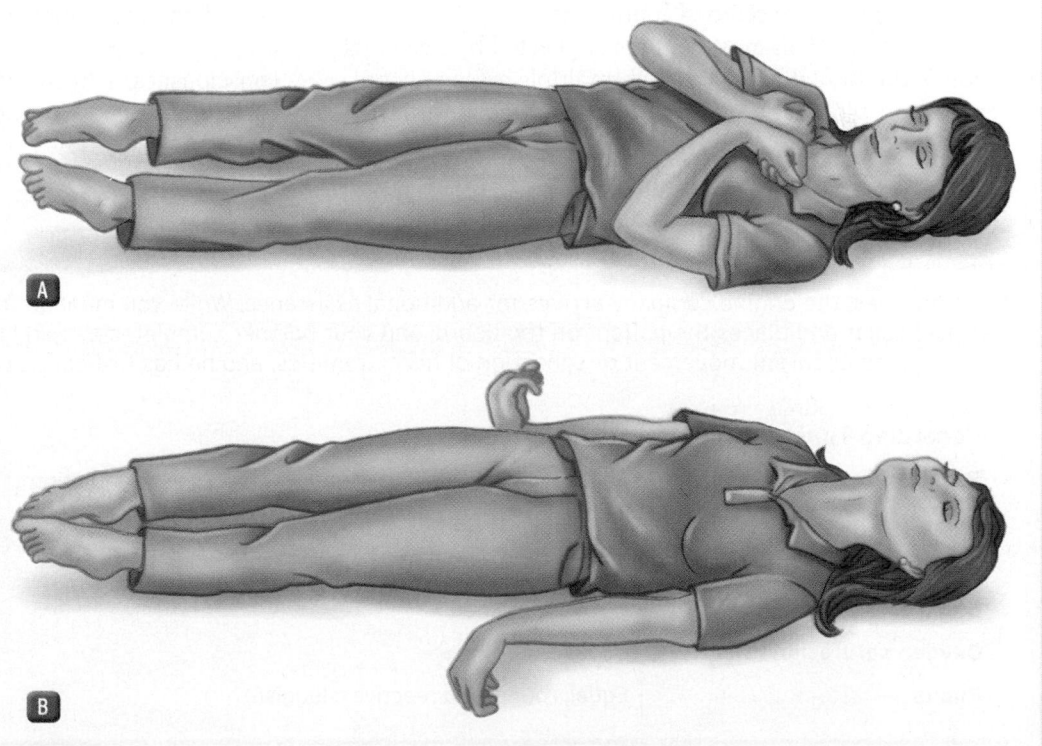

Figure 30 Posturing indicates significant ICP. **A.** Decorticate (flexor) posturing. You can remember this by thinking of the arms being pulled into the "core" of the body. **B.** Decerebrate (extensor) posturing.

Retrograde amnesia, a loss of memory relating to events that occurred before the injury, or anterograde (posttraumatic) amnesia, a loss of memory relating to events that occurred after the injury, may follow a concussion.

Diffuse Axonal Injury Diffuse axonal injury (DAI) is associated with or similar to a concussion. Unlike a concussion, however, this more severe diffuse brain injury is often associated with a poor prognosis. DAI involves stretching, shearing, or tearing of nerve fibers with subsequent axonal damage. An axon is a long, slender extension of a neuron (nerve cell) that conducts electrical impulses away from the neuronal soma (cell body) in the brain.

DAI most often results from high-speed, rapid acceleration-deceleration forces (such as motor vehicle crashes, significant falls). The severity and, thus, the prognosis of DAI depends on the degree of axonal damage (ie, stretching versus shearing or tearing); DAI is classified as being mild, moderate, or severe Table 7.

Focal Brain Injuries

A focal brain injury is a specific, grossly observable brain injury (ie, it can be seen on a CT scan). Such injuries include cerebral contusions and intracranial hemorrhage.

Cerebral Contusion In a cerebral contusion, brain tissue is bruised and damaged in a local area. Because a cerebral contusion is associated with physical damage to the brain, greater neurologic deficits (such as prolonged confusion, loss of consciousness) are more commonly observed than with a concussion. The same mechanisms of injury that cause concussions—acceleration-deceleration forces and direct blunt head trauma—also cause cerebral contusions.

The area of the brain most commonly affected by a cerebral contusion is the frontal lobe, although multiple areas of contusion can occur, especially following coup-contrecoup injuries.

As with any bruise, the reaction of the injured tissue will be to swell. This swelling inevitably leads to increased ICP and the negative consequences that accompany it.

Intracranial Hemorrhage The closed box of the skull has no extra room for accumulation of blood, so bleeding inside the skull also increases ICP. Bleeding can occur between the skull and dura mater, beneath the dura mater but outside the brain, within the parenchyma (tissue) of the brain itself (intracerebral space), or into the CSF (subarachnoid space).

An epidural hematoma is an accumulation of blood between the skull and dura mater; it occurs in approximately 0.5% to 1% of all head injuries Figure 31. An epidural hematoma is nearly always the result of a blow to the head that produces a linear fracture of the thin temporal bone. The middle meningeal artery courses along a groove in that bone, so it is prone to disruption when the temporal bone is fractured. In such a case, brisk arterial bleeding into the epidural space will result in rapidly progressing symptoms.

Often, the patient loses consciousness immediately following the injury; this is often followed by a brief period of consciousness ("lucid interval"), after which the patient lapses back into unconsciousness. Meanwhile, as ICP increases, the

YOU are the Medic | PART 3

Within minutes, the engine company arrives for additional assistance. While you manage the airway, the engine crew places a cervical collar and places the patient on the board, and your partner completes a rapid head-to-toe exam. He tells you the patient has no apparent movement or sensation of his extremities, and he has lost control of his bowel and bladder.

Recording Time: 5 Minutes

Respirations	Shallow and labored, assisting with bag-mask ventilation
Pulse	50 beats/min
Skin	Wet and flushed
Blood pressure	Not yet obtained
Oxygen saturation (Spo$_2$)	86%
Pupils	Equal, round, and reactive (sluggish)

5. Why is the patient bradycardic and hypotensive?

6. How would you manage these vital signs?

Table 7 Diffuse Axonal Injury

Type of DAI	Pathophysiology	Incidence	Signs and Symptoms	Prognosis
Mild DAI	Temporary neuronal dysfunction; minimal axonal damage	Most common result of blunt head trauma; concussion is an example	Loss of consciousness (brief, if present); confusion, disorientation, amnesia (retrograde and/or anterograde)	Minimal or no permanent neurologic impairment
Moderate DAI	Axonal damage and minute petechial bruising of brain tissue; often associated with a basilar skull fracture	20% of all severe head injuries; 45% of all diffuse axonal injuries	Immediate loss of consciousness: secondary to involvement of the cerebral cortex or the reticular activating system of the brainstem; Residual effects: persistent confusion and disorientation; cognitive impairment (eg, inability to concentrate); frequent periods of anxiety; uncharacteristic mood swings; sensory/motor deficits (such as altered sense of taste or smell)	Survival likely, but permanent neurologic impairment common
Severe DAI	Severe mechanical disruption of many axons in both cerebral hemispheres with extension into the brainstem; formerly called "brainstem injury"	16% of all severe head injuries; 36% of all diffuse axonal injuries	Immediate and prolonged loss of consciousness; posturing and other signs of increased ICP	Survival unlikely; most patients who survive never regain consciousness but remain in a persistent vegetative state

oculomotor nerve (third cranial nerve) is compressed against the tentorium, and the pupil on the side of the hematoma becomes fixed and dilated. Death will follow rapidly without surgery to evacuate the hematoma.

A **subdural hematoma** is an accumulation of blood beneath the dura mater but outside the brain **Figure 32**. It usually occurs after falls or injuries involving strong deceleration forces and occurs in approximately 5% of all head injuries. Subdural hematomas are more common than epidural hematomas and may or may not be associated with a skull fracture. Bleeding within the subdural space typically results from rupture of the veins that bridge the cerebral cortex and dura.

A subdural hematoma is associated with venous bleeding, so this type of hematoma—and the signs of increased ICP—typically develops more gradually than with an epidural hematoma. The patient with a subdural hematoma often experiences

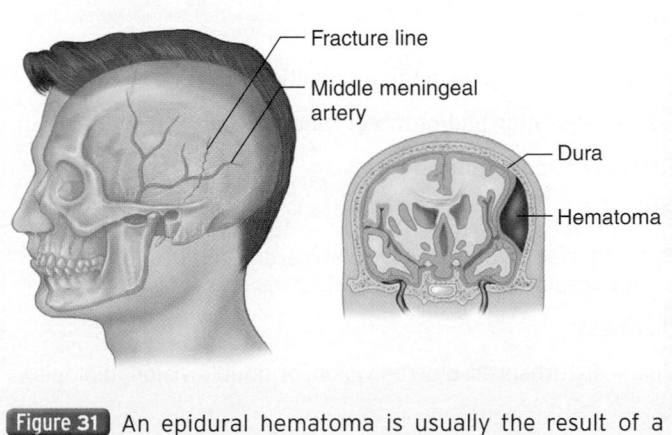

Figure 31 An epidural hematoma is usually the result of a blow to the head that produces a linear fracture of the temporal bone and damages the middle meningeal artery. Blood accumulates between the dura mater and the skull.

Fracture line
Middle meningeal artery
Dura
Hematoma

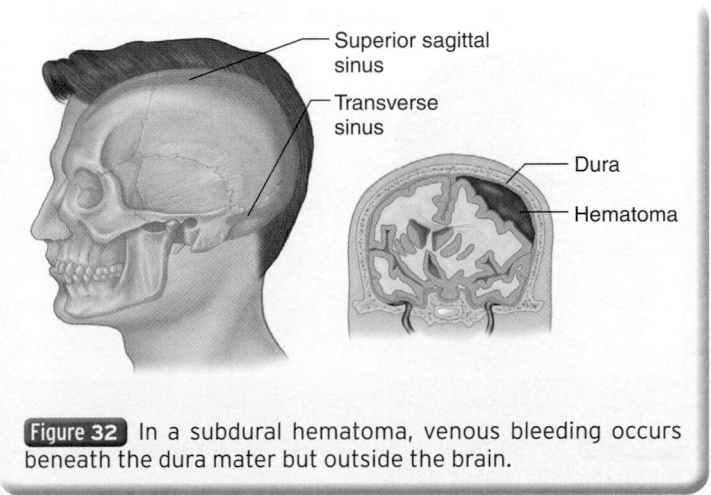

Figure 32 In a subdural hematoma, venous bleeding occurs beneath the dura mater but outside the brain.

Superior sagittal sinus
Transverse sinus
Dura
Hematoma

a fluctuating level of consciousness, focal neurologic signs (such as unilateral hemiparesis), or slurred speech.

Subdural hematomas are classified as acute (clinical signs developing within 24 hours following injury) or chronic (symptoms may not appear for as long as 2 weeks). Chronic subdural hematomas are more common in elderly patients, patients with alcoholism, patients with bleeding diatheses (such as hemophilia), and patients taking anticoagulants (such as warfarin).

An <u>intracerebral hematoma</u> involves bleeding within the brain tissue itself **Figure 33**. This type of injury can occur following a penetrating injury to the head or because of rapid deceleration forces.

Many small, deep intracerebral hemorrhages are associated with other brain injuries, such as DAI. The progression of increased ICP and neurologic deficit depends on several factors, including the presence of other brain injuries, the region of the brain involved (frontal and temporal lobes are most common), and the size of the hemorrhage. Once symptoms appear, the patient's condition often deteriorates quickly. Intracerebral hematomas have a high mortality rate, even if the hematoma is surgically evacuated.

In a <u>subarachnoid hemorrhage</u>, bleeding occurs into the subarachnoid space, where the CSF circulates. It results in bloody CSF and signs of meningeal irritation (such as nuchal rigidity, headache). Common causes of a subarachnoid hematoma include trauma or rupture of an aneurysm or arteriovenous malformation.

The patient with a subarachnoid hematoma typically presents with a sudden, severe headache. This headache is often localized initially but later becomes diffuse secondary to increased meningeal irritation. As bleeding into the subarachnoid space increases, the patient experiences the signs and symptoms of increased ICP: decreased level of consciousness, pupillary changes, posturing, vomiting, and seizures. A sudden, severe subarachnoid hematoma usually results in death. People who survive often have permanent neurologic impairment.

Finally, bleeding between the periosteum of the skull and the galea aponeurosis is called a <u>subgaleal hemorrhage</u>. It can be seen in conjunction with injuries to the skull and scalp. It is difficult to appreciate because a large amount of blood may

be spread out over the entire surface of the skull. In the newborn and infant population, it can result in enough blood loss to precipitate hypovolemia. In this age group, the accumulation of blood may make it difficult or impossible to reference the fontanelles and suture lines of the skull. It is often described as a boggy mass that is moveable and compressible on palpation. In contrast, a <u>supragaleal hematoma</u> will often be defined as a firmer, nodular mass occasionally with the idiom "goose egg" used to describe it.

■ Assessment and Management

Signs and symptoms of head injury are listed in **Table 8**. Prehospital assessment and management of the head-injured patient should be guided by factors such as the severity of the injury

> ### Words of Wisdom
>
> The most important single sign in the evaluation of a head-injured patient is a changing state of consciousness.

Table 8 Signs and Symptoms of Head Injury

Lacerations, contusions, or hematomas to the scalp
Soft area or depression noted on palpation of the scalp
Visible fractures or deformities of the skull
Battle sign or raccoon eyes
CSF rhinorrhea or otorrhea
Pupillary abnormalities   ■ Unequal pupil size   ■ Sluggish or nonreactive pupils
A period of unresponsiveness
Confusion or disorientation
Repeatedly asking the same question(s) (perseveration)
Amnesia (retrograde and/or anterograde)
Combativeness or other abnormal behavior
Numbness or tingling in the extremities
Loss of sensation and/or motor function
Focal neurologic deficits
Seizures
Cushing triad: hypertension, bradycardia, and irregular or erratic respirations
Dizziness
Visual disturbances, blurred vision, or double vision (diplopia)
Seeing "stars"
Nausea or vomiting
Posturing (decorticate and/or decerebrate)

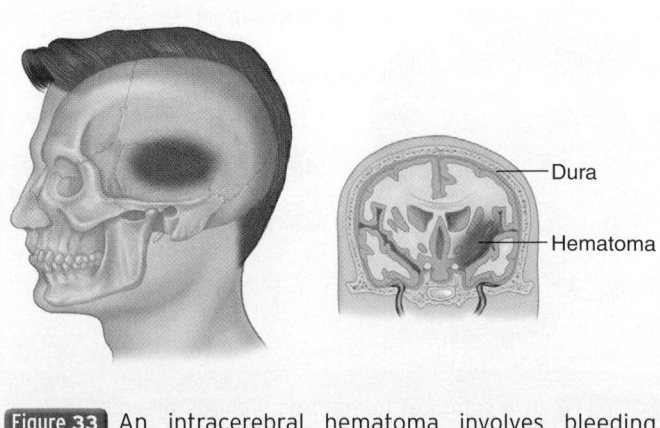

Figure 33 An intracerebral hematoma involves bleeding within the brain tissue itself.

and the patient's level of consciousness. As with any patient, your treatment priorities must be based on what will kill the patient *first*.

Thermal Management

Do not allow the patient to become overheated. Patients with a head injury, unlike those with shock, can develop a high body temperature (<u>hyperpyrexia</u>), which in turn may worsen the condition of the brain. Do not cover the patient with blankets if the ambient temperature is 70°F (21°C) or higher.

Controversies

There has been some thought that localized hypothermia may benefit patients with acute head injuries because hypothermia increases intracranial pressure. However, multiple studies and trials of patients with head injuries have shown that hypothermic therapy did not improve outcomes, and that rewarming patients can create additional problems.

Treatment of Associated Injuries

If the patient has an open fracture of the skull with brain tissue oozing out, cover it *lightly* with a sterile dressing that has been moistened with sterile saline. Likewise, for leakage of CSF from the ears or nose, apply loose sterile dressings, just to keep the area clean. Objects impaled in the skull should be stabilized in place and protected from being jarred.

Pharmacologic Therapy

Pharmacologic therapy, other than that used to facilitate intubation or treat seizures, is usually not indicated for brain-injured patients in the prehospital setting. However, if transport will be prolonged, medical control may order the administration of certain medications, such as mannitol (Osmitrol) and/or furosemide (Lasix) to reduce cerebral edema and decrease ICP.

Seizures in a brain-injured patient must be terminated as soon as possible because they provoke further increases in ICP or body temperature. Benzodiazepines, such as diazepam (Valium) or lorazepam (Ativan), should be used to control seizure activity in brain-injured patients. Follow local protocol or contact medical control regarding the doses of these drugs.

Once at the hospital, there are neuroprotective agents that the brain-injured patient may receive. At this time, these are not administered in the prehospital setting, but that could change in the future.

Pathophysiology, Assessment, and Management of Scalp Lacerations

Scalp lacerations can vary between minor to serious. Because of the scalp's rich blood supply, even small lacerations can quickly lead to significant blood loss **Figure 34**. Because these are typically visually graphic injuries with a large amount of blood, be certain to conduct a thorough evaluation and do not become distracted or too focused on the scalp injury at the risk of missing

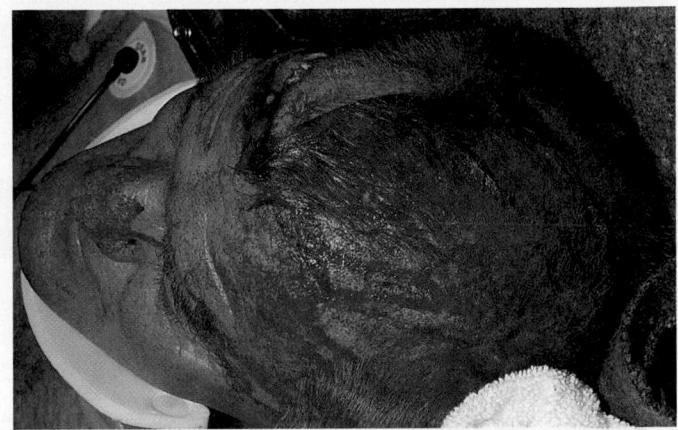

Figure 34 The scalp has a rich blood supply, so even small lacerations can lead to significant blood loss.

a more significant underlying injury. Hypovolemic shock in adults is rarely caused by scalp lacerations alone; this is a more common occurrence in children. However, bleeding from the scalp can contribute to hypovolemia in any patient, especially one with multiple injuries. If the adult patient is exhibiting signs of hypovolemic shock and it persists after addressing the scalp laceration, continue to look for other possible causes of the volume loss. In addition, because scalp lacerations usually result from direct blows to the head, they often indicate deeper, more severe injuries.

Assessment and Management

When you are assessing the laceration, consider the mechanism as one of the key pieces of information in deciding how best to proceed in treatment. If you were to apply direct pressure to a laceration that overlies a skull fracture in which the bone ends can be moved, the resulting injury to the brain or meninges could be devastating and have long-term consequences. Inspect the laceration for indications of missing tissue (avulsions) and possible impaled objects or residual contaminants. Keep in mind that both subgaleal and supragaleal hematomas may mask the presence of a depressed skull fracture; therefore, determining the mechanism will be paramount. Evaluate the wound for signs of continued bleeding and reevaluate often as the vital signs return to normal baseline, because bleeding may reoccur when sympathetic stimulation has receded. If determination of the primary mechanism is impossible, it is best to assume that skull involvement is present.

In isolated lacerations not involving suspected fractures of the skull, stopping the bleeding is the primary course of action. Application of direct pressure is the best procedure for minor to moderate lacerations. In the setting of significant lacerations, direct pressure may not be enough to control the blood loss. Pressure dressings and hemostatic agents may be required to control the bleeding. When you suspect that your patient has skull instability, your protocol may allow you to move directly to the use of hemostatic agents. In the prehospital setting, if time and other injuries do not prevent it, a quick cleansing rinse, preferably with sterile saline, can help to reduce the incidence of significant infection. It is not recommended to explore the injury because this may cause disruption of clot formation and reinitiate bleeding, and you may disturb bone fragments in patients with skull involvement.

Pathophysiology, Assessment, and Management of Spine Injuries

Spinal cord injury (SCI) is one of the most devastating injuries encountered by prehospital providers. Unfortunately, treatment options for SCIs are currently limited, with therapy relying heavily on rehabilitation over acute intervention. Preventive measures directed toward reducing the incidence of primary and secondary SCIs are the health care provider's best option for decreasing the morbidity and mortality associated with SCI.

In the United States, an estimated 11,000 new cases of SCI occur each year. The prevalence (existing cases) of SCI in the United States is 183,000 to 230,000 people. The average age at the time of injury is 32.1 years; 80% of patients are younger than 40 years and 55% are between ages 16 and 30 years. The National Spinal Cord Injury Database recognizes 38 separate causes of injury that are classified into five major categories: motor vehicle crashes (35% to 40%); acts of violence (24.5%); falls, especially in the elderly (21.8%); recreational/athletic activities, especially diving (7.2%); and other causes, including diseases such as polio, spina bifida, and Friedreich ataxia.

The overall in-hospital mortality rate is 7% for isolated SCI. In the first few months after injury, the mortality rate is as high as 20%, a rate that increases with age. The leading causes of death for SCI patients who are discharged from the hospital are pneumonia, pulmonary embolism, and septicemia.

Words of Wisdom

Patients with spinal cord injury face dramatic changes in lifestyle. A simple walk in the park, a trip to the shopping mall, or the commute to work becomes much more difficult. Caring for the patient with a spinal cord injury also brings significant financial costs.

Mechanism of Injury

Acute injuries of the spine are classified according to the associated mechanism, location, and stability of the injury. Vertebral fractures can occur with or without associated SCI. Stable fractures pose less risk to the spinal cord. Unstable injuries involve multiple columns of the spine and are often associated with damage to portions of the vertebrae and ligaments that directly protect the spinal cord and nerve roots. Unstable injuries carry a higher risk of complicating SCI and progression of injury without appropriate treatment.

Flexion Injuries

Flexion injuries result from forward movement of the head, typically as the result of rapid deceleration (eg, in a motor vehicle

crash) or from a direct blow to the occiput **Figure 35**. At the level of C1–C2, these forces can produce an unstable dislocation with or without an associated fracture. A dislocation can be complete or partial; when partial, this is termed a subluxation. Farther down the spinal column, flexion forces are transmitted anteriorly through the vertebral bodies and can result in an anterior wedge fracture. Depending on their severity, anterior wedge fractures can be stable or unstable. Loss of more than half the original size of the vertebral body or multiple levels of injury suggest relatively increased instability.

Hyperflexion injuries of greater force can result in teardrop fractures—avulsion fractures of the anterior-inferior border of the vertebral body. The injuries to ligaments associated with teardrop fractures raise concern for possible SCI and qualify as unstable fractures. Severe flexion can also result in a potentially unstable dislocation of vertebral joints. This situation does not involve fracture but can severely injure the ligaments. Strong forces can result in the anterior displacement of facet joints. A bilateral facet dislocation is an extremely unstable injury.

Patients can also experience lateral bending, which is similar to a flexion-extension injury. In flexion-extension, the patient's head moves from front to back and is overstretched on one side while being overcompressed on the opposite side. With lateral bending, the patient experiences the same type of injury, but from left to right rather than from front to back.

Rotation With Flexion

The only area of the spine that allows for significant rotation is C1–C2. Injuries to this area are considered unstable due to its high cervical location and scant bony and soft-tissue support. Rotation-flexion injuries often result from high acceleration forces. Rotation with abrupt flexion can produce a stable dislocation in the cervical spine **Figure 36**. In the thoracolumbar spine, rotation-flexion forces typically cause fracture rather than dislocation.

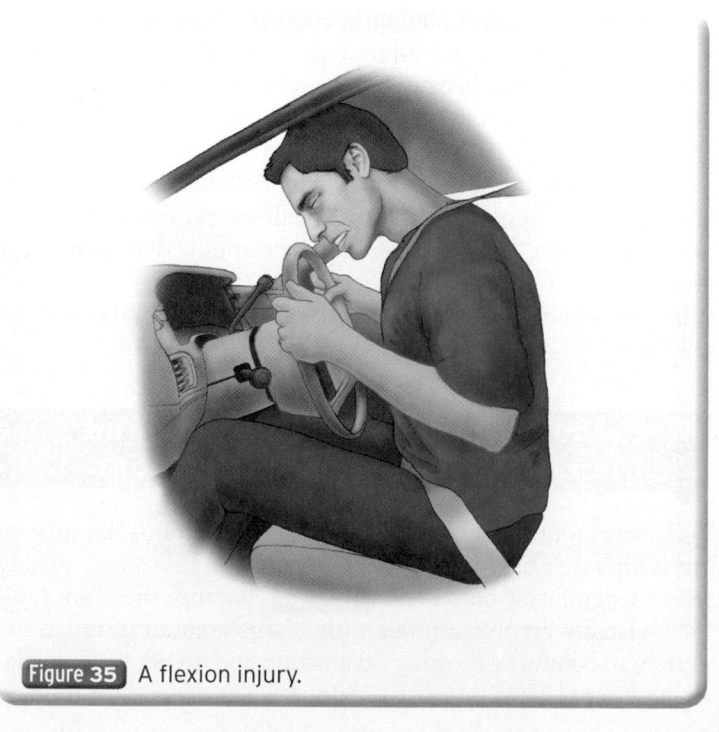

Figure 35 A flexion injury.

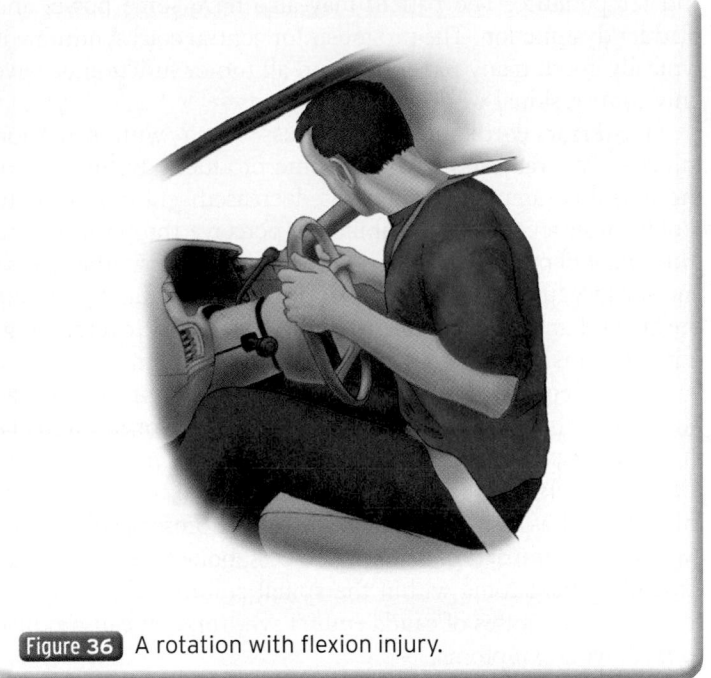

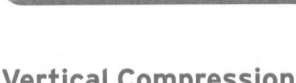 A rotation with flexion injury.

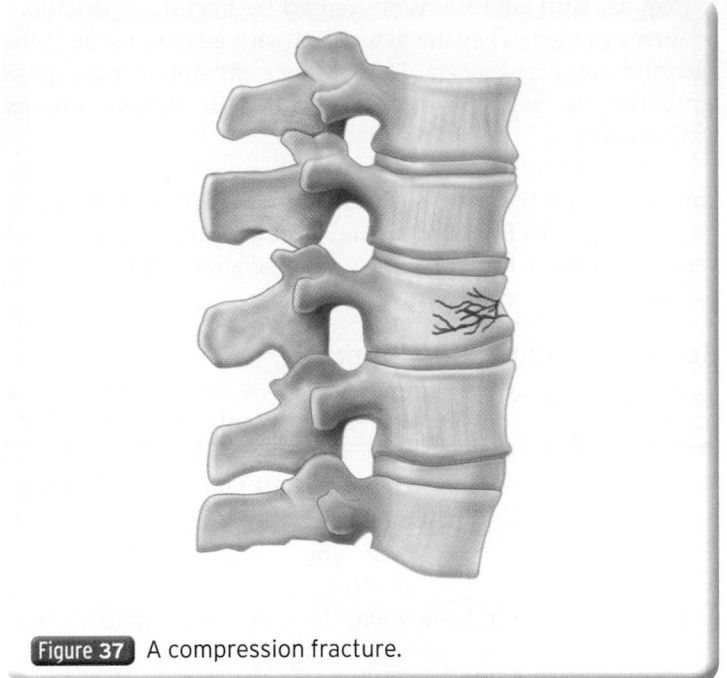

Figure 37 A compression fracture.

Vertical Compression

<u>Vertical compression</u> forces are transmitted through vertebral bodies and directed either inferiorly through the skull or superiorly through the pelvis or feet. They typically result from a direct blow to the crown (parietal region) of the skull or rapid deceleration from a fall through the feet, legs, and pelvis. Forces transmitted through the vertebral body cause fractures, ultimately shattering and producing a "burst" or compression fracture without associated SCI **Figure 37** . Compression forces can cause the herniation of disks, subsequent compression on the spinal cord and nerve roots, and fragmentation into the canal.

Although most fractures resulting from these injuries are stable, primary SCI can occur when the vertebral body is shattered and fragments of bone become embedded in the cord. Some compression injuries may be associated with significant retropharyngeal edema, and serious airway compromise is a consideration.

Hyperextension

<u>Hyperextension</u> of the head and neck can result in fractures and ligamentous injury of variable stability **Figure 38** . The hangman's fracture (C2), or distraction, results from hyperextension due to rapid deceleration of the skull, atlas, and axis as a unit. The resulting bilateral pedicle fracture of C2 is an unstable fracture but is rarely associated with SCI. A teardrop fracture of the anterior-inferior edge of the vertebral body results from hyperextension, resulting in rupture or tear of the anterior longitudinal ligament. The injury is stable with the head and neck in flexion, but unstable in extension due to loss of structural support.

■ Categories of Spinal Cord Injuries

Primary Spinal Cord Injury

<u>Primary spinal cord injury</u> is injury that occurs at the moment of impact. Penetrating trauma typically results in transection of nonregenerative neural elements and complete injuries. Blunt trauma

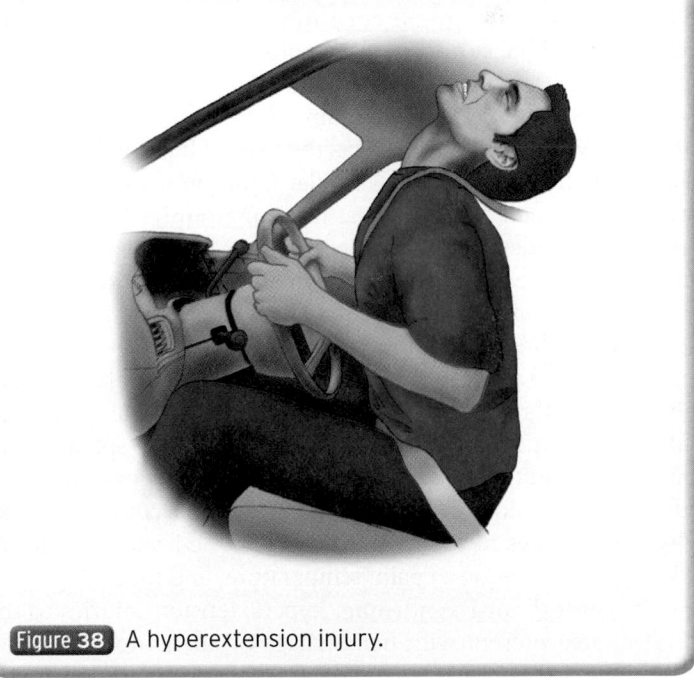

Figure 38 A hyperextension injury.

may displace ligaments and bone fragments, resulting in compression of points of the spinal cord or an incomplete dislocation of the vertebral body. Hypoperfusion and ischemia may also result from this type of injury to the spinal vasculature. Necrosis from prolonged ischemia leads to permanent loss of function.

Spinal cord concussion, which is characterized by a temporary dysfunction that lasts from 24 to 48 hours, accounts for 3% to 4% of all SCIs. Cord concussion is considered an incomplete injury and may present in patients with simple compression fractures or in those without radiologic evidence of a fracture. The temporary dysfunction may be due to a short-duration shock or pressure wave within the cord.

Spinal cord contusions are caused by fracture, dislocation, or direct trauma. They are associated with edema, tissue damage, and vascular leakage. Hemorrhagic disruption may cause temporary to permanent loss of function despite normal radiographs.

Cord laceration usually occurs when a projectile or bone enters the spinal canal. Such an injury is likely to result in hemorrhage into the cord tissue, swelling, and disruption of some portion of the cord and its associated communication pathways.

Secondary Spinal Cord Injury

Secondary spinal cord injury occurs when multiple factors permit a progression of the primary SCI; the ensuing cascade of inflammatory responses may result in further deterioration. These effects can be exacerbated by exposing neural elements to further hypoxemia, hypoglycemia, and hypothermia. Although some SCI may be unavoidable, you should minimize further injury through stabilization—that is, through spinal motion restriction and neutral alignment. In addition, minimizing heat loss and maintaining oxygenation and perfusion are key elements in the care of a patient with a possible SCI.

Regardless of the mechanism of injury, all SCIs are classified as complete or incomplete depending on the degree of damage. **Complete spinal cord injury** involves complete disruption of all tracts of the spinal cord, with permanent loss of all cord-mediated functions below the level of transection. The patient will have no sensation, pain, or movement below the site of injury. When the injury affects the patient high in the cervical spine, quadriplegia results. A similar injury in the high thoracic area would result in paraplegia. In an **incomplete spinal cord injury**, the patient retains some degree of cord-mediated function. The degree of SCI is best determined 24 hours after the initial injury; the initial dysfunction may be temporary, and there is some potential for recovery.

Anterior cord syndrome results from the displacement of bony fragments into the anterior portion of the spinal cord, often due to flexion injuries or fractures. The anterior spinal artery provides blood to the anterior two thirds of the spinal cord; disruption of this flow will present as an anterior cord syndrome. Physical findings include paralysis below the level of the insult with loss of sensation to pain, temperature, and touch.

In **central cord syndrome**, hyperextension injuries to the cervical area present with hemorrhage or edema to the central cervical segments. This type of damage is rarely associated with fractures or bone disruption but more often occurs in conjunction with tears to the anterior longitudinal ligament. Central cord syndrome is frequently seen in older patients, who may already have a significant degree of cervical spondylosis and stenosis due to arthritic changes. A brief episode of hyperextension can exert pressure on the spinal cord within the relatively diminished spinal canal. Within the central cord, motor (efferent) fibers are distributed in a unique fashion, with more cervical and thoracic motor and sensory tracts than in the periphery of the cord. The patient with central cord syndrome will present with greater loss of function in the upper extremities than in the lower extremities, with variable loss of sensation to pain

and temperature. The patient may also have some bowel and bladder dysfunction. The prognosis for central cord syndrome is typically good; many patients regain all motor function or have only some residual weakness in the hands.

Posterior cord syndrome is associated with extension injuries. This relatively rare syndrome produces dysfunction of the dorsal columns, presenting as decreased sensation to light touch, proprioception (the ability to perceive the position and movement of one's body), and vibration, while most other motor and sensory functions remain intact. Recovery of function is less prevalent than with central cord syndrome, but the overall prognosis remains good with therapy and rehabilitation.

Cauda equina syndrome is defined as a compression of the bundle of nerve roots that resembles a horse's tail or *cauda equine* in Latin, located at the end of the spinal cord. This region is in the lower back, technically inferior to the spinal cord, which terminates at L1 as the conus medullaris. In the presence of trauma, swelling after impact, penetrating objects, bone fragments, or an expanding hematoma within the spinal column in the lumbar region are the causes of cauda equina syndrome. It can produce the following symptoms:

- Severe low back pain
- Myalgia, paresthesia, or myasthenia in one or both legs
- Loss of or altered sensations in the legs, buttocks, inner thighs, backs of the legs, or feet that are severe or worsen. Your patient may report trouble feeling anything in the areas of the body that would sit in a saddle (called saddle anesthesia).
- Acute bladder or bowel dysfunction, such as retention or incontinence, which indicates perineal anesthesia, is clinically diagnostic for cauda equina syndrome. In the trauma center setting, digital rectal tone is evaluated to determine innervation of the entire length of the spinal cord. The absence of rectal tone on this exam is suggestive for SCI or cauda equina syndrome.

Brown-Séquard syndrome occurs typically after penetrating trauma and is accompanied by functional hemisection of the cord and complete damage to all spinal tracts on the involved side. Injury to the corticospinal motor tracts causes motor loss on the same side as the injury, but below the lesion. Damage to the dorsal column causes loss of sensation to light touch, proprioception, and vibration on the same side as the injury (below it). Disruption of the spinothalamic tracts causes loss of sensation to pain and temperature on the opposite side of injury, below the lesion.

Spinal shock refers to the temporary local neurologic condition that occurs immediately after spinal trauma. Swelling and edema of the cord begin within 30 minutes of the initial insult and can lead to a physiologic transection, mechanically disrupting all nerve conduction distal to the injury. The patient may present with variable degrees of acute spinal injury, potentially with flaccid paralysis, flaccid sphincters, and absent reflexes. Sensory function below the level of injury will be impaired, as will thermoregulation and visceral sensation below the lesion, resulting in bowel distention from a loss of peristalsis. Spinal shock usually subsides in hours to weeks, depending on the severity of injury.

<u>Neurogenic shock</u> results from the temporary loss of autonomic function, which controls cardiovascular function, at the level of injury. Marked hemodynamic and systemic effects are seen: hypotension occurs due to absent or impaired peripheral vascular tone with the loss of alpha receptor stimulation; blood pools in the enlarged vascular space, causing a relative hypovolemia and making the patient extremely sensitive to sudden position changes; and cardiac preload decreases, resulting in decreased stroke volume and cardiac output. Bradycardia results as well. The adrenal gland loses its sympathetic stimulation and does not produce epinephrine or norepinephrine. Hypothermia and absence of sweating are also seen because of the loss of sympathetic stimulation. The classic case of neurogenic shock is a hypotensive, bradycardic patient whose skin is warm, flushed, and dry below the level of the spinal lesion. The patient may also have paralytic ileus, which is paralysis of the small bowel. If this

Special Populations

Spinal cord injury without radiographic abnormalities (SCIWORA) can occur in children because their vertebrae lie flatter on top of each other; in adults, the vertebrae are more curved. A child's vertebrae can easily dislocate and quickly relocate back into their normal positions. The radiograph of a child who has experienced SCIWORA may have no evidence of fracture and will show a perfectly aligned vertebral column, yet the cord itself has been compressed or transected. SCIWORA cannot be diagnosed in the prehospital setting. Even in the emergency department, sophisticated studies such as MRI may be required **Figure 39**.

Of note, patients with Down syndrome are more prone to SCIWORA because they are predisposed to atlantoaxial instability (AAI); 13% of people with Down syndrome have asymptomatic AAI, and 2% have spinal cord compression due to the disorder. AAI is defined as excessive mobility of the articulation of the atlas (C1) and the axis (C2). This may lead to subluxation of the cervical spine. Radiographs are necessary in order to make a diagnosis.

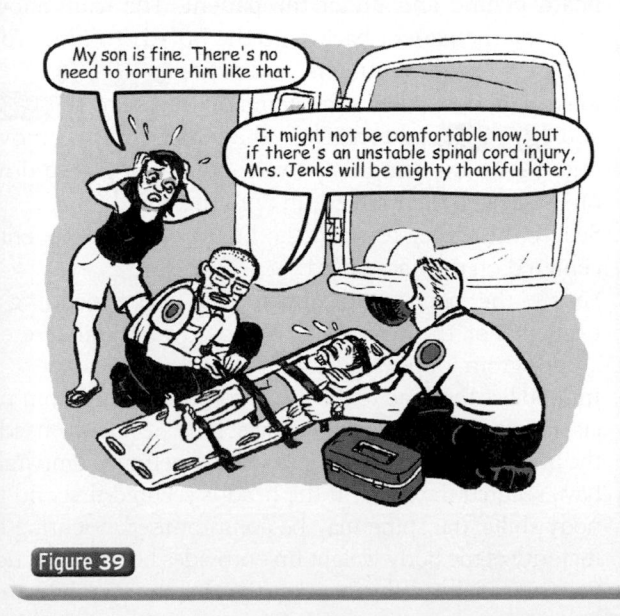

Figure 39

Special Populations

When you are managing patients with potential spinal injuries, remember the general considerations for pediatric, geriatric, and bariatric patients discussed in the chapter, *Patients With Special Challenges*. For example, obese patients have special concerns related to airway management and transport, whereas geriatric patients can experience devastating injuries from trauma that would be relatively minor for an adult patient. In all three groups, it can be difficult to determine the exact location of pain: geriatric patients have decreased pain sensation, pediatric patients cannot necessarily verbalize the exact location of their pain, and bariatric patients may be more difficult to palpate in areas where there is more tissue.

is the case, the patient will have hypoactive (slow) bowel sounds. If you note this finding, include it in your report to the receiving facility and in your documentation.

Assessment and Management

Limiting the progression of secondary SCI is a major goal of prehospital management of SCI. You should be familiar with the circumstances that commonly produce SCI and try to determine, through history-taking and examination of the scene, whether any of these circumstances exist.

As discussed earlier in the section on patient assessment, backboard placement and neurologic examination are important steps in the assessment process of a patient with SCI.

Current principles of spine trauma management include recognition of potential or actual injury, appropriate immobilization (ie, spinal motion restriction), and reduction or prevention of the incidence of secondary injury. The primary goal of spinal immobilization is to prevent further injuries. Unfortunately, studies have shown that complete spinal immobilization can be painful, especially at pressure points of the occiput and lumbrosacral areas, and can produce a restriction on ventilation. Spinal motion restriction also increases the risk for aspiration. Rigid cervical collars have been implicated as contributing to elevated ICP. Prolonged scene times can also be an issue, as with any trauma patient. The goal of all EMS providers, no matter what level, should be to spend no more than 10 minutes on the scene before the patient is transported to the most appropriate facility unless lengthy extrication is taking place or the team is awaiting air evacuation **Figure 40**.

Although a definitive prehospital clinical spine clearance protocol has not yet been established, current practices reflect the principles of hospital-based models. Specific criteria to determine whether complete immobilization is necessary should be reviewed by medical directors for efficacy. If the patient has no neurologic deficit; is not under the influence of alcohol, drugs, or medications; has no distracting injuries; has no motor or sensory deficit; and has no pain or tenderness on movement or palpation, then he or she may not require immobilization. If there is any doubt, the patient should be immobilized. As always, follow local protocols as determined by the medical director.

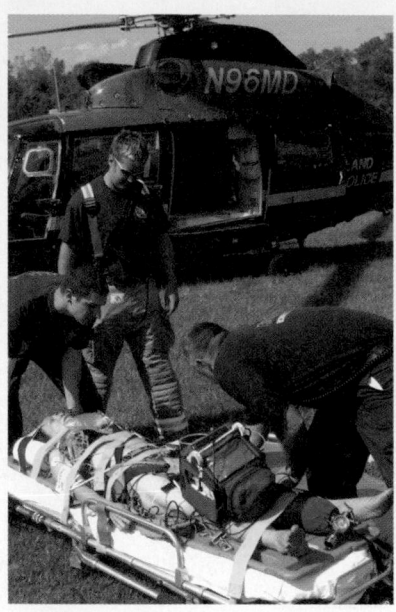

Spinal Splinting Procedures

For splinting purposes, the spine should be considered one long bone articulating with the head and the pelvis at either end. Thus, you cannot isolate and splint at only one level of the spinal column; there is simply *no such thing as partial spinal immobilization.*

Supine Patients A supine patient can be effectively immobilized by securing him or her to a long backboard. The preferred procedure for moving a patient from the ground

Special Populations

When you are immobilizing pregnant patients, tilt the backboard 15 to 20 inches to the left using a pillow or blankets.

to a backboard is the four-person log roll that should be performed whenever you suspect a spinal injury. In other cases, you may choose to slide the patient onto a backboard or use a scoop stretcher. The patient's condition, the scene, and available resources will dictate which method you choose. Ideally, the patient should be log rolled away from the side of injury. Another technique that limits movement of the spine is the use of a scoop stretcher to lift a patient a few inches off the floor or ground while crew members slide a long backboard under the patient.

Your job is to ensure that the head, torso, and pelvis move as a unit, with your teammates controlling the movement of the body. If necessary, you may recruit bystanders to the team, but instruct them fully before moving the patient.

To immobilize a patient on a backboard, follow these steps:

1. Take standard precautions, and then begin manual in-line stabilization from a kneeling position at the patient's head. Hold the head firmly with both hands. The paramedic at the head directs all patient movement.
2. Support the lower jaw with your index and middle fingers, and support the head with your palms. If the patient's head is not facing forward, gently move it until the patient's eyes are looking straight ahead and the head and torso are in line (neutral alignment). Never twist, flex, or extend the head or neck excessively. Do not remove your hands from

Special Populations

In most instances, a toddler can be immobilized in a child seat. If the child and seat need to be placed in a supine position, the child must be extricated from the car seat to avoid placing extra pressure on the abdomen and reducing the lung expansion.

the patient's head until the patient is properly secured to a backboard and the head is immobilized.

3. Assess distal PMS function in each extremity.
4. Apply an appropriately sized cervical collar. A cervical collar is used in addition to—not instead of—manual in-line cervical spine (also called c-spine) immobilization. Select the collar based on the manufacturer's specifications, and make sure it fits correctly. An improperly sized immobilization device could cause further injury. If you do not have the correct size, use a rolled towel; tape it to the backboard around the patient's head, and provide continuous manual support. Place the chin support snugly underneath the chin. While you are maintaining manual in-line stabilization, wrap the collar around the neck and secure the collar to the far side of the chin support. Recheck that the patient is in a neutral in-line position.
5. The other team members should *position the immobilization device* (backboard) and place their hands on the far side of the patient to increase their leverage. Instruct them to use their body weight and their shoulder and back muscles to ensure a smooth, coordinated pull, concentrating their pull on the heavier portions of the patient's body **Figure 41A**.
6. On command from the paramedic at the patient's head, the rescuers should *roll the patient* toward themselves. One rescuer should then quickly examine the back while the patient is rolled on the side, and then slide the backboard behind and under the patient. The team should then roll the patient back onto the board, avoiding rotation of the head, shoulders, and pelvis **Figure 41B**.
7. Make sure the patient is centered on the board **Figure 41C** and **Figure 41D**. Alternatively, the patient may be moved onto the board using only two moves: first placed down on the board, then pulled up onto the board.
8. Secure the upper torso to the board once the patient is centered on the backboard.
9. Secure the pelvis and upper legs, using padding as needed. For the pelvis, use straps over the iliac crests and/or groin loops (leg straps).
10. Immobilize the head to the board by positioning a commercial immobilization device or towel rolls. Secure the head to the board only after spider straps or something comparable have secured the torso. If the head is secured first and the body shifts, the spine may be compromised. Securing the majority of the body weight first provides better protection.
11. Secure the head by taping the head immobilization device across the forehead. To prevent airway problems and maintain access to the airway, do not tape over the

throat or chin. Instead, tape across the cervical collar just under the chin without covering the opening **Figure 41E**.

12. Pad the voids **Figure 41F**.
13. Check and readjust straps as needed to ensure that the entire body is snugly secured and will not slide during movement of the board or patient transport.
14. Reassess distal PMS function in each extremity, and continue to do so periodically.

Do not force the head into a neutral, in-line position if the patient has muscle spasms in the neck; increased pain with movement (ie, interlocked facets); numbness, tingling, or weakness; or a compromised airway or ventilation. In these situations, immobilize the patient in the position in which you found him or her.

The patient should be maintained in the neutral position unless pain or resistance to movement prevents it, in which case you should maintain the patient in the position found.

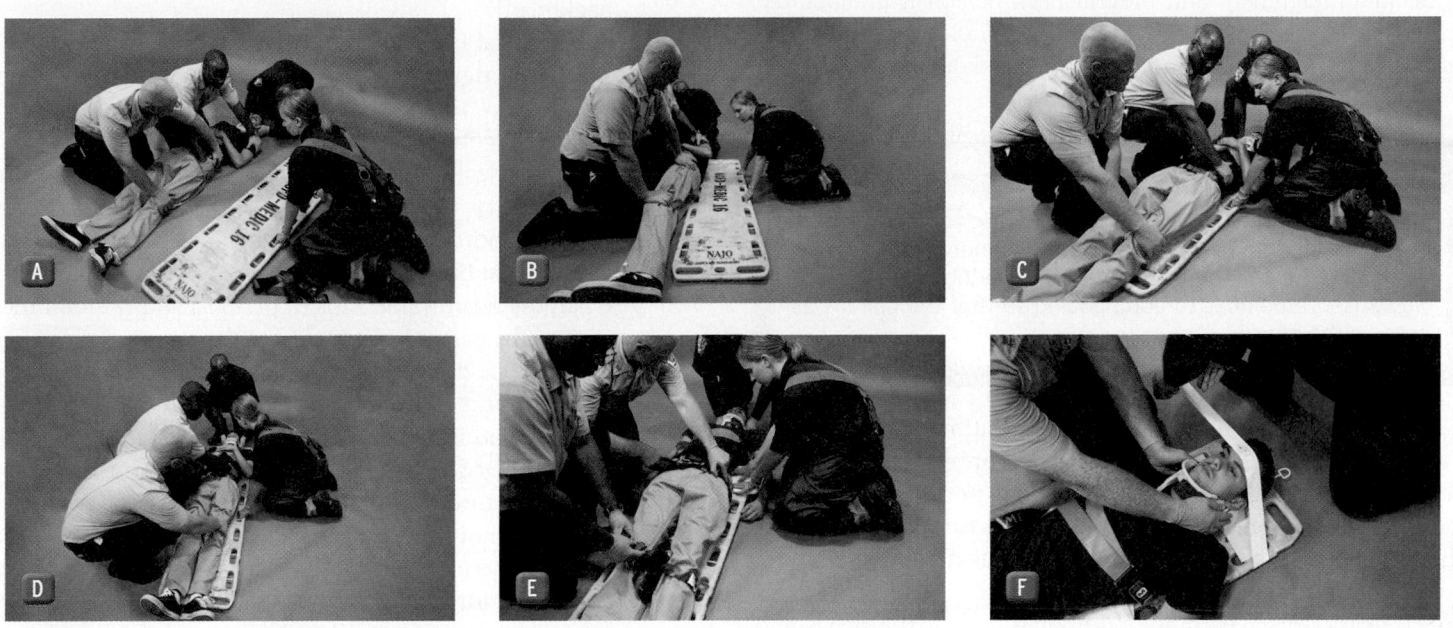

Figure 41 Immobilizing a patient to a long backboard. **A.** Placing hands on the far side of the patient. **B.** Rolling the patient and examining the back. **C.** Roll the patient onto the board. **D.** Move and center the patient up onto the board. **E.** Securing the upper and lower torso and padding the voids. **F.** Securing the head.

YOU *are the Medic* PART 4

While en route to the hospital, you intubate the patient while your partner establishes two large-bore IV lines and begins fluid resuscitation. In the ambulance, you are better able to see that his skin is flushed, and he also has an abrasion to his right forehead at the hairline. No other apparent injuries are found. Sinus bradycardia is noted on the monitor.

Recording Time: 17 Minutes	
Respirations	Assisted via bag-mask ventilation and ETT
Pulse	42 beats/min
Skin	Flushed
Blood pressure	70/p
Oxygen saturation (Spo$_2$)	Unable to obtain
Pupils	Equal, round, and reactive (sluggish)

7. What other immediate treatments are required?

8. On the basis of the events, what additional factors could complicate the patient's outcome?

Neutral positioning provides the most space for the spinal cord and may reduce cord hypoxia and excess pressure on the tissue. Do not place pillows under the patient's head. MRI studies, however, have revealed that the adult cervical spinal canal is anatomically aligned if the head is elevated by padding under the occiput with a folded towel or pad. About 80% of adult patients placed flat on a long backboard will be in extension and will require $1/2$ to 2 inches of padding to achieve neutral positioning. Pediatric patients have relatively larger heads, so they need padding under the torso to maintain alignment and prevent neck flexion if immobilized on an adult backboard. Newer pediatric backboards include a recessed portion that accommodates the head or torso padding.

Special Populations

Do not accept the labeled sizes ("pediatric" or "infant") for cervical collars. Measure each patient individually. Never place tape across the child's neck; it may obstruct the airway. Also, remember to add padding so that the child is as wide as the board.

Patients who are found in a prone position or on their side should be log rolled into the supine position with the head and neck manually stabilized in the position in which they were found, and then immobilized as described earlier. One rescuer should take control of the cervical spine using a crossed-hand position to roll the patient. The second rescuer should be positioned at the torso, with any additional help at the pelvis and legs. The rescuer at the head counts, and the patient is rolled as a unit into a supine position. Assessment and immobilization should then continue as usual.

Seated Patients Patients found in a sitting position (eg, after a motor vehicle crash) who are without cardiorespiratory compromise but require spine immobilization should also be approached with manual stabilization of the head and neck. A rigid cervical collar should be measured and placed appropriately, and a vest-type board should be used to facilitate the transfer of the patient onto a long backboard. Exceptions to this rule include the following situations in which you do not have time to first secure the patient to the short board:

- You or the patient is in danger.
- You need to gain immediate access to other patients.
- The patient's injuries justify urgent removal.

Words of Wisdom

Never release manual in-line neck stabilization until the patient's entire spine is properly immobilized. A patient's cervical spine is not considered properly immobilized until lateral immobilization is securely in place. Cervical collars will not eliminate neck movement entirely. The collar simply reminds both the patient and the EMS provider that there is a potential vertebral or spinal problem and to take special caution.

In these situations, your team should lower the patient directly onto a long backboard, using the rapid extrication technique discussed later in this chapter. Provide manual stabilization of the cervical spine as you move the patient. Rapid extrication is indicated only in cases of life- or limb-threatening injury. In all other cases, follow these steps to immobilize a seated patient:

1. Stabilize the head and then maintain manual in-line stabilization until the patient is secured to the long backboard.
2. Assess distal PMS function in each extremity.
3. Apply the rigid cervical collar. Because the cervical collar does not provide complete stabilization of the cervical spine, continue manual stabilization of the patient's head and neck until the patient is fully immobilized on a backboard.
4. Insert a short board between the patient's upper back and the seat back.
5. Open the board's side flaps (if present) and position them around the patient's torso, snug to the armpits **Figure 42A**.
6. Once the device is properly positioned, secure the upper torso straps.
7. Position and fasten both groin loops (leg straps). Pad the groin as needed. Check all torso straps and make sure they are secure. Make any adjustments necessary without excessive movement of the patient.
8. Pad any space between the patient's head and the device.
9. Secure the forehead strap or tape the head securely, then fasten the lower head strap around the rigid cervical collar **Figure 42B**.
10. Place the long backboard next to the patient's buttocks, perpendicular to the trunk.
11. Turn the patient parallel to the long board, and slowly lower him or her onto it.
12. Lift the patient and the vest-type board together as a unit (without rotating the patient), and slip the long backboard under the patient and device **Figure 42C**.

Special Populations

Osteoporosis in the thoracic and lumbar spine contributes to a high rate of injury in older patients. Three types of fractures are commonly encountered in these patients:

- Compression fractures—stable injuries that often result from minimal trauma, eg, simply bending over, rising from a chair, or sitting down forcefully.
- Burst fractures—unstable fractures that typically result from a high-energy mechanism of injury such as a motor vehicle crash or a fall from a substantial height. They may lead to neurologic injury secondary to shifting of the vertebrae with damage to the spinal cord.
- Seat belt-type fractures—involve flexion and cause a fracture through the entire vertebral body and bony arch. These injuries typically result from an ejection or in people who are wearing only a lap belt without a shoulder harness.

13. Release the leg straps and loosen the chest strap to allow the legs to straighten and give the chest room to fully expand.
14. Secure the short board and long backboard together. Do not remove the vest-type board from the patient.
15. Reassess distal PMS function in all four extremities. Note your findings on the patient care report, and prepare for transport **Figure 42D**.

Rapid Extrication With the rapid extrication technique, the patient can be moved from sitting in a car to lying supine on a backboard in approximately 2 minutes. You should use the rapid extrication technique in the following situations:

- The vehicle or scene is unsafe.
- The patient cannot be properly assessed before being removed from the car.
- The patient needs immediate intervention that requires a supine position.
- The patient's condition requires immediate transport to the hospital.
- The patient blocks your access to another seriously injured patient.

In such cases, the delay that results from applying a short board or a vest-type board is contraindicated and unacceptable. Unfortunately, the manual support and immobilization that you provide when using the rapid extrication technique carry a greater risk of spine movement. You should not use the rapid extrication technique if no urgency exists.

The rapid extrication technique requires a team of three providers who are knowledgeable and practiced in the procedure. Follow these steps:

1. The first rescuer provides manual in-line stabilization of the patient's head and cervical spine from behind. Support may be applied from the side, if necessary, by reaching through the driver's door.
2. The second rescuer serves as a team leader and gives the commands to coordinate the team's moves until the patient is supine on the backboard. Because the second rescuer lifts and turns the patient's torso, he or she must be physically capable of moving the patient. The second rescuer works from the driver's doorway. If the first rescuer is also working from that doorway, the second rescuer should stand closer to the door hinges toward the

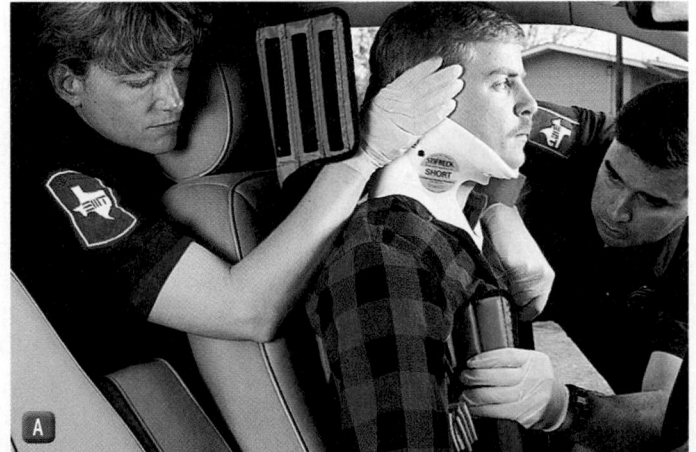
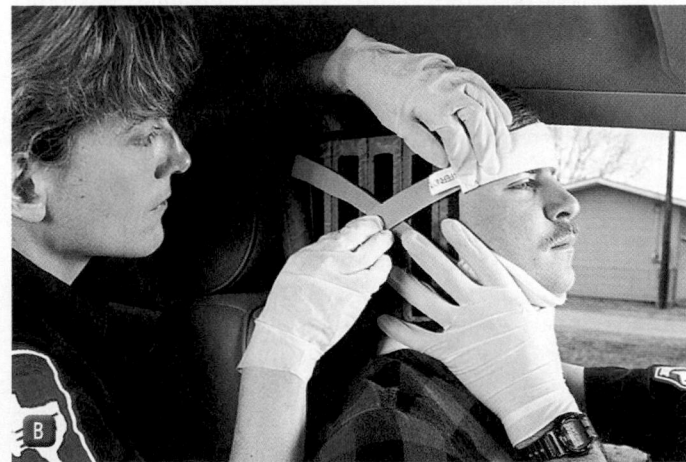
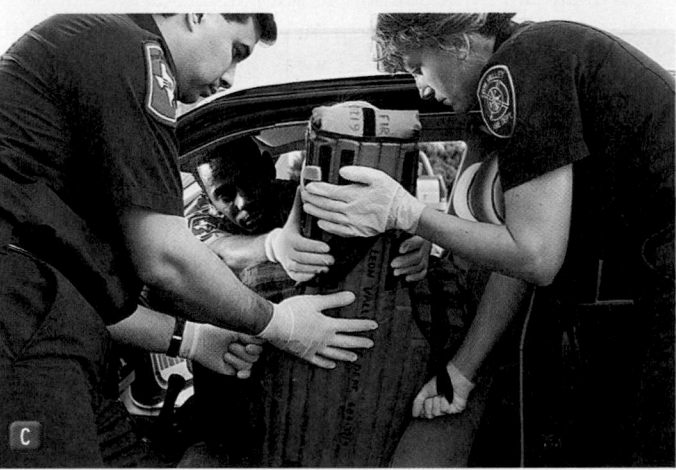
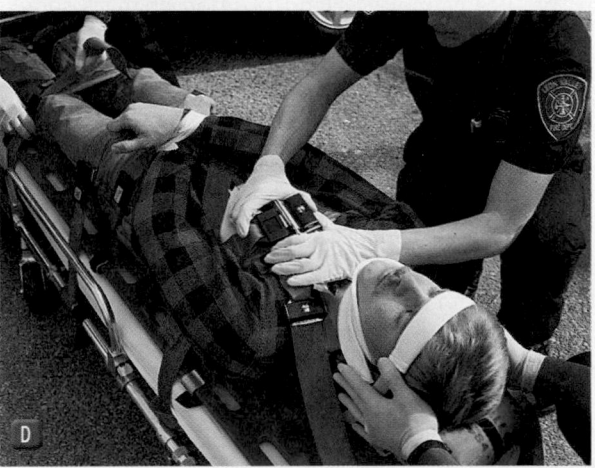

Figure 42 Immobilizing a patient found in a sitting position. **A.** Positioning around the patient's torso. **B.** Securing the head straps. **C.** Lowering the patient onto the backboard. **D.** Securing immobilization devices.

Special Populations

To immobilize kyphotic patients, several blankets and pillows or vacuum splints may be required to provide support to the head and upper back. Make sure that the empty spaces under the patient's knees or lumbar spine are padded as well.

front of the vehicle. The second rescuer applies a rigid cervical collar and performs the primary assessment.

3. The second rescuer provides continuous support of the patient's torso until the patient is supine on the backboard. Once the second rescuer takes control of the torso, usually in the form of a body hug, he or she should not let go of the patient for any reason. Some type of cross-chest shoulder hug usually works well, but you must decide which method will work best for any given patient. You cannot simply reach into the car and grab the patient because this will twist the patient's torso. You must rotate the patient as a unit.

4. The third rescuer works from the front passenger seat and rotates the patient's legs and feet as the torso is turned, ensuring that they are free of the pedals and any other obstruction. The third rescuer should first carefully move the patient's nearer leg laterally, without rotating the patient's pelvis and lower spine. The pelvis and lower spine rotate only as the third rescuer moves the second leg during the next step. Moving the nearer leg first makes it much easier to move the second leg in concert with the rest of the body. Once the third rescuer moves the legs together, they should be moved as a unit Figure 43A .

5. The patient is rotated 90° so that his or her back faces out the driver's door and the feet are on the front passenger's seat. This coordinated movement is done in three or four short, quick, one eighth to one quarter turns. The second rescuer coordinates the sequence of moves and the first rescuer directs each quick turn by saying, "Ready, turn" or "Ready, move." Hand position changes should be made between moves.

6. In most cases, the first rescuer will be working from the back seat. At some point, either because the doorpost is in the way or because he or she cannot reach farther from the back seat, the first rescuer will be unable to follow the torso rotation. At that time, the third rescuer should assume temporary manual in-line stabilization of the head and neck until the first rescuer can regain control of the head from outside the vehicle. If a fourth rescuer is present, the fourth rescuer stands next to the second rescuer. The fourth rescuer takes control of the head and neck from outside the vehicle without involving the third rescuer. As soon as the change has been made, the rotation can continue Figure 43B .

7. Once the patient has been fully rotated, the backboard is placed against the patient's buttocks on the seat. Do not try to wedge the backboard under the patient. If only three rescuers are present, place the backboard within

arm's reach of the driver's door before the move so that the board can be pulled into place when needed; the far end of the board can be left on the ground. When a fourth rescuer is available, the first rescuer exits the rear seat of the car, places the backboard against the patient's buttocks, and maintains pressure in toward the vehicle from the far end of the board. When the door opening allows, some rescuers prefer to insert the backboard onto the car seat before the patient is rotated.

8. As soon as the patient has been rotated and the backboard is in place, the second and third rescuers lower the patient onto the board while supporting the head and torso so that neutral alignment is maintained. The first rescuer holds the backboard until the patient is secured Figure 43C .

9. The third rescuer moves across the front seat to be in position at the patient's hips. If the third rescuer stays at the patient's knees or feet, he or she will be ineffective in helping to move the body's weight. The knees and feet follow the hips.

10. The fourth rescuer maintains in-line support of the head and takes over giving the commands. If a fourth rescuer is not present, you can direct a volunteer to assist you. The second rescuer maintains the direction of the extrication; this rescuer stands with his or her back to the door, facing the rear of the vehicle. The backboard should be immediately in front of the third rescuer. The second rescuer grasps the patient's shoulders or armpits. On command, the second and third rescuers slide the patient 8 to 12 inches along the backboard, repeating this slide until the patient's hips are firmly on the backboard.

11. The third rescuer gets out of the vehicle and moves to the opposite side of the backboard, across from the second rescuer. The third rescuer takes control at the shoulders, and the second rescuer moves back to take control of the hips. On command, these two rescuers move the patient along the board in 8- to 12-inch slides until the patient is completely on the board Figure 43D .

12. The first (or fourth) rescuer continues to maintain manual in-line support of the patient's head. The second and third rescuers grasp their side of the board, and then carry it and the patient away from the vehicle onto the prepared stretcher nearby.

Words of Wisdom

Occasionally patients who have just sustained a potential spine injury and are standing up at a crash scene need to be immobilized. Use of the standing takedown technique is strongly recommended. Immobilization to the backboard is not performed while patients are in the standing position because many of these patients will not stand still for the amount of time it takes to complete the immobilization. Some may be dizzy, weak, or intoxicated. Patients who have sustained head trauma may have a head injury. Also, if the backboard is applied and the patient is then placed in the supine position, the straps and padding may loosen as the patient lies down.

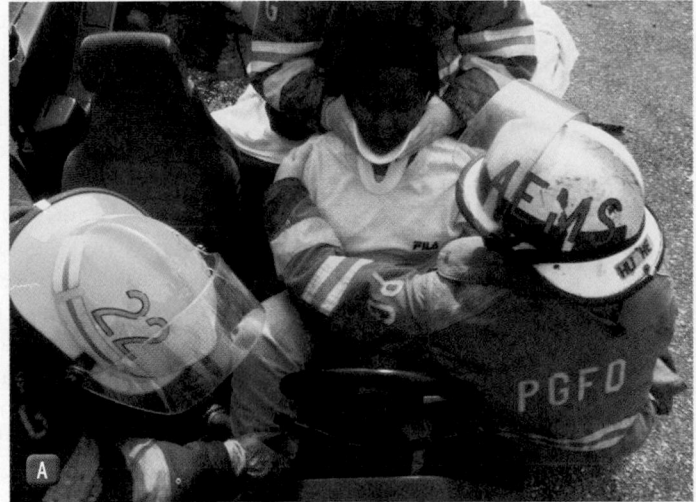
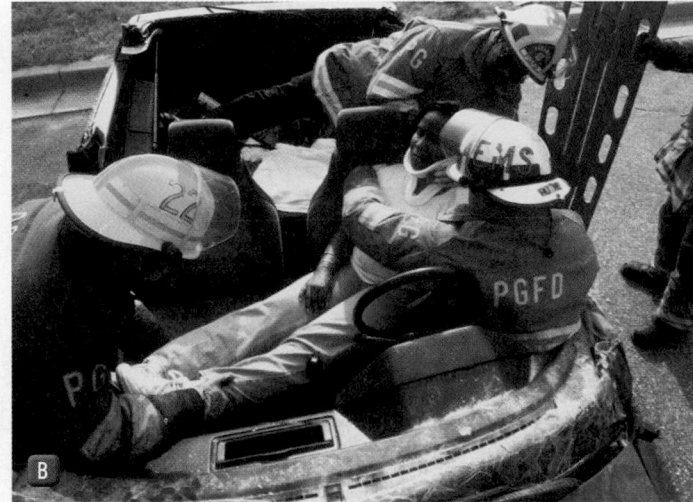
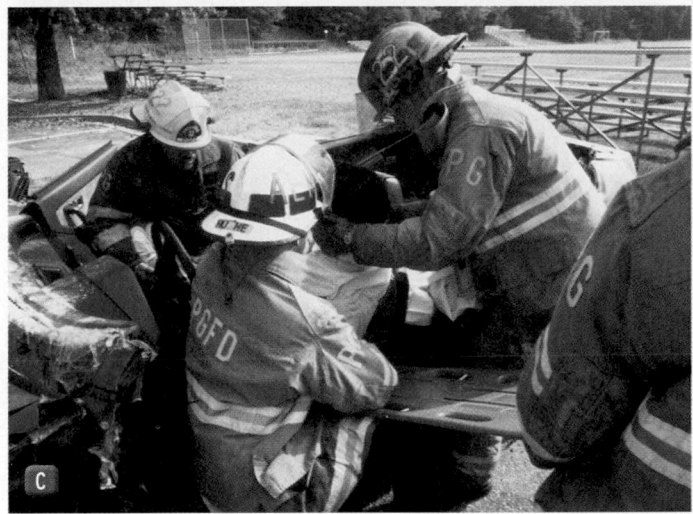
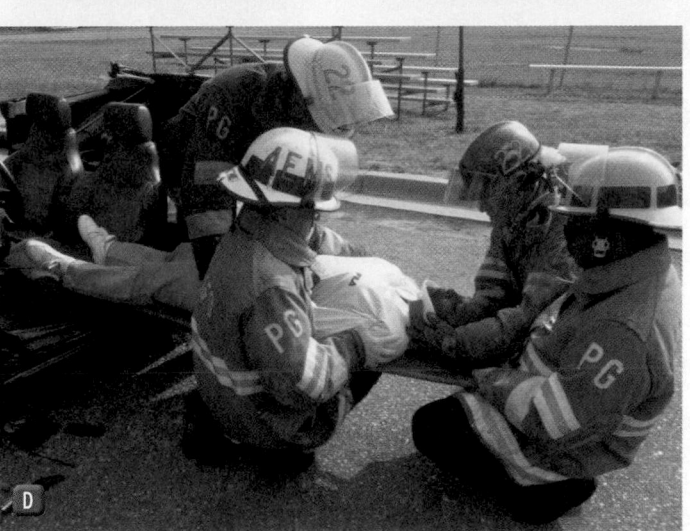

Figure 43 Rapid extrication technique. **A.** Moving the patient's legs without moving the pelvis or spine. **B.** Rotating the patient as a unit. **C.** Placing the backboard on the seat. **D.** Sliding the patient onto the board.

In some cases, you will be able to rest the head end of the backboard on the stretcher while the patient is moved onto the backboard; in others, you will not. Once the backboard and patient have been placed on the stretcher, you should begin life-saving treatment immediately. If you used the rapid extrication technique because the scene was dangerous, you and your team should immediately move the stretcher a safe distance away from the vehicle before you assess or treat the patient.

The steps of the rapid extrication technique must be considered a general procedure to be adapted as needed. Every situation will be different—a different car, a different size and priority patient, and a different crew. Your resourcefulness and ability to adapt are necessary elements of a successful rapid extrication.

Standing Patients Ambulatory patients found on the scene may require immobilization after examination and determination of mechanism and reliability. If you suspect underlying head,

neck, or spine injuries, carefully take down the patient using the standing takedown (described below), then immobilize the patient to a long backboard. This will require a minimum of three rescuers, undertaking the following steps:

1. Establish manual, in-line stabilization, apply a rigid cervical collar, and instruct the patient to remain still.
2. Position the board upright, directly behind the patient.
3. Two rescuers stand on either side of the patient; the third is directly behind the patient, maintaining immobilization.
4. The two rescuers grasp the handholds at shoulder level or slightly above by reaching under the patient's arms while standing at either side **Figure 44A**.
5. Prepare to lower the patient to the ground **Figure 44B**.
6. Carefully lower the patient as a unit under the direction of the rescuer at the head. The rescuer at the head must make sure the patient's head stays against the board and then carefully rotate his or her hands while the patient is being lowered to maintain in-line stabilization **Figure 44C**.

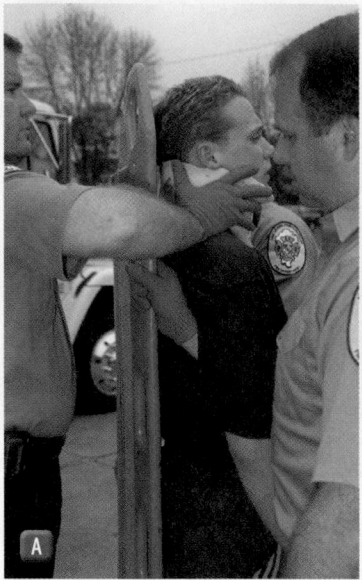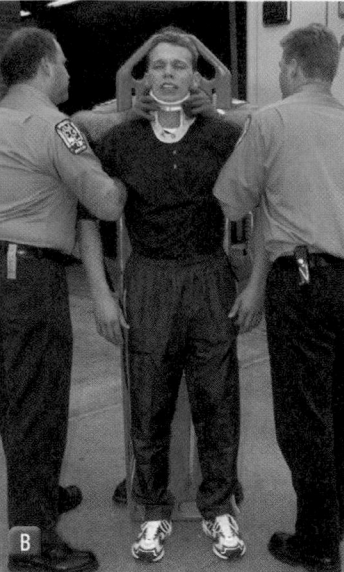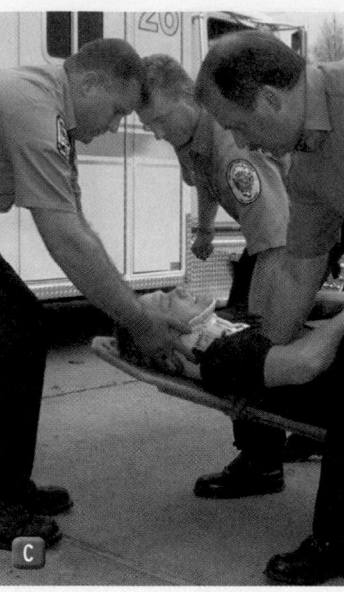

Figure 44 Immobilizing a patient found in a standing position. **A.** Positioning rescuers at the sides of the backboard. **B.** Preparing to lower the patient. **C.** Lowering the patient to the ground. Once the patient's head is on the board, do not lift it off the board!

Packaging and Removal of Injured Patients From the Water

Whatever the type of accident, the principles of packaging and removal are the same: Keep the head, neck, and trunk in alignment. When the patient may have sustained a spine injury in a confirmed diving accident, spinal immobilization must be initiated even before the patient is removed from the water. In the following cases, you should assume the patient has a spinal injury and proceed with spinal immobilization:

- Diving injury
- Boating injury
- Watercraft injury
- Falls from heights such as cliffs or bridges

If respiratory arrest is suspected, ventilation can be done while still in the water; in case of cardiac arrest, however, the rescuer should quickly evaluate the mechanism of injury. If a spine injury is not obvious, immediately remove the patient from the water and begin CPR. However, if there is any indication of a spine injury, follow these steps to stabilize the patient in the water:

1. If the patient is prone in the water, approach the patient from the top of the head, and place your arm under the body so that the head is supported on your arm and the chest on your hand. Place your other arm across the head and back to splint the head and neck between your arms. Continuing to support the patient's head and neck in that fashion, take a step backward and smoothly turn the patient to the supine position **Figure 45A**.

    Two rescuers are usually required to turn the patient safely, but in some cases one rescuer will suffice. Always rotate the entire upper half of the patient's body as a single unit. Twisting only the head, for example, may aggravate any injury to the cervical spine.

2. Open the airway and begin ventilation. Immediate ventilation is the primary treatment of all drowning and submersion patients. As soon as the patient is face up in the water, use a pocket mask if it is available. Have the other rescuer support the head and trunk as a unit while you open the airway and begin artificial ventilation **Figure 45B**.

3. Float a buoyant backboard under the patient as you continue ventilation.

4. Secure the head and trunk to the backboard to eliminate motion of the cervical spine. Do not remove the patient from the water until this step is complete **Figure 45C**.

5. Remove the patient from the water, on the backboard.

6. Remove wet clothes, and cover the patient with a blanket. Give supplementary oxygen if the patient is breathing adequately; give positive-pressure ventilation if the patient is apneic or breathing inadequately. Begin CPR if there is no pulse. Effective chest compressions cannot be performed when the patient is still in the water **Figure 45D**.

7. Consider using an advanced airway device to maintain the airway if needed. Place the patient on a cardiac monitor and treat dysrhythmias according to the ACLS algorithms (discussed in other chapters).

Patients Wearing Helmets

Helmets are a relatively common finding in motor vehicle and sports-related injuries. The use of helmets has been shown to reduce both the incidence and the severity of brain injuries associated with trauma, and their use is widely encouraged. Most helmets consist of an inner foam layer surrounded by a durable plastic shell. Helmets can inhibit full exposure of the patient and could hinder your efforts at airway management and spinal stabilization. Unfortunately, the removal of most types of helmets can result in some spinal motion even under the best circumstances. However, a securely fitting helmet can provide a degree of stabilization and under the proper circumstances can actually assist in maintaining the spine in a neutral position.

The Inter-Association Task Force for the Appropriate Care of the Spine-Injured Athlete (convened in 1999) recommended helmet removal in the following situations:

- The helmet and chin strap fail to hold the head securely, as with a loose-fitting helmet.

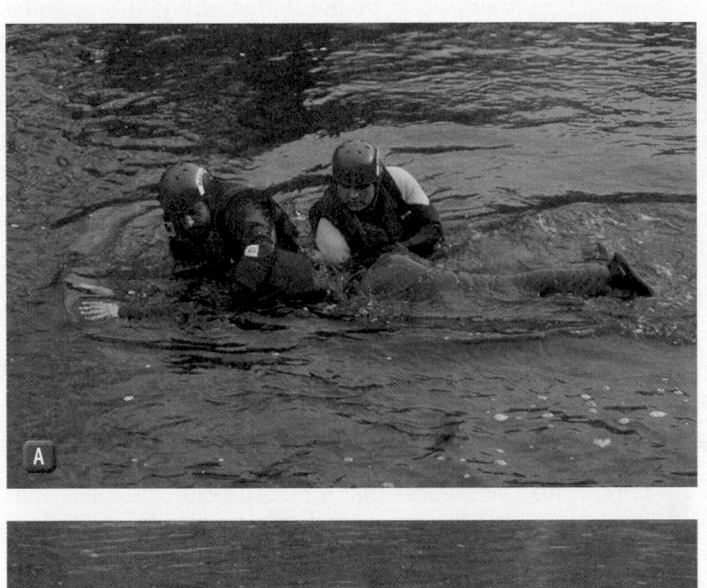
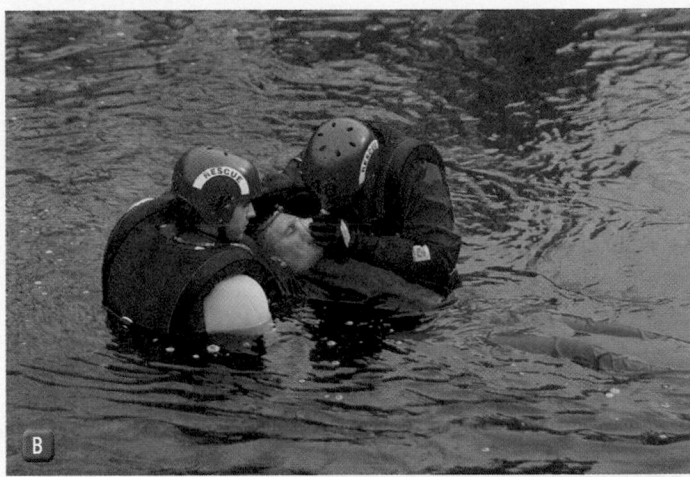
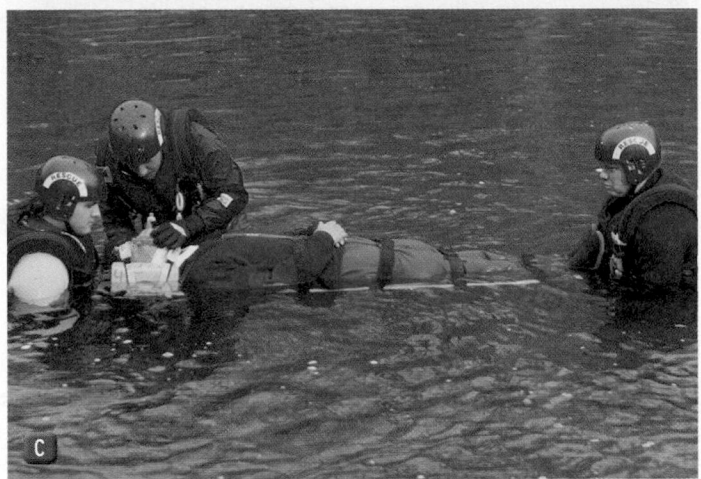
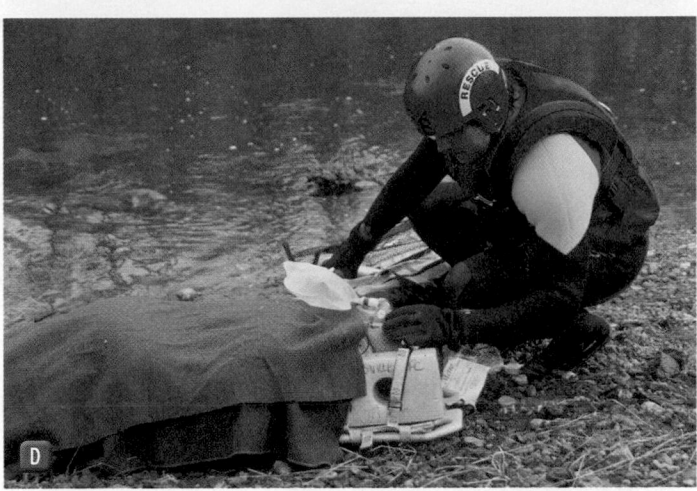

Figure 45 Stabilizing a suspected spine injury in the water. **A.** Turning the patient to a supine position in the water. **B.** Providing artificial ventilation. **C.** Securing the patient to a backboard. **D.** Providing care once out of the water.

- The helmet and chin strap design prevent adequate airway control, even after the removal of a face mask.
- A helmet with a face mask cannot be removed after a reasonable amount of time.
- The helmet prevents proper immobilization for transport.

Only providers who are familiar with the procedure should attempt helmet removal. A single rescuer should not attempt helmet removal because the maneuver requires two providers:

1. Kneel at the patient's head. Leave enough room between your knees and the helmet so that you can remove the helmet. Your partner should kneel on one side of the patient, at the shoulder area.
2. Stabilize the helmet by placing your hands on either side of it, with your fingers on the patient's lower jaw to prevent movement of the head. Once your hands are in position, your partner can loosen the face strap.
3. Your partner should open the face shield, if there is one, and assess the patient's airway and breathing. Remove eyeglasses if the patient is wearing them.

4. Once the strap is loosened, your partner should place one hand on the patient's lower jaw at the angle of the jaw and the other behind the head at the back of the helmet. You may then pull the sides of the helmet away from the patient's head **Figure 46A**.
5. Gently slip the helmet partly off the patient's head, stopping when the helmet reaches the halfway point.
6. Your partner then slides his or her hand from the back of the helmet to the occiput, preventing the head from falling back once the helmet is completely removed **Figure 46B**.
7. Once your partner's hand is in place, remove the helmet and provide manual in-line cervical spine stabilization **Figure 46C**.
8. Apply a rigid cervical collar and secure the patient to the backboard.
9. With large helmets or small patients, you may need to add padding under the shoulders to prevent flexion of the neck. If the patient is wearing shoulder pads or a heavy jacket, you may need to pad behind the head to prevent extension of the neck.

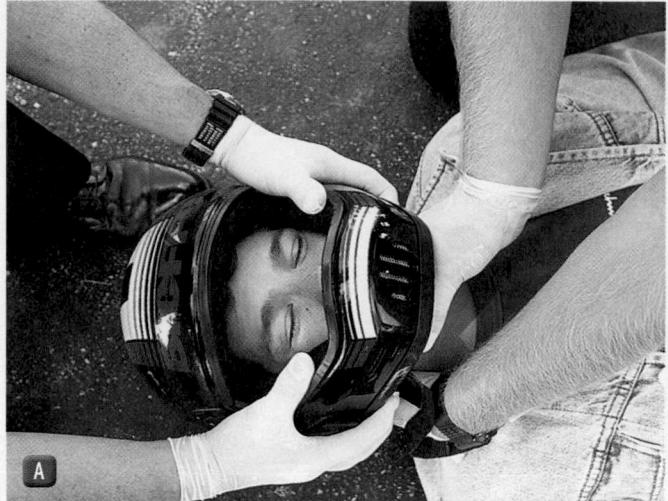

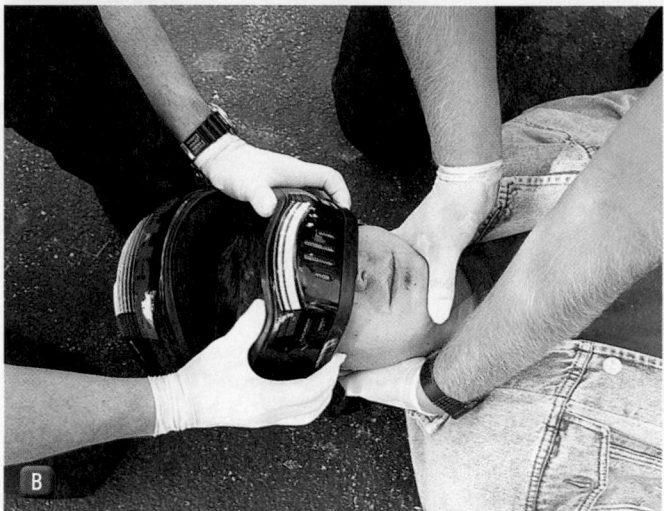

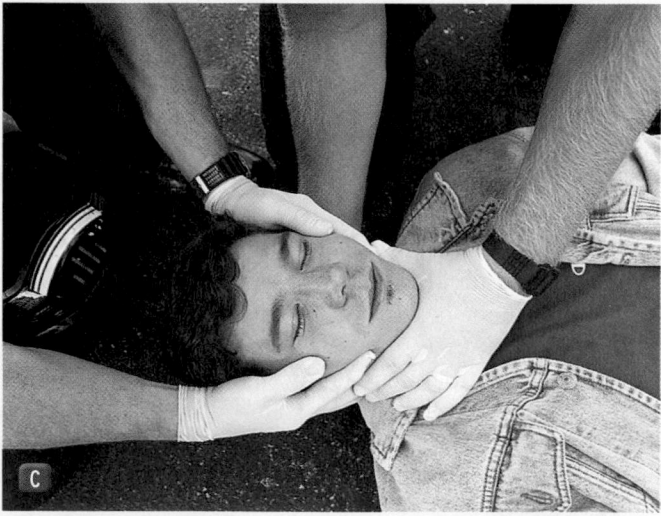

Figure 46 Removing a helmet. **A.** Spread the helmet to clear the ears while the other rescuer stabilizes the neck. **B.** Remove the helmet carefully, clearing the nose. **C.** Now take over manual in-line cervical spine stabilization.

You do not need to remove a helmet if you can access the patient's airway, the head is snug inside the helmet, and the helmet can be secured to an immobilization device. If the patient is wearing padding, keep in mind that the padding and the helmet may work together to provide alignment of the spine. Removal of one without removing the other may cause inadvertent misalignment. If you are able to remove the face mask of the helmet to control the airway and the posterior padding does not prevent treatment, it may be better to leave both of these protection devices in place until after the spine has been cleared using radiographic modalities.

Words of Wisdom

When you encounter a patient with a helmet, note whether he or she is wearing a special removal device in the helmet, such as the Eject Helmet Removal System. This device contains a small air bladder that is placed inside the top of the helmet. An air tube descends from the bladder down the right side of the helmet. Should it become necessary for an emergency provider to remove the helmet, he or she must first cut the helmet's chin strap and remove the patient's goggles or eyeglasses. The provider attaches the inflator bulb to the Eject tube connector, inflating the bladder to gently lift the helmet off the patient's head.

■ Pharmacotherapy of Spinal Cord Injury

Short-acting, reversible sedatives are recommended for the acute agitated patient after a correctible cause of agitation (eg, hypoxia) has been excluded. The risk of secondary injury due to movements from acute agitation must be balanced with potential airway and ventilatory compromise as well as a reliable neurologic exam. Pain medication may also be necessary.

Corticosteroids are anti-inflammatory agents that are sometimes still used in the acute phase of SCI. However, many recent protocols avoid their use as they are more likely to lead to significant complication than to improved outcome, particularly in cases of penetrating trauma.

■ Complications of Spinal Cord Injury

The complications of SCI are a consistent cause of the high morbidity and mortality—and high financial cost—associated with this type of injury. Many of the acute-phase complications of SCI have already been addressed in this chapter, such as the potential for aspiration or respiratory arrest, especially with high cervical injuries. Lower cervical lesions may preserve the diaphragm, but the loss of intercostal muscles ultimately impairs coughing and deep breathing, predisposing the patient to atelectasis and pneumonia. Deep vein

Controversies

Considerable controversy exists regarding whether to remove helmets in the field. The key considerations boil down to the urgency of airway management, the fit of the helmet, and the best-trained hands to take it off.

thrombosis and pulmonary embolism are late complications that may result from immobility and can become potentially life threatening.

<u>Autonomic dysreflexia</u>, also called autonomic hyperreflexia, is typically a late complication of SCI but can occur acutely. This potentially life-threatening emergency most commonly occurs with injuries above T4–T6 and results from the loss of parasympathetic stimulation. Patients present clinically with evidence of a massive, uninhibited, uncompensated cardiovascular response due to some stimulation of the sympathetic nervous system below the level of injury (Table 9). The irritated area sends a signal that is not able to reach the brain, and unabated sympathetic nervous system stimulation results in vasoconstriction as evidenced by cool, pale extremities, systolic blood pressures of greater than 200 mm Hg, and diastolic blood pressures of 130 mm Hg or greater. Hypertension leads to parasympathetic stimulation from activation of the vasomotor center in the medulla. Vagal compensation causes bradycardia and vasodilation of peripheral and visceral vessels above the level of the lesion, although vessels below the SCI remain constricted. Selective vasodilation results in flushed, diaphoretic skin and nasopharyngeal vessel congestion.

Autonomic dysreflexia can be precipitated by any noxious stimuli below the level of a cervical or high thoracic SCI. Common precipitators include skin lesions such as insect bites, constrictive clothing, or sharp objects compressing the skin. Sharp objects should be removed from pockets or seat cushions. Localized wounds such as lacerations, abrasions, decubitus ulcerations, or ingrown toenails are often the source of stimulation. Irritation from skin lesions should be minimized with cold packs. Distention of the bladder due to obstructed urine outflow from spasm or kinked indwelling catheters as well as bladder infection, constipation, or bowel impaction must be suspected. Catheters should be irrigated and obstructions removed. In men, tight condom catheters can pinch genitalia and should be checked and removed if necessary. In women, menstrual cramps or pregnancy can be a source of the stimulation.

Management of autonomic dysreflexia is usually not a prehospital intervention. If the source cannot be found or minimized to an effective extent, it may be necessary to reduce blood pressure with vasodilators.

Controversies

Classic education holds that intervertebral disks have no sensory nerve fibers. In reality, sensory nerves extend into the disk over at least one third the radius of the outer rim, the anulus fibrosus. In the clinical setting, it is impossible to tell whether low back pain is coming solely from the irritation of these nerves. However, this etiology is always a possibility, even if MRI and CT scans show no damage. Injury to these nerves occurs at a microscopic level that is undetectable on standard tests.

Nontraumatic Spinal Conditions

Back pain is one of the most common physical complaints in emergency departments throughout the United States. An estimated 60% to 90% of the US population is afflicted with some form of low back pain. Expenses related to back pain are high due to the extensive costs of therapy and lost wages from missed work days. Upright posture brings a significant amount of weight to bear on the lumbar spine—specifically at L4–L5, where the natural bend in the spine's curvature changes. As a consequence, most people are susceptible to injury or degenerative disease. Spinal tumors can also be a cause of pain and debilitation. Occupations that require repetitive lifting, exposure to vibrations from vehicles or industrial machinery, and comorbid diseases such as osteoporosis are all risks for developing low back pain. Most cases of low back pain are idiopathic, and making a precise diagnosis can be difficult.

When you are evaluating nontraumatic back pain, it is important to consider disease processes that can result in significantly debilitating lesions, including SCI (Table 10). In the absence of trauma, the patient who presents with the complaint of low back pain must be assessed with you keeping the anatomy and neurophysiology of the spine and spinal cord in mind. Pay particular attention to the medications the patient is taking because patients with chronic back pain and tumors may require high levels of narcotics to control the intense pain.

Pain may result from <u>strain</u> or <u>sprain</u> of paravertebral muscles and supporting ligamentous structures without significant injury to nerve elements. Older patients (especially women) with a history of osteoporosis are at high risk for spontaneous compression fractures of the spine; these typically stable fractures are not associated with SCI. Furthermore, tumors in the spine from a variety of metastatic carcinomas can cause

Table 9 Signs and Symptoms of Autonomic Dysreflexia
Hypertension
Headache
Nasal congestion
Dilation of the pupils
Anxiety
Bradycardia
Rebound hypotension
Flushing and sweating above SCI
Erect hairs above SCI
Chills without fever
Bronchospasm
Seizures, stroke, and death

Table 10 Common Causes of Low Back Pain

Muscle or ligament strains
Fractures
Osteomyelitis–bone infection
Degenerative joint/disk disease
Spondylolysis
Bursitis/synovitis
Disk herniation
Tumor

Words of Wisdom

Spondylolysis is a structural defect of the spine involving the lamina or vertebral arch. It usually occurs between the superior and inferior articulating facets. In most people, it is congenital and therefore chronic. A radiograph is necessary to confirm spondylolysis.

pathologic spine fractures, with extension of bone fragments or the tumor itself into the spinal canal causing SCI.

Degenerative disk disease is a common entity in patients older than 50 years. Over time, biomechanical alterations of the intervertebral disk will result in loss of height and reduce the shock-absorbing effect of the disk. Significant narrowing may result in variable segment stability.

Disk herniation may be caused by some degree of trauma in patients with preexisting disk degeneration. It typically affects men between ages 30 and 50 years, and may result from poor lifting technique. Herniation most commonly occurs at L4–L5 and L5–S1 but may also occur in C5–C6 and C6–C7. Patients will present with pain, usually with straining; they may have tenderness of the spine and often have limited range of motion. Alterations in sensation and motor functions may exist as well. Cervical herniations may present with upper extremity pain or paresthesias that worsen with neck motion. Motor weakness may also occur due to spinal cord compression.

Definitive diagnosis of back pain may require multiple modalities of radiographic imaging. Prehospital management of low back pain in the absence of trauma is primarily palliative, directed at decreasing any pain or discomfort with movement. Patients who experience significant pain with movement or have neurologic deficits may benefit from spinal immobilization to prevent irritation of neural elements. Be aware that immobilization may also be associated with increased back pain, however.

Words of Wisdom

Some patients with acute low back spasm are literally paralyzed with pain. To move them, use a "scoop-type" metal stretcher that fits under the patient. Administration of IV diazepam may be extremely helpful in relieving severe muscle spasm.

■ Injury Prevention

Prevention of head and spine trauma includes general safety measures that can decrease overall risk of injury. Driving safely can reduce the likelihood of spinal injury, a multitude of other injuries, and death. Motorcycles and all-terrain vehicles should not be ridden by two persons on the same vehicle; there should only be one rider. Finally, adhering to posted safety alerts, such as those regarding safe diving at swimming pools, can also help reduce the occurrence of injuries.

YOU *are the Medic* | SUMMARY

1. Given the updated information, what should you consider doing?

If you have not already done so, it would be appropriate to request additional resources because this patient's condition is critical and he will require spinal precautions.

2. What safety concerns do you have?

Dim lighting, slick surfaces, and the pool are all causes for concern. With the presence of an emotional crowd, you should maintain situational awareness. Although the police have deemed the scene as safe, it is your and your partner's responsibility to remain aware of your surroundings.

3. What injuries do you suspect?

Given the nature of the scene and the primary assessment of your patient, it is highly likely that he has a high cervical spine fracture.

4. What interventions are required?

Airway stabilization and spinal precautions are immediately indicated. Additionally, if the patient is unable to oxygenate well, the use of a bag-mask device with high-flow oxygen and airway adjuncts is warranted. As with any call, start with the basics.

5. Why is the patient bradycardic and hypotensive?

The patient has neurogenic shock. The cervical spinal cord injury has disrupted the communication of the brain and the body. The sympathetic nervous system has been blocked, resulting in vasodilation and bradycardia.

6. How would you manage these vital signs?

Establish intravenous access with two large-bore catheters and provide a 20 mL/kg bolus of crystalloids such as normal saline or lactated Ringer's. Do not be surprised if this fails to improve the patient's blood pressure because these patients will likely require vasopressors such as dopamine or norepinephrine. To improve cardiac effects, administering atropine or performing transcutaneous pacing can be considered. The routine use of IV glucocorticoids such as methylprednisolone (Solu-Medrol) is controversial, and as with all interventions, should be done according to local protocols.

7. What other immediate treatments are required?

The patient is at high risk for hypothermia, not only because his blood vessels are dilated due to lack of sympathetic tone, but also because he is wet and naked. Dry the patient, cover him with blankets, and ensure the ambulance is warm. Hypothermia impairs hemoglobin from off-loading oxygen, worsening the patient's condition.

8. On the basis of the events, what additional factors could complicate the patient's outcome?

The presence of alcohol and possibly drugs not only cloud a patient's judgment but make it difficult for a patient to be aware of all injuries. Therefore, the information you obtain from the patient history is most likely unreliable. Additionally, with all shallow water diving incidents, head injuries as well as spinal trauma must be considered.

YOU are the Medic   SUMMARY, continued

EMS Patient Care Report (PCR)

Date: 05-01-11	Incident No.: 7728	Nature of Call: Diving injury		Location: Clarke County Swimming Pool	
Dispatched: 0130	En Route: 0133	At Scene: 0135	Transport: 0152	At Hospital: 0207	In Service: 0222

Patient Information

Age: 19 Sex: M Weight (in kg [lb]): 75 kg (165 lb)	Allergies: No known drug allergies Medications: None Past Medical History: None Chief Complaint: Unresponsive

Vital Signs

Time: 0135	BP:	Pulse: 50	Respirations: Fast	Spo$_2$: 86
Time: 0140	BP: 70/p	Pulse: 42	Respirations:	Spo$_2$: None
Time: 0152	BP: 72/p	Pulse: 40	Respirations:	Spo$_2$: None
Time: 0145	BP: 70/p	Pulse: 42	Respirations:	Spo$_2$: None

EMS Treatment
(circle all that apply)

Oxygen @ __15__ L/min via (circle one): NC NRM Bag-mask device With high-flow oxygen	Assisted Ventilation: Yes	Airway Adjunct: OPA followed by ETI	CPR
Defibrillation	Bleeding Control: No external hemorrhage noted	Bandaging: 4 × 4 to head abrasion	Splinting: Long backboard	Other

Narrative

Dispatched to an unknown incident at Clarke County Swimming Pool. Arrived to find 19-year-old male lying face up next to the pool in obvious respiratory distress. According to witnesses, pt dove headfirst into the pool; under water for approximately 30 seconds; pt was pulled from the water by witnesses; according to witnesses, pt consumed "a couple beers" at approximately 2400 hours; no known drug allergies, no known PMH.

  Pt unresponsive, skin, wet/flushed. Addressed ABCs w/cervical spine precautions. Suspect possible head injury/c-spine injury with neurogenic shock. Called for additional assistance.

HEENT—quarter-sized abrasion to right forehead, no major bleeding, otherwise atraumatic, PEARRL (sluggish) 4 mm, no tracheal deviation or JVD, cx accessory muscle use present, breath sounds diminished bilaterally, equal excursion, no apparent trauma, abdomen, soft, no distention/rigidity, pelvis stable, loss of bowel and bladder; no motor function or reflexes present in upper or lower extremities, weak, slow pulses present in upper extremities only; back no obvious injuries noted.

  Immobilized on LSB with p/m/s assessed before and after with no changes. Moved to ambulance. Vital signs as noted above. ETI with 8.0 mm ETT depth of 21 at the teeth. Two large-bore IVs with 1,500-mL NS bolus administered. Orders for dopamine 15 mcg/kg/min. Released to trauma center staff. **End of report**

Prep Kit

- The skull is a rigid, unyielding box that does not accommodate a swelling brain or accumulations of blood.

- Be familiar with high-risk mechanisms of injury that can cause head injury, brain injury, and spinal cord injury, such as motor vehicle crashes, falls, and penetrating trauma. Full spinal motion restriction should be applied unless there is a compelling reason not to.

- Airway is a priority; maintain the head and neck in neutral alignment while you are suctioning and performing airway management. Consider endotracheal intubation in patients with spinal injuries, but remember that endotracheal intubation requires special precautions in patients with head injuries because it may precipitate a dangerous rise in intracranial pressure.

- Control major bleeding without placing pressure on a potential underlying fracture. Provide fluid resuscitation, but restrict use of IV fluids in patients with severe closed head injuries to minimize cerebral edema; however, avoid hypotension.

- Transport patients with severe injuries promptly to a trauma center. Use lights and siren cautiously; a siren could precipitate seizures and exacerbate intracranial pressure.

- Level of consciousness should continuously be assessed, including repeat assessments of the Glasgow Coma Scale score and pupillary assessment. Secondary assessment may include a full-body exam and a neurologic exam.

- Head injuries include skull fractures (linear, depressed, basilar, and open) and traumatic brain injury (cerebral concussion, diffuse axonal injury, cerebral contusion, and intracranial hemorrhage).

- Normal intracranial pressure is 0 to 15 mm Hg in adults. Increased intracranial pressure can squeeze the brain against the interior of the skull and/or press it into sharp edges within the cranium. If severely increased intracranial pressure is not promptly treated, cerebral herniation will occur.

- Cerebral perfusion pressure is the pressure of blood flowing through the brain; it is the difference between the mean arterial pressure and intracranial pressure.

- If the cerebral perfusion pressure drops below 60 mm Hg in the adult, cerebral ischemia will likely occur, increasing the risk of permanent brain damage or death.

- Begin treatment of a head-injured patient by stabilizing the cervical spine, opening the airway with the jaw-thrust maneuver, and assessing the ABCs.

- All head-injured patients should receive 100% oxygen as soon as possible. If the patient is breathing adequately, apply a nonrebreathing mask set at 15 L/min. If the patient is breathing inadequately, assist ventilation and consider intubation.

- Ventilate a brain-injured adult at a rate of 10 breaths/min. Avoid routine hyperventilation unless signs of cerebral herniation are present. Hyperventilation in a brain-injured adult is defined as a ventilation rate of 20 breaths/min.

- Restrict IV fluids in a head-injured patient unless hypotension (systolic blood pressure of less than 90 mm Hg) is present. Hypotension in a brain-injured patient should be treated with crystalloid fluid boluses in a quantity sufficient to maintain a systolic blood pressure of at least 90 mm Hg.

- Frequently monitor a head-injured patient's level of consciousness, and document your findings. The Glasgow Coma Scale is an effective, reliable tool. Assessment using the Glasgow Coma Scale must be repeated frequently if the score is to be a reliable indicator of the patient's clinical progression.

- Intubation of a brain-injured patient may require pharmacologic adjuncts (such as sedation, neuromuscular blocking drugs).

- Seizures may occur in a brain-injured patient and can aggravate intracranial pressure and cause or worsen cerebral ischemia. Treat seizures with a benzodiazepine (such as diazepam, lorazepam).

- A brain-injured patient's survival depends on recognition of the injury, prompt and aggressive prehospital care, and rapid transport to a trauma center that has neurosurgical capabilities. Consider air transport if ground transport time will be prolonged.

- Do not become distracted by scalp lacerations. Once life threats are managed, evaluate the wound for continued bleeding. With isolated fractures not involving suspected skull fracture, apply direct pressure and use a pressure dressing or hemostatic agent if required.

- Spinal cord injuries are among the most devastating injuries encountered by prehospital providers. In order to decipher the often subtle findings associated with a spinal cord injury, you need to understand the form and function of spinal anatomy.

- Acute injuries of the spine are classified according to the associated mechanism, location, and stability of injury.

- Vertebral fractures can occur with or without associated spinal cord injury.

- Stable fractures typically involve only a single column and pose a lower risk to the spinal cord.

- Primary spinal cord injury occurs at the moment of impact. Secondary spinal cord injury occurs when multiple factors permit a progression of the primary spinal cord injury. The ensuing cascade of inflammatory responses may result in further deterioration.

- Limiting the progression of secondary spinal cord injury is a major goal of prehospital management of spinal cord injury.

- Current principles of spine trauma management include recognition of potential or actual injury, appropriate immobilization, and reduction or prevention of the incidence of secondary injury.

- Short-acting, reversible sedatives are recommended for the acute patient after a correctible cause of agitation has been excluded.

- The use of corticosteroids in the acute phase of spinal cord injury is controversial.

- The complications of spinal cord injury are a consistent cause of the high morbidity and mortality associated with this type of injury.

- Back pain is one of the most common physical complaints to present to emergency departments throughout the United States. Most cases of low back pain are idiopathic and difficult to precisely diagnose.

■ Vital Vocabulary

anterior cord syndrome A condition that occurs with flexion injuries or fractures, resulting in the displacement of bony fragments into the anterior portion of the spinal cord; findings include paralysis below the level of the insult and loss of pain, temperature, and touch sensation.

anterograde (posttraumatic) amnesia Loss of memory relating to events that occurred after the injury.

arachnoid The middle membrane of the three meninges that enclose the brain and spinal cord.

auditory ossicles The bones that function in hearing and are located deep within cavities of the temporal bone.

autonomic dysreflexia A potentially life-threatening late complication of spinal cord injury in which a massive, uninhibited, uncompensated cardiovascular response occurs due to stimulation of the sympathetic nervous system below the level of injury; also known as autonomic hyperreflexia.

autoregulation An increase in mean arterial pressure to compensate for decreased cerebral perfusion pressure; compensatory response of the body to shunt blood to the brain; manifests clinically as hypertension.

axon Long, slender extension of a neuron (nerve cell) that conducts electrical impulses away from the neuronal soma.

Babinski reflex When the toe(s) moves upward in response to stimulation to the sole of the foot. Under normal circumstances, the toe(s) moves downward.

basal ganglia Structures located deep within the cerebrum, diencephalon, and midbrain that have an important role in coordination of motor movements and posture.

basilar skull fractures Usually occur following diffuse impact to the head (such as falls, motor vehicle crashes); generally result from extension of a linear fracture to the base of the skull and can be difficult to diagnose with a radiograph (x-ray).

Battle sign Bruising over the mastoid bone behind the ear commonly seen following a basilar skull fracture; also called retroauricular ecchymosis.

Biot respirations Characterized by an irregular rate, pattern, and volume of breathing with intermittent periods of apnea; also called ataxic respirations.

brain Part of the central nervous system located within the cranium; contains billions of neurons that serve a variety of vital functions.

brainstem The midbrain, pons, and medulla, collectively.

Brown-Séquard syndrome A condition associated with penetrating trauma with hemisection of the spinal cord and complete damage to all spinal tracts on the involved side.

cauda equina The location where the spinal cord separates, composed of nerve roots.

cauda equina syndrome A neurologic condition caused by compression of the bundle of nerve roots located at the end of the spinal cord.

central cord syndrome A condition resulting from hyperextension injuries to the cervical area that cause damage with hemorrhage or edema to the central cervical segments; findings include greater loss of function in the upper extremities with variable sensory loss of pain and temperature.

central nervous system (CNS) The system containing the brain and spinal cord.

central neurogenic hyperventilation Deep, rapid respirations; similar to Kussmaul, but without an acetone breath odor; commonly seen following brainstem injury.

cerebellum The region of the brain essential in coordinating muscle movements in the body; also called the athlete's brain.

cerebral concussion Occurs when the brain is jarred around in the skull; a mild diffuse brain injury that does not result in structural damage or permanent neurologic impairment.

cerebral contusion A focal brain injury in which brain tissue is bruised and damaged in a defined area.

cerebral cortex The largest portion of the cerebrum; regulates voluntary skeletal movement and one's level of awareness—a part of consciousness.

cerebral edema Cerebral water; causes or contributes to swelling of the brain.

cerebral perfusion pressure (CPP) The pressure of blood flow through the brain; the difference between the mean arterial pressure (MAP) and intracranial pressure (ICP).

cerebrospinal fluid (CSF) Fluid produced in the ventricles of the brain that flows in the subarachnoid space and bathes the meninges.

cerebrum The largest portion of the brain; responsible for higher functions, such as reasoning; divided into right and left hemispheres, or halves.

Cheyne-Stokes respirations The respirations that are fast and then become slow, with intervening periods of apnea; commonly seen following brainstem injury.

choroid plexus Specialized cells within the hollow areas in the ventricles of the brain that produce cerebrospinal fluid.

complete spinal cord injury Total disruption of all tracts of the spinal cord, with all cord-mediated functions below the level of transection lost permanently.

coronal suture The point where the parietal bones join with the frontal bone.

coup-contrecoup injury Dual impacting of the brain into the skull; coup injury occurs at the point of impact; contrecoup injury occurs on the opposite side of impact, as the brain rebounds.

cranial vault The bones that encase and protect the brain, including the parietal, temporal, frontal, occipital, sphenoid, and ethmoid bones; also called the cranium or skull.

cribriform plate A horizontal bone perforated with numerous foramina for the passage of the olfactory nerve filaments from the nasal cavity.

crista galli A prominent bony ridge in the center of the anterior fossa and the point of attachment of the meninges.

critical minimum threshold Minimum cerebral perfusion pressure required to adequately perfuse the brain; 60 mm Hg in the adult.

Cushing triad Hypertension (with a widening pulse pressure), bradycardia, and irregular respirations; classic trio of findings associated with increased intracranial pressure.

decerebrate (extensor) posturing Abnormal posture characterized by extension of the arms and legs; indicates pressure on the brainstem.

decorticate (flexor) posturing Abnormal posture characterized by flexion of the arms and extension of the legs; indicates pressure on the brainstem.

depressed skull fractures Result from high-energy direct trauma to a small surface area of the head with a blunt object (such as a baseball bat to the head); commonly result in bony fragments being driven into the brain, causing injury.

dermatomes Areas of the body innervated by sensor components of spinal nerves.

diencephalon The part of the brain between the brainstem and the cerebrum that includes the thalamus, subthalamus, and hypothalamus.

diffuse axonal injury (DAI) Diffuse brain injury that is caused by stretching, shearing, or tearing of nerve fibers with subsequent axonal damage.

diffuse brain injury Any injury that affects the entire brain.

dura mater The outermost layer of the three meninges that enclose the brain and spinal cord; it is the toughest meningeal layer.

epidural hematoma An accumulation of blood between the skull and dura.

facet joint The joint on which each vertebra articulates with adjacent vertebrae.

flexion injury A type of injury that results from forward movement of the head, typically as the result of rapid deceleration, such as in a car crash, or with a direct blow to the occiput.

focal brain injury A specific, grossly observable brain injury.

fontanelles The soft spots in the skull of a newborn and infant where the sutures of the skull have not yet grown together.

foramen magnum The large opening at the base of the skull through which the spinal cord exits the brain.

foramina Small natural openings, perforations, or orifices, such as in the bones of the cranial vault; plural of foramen.

frontal lobe The portion of the brain that is important in voluntary motor actions and personality traits.

galea aponeurotica Tough, tendinous layer of the scalp.

Glasgow Coma Scale (GCS) A widely accepted method of assessing level of consciousness that is based on three independent measurements: eye opening, verbal response, and motor response.

hard palate The bony anterior part of the roof of the mouth.

head injury A traumatic insult to the head that may result in injury to soft tissue, bony structures, or the brain.

herniation Process in which tissue is forced out of its normal position, such as when the brain is forced from the cranial vault, either through the foramen magnum or over the tentorium.

hyperesthesia Hyperacute pain to touch.

hyperextension Extension of a limb or other body part beyond its usual range of motion.

hyperpyrexia A high body temperature.

hypothalamus The most inferior portion of the diencephalon; responsible for control of many body functions, including heart rate, digestion, sexual development, temperature regulation, emotion, hunger, thirst, and regulation of the sleep cycle.

incomplete spinal cord injury Spinal cord injury in which there is some degree of cord-mediated function; initial dysfunction may be temporary and there may be potential for recovery.

intracerebral hematoma Bleeding within the brain tissue (parenchyma) itself; also referred to as an intraparenchymal hematoma.

intracranial pressure (ICP) The pressure within the cranial vault; normally 0 to 15 mm Hg in adults.

lambdoid suture The point where the occipital bones attach to the parietal bones.

lamina Arise from the posterior pedicles and fuse to form the posterior spinous processes.

limbic system Structures within the cerebrum and diencephalon that influence emotions, motivation, mood, and sensations of pain and pleasure.

linear skull fractures Account for 80% of skull fractures; also referred to as nondisplaced skull fractures; commonly occur in the temporal-parietal region of the skull; not associated with deformities to the skull.

mastoid process A cone-shaped section of bone at the base of the temporal bone.

mean arterial pressure (MAP) The average (or mean) pressure against the arterial wall during a cardiac cycle.

medulla Continuous inferiorly with the spinal cord; serves as a conduction pathway for ascending and descending nerve tracts; coordinates heart rate, blood vessel diameter, breathing, swallowing, vomiting, coughing, and sneezing.

meninges A set of three tough membranes, the dura mater, arachnoid, and pia mater, that encloses the entire brain and spinal cord.

myotomes Regions of the body innervated by the motor components of spinal nerves.

nasal cavity The chamber inside the nose that lies between the floor of the cranium and the roof of the mouth.

nerve root injury Injury to a nerve at the level of the spinal cord.

neurogenic shock Shock caused by massive vasodilation and pooling of blood in the peripheral vessels to the extent that adequate perfusion cannot be maintained.

neuronal soma The body of a neuron (nerve cell).

occipital condyles Articular surfaces on the occipital bone in which the skull articulates with the atlas on the vertebral column.

occipital lobe The portion of the brain that is responsible for the processing of visual information.

olfactory nerves Nerves that participate in the transmission of scent impulses.

palatine bone An irregularly shaped bone found in the posterior part of the nasal cavity.

parasympathetic nervous system Subdivision of the autonomic nervous system; involved in control of involuntary, vegetative functions, mediated largely by the vagus nerve through the chemical acetylcholine.

parietal lobe The portion of the brain that is the site for reception and evaluation of most sensory information, except smell, hearing, and vision.

pedicles Thick lateral bony struts that connect the vertebral body with the spinous and transverse processes and make up the lateral and posterior portions of the spinal foramen.

periorbital ecchymosis Bruising under or around the orbits that is commonly seen following a basilar skull fracture; also called raccoon eyes.

peripheral nerve injury Injury to a nerve anywhere in the body that is outside of the spinal cord.

pia mater The innermost and thinnest of the three meninges that enclose the brain and spinal cord; rests directly on the brain and spinal cord.

plexus A cluster of nerve roots that permits peripheral nerve roots to rejoin and function as a group.

pons Lies below the midbrain and above the medulla and contains numerous important nerve fibers, including those for sleep, respiration, and the medullary respiratory center.

posterior cord syndrome A condition associated with extension injuries with isolated injury to the dorsal column; presents as decreased sensation to light touch, proprioception, and vibration while leaving most other motor and sensory functions intact.

posterior spinous process Formed by the fusion of the posterior lamina, this is an attachment site for muscles and ligaments.

primary brain injury An injury to the brain and its associated structures that is a direct result of impact to the head.

primary spinal cord injury Injury to the spinal cord that is a direct result of trauma—for example, transection of the spinal cord from penetrating trauma or displacement of ligaments and bone fragments, resulting in compression of the spinal cord.

proprioception The ability to perceive the position and movement of one's body or limbs.

raccoon eyes Bruising under or around the orbits that is commonly seen following a basilar skull fracture; also called periorbital ecchymosis.

reticular activating system (RAS) Located in the upper brainstem; responsible for maintenance of consciousness, specifically one's level of arousal.

retrograde amnesia Loss of memory relating to events that occurred before the injury.

rotation-flexion injury A type of injury typically resulting from high acceleration forces; can result in a stable unilateral facet dislocation in the cervical spine.

sagittal suture The point of the skull where the parietal bones join.

secondary brain injury The "after effects" of the primary injury; includes abnormal processes such as cerebral edema, increased intracranial pressure, cerebral ischemia and hypoxia, and infection; onset is often delayed following the primary brain injury.

secondary spinal cord injury Injury to the spinal cord, thought to be the result of multiple factors that result in a progression of inflammatory responses from primary spinal cord injury.

skull The structure at the top of the axial skeleton that houses the brain and consists of 28 bones that comprise the auditory ossicles, the cranium, and the face.

spinal clearance The act of declaring that a spinal injury is not present.

spinal cord The part of the central nervous system that extends downward from the brain through the foramen magnum and is protected by the spine.

spinal shock The temporary local neurologic condition that occurs immediately after spinal trauma; swelling and edema of the spinal cord begin immediately after injury, with severe pain and potential paralysis.

sprain Stretching or tearing of ligaments.

strain Stretching or tearing of muscle or tendon.

subarachnoid hemorrhage Bleeding into the subarachnoid space, where the cerebrospinal fluid circulates.

subarachnoid space The space located between the pia mater and the arachnoid.

subdural hematoma An accumulation of blood beneath the dura but outside the brain.

subgaleal hemorrhage Bleeding between the periosteum of the skull and the galea aponeurosis.

subluxation A partial dislocation.

subthalamus The part of the diencephalon that is involved in controlling motor functions.

supragaleal hematoma Bleeding between the subgaleal area of the skull and the galea aponeurosis.

sympathetic nervous system Subdivision of the autonomic nervous system that governs the body's fight-or-flight reactions by inducing smooth muscle contraction or relaxation of the blood vessels and bronchioles.

temporal lobe The portion of the brain that has an important role in hearing and memory.

tentorium A structure that separates the cerebral hemispheres from the cerebellum and brainstem.

thalamus The part of the diencephalon that processes most sensory input and influences mood and general body movements, especially those associated with fear or rage.

transverse spinous process The junction of each pedicle and lamina on each side of a vertebra; these project laterally and posteriorly and form points of attachment for muscles and ligaments.

traumatic brain injury (TBI) A traumatic insult to the brain capable of producing physical, intellectual, emotional, social, and vocational changes.

trismus Clenching of the teeth owing to spasm of the jaw muscles.

ventricles Specialized hollow areas in the brain.

vertebral body Anterior weight-bearing structure in the spine made of cancellous bone and surrounded by a layer of hard, compact bone that provides support and stability.

vertical compression A type of injury typically resulting from a direct blow to the crown of the skull or rapid deceleration from a fall through the feet, legs, and pelvis, possibly causing a burst fracture or disk herniation.

zygomatic arch The bone that extends along the front of the skull below the orbit.

Assessment in Action

It is 8:45 AM when you are dispatched for a LifeLine activation at 310 Summit Point Avenue. You arrive to a secured residence with no evidence that it is occupied. You have been here several times for "false activations," and after knocking on the door and looking in all of the windows, you see no one and believe this is another false alarm. Just as you are notifying dispatch, a concerned family member runs up to you saying, "I know she's in there! She calls me every morning at 8:00 AM, and I haven't heard from her today."

Because you cannot gain entry into the house, you place a call for law enforcement assistance. The police arrive, break a locked window, and gain entry into the home. As you and your partner enter the home, you hear cries for help. You find an elderly woman in the upstairs bathroom with a hematoma to her forehead and no other obvious injuries. She tells you she slipped and struck the front of her head on the bathtub. Now she's having trouble "making her arms work."

1. Which of the following syndromes is your patient exhibiting?
   A. Anterior cord syndrome
   B. Central cord syndrome
   C. Posterior cord syndrome
   D. Brown-Séquard syndrome

2. What other signs and symptoms may the patient exhibit?
   A. Loss of bowel and bladder function
   B. Loss of sensation to pain
   C. Loss of sensation to temperature
   D. All of the above

3. What history may this patient have that could exacerbate her injury?
   A. Acute myocardial infarction
   B. Type 1 diabetes
   C. Type 2 diabetes
   D. Spondylosis

4. The patient's complaint about her arms can be attributed to disturbance of the:
   A. motor fibers.
   B. efferent fibers.
   C. Both A and B
   D. Neither A nor B

5. The prognosis for the patient's injury pattern includes:
   A. complete paralysis.
   B. death.
   C. weakness in the hands.
   D. weakness in the feet.

6. This type of injury is typically seen in:
   A. cervical or thoracic fractures.
   B. subluxations.
   C. tears to the supporting ligaments.
   D. young patients.

Additional Questions

7. How can routine calls place providers and patients at risk?

8. What are the legal implications of forced entry into a home?

9. When you are applying spinal precautions to an elderly patient, what considerations should be made?

Chest Trauma

National EMS Education Standard Competencies

Trauma

Integrates assessment findings with principles of epidemiology and pathophysiology to formulate a field impression to implement a comprehensive treatment/disposition plan for an acutely injured patient.

Chest Trauma

Recognition and management of

- Blunt vs penetrating mechanisms (pp 1698-1699)
- Open chest wound (pp 1706-1713)
- Impaled object (pp 1699-1701)

Pathophysiology, assessment, and management of

- Blunt vs penetrating mechanisms (pp 1698-1699)
- Hemothorax (p 1712)
- Pneumothorax (pp 1706-1712)
  - Open (pp 1707-1708)
  - Simple (pp 1706-1707)
  - Tension (pp 1708-1712)
- Cardiac tamponade (pp 1713-1714)
- Rib fractures (p 1705)
- Flail chest (pp 1703-1705)
- Commotio cordis (pp 1715-1716)
- Traumatic aortic disruption (pp 1716-1717)
- Pulmonary contusion (pp 1712-1713)
- Blunt cardiac injury (p 1715)
- Tracheobronchial disruption (p 1719)
- Diaphragmatic rupture (pp 1718-1719)
- Traumatic asphyxia (pp 1719-1720)

Knowledge Objectives

1. Review the anatomy and physiology of the chest. (pp 1695-1698)
2. Understand the mechanics of ventilation in relation to chest trauma. (pp 1698-1699)
3. Describe the assessment process for patients with chest trauma. (pp 1699-1703)
4. Discuss the significance of various signs and symptoms of chest trauma, including changes in pulse rate, dyspnea, jugular vein distention, muffled heart sounds, changes in blood pressure, diaphoresis or changes in pallor, hemoptysis, and changes in mental status. (pp 1699-1701)
5. Discuss the emergency medical care of a patient with chest trauma. (p 1703)
6. Discuss the pathophysiology, assessment, and management of chest wall injuries, including flail chest, rib fractures, sternal fractures, and clavicle fractures. (pp 1703-1706)
7. Discuss the pathophysiology, assessment, and management of lung injuries, including simple pneumothorax, open pneumothorax, tension pneumothorax, hemothorax, and pulmonary contusion. (pp 1706-1713)
8. Discuss the pathophysiology, assessment, and management of myocardial injuries, including cardiac tamponade, myocardial contusion, myocardial rupture, and commotio cordis. (pp 1713-1716)
9. Discuss the pathophysiology, assessment, and management of vascular injuries, including traumatic aortic disruption and penetrating wounds of the great vessels. (pp 1716-1718)
10. Discuss the pathophysiology, assessment, and management of other chest injuries, including diaphragmatic injury, esophageal injury, tracheobronchial injuries, and traumatic asphyxia. (pp 1718-1720)

Skills Objectives

1. Describe the steps to take in the assessment of a patient with suspected chest trauma. (pp 1699-1703)
2. Demonstrate the management of a patient with a tension pneumothorax using needle decompression. (pp 1709-1712, Skill Drill 1)

Introduction

Chest (thoracic) trauma is not a disease of modern society. For as long as humans have been capable of falling or injuring one another, damage to the thoracic cavity has been a significant concern in the management of the trauma patient. As more rapid forms of transportation and more lethal weapons continue to evolve, the incidence and severity of thoracic trauma are not likely to diminish, nor is the need for its rapid assessment and treatment.

Today, thoracic trauma accounts for a significant number of serious injuries and fatalities. According to the Centers for Disease Control and Prevention (CDC) Figure 1, thoracic trauma causes more than 700,000 emergency department visits and more than 18,000 deaths in the United States annually. The National Trauma Data Bank (NTDB) reported 135,733 traumatic incidents involving the thoracic region in 2010, representing 10.7% of all reported traumatic cases. Only traumatic brain injuries account for more deaths among trauma victims. An estimated one in four trauma deaths is directly due to thoracic injuries, and thoracic trauma is a contributing factor in another 25% of trauma patients who die of their injuries.

Given the specific organs that are housed within the thoracic cavity, it is not surprising that these injuries can be so deadly. In addition, the mechanism producing these injuries often involves a great deal of force transmitted to the body.

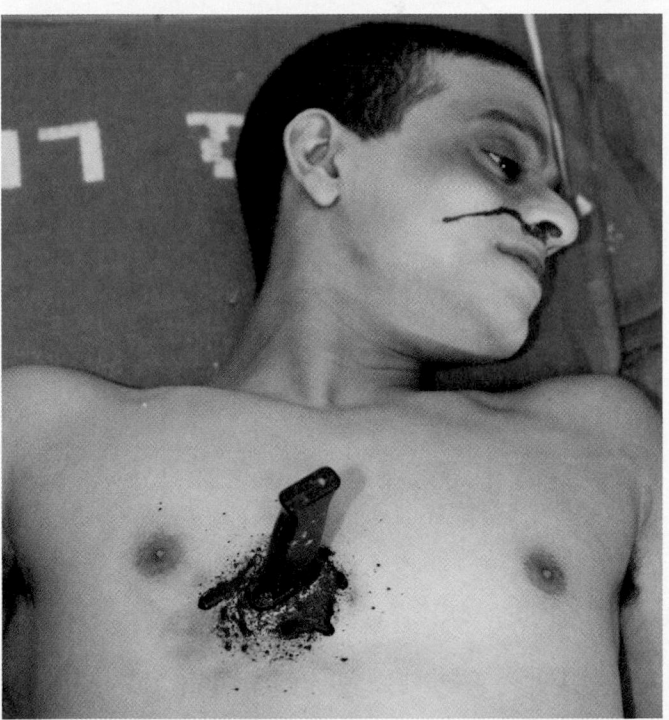

Figure 1 Today, thoracic trauma accounts for a significant number of serious injuries and fatalities.

Words of Wisdom

Thoracic injuries, whether severe or seemingly minor, often give rise to elusive findings that are overshadowed by associated injuries.

Anatomy

The **thorax** consists of a bony cage overlying some of the most vital organs in the human body. The dimensions of the thorax are defined posteriorly by the thoracic vertebrae and ribs, inferiorly by the diaphragm, anteriorly and laterally by the ribs, and superiorly by the **thoracic inlet** Figure 2.

The dimensions of this area of the body are of great importance in the physical assessment of the patient. Although the thoracic cavity extends to the twelfth rib posteriorly, the diaphragm inserts into the anterior thoracic cage just below the fourth or fifth rib. With the movement of the diaphragm during respiration, the size and dimensions of the thoracic cavity will vary, which could in turn affect the organs or cavities (thoracic versus abdominal) in case of blunt or penetrating injury Figure 3.

The bony structures of the thorax include the sternum, clavicle, scapula, thoracic vertebrae, and 12 pairs of ribs. The **sternum** consists of three separate portions: the superior **manubrium**, the central

YOU *are the Medic*   PART 1

Your unit is dispatched to meet with law enforcement personnel on the scene of a stabbing. When you arrive, an officer meets you and directs you to the patient. As you approach the patient, you see a man who appears to be about 40 years old. He is sitting upright, with his back against a wall and is conscious. The officer tells you that the patient is extremely intoxicated. A knife is protruding from his left anterior chest, just below the middle of the clavicle. The patient is actively trying to pull the knife out, with little success.

1. What is your primary concern for this patient?
2. What anatomic structures could be damaged in relation to the position of the knife?

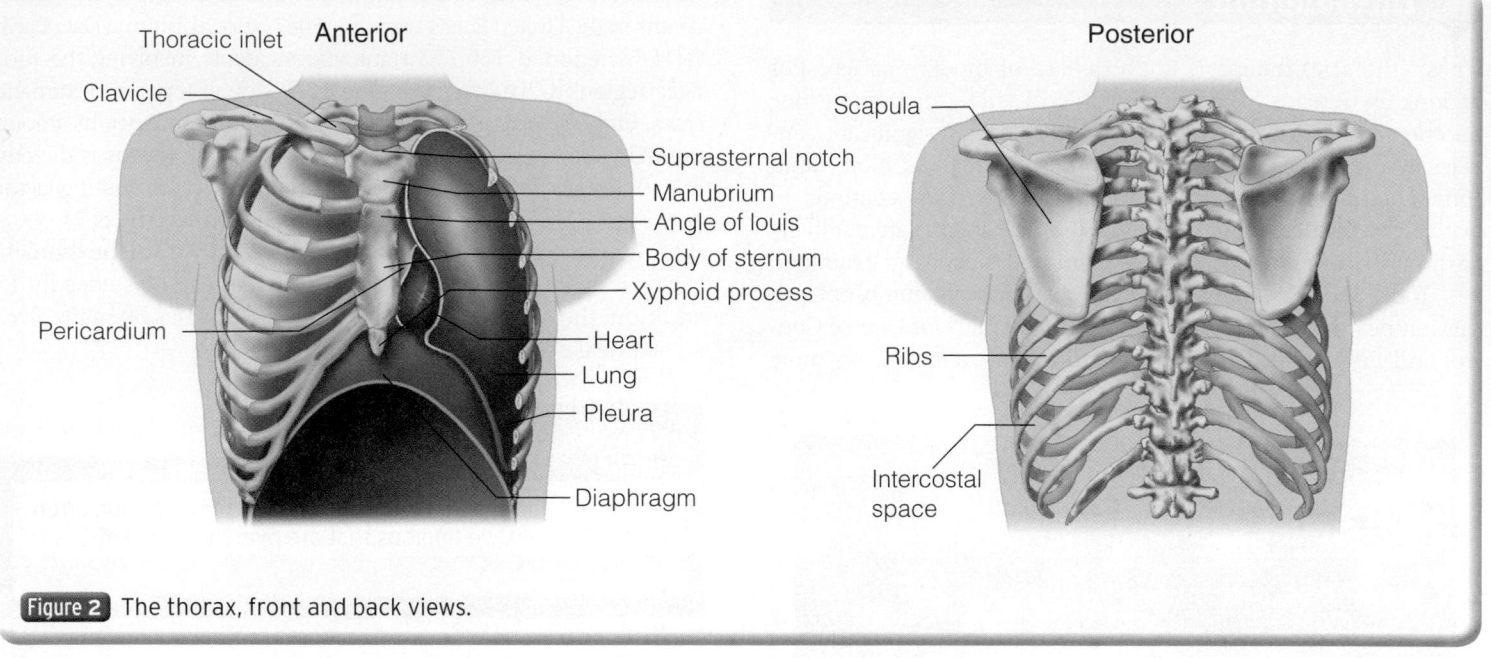

Figure 2 The thorax, front and back views.

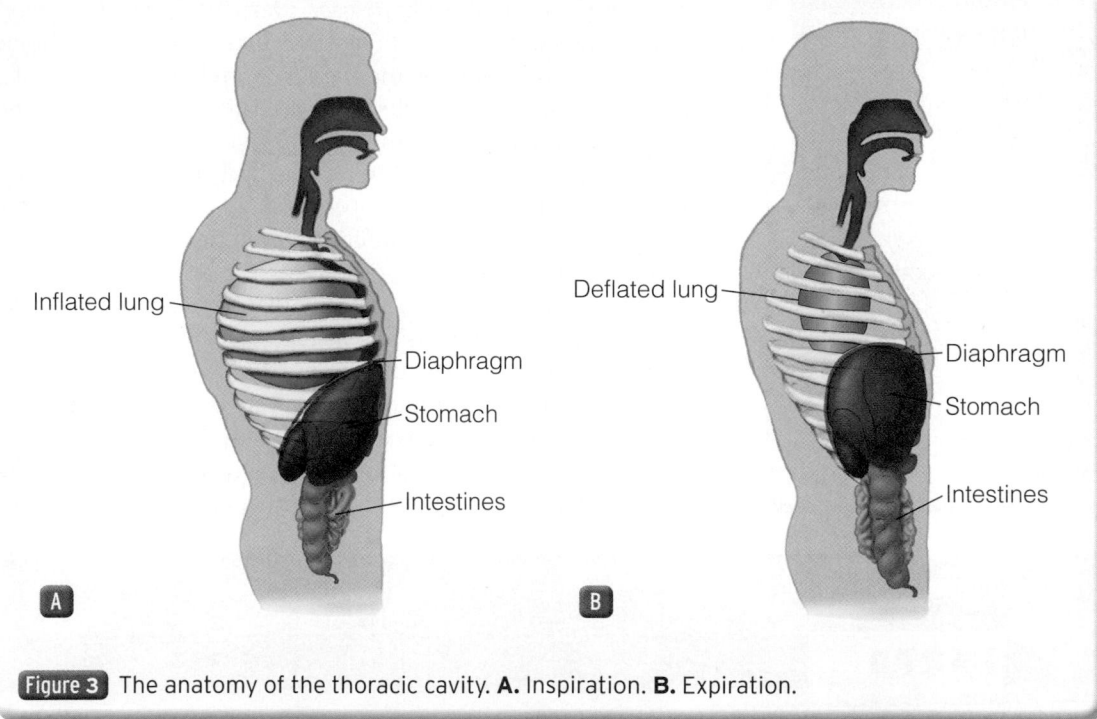

Figure 3 The anatomy of the thoracic cavity. **A.** Inspiration. **B.** Expiration.

sternal body, and the inferior **xiphoid process**. The space superior to the manubrium is termed the **suprasternal notch**; the junction of the manubrium and sternal body is referred to as the **angle of Louis**.

The **clavicle** is an elongated, S-shaped bone that connects to the manubrium medially and overlies the first rib as it proceeds laterally toward the shoulder. Beneath the clavicle lie the subclavian artery and vein. Laterally, the clavicle connects to the acromion process of the **scapula**, the triangular bone that overlies the posterior aspect of the upper thoracic cage.

Each of the 12 matched pairs of ribs attaches posteriorly to the 12 thoracic vertebrae. Anteriorly, the first seven pairs of ribs attach directly to the sternum via the costal cartilage. The costal cartilage then continues inferiorly from the seventh rib and provides an indirect connection between the anterior portions of the eighth, ninth, and tenth ribs and the sternum. The eleventh and twelfth ribs have no anterior connection and, therefore, are known as the "floating ribs."

Between each rib lies an **intercostal space**. These spaces are numbered accord-ing to the rib superior to the space (ie, the space between the second and third ribs is the second intercostal space). These spaces house the intercostal muscles and the **neurovascular bundle**, which consists of an artery, vein, and nerve that run on the bottom aspect of each individual rib.

The central region of the thorax is the **mediastinum**, which contains the heart, great vessels, esophagus, lymphatic channels, trachea, mainstem bronchi, and paired vagus and phrenic nerves. The heart resides within a tough fibrous sac called the **pericardium**. Much like the pleura, the pericardium has two surfaces—the inner visceral layer, which adheres to the heart and forms the epicardium, and the outer parietal layer, which comprises the sac itself. The pericardium that covers the inferior aspect of the heart is directly attached to the diaphragm. The heart is positioned so that the most anterior portion is the right ventricle, which has relatively thin chamber walls. The pressure within the right ventricle is approximately one fourth of the pressure within the left ventricle. Most of the heart is protected anteriorly by the sternum. With each beat, the apex of the heart can be felt in the fifth intercostal space along the midclavicular line, a phenomenon known as cardiac impulse. The average cardiac output for an adult (heart rate times the stroke volume) is $70 \times 70 = 4,900$ mL/min, though it varies depending on the patient's size.

The aorta is the largest artery in the body. As it exits the left ventricle, it ascends toward the right shoulder before turning to the left and proceeding inferiorly toward the abdomen. This artery has three points of attachment—the anulus at its origin from the aortic valve, the ligamentum arteriosum, and the aortic hiatus. These attachments represent sites of potential injury when the vessel is subject to significant shearing forces, such as those seen during sudden deceleration mechanisms.

The lungs occupy most of the space within the thoracic cavity. Like the pericardium, the lungs are lined with a dual layer of connective tissue known as the **pleura**. The parietal pleura lines the interior of each side of the thoracic cavity. The visceral pleura lines the exterior of each lung.

A small amount of viscous fluid separates the two layers of pleura. This fluid allows the two layers of connective tissue to move against each other without friction or pain. It creates a surface tension that holds the layers together, thereby keeping the lung from collapsing away from the thoracic cage on exhalation. If this space becomes filled with air, blood, or other fluids, the surface tension is lost and the lung collapses.

The **diaphragm**, the primary muscle of breathing, forms a barrier between the thoracic and abdominal cavities. It works in conjunction with the intercostal muscles to increase the size of the thoracic cavity during inspiration, creating the negative pressure that pulls air in via the trachea. In times of distress, this breathing effort can be aided by other accessory muscles of the thoracic cavity, including the trapezius, latissimus dorsi, rhomboids, pectoralis, and sternocleidomastoid **Figure 4** .

Physiology

The primary physiologic functions of the thorax and its contents are to maintain oxygenation and ventilation and (via the heart) to maintain circulation.

The process of breathing includes both the delivery of oxygen (O_2) to the body and the elimination of carbon dioxide (CO_2) from the body. Whereas these processes are often accomplished simultaneously, they are, in fact, different aspects of the breathing process.

First, however, the brain must stimulate the person to breathe. This stimulation occurs via chemoreceptors that are located in the carotid sinus and aortic arch. These chemoreceptors analyze the arterial blood. When the level of CO_2 gets too high, the receptors send a message to the brain, which responds by increasing the respiratory rate in an effort to "blow off the CO_2." Some patients with end-stage chronic obstructive pulmonary disease (COPD) may employ a secondary mechanism called hypoxic drive for this function because they retain excess CO_2 on a chronic basis.

As the diaphragm contracts downward, the intercostal and accessory muscles pull the chest wall out and away from the center of the body. The resulting negative pressure within the thoracic cavity draws air in through the mouth and nose, down the trachea, passing through smaller and smaller bronchioles until finally it reaches the alveolar spaces. The new air both mixes with and replaces the air contained within the alveoli.

While respiration is occurring, blood is being delivered via the pulmonary circulation to the capillaries that lie adjacent to the alveoli. This blood has returned to the heart after traversing the body, having delivered its oxygen to the cells and removed the cellular waste products such as CO_2. As a result, the

Special Populations

Pediatric and geriatric patients have anatomic and physiologic differences. For example, the incidence of rib fractures varies with age. The ribs of children are pliable, so they may injure underlying structures without being fractured. In older patients, the brittle nature of the bones makes the ribs more likely to fracture.

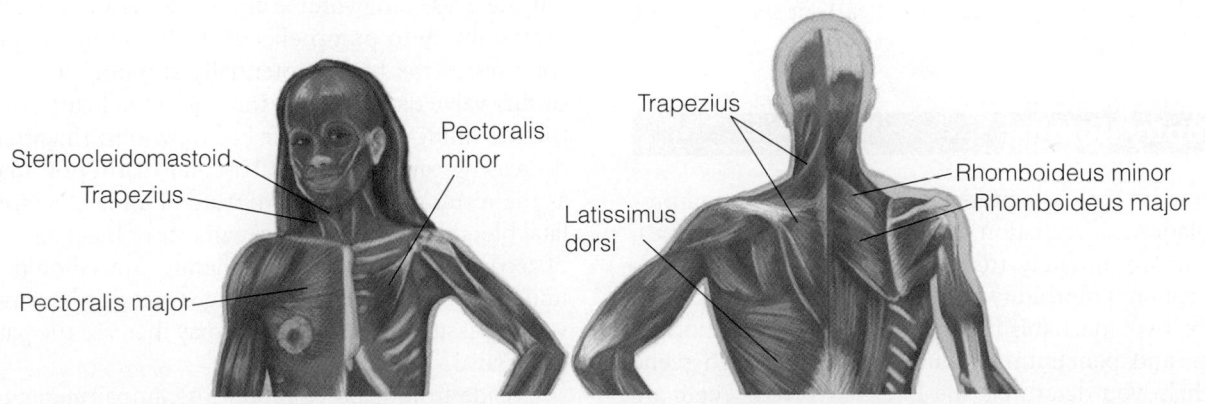

Figure 4 The muscles of the thoracic cavity include the trapezius, latissimus dorsi, rhomboid, pectoralis, and sternocleidomastoid muscles.

blood entering the capillaries adjacent to the alveoli has a low O_2 concentration and a high CO_2 concentration.

The process of oxygenation includes the delivery of O_2 from the air to the blood, where it is carried to cells and tissues throughout the body. Because the air entering the alveoli contains a higher concentration of O_2 (ranging from 21% in room air to as much as 100% in a nonrebreathing mask or bag mask under ideal circumstances) than the blood in the nearby capillaries, the O_2 will follow its concentration gradient and enter the blood. Most of the O_2 binds to hemoglobin within the red blood cells, and the O_2 returns to the heart with the blood, where it is then pumped throughout the body.

Ventilation is the process by which CO_2 is removed from the body. The air in the environment contains little CO_2 (0.033%). As a result, when air enters the alveoli, it contains little CO_2 compared with the blood in the nearby capillaries. The CO_2 diffuses down its concentration gradient, leaving the blood and entering the air within the alveoli.

As the diaphragm and the chest wall relax, positive pressure is created within the thorax. The air from which O_2 has been absorbed and into which CO_2 has been diffused is then exhaled. With each subsequent respiration (inhalation and exhalation), the process is repeated.

Proper functioning of the heart is essential to the delivery of blood to the body's tissues. As blood returns from the body via the inferior and superior vena cavae, it is pumped from the right side of the heart to the lungs, where the processes of oxygenation and ventilation take place. As oxygenated blood returns from the lungs, it enters the left side of the heart and is then pumped out to the body.

The ability to pump blood depends on having a functional pump (the heart), an adequate volume of blood to be pumped, and a lack of resistance to the pumping mechanism (afterload)—factors that collectively determine the cardiac output. Cardiac output is the volume of blood delivered to the body in 1 minute. The volume is identified by counting the number of times the heart beats in a minute (heart rate) and determining the amount of blood delivered to the body with each beat (stroke volume). Thus cardiac output equals the heart rate (beats/min) multiplied by the stroke volume (milliliters of blood per beat). Any injury that limits the heart's pumping ability, the delivery of blood to the heart, the blood's ability to leave the heart, or the heart rate will affect cardiac output.

■ Pathophysiology

Traumatic injury to the chest presents the possibility of compromise of ventilation, oxygenation, or circulation. These injuries, if missed or inappropriately treated, could contribute significantly to the patient's morbidity or even cause death.

There are two mechanisms of injury (MOIs) in thoracic trauma: blunt and penetrating. Conducting a thorough scene size-up will help you determine the forces involved. There are also two basic injury patterns of chest injuries: open and closed. As the name implies, a closed chest injury is one in which the skin overlying the injury remains intact. This type of injury is generally caused by blunt trauma, such as when a driver strikes a steering wheel in a motor vehicle crash or is struck by a falling object. The force is distributed over a large area. Visceral injuries occur from deceleration, shearing forces, compression, or rupture. In an open chest injury, the chest wall itself is penetrated by some object, such as a knife, a bullet, or a piece of metal. Penetrating injuries distribute the forces of injury over a smaller area; however, the trajectory of a bullet is often unpredictable and all thoracic structures are at risk.

In blunt trauma, a blow to the chest may fracture the ribs, the sternum, or whole areas of the chest wall; bruise the lungs and the heart; and even damage the aorta. Although the skin and chest wall are not penetrated in a closed injury, broken ribs may lacerate the intrathoracic organs. Indeed, vital organs can actually be torn from their attachment in the chest cavity without any break in the skin.

Blast injuries may be classified as blunt or penetrating. The shock wave during the primary blast compresses organs similar to blunt trauma, and, during the secondary phase, objects may be thrown and penetrate the body.

Special Populations

Pediatric and geriatric patients have differences for you to consider during the assessment process. For example, pediatric signs of pneumothorax or hemothorax are often subtle, and you may not see signs of jugular vein distention as you would in an adult. A geriatric patient experiencing blunt trauma would have considerably higher mortality and morbidity rates than other populations. Consider such differences during the assessment of various populations.

Thoracic trauma may impair cardiac output, decreasing blood pressure and perfusion to vital organs. Considering the contents of the thoracic cavity, any injury to the chest has the potential to be lethal. Trauma may result in blood loss, pressure changes, vital organ damage, or any combination of these. Bleeding into the thoracic cavity significantly increases the chance of hypovolemia and hypoxia. Increased intrapleural pressures not only decrease lung volume and oxygenation, but also impair the heart's ability to pump effectively. Blood in the pericardial sac compresses the heart, potentially stopping it altogether. Myocardial valve damage from trauma to the heart can disrupt ventricular filling, allowing for backflow into the atria and further decreasing cardiac output. Vascular disruption may also occur as the result of trauma. A rupture of a major vessel can lead to fatal blood loss, and even a small tear or blockage can cause lack of oxygenation and tissue ischemia. You should have a good understanding of the underlying structures because it increases your assessment abilities and it may increase the patient's chance of survival.

Aside from massive blood loss, impairments in ventilatory efficiency may also be rapidly fatal. Any injury that compromises the chest bellows action decreases air exchange and subsequent oxygenation. A patient experiencing severe chest pain tends to breathe shallowly in an attempt to decrease the discomfort created by movement. This further reduces minute volume, the volume of air exchanged between the lungs and environment in 1 minute. Air entering the pleural space as the result of an open or closed pneumothorax, a tracheal tear, or other damage compresses the lungs and decreases tidal volume. This problem also occurs when blood collects in the thoracic cavity and prevents full expansion of the lungs. Various injuries caused by chest trauma, such as rib fractures and diaphragmatic injury, result in fewer pressure changes and, therefore, less movement of air, which further decreases the amount of o_2 available for gas exchange.

Other complications are also capable of impairing gas exchange. **Atelectasis** is alveolar collapse that prevents the use of that portion of the lung for ventilation and oxygenation. Atelectasis significantly reduces the surface area available for gas exchange. The more alveoli that are damaged, the less gas exchange occurs. Bruised lung tissue may produce marked hypoxemia as fluid accumulates and impairs gas exchange. Disruption of the respiratory tract occurring from rupture or tearing of any of the respiratory structures prevents o_2 from reaching the alveoli, further impairing gas exchange.

Patient Assessment

Scene Size-up

When you arrive on the scene, your first responsibility is to ensure the safety of both you and your partner. Make sure that the scene is safe to enter and follow standard precautions, using the appropriate personal protective equipment. After you identify the number of patients, triage those patients, and request any additional resources needed, try to determine the MOI. Remember that chest injuries are common in motor vehicle crashes, falls, and assaults.

Primary Assessment

Form a General Impression

As you approach the patient, you will form a general impression of the patient's condition. It is important to assess the patient's level of consciousness using AVPU. Responsive patients may be able to tell you their chief complaint. Note not only what they say, but also how they say it.

Difficulty speaking may indicate several problems, and chest injury is an important one. Perform a rapid scan of the patient. Look for obvious injuries, the appearance of blood, and difficulty breathing. Look for cyanosis, irregular breathing, and chest rise and fall on only one side. Observe the neck, looking for accessory muscle use while breathing; also look for extended or engorged external jugular veins. If no obvious problems are seen, begin looking for them by focusing on the ABCs. The initial general impression will help you develop an index of suspicion for serious injuries and determine your sense of urgency for medical intervention. A good question

to ask yourself is "How sick is this patient?" Patients with significant chest injuries will "look" sick and are often frightened or anxious. Keep in mind that you are rapidly searching for life threats and you will repeat the physical examination in a more detailed manner later in the assessment if time and patient condition allow.

Airway and Breathing

Assess the patient's airway status while providing manual in-line immobilization of the cervical spine. Assess for injuries that may result in either obstruction or impairment of the airway. The most common cause of airway obstruction is the tongue's posterior displacement in the setting of altered mental status. Other foreign bodies that may obstruct the airway include the patient's teeth, dentures, blood, mucus, or vomitus. Additionally, the trauma may either directly injure the airway or result in secondary obstruction due to inflammation or edema.

Patients with airway compromise may present in a variety of ways, depending on the severity of the impairment, its duration, and other associated injuries. The airway itself may manifest signs of obstruction—for example, stridor, hoarseness or other changes in the voice, gurgling or snoring respirations, or coughing. Patients may also demonstrate signs of either hypoxia or hypercarbia. Alterations in mental status may range from anxiety to stupor to unresponsiveness. Abnormal respiratory findings may include tachypnea, coughing, hemoptysis, accessory muscle use, and retractions.

When a patient has airway impairment, you must take immediate action to remedy the situation. Any patient with an airway issue should be assumed to have a simultaneous cervical spine injury and should be manually immobilized. Because of the potential for compromising the cervical spine, the head tilt–chin lift maneuver should be avoided in favor of the jaw-thrust maneuver. Suction, basic airway adjuncts (ie, oropharyngeal or nasopharyngeal airways), advanced airway adjuncts (ie, endotracheal intubation, king LT, laryngeal mask airway, or a Combitube), or surgical airway management should be used as needed to ensure adequate airway management and protection.

Words of Wisdom

Noisy breathing is obstructed breathing.

Once the airway has been assessed and managed appropriately, your assessment should turn to the patient's breathing. The goal here is to identify and manage any impairment of the patient's oxygenation and ventilation. Such problems may result from deficiencies in diffusion due to pulmonary injuries, preexisting disease, or deficiencies in air movement due to pulmonary, musculoskeletal, or neurologic impairments.

To adequately assess the patient's breathing, the patient's clothing must be removed to expose the thoracic cavity. Taking a systematic approach to assessment will then help you to identify both obvious and subtle injuries or impairments.

Begin with an inspection of the patient's thorax. Consider the contour, appearance, and symmetry of the chest wall. Signs of soft-tissue injury (contusions, abrasions, lacerations, or deformity) suggest the possibility of an underlying injury. Paradoxical motion of a section of the chest wall, retractions, subcutaneous air or edema, impaled objects, or penetrating injuries also suggest an underlying injury with the potential to compromise the patient's breathing. If you determine the patient has paradoxical movement of the chest wall or penetrating trauma, address this life threat at once. When further dressings can be applied, you should apply an occlusive dressing to all penetrating injuries to the chest. Continued treatments of these types of injuries will often depend on local protocols.

Consider the adequacy of both ventilation and oxygenation. To assess ventilation, examine the patient's respiratory rate, depth, and effort. Reliance on accessory muscles or findings such as nasal flaring suggest ventilatory compromise. Inadequate oxygenation may be inferred from findings such as cyanosis or altered mental status.

Apply O_2 with a nonrebreathing mask at 15 L/min. Provide positive-pressure ventilations with 100% O_2 if breathing is inadequate based on the patient's level of consciousness and breathing rate and quality. As a note of caution, remember that when you are providing positive-pressure ventilation, you are overcoming the normal physiologic functions, and, if your patient has a pneumothorax (collapsed lung), you can quickly exacerbate the injury. Be diligent with auscultation of breath sounds, and evaluate the effectiveness of your ventilatory support with signs of circulation to the skin. Be aware of decreasing O_2 saturation (Spo_2) values because they may indicate the development of hypoxia. Watch for signs of an impending tension pneumothorax, such as increasingly poor compliance during ventilation.

The final steps in the assessment of the patient's breathing entail the palpation, percussion, and auscultation of the chest. While you are palpating the chest, assess for any evidence of point tenderness, bony instability, **crepitus**, **subcutaneous emphysema**, edema, and tracheal position. Percussion can help to identify either hyperresonance (suggesting increased air within the cavity) or dullness (suggesting blood within the cavity). Auscultation includes the usual assessment for adventitious lung sounds (ie, wheezing, crackles or rales, rhonchi) plus confirmation that lung sounds are present in all lung fields.

Words of Wisdom

A patient's blood pressure can serve as a clinical guide to patient assessment and management. Hypotension alone or in combination with tachycardia may suggest hypovolemia. In a patient with thoracic trauma, however, consideration must be given to both tension pneumothorax and pericardial tamponade as sources of this clinical finding. Regardless of the etiology of the hypotension, this finding suggests a critically injured patient in need of immediate transport, ideally to a trauma center.

Circulation

The next step in the assessment involves evaluating your patient's circulatory status. The first insight into the adequacy of the patient's circulation is his or her mental status. Once you have corrected any hypoxia or ventilatory cause leading to altered mental status, circulatory impairment should be suspected when your patient presents in a restless, agitated, confused, irrational, or comatose state. If the patient is well oxygenated and ventilating adequately, these signs may indicate inadequate cerebral perfusion.

A rapid assessment of your patient's pulses can provide a great deal of information about the patient's circulatory status. For example, absent peripheral pulses suggest that the blood pressure is low. The pulses should be assessed for their rate, quality, rhythm, location, and respiratory-induced changes.

Whereas tachycardia is frequently associated with hypovolemia, this is not always the case. Pain, hypoxia, psychological stress related to the incident, and other factors may manifest in tachycardia. A low heart rate does not exclude the possibility of hypovolemia or shock. Neurogenic shock, severe hypoxia, Cushing reflex, use of beta blockers, and myocardial injury may all result in bradycardia and mask simultaneous hypovolemia. Similarly, while a "thready" or "weak" pulse quality may suggest volume loss, its presence does not guarantee such a state and its absence does not exclude it.

An irregular pulse first raises the possibility of ectopic activity, suggesting hypoxia or hypoperfusion. An irregular pulse noted during the primary assessment should raise your suspicion of serious underlying injuries or shock. Although an ECG monitor may be applied to evaluate the rhythm at this time, this step is recommended only if it does not cause any delay in completing the primary assessment (eg, your partner could perform this task while you continue the primary assessment).

Jugular vein distention (JVD) suggests increased intravenous pressure—perhaps resulting from a tension pneumothorax, volume overload, right-sided heart failure, or cardiac tamponade **Figure 5** . Because true JVD is measured with the

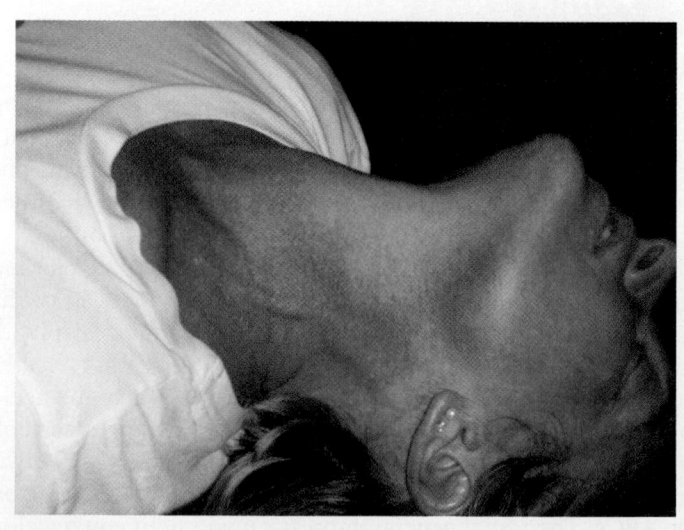

Figure 5 Jugular vein distention.

patient in a 45° semi-Fowler's position, it may be difficult to assess when cervical spine precautions have been implemented. Nevertheless, a lack of JVD in the supine position in combination with other physical findings (eg, tachycardia, altered mental status, thready pulses, poor skin perfusion) may suggest a hypovolemic state Figure 6 .

Auscultation of the heart sounds is another important part of the circulatory assessment. For patients with potential intrathoracic injuries, note whether their heart sounds are easily heard or whether they are muffled. Performing such an assessment may prove difficult in the back of a moving or running ambulance or because of other noise on the scene. Even so, the presence of muffled heart tones is an important diagnostic clue to the presence of either a tension pneumothorax (because of its resultant mediastinal shift) or a cardiac tamponade.

Even if the assessment of the patient's circulatory status suggests hypovolemic shock, you should recognize that the cause of that state may not lie within the thorax. Only one in four patients with a combination of thoracic trauma and shock will have a significant source of hemorrhage within the chest. For this reason, after completing the primary assessment, managing any immediate life-threatening conditions, and prioritizing the patient, you must obtain the patient's history and perform a complete physical examination to identify other significant injuries.

Words of Wisdom

It is not necessary to make a specific diagnosis to appreciate that a patient is critically injured.

Transport Decision

Priority patients are considered patients who have a problem with their airway, breathing, and/or circulation. Sometimes the priority is obvious, and the decision to transport quickly is also easy. At other times, what is happening outside the body may not provide obvious clues to the seriousness of what is happening inside the body. Pay attention to subtle clues such as the appearance of the skin, level of consciousness, or a sense of impending doom in the patient. These symptoms are not as dramatic as a large gash across the chest or air being sucked into the chest; however, they can be equally important indicators of a life-threatening condition. When you find signs of poor perfusion or inadequate breathing, transport quickly and perform the remainder of the assessment en route to the emergency department. A delay on the scene to perform a lengthy assessment will reduce the chances of survival for your patient. With chest injuries, when in doubt, transport rapidly to a hospital. Table 1 lists the "deadly dozen" chest injuries.

■ History Taking

Depending on the severity of the injuries identified up to this point, history taking may need to be done en route to the emergency department.

A relevant patient history should be obtained, including a SAMPLE history. Ask the usual questions related to the patient's symptoms, allergies, medications, past medical history, and last oral intake. Questions about the events surrounding the incident should focus on the MOI: the speed of the vehicle or height of the fall, the use of safety equipment (helmet, air bag, seat belt,

Words of Wisdom

Any injury below the level of the nipples should be presumed to be an abdominal injury as well as a chest injury.

Table 1 Life-Threatening Chest Injuries

Immediately life-threatening chest injuries that must be detected and managed during the primary assessment:

1. Airway obstruction
2. Bronchial disruption
3. Diaphragmatic tear
4. Esophageal injury
5. Open pneumothorax
6. Tension pneumothorax
7. Hemothorax
8. Flail chest
9. Cardiac tamponade

Potentially lethal chest injuries that may be identified during the secondary assessment:

10. Traumatic aortic disruption
11. Myocardial contusion
12. Pulmonary contusion

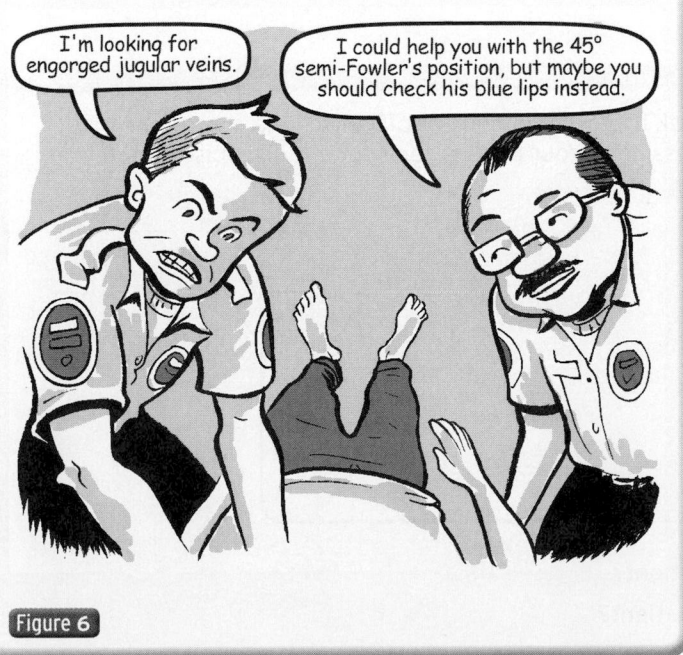

Figure 6

life jacket), the type of weapon used, the number of penetrating wounds, and so on.

Secondary Assessment

The secondary assessment, which may be performed en route to the hospital for patients with a significant MOI, should include a complete head-to-toe assessment of the patient. This examination allows you to identify any physical injuries as well as reassess injuries identified in the primary assessment. For the chest trauma patient, pay particular attention to the patient's cervical spine, back, and abdomen, as well as the neurologic and circulatory function in the patient's extremities.

Look for injuries with the potential to compromise the ABCs—namely, aortic transections, great vessel injuries, bronchial disruptions, myocardial contusions, pulmonary contusions, simple pneumothoraces, rib fractures, and sternal fractures. If you have not already done so, obtain a full set of vital signs—including pulse rate, blood pressure, respirations, O_2 saturation, and mental status. The use of monitoring equipment such as capnography and pulse oximetry can aid in the assessment. It is advisable to use the pulse oximeter on any patient with a chest injury to establish a baseline measurement and to help you recognize any downward trends that indicate the patient's condition is worsening.

In a patient who has an isolated injury to the chest with a limited MOI, such as in a stabbing, you should focus your assessment on the isolated injury, the patient's complaint, and the body region affected. However, it is important in patients with a chest injury not to focus only on a chest wound. With significant trauma, you should quickly assess the entire patient from head to toe. While you are assessing the skin, look for ecchymosis and other evidence of trauma. Ensure that wounds are identified and control of the bleeding has been established. Note the location and extent of the injury. Assess all underlying systems. Examine the anterior and posterior aspects of the chest wall, and be alert to changes in the patient's ability to maintain adequate respirations.

If there is significant trauma (such as blunt trauma or a gunshot wound) likely affecting multiple systems, perform a full-body scan looking for DCAP-BTLS to determine the nature and extent of thoracic injury. This examination will help you to determine all of the injuries and the extent of the injuries. Inspection or visualization of the region looking for deformities, such as asymmetry of the left and right sides of the chest or shoulder girdle, may reveal the presence of multiple rib fractures, crush injuries, or significant chest wall injury. Identification of discrete areas of contusion or abrasion may pinpoint a specific point of impact. The presence of puncture wounds or other penetrating injuries indicates a possible open chest injury that should be managed accordingly. Be alert for associated burns, which may alter respiratory mechanics. Palpate for tenderness to localize the injury and the presence of fractures. Look for lacerations and local swelling. Application of this systematic approach to patient assessment minimizes the chance of missing significant injury.

Reassessment

When you are reassessing the chest trauma patient, obtain repeated assessments of the patient's vital signs, oxygenation, circulatory status, and breath sounds. Because the progression from pneumothorax to tension pneumothorax can occur quite rapidly, all patients with a presumptive diagnosis of a pneumothorax should be considered to be in unstable condition and reassessed at least every 5 minutes for worsening dyspnea, tachycardia, and the development of JVD. Similarly, other chest injuries may suggest the presence of more serious underlying pathologic conditions. Because these injuries may have

YOU are the Medic   PART 2

You observe that the patient has labored, shallow breathing. You ask the law enforcement officer to help control the patient's hands while you and your partner conduct a primary assessment. Your partner feels for a radial pulse and reports that it is rapid and weak. There is no blood coming from the wound.

Recording Time: 1 Minute	
Appearance	Awake
Level of consciousness	Disoriented
Airway	Open
Breathing	Labored and shallow
Circulation	Poor

3. What immediate treatment do you need to provide to this patient?

4. What steps will you take in your further assessment of this patient?

been overlooked during the primary assessment, you need to maintain a high degree of clinical suspicion during the on-scene treatment and transport of these patients.

Emergency Medical Care

As with any trauma patient, your management of patients with identifiable chest injuries must focus on maintaining the airway, ensuring oxygenation and ventilation, supporting the circulatory status, and expeditiously transporting the patient to an appropriate facility.

With one exception, airway management of the patient with chest trauma should proceed the same as with any other trauma patient. The jaw-thrust maneuver should be used rather than the head tilt–chin lift, because the former technique better limits cervical spine motion. Nasal airways should be avoided in patients with signs of facial injury. Instead, endotracheal intubation should be performed while maintaining manual in-line immobilization of the cervical spine. When a patient with chest trauma has a possible tracheal injury, however, endotracheal intubation should be reconsidered. With a partial tracheal tear, you run the risk of completing the tracheal tear when you are passing the endotracheal tube, a complication that can result in an unmanageable airway. Consequently, when you suspect your patient has a partial tracheal tear, you should use the least invasive airway management technique possible.

As part of airway management, you must ensure that the patient maintains adequate oxygenation and ventilation. Oxygenation is accomplished by providing patients with high-flow O_2 via a nonrebreathing mask or, if necessary, with bag-mask ventilation. Ventilation is a more delicate issue in light of the potential complications that can arise from underlying thoracic injuries; therefore, you must provide ventilatory assistance in a highly vigilant fashion. Delivery of positive pressure could potentially hasten the expansion of a pneumothorax, convert a pneumothorax into a tension pneumothorax, or increase the dissection of air through a tracheobronchial injury. Positive-pressure ventilation should not be withheld, however; rather, it should be delivered in a manner that minimizes the degree of pressure used. Watch your patient's chest closely—you are looking for visible chest rise without excessive overinflation!

Assessment of the ability of the circulatory system to provide oxygenation and ventilation to the body tissues is the next step in the management of any trauma patient. The patient whose circulatory status is compromised (as evidenced by tachycardia, hypotension, or end-organ dysfunction) requires supportive measures until definitive care can be delivered. Placing the patient in a supine or Trendelenburg position will deliver blood otherwise held in the venous system of the lower extremities to the central circulation. The provision of judicious intravenous fluids may also help to expand the intravascular volume while maintaining the oxygen-carrying capacity of the blood.

Pharmacologic agents have a limited role in the management of a trauma patient. With the exception of those medications necessary to ensure appropriate airway management, the only drugs currently used are agents for pain management. Narcotic and nonnarcotic analgesics are essential components of the appropriate and compassionate treatment of any trauma patient. As a responsible paramedic, you will take the proper steps to minimize the pain of your patients, although you may often be limited by local protocols, short transport times in more urban settings, and the clinical status of the patient (including appropriate concern about narcotic suppression of the respiratory drive in thoracic trauma patients). Nonpharmaceutical approaches may include appropriate splinting, application of cold packs, and careful handling.

Words of Wisdom

Treatment of pain and anxiety can help with packaging and transport of the patient, thus minimizing secondary injury.

Finally, the global assessment and management of patients with chest trauma includes deciding the appropriate facility to which the patient should be transported. Trauma centers designated to provide multisystem evaluation and management of trauma patients would be the first choice for most patients with chest trauma, particularly those with potentially life-threatening injuries. Sometimes, however, such facilities may not be readily available or may be physically too distant to allow for timely transport (eg, in a rural environment).

The principle of the Golden Period is the time during which treatment of shock or traumatic injuries is most critical and the potential for survival is best.

Words of Wisdom

There are a select few injuries that you must be able to quickly identify and treat during your assessment of the patient's breathing—namely, open pneumothorax and tension pneumothorax. These injuries, if missed, may claim the patient's life.

Pathophysiology, Assessment, and Management of Chest Wall Injuries

Flail Chest

Flail chest, a major injury to the chest wall, may result from a variety of blunt force mechanisms such as falls, motor vehicle crashes, and assaults **Figure 7**. It occurs in as many as 20% of admitted trauma patients. The associated mortality rates range

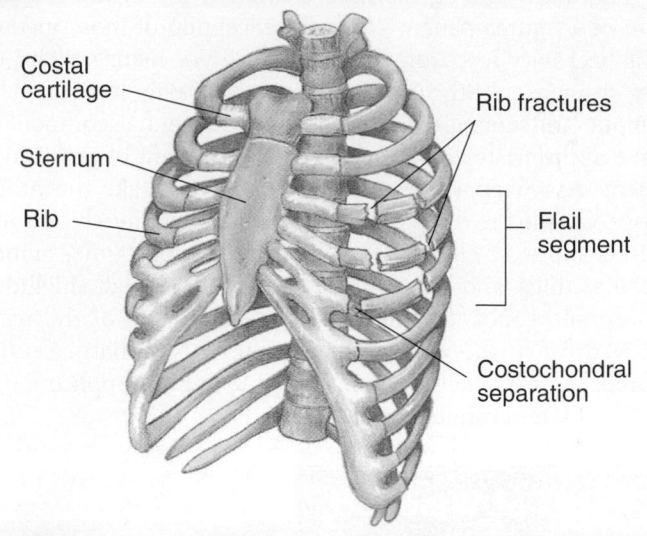

Figure 7 In flail chest injuries, two or more adjacent ribs are fractured in two or more places. A flail segment will move paradoxically when the patient breathes.

from 50% to even higher rates in patients older than 60 years. Mortality rates are directly related to the underlying and associated injuries. Patients are more likely to sustain a mortal injury if they are elderly, have seven or more rib fractures or three or more associated injuries, present with shock, or have associated head trauma.

A flail segment is defined as two or more adjacent ribs that are fractured in two or more places. The segment between those two fracture sites becomes separated from the surrounding chest wall, leaving it free to succumb to the underlying pressures—hence the name "free-floating segment." Both the location and the size of the segment can affect the degree to which the flail segment impairs chest wall motion and subsequent air movement. In a flail sternum (the most extreme case), the sternum is completely separated from the ribs because of fractures or ruptured costal cartilage. This type of injury results in mechanical dysfunction of both sides of the chest and more severe respiratory impairment.

Once a flail segment has occurred, the underlying physiologic pressures cause paradoxical movement of the segment when compared with the rest of the chest wall. Expansion of the chest wall on inspiration results in negative pressure within the thoracic cavity, which in turn draws the flail segment in toward the center of the chest. As the chest relaxes or is actively contracted (depending on the degree of dyspnea), the resulting positive pressure forces air from the lungs and also forces the flail segment out away from the thoracic cavity. Because of these movements, the lung tissue beneath the flail segment is not adequately ventilated. A flail segment can quickly become life-threatening, which explains why it is managed during the primary assessment of the patient. Initial identification of the flailed section might not be immediately apparent due to the intercostal muscle "splinting" the area, thus making paradoxical movement a late sign of flailed

segments. Proper assessment of this area includes palpation of the injury site for fractures of the rib cage and the presence of crepitus (bone ends grating together). Typical management involves the use of positive-pressure ventilation as well as positive end-expiratory pressure (PEEP) when you are assisting ventilations for the patient.

> ### Words of Wisdom
>
> Pulmonary contusion is the main cause of hypoxemia seen with flail chest injuries.

The blunt force trauma that causes the flail segment can also produce a **pulmonary contusion**, an injury to the underlying lung tissue that inhibits the normal diffusion of O_2 and CO_2 **Figure 8**. Three physical mechanisms contribute to the formation of a pulmonary contusion: implosion, inertial effects, and the Spalding effect. In the implosion effect, positive pressure created by the trauma compresses the gases within the lung, which quickly re-expand. If this re-expansion is too great, the lung tissue will sustain an implosion injury. Inertial effects are created by tissue density differences between the alveoli and the larger bronchioles. These tissues accelerate and decelerate at different rates, causing them to tear and hemorrhage. With the Spalding effect, the pressure waves generated by either penetrating or blunt trauma disrupt the capillary-alveolar membrane, resulting in hemorrhage.

If the blunt force that fractures the ribs drives those bone fragments farther into the body, a pneumothorax or hemothorax may result. In addition, the pain associated with the fractures may prevent the patient from taking in adequate tidal volume because he or she is consciously trying to minimize the movement of that segment of the chest. This "self-splinting" action uses the

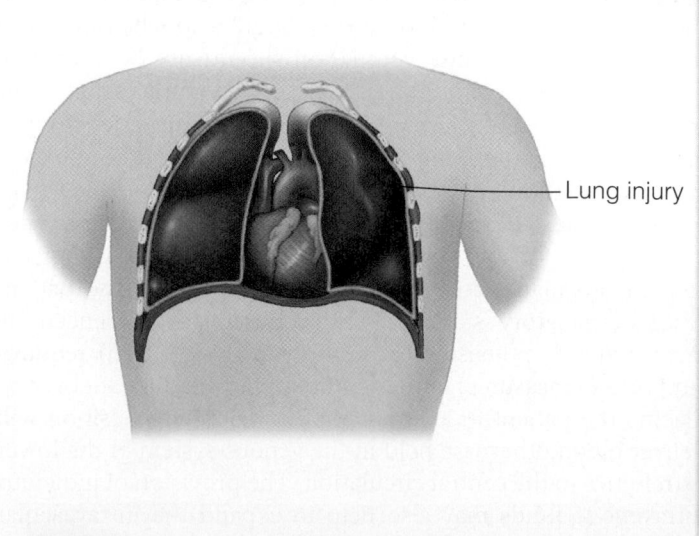

Figure 8 A pulmonary contusion is an injury to underlying lung tissue that inhibits diffusion.

intercostal muscles and purposefully limits chest wall movement to minimize pain. Unfortunately, this action further limits the pulmonary system's ability to compensate for the injury.

Assessment and Management

Physical assessment is the key to identifying a patient with a flail segment. Beginning with general inspection of the chest, you will note evidence of soft-tissue injury to the chest. On further examination, you may observe paradoxical chest wall movement, although the patient's efforts to splint the injury may prevent its visibility.

On palpation, crepitus and tenderness may be noted at the site, and dissection of air into the tissues should raise your clinical suspicion for this injury and an underlying pneumothorax. Auscultation will reveal decreased or even absent breath sounds on the affected side, depending on the degree of underlying injury, splinting, and pneumothorax.

As the injury begins to affect the patient's physiology, the expected signs and symptoms of hypoxia, hypercarbia, and pain will become apparent. The patient will most likely have one or more of the following associated findings: complaints of pain, tenderness on palpation, splinting, shallow breathing, agitation/anxiety (hypoxia) or lethargy (hypercarbia), tachycardia, and cyanosis.

Words of Wisdom

If a patient requires ventilatory support, it is much safer to apply it "prophylactically" before actual ventilatory failure develops.

Flail segments pose a threat to the patient's ability to breathe and should be treated immediately. When the patient has progressive respiratory failure, intubation and positive-pressure ventilation are indicated. Intubating the patient uses positive-pressure ventilation as a means of expanding the collapsed alveoli. That portion of the lung parenchyma is then able to contribute to the oxygenation and ventilation of the patient.

If intubation is not required, you must provide the patient with supplementary O_2 in the form of high-flow O_2 via a nonrebreathing mask. This action will increase the partial pressure of O_2 delivered to the functional parts of the lung, thereby increasing O_2 delivery to the body as a whole.

Stabilizing a flail segment is a controversial issue. Current guidelines suggest that providing positive-pressure ventilation provides internal stabilization and increases oxygenation and ventilation for management of a pulmonary contusion. However, some recent studies have shown that patients may benefit from early operative stabilization that may possibly reduce further acute complications. Follow local protocols.

■ Rib Fractures

Rib fractures—the most common thoracic injuries—are seen in more than half of all thoracic trauma patients. Even when the patient experiences no underlying or associated injury, the pain produced by the broken ribs can result in significant morbidity because it contributes to inadequate ventilation, self-splinting, atelectasis, and the possibility of infection (pneumonia) due to inadequate respiration.

When you are examining the chest of a patient who has sustained either blunt or penetrating injury, palpate for subcutaneous emphysema (air under the skin), which can indicate a potential pneumothorax. It has been described as a "snap, crackle, pop" sensation under the skin or a feeling like popping the plastic bubbles in the wrap used to protect fragile items during shipping.

In blunt trauma, the force applied to the thoracic cage results in a fracture of the rib in one of three areas: the point of impact, the edge of the object, or the posterior angle of the rib (weak point). Because they are less well protected by other bony and muscular structures, ribs four through nine are the most commonly fractured.

The ribs are part of a ring that helps to expand and contract the thoracic cavity. Because a fracture of one or more ribs destroys the integrity of this ring, the patient's ability to adequately ventilate is diminished. Just as importantly, the patient will attempt to limit the pain caused by these injuries by using shallow breathing. This tendency results in atelectasis and may lead to hypoxia or pneumonia.

The presence of rib fractures should also make you suspicious for other associated injuries. When the clinical examination suggests a fracture of ribs four through nine, you should be concerned about associated aortic injury, tracheobronchial injury, pneumothorax, vascular injury, or other more serious injuries. Similarly, fractures of the lower ribs (9 through 11) should raise your concern for an associated intra-abdominal injury.

Assessment and Management

Patients with rib fractures typically report pleuritic chest wall pain and mild dyspnea. The physical examination may reveal chest wall tenderness and overlying soft-tissue injury. Crepitus and subcutaneous emphysema may also be noted. When you are assessing the adequacy of the patient's respiratory effort, watch for shallow ventilations as the patient attempts to limit the movement of the affected area of the thoracic cage. The patient may also lean toward the injury site to reduce muscular tension on the fracture(s).

The management of rib fractures focuses on the ABCs and evaluating the patient for other, more lethal injuries. Administer supplemental O_2 and gently splint the patient's chest wall by having the patient hold a pillow or blanket against the area; this measure may allow the patient to take deeper breaths, something that should be encouraged despite the pain. Intravenous analgesics may also assist in this regard.

■ Sternal Fractures

Approximately one in 20 patients with blunt thoracic trauma will sustain a sternal fracture. Although this injury is of little consequence by itself, it is associated with other injuries that cause more than one fourth of patients with this fracture to die. Specifically, findings of myocardial contusions, flail sternum, pulmonary contusions, head injuries, intra-abdominal injuries, and myocardial rupture increase the likelihood of death.

Words of Wisdom

The sternum is a thick bone. If the thorax receives enough force to fracture the sternum, you must assume that the same force was transmitted to the heart, great vessels, lungs, and diaphragm.

Assessment and Management

On examination, the patient with a sternal fracture will report pain over the anterior part of the chest. Palpation of the area may reveal tenderness, deformity, crepitus, overlying soft-tissue injury, and the possibility of a flail segment. Given the risk of an underlying myocardial contusion, ECG rhythm analysis should be performed.

The treatment of sternal fractures is supportive only. Assess the patient's ABCs, and manage associated injuries accordingly. Analgesics in doses sufficient to provide pain relief without suppressing the respiratory drive may aid the patient's ventilatory efforts.

Words of Wisdom

Be alert for the development of a pneumothorax in a patient with a sternal fracture.

Clavicle Fractures

The clavicle, or collarbone, is one of the most commonly fractured bones in the body. Fractures of the clavicle occur most often in children when they fall on an outstretched hand, and are commom in cycling crashes and snowboarding. They can also occur with crushing injuries of the chest.

Assessment and Management

A patient with a fracture of the clavicle will report pain in the shoulder and will usually hold the arm across the front of his or her body. A young child often reports pain throughout the entire arm and is unwilling to use any part of that limb. These complaints may make it difficult to localize the point of injury, but, generally, swelling and point tenderness occur over the clavicle. Because the clavicle is subcutaneous, the skin will occasionally "tent" over the fracture fragment. The clavicle lies directly over major arteries, veins, and nerves; therefore, fracture of the clavicle may lead to neurovascular compromise.

Fractures of the clavicle and scapula and acromioclavicular separations can be splinted effectively with a sling and swathe. A sling is any bandage or material that helps support the weight of an injured upper extremity, relieving the downward pull of gravity on the injured site. To be effective, a sling must apply gentle upward support to the olecranon process of the ulna (at the elbow). The knot of the sling should be tied to one side of the neck so that it does not press uncomfortably on the cervical spine.

Pathophysiology, Assessment, and Management of Lung Injuries

Simple Pneumothorax

Small pneumothoraces that are not under tension are a frequent occurrence in the blunt trauma patient, occurring in almost half of patients with thoracic trauma. Patients with penetrating trauma to the chest almost always have a **pneumothorax**—that is, the accumulation of air or gas in the pleural cavity Figure 9 . In this condition, air enters through a hole in the chest wall (that seals itself after air has entered the pleural space) or the surface of the lung as the patient attempts to breathe, causing the lung on that side to collapse as pressure continues to build in the pleural cavity.

Depending on the size of the hole and the rate at which air fills the cavity, the lung may collapse in a few seconds, a few hours, or not at all. If the chest wall hole is at least two thirds the size of the trachea, more air will enter from the atmosphere, creating a sucking sound. The larger the hole, the more rapidly the lung will collapse. Delayed or improper treatment of a simple pneumothorax may lead to a tension pneumothorax. Some low-velocity wounds may self-seal, remedying the problem.

Assessment and Management

The presentation and physical findings in a patient with a simple pneumothorax depend on the size of the pneumothorax and the degree of resulting pulmonary compromise. With a small pneumothorax, the patient may report only mild dyspnea and pleuritic chest pain on the affected side, and in young and fit patients, the simple pneumothorax may be well tolerated with no need for you to decompress the chest. Diminished or

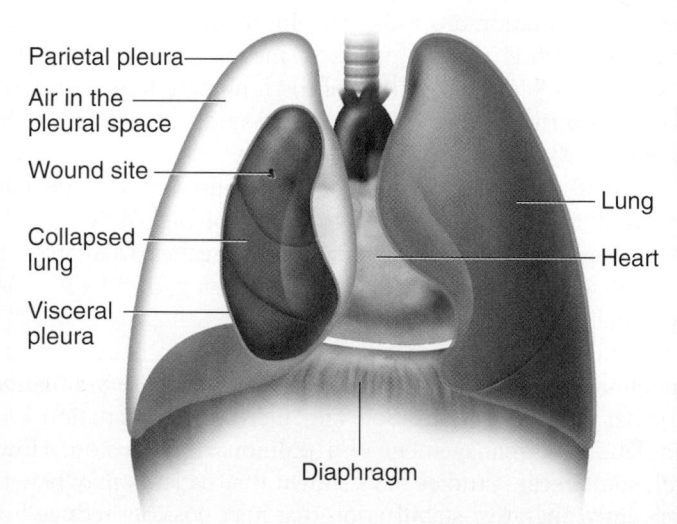

Parietal pleura

Air in the pleural space

Wound site

Collapsed lung

Visceral pleura

Lung

Heart

Diaphragm

Figure 9 Pneumothorax occurs when air leaks into the space between the pleural surfaces from an opening in the chest or the surface of the lung. The lung collapses as air fills the pleural space.

unequal breath sounds may be heard on auscultation, a finding that is best heard anteriorly if the patient is in the supine position or in the apices if the patient is upright. (Air will accumulate at the highest point and diminish lung sounds in that area.) Hyperresonance may also be found on the affected side.

As the pneumothorax increases in size, the degree of compromise likewise increases. Patients with larger pneumothoraces will report increasing dyspnea and demonstrate signs of more serious respiratory compromise and hypoxia: agitation, altered mental status, tachypnea, tachycardia, cyanosis, lowered pulse oximetry readings, **pulsus paradoxus** (a drop in blood pressure), and absent breath sounds on the affected side.

The management of the patient with a simple pneumothorax begins with you covering large open wounds immediately using a nonporous dressing secured on three sides. Maintain the ABCs and provide high-concentration O_2. Supplemental O_2 aids the patient in overcoming any degree of hypoxia that may exist. Positive-pressure ventilation will aggravate the condition, possibly resulting in tension pneumothorax. The most critical intervention for these patients is for you to conduct repeated assessments to ensure that the injury has not progressed to a tension pneumothorax. If signs and symptoms show the development of a tension pneumothorax, "burping" or removing the dressing may be needed to allow for the release of the trapped air within the thoracic cavity. Most pneumothoraces result from a small pulmonary injury that seals itself off, preventing further air loss. For those that do progress, however, rapid recognition and management of this condition can be lifesaving.

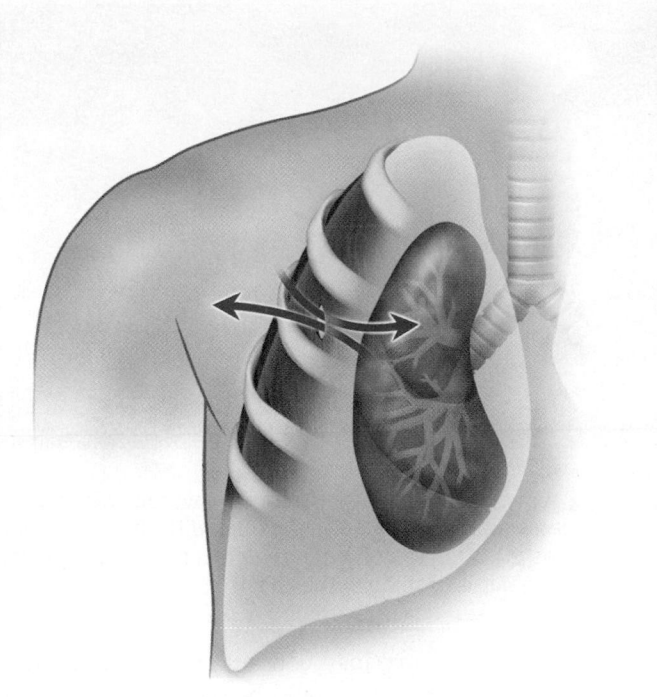

Figure 10 With a sucking chest wound, air passes from the outside into the pleural space and back out with each breath, creating a sucking sound. The size of the defect does not need to be large to compromise ventilation.

Open Pneumothorax

An **open pneumothorax** occurs when a defect in the chest wall allows air to enter the thoracic space. It results from penetrating chest trauma—for example, gunshot/knife wounds or other impaled objects. The penetrating injury creates a link between the external environment and the pleural space. With each inspiration, the negative pressure created within the thoracic cavity draws more air into the pleural space, resulting in a pneumothorax. As the pneumothorax increases in size, the lung on the involved side loses its ability to expand. Also, if the "hole" is larger than the glottic opening, the air is more likely to enter the chest wall rather than entering via the trachea. As a consequence, the respiratory effort moves air in through the chest wound rather than through the lung, creating the "sucking chest wound" **Figure 10**.

The collapse of the involved lung creates a mismatch between ventilation and perfusion. If you assume that the pulmonary vasculature on the involved side remains intact, the heart will continue to perfuse the involved lung while the pneumothorax prevents adequate ventilation. The result is an inability to deliver O_2 to the involved lung (hypoxia) and an inability to eliminate CO_2 (hypercarbia).

Assessment and Management

On physical assessment of a patient with an open pneumothorax, exposure of the chest will reveal a chest wall defect or impaled object. If air is being drawn into the chest by the negative inspiratory pressure, a "sucking chest wound" may be noted. If air is being forced out of the chest with the positive pressure of expiration, the result may be a bubbling wound. The movement of air in and out of the open wound may also lead to dissection of that air within the subcutaneous tissue, resulting in subcutaneous emphysema.

With any injury that has the potential to violate the integrity of the thoracic cavity, your assessment should focus on evaluating the patient for the presence of a pneumothorax. Due to the decreased ability to oxygenate and ventilate, the patient will experience tachycardia, tachypnea, and restlessness. These symptoms may be simply a manifestation of the pain from the injury, but other findings may confirm an underlying pneumothorax.

As the air within the interpleural space (the pneumothorax) increases, the patient's breath sounds will diminish on the affected side. Because this expanding volume consists of air, percussion of the chest will aid in the assessment by demonstrating a hyperresonant sound. These physical findings should confirm your suspicion of an open pneumothorax.

Sucking chest wounds must be treated immediately **Figure 11**. The injury should first be converted to a closed injury to prevent further expansion of the pneumothorax. To do so, immediately place your gloved hand over the injury and then replace that hand with an occlusive dressing or a commercial chest seal such as the Asherman Chest Seal. Because of the possibility that

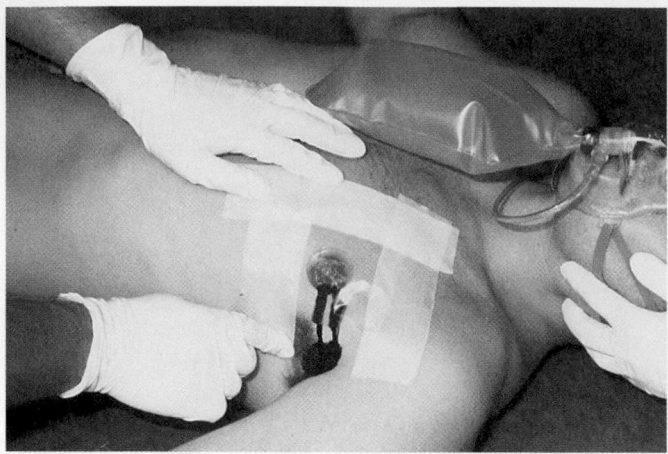

Figure 11 A sucking chest wound can be covered with a large airtight dressing that seals on three sides with the fourth side left open as a flutter valve. A commercial chest seal can also be used to seal the opening in the chest.

an underlying lung injury may continue to contribute to the pneumothorax, this dressing should be secured on three sides to facilitate the release of increased pressure, should it develop.

All patients with open pneumothoraces, regardless of their oxygenation status as determined by pulse oximetry, should be placed on high-flow supplemental O_2 via a nonrebreathing mask. If oxygenation or ventilation remains inadequate, endotracheal intubation may be required. You may use sedation or neuromuscular blockade to facilitate this process, depending on your local protocols.

An open pneumothorax rarely progresses to a tension pneumothorax. If it does, you should remove the patient's occlusive dressing or commercial chest seal to allow the pneumothorax to "vent" through the opening in the thoracic cavity.

If this measure does not relieve this life-threatening condition, treatment should progress as described in the next section.

■ Tension Pneumothorax

A **tension pneumothorax** is a life-threatening condition that results from continued air accumulation within the interpleural space **Figure 12**. A tension pneumothorax may result from an open or closed injury. Air may enter the pleural space from an open thoracic injury, an injury to the lung parenchyma due to blunt trauma (the most common cause of tension pneumothorax), barotrauma due to positive-pressure ventilation, or tracheobronchial injuries due to shearing forces. Although the exact incidence of this injury is unknown, many patients transported to Level 1 regional trauma centers in cardiac arrest receive emergent treatment for this condition secondary to blunt trauma.

An injury to the lung can cause a one-way valve to develop, allowing air to move into the pleural space but not to exit from it. As it continues to accumulate, the air exerts increasing pressure against the surrounding tissues. This growing pressure compresses the involved lung, diminishing its ability to oxygenate blood or eliminate CO_2 from the blood. Eventually, the pressure increase causes the lung to collapse on the affected side and the mediastinum to shift to the contralateral side. The lung collapse leads to right-to-left intrapulmonary shunting and hypoxia. A reduction in cardiac output occurs as the increased intrathoracic pressure causes compression of the heart and vena cava, reducing preload by decreasing venous return to the heart.

This pressure increase may even exceed the pressure within the major venous structures, decreasing venous return to the heart, diminishing preload, and eventually resulting in a shock state. As venous return decreases, the patient's body attempts to compensate by increasing the heart rate in an attempt to maintain cardiac output.

YOU *are the Medic* **PART 3**

Your partner has placed a nonrebreathing mask at 15 L/min on the patient. You listen to lung sounds and find them absent on the left upper lobe with crackles in the left base. The right lung sounds are within normal limits.

Recording Time: 5 Minutes	
Respirations	24 breaths/min
Pulse	120 beats/min, weak
Skin	Cool, pale, moist
Blood pressure	92/70 mm Hg
Oxygen saturation (Spo₂)	95% at 15L/min via nonrebreathing mask
Pupils	Equal and reactive to light

5. Do you remove the knife or bandage it in place?

6. What additional findings would you be looking for in a focused assessment of the chest?

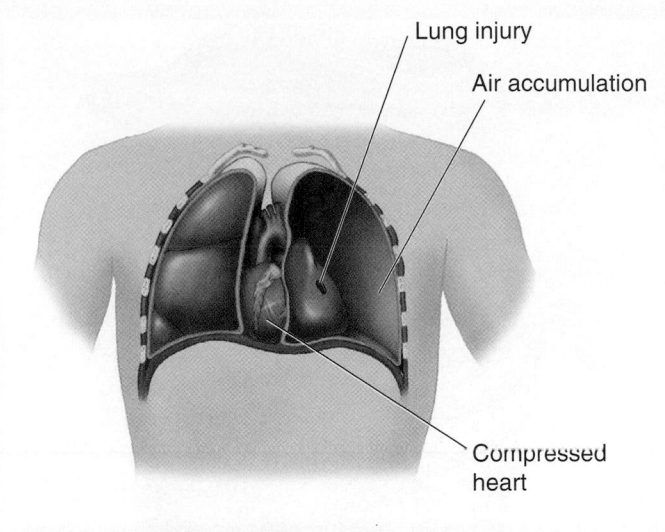

Lung injury

Air accumulation

Compressed heart

Figure 12 In a tension pneumothorax, air accumulates in the pleural space, eventually causing compression of the heart and great vessels.

Assessment and Management

The classic signs of a tension pneumothorax are an absence of breath sounds on the affected side, unequal chest rise, pulsus paradoxus, tachycardia and dysrhythmias such as progression to ventricular tachycardia and ventricular fibrillation, JVD, narrow pulse pressure, and tracheal deviation. Whereas tachycardia may not be a unique finding in the trauma patient, tension pneumothorax induces this change—not because of a hypovolemic state, but rather because of the inability of blood to easily return to the heart from the venous system. The increasing pressure within the thoracic cavity leads to the accumulation of blood within the great vessels just outside the thoracic cavity. As the pressure is translated into the most superficial of these veins—the jugular veins—they become distended with blood. Such JVD is usually a late sign of tension pneumothorax.

During normal inspiration, the negative pressure within the chest decreases blood return, particularly from the legs if the patient is standing, to the heart, thus decreasing preload and slightly decreasing systolic blood pressure (typically less than 10 mm Hg). In pathological conditions such as tension pneumothorax or pericardial tamponade where the right ventricle is functionally being compressed, the effect on preload of inspiration is magnified, and a drop in blood pressure associated with creating negative intrathoracic is more pronounced. This condition is known as pulsus paradoxus. In many cases, the radial pulse will actually be palpable with expiration and nonpalpable on inspiration, despite irrefutable evidence of cardiac contraction by stethoscope or ECG.

The jugular veins, which exit the thoracic cavity from beneath the clavicles and cross over the sternocleidomastoid muscles as they move superiorly, are considered to be distended when they are engorged to a level 1 to 2 cm above the clavicle. This assessment is properly done with the patient in a 45° Fowler's position; however, this is something that cannot be accomplished during the primary assessment of the patient in the field.

Because of the mediastinal shift caused by the increasing pressure, palpation or visualization of the trachea may manifest in a deviation of the trachea away from the affected side. However, this late finding in a tension pneumothorax may not be present despite the rapid decompensation of the patient's clinical status. For this reason, you must be vigilant in watching for the cardiopulmonary findings associated with a tension pneumothorax and not rely on the presence of all the classic physical findings in making the diagnosis.

The accumulation of air within the pleural space decreases the lung volume and diminishes the breath sounds on the affected side when you auscultate the chest. Because air causes the loss of breath sounds on that side, the chest will be resonant (like a bell) when percussed, as opposed to the dull sensation expected with fluid or blood.

Due to the injury and the collapsing lung, a patient with a tension pneumothorax often reports pleuritic chest pain and dyspnea. The resulting hypoxia may cause the patient to become anxious, tachycardic, tachypneic, and even cyanotic.

Hypotension, as a late finding of tension pneumothorax, should not be used to either confirm or exclude the possibility of a tension pneumothorax. Its presence may suggest that the pneumothorax has produced such significant pressure as to severely impede preload, or it may represent a simultaneous shock state due to other injuries. Normal blood pressure suggests that, when other signs of a tension pneumothorax are present, the heart is adequately compensating for the diminished venous return.

Words of Wisdom

Shock (a late sign), decreased breath sounds, and hyperresonance to percussion on the same side of the chest mean a tension pneumothorax is present until proven otherwise.

All patients presenting with signs of a tension pneumothorax should immediately be placed on high-flow supplemental O_2 (12 to 15 L/min) via a nonrebreathing mask. Inspect the chest and cover open wounds with a nonporous or occlusive dressing. If signs of tension are present, lift one corner of the dressing to allow air to escape.

In a patient who has a closed tension pneumothorax and clinical findings that suggest immediate relief of the elevated pressures is needed, you must accomplish this through a **needle decompression**, also referred to as a needle thoracentesis or pleural decompression. The steps for performing a needle decompression are described in **Skill Drill 1**:

Skill Drill 1

1. Assess the patient to ensure that the presentation matches that of a tension pneumothorax **Step 1**:
   - Difficult ventilation despite an open airway
   - Jugular vein distention (may not be present with associated hemorrhage)
   - Absent or decreased breath sounds on the affected side
   - Hyperresonance to percussion on the affected side
   - Tracheal deviation away from the affected side (this late sign is not always present)
   - Pulsus paradoxus
   - Tachycardia

2. Prepare and assemble all necessary equipment:
   - Large-bore IV catheter, preferably 10- to 14-gauge and at least 2 inches long
   - Alcohol or povidone iodine (Betadine) preps
   - Flutter valve: cut off one finger of a glove to use as a substitute if you do not have a commercial device available.
   - Adhesive tape
3. Obtain orders from medical control if needed by your service's protocols `Step 2`.
4. Locate the appropriate site `Figure 13` `Step 3`. Find the second or third rib because you will need to insert the needle just above the third rib into the intercostal space at the midclavicular line on the affected side. If there is significant trauma to the anterior portion of the chest, use the intercostal space between the fourth and fifth ribs at the midaxillary line on the affected side. However, the midclavicular line approach is preferred because it is usually easier to access with less chance of dislodging the needle.
5. Cleanse the appropriate area using aseptic technique `Step 4`.
6. Make a one-way valve, or flutter valve, by inserting the catheter through the end of the finger of a medical glove, cut off from the glove `Step 5`. Or, use a commercially prepared device.

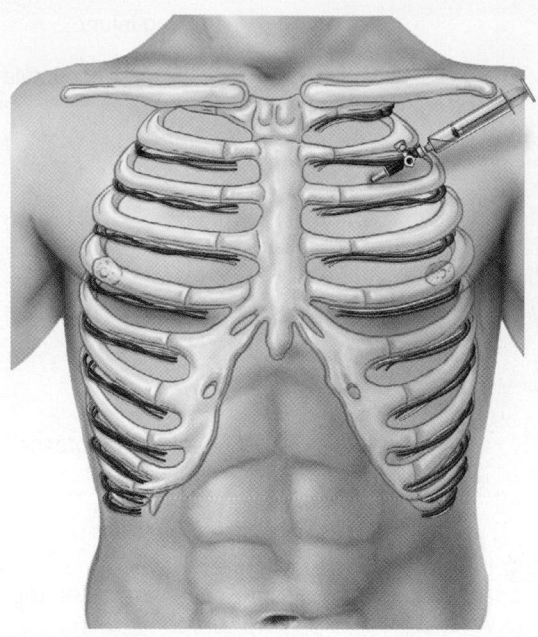

Figure 13 Correct placement of the needle for decompression. The positions of nerves, arteries, and veins are shown in relation to the ribs.

Words of Wisdom

Patients with a pneumothorax, tension pneumothorax, hemothorax, or hemopneumothorax may need a chest tube inserted. A chest tube is a flexible plastic tube that is inserted through the side of the chest into the pleural cavity to remove air, fluid, or pus from the pleural cavity `Figure 14`. It was traditionally attached to an underwater seal to create a one-way system allowing for air or fluid to drain from the chest with each exhalation, reestablishing the interpleural negative pressure and reinflating the lung. Modern systems no longer use a water chamber, but they do have the same effect.

Whereas insertion of a chest tube is not commonly within a paramedic scope of practice, the monitoring and transport of a patient with an existing chest tube is within the National Standards.

When monitoring and transporting a patient with a chest tube in place:

- Make sure all connections are taped or banded with wire to prevent accidental separation.
- Ensure that the dressing over the insertion site is securely taped and occlusive. Use a felt-tip marker to mark the depth of the tube; if there are markings, note the depth of the tube on the transfer chart. Make sure the tube is sutured, wired, or taped so it cannot be accidently pulled out.
- Maintain the drainage unit below the level of the chest at all times during transport. Many units have bed hangers so that the unit can be hung on the stretcher. If there is water in the unit, keep it upright at all times. If attached to a suction device, find out if the suction can be discontinued for transport; if not, attach it to portable suction.
- Tubing should be kept coiled to prevent kinks or dependent loops.

- Assess and document bubbling in the water seal (does not have to be continuous), any output in the collection chamber, and its type (eg, blood).
- Do not clamp tubes for transport. This could cause a tension pneumothorax.
- Continuous bubbling may be a sign of tracheobronchial laceration. Large amounts of bloody drainage need to be balanced by transfusion.

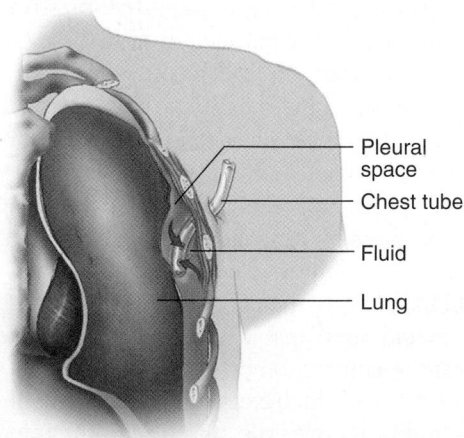

Pleural space
Chest tube
Fluid
Lung

Figure 14 A chest tube is inserted through the side of the chest into the pleural space.

Skill Drill 1

Needle Decompression (Thoracentesis) of a Tension Pneumothorax

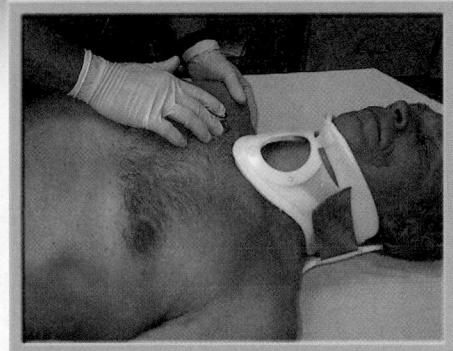

Step 1 Assess the patient.

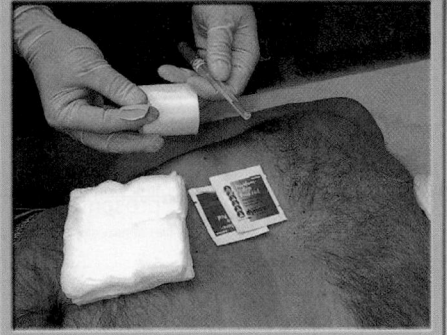

Step 2 Prepare and assemble all necessary equipment. Obtain orders from medical control.

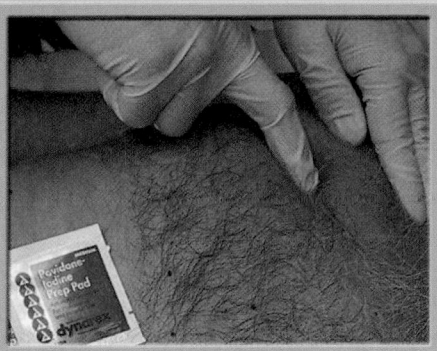

Step 3 Locate the appropriate site between the second and third rib.

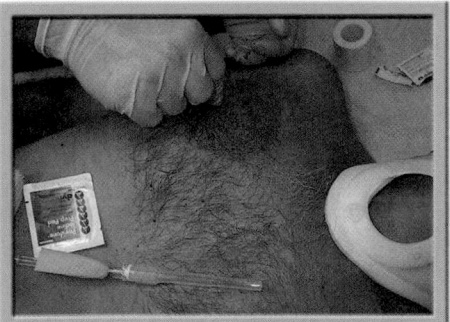

Step 4 Cleanse the appropriate area using aseptic technique.

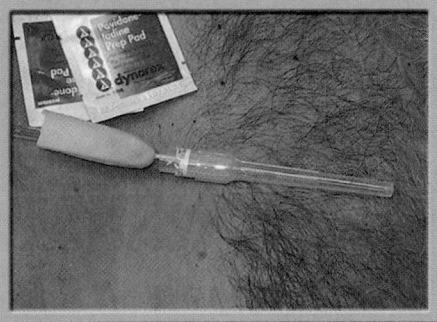

Step 5 Make a one-way valve or flutter valve.

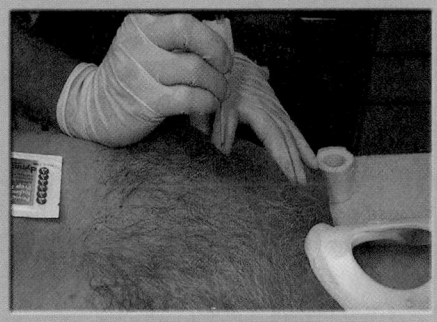

Step 6 Insert the needle at a 90° angle, and listen for the release of air.

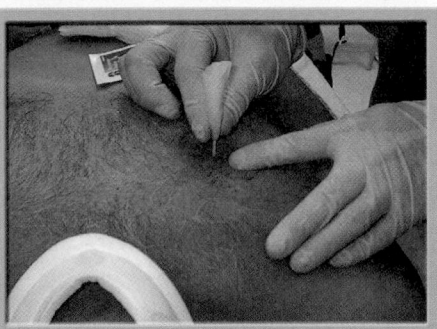

Step 7 Remove the needle. Properly dispose of the needle in the sharps container.

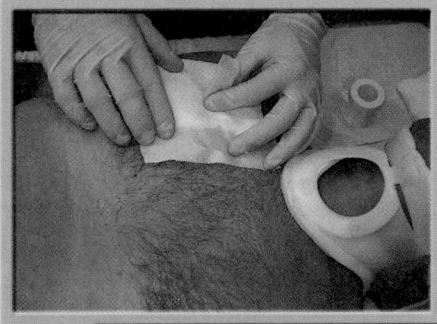

Step 8 Secure the catheter in place. Monitor the patient closely for recurrence of the tension pneumothorax.

7. Insert the needle at a 90° angle, and listen for the release of air **Step 6** . Insert the needle just superior to the third rib, midclavicular, or just above the sixth rib, midaxillary. (The nerves, arteries, and veins run along the inferior borders of each rib.)

8. Remove the needle, and place the needle in the sharps container **Step 7** .

9. Secure the catheter in place in the same manner you would use to secure an impaled object.

10. Monitor the patient closely for recurrence of the tension pneumothorax Step 8. This procedure may need to be repeated several times before arrival at the emergency department.

The performance of a needle decompression is not without risk. If the needle is improperly placed (ie, not inserted over the top of the rib), injury to the intercostal vessels may result in significant hemorrhage. Similarly, passing the needle into the chest may injure the lung parenchyma. However, failure to treat tension pneumothorax will cause the patient to progress to pulseless electrical activity and cardiopulmonary arrest.

■ Hemothorax

A **hemothorax** occurs when the potential space between the parietal and visceral pleura is violated and blood begins to accumulate within this space Figure 15. Hemothorax occurs in approximately 25% of patients with chest trauma. Although it is most commonly caused by tears of lung parenchyma, it may also result from penetrating wounds that puncture the heart or major vessels within the mediastinum or from blunt trauma with deceleration shearing of major vessels. Rib fractures and injuries to the lung parenchyma are the most common sources of injury in the case of a hemothorax. Other causes include injury to the liver, spleen, aorta, internal mammary arteries, intercostal arteries (which can lose up to 50 mL of blood per minute), and other intrathoracic vessels. Due to the location of these injuries, control of bleeding will be impossible with the usual practices and the amount of circulating blood can be greatly reduced, causing hypovolemic shock.

The collection of blood within the pleural space compresses and displaces the surrounding lung, limiting the patient's ability to adequately oxygenate and ventilate. Unlike a pneumothorax, this injury has the added potential of causing hypovolemia. A **hemopneumothorax** occurs when both blood and air are present in the pleural space Figure 16.

A massive hemothorax is defined as accumulation of more than 1,500 mL of blood within the pleural space. For the average adult, this amount represents a nearly 25% to 30% blood volume loss, meaning that the patient's condition will have

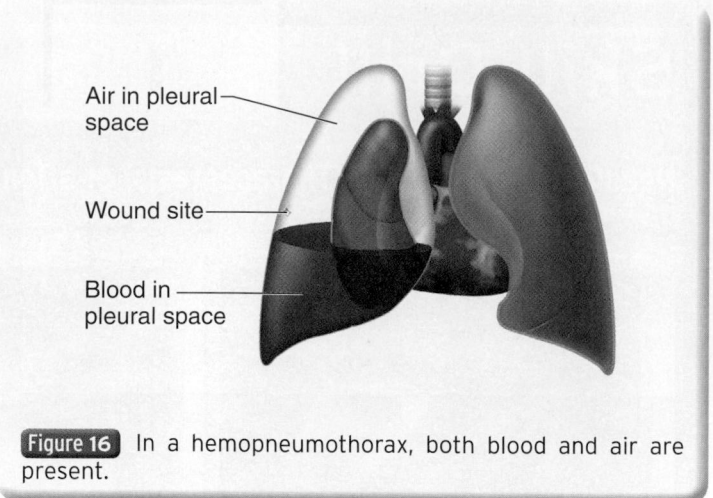

Figure 16 In a hemopneumothorax, both blood and air are present.

Air in pleural space

Wound site

Blood in pleural space

progressed to decompensated shock. Because each lung can hold up to 3,000 mL, it is possible for a patient to completely bleed out into the thoracic cavity.

Assessment and Management

Physical assessment of a massive hemothorax will reveal signs of both ventilatory insufficiency (hypoxia, agitation, anxiety, tachypnea, dyspnea) and hypovolemic shock (tachycardia, hypotension, pale and clammy skin). The physical findings that help to differentiate this hemothorax from other injuries include the lack of tracheal deviation, possible bloody sputum (hemoptysis), and dullness that may be noted on percussion of the affected side of the chest. Neck veins will be flat with associated hypovolemia and distended if there is increased intrathoracic pressure.

The prehospital management of a suspected hemothorax is supportive with rapid transport to the appropriate facility. If the airway does not require intervention, place the patient on high-flow supplemental O_2 via a nonrebreathing mask. Initiate two large-bore peripheral IVs, with fluid resuscitation being guided by local protocols and directed at limiting the duration of hypotension. Hypovolemic shock with hypotension that persists for more than 30 minutes raises the mortality from 1 in 10 patients to as high as 1 in 2 patients. For patients older than 65 years, that risk jumps dramatically, to 9 out of 10 patients.

Words of Wisdom

The major problem following the occurrence of a massive hemothorax is the development of hypovolemic shock and respiratory compromise.

■ Pulmonary Contusion

The position of the lungs just beneath the thoracic cage places them at increased risk for injury with thoracic trauma. As the lung tissue is compressed against the chest wall by force or by the positive pressure within the chest during a thoracic injury,

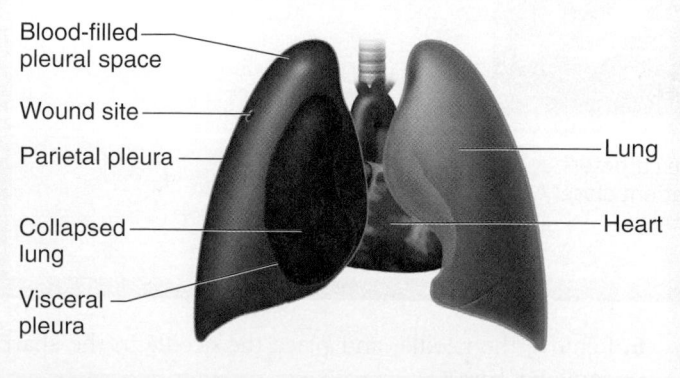

Blood-filled pleural space

Wound site

Parietal pleura

Collapsed lung

Visceral pleura

Lung

Heart

Figure 15 A hemothorax is a collection of blood in the pleural space produced by bleeding within the chest.

alveolar and capillary damage results. This trauma may affect the lungs in a localized area such as a patient with a penetrating injury, or a diffuse area, as in the case of a patient who sustained blunt force trauma to the chest. It leads immediately to a loss of fluid and blood into the involved tissues, followed by white blood cell migration into the area, and, eventually, local tissue edema.

This local tissue injury and edema dilute the local surfactant in the alveoli, diminishing their compliance and causing alveolar collapse (atelectasis). The edema also reduces the delivery of O_2 across the capillary-alveolar interface, resulting in hypoxia. The hypoxia then worsens the situation by thickening the mucus produced, which may in turn lead to bronchiolar obstruction, air trapping, or an increase in physiologic dead air space and further atelectasis.

If the contusion is large, the body compensates by vasoconstricting pulmonary blood flow and increasing cardiac output. This is an attempt to shunt blood from the injured area and increase its delivery to pulmonary tissue that may be able to oxygenate the blood. This pulmonary shunting decreases the functional reserve capacity and leads to mixed venous blood being returned to the heart, further worsening the hypoxemia.

Assessment and Management

The assessment of the patient with a pulmonary contusion may not initially reveal the presence or severity of the injury because it may take 24 hours before the severity of the injury becomes clinically evident. Because not every trauma patient presents immediately for medical treatment (eg, cases involving domestic violence, assaults, injuries that occur while intoxicated, patients in remote areas who are not immediately located, or search and rescue operations), it is important to be familiar with the clinical presentation of this injury.

Hypoxia and CO_2 retention lead to respiratory distress, dyspnea, tachypnea, agitation, and restlessness. Due to the capillary injury and the hemorrhage into the pulmonary parenchyma, the patient may present with hemoptysis (coughing up blood). Evidence of overlying injury may include contusions, tenderness, crepitus, or paradoxical motion. Auscultation may reveal wheezes, rhonchi, rales, or diminished lung sounds in the affected area. In severe cases, cyanosis and low O_2 saturations may be found.

The treatment of pulmonary contusion begins with the assessment and, as needed, management of the patient's airway. Both high-concentration O_2 and positive-pressure ventilation may be used to overcome the pathologic changes described earlier. Because edema may exacerbate the injury, use caution when you are administering IV fluids. The use of IV fluids should be controlled with small fluid boluses at a time to improve cardiac output; overhydration is contraindicated in this setting. In some cases, the administration of small amounts of analgesics may aid the patient in maximizing ventilatory function without suppressing ventilatory drive by reducing pain associated with this injury.

■ Pathophysiology, Assessment, and Management of Myocardial Injuries

■ Cardiac Tamponade

Cardiac tamponade is defined as excessive fluid in the pericardial sac, causing compression of the heart and decreased cardiac output **Figure 17**. Cardiac tamponade may also be referred to as pericardial tamponade. The hemodynamic

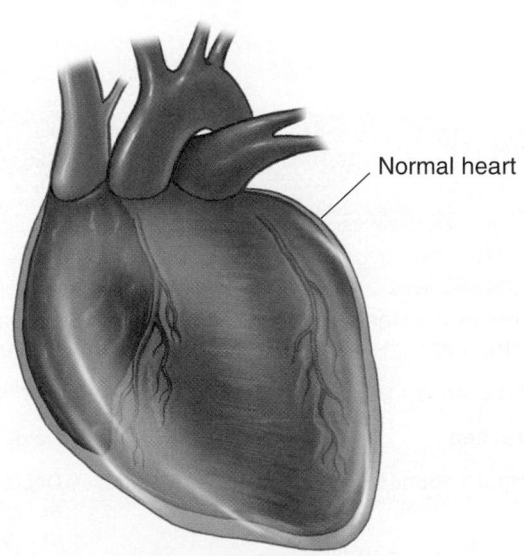 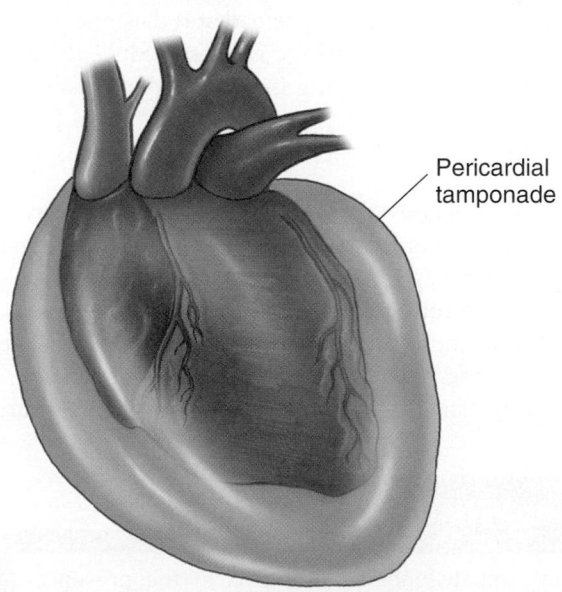

Normal heart

Pericardial tamponade

Figure 17 Cardiac tamponade is a potentially fatal condition in which fluid builds up within the pericardial sac, compressing the heart's chambers and dramatically impairing its ability to pump blood.

effects of cardiac tamponade are determined by the size of the perforation in the pericardium, the rate of hemorrhage from the cardiac wound (dependent on the type of vessel artery vs. vein), and the chamber of the heart involved (the right ventricle is most often penetrated due to its anatomic position). The injury is more commonly caused by a penetrating mechanism, but is also caused by blunt injuries to the chest. Few patients with blunt thoracic trauma experience cardiac tamponade, whereas almost all patients with cardiac stab wounds develop this condition.

The mortality associated with tamponade varies, with high-velocity injuries (gunshots) carrying a higher risk of death than low-velocity injuries (stabbings). If cardiac tamponade is the only injury, mortality is greatly reduced.

Cardiac tamponade can occur in both medical and trauma patients. In the medical setting, inflammatory processes (ie, pericarditis, uremia, myocardial infarction) lead to the slow collection of fluid within the pericardial sac and the gradual distention of the parietal pericardium. Through this process, 1,000 to 1,500 mL of fluid may accumulate in the pericardial sac. Conversely, the bleeding in the trauma patient is rapid, with blood loss from the coronary vasculature or the myocardium itself quickly collecting between the visceral and parietal pericardium. Because the parietal pericardium is not able to rapidly stretch due to its fibrous tissue, an accumulation of as little as 50 mL of blood can cause a reduction in cardiac output.

As the pericardium fills, the continued bleeding increases the pressure within the pericardium. The more pliable structures within the pericardium—namely, the atria and the vena cavae—become compressed, which drastically reduces the preload being delivered to the heart and thereby diminishes stroke volume. The heart initially attempts to compensate for this reduction in preload by increasing the heart rate. This attempt to maintain cardiac output is only temporary because the continued bleeding will further restrict preload and diastolic filling. The pressure within the pericardial sac will also reduce the perfusion in the myocardium, resulting in global myocardial dysfunction. The combination of these two processes leads to the development of hypotension.

Assessment and Management

Beck triad is the classic combination of physical findings found in 30% of patients diagnosed with cardiac tamponade. It includes muffled heart tones, hypotension, and JVD.

Another classic finding in cardiac tamponade (albeit one that is not always present) is the ECG finding of electrical alternans. As fluid accumulates within the pericardial sac, the heart begins to oscillate with each beat. As the heart swings back and forth within the pericardium, its electrical axis changes. Electrical alternans is not commonly seen in acute cardiac tamponade and must be differentiated from bigeminal ectopy, but it is a classic sign of cardiac tamponade. Cardiac output is affected due to an increase in diastolic pressure, and as the condition progresses, a narrowing of pulse pressures will result.

The reduced cardiac output, hypoperfusion, and hypotension observed in cardiac tamponade produce the findings typical of a patient in shock: weak or absent peripheral pulses, diaphoresis, dyspnea, cyanosis, altered mental status, tachycardia, tachypnea, and agitation. Although these symptoms by themselves do not suggest or exclude the presence of cardiac tamponade, identifying them can flesh out the physical assessment.

Physical findings in a patient with cardiac tamponade are not significantly different than those of a tension pneumothorax—namely, hypotension, JVD, tachycardia, altered mental status, and signs of tissue hypoperfusion. One way to differentiate between the two is to remember that in cardiac tamponade, the breath sounds will be equal and the trachea will be midline because the lungs are not affected. **Table 2** compares the physical findings of these two emergencies.

The treatment of the patient with cardiac tamponade begins by assessing and managing the ABCs, ensuring adequate O_2 delivery, and establishing IV access. Provide a rapid fluid bolus to maintain cardiac output. Administering IV fluids may slow the patient's deterioration by momentarily increasing preload. The ultimate treatment for cardiac tamponade is **pericardiocentesis**, which involves inserting a needle attached to a syringe into the chest far enough to penetrate the pericardium to withdraw fluid **Figure 18**. The patient with a cardiac tamponade should be transported rapidly to a trauma center for pericardiocentesis. Definitive management occurs in the operating room, in the hands of a cardiothoracic surgeon.

Words of Wisdom

Hypotension and distended neck veins in the presence of normal lung sounds (which rules out pneumothorax), combined with an appropriate history, suggest cardiac tamponade.

Table 2   **Physical Findings of Cardiac Tamponade Versus Tension Pneumothorax**

Physical Finding	Cardiac Tamponade	Tension Pneumothorax
Presenting sign/symptom	Shock	Respiratory distress
Neck veins	Distended	Distended
Trachea	Midline	Deviated
Breath sounds	Equal on both sides	Decreased or absent on side of injury
Chest percussion	Normal	Hyperresonant on side of injury
Heart sounds	Muffled	Typically normal

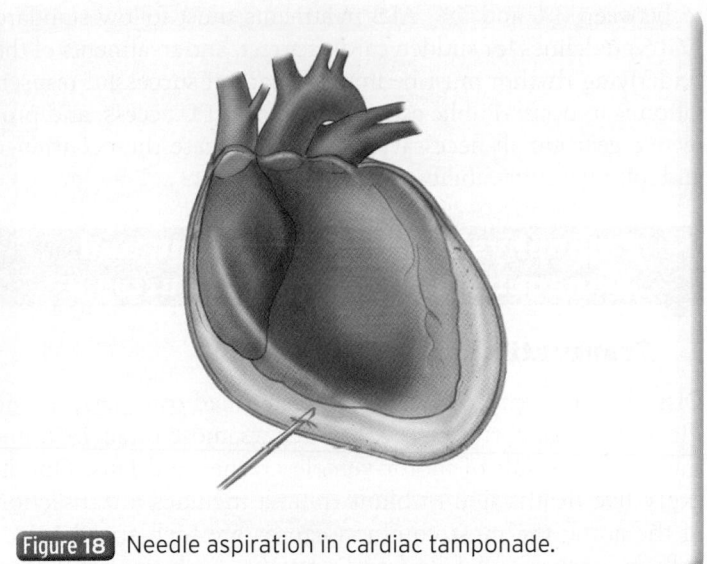

Figure 18 Needle aspiration in cardiac tamponade.

(PVCs), a new right bundle branch block, AV blocks, nonspecific ST-segment and T-wave changes, and ventricular tachycardia or fibrillation. In the event of a coronary artery injury (likely the right coronary artery), ischemic changes consistent with those seen in myocardial infarction may also occur.

The treatment of patients with possible myocardial contusion begins with nonspecific, supportive care, including O_2 administration, frequent assessment of vital signs, cardiac monitoring, and establishing IV access. Fluid resuscitation should be instituted as needed to maintain the patient's blood pressure. Unless allowed by local protocols, consultation with online medical control should precede the administration of antidysrhythmic agents to trauma patients.

Myocardial Contusion

The heart's anterior and unprotected position just behind the sternum puts it in a potentially precarious position during a blunt force mechanism. At speeds of greater than 20 to 35 miles per hour, the sudden deceleration of the chest wall may cause the heart to move forward until it collides with the posterior aspect of the sternum, leading to the blunt cardiac injury known as **myocardial contusion**. This type of injury is characterized by local tissue contusion and hemorrhage, edema, and cellular damage within the involved myocardium. Direct damage to the epicardial vessels (coronary arteries and veins) may compromise the blood flow to the heart. Damage to the myocardium tissue at a cellular level may result in ectopic activity, re-entry pathways, and dysrhythmias.

Complications of myocardial contusions are similar to the complications seen in patients who experience a myocardial infarction. With this in mind, you will need to quickly obtain a 12- or 15-lead ECG to determine the degree of cardiac dysfunction. Dysrhythmias may occur (although they are uncommon in children) due to cellular membrane injury and changes in the myocardial action potential. Structural changes may include the development of a ventricular septal defect, myocardial rupture or aneurysm formation, and coronary artery occlusion.

Assessment and Management

Sharp, retrosternal chest pain is the most common complaint among patients with myocardial contusion. Inspection of the area may reveal soft-tissue or bony injury in the area. Crackles or rales (due to pulmonary edema from left ventricular dysfunction) may be heard on auscultation.

The ECG in a patient with a myocardial contusion is often abnormal. Sinus tachycardia is the most common ECG abnormality seen in patients with a cardiac contusion. Additional ECG changes may include atrial fibrillation or flutter, premature atrial contractions (PACs) or premature ventricular contractions

Myocardial Rupture

Myocardial rupture is an acute perforation of the ventricles, atria, intraventricular septum, intra-atrial septum, chordae, papillary muscles, or valves. The application of severe blunt force to the chest compresses the heart between the sternum and the vertebrae, which can rupture the myocardium. In penetrating trauma, a foreign object or bony fragment may be propelled into the heart, resulting in a laceration of the myocardial wall. Whether it occurs from a penetrating injury or blunt trauma, a ruptured myocardium is a life-threatening condition.

Assessment and Management

Remember that myocardial rupture is life-threatening. Patients may present with acute pulmonary edema or signs of cardiac tamponade. Unless the latter is present and a pericardiocentesis can be done, patients with myocardial rupture should receive supportive care and be rapidly transported to a facility where a thoracotomy can be performed.

Commotio Cordis

If the thorax receives a direct blow during the critical portion of the heart's repolarization period, the result may be immediate cardiac arrest. **Commotio cordis** is ultimately the result of the chest wall impact directly over the heart, especially directly over the left ventricle. Impacts to the chest that are not directly over the heart will not cause commotio cordis.

Commotio cordis (Latin for commotion or disturbance of the heart) commonly occurs in Caucasian boys between ages 4 and 16 years and is the second most common cause of sudden cardiac death in young male athletes. Approximately 50% of the reported cases occurred during competitive sports, whereas the other cases occurred as the result of typical accidents or motor vehicle crashes involving direct impacts to the chest. According to the National Commotio Cordis Registry, the majority of athletes were between ages 10 and 25 years; 26% were younger than age 10 years, and 9% were older than age 25 years. This phenomenon has been documented to have occurred following blunt or nonpenetrating chest trauma to the anterior aspect of the chest. Commotio cordis may occur during sports where contact with high-speed objects occurs, including softball, baseball, lacrosse, polo, rugby, boxing, football, or hockey or from items such as bats, snowballs, fists, and even from kicks and punches during kickboxing, boxing, or karate.

Assessment and Management

Patients who are unresponsive, apneic, and pulseless may be experiencing commotio cordis. Many of these patients are cyanotic, and tonic-clonic (grand mal) seizures have been evident in some. Chest wall contusions and localized bruising that correspond to the site of chest impact are also indicators.

Due to increased awareness of this condition and preparation such as CPR and automated external defibrillators (AEDs) being accessible at sporting events, survival rates have increased to approximately 35% over the past decade (National Commotio Cordis Registry). Factors such as delays in CPR and AED access of more than 3 minutes will decrease survival rates

to between 3% and 5%. ALS treatments must follow standard ACLS guidelines for sudden cardiac arrest, and treatments of the underlying rhythm must be initiated early if successful resuscitation is to occur. Public awareness, CPR, AED access, and protective gear are all necessary items to decrease the occurrence and improve survivability of this type of event.

■ Pathophysiology, Assessment, and Management of Vascular Injuries

■ Traumatic Aortic Disruption

Dissection or rupture of the aorta, also called traumatic aortic disruption or aortic dissection, occurs most often in blunt trauma as a result of motor vehicle crashes and falls. One in every five deaths due to blunt trauma includes a transection of the aorta; the most common causes are high-speed motor vehicle crashes and falls from a height. Each year, 5,000 to 8,000 people in the United States die as a result of aortic or great vessel rupture. Given that the body's entire blood volume passes through this vessel, the high mortality associated with such an injury comes as no surprise. Of those patients who experience an aortic injury, only a few will survive until EMS units arrive; most of the patients reached by EMS personnel can survive with prompt management including surgical intervention.

The most widely accepted theory of how this injury evolves holds that the aorta is injured at its fixed points due to shearing forces. The high-velocity, high-energy impacts that result in these injuries cause the aortic arch to swing forward. The resulting tension, along with rotation and torque on the area, causes the descending aorta to rupture at its point of attachment to the posterior thoracic wall **Figure 19** .

YOU *are the Medic*   PART 4

You and your partner place the patient in full spinal precautions, bandage the knife in place, and move him to the back of your ambulance for further assessment. Further assessment of the chest reveals no signs of subcutaneous emphysema, muffled heart tones, or rib fractures. You apply the cardiac monitor and find a sinus tachycardia with no ectopy at a rate of 120 beats/min.

Recording Time: 10 Minutes	
Respirations	24 breaths/min
Pulse	120 beats/min, weak
Skin	Cool, pale, moist
Blood pressure	90/72 mm Hg
Oxygen saturation (Spo$_2$)	96% at 15L/min via nonrebreathing mask
Pupils	Equal and reactive to light

7. What is the next treatment you should consider for this patient?

8. How often should you reassess this patient?

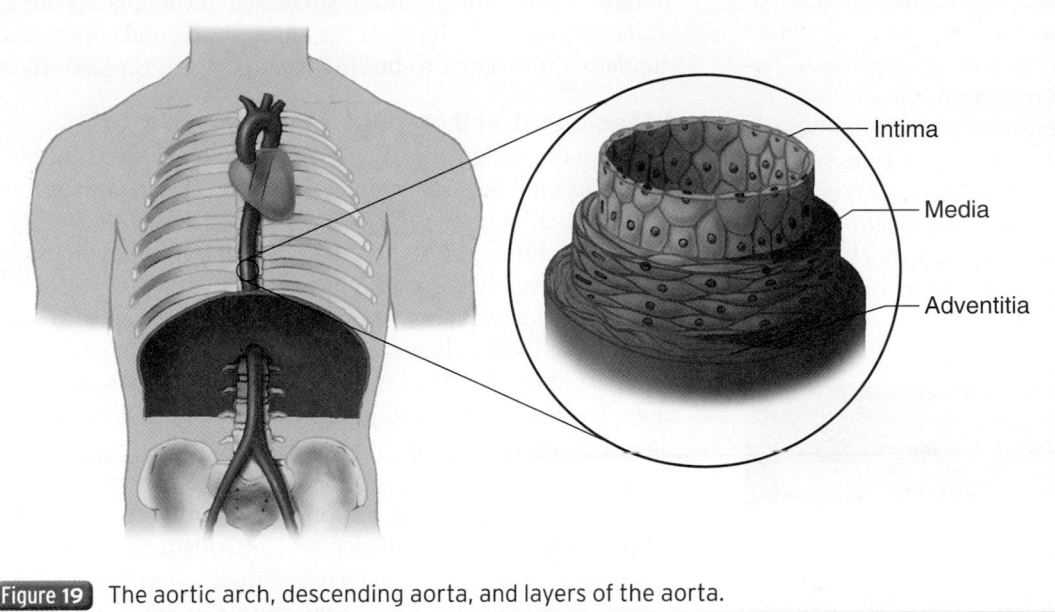

Figure 19 The aortic arch, descending aorta, and layers of the aorta.

Intima

Media

Adventitia

Because of the high energy involved with aortic injuries, associated injuries are to be expected. They may include multiple rib fractures, flail segment, sternal or scapular fracture, pericardial tamponade, hemothorax or pneumothorax, and clavicle fracture.

The prehospital management of potential aortic injuries is symptomatic. After assessment and management of the ABCs, the patient should receive gradual IV hydration for the treatment of hypotension. Aggressive fluid administration may result in sudden changes in the intra-aortic pressure that could worsen the injury. Do not use pressor agents. Expedited transport to a trauma center with an available cardiothoracic surgeon is essential.

The aorta includes three layers—the intima, the media, and the adventitia. If the injury tears the intima, the high pressure within the aorta allows the blood to dissect along the media. More severe injuries damage all three layers of the aorta, allowing blood to leak from the aorta into the surrounding tissues. If these tissues cannot stop the bleeding, the patient can survive only with prompt intervention. Otherwise, the injury will be fatal.

Assessment and Management

Depending on the exact nature of the injury, the symptoms and physical exam findings in cases of traumatic aortic disruption or transection will vary from a patient in unstable condition to one with no physical complaints. However, most patients will report tearing pain behind the sternum or in the scapula. Other findings may include signs of hypovolemic shock, dyspnea, and altered mental status. If a hematoma forms in the area of the esophagus, trachea, or larynx, the patient may present with dysphagia, stridor, and hoarseness, respectively. The patient may also have difficulty swallowing. A harsh murmur may be noted due to the turbulence created as the blood passes the site of the injury to the intima in the aorta.

Recognition of traumatic aortic disruption often comes from a high index of suspicion based on the MOI because a high percentage of patients have no signs of external chest trauma. Assessment of the patient's pulses in all extremities is an important key to the identification of these injuries. As the disruption compresses the aorta and progresses along its branch vessels, blood flow to the extremities may be compromised. This phenomenon results in diminished pulses compared with those closer to the site of the injury. On exam, you will note a stronger pulse (and higher blood pressure) in the right arm than in the left arm or the lower extremities. Hypotension and signs of shock may be present.

Controversies

It has long been taught that the presence of first or second rib fractures (which are often a radiographic finding rather than a physical exam finding) suggests that there is an increased chance that aortic injuries may be present, but this association has lately come into question.

Great Vessel Injury

With the exception of the aorta, the great vessels are located in areas that offer protection from adjacent bony structures and other tissues. As a consequence, injury to these vessels is much more likely with penetrating trauma. In rare instances, blunt trauma may damage the overlying structures or produce a severe rotational injury (such as that caused by machinery).

Some great vessel injuries may result in occlusion or spasm of the involved artery. These injuries will present with ischemic changes (pain, pallor, paresthesias, pulselessness, paralysis) in areas in which the blood supply is coming from the involved artery.

Assessment and Management

If the vessel is not injured in such a way that bleeding is prevented, the patient with a great vessel injury will present with

Words of Wisdom

Suspect aortic rupture in any accident involving powerful deceleration forces.

signs and symptoms of hypovolemic shock, hemothorax, or cardiac tamponade. If the bleeding results in formation of a hematoma, the compression of adjacent structures (ie, esophagus, trachea) may produce additional signs and symptoms.

The management of potential injuries to the great vessels is no different from the management of any other form of acute blood loss. Establish an IV line to provide hydration en route to the trauma center, and treat pericardial tamponade immediately if it is found. Do not use a pneumatic antishock garment because it will increase the pressures within the involved vessels and may contribute to greater blood loss.

Pathophysiology, Assessment, and Management of Other Thoracic Injuries

Diaphragmatic Injuries

Diaphragmatic injury occurs in a relatively small percentage of all trauma patients, yet the potential for this injury has prompted a change in the management of penetrating trauma in recent years. For example, some surgeons manage penetrating trauma between the midaxillary lines, below the clavicle, and above the iliac crests by undertaking surgical exploration to ensure that the diaphragm is intact. This conservative approach reflects the possibility that a missed diaphragmatic injury may result in significant complications in the years following the injury.

Words of Wisdom

Blunt disruptions of the diaphragm are usually associated with herniation of all or part of the liver into the right side of the chest and the stomach into the left side of the chest. The hiatius is the weakest point and hiatal hernias are common.

Injury to the diaphragm may result from direct penetrating injury or blunt force trauma leading to diaphragmatic rupture. Because the diaphragm is protected by the liver on the right side, most diaphragmatic injuries (particularly those due to blunt trauma) occur on the left side. Once the diaphragm has been injured, the healing process is inhibited by the natural pressure differences between the abdominal and thoracic cavities.

Injury to the diaphragm and the associated physical findings have been separated into three phases: acute, latent, and obstructive. The acute phase begins at the time of injury and ends with recovery from other injuries (which may overshadow the diaphragmatic injury and serves to explain why less than one fourth of these injuries are identified during the acute phase). In the latent phase, the patient experiences intermittent abdominal pain due to the periodic herniation or entrapment of abdominal contents in the defect. The obstructive phase occurs when any abdominal contents herniate through the defect, cutting off their blood supply (infarct) in the process.

A rare but ultimate complication of a diaphragmatic injury is the herniation of sufficient abdominal contents into the thoracic cavity. The resulting increased intrathoracic pressure both compresses the lung on the affected side and compromises circulatory function; this finding is called a tension gastrothorax.

Assessment and Management

Although diaphragmatic injuries are not likely to be identified in the prehospital setting, you should still maintain clinical suspicion for such injuries **Figure 20**. You are most likely to care for the patient during the acute phase, but delayed presentations in the obstructive phase are also possible.

In the acute phase, the patient may present with hypotension, tachypnea, bowel sounds in the chest, chest pain, or absence of breath sounds on the affected side. These signs indicate a large diaphragmatic injury that may be followed by herniation of the abdominal contents into the thoracic cavity.

In the obstructive phase, as the blood supply to the herniated organs becomes compromised, symptoms will include nausea, vomiting, abdominal pain, constipation, dyspnea, and abdominal distention. In many cases, these symptoms are severe and unrelenting. The most severe findings may be consistent with a tension gastrothorax.

In both the acute and obstructive phases, management of diaphragmatic injury focuses on maintaining adequate oxygenation and providing rapid transport to the hospital. Elevate the head of the backboard to keep the abdominal contents in the

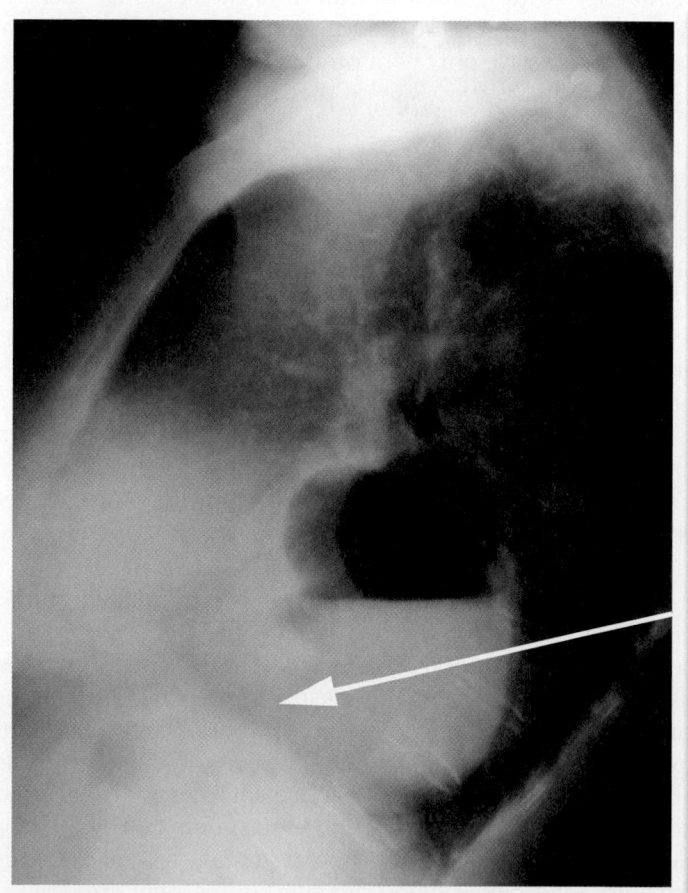

Figure 20 Radiograph of a diaphragmatic rupture. The shadow shows the stomach herniated through the diaphragmatic rupture.

abdominal cavity, and provide positive-pressure ventilation for hypoventilation. In prehospital systems that allow for such procedures, nasogastric tube placement may improve the patient's condition by decompressing the involved gastrointestinal organs.

> ### Words of Wisdom
>
> Use of nitrous oxide should be avoided in patients with a possible diaphragmatic injury because it can greatly increase the volume of gas within entrapped viscera.

Esophageal Injuries

Esophageal injuries are one of the most rapidly fatal injuries to the gastrointestinal tract, particularly if the diagnosis is not made early. Fortunately, even with penetrating trauma, such injuries are rare. Because of the location of the esophagus, however, it is often associated with other significant injuries.

Assessment and Management

Esophageal injuries often present with other thoracic and spinal injuries due to the location of the esophagus within the thorax. The patient may experience pleuritic chest pain, and particularly pain that is made worse by swallowing or flexion of the neck. Subcutaneous emphysema may occur, but more than half of esophageal injury patients with this finding have an associated tracheal injury.

No specific therapy for esophageal injuries is possible in the prehospital setting. Definitive care occurs once the patient is evaluated in the hospital and an appropriate surgical consultation is achieved. In the meantime, you should ensure that the patient is given nothing orally to help minimize complications related to this injury.

Tracheobronchial Injuries

Injuries to the major airways are rare. In most instances, they are caused by penetrating injuries, but they may occasionally be seen in severe deceleration injuries. Tracheobronchial injuries have a high mortality rate due to the associated airway obstruction.

As with aortic injuries, the site of a tracheobronchial injury is often close to a point of attachment—namely, the carina. The injury to the trachea or mainstem bronchi allows for rapid movement of air into the pleural space, resulting in a pneumothorax. As this injury progresses to a tension pneumothorax, a needle thoracentesis is often insufficient because the rate of air entry into the pleural space exceeds the rate at which the air can escape from the inserted angiocath.

Assessment and Management

The clinical presentation of tracheobronchial injuries may vary from mildly symptomatic to severe respiratory compromise.

Expected physical findings include hoarseness, dyspnea and tachypnea, respiratory distress, and hemoptysis. Look for findings of a pneumothorax or tension pneumothorax.

> ### Words of Wisdom
>
> Patients who have been aggressively and improperly restrained by law enforcement personnel, by EMS personnel, or in an altercation situation may experience traumatic asphyxia.

The treatment of a patient with a suspected tracheobronchial injury centers on adequate assessment and management of the patient's ABCs. The patient with a tenuous airway who can be managed with bag-mask ventilation should not be intubated, because introducing an endotracheal tube may complete a partial tracheal injury and result in complete airway obstruction. Similarly, because of the rapid loss of air into the pleural space, high ventilatory pressures should be avoided when you are providing positive-pressure ventilation (bag the patient gently and slowly).

Traumatic Asphyxia

Traumatic injuries that suddenly and forcefully compress the thoracic cavity may induce **traumatic asphyxia** **Figure 21** . Traumatic asphyxia may result from an unrestrained driver hitting a steering wheel or a pedestrian who is compressed between a vehicle and a wall. The sudden compression of the chest causes pressure to be translated into the major veins of the head, neck, and kidneys. This massive increase in pressure then passes into the capillary beds, resulting in their rupture.

Assessment and Management

Traumatic asphyxia is characterized by a series of dramatic physical findings. Patients will have cyanosis of the head, the upper

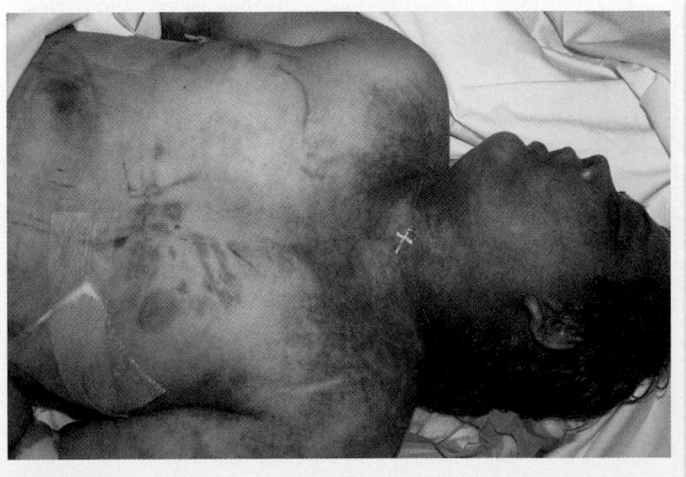

Figure 21 Traumatic asphyxia.

extremities, and the torso above the level of the compression. Ocular hemorrhage may be mild, such as bleeding into the anterior surface of the eye (**subconjunctival hematoma**), or extremely dramatic, causing the eyes to protrude from their normal position (**exophthalmos**). Other facial structures, including the tongue and lips, may also become dramatically swollen and cyanotic.

Although the term "asphyxia" implies a uniformly fatal outcome for patients, this is not always the case. Given the significant force required to produce traumatic asphyxia, however, your suspicion for associated injuries should be quite high. Do not let the dramatic physical findings in the head and neck distract you from those injuries that are immediately life-threatening.

After other life-threatening injuries are managed, the treatment of patients exhibiting traumatic asphyxia is relatively brief. In the absence of intubation, provide high-flow supplemental O_2 via a nonrebreathing mask. Take cervical spine precautions, including spinal immobilization. IV access should be obtained with two large-bore IV lines. Transport to the nearest appropriate trauma center.

YOU *are the Medic*   SUMMARY

1. What is your primary concern for this patient?

Your immediate concern is the overall presentation of the patient. Does your rapid scan reveal any obvious life threats? Is he conscious? Does he have obvious breathing difficulty or evidence of injury? Does he appear pale, cyanotic, red, or gray? Is he alert and oriented or confused? You already know the cause of injury and that the patient is intoxicated. What you do not know is what damage has been done and how it is affecting the patient.

2. What anatomic structures could be damaged in relation to the position of the knife?

The structures located in the vicinity of the knife blade are the left lung, heart, aorta, and the pleural layers. You should not assume the length of the knife blade as being long or short. You should not assume any single structure in the vicinity of the wound is not damaged.

3. What immediate treatment do you need to provide to this patient?

Immediate treatment is centered on maintaining the patient's airway and providing oxygen. You can be reasonably confident there is damage to the respiratory system due to the location of the knife. You will need to conduct a focused assessment to determine the extent of the damage.

4. What steps will you take in your further assessment of this patient?

The breathing assessment begins with an inspection of the patient's thorax. Consider the contour, appearance, and symmetry of the chest wall. Signs of soft-tissue injury (contusions, abrasions, lacerations, or deformity) suggest the possibility of an underlying injury. Paradoxical motion of a section of the chest wall, retractions, subcutaneous air or edema, impaled objects, or penetrating injuries also suggest an underlying injury with the potential to compromise the patient's breathing. Consider the adequacy of both ventilation and oxygenation. To assess ventilation, examine the patient's respiratory rate, depth, and effort. The final steps in the assessment of the patient's breathing entail the palpation, percussion, and auscultation of the chest. Auscultation of the heart sounds is another important part of the circulatory assessment. For patients with potential intrathoracic injuries, note whether the heart sounds are easily heard or whether they are muffled. Performing such an assessment may prove difficult in the back of a moving or running ambulance or because of other noise on the scene. Even so, the presence of muffled heart tones is an important diagnostic clue to the presence of either a tension pneumothorax (because of its resultant mediastinal shift) or a pericardial tamponade.

5. Do you remove the knife or bandage it in place?

The best course of treatment is to leave the knife in the chest and bandage it in place. You have no idea what structures could be damaged by pulling the knife out of the chest.

6. What additional findings would you be looking for in a focused assessment of the chest?

The final steps in the assessment of the patient's breathing entail the palpation, percussion, and auscultation of the chest. While palpating the chest, assess for any evidence of point tenderness, bony instability, crepitus, subcutaneous emphysema, edema, and tracheal position. Percussion can help to identify either hyperresonance (suggesting increased air within the cavity) or dullness (suggesting blood within the cavity).

7. What is the next treatment you should consider for this patient?

The patient whose circulatory status is compromised (as evidenced by tachycardia, hypotension, or end-organ dysfunction) requires supportive measures until definitive care can be delivered. Placing the patient in a supine or Trendelenburg position will deliver blood otherwise held in the venous system of the lower extremities to the central circulation. The provision of judicious IV fluids may also help to expand the intravascular volume while maintaining the oxygen-carrying capacity of the blood.

8. How often should you reassess this patient?

In your reassessment of the thoracic trauma patient, obtain repeated assessments of the patient's vital signs, oxygenation, circulatory status, and breath sounds. Because the progression from pneumothorax to tension pneumothorax can occur quite rapidly, all patients with a presumptive diagnosis of a pneumothorax should be considered to be in unstable condition and reassessed at least every 5 minutes for worsening dyspnea, tachycardia, and the development of jugular vein distention.

YOU are the Medic   SUMMARY, continued

EMS Patient Care Report (PCR)

Date: 05-22-11	Incident No.: 73577	Nature of Call: Stabbing		Location: 1040 Main Street	
Dispatched: 0115	En Route: 0116	At Scene: 0121	Transport: 0135	At Hospital: 0142	In Service: 0200

Patient Information

Age: 40 **Sex:** M **Weight (in kg [lb]):** 91 kg (200 lb)	**Allergies:** Unknown **Medications:** Unknown **Past Medical History:** Unknown **Chief Complaint:** Stabbing to left upper chest

Vital Signs

Time: 0226	BP: 92/70	Pulse: 120	Respirations: 24	Spo$_2$: 95%
Time: 0131	BP: 90/72	Pulse: 120	Respirations: 24	Spo$_2$: 96%
Time:	BP:	Pulse:	Respirations:	Spo$_2$:

EMS Treatment
(circle all that apply)

Oxygen @ __15__ L/min via (circle one): NC (NRM) Bag-mask device	Assisted Ventilation	Airway Adjunct:	CPR
Defibrillation	**Bleeding Control**	(Bandaging)	**Splinting**	**Other:** (Spinal immobilization; IV line with saline)

Narrative

Arrived to find approx 40-year-old male with a knife protruding from his left upper chest ½ inch below mid-clavicle. Only the handle of the knife is visible. Law enforcement is present and reports the pt is intoxicated. Pt is conscious and disoriented, actively trying to remove the knife. Officer assisted with restraining pt hands until assessment could be made. Oxygen via nonrebreathing mask @ 15 L/min applied. pt chest wall is intact with no bleeding from the wound noted. Lung sounds absent in the left upper lobe and crackles in all left lower fields. Right lung sounds are within normal limits. Knife secured in place with a bulky dressing. Pt secured to a long backboard with spinal precautions. IV normal saline established with 16 gauge in left antecubital vein. pt transported to the trauma center with no change in condition. Report to Dr. Morrison on arrival. **End of report**

Prep Kit

- The thorax contains the ribs, thoracic vertebrae, clavicle, scapula, sternum, heart, lungs, diaphragm, great vessels (including the aorta), esophagus, lymphatic channels, trachea, mainstem bronchi, and nerves.

- Oxygenation and ventilation (delivery of oxygen and removal of carbon dioxide) take place within the thorax, as well as some aspects of circulation.

- Injuries to the thorax can cause air or blood to enter the lungs, or may prevent the organs from being able to move properly, inhibiting oxygenation and ventilation.

- Begin the assessment of a thoracic trauma patient as you would any other patient—with a scene size-up and assessment of the ABCs.

- When you are assessing breathing, note any signs of injury to the thorax, which could indicate additional underlying injuries. Look for paradoxical motion, retractions, subcutaneous emphysema, impaled objects, or penetrating injuries.

- Consider the adequacy of ventilation and oxygenation. Watch for signs of hypoxia, an irregular pulse, changes in blood pressure, and jugular vein distention.

- Because the mechanism of injury that caused the thoracic problem may have been traumatic, always consider cervical spine stabilization in such cases.

- Several types of chest injuries may have similar signs and symptoms, such as hypoxia, pain, tachycardia, cyanosis, and shock. Managing the various chest injuries involves several common steps: maintaining the airway, ensuring oxygenation and ventilation, supporting circulatory status, and transporting quickly. Learning the subtle differences between various chest injuries will help you manage them more specifically.

- Chest wall injuries include flail chest, rib fractures, sternal fractures, and clavicle fractures.

- In flail chest, two or more ribs are broken in two or more places. It can result in a free-floating segment of rib that moves paradoxically when compared with the rest of the chest wall. As a result, the lung tissue beneath the flail segment is not adequately ventilated.

- Management of flail chest includes airway management and possibly positive-pressure ventilation, if the patient experiences respiratory failure. Intubation may also be necessary.

- Rib fractures produce significant pain and can prevent adequate ventilation. Sternal and clavicle fractures are also problematic because they are usually associated with other serious injuries.

- Management of rib fractures should focus on the ABCs and gentle splinting of the patient's chest by having the patient hold a pillow or blanket against the area.

- Lung injuries include simple pneumothorax, open pneumothorax, tension pneumothorax, hemothorax, and pulmonary contusion.

- A pneumothorax occurs when air leaks into the space between the pleural surfaces from an opening in the chest or the surface of the lung. The lung collapses as air fills the pleural space. The result is a mismatch between ventilation and perfusion.

- Management of a pneumothorax begins with the ABCs and administration of high-concentration oxygen. Cover a sucking chest wound with a nonporous dressing.

- A tension pneumothorax is a life-threatening condition and results from collection of air in the pleural space. The air exerts increasing pressure on surrounding tissues as it accumulates, compromising ventilation, oxygenation, and circulation.

- Patients with a tension pneumothorax should be placed on high-flow supplemental oxygen via a nonrebreathing mask. Cover open wounds with a nonporous or occlusive dressing. If signs of tension are present, lift one corner of the dressing to allow air to escape. In the event of a closed tension pneumothorax, immediate relief of the elevated pressures must then be accomplished through a needle decompression.

- A hemothorax is the accumulation of blood between the parietal and visceral pleura. It results in compression of structures around the collection of blood and compromises ventilation, oxygenation, and circulation.

- If the airway of a patient with a hemothorax does not require intervention, place the patient on high-flow supplemental oxygen via a nonrebreathing mask. Initiate two large-bore peripheral IVs, with fluid resuscitation being guided by local protocols and directed at limiting the duration of hypotension.

- A hemopneumothorax is the collection of both blood and air in the pleural space.

- A pulmonary contusion occurs from compression of the lung. It results in alveolar and capillary damage, edema, and hypoxia.

- For patients with a pulmonary contusion or cardiac tamponade, assess and manage the ABCs and consider administering IV fluids.

- Myocardial injuries include cardiac tamponade, myocardial contusion, myocardial rupture, and commotio cordis.

- Cardiac tamponade occurs when excessive fluid builds up in the pericardial sac around the heart. The heart becomes compressed and stroke volume is compromised.

- The treatment of the patient with cardiac tamponade begins by managing the ABCs, ensuring adequate oxygen delivery, and establishing IV access. Provide a rapid fluid bolus to maintain cardiac output. Pericardiocentesis is the ultimate treatment option for this condition, a risky technique that is rarely performed by paramedics.

- Myocardial contusion is essentially blunt trauma to the heart. Hemorrhage, edema, and cellular damage result, and dysrhythmias may occur.

- Management of patients with a myocardial contusion should be supportive, but also includes cardiac monitoring and establishing IV access. Fluid resuscitation should be instituted as needed to maintain the patient's blood pressure. Consultation with online medical control may precede the administration of antidysrhythmic agents.

- Myocardial rupture is perforation of one or more elements of the anatomy of the heart, such as the ventricles, atria, or valves. It can occur from blunt or penetrating trauma.

- Patients with myocardial rupture should receive supportive care and be rapidly transported to a trauma center where a thoracotomy can be performed.

- Commotio cordis occurs from a direct blow to the chest during a critical portion of the heart's repolarization period, resulting in possible cardiac arrest.

- ALS treatments for commotio cordis must follow standard ACLS guidelines for sudden cardiac arrest and treatments of the underlying rhythm must be initiated early if successful resuscitation is to occur.

- Vascular injuries include traumatic aortic disruption and great vessel injury.

- Traumatic aortic disruption is literally ripping of the aorta. Injuries to other great vessels may cause similar problems of potentially fatal bleeding.

- Care for patients with traumatic aortic disruption focuses on symptom control. After assessment and management of the ABCs, the patient should receive gradual IV hydration for the treatment of hypotension. Management of patients with great vessel injuries is no different from those with acute blood loss.

- Other thoracic injuries include diaphragmatic injuries (abdominal contents may herniate through the injury and cut off the blood supply); esophageal injuries, which can be rapidly fatal; tracheobronchial injuries (injury to the airways); and traumatic asphyxia (sudden compression of the chest leading to pressure on the head, neck, and kidneys, causing capillary beds to rupture).

Prep Kit, continued

■ Vital Vocabulary

angle of Louis Prominence on the sternum that lies opposite the second intercostal space.

atelectasis Alveolar collapse that prevents use of that portion of the lungs for ventilation and oxygenation.

cardiac tamponade A condition in which the atria and right ventricle are collapsed by a collection of blood or other fluid within the pericardial sac, resulting in a diminished cardiac output.

clavicle An S-shaped bone, also called the collarbone, that articulates medially with the sternum and laterally with the shoulder.

commotio cordis An event in which an often fatal cardiac dysrhythmia is produced by a sudden blow to the thoracic cavity.

crepitus A grating sensation made when two pieces of broken bone rub together or subcutaneous emphysema is palpated.

diaphragm Large skeletal muscle that plays a major role in breathing and separates the chest cavity from the abdominal cavity.

exophthalmos Protrusion of the eyes from the normal position within the socket.

flail chest An injury that involves two or more adjacent ribs fractured in two or more places, allowing the segment between the fractures to move independently of the rest of the thoracic cage.

hemopneumothorax A collection of blood and air in the pleural cavity.

hemothorax The collection of blood within the normally closed pleural space.

intercostal space The space between two ribs, named according to the number of the rib above it, that contains the intercostal muscles and neurovascular bundle.

jugular vein distention (JVD) A prominence of the jugular veins due to increased volume or increased pressure within the central venous system or the thoracic cavity.

manubrium The superior segment of the sternum; its lower border defines the angle of Louis.

mediastinum Space within the chest that contains the heart, major blood vessels, vagus nerve, trachea, and esophagus; located between the two lungs.

myocardial contusion Blunt force injury to the heart that results in capillary damage, interstitial bleeding, and cellular damage in the area.

myocardial rupture An acute traumatic perforation of the ventricles, atria, intraventricular septum, intra-atrial septum, chordae, papillary muscles, or valves.

needle decompression Also referred to as a needle thoracentesis, this procedure introduces a needle or angiocath into the pleural space in an attempt to relieve a tension pneumothorax.

neurovascular bundle A closely placed grouping of an artery, vein, and nerve that lies beneath the inferior edge of a rib.

open pneumothorax The result of a defect in the chest wall that allows air to enter the thoracic space.

pericardial sac The potential space between the layers of the pericardium.

pericardiocentesis A procedure in which a needle or angiocath is introduced into the pericardial sac to relieve cardiac tamponade.

pericardium Double-layered sac containing the heart and the origins of the superior vena cava, the inferior vena cava, and the pulmonary artery.

pleura Membrane lining the outer surface of the lungs (visceral pleura), the inner surface of the chest wall, and the thoracic surface of the diaphragm (parietal pleura).

pneumothorax The collection of air within the normally closed pleural space.

pulmonary contusion Injury to the lung parenchyma that results in capillary hemorrhage into the tissue.

pulsus paradoxus A drop in the systolic blood pressure of 10 mm Hg more than during inspiration; commonly seen in patients with cardiac tamponade or severe asthma.

scapula A large, flat, triangular bone along the posterior thorax that articulates with the clavicle and humerus.

sternum Also known as the breastbone, this bony structure along the midline of the thorax provides a point of anterior attachment for the thoracic cage.

subconjunctival hematoma The collection of blood within the sclera of the eye, presenting as a bright red patch of blood over the sclera but not involving the cornea.

subcutaneous emphysema A physical finding of air within the subcutaneous tissue.

suprasternal notch The indentation formed by the superior border of the manubrium and the clavicles, often used as a landmark for procedures such as subclavian vein access.

tension pneumothorax A life-threatening collection of air within the pleural space; the volume and pressure have both collapsed the involved lung and caused a shift of the mediastinal structures to the opposite side.

thoracic inlet The superior aspect of the thoracic cavity, this ring-like opening is created by the first vertebral vertebra, the first rib, the clavicles, and the manubrium.

thorax The part of the body between the neck and the diaphragm, encased by the ribs.

traumatic aortic disruption Dissection or rupture of the aorta.

traumatic asphyxia A pattern of injuries seen after a severe force is applied to the thorax, forcing blood from the great vessels and back into the head and neck.

xiphoid process An inferior segment of the sternum often used as a landmark for cardiopulmonary resuscitation.

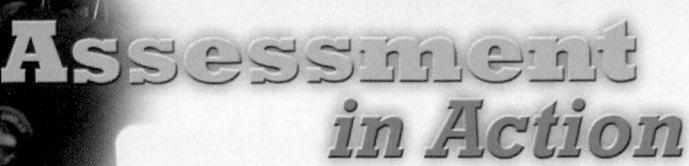

Assessment in Action

Your unit is dispatched to a local soccer field for a player down. When you arrive on scene, a man in his 20s appears to be in a great deal of pain. The patient is conscious and lying supine on the ground holding his chest. The coach states the patient was hit in the chest by an opposing player's head. The patient fell to the ground but did not lose consciousness.

1. What is the most common thoracic injury?
   A. Pulmonary contusion
   B. Rib fractures
   C. Flail chest
   D. Penetrating trauma

2. When you assess this patient you find his respiratory rate and quality is rapid and shallow. You suspect the patient is limiting his chest expansion due to pain. If the patient continues this respiratory pattern, what condition may develop?
   A. Pulmonary contusion
   B. Subcutaneous emphysema
   C. Atelectasis
   D. Cardiac contusion

3. When you are assessing the patient's chest, you find extensive bruising and instability over the right lower ribs. What other type of injury may you want to consider?
   A. Abdominal injuries
   B. Cardiac contusion
   C. Pelvic injuries
   D. Flail segment

4. Air in the pleural cavity is known as:
   A. hemothorax.
   B. cardiac contusion.
   C. pulmonary contusion.
   D. pneumothorax.

5. What is the most effective way to stabilize rib fractures in a conscious, cooperative patient?
   A. Tighten the backboard straps across the patient's chest
   B. Tape the patient's chest
   C. Sandbag application
   D. Self-splinting

Additional Questions

6. Describe the mechanism in which barotrauma causes a pneumothorax.

7. Describe the steps in assessing jugular vein distention.

Abdominal and Genitourinary Trauma

National EMS Education Standard Competencies

Trauma

Integrates assessment findings with principles of epidemiology and pathophysiology to formulate a field impression to implement a comprehensive treatment/disposition plan for an acutely injured patient.

Abdominal and Genitourinary Trauma

Recognition and management of

- Blunt versus penetrating mechanisms (pp 1734-1737, 1741-1742)
- Evisceration (pp 1739-1740, 1741)
- Impaled object (pp 1741-1742)

Pathophysiology, assessment, and management of

- Solid and hollow organ injuries (pp 1742-1743)
- Blunt versus penetrating mechanisms (pp 1734-1737, 1741-1742)
- Evisceration (pp 1739-1740, 1741)
- Injuries to the external genitalia (pp 1746-1747)
- Vaginal bleeding due to trauma (see chapter, *Gynecologic Emergencies*) (pp 1746-1747)
- Sexual assault (see chapter, *Gynecologic Emergencies*) (pp 1746-1747)
- Vascular injury (pp 1743-1744)
- Retroperitoneal injuries (p 1743)

Knowledge Objectives

1. Describe the anatomy and physiology of the abdomen, including an explanation of abdominal quadrants and boundaries. (pp 1728-1734)
2. List the vascular structures contained in the abdomen. (pp 1730-1731)
3. Discuss the solid and hollow organs of the abdomen. (pp 1730-1731)
4. Describe the anatomy and physiology of the female and male genitourinary systems, and distinguish between hollow and solid organs. (pp 1731-1732)
5. Define and discuss closed abdominal injuries, providing examples of the mechanisms of injury that are likely to cause this type of trauma in a patient. (p 1734)
6. Define and discuss open abdominal injuries, including ways to distinguish low-velocity, medium-velocity, and high-velocity injuries, and provide examples of the mechanisms of injury that would cause each. (pp 1734-1735)

7. Discuss the assessment of a patient who has experienced an abdominal or genitourinary injury. (pp 1737-1741)
8. Discuss special considerations related to patient privacy when assessing a patient with a genitourinary injury. (pp 1737-1738)
9. Discuss the emergency medical care of a patient who has sustained a closed abdominal injury. (pp 1741-1742)
10. Discuss the emergency medical care of a patient who has sustained an open abdominal injury, including penetrating injuries and abdominal evisceration. (pp 1741-1742)
11. Describe the different ways solid organs of the abdomen, including the liver, spleen, pancreas, and diaphragm can be injured, and list the signs and symptoms a patient might exhibit depending on the organ(s) involved. (pp 1742-1743)
12. Describe the different ways hollow organs of the abdomen, including the small intestine, large intestine, and stomach can be injured, and list the signs and symptoms a patient might exhibit depending on the organ involved. (p 1743)
13. Describe how retroperitoneal injuries can occur, and the signs and symptoms associated with these. (p 1743)
14. Discuss abdominal vascular injuries, and the signs and symptoms associated with these. (pp 1743-1744)
15. Describe duodenal injury, and the signs and symptoms associated with it. (p 1744)
16. Discuss the types of traumatic injuries that may be sustained by the organs of the male and female genitourinary systems, including the kidneys, urinary bladder, ureters, urethra, and internal and external genitalia. (pp 1744-1747)
17. Discuss the assessment and emergency medical care of a patient who has sustained a genitourinary injury related to the kidneys, urinary bladder, ureters, urethra, and internal and external genitalia. (pp 1745-1747)

Skills Objectives

1. Demonstrate proper emergency medical care of a patient who has experienced a blunt abdominal injury. (pp 1741-1742)
2. Demonstrate proper emergency medical care of a patient who has a penetrating abdominal injury with an impaled object. (pp 1741-1742)
3. Demonstrate how to apply a dressing to an abdominal evisceration wound. (p 1741)

■ Introduction

The abdominal cavity is the largest cavity in the body. Because this cavity extends from the diaphragm to the pelvis, the evaluation and management of patients with abdominal trauma can be challenging. There is great variability in the presentation of conditions, which are rarely resolved in the prehospital setting. Abdominal injuries may be life threatening; therefore, patient assessment should be rapid so management and transport to an appropriate facility can be started.

The abdominal cavity contains several vital organ systems such as the digestive, urinary, and genitourinary systems. These organ systems are vulnerable to trauma partly because of their location, but they also lack some of the protective structures afforded by the skeletal system. Abdominal trauma may be caused by blunt or penetrating force and ranges from minor single-system injuries to the more complicated and potentially devastating multisystem injuries. Abdominal injuries are difficult to prevent because the risk of people being involved in crashes and sustaining other forms of trauma cannot be eliminated. Factors such as an empty bladder and toned abdominal muscles can help decrease potential damage should trauma occur to the abdomen.

Because of the broad spectrum of abdominal injuries, assessment and interventions should be performed quickly and cautiously. Delays in the recognition and management of abdominal injuries can have disastrous consequences. Assessments in the field can be difficult because of other system injuries that may lead to changes in a patient's mental status and sensation. For example, an unresponsive patient or a patient who does not feel pain after spinal trauma may not be able to communicate, leaving the determination of existing injuries to be based solely on presenting signs and the mechanism of injury (MOI). Sometimes it is difficult to perform a proper assessment on a patient who is intoxicated, has used illicit drugs, has injury to the brain or spinal cord, or has sustained injury to adjacent structures such as the pelvis or ribs.

According to the National Center for Injury Prevention and Control, trauma is the leading cause of death in people ages 1 to 44 years. Blunt abdominal trauma is the leading cause of morbidity and mortality in all age groups. In recent years, there has been a concerted effort to reduce morbidity and mortality resulting from abdominal trauma. This process has taken shape at several different levels. The education of prehospital providers in recognizing the need for rapid transport has made a significant reduction in the time from injury to definitive care. The advances in hospital care, such as improved diagnostic equipment (eg, ultrasound), surgical techniques, and postoperative care have also improved patient outcomes. Furthermore, trauma system development has played a large role in providing advanced interventions and detection of traumatic injuries.

Trauma to the genitourinary (GU) system—ie, the kidneys, ureters, bladder, and male and female reproductive organs—may result from either blunt or penetrating trauma. Such injuries

YOU *are the Medic*   **PART 1**

You are the second unit dispatched to the scene of a motor vehicle crash. On arrival, you find the vehicle has sustained front-end damage from striking a utility pole. There are approximately 20 inches of frontal intrusion. The driver and driver's side rear seat passenger are still in the vehicle. You notice that the driver's side air bag deployed. The first crew arrived on scene seconds before your crew and is caring for the driver. Your crew is assigned the care of the rear seat passenger.

Your patient is a 5-year-old boy who was not restrained in a booster seat or car seat, but was wearing an adult seat belt. As you access the child, you find him slouched down in the rear seat, and he is alert and crying. He appears pale and scared, and you observe facial grimacing.

Recording Time: 1 Minute	
Appearance	Eyes open; slouched down in seat (slid partially under seat belt)
Level of consciousness	Alert and crying
Airway	Patent; patient is crying
Breathing	Rapid and shallow
Circulation	Rapid radial pulse

1. What are your immediate concerns?
2. What are your immediate treatment priorities?
3. What are your early communication and transport plans?

are found in 10% to 20% of major trauma patients and 2% to 5% of all trauma patients. Eighty percent of all injuries to the GU system involve the kidneys. You should consider trauma to the GU system whenever a patient has sustained injuries to the lower rib cage, abdomen, pelvis, or upper legs.

Words of Wisdom

Unrecognized abdominal injury remains a cause of preventable death after trauma to the trunk of the body.

The purpose of this chapter is to supply the information necessary for you to assess and begin managing the trauma patient as quickly and with as much confidence as possible. This chapter provides the concepts and vocabulary for the effective understanding and communication of critical data that will improve the assessment of the trauma mechanism. Your field account from the scene is the only source of information for physicians and surgeons to help them understand the events and mechanism that led to any given trauma presentation. This information is critical in visualizing and searching for injuries that may not be obviously apparent on physical examination, as is often seen with abdominal trauma.

Anatomy and Physiology

Anatomic Regions

Knowledge of the anatomic boundaries of the abdomen is important when you are looking for potential injury patterns, such as hollow organ injury, vascular injury, solid organ injury, or injuries to the retroperitoneal area. The oval-shaped abdominal cavity extends from the dome-shaped diaphragm, a large muscle separating the thoracic cavity from the abdomen, to the pelvic brim. The pelvic brim stretches at an angle from the intervertebral disks between L5 and S1 to the pubic symphysis.

The abdomen is divided into three sections, the anterior abdomen, the flanks, and the posterior abdomen or back **Figure 1**. The outer boundary of the abdominal cavity is the abdominal wall on the front of the body and the peritoneal surface on the back of the body. The abdomen extends upward into the lower thorax at about the level of the nipples or the fourth intercostal space. The anterior part of the abdomen is located under the diaphragm, a thin sheet of muscle, and is enclosed by the lower ribs. The abdomen extends inferiorly from the nipples, to the inguinal ligaments and pubic symphysis pubis, inferiorly, and laterally to the anterior of the axillary line. The flanks include the regions between the anterior and posterior axillary lines from the sixth intercostal space to the iliac crest. The back extends posteriorly between the posterior axillary lines, from the tip of the scapula to the iliac crests. The flanks and the back are protected by thick abdominal wall muscles that protect that region from low-velocity penetrating trauma.

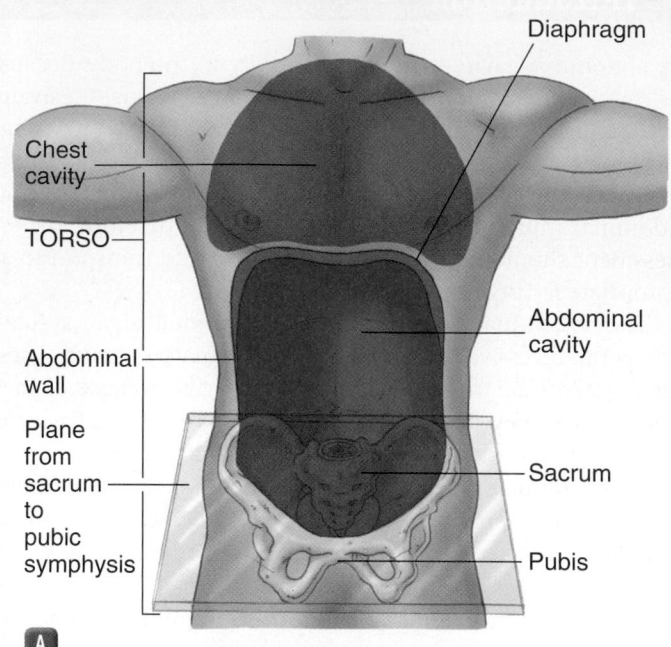

A

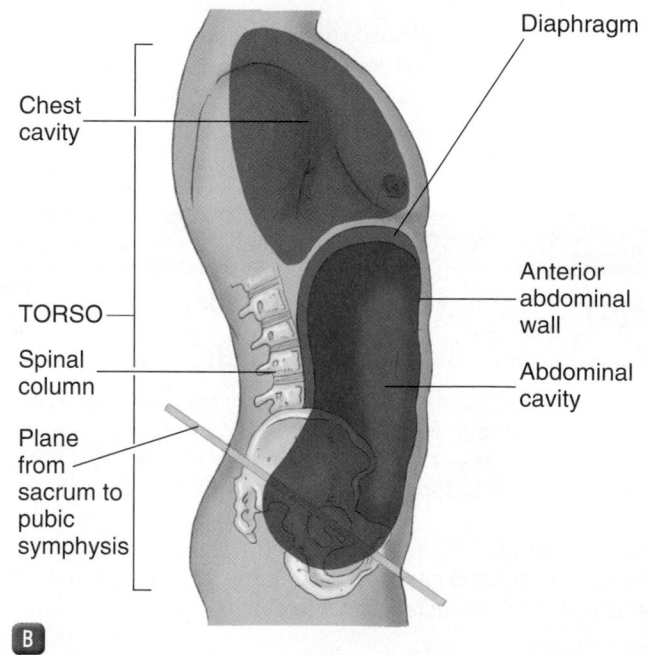

B

Figure 1 The external abdomen consists of the anterior abdomen, the flanks, and the back (retroperitoneal area). The boundaries of the abdomen are the anterior and posterior abdominal cavity walls, the diaphragm, and an imaginary plane from the pubic symphysis to the sacrum. **A.** Anterior view. **B.** Lateral view.

To describe a location in the abdomen, or a source of pain found when you are conducting your assessment, the quadrant system is generally used **Figure 2**. If you were to place a large imaginary "+" sign with the center directly on the umbilicus (navel) with the vertical axis extending from the pubic symphysis

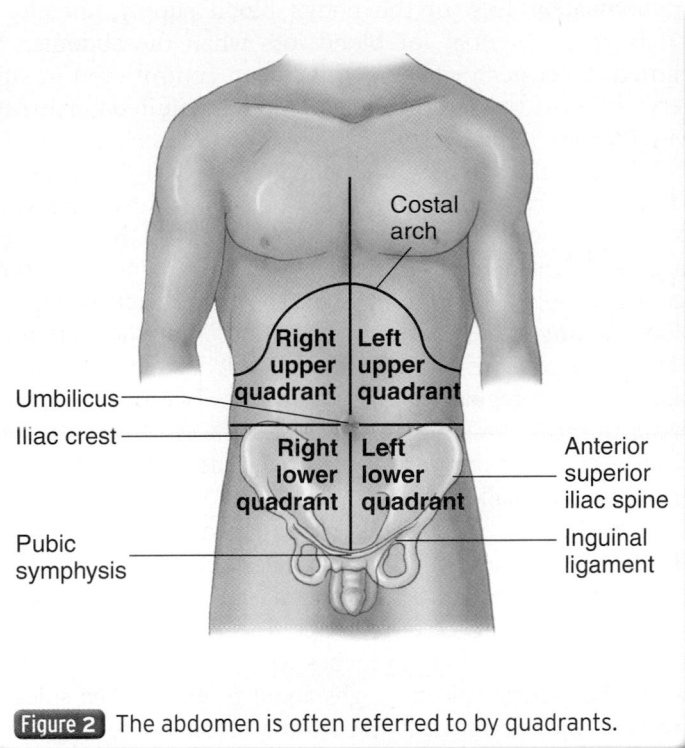

Costal arch

Umbilicus

Iliac crest

Right upper quadrant | **Left upper quadrant**

Right lower quadrant | **Left lower quadrant**

Pubic symphysis

Anterior superior iliac spine

Inguinal ligament

Figure 2 The abdomen is often referred to by quadrants.

to the xiphoid process and the horizontal axis extending to both flanks, this would create four quadrants. These four regions are as follows: the right upper quadrant (RUQ), the right lower quadrant (RLQ), the left lower quadrant (LLQ), and the left upper quadrant (LUQ). The area around the umbilicus is referred to as the **periumbilical** area.

The abdominal cavity is lined with a membrane called the **peritoneum**, which is similar to the pleura that line the thoracic cavity. The **mesentery** is a membranous double fold of tissue in the abdomen that attaches various organs to the body wall. The internal abdomen is structurally divided into three regions: the peritoneal space, the retroperitoneal space, and the pelvis **Figure 3**.

The **peritoneal space** is sometimes described as a division of two parts, upper and lower. The upper peritoneal cavity, also known as the thoracoabdominal component of the abdomen, is covered by the lower part of the thorax. You will find the diaphragm, liver, spleen, stomach, gallbladder, and transverse colon located here. At the peak of a full expiration, the diaphragm rises to the fourth intercostal space. The lower peritoneal cavity contains the small bowel, sigmoid colon, parts of the descending and ascending colon, and, in women, the internal reproductive organs. All of these structures are encased in the peritoneum.

The **retroperitoneal space** is the area posterior to the peritoneal lining of the abdomen, and contains the abdominal aorta, inferior vena cava, pancreas, kidneys, ureters, and most of the duodenum and the posterior aspects of the descending and ascending colon, as well as the retroperitoneal components of the pelvic cavity. The rectum, ureters, bladder, iliac vessels, pelvic vascular plexus, major vascular structures, pelvic skeletal structures, and reproductive organs lie in the pelvis.

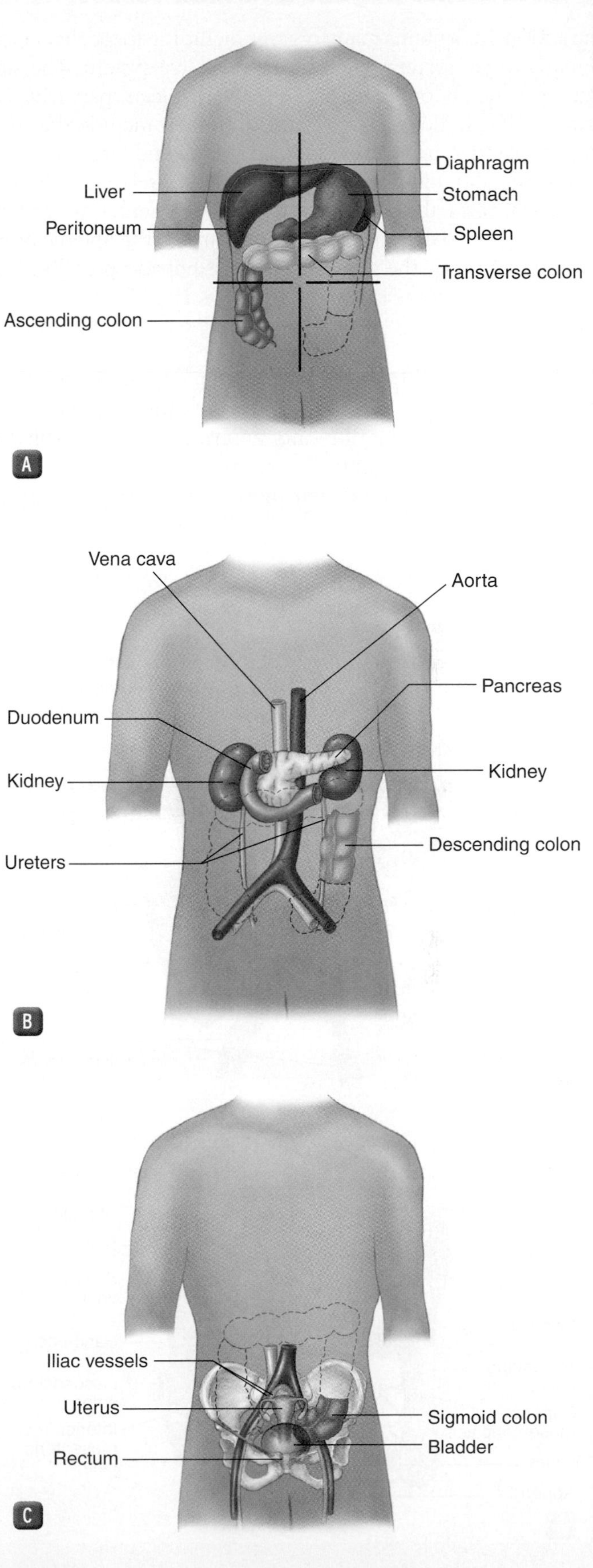

Liver — Diaphragm

Peritoneum — Stomach

— Spleen

— Transverse colon

Ascending colon

A

Vena cava — Aorta

Duodenum — Pancreas

Kidney — Kidney

— Descending colon

Ureters

B

Iliac vessels

Uterus — Sigmoid colon

— Bladder

Rectum

C

Figure 3 Different organs of the abdomen are contained in the peritoneum **(A)**, the retroperitoneal space **(B)**, and the pelvis **(C)**.

Abdominal Organs and Vital Vessels

The abdomen contains many organs, including those that belong to many organ systems such as the digestive system. The solid organs of the abdomen include the liver, spleen, pancreas, and kidneys. The hollow organs of the abdomen include the stomach, gallbladder, urinary bladder, and small and large intestines. Finally, the abdomen includes many vital vessels, including the abdominal aorta, the superior and inferior mesenteries, the renal artery, the gonadal arteries, the gastric artery, the splenic artery, the hepatic artery, the iliac arteries, the hepatic portal system, and the inferior venae cavae **Figure 4**.

Solid Organs

The liver is a solid organ, and is the largest organ in the abdomen. It lies in the right upper quadrant (extending to the epigastrium), superior and anterior to the gallbladder and the hepatic and cystic ducts, and superior to the stomach. The liver has a significant blood supply provided by the hepatic artery and the hepatic-portal vein. The liver contains

approximately 13% of the body's blood supply; therefore, it has great potential for blood loss when the abdomen is injured. Liver hemorrhage is difficult to control even in surgery; therefore a blood transfusion is often required in patients with injuries to the liver.

The functions of the liver are many. The liver detoxifies the blood by removing drugs and other poisonous substances such as ammonia, which it converts into urea, which is then excreted in urine. It has functions that relate to the blood, including processing hemoglobin before it is stored or used, and regulating blood clotting. It has an immune function; it produces immune factors and removes bacteria from the bloodstream. Finally, it plays a role in regulating fats; it produces bile (which is necessary to break down ingested fats), produces cholesterol, and produces proteins that carry fats through the body to ultimately drain into the small intestine.

Like the liver, the spleen is a solid organ in the peritoneum. This highly vascular organ lies in the left upper quadrant, behind the stomach and under the diaphragm, and is partially protected by the left lower rib cage. Its shape resembles a catcher's mitt. It is about 5 inches long, 3 inches wide, and 1.5 inches thick. A healthy, average spleen weighs about 6 ounces. The spleen's functions include filtering and storing blood. Malformed, old, or damaged red blood cells are filtered out and broken down by macrophages. Iron is stored in the spleen until it is returned to the bone marrow for the production of hemoglobin. When the body needs extra blood—for example, following trauma—the spleen can provide blood to the circulatory system. Finally, the spleen also plays an important role in the immune system by detecting potentially pathogenic organisms and, along with the lymph nodes, producing lymphocytes that produce antibodies that weaken or kill bacteria.

The pancreas is an organ located in the retroperitoneal space in the middle of the abdomen under the liver and behind the stomach. Acinar cells are the exocrine cells of the pancreas that produce and secrete enzymes into the duodenum that aid in digestion along with bile from the gallbladder. The pancreas also secretes the hormone insulin from the islets of Langerhans, which is responsible for helping glucose enter the cells.

Hollow Organs

The stomach is an intraperitoneal hollow organ that lies in the left upper quadrant and epigastric region. It is concave (the lesser curvature) on its right side, and convex (the greater curvature) on its left side. The esophagus passes through the diaphragm and opens via the cardia into the stomach. The uppermost part of the stomach is called the fundus, and it is able to adapt to varying amounts of food. This is also where gas bubbles rise to, particularly after a meal. The largest part of the stomach is known as the body. It serves primarily as the storage area for ingested food and liquid. The lower part of the stomach is known as the antrum, and is somewhat funnel-shaped, with its narrow end connecting to the pyloric canal, which empties into the duodenum.

There are three layers of the stomach wall **Figure 5**. The external layer, called the longitudinal muscle, is continuous with the longitudinal muscle of the esophagus. These muscles fibers are divided at the cardia into two broad bands. The middle, or

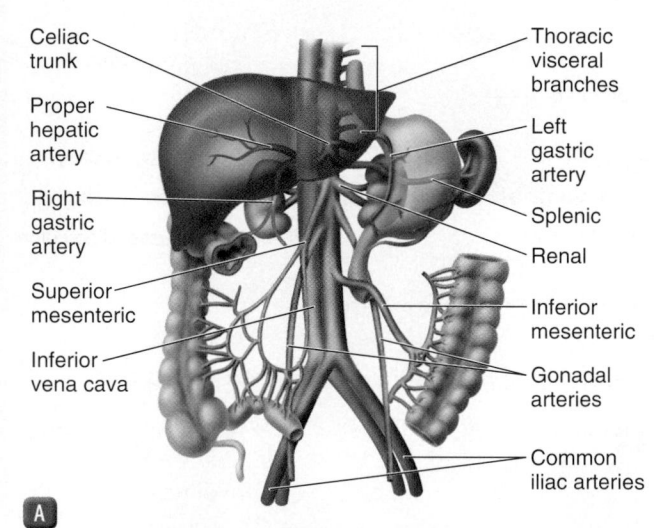

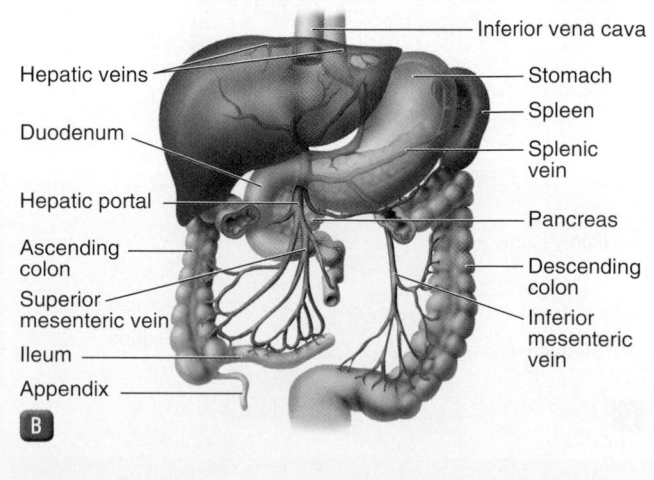

Figure 4 **A.** Arteries of the abdomen. **B.** Veins of the abdomen.

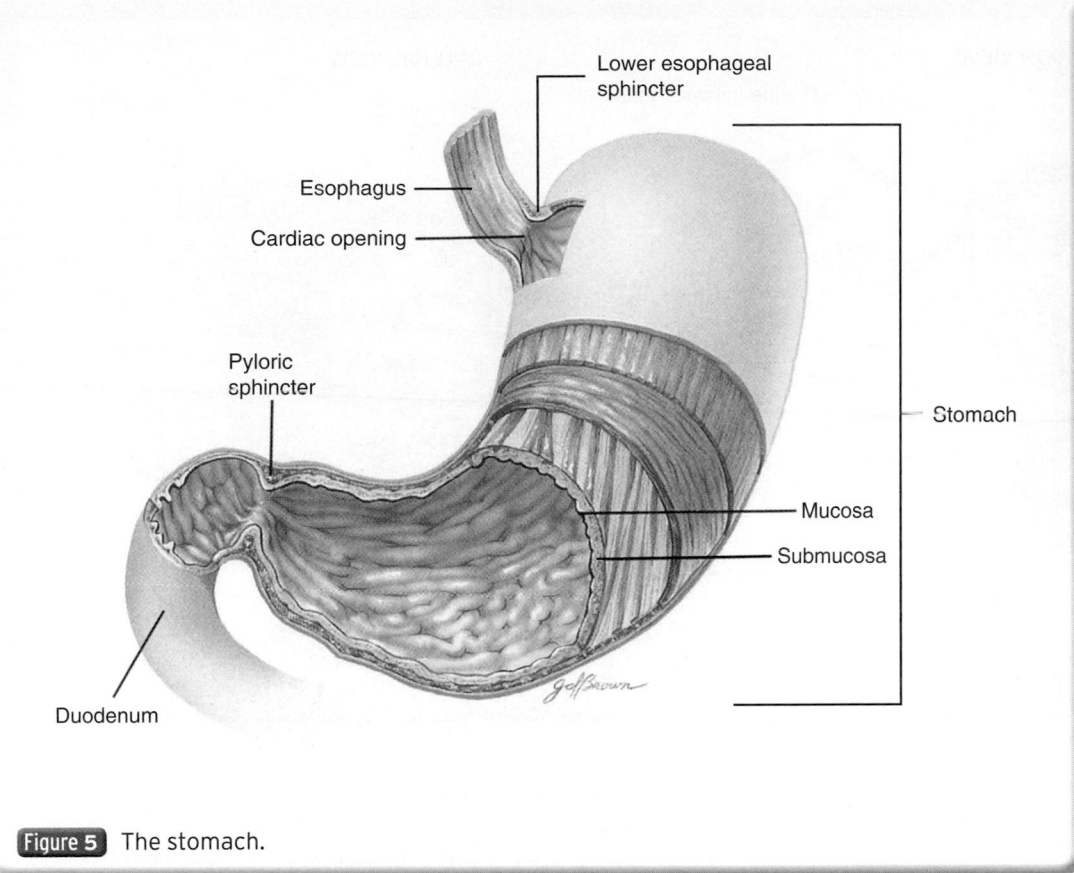

Figure 5 The stomach.

circular layer, the strongest of the three layers, completely covers the stomach. This circular muscle becomes significantly thicker to form the pyloric sphincter. The inner layer, or oblique layer, is the strongest in the fundus region and becomes progressively weaker toward the pylorus. Blood is supplied to the stomach via the celiac trunk that branches from the abdominal portion of the aorta. Blood from the stomach is returned to the venous system via the portal vein, which carries blood to the liver. The nerve supply is provided by the sympathetic (celiac or solar plexus) and parasympathetic (vagus nerve or 10th cranial) divisions of the autonomic nervous system. The stomach contains acid that assists in the digestive process. The gastric juice that is secreted is a mixture of water, hydrochloric acid (strong enough to dissolve metal and has a pH of 1.5 to 3), organic substances (mucus, pepsin, and protein), and electrolytes (potassium, sodium, bicarbonate, sulfate, and phosphate).

The gallbladder is a saclike organ located on the lower surface of the liver that acts as a reservoir for bile, one of the digestive enzymes produced by the liver. The liver continually secretes bile, and the gallbladder stores 50 mL of it, where it becomes more concentrated, until it is released through the cystic duct into the duodenum during the digestive process.

The small and large intestines run from the end of the stomach to the anus. The majority of the intestines are in the intraperitoneal area. They digest and absorb water and nutrients. The first part of the small intestine, the **duodenum**, is retroperitoneal. It is 9 to 11 inches (approximately 3 meters) long and forms a C-shaped curve around the head of the pancreas. The duodenal bulb is the widest part of the small intestine. As contents pass through the stomach, they move through the **pylorus**, a circumferential muscle at the end of the stomach that acts as a valve between the stomach and the duodenum. The cecum is a pouch at the junction of the small intestine and large intestine. In our human ancestors, the cecum was larger but has grown smaller throughout evolution to form the appendix.

The large intestine, also called the colon, receives approximately 10 L of water per day. Approximately 1.5 L are from food, and 8.5 L from secretions. About 95% of this water is reabsorbed. The large intestine also absorbs sodium (Na+) and other ions and excretes other metallic ions into wastes. If water is not absorbed, diarrhea can result, causing dehydration and ion loss. The intestines also absorb vitamin K produced by colon bacteria. The last 20 cm (approximately 8 inches) of the large intestine is the rectum. Finally, stool passes through the rectum and out of the body through the anus. The feces are composed of approximately 75% water and 25% solids. Approximately one third of the solids are intestinal bacteria, and two thirds are undigested materials.

■ Organs of the Genitourinary System

The abdomen also contains organs of the urinary system. The kidneys are located in the retroperitoneal space. They filter blood and excrete body wastes in the form of urine. The kidneys are discussed in greater detail in the chapter, *Genitourinary and Renal Emergencies*. The urinary bladder, a hollow, muscular sac situated in the pelvis along the midline, stores urine until it is excreted. The ureters are a pair of thick-walled, hollow tubes that carry urine from the kidneys to the urinary bladder.

The abdomen also contains organs of the reproductive system. The female reproductive system **Figure 6** contains the uterus, a pear-shaped organ located in the midline of the lower abdomen that allows the implantation, growth, and nourishment of a fetus during pregnancy. The female reproductive system also contains the ovaries (the female reproductive organs), located one on each side of the lower abdominal quadrants. The ovaries produce the precursors to mature eggs, and produce hormones that regulate female reproductive function. These organs can also be injured from crushing and compression forces as well as shearing injuries that may result when a restraint device, such as a lap belt or shoulder belt, are worn improperly.

The male reproductive system **Figure 7** contains the penis, the male external reproductive organ, as well as the testes,

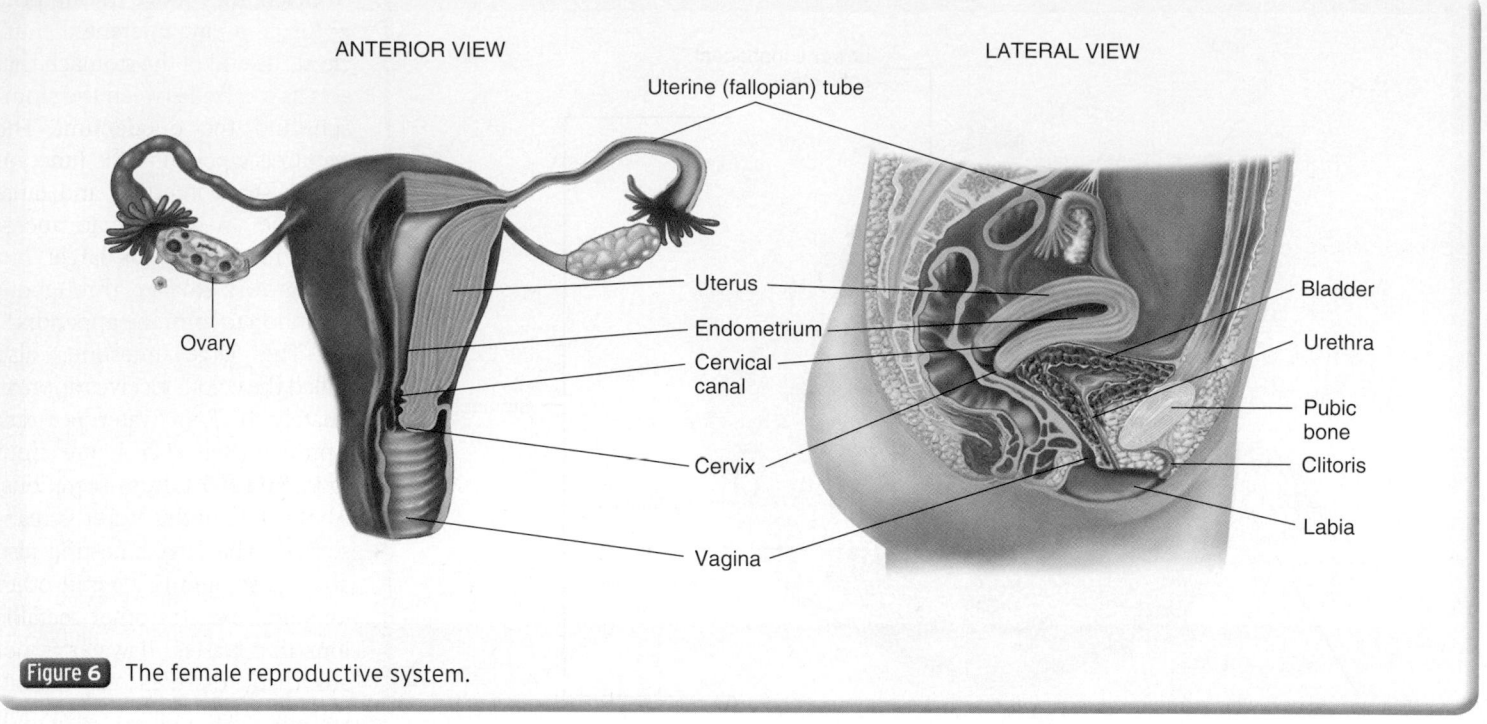

ANTERIOR VIEW

LATERAL VIEW

Uterine (fallopian) tube

Uterus

Endometrium

Cervical canal

Cervix

Ovary

Vagina

Bladder

Urethra

Pubic bone

Clitoris

Labia

Figure 6 The female reproductive system.

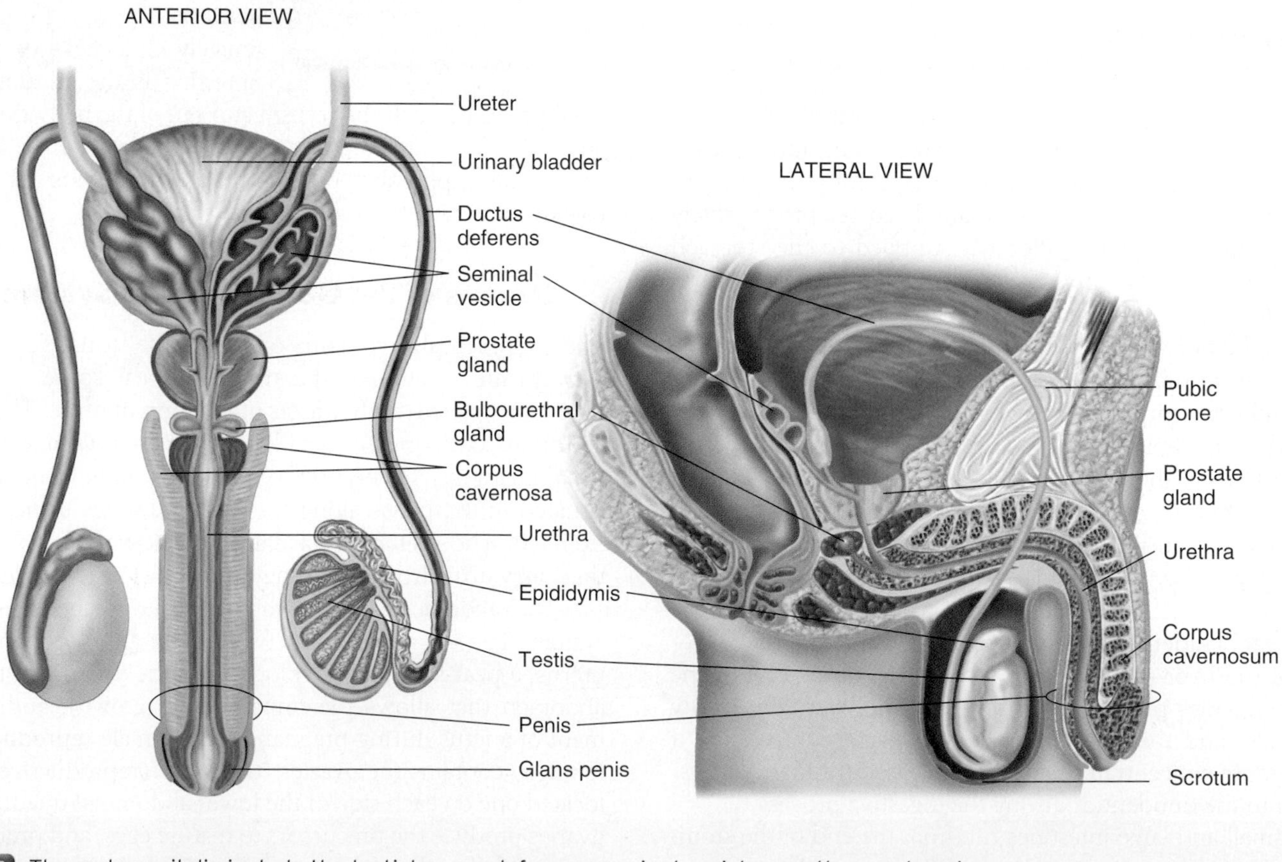

ANTERIOR VIEW

LATERAL VIEW

Ureter

Urinary bladder

Ductus deferens

Seminal vesicle

Prostate gland

Bulbourethral gland

Corpus cavernosa

Urethra

Epididymis

Testis

Penis

Glans penis

Pubic bone

Prostate gland

Urethra

Corpus cavernosum

Scrotum

Figure 7 The male genitalia include the testicles, vas deferens, seminal vesicles, urethra, and penis.

also known as the testicles. The testes produce sperm and secrete male hormones such as testosterone. The testicles have two layers of covering—the tunica albuginea and the tunica vaginalis—and are held outside the body in the scrotal sac. The testicles can be retracted into a more protected position by the cremaster muscles.

The Diaphragm

One additional structure in the abdomen is the diaphragm—the domed-shaped muscle that separates the thoracic cavity from the abdominal cavity. It curves from its point of attachment in the flanks at the 12th rib and peaks in the center at the 4th intercostal space.

Physiology

When abdominal trauma occurs, the internal body locations where enough blood can be lost to cause shock include the abdomen, retroperitoneal space, and muscle compartments of the proximal lower extremities (as well as surfaces surrounding the patient, as a result of bleeding from open wounds) Figure 8 . Because the abdomen and retroperitoneum can accommodate large amounts of blood, the bleeding may produce few signs and symptoms of the trauma. Even the patient's vital signs and physical exam may not indicate the extent of the bleeding.

The organs that are most frequently injured after sustaining blunt trauma are the spleen (in approximately 50% of the cases), followed by the liver (in approximately 40%). Because of its size, the liver is the organ that is most frequently injured in penetrating trauma. Solid organs, such as the liver or spleen, can easily be crushed by external blunt trauma. They both have a large

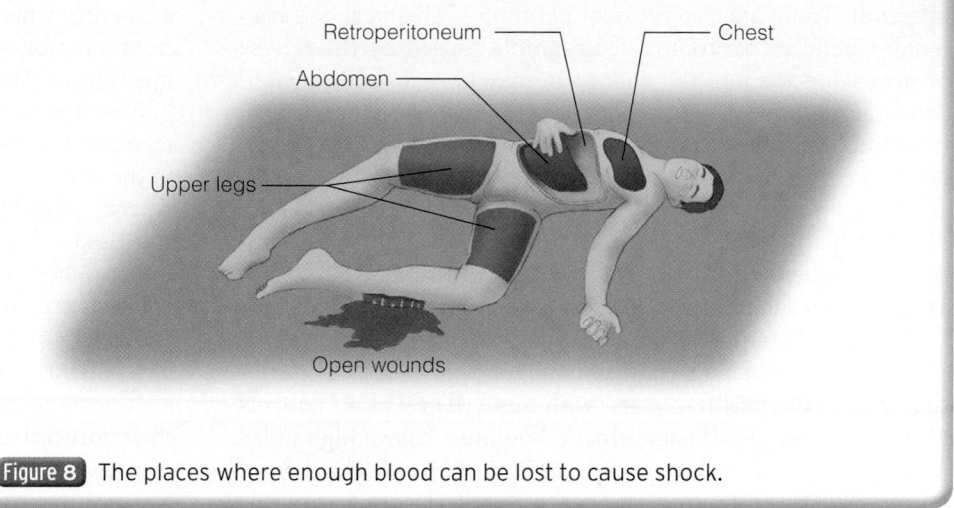

Figure 8 The places where enough blood can be lost to cause shock.

blood supply and can bleed profusely. If a trauma patient has unexplained symptoms of shock, you should suspect abdominal trauma.

Hollow organs are more resilient to blunt trauma and less likely to be injured by trauma unless they are full. However, when a hollow organ is full, it is likely to be injured and can burst in the same way a chemical cold pack breaks when you apply pressure to the outer bag. The danger of bursting hollow organs is that they hold toxins (such as urine, feces, bile, or stomach acids) that can spill out into the abdominal cavity. This spillage can cause <u>peritonitis</u>, an inflammation of the lining of

YOU are the Medic   PART 2

The patient is alert, crying, and difficult to console. The child tells you he is unsure "what happened," but is able to answer questions appropriate for his age. His skin is cool, pale, and slightly moist.

Before moving your patient, you perform a primary assessment and a rapid trauma assessment and find that he is guarding his abdomen. He cries loudly when you palpate his left upper quadrant.

Recording Time: 5 Minutes	
Level of consciousness	Alert, crying with appropriate verbal responses
Skin	Cool, pale, and slightly moist
Pulse	155 beats/min; weak and regular
Blood pressure	82/55 mm Hg
Respirations	40 breaths/min
Oxygen saturation (Spo$_2$)	98% while receiving 12 L/min via nonrebreathing mask

4. What do these signs indicate to you?

5. What does abdominal guarding usually indicate?

6. What can you conclude from the patient's vital signs?

the abdomen (the peritoneum). Peritonitis is a life-threatening infection. There are two types of peritonitis: chemical and bacterial. Chemical peritonitis, for example caused by the release of stomach acids into the abdomen, may have a sudden onset. Bacterial peritonitis—caused, for example, by the release of feces into the abdomen—may develop more slowly, over several hours. Peritonitis can also be classified as primary or secondary. Primary peritonitis occurs when infection travels from the blood or lymph nodes into the peritoneum. Secondary peritonitis occurs when infection travels from the gastrointestinal or biliary tract into the peritoneum. Of the two, secondary peritonitis is much more common.

The management of trauma in the hospital has changed substantially in the past few years, with more than 95% of patients receiving nonsurgical management. You must have a high index of suspicion and a clear understanding of the mechanism of injury (MOI) your trauma patient was exposed to.

■ Mechanism of Injury

Trauma is a significant cause of death in adults and is the leading cause of death in patients ages 1 to 44 years, and according to the National Vital Statistics System of the Centers for Disease Control and Prevention, it is the fifth leading of cause of death for all ages. About 80% of all significant traumas involve the abdomen; however, the exact definition of the term "significant" is not clear in the literature, with most of the trauma statistics coming from regional trauma centers. Unrecognized abdominal trauma is the leading cause of unexpected deaths because it results in a delay in surgical intervention. Other causes of trauma include injuries to pedestrians from being struck by a motor vehicle, and assaults.

■ Blunt Trauma

At least two thirds of all abdominal injuries involve **blunt trauma**, most of which occur during motor vehicle crashes **Figure 9**, with a resulting mortality rate of about 5%. A direct

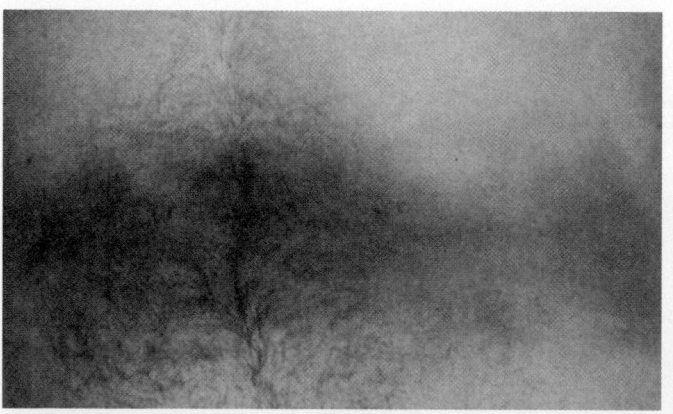

Figure 9 Blunt trauma occurs most frequently in vehicle crashes, and typically leads to closed abdominal injury—the internal organs are injured, but the skin remains intact.

blow to the abdomen, such as contact with the lower rim of a steering wheel or a door intruding into the passenger space from a motor vehicle crash, can cause compression and crushing injuries. These forces can deform solid organs and can cause hollow organs to rupture, spilling their contents into the abdomen and resulting in an increased risk of infection. Blunt trauma to the abdomen results from compression or deceleration forces and can often lead to a **closed abdominal injury**—one in which soft-tissue damage occurs inside the body, but the skin remains intact. When you are assessing the abdominal region in a patient who has received blunt trauma, consider three common MOIs: shearing, crushing, and compression. In the rapid deceleration of a patient during a motor vehicle crash or fall from a height, a shearing force can be created as the internal organs continue their forward motion. This causes hollow, solid, and visceral organs and vascular structures to tear, especially at their points of attachment to the abdominal wall. Organs that shear or tear include the liver, kidneys, small and large intestines, and spleen. In motor vehicle crashes, this MOI has been described as the third collision (such as the car into the wall, the patient into the steering column, and the internal organs into the patient's inner rib cage). Consider abdominal bleeding if the patient reports abdominal pain and you note rigidity during your assessment. Other signs that may indicate intra-abdominal bleeding after blunt trauma include referred shoulder pain or unexplained hypotension. Suspect intra-abdominal bleeding when multiple traumas are present, especially if hypotension is unexplained.

Crush injuries are the result of external factors at the time of impact; they differ from decelerating injuries occurring before impact. When abdominal contents are crushed between the anterior abdominal wall and the spinal column (or other structures in the rear), crushing occurs. Solid organs like the kidneys, liver, and spleen are at the greatest risk of injury from this mechanism. Direct application of crushing forces to the abdomen would come from objects like the dashboard, the front hood of a car (in a vehicle-pedestrian crash), or from falling objects. Additionally, these injuries can be caused by a restraining device that has not been properly attached or worn or by the steering wheel striking the abdominal cavity of an unrestrained driver as the person is propelled forward.

The last MOI to consider is compression injury resulting from a direct blow or external compression from a fixed object (such as a lap belt or air bag). These compression forces will deform hollow organs, increasing the pressure within the abdominal cavity. This dramatic change in abdominal pressure can cause a rupture of the small intestine or diaphragm. Rupture of organs can lead to uncontrollable hemorrhage and peritonitis.

■ Penetrating Trauma

Penetrating trauma results most commonly from low-velocity (< 200 ft per second) gunshot or stab wounds, resulting in tissue damage by lacerating or cutting. Penetrating trauma causes an **open abdominal injury**—one in which a break in the surface of the skin or mucous membrane exposes deeper tissue to potential contamination. In general, gunshot wounds cause more injury than stab wounds because bullets travel deep into the body and have more kinetic energy, increasing the damage lateral to the track of the missile due to temporary cavitation. Gunshot wounds most commonly involve injury to the small bowel, colon, liver, and vascular structures; the extent of injury is less predictable than the injury caused by stab wounds because gunshot wounds depend mostly on the characteristics of the weapon and the characteristics of the bullet. In penetrating trauma from stab wounds, the liver, small bowel, diaphragm, and colon are the organs most frequently injured.

The extent of damage from a penetrating injury is often a function of the energy that has been imparted to the body. Remember the following equation:

$$\text{Kinetic energy} = \frac{\text{Mass}}{2} \times \text{Velocity}^2$$

or

$$KE = \frac{mv^2}{2}$$

Thus the permanent injury as well as the temporary injury from the tract of the projectile can be considerable with high-velocity penetrations. The velocity delivered during penetrating trauma is typically divided into three levels; low velocity (less than 200 ft per second) such as from a knife, ice pick, or handgun; medium velocity (200 to 2,000 ft per second) such as from a 9-mm gun or shotgun; and high velocity (more than 2,000 ft per second) such as from a high-powered sporting rifle or military weapon. The trajectory or direction the projectile traveled and the distance it had to travel, as well as the profile of the bullet, can contribute considerably to the extent of the injury.

Words of Wisdom

Always remember the concept of associated injuries. On the basis of the MOI, some of the following syndromes are common:

- Fractures of the lower rib cage → suspect spleen and/or liver injuries
- Upper abdominal injuries → suspect chest trauma
- Pelvic fractures → suspect intra-abdominal trauma (bladder laceration)
- Penetrating wounds at or below the nipple line → suspect intra-abdominal injury

Motor Vehicle Crashes

In motor vehicle crashes there are five typical patterns of impact (frontal, lateral, rear, rotational, and rollover) that are discussed in depth in the chapter, *Trauma Systems and Mechanisms of Injury*. Each of these different mechanisms, with the exception of the rear impact, has the potential to cause significant injury to abdominal organs. In a rear-impact crash, the patient is less likely to have an injury to his or her abdomen if he or she has been restrained properly. However, if restraints are improperly worn or not used at all, the potential for injury is great.

Rollover impacts present the greatest potential to inflict lethal injuries. Unrestrained occupants may change direction

several times with an increased risk of ejection from the vehicle. The occupants involved in a rollover may collide with each other as well as with the vehicle interior, producing a wide range of probable injuries. If one of the following is present, consider transporting the patient to a trauma center:

- Ejection from *any* vehicle (car, motorcycle, or all-terrain vehicle)
- Death of another patient in the same vehicle
- Falls of greater than 15 ft to 20 ft or three times the patient's height
- Vehicle rollover with unrestrained driver or occupants
- High-speed vehicle crash (35 miles per hour or greater)
- Vehicle-pedestrian crash
- Motorcycle crash
- Penetrating wounds to the head, chest, or abdomen

Seat belts have prevented many thousands of injuries and saved many lives, including those of people who would have otherwise been ejected from the vehicle. However, seat belts occasionally cause blunt injuries to the abdominal organs. When worn properly, a seat belt lies below the anterior superior iliac spines of the pelvis and against the hip joints. If the belt lies too high, it can squeeze abdominal organs or great vessels against the spine when the car suddenly decelerates or stops **Figure 10**. Occasionally, fractures of the lumbar spine have been reported.

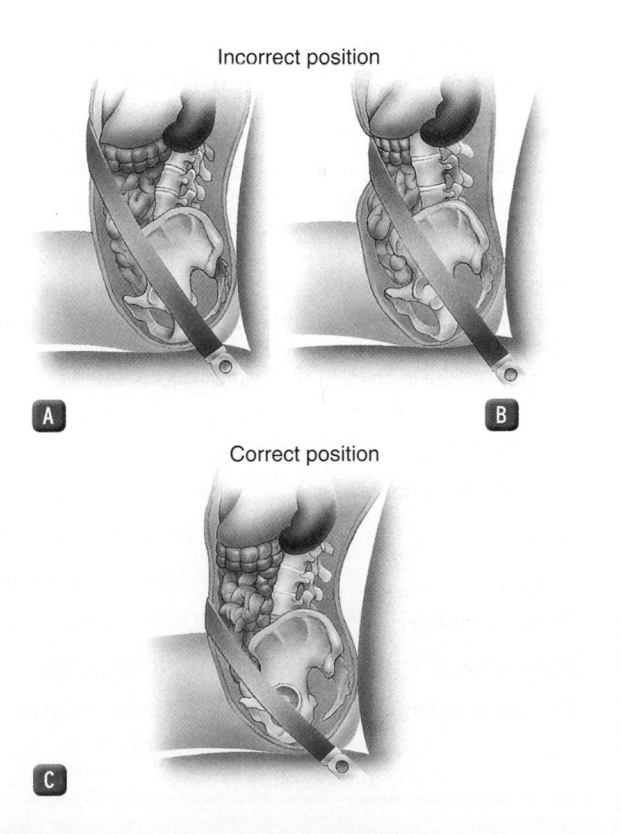

Incorrect position

A   B

Correct position

C

Figure 10 **A** and **B** show improper positioning of seat belts. The proper position for a seat belt is below the anterior superior iliac spines of the pelvis and against the hip joints, as shown in **C**.

Motorcycle Falls or Crashes

With the popularity of motorcycles and the production of high-performance racing bikes that are most attractive to younger and inexperienced riders, motorcycle crashes continue to increase. In a motorcycle crash, any structural protection from a steel cage, as is the case in an automobile, does not exist. The motorcyclist's only protection is those protective devices worn by the rider, such as the helmet and abrasion-resistant or leather pants, gloves, jacket, and boots. Although helmets are designed to protect against impact to the head, they transmit any impact to the cervical spine so they do not protect against severe cervical injury. You should consider transport to a trauma center with crashes occurring at speeds of greater than 20 mph or with separation of the rider from the motorcycle.

Falls From Heights

When an adult falls from a height, the fall usually occurs in the context of criminal activity, attempted suicide, or intoxication. The position or orientation of the body at the moment of impact will help determine the type of injuries sustained and their survivability. The surface onto which the person has fallen and the degree to which that surface can deform (plasticity) under the force of the falling body can help in dissipating the forces of sudden deceleration. Remember that a fall produces acceleration downward at 9.8 m/sec^2. If a person falls for 2 seconds, the speed at impact is nearly 20 m/sec. A person falling from a second story (24 ft) will reach a velocity of 39 feet per second (fps) and experience an impact force of 95 g on impact. Height plus stopping distance predict the magnitude of deceleration forces. Consider immediate transport to a trauma center with falls of greater than 20 ft.

Blast Injuries

Although most commonly associated with military conflict, blast injuries are also seen in civilian practice in mines, shipyards, chemical plants, and increasingly in association with terrorist activities. Blast injuries, particularly those from weapons designed specifically for antipersonnel effects (such as mines or grenades) can generate fragments traveling at velocities of 4,500 fps. This is nearly double the velocity of a projectile from a high-speed rifle. Any energy transmitted from a blast fragment will cause extensive and disruptive damage to tissue. People who are injured in explosions may be injured by any of four different mechanisms: primary, secondary, tertiary, and quaternary. The primary blast injury is an injury from the direct effects of the pressure wave and is most injurious to gas-containing organs. The tympanic membrane is the most vulnerable structure to the effects of the primary blast; if the pressure from the wave is more than 2 atmospheres, the tympanic membrane can rupture.

YOU *are the Medic* PART 3

As a precaution, you initiate spinal immobilization using specialized pediatric equipment. Oxygenation is supported by the placement of oxygen via nonrebreathing mask at 12 L/min. The child's mother (driver) is notified of your transport plan to a pediatric trauma center.

En route, you establish a large-bore IV. Medical direction is consulted regarding fluid resuscitation. You complete your secondary assessment, remaining suspicious about his left upper quadrant abdominal pain and guarding. You observe a 6- × 2-inch contusion, likely from the inappropriately placed seat belt, to his left upper quadrant. The patient also reports pain in his left shoulder. No other trauma injuries are noted during your secondary assessment.

Recording Time: 10 Minutes	
Level of consciousness	Alert with appropriate verbal responses for age
Skin	Cool, pale, and slightly moist
Pulse	165 beats/min; weak and regular
Blood pressure	60/35 mm Hg
Respirations	42 breaths/min
Oxygen saturation (Spo$_2$)	98% while receiving 12 L/min via nonrebreathing mask
Pupils	PEARRL

7. What does left upper quadrant tenderness suggest?

8. Why should this patient be transported to a pediatric trauma center?

9. What may the left shoulder pain indicate?

Lung tissue can develop evidence of contusion, edema, and rupture. Rupture of the pulmonary veins produces the potential for air embolism and sudden death. Intraocular hemorrhage and retinal detachments are common manifestations. The secondary blast injury is caused by debris or fragments from the explosion striking the person. The tertiary blast injury is produced when a person is propelled through the air and strikes another object. Secondary and tertiary blast injuries can cause trauma similar to penetrating and blunt mechanisms, respectively. There are also injuries called quaternary blast injuries or miscellaneous blast injuries that include burns and respiratory injuries from inhaling hot gases or chemicals and exacerbation of existing conditions including asthma, chronic obstructive pulmonary disease, hypertension, angina, and hyperglycemia.

Words of Wisdom

Part of the abdomen is in the chest!

General Pathophysiology

Hemorrhage is a major concern in patients with abdominal trauma. It can occur when there is external or internal blood loss. When you are caring for patients with abdominal trauma, especially blunt abdominal trauma, the estimation of the volume of blood lost is difficult. Signs and symptoms will vary greatly depending on the volume of blood lost and the rate at which the body is losing blood. Key indicators of hemorrhagic shock will become apparent with the assessment of the neurologic and cardiovascular systems.

As hypovolemia increases, the patient will have initial agitation and confusion. The heart compensates early for this loss by an increase in heart rate (tachycardia) and stroke volume. As hypoperfusion continues, the coronary arteries can no longer meet the increased demands of the myocardium, which leads to ischemia and heart failure. The symptoms of cardiac dysfunction are demonstrated by the presence of chest pain, tachypnea with adventitious (abnormal) lung sounds, and dysrhythmias. If left untreated, hypoperfusion will result in anaerobic metabolism and acidosis.

Injuries to hollow or solid organs can result in the spillage of their contents into the abdominal cavity. When the enzymes, acids, or bacteria leak from hollow organs into the peritoneal or retroperitoneal space, they cause irritation of the nerve endings. These nerve endings are found in the fascia of the surrounding tissues. As the inflammation affects deeper nerve endings (such as the endings of the afferent nerves), localized pain will result. Pain is localized if the extent of the contamination is confined; pain becomes generalized if the entire peritoneal cavity is involved.

Patient Assessment

During the evaluation of the abdominal cavity, you must look for evidence of hemorrhage (shock) or spillage of bowel contents (pain or tenderness) into the abdominal space. You should have a high index of suspicion and understand that intra-abdominal injuries are likely with trauma to the chest or abdomen. Your priorities in resuscitation begin with providing adequate tissue perfusion and oxygen delivery. In 10% of mortalities after trauma, the abdominal injury proves to be the primary cause of death; however, in a substantial number of cases, the exact cause of death is not clear.

The evaluation of a patient who has abdominal trauma must be systematic, keeping the entire patient in mind and prioritizing injuries accordingly. Approximately 20% of all patients with significant **hemoperitoneum**—collection of blood in the abdominal cavity—have a benign abdominal exam on first assessment. The abdomen should be examined closely for bruising, road rash, localized swelling, lacerations, distention, or pain Figure 11 . Clues to intra-abdominal trauma will include symptoms of shock not proportional to obvious external evidence or estimated blood loss. Retroperitoneal hemorrhage may be present because of damaged muscle, lacerated or avulsed kidneys, and injuries to the vessels of the supporting mesentery. All abdominal organs have a generous blood supply, making them susceptible to significant bleeding as a result of blunt forces causing a shearing-type injury. An injury to the abdomen can be fatal primarily because of hemorrhage. The injury can be slow to develop, and may be subtle and difficult to locate and assess.

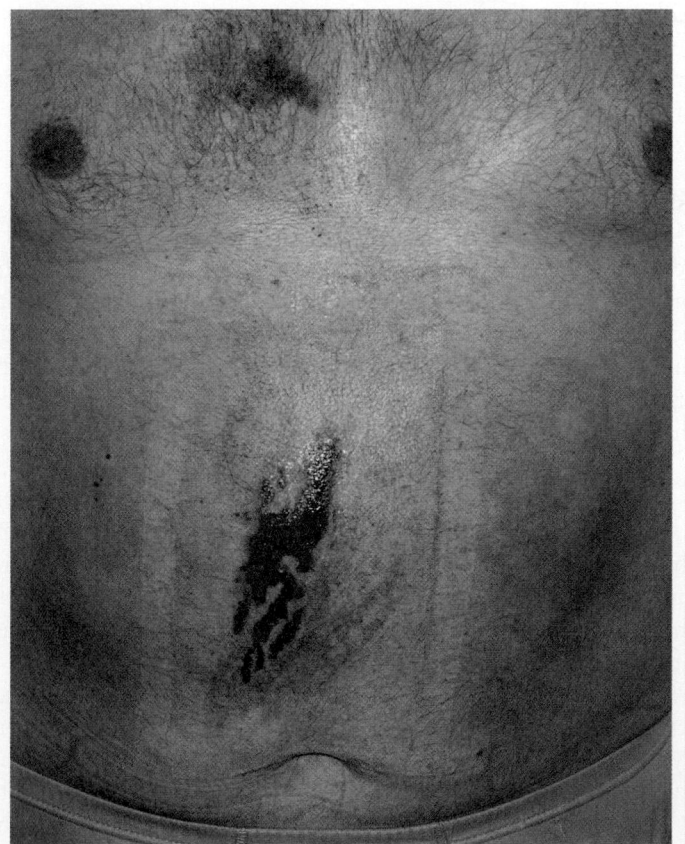

Figure 11 Examine the abdomen closely for bruising, road rash, localized swelling, lacerations, distention, and pain.

Finally, when you are assessing a genitourinary injury, there is a potential for embarrassing the patient. Maintain a professional presence at all times when assessing and treating these injuries. Remember to provide privacy for the patient during the assessment process. Look for blood first on the patient's undergarments and only inspect the external genitalia when the patient reports pain or there are external signs of injury.

Scene Size-up

As with all other aspects of prehospital care, scene safety remains the priority before providing any patient care. It is always important to remember that if a patient has penetrating or blunt trauma, some external force caused this injury (such as a gun, knife, or the baseball bat in the corner of the room!). These situations could also potentially be dangerous to the paramedic.

Primary Assessment

Form a General Impression

Quickly assess the patient's condition with a simple inspection, noting the manner in which he or she is lying. Movement of the body or the abdominal organs irritates the inflamed peritoneum, causing additional pain. To minimize this pain, patients may lie still, usually with the knees drawn up, and breathe using rapid and shallow breaths. For the same reason, they may contract abdominal muscles (guarding). Therefore, quiet, still patients may have severe injuries, whereas a patient who is moving around is less likely to have peritonitis.

Airway and Breathing

Once you have determined that the scene is safe and formed a general impression, the first patient priorities are those of the primary assessment: mental status, airway, breathing, circulation, and prioritizing the patient. As you work your way through the primary assessment, keep in mind that more subtle signs and symptoms are often uncovered during history taking and the secondary assessment.

Remember to keep the airway clear of vomitus so that it is not aspirated into the lungs, especially in a patient who is unresponsive or has an altered level of consciousness. Turn the patient to one side, using spinal precautions if necessary, and try to clear any material from the throat and mouth. Note the nature of the vomitus: undigested food, blood, mucus, or bile.

Quickly assess the patient for adequate breathing. A distended abdomen or pain may prevent adequate inhalation. When these guarded respirations decrease the effectiveness of the patient's breathing, providing supplemental oxygen with a nonrebreathing mask will help improve oxygenation. If the patient's level of consciousness is decreased and respirations are shallow, consider supplementing respirations with a bag-mask device. Use airway adjuncts as necessary to ensure a patent airway and assist with breathing.

Circulation

Superficial abdominal injuries usually do not produce significant external bleeding. Internal bleeding from open or closed abdominal injuries, however, can be profound. Trauma to the kidneys, liver, and spleen can cause significant internal bleeding. Evaluate the patient's pulse and skin color, temperature, and condition to determine the stage of shock. If you suspect shock, treat the patient for shock according to your protocols. Wounds should be covered and bleeding controlled as quickly as possible.

When you are caring for a potential genitourinary emergency, remember that the genitourinary system is very vascular and can be a significant source of bleeding. Quickly assess the patient's pulse rate and quality; determine the skin condition, color, and temperature; and check the capillary refill time. These assessments will help you determine the presence of circulatory problems or shock. Closed injuries do not have visible signs of bleeding. Because the bleeding is occurring inside the body, shock may be present. Your assessment of the pulse and skin will give you an indication as to how aggressively you need to treat your patient for shock.

If visible significant bleeding is seen, you must begin the steps necessary to control bleeding. Significant bleeding is an immediate life threat and must be controlled quickly using appropriate methods. In dark environments, bleeding can be difficult to see. Thick clothing may also hide bleeding. After you consider the MOI and form suspicions as to where bleeding may occur, expose that part of the body.

Transport Decision

Because of the nature of abdominal injuries, a short on-scene time and quick transport to the hospital are generally indicated. Abdominal pain together with an MOI that suggests injury to the abdomen or flank is a good indication for rapid transport. Because it is not possible to diagnose organ rupture in the field, do not delay transport when internal injuries are possible. The condition of a patient with visible significant bleeding or signs of significant internal bleeding may quickly become unstable. Treatment should be directed at quickly addressing life threats and providing rapid transportation to the closest appropriate hospital.

Patients with abdominal injuries should be evaluated at the highest level of trauma center available because of the hidden or occult nature of most abdominal injuries. Transport to a trauma center is indicated for any patient who has an MOI that produces a high index of suspicion and who has any visible significant trauma, whether blunt or penetrating. Follow local protocols when you are considering a lower level of care such as acute care sites and clinics. Only the lowest levels of MOI should be considered eligible for these types of facilities.

A patient with a genitourinary system injury should be taken to a trauma center for evaluation and treatment. Any injury to this system can prove to be life altering and often requires a medical specialist to provide specialized care. When possible and protocols allow, transport the patient to a facility capable of treating this subset of injuries.

History Taking

Try to obtain as many details about an injury as possible, keeping in mind that trauma patients should be transported to the hospital quickly. In other words, in addition to getting information about the patient (such as the SAMPLE history), it is important to obtain details on how the injury occurred, whether from the patient, witnesses, police, or other EMS providers.

When a patient has blunt trauma caused by a motor vehicle crash, determine the types of vehicles involved, the speed at which they were traveling, and how the vehicles collided. You should also try to find out other information about the event, such as the use of seat belts, the deployment of air bags, and the patient's position in the vehicle.

When a patient has sustained penetrating trauma, it is helpful to identify the type of weapon used; however, this is often impossible because assailants usually leave with their weapon. In a gunshot case, determine the type of gun and the number of shots, if possible. Also try to ascertain an estimated distance between the victim and the assailant whenever possible. In patients with stab wounds, determine the type of knife, the possible angle of the entrance wound, and the number of stab wounds. Patient care, however, always remains the priority.

Secondary Assessment

The first step during the physical exam is inspection of the abdomen—this is critical. This means you will need to expose the abdomen and inspect for signs of trauma (such as DCAP-BTLS). Often the injury to the abdomen involves ecchymosis, abrasions, or lacerations. When you are removing the patient's clothing, note whether there is the presence of blood from the vagina or rectum. If blood is noted, be sure to inspect those areas more closely during your physical exam.

Blood, gastrointestinal contents, and urine that have spilled into the peritoneum may produce peritonitis that could result in decreased or absent abdominal sounds. Auscultation of bowel sounds is not a useful assessment tool in the prehospital setting, but it may be used to confirm the presence or absence of bowel sounds—information that the receiving hospital will find useful. The next steps in the abdominal exam are percussion and palpation. With these maneuvers, look for tenderness and signs of peritonitis (such as the patient guarding his or her abdomen or experiencing pain while being gently moved to the stretcher). Involuntary muscle guarding is a reliable sign of peritoneal irritation. Carefully palpate the entire abdomen, beginning with the quadrant that is farthest away from the injury, while assessing the patient's response and noting abdominal masses and deformities. Examination of the pelvic structures is made difficult by the overlying bones.

During your physical exam, also note whether the patient has hematuria (blood in the urine). This is a cardinal sign of renal and urinary tract injury, which can occur when renal or urinary vessels rupture, or when blood is able to enter the urine during glomerular filtration. Note the color of the urine—a darker brown suggests bleeding in the upper urinary tract, whereas a brighter red is most likely due to bleeding in the lower portion of the tract.

The presence of a pregnant uterus should also be determined. Traumatic injuries to pregnant patients can be further complicated by the physiologic changes experienced by the patient. Some changes can mimic shock. For example, the pregnant patient's heart rate can increase by as much as 20 beats/min, blood volume increases by 50% during mid-pregnancy, and a pregnant woman can experience relative anemia from hemodilution. Due to the increase in blood flow to the uterus, the risk for massive blood loss is greatly increased with trauma to the bony pelvis. At term, the placenta/uterus can perfuse approximately 600 to 800 mL of blood per minute.

Management of pregnant patients should always start with the ABCs. There is a higher risk of aspiration and increase in gastric acidity. All pregnant patients should receive maximum oxygenation because of increased oxygen consumption and reduced reserve. Hypoxia can cause a 30% reduction in uterine blood flow. It has been shown that warm lactated Ringer's solution can restore fetal oxygenation better than other crystalloids. Also, remember that if the pregnant patient is more than 20 weeks' gestation, she should be tilted at least 15° to her left to prevent vena cava syndrome. If the patient is secured to a long backboard, towel rolls can be placed under the backboard to accomplish the tilting.

Finally, several newer technologies are useful when assessing abdominal trauma in the prehospital environment. The use of portable ultrasound machines has been being studied for several years. An exam with a FAST ultrasound, which stands for Focused Assessment with Sonography for Trauma, also can be used early in the patient's evaluation, and has been shown to decrease scene time, treatment costs, and the length of hospital stays.

Another technology entering the arena of prehospital care is telemedicine, which allows physicians from remote areas (such as base medical centers) to receive and review images and diagnostic data from rural EMS providers on scene or en route.

A common misconception is that patients without abdominal pain or abnormal vital signs are unlikely to have serious intra-abdominal injuries. Keep in mind that peritonitis can take hours to days to develop. Similarly, nonspecific symptoms such as hypotension, tachycardia, and confusion may not develop until the patient has lost more than 40% of his or her circulating blood volume. Always maintain a high index of suspicion in any patient who has an MOI consistent with abdominal trauma, regardless of the examination findings. Abdominal distention is a late indication of abdominal trauma. Patients must have a significant volume of blood enter the abdominal cavity to fill it and produce distention.

Special Populations

Because older people usually have a more flaccid abdominal wall (containing less muscle and more fat) than younger people, apply increased pressure when you are palpating the abdomen to assess for injury. You should suspect that any older trauma patient who reports abdominal pain has an internal organ injury.

As part of the physical exam of a trauma patient, you may be faced with a number of challenges associated with abdominal trauma. You may discover the presence of an abdominal evisceration—displacement of an organ outside the body, or an impaled object. Management of these situations will be discussed later in this chapter.

If you suspect injury to the diaphragm, focus on the airway, breathing, and circulatory status of the patient. Remember that the diaphragm plays a large role in the mechanical process of breathing. Signs and symptoms of a diaphragmatic rupture can include abdominal pain, acute respiratory distress, decreased breath sounds, abdominal sounds in the chest, subcutaneous emphysema, and a sunken abdomen or an abdomen that appears empty. Examine the patient's neck and chest, paying particular attention to the trachea (tracheal deviation due to mediastinal shift), symmetry of the chest during expansion, and absence of breath sounds.

Assess the patient's pain. There are two types: somatic pain and visceral pain. **Somatic pain** comes from skin and muscle, as well as joints, ligaments, and tendons. It is often described as sharp and localized to the area of injury. Bleeding, swelling, and cramping may exist with somatic pain. This pain usually responds well to medications such as opioids and nonsteroidal anti-inflammatory drugs.

Visceral pain comes from organs inside the body with injury or illness. This type of pain travels from pain receptors in the nerves running throughout the body. The pain receptors transfer the information to the brain where the pain is then perceived. Visceral pain can radiate to other locations such as the back and chest. There are three main areas where visceral pain is felt: the thorax, abdomen, and pelvis. The receptors in these cavities respond to stretching, oxygen deprivation, and swelling. Visceral pain is often described as a deep ache with cramping. Opioids are the most effective for this type of pain.

Words of Wisdom

Cullen sign is a black-and-blue discoloration (ecchymosis) in the umbilical region caused by peritoneal bleeding. Grey Turner sign includes ecchymosis present in the lower abdominal and flank regions. They are both caused by intra-abdominal bleeding found 12 to 24 hours after the initial injury. The presence of these signs is helpful, but their absence does not rule out life-threatening abdominal hemorrhage.

At this point, you will have completed the primary assessment as well as the rapid exam. The next step is for you to perform a thorough full-body exam (head-to-toe physical exam) when you have a patient who has abdominal trauma and a significant MOI. However, this head-to-toe physical exam should be conducted en route to the emergency department (ED) to avoid any unnecessary delays. Basically, a full-body exam assesses the same structures as the rapid exam, except more methodically. Close examination may uncover additional findings that were either not picked up during the rapid exam or are only now starting to develop (such as hematoma, bruises, or tender areas). As long as you can ensure that the problems found in the primary assessment have been attended to, and there is time en route, perform a very thorough physical exam on your patient.

Words of Wisdom

An injury to the chest anywhere below the nipples should also be considered an injury to the abdomen.

Reassessment

Reassessment includes performing the primary assessment again, as well as retaking vital signs and checking interventions on the patient.

Pertinent field documentation of the abdominal trauma assessment should include the following: whether or not seat belts were worn, which type, and their position on the patient; the location, intensity, and quality of pain; whether or not nausea or vomiting is present; the contour of the abdomen; any ecchymosis or open areas present on the soft-tissue inspection; the presence or absence of rebound tenderness, guarding, rigidity, spasm, or localized pain; any changes in the level of consciousness and serial vital signs; other injuries found; the presence or absence of alcohol, narcotics, or any type of analgesic; and the results of your reassessment.

Emergency Medical Care

In general, the prehospital management of patients who have abdominal trauma is straightforward. As always, ensuring an open airway while taking spinal precautions is the first step. Administer high-concentration oxygen to the patient via a nonrebreathing mask. Establish IV access with two large-bore lines, and start replacing fluid with lactated Ringer's solution or normal saline to maintain a systolic blood pressure of 90 to 100 mm Hg (lactated Ringer's solution is the preferred crystalloid). Do not delay transport to initiate IV therapy; establish IV lines whenever possible during transport. Minimize external hemorrhage by applying pressure dressings. Apply a cardiac monitor and pulse oximetry as well as capnography, if possible. Transport the patient to the appropriate hospital or regional trauma center, depending on your local transport protocols. Note that the assessment should also not delay patient care and transport. Repeated abdominal examinations are the key to discovering a patient's worsening condition before vital signs change.

Words of Wisdom

A distended, tender abdomen after injury means internal bleeding and significant blood loss. Treat for shock and transport immediately.

Administering pain medication is somewhat controversial because it may mask symptoms and often is contraindicated because of the patient's hypotension. In most instances, it may be appropriate to consult with medical direction en route to the hospital to discuss analgesia. While historically it was thought best not to mask the pain until the patient was diagnosed in the ED, today many medical directors feel that pain management is a more humane approach, and will order an analgesic such as Fentanyl.

Evisceration

An evisceration is protrusion of abdominal organs through a wound in the abdominal wall **Figure 12**. The protrusion may be small or large. Generally, little pain is associated with this type of injury; do not apply any material that will adhere to the abdominal structures. Do not attempt to place the organ back into the body. Apply a normal saline-soaked sterile dressing over the top of the evisceration. Cover to keep warm. Transport the patient immediately to the closest appropriate hospital. Strangulation of the bowel by the abdominal wall causes decreased blood flow to the protruding part and can cause death to that part of the bowel. Early symptoms are localized pain, nausea, and vomiting. Also, the patient can experience peritonitis if the bowel is leaking fluids into the abdominal cavity. Patients may feel more comfortable with their knees bent. Encourage the patient not to cough or bear down, and consider providing pain relief.

Impaled Objects

You may encounter a patient who has an impaled object **Figure 13**. Stabilize the impaled object and transport the patient in the position in which he or she was found. Stabilization of an impaled object can be impractical under some field conditions, but effective stabilization and safe transportation can help

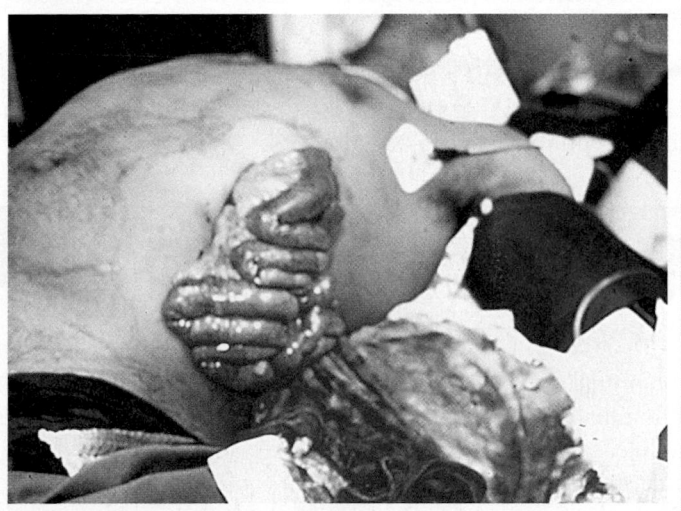

Figure 12 An abdominal evisceration is an open abdominal wound from which internal organs or fat protrude.

YOU *are the Medic* | PART 4

On arrival at the hospital, the patient's condition is immediately evaluated by the trauma team, and a CT scan of the abdomen, head, neck, chest, and spine is completed. According to the attending physician, there is no injury to the head, chest, neck, or spine, but the abdominal CT scan reveals hemorrhage from the spleen. The patient is evaluated by the trauma team and taken emergently to the operating room for removal of his bleeding spleen.

10. Why is it important to transport trauma patients (especially those with abdominal trauma) to trauma centers?

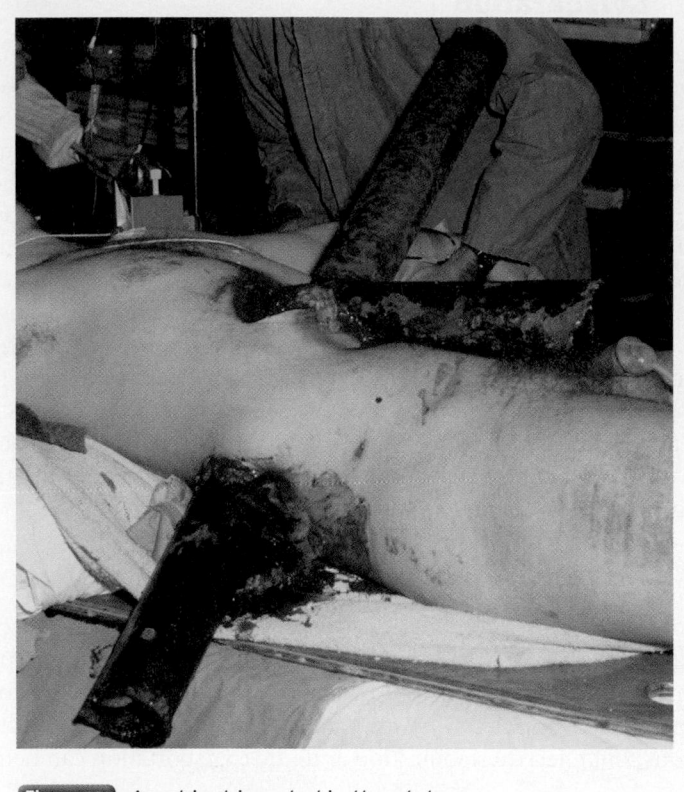

Figure 13 An object impaled in the abdomen.

reduce serious tissue damage. Additionally, significant infection often develops in this type of wound, so early intervention with sterile techniques should be employed.

■ Pathophysiology, Assessment, and Management of Specific Injuries

■ Pathophysiology

Abdominal trauma can be life threatening. Injuries of the abdominal organs, especially those in the retroperitoneal area, can bleed profusely and can hold a large amount of blood. Solid organs such as the kidneys and liver can bleed profusely when torn or cut, as do the major blood vessels that run through the abdominal cavity.

Injuries to hollow organs such as the stomach, although not likely to result in shock, produce a serious risk of infection. The bowel can spill its contents into the abdominal cavity, causing peritonitis and systemic infection. The main causes of death that result from abdominal trauma are hemorrhage and systemic infection.

Injuries to Solid Abdominal Organs

The solid organs in the abdomen include the liver, spleen, kidneys, and pancreas. When a solid organ in the abdomen is injured during blunt or penetrating trauma, the organ releases blood into the peritoneal cavity. This can cause nonspecific signs such as tachycardia and hypotension. Findings relate to the size of the injury and the time since the injury occurred.

Liver Injuries The liver is the largest organ in the abdominal cavity and the most vascular, receiving 25% of the cardiac output. Because of its size and location, it is the most vulnerable organ in the abdomen. The superior border of the liver can be as high as the patient's nipples, so a liver injury must be suspected in all patients who have right-sided chest trauma as well as abdominal trauma. Suspect injury if there are fractures to the 7th through 9th ribs overlying the liver. Also, the ligament in front of the liver (ligamentum teres) can slice the liver in situations involving sudden deceleration. Five percent of adult trauma patients admitted to the ED have liver injuries, and they are the most common injury in children admitted to the ED. The liver can be contused or lacerated, and a hematoma can develop. Suspect laceration when penetrating trauma involves the right upper abdomen or right lower chest.

Spleen Injuries Falls and motor vehicle crashes can injure the spleen. However, less obvious injury patterns in activities such as sports (for instance, tackling in football or checking in lacrosse) can also cause injury to the spleen. It is the most commonly injured organ in blunt abdominal trauma in adults and is the second most injured abdominal organ in children. There are case reports of patients who sustained a ruptured spleen even though the contact was relatively minor. This is especially true if the spleen is enlarged from mononucleosis or other underlying disease. Approximately 5% of circulating blood filters through the spleen every minute. It gets direct vascular supply from the aorta, and its drainage goes directly into the inferior vena cava. When the spleen ruptures, blood spills into the peritoneum, which can ultimately cause shock and death. The spleen, like the liver, can bleed profusely. A ruptured spleen can be life threatening. Unlike the liver, penetrating trauma does not present as much of an immediate threat of shock unless a major blood vessel supplying the organ is lacerated. Suspect spleen lacerations when fractures of the 9th through 10th ribs on the left side are present or when the patient reports left upper quadrant tenderness, hypotension, and tachycardia. It is common for the patient to report left shoulder pain, but this sign does not appear until 1 to 2 hours after the injury.

Pancreas Injuries Pancreatic injury occurs in less than 5% of all major abdominal traumas. Because of the anatomic position of the pancreas in the retroperitoneum, it is relatively well protected. It typically takes a high-energy force to damage the pancreas. These high-energy forces are most commonly produced by penetrating trauma (for example, from a bullet) but can also be caused by blunt trauma (such as from a steering wheel or handlebars from a motorcycle). In blunt trauma, an unrestrained driver who hits the steering column or a bicyclist who hits the handlebars is at risk of pancreatic injury. Patients tend to present with vague upper and mid-abdominal pain that can radiate into the back. The patient may have peritoneal irritation hours after the injury, revealing the presence of traumatic pancreatitis. Patients have been known to develop a form of diabetes after a severe injury to the pancreas.

Diaphragm Injuries The diaphragm plays the primary role in a patient's ventilatory process. Any injury to the diaphragm will cause signs and symptoms of ventilatory compromise. Diaphragmatic injuries or ruptures are not isolated incidents; patients often have associated thoracic, abdominal, head, and extremity injuries.

Injuries to the diaphragm are rare, and result both from blunt trauma (typically high-speed motor vehicle crashes) and from penetrating trauma. A lateral impact during a motor vehicle crash is most likely to cause a diaphragmatic rupture because of the twisting or distortion of the chest wall that may shear or tear the diaphragm. In frontal motor vehicle crashes, the patient may strike the steering wheel or column. This may cause a significant change in abdominal pressure, which may also tear the diaphragm.

Injuries to Hollow Intraperitoneal Organs

The hollow organs of the abdomen include the small and large intestines, stomach, and bladder. Hollow visceral injuries produce most of their symptoms from peritoneal contamination. When a hollow organ such as the stomach or bowel is injured, it releases its contents into the abdomen. These contents may irritate the abdomen, producing symptoms. When the patient has the seat belt sign—a contusion or abrasion across the lower abdomen—this usually means that he or she also has intraperitoneal injuries.

Injuries to the Small and Large Intestines The intestines are most commonly injured from penetrating trauma, although they can be injured from severe blunt trauma as well. When ruptured, the intestines spill their contents (which contain fecal matter and a large amount of bacteria) into the peritoneal or retroperitoneal cavities, resulting in peritonitis. Blunt trauma to the abdominal wall most commonly causes injury to the duodenum because of its location and ligamentous attachment. It can present as back

pain. Penetrating trauma will cause injury to the small bowel, then the stomach and large intestine. The most common cause is the seat belt, because the lap belt lies along the lower quadrant of the abdominal cavity. Symptoms will be caused by the contents rather than the blood loss. Rupture of the stomach causes rapid burning epigastric pain, rigidity, and rebound tenderness. Small-bowel and colon injury may only present with generalized pain.

Stomach Injuries Most injuries to the stomach result from penetrating trauma; the stomach is rarely injured from blunt trauma. When rupture of the stomach does occur after blunt trauma, it is usually associated with a recent meal or inappropriate use of a seat belt. Trauma to the stomach frequently results in the spillage of acidic material into the peritoneal space, creating a chemical irritation that produces abdominal pain and peritoneal signs relatively quickly, although patients taking antacid medications may have delayed symptoms.

Retroperitoneal Injuries

Structures contained within the retroperitoneal cavity are the pancreas, kidneys, vascular structures, and part of the small intestine. Injuries confined to the retroperitoneum can be very difficult to diagnose. In general, they are in an area that is remote from physical examination, and an injury initially does not present with signs and symptoms of peritonitis.

Because the blood or other contaminants are held in the retroperitoneal space, they do not frequently cause abdominal pain, peritoneal signs, or abdominal distention. Occasionally, retroperitoneal bleeding can lead to ecchymosis of the flanks (Grey Turner sign) or around the umbilicus (Cullen sign). This ecchymosis is usually delayed hours to days, however, and is unreliable in the prehospital setting.

Vascular Injuries

Besides the kidneys, the vascular structures found in the retroperitoneal space include the descending aorta (and its branches), the superior phrenic artery, the inferior phrenic artery, the inferior vena cava, and the mesenteric vessels. Injuries to these structures occur with both blunt and penetrating trauma, but penetrating trauma is the major cause. Penetrating trauma that causes injury to the great vessels of the abdomen will also be associated with injuries to multiple intra-abdominal organs. Blunt trauma can cause injuries to vascular structures in the intraperitoneal space because they are sheared from their points of attachment. Vascular injuries are often masked by other injuries. The significance of the injury depends on how many vessels were injured and the length of time that has passed since the injury occurred. Bleeding stemming from veins can be more serious than arterial bleeding, which can occlude the lumen of the artery.

The patient could have an abdominal aortic aneurysm that has developed and become worse as a result of abdominal trauma. The specifics on abdominal aortic aneurysm are discussed in the chapter, *Cardiovascular Emergencies*.

Duodenal Injuries

In abdominal trauma, the duodenum can rupture, spilling its contents into the retroperitoneum, usually because of high-speed deceleration injuries. Contamination of the retroperitoneum with duodenal contents may ultimately produce abdominal pain or fever, although symptoms will not likely develop for hours to days. Abdominal pain, nausea, and vomiting may develop, although belatedly. Because of the delayed presentation and variable symptoms, a high degree of suspicion for duodenal injury must be maintained in any abdominal trauma, but especially in high-speed deceleration crashes. As a result of the duodenum's close proximity to multiple organs, it is unlikely that it will be injured by itself. A duodenum injury should be suspected in children who are thrown from a bicycle and strike their abdomen on the handlebars.

Kidney Injuries

Renal (kidney) trauma is seen in less than 5% of all trauma patients, with about 75% of such cases involving patients younger than age 45 years. Injuries to the kidneys generally involve large forces, eg, falls from height, high-speed motor vehicle crashes, or sports-related injuries. Suspect injury with fractures of the 11th and 12th ribs or flank tenderness.

Blunt renal trauma results when the kidney becomes compressed against the lower ribs or lumbar spine (as is seen in sports injuries, also known as kidney punch) or when the upper abdomen becomes compressed just below the rib cage (such as when a child is run over by a car). Contact sports such as football, soccer, hockey, boxing, and rugby are some of the more common culprits in renal injury **Figure 14**. A ruptured kidney will usually present with pain on inspiration in the abdomen and flank areas. Gross hematuria will almost always be present.

Penetrating renal trauma can occur with gunshot or stab wounds in the abdomen or lower chest. A high suspicion for significant injury must be maintained regardless of the site of the entry wound. Penetrating renal trauma is more likely to be associated with injury to the liver, lung, and spleen. For instance, the upward motion of stabbing may cause a renal laceration as well as a pneumothorax. A gunshot wound may result in direct injury to the kidney, but produce greater surrounding tissue destruction due to the expanding cavity created by the traveling bullet.

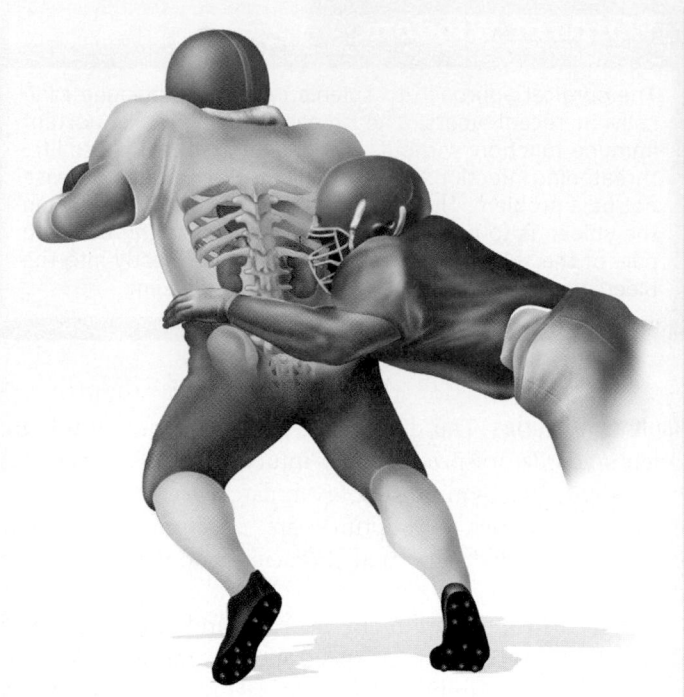

Figure 14 A football tackle that results in blunt trauma to the lower rib cage or flank can cause renal injury.

Ureter Injuries

Ureteral injuries are difficult, if not impossible, to identify in the prehospital setting. However, they rarely lead to an immediate life-threatening condition. A high index of suspicion should remain, just the same.

Bladder and Urethra Injuries

Trauma to the bladder or urethra is often associated with other significant injuries. For instance, 27% of urethral injuries occur in conjunction with other intra-abdominal injuries.

A blunt or penetrating injury to the bladder may result in bladder rupture or laceration, usually as a result of blunt trauma. The likelihood of a bladder injury varies by the severity of the mechanism, but also by the degree of the bladder distention. The fuller the bladder the greater the opportunity for injury. A seat belt that causes contusions to the lower abdomen may also cause blunt trauma to the bladder. This type of injury is seen more frequently in drunk drivers, who are more likely to have a full bladder.

Bladder injuries are usually associated with pelvic injuries from motor vehicle crashes, falls from heights, and physical assaults to the lower abdomen. These MOIs may cause a pelvic fracture to perforate the bladder.

Bladder rupture is associated with a high mortality rate because the trauma required to pierce the bladder frequently damages other organs or vascular structures. If a bladder rupture results from sudden deceleration forces, such as those occurring in motor vehicle crashes, urine may be spilled into either part of the abdominal cavity, leading to intraperitoneal, extraperitoneal, or retroperitoneal rupture.

Assessment

Because signs such as tachycardia and hypotension may not develop until a patient has lost a significant volume of blood, normal vital signs do not rule out the possibility that there has been a significant intra-abdominal injury. Bleeding into the peritoneal cavity from solid organ injuries can also produce abdominal tenderness or distention even though the distention may not be evident until the patient has lost nearly all the blood in the abdomen. Palpation of the abdomen may reveal localized or generalized tenderness, rigidity, or rebound tenderness, all of which suggest a peritoneal injury.

When the liver is injured, it releases blood and bile into the peritoneal cavity. The blood loss can be massive, resulting in abdominal distention, hypotension, tachycardia, shock, and even death. In addition, the release of bile into the peritoneum can produce abdominal pain and peritonitis along with **Kehr sign** (pain in the shoulder as a result of the presence of blood or other irritants in the peritoneal cavity) as blood accumulates around the diaphragm.

As with other intra-abdominal organ injuries, the signs and symptoms of splenic rupture are nonspecific, and as many as 40% of patients have no symptoms. Some patients report only pain in the left shoulder (Kehr sign) because of referred pain from diaphragmatic irritation Figure 15.

Injuries to the pancreas have subtle or absent signs and symptoms initially and should be suspected in any rapid deceleration injury. Over the course of hours to days, pancreatic injuries result in the spillage of enzymes into the retroperitoneal space, damaging surrounding structures and leading to infection and retroperitoneal abscess. Injury should be suspected after a localized blow to the midabdomen. These patients usually experience a vague upper and midabdominal pain that radiates to the back. Peritoneal signs may develop several hours after the injury.

Assessment findings in a patient with vascular injuries depend on whether or not the bleeding is contained (a hematoma) or there is active hemorrhage. In active hemorrhage, the patient will present with significant hypotension, tachycardia, and shock.

The most frequent presentation of blunt renal trauma is flank pain and **hematuria** (blood in the urine), which usually

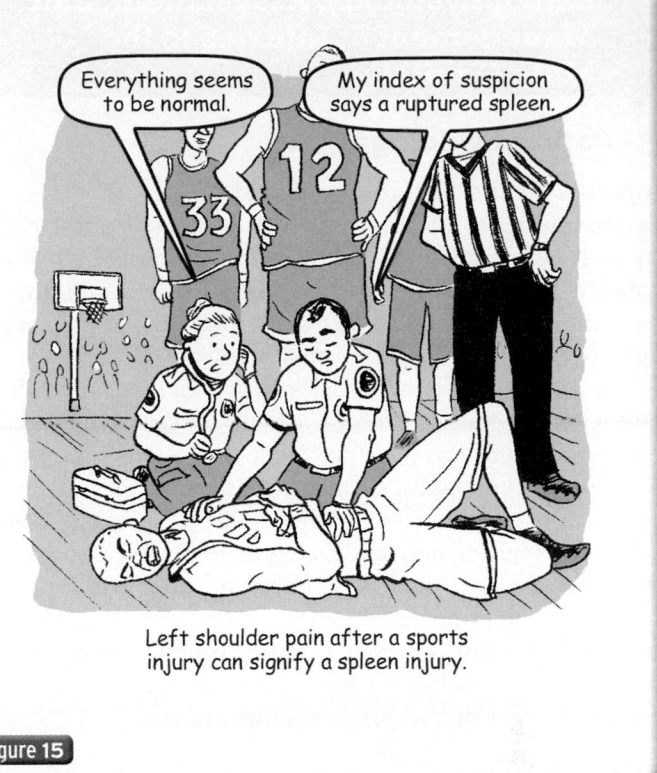

Left shoulder pain after a sports injury can signify a spleen injury.

Figure 15

goes undetected until evaluation in the ED. Suspicion for renal injuries should be high whenever a patient has obvious hematomas or ecchymoses over the upper abdomen, lateral aspects of the middle back, or lower rib cage. Fractures of the lower rib cage should also raise the suspicion for renal trauma.

Bladder injury should be suspected in any patient with trauma to the lower abdomen or pelvis. Bladder injury may also be suspected in the prehospital setting if a patient reports an inability to urinate, blood is noted at the penile opening during history taking and secondary assessment, or the patient has tenderness on palpation of the suprapubic region. The signs and symptoms of bladder injuries are generally nonspecific but may present as gross hematuria, suprapubic pain and tenderness, difficulty voiding, and abdominal distention, guarding, or rebound tenderness. The presence of signs of peritoneal irritation may also indicate the possibility of an intraperitoneal bladder rupture.

Finally, ultrasound is being used more extensively in the ED and may be used in the field under limited circumstances.

Management

As mentioned previously, it is crucial for you to have a high index of suspicion when the MOI suggests possible internal abdominal damage. Management of solid organ injuries includes rapid transport, with close monitoring for changes in vital signs and patient condition.

Care of bladder and urethra injuries follows basic trauma principles; secure the airway, address breathing issues, support the circulatory system, and immobilize the spine if necessary.

Pathophysiology, Assessment, and Management of Injuries to the Male Genitalia

Pathophysiology

Injuries to the Testicle or Scrotal Sac

Severe injuries to the testicles are rare because of their mobility and natural position. Although loss of fertility is the major concern when a patient sustains a testicular injury, the exact outcome depends on whether the testicle can be preserved via definitive treatment in the hospital setting.

Blunt trauma to the testicles or scrotal sac can result from motor vehicle crashes, physical assaults, or sports injuries. Blunt testicular trauma can result in simple contusions, rupture of the testicle, and, in rare cases, torsion (twisting) of the testicle. More than half of all testicular ruptures occur in sports participants. Testicular injuries frequently present following trauma to the thighs, buttocks, penis, lower abdomen, and pelvis.

Penetrating trauma to the testicles or scrotal sac may result from stab wounds, gunshot wounds, blast wounds, or animal bites. You should have a high suspicion for other associated injuries in cases of obvious penetrating trauma.

Penis Injuries

The penis is a vital organ for both proper urination and sexual function. Injuries to the penis may result from blunt or penetrating trauma but also may arise from sexual behavior or self-mutilation. Physiologically, the penis becomes erect when blood fills the corpus cavernosa. Priapism—a painful, tender, persistent erection—can have nontraumatic causes, such as sickle cell disease.

A fractured penis may occur when an erect penis is accidentally impacted against the partner's pubic symphysis or bent too far via self-manipulation.

Penetrating trauma to the penis most often results from gunshot wounds. Also, reports in the medical literature describe self-mutilation or amputation of the penis. Typically this type of injury occurs in patients with significant psychiatric disorders.

Assessment

Contusions of the testicles or scrotal sac result in painful hematomas that may respond to application of ice packs. Rupture of the testicle is difficult to identify in the prehospital setting, although tender scrotal swelling should be a presenting complaint. Similarly, you will not be able to determine if a particular blunt trauma has resulted in a testicular torsion. Although serious injury to the testicles is rare, it does not require much force to cause intrascrotal bleeding. If enough bleeding or concomitant swelling occurs, pressure necrosis (tissue death) may result. For this reason, you should not ignore testicular complaints even in the face of other trauma, and should communicate this concern to the ED staff.

In the case of a penile fracture, the wall of the corpora cavernosa is torn; pain and a large hematoma are the presenting signs and symptoms.

When there is penetrating trauma to the penis, attention should be paid to controlling hemorrhage and assessing the patient for other injuries associated with the trauma.

Special Populations

In the pediatric population, penile contusions have been reported to occur when a toilet seat falls unexpectedly and compresses the child's penis. Ice packs can help decrease swelling. Note that penile trauma in a child may be a sign of abuse, and an evaluation for other injuries may be warranted.

Management

Scrotal lacerations or avulsions should be treated with proper attention to any hemorrhage or testicular evisceration. Gentle compression and the application of ice packs may help decrease bleeding, swelling, and pain. Provide pain relief as well as emotional support.

A scrotal laceration may serve as a portal through which bacteria can enter the scrotum or perineum. The resulting infection, called Fournier gangrene, causes necrosis of the muscle and other subcutaneous tissue within the scrotum. The scrotum may feel spongy, and the accumulation of gas in the scrotal sac may produce the distinctive sounds of crepitus. The scrotal tissues will become gray-black, drainage will occur at the wound site, and fever and scrotal pain will be present. This is a true emergency, and prompt transport to the hospital is indicated. If left untreated, the infection can enter the bloodstream, causing systemic sepsis.

In the case of an amputation, attempts should be made to recover the amputated penis because surgical repair is often possible.

A number of reports have described people who have placed objects around the penis, testicles, or both. Inability to remove the object can result in incarceration of the organ, with tissue death being the most feared consequence. No attempt to remove the object should be made in the field. Instead, the patient should be transported to the hospital for proper evaluation and treatment, which may necessitate the use of cutting devices or aspiration of the distal edema.

Pathophysiology, Assessment, and Management of Injuries to the Female Genitalia

Pathophysiology

Vaginal trauma may be the result of blunt or penetrating trauma or may be self-inflicted. Blunt trauma may result from motor vehicle crashes in which high-energy impacts cause significant abdominal and pelvic trauma or from saddle-type injuries, eg, falling on the handlebars of a bicycle. Lacerations to the vaginal wall can occur, as well as uterine rupture or ovarian contusion. Trauma to the external genitalia may produce contusions to the vulva or labia.

Penetrating trauma to the reproductive organs may result from stabbings to the lower pelvis or gunshot wounds. Because the path of a bullet cannot be predicted from the entry wound alone, any injuries to the abdomen or upper legs may have also damaged the reproductive organs.

Self-inflicted trauma has been reported in female children and in psychiatric patients who insert foreign bodies into their genitalia.

Assessment

Signs of trauma may include hematomas and ecchymoses in the lower pelvic area and on the external female genitalia, bleeding from the vagina, and tenderness on palpation of the lower pelvis. The assessment may reveal clues of sexual assault; this topic is covered in the chapter, *Gynecologic Emergencies*.

Management

Use compression to stem any external hemorrhage, and administer replacement fluids to treat the hypotensive patient. Use any pain medication with extreme caution in the hypotensive patient.

Occasionally, women of reproductive age can cause vaginal lacerations by using devices or tools to remove tampons, pads, and other products that they could not digitally remove from the vaginal canal. Do not attempt to remove any objects; immediately transport the patient for treatment at the hospital. Finally, remember emotional considerations and be familiar with your reporting requirements for assault.

Words of Wisdom

Pelvic fractures may result from blunt trauma from motor vehicle crashes, motorcycle crashes, or from vehicles striking pedestrians. Pelvic fractures are commonly associated with internal abdominal injuries; signs and symptoms include pain in the pelvis, groin, or hips; hematomas or contusions to the pelvic region; obvious external bleeding; or hypotension without obvious external bleeding. Pelvic fractures are covered in the chapter, *Orthopaedic Trauma*.

YOU are the Medic | SUMMARY

1. What are your immediate concerns?

Immediate concerns may include spinal cord injuries, occult abdominal trauma, and injuries to the airway. The patient slid under the adult seat belt, potentially causing blunt force trauma to his abdomen and trauma to his chest and neck.

2. What are your immediate treatment priorities?

Immediate treatment priorities include spinal precautions and supporting airway and breathing.

3. What are your early communication and transport plans?

Effective early communication with the receiving facility and transport to a pediatric trauma center will improve this pediatric patient's prognosis. Depending on your location you may consider transport by air.

4. What do these signs indicate to you?

His cool, pale, and moist skin could be a result of peripheral-vascular shunting as seen in the early stages of shock. When the sympathetic nervous system stimulates the release of epinephrine and norepinephrine from the adrenal glands, peripheral vasoconstriction occurs and the sweat glands are opened.

5. What does abdominal guarding usually indicate?

The presence of abdominal pain and guarding suggests occult abdominal trauma.

6. What can you conclude from the patient's vital signs?

The patient's blood pressure is in the low normal range for age and the pulse rate is rapid for his age. The patient's tachycardia

could be caused by the body's attempt to compensate. Considering his abdominal exam findings, the tachycardia could be a sign of shock in this patient.

7. What does left upper quadrant tenderness suggest?

Left upper quadrant tenderness may indicate injury to the spleen, diaphragm, pancreas, or stomach.

8. Why should this patient be transported to a pediatric trauma center?

Trauma patients in all age groups benefit from transport to trauma centers. Transport of this pediatric patient to a pediatric trauma center will improve this patient's chance of survival. Depending on your location you may consider transport by air.

9. What may the left shoulder pain indicate?

The left shoulder pain could be Kehr sign—referred pain indicative of a splenic injury. However, it may also just indicate musculoskeletal injury such as a sprain or strain.

10. Why is it important to transport trauma patients (especially those with abdominal trauma) to trauma centers?

Trauma centers have the specialized staff, equipment (eg, imaging devices), and resources to provide the best care for trauma patients. It has been demonstrated that trauma patients have better chances of survival when they are treated at trauma centers. The closest hospital may not have the appropriate imaging devices and staff ready to diagnose and treat this patient.

YOU *are the Medic* | SUMMARY, *continued*

EMS Patient Care Report (PCR)

Date: 10-20-11	Incident No.: 126	Nature of Call: MVC		Location: Pine & Chestnut	
Dispatched: 1304	En Route: 1305	At Scene: 1311	Transport: 1321	At Hospital: 1336	In Service: 1406

Patient Information

Age: 5 Sex: M Weight (in kg [lb]): 17 kg (34 lb)	Allergies: No known drug allergies Medications: None Past Medical History: None Chief Complaint: Left upper quadrant abdominal pain

Vital Signs

Time: 1316	BP: 82/55	Pulse: 155	Respirations: 40	Spo₂: 98%
Time: 1322	BP: 60/35	Pulse: 165	Respirations: 42	Spo₂: 98%
Time:	BP:	Pulse:	Respirations:	Spo₂:

EMS Treatment
(circle all that apply)

Oxygen @ __12__ L/min via (circle one): NC (NRM) Bag-mask device	Assisted Ventilation	Airway Adjunct	CPR
Defibrillation	Bleeding Control	Bandaging	Splinting	(Other:) Spinal immobilization, IV NS lock 20 GA left AC

Narrative

Pt is a 5-year-old male, rear driver's side passenger, involved in an MVC, vehicle vs. utility pole. On arrival, vehicle reveals about 20 inches of intrusion to front and broken windshield. No passenger air bag deployment and no car seat or booster seat used. Found pt alert, crying, and slouched under adult seat belt restraint. Pt difficult to console, but complains of left upper quadrant pain. Fitted with c-collar and immobilized on pediatric long backboard and loaded in ambulance. En route VS repeated and pt complains of left shoulder pain. Left upper quadrant reveals tenderness, a 6 × 2 inch contusion and swelling. Left shoulder unremarkable. No other associated trauma injuries noted. Contacted medical direction and Dr. Smith recommended no fluid volume resuscitation. Transported pt to Cardinal Glennon Children's Hospital room # 14 and report given to Julia, RN. No pt belongings transported. ED staff notified of mother's transport location and contact information. **End of report**

Prep Kit

■ Ready for Review

- Unrecognized abdominal trauma is the leading cause of unexpected death in trauma patients. Recognizing abdominal injuries and providing rapid transport is one of the best contributions you can make to a patient who has these injuries.

- The abdomen contains many vital organs and structures, including the kidneys, liver, spleen, pancreas, diaphragm, small and large intestines, stomach, bladder, and several great vessels.

- The quadrant system is generally used to describe a location in the abdomen. The four quadrants consist of the right upper quadrant (RUQ), the right lower quadrant (RLQ), the left lower quadrant (LLQ), and the left upper quadrant (LUQ).

- The peritoneum is a membrane that lines the abdominal cavity. Abdominal trauma can lead to peritonitis, an inflammation of the peritoneum that results from either blood or hollow organ contents spilling into the abdominal cavity. This is a life-threatening infection.

- The retroperitoneal space is the area behind the peritoneum and contains the aorta, vena cava, pancreas, kidneys, ureters, and portions of the duodenum and large intestine.

- When a patient has experienced trauma to the chest or abdomen, you should suspect that he or she also has additional internal abdominal injuries. Also suspect abdominal trauma in patients who have unexplained symptoms of shock.

- Injury to the abdomen may be slow to develop, and can be fatal. An injury may be subtle and difficult to locate and assess.

- Solid organs such as the liver and spleen have a large blood supply and can easily be crushed by blunt trauma. The abdomen and retroperitoneum can accommodate large amounts of blood but produce few signs and symptoms.

- Injury to hollow organs can cause the release of toxins such as urine, bile, or stomach acid into the abdominal cavity, causing major peritonitis.

- At least two thirds of all abdominal injuries involve blunt trauma, occurring often during motor vehicle crashes.

- Penetrating trauma most commonly results from stab wounds or low-velocity gunshot wounds. Penetrating trauma causes open abdominal injury.

- During patient assessment, note the manner in which the patient is lying; patients who are quiet or still should increase your index of suspicion of injuries. Prioritize the ABCs, remembering that a distended abdomen can prevent adequate inhalation, and internal unseen injuries can lead to shock. Assessment findings of the pulse and skin will give you an indication as to how aggressively you need to treat for shock.

- Assessment should never delay patient care and transport! Short on-scene time and quick transport to a trauma center are generally indicated. Evaluate more subtle signs and symptoms during history taking and the secondary assessment.

- Try to obtain as many details about an injury as possible. Also note the use of seat belts, deployment of air bags, and the patient's position in the vehicle. If a weapon was involved, note the type of weapon if this information is available.

- Peritonitis can take hours to days to develop. Shock, tachycardia, and confusion may not develop until the patient has lost a significant amount of blood. Maintain a high index of suspicion for a patient who has a mechanism of injury consistent with abdominal trauma, regardless of vital signs and other findings.

- Generally, management of patients with abdominal trauma is straightforward:
  - Ensure a secure airway.
  - Establish intravenous access and fluid replacement without delaying transport.
  - Minimize hemorrhaging with pressure dressings.
  - Apply a cardiac monitor and oxygen therapy, and then transport.
    - Kidney trauma can cause flank pain and hematuria. Management is the same as for other types of abdominal trauma.
    - Suspect a bladder injury in any patient who has trauma to the lower abdomen or pelvis. Symptoms include inability to urinate, blood at the urethral opening, and tenderness of the suprapubic region. Management follows basic trauma principles.
    - Blunt trauma to the testicles can cause painful hematomas, testicular rupture, or testicular torsion. The scrotum may be tender and swollen. Lacerations or avulsions should be treated with gentle compression and ice packs.
    - Blunt trauma to the penis can cause a large hematoma and pain. Management follows basic trauma principles.
    - Vaginal trauma can cause hematomas and ecchymoses in the lower pelvic area and on the external female genitalia, bleeding from the vagina, and tenderness on palpation of the lower pelvis.

- Pelvic fractures can result in damage to the major vascular structures, which can cause life-threatening hemorrhage.

- Because of the forces required to break the pelvis, if the patient has a pelvic fracture, suspect multisystem trauma.

Prep Kit, continued

Vital Vocabulary

blunt trauma Injury resulting from compression or deceleration forces, potentially crushing an organ or causing it to rupture.

closed abdominal injury An injury in which there is soft-tissue damage inside the body, but the skin remains intact.

duodenum The first part of the small intestine.

evisceration Displacement of an organ outside the body.

hematuria Blood in the urine.

hemoperitoneum The presence of extravasated blood in the peritoneal cavity.

Kehr sign Left shoulder pain that may indicate a ruptured spleen.

mesentery A membranous double fold of tissue in the abdomen that attaches various organs to the body wall.

open abdominal injury An injury in which there is a break in the surface of the skin or mucous membrane, exposing deeper tissue to potential contamination.

penetrating trauma An injury in which the skin is broken; direct contact results in laceration of the structure.

peritoneal space The area in the abdomen encased in the peritoneum, and which consists of an upper and lower part.

The upper portion contains the diaphragm, liver, spleen, stomach, gallbladder, and transverse colon. The lower portion contains the small bowel, sigmoid colon, parts of the descending and ascending colon, and, in women, the internal reproductive organs.

peritoneum A membrane in the abdomen encasing the liver, spleen, diaphragm, stomach, and transverse colon.

peritonitis Inflammation of the peritoneum that results from either blood or hollow organ contents spilling into the abdominal cavity.

periumbilical Pertaining to the area around the umbilicus.

pylorus A circumferential muscle at the end of the stomach that acts as a valve between the stomach and duodenum.

retroperitoneal space The area in the abdomen containing the aorta, vena cava, pancreas, kidneys, ureters, and portions of the duodenum and large intestine.

somatic pain Localized pain, usually felt deeply, which represents irritation or injury to tissue, causing activation of peripheral nerve tracts.

visceral pain Crampy, aching pain deep within the body, the source of which is usually difficult to pinpoint; common with genitourinary problems.

Assessment in Action

You are dispatched to the scene of a 19-year-old man who has been assaulted. When you arrive you find the patient sitting on the sidewalk. A police officer at the scene is holding pressure to the patient's right upper abdomen with a blood-soaked gym towel. You observe no other obvious trauma injuries.

Your partner takes over control of applying pressure to the patient's abdomen with a sterile trauma dressing. As the bloody towel is replaced, you note a 2-inch deep laceration to the right upper quadrant with constant slow bleeding. The patient is alert and oriented and states, "I got stabbed!" He is only reporting right upper abdominal pain and denies associated trauma injuries. The patient appears pale and diaphoretic and asks to lie down. His vital signs are as follows: respirations, 24 breaths/min; pulse, 136 beats/min; blood pressure, 86/56 mm Hg; and pulse oximetry, 97% on room air. The patient is placed on the stretcher in a supine position as requested. En route a full-body exam is performed and found to be unremarkable except for his abdominal laceration/penetration. His abdomen is rigid, distended, and tender to the right upper quadrant. Bleeding is controlled with manual pressure only. Two large-bore IVs are initiated and oxygen is applied. The patient is transported to the closest trauma center.

1. Which of the following are considered solid organs of the abdomen?
   A. Liver, spleen, kidneys, and pancreas
   B. Liver and spleen
   C. Large intestine, small intestine, and kidneys
   D. Liver, spleen, kidneys, and intestines

2. On the basis of the patient's wound, what type of injury should you suspect?
   A. Lacerated liver
   B. Ruptured spleen
   C. Contusion of the heart
   D. Ruptured appendix

3. On-scene care of a patient who has signs of shock from abdominal injury should include which of the following?
   A. Comprehensive physical exam
   B. Initiation of IV fluid therapy
   C. Reassessment
   D. Oxygen administration

4. The abdominal cavity is lined with a membrane called the:
   A. retroperitoneal space.
   B. pylorus.
   C. peritoneum.
   D. periumbilical.

5. The liver is a highly vascular organ that lies in the _____ quadrant.
   A. right upper
   B. right lower
   C. left upper
   D. left lower

6. Rupture of an organ can lead to hemorrhage and:
   A. peritoneum.
   B. peritonitis.
   C. hemoperitoneum.
   D. internal bleeding.

7. Signs of abdominal hemorrhage may include:
   A. tender abdomen, hypertension, and bradycardia.
   B. tachycardia, hypertension, and distention.
   C. periumbilical ecchymosis, distention, bradycardia, and shock.
   D. distention, hypotension, tachycardia, and shock.

Additional Questions

8. Discuss the value of performing percussion of the abdomen as part of the prehospital abdominal exam.

9. Is auscultation of bowel sounds useful in assessing for abdominal trauma?

Orthopaedic Trauma

National EMS Education Standard Competencies

Trauma

Integrates assessment findings with principles of epidemiology and pathophysiology to formulate a field impression to implement a comprehensive treatment/disposition plan for an acutely injured patient.

Orthopaedic Trauma

Recognition and management of

- Open fractures (pp 1764-1766)
- Closed fractures (pp 1764-1766)
- Dislocations (pp 1766-1768)
- Amputations (p 1769)

Pathophysiology, assessment, and management of

- Upper and lower extremity orthopaedic trauma (p 1754)
- Open fractures (pp 1764-1766; 1782-1789)
- Closed fractures (pp 1764-1766; 1782-1789)
- Dislocations (pp 1766-1768; 1789-1792)
- Sprains/strains (p 1768)
- Pelvic fractures (pp 1784-1786)
- Amputations/replantation (p 1769)
- Compartment syndrome (pp 1780-1781)
- Pediatric fractures (p 1779)
- Tendon laceration/transection/rupture (Achilles and patellar) (pp 1768; 1792)

Medicine

Integrates assessment findings with principles of epidemiology and pathophysiology to formulate a field impression and implement a comprehensive treatment/disposition plan for a patient with a medical complaint.

Nontraumatic Musculoskeletal Disorders

Anatomy, physiology, pathophysiology, assessment, and management of

- Nontraumatic fractures (pp 1792-1795)

Anatomy, physiology, epidemiology, pathophysiology, psychosocial impact, presentations, prognosis, and management of common or major nontraumatic musculoskeletal disorders

- Disorders of the spine (p 1793)
- Joint abnormalities (pp 1793-1794)
- Muscle abnormalities (p 1794)
- Overuse syndromes (pp 1794-1795)

Knowledge Objectives

1. Describe the incidence, morbidity, and mortality of musculoskeletal injuries. (p 1754)
2. Discuss the anatomy and physiology of the musculoskeletal system. (pp 1754-1763)
3. Predict injuries based on the mechanism of injury, including:
   a. Direct (pp 1763-1764)
   b. Indirect (p 1764)
   c. Pathologic (pp 1763-1764)
4. Describe age-associated changes in the bones. (p 1758)
5. Discuss the general pathophysiology of musculoskeletal injuries, including fractures, ligament injuries, dislocations, muscle injuries, tendon injuries, and injuries that may signify fractures. (pp 1764-1769)
6. Discuss fracture classifications, including linear, transverse, oblique, spiral, impacted, comminuted, segmental, complete, incomplete, nondisplaced, and displaced. (pp 1765-1766)
7. Discuss the pathophysiology of open versus closed fractures. (p 1765)
8. Discuss the signs and symptoms of a fracture. (pp 1765-1766)
9. Describe the process of assessing a patient with a musculoskeletal injury. (pp 1769-1774)
10. Discuss the assessment findings associated with musculoskeletal injuries. (pp 1769-1770)
11. List the six "P"s of musculoskeletal injury assessment. (p 1771)
12. List the primary signs and symptoms that can indicate less obvious extremity injury. (pp 1769-1774)
13. List the other signs and symptoms that can indicate less obvious extremity injury. (pp 1769-1774)
14. Discuss the need for assessment of pulses, motor, and sensation before and after splinting. (pp 1775-1779)
15. Identify the need for rapid intervention and transport when dealing with musculoskeletal injuries. (p 1770)
16. Discuss the general emergency care principles used in managing musculoskeletal injuries. (pp 1774-1779)
17. Discuss the relationship between volume of hemorrhage and open or closed fractures. (p 1774)
18. Discuss methods of pain control for a patient with a musculoskeletal injury. (pp 1774-1775)
19. Discuss the general guidelines of splinting. (pp 1775-1779)
20. Discuss the pathophysiology, assessment, and management of complications of musculoskeletal injuries, including vascular injuries, neurovascular injuries, compartment syndrome, crush injuries, and thromboembolic disease. (pp 1780-1782)
21. Discuss the pathophysiology, assessment, and management of specific fractures, including shoulder girdle fractures, midshaft humerus fractures,

elbow fractures, forearm fractures, wrist and hand fractures, pelvic fractures, hip fractures, femoral shaft fractures, knee fractures, tibia and fibula fractures, ankle fractures, and calcaneus fractures. (pp 1782–1789)

22. Describe the special considerations involved in femur fracture management. (pp 1787–1788)

23. Discuss the pathophysiology, assessment, and management of pediatric fractures. (p 1779)

24. Discuss the pathophysiology, assessment, and management of specific joint injuries and dislocations, including those to the shoulder girdle, elbow, wrist and hand, finger, hip, and knee. (pp 1789–1792)

25. Explain the importance of manipulating a knee dislocation or fracture with an absent distal pulse. (pp 1791–1792)

26. Describe the procedure for reduction of a shoulder, finger, or ankle dislocation or fracture. (pp 1782, 1783–1784, 1788, 1790, 1791)

27. Discuss the pathophysiology, assessment, and management of bony abnormalities, including osteomyelitis and tumors. (p 1793)

28. Discuss the pathophysiology, assessment, and management of disorders of the spine, including cauda equina syndrome. (p 1793)

29. Discuss the pathophysiology, assessment, and management of joint abnormalities, including arthritis, septic arthritis, gout, rheumatoid arthritis, and osteoarthritis. (pp 1793–1794)

30. Discuss the pathophysiology, assessment, and management of muscle abnormalities, including myalgia and myositis. (pp 1794, 1795)

31. Discuss the pathophysiology, assessment, and management of overuse injuries, including tendinitis, bursitis, carpal tunnel syndrome, and polyneuropathy. (pp 1794–1795)

32. Discuss the pathophysiology, assessment, and management of soft-tissue infections, including fasciitis, gangrene, paronychia, and flexor tenosynovitis of the hand. (p 1795)

Skills Objectives

1. Demonstrate performing a motor function and sensory exam. (pp 1771–1774, Skill Drill 1)

2. Demonstrate how to properly splint an injured extremity. (pp 1775–1779)

Introduction

Musculoskeletal injuries are one of the most common reasons that patients seek medical attention. Complaints related to the musculoskeletal system lead to almost 60 million visits to physicians annually in the United States, more than for any other reason. Some of these injuries will result in some type of musculoskeletal impairment, leading to millions of missed days of work or school and costing hundreds of billions of dollars yearly. An estimated 70% to 80% of all patients with multiple system trauma may have one or more musculoskeletal injuries. Some areas of public policy, legislative changes, and public education have been effective in reducing the injury problem. For example, efforts related to cell phone use by drivers, seat belt use in motor vehicles, and falls in older people have had positive impacts.

Injuries related to the musculoskeletal system are usually easily identifiable because of the associated pain, swelling, and deformity. Although these injuries are rarely fatal, they often result in short- or long-term disability. By providing prompt temporary measures, such as splinting and analgesia, paramedics may help reduce the period during which patients are disabled. However, despite the sometimes dramatic appearance of these injuries, you should not focus on the musculoskeletal injury without first determining that no life-threatening injury exists. *Never forget the ABCs!*

Anatomy and Physiology of the Musculoskeletal System

The musculoskeletal system gives the body its shape and allows for its movement. It is essential that you understand its basic anatomy and physiology.

Functions of the Musculoskeletal System

The musculoskeletal system performs many important functions within the body. Bones help *support* the soft tissues of the body and form a framework that gives the human body its shape and allows it to maintain an erect posture. *Movement* is generated because muscles are attached to bones by <u>tendons</u>. (Reminder: Muscles-To-Bones [MTB] means Muscles–Tendons–Bones.) When a muscle contracts, the force generated by the muscle is transferred to a bone on the opposite side of the <u>joint</u> from the muscle, leading to motion. Bones also offer *protection* to the more fragile organs and structures beneath them—for example, the skull's protection of the brain, the rib cage's protection of the heart and lungs, and the spinal column's protection of the spinal cord.

Another important function of the musculoskeletal system is <u>hematopoiesis</u>—the process of generating blood cells. In adults, it most commonly occurs in the red bone marrow of the sternum, ribs, vertebral bodies, pelvis, and the proximal portions of the femur and humerus. Each day, the body produces

YOU *are the Medic* PART 1

You are dispatched to the scene of a private residence for a 24-year-old male roofer who fell off a ladder while carrying up some shingles. Coworkers witnessed the fall and tell you that he fell about 15 to 20 feet, landing feet-first on the lawn.

When you arrive you find the patient lying supine on the grass next to the ladder. He is alert and seems to be slow to answer all questions. He recalls the event and describes feeling light-headed when he was climbing up the ladder before he fell. He reports feeling sleepy and weak and has lower back pain, bilateral lower extremity pain, and bilateral wrist pain.

Recording Time: 1 Minute	
Appearance	Eyes open to voice
Level of consciousness	V (Responsive to verbal stimuli)
Airway	Patent with clear speech
Breathing	Nonlabored and shallow
Circulation	Rapid radial pulse; no obvious external bleeding

1. What are your initial assessment and treatment priorities?
2. What other information would you obtain about the patient and the incident?
3. What are your early communication and transport plans?

new red blood cells, white blood cells, and platelets from the stem cells that are present in the bone marrow, thereby replacing those that have been lost or that are no longer functional.

■ The Body's Scaffolding: The Skeleton

The integrated structure formed by the 206 bones of the body is called the skeleton. It may be divided into two distinct portions: the <u>axial skeleton</u> and the <u>appendicular skeleton</u>. The axial skeleton is composed of the bones of the central part, or axis, of the body; its divisions include the vertebral column, skull, ribs, and sternum. The skull is composed of the cranium, basilar skull, face, and inner ear Figure 1 .

The spine is composed of 33 spinal vertebrae: 7 cervical, 12 thoracic, 5 lumbar, 5 sacral, and 4 coccygeal. Moving anteriorly, the thorax is formed by the sternum and 12 pairs of ribs. The appendicular skeleton is divided into the <u>pectoral girdle</u>, the <u>pelvic girdle</u>, and the bones of the upper and lower extremities.

Shoulder and Upper Extremities

The pectoral girdle Figure 2 , also referred to as the shoulder girdle, consists of two scapulae and two clavicles. The <u>scapula</u> (shoulder blade) is a flat, triangular bone held to the rib cage posteriorly by powerful muscles that buffer it against injury. The <u>clavicle</u> (collarbone) is a slender, S-shaped bone attached by ligaments at the medial end to the sternum and at the lateral end to the raised tip of the scapula, called the <u>acromion</u>. The clavicle acts as a strut to keep the shoulder propped up; however, because it is slender and very exposed, this bone is vulnerable to injury.

The upper extremity Figure 3 joins the shoulder girdle at the glenohumeral joint. The proximal portion contains the <u>humerus</u>, a bone that articulates proximally with the scapula

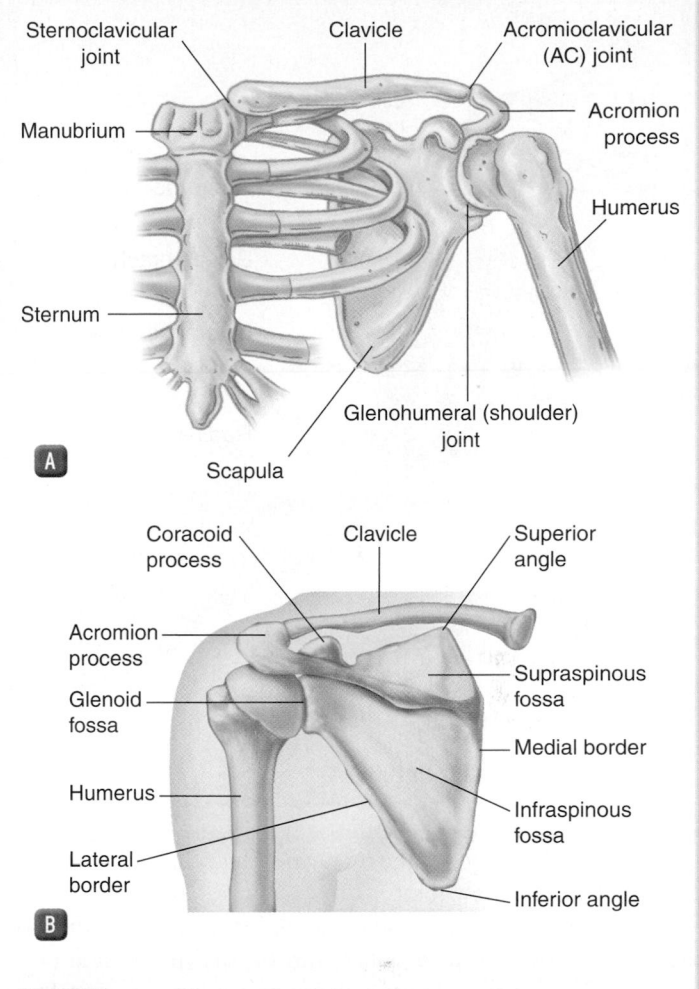

Figure 2 The pectoral girdle. **A.** Anterior view, including the clavicle. **B.** Posterior view, including the scapula.

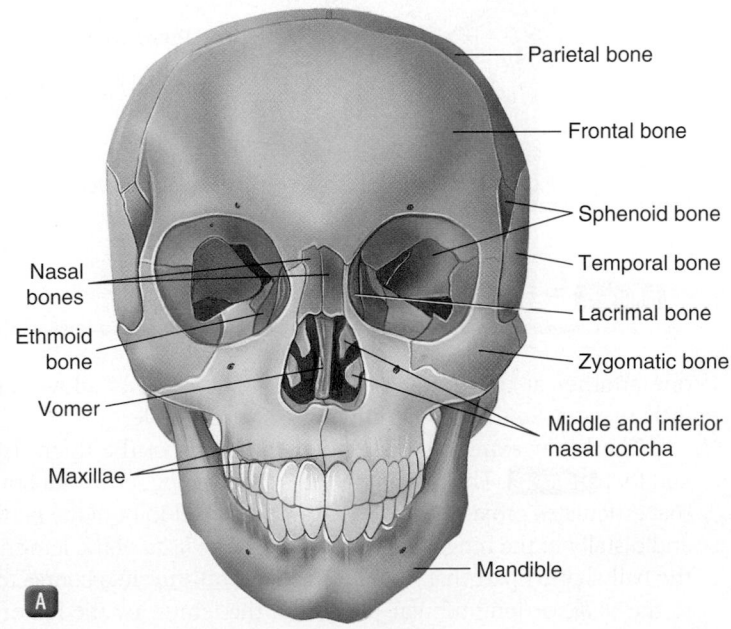

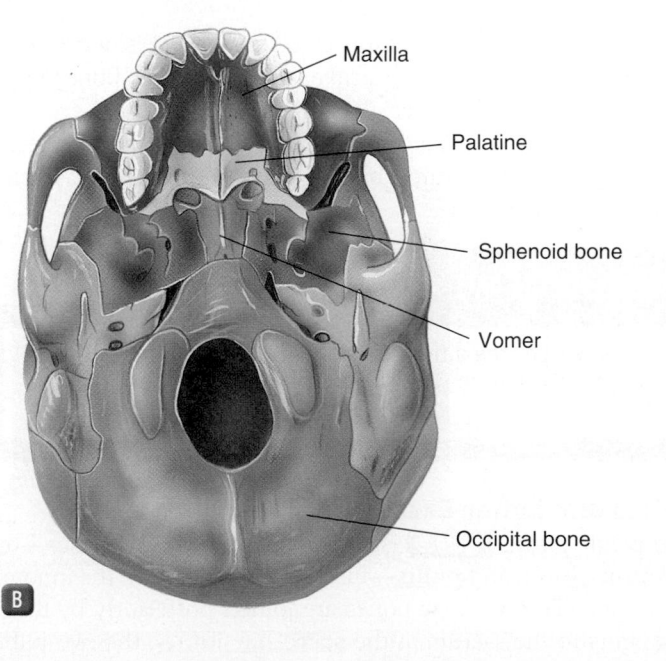

Figure 1 The skull and its components. **A.** Front view. **B.** Bottom view.

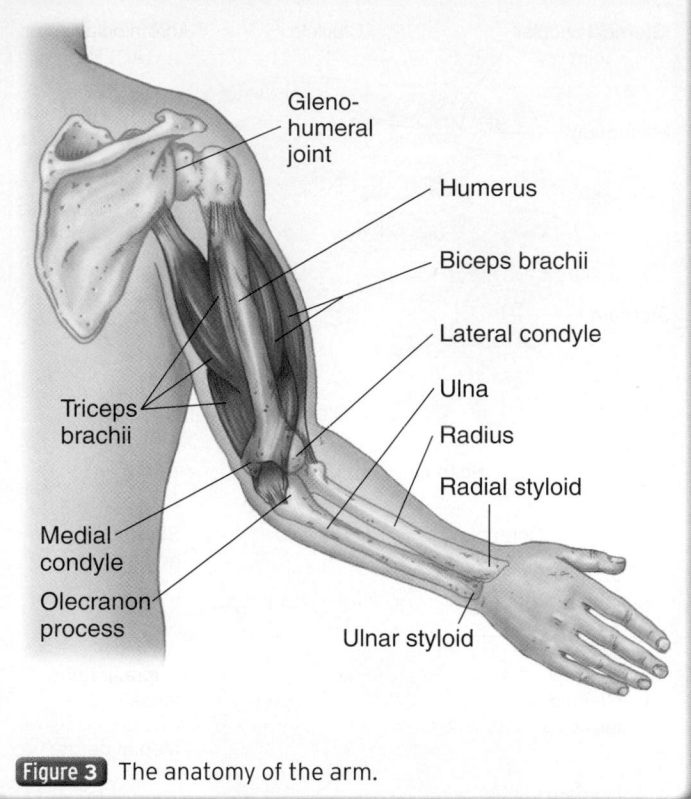

Figure 3 The anatomy of the arm.

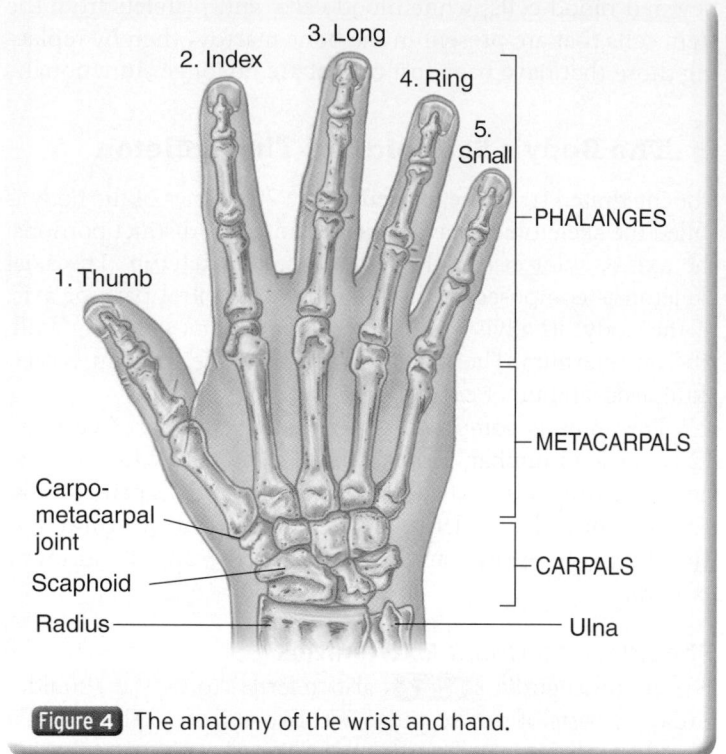

Figure 4 The anatomy of the wrist and hand.

and distally with bones of the forearm—the radius and ulna—to form the hinged elbow joint.

The **radius** and **ulna** make up the forearm. The radius, the larger of the two forearm bones, lies on the *thumb* side of the forearm. Distally, the ulna is narrow and is on the little-finger side of the forearm. It serves as the pivot around which the radius turns at the wrist to rotate the palm upward (**supination**) or downward (**pronation**). Because the radius and the ulna are arranged in parallel, when one is broken, the other is often broken as well.

The hand **Figure 4** contains three sets of bones: wrist bones (**carpals**), hand bones (**metacarpals**), and finger bones (**phalanges**). The carpals, especially the scaphoid, are vulnerable to fracture when a person falls on an outstretched hand. Phalanges are more apt to be injured by a crushing injury, such as being slammed in a car door.

Words of Wisdom

To remember the difference between supination and pronation, think of soup. The SUPinated hand can hold a cup of SOUP.

Pelvis and Lower Extremities

The pelvic girdle **Figure 5** is actually three separate bones—the **ischium**, **ilium**, and **pubis**—fused together to form the innominate bone. The two iliac bones are joined posteriorly by tough ligaments to the sacrum at the **sacroiliac joints**; the two pubic bones are connected anteriorly by equally tough ligaments to

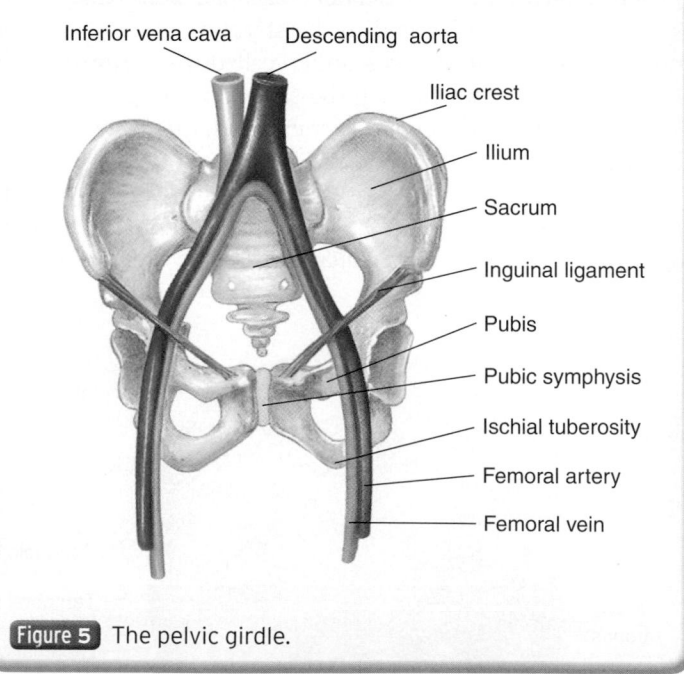

Figure 5 The pelvic girdle.

one another at the **pubic symphysis**. These joints allow very little motion, so the pelvic ring is strong and stable.

The lower extremity consists of the bones of the thigh, leg, and foot **Figure 6**. The **femur** (thighbone) is a long, powerful bone that articulates proximally in the ball-and-socket joint of the pelvis and distally in the hinge joint of the knee. The *head* of the femur is the ball-shaped part that fits into the **acetabulum**. It is connected to the *shaft*, or long tubular portion of the femur, by the femoral *neck*. The femoral neck is a common site for fractures, generally referred to as hip fractures, especially in the older population.

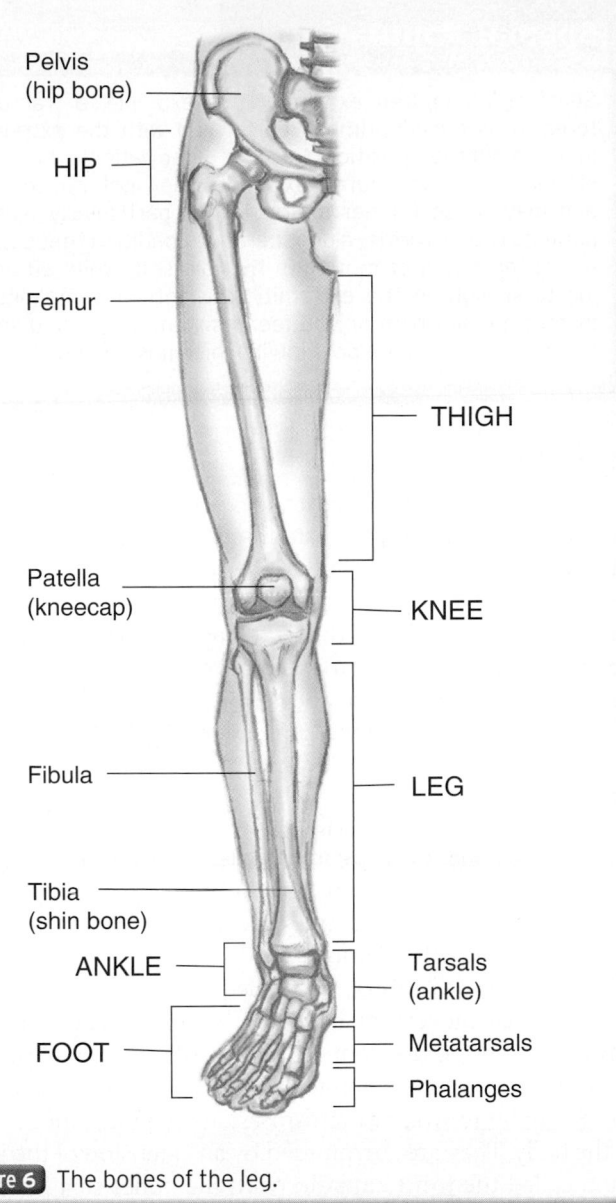

Pelvis
(hip bone)

HIP

Femur

THIGH

Patella
(kneecap)

KNEE

Fibula

LEG

Tibia
(shin bone)

ANKLE

Tarsals
(ankle)

FOOT

Metatarsals

Phalanges

Figure 6 The bones of the leg.

The lower leg consists of two bones: the **tibia** and the **fibula**. The tibia (shinbone) forms the inferior component of the knee joint. Anterior to this joint is the **patella** (kneecap), a bone that is important for knee extension. The tibia runs down the front of the lower leg, where it is vulnerable to direct blows, and can be felt just beneath the skin. The much smaller fibula runs posteriorly and laterally to the tibia. The fibula is not a component of the knee joint, but it does make up the lateral border of the ankle joint (lateral **malleolus**) at its distal articulation.

Words of Wisdom

Here's a tip to help remember which bones are carpal (hand bones) and which bones are tarsal (foot bones): "I steer my CAR (pal) with hands and walk through TAR (sal) with my feet."

The foot consists of three classes of bones: *ankle bones* (**tarsals**), *foot bones* (**metatarsals**), and *toe bones* (phalanges) **Figure 7**. The largest of the tarsal bones is the heel bone, or **calcaneus**, which is subject to injury when a person falls from a height and lands on the feet.

■ Characteristics and Composition of Bone

Bone Shapes

Bones may be classified based on their shape. **Long bones** are longer than they are wide; examples include the femur, humerus, tibia, fibula, radius, and ulna. **Short bones** are nearly as wide as they are long; they include the phalanges, metacarpals, and metatarsals. **Flat bones** are thin, broad bones; they include the sternum, ribs, scapulae, and skull. **Irregular bones** do not fit into one of the other categories but rather have a shape that is designed to perform a specific function, such as the bones of the vertebral column and the mandible. **Round bones** are generally found in proximity to a joint and help with movement. They are often referred to as sesamoid bones because of their location within a tendon. The patella is the largest of the round bones.

Typical Long Bone Architecture

Long bones have several distinct regions and anatomic features **Figure 8**. These bones can grow to such long lengths because of the presence of the growth plate, or **physis**, in children. Once a person reaches adulthood, the growth plate closes and the mature adult bone is complete. The long bone is divided into three regions: the **diaphysis**, the **epiphysis**, and the **metaphysis**.

The articular surfaces of a long bone come in contact with other bones to form **articulations** (joints). These regions of the bone are covered by articular **cartilage**, a substance that acts as a cushion to protect the bone from damage and wear.

The portion of bone that is not covered by articular cartilage is, instead, covered by the **periosteum**. The periosteum is a dense, fibrous membrane contains capillaries and cells that are important for bone repair and maintenance. In the inner portion

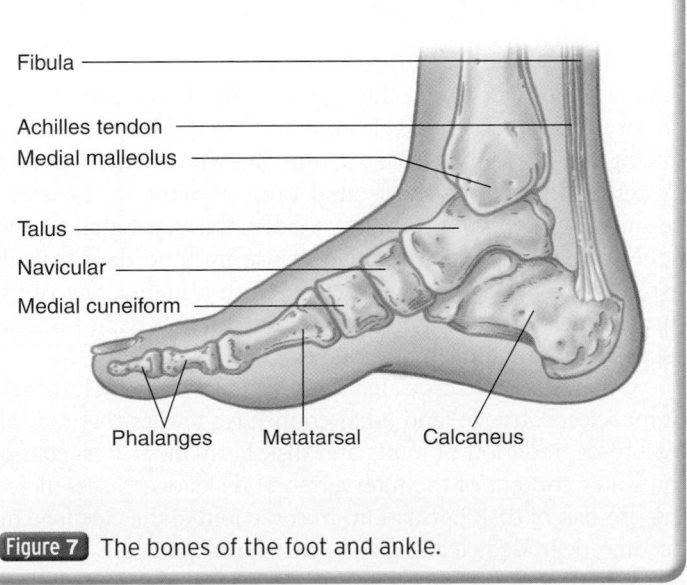

Fibula

Achilles tendon

Medial malleolus

Talus

Navicular

Medial cuneiform

Phalanges   Metatarsal   Calcaneus

Figure 7 The bones of the foot and ankle.

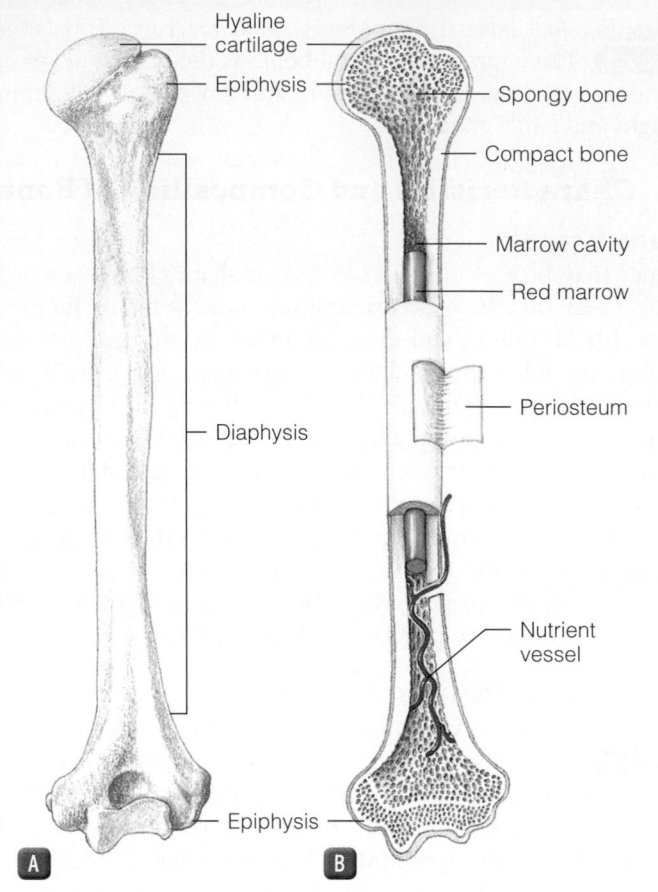

Figure 8 Anatomy of the long bone. **A.** The humerus. Notice the long shaft and dilated ends. **B.** Longitudinal section of the humerus showing compact bone, spongy bone, and marrow.

of the long bone, blood comes from the nutrient artery of the bone. Once it penetrates the bone's outer cortex, the artery enters the **medullary canal**, the hollow inner portion of the shaft that is lined by the **endosteum** (similar to the periosteum, but on the inside) and contains yellow (fatty) marrow in adults.

Age-Associated Changes in Bone

Bone ages just like any other tissue of the body, decreasing in density after age 35 years, leading to a loss of height, and producing changes in facial structure. In women, this decrease in density is further accelerated once menopause is reached because of the loss of estrogen, a hormone that helps promote bone formation. A significant decrease in bone density, called **osteoporosis** **Figure 9**, is associated with a higher risk of fracture. People with osteoporosis are at risk for incurring a fracture, especially in the hip, spine, and wrist.

Other changes associated with aging of bone include aging of muscles, cartilage, and other connective tissues that may also lead to degradation of joints and disk herniation. For example, the water content of the intervertebral disks decreases, increasing the risk of disk herniation. In some joints, the cartilage may become degraded, leading to arthritis and pain; in others, the cartilage becomes calcified, leading to restricted motion.

Joints

When two bones come together, they articulate with one another to form a joint. Some joints are fused and allow for no motion, such as the joints of the skull. Other joints allow for motion by permitting movement between the two bones, typically within a certain plane of motion that is defined by the structure of the bones that form it. The various motions that a joint may allow include flexion, extension, **abduction**, **adduction**, rotation, circumduction, pronation, and supination **Figure 10**.

Types of Joints

The three general types of joints are fibrous, cartilaginous, and synovial **Figure 11**. **Fibrous joints**, also referred to as synarthroses or fused joints, contain dense fibrous tissue that does not allow for movement. Examples include the bones of the skull and the distal tibiofibular joint.

Cartilaginous joints, also called amphiarthroses, allow for very minimal movement between the bones. The pubic symphysis and the joints connecting the ribs to the sternum are examples of this type of joint.

Synovial joints, or diarthroses, are the most mobile joints of the body. They are surrounded by an extension of the periosteum called the **joint capsule**, with the bones that form them being held in place by very strong **ligaments**. Within the joint are the articular cartilage and the **synovial membrane**, which secretes synovial fluid into the joint cavity for lubrication.

Bursa

A **bursa** is a padlike sac or cavity located within the connective tissue, usually in proximity to a joint. It may be lined with a synovial membrane and typically contains fluid that helps reduce the amount of friction between a tendon and a bone or between a tendon and a ligament. Examples include the olecranon bursa of the elbow and the prepatellar bursa of the knee. Bursitis is inflammation of a bursa.

Words of Wisdom

The acronym MTB (muscles-tendons-bone) can help you remember that tendons connect muscles to bone.

The acronym BLB (bones-ligaments-bones) can help you remember that ligaments connect bones to other bones.

These inelastic bands of connective tissue have a structure similar to that of tendons.

Cartilage consists of fibers of collagen embedded in a gelatinous substance. This flexible connective tissue forms the smooth surface over bone ends where they articulate, provides cushioning between vertebrae, gives structure to the nose and external ear, forms the framework of the larynx and trachea, and serves as the model for the formation of the skeleton in children. Cartilage has a very limited neurovascular supply—it receives nutrients through diffusion from the outer covering of the cartilage or from the synovial fluid—so it does not heal well if it is injured.

The Moving Forces: Muscles

Muscles are composed of specialized cells that contract (shorten) when stimulated to exert a force on a part of the body. Three types of muscle are found in the body: cardiac muscle, skeletal muscle, and smooth muscle **Figure 12** .

Skeletal Muscle

Skeletal muscle **Figure 13** is also called **voluntary muscle**, because its contractions are largely under voluntary control, or **striated muscle**, because striations can be seen in it during microscopic examination. Skeletal muscle includes all of the muscles attached to the skeleton and forms the bulk of the tissue of the arms and legs. It is also found along the spine and buttocks. By maintaining a state of partial contraction, this type of muscle allows the body to maintain its posture and to sit or stand. It varies greatly in size and shape, from thin strands to the large muscles of the thigh and back. It also constitutes the muscles of the tongue, soft palate, scalp, pharynx, upper esophagus, and eye. About 40% to 50% of normal body weight is skeletal muscle, as it has a high water content. In addition, because of its high metabolic rate and demand for energy and oxygen, skeletal muscle has a very rich blood supply, which causes it to bleed significantly when injured.

Skeletal muscles are profoundly affected by the amount of training and work to which they are subjected. Unused muscles tend to **atrophy** (shrink or waste away), whereas physical training promotes **hypertrophy** (increase in size).

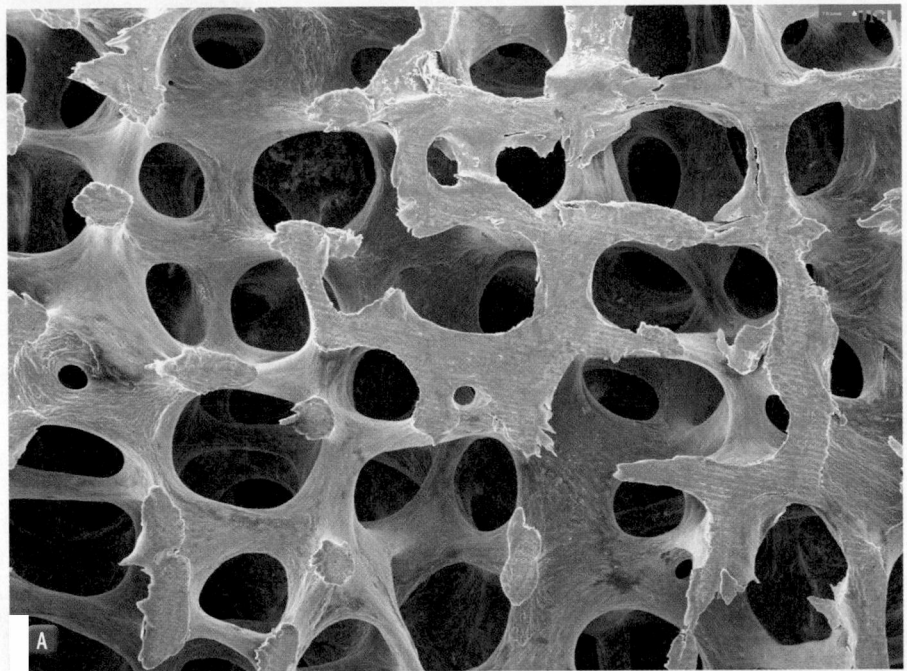
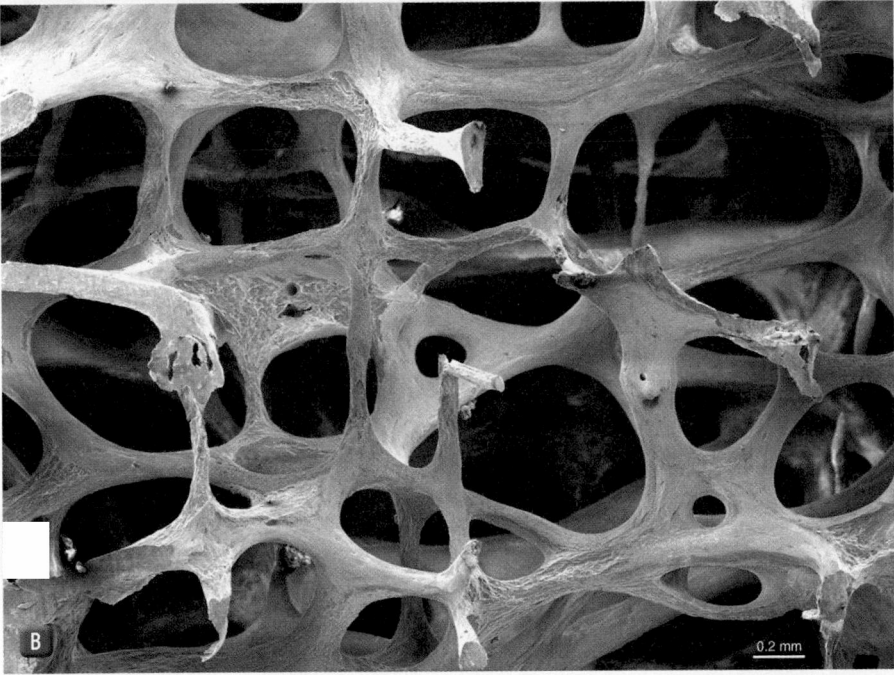

Figure 9 The structural difference between normal and osteoporotic bone. **A.** Normal bone in a 29-year-old woman. **B.** Osteoporotic bone in a 92-year-old woman.

Skeletal Connecting and Supporting Structures

Tendons connect muscle to bone. These flat or cordlike bands of connective tissue are white and have a glistening appearance.

Ligaments connect bone to bone and help maintain the stability of joints and determine the degree of joint motion.

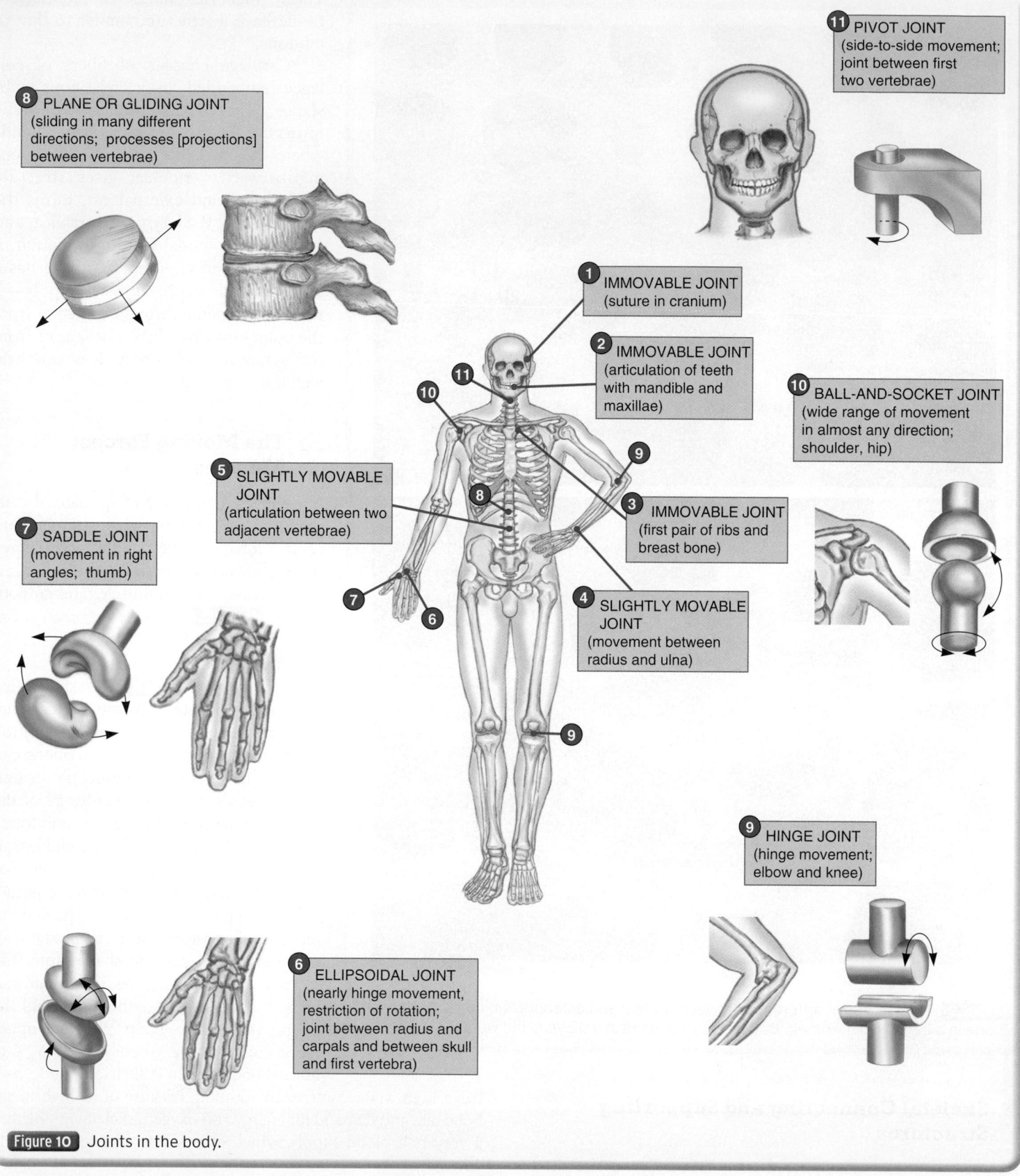

8 PLANE OR GLIDING JOINT (sliding in many different directions; processes [projections] between vertebrae)

11 PIVOT JOINT (side-to-side movement; joint between first two vertebrae)

1 IMMOVABLE JOINT (suture in cranium)

2 IMMOVABLE JOINT (articulation of teeth with mandible and maxillae)

10 BALL-AND-SOCKET JOINT (wide range of movement in almost any direction; shoulder, hip)

5 SLIGHTLY MOVABLE JOINT (articulation between two adjacent vertebrae)

7 SADDLE JOINT (movement in right angles; thumb)

3 IMMOVABLE JOINT (first pair of ribs and breast bone)

4 SLIGHTLY MOVABLE JOINT (movement between radius and ulna)

9 HINGE JOINT (hinge movement; elbow and knee)

6 ELLIPSOIDAL JOINT (nearly hinge movement, restriction of rotation; joint between radius and carpals and between skull and first vertebra)

Figure 10 Joints in the body.

Skeletal muscles are attached to bones by tendons. Tendons cross joints to create a pulling force between two bones when a muscle contracts. The biceps muscle, for example, has its origin on the scapula; the biceps tendon passes over the head of the humerus, where it fuses with the body of the biceps muscle; at the distal end of the biceps, a tendon passes over the anterior surface of the elbow and inserts on the radius. Thus, when the biceps muscle contracts, the force causes the elbow to bend (flex).

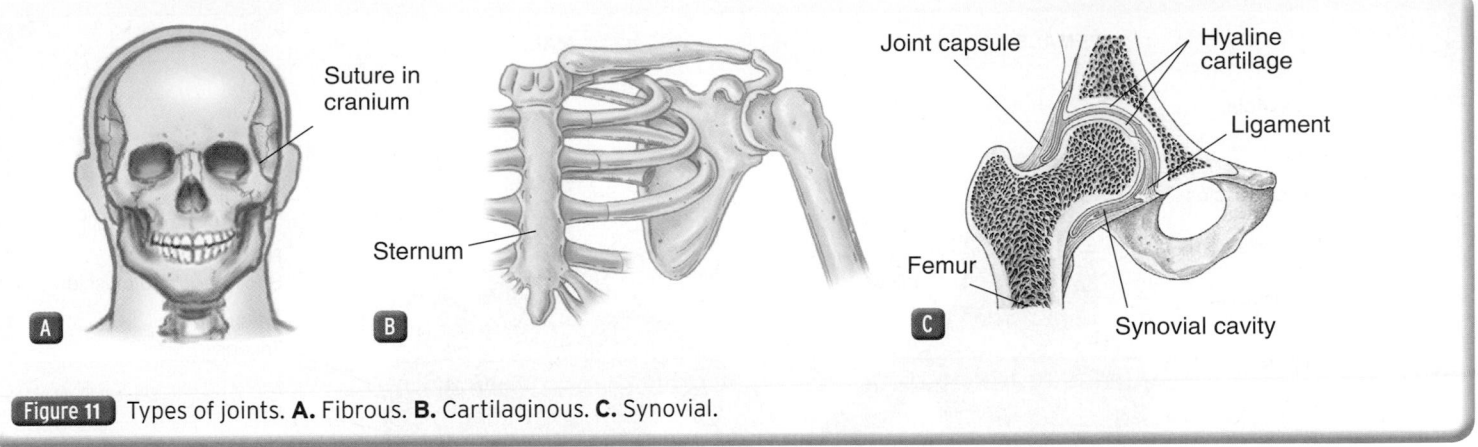

Figure 11 Types of joints. **A.** Fibrous. **B.** Cartilaginous. **C.** Synovial.

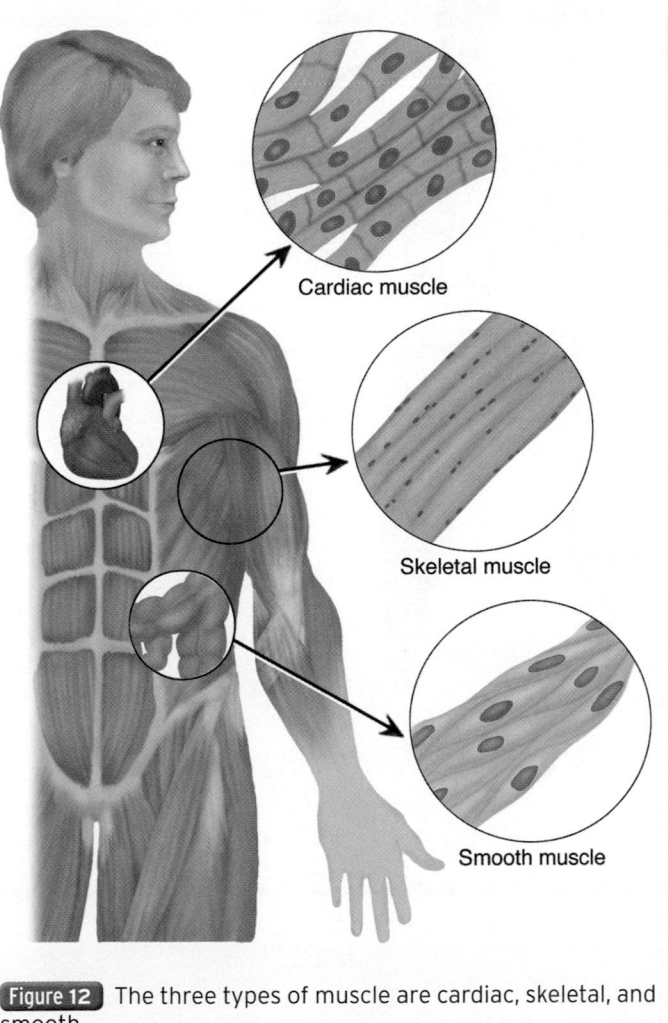

Figure 12 The three types of muscle are cardiac, skeletal, and smooth.

Muscle contraction requires energy. This energy is derived from the metabolism of glucose and results in the production of **lactic acid** (lactate). Lactic acid, in turn, must be converted into carbon dioxide and water, a process that requires oxygen. For that reason, vigorous muscular activity is often followed by an increased respiratory rate, which increases oxygen delivery to and carbon dioxide removal from the tissues.

The sensation of **muscle fatigue** occurs when the energy supply to the muscle is inadequate to meet the energy demands. If muscle fatigue occurs as a result of excessive muscular activity, rest produces quick recovery. If fatigue occurs from a lack of oxygen or essential nutrients or electrolytes (such as sodium or calcium), however, rest will not lead to such a quick recovery.

Muscle Innervation

Skeletal muscle is innervated by **somatic motor neurons**. These neurons transmit electrical stimuli to a muscle that cause it to contract. The combination of the muscle and the neuron that innervates it constitutes a motor unit. A motor unit that receives a signal to contract responds as forcefully as possible or does not contract at all: It is an all-or-nothing response. To generate a more forceful contraction, more neurons need to signal more muscle cells to contract, a process called **recruitment**.

Innervation of the upper extremities arises from the brachial plexus. The brachial plexus is formed by a network of nerves that originate from the spinal cord at the C5–T1 levels. After the fibers of these nerves network with one another, five distinct nerves are formed: the axillary, radial, musculocutaneous, ulnar, and median. Innervation of the lower extremities is provided by the lumbar and lumbosacral plexuses, which are formed by the spinal nerves that originate from L1–S4. The networking of nerves within these two plexuses leads to the formation of multiple distinct nerves, including the sciatic nerve, which branches in the popliteal fossa to form the peroneal and tibial nerves, and the femoral nerve.

Musculoskeletal Blood Supply

When a person has a musculoskeletal injury, the arteries that supply the injured region may also be damaged. Therefore, it is important to realize which arteries are present in each part of the extremity **Figure 14**.

The upper extremity's blood supply originates from the **subclavian artery**. When the subclavian artery reaches the **axilla**, it is referred to as the **axillary artery**. After giving off several branches that supply the shoulder region with blood, the artery leaves the axilla and becomes the **brachial artery**. After the brachial artery passes through the elbow, it divides

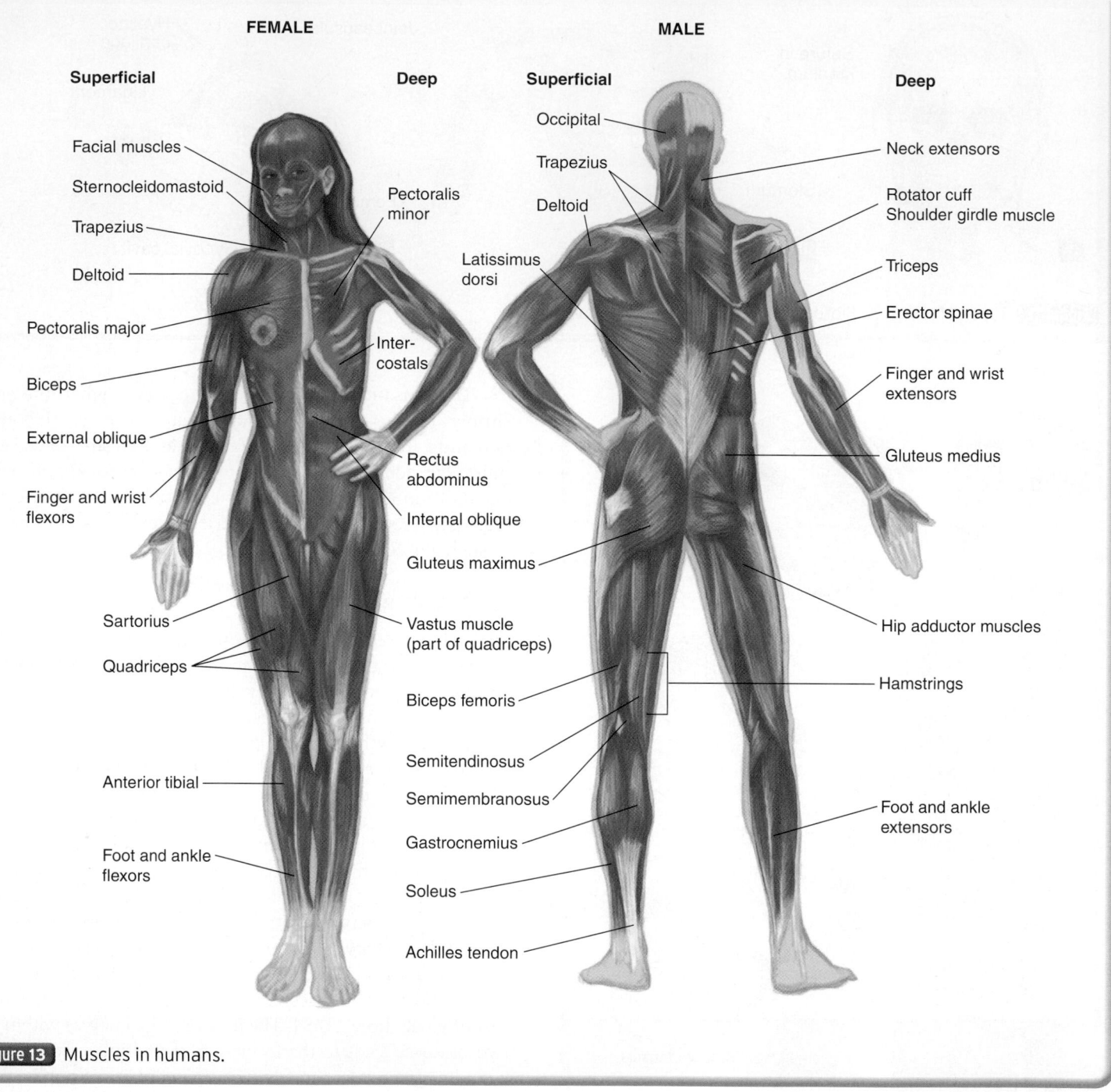

Figure 13 Muscles in humans.

into the <u>radial artery</u> and <u>ulnar artery</u>. In the hand, the radial and ulnar arteries form superficial and deep arcades of blood vessels that branch to form the arteries of each finger, the <u>digital arteries</u>.

In the lower extremity, the blood supply originates from the external iliac artery. When the external iliac artery reaches the leg, it becomes the <u>femoral artery</u>. When it reaches the knee, the femoral artery turns posteriorly and laterally and is referred to as the <u>popliteal artery</u>. The popliteal artery divides into the <u>anterior tibial artery</u> and <u>posterior tibial artery</u>. The anterior tibial artery travels along the anterior and

lateral surface of the tibia until it reaches the ankle, where it proceeds along the <u>dorsal</u> surface of the foot toward the great toe and becomes the dorsalis pedis artery. The posterior tibial artery travels along the posterior aspect of the tibia until it reaches the ankle, where it follows a path just behind the medial malleolus until it reaches the <u>plantar</u> aspect of the foot. Within the foot, arcades of arteries supply the various structures with blood and give off branches that form the digital arteries of the toes. Interestingly, though everyone has a dorsalis pedis pulse, it is not easily palpable in about 15% of the population.

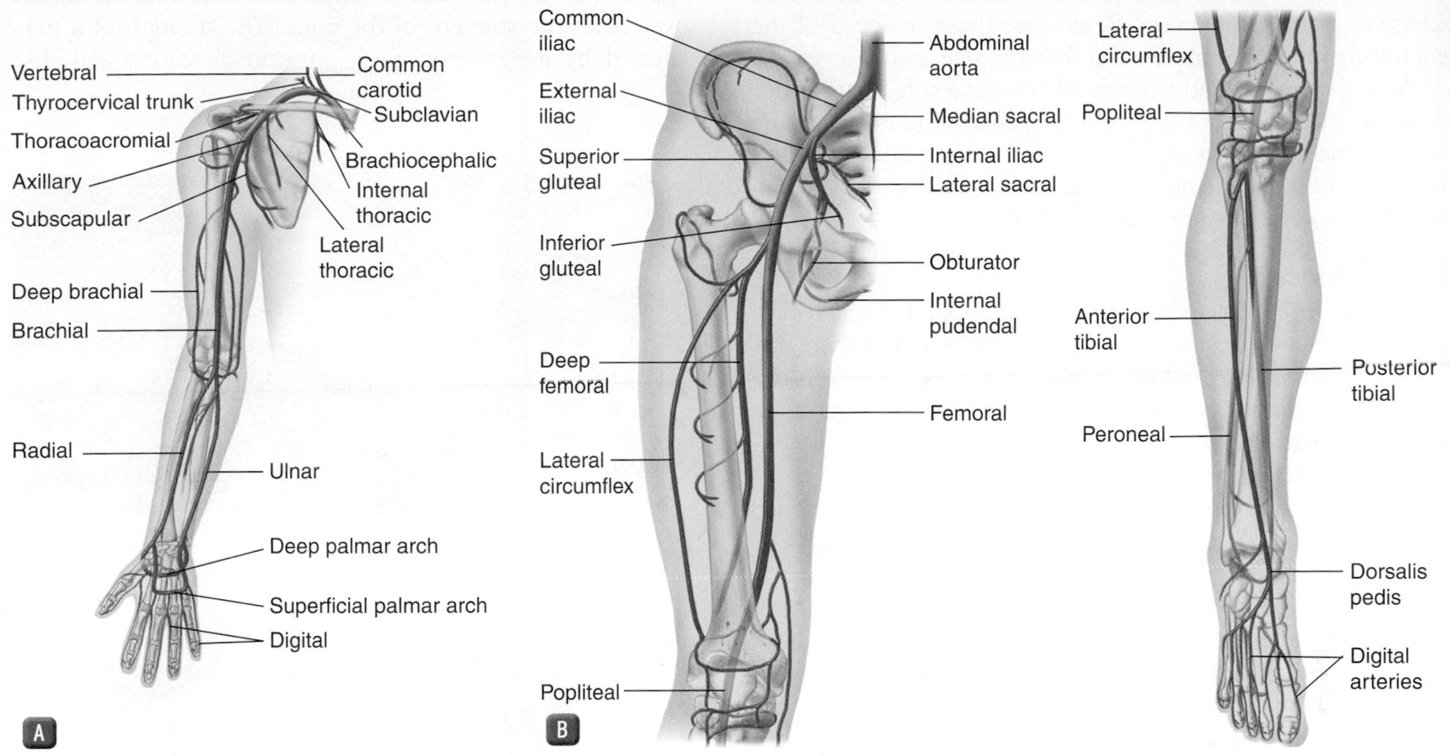

Figure 14 diagram labels:

A. (Upper extremity)
- Vertebral
- Thyrocervical trunk
- Thoracoacromial
- Axillary
- Subscapular
- Common carotid
- Subclavian
- Brachiocephalic
- Internal thoracic
- Lateral thoracic
- Deep brachial
- Brachial
- Radial
- Ulnar
- Deep palmar arch
- Superficial palmar arch
- Digital

B. (Lower extremity)
- Common iliac
- External iliac
- Superior gluteal
- Inferior gluteal
- Deep femoral
- Lateral circumflex
- Popliteal
- Abdominal aorta
- Median sacral
- Internal iliac
- Lateral sacral
- Obturator
- Internal pudendal
- Femoral
- Lateral circumflex
- Popliteal
- Anterior tibial
- Peroneal
- Posterior tibial
- Dorsalis pedis
- Digital arteries

Figure 14 The arterial supply of the extremities. **A.** Upper extremities. **B.** Lower extremities.

Special Populations

In the geriatric patient, fractures and dislocations may be associated with osteoarthritis or the normal atrophy and weakening processes associated with aging. Signs of abuse are most likely detected by you conducting a thorough patient history and looking for environmental clues.

■ Patterns and Mechanisms of Musculoskeletal Injury

Skeletal injuries result from blunt and penetrating trauma. In some cases, a force that might not generally cause harm to healthy bone produces a fracture. Such a <u>pathologic fracture</u> occurs when a medical condition causes the bone to become abnormally weak. In adults and children, motor vehicle crashes, falls, and athletic activities are common causes of injury. Among children, intentional trauma or abuse is a common cause of fractures and musculoskeletal injuries.

Sports account for a significant number of musculoskeletal injuries **Figure 15**.

■ Injury Forces and Motions

Direct Force

An object that strikes a person will transfer its energy to its point of impact. This energy is first absorbed by the soft tissues in the region of the impact. When the amount of force is so great that the soft tissues cannot fully dissipate it, a fracture occurs.

Penetrating injuries may also lead to a fracture or other musculoskeletal injury. A high-velocity injury, such as that

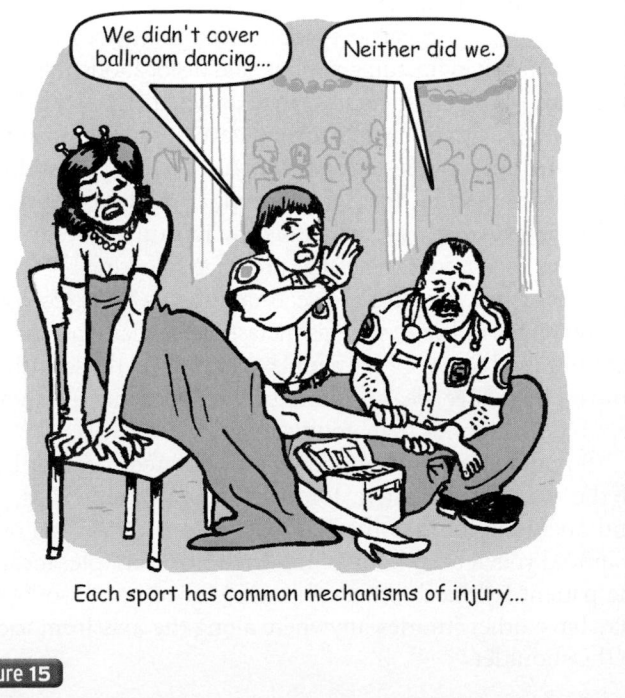

We didn't cover ballroom dancing...

Neither did we.

Each sport has common mechanisms of injury...

Figure 15

caused by a high-power rifle, typically shatters bone and causes extensive soft-tissue damage. Remember that the speed of the penetrating object has more effect than the size of that object.

An impalement injury commonly causes a soft-tissue injury similar to that seen in a low-velocity penetrating injury. If the impaled object happens to strike a bone, it may cause a fracture. In any case of impalement, it is essential to stabilize the object to protect the soft tissues from further injury.

Indirect Force

An <u>indirect injury</u> occurs when a force is applied to one region of the body but causes an injury in another region of the body. In this type of injury, the force is transmitted through the skeleton until, at some point, it reaches an area that is structurally weak in comparison with the other parts of the musculoskeletal system through which the force has traveled.

For example, a hip fracture may occur when a person's knee strikes the dashboard during a motor vehicle crash. In this case, the force is applied to the knee and travels proximally along the femur. When this force reaches the femoral neck, it causes the femoral neck to fracture.

Forces may be transmitted along the entire length of a bone or through several bones in series and may cause an injury anywhere along the way. Thus, a person falling on an outstretched hand may have one or more injuries as the result of forces transmitted proximally from the point of impact: (1) fracture of the scaphoid bone of the hand (direct blow); (2) fracture of the distal ulna and radius (Colles fracture; **Figure 16**); (3) fracture-dislocation of the elbow; (4) fracture-dislocation of the shoulder; or (5) fracture of the clavicle.

<u>Twisting injuries</u>, like those that commonly occur in football or skiing, result in fractures, sprains, and dislocations. Typically, the distal part of the limb remains fixed, as when cleats or a ski holds the foot to the ground, while torsion develops in the proximal section of the limb; the resulting force causes tearing of tendons and ligaments and spiral fractures of bone. <u>Fatigue fractures</u>, also called <u>march fractures</u>, are caused by repetitive stress and most commonly occur in the feet after prolonged walking.

Pathologic fractures are seen in patients with diseases that weaken areas of bone, such as metastatic cancer, and may occur with minimal force. Older people, particularly those with osteoporosis, also have weaker, more brittle bones and are more susceptible to fractures than younger people.

Some injuries are commonly encountered together because of the way the causative forces are transmitted; thus, if you find one, look for the others **Table 1**. Pain and swelling over the scaphoid (navicular) bone of the wrist, for example, means that the patient fell hard against an outstretched hand, so he or she may have other injuries anywhere along the axis from the hand to the shoulder.

◼ **Pathophysiology**

◼ **Fractures**

A <u>fracture</u> is a break in the continuity of a bone. Fractures occur when the magnitude of the force applied to a bone (a single

application or an accumulation of repetitive applications) overcomes the strength of the bone. The strength of a bone is affected by age, osteoporosis, nutritional status, and disease processes.

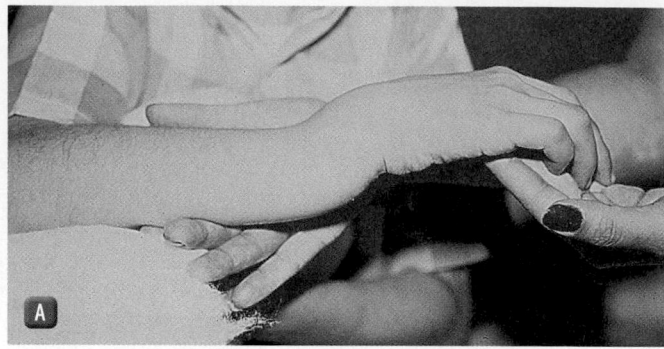

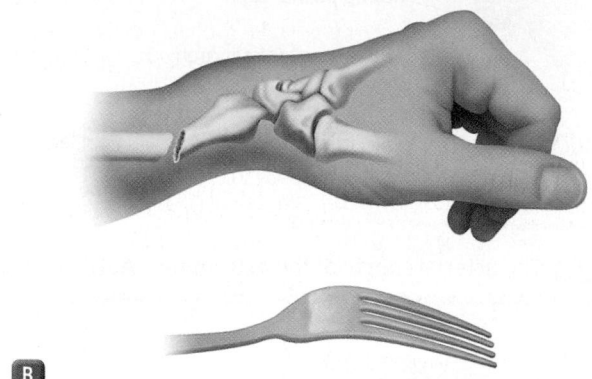

Figure 16   **A.** Fractures of the distal radius produce a characteristic Colles fracture (silver fork deformity). **B.** An artist's illustration of the injury.

Table 1 Musculoskeletal Injuries That Commonly Occur Together	
If You Find	**Look For**
Scapular fracture	Rib fracture, pulmonary contusions, pneumothorax
Scaphoid fracture	Wrist, elbow, or shoulder fracture
Pelvic fracture	Lumbosacral spine and other long bone fractures, intra-abdominal or genitourinary injury
Hip dislocation	Fracture of the acetabulum or femoral head
Femoral fracture	Dislocation of ipsilateral hip
Patellar fracture	Fracture-dislocation of ipsilateral hip
Knee dislocation	Tibial fracture; distal pulse may be absent
Calcaneal fracture	Fracture of the ankle, leg, hip, pelvis, spine, and the other calcaneus

Fracture Classification

Fracture Type A fracture may be classified based on the direction that the fracture line travels through a bone, number of fractures on the bone, or number of cortices (layers) involved **Figure 17** **Table 2**.

Fracture Classification Based on Displacement Fractures may be classified based on the type of displacement **Table 3**.

Angulation of a fracture means that each end of the fracture is not aligned in a straight line and that an angle has formed

between them. Angulation may occur in the frontal plane, sagittal plane, or both.

Open Versus Closed Fractures In an **open fracture** **Figure 18**, sometimes called a **compound fracture**, a break in the overlying skin allows the fracture to communicate with the outside environment. In a **closed fracture** **Figure 19**, the skin over the fracture site remains intact.

In addition to having a higher risk of infection, open fractures have the potential for more blood loss than a closed fracture for two reasons. First, open fractures usually result from high-energy injuries, so they typically involve more soft-tissue damage. Second, in most fractures, the periosteal vessels and the vessels supplying the surrounding soft tissues are disrupted, leading to the formation of a hematoma. In a closed fracture, the increased interstitial pressure within the hematoma compresses the blood vessels, limiting the size of the hematoma. For example, in a closed femur fracture, the blood loss may exceed 1 liter before enough pressure develops to tamponade the bleeding. In contrast, open fractures allow much of the blood to escape, so tamponade does not occur as readily or at all.

Signs and Symptoms of a Fracture

The primary symptom of a fracture is *pain* that is usually well localized to the fracture site. In addition, the patient may report hearing a snap or feeling a break. Signs of fracture detected on physical examination include the following:

- *Deformity* is one of the most reliable signs of a fracture. The limb may be found in an unnatural position or show motion at a place where there is no joint. Compare the deformed limb with the extremity on the other side **Figure 20**.
- *Shortening* occurs in fractures when the broken ends of a bone override one another. It is characteristic of femur fractures, for example, because the broken femur can no longer serve as a strut to oppose spasm in the powerful thigh muscles.
- Visual inspection will usually reveal *swelling* at the fracture site due to bleeding

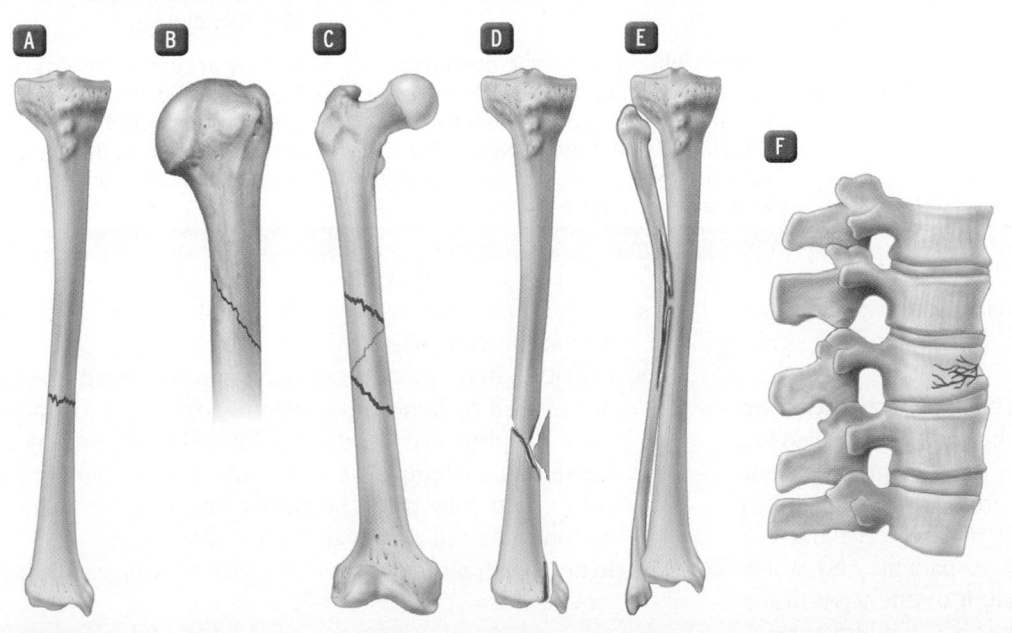

Figure 17 Types of fractures. **A.** Transverse fracture of the tibia. **B.** Oblique fracture of the humerus. **C.** Spiral fracture of the femur. **D.** Comminuted fracture of the tibia. **E.** Greenstick fracture of the fibula. **F.** Compression fracture of a vertebral body.

Table 2 Fracture Classification Based on Fracture Type

Category	Type of Fracture	Description	Common Causes
Direction the fracture line travels through a bone	Linear fracture	Parallel to the long axis of the bone	Low-energy stress injuries
	Transverse fracture	Straight across a bone at right angles to each cortex	Direct, low-energy blow
	Oblique fracture	At an angle across the bone	Direct or twisting force
	Spiral fracture	Encircles the bone	Twisting injury
	Impacted fracture	End of one bone becomes wedged into another bone	Fall from a significant height
Number of fractures on one bone	Comminuted fracture	> 2 fracture fragments located in one area of the bone.	High-energy injury (such as crush injury)
	Segmental fracture	< 2 fracture fragments, but breaks occur in different parts of the bone.	High-energy injury
Number of cortices injured	Complete fracture	Break through both cortices	High-energy injury
	Incomplete fracture	Break through one cortex	Low-energy injury
	▪ Greenstick fracture	Typically occurs in the proximal metaphysis or diaphysis of the tibia, radius, or, when this fracture occurs in the shaft, the cortex on the convex side of the deformity is broken, but the cortex on the concave side remains intact.	Occurs exclusively in children.
	▪ Buckle fracture (torus fracture)	Occurs in the metaphysis of long bones in response to excessive compression loading on one side of the bone; the compressed cortex buckles, and the opposite cortex is pulled away from the physis.	Unique to children; most commonly seen in the distal radius, usually resulting from a fall on an outstretched hand.
	▪ Bowing fracture	When a compression force is applied to a bone, numerous small fractures on the compressed side of the bone cause it to bend.	Often occurs in children and young adults; most commonly affects the radius, ulna, tibia, fibula, or clavicle.
	▪ Fatigue fracture (stress fracture)	Occurs when the muscle develops faster than the bone and places exaggerated stress on the less-developed bone; may also be due to repetitive small injuries that eventually lead to bone failure.	Usually occurs in the legs or feet of people who engage in strenuous, repetitive activities (such as dancers, joggers, military recruits).

from the broken bone and the accumulation of fluid. As blood infiltrates the tissues around the broken bone ends, *ecchymosis* will become apparent.

- *Guarding* and *loss of use* characterize most fractures. The patient will try to keep a fractured bone still and will avoid putting any stress on it. Sometimes the measures a patient takes to protect a fractured bone from movement are so characteristic that one can almost diagnose the fracture without examining the extremity. A patient who walks to the ambulance holding the dorsum of one wrist in the other hand, for example, likely has a Colles fracture. A patient standing with the head cocked toward a "knocked-down shoulder" probably has a fracture of the clavicle on the side to which the head is leaning.

- A fractured bone is almost invariably *tender to palpation* over the fracture site.
- Palpation may reveal **crepitus**, a grating sound or sensation caused by bone ends touching, over the broken bone ends. Crepitus may be noted as an incidental finding during splinting attempts. Do *not* try to elicit this sign, because your efforts may result in further injury to the bone and surrounding soft tissues and cause severe pain.
- In an open fracture, *exposed bone ends* may be visible in the wound.

■ Ligament Injuries and Dislocations

The shapes of the bones that form a joint and the tightness of the ligaments that hold them in place are key factors in determining a

Table 3	Fracture Classification Based on Displacement	
Type of Fracture	Description	Common Causes
Nondisplaced fracture	Bone remains aligned in its normal position, despite the fracture.	Low-energy injury
Displaced fracture	Ends of the fracture move from their normal positions.	High-energy injury
▪ **Overriding**	Muscles pull the distal fracture fragment alongside the proximal one, leading them to overlap; the limb becomes shortened.	Only occurs when a fracture is fully displaced and there is no bone contact
▪ **Distraction injury**	A powerful tensile force is rapidly applied to a bone, causing it to fracture–the bone ends are pulled apart.	Industrial equipment, machinery
▪ Impacted fracture (impaction injury)	A massive compressive force is applied to a bone, causing it to become wedged into another bone.	More likely to happen in **cancellous bone**
▪ **Avulsion fracture**	A powerful muscle contraction causes the insertion site of the muscle to be fractured off of the bone.	Sudden "jerking" of a body part
▪ **Depression fracture**	Blunt trauma to a flat bone (such as the skull) causes the bone to be pushed inward.	Blunt injury

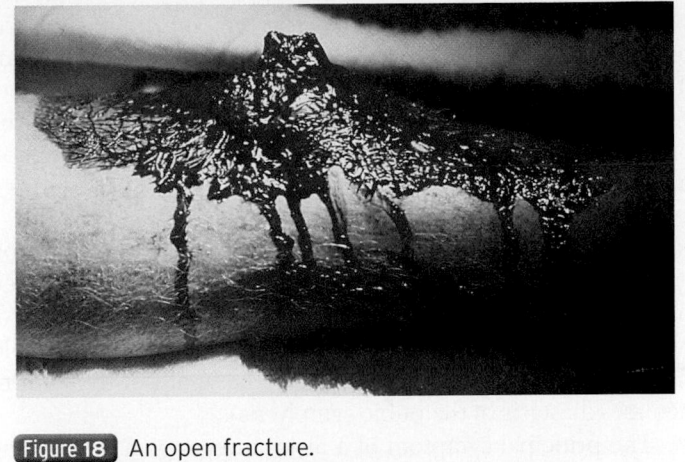

Figure 18 An open fracture.

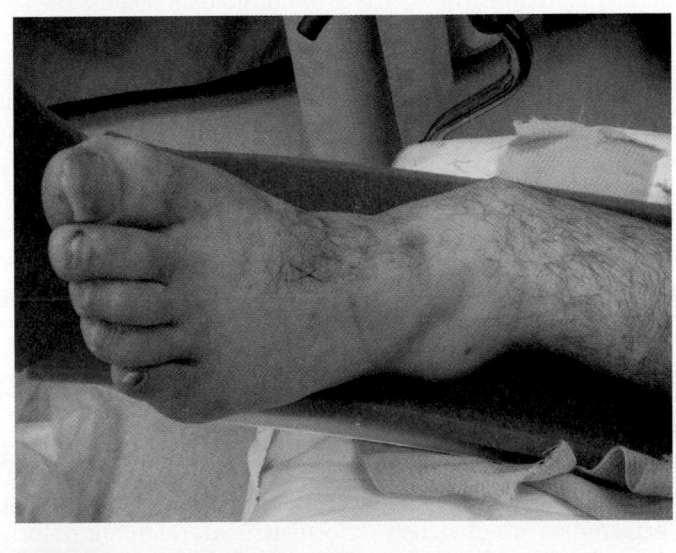

Figure 19 A closed fracture.

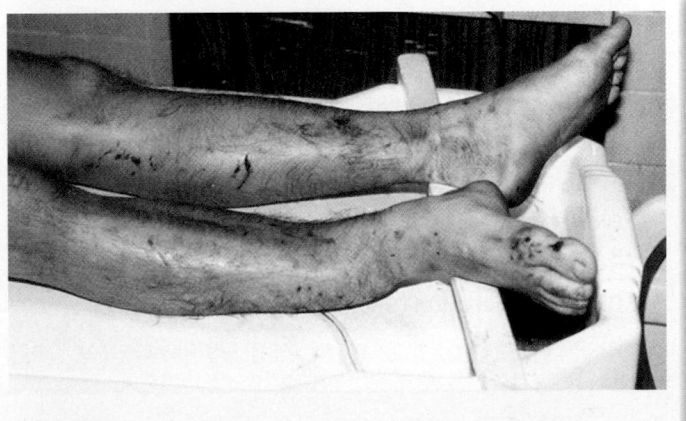

Figure 20 Obvious deformity is a sign of bone fracture.

joint's **range of motion (ROM)**. When forced beyond their normal limit, the bones that form a joint may break or become displaced, and the supporting ligaments and joint capsule may tear.

Dislocations, Subluxations, and Diastases

In a **dislocation**, a bone is totally displaced from the joint. Typically, at least part of the supporting joint capsule and some of the joint's ligaments are disrupted. Dislocations occur when a body part moves beyond its normal range of motion and the articular surfaces are no longer intact. The dislocated bones are then locked in place by muscle spasms. Evaluation of the patient usually reveals an obvious and significant deformity, a significant decrease in the joint's ROM, and severe pain. In all cases of a dislocation, a fracture should be suspected until ruled out by radiographs.

The partial dislocation of a joint is a **subluxation**. In this type of injury, the articular surfaces of the bones that form the joint are no longer completely in contact. In some cases, part of the joint capsule and supporting ligaments may be damaged. Despite the subluxation, the patient may be able to move the joint to some degree. Failure to recognize and treat a subluxation may lead to persistent joint instability and pain. A **luxation** is a complete dislocation.

When the ligaments that hold two bones in a fixed position with respect to one another are disrupted and the space between them increases, a situation known as a **diastasis** occurs. An example of this would be an injury to the ligaments that hold the pubic symphysis together, causing the width of the joint to increase (diastasis of the pubic symphysis).

The principal symptom of a dislocation is pain or a feeling of pressure over the involved joint, plus loss of motion of the joint. A patient with a posterior dislocation of the shoulder, for example, is unable to raise the arm but holds it against the side instead. Sometimes the joint will seem "frozen." The principal sign of dislocation is deformity.

A dislocation is considered an urgent injury because of its potential to cause **neurovascular compromise** distal to the site of injury. If the dislocated bone presses on a nerve, there may be numbness or weakness distally; if an artery is compressed, there may be absent distal pulses (such as in a knee dislocation). For these reasons, you should always assess the patient's neurovascular status distal to the site of dislocation (check pulse and motor and sensory functions [PMS]) prior to splinting as well as after splinting.

Sprains

Sprains are injuries in which ligaments are stretched or torn. They usually result from a sudden twisting of a joint beyond its normal range of motion that also causes a temporary subluxation. The majority of sprains involve the ankle or the knee because most occur after a person misjudges a step or landing. Evasive moves, like those done during a sporting event, commonly cause sprains in athletes.

Sprains are typically characterized by pain, swelling, and discoloration over the injured joint and unwillingness to use the limb. In contrast with fractures and dislocations, sprains usually do not involve deformity and joint mobility is usually limited by pain, not by joint incongruity Figure 21 .

■ Muscle and Tendon Injuries

Muscle and tendon injuries include strains, Achilles tendon rupture, and injuries related to inflammatory processes, such as bursitis and tendinitis, discussed later in this chapter.

A **strain** (pulled muscle) is an injury to a muscle and/or tendon that results from a violent muscle contraction or from excessive stretching. Often no deformity is present and only minor swelling is noted at the site of injury. Some patients may report increased pain with passive movement of the injured extremity.

YOU are the Medic   PART 2

The patient remains slow to respond, but alert and oriented to person, place, and time. His bilateral wrists and both lower extremities are obviously deformed. Bilateral femur deformity is observed. His skin is pale, cool, and slightly moist.

Before moving your patient, you splint his bilateral legs, fit him with a cervical collar, and initiate spinal precautions. His back reveals deformity and pain at L-4 and L-5. The patient tells you that he has type 1 diabetes and has been feeling light-headed intermittently over the past couple of days. You obtain his blood glucose level, which is 51 mg/dL.

Recording Time: 5 Minutes	
Level of consciousness	Alert (oriented to person, place, and day)
Skin	Cool, pale, and slightly moist
Pulse	116 beats/min; weak and regular
Blood pressure	104/60 mm Hg
Respirations	24 breaths/min
Oxygen saturation (Spo$_2$)	98% on room air
Blood glucose	51 mg/dL

4. What do these physical findings indicate to you?

5. Why is a history of type 1 diabetes significant?

6. What can you conclude from the patient's vital signs?

7. Why is a blood glucose reading of 51 mg/dL significant?

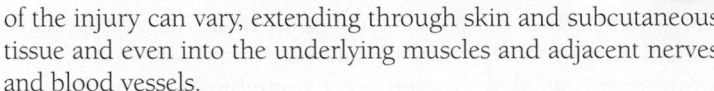

Words of Wisdom

To help remember that a strain involves a tendon, note that the word "strain" includes a "T" (for tendon). The word "sprain" does not include a "T"; sprains do not involve tendons, but rather ligaments.

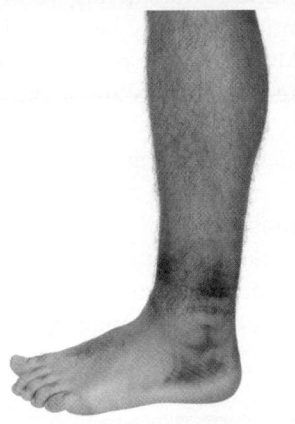

Figure 21 Swelling around an ankle from an injury. It is often not possible without x-ray imaging to determine whether a patient has a fracture.

Because it may be difficult to differentiate among the various types of injuries in the field, it is best to err on the side of caution and treat every severe sprain as if it were a fracture.

■ Injuries That May Signify Fractures

Amputations

An **amputation** is the separation of a limb or other body part from the remainder of the body **Figure 22**. The amputation may be incomplete, leaving only a small segment of tissue connecting the part, or it may be complete, causing the part to be fully separated. Hemorrhage from complete or incomplete amputations can be severe and life threatening. Fractures may also be present with amputations. Amputations are discussed in more detail in the chapter, *Soft-Tissue Trauma*.

Lacerations

A laceration is a smooth or jagged cut caused by a sharp object or a blunt force that tears the tissue. The depth of the injury can vary, extending through skin and subcutaneous tissue and even into the underlying muscles and adjacent nerves and blood vessels.

Lacerations involved in damaged arteries or veins may result in severe bleeding. The presence of lacerations may also be a sign of an underlying fracture.

Deep lacerations may injure the muscle nerves, or vasculature, so distal PMS functions should always be evaluated.

■ Patient Assessment

When you are assessing an injured patient, *do not be distracted by visually impressive injuries!* It is essential to complete the primary assessment of the patient before focusing on the extremities. In cases of musculoskeletal injuries, patients may be classified based on the presence or absence of associated injuries:

- Life- or limb-threatening injury or condition, including life- or limb-threatening musculoskeletal trauma
- Life-threatening injuries and only simple musculoskeletal trauma
- Life- or limb-threatening musculoskeletal trauma and no other life-threatening injuries
- Isolated, non–life- or non–limb-threatening injuries

■ Scene Size-up

As with all patients, you should conduct a scene size-up, focusing on safety and standard precautions. Consider the mechanism of injury (MOI), as well as whether spinal stabilization will be needed, and the potential hazards that may be present at such a scene. Once on scene, observe for hazards and don standard precautions appropriate for the MOI. A mask, gown, and eye protection may be needed for severe MOIs or when there is the possibility of hidden bleeding. Finally, request additional resources as needed.

■ Primary Assessment

Perform a primary assessment focusing on the patient's mental status, ABCs, and priority. If the primary assessment indicates that the patient has no immediately life-threatening condition and only localized musculoskeletal trauma, continue with history taking and a secondary assessment. If the patient has a significant MOI, complete a rapid exam and perform a full-body exam en route to the emergency department. The priorities throughout the assessment and management of musculoskeletal injuries should include identifying the injuries, preventing further harm or damage to the injured structures and surrounding tissues, supporting the injured area, and administering pain medication if necessary.

Form a General Impression

Evaluate the patient's level of consciousness and orientation. Check for responsiveness using the AVPU (Awake and alert, responsive to Verbal stimuli or Pain, or Unresponsive) scale. Generally you can assess a patient's mental status by asking

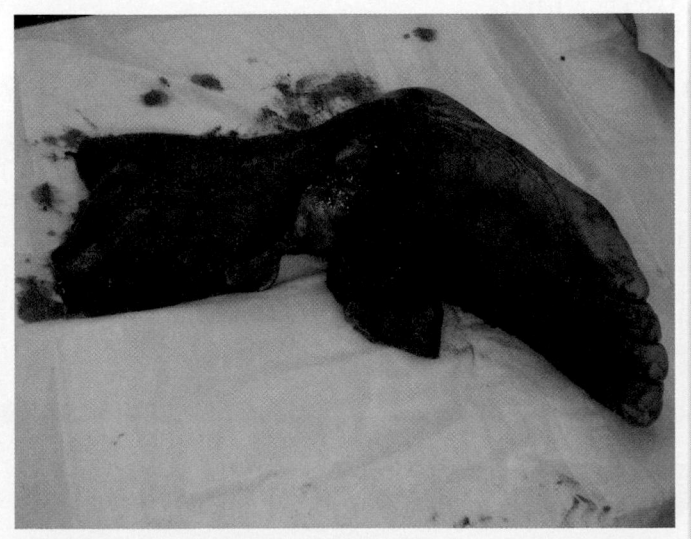

Figure 22 An amputation involving a leg.

the patient about his or her chief complaint. An unresponsive patient may indicate a life-threatening condition. You should administer high-flow oxygen via a nonrebreathing mask (or a bag-mask device, if indicated) to all patients whose level of consciousness is less than alert and oriented and provide immediate transport to the emergency department.

The patient's emergency may be simple and usually not life threatening; however, some situations will include multiple problems, only one of which involves musculoskeletal injuries. If there was significant trauma and multiple body systems are affected, the musculoskeletal injuries may be a lower priority. Do not waste scene time on prolonged musculoskeletal assessment or splinting. Use a long backboard as a "full-body" splint and complete additional assessment of musculoskeletal injuries during transport.

Airway and Breathing

Musculoskeletal injuries are rarely an immediate threat to life. A fracture can wait. The airway cannot. Even though an injury to the arm or leg may be obvious, take the time to evaluate the adequacy of the airway and breathing. Very little else matters if the patient's airway and breathing are inadequate. Problems such as injuries to the head, injuries to the spine, intoxication, or other related illnesses and injuries may cause inadequate breathing. Evaluating the chief complaint and MOI will help you to identify whether the patient has an open airway and whether breathing is present and adequate.

If a spinal injury is suspected, take the appropriate precautions and prepare for stabilization.

Circulation

Determine whether the patient has a pulse, has adequate perfusion, or is bleeding. Hypoperfusion will most likely be your primary concern. If the skin is pale, cool, or clammy and capillary refill time is slow, treat your patient for shock immediately. Maintain a normal body temperature. If musculoskeletal injuries in the extremities are suspected, they must be at least initially stabilized, if not splinted, prior to moving. Eliminating this cause of shock may need to be done later in your assessment. Assess for pulses proximal to the injury and note any circulatory changes before and after any manipulation as well as frequently during transport.

Note whether fractures have broken through the skin; this can cause external bleeding. Handle injured extremities carefully so that a closed fracture does not become an open fracture. If external bleeding is present, bandage the extremity, using sterile dressings to cover the wound and bone to reduce the potential for bone infection. The bandage should be secure enough to control bleeding without restricting circulation distal to the injury. Monitor bandage tightness by assessing the circulation, sensation, and movement distal to the bandage. Swelling from fractures and internal bleeding may cause bandages to become too tight. If bleeding cannot be controlled, you should quickly proceed to apply a tourniquet.

Transport Decision

If the patient you are treating has an airway or breathing problem or significant bleeding, provide rapid transport to the hospital for treatment. A patient who has a significant MOI but whose condition appears otherwise stable should also be transported promptly to the closest appropriate hospital. Patients with bilateral fractures of the long bones (humerus, femur, or tibia) have been subjected to a high amount of kinetic energy, which should dramatically increase your index of suspicion for serious unseen injuries. When a decision for rapid transport is made, you can use a backboard as a splinting device to splint the whole body rather than splinting each extremity individually. If you take time to splint the patient's arms and legs individually, you may delay the prompt surgical intervention that may be needed for other injuries when a significant MOI has occurred. Individual splints should be applied en route if the ABCs are stable and time permits.

Patients with a simple MOI, such as twisting of an ankle or dislocating a shoulder, may be further assessed and their condition stabilized on scene prior to transport if no other problems exist. Handle fractures carefully while preparing for transport. Careful handling is necessary to limit pain and prevent sharp bone ends from breaking through the skin or damaging nerves and blood vessels in the extremity.

■ History Taking

Obtain the patient's medical history using the standard SAMPLE format. This history should also identify any preexisting musculoskeletal disorders and attempt to learn more about the injury. Some information obtained will be relevant to the injury (such as the patient having osteoporosis, or taking anticoagulant medications).

Obtain information about the incident that led to the injury from the patient and any bystanders who witnessed it. In particular, determine the condition and position of the patient immediately before the incident, the details of the incident, and the patient's position after the incident. Also, ask the patient for a subjective description of the injury: How did this happen? Did you hear a pop? Do you have pain? What functional limitations do you now have?

Special Populations

Children with fractures may not want you to see, touch, or splint the injured extremity. You should always be honest with children about what you are doing and whether it will hurt. In particular, splinting is a necessary and sometimes painful intervention for a child with a fracture. Once the splint is in place, cold packs are applied, and analgesia is considered, the child will likely have less pain because the fracture is stabilized.

■ Secondary Assessment

When examining the patient, obtain a baseline set of vital signs. The focus can then shift to evaluating the injured extremity. One of the simplest ways to assess an extremity is to compare one side with the other, noting any discrepancy in length, position, or skin color. Next, complete an exam noting DCAP-BTLS (Deformity, Contusions, Abrasions, Penetrating injury–Burns, Tenderness, Lacerations, Swelling) as you observe and palpate the soft tissue from head to toe and assess the patient for limitations, such as inability to move a joint. While performing the exam, be sure to cover the <u>6 Ps of musculoskeletal assessment</u>: Pain, Paralysis, <u>Paresthesias</u> (numbness or tingling), Pulselessness, Pallor (pale or delayed capillary refill in children), and Pressure.

Pain

A person experiences acute pain when peripheral pain receptors (nociceptors) convert painful stimuli into electrical impulses that are transmitted via the peripheral nerve fibers to the spinal cord. The signal ascends along the spinal cord to the pain-sensing region of the brain. When a tissue is injured, various chemical mediators are released that facilitate the conduction of the painful stimulus to the brain.

When assessing a patient's pain, remember the OPQRST mnemonic: Onset of the pain; Provoking or Palliating factors; Quality of the pain (such as sharp, pressure, crampy); Region of the pain, including its primary location and areas where pain radiates or refers; Severity of the pain; and the Time (duration) that the patient has been experiencing pain. It is also useful to have the patient quantify the severity of the pain by using a scale of 1 to 10 or with visual images such as faces that appear to be happy or in pain (see chapter, *Pediatric Emergencies*).

Inspection

When you are inspecting an injured extremity, always evaluate the joint above and the joint below the site of injury because the injuring force may have affected these sites as well. In particular, compare the injured side with the uninjured side. While inspecting a patient's injuries, look for the following signs:

- Deformity, including asymmetry, angulation, shortening, and rotation
- Skin changes, including contusions, abrasions, avulsions, punctures, burns, lacerations, and bone ends
- Swelling
- Muscle spasms
- Abnormal limb positioning
- Increased or decreased ROM
- Color changes, including pallor and cyanosis
- Bleeding, including estimating the amount of blood loss

Palpation

Palpation of an injured extremity should include the injury site and the regions above and below it. Regions of <u>point tenderness</u> (those that the patients identifies as painful) should be identified. Reassess any tender areas frequently to determine whether there are changes in the location or severity of the pain or tenderness. Note that while point tenderness is one of the best indicators of an injury, it may be absent in patients who are intoxicated or who have an injury to the spinal cord.

When you are palpating an injured site, attempt to identify instability, deformity, abnormal joint or bone continuity, and displaced bones. Feel for crepitus, which is commonly found at the site of a fracture. Palpate distal pulses on all extremities, with special attention to comparing the strength of the pulses in the injured extremity with those in a normal one.

On occasion, an arterial injury may be identified while palpating an extremity. Signs of an arterial injury include a pulsatile expanding hematoma, diminished distal pulses, a palpable thrill (vibration) over the site of injury that correlates with the patient's heartbeat, and difficult-to-control bleeding.

The purpose of palpating the pelvis is to identify instability and point tenderness. Apply pressure over the pubic symphysis to evaluate for tenderness and crepitus. Next, press the iliac wings toward the midline and then posteriorly. Any gross instability found during this examination should be reported to hospital personnel because it may indicate a severe pelvic injury. Do not repeatedly examine the pelvis if instability is found because the manipulation may disrupt blood clots and cause further bleeding.

The upper and lower extremity exam should include palpation of the entire length of each arm and leg to identify any sites of injury. The most efficient way to accomplish this is to place your hands around the extremity and squeeze. Repeat this procedure every few centimeters until you reach the end of the extremity. When evaluating the upper extremities, always examine the cervical spine and shoulder because complaints within the arm may be caused by a more proximal disorder. Likewise, with the lower extremities, always conduct an exam of the pelvis and hip if the patient complains of pain in the leg.

Motor Function and Sensory Exam

In the case of a musculoskeletal injury, it is essential to assess a patient's distal pulse as well as motor and sensory function. A motor function exam should be performed whenever a patient has an injury to an extremity, provided the patient does not also have a life-threatening injury. When you are assessing motor function, consider the preinjury level of function. In some cases, weakness or motor deficits may be due to prior injuries or medical problems. For this reason, you should perform a careful review of the patient's history whenever a patient reports being weak or unable to move an extremity.

While you are performing a motor exam, carry out each test with and without resistance because some patients may be too weak to overcome any outside resistance. Also, perform the test on both sides of the body simultaneously so that each extremity can be compared.

A sensory exam should be performed on all patients who have an injury or complaint related to an extremity, assuming that it does not take attention away from a potentially fatal condition. The sensory exam and history should attempt to identify any preexisting deficits in function or other disorders, including diabetes and nerve disorders that may cause changes in sensation. It is important to assess not only for the presence or absence of sensation, but also for the quality and symmetry of sensation.

To perform a sensory exam, first ask the patient if he or she feels any abnormal sensations, such as numbness, tingling, or burning. Next, conduct a gross sensory exam by lightly touching the injured extremity and the unaffected side simultaneously; have the patient report whether the two sides feel the same or different. In some cases, a patient may report an abnormally severe sensation of pain when just lightly touched. Such hyperesthesia may be a sign of an injury to the spinal cord.

To perform a motor function and sensory exam, follow the steps shown in Skill Drill 1 :

Skill Drill 1

1. Have the patient flex his or her arms at the elbow to test musculocutaneous nerve motor function Step 1 .
2. Evaluate the patient's ability to extend the arms at the elbow to test radial nerve motor function Step 2 .
3. Have the patient extend the thumbs (thumbs up) to test radial nerve motor function Step 3 .
4. Assess the patient's ability to make an "okay" sign to test median nerve motor function Step 4 .
5. Check the patient's ability to spread his or her fingers apart to test ulnar nerve motor function Step 5 .
6. Instruct the patient to extend his or her legs at the knee to test femoral nerve motor function Step 6 .
7. Have the patient plantarflex his or her feet to test tibial nerve motor function Step 7 .
8. Assess the patient's ability to <u>dorsiflex</u> the feet to test deep peroneal nerve motor function Step 8 .
9. Check light touch over the lateral surface of the shoulder (over the deltoid) to test axillary nerve sensory function Step 9 .
10. Evaluate light touch on the anterolateral surface of the forearm to test musculocutaneous nerve sensory function Step 10 .
11. Assess light touch on the dorsal surface of the web space of the thumb to test radial nerve sensory function Step 11 .

Skill Drill 1

Performing a Motor Function and Sensory Exam

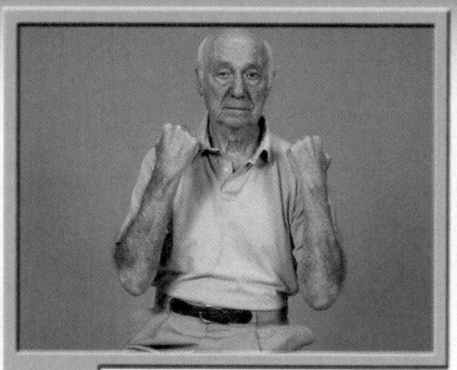

Step 1 Have the patient flex his or her arms at the elbow.

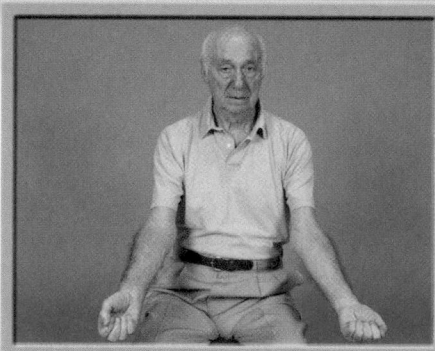

Step 2 Have the patient extend the arms at the elbow.

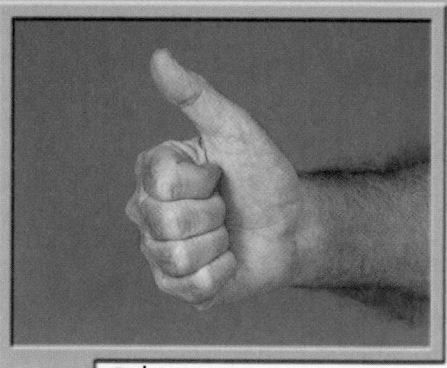

Step 3 Have the patient extend the thumbs (thumbs up).

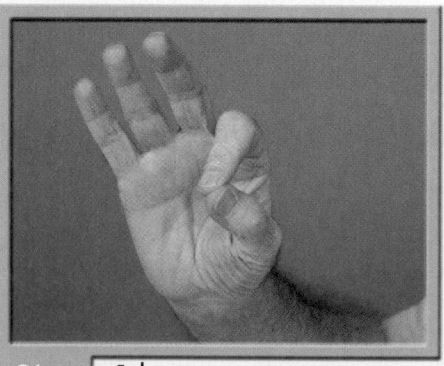

Step 4 Have the patient make an "okay" sign.

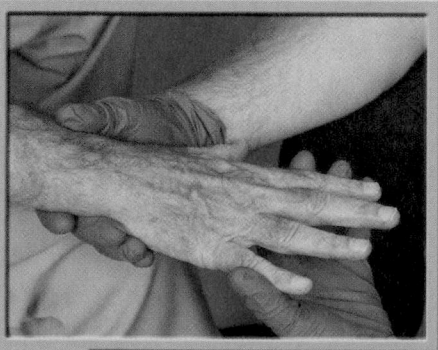

Step 5 Have the patient spread his or her fingers apart.

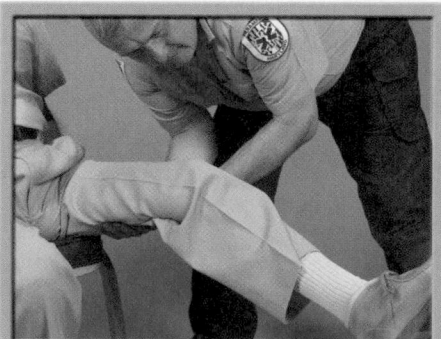

Step 6 Instruct the patient to extend his or her legs at the knee.

Continues

Skill Drill 1

Performing a Motor Function and Sensory Exam *(continued)*

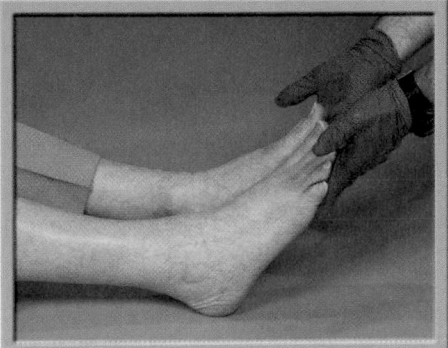

Step 7 Have the patient flex his or her feet and ankles downward.

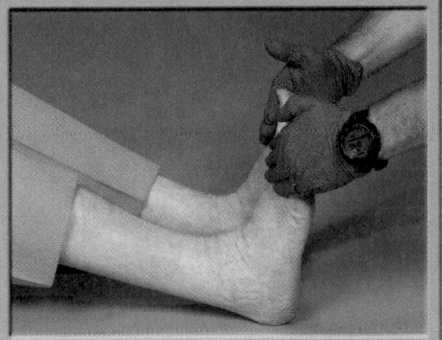

Step 8 Instruct the patient to flex the feet and ankles upward.

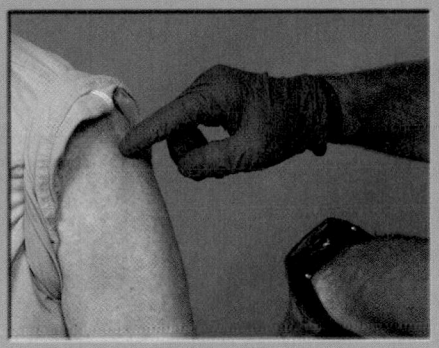

Step 9 Evaluate light touch over the lateral surface of the shoulder (over the deltoid).

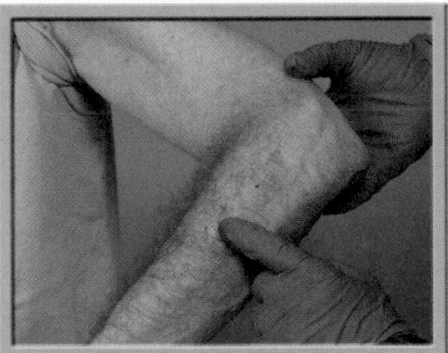

Step 10 Evaluate light touch on the anterolateral surface of the forearm.

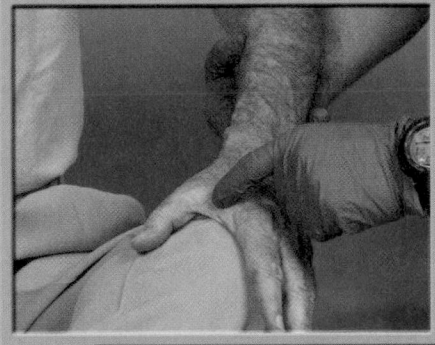

Step 11 Assess light touch on the dorsal surface of the web space of the thumb.

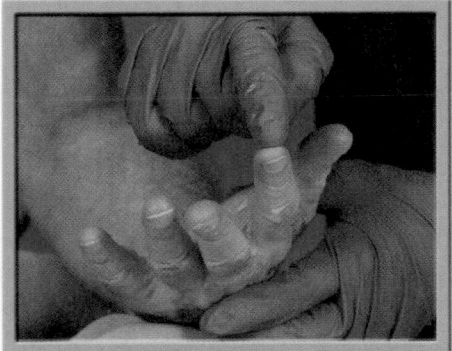

Step 12 Lightly touch the volar surface of the distal thumb, index, and middle fingers.

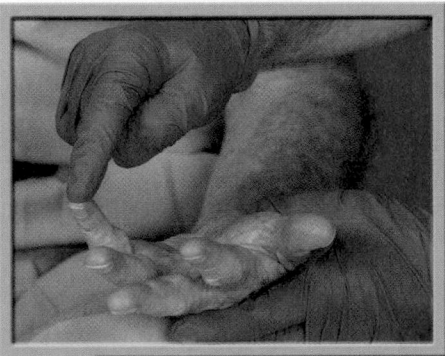

Step 13 Lightly touch the distal volar surface of the small finger.

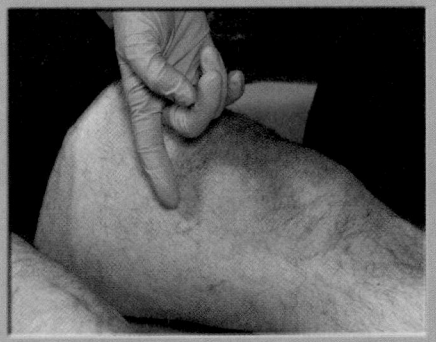

Step 14 Examine the patient's sense of light touch over the anteromedial surface of the thigh.

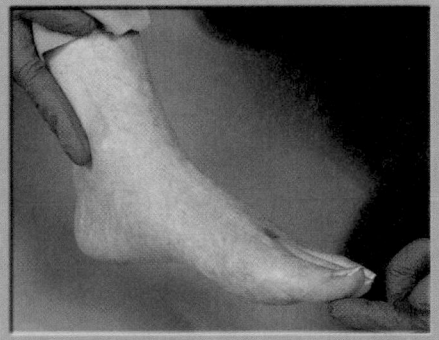

Step 15 Evaluate light touch on the plantar surface of the toes.

Continues

Skill Drill 1

Performing a Motor Function and Sensory Exam (continued)

Step 16 Assess light touch in the web space between the great toe and the second toe.

12. Lightly touch the **volar** surface of the distal thumb, index, and middle fingers to test median nerve sensory function (Step 12).
13. Lightly touch the distal volar surface of the small finger to test ulnar nerve sensory function (Step 13).
14. Examine the patient's sense of light touch over the anteromedial surface of the thigh to test femoral nerve sensory function (Step 14).
15. Evaluate light touch on the plantar surface of the toes to test tibial nerve sensory function (Step 15).
16. Assess light touch in the web space between the great toe and the second toe to test peroneal nerve sensory function (Step 16).

Reassessment

The overall goal in the treatment of a musculoskeletal injury is to identify the type and extent of the injury and to provide treatment that maximizes the normal healing process of the injured structure. This process begins in the field with a thorough assessment of the patient and proper stabilization of injuries to prevent further harm.

Emergency Medical Care

General treatment of fractures includes controlling external bleeding and preventing infection in open fractures, managing internal bleeding (shock considerations), and immobilizing the limb.

Documentation and Communication

Always document the findings of a neurovascular exam, even if they are normal. When an abnormality is identified, document the specific deficit—for example, the patient was unable to extend the thumb or the wrist.

General treatment of sprains is similar to that of fractures and includes the following (numbers 1 through 4 form the mnemonic ICES):

1. **Immobilize.** Immobilize or splint injured area
2. **Chill.** Use ice or a cold pack over the injury
3. **Elevate.**
4. **Splint.** Splint with an elastic bandage (usually applied at the hospital once radiography rules out a fracture).
5. Reduced or protected weight bearing
6. Pain management as soon as practical

Volume Deficit Due to Musculoskeletal Injuries

Fractures may lead to significant blood loss from damage to vessels within the bone and musculature around the bone and, in some cases, from damage to large blood vessels in the region of the fracture. When you are caring for patients with fractures, undertake interventions such as applying direct pressure, splinting, and administering intravenous (IV) fluids to prevent hypotension and unstable condition of the patient. Table 4 lists the potential blood loss from various fracture sites and may serve as a guideline for estimating the amount of resuscitation required. The goal of prehospital management should be to keep the patient's volume, vital signs, and mental status normal.

Pain Control

A patient who has sustained a musculoskeletal injury may experience pain for a number of reasons. Pain may be caused by a fracture or continued movement of an unstable fracture, muscle

Table 4 Potential Blood Loss From Fracture Sites

Fracture Site	Potential Blood Loss (mL)
Pelvis	1,500–3,000
Femur	1,000–1,500
Humerus	250–500
Tibia or fibula	250–500
Ankle	250–500
Elbow	250–500
Radius or ulna	150–250

spasm, soft-tissue injury, nerve injury, or muscle ischemia. Orthopaedic injuries are often extremely painful, so the goal of prehospital pain control should be to diminish the patient's pain to a tolerable level.

A number of interventions may be performed in the field to control pain from a musculoskeletal injury. The first step is to assess the level of pain. Establishing a baseline level of pain and reassessing it after each intervention allow you to determine the effectiveness of the treatment being provided. Simple methods for controlling pain include splinting, resting and elevating the injured part, and applying ice or heat packs.

When simple procedures do not effectively control a patient's pain, consider the administration of an analgesic or antispasmodic agent. Analgesics used in the field include narcotics, such as fentanyl and morphine, and nitrous oxide; antispasmodic agents include diazepam and lorazepam. These agents should be reserved for patients in hemodynamically stable condition who have an isolated musculoskeletal injury. It is important to obtain vital signs before and after administering any medication for pain and spasm and to monitor the patient's respiratory status for signs of respiratory depression. After pain medication is administered, reassess the patient's pain to ensure that pain relief is adequate.

Administering pain medication before splinting may allow the extremity to be stabilized more effectively. Remember, *it hurts* to have an injured extremity held in the proper position for splinting. Pain medication may make it possible for the patient to tolerate that position longer and allow the splint to be applied properly.

Cold and Heat Application

Cold packs are useful for treating patients during the initial 48 hours following an injury and are very effective at decreasing pain and swelling. Cooling the injured area causes vasoconstriction of the blood vessels in the region and decreases the release of inflammatory mediators. As a result, swelling and inflammation are reduced when cold packs are used during the acute stage of an injury.

Conversely, heat therapy should generally be avoided during the initial 48 to 72 hours following an injury because it may actually increase pain and swelling during this period. Once the acute phase of the injury ends and the damaged blood vessels become clotted, heat packs are useful for increasing blood flow to the region to decrease stiffness and to promote healing. As a consequence, heat packs may be beneficial for patients who report an injury that occurred several days before contacting paramedics.

Splinting

Splinting is intended to provide support to and prevent motion of the broken bone ends **Figure 23**. Correctly splinting an injured extremity not only decreases the pain a patient experiences, but also reduces the risk of further damage to muscles, nerves, blood vessels, and skin. In addition, splinting helps to control bleeding by allowing clots to form where vessels were damaged. When a patient with multiple orthopaedic injuries

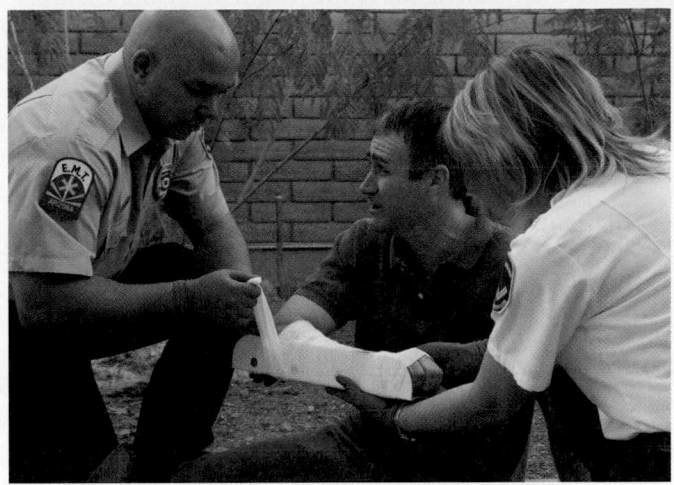

Figure 23 Splinting reduces pain and helps prevent additional damage to the extremity.

must be transported immediately, you will not have time to splint each fracture one by one. The best way to stabilize multiple fractures when the patient's overall condition is critical is to splint the axial skeleton by using a long backboard and straps or an alternative device, such as a vacuum mattress. This will serve three purposes: (1) it will protect against a spinal injury; (2) it will reduce the movement of injured extremities by securing them to the board; and (3) it will save time at the scene.

Principles of Splinting

Splinting is one of the most crucial skills to learn when caring for patients with musculoskeletal injuries. Failure to properly splint an injured extremity leads to unnecessary discomfort and the possibility of further injury or harm. Allowing a closed fracture in the distal tibia to become an open fracture owing to mishandling or improper splinting will result in the need for surgery and a hospital stay and may increase the patient's rehabilitation time. Keep the following points in mind when applying a splint:

1. The injured area must be adequately visualized before splinting. Remove clothing as necessary so that you can inspect the area thoroughly.
2. Assess and *record* distal PMS functions before and after splinting.
3. Cover all wounds with a dry, sterile dressing before applying the splint. To prevent infection following an open fracture, you should brush away any obvious debris on the skin surrounding an open fracture before applying a dressing. Do not enter or probe the open fracture site in an attempt to retrieve debris because this may lead to further contamination. Do not attempt to push exposed bone ends back under the skin.
4. Do not move the patient before splinting unless an immediate hazard exists.
5. *For fractures*, the splint must immobilize the bone ends and the two adjacent joints. *For dislocations*, the splint

must extend along the entire length of the bone above and the entire length of the bone below the dislocated joint.

6. Pad the splint well to prevent local pressure and to provide optimal motion restriction.

7. Support the injured site manually with one hand above and one hand below the injury, and minimize movement until the splint is applied and secured.

8. If a long bone fracture is severely angulated, gently apply longitudinal traction (tension) to attempt to realign the bone and improve circulation. Use a smooth, firm grip to apply manual traction, and take care to avoid any sudden, jerky movements of the limb. *Do not attempt to straighten fractures involving joints without first obtaining medical direction.* In fact, there is no need to straighten or manipulate the joint unless it has no distal pulse.

9. Splint the knee straight if not directly injured and angulated; splint the elbow at a right angle. (The patient may not be able to tolerate this procedure, and rapid transport should be initiated.)

10. If the patient reports severe pain or is resistant to movement, discontinue applying traction, splint in the position of deformity, and carefully monitor the distal neurovascular status (PMS).

11. Splint firmly, but not so tightly as to occlude the distal circulation.

12. If possible, do not cover fingers and toes with the splint to allow for monitoring of skin CTC (color, temperature, and condition).

13. If possible, apply cold packs and elevate the splinted limb to minimize swelling.

14. When the patient has a life-threatening injury, individual splint application for possible fractures must not delay transportation and might not be accomplished.

Note that there is no part of the body that cannot be splinted using a long backboard.

Types of Splints

Any device used to immobilize a fracture or dislocation is considered a splint. Commercially available splints include board splints, inflatable or vacuum splints, and traction splints. Lack of a commercially made splint should never prevent proper immobilization of an injured patient; multiple casualties may tax the resources of even the best-equipped ambulance, requiring improvisation.

Rigid Splints A rigid splint is any inflexible device that may be attached to a limb to maintain stability—a padded board, a piece of heavy cardboard, or an aluminum "ladder" or SAM splint molded to fit the extremity. More elaborate rigid splints are designed to quickly fit around two or three sides of an

extremity and be secured with self-adhesive (Velcro) straps or cravats. Some rigid splints are made of a radiolucent material that allows radiographs to be obtained without removal of the splint. Whatever its construction, the splint must be generously padded to ensure even pressure along the extremity and long enough to be secured well above and below the fracture site (beyond the proximal and distal joints).

When you are applying a rigid splint, grasp the extremity above and below the fracture site, and apply gentle traction. Another provider should then place the splint alongside the limb. While one provider maintains traction, the other wraps the limb and splint in self-adhering bandages that are tight enough to hold the splint firmly to the extremity but not so tight as to occlude circulation **Figure 24**. (If the splint has its own straps that are used to secure it to the extremity, this step is not required.) Leave the fingers or toes out of the bandage so that distal circulation can be monitored.

Sling and Swathe An arm sling may be fashioned from a triangular bandage and is useful to stabilize injuries that involve the shoulder or as an adjunct to a rigid splint of the upper extremity. The sling holds the injured part against the chest wall and takes some of the weight off the injured area. (A quick alternative is for you to simply pin the arm to the patient's jacket.)

To apply a sling, place the splinted extremity in a comfortable position across the chest and lay the long edge of a triangular bandage along the patient's side opposite the injury. Bring the bottom edge of the bandage up and over the forearm and tie it *at the side* of the neck to the other end. Tie or pin the pointed end of the sling, at the elbow, to form a cradle. Secure the sling so that the hand is carried higher than the elbow and the fingers

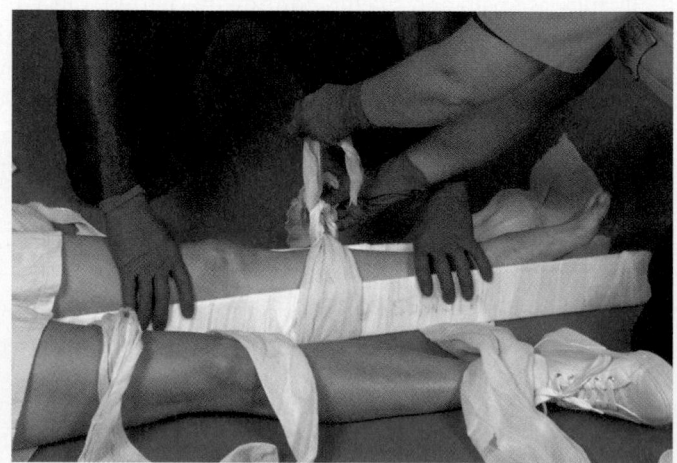

Figure 24 In applying a rigid splint, wrap the limb and splint so that the splint is firmly in place but does not cut off circulation.

are visible for checking peripheral circulation **Figure 25**. If the patient is large, tie two cravats together using a square knot, to give you more material. Cushion the sling with gauze pads to secure the splint and increase patient comfort.

An arm that is splinted with a sling can be further stabilized by adding a swathe. Create a swathe by using one or more triangular bandages to secure the arm firmly to the chest wall. This technique is particularly useful for injuries to the clavicle and for anterior dislocations of the shoulder. Do not use a sling if the patient has a neck injury. Be careful not to secure the swathe so tight as to reduce chest expansion during respirations.

Pneumatic Splints Pneumatic splints (also known as air splints or inflatable splints) are useful for stabilizing fractures involving the lower leg or forearm. They are not effective for angulated fractures or for fractures that involve a joint because they will forcefully attempt to straighten the fracture or joint. Likewise, air splints should not be used on open fractures in which the bone ends are exposed.

Air splints offer two distinct advantages: they can help slow bleeding and minimize swelling by applying pressure over fracture sites to decrease small-vessel bleeding.

The method of application for an air splint depends on whether it is equipped with a zipper. If it is not, gather the splint

on your own arm so that its proximal edge is just above your wrist. Grasp the patient's hand or foot while an assistant maintains proximal countertraction, then slide the air splint over your hand and onto the patient's extremity. Position the air splint so that it is free of wrinkles. Then, while you continue to maintain traction, instruct your assistant to inflate the splint with a commercially available device that is compatible with the splint system. Do *not* use a compressed air tank to inflate an air splint. If the air splint has a zipper, apply it to the injured area while an assistant maintains traction proximally and distally; then zip it up and inflate **Figure 26**. In either case, inflate the splint just to the point at which finger pressure will make a slight dent in the splint's surface.

You must watch air splints carefully to ensure that they do not lose pressure or become overinflated. Overinflation is particularly likely when the splint is applied in a cold area and the patient is subsequently moved to a warmer area because the air inside the splint will expand as it gets warmer, possibly increasing pressure and causing pulses to cease. Air splints will also expand when going to a higher altitude if the patient compartment is unpressurized, a factor that must be considered when patients are transported by air ambulance.

If a patient has injuries to the lower extremities or pelvis, you may be able to use a pneumatic antishock garment (PASG) as a splinting device, if local protocol allows. Situations in which use of a PASG is allowed vary widely by locale. Many EMS systems no longer use this device because of problems reported with its use. Be sure to check with medical control in every case. The PASG is relatively contraindicated for treatment of shock but may have some value as a splinting device in rare circumstances.

Do not use the PASG if any of the following conditions exist:

- Pregnancy
- Pulmonary edema
- Acute heart failure
- Penetrating chest injuries
- Groin injuries
- Major head injuries
- A transport time of less than 30 minutes

In these situations, the PASG may worsen or complicate the patient's condition. Consult with medical control if you

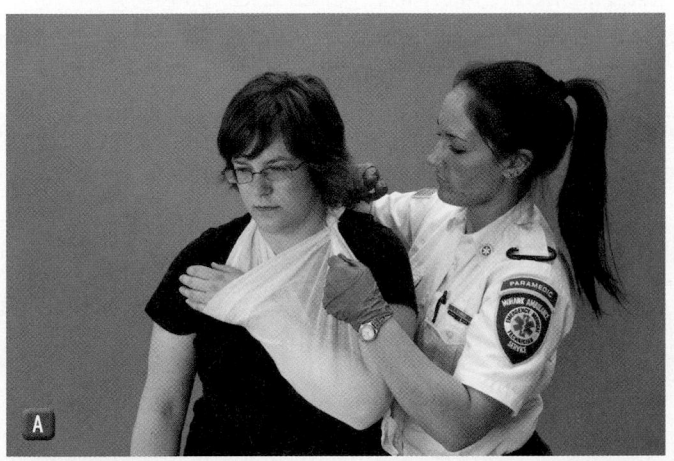

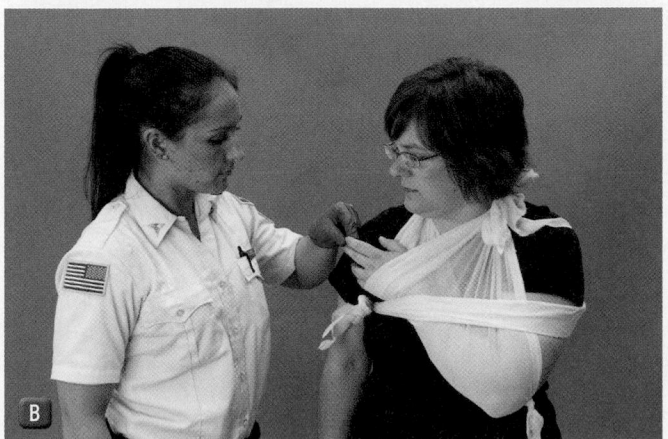

Figure 25 **A.** Apply the sling so that the knot is tied at one side of the neck. **B.** Secure the sling. Leave the fingers exposed to allow for circulation checks.

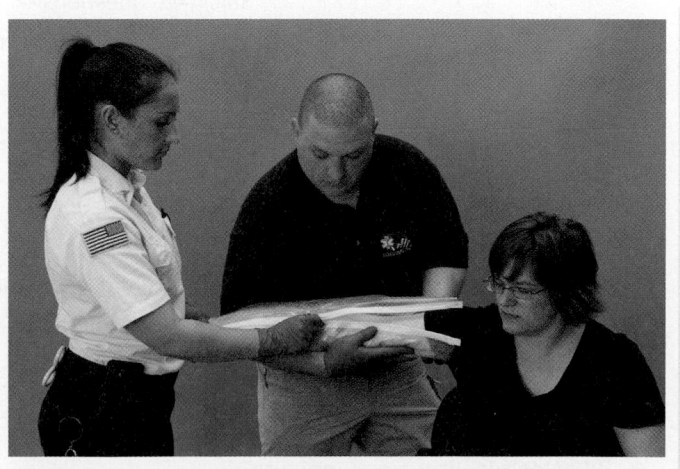

Figure 26 Positioning an air splint that features a zipper.

think prolonged use or use in unusual circumstances may be necessary. When applying the PASG, you should carefully inflate the device in increments. As a general rule, gradually inflate the legs of the PASG before inflating the abdominal portion. If you are using the device to stabilize a possible pelvic fracture, you must inflate all compartments. Always document all obvious injuries and deformities before application of the PASG.

Do not remove a PASG in the field. It must be deflated gradually in the hospital under careful supervision by a physician. Before handing off your patient to hospital personnel, report the patient's blood pressure, the time you applied the PASG, and the results.

Vacuum Splints A vacuum splint consists of a sealed mattress that is filled with air and thousands of small plastic beads. The mattress is laid out on the stretcher, and the patient is placed on top of it and allowed to settle into a comfortable position. A suction pump attached to the mattress is then used to evacuate the air from inside the mattress. The resulting vacuum inside the mattress compresses the beads in such a way that the whole splint becomes rigid, much like a plaster cast that has been molded to conform to the contours of the patient's entire posterior surface.

The vacuum mattress is an excellent splint, but there are a few factors that may limit its broad appeal. The splint is quite bulky, so it not only takes up a lot of storage room in the vehicle, but also can be difficult to work with in cramped quarters.

Furthermore, like all vacuum splints, it requires a mechanical suction pump, yet another piece of equipment to grab.

A smaller vacuum splint is available to splint individual limbs. This type of splint is applied by positioning the injured limb on the splint and then evacuating the air from inside of it. The result is a splint that is molded to the extremity Figure 27. This type of vacuum splint requires less space than a mattress-style vacuum splint but is still relatively expensive compared with standard rigid splints.

Pillow Splints A pillow is an effective means to stabilize an injured foot or ankle. Simply mold an ordinary pillow around the affected foot and ankle in a position of comfort, then secure the pillow in place with several cravats. Pillows can also be molded around an injured knee or elbow and are invaluable for padding backboards when they are used to stabilize patients with dislocated hips.

Traction Splints Following a femur fracture, the strong muscles of the thigh go into spasm and often lead to significant pain and deformity. Traction splints provide constant pull on a fractured femur, thereby preventing the broken bone ends from overriding as a result of unopposed muscle contraction. In addition, these splints help maintain alignment of the fracture pieces and provide effective stabilization of the fracture site. As a result, patients are likely to experience less pain.

YOU are the Medic | PART 3 |

Before moving your patient into the ambulance, you reassess his most distal pulses as well as sensation and motor function. Oxygenation is supported via nasal cannula at 4 L/min.

En route to a trauma center, a large-bore IV line is established. Medical direction is consulted regarding fluid resuscitation and glucose administration. Dextrose 50%, 25 grams via IV push, is administered per protocol. You complete your secondary assessment, remaining suspicious about continued hemorrhage from multiple long-bone fractures and impending shock. The patient's abdomen remains unremarkable. The patient responds more rapidly to questions and states he feels less "sleepy" after the glucose administration. His bilateral wrists are splinted. He now reports pain to his wrists and legs.

Recording Time: 15 Minutes	
Level of consciousness	Verbal, still oriented only to person and place; able to respond quickly to questions
Skin	Cool, pale, and slightly moist
Pulse	128 beats/min; weak and regular
Blood pressure	84/44 mm Hg
Respirations	24 breaths/min
Oxygen saturation (Spo$_2$)	98% while receiving 4 L/min via nasal cannula
Pupils	PEARRL
Pain scale	Visual Analog Scale; pain is an "8" on "0–10" scale.
Blood glucose	126 mg/dL (after glucose administration)

8. Why should this patient be transported to a trauma center?

9. What do his vital signs indicate?

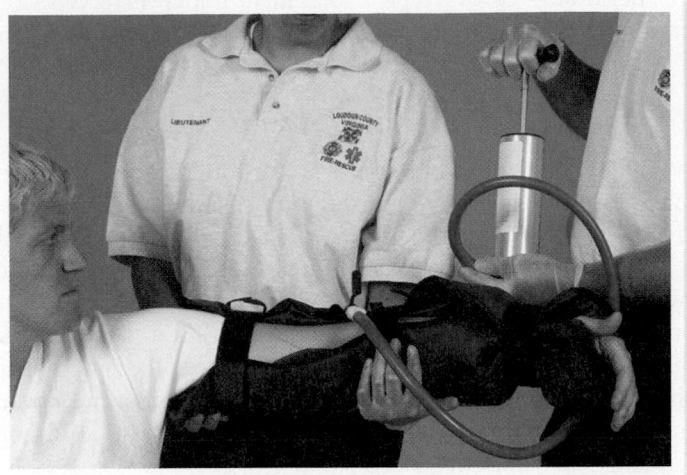

Figure 27 Applying a vacuum splint to a limb.

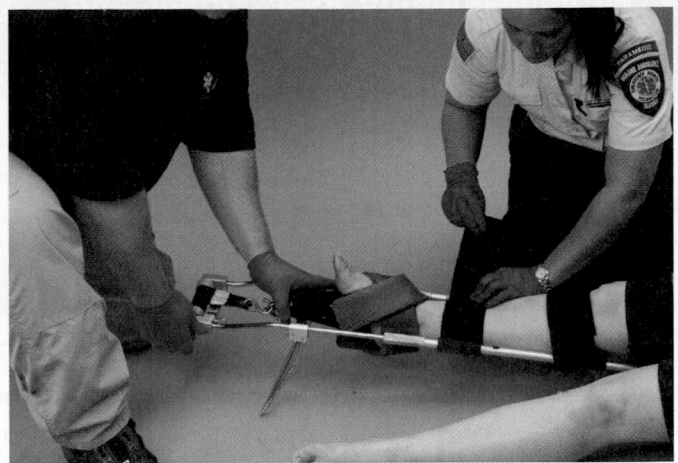

Figure 28 Applying a Hare traction splint. One rescuer connects the straps and another checks distal pulse, motor function, and sensation.

Special Populations

Because vacuum mattresses conform to the body, they may be useful for older patients who have abnormal curvatures of the spine and are suspected of having spinal column injuries.

Traction splints also reduce blood loss. Normally, the thigh is shaped like a cylinder. In a femur fracture, the thigh is shortened and becomes spherical. The volume of a sphere can be substantially greater than that of a cylinder, so a person with an untreated femur fracture can accumulate more blood in the thigh than a person whose thigh is pulled out to length by a traction splint.

Traction splints are indicated for the treatment of most closed femur fractures. They should not be used when the patient has an additional fracture below the knee on the same extremity, and they should not be used on open femur fractures. The most commonly used traction splints are the Sager and the Hare traction splints. The basic principles of application are the same for both. After assessing the injured extremity for distal PMS functions, place the splint next to the uninjured leg to determine the proper length. The traction splint should extend 6 to 10 inches beyond the foot.

Support and stabilize the leg to minimize movement while another rescuer applies the ankle hitch. When the hitch is secure, the second rescuer will apply gentle longitudinal traction using enough force to realign the extremity. The initial rescuer can then place the splint into position and connect the upper attachment point of the splint and then the ankle hitch Figure 28. Then secure the velcro straps. After applying the splint, reassess PMS functions before securing the patient and splint for transport.

Buddy Splinting Buddy splinting is used to splint injuries that involve the fingers or toes. With this technique, an adjacent uninjured finger or toe serves as a splint to the injured one. To buddy splint, tape the injured digit to an uninjured one. Place a gauze pad between the digits that are taped together, and ensure

that the tape does not pass over joints. Make sure the tape is not so tight as to cut off circulation.

■ Pathophysiology, Assessment, and Management of Pediatric Fractures

Children's bones grow significantly and contain growth plates (ossification centers) made of cartilage. Because these growth plates are relatively weak, the bones of growing children are weaker than their ligaments and tendons, making fractures more common than sprains. Joint dislocations do not usually occur without an associated fracture.

A growth plate may fracture even with a low-energy MOI. Signs and symptoms may not include the level of tenderness, swelling, and bruising usually associated with a broken bone.

Pelvic fractures are uncommon in young children and usually only occur with high-energy MOIs. The risk for pelvic fracture increases in adolescence, when the skeleton and MOIs become more like those of adults.

■ Assessment and Management

When you are assessing a pediatric patient with a musculoskeletal injury, remember to consider whether the MOI suggests possible abuse. Observe the interaction between the parent and child. Also, your approach may need to be adjusted to one that is appropriate for the child's age. Different ages may react differently to trauma. As always, assess pulses and motor and sensory function distal to the site of the injury, and assess for comorbidity.

Stabilize all sprains or strains and suspect fractures; growth plate injuries may result in poor bone growth. Immobilize the injured part in the same way as you would for an adult, and use cold packs to reduce swelling.

Transport the injured child with a family member. If a family member is not present, remember rules of consent. Always inform someone—family member, teacher, or guardian—of the transport location.

Pathophysiology, Assessment, and Management of Complications of Musculoskeletal Injuries

Musculoskeletal injuries can lead to numerous complications—not just those involving the musculoskeletal system, but also systemic changes or illness. It is essential to not focus all of your attention on the musculoskeletal injury: keep in mind that there is a patient attached to the injured extremity!

The likelihood of having a complication is often related to the strength of the force that caused the injury, the injury's location, and the patient's overall health. Any injury to a bone, muscle, or other musculoskeletal structure is likely to be accompanied by bleeding. In general, the greater the force that caused the injury, the greater the hemorrhage that will be associated with it.

Following a fracture, the sharp ends of the bone may damage muscles, blood vessels, arteries, and nerves, or the ends may penetrate the skin and produce an open fracture. A significant loss of tissue may occur at the fracture site if the muscle is severely damaged or if the bone's penetration of the skin causes a large defect.

Long-term disability is one of the most devastating consequences of a musculoskeletal injury. In many cases, a severely injured limb can be repaired and made to look almost normal. Unfortunately, many patients cannot return to work for long periods because of the extensive rehabilitation required and because of chronic pain. Paramedics have a critical role in mitigating the risk of long-term disability. By preventing further injury, reducing the risk of wound infection, minimizing pain by the use of cold packs and analgesia, and transporting patients with musculoskeletal injuries to an appropriate medical facility, they help reduce the risk or duration of long-term disability.

Vascular and Neurovascular Injuries

When blood vessels are damaged following a musculoskeletal injury, loss of blood flow can occur in the body part supplied by that vessel. This is called **devascularization**.

Additionally, neurovascular injuries can occur. The skeletal system normally protects the neurovascular structures within the limbs from injury. These critical structures typically lie deep within the limb and close to the skeleton. For example, the brachial plexus is situated within the axilla and the inner aspect of the arm, shielded from injury by the shoulder girdle. When the shoulder girdle or proximal humerus is fractured, displaced fracture fragments may lacerate or impale the nerves of the plexus, leading to a neurologic deficit. Neurovascular injuries are also likely to occur following a joint dislocation because the nerves and vessels in the region of a joint tend to be more securely tethered to the soft tissues and are less likely to escape injury.

Assessment and Management

The types of injuries that a blood vessel may sustain include a contusion of the vessel wall, laceration, kinking or bending, and formation of pseudoaneurysms. In addition, a blood vessel may thrombose (become occluded by a clot) when the injury causes blood flow to become very slow.

Regardless of the type of vascular injury involved, it is important to assess and reassess pulses, control bleeding, and maintain adequate intravascular volume by using IV fluid.

Compartment Syndrome

Within a limb, groups of muscles are surrounded by an inelastic membrane called **fascia**. Thus, the muscles are confined to an enclosed space, or compartment, that can accommodate only a limited amount of swelling. When bleeding (hematoma) or swelling occurs within a compartment as the result of a fracture or severe soft-tissue injury, the pressure within it rises. Pressure that is too high may impair circulation and lead to pain, sensory changes, and progressive muscle death. This condition, known as **compartment syndrome**, is one of the most devastating consequences of a musculoskeletal injury.

External and internal factors can lead to the development of compartment syndrome. External factors include bandages, splints, casts, and a PASG that are applied too tightly and restrict circulation. A number of internal factors can also increase the amount of material within a compartment. For example, bleeding within a compartment may occur because of a fracture, dislocation, crush injury, vascular injury, soft-tissue injury, bleeding disorder, or snake bite (though this is unusual). Alternatively, fluid leakage or edema may occur secondary to ischemia, excessive exercise, trauma, burns, or any condition associated with the leakage of proteins and fluid from vessels into the interstitial space. Circulatory problems, including compartment syndrome, can result from a plaster cast that is too tight around a swollen limb. A common misconception is that open fractures are safe from compartment syndrome—not true.

Assessment

Signs and symptoms of compartment syndrome include early and late findings. Typically, the first complaint is a searing or burning *pain* that is localized to the involved compartment and out of proportion to the injury. This pain is often severe and typically not relieved with pain medication, including narcotics. When you examine the patient, passive stretching of an ischemic muscle will result in severe pain. In the lower extremities, test for this condition by flexing and extending the great toe and by dorsiflexion and plantar flexion of the foot. In the upper extremity, use finger and hand flexion and extension.

During examination of the patient, the affected area may feel very firm and there may be skin pallor. Typical neurologic changes include paresthesias, such as a burning sensation, numbness, or tingling, and paralysis of the involved muscles, which occurs late in the condition. Another late sign of compartment syndrome is pulselessness. If a plaster cast has been applied, be sure to check pulses, and sensory and motor function distal to the cast terminus. By the time the pressure within the compartment reaches the point where it totally occludes the artery passing through it, significant muscle necrosis has probably occurred.

Management

The goal of prehospital care is to deliver the patient to an emergency facility before the extremity is pulseless. Thus, management should include elevating the extremity to heart level (not above!), placing cold packs over the extremity, and opening or loosening constrictive clothing and splint material. Apply high-flow oxygen and give a bolus of an isotonic crystalloid solution to help the kidneys flush out toxins from resulting rhabdomyolysis, which is discussed in the next section.

> ### Words of Wisdom
>
> A patient who shows evidence of compartment syndrome must be transported on an emergency basis to the hospital. There is no treatment for this syndrome other than surgery—do not delay transport.

Crush Syndrome

Crush syndrome occurs because of a prolonged compressive force that impairs muscle metabolism and circulation—actually, following the extrication or release of an entrapped limb. When muscles are crushed beyond repair, tissue necrosis develops and leads to release of harmful products, a process known as rhabdomyolysis. This condition happens not only in trauma patients, but also in patients who have been lying on an extremity for an extended period (4 to 6 hours of compression)—for example, when a drug overdose or stroke victim is not found for an extended period.

After a muscle is compressed for 4 to 6 hours, the muscle cells begin to die and release their contents into the localized vasculature. When the force compressing the region is released, blood flow is reestablished and the material from the cells that was released into the local vasculature quickly returns to the systemic vasculature. The primary substances that are of concern are lactic acid, potassium, and myoglobin. The release of these substances into the circulation is likely to result in decreased blood pH (a condition known as acidemia), hyperkalemia, and renal dysfunction.

Assessment and Management

Treatment of crush syndrome, which aims to prevent complications due to toxin release, should always be performed with medical direction. A number of steps must be taken *before* releasing the compressing force. As with all patients, assess the ABCs in case of suspected crush syndrome. Ensure that the patient is being given high-flow supplemental oxygen, and then administer a bolus of crystalloid solution to increase the intravascular volume and to protect the kidneys from the forthcoming myoglobin load. Establish cardiac monitoring to evaluate for electrocardiographic (ECG) changes related to hyperkalemia (such as peaked T waves, widening QRS complex, prolonged PR interval, dysrhythmia). To protect against the surge of potassium, a nebulizer treatment with albuterol may be given during extrication (beta-2 agonists promote the movement of potassium into cells). Once the patient is freed, if the ECG shows changes consistent with hyperkalemia, administer calcium to stabilize the myocardium; also give sodium bicarbonate to promote the intracellular shift of potassium. Insulin may also be given intravenously with dextrose, in the hospital, to facilitate the intracellular movement

of potassium. Compressive devices such as a PASG should not be applied.

Thromboembolic Disease

Thromboembolic disease, including deep vein thrombosis (DVT) and pulmonary embolism, is a significant cause of death following musculoskeletal injuries, especially injuries to the pelvis and lower extremities that lead to prolonged immobilization.

Assessment and Management

Signs and symptoms of DVT include disproportionate swelling of an extremity, discomfort in an extremity that worsens with use, and warmth and erythema of the extremity. When a DVT dislodges, it may cause a pulmonary embolism—a blood clot that occludes a portion or all of the pulmonary arteries **Figure 29**.

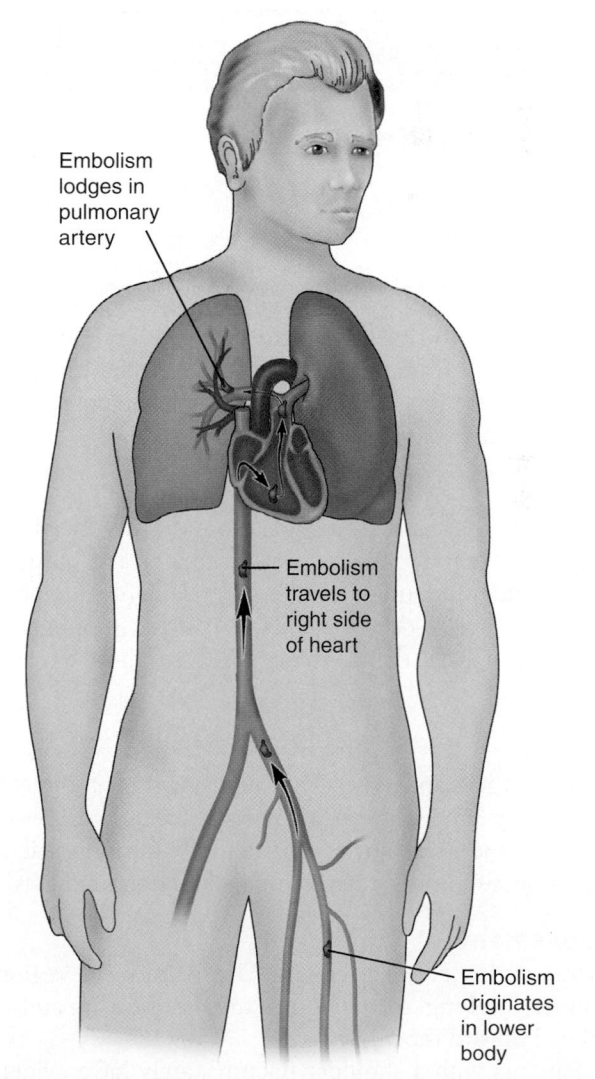

Embolism lodges in pulmonary artery

Embolism travels to right side of heart

Embolism originates in lower body

Figure 29 When a portion of a deep vein thrombosis dislodges, it may travel to the pulmonary arteries and inhibit blood flow from the heart to the lungs.

Signs and symptoms of a pulmonary embolism include a sudden onset of dyspnea, pleuritic chest pain (either side), dyspnea, tachypnea, tachycardia, low-grade fever right-sided heart failure, shock, and, in some cases, cardiac arrest.

In addition to the risk of DVT, patients with long bone or pelvic fractures are at risk for developing a fat embolism. In this condition, fat droplets become lodged in the vasculature of the lungs. Affected patients have inflammation of the vasculature of the lungs and other blood vessels where fat is deposited. Generally, symptoms begin within 12 to 72 hours of injury; they include tachycardia, dyspnea, tachypnea, pulmonary congestion, fever, petechiae, change in mental status, and organ dysfunction.

Treatment for thromboembolic disease in the field is limited to maintaining an airway, adequate oxygenation, and intravascular volume and rapid transportation to an emergency department.

Pathophysiology, Assessment, and Management of Specific Fractures

Shoulder Girdle

The shoulder girdle consists of the clavicle, shoulder, and scapula.

Clavicle

Clavicle fractures are very common and often occur in children. In most cases, the clavicle fractures in the middle third of the bone, typically from a fall onto an outstretched hand or from direct lateral trauma to the shoulder (as in contact sports, snowboarding, and cycling).

Shoulder

Fractures of the shoulder include those that involve the <u>glenoid fossa</u> of the scapula, the humeral head, and the humeral neck. Most shoulder fractures are caused by a fall onto an outstretched hand and usually occur in elderly patients (younger patients tend to dislocate the shoulder because they have stronger bones).

Scapula

Injuries to the scapula usually result from violent, direct trauma. Therefore, when a scapular injury is suspected, it is essential to look for associated injuries—particularly intrathoracic injuries, such as pneumothorax, hemothorax, and fractured ribs.

Assessment

Patients with a clavicle fracture have pain in the region of the shoulder, swelling, unwillingness to raise the arm, and tilting of the head toward the injured side.

Patients with a shoulder fracture rarely have evidence of a significant deformity, but instead have considerable swelling, ecchymosis, and pain with movement of the arm. In some cases, an associated injury to the brachial plexus may be identified during the neurologic examination.

Signs and symptoms of a scapular fracture include pain that increases with arm abduction and swelling in the region of the

scapula. Potential complications include axillary artery or nerve injury, brachial plexus injury, pulmonary contusion, and clavicle fractures.

Management

Fractures in the shoulder region may usually be treated by using a sling and swathe. These bindings should be applied to maintain the extremity in the position of comfort, often keeping the arm against the chest wall to allow the body to act as a splint. In cases of suspected scapula fractures, full spinal stabilization will often be warranted given the amount of force required to cause a fracture.

Midshaft Humerus Fractures

Fractures of the shaft of the humerus usually occur in younger patients secondary to high-energy injuries, such as motor vehicle crashes. Unlike fractures that occur more proximally, these injuries typically have substantial deformity.

Assessment

Examination of the extremity usually reveals a significant amount of swelling, ecchymosis, gross instability of the region, and crepitus. If the force that caused the injury is severe enough, the nerves and blood vessels in the upper arm may also be damaged. Of particular concern is the radial nerve, which may be injured by the force itself or could become entrapped within the fracture site. The classic sign of a radial nerve injury is wrist drop.

Management

If the fracture is angulated, longitudinal traction may be applied to correct the deformity, but efforts should be halted if the patient's pain is too severe or if neurovascular status worsens. Once the extremity is in the desired position, apply a rigid splint that extends from the axilla to the elbow. Next, apply a sling and swathe to stabilize the arm to the chest wall, and place cold packs over the fracture site to decrease the patient's pain and swelling.

Elbow

Distal Humerus

<u>Supracondylar fractures</u> of the humerus occur often in children. The typical mechanism is a fall onto an outstretched hand with the elbow in extension, thereby breaking the distal humerus; as a result, the distal fragment of the humerus is pushed posteriorly and the humeral shaft is pulled anteriorly, where it compresses the brachial artery and the radial and median nerves. If the brachial artery is compromised, the patient could develop compartment syndrome in the forearm. When this complication occurs, the patient is at risk for a <u>Volkmann ischemic contracture</u>, a condition in which muscles of the forearm degenerate from prolonged ischemia. The patient's muscles that allow for movement of the fingers become contracted and nonfunctional, and the patient loses the ability to use the hand.

Proximal Radius and Ulna

Radial head fractures may result from a fall onto an outstretched hand or from a direct blow to the bone. Similar to distal humerus fractures, these injuries may lead to an injury of the nerves or blood vessels in proximity to the fracture site. Therefore, a careful neurovascular examination should be performed.

Assessment and Management

Patients with a distal humerus fracture will report pain in the area of the elbow and typically have a significant degree of swelling and ecchymosis.

Radial head fractures cause the patient to have significant pain when he or she attempts supination or pronation. In either case, the patient is likely to have pain and ecchymosis in the region of the injury.

Treatment of injuries in the region of the elbow is the same regardless of the exact location of the injury. The injured extremity must be repeatedly assessed for evidence of compartment syndrome. Before splinting the extremity, it is mandatory to document a neurovascular exam. The injured extremity should be splinted in the position that it is found if the patient has a strong distal pulse, and cold packs should be used only if there is no evidence of compartment syndrome. If the patient has an absent distal pulse or neurologic deficits, consult with the appropriate medical facility to determine whether you should attempt fracture reduction. In any event, the patient must be transported urgently to the closest appropriate medical facility for definitive treatment.

■ Forearm

Fractures of the forearm may involve the radius, the ulna, or, more commonly, both. Injury may result from a direct blow to the bone, the classic example of which is the nightstick fracture of the ulna. In other cases, injury occurs because of a fall onto an outstretched hand, as in the case of a Colles fracture, also called a silver fork fracture. This fracture typically occurs in older patients with osteoporosis who have fallen but may be found in younger patients as well.

Assessment and Management

A patient with a Colles fracture usually has a dorsally angulated deformity of the distal forearm (the "**silver fork deformity**") and pain and swelling near the injured site.

A variety of splints may be used to secure a forearm fracture. Regardless of the type, the splint should provide stabilization of the entire forearm and, in cases of more proximal fractures, the elbow. Apply cold packs to the injury site to decrease pain and swelling. Frequent neurovascular exams are warranted to monitor for evidence of compartment syndrome and acute carpal tunnel syndrome.

■ Wrist and Hand

Injuries to the wrist and hand may lead to significant long-term disability, especially in people who rely on the use of their hands to earn a living. Sometimes these injuries occur while working at the job or at home; in other cases they result from a fall or during a sporting event. Careful splinting of the injured site is essential to help reduce the risk of long-term disability.

Scaphoid

The **scaphoid**, also called the carpal navicular, is located just distal to the radius. It may be injured from a fall onto an outstretched hand. The major complication of a scaphoid fracture is **avascular necrosis** of the bone, or poor fracture healing because of the limited blood supply to this bone.

Boxer's Fracture

A **boxer's fracture** is a fracture of the neck of the fifth metacarpal (small finger). It commonly occurs after punching a hard object, such as a wall or a door.

Metacarpal Shaft

Fractures of the metacarpals may result from a crush injury or from direct trauma.

Mallet Finger (Baseball Fracture)

A **mallet finger** occurs when a finger is jammed into an object, such as a baseball or basketball, resulting in an avulsion fracture of the extensor tendon.

Assessment

The classic finding for a scaphoid fracture is pain and tenderness in the anatomic snuffbox. To identify the anatomic snuffbox on yourself, extend your thumb. Two tendons will be visible at the base of the thumb on the radial aspect of the wrist. The region between these two tendons is the **snuffbox** Figure 30 .

The patient with a boxer's fracture typically has pain over the ulnar aspect of the hand and may have noticeable swelling.

Assessment of the injured hand with metacarpal fractures may reveal abnormal rotation or alignment of the fingers, swelling of the palm, and pain and tenderness in the region of injury. You should assess the neurovascular function of the hand and fingers following a crush injury because development of compartment syndrome is possible within the hand.

The patient with mallet finger will not be able to extend the distal phalynx of the finger and will maintain it in a flexed position.

Management

Splint the injured hand in the position of function by placing the wrist in about 30° of dorsiflexion with fingers slightly

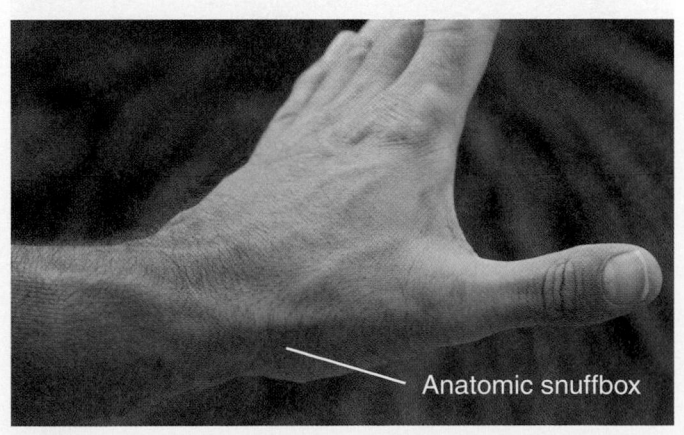

Anatomic snuffbox

Figure 30 The region between the two tendons shown is the anatomic snuffbox.

flexed (a roll of gauze approximately 2 to 3 inches in diameter accomplishes this nicely). Next, secure the extremity to an armboard or other rigid splint that extends proximally to the elbow and is slightly elevated to help reduce swelling **Figure 31**. For injuries that are isolated to the digits, use a foam-padded flexible aluminum splint to splint the injured digit, if available. In the case of penetrating injuries, regardless of whether a fracture is present, apply bulky dressings to the site of injury and splint the injured hand in the position of function.

▌ Pelvis

Pelvic fractures are relatively uncommon injuries, accounting for fewer than 3% of all fractures. Despite their low incidence, these injuries are responsible for a significant number of deaths in blunt trauma patients. The risk of death following a pelvic fracture ranges from 8% to 50%, depending on the severity of the injury; when the fracture is open, the mortality rate rises to 25% to 50%. Death after a pelvic fracture commonly results from massive hemorrhage caused by damage to the arteries and veins of the pelvis.

Disruptions of the pelvic ring occur secondary to high-energy trauma. The majority of pelvic fractures are a result of blunt trauma from motor vehicle collision, motorcycle crashes, or vehicles striking pedestrians. Pelvic fractures may also result from crush injuries and falls from a significant height. Because of the forces required to break the pelvis, suspect multisystem trauma, including abdominal trauma and head injury, if your patient has a pelvic injury (until proven otherwise) **Figure 32**.

A number of structures within the pelvis are at risk for injury when it is fractured—the bladder, urethra, rectum, vagina, and sacral nerve plexus. The blood vessels that are most prone to damage are the veins within the pelvis, but there may be damage to the internal or external iliac vessels and to arteries in the lumbar region. The nerves at greatest risk of injury are those in the lumbar and sacral regions and the sciatic and femoral nerves.

There are four main types of pelvic fractures, listed in **Table 5**. Specific types of fractures are discussed in the next sections.

Lateral Compression Pelvic Ring Disruptions

__Lateral compression__ injuries result from an impact on the side of the body (such as being struck by a car from the side or falling from a significant height and landing on one side of the body). The side of the pelvis that sustains the impact becomes internally rotated around the sacrum, and the actual volume within the pelvis decreases **Figure 33**. It does not usually result in an unstable pelvis. Because the volume in the pelvis is reduced, not increased, life-threatening hemorrhage is less common in such

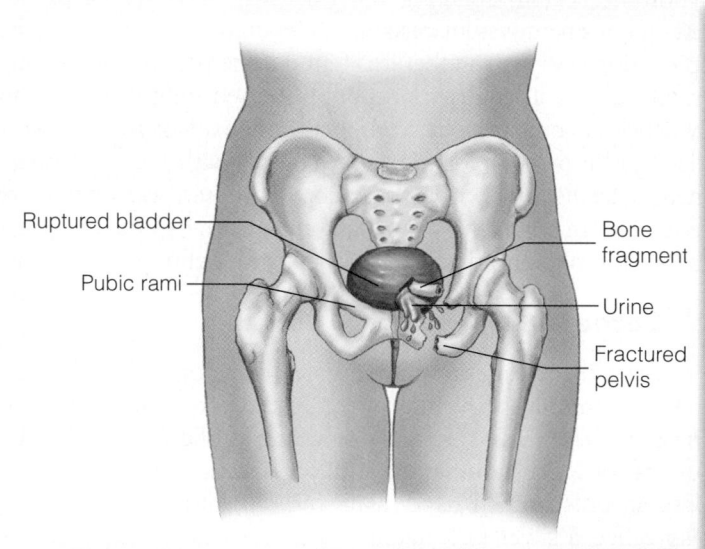

Ruptured bladder

Pubic rami

Bone fragment

Urine

Fractured pelvis

Figure 32 Pelvic fractures occasionally cause laceration of the bladder as a result of penetration by bony fragments. Externally, pelvic fractures can cause severe bruising and swelling.

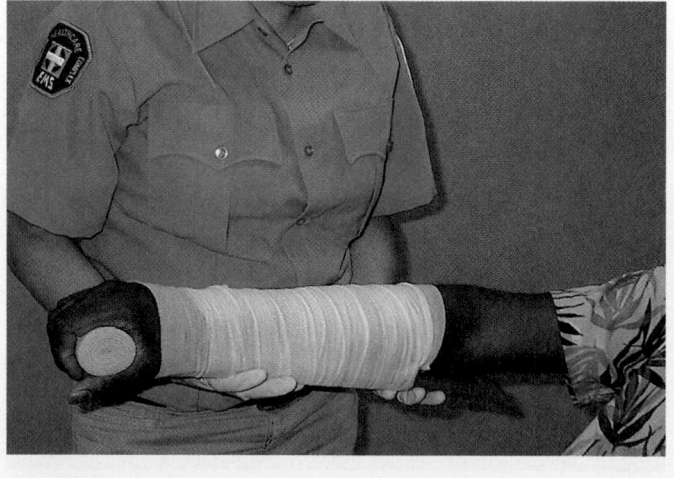

Figure 31 Splinting the hand and wrist.

Table 5	**Types of Pelvic Fractures**
Type	**Fractures in Category**
Type I	<ul><li>Avulsion fractures</li><li>Fracture of pubis or ischium</li><li>Fracture of iliac wing</li><li>Fracture of sacrum</li><li>Fracture of coccyx</li></ul>
Type II	<ul><li>Single fracture of pelvic ring (including unilateral fractures of both pelvic rami)</li><li>Subluxation of the pubic symphysis</li><li>Fracture near the sacroiliac joint</li></ul>
Type III	<ul><li>Multiple breaks of pelvic ring</li></ul>
Type IV	<ul><li>Involve acetabulum</li></ul>

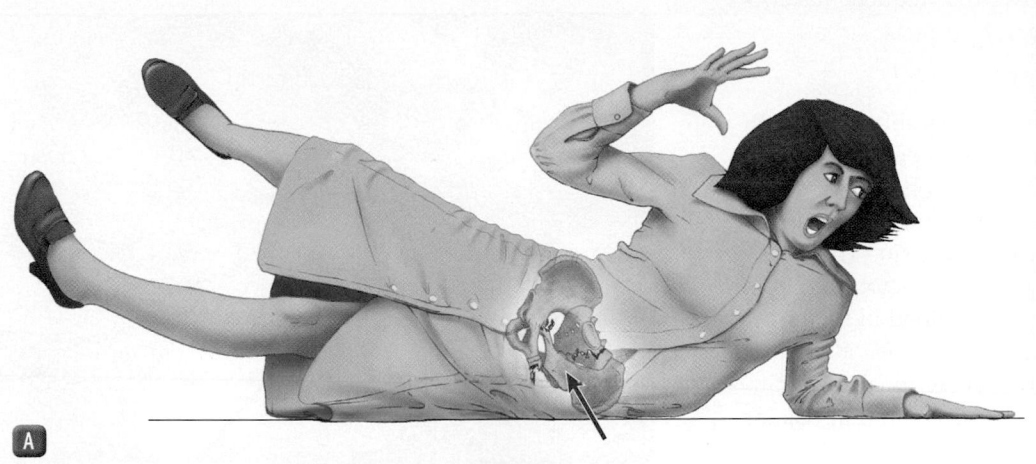

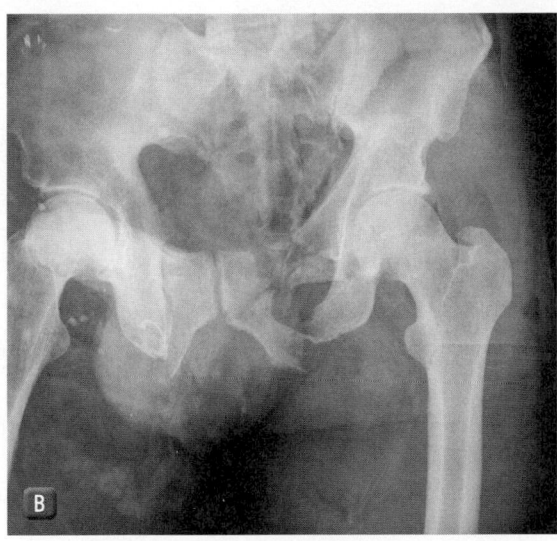

Figure 33 **A.** A lateral compression injury to the pelvis. **B.** A radiograph of a lateral compression injury.

head, with disruption of the bony or ligamentous structures. Thus, this kind of injury has anterior and posterior components. The anterior component involves a fracture of the rami or disruption of the pubic symphysis. The posterior component involves a fracture of the ilium or sacrum or a disruption of the sacroiliac joint. This unstable fracture results in an increase in pelvic volume.

Straddle Fracture

A <u>straddle fracture</u> occurs after a fall when a person lands in the region of the perineum and sustains bilateral fractures of the inferior and superior rami. This injury does not interfere with weightbearing, but it does carry a risk owing to its associated complications, particularly those of the lower genitourinary system.

Open Pelvic Fractures

Although penetrating trauma to the pelvis may result in bony fractures, the more worrisome injury is to the major vascular structures, which can cause life-threatening hemorrhage. Such an injury is defined by the presence of a laceration of the skin in the pelvic region, vagina, or rectum. Open fractures (not to be confused with open-book fractures) are uncommon and may result from either penetrating or blunt trauma, caused by a high-velocity injury. This causes subsequent massive hemorrhage and has a mortality rate of 25%

cases. However, lateral compression is often associated with injuries in other regions of the body.

Anterior-Posterior Compression Pelvic Ring Disruptions

These injuries may occur following a head-on motor vehicle crash, motorcycle crash, or fall or in a pedestrian who is struck head-on by a vehicle. The force of the impact compresses the pelvis in the anterior-to-posterior direction, causing the pubic symphysis and posterior supporting ligaments to be disrupted and tear apart. The pelvis then spreads apart and opens like a book—therefore the name <u>open-book pelvic fracture</u>. Such an injury has the potential for massive blood loss because the volume of the pelvis is greatly increased.

Vertical Shear

<u>Vertical shear</u> injuries occur when a major force is applied to the pelvis from above or below, such as when a person falls from a significant height and lands on the feet. On landing, the force is transmitted through the legs to the pelvis, leading to the complete displacement of one or both sides of the pelvis toward the

Words of Wisdom

There is an old medical school scenario of a patient who was shot in the head who is hypotensive. The puzzle is, "What's wrong with the patient?" The answer, as we have learned in this chapter, is that the patient was probably shot in the belly with a second bullet! Always remember that hemorrhaging will continue until controlled in the operating room under "bright lights and cold steel." Survival may be determined by the length of time from the injury to definitive surgical control of the hemorrhage. Delays in the field may have a negative impact on the patient's long-term survival. So, if you are not the solution to this patient's problem, don't add to the problem. Get the patient to the trauma center!

to 50%. When the patient does survive, the frequent result is chronic pain and permanent disability.

Assessment

Patients with pelvic ring disruptions who have a stable injury, such as a minimal lateral compression injury, may report pain in the pelvis and difficulty bearing weight. Patients with a more severe injury may show evidence of profound shock, gross pelvic instability, and diffuse pelvic and lower abdominal pain. There may also be bruising or lacerations in the perineum, scrotum, groin, suprapubic region, and flank and hematuria (blood in the urine) or blood coming from the meatus of the penis, vagina, or rectum.

The patient with a vertical shear is likely to have significant shortening of the limb on the affected side and is at risk for massive hemorrhage into the pelvis.

Even small amounts of blood found during a vaginal or rectal exam should raise your suspicion for an open pelvic fracture.

However, properly evaluating and treating a patient is more important than identifying the specific type of pelvic fracture. Assessment of the patient with a possible pelvic fracture should begin as in any other trauma patient—with a primary assessment of the mental status and ABCs, taking spinal precautions. During the rapid exam of the patient, you should search for injuries typically associated with pelvic fractures. Assess the pelvis for bleeding, lacerations, bruising, and instability. To assess for instability, apply pressure over the iliac wings in a medial direction and in a posterior direction. Once instability of the pelvis is identified, the pelvis should not be reassessed for instability to avoid causing increased bleeding.

A search for entry and exit wounds for a penetrating trauma is helpful, but an extended search should never delay quick transport and treatment of hypotension.

Management

Treatment should include careful monitoring of the ABCs, spinal stabilization, and IV access with at least one (if not two) large-bore catheters. Patients with open-book pelvic fractures will require IV fluids with lactated Ringer's solution or normal saline but may still remain hypotensive in the field. Management of the pelvic injury is aimed at reducing the amount of bleeding and decreasing the degree of instability. It is often appropriate to seek medical direction for the management of these patients, especially for determining how to best stabilize the pelvis. Methods used to accomplish this may include application of a pelvic binder or simply tying a sheet around the pelvis. Applying pressure to the iliac wings and forcing them to shift toward the midline reduces the potential space within the pelvis, which may allow for tamponade of the bleeding vessels.

Follow the steps below to apply a pelvic binder **Figure 34**:

1. Log roll the patient on a backboard to get the binder into position behind the pelvis. Alternatively, the binder can be placed onto the board prior to moving the patient onto the backboard.
2. Make sure the binder is positioned over the trochanters and below the ribs and top of the iliac wings so it does not impede breathing when tightened.

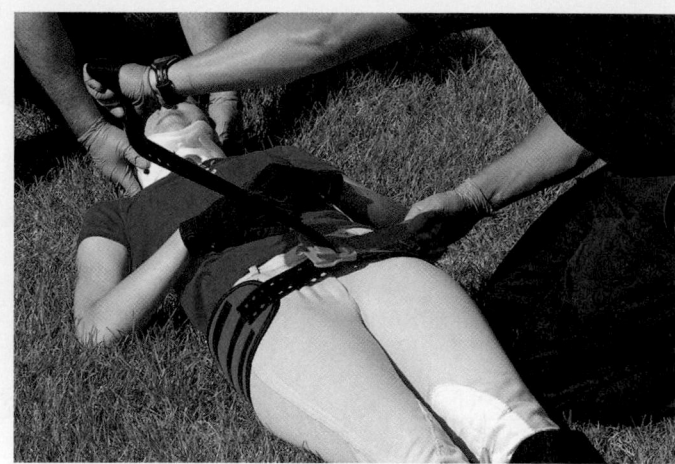

Figure 34 Application of a pelvic binder is one of the best ways to stabilize the pelvis and control hemorrhage.

3. Connect the two sides of the binder together anteriorly using the Velcro straps.
4. Apply gentle but firm pressure from either side of the patient to close down the pelvic volume by pushing the two sides of the unstable disrupted pelvis together.
5. Perform definitive tightening of the binder to hold the reduced position of the pelvic ring.
6. Check to be sure that the patient is still able to breathe easily and that the binder is not impeding chest excursion with ventilation. If it is, open the binder immediately and reposition it lower.

Once packaged, the patient should be rapidly transported to a trauma center, and IV fluid should be administered to maintain adequate tissue perfusion, but hypertension should be avoided because too much fluid can exacerbate bleeding and disrupt the natural hemostasis.

The PASG is a controversial treatment that can be used to stabilize the pelvis during rapid transports. It can potentially decrease pain by causing less movement of the fractured bones and decrease bleeding by reducing pelvic volume, although some emergency medicine specialists believe that the PASG may increase bleeding by putting pressure on pelvic vessels.

▌ Hip

A hip fracture involves a fracture of the femoral head, femoral neck, intertrochanteric region, or proximal femoral shaft. Fractures of the femoral head are uncommon injuries that are usually associated with a hip dislocation. Femoral neck and **intertrochanteric fractures** typically occur in older patients with osteoporosis who have fallen and sustained direct trauma to the hip. They may occur in younger patients with healthy bone, typically as the result of a high-energy mechanism. Proximal femoral shaft fractures can occur in patients of any age and result from a high-energy mechanism.

Assessment

Patients with a hip fracture will report pain in the affected hip, especially with attempts at movement, and report an inability to bear weight. They may also report hearing or feeling something snap. If the fracture is displaced, the patient almost always has an externally rotated and shortened leg. If there is no displacement, the leg may appear normal. Examination of the injury site usually finds tenderness to palpation, and there may be noticeable swelling, deformity, or ecchymosis.

Management

The treatment of hip fractures depends on the MOI. Hip fractures in older patients who sustained a low-energy injury, such as a fall from a standing position, do not require traction splints. Treat these injuries by supporting the injured extremity in the position in which it is found. This may be accomplished by placing pillows or blankets under the affected extremity and securing them in place **Figure 35**.

In younger patients and in those with high-energy injuries, treat the patient as you would any other trauma patient: fully immobilize the patient, establish vascular access, monitor for shock, and transport to a trauma center. Consider using a PASG if dictated per local protocol.

Definitive treatment of a hip fracture almost always requires surgery. If possible, the bone is repaired with plates, rods, or screws. Sometimes, however, the hip must be replaced.

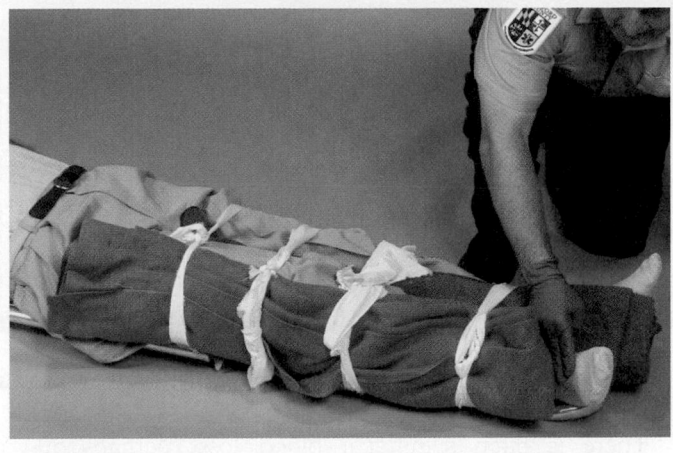

Figure 35 An acceptable method for splinting a hip fracture.

Femoral Shaft

Femoral shaft fractures occur following high-energy impacts. Thus, the presence of a fracture of the femoral shaft should alert you to the risk of other injuries.

Assessment and Management

Patients with femoral shaft fractures will report severe pain. The fracture may be severely angulated or lead to significant

---

YOU are the Medic   PART 4

En route you reassess his splints and distal pulses, motor function, and sensation to his lower extremities. His pedal pulses are absent bilaterally and he is unable to move his toes and cannot feel you touch them. After consulting with medical direction, you administer a 500-mL normal saline bolus and reassess his condition. You receive an order to administer 50 mg of fentanyl IVP every 15 minutes as necessary and as vital signs permit. His pain improves and he thanks you for your care. Blankets are placed to keep him warm. His blood glucose level is now 122 mg/dL. On arrival at the hospital, the patient's pedal pulses and sensation to his toes return.

Recording Time: 20 Minutes	
Level of consciousness	Remains alert and oriented to person, place, and time
Skin	Cool, pale, and dry
Pulse	110 beats/min; weak and regular (after fluid bolus)
Blood pressure	95/56 mm Hg
Respirations	20 breaths/min
ECG	Sinus tachycardia
Oxygen saturation (Spo$_2$)	98% while receiving 4 L/min via nasal cannula
Pupils	PEARRL
Pain scale	Visual Analog Scale; pain is a "3" on "0–10" scale
Blood glucose	122 mg/dL

10. What do absent pedal pulses, absent motor function, and lack of sensation in the toes indicate?

11. Why is it important to treat the patient's pain?

limb shortening, or it may be open. Examination may identify significant thigh edema, bruising, crepitus, and muscle spasm.

There is often significant blood loss (perhaps 500 to 1,500 mL) at the fracture site. In addition, damage to the neurovascular structures of the thigh is possible. Femoral shaft fractures also place the patient at risk for fat emboli.

Management of femoral shaft fractures includes monitoring for evidence of shock, full spinal immobilization, and establishing vascular access. Place the injured extremity in a traction splint or use a PASG, to achieve stability and hemorrhage control. Because these injuries may be extremely painful, consider the administration of pain medication.

Knee

Fractures of the knee may involve the distal femur, proximal tibia, or patella. An injury to this region may result from a direct blow to the knee, an axial load of the leg, or powerful contractions of the quadriceps.

Assessment and Management

Assessment of the patient generally reveals significant pain in the knee, decreased ROM, pain with movement and weightbearing, ecchymosis, swelling, and, in the case of displaced fractures, deformity.

Management of knee fractures depends on the position of the leg and the status of distal pulses. If the patient has a good distal pulse, splint the extremity in the position that it is found. If there is no distal pulse, seek medical consultation to determine whether you should attempt manipulation before transportation. In all cases, elevate the leg to the heart level and apply cold packs. Frequent neurovascular checks are mandatory, given the high incidence of compartment syndrome and neurovascular injury in cases of knee fracture.

Tibia and Fibula

Fractures of the tibia and/or fibula may result from direct trauma to the lower leg or from application of rotational or compressive forces.

Assessment and Management

These injuries often present with significant deformity and soft-tissue injury. Complications may include compartment syndrome, neurovascular injury, infection, poor healing, and chronic pain.

Apply a rigid, long leg splint, and administer pain medication as necessary. If there is gross angulation, attempt to align the leg after administering pain medication, documenting the premanipulation and postmanipulation neurovascular status. Monitor the patient for evidence of compartment syndrome, elevate the extremity to heart level, and apply cold packs.

Ankle

Fractures of the ankle **Figure 36** usually result from sudden, forceful movements of the foot that damage the malleoli and sometimes produce dislocation (called a fracture-dislocation). In other cases, an axial load is transmitted through the foot and causes the <u>talus</u> (the bone of the foot that articulates with the tibia) to impact the distal tibia, leading to a fracture.

Assessment and Management

Signs and symptoms of an ankle fracture include pain, deformity, and swelling. Ankle fractures may lead to damage of the nerves and blood vessels that supply the foot, the development of compartment syndrome, and chronic ankle pain and arthritis.

Ankle fractures should be stabilized using a commercially available splint or a pillow splint. The toes should be exposed to allow for frequent checks of distal neurovascular function. Elevate the extremity to the heart level, and apply cold packs to reduce swelling.

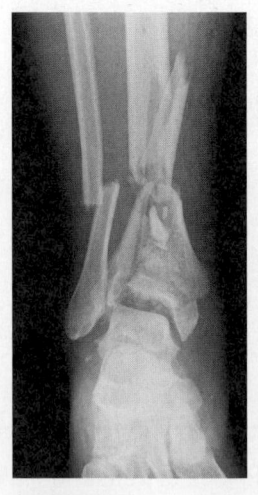 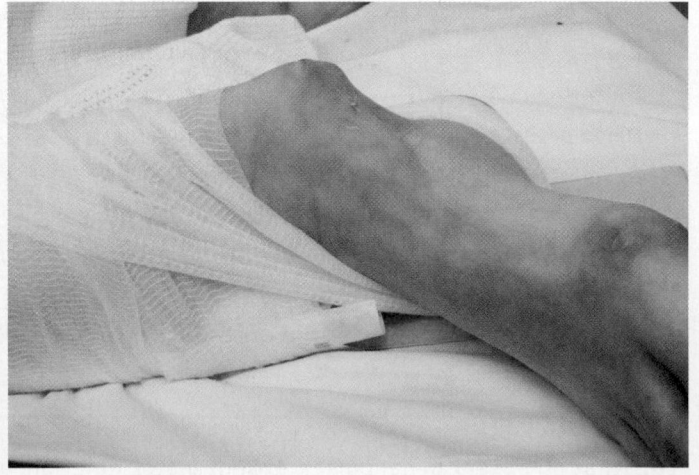

Figure 36 Two views of a severe fracture of the ankle.

If an ankle fracture-dislocation is associated with a pulseless foot, medical direction may recommend that you attempt reduction. To reduce a fracture-dislocation of the ankle, first relax the calf muscles to allow the foot to move more freely by flexing the patient's leg at the knee. With the leg flexed, grasp the heel and the foot just proximal to the toes and apply gentle traction. Next, rotate the foot back into its normal position without forcing it. If this procedure is successful, reassess the distal neurovascular status and splint the extremity in the reduced position, using care not to allow the ankle to dislocate again. If the fracture-dislocation cannot be reduced, notify medical control and expedite transportation after splinting the ankle in the position in which it was found.

Words of Wisdom

Whenever an open fracture is reduced, there is a risk that blood will be splashed. Always wear safety glasses and a gown, in addition to gloves, when splinting or manipulating an open fracture.

■ Calcaneus

The calcaneus may be fractured when a patient jumps from a height and lands on the feet or when a powerful force is applied directly to the heel.

Assessment and Management

These injuries present with foot pain, swelling, and ecchymosis and should alert providers to the possibility of injuries in the knee, pelvis, and spine.

When a calcaneus fracture is suspected, splint the injured extremity with a pillow and apply ice packs to help decrease swelling. Any patient with a suspected calcaneus fracture requires spinal stabilization given the high risk of an associated spinal injury, particularly bilateral fractures (parachutist fracture).

■ Pathophysiology, Assessment, and Management of Ligament Injuries and Dislocations

■ Shoulder Girdle Injuries and Dislocations

Acromioclavicular Joint Separation

Separation of the acromioclavicular (AC) joint **Figure 37** usually occurs from a direct blow to the superior aspect or point of the shoulder, as may happen during contact sports and falls.

Posterior Sternoclavicular Joint Dislocation

Posterior dislocation of the clavicle at its junction with the sternum most often occurs as a result of a direct blow to the clavicle but is sometimes seen after strong pressure is applied to the posterior shoulder (as when a football player ends up at the bottom of a pile-up). This injury is rarely difficult to identify because there is pain and swelling at the sternoclavicular joint. What makes this a potentially dangerous and even potentially fatal injury is not the dislocation itself, but the possible damage

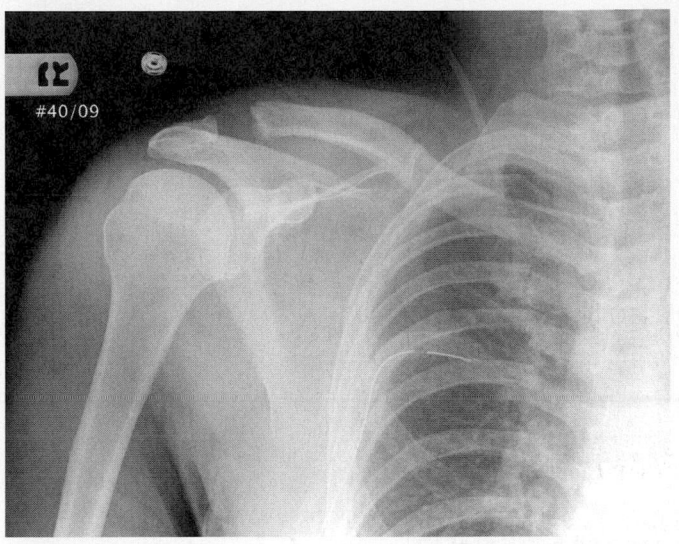

Figure 37 Separation of the AC joint. This space is wider than it should normally be.

to underlying structures—specifically, the trachea, esophagus, jugular vein, subclavian vein and artery, carotid artery, and other vascular structures.

Shoulder Dislocation

Roughly 90% of shoulder dislocations are anterior dislocations. Usually, anterior shoulder dislocations are caused by a fall onto an outstretched arm that is abducted and externally rotated.

Assessment

Patients with AC joint separation generally report pain and tenderness in the region of the AC joint, and the prominence of the distal clavicle may lead to a noticeable protrusion.

Any symptoms of a posterior dislocation of the clavicle that suggest an underlying injury—such as dyspnea, pain on swallowing, a sensation of choking, loss of pulses, or a sensory deficit in the upper extremity on the same side—are danger signals and should prompt rapid transport of the patient a trauma center.

Patients experiencing shoulder dislocation report severe pain and have significantly decreased ROM at the shoulder. The arm is usually abducted and externally rotated, and any efforts at moving it result in extreme pain **Figure 38**. A prominent bulge from the acromion is often noted on the anterior surface of the shoulder, the humeral head may be palpable, and the patient may experience frequent and painful muscle spasms.

Posterior shoulder dislocations are much less common and are often caused by massive muscle contractions such as those seen with electrical shocks and seizures. These injuries present with the same reports of pain and limited motion, but the arm is maintained in internal rotation and adduction.

In some patients, a shoulder dislocation will produce a tear of the rotator cuff or a fracture of the glenoid. Some patients may have a concomitant injury to the brachial plexus, axillary artery, or axillary vein. The axillary nerve is also prone to injury during a shoulder dislocation; assess sensation over the deltoid

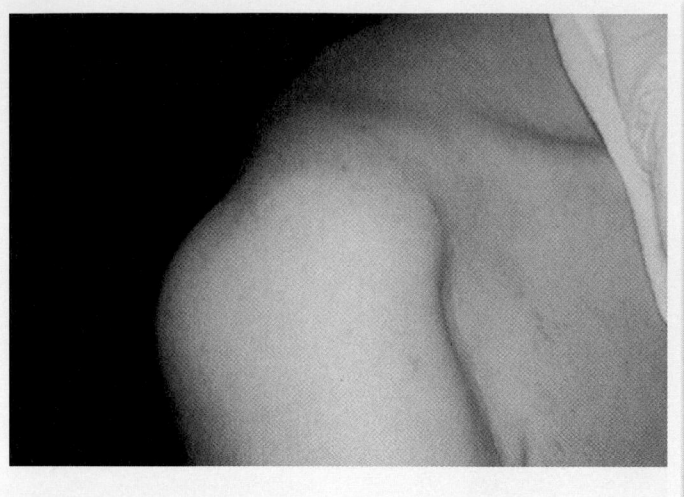

Figure 38 The typical appearance of an anterior shoulder dislocation.

muscle to determine whether there is a sensory deficit in the distribution of this nerve. Patients with a shoulder dislocation are also at risk for future dislocations, especially during the first 2 years following the injury and if the patient is young.

Management

In cases of an AC joint separation, a sling and swathe will often provide significant pain relief. In case of a posterior sternoclavicular joint dislocation, position the patient supine with the arm on the affected side abducted and place a rolled towel under the shoulder blade, a position that may take some of the pressure off the structures beneath the sternoclavicular joint. Pay close attention to the patient's airway, and keep airway equipment readily available.

For a dislocated shoulder, splint the injured extremity in the position in which it was found by using blankets, pillows, and, when possible, a sling and swathe. When applying the swathe, it may be necessary to connect two cravats together so as to encircle the patient's body, extremity, and pillows or blankets. Given the likelihood of muscle spasm and pain, use of pain medication and antispasmodic agents may be necessary. Perform neurovascular assessments frequently to monitor for changes in function.

▮ Elbow Dislocation

Elbow dislocations are medical emergencies because of the high risk of neurovascular injury. The vast majority of elbow dislocations are posterior injuries that result from a fall onto an outstretched hand or from hyperextension of the elbow joint.

Subluxation of the radial head is also referred to as **nursemaid's elbow**. It commonly occurs in children younger than 6 years and is caused by a sudden pull on the child's arm.

Assessment and Management

Patients usually report significant pain in the region of the elbow and may have a large degree of swelling and ecchymosis. A palpable deformity may be present at the elbow from the

prominence of the <u>olecranon</u> process **Figure 39**, and there is typically locking or resistance to movement of the joint. Major complications of an elbow dislocation include an associated fracture in the region of the joint, brachial artery injury, median nerve injury, and injury to the ulnar nerve.

Clinically, for patients with radial head subluxation, the injured arm is held in flexion and the child will often refuse to move the hand or elbow on the injured side. In general, there is only mild swelling in the region of the elbow.

When you suspect a dislocation or subluxation in the elbow, splint the injured extremity in the position in which it was found. A sling and swathe may be applied to provide additional stabilization to the injured elbow.

▮ Wrist and Hand Dislocation

The wrist can become dislocated when it is hyperextended beyond its normal ROM.

Assessment and Management

A patient with a wrist or hand dislocation will have pain, swelling, and deformity, much like that seen with fractures. Treatment for fractures and dislocations, sprains, and strains of the wrist or hand is essentially the same.

Use a padded board or pillow splint with a sling and swathe to stabilize a dislocated hand or wrist. As always, use cold packs and elevation, and consider administering pain relief. If possible, the hand should be placed in the position of function and a roll of gauze placed in the curled palm.

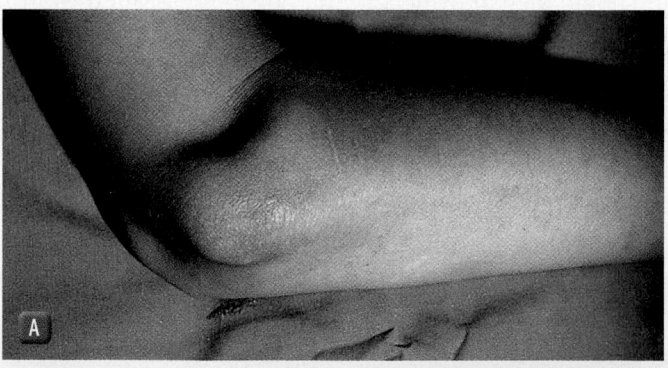

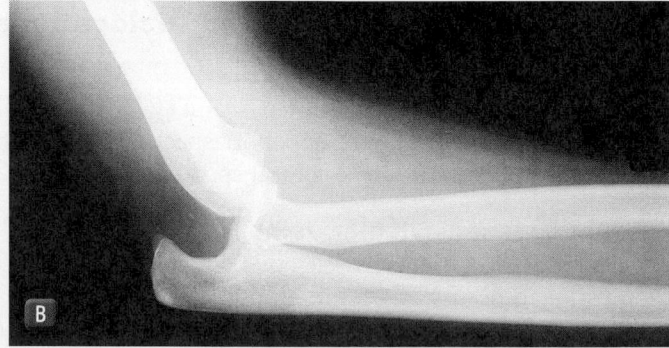

Figure 39 A posteriorly dislocated elbow. **A.** The clinical appearance of an elbow dislocation. **B.** Radiographic appearance of the same elbow.

Finger Dislocation

Finger dislocations are caused by a sudden "jamming" force or from extension of the fingers beyond the normal ROM.

Assessment and Management

There is generally pain and deformity at the affected joint, and there may be compromise of the neurovascular structures of the digit, leading to paresthesias.

Manage the dislocated finger by splinting the entire hand in the position of function and using soft dressings as needed to support the digit, or simply tape the fingers together (buddy system). Do not attempt to relocate the injured digit in the field unless you are directed to do so by medical control. To reduce a dislocated digit, if the digit is dislocated to the dorsal side, extend the digit; if it is dislocated to the volar side, flex the digit. Next, use gentle longitudinal traction to bring the digit back into its normal position. It may be helpful to apply pressure at the dislocated joint to push the distal part into position. Following reduction, the neurovascular status of the digit should be reassessed and the digit should be fully immobilized to prevent it from dislocating again.

Hip Dislocation

More than 90% of all hip dislocations involve posterior dislocation. The majority of these dislocations occur due to deceleration injuries, in which a flexed knee strikes an immobile object with a great degree of force **Figure 40**.

When a patient has a posterior hip dislocation, the leg of the affected side is typically found in flexion, adduction, and internal rotation, and it is noticeably shorter. Patients report severe pain and inability to move the leg, and significant soft-tissue swelling may be evident. Complications arising from such injuries include sciatic nerve injury, avascular necrosis of the hip, and associated fractures of the acetabulum.

Anterior hip dislocations usually follow a forceful spreading injury that occurs while the hip is flexed. The affected leg is usually flexed, abducted, and externally rotated, and the patient reports severe pain. Major complications of this type of injury include injury to the femoral artery or nerve and avascular necrosis of the hip.

Assessment and Management

Because the majority of hip dislocations are associated with a high-energy mechanism, a full-body exam should be conducted and the patient fully stabilized. Splint the injured extremity in the position in which it is found by using blankets and pillows. Perform and document frequent neurovascular checks on your patient care report. Once at the hospital, the patient generally requires sedation and muscle relaxants to allow the hip to be repaired.

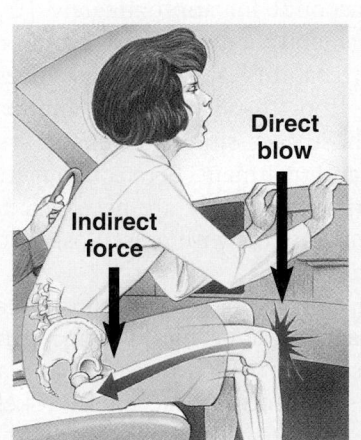

Figure 40 When a flexed knee strikes a dashboard, the force may be transmitted to the femur, causing it to be driven posteriorly. The hip may dislocate, and the acetabulum may fracture.

Knee Dislocation

Dislocations of the knee are true emergencies that may threaten the limb. When the knee is dislocated, the ligaments that provide support to it may be damaged or torn. The knee may be dislocated by high-energy trauma (as in motor vehicle crashes), or it may dislocate secondary to powerful twisting forces (as when athletes attempt to avoid another player). In most cases, the knee will spontaneously replace itself following the injury and there may be no obvious evidence of injury.

The direction of dislocation refers to the position of the tibia with respect to the femur. Anterior knee dislocations, which result from extreme hyperextension of the knee, are the most common, occurring in almost half of all cases. Commonly, the anterior and posterior cruciate ligaments are damaged, but there is also a high risk of injury to the popliteal artery.

In posterior dislocations, a direct blow to the knee forces the tibia to shift posteriorly. There is also the possibility of damage to the cruciate ligaments and injury to the popliteal artery.

Medial dislocations result from a direct blow to the lateral part of the leg. Because the deforming force causes the medial aspect of the knee to stretch apart, there is a high likelihood of injury to the medial collateral and cruciate ligaments. When the force is applied from the medial direction, a lateral dislocation occurs and the lateral part of the knee is stretched apart, injuring the lateral collateral ligament. Lateral and medial dislocations happen less commonly and have a lesser risk of injuring the popliteal artery.

Assessment and Management

Patients with a knee dislocation will typically report pain in the knee and report that the knee "gave out." If the knee did not spontaneously replace itself there may be evidence of significant deformity and decreased ROM. Complications may include limb-threatening popliteal artery disruption; injuries to the popliteal, peroneal, and tibial nerves; and joint instability. Do not confuse this injury with a relatively minor patella dislocation.

In all cases of knee dislocation, distal neurovascular function must be assessed frequently and will often guide the management. If a pulse is palpable in the foot, splint the knee in the position in which it is found. If there is no palpable pulse, you may need to reduce the knee to restore circulation. A number of factors, including time to the hospital and duration of dislocation, will affect this decision, so you should always seek medical direction before reducing a dislocated knee.

To reduce a dislocated knee, apply longitudinal traction to the tibia in the direction of the foot. While the first rescuer is applying traction, a second provider should apply pressure to the distal femur and proximal tibia. If the knee is dislocated anteriorly, apply pressure to the femur in the anterior direction and to the tibia in the opposite direction. In the case of a posterior dislocation, apply pressure in the opposite manner, with the tibia pressed anteriorly and the femur pressed posteriorly. Once the reduction has been accomplished, check the patient's neurovascular status and splint the leg securely. If the attempt at reduction fails, splint the knee in the position in which it is found and undertake rapid transportation to an appropriate facility.

Tendon Lacerations, Transections, and Ruptures

Knee Injury
The knee can be twisted during sports, resulting in potential laceration, transection, or rupture of the anterior cruciate ligament, the posterior cruciate ligament, the lateral collateral ligament, or the medial collateral ligament. Compression injury can result from a direct blow to the knee. Lateral and medial sprains can occur from abnormal twisting.

In addition, the knee can be hyperextended (stretched beyond its usual ROM) or can experience a torsion injury when the foot is fixed but the body pulls in another direction.

Shoulder Injury
Sternoclavicular sprain can occur from a direct blow, or from twisting of a posteriorly extended arm. Also, rotator cuff injury can occur from a violent pull on the arm, an abnormal rotation, or a fall on an outstretched arm. Rotator cuff injuries are often associated with chronic degenerative changes on the undersurface of the acromion.

Assessment and Management
Special assessment findings include muscle weakness, pain, edema, and loss of ROM. You should treat these as joint injuries and splint in place.

Principles of treating tendon injuries are the same as those used in treating other musculoskeletal injuries. Compare the symmetry of the injured limb with the opposite limb. Determine the extremity's ROM. Use cold packs, elevate the extremity, assess PMS function distal to the injury site, and stabilize if needed. As always, provide psychological support to the patient, and adjust your approach when working with a pediatric patient. If an athletic trainer is on site, he or she may have specialized knowledge of sports injuries and may be able to provide additional assistance.

Achilles Tendon Rupture

A rupture of the Achilles tendon usually occurs in athletes older than 30 years who are involved in start-and-stop sports such as basketball or football.

Assessment and Management
The most immediate indications are pain from the heel to the calf and a sudden inability for **plantar flexion** of the foot. As

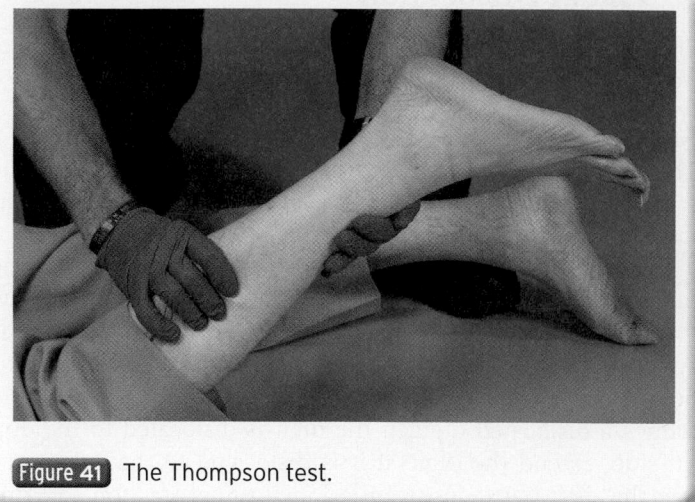

Figure 41 The Thompson test.

time passes, the calf muscles begin to contract proximally and a deformity within the calf may develop. The **Thompson test** can be performed in the field to identify an Achilles tendon rupture. To perform this test, have the patient assume a prone position and then squeeze the calf muscles of the injured leg **Figure 41**. If the foot plantarflexes while squeezing, the tendon is most likely intact. If there is no movement of the foot, the Achilles tendon has likely been torn.

Management of an Achilles tendon injury includes ICES and pain control. These injuries are treated with surgery or multiple casts and can require up to 6 months for recovery.

Pathophysiology, Assessment, and Management of Nontraumatic Musculoskeletal Disorders

Musculoskeletal complaints account for approximately 10% of all medical complaints in general medical practice and are one of the leading causes of disability in the United States. These complaints can range from those requiring minimal treatment and evaluation to those necessitating extensive systematic testing, examination, and treatment. Both a systematic physical examination and thorough history are necessary to appropriately evaluate and treat patients with musculoskeletal problems.

Patients presenting with nontraumatic musculoskeletal disorders generally do not have an acute life-threatening condition, although frequently a concern for the neurovascular status of an affected limb exists. Nontraumatic musculoskeletal disorders can be complex medical issues encompassing aspects of rheumatology, neurology, oncology, hematology, and infectious diseases. Generally these patients have a history of musculoskeletal disorders and are already under a physician's care. It is important to ask whether the patient is following the advice given, that is, is the patient compliant with medications and physical therapy.

Bony Abnormalities

Osteomyelitis

Osteomyelitis is a bacterial infection of the bone. It can be caused by systemic or local infections, and can develop in people with weakened immune systems, such as those with diabetes, the elderly, or drug addicts. Any open wound over a bone or decubitus ulcer can lead to an infection, resulting in osteomyelitis.

The signs and symptoms of osteomyelitis are the same as in any infection. These can include fever, chills, erythema over the site, swelling, and pain. It can be a slow or rapid onset.

EMS treatment is recognition, splinting, and transport. The patient will need antibiotics and often surgery to treat the disease.

Tumors

A tumor is a growth of abnormal tissue. Bone tumors can cause pathologic fractures in the bone as they increase in size. These tumors can be benign or malignant. The most common primary tumors of the bone are multiple myelomas, Ewing's sarcoma (mostly found in children and adolescents), osteosarcoma, and chondrosarcoma.

Usually there will be pain in the affected area. There may be signs of infection such as night sweats or difficulty in using the affected extremity, but there may be no pain or discomfort at all. Swelling or a mass of tissue at the bone site is possible. You should compare the extremities for asymmetry. Splint the area of concern and transport for further evaluation.

Disorders of the Spine

Back pain affects up to 90% of the population at some point and is a common presenting complaint for patients who call for EMS. Most of these patients will have no definite physical or historical cause for their complaint. Back pain is assessed into three categories: acute (less than 6 weeks in duration), subacute (from 6 to 12 weeks), and chronic (greater than 12 weeks). Because most back pain resolves within 4 weeks, pain lasting longer than 4 weeks warrants additional examination. Patients whose conditions fall into the chronic category who are younger than 18 years have a higher incidence of congenital abnormalities, while those older than 50 years have a greater chance of the pain having an intraabdominal, tumor, or vascular cause.

Due to exertional stress or overloading, patients may present with a variety of muscular back sprains and strains of varying severity. These patients should be assessed for any associated trauma and transported in a position of comfort.

Assessment of the patient with lower back pain should consist of obtaining a history including a SAMPLE history, examination of the ABCs, and evaluation of pain levels. A typical finding with a spinal disorder is a diminishing pain level with decreased movement. A patient who is writhing in pain suggests the potential for a more severe underlying process, such as abdominal aortic aneurysm or epidural abscess.

Physical examination of the back should include looking for contusions or abrasions consistent with trauma, warmth or drainage suggesting infection, and point tenderness with percussion along the spine, indicating possible bacterial infection.

Pain increasing with leg straightening while supine may indicate a lower back herniated disk, particularly if the pain radiates to below the level of the knee.

Any patient with a suspected nontraumatic spinal disorder should undergo a neurologic and function examination prior to movement. Patients with scoliosis or kyphosis could require you to adapt your transportation modalities.

Cauda Equina Syndrome

Cauda equina syndrome is caused by spinal cord compression due to a tumor, herniated disk, infection, or hematoma. A differentiating factor between back pain and cauda equina is the presence of neurologic involvement.

The most common sensory deficit in cauda equina cases is in the buttocks, perineum, and posterior-superior thighs in a "saddle–like" distribution pattern. Often these patients will report urinary retention or sudden loss of bowel or bladder incontinence. Any patient presenting with back pain and bowel or bladder symptoms of any type warrants urgent transport to an emergency department and consultation with a spine surgeon.

Spinal Stenosis

Spinal stenosis is a narrowing of the spinal canal that can occur at single or multiple levels.

Patients with spinal stenosis will report back pain usually exacerbated by prolonged standing and extension, and relieved by rest and spinal flexion.

These patients should be placed in a position of comfort if transport is required.

Joint Abnormalities

Arthritis

Arthritis means inflammation of a joint. Arthritic complaints are a common cause of pain leading to activation of EMS. Arthritis can have multiple etiologies and presentations and can lead to joint destruction, sepsis, and death in the worst cases. The three most common types of arthritis are osteoarthritis (OA), rheumatoid arthritis (RA), and gouty arthritis.

Osteoarthritis (OA) is a disease of the joints that occurs as they age and begin to wear. In general, the risk of developing OA increases with age, but other factors also increase the risk, such as obesity and prior joint injury.

Rheumatoid arthritis (RA) is a systemic inflammatory disease that affects joints and other body systems. RA can be a mild and nonprogressive disease, or can be a full-blown, fatal illness. In RA, significant bone erosion at the affected joints makes them more susceptible to fractures and dislocations. Of particular concern is the cervical spine, which is at high risk of subluxating following trauma or during intubation.

Gout, or crystal-induced arthritis, is a condition in which the body has difficulty eliminating uric acid (hyperuricemia), and the result is buildup of the salts of uric acid. When the concentration of uric acid in the blood becomes too great, the uric acid may crystallize within the synovial fluids of a joint.

<u>Septic arthritis</u> typically involves the knee, shoulder, hip, ankle, elbow, wrist, or knee. This condition is caused by a bacterial infection such as *Streptococcus* or *Staphylococcus*.

OA is characterized by pain and stiffness, which typically get worse with use, and "cracking" or "crunching" of the affected joints. The spine, hands, knees, and hips are the most commonly affected sites.

For the patient with RA, inflammation of almost any joint combination is possible; however, symmetric involvement of the hands, feet, or wrists are most common. Its onset can be either insidious or acute.

The patient with gout will have a hot, red, swollen joint with decreased ROM. Greater than 50% of cases involve the big toe, although the ailment can present in multiple other locations, such as fingers, elbow joints, and as kidney stones.

Patients with septic arthritis may have a history of IV drug use and a fulminant presentation of a marked toxicity, fever, and altered level of consciousness. In elderly patients septic arthritis can have a more insidious onset with malaise, anorexia, and lack of fever. Multiple joint involvements occur in approximately 10% of patients.

Treatment of OA involves low-impact physical therapy, pain control, anti-inflammatory medications, joint injections, and, in severe cases, joint replacement surgery.

Give extra attention to the cervical spine of a patient with RA to prevent further injury. Primary medical treatment typically includes use of various nonsteroidal anti-inflammatory drugs (NSAIDs).

> ### Special Populations
>
> There are multiple forms of juvenile arthritis; however, the causes are unknown. Diagnosis is based on medical history and a continuous observation of the patient. Treatment will be based on the patient's history and presentation, and will primarily be supportive. In extreme cases, pain management may be considered.

Prehospital treatment of gout involves stabilization, pain relief (NSAIDs and corticosteroids), and transportation to an emergency department, where the fluid in the joint can be aspirated to search for the characteristic crystals of gouty arthritis. Primary treatment then relies on dietary and lifestyle changes to reduce uric acid levels.

Slipped Capital Femoral Epiphysis

<u>Slipped capital femoral epiphysis (SCFE)</u> is a problem in the hip that affects the epiphysis of the femur. It occurs in children and adolescents. It is also more prominently found in overweight children compared with children of normal weight. SCFE is considered a pediatric disease.

Unless there are signs of trauma, SCFE is a gradual-onset condition. The most common signs are difficulty in walking and a noticeable limp. Sometimes the patient will not be able to bear any weight on the limb. There may be pain at the hip, and normal flexion and rotation will be painful and limited.

■ Muscle Disorders

Muscle disorders can present in a wide variety of ways, from simple overuse syndromes to serious viral illnesses. The term <u>myalgia</u> refers to muscle pain that is a symptom of some other underlying issue. The most common cause is simple stress or straining of the muscle, but may involve viral infections, nutritional deficiencies, or metabolic myopathy. Medication-induced myalgia can be caused by vaccinations, angiotensin-converting enzyme inhibitors, cholesterol-lowering medication, and cocaine use. Diseases resulting in a symptom of myalgia can range from the common flu, Lyme disease, malaria, roundworm (trichinosis), lupus, and muscle abscesses.

As mentioned, the most common cause of myalgia is a repetitive strain injury or muscle overuse. These can be caused by ergonomic conditions such as repetitive motion for extended periods of time or prolonged use of a body part in a less than optimal position. A common symptom is short periods of intense pain in a diffuse area of the body. The pain typically gets worse with activity and can subside with rest. Treatment primarily relies on cessation of activity and NSAID treatment for inflammation and pain.

■ Overuse Syndromes

Tendinitis and Bursitis

When a muscle is subjected to frequent, repetitive use, its tendon or nearby bursa is at risk for becoming inflamed. When inflammation of the tendon causes pain, the patient is said to have <u>tendinitis</u>. When a bursa becomes painful and inflamed, it is called <u>bursitis</u>.

With tendinitis, there will typically be point tenderness on the inflamed tendon, with pain often increasing if the person performs the movement that led to the inflammation. Patients with bursitis often complain of pain in the region of the inflamed bursa, especially with motions that cause the space where the bursa sits to become smaller. Examination of the site may reveal tenderness, swelling, erythema, and warmth.

Tendinitis and bursitis are treated with ICES and pain relievers. In many cases, in-hospital treatment also includes corticosteroid injections.

Carpal and Cubital Tunnel Syndromes

In contrast with the diffuse, nonanatomically specific form of most myalgias, syndromes such as <u>carpal tunnel syndrome</u> or <u>cubital tunnel syndrome</u> present with specific anatomic symptoms that are more readily identifiable. The symptoms of carpal tunnel syndrome are caused by compression of the median nerve at the wrist where it passes through the carpal canal. This compression can be caused by inflammation and swelling of tissue around the canal, by narrowing of the canal, or by pressure from outside the canal. Similarly, in cubital tunnel syndrome, also known as ulnar nerve entrapment, the ulnar nerve is compressed at the cubital tunnel along the outer edge of the elbow.

Patients with carpal tunnel syndrome have numbness and tingling in the hands, in particular to the index, thumb, and middle fingers that are innervated by the median nerve. Cubital tunnel syndrome exhibits burning, numbness, tingling, and possible partial loss of function of the "pinkie" finger, and in the medial aspect of the ring finger.

Prehospital management of both cubital and carpal tunnel syndromes includes recognition, splinting, and transport. Definitive treatment of both syndromes includes rest of the affected extremity, removal of the underlying cause (typically occupational or positional), and possibly physical therapy. In the worst cases, surgical decompression of the canal may be required.

Polyneuropathy

In contrast to the nerve compression of tunnel syndromes, peripheral neuropathy, or peripheral nerve syndrome, stems from actual nerve damage of the peripheral nervous system. Causes are potentially numerous, and in a majority of cases the pathophysiology is not well understood. In the prehospital environment, it is important for you to obtain a comprehensive history to help determine onset, duration, patterns, and symmetry of symptoms; this information ultimately helps a physician in beginning to make a diagnosis and initiate treatment of the patient with peripheral neuropathy.

Polyneuropathy occurs when there is simultaneous dysfunction of multiple peripheral nerves. Symptoms can present as motor, sensory, or both. Polyneuropathies can develop over days to weeks, and are considered to be an acute condition. The most significant polyneuropathy is Guillain-Barré syndrome. This syndrome has an unclear etiology, but results in inflammation and demyelination of peripheral nerves. Typically, the patient has a recent history of illness such as an upper respiratory tract infection, surgery, or vaccination. Motor weakness begins proximally and progresses during a period of days to weeks in an ascending fashion to full motor paralysis. The illness typically peaks in 10 to 14 days; however, recovery can take months, and full recovery is sometimes not possible.

Poliomyelitis is a polyneuropathy affecting the musculoskeletal system in a less organized and more centralized pattern than Guillain-Barré syndrome. It produces asymmetric paralysis primarily of the lower extremities and by definition does not include sensory loss. The greatest risk in poliomyelitis is of respiratory muscle paralysis. Progression of paralysis stops when the patient becomes afebrile. Due to effective vaccination programs, poliomyelitis is exceeding rare in the United States today.

Most cases of polyneuropathy that you will see will be acute cases. Because the causes are often unknown, PPE is essential. ABCs, current history, and transport are mandated so that a definitive diagnosis can be reached at the hospital. Pain management should be considered.

◼ Soft-Tissue Infections

Myositis

Myositis, or inflammation of the muscle, can be caused by injury or infection. It can also be caused by overuse of a muscle. In some cases it is considered to be an autoimmune disorder.

Treatment will be based on the patient's complaint and history. Some signs to look for include signs of infection (fever), muscle weakness, and fatigue on exertion. These symptoms generally will not be considered life threatening. Treatment is based on patient presentation. Transport the patient to the hospital for definitive diagnosis.

Fasciitis

Fasciitis is inflammation of the fascia. The most serious form of this condition is called necrotizing fasciitis, "the flesh eating" disease. It is rare, but 25% of people who get this disease will die from it. It is an infection caused by bacteria.

Recognition of this disease by EMS personnel is particularly difficult but critical because early intervention is crucial. Look for a history of vector transmission, insect bites, or jellyfish stings. Skin at the site may be reddened and warm; additional symptoms include fever, night sweats, chills, vomiting, and diarrhea. It is important to take standard precautions and properly handle contaminated articles, such as clothing, to limit exposure. Transport to the hospital for diagnosis.

Gangrene

Gangrene is caused when blood supply delivery to tissue is interrupted or stopped. Gangrene is referred to as "wet" or "dry." Wet gangrene causes sepsis and the patient can die within hours. Dry gangrene can take months to develop. Gangrene is usually caused by diseases such as diabetes or atherosclerotic peripheral vascular disease. Smokers are more likely to develop symptoms because their peripheral vasculature is compromised. Gangrene can also be caused by traumatic injuries such as burns, frostbite, or wounds.

Gangrene should be suspected if the patient has chronic risk factors such as diabetes and there is numbness, coolness, or swelling of an extremity. Also, gangrene (particularly wet gangrene) has a very bad odor. Late signs of gangrene also will be characterized by discoloration of the limb to black, blue, or red. Treatment involves transporting to a suitable facility, and also being sure to take standard precautions. Treatment in the hospital may involve amputation or surgical debridement of the affected area. Antibiotics may also be used.

Paronychia

Paronychia is the most common infection of the hand in the United States. It is a bacterial infection located near the nail plate. If not recognized and treated, it can spread through the hand and into the circulatory and lymphatic systems.

A small pustule or redness, with or without pus, will be present. There may be an abscess at the site. Transport for antibiotic therapy or lancing of the abscess.

Flexor Tenosynovitis of the Hand

Flexor tenosynovitis of the hand is caused by an infection that is usually the result of penetrating trauma to the hand. It involves the sheath of the tendons that flex the fingers. Signs include inability to extend the involved finger, pain, and swelling along the path of the tendon. It also occurs chronically in patients with a history of RA. It can also occur due to overuse of the hand.

The presentation of this condition may be swelling, redness, and limited mobility in the hand. Pay particular attention to patients with a history of RA. Transport the patient so he or she can receive definitive treatment for the infection and possible orthopaedic intervention.

YOU are the Medic SUMMARY

1. What are your initial assessment and treatment priorities?

Initial assessment priorities include assessing for head and spinal cord injuries, occult abdominal trauma, and bleeding from multiple fractures. The patient is feeling sleepy and weak and has a rapid radial pulse. Therefore treatment priorities will focus on treatment for possible shock. In addition, treatment priorities include spinal precautions and supporting airway and breathing.

2. What other information would you obtain about the patient and the incident?

It is important to attempt to understand why the patient fell. What does the patient recall regarding the event? Are alcohol or drugs involved? Or can any information be revealed from the patient's medical history or recent health complaints?

3. What are your early communication and transport plans?

Effective early communication with the receiving facility and transport to a trauma center will improve this patient's outcome. Depending on your location, you may consider transport by air.

4. What do these physical findings indicate to you?

His pale, cool, moist skin could be a result of peripheral-vascular shunting as seen in early stages of shock. When the sympathetic nervous system stimulates the release of epinephrine and norepinephrine from the adrenal glands, peripheral vasoconstriction occurs and the sweat glands are opened. Deformity to his bilateral wrists, femurs, and lower extremities are most likely due to fractures.

5. Why is a history of type 1 diabetes significant?

The history of type 1 diabetes may explain the report of feeling light-headed during the past few days and may have contributed to the same complaint experienced before he fell. His blood glucose level should be checked.

6. What can you conclude from the patient's vital signs?

The patient's blood pressure is normal, but his pulse rate is rapid. The patient's tachycardia could be caused by the body's attempt to compensate for blood loss. Considering his physical exam findings, the tachycardia could be a sign of shock.

7. Why is a blood glucose reading of 51 mg/dL significant?

According to the American Diabetic Association, a normal random glucose level should be between 70 and 125 mg/dL. Therefore his blood glucose level is too low. This would explain his feeling of light-headedness and possibly the cause of him falling off the ladder. The finding that his mental status improved after the IV administration of glucose also supports this thinking.

8. Why should this patient be transported to a trauma center?

Trauma patients in all age groups benefit from transport to trauma centers. Transport of this patient to a trauma center will improve this patient's outcome. Depending on your location you may consider transport by air.

9. What do his vital signs indicate?

The level of tachycardia has increased, indicating that the body is compensating for shock. The patient is now hypotensive, indicating that internal bleeding from multiple long bone fractures is significant.

10. What do absent pedal pulses, absent motor function, and lack of sensation to the toes indicate?

Absent pedal pulses, absent motor function, and lack of sensation to his toes may indicate neurovascular damage to his extremities. It may also be a result of poor peripheral circulation secondary to his hypotension.

11. Why is it important to treat the patient's pain?

It is very important to make the patient comfortable and treat his pain because pain causes unfavorable physiologic changes in perception and vital signs. However, careful monitoring is required when narcotic analgesics are given to trauma patients with probable internal hemorrhage. Remember that side effects of narcotic analgesics include respiratory depression, bradycardia, and hypotension.

YOU are the Medic   SUMMARY, continued

EMS Patient Care Report (PCR)

Date: 10-15-11	Incident No.: 128	Nature of Call: Fall		Location: 12301 Matthews Lane	
Dispatched: 1304	En Route: 1305	At Scene: 1311	Transport: 1327	At Hospital: 1342	In Service: 1412

Patient Information

Age: 24 Sex: M Weight (in kg [lb]): 75 kg (150 lb)	Allergies: No known drug allergies Medications: Humulin and Novolog Past Medical History: Type 1 diabetes Chief Complaint: Bilateral wrist, thigh, and lower extremity pain

Vital Signs

Time: 1316	BP: 104/60	Pulse: 116	Respirations: 24	Spo$_2$: 98%
Time: 1321	BP: 94/53	Pulse: 122	Respirations: 24	Spo$_2$: 98%
Time: 1326	BP: 84/44	Pulse: 128	Respirations: 24	Spo$_2$: 98%
Time: 1331	BP: 95/56	Pulse: 110	Respirations: 20	Spo$_2$: 98%

EMS Treatment
(circle all that apply)

Oxygen @ __4__ L/min via (circle one): (NC) NRM Bag-mask device	Assisted Ventilation	Airway Adjunct:	CPR
Defibrillation	Bleeding Control	Bandaging	(Splinting:) Wrists, femurs, & lower extremities	(Other:) IV NS lock #16 GA left AC Cervical stabilization 50 mg fentanyl IVP Blankets

Narrative

Pt 24-year-old male roofer who fell about 20 feet, landing on his feet impacting the lawn. On arrival found pt lying supine on ground alert and oriented x 3, but slow to answer questions. Skin is pale, cool, and moist. Obvious deformity observed to bilateral wrists, bilateral femurs, and bilateral lower extremities. Pt recalls entire event and denies LOC, neck pain, numbness/tingling in extremities, headache, nausea/vomiting, abdominal pain, chest pain, or dyspnea, but states he was "light-headed" while climbing the ladder before he fell. Complains of bilateral wrist pain, bilateral femur pain, low back pain, and bilateral lower extremity pain. Pain an "8" on "0-10" scale. Fitted pt with c-collar and immobilized to long backboard. After splinting, pedal pulses are absent, sensation to toes is absent, and the pt is unable to move his toes upon command. Blood glucose 51 mg/dL. D$_{50}$ 25 grams IVP given per protocol. Improved to 126 mg/dL. En route medical direction is called and spoke to Dr. Hartmann who advised a 500-mL NS IV bolus and gave orders for fentanyl 50 mcg IVP PRN and as vital signs permit. Fentanyl 50 mcg IVP given and 500-mL NS IV bolus given. Pain now a "3" on "0-10" scale and blood glucose is 122 mg/dL. Transported pt to St. Anthony's Hospital room #14 and report given to Julia, RN. No pt belongings transported. **End of report**

Prep Kit

- Injuries and complaints related to the musculoskeletal system are one of the most common reasons that patients seek medical attention.

- Musculoskeletal injuries are sometimes very dramatic, but attention should not be focused on them until life-threatening conditions have been addressed.

- You have a vital role in reducing the complications associated with musculoskeletal injuries by promptly and effectively splinting injured extremities.

- Assume the existence of a fracture whenever a patient who reports a musculoskeletal injury has deformity, bruising, decreased range of motion, or swelling.

- Always perform and record an accurate neurovascular examination before and after splinting an injured extremity.

- Check penetrating injuries for underlying fractures or other musculoskeletal injury.

- Musculoskeletal injuries are likely to be accompanied by hemorrhage.

- When a dislocation is associated with absent distal pulses, obtain medical direction to determine whether the injury should be reduced.

- Look for injuries to the chest and abdomen, and fully stabilize the spine when patients have evidence of a high-energy injury, such as a femoral shaft or scapular fracture.

- Because fractures may be associated with significant blood loss, resuscitation with IV fluid may be necessary.

- Pelvic fractures are potentially lethal injuries owing to the massive potential for blood loss.

- Posterior sternoclavicular joint dislocations are potentially fatal due to possible damage to underlying structures.

- *Never forget the ABCs!* Do not become distracted; the fracture can wait if airway, breathing, or circulation problems are noted.

- Pediatric fractures are different in that the bones of children contain growth plates that are weaker and make children more susceptible to fractures than sprains. Joint dislocations do not usually occur without an associated fracture. Such an injury can occur from a low-energy mechanism of injury (MOI), and the usual tenderness, swelling, and bruising may not be present.

- Remember to consider whether the MOI suggests possible abuse. Observe the relationship between the parent and child. Adjust your approach to one that is appropriate for the child's age.

- Musculoskeletal injuries can lead to numerous complications, including vascular injuries, neurovascular injuries, compartment syndrome, crush syndrome, and thromboembolic disease.

- Blood vessels can be damaged following a musculoskeletal injury. Loss of blood flow to the area of the musculoskeletal injury is called devascularization.

- Neurovascular injuries include impalement or laceration of nerves of a plexus, leading to a neurologic deficit. Neurovascular injuries can also occur following a joint dislocation.

- Compartment syndrome occurs when bleeding or swelling increases within a compartment to the point that the pressure within that compartment impairs circulation. This can cause pain, sensory changes, and muscle death.

- Crush syndrome occurs when a prolonged compressive force impairs muscle metabolism and circulation. When the compressive force is released, toxins enter the patient's circulation.

- Nontraumatic musculoskeletal disorders can be highly complex medical issues encompassing aspects of rheumatology, neurology, oncology, hematology, and infectious diseases. Nontraumatic musculoskeletal disorders include bony abnormalities such as osteomyelitis and tumors, disorders of the spine including low back pain and disc disorders, joint abnormalities, muscle abnormalities, overuse syndromes, and soft-tissue infections.

- Slipped capital femoral epiphysis (SCFE) is a problem in the hip that affects the epiphysis of the femur. It occurs in children and adolescents. The most common sign is difficulty in walking and possible pain at the hip. Transport these patients for evaluation.

- Types of arthritis include osteoarthritis, rheumatoid arthritis, gout, and septic arthritis. Gout can be treated with immobilization, pain relief, and transport.

- Muscle disorders include myalgia and myositis. Myalgia is muscle pain that is a symptom of some other underlying issue. Myositis is inflammation of the muscle. Treatment will be based on the patient's complaint and history. Transport for definitive diagnosis.

- Tendinitis and bursitis are overuse syndromes, which occur from frequent and repetitive use which results in inflammation. Tendinitis and bursitis are treated with ICES, pain relievers, and steroid injections.

- Paramedics may encounter patients with numbness, tingling, or pain in their wrist or hand. This can be from carpal tunnel syndrome or cubital tunnel syndrome. Prehospital treatment includes recognition, splinting, and transport.

- Polyneuropathy, or peripheral nerve syndrome, stems from actual nerve damage of the peripheral nervous system. Good history taking is important to provide a basis for a physician to begin diagnosis and treatment. Also, prehospital pain management should be considered.

- Soft-tissue infections include fasciitis, gangrene, paronychia, and flexor tenosynovitis of the hand.
- Fasciitis is inflammation of the fascia. The most serious form is necrotizing fasciitis. Recognition of this by EMS personnel is difficult but critical. Look for a history of vector transmission, insect bites, or jellyfish stings. Take standard precautions, properly handle contaminated articles, and transport to the hospital for diagnosis.
- Gangrene is caused when blood supply to tissue is interrupted or stopped. Suspect gangrene if the patient has chronic risk factors such as diabetes and there is numbness, coolness, or swelling of an extremity, and there is a very bad odor. Take standard precautions and transport.
- Paronychia is a bacterial infection located near the nail plate. If not recognized and treated, it can spread through the hand and into the circulatory and lymphatic systems. It is seen as a small pustule or redness, with or without pus. Provide transport.
- Flexor tenosynovitis of the hand is caused by an infection that is usually the result of penetrating trauma to the hand. Symptoms include swelling, redness, and limited mobility in the hand. Pay particular attention to patients with a history of rheumatoid arthritis, and provide transport.

■ Vital Vocabulary

__6 Ps of musculoskeletal assessment__ Pain, Paralysis, Parasthesias, Pulselessness, Pallor, and Pressure.

__abduction__ Movement *away* from the midline of the body.

__acetabulum__ The cup-shaped cavity in which the rounded head of the femur rotates.

__acromion__ Lateral extension of the scapula that forms the highest point of the shoulder.

__adduction__ Movement *toward* the midline of the body.

__amputation__ Severing of a part of the body.

__angulation__ The presence of an abnormal angle or bend in an extremity.

__anterior tibial artery__ The artery that travels through the anterior muscles of the leg and continues to the foot as the dorsalis pedis.

__appendicular skeleton__ The part of the skeleton comprising the upper and lower extremities.

__arthritis__ Inflammation of the joints.

__articulations__ The locations where two or more bones meet; *joints*.

__atrophy__ Wasting away of a tissue.

__avascular necrosis__ Tissue death resulting from the loss of blood supply.

__avulsion fracture__ A fracture that occurs when a piece of bone is torn free at the site of attachment of a tendon or ligament.

__axial skeleton__ The part of the skeleton comprising the skull, spinal column, and rib cage.

__axilla__ The armpit.

__axillary artery__ The artery that runs through the axilla, connecting the subclavian artery to the brachial artery.

__bowing fracture__ An incomplete fracture typically occurring in children in which the bone becomes bent as the result of a compressive force.

__boxer's fracture__ A fracture of the head of the fifth metacarpal that usually results from striking an object with a clenched fist.

__brachial artery__ The artery that runs through the arm and branches into the radial and ulnar arteries.

__buckle fracture__ A common incomplete fracture in children in which the cortex of the bone fractures from an excessive compression force; also called a torus fracture.

__buddy splinting__ Securing an injured digit to an adjacent uninjured one to allow the intact digit to act as a splint.

__bursa__ A fluid-filled sac located adjacent to joints that reduces the amount of friction between moving structures.

__bursitis__ Inflammation of a bursa.

__calcaneus__ The heel bone; the largest of the tarsal bones.

__cancellous bone__ Trabecular or spongy bone.

__carpal tunnel syndrome__ Compression of the median nerve at the wrist where it passes through the carpal canal, causing numbness and tingling in the hand, and possibly pain.

__carpals__ The eight small bones of the wrist.

__cartilage__ Tough, elastic substance that covers opposable surfaces of moveable joints and forms part of the skeleton.

__cartilaginous joints__ Joints that are spanned completely by cartilage and allow for minimal motion.

__cauda equina syndrome__ A neurologic condition caused by spinal cord compression.

__clavicle__ The collarbone.

__closed fracture__ A fracture in which the skin is not broken.

__comminuted fracture__ A fracture in which the bone is broken into three or more pieces.

__compartment syndrome__ An increase in tissue pressure in a closed fascial space or compartment that compromises the circulation to the nerves and muscles within the involved compartment.

__complete fracture__ A fracture in which the bone is broken into two or more completely separate pieces.

__compound fracture__ An open fracture; a fracture beneath an open wound.

__crepitus__ A grating sensation felt when moving the ends of a broken bone.

__crush syndrome__ A condition that arises after a body part that has been compressed for a significant period is released, leading to the entry of potassium and other metabolic toxins into the systemic circulation.

cubital tunnel syndrome Compression of the ulnar nerve at the tunnel along the outer edge of the elbow, causing numbness, tingling, and possible partial loss of function of the little finger and medial aspect of the ring finger.

deep vein thrombosis (DVT) The formation of a blood clot within the larger veins of an extremity, typically following a period of prolonged stabilization.

depression fracture A fracture in which the broken region of the bone is pushed deeper into the body than the remaining intact bone.

devascularization The loss of blood to a part of the body.

diaphysis The shaft of a long bone.

diastasis An increase in the distance between the two sides of a joint.

digital arteries The arteries that supply blood to the fingers and toes.

dislocation The displacement of a bone from its normal position within a joint.

displaced fracture A break in which the ends of the fractured bone move out of their normal positions.

distraction injury An injury that results from a force that tries to increase the length of a body part or separate one body part from another.

dorsal Referring to the back or posterior side of the body or an organ.

dorsiflex To bend the foot or hand backward.

endosteum The inner lining of a hollow bone.

epiphysis The end region of a long bone extending between the metaphysis and the articulate (joint) surface.

fascia A strong, fibrous membrane that covers, supports, and separates muscles.

fasciitis Inflammation of the fascia.

fatigue fractures Fractures that result from multiple compressive loads.

femoral artery The main artery supplying the thigh and leg.

femoral shaft fractures A break in the diaphysis of the femur.

femur The proximal bone of the leg that extends from the pelvis to the knee.

fibrous joints The joints that contain dense fibrous tissue and allow for no motion.

fibula The smaller of the two bones of the lower leg.

flat bones Bones that are thin and broad, such as the scapula.

flexor tenosynovitis of the hand A closed-space infection of the hand.

fracture A break or rupture in the bone.

gangrene Dying or dead tissue due to nonsupply of blood to the tissues.

glenoid fossa Socket in the scapula in which the head of the humerus rotates.

gout A painful disorder characterized by the crystallization of uric acid within a joint.

greenstick fracture A type of fracture occurring most frequently in children in which there is incomplete breakage of the bone.

hematopoiesis The generation of blood cells.

humerus The bone of the upper arm.

hypertrophy An increase in size.

hyperuricemia High levels of uric acid in the blood.

ilium The broad, uppermost bone of the pelvis.

impacted fracture A broken bone in which the end of one bone becomes wedged into another bone, as could be the case in a fall from a significant height.

incomplete fracture A fracture in which the bone does not fully break.

indirect injury An injury that results from a force that is applied to one region of the body but leads to an injury in another area.

intertrochanteric fractures Fractures that occur in the region between the lesser and greater trochanters.

irregular bones Bones with unique shapes that allow them to perform a specific function and that do not fit into the other categories based on shape.

ischium The lowermost dorsal bone of the pelvis.

joint The point at which two or more bones articulate, or come together.

joint capsule A saclike envelope that encloses the cavity of a synovial joint.

lactic acid A metabolic end product of the breakdown of glucose that accumulates when metabolism proceeds in the absence of oxygen.

lateral compression A force that is directed from the side toward the midline of the body.

ligaments Tough bands of tissue that connect bone to bone around a joint or support internal organs within the body.

linear fracture A fracture that runs parallel to the long axis of a bone.

long bones Bones that are longer than they are wide.

luxation A complete dislocation.

malleolus The large, rounded, bony protuberance on either side of the ankle joint.

mallet finger An avulsion fracture of the extensor tendon of the distal phalynx caused by jamming a finger into an object.

march fractures *See* fatigue fractures.

medullary canal The hollow center portion of a long bone.

metacarpals The five bones that form the palm and back of the hand.

metaphysis The region of the long bone between the epiphysis and diaphysis.

metatarsals The five long bones extending from the tarsus to the phalanges of the foot.

muscle fatigue The condition that arises when a muscle depletes its supply of energy.

myalgia Muscle pain.

myositis Inflammation of the muscle, usually caused by infection.

neurovascular compromise The loss of the nerve supply, blood supply, or both to a region of the body, typically distal to a site of injury; characterized by alterations in sensation, including numbness and tingling, or by a loss or decrease of motor function; vascular compromise is indicated by weak or absent pulses, poor skin color, and cool skin.

nondisplaced fracture A break in which the bone remains aligned in its normal position.

nursemaid's elbow The subluxation of the radial head that often results from pulling on an outstretched arm.

oblique fracture A fracture that travels diagonally from one side of the bone to the other.

olecranon The proximal bony projection of the *ulna* at the elbow; the part of the ulna that constitutes the "funny bone."

open-book pelvic fracture A life-threatening fracture of the pelvis caused by a force that displaces one or both sides of the pelvis laterally and posteriorly.

open fracture Any break in a bone in which the overlying skin has been damaged.

ossification center Areas where cartilage is transformed through calcification into a new area of bone.

osteoarthritis (OA) The degeneration of a joint surface caused by wear and tear that lead to pain and stiffness.

osteoporosis A condition characterized by decreased bone density and increased susceptibility to fractures.

overriding The overlap of a bone that occurs from the muscle spasm that follows a fracture, leading to a decrease in the length of the bone.

paresthesias Abnormal sensations such as burning, numbness, or tingling.

paronychia Infection of the area around the fingernail bed.

patella The kneecap.

pathologic fracture A fracture that occurs in an area of abnormally weakened bone.

pectoral girdle The shoulder girdle.

pelvic girdle The large bone that arises in the area of the last nine vertebrae and sweeps around to form a complete ring.

periosteum The fibrous tissue that covers bone.

phalanges The bones of the fingers or toes.

physis The growth plate in long bones.

plantar Referring to the sole of the foot.

plantar flexion Bending of the foot toward the ground.

point tenderness The tenderness that is sharply localized at the site of the injury, found by gently palpating along the bone with the tip of one finger.

polyneuropathy A type of disorder in which multiple nerves become dysfunctional.

popliteal artery The artery in the area or space behind the knee joint.

posterior tibial artery The artery that travels through the calf muscles to the plantar aspect of the foot.

pronation The act of turning the palm of the hand backward or downward, performed by internal rotation of the forearm.

pubic symphysis The midline articulation of the pubic bones.

pubis One of two bones that form the anterior portion of the pelvic ring.

pulmonary embolism Obstruction of a pulmonary artery or arteries by solid, liquid, or gaseous material swept through the right side of the heart into the lungs.

radial artery The artery pertaining to the wrist.

radius The bone on the thumb side of the forearm.

range of motion (ROM) The arc of movement of an extremity at a joint in a particular direction.

recruitment The process of signaling additional muscle fibers to contract to create a more forceful contraction.

rhabdomyolysis The destruction of muscle tissue leading to a release of potassium and myoglobin.

rheumatoid arthritis (RA) An inflammatory disorder that affects the entire body and leads to degeneration and deformation of joints.

round bones The small bones that are found adjacent to joints that assist with motion.

sacroiliac joints The points of attachment of the *ilium* to the sacrum.

scaphoid The wrist bone that is found just beyond that most distal portion of the radius.

scapula The shoulder blade.

segmental fracture A bone that is broken in more than one place.

septic arthritis Inflammation of a joint based on a bacterial or fungal infection.

short bones The bones that are nearly as wide as they are long.

silver fork deformity The dorsal deformity of the forearm that results from a Colles fracture.

skeletal muscle Muscle that is attached to bones and usually crosses at least one joint; striated or voluntary muscle.

slipped capital femoral epiphysis (SCFE) A dislocation of the epiphyseal end of the femur, usually found in children and adolescents.

snuffbox The region at the base of the thumb where the scaphoid may be palpated.

somatic motor neurons The nerve fibers that transmit impulses to a muscle.

spinal stenosis Narrowing of the spinal canal, causing back pain that worsens with standing or walking.

spiral fracture A break in a bone that appears like a spring on a radiograph.

sprains Injuries, including a stretch or a tear, to the ligaments of a joint that commonly lead to pain and swelling.

straddle fracture A fracture of the pelvis that results from landing on the perineal region.

strain Stretching or tearing of a muscle by excessive stretching or overuse.

stress fracture A fracture that results from exaggerated stress on the bone caused by unusually rapid muscle development.

striated muscle Skeletal muscle that is under voluntary control.

subclavian artery The artery that travels from the aorta to each upper extremity.

subluxation A partial or incomplete dislocation.

supination To turn the forearm laterally so that the palm faces forward (if standing) or upward (if lying supine).

supracondylar fractures Fractures of the distal humerus that occur just proximal to the elbow.

synovial joints Joints that permit movement of the component bones.

synovial membrane The lining of a joint that secretes synovial fluid into the joint space.

talus The bone of the foot that articulates with the tibia.

tarsals The ankle bones.

tendinitis Inflammation of a tendon that most commonly results from overuse.

tendons The fibrous portions of muscle that attach to bone.

Thompson test Squeezing of the calf muscle to evaluate for plantar flexion of the foot to determine whether the Achilles tendon is intact.

thromboembolic disease The condition in which a patient has a deep vein thrombosis or pulmonary embolism.

tibia The shinbone.

torus fracture *See* buckle fracture.

transverse fracture A fracture that runs in a straight line from one edge of the bone to the other and that is perpendicular to each edge.

twisting injuries Injuries that commonly occur during athletic activities in which an extremity rotates around a planted foot or hand.

ulna The larger bone of the forearm, on the side opposite the thumb.

ulnar artery The artery of the forearm that travels along its medial aspect.

vertical shear The type of pelvic fracture that occurs when a massive force displaces the pelvis superiorly.

volar Pertaining to the palm or sole; referring to the flexor surfaces of the forearm, wrist, or hand.

Volkmann ischemic contracture Contraction of the fingers and, sometimes, the wrist, with loss of muscular power with death and resultant contracture of the forearm musculature, that sets in rapidly after severe injury around the elbow joint.

voluntary muscle Muscle that can be controlled by a person.

Assessment in Action

You are dispatched to the scene of a 69-year-old woman who fell while dancing at her grand-daughter's wedding reception. When you arrive, you find the patient lying supine on the dance floor holding her right hip and grimacing in pain. According to the patient, she was dancing when she felt a "pop" in her right hip and then she fell, hitting her right leg on the wooden dance floor. She states she has a history of osteoporosis.

You observe that the right leg is abnormally rotated and shortened in contrast to the left leg. Pedal pulses are strong and regular bilaterally, and she has normal sensation to her toes but is unable to move them upon command. The patient is alert and oriented and states "my hip really hurts." She is reporting only intense right hip pain and denies associated trauma injuries. The patient's skin is pink, warm, and dry. Her vital signs are as follows: respirations, 24 breaths/min; pulse, 112 beats/min; and blood pressure, 126/68 mm Hg. A pulse oximetry reading is 98% on room air. The patient is placed on the stretcher in a supine position as requested with her right leg and hip supported with pillows and blankets. Her right femur and hip reveal swelling and ecchymosis. En route, a full-body exam is performed and found to be unremarkable except for her right hip deformity. A large-bore IV line is initiated and oxygen is applied. Medical direction is contacted and a narcotic analgesic is administered for pain. The patient is transported to the closest trauma center.

1. What type of fracture may be experienced in elderly patients?
   A. Pathologic fractures
   B. Fatigue fractures
   C. March fractures
   D. Twisting fractures

2. Which of the following occurs when the broken ends of a bone override one another?
   A. Lengthening
   B. Rupturing
   C. Shortening
   D. Dislocation

3. Swelling at the fracture site is due to:
   A. twisting of the bones.
   B. poor blood return.
   C. interruptions in nervous system stimulation.
   D. bleeding from the broken bone ends.

4. The clinical term that describes blood collecting under the skin is called:
   A. hemoptysis.
   B. pertussis.
   C. ecchymosis.
   D. hematemesis.

5. Palpation may reveal _____, which is described as a grating sensation over the broken bone ends.
   A. crepitus
   B. contusion
   C. ecchymosis
   D. paresthesia

6. A fracture or dislocation may result in a significant decrease in the:
   A. patient's blood glucose level.
   B. range of motion (ROM).
   C. red blood cell production.
   D. internal bleeding.

7. Fractures that cause a break in the overlying skin are called:
   A. closed fractures.
   B. distended fractures.
   C. wild fractures.
   D. open fractures.

Additional Questions

8. How should paramedics manage musculoskeletal injuries in the field when they cannot be differentiated as sprains, strains, or fractures?

9. What is the best approach to assessing musculoskeletal injuries?

Environmental Emergencies

National EMS Education Standard Competencies

Trauma

Integrates assessment findings with principles of epidemiology and pathophysiology to formulate a field impression to implement a comprehensive treatment/disposition plan for an acutely injured patient.

Environmental Emergencies

Recognition and management of
- Submersion incidents (pp 1821-1830)
- Temperature-related illness (pp 1808-1821)

Pathophysiology, assessment, and management of
- Near drowning (pp 1821-1824)
- Temperature-related illness (pp 1808-1821)
- Bites and envenomations (pp 1833-1840)
- Dysbarism
  - High-altitude (pp 1830-1832)
  - Diving injuries (pp 1824-1830)
- Electrical injury (pp 1832-1833)
- Radiation exposure (see chapter, *Burns*)
- High-altitude illness (pp 1830-1832)

Knowledge Objectives

1. Describe four factors that affect how a person deals with exposure to a cold or hot environment and how each one relates to emergency medical care. (p 1805)
2. Explain the four different ways a body can lose heat and ways the rate and amount of heat loss or gain can be modified in an emergency situation. (pp 1807-1808)
3. Describe the various forms of illnesses caused by heat exposure, including their signs and symptoms, and give examples of persons who are at the greatest risk of developing one of them. (pp 1808-1814)
4. Describe the process of providing emergency care to a patient who has sustained a heat injury, including assessment of the patient, review of signs and symptoms, and management of care. (pp 1808-1814)
5. Define and discuss hypothermia, including the signs and symptoms of its four different stages and the risk factors for developing it. (pp 1816-1820)
6. Explain local cold injuries and their underlying causes. (pp 1814-1816)
7. Describe the process of providing emergency care to a patient who has sustained a local cold injury, including assessment of the patient, review of signs and symptoms, and management of care. (pp 1814-1816)
8. Explain the importance of following regional and state protocols when rewarming a patient who is experiencing moderate or severe hypothermia. (pp 1819-1821)
9. Define drowning and discuss its incidence, risk factors, and prevention. (pp 1821-1824)

10. Describe the various types of diving emergencies, how they may occur, and their signs and symptoms. (pp 1824-1830)
11. Describe the process of providing emergency care to a patient who has been involved in a drowning or diving emergency, including assessment of the patient, review of signs and symptoms, and management of care. (pp 1822-1824, 1825-1830)
12. Discuss the types of dysbarism injuries that may be caused by high altitudes, including their signs and symptoms and emergency medical treatment in the field. (pp 1830-1832)
13. Discuss lightning injuries, including their incidence, risk factors, assessment, and emergency medical treatment. (pp 1832-1833)
14. Identify the species of spiders found in the United States that may cause life-threatening injuries, and then describe the process of providing emergency care to patients who have been bitten by each type. (pp 1837-1838)
15. Discuss the emergency medical care of patients who have been stung by hymenoptera and scorpions, and bitten by ticks, including steps the paramedic should follow if a patient develops a severe reaction to the sting or bite. (pp 1834-1835, 1839-1840)
16. Identify the species of snakes found in the United States that are venomous, and then describe the process of providing emergency care to patients who have been bitten by each type and are showing signs of envenomation. (pp 1835-1837)
17. Discuss the emergency medical care of a patient who has been bitten by a tick, and of a patient who experiences paralysis thereafter. (pp 1839-1840)

Skills Objectives

1. Demonstrate the emergency medical treatment of local cold injuries in the field. (pp 1814-1816)
2. Demonstrate using a warm-water bath to rewarm the limb of a patient who has sustained a local cold injury. (pp 1815-1816)
3. Demonstrate how to treat a patient with heat cramps. (pp 1809-1810)
4. Demonstrate how to treat a patient with heat exhaustion. (pp 1810-1811)
5. Demonstrate how to treat a patient with heatstroke. (pp 1811-1814)
6. Demonstrate how to care for a patient who is suspected of having an air embolism or decompression sickness following a diving emergency. (pp 1828-1829)
7. Demonstrate how to care for a patient who has been struck by lightning. (pp 1832-1833)
8. Demonstrate how to care for a patient who has been bitten by a black widow or brown recluse spider. (pp 1837-1839)
9. Demonstrate how to care for a patient who has been bitten by a pit viper and is showing signs of envenomation. (pp 1835-1837)
10. Demonstrate how to care for a patient who has been bitten by a coral snake and is showing signs of envenomation. (pp 1835-1837)
11. Demonstrate how to care for a patient who is experiencing altitude illness. (pp 1830-1832)
12. Demonstrate how to care for a patient who has been bitten by a tick. (pp 1839-1840)

Introduction

According to the Centers for Disease Control and Prevention, 4,607 people in the United States died of hypothermia-related causes from 1999 to 2002. During 1999 to 2003, 3,442 deaths were reported as resulting from exposure to extreme heat. The heat wave that afflicted Europe in the summer of 2003 was estimated to have caused as many as 70,000 deaths. **Environmental emergencies** are medical conditions caused or worsened by the weather, terrain, or unique atmospheric conditions present at high altitude or underwater. Most EMS providers would recognize the obvious problem of a child who has fallen into an icy lake. The challenge lies in recognizing patients with environmental emergencies in the unusual settings of endurance sports events or at mass gatherings, and even acutely confused older patients Figure 1.

Unique to environmental emergencies are the conditions that directly cause harm or complicate treatment and transport considerations. Wind, rain, snow, temperature extremes, and humidity may all affect the body's ability to adapt to its environment. Unprepared hikers can experience cold illnesses during summer rainstorms as easily as overdressed snow sports enthusiasts can die of heat illnesses during strenuous outings. The locations of these outings can also have a huge impact on the ability to know about, respond to, and rescue people in remote settings Figure 2.

Certain common risk factors predispose people to environmental emergencies. In addition, young and older people have unique disadvantages when it comes to thermoregulation. Conditions such as diabetes, cardiac disease (for example, coronary artery disease, congestive heart failure), restrictive lung disease, thyroid disease, and psychiatric illnesses can alter the body's

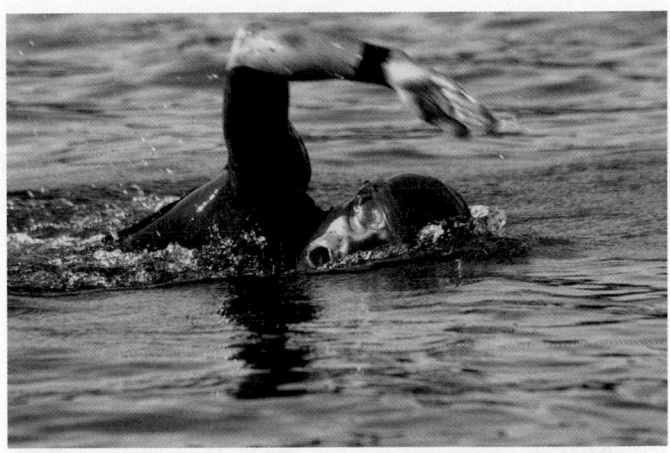

Figure 1 Environmental emergencies can occur in a variety of settings, including endurance sports events.

YOU *are the Medic* PART 1

You are dispatched to the scene of a private residence for a 20-year-old man who came stumbling home after falling through the ice while out riding his snowmobile. His mother tells you he walked home, approximately half a mile. She states she had him remove his clothes; she then wrapped him in a warm blanket and gave him some hot coffee. She went to prepare a warm bath when she heard a "thud" in the kitchen. When she entered the kitchen, she found him sitting on the floor and he "wasn't acting right," so she called EMS. The current ambient temperature outside is 36°F.

When you arrive, you find the patient sitting on the kitchen floor alert and shivering. He responds to your voice but has difficulty answering questions. His face is pink, but his lips are dusky. He recalls the event and denies any injuries, but reports "aching all over" and "feeling weak and sleepy."

Recording Time: 1 Minute	
Appearance	Eyes open and shivering
Level of consciousness	V (responsive to verbal stimuli)
Airway	Patent with clear speech
Breathing	Nonlabored, slow, and shallow
Circulation	Rapid radial pulse; no obvious external bleeding

1. What are your assessment and treatment priorities?
2. What other information would you obtain about the patient and the incident?
3. What are your early communication and transport plans?

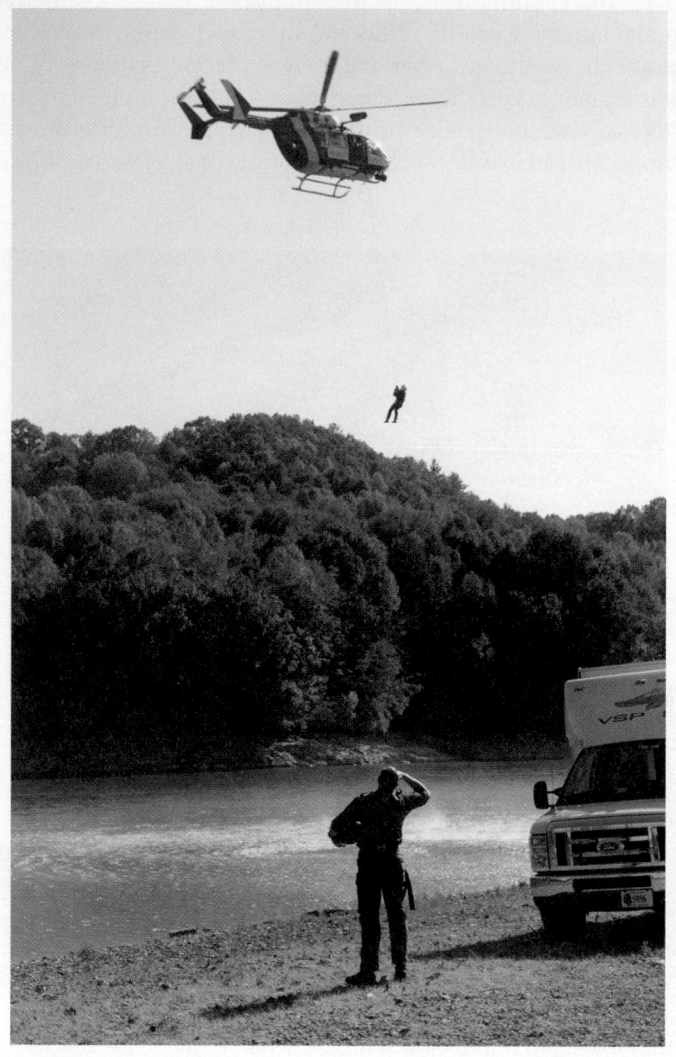

Figure 2 Environmental emergencies can occur in remote settings where rescue can be challenging.

ability to compensate for environmental extremes. A patient who is dehydrated can be at risk. Finally, the patient's overall health and fitness status and ability to acclimatize (that is, physiologically adjust to the new environment) can mean the difference between life and death.

This chapter first describes the techniques that the healthy body uses to respond to changes in temperature. It then assesses factors that can interfere with the body's ability to shed or gain heat, thereby increasing a person's risk of experiencing an environmental emergency. Next, it examines the pathophysiology, assessment, and management of environmental illnesses.

■ Anatomy and Physiology

■ Homeostasis and Body Temperature

Homeostasis refers to body processes that balance the supply and demand of the body's needs. Ensuring the balance between heat production and heat dissipation (thermoregulation) is the

job of thermosensitive neurons in the anterior hypothalamus. The hypothalamus—the "master thermostat" in the brain—operates according to the principle of negative feedback control: A rise in core body temperature elicits responses that increase heat loss and shut off normal heat production pathways (thermogenesis); a fall in core body temperature prompts heat production and conservation and turns off normal heat-liberating pathways (thermolysis) **Figure 3**.

Words of Wisdom

Do not become a victim yourself. Stay hydrated, dress for the weather, and store oral fluids in a cooler in your rig.

The human body defends a constant core temperature of approximately 98.6°F (37°C) that represents a balance between the heat produced or absorbed by the body and the heat released to the outside. At this temperature, the metabolic reactions of the body proceed at their optimal level. Temperatures in the core (the brain and thoracoabdominal organs) remain relatively constant. The temperature of the periphery (the skin and extremities) can fluctuate a great deal, so this part of the body has a major role in thermoregulation. The lowest body temperature at which human survival of accidental hypothermia has been reported is 56.7°F (13.7°C). More generally, hypothermia is commonly defined as a core body temperature (CBT) starting at 95°F (35°C) and heatstroke at 104°F (40°C). CBT is defined

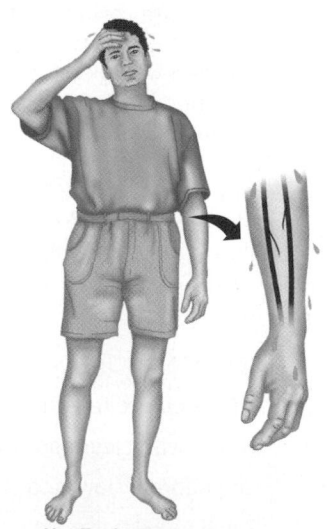
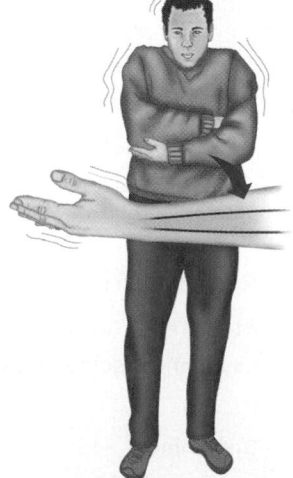

Hot Environment
- Hypothalamus stimulated
- Blood vessels dilate, maximizing heat loss from skin
- Body sweats, causing evaporation and cooling

Body temperature decreases

Cold Environment
- Hypothalamus stimulated
- Blood vessels constrict, minimizing heat loss from skin
- Muscles shiver, generating heat

Body temperature increases

Figure 3 Like a car thermostat, the hypothalamus notes a rise or fall in core body temperature and elicits responses to regulate it.

as the temperature in the part of the body comprising the heart, lungs, brain, and abdominal viscera.

In the field, the oral temperature is commonly used and is a suitable measurement for general medical conditions such as suspected pneumonia. It can vary dramatically from the CBT if the patient has been mouth breathing or drinking hot or cold liquids. The axillary temperature, taken in the armpit, is about 1°F cooler than the oral temperature. Likewise the rectal temperature is about 1°F hotter. In field situations, the most accurate means of determining CBTs is to use a rectal thermometer capable of measuring extremes of temperatures. This can be done with a mercury or electronic thermometer; however, accurate measurement of core body temperature in the prehospital environment is highly unlikely to ever impact treatment. Tympanic temperatures, which are taken with a device that measures the heat reflected off the eardrum, as well as various commercial devices for measuring skin temperatures, are somewhat less reliable Figure 4 .

Thermoregulatory Mechanisms

The body's main thermoregulatory center is located in specialized tissue found in the hypothalamus. The thermogenic (heat-generating) tissues in the hypothalamus are mediated by the sympathetic nervous system; the thermolytic (heat-liberating) tissues are mediated by the parasympathetic nervous system. The hypothalamus receives signals from peripheral warm and cold thermoreceptors (located primarily in the skin and muscles) and central receptors (triggered by changes in blood temperature; located in the core).

At rest, the body produces heat chiefly by the metabolism of nutrients (carbohydrates, fats, and rarely proteins), with the subsequent liberation of primarily water and carbon dioxide. The liver and skeletal muscles are the major contributors to the **basal metabolic rate (BMR)**, the heat energy produced at rest from normal body metabolic reactions. The BMR of the average 70-kg adult is in the range of 60 to 70 kilocalories per hour. Many factors affect this rate, including age, gender, stress, and hormones. The most important factor, however, is body surface area. As the ratio of body surface area to body volume increases, heat loss to the environment increases. Thus, when two people have the same weight, the shorter person will have a higher BMR.

Exertion also affects the metabolic rate. For example, a brisk walk can produce heat totaling 300 kcal/h. The recommended daily caloric intake is around 2,000 to 2,500 kcal (a food "calorie" is actually a kilocalorie). Men's bodies require slightly higher calorie intake than women's (for example, a moderately active woman between ages 19 and 30 requires 2,000 to 2,200 calories per day, while a man in the same category requires 2,600 to 2,800 calories).

Some of the heat generated by metabolism and glycogen breakdown for muscular work is used to warm the body; the excess is dissipated, ordinarily by taking advantage of the temperature gradient between the body and the outside environment. If the environmental temperature is higher than the body temperature, there is a third potential source of body heat: absorption of heat from the outside. Standing in bright sunshine on a hot, breezeless day, for example, can add up to 150 kcal/h to the internal heat load.

Lastly, the skin plays a vital role in body temperature regulation. Although the mechanisms are quite complicated, the body has the ability to both conserve and liberate large amounts of heat energy through the skin. In an effort to liberate heat, blood flow to the skin can involve up to 8 liters per minute and 60% of cardiac output. In cold situations, blood flow can approach zero in specific areas.

Physiologic Responses to Heat and Cold

Thermolysis

The body reacts to its daily production of heat energy and to hot environmental conditions in much the same way—**thermolysis**, the release of stored heat and energy from the body. An increase in the CBT causes the hypothalamus to send signals via efferent pathways in the autonomic nervous system, causing vasodilation and sweating.

Because of cutaneous vasodilation, the effective volume of the vascular system is increased (when the diameter of a tube, such as an artery, is increased, its volume increases); the heart must increase its output to compensate for this effect. The pulse rate and stroke volume increase, but the work of the heart is markedly increased. If vasodilation increases dramatically, the person may have a complete loss of vasomotor control (that is, the ability of the arteries to constrict in response to sympathetic stimulation). In that case, blood pools in the periphery, and the patient could experience neurogenic shock.

When warmed blood from the core and overheated muscles heads for the peripherally dilated cutaneous vessels, it may be cooled in four major ways (in addition to behavioral changes, such as slowing down or seeking shade):

- **Radiation**, the transfer of heat via electromagnetic waves, accounts for more than 65% of heat loss in a cooler setting. Heat loss through the head is especially notable. If the ambient temperature is high (68°F or greater), body heat will be gained.

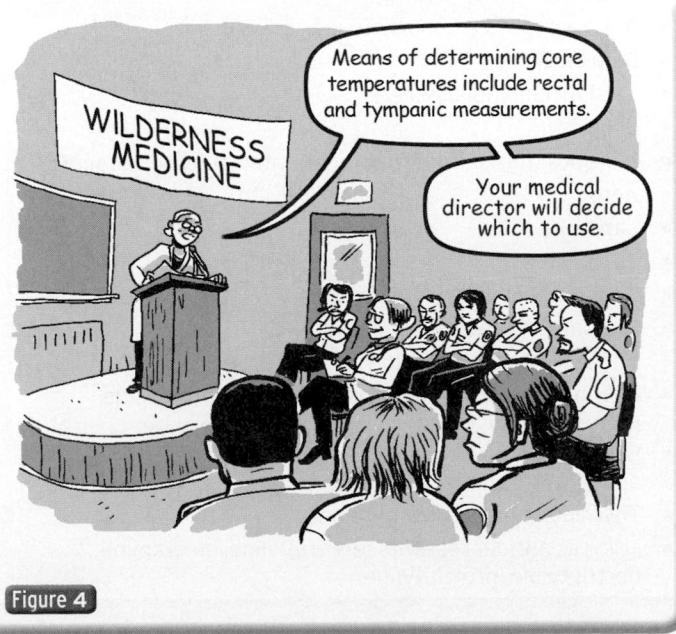

Means of determining core temperatures include rectal and tympanic measurements.

Your medical director will decide which to use.

WILDERNESS MEDICINE

Figure 4

- <u>Conduction</u> is the transfer of heat from a hotter object to a cooler object by direct physical contact. Air is a poor conductor of heat (only 2% of body heat is lost to it), whereas the ground is a good conductor. Water is the best conductor. A person who falls into a cold lake will lose heat 25 times faster than a dry person exposed to air of the same temperature. Clothing soaked with rain, snow, or perspiration can be just as dangerous.

- <u>Convection</u> refers to the transfer of energy that takes place when moving air (or liquids) disturbs molecules next to an object. It can be thought of as a property that aids in conduction. A person instinctively uses this principle when blowing on hot food to cool it. Likewise, air moving across the body surface can pick up heat and carry it away. The faster the air is moving, the faster it can remove heat from the body. The **wind chill factor** measures the chilling effect of a given temperature at a given wind speed. For example, the chilling effect of a 30°F temperature with a 35 mph wind is –4°F.

- <u>Evaporation</u>, the conversion of a liquid to a gas, liberates 1 kcal per 1.7 mL of sweat. Sweating and heat dissipation by evaporation normally account for about 30% of cooling. Evaporation is the main mode of cooling in higher temperatures until a high humidity level slows the rate of evaporation. It has a minor role via respiration. This phenomenon is also behind the evaporative method of cooling for heatstroke patients. In cold conditions, wet clothes can cause heat loss by conduction and, as they dry, further heat loss by evaporation.

These four mechanisms require a thermal gradient between the body and its surroundings; that is, the mechanisms work only as long as the temperature of the skin surface is higher than that of the outside environment (and metabolism does not produce an overwhelming heat load). When the outside temperature approaches or exceeds skin surface temperature, however, heat loss by radiation and convection diminishes and finally ceases. When the environmental temperature exceeds the skin temperature, the body absorbs heat. In those circumstances, the increase in blood flow to the skin becomes counterproductive because it promotes increased heat absorption.

The only way the body can dissipate heat when the ambient temperature approaches body temperature is by the evaporation of sweat, up to a point. A healthy adult can sweat a maximum of about 1 L/h but cannot maintain that rate for more than a few hours at a time. Furthermore, for effective evaporation of sweat, the ambient air must be relatively unsaturated with water. As the relative humidity increases, the rate of evaporation decreases; effective sweat evaporation ceases when the relative humidity reaches about 75%.

Thermogenesis

In a cold environment, the skin serves as the body's thermostat. If your skin is cold, your body will shiver even if your CBT is not lowered. <u>Thermogenesis</u>, the production of heat and energy for the body, is the main method of dealing with cold stressors. In addition to normal heat production from the BMR and physical exertion, the hypothalamic center and sympathetic nervous system can increase muscle tone and initiate shivering in the short term and increase thyroid levels in the long term. The hypothalamus also stimulates peripheral vasoconstriction, thereby shunting blood to the core. The eccrine sweat glands receive cholinergic stimuli to decrease sweating. The thicker the outer shell, the better the insulation. All other factors being equal, heavier people are more effectively insulated from the cold. This conservation of heat for the sake of the core continues until the body's ability to generate heat becomes overwhelmed, resulting in hypothermia.

■ Pathophysiology, Assessment, and Management of Heat Illness

<u>Heat illness</u> is an increase in CBT due to inadequate thermolysis. The fundamental problem is the inability to get rid of the heat buildup in the body, often because of hot and humid conditions. A person's general state of health, clothing, mobility, age, preexisting illnesses, and certain medications Table 1 can add to the problem. When the thermoregulatory system is taxed beyond its limits or fails for any reason, the CBT soars, sometimes rising from normal to about 106°F (41°C) in less than 15 minutes (beyond the upper limit of 104°F [40°C] for heatstroke). That is the situation in heatstroke, for example.

Table 1 Medications Contributing to Heat Illness

- Alcohol
- Alpha agonists
- Amphetamines
- Anticholinergic medications (atropine sulfate, scopolamine, benztropine mesylate, belladonna, and synthetic alkaloids)
- Antihistamines
- Antiparkinsonian agents
- Antipsychotics (such as haloperidol)
- Beta blockers
- Calcium channel blockers
- Cocaine
- Diuretics (furosemide, hydrochlorothiazide, bumetanide)
- Heroin
- Laxatives
- Lithium
- Lysergic acid diethylamide (LSD)
- Monoamine oxidase inhibitors
- Phencyclidine hydrochloride
- Phenothiazines (prochlorperazine, chlorpromazine, promethazine)
- Sympathomimetic medicines (amphetamines, epinephrine, ephedrine, cocaine, norepinephrine)
- Thyroid agonists (levothyroxine)
- Tricyclic antidepressants (amitriptyline, imipramine, nortriptyline, protriptyline)

Risk Factors for Heat Illness

Certain factors increase a person's risk for ill effects from any given heat stress; the factors are summarized in Table 2 . Older people are at particular risk because they do not adjust as well to the heat: they perspire less; they acclimatize more slowly; they feel thirst less readily in response to dehydration; and decreased mobility can affect the ability to obtain fluids. Older people are also more likely to have chronic conditions, such as diabetes and cardiovascular disease, which can dramatically interfere with normal heat regulation. In addition, they are more apt to be taking medications that disrupt the body's mechanisms for dissipating heat.

Numerous medications can affect the body's ability to regulate its temperature. Diuretics may result in dehydration and electrolyte disturbances. These conditions may then interfere with peripheral vasodilation needed for heat transfer. Beta blockers can lessen a tachycardic response to heat stress, as can normal age-related decreases in maximum pulse rate. Acclimatization has numerous adaptive physiologic effects. It can decrease the likelihood of heat illness, but it takes days of a person performing controlled, progressive exertion in a hot environment to be effective.

Among young and healthy people, infants and young children are most vulnerable to heat stress when exposed to a hot environment. Children, compared with adults, have proportionately higher metabolic heat production, have a CBT that rises faster during dehydration, and do not dissipate heat as well owing to their smaller organ and vascular systems. Athletes and military recruits engaging in heavy exertion in hot conditions are also at increased risk.

The following subsections discuss the major types of heat illness Table 3 .

Heat Cramps

Pathophysiology

Heat cramps are acute, involuntary, painful muscle spasms, usually in the lower extremities, the abdomen, or both, that occur because of profuse sweating and subsequent sodium losses in sweat. Three factors contribute to heat cramps: salt depletion, dehydration, and muscle fatigue. Heat cramps most often afflict people in good physical condition—for example, athletes, military personnel, and physical laborers. A recent study of US college football players showed a twofold increase in sweat sodium losses in athletes prone to heat cramps. Usually a person exerting himself or herself in a hot environment will become thirsty and increase fluids intake. But if the person is sweating heavily, he or she is losing fluids and salt through the

Table 2 Factors That Predispose to Heat Illness

Factors That Increase Internal Heat Production	Factors That Interfere With Heat Dissipation
<ul><li>Physical exertion</li><li>Response to infection (fever)</li><li>Hyperthyroidism</li><li>Agitated and tremulous states (Parkinson, psychosis, mania, drug withdrawal–opiate and alcohol)</li><li>Drug overdoses (such as sympathomimetics, cocaine, caffeine, lysergic acid diethylamide [LSD], phencyclidine hydrochloride, methamphetamine, ecstasy)</li></ul>	<ul><li>High ambient temperature</li><li>High humidity</li><li>Obesity (insulation effect, less efficient dissipation)</li><li>Impaired vasodilation</li><li>Diabetes</li><li>Alcoholism</li><li>Drugs: diuretics, tranquilizers, beta blockers, antihistamines, phenothiazines, antidepressants</li><li>Impaired ability to sweat (cystic fibrosis, skin diseases, healed burns)</li><li>Heavy or tight clothing (especially personal protective equipment)</li></ul>
Factors That Increase Heat Absorption	**Factors That Impair the Body's Response to Heat Stress**
<ul><li>Confined, unventilated, hot living quarters</li><li>Working in hot conditions</li><li>Being in parked automobiles in summer</li></ul>	<ul><li>Dehydration (including recent GI or respiratory infections)</li><li>Prior episode of heatstroke</li><li>Hypokalemia</li><li>Cardiovascular disease</li><li>Previous stroke or other central nervous system lesion</li></ul>

Table 3 Comparing Conditions Resulting from Heat Stress

Variable	Heat Cramps	Heat Exhaustion	Heatstroke
Pathophysiology	Sodium and water loss	Sodium and water loss, hypovolemia	Failure of heat-regulating mechanisms
Mental status	Normal	Normal or mild confusion	Altered, delirium, seizures
Temperature	May be mildly elevated	Usually mildly elevated	>104°F (40°C)
Skin	Cool, moist	Pale, cool, moist	Dry, hot, but sweating may persist, especially with exertional heatstroke
Muscle cramping	Severe	May or may not be present	Absent

skin. If the person drinks plain water, he or she will not replace sweat sodium losses **Figure 5**. Hence, the rehabilitation sector at a fire should have approved electrolyte solutions available instead of just plain water.

Assessment

Heat cramps usually start suddenly during strenuous and/or prolonged physical activity. They may be mild, characterized by only slight abdominal cramping and tingling in the extremities. More often, however, they present with severe, incapacitating pain in the extremities and abdomen. The patient may become hypotensive and nauseated but remains alert. The pulse is generally rapid, the skin pale and moist, and the temperature normal.

Management

Treatment of heat cramps aims to eliminate the exposure and restore lost salt and water to the body:

- Move the patient to a cool environment. Have the patient lie down if he or she feels faint.
- If the patient is not nauseated, give one or two glasses of a salt-containing solution (such as lemonade with 1/2 teaspoon of salt added or a commercial sports drink) **Figure 6**. Instruct the patient to drink the solution slowly. Have the patient munch on salty chips or pretzels. Salt tablets can irritate the stomach lining and may precipitate or worsen nausea.
- If the patient is too nauseated to take liquids by mouth, insert an intravenous (IV) catheter and infuse normal saline rapidly. (Consult medical control for the IV rate.)
- Do not massage the cramping muscles. That tactic may actually aggravate the pain.
- As the patient's salt balance is restored, the symptoms will abate and the patient may want to resume activity. In the field, this decision is best made with medical control.

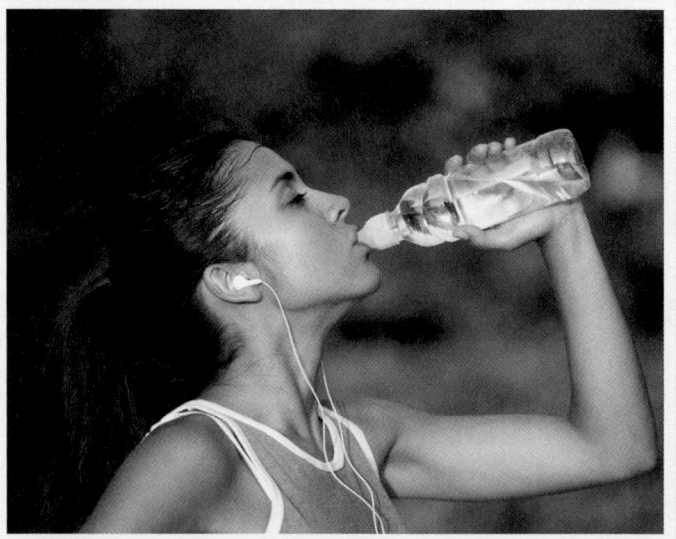

Figure 5 If you drink plain water, you will not replace sweat salt losses.

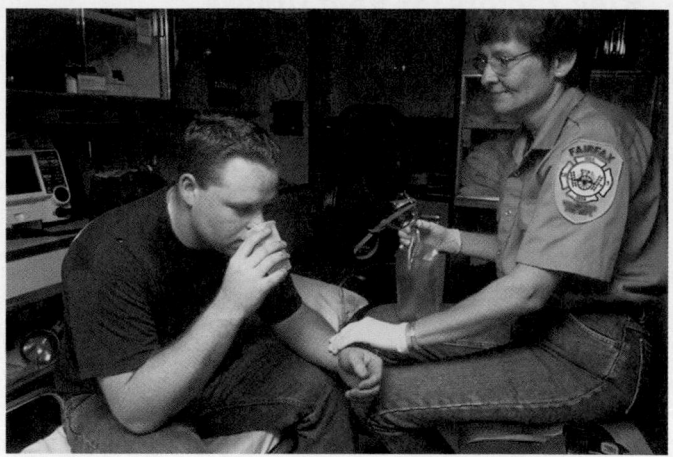

Figure 6 Give the patient with heat cramps one or two glasses of a salt-containing solution if he or she is not nauseated.

◼ Heat Syncope

Pathophysiology

Heat syncope is an orthostatic syncopal, or near-syncopal, episode that typically occurs in nonacclimated people who may be under heat stress. Whereas the elderly are certainly at higher risk, they are also at higher risk for cardiac syncope and atypical acute coronary syndromes, and due caution is advisable. Heat syncope can occur with prolonged standing, as in mass outdoor gatherings, or when standing suddenly from a sitting or lying position. One of the body's thermoregulatory functions is peripheral vasodilation. The causes are thought to be an upright posture in which gravity causes dependent pooling of blood, which can also possibly be exacerbated by some degree of dehydration and/or hypokalemia.

Assessment and Management

Treatment involves placing the patient in a supine position and replacing fluid deficits. If the patient does not recover quickly in the supine position, suspect heatstroke, heat exhaustion, cardiac syncope, or atypical acute coronary syndromes.

◼ Heat Exhaustion

Pathophysiology

Heat exhaustion is a clinical syndrome thought to represent a milder form of heat illness on a continuum leading to heatstroke. Its hallmarks are volume depletion and heat stress. Classically, two forms are described: water-depleted and sodium-depleted. Water-depleted heat exhaustion occurs primarily in geriatric patients owing to immobility, medications that contribute to dehydration, and decreased thirst sensitivity and in active younger workers or athletes who do not adequately replace fluids in a hot environment. Sodium-depleted heat exhaustion may take hours or days to develop and results from huge sodium losses from sweating but replacing only free water, not sodium.

A concept closely related to sodium-depleted heat exhaustion is **exercise-associated hyponatremia**. Studies from the Boston Marathon, the Grand Canyon National Park, and the military point to a common thread: prolonged exertion usually in a hot environment coupled with excessive fluid intake. Most victims have too much water in their body in relationship to total sodium. Recent evidence also points to arginine vasopressin (AVP) as a contributing factor (AVP is a hormone that increases water absorption in the kidneys). According to experts, the first symptoms are often nonspecific and include nausea, vomiting, weight gain, and headache. As the severity worsens, mental status changes (confusion, agitation, disorientation) become common. Cerebral edema, pulmonary edema, respiratory distress, seizures, coma, and death may ensue if the condition goes untreated or unrecognized.

You should always remain alert for older, debilitated patients (who may simply be hyponatremic without the exercise-induced component) and patients who participate in extreme endurance sports of greater than 3 hours duration, such as marathons and Ironman competitions. The Second International Exercise-Associated Hyponatremia Consensus Development Conference, held in 2007, recommends "any athlete with exercise-associated hyponatremia encephalopathy should be immediately treated with a bolus infusion of 100 mL of 3% NaCl to acutely reduce brain edema. Up to two additional 100-mL 3% NaCl bolus infusions should be administered at 10-minute intervals if there is no clinical improvement." These experts also state that a means of measuring serum sodium on site should be available.

Assessment

Symptoms of heat exhaustion can be nonspecific and may include headache, fatigue, weakness, dizziness, nausea, vomiting, and, sometimes, abdominal cramping. The patient is usually sweating profusely, and the skin is pale and clammy. The core temperature may be normal or slightly elevated (less than 104°F [40°C]). Tachycardia is present, although this response may be blunted if the patient is taking a beta blocker. Respirations are fast and shallow. Tachypnea may produce symptoms of hyperventilation: carpopedal spasm, perioral numbness, and a low end-tidal carbon dioxide level. Blood pressure may be decreased due to peripheral pooling of blood or volume depletion; if not decreased at rest, blood pressure will almost certainly drop when the patient tries to sit or stand from a recumbent position (**orthostatic hypotension**). If the patient reports brown urine, suspect rhabdomyolysis (the destruction of muscle tissue leading to a release of potassium and myoglobin).

Heat exhaustion is sometimes mistaken for "summer flu," and the condition may be misdiagnosed. If left untreated, heat exhaustion may progress to heatstroke. Elderly patients with primary gastrointestinal (GI) infections (nausea/vomiting and diarrhea) may be mistaken for experiencing heat exhaustion especially if they are found in a hot environment. However, be cautious because GI symptoms can also occur with heatstroke.

Management

The treatment of heat exhaustion is aimed at removing the patient from exposure to heat and repairing the derangement in fluid and electrolyte balance:

- Move the patient to a cool environment; remove excess clothing, and place supine with legs elevated.
- If the patient's temperature is elevated, sponge, spray, or drip the patient with tepid water and fan gently to make him or her more comfortable—but do not overdo it. Heroic measures to lower body temperature rapidly are unnecessary, and chilling the patient can cause shivering and thermogenesis.
- Consider specially designed cooling chairs for hand and forearm immersion in cold water for rehabilitation at fire scenes, mass gatherings, and endurance sports.
- Oral hydration with sports drinks may be appropriate. If nausea and vomiting are present, start a normal saline IV line and draw blood for electrolyte determinations. Use the pulse rate and blood pressure to guide the fluid amounts administered.
- If exercise-associated hyponatremia is suspected, do not give fluids by mouth. Instead, draw blood for checking the blood sodium level and administer IV normal saline or hypertonic saline depending on local circumstances.
- Monitor cardiac rhythm, vital signs, temperature, and end-tidal carbon dioxide.
- If you cannot determine whether the patient has heat exhaustion or heatstroke, treat for heatstroke. You may also want to consider administration of an antiemetic (ie, ondansetron [Zofran]).

Controversies

The actual diagnosis of heat exhaustion versus heatstroke can be challenging, and there is a great deal of overlap in signs and symptoms. This determination is further complicated if the patient already has a preexisting altered mental status and the fact that the patient may continue to sweat. The safest and easiest way to differentiate between the two conditions is to remember that heatstroke involves an elevated temperature and an altered mental status.

Heatstroke

Pathophysiology

Of all heat illnesses, **heatstroke** is the least common but the most deadly. It is caused by a severe disturbance in the body's thermoregulation and is a profound emergency, with mortality rates as high as 10% in treated patients and 30% to 80% in untreated patients. Emergency medicine physicians typically rely on two findings to make this diagnosis: core temperature of more than 104°F (40°C) and altered mental status.

As would be expected, the pathophysiologic consequences are related to the effects of elevated temperatures on the body's cells. This is evidenced by disruption of cell membranes, adenosine triphosphate transport channels, enzymes, breakdown of muscle cells (as evidenced by the presence of elevated serum creatine phosphokinase and presence of the muscle protein myoglobin in the urine), and electrolyte disturbances. Heat-labile proteins break down and lead to edema and hemorrhage. This increased vascular permeability leads to decreased cardiac output, hypotension, and shock. Loss of sweating is a consequence, not a cause of heatstroke.

Two heatstroke syndromes are distinguished: classic and exertional Table 4 . **Classic heatstroke** (passive heatstroke), which usually occurs during heat waves, is most likely to strike very old, very young, or bedridden people. Patients with chronic illnesses, such as diabetes or heart disease, are particularly susceptible, as are people with alcoholism and patients taking certain medications (diuretics, sedatives, anticholinergics). In this syndrome, high environmental temperatures initially elicit thermolysis, but the CBT eventually soars, and the typical signs and symptoms of heatstroke appear. Some research has shown that being confined to a bed, not leaving home daily, and not being able to care for oneself were the greatest risk factors of death during heat waves. Preexisting psychiatric illness tripled the risk of death followed by cardiovascular and pulmonary diseases.

Exertional heatstroke is typically an illness of young and fit people exercising in hot and humid conditions. When the ambient temperature approaches body temperature, radiation and convection are no longer effective means of shedding excess heat. If the relative humidity rises above 75%, evaporative cooling becomes ineffective. Persons who continue exercising in such conditions will continue generating heat without any means of

releasing that heat. They often sweat profusely. Heat will then build up within the body, causing the CBT to skyrocket. This is a common scenario with high school or college athletes, military recruits, and others participating in intense, prolonged activity in hot and/or humid conditions.

Table 4 Classic Versus Exertional Heatstroke

Characteristic	Classic Heatstroke	Exertional Heatstroke
Age	Older	Younger
General health	Chronic diseases, schizophrenia	Healthy person
Medications	Beta blockers, diuretics, anticholinergics	Often none, consider stimulant abuse
Activity	Very little to bedridden	Strenuous
Sweating	May be absent	Present
Skin	Hot, red, dry	Moist, pale
Blood glucose level	Normal	Hypoglycemic
Rhabdomyolysis	Rare	Common
Acute renal failure	Rare	Common

YOU are the Medic PART 2

The patient remains slow to respond, but is alert and oriented to person, place, and time. He continues to shiver as you dry him off, examine him, and cover him with dry blankets. His skin is pale, cold, and slightly moist.

Before moving your patient, you fit him with a cervical collar and initiate spinal precautions. His head, neck, and back are unremarkable. Besides his report that he is "aching all over," he reports pain to his hands, fingers, feet, and toes. He has absent distal pulses, is unable to move his toes on command, and cannot feel you touch his toes. His fingers and toes are soft to the touch. He moves his lower extremities on command, but they are weak and uncoordinated. The patient reveals no health history.

Recording Time: 10 Minutes	
Level of consciousness	Alert (oriented to person, place, and day), but slow to respond
Respirations	10 breaths/min; slow and shallow
Pulse	104 beats/min; weak and irregular
Skin	Cold, pale, and slightly moist
Blood pressure	80/40 mm Hg
Oxygen saturation (Spo$_2$)	95% on room air

4. What do these physical findings indicate to you?

5. Why is his shivering significant?

6. What can you conclude from the patient's vital signs?

Assessment

Both types of heatstroke present with similar signs and symptoms, which may or may not be recognized as the consequence of heat exposure. Patients most likely will not be able to give a coherent history because they will be confused, delirious, or comatose. Often the earliest signs of heatstroke are changes in behavior—irritability, combativeness, signs the patient is hallucinating—which may mislead bystanders and EMS workers into thinking the patient is having a behavioral or substance-related emergency. Older patients with heatstroke may present with signs resembling those of a suspected stroke, including trouble walking, talking, or using an arm or leg. Other central nervous system disturbances that commonly occur are seizures and constricted pupils.

Words of Wisdom

Suspect heatstroke and check a core temperature in any person behaving strangely in a hot environment.

The diagnostic vital sign is, of course, a markedly elevated temperature, usually of greater than 104°F (40°C). However, it may be lower and thus misleading if any cooling techniques have been undertaken by bystanders. You should never assume that a temperature of 104°F (40°C) is required for the diagnosis of heatstroke. Signs of a hyperdynamic state are usually present: tachycardia, hyperventilation with a lowered end-tidal carbon dioxide, and lowered peripheral vascular resistance from efforts of the body to cool itself with vasodilation. Heatstroke is characterized by some degree of dehydration that worsens the problem by decreasing the body's ability to get the hotter core blood to the periphery for thermolysis. Blood pressure can be normal or decreased depending on the level of dehydration. The skin can be dry, red, and hot in classic heatstroke or pale and sweaty in exertional heatstroke. However, the presence or absence of sweating is not important! If the patient's temperature is markedly elevated and he or she has an altered mental status, assume heatstroke regardless of whether the patient is sweating or not.

The diagnosis of heatstroke is easy to miss. It may develop rapidly in a patient whose heat exhaustion was mistaken for the flu, or it may present as coma of unknown origin. Unless you keep the possibility of heatstroke constantly in mind during the hot months of the year and assess the patient's temperature as part of the vital signs, you may waste precious time searching for some other cause of the patient's symptoms.

Fever and Conditions That Mimic Heatstroke New paramedics may face a perplexing challenge: Why is this nursing home patient's temperature elevated? Is it heatstroke, a febrile illness, or sepsis? Neurologic changes can be present in all three situations. The history, however, may suggest infectious causes. For example, is there a change in the urine color in a catheter bag, a recent complaint of cough and dyspnea, or an obvious skin infection? Complaints of a fever, rash, photophobia, and stiff neck may point to meningitis. An intermittent shaking chill also favors infectious causes of increased temperature.

A fever can signal that the body is fighting an infection by inhibiting reproduction of harmful toxins. Pyrogens (proteins secreted by infective organisms and the body's immune system) act on the hypothalamus by increasing the thermal set point, which results in a fever. The body then uses its thermoregulatory tools to maintain the new temperature setting. The patient with a reset temperature may adapt to this change by wearing more clothes, and sometimes the body creates more heat via shivering. Although aspirin and nonsteroidal anti-inflammatory drugs can lower a fever (by blocking prostaglandins), they are dangerous to use when you are treating heat illnesses.

Anticholinergic poisoning presents with an elevated temperature; dry, red skin; mental status changes; and tachycardia. Anticholinergic poisonings usually cause dilated pupils, whereas patients with heatstroke usually have constricted pupils.

Two rare syndromes cause hyperthermia. <u>Neuroleptic malignant syndrome (NMS)</u> is caused by antipsychotic and some antiemetic medications and patients present with <u>hyperthermia</u>, muscular rigidity, altered mental status, and a hyperdynamic state. <u>Malignant hyperthermia</u> can occur as a result of common anesthesia medications (notably succinylcholine) and presents similarly to NMS. Researchers are exploring a common genetic contributor to malignant hyperthermia and heatstroke.

Management

If you are unsure about what exactly is causing the patient's elevated temperature, the prudent step is for you to treat for heatstroke because of the deadly consequences of missing the diagnosis. Online medical control may also help you with treatment plans.

Heatstroke treatment requires two things: removing the patient from the offending environment and rapid cooling. The main methods used for rapid cooling are ice water or cold water body immersion and evaporative cooling by spraying cold or cool water over the patient accompanied by the use of fans to promote convection. Recent research related to exertional heatstroke found that ice water immersion, more than cold water immersion, is the most rapid means of cooling patients. Further, dousing patients with water or spraying them with a mist and fanning them was found to be acceptable. Ineffective methods included ice packs alone or in combination with fanning, fanning without use of water, and cooling blankets. Current evidence suggests that concerns about shivering and raising CBT are unfounded. Evidence-based guidelines from the American College of Sports Medicine reiterated the importance of cooling first, then providing transport. Obvious limitations include the need for ice and responsive patients not tolerating this measure well. A summary of treatment for heatstroke is as follows:

- Evaluate the ABCs, administer supplemental oxygen, consider sedation if the patient is agitated or combative, and be prepared to intubate.
- Move the patient to a cool environment, and strip the patient. Cooling efforts should continue until the rectal temperature has fallen below about 102°F (39°C).

- Cool as rapidly as possible by the most expeditious means available:
  - Consider ice water immersion because it is the fastest cooling method. Cooling with ice water–soaked blankets and fanning is nearly as effective as immersion. Pay close attention to airway status and watch for seizures.
  - Spray the patient with cold or cool water while fanning constantly to promote rapid evaporation. The ambulance should carry a portable fan during the summer months for this purpose or use a fire department ventilation fan.
- Start an IV line, administer normal saline, and check the blood glucose level. Be careful with fluids—pulmonary edema is a known complication of heatstroke. Remember that cooling promotes peripheral vasoconstriction that can raise the blood pressure.
- Monitor cardiac rhythm, and remember that rhabdomyolysis can occur with resultant hyperkalemia.
- Be prepared to treat seizures with common antiseizure medicines (lorazepam, midazolam, or diazepam).

Prevention of Heat Illness Military organizations have understood the effects of heat illness for decades. They were one of the first groups to understand the importance of acclimatization. More modern contributions have included standards for conducting training in hot environments. Heat stress indices are a variety of scientific measurements that allow for an estimation of the effect of variables such as temperature, humidity, and wind speed on the ability to work in hot environments. These indices have applications not just for the military but are regulated for numerous industries and even scholastic sports. One of the most widely used is the wet-bulb globe temperature index. This equation takes into account three things. First is the wet bulb temperature, which is measured by placing moistened material over the end of the thermometer (simulating natural sweating) while the thermometer is exposed to the sun or wind. Second is the air or dry bulb temperature, which is shielded from sun. Lastly, the black globe temperature is basically a thermometer inside a small black ball, which estimates the effect of solar radiation (direct sunlight).

The following measures can help protect you, your colleagues, and the communities you serve from heat illness:

1. Acclimatize whenever possible. Maintain personal fitness.
2. Limit time spent in heavy activity in PPE (eg, wildland duties in bunker gear), especially during the hottest parts of the day or season. Paramedics working in hot climates should have appropriate summer uniforms.
3. Maintain hydration, eat appropriately, and rest. Avoid beverages with a high sugar and/or caffeine content. Some ambulances are equipped with an onboard refrigerator for hot weather. Otherwise, carry a portable cooler, fill it about half full with crushed ice, and stock it with sports drinks or other salt-containing drinks for patients and the crew.
4. Develop or research standards on activities in hot weather from professional organizations (National Fire Protection Agency, Occupational Safety and Health Administration, American College of Sports Medicine).

5. Improve your own physical fitness, both in terms of cardiovascular endurance and muscular strength.
6. Conduct community-based programs aimed at high-risk populations—for example, nursing home risk assessments and prevention programs.

Be alert for early symptoms of heat illness, such as headache, nausea, cramps, and dizziness. If you experience any of those symptoms, get out of the hot environment immediately and get medical attention.

Pathophysiology, Assessment, and Management of Cold Injuries

Local Cold Injury/Frostbite

Pathophysiology

Most injuries from the cold are localized to the extremities or exposed parts of the body, such as the tips of the ears, nose, upper cheek, and tips of the fingers or toes **Figure 7**. Local freezing injuries fall under the general heading of frostbite. **Frostbite** is an ischemic injury that is classified as superficial or deep depending on whether tissue loss occurs.

A mild form of frostbite, sometimes called **frostnip**, develops slowly and generally is not painful; however, the patient may report numbness. It is common among people who participate in winter sports. This problem is easily treated by placing

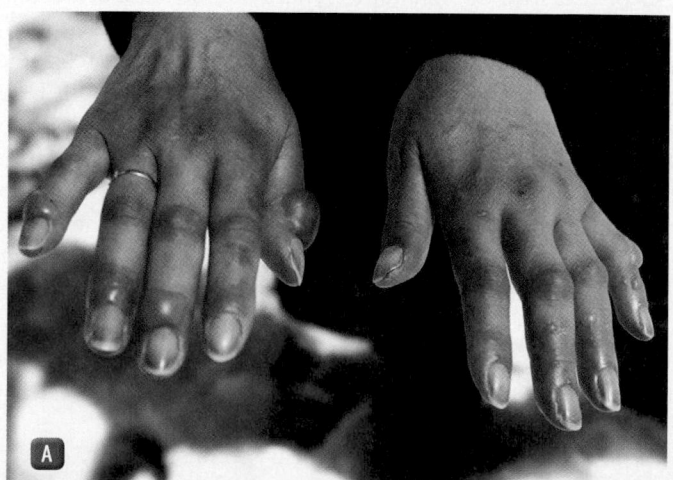

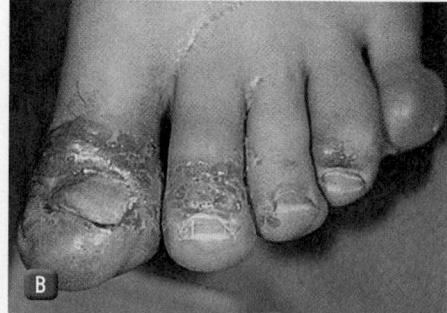

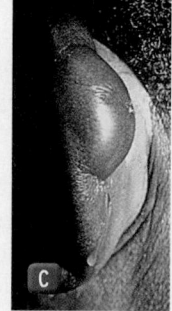

Figure 7 The extremities (**A** and **B**) and the ears (**C**) are particularly susceptible to frostbite.

a warm hand firmly over the chilled nose or ear. If the fingers have frostnip, they can be warmed by placing them into the armpit. The return of warmth to a frost-nipped area is usually signaled by some redness and tingling. A warming technique called windmilling involves rapidly making a large circle with your arm and hand, starting with your hand next to your side, raising it backward and up until you are reaching straight up, and moving it rapidly down frontward. This technique forces blood into the cold hand.

Deeper degrees of frostbite involve freezing of tissues and can occur in ambient temperatures that are well below the freezing point. This freezing injury cascade starts with initial freezing of tissues with microvasoconstriction and local fluid shifting. Cells are composed chiefly of water, so when they are subjected to low enough temperatures, the water within them turns into ice crystals, causing cellular shrinkage and a hyperosmolar state. This problem is further complicated by increased viscosity accompanied by "sludging," poor flow, capillary leakage due to osmotic imbalance, and resultant thrombus and ischemic injury.

Risk Factors for Frostbite Several factors predispose a person to frostbite:

- Cold exposure without adequate clothing
- Impeding the circulation to the extremities:
  - Wearing restrictive or tight clothing
  - Smoking, which constricts arteries
  - Drinking alcohol, which helps peripherally dilate blood vessels and causes diuresis
- Fatigue, dehydration, or hunger
- Coming in direct contact with cold objects (conduction)
- Hypothermia (experiencing generalized hypothermia is the most likely way to sustain a local cold injury)

Assessment

Superficial Frostbite The most common symptom of <u>superficial frostbite</u> is an altered sensation: numbness, tingling, or burning. The skin typically appears white and waxy and has been compared with frozen halibut **Figure 8**. Because it is frozen, the skin is firm to palpation, but the underlying tissues remain soft. Once thawing occurs, the injured area turns cyanotic, and the patient experiences a hot, stinging sensation. Capillary leakage produces edema in the frostbitten area, though development of blisters (blebs) is more characteristic of deep frostbite. Dull or throbbing pain may persist for days or weeks after the injury.

Deep Frostbite <u>Deep frostbite</u> usually involves the hands or the feet. A frozen extremity looks white, yellow-white, or mottled blue-white, and it is hard, cold, and without sensation. The major tissue damage occurs not from the freezing of the tissues, but rather when the tissues thaw out, particularly if thawing occurs gradually. When tissues thaw slowly, partial refreezing of melted water may occur. Because these new ice crystals tend to be much larger than those formed during the original freeze, they cause even greater tissue damage. As thawing occurs, the injured area turns purple and becomes excruciatingly painful. <u>Gangrene</u> (permanent cell death) may

set in within a few days, requiring amputation of all or part of the injured limb **Figure 9**.

Management

The prehospital treatment of superficial frostbite does not differ significantly from that of deep frostbite. Usually it is difficult to determine the depth of the injury when you first see it. As the affected area is rewarmed, what was mild or little pain can become excruciating as the second phase of frostbite damage occurs: reperfusion injury. The most important factors at this time are distance to the hospital and whether the injured extremity has been partially or completely thawed before your arrival at the scene. If the extremity is still frozen when you reach the patient, you may opt to leave it frozen until the patient arrives at the hospital because rapid rewarming is difficult to carry out

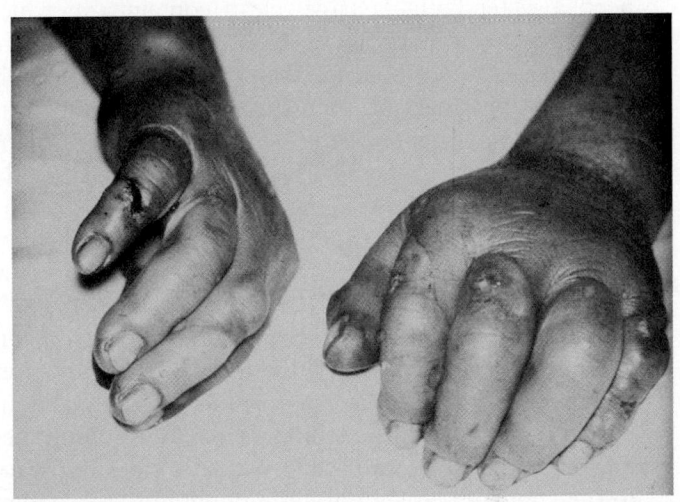

Figure 8 Frostbitten parts are hard and usually waxy to the touch.

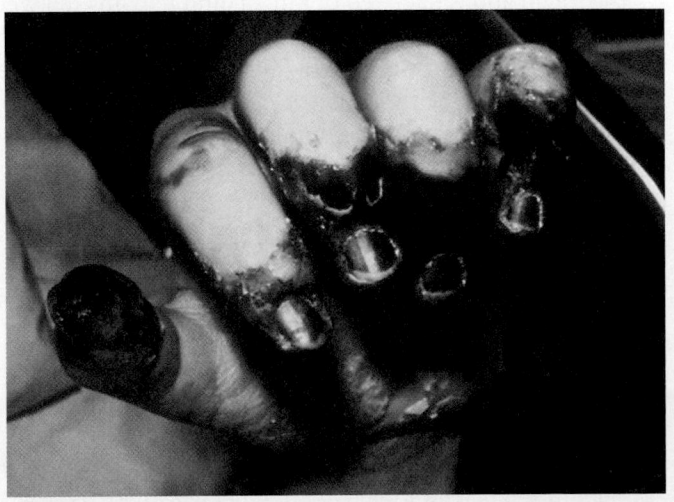

Figure 9 Gangrene can occur when tissue is frozen and chemical changes occur in the cells.

properly in the field. Contact medical control to discuss various options.

General principles include the following:

- Get the patient out of the cold. Take the patient indoors or into a heated ambulance depending on circumstances. Remove wet clothing.
- Do not rub or massage the frostbitten area; massage will cause further damage to injured tissues.
- Transport the patient to the hospital with the injured area elevated.
- Administer pain medicines as needed.
- Cover blisters with a dry, sterile dressing.
- Consider rewarming only if the potential to refreeze does not exist.

Principles of rewarming are as follows:

1. If rewarming is agreed to by medical control, rewarm the injured extremity before transport. To do so, you will need a water bath—a large, clean container in which the extremity can be immersed without touching the container's side or bottom. Water should be heated in a second container and then stirred into the water bath until the temperature of the bath is between 98°F and 100°F (about 37°C and 39°C). While you are heating the water, administer IV analgesia such as fentanyl or morphine. The patient will experience severe pain as the limb thaws out, and you want to mitigate that pain as much as possible.

2. When the water bath has reached the appropriate temperature, gently immerse the injured extremity. Keep a thermometer in the water. When the water temperature falls below 98°F (37°C), temporarily remove the injured extremity from the bath while you add more hot water to the container. Stir the water around and keep adding more hot water until the bath is again in the appropriate temperature range; then reimmerse the injured extremity.

   The rewarming procedure typically takes 10 to 30 minutes. It is complete when the frozen area is warm to the touch and is deep red or bluish (and remains red when you remove the limb from the water bath). While rewarming is in progress, the patient should be kept warm, preferably indoors, with insulated clothing and blankets. Do not permit the patient to smoke because nicotine causes vasoconstriction and, therefore, interferes with blood flow to the injured area. Do not allow the patient to ingest anything by mouth.

3. Once rewarming is complete, dry the extremity and gently apply sterile dressings. Use sterile gauze to separate frostbitten fingers and toes.

Words of Wisdom

Do not attempt rewarming in the field if there is any possibility of refreezing or if the patient must walk on the frostbitten foot.

Trench Foot and Chilblains

Trench foot involves a process similar to frostbite but can occur at temperatures as high as 60°F. It is caused by prolonged exposure to cool, wet conditions. The mechanism of injury can be explained by conduction: Wet feet lose heat 25 times faster than dry feet. Vasoconstriction and an ischemic cascade similar to that seen with frostbite then set in. Prevention—keeping the feet dry and warm—is the best treatment.

Chilblains describe itchy reddish or purple lesions usually on the face or extremities. These are believed to represent longer exposure to temperatures just above freezing.

Treatment is removal from environmental extremes and room temperature rewarming.

Hypothermia

Pathophysiology

Hypothermia is defined as a decrease in CBT generally starting at 95°F (35°C), owing to inadequate thermogenesis and/or excess environmental cold stress. This definition is somewhat arbitrary because pathophysiologic mechanisms start sooner than 95°F (35°C). Moreover, other experts define it as a CBT below 93.2°F (34°C). Extreme cold weather does not need to be present for a person to become hypothermic. For example, a geriatric patient with alcoholism who has had a stroke and is now living alone can become hypothermic in a home heated to 60°F. Other examples include an unprepared hiker caught in a summer wind and rainstorm or a person who becomes submerged in icy water **Figure 10**.

Hypothermia is sometimes also called accidental hypothermia to distinguish it from therapeutic or induced hypothermia, which is a key step in the last link in the chain of survival for comatose patients with return of spontaneous circulation.

The body regulates cold stress by increasing thermogenesis, decreasing thermolysis, and pursuing adaptive behavioral changes. Simply put, vasoconstriction produces peripheral tissue ischemia. Continued drops in temperature cause the

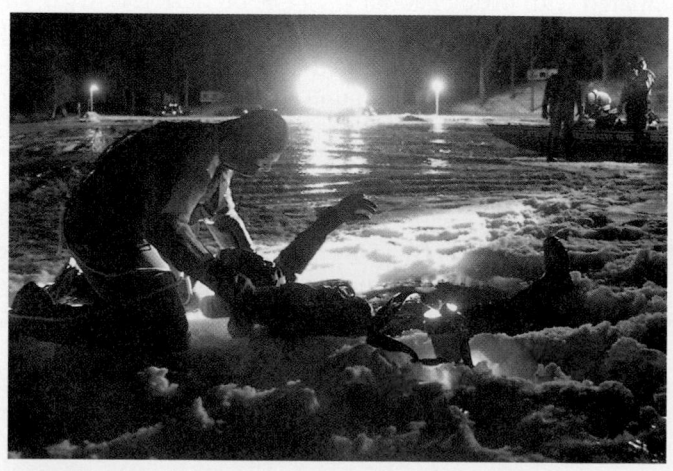

Figure 10 Patients who have been submerged in cold water are at high risk for hypothermia.

hypothalamic center to stimulate shivering. If cold continues, vasoconstriction is lost and then vasodilation occurs with loss of core heat to the periphery. Table 5 summarizes the factors contributing to thermoregulation and hypothermia.

Risk Factors for Hypothermia People at risk for hypothermia have increased thermolysis, decreased thermogenesis, impaired thermoregulation, or other contributing factors. Many issues can lead to the development of a hypothermic condition, including cold temperatures, fatigue, improper gear for adverse conditions, wetness, dehydration, malnutrition, and the length of exposure and intensity of weather conditions Table 6.

Research has shown that alcohol is by far the most common cause of heat loss in urban settings. It predisposes the patient to hypothermia by impairing shivering thermogenesis (decreased thermogenesis) and by promoting cutaneous vasodilation (increased thermolysis), which hinders the body's attempts to create an insulating shell around its warm core. Liver disease, which leads to inadequate glycogen stores, and the subnormal nutritional status of most people with alcoholism further impair metabolic heat generation. Finally, alcohol impairs judgment, which often leads to inappropriate behavior in cold conditions. Impaired thermoregulation can also occur with therapeutic use or overdoses of sedative medications, tricyclic antidepressants, and phenothiazines, primarily by interfering with central nervous system (CNS)-mediated vasoconstriction.

Older people often cannot generate heat effectively because of reduced muscle mass and a diminished shivering response. Atrophy of subcutaneous fat cells also reduces an elderly patient's insulation against heat loss. Medications commonly prescribed to older people may interfere with vasoconstriction as well. Hypothyroidism and malnutrition may further contribute to an older person's vulnerability (decreased thermogenesis).

Words of Wisdom

Simply covering a patient hit by a car and lying in the street is not good enough; body heat continues to be conducted away into the cold pavement. Quickly remove the patient from the street onto a blanket or padded backboard, and move to the ambulance.

The most important of the other factors contributing to hypothermia is trauma. Hypotension and hypovolemia can interfere with normal thermoregulation. Patients with CNS trauma, shock, and burns will not be able to mount a shivering response owing to the nature of their injuries. Last, hypothermia in trauma patients can lead to lethal coagulation problems and acidosis. If you are wearing protective gear in the cold, make sure your ambulance is preheated, ask the patient if he or

Table 5 Factors Contributing to Thermoregulation and Hypothermia

If thermogenic factors plus heat retention factors are less than cold factors, then hypothermia results.

Thermogenic Factors	Heat Retention Factors	Cold Factors
Muscular exertion	Vasoconstriction	Radiation ■ Temperature ■ Surface areas
Shivering (↑ BMR 2-5 times)	Body surface area	Convection ■ Windchill
Energy stores	Adipose tissue	Conduction ■ Wetness

Table 6 Factors That Predispose to Cold Illness

Factors That Increase Heat Loss	Factors That Impair Thermoregulatory Mechanisms	Factors That Decrease Heat Production	Miscellaneous Causes
■ Cold water drowning ■ Wet clothes ■ Windchill ■ Impaired judgment from drugs or alcohol ■ Vasodilation from: - Alcohol - Acute spinal cord injury ■ Diabetic peripheral neuropathies	■ Dehydration ■ Parkinson disease or dementias ■ Multiple sclerosis ■ Anorexia nervosa ■ Central nervous system bleeding or ischemia, spinal cord injury with neurogenic shock ■ Multisystem trauma ■ Drugs interfering with vasoconstriction: - Alcohol - Benzodiazepines - Phenothiazines - Tricyclic antidepressants	■ Hypothyroidism ■ Age extremes ■ Hypoglycemia ■ Malnutrition ■ Inability to shiver and immobility	■ Sepsis ■ Meningitis ■ Overzealous heatstroke treatment

she is cold, and do what you can to conserve the patient's body heat **Figure 11**.

Assessment

The National Institutes of Health has initiated a public awareness campaign informing the public to watch for "umbles"—stumbles, mumbles, fumbles, and grumbles. These behaviors are good indicators of how the cold affects the cerebral and cognitive functioning of patients in the early stages of hypothermia.

The 2010 American Heart Association Advanced Cardiac Life Support (ACLS) guidelines define mild hypothermia as a CBT of greater than 93.2°F (34°C), moderate between 86°F to 93.2°F (30°C to 34°C) and below this is considered severe hypothermia. In the early stage of hypothermia, the CBT is more than 95°F, but the patient shows obvious signs and symptoms of hypothermia. Fortunately, the body may compensate for this condition through thermogenesis until the patient finds a way to increase heat production or the glycogen energy stored in the muscles and liver is exhausted.

Hypothermia may also be classified according to the time to onset. Acute occurs rapidly (as in cold water submersion), subacute over a short period of (as in exposure to cold conditions during a short time), and chronic that may occur over days (for example, an urban homeless person or a poorly heated home with an elderly resident). In yet another classification, primary hypothermia is caused by cold exposures, whereas secondary hypothermia is due to problems such as severe sepsis.

In mild hypothermia, the hypothalamic-induced shivering is in full force and the "umbles" are noticeable. Often, however, the initial symptoms are vague. Older people may simply have a more flat affect, be slightly more confused, or develop symptoms suggestive of a possible stroke, including dysarthria and **ataxia**. No strong correlation has been observed between signs or symptoms and a specific CBT.

The net effect of hypothermia is to slow things down, but different body systems react in different ways. The overall slowdown of function is most dramatically apparent in the CNS, where just about everything slows—thinking, feeling, and speaking. A hypothermic patient is typically apathetic and often shows impaired reasoning ability. Speech is slow and may be slurred; coordination is impaired; and the gait is ataxic. These signs and symptoms may closely resemble those associated with stroke, head injury, acute psychiatric disturbance, or alcohol intoxication, which most likely explains why many cases of hypothermia are initially misdiagnosed.

In the cardiovascular system, hypothermia induces several changes. Initially, as peripheral vasoconstriction shunts blood to the body core, the body's volume receptors interpret the increased flow as an increase in volume. The sodium reabsorption mechanism becomes impaired, leading to maintenance of urine output (**cold diuresis**). At the same time, cooling of the tissues induces a flow of water from the intravascular to the extravascular spaces. The net effects are to increase the viscosity of the blood, thereby impairing circulation, and to produce a state of hypovolemia. Meanwhile, the heart is being affected by the drop in body temperature. Cold initially speeds up the heart, then slows the rate and disrupts the electric conduction system. At a CBT of approximately 90°F (32.2°C), the body experiences cardiac dysrhythmias, including atrial fibrillation. A unique Osborn wave may be observed if shivering does not obscure the tracing **Figure 12**. Of special concern is ventricular fibrillation (V-fib), to which a hypothermic heart becomes susceptible at a CBT of around 82.4°F (28°C). The 2010 American Heart Association ACLS guidelines suggest attempting defibrillation once. If V-fib persists, the advice and evidence is unclear and treatment may include repeated attempts in conjunction with rewarming strategies.

Initially, the respiratory rate speeds up, but later it slows, leading to a decrease in minute volume. Tracheobronchial secretions increase, and bronchospasm may occur. Noncardiogenic pulmonary edema may occur, especially in elderly patients. At 90°F (32.2°C), hypoventilation is profound,

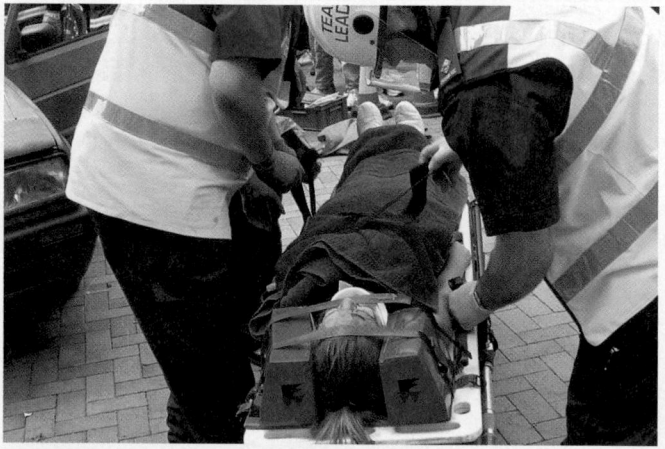

Figure 11 Trauma patients need to be moved to the backboard or stretcher as soon as is safe and medically appropriate. A blanket should be used to conserve body heat.

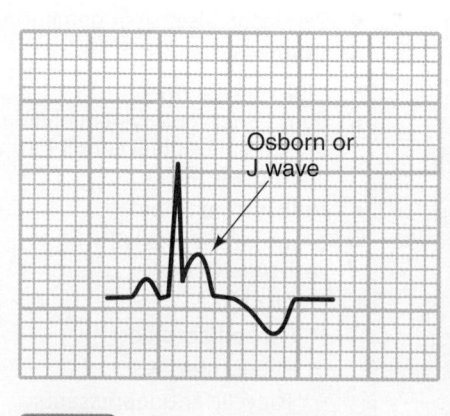

Osborn or J wave

Figure 12 Osborn or J wave.

protective airway reflexes decline, and oxygen consumption decreases by about half.

The muscular system also slows down in response to cold. Although the initial muscular reaction to cold is shivering, that reaction can cause challenges because while it generates heat, it also makes skilled movements more difficult. Shivering, in any case, ceases around 91°F (32.8°C). Thereafter, cold muscles become progressively weaker and stiffer, impairing the exposed person's ability to save himself or herself.

Finally, cold affects the body's metabolism. Shivering can deplete the body of glucose, leading to hypoglycemia. Meanwhile, insulin levels fall, making further glucose metabolism impossible, so the body switches to the metabolism of fat. The liver's metabolism of drugs is also affected by the cold. Because medications are metabolized more slowly than normal, the effects of those drugs last much longer.

Management

This section first discusses general care and then explains how to manage cardiac arrest in a hypothermic patient. General care is aimed at preserving further heat loss and rewarming. The patient should be stripped of wet clothes and insulated from further heat loss. The 2010 American Heart Association ACLS guidelines divide hypothermia into three classes and base treatment on the CBT and the presence (or absence) of a perfusing rhythm. Figure 13 summarizes and adapts these recommendations for prehospital care.

Breathing Patients with a Pulse

Mild Hypothermia Cases: 93.2°F (34°C) The treatment is passive rewarming that involves removing wet clothing, drying the patient's skin, moving the patient into a warmed ambulance, and using warm blankets or "space" blankets to prevent further conductive heat loss. Depending on the patient's location and the relative ease of transport, you may have to promote heat generation by feeding the patient, giving warm fluids (not caffeine or alcohol), and getting the patient to move about.

Moderate Hypothermia Cases: 86°F to 93.2°F (30°C to 34°C) Assuming the patient has a perfusing rhythm, the treatment is active external rewarming because passive rewarming will generally not be sufficient. This approach involves the use of several means to directly warm the patient's skin, including heating blankets or radiant heat from hot packs placed in the groin, neck, and axillae; and forced hot air. Technically the use of warmed IV fluids at temperatures from 102°F to 105°F is considered active core rewarming. It is prudent to administer a fluid bolus (unless otherwise contraindicated) to counter the hypovolemia commonly encountered in hypothermia. Commercial warming devices that use special blankets and a heated fan unit can warm patients at a rate of up to 4.3°F per hour, which is much faster than warm blankets (2.2°F). Carefully monitor the patient for direct thermal tissue injury and hemodynamic changes because active external rewarming measures can cause **afterdrop**. Afterdrop, the continued lowering of the CBT even after the patient is removed from the cold, is more common in patients with chronic hypothermia and hypothermia complicated by frostbitten extremities. In theory it is caused by rewarming peripheral blood before the core is warmed, leading to peripheral vasodilation (rewarming shock), although inadequate fluid resuscitation may also play a role.

Paramedics working in regions in which winter wilderness rescue operations are routine should carry specialized gear for prehospital management of hypothermia. The hydraulic sarong, for example, is a thin, double-layered blanket with a network of plastic tubing running between the two layers Figure 14 . This blanket is wrapped around the hypothermic patient, and water heated over a camp stove is pumped through the tubing. Other devices have been developed to help deliver heated, humidified supplemental oxygen to aid in core rewarming. Note that the oxygen must be heated *and* humidified to be effective, which generally requires the use of commercial devices.

Severe Hypothermia Cases: Less Than 86°F (30°C) The active core rewarming sequence used to treat severe hypothermia is accomplished in-hospital using the following modalities: warm IV fluids; warm, humid oxygen; body cavity lavage (peritoneal or thoracic); extracorporeal rewarming; and esophageal rewarming tubes. Cardiopulmonary bypass and continuous arteriovenous rewarming are the most rapid methods, but require specialized equipment and personnel. Rewarming should continue until the CBT is greater than 95°F (35°C), spontaneous circulation returns, or resuscitative efforts cease.

Patients with No Pulse or Not Breathing

The 2010 BLS guidelines recommend CPR if no signs of life are present. Rhythm identification should be rapidly accomplished. As mentioned previously, one attempt at defibrillation seems prudent. Other authorities argue that if there is an organized rhythm on the ECG, then CPR should be withheld because it represents a viable rhythm; follow your local guidelines. Establish IV access. Infuse warm normal saline. Attempt to insert an advanced airway, and ventilate with warm, humid oxygen. Commercial devices are available for both IV fluids and oxygen delivery. The 2010 American Heart Association ACLS guidelines suggest that "it may be reasonable to consider administration of a vasopressor during cardiac arrest according to the standard ACLS algorithm concurrent with rewarming strategies."

Withholding and Cessation of Resuscitative Efforts

In the field, patients with obvious lethal traumatic injuries or those so solidly frozen as to block the airway or chest compression efforts generally are dead. If submersion preceded the arrest, successful resuscitation is unlikely, with the possible exception of persons who have been immersed in icy waters. Trauma, alcohol overdose, and drug overdose could have led to hypothermia in the first place and can hamper resuscitation efforts. Try to factor these conditions into your treatment decisions and seek medical control input. For example, a heroin user who was found outdoors and quickly recovers after naloxone administration should have a temperature check and should not be left at the scene.

Some providers believe that patients who appear dead after prolonged exposure to cold temperatures are not dead until

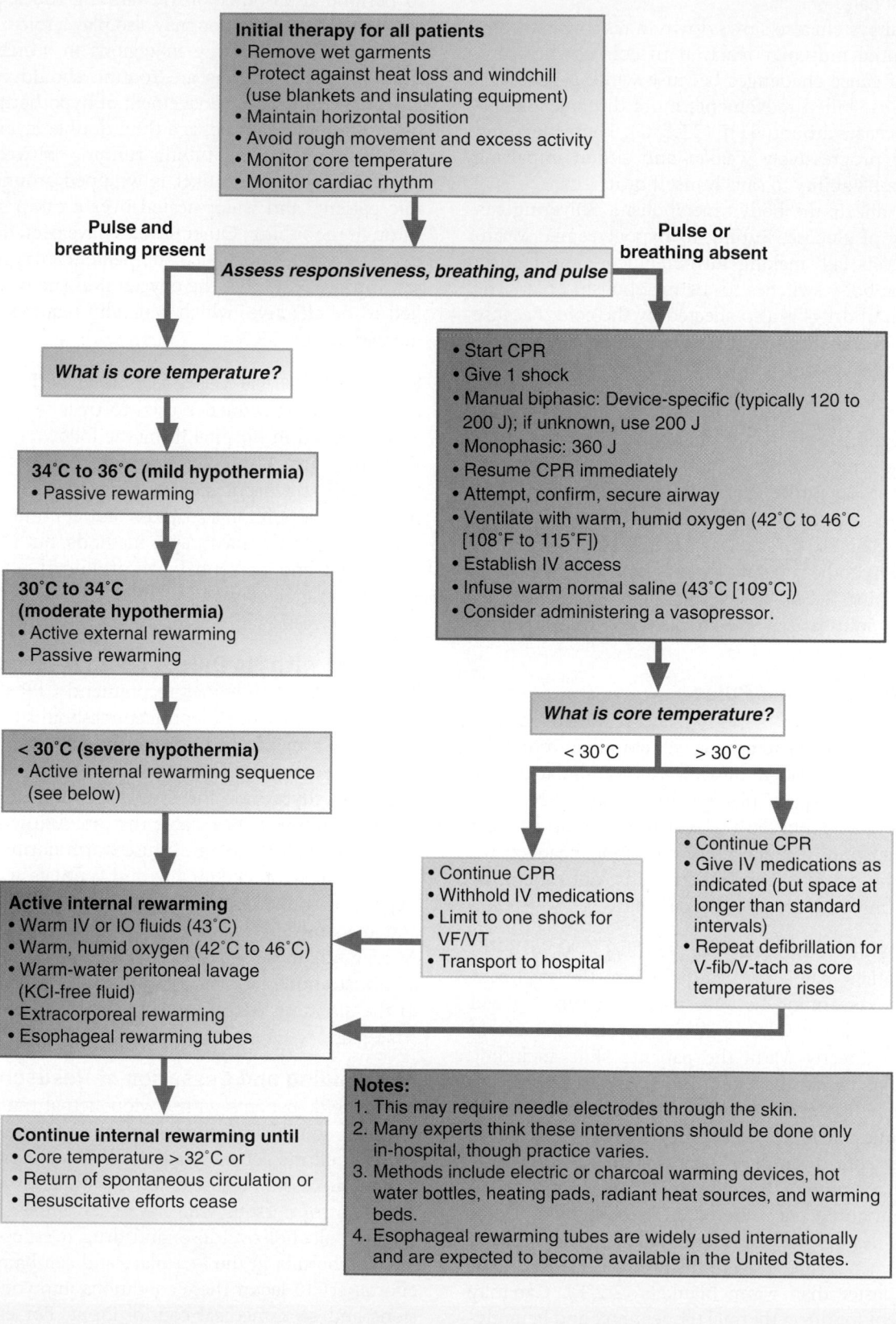

Initial therapy for all patients
- Remove wet garments
- Protect against heat loss and windchill (use blankets and insulating equipment)
- Maintain horizontal position
- Avoid rough movement and excess activity
- Monitor core temperature
- Monitor cardiac rhythm

Pulse and breathing present ← *Assess responsiveness, breathing, and pulse* → **Pulse or breathing absent**

What is core temperature?

34°C to 36°C (mild hypothermia)
- Passive rewarming

30°C to 34°C (moderate hypothermia)
- Active external rewarming
- Passive rewarming

< 30°C (severe hypothermia)
- Active internal rewarming sequence (see below)

Active internal rewarming
- Warm IV or IO fluids (43°C)
- Warm, humid oxygen (42°C to 46°C)
- Warm-water peritoneal lavage (KCl-free fluid)
- Extracorporeal rewarming
- Esophageal rewarming tubes

Continue internal rewarming until
- Core temperature > 32°C or
- Return of spontaneous circulation or
- Resuscitative efforts cease

- Start CPR
- Give 1 shock
- Manual biphasic: Device-specific (typically 120 to 200 J); if unknown, use 200 J
- Monophasic: 360 J
- Resume CPR immediately
- Attempt, confirm, secure airway
- Ventilate with warm, humid oxygen (42°C to 46°C [108°F to 115°F])
- Establish IV access
- Infuse warm normal saline (43°C [109°C])
- Consider administering a vasopressor.

What is core temperature?

< 30°C

> 30°C

- Continue CPR
- Withhold IV medications
- Limit to one shock for VF/VT
- Transport to hospital

- Continue CPR
- Give IV medications as indicated (but space at longer than standard intervals)
- Repeat defibrillation for V-fib/V-tach as core temperature rises

Notes:
1. This may require needle electrodes through the skin.
2. Many experts think these interventions should be done only in-hospital, though practice varies.
3. Methods include electric or charcoal warming devices, hot water bottles, heating pads, radiant heat sources, and warming beds.
4. Esophageal rewarming tubes are widely used internationally and are expected to become available in the United States.

Figure 13 Prehospital hypothermia treatment algorithm.

"warm and dead." The effects of hypothermia may essentially protect the brain and organs if hypothermia develops quickly, a fact that is being used to successfully treat some cardiac arrest patients. Sometimes it may be impossible to know which came first—a cardiac arrest and then hypothermia or vice versa. In those situations, it is prudent to attempt resuscitation.

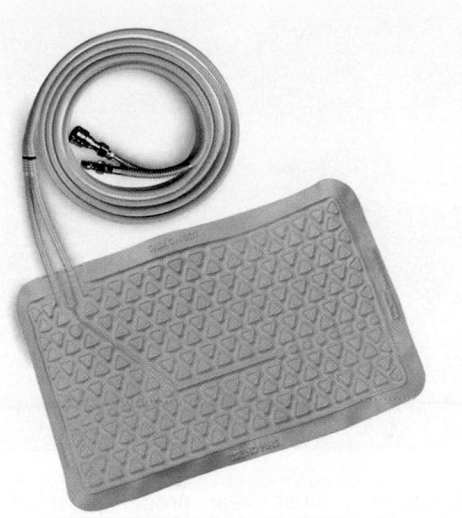

Figure 14 The hydraulic sarong can be wrapped around a patient with hypothermia and warms the patient via warm water fed through tubes.

Controversies

There is a widespread belief that rough handling of a hypothermic patient may cause the heart rhythm to change to V-fib. Although people in severe hypothermia are prone to a V-fib arrest, it has not been clearly demonstrated that intubation or roughly handling the patient causes V-fib. In fact, Danzl's multicenter hypothermia survey showed no case of V-fib in 117 hypothermic patients who were intubated. Do not let your concern for possible V-fib prevent you from inserting an advanced airway or moving the patient.

■ Pathophysiology, Assessment, and Management of Drowning

■ Pathophysiology

According to the Centers for Disease Control and Prevention, 3,443 fatal unintentional drownings occurred in the United States in 2007, making an average of about 10 people per day. In the United States, drowning is the second leading cause of injury-related death among children younger than 15 years. The numbers in the United States have improved significantly over the last century due to improved prevention and education, although they remain unchanged over the past decade.

The first task in understanding drowning is to define this condition. In 2005, the World Health Organization adopted the definition of the First World Congress on Drowning held in 2002, which will be used here: **Drowning** is the process of experiencing respiratory impairment from submersion or immersion in liquid. Drowning outcomes include death, morbidity, and near morbidity. Terms such as near-drowning, wet, dry, and secondary drowning are confusing and while previously popular have no effect on care and should no longer be used.

People may live or die based on what happens when a liquid-air interface occurs at the airway's entrance. Consequently, the drowning continuum progresses from breath holding, to **laryngospasm**, to the accumulation of carbon dioxide and the inability to oxygenate the lungs, to subsequent respiratory and cardiac arrest from multiple-organ failure due to tissue hypoxia. The patient can be resuscitated at any point along this continuum and generally speaking, the earlier the resuscitation takes place, the better the success rate.

Table 7 lists the risk factors for drowning. Note that toddlers typically drown in bathtubs, school-age children in pools, and teens in lakes or rivers. Comorbidities such as a seizure disorder or medical/physical handicaps may also contribute to drowning in an apparently safe environment such as a bathtub.

Drowning generally follows a predictable sequence starting when the victim cannot keep his or her face out of the liquid medium:

- The length of breath holding depends on the victim's state of health and fitness, his or her level of panic, and the water temperature; duration of breath holding is shorter in colder water.
- As water enters the mouth and nose, coughing and gasping ensue, and the victim may swallow considerable amounts of water. While some theoretic differences distinguish saltwater and freshwater drownings, this information is not clinically useful while you are resuscitating a patient. Both freshwater and saltwater can lead to pulmonary injuries, but the water composition does not significantly affect electrolytes or blood volume, as was previously thought.
- Water in the pharynx and laryngeal areas leads to spasms of the laryngeal muscles (laryngospasm).
- Laryngospasm leads to asphyxia—that is, a combination of hypoxemia and hypercarbia—and the patient may lose consciousness. Hypoxemia stimulates the body to shift from aerobic to anaerobic metabolism, with the ensuing production of lactate and development of metabolic acidosis.
- Eventually laryngospasm ceases and various amounts of water begin to enter the lungs.
- It is believed that the initial hypoxic insult occurs from apnea; however, as time progresses, the lungs are injured directly in a process called **acute lung injury**. Here the lung tissue is directly damaged via complex biochemical processes (including dysfunction of basement membranes,

Table 7 Risk Factors for Drowning

- Male sex
- Younger than 20 years (even higher for < 5 years)
- Preexisting conditions, such as seizure disorder, mental/physical handicaps
- Alcohol use
- Ineffective safety barriers (gates, locks, or use of a solar panel on a pool)
- Hyperventilation (see diving section on shallow water blackout syndrome)

and surfactant and cytokine damage leading to problems with the normal alveolar-capillary interface including fluid-filled airspaces and alveolar collapse). The net result is poor lung compliance and difficulty effectively ventilating and oxygenating the victim. This leads to hypoxic brain damage, and all the deleterious effects of hypoxia on the myocardium including dysrhythmias and cardiac arrest may occur.

Assessment

In general terms, the resuscitation of a victim of a drowning is the same as that for any other patient in respiratory or cardiac arrest, albeit with a few new logistic problems.

First, you must reach the victim. People who have specialized training and experience in water rescue are best able to accomplish this task Figure 15 . Many fire departments and law enforcement agencies have water rescue teams, as does the US Coast Guard.

When you reach the victim, the steps of treatment follow the usual sequence of ABCs. The first priority is establishing

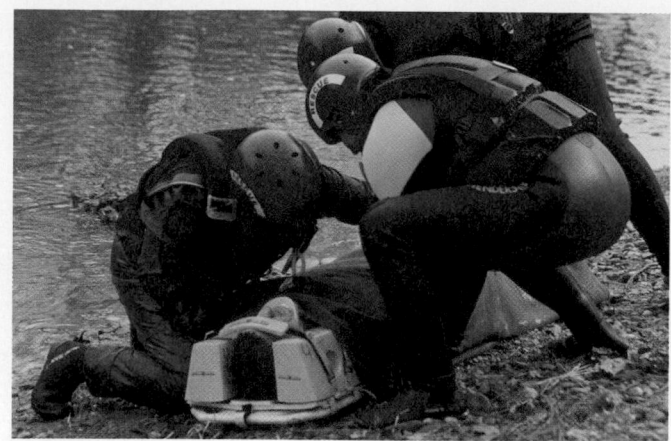

Figure 15 Rescuers must wear proper personal protective equipment, including a personal flotation device, when performing a water rescue.

YOU are the Medic   PART 3

Before moving the patient into the ambulance, you reassess his most distal pulses, sensation, and motor function. Oxygenation is supported by the placement of oxygen via a nasal cannula at 4 L/min.

En route you complete your secondary assessment, remaining suspicious about a possible head injury. Except for his frostbitten upper and lower extremities, his exam is unremarkable. The patient's fingers and toes remain soft, but sensation remains absent. The hands, fingers, toes, and feet are wrapped with bulky dressings to protect them. The patient rates his pain an "8" on a "0 to 10" scale. A large-bore IV line is established. The patient's blood glucose level is 48 mg/dL. Medical direction is consulted regarding fluid resuscitation, pain management, and glucose administration. Warm IV fluids are infused and a 500-mL normal saline bolus PRN is ordered. Dextrose 50% 25 grams IVP is administered, and morphine sulfate 2 mg IVP is given every 15 minutes PRN and as vital signs permit, titrated to effect. Heat packs are placed to his groin, neck, and axillae and the heat is turned up in the back of the ambulance. You transport the patient to a trauma center.

Recording Time: 20 Minutes	
Level of consciousness	Alert, still oriented to person, place, and day; able to respond quickly to questions
Respirations	12 breaths/min
Pulse	104 beats/min; weak and irregular
Skin	Cold, pale, and slightly moist
Blood pressure	89/54 mm Hg
Temperature	Oral, 87°F (30.6°C); rectal, 91°F (32.8°C)
ECG	Atrial flutter
Oxygen saturation (Spo$_2$)	98% while receiving 4 L/min via nasal cannula
Pupils	PEARRL
Pain scale	Visual analog scale; pain is an "8" on "0 to 10" scale

7. Why is the blood glucose reading of 48 mg/dL significant?

8. Would you support the patient drinking warm fluids?

9. What is the significance of his dysrhythmia?

the airway. Cervical spine precautions should then be taken if necessary. The 2010 American Heart Association ACLS guidelines recommend against routine cervical spine stabilization because this may hamper patient transport and care. The exceptions are patients who have a history of diving or using a waterslide, signs of injury, and alcohol intoxication.

Management

Continue rescue breathing until the patient is on land. Once the patient is on a solid surface, start supplementary oxygen and at the same time quickly determine whether the patient has a pulse. A drowning victim in accordance with 2010 American Heart Association ACLS guidelines continues to be treated according to the traditional ABC guidelines, as opposed to the CAB approach used in most resuscitations. Once two breaths have been given, chest compressions are then started and continued in accordance with ACLS and Pediatric Advanced Life Support guidelines: establish IV access, administer indicated medications such as epinephrine, perform cardiac monitoring, and defibrillate any shockable rhythms. Note that only the patient's chest needs to be dried prior to AED placement; the entire body does not need to be dried. Additional drying of the patient can be performed when it will not delay further defibrillation attempts.

Do not perform manual abdominal thrusts (Heimlich maneuver) to remove water from the lungs because they may displace water from the stomach into the lungs, increasing the risk of pneumonitis and subsequent lung infections. Suction may be used to clear the airway. Early advanced airway placement is indicated if BLS airway interventions fail.

Studies show that most drowning victims receiving rescue breathing or compressions will vomit; remove vomit from the mouth via suction, finger swipes, or other devices such as towels. Consider placing the patient on his or her side (or log rolling if on a backboard) to avoid aspiration.

During normal, spontaneous breathing, the pressure in the airways at the end of exhalation is effectively zero. As a result, some alveoli normally collapse during the expiratory phase of the respiratory cycle. When there is widespread atelectasis and shunt—as in drowning—it is desirable to maintain some positive pressure at the end of exhalation to keep the alveoli open and to drive any fluid that may have accumulated in the alveoli back into the interstitium or capillaries. The technique called positive end-expiratory pressure (PEEP) focuses on maintaining some degree of positive pressure at the end of the expiratory phase of respiration. In the field, PEEP is indicated for intubated patients who must be transported over long distances to the hospital after submersion or who have other conditions that produce significant shunt. Several commercial devices are designed to allow PEEP via an endotracheal (ET) tube. In addition, portable ventilators usually have a PEEP setting.

If an ET tube has been inserted (not before insertion!), insert a nasogastric tube to decompress the stomach (discussed in the chapter, *Airway Management and Ventilation*). If a pulse is absent, implement ALS measures similar to those used in any other case of cardiopulmonary arrest: Establish IV access, administer epinephrine, and perform cardiac monitoring and defibrillation as indicated.

Patients rescued from submersion are prone to bronchospasm from the irritation to their airways. If you hear wheezes, administer a beta-2 adrenergic drug, such as albuterol by nebulizer, as you would for a patient having an acute asthmatic attack. However, avoid corticosteroids because they are associated with adverse outcomes in drowning victims.

Do not give up on the victim of submersion, especially if the patient is a child and the incident occurred in icy water. Successful resuscitations with complete neurologic recovery have been reported even in cases in which the victim had been submerged for more than 1 hour in icy water. This is because hypothermia decreases the body's metabolic demand, likely protecting the body and brain from the effects of prolonged hypoxia. However, because hypothermia is more often dangerous than protective, remember to consider the effects of hypothermia on a drowning patient, including using the hypothermia algorithm. Do not forget to search for comorbidities, including trauma, hypoglycemia, acute coronary syndrome, cerebrovascular accident, or alcohol or drug intoxication.

Studies indicate that the length of submersion and the response to field resuscitation are major predictors of outcome. In other words, if patients are awake on hospital arrival, they will most likely have a better outcome.

Paramedics have a unique opportunity to participate in injury prevention activities. This can be as simple as commenting on pool safety practices during a call, to more formal participation in community education and prevention programs. Table 8 summarizes the management of drowning.

Postresuscitation Complications
Adult respiratory distress syndrome, hypoxic brain injury, multi-organ failure and sepsis syndromes are common complications

Table 8 Management of Drowning
▪ Rescuers trained and practiced in doing so should perform the water rescue.
▪ Protect the cervical spine in cases of obvious trauma, diving, waterslides, or alcohol intoxication.
▪ Ensure basic life support measures are being carried out with an emphasis on airway and oxygenation.
▪ Anticipate vomiting; have suction immediately available.
▪ Administer supplemental oxygen and intubate if needed.
▪ Establish IV access.
▪ Measure core temperature; prevent or treat hypothermia.
▪ Administer a beta-2 adrenergic for wheezing.
▪ Monitor end-tidal carbon dioxide and pulse oximetry.
▪ Insert a nasogastric tube in intubated patients.
▪ Transport every drowning patient to the hospital, including patients who seem to recover at the scene.

that can occur hours to days after a submersion. These factors highlight the importance of an emergency department evaluation of submersion victims. Their symptoms may be subtle (slight cough, mild tachypnea), or they may be asymptomatic. Those who walk and talk, then deteriorate, are said to have experienced postsubmersion syndrome.

■ Pathophysiology, Assessment, and Management of Diving Injuries

There are 5 million recreational scuba divers in the United States, not to mention people engaged in diving for commercial and military purposes, and about 200,000 Americans receive scuba instruction every year. Paramedics who work in coastal or lakefront areas in which diving is popular are likely to encounter a diving casualty; therefore, they should become familiar with diving medicine.

Four modes of diving are distinguished:

- **Scuba diving.** The most popular form of diving, scuba diving is named for the <u>self-contained underwater breathing apparatus</u> that the diver carries on his or her back.
- <u>Breath-hold diving</u>. Also called free diving, it does not require any equipment, except sometimes a snorkel.
- <u>Surface-tended diving</u>. Air is piped to the diver through a tube from the surface.
- <u>Saturation diving</u>. The diver remains at depth for prolonged periods.

All divers, irrespective of the type of diving they do, are subject to the increased ambient pressures that occur underwater. Injury results from the physical effect of these pressures on the body. In order for you to understand these changes, it is important to review how gases act under different physical conditions.

■ General Pathophysiology: Physical Principles of Pressure Effects

Pressure, which is defined as force per unit area, may be expressed in a number of ways. The weight of air at sea level, for example, can be expressed as 14.7 pounds per square inch (psi), as 760 mm Hg, or as 1 <u>atmosphere absolute (ATA)</u>. The latter system—measurement in ATA—is used most commonly in diving medicine. Because water is much denser than air, relatively small changes in depth produce large changes in pressure. For every 33 <u>feet of seawater (fsw)</u>, the pressure increases 1 ATA. The depth of the dive can be used to estimate the pressure to which the diver was exposed: At sea level, the pressure is 1 ATA; at a depth of 33 fsw, the pressure is 2 ATA; at 66 fsw, it is 3 ATA; and so forth. The majority of scuba diving is done at depths between 60 and 120 fsw (3 to 5 ATA).

Liquids such as water are not compressible—that is, their volumes do not change with pressure. Because the body and its tissues are composed primarily of water, their volumes are not significantly affected by the pressure changes experienced in descent or ascent through water. Gas-filled organs are another matter, however, because gases *are* compressible and follow several physical laws:

- <u>Boyle's law</u> states that at a constant temperature, the volume of a gas is inversely proportional to its pressure (if you double the pressure on a gas, you halve its volume):

$$PV = K$$

where P = pressure, V = volume, and K = a constant. As a diver descends (and the pressure goes up), gas volume is reduced; as the diver ascends (pressure goes down), gas volume increases. As shown in **Figure 16**, this effect is most extreme near the water's surface. This law explains the barotrauma that can occur in gas-filled spaces in the body (including lungs, GI tract, sinuses, and parts of the ear).

- <u>Dalton's law</u> deals with the pressures exerted by mixtures of different gases. Dalton's law states that each gas in mixture exerts the same <u>partial pressure</u> that it would exert if it were alone in the same volume and that the total pressure of a mixture of gases is the sum of the partial pressures of all gases in the mixture. Thus, for fresh air:

$$P_{total} = P_{O_2} + P_{CO_2} + P_{N_2}$$

When total pressure increases, the partial pressure of each gas increases proportionally. This law helps explain <u>nitrogen narcosis</u>, oxygen toxicity, and the dangers of contamination in pressurized breathing systems. Because the relative percentage of each gas remains constant at different pressures, it also explains why pulse oximetry readings in divers with nitrogen narcosis remain unaffected.

- <u>Henry's law</u> states that the amount (concentration) of gas dissolved in a liquid is directly proportional to the partial pressure of the gas above the liquid:

$$P = kC$$

Where P is partial pressure of the gas above the liquid, k is a constant, and C is concentration of gas in the liquid. A classic example of this law is when a sealed bottle that has dissolved carbon dioxide is opened. The opened bottle allows carbon dioxide to escape, lowering the partial pressure (P) of the gas. This forces the concentration of carbon dioxide in the soda to decrease as well, and the extra carbon dioxide escapes as bubbles. This law explains decompression sickness (the "bends").

Fresh air is composed of about 79% nitrogen and 21% oxygen. Nitrogen is an inert fat-soluble gas (it prefers to dissolve in fatty or lipid-rich tissues including the nervous system). Nitrogen in the body follows the laws described above. Per Boyle's law, the volume of nitrogen decreases as pressure increases (during descent) and its volume increases as pressure decreases (during ascent) leading to barotrauma. Per Dalton's law, the partial pressure of nitrogen increases as total pressure increases. Nitrogen at a high enough partial pressure becomes an anesthetic, leading to nitrogen narcosis at depths of around 100 fsw. Per Henry's law, as pressure

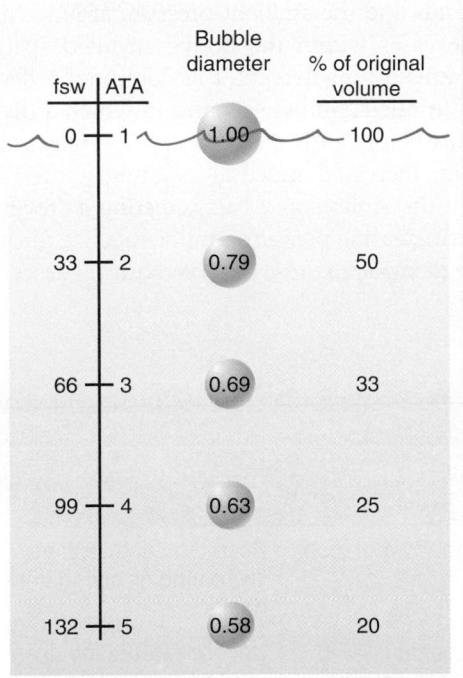

fsw	ATA	Bubble diameter	% of original volume
0	1	1.00	100
33	2	0.79	50
66	3	0.69	33
99	4	0.63	25
132	5	0.58	20

Figure 16 Boyle's law: As a bubble descends through water, its volume changes in inverse proportion to the ambient temperature.

decreases during ascent, nitrogen comes out of solution in the blood and may cause bubbles in tissue, leading to decompression sickness, or the bends. Oxygen also follows these laws, and it can cause oxygen toxicity at depths via the same mechanism as nitrogen narcosis. However, because oxygen is taken up and metabolized by the body, oxygen does not contribute to decompression sickness.

To avoid the problems listed above, commercial divers use a decompression schedule in order to allow gases time to equilibrate. Recreational divers usually adhere to a "no-decompression" limit (a table outlining safe times at various depths) so they do not have to decompress on surfacing. Use of enriched Nitrox gas, which is a gas with a lower nitrogen and higher oxygen concentration, decreases the risk of nitrogen narcosis and decompression illness (DCI) (these illnesses will be discussed later), but it increases the risk of oxygen toxicity. Dive tables and dive computers provide guidelines for divers regarding when to take decompression stops during the dive, but they are not perfect. Even if divers follow recommended tables or use the appropriate gas mixture, they may still be at risk for any type of diving injury.

General Assessment: Diving History

It is important for you to obtain as many details as you can about the dive and the onset of the patient's symptoms. As you obtain the diving history, it is helpful to use a special form that records the following information:

- When did symptoms start (during ascent or descent)? Decompression sickness will usually manifest within the first hour of surfacing and usually within 24 hours. If the patient flew after diving, consider decompression sickness up to 72 hours afterwards. Symptoms occurring within 10 minutes of surfacing suggest air embolism, especially when they are accompanied by a loss of consciousness.
- What type of diving was done and what type of equipment was used?

- What type of tank was used (compressed air or a Nitrox system [combination of nitrogen and oxygen] with distinctive yellow and green stripes on the tank or a different mixed gas)?
- Where is the diving site, and what was the water temperature?
- How many dives were made during the past 72 hours, and what were the depth, bottom time, and surface interval for each?
- Was a dive computer used?
- Were safety stops used?
- Were there any attempts at in-water decompression (considered risky)?
- Were there any dive complications?
- What were predive and postdive activities?

Injuries at Depth

Pathophysiology

Nitrogen narcosis ("rapture of the deep" or "narc'ed") is a state of altered mental status caused by breathing compressed nitrogen-containing air at depth. The human body does not use nitrogen for metabolism; thus, in a breathing gas mixture, nitrogen dilutes the concentration of oxygen. Nitrogen, which makes up 79% of fresh air, will also make up 79% of compressed air according to Dalton's law. When the pressure increases, the partial pressure of nitrogen increases as well. At a partial pressure of about 3.2 ATA, reached at about 100 ft, nitrogen begins to have anesthetic properties and divers may begin to feel the effects of nitrogen narcosis. It becomes more pronounced at 150 fsw, and is why sport divers should not use compressed air only for dives of greater than 120 ft.

Assessment

Signs and symptoms include a euphoric feeling; inappropriate behavior at depth, including lack of concern for safety, apparent stupidity or inappropriate laughter; and tingling of the lips, gums, and legs. A diver may suddenly become panicked and spit out the regulator or surface too quickly. Divers report that they are able to better tolerate breathing compressed air as their diving experience increases.

Management

The only effective way to counteract the narcotic effect of nitrogen is to lower the nitrogen partial pressure through controlled ascent or use a mixed gas for diving with a decreased nitrogen percentage.

Injuries During Descent and Ascent

Barotrauma

Pathophysiology The major problem divers encounter during descent is barotrauma ("squeeze"). This injury results from a pressure imbalance between gas-filled spaces inside the body and the external atmosphere. Barotrauma can result from two different mechanisms: compression of gases within body spaces during descent or expansion of gases within those spaces during ascent (discussed later). Barotrauma can affect any gas-filled space in the body, including the sinuses, the inner and middle ears, and even teeth. **Table 9** summarizes the types of barotrauma.

A person who is scuba diving is generally protected from barotrauma by breathing compressed air that matches the pressure of the surrounding environment. Thus, as long as the air-filled cavities of the body can equilibrate freely, they will not implode. This no longer holds true if there is an obstruction, such as with a sinus or ear infection.

As the diver ascends and the ambient pressure around him or her decreases, the gases within the body's air-filled spaces expand. As in barotrauma during descent, this commonly affects the ears and sinuses. In one common scenario in which a diver has used decongestants before a dive, the medication may wear off before ascent. The increased mucosal swelling allows air to become trapped in the sinuses and ears, creating a "reverse squeeze" in which the increasing pressure cannot equalize during ascent. Symptoms are identical to those observed during descent.

Table 9 Diving Injuries (Types of Barotrauma)

Mechanisms and Pathophysiology	Body Region	Condition	Clinical Features	Treatment
During *descent*: compression of gas in closed spaces	Ear	External ear squeeze (*barotitis externa*)	Otalgia, bloody otorrhea	Keep ear canal dry; no swimming or diving until healed
		Middle ear squeeze (*barotitis media*)	Severe ear pain, tympanic membrane can rupture; emesis, vertigo, nystagmus; self-limited facial nerve palsy	Decongestants; no diving until healed, may need IV antinausea medications
		Inner ear squeeze	Tinnitus, vertigo, hearing loss; emesis, pallor, diaphoresis	May need IV antinausea medications, decongestants; surgical repair
	Paranasal sinuses	Sinus squeeze	Severe pain over affected sinuses and upper teeth, epistaxis	Topical and oral decongestants
	Face	Face mask squeeze	Ecchymoses and petechiae of skin beneath face mask; scleral/conjunctival hemorrhage	Cold compresses, prevent by forced exhalation through nose
During *ascent*: expansion of gas in closed spaces	Gastrointestinal tract	"Gas in gut" (*aerogastralgia*)	Colicky belly pain, belching, flatulence; rare pneumoperitoneum	Rare reports of rupture; usually, no care needed
	Lungs	Pulmonary barotrauma "burst lung," pulmonary overpressurization syndrome (POPS)	Dyspnea, dysphagia, hoarseness, substernal pain; subcutaneous emphysema around neck; pneumothorax, syncope	100% oxygen; decompress pneumothorax
		Arterial gas embolism (AGE)–complication of POPS	Altered mental status, vertigo, dizziness, seizures, dyspnea, pleuritic chest pain, sudden loss of consciousness on surfacing; sudden death	100% oxygen; transport supine, avoid Trendelenburg position; hyperbaric therapy; consider steroids
Decompression sickness	Skin		Pruritus, subcutaneous emphysema, swelling, rashes	100% oxygen; observe for complications

Continues

Table 9 Diving Injuries (Types of Barotrauma), continued

Mechanisms and Pathophysiology	Body Region	Condition	Clinical Features	Treatment
	Joints and muscles	Bends ("pain-only bends")	Arthralgias, especially in elbows and shoulders, relieved by pressure	100% oxygen, analgesia; observe
	Cerebrum		Multiple sensory and motor disturbances	100% oxygen, hyperbaric therapy; IV fluids
	Cerebellum	The "staggers"	Unsteadiness, incoordination, vertigo	100% oxygen, hyperbaric therapy; IV fluids
	Spinal cord		Paraplegia, paraparesis, bladder dysfunction (inability to void), back pain	100% oxygen, hyperbaric therapy; IV fluids
	Lungs	Venous air embolism (the "chokes")	Chest pain, cough, dyspnea, signs of pulmonary embolism	100% oxygen, hyperbaric therapy; IV fluids
Dissolved nitrogen	Central nervous system	Nitrogen narcosis ("rapture of the deep")	Symptoms like those of alcohol intoxication	Controlled ascent to shallower water
Hyperventilation before dive	Central nervous system	Shallow water blackout (in breath-hold dives)	Loss of consciousness just before reaching surface	100% oxygen; assisted breathing

Assessment and Management If there is a blockage in the eustachian tube, which connects the middle ear with the nasopharynx, or if the diver cannot equalize ear pressures with a Valsalva maneuver, the pressure in the middle ear cannot be equalized with that of the outside water. A characteristic "middle ear squeeze" syndrome then develops with severe ear pain. If the tympanic membrane ruptures, nausea, vomiting, and vertigo may occur. This effect is especially likely in colder waters. At depths, this reaction may cause panic, rapid ascent, and the problems associated with such an ascent. Treatment involves a loose dressing for ear bleeding; some patients may require IV antiemetics or sedatives. Note that some symptoms, such as hearing loss and vertigo, may be a sign of decompression sickness.

Pulmonary Overpressurization Syndrome (POPS)

Pathophysiology A more dangerous form of barotrauma can occur when divers fail to exhale during an ascent, and pressure in the lungs is increased. The lung volume of scuba divers who have inhaled to their total lung capacity at a depth of 33 fsw (1 ATA) doubles by the time divers reach the surface if they were to hold their breath during ascent. This is likely to occur in an emergency ascent, for example, when divers panic due to difficulty with their equipment and give in to the instinctive impulse to hold their breath under water. The result is one of the worst forms of barotrauma of ascent—**pulmonary overpressurization syndrome (POPS)**, also known as "burst lung." It can cause pneumothorax, mediastinal and subcutaneous emphysema, alveolar hemorrhage, and a lethal **arterial gas embolism (AGE)**, discussed in the next section. Because the relative pressure and volume changes are greatest near the surface of the water, a small overpressurization—that produced by breath holding for the last 6 ft of ascent, for example—can suffice to rupture alveoli. For that reason, all diving students are trained to exhale constantly as they are ascending so as to vent air from their lungs. People with chronic obstructive pulmonary disease (COPD) and asthma are at a slightly increased risk owing to their already altered air movement dynamics.

Assessment and Management When alveoli rupture, the signs and symptoms depend in part on where the escaping air ends up. Most commonly, it leaks into the mediastinum and beneath the skin, causing mediastinal and subcutaneous emphysema. The patient may report a sensation of fullness in the throat, pain on swallowing (**odynophagia**), dyspnea, or substernal chest pain. When the patient speaks, he or she may be hoarse or have a brassy quality to the voice. Physical examination may reveal palpable subcutaneous air above the clavicles. Sometimes a crunching noise that is synchronous with the heartbeat may be audible by auscultation (called Hamman's crunch). Another less common result of alveolar rupture is pneumothorax; therefore, you should always look for unequal breath sounds, low pulse oximetry values, and hyperresonance on the affected side of the chest.

The prehospital treatment of a patient with pulmonary barotrauma depends—at least in terms of urgency—on whether the patient has an arterial gas embolism (discussed next). A diver with only pneumomediastinum and subcutaneous emphysema will most likely be managed symptomatically in the hospital. A pneumothorax may require needle decompression or a chest tube. In the field, provide 100% oxygen (by nonrebreathing mask; if you must bag the patient be careful—that is, do not give PEEP to a patient with POPS!) because it increases oxygen's partial pressure and may decrease bubble size and speed up "off-gassing."

Arterial Gas Embolism

Pathophysiology By far the most dangerous possible consequence of POPS is AGE, which is second only to drowning as a cause of death among divers. Air bubbles from ruptured alveoli enter the pulmonary capillaries and coalesce into increasingly larger bubbles as they travel through the pulmonary veins back to the left side of the heart. From the left ventricle, these bubbles may enter the coronary arteries, producing all of the effects of acute myocardial infarction, including cardiac arrest. The vast majority of air emboli, however, rise to the head, generally the highest point in the diver's body, where they cause stroke-like symptoms within the cerebral circulation.

Assessment The clinical picture of a patient with AGE tends to be dramatic. Symptoms usually appear within seconds or minutes (most commonly within 10 minutes) after surfacing and may involve just about any cerebral function. There is usually a history of panic or an uncontrolled ascent, although it can occur in shallow water. The patient may experience weakness or paralysis of one or more of the extremities, seizure activity, or unresponsiveness. A variety of other neurologic symptoms—including paresthesias, visual disturbances, deafness, and changes in mental status—are also reported.

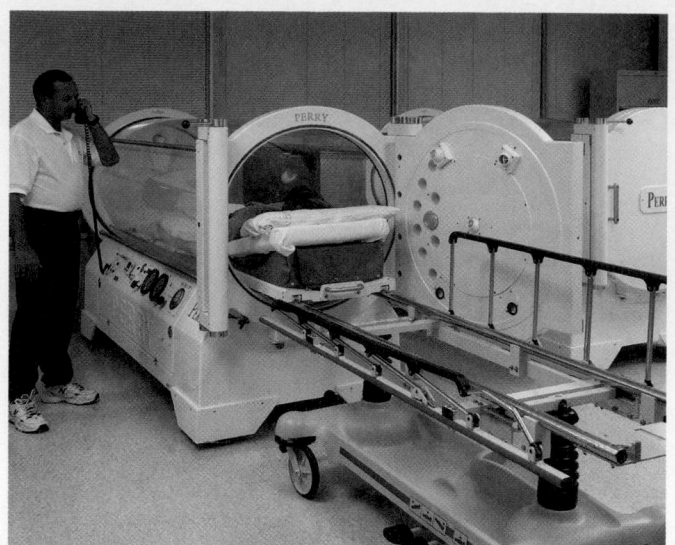

Figure 17 A hyperbaric chamber, usually a small room, is pressurized to more than atmospheric pressure and used in the treatment of decompression sickness and air embolism.

Words of Wisdom

Any diver who loses consciousness right after a dive has experienced an air embolism until proved otherwise.

Management If you suspect an AGE, transport the patient to a hyperbaric chamber facility as soon as possible for recompression **Figure 17**. Treatment of a suspected AGE is summarized below:

- Ensure an adequate airway. Intubate an unresponsive patient with an advanced airway, but remember to fill air balloons with saline—not air—to allow for hyperbaric therapy.
- Administer 100% supplemental oxygen by nonrebreathing mask.
- Transport in a supine position; avoid Trendelenburg. Monitor/treat for hypothermia if appropriate.
- Ground transport is preferred to air owing to cabin pressures, but in general, the most expeditious form of transportation to a center capable of hyperbaric oxygen therapy should be utilized.
- Establish IV access, and administer normal saline solution.
- Monitor cardiac rhythm, and be prepared to treat dysrhythmias.
- Have drugs ready for immediate use if needed:
  - Seizures may require sedatives (lorazepam, midazolam, or diazepam).

- Dopamine infusion (10 µg/kg/min) may be needed for hypotension.
- Follow local protocols for direct referral to a hyperbaric chamber facility.
- Lidocaine and steroid administration are controversial—follow local protocols.

Decompression Sickness

Pathophysiology Decompression sickness (DCS) refers to a broad range of signs and symptoms caused by nitrogen bubbles in blood and tissues coming out of solution during ascent. Bubbles do their damage in two ways: by interfering mechanically with tissue perfusion and by triggering chemical changes within the body. The ensuing multisystem disorder can potentially affect almost every organ in the body. Because nitrogen is highly lipid-soluble, the CNS and the spinal cord are more susceptible to DCS.

As a diver descends, increasing quantities of nitrogen and oxygen become dissolved in the blood (per Henry's law) and are then carried to the tissues, where oxygen is metabolized but nitrogen remains. As the diver ascends and ambient pressure decreases, the reverse process occurs: Nitrogen begins to diffuse out of the tissues. If the ascent is slow enough, the amount of nitrogen in the tissues will equilibrate with that in the alveoli and escape harmlessly with each breath. If the ascent takes place more rapidly than nitrogen can be removed, however, the diver's tissues will literally begin to bubble. This effect can be worsened if the diver undertakes multiple dives in a short time without allowing for nitrogen off-loading after each dive.

Other risk factors for DCS include obesity (more fatty tissues), dehydration, fatigue, and flying (going to higher altitude) within 12 to 14 hours of diving. Note that the activity of diving alone can lead to dehydration because it often involves activity in tropical climates while breathing dry air. Another risk factor for severe neurologic DCS is the presence of a patent foramen ovale, which affects as much as one third of the general population. This congenital defect arises when the foramen ovale between the atria fails to close at birth; it may allow nitrogen bubbles to travel from the pulmonary circulation directly into the systemic circulation, leading to increased damage of the CNS and proximal spinal cord.

Assessment Decompression sickness is classified as type I or type II. Type I refers to mild forms of DCS that involve only the skin, lymphatic system, and musculoskeletal system. Joint pain, the most common symptom, causes the patient to "bend" over in pain. The skin may become mottled and pruritic. The patient may be fatigued and weak. Lymph dysfunction is rarely seen and can lead to edema. Type II includes all the other organs, including pulmonary, cardiovascular, and nervous systems, and is more dangerous. A much more informative way to describe DCS is to specify the systems affected and the precise symptoms (see Table 9).

Management You may not always be able to distinguish between DCS and AGE in the field, especially when the patient has neurologic symptoms **Figure 18**. The term DCI is sometimes used to refer to both DCS and AGE. As a general rule, symptoms produced by air embolism usually reflect cerebral dysfunction, whereas the spinal cord is more likely to be involved in DCS. A loss of consciousness points to AGE. In terms of prehospital treatment, management in either case is basically the same: administer 100% oxygen, manage acute problems such as dysrhythmias and seizures, and transport the patient to a hyperbaric facility in optimal condition even if symptoms appear to resolve. Treatment of DCS is summarized as follows:

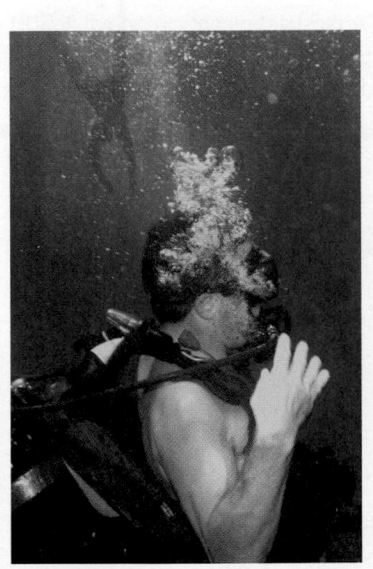

Figure 18 Decompression sickness (the "bends") affects divers who ascend to the surface too quickly.

- Ensure an adequate airway.
- Administer 100% supplemental oxygen by nonrebreathing mask.
- Insert an IV line for normal saline, and administer fluids at the rate ordered. (For long-range transport of a catheterized patient, adjust fluids to produce a urine output of 1 to 2 mL/kg/h.)
- Do not use nitrous oxide/oxygen (Nitronox) for analgesia!
- Arrange for transport per protocol to a hyperbaric facility. If you do not know where the facility is, contact the Divers Alert Network (DAN) for assistance: (919) 684-8111.

Hyperbaric Oxygen Therapy Hyperbaric oxygen therapy involves intermittent inhalation of pure oxygen under a pressure of greater than 1 ATA. This treatment mechanically reduces bubble size, reduces nitrogen content, and increases oxygen delivery to ischemic tissues. Treatment pressures and times are dictated by established tables such as the US Navy Treatment Tables. Hyperbaric oxygen is indicated in patients with AGE and DCS as well as carbon monoxide poisoning and some other subacute or chronic medical conditions. It is also used in routine decompression of industrial divers. Hyperbaric oxygen does have some risks: it can convert a pneumothorax into a tension pneumothorax if there is no chest tube. It can cause seizures due to oxygen toxicity, and it can cause barotrauma via the same mechanism as diving. Care is recommended with pregnant patients and those with lung disease such as asthma or COPD, fever, or seizure disorders due to the potential for barotraumas or seizures. However, in the setting of a patient with a possible AGE or DCS, the benefits of hyperbaric oxygen treatment may certainly outweigh the risks.

■ Other Gas-Related Problems

Pathophysiology

Most recreational divers breathe compressed air. Tanks that hold various mixtures of nitrogen and oxygen allow divers to remain underwater for longer periods. Such divers are less likely to develop DCS because they are breathing less nitrogen. Conversely, these divers are more prone to oxygen toxicity, which constitutes a CNS emergency. Air with an oxygen concentration of 21% can cause toxicity at about a depth of 200 ft.

Assessment

An affected diver may experience dizziness, lack of coordination, confusion, twitching or paresthesia symptoms, and underwater seizures.

Management

Evacuation from the water involves a controlled ascent to the surface by the diver or dive partner while ensuring the diver continues to maintain an airway and have access to air during ascent. Whereas DCS may be a concern after an emergent ascent, the risk of AGE is actually not increased when a seizing or postictal patient is brought to the surface.

On rare occasions, a scuba tank may be filled with contaminated air, especially if the compressor that fills the tank malfunctions. Carbon monoxide and carbon dioxide will affect the diver early in the dive—a characteristic that helps distinguish this condition from DCS. Treatment, once back in the boat or on the shore, involves 100% oxygen and supportive therapy; hyperbaric oxygen therapy in pregnant patients or those with significant exposure has been shown to decrease long-term neurologic consequences of carbon monoxide poisoning.

■ Shallow Water Blackout

Pathophysiology

Shallow water blackout is a condition that may be seen by paramedics in any part of the country, even in desert states. The blackout most frequently occurs in adolescent boys who are competing to see who can remain the longest underwater. One way of extending a person's underwater endurance is to hyperventilate just before diving beneath the surface. Hyperventilation decreases Pa_{CO_2} and causes cerebral vasoconstriction. Meanwhile, as the swimmer descends, his or her Pa_{O_2} increases. Because the Pa_{CO_2} is relatively low, the swimmer's respiratory drive is suppressed, so he or she can remain underwater longer than normal while oxygen continues to be removed from the alveoli. The swimmer remains conscious because cerebral function is maintained by the increased Pa_{O_2} at depth. On surfacing, however, ambient pressure rapidly decreases, the Pa_{O_2} plummets, and hypoxemia combined with cerebral vasoconstriction causes blackout just before reaching the surface.

Assessment and Management

Treatment is the same as for any other case of drowning. When the patient regains consciousness, however, you need to explain the seriousness of what just happened. Explain to the victim and any other participants that hyperventilation before a breath-hold dive is a dangerous activity that can result in death.

■ Getting Help for Diving Injuries

A valuable resource for emergency medical personnel dealing with underwater diving accidents is the DAN, which provides a 24-hour emergency consultation service at (919) 684-8111.

Calls are received at DAN headquarters at Duke University Medical Center, Durham, North Carolina, and the caller is immediately connected with a physician experienced in diving medicine who can assist with diagnosis, provide advice for early management of the accident, and supervise referral to an appropriate recompression chamber when necessary. The DAN also produces many excellent training and continuing medical education resources that are available on its website.

Documentation and Communication

In case of a diving emergency, pass along the following information to the emergency department: how long the diver was at the bottom, how many dives were performed, whether the patient was carrying a computer that recorded dive-related data, whether there was a decompression stop before fully ascending, and how deep the diver was.

■ Pathophysiology, Assessment, and Management of Altitude Illness

Altitude is considered to be a terrestrial elevation above 1,500 m (5,000 ft) because this is the level where the body normally begins to have physiologic changes due to the hypobaric hypoxia

YOU are the Medic — PART 4

En route you reassess the patient's distal pulses, motor function, and sensation to his upper and lower extremities. His pedal pulses are now present bilaterally. He is unable to move his fingers and toes, but they remain cold and he cannot feel you touch them. After consulting with medical direction, you administer an additional 500-mL warm normal saline bolus and reassess. The patient's shivering has ceased. His pain has improved and he thanks you for your care. Blankets and heat packs are replaced to keep him warm. On arrival at the hospital, the patient's sensation to his toes returns.

Recording Time: 30 Minutes	
Level of consciousness	Alert, still oriented to person, place, and time; able to respond quickly to questions
Respirations	14 breaths/min
Pulse	104 beats/min; strong and regular
Skin	Cool, pale, and dry
Blood pressure	110/64 mm Hg (after 1,000 mL of warm normal saline)
Temperature	Oral, 90°F (32.2°C); rectal; 93°F (33.9°C)
ECG	Normal sinus rhythm
Oxygen saturation (Spo$_2$)	98% while receiving 4 L/min via nasal cannula
Pupils	PEARRL
Pain scale	Visual analog scale; pain is a "4" on "0 to 10" scale

10. What are your reassessment priorities?

11. Why is it important to treat the patient's pain?

it is exposed to. Altitude illness is a problem of hypobaric hypoxia—that is, low partial pressure of oxygen leading to hypoxia. As per Dalton's law that was discussed in the section on diving, the amount of a gas that is available for the body to use is determined by the partial pressure driving that gas. As a person ascends in elevation, atmospheric pressure decreases, and therefore the partial pressure of oxygen decreases (hypobaric). This results in a decreasing amount of oxygen available for the body to use. Whereas the partial pressure of oxygen in the atmosphere decreases with increasing altitude, it remains a constant 21% of the makeup of atmospheric gases. For example, the partial pressure of arterial oxygen (Pao$_2$) is 103 mm Hg at sea level but only 81 mm Hg in Denver (elevation 5,280 ft). Barometric pressure also varies according to how far from the equator you are located (it is lower the farther you are from it) and is typically lower in the winter. Interestingly, local changes in barometric pressures can alter the "relative altitude" by 500 to 2,500 ft.

Pathophysiology

Altitude illnesses are illnesses caused by the effects of hypobaric (low atmospheric pressure) hypoxia on the CNS and pulmonary system as a result of unacclimatized people ascending to a higher altitude. It runs the gamut from the common acute mountain sickness (AMS) to the rare deaths from high-altitude cerebral edema (HACE) and high-altitude pulmonary edema (HAPE).

Altitude illness typically occurs in people who rapidly ascend to heights above 8,000 ft but can occur at altitudes as low as 6,500 ft. Symptoms usually occur within 6 to 10 hours. The incidence of altitude illness is directly related to both how high people ascend as well as how quickly they arrive at that elevation. If people ascend slowly enough, their body will acclimatize to altitude and no illness will develop. Altitude illness develops when people ascend higher or faster than their body can acclimatize to the altitude. Studies have shown that among skiers who go from sea level to higher elevations and sleep at around 8,500 ft, there is a 25% chance of developing AMS. AMS is even more common among climbers of Mt. Rainier (who typically go from sea level to 14,400 ft in as little as 18 to 24 hours), averaging 67% of all climbers. If you go fast and high, you will get sick; if you go slowly enough, you will not get sick.

In a simplified description, the body adjusts or acclimatizes to altitude by defending the amount of oxygen available for delivery to the tissues. The first response to hypobaric hypoxia is hyperventilation; this allows for the blowing off of carbon dioxide in exchange for holding onto oxygen. However, this quickly leads to a respiratory alkalosis, for which the body must compensate in order to continue to hyperventilate. This is done by the kidneys secreting bicarbonate in the urine. This causes a compensatory metabolic acidosis and the body can continue to hyperventilate. Other changes such as the increased production of red cells and changes at the cellular level to improve oxygen transfer also occur, but take several days to a week.

Hypoxia is the main culprit behind the pathophysiologic responses observed in altitude illness, but the exact mechanism remains poorly understood. The hypoxia is believed to initiate a complex series of reactions (often sympathetically mediated) that result in overperfusion to the brain and lungs, with resultant increases in capillary pressures, leakage, and then cerebral and pulmonary edema. HAPE, while part of the spectrum of altitude illness, results from marked vasospasm of the pulmonary arteries; this results in a high pressure driving fluid from the pulmonary vasculature into the lungs and causing pulmonary edema. HAPE does not result from a volume overload state (as can be seen in cardiogenic pulmonary edema). The treatments for HAPE therefore differ markedly from standard pulmonary edema, and nitroglycerin and furosemide (Lasix) are not used to treat HAPE.

Risk Factors for Altitude Illness

Several factors predispose a person to altitude illnesses. The most important risk factor is a prior history of AMS. In cases where people have previously become ill, they should slow their ascent and/or use prophylactic medicines to decrease the likelihood of illness. Normal residence below 3,000 ft, obesity, and rapid or high ascents also increases the risk of developing altitude illness **Figure 19**. Physical fitness is not a factor. Age does not matter with the exception that there is some suggestion that the elderly may be less likely to develop such an illness. The susceptibility to altitude illness is individually variable and not predictable other than by a past history of altitude exposure.

Assessment

When people ascend to an elevation higher or faster than their body can acclimatize, altitude illness develops. Altitude illness is a spectrum of illness ranging from mild AMS to life threatening HACE and HAPE. AMS is a clinical diagnosis; there are no specific physical findings that define it. HACE and HAPE have a combination of historic and physical findings that define them. The following definitions of altitude illness have been internationally established:

- **Acute mountain sickness (AMS)**. Headache plus at least one of the following: fatigue or weakness, gastrointestinal symptoms (nausea, vomiting, or loss of appetite),

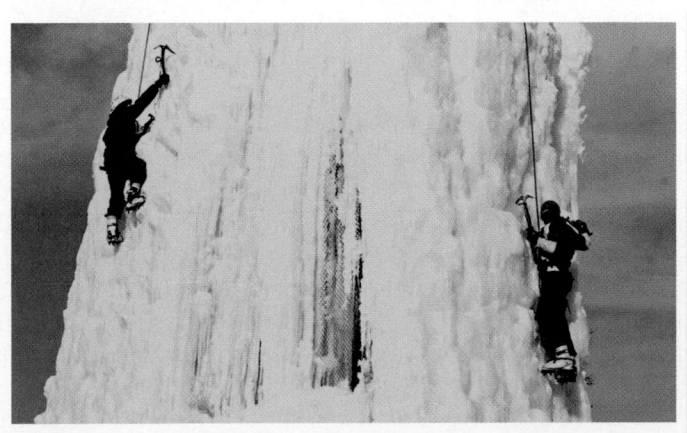

Figure 19 Rapid or high ascents increase the risk of developing altitude illness.

dizziness or light-headedness, or difficulty sleeping. The headache is often described as throbbing that is worse over the temporal or occipital areas and is exacerbated by the Valsalva maneuver.

- **High-altitude pulmonary edema (HAPE)**. At least two of the following symptoms: dyspnea at rest, cough, weakness or decreased exercise performance, or chest tightness or congestion. Also, at least two of the following signs: central cyanosis, audible rales or wheezing in at least one lung field, tachypnea, or tachycardia.
- **High-altitude cerebral edema (HACE)**. HACE requires the presence of a change in mental status and/or ataxia in a person with AMS or the presence of mental status changes and ataxia in a person without AMS.

Other conditions can mimic AMS, and the emergence of symptoms 4 or more days after being at higher elevations, a lack of a headache, or the failure of descent to improve signs or symptoms points to other causes.

■ Management

The mainstay of management of all altitude illness includes oxygen, descent, and evacuation, though the specifics of each illness vary. Prevention is best accomplished via acclimatization, and/or the use of acetazolamide in those persons likely to be susceptible for developing altitude illness given a planned ascent rate. A standard for slow ascent is to ascend sleeping altitude only 300 meters per day once over 2,500 meters in elevation. This is of course a slow ascent rate. Acetazolamide is a carbonic anhydrase inhibitor, which means it causes the kidneys to secrete bicarbonate. This causes a metabolic acidosis that the body compensates for by hyperventilating to create a respiratory alkalosis. Acetazolamide thus helps the body to acclimatize by causing the needed physiologic changes, though in reverse. Acetazolamide also decreases cerebrospinal fluid production, so it may cause some affect through decreasing minimal cerebral edema. Side affects commonly seen are diffuse and migratory paresthesias, mild diuresis, and because it hydrolyzes carbon dioxide on the tongue, it makes all carbonated beverages taste bad. Acetazolamide is a sulfa-based drug, so it should be avoided in people who develop anaphylaxis to sulfa-based antibiotics. Acetazolamide is also the only drug with an FDA approval for prevention and treatment of altitude illness.

The treatment of AMS can be both symptomatic and physiologic. Acetaminophen or aspirin can be used for headache. Antiemetics such as prochlorperazine (Compazine) or ondansetron (Zofran) can be used for nausea. Acetazolamide both treats AMS and helps the body to acclimatize to altitude. Oxygen, if available, is helpful. A patient with AMS does not mandatorily need to descend (though descent will rapidly improve AMS), but should not ascend further until the symptoms have resolved.

Descent and oxygen are the mainstays of HAPE treatment. A patient with HAPE should descend immediately. The use of medications for HAPE as adjunctive treatment is limited to those patients where descent and oxygen are not readily available or when these are not resulting in a rapid improvement in the patient. The failure of significant descent and oxygen to improve HAPE should also cause you to consider a different cause of the pulmonary symptoms.

Because a primary physiologic change causing HAPE is elevated pulmonary arterial pressure, the medications used to treat and prevent HAPE are predominantly pulmonary artery vasodilators. Nifedipine remains the gold standard for prevention and adjunctive treatment of HAPE. The phosphodiesterase inhibitors sildenafil and tadalafil are used for treatment of pulmonary hypertension and are becoming more popular for use in prevention and treatment of HAPE. Salmeterol has also been shown to be beneficial in preventing HAPE. Albuterol has not been studied but should be as effective as salmeterol. Dexamethasone has also been shown in a small well-done study to be effective in preventing HAPE, though its use has not become routine. Remember, HAPE is not a fluid overload problem, so nitrates and furosemide (Lasix) should not be used.

HACE treatment involves oxygen, mandatory descent, and use of dexamethasone. Whereas the former two are the most important, it has become standard procedure for dexamethasone to be given as soon as possible. A dose of 8 mg is given by any accessible route followed by 4 mg every 6 hours during descent/evacuation.

Portable Hyperbaric Chambers

Another adjunct useful for prehospital treatment of altitude illness when descent cannot be carried out is the use of the portable hyperbaric chamber. These are available as the Gamow bag, the PAC, and the Certec bag. The patient is placed inside these bags and air is pumped in under pressure by foot pump or electric pump. The increased pressure around the patient provides the equivalent of the patient having descended several hundred to several thousand feet. These bags are even more effective when the patient is placed on oxygen inside the bag. They are, however, cramped, claustrophobic for the patient, and make it difficult to treat a patient once they are locked inside.

■ Pathophysiology, Assessment, and Management of Lightning Strike

■ Pathophysiology

It is important for prehospital personnel to know how to care for patients injured by a lightning strike because it is the leading cause of "environmental" death in the US. In fact, 50 to 300 deaths a year in the US are attributed to lightning, with Florida being the leading state for lightning strikes. Lightning strike morbidity is even higher, with between three to five times more people being struck than are killed, though this number may be higher because the actual number struck remains unknown. Lightning strikes are not like industrial electrical injuries, and should not be treated similarly. Lightning is neither an AC nor DC current; it is a massive unidirectional flow of electrons, with voltages in the millions, up to 30 million or more volt range. As opposed to industrial injuries from high voltage, however, the duration of the current is miniscule, on the order of only one thousandth or even ten thousandth of a second; thus much of this energy is not typically transferred into the victim but rather flows over them.

The most common cause of lightning injury is a side splash injury in which lightning hits an object and then spreads out from that point, though it can also strike a person directly.

The energy from a bolt of lightning may act as a giant depolarizing charge to the entire body. This can cause asystole and respiratory arrest both via diaphragm depolarization as well as a brainstem-induced central apnea. After this depolarization, the heart, due to its automaticity, will usually resume a sinus rhythm spontaneously. However, the body's respiratory effort does not spontaneously restart, and if the patient remains apneic, the heart will then go into a secondary hypoxic arrest. Thus, if CPR is instituted promptly, most lightning strike victims will survive. However, while correct prehospital treatment results in a low death rate from lightning strike, morbidity is high; as many as 75% of people struck by lightning will have some long-term complication. Clinically significant burns are not usually seen with lightning strikes unless victims have metal objects on them that can heat up and can cause thermal burns (large metal belt buckles for example), or if they are wet and the water is converted to steam causing steam burns. Lightning strike victims may have a "Lichtenberg figure" **Figure 20** . This is pathognomonic of a lightning strike, though it is not an actual burn, but rather caused by the electron shower on the skin. Lightning strike victims may also have been thrown by the strike and should be evaluated for trauma.

Words of Wisdom

The most common time for lightning is 3 to 6 PM local time. The most dangerous time for lightning is the time just before and just after the storm has occurred.

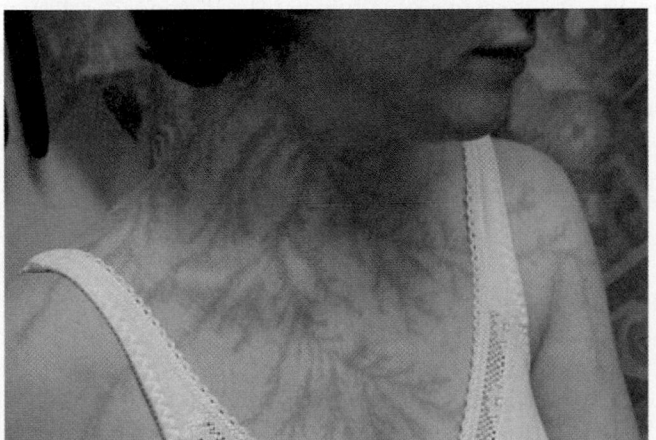

Figure 20 A Lichtenberg figure, pathognomonic of a lightning strike. It is caused by the electron shower over the skin and can last for hours to days.

Table 10 Prevention Techniques to Avoid Being Struck by Lightning

- Avoid open areas where you become the tallest object around.
- Avoid extremes of high or low ground.
- Avoid direct contact with metal or current-carrying objects.
- Avoid seeking shelter under a lone tree or in the middle of an open area.
- Seek shelter amidst trees of uniform size.
- If caught alone in an open area, keep the feet together and squat close to the ground. If legs are spread apart this theoretically provides the path of least resistance for current to run up one leg, through the body, and down the other leg, which is a path of lower resistance than through the ground.
- If caught with a group in an open area, spread out to prevent the splash effect of a lightning strike, but remain within eyesight. Each person should keep the feet and knees together and squat close to the ground.
- Being inside of a metal vehicle is extremely safe because electricity flows around the metal vehicle without entering the vehicle itself. The safety has nothing to do with the insulating effect of rubber tires. A metal vehicle would be just as effective if it were sitting on the ground on its rims. In a lightning storm, stay in your rig.
- The 30-30 rule: if the time from lighting until thunder is 30 seconds or less, make sure you are under cover. Do not leave until 30 minutes after the storm has passed. Remember the most dangerous time is just before arrival of the storm and just afterwards.

Table 10 lists prevention techniques to avoid being struck by lightning.

■ Assessment and Management

Assessment and management of injuries resulting from lightning strikes are covered in the chapter, *Burns*. Recall that the initial approach and triage of lightning victims is different than encountered in other situations. It is best summed up as "reverse triage": If patients have any signs of life, they will likely recover and can be attended to secondarily; those who appear dead are the ones who must be attended to first. A lightning strike induces cardiac and respiratory arrest. As mentioned, the heart will often restart spontaneously; however, respirations will not, and the victim therefore becomes hypoxic, preventing the heart from recovering. If CPR/rescue breathing is given, hypoxia may be prevented and the heart may restart. All victims of lightning strike need to be evaluated at a medical facility.

■ Pathophysiology, Assessment, and Management of Envenomation: Bites and Stings

There are literally thousands of creatures that produce and secrete venom in the continental United States. Fortunately, most of them do not have an effective method of injecting or spreading that venom to humans. The commonly encountered venomous creatures that you need to be aware of are the following:

- Insects of the hymenoptera species (bees, wasps, hornets, and fire ants)
- Snakes of the *Elapidae* and *Crotalid* species
- Spiders of the *Latrodectus mactans* (black widow), *Loxosceles reclusa* (brown recluse), and *Tegenaria agrestis* (hobo) variety
- Scorpions of the *Centruroides* species

The most frequent cause of mortality from all bites and **envenomations** is not the venom itself but an anaphylactic reaction to it. Anaphylaxis can occur with exposure to any venom, but is most commonly seen with hymenoptera envenomation, and thus the most deaths related to envenomation result from hymenoptera bites. Anaphylaxis is covered in the chapter, *Immunologic Emergencies*. The important point is that treatment of anaphylaxis due to bites and envenomations is no different than treatment of anaphylaxis from any other cause.

The mainstay of treatment of all envenomations that do not involve anaphylaxis is the management of the ABCs and transport. There are no antivenins commonly used prehospitally in the United States. Vascular access should be obtained for all transported patients. Do not overlook scene safety; the venomous creatures may still be around. It is also not uncommon for the patient or friends to have captured the offending creature and placed it in a bag or container with the intention of bringing it to the hospital for identification. Be careful how you handle the bag or container because some creatures, even when dead (*crotalids*), can cause envenomation.

■ Hymenoptera

Pathophysiology

As mentioned, the most common cause of envenomation-related deaths in the United States is the hymenoptera order, which includes European (honey) bees (*Aphidae*); yellow jackets, wasps, hornets (*Vespidae*); and fire ants (*Formicidae*) **Figure 21**.

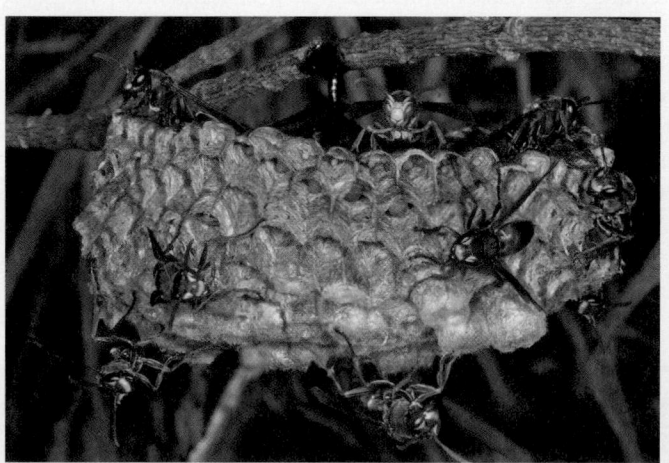

Figure 21 Hymenoptera stings include those from bees, wasps, hornets, yellow jackets, and ants.

There are estimated to be greater than 1 million hymenoptera stings annually in the United States, 3% of which require treatment for anaphylaxis. Among the hymenoptera there is a degree of cross reaction in the venom of all three of these subfamilies with each other. Therefore, a person who becomes anaphylactic after a bee sting could also become anaphylactic to a fire ant bite. In the case of stinging by a honeybee, the stinger/venom sac is pulled from the bee's body and remains attached to the skin. This only rarely occurs with any of the other subfamilies.

Assessment

The venom of hymenoptera is a complex mixture of proteins that cause a local reaction with symptoms of erythema, swelling, and pruritus. Melittin is a protein in the venom that causes the immediately painful feeling of a sting. It works through a direct effect on skin pain receptors. The more severe hymenoptera sting reactions, when they occur, are immunoglobulin-E mediated. In a quarter of those people stung, a local reaction develops, and can become quite extensive over the day or two following the sting. It is exceedingly rare for an infection to develop after a hymenoptera sting. Erythema and swelling, often with associated pruritus that begins within a day of the sting, is a local reaction and not an infection.

Anaphylaxis after a hymenoptera sting occurs rapidly, typically within 10 minutes, 95% of the time within 60 minutes, though rarely up to 4 hours.

Management

If the patient has no history of allergy to bee stings and does not have a systemic reaction, transport to the hospital is usually unnecessary. When this decision is made, advise the patient of the warning signs of anaphylaxis and the urgency of calling 9-1-1 in such an event. Instruct the patient to have the wound checked by a physician if it does not improve markedly within 24 hours. Infection is likely after the stings of fire ants, which roam the southeastern United States throughout the late spring and early summer. Fire ant stings typically produce small pustules at the sting site about 6 hours after the sting. When the pustules are broken open—oftentimes when the patient starts to scratch—the affected area is vulnerable to secondary infection.

Treatment of a hymenoptera sting focuses primarily on pain relief and minimization of the risk of infection. First, determine whether the stinger and venom sac are still attached to the skin. If so, remove the stinger as rapidly as possible using the most readily available technique. Previously it was recommended that one use a scalpel blade to gently scrape the stinger and venom sac from the wound. This was suggested as it was felt using an improper technique would inadvertently release additional venom into the skin during removal. It has subsequently been found that rapid removal is by far more important than how this is accomplished.

After removing the stinger, clean the wound thoroughly with soap and water or an antiseptic solution such as povidone-iodine. Local reactions are treated with cool compresses and elevation. Antihistamines are also used for symptomatic treatment. Antihistamines can be given orally as well as in the topical form sprayed onto the sting site. In small localized reactions, topical hydrocortisone can be used.

Specific treatment of fire ant stings includes moving the patient (and crew) away from the site, brushing off ants, and providing supportive care.

Snake Bites

Pathophysiology

There are two families of snakes in the US that are of concern for envenomation: the *Viperidae*, which cause 99% of all bites and the *Elapidae*, which cause the remaining 1%. There are approximately 10,000 snake bites in the US every year, with only 2,000 people presenting for actual treatment for the envenomation. Whereas morbidity can be significant, fatalities are rare, with only four to five seen per year. Bites are seen most commonly in the southeastern United States and Texas has the greatest number of recorded snake fatalities.

Pit viper venom contains hemolytic and proteolytic enzymes that lead to extensive local tissue damage in addition to systemic effects. This explains the medically important consequences of these bites; namely, the injection of these hemotoxic substances creates soft-tissue swelling and necrosis, local and then systemic bleeding, and clotting problems. In contrast, coral snakes possess potent neurotoxic venom that leads to paresthesias, fasciculations, weakness, respiratory difficulty, and other strokelike symptoms, but little in the way of direct local tissue injury.

Crotalids: Pit Vipers *Vipiridae*, subfamily *Crotalidae*, are the "pit vipers" and the cause of the greatest number of bites and morbidity. The name pit viper is derived from the heat-sensing pits that are located between the eye and the nostril Figure 22 . Other common findings in all crotalids include elliptical eyes and a single row of subcaudal plates (scales on the underside of the snake near the tail). Commonly encountered pit vipers include rattlesnakes (timber rattler, prairie rattler, and the eastern and western diamondback), cottonmouths (water moccasins), and copperheads. Eastern and western diamondbacks cause the greatest morbidity and mortality from snake bite.

Elapids: Coral Snakes There are three main coral snakes of concern in North America: the eastern coral snake, the Texas coral snake, and the Sonoran coral snake. Fortunately, it is difficult for the coral snake to inject its venom because its fangs are small. Envenomation typically occurs only in those persons who are handling the snake because the snake needs to stay attached to cause envenomation. The envenomation causes few local symptoms and it may be several hours before systemic symptoms develop. For this reason, any patient with a possible elapid bite needs to be transported. In the continental United States only, the elapid can be described by its banding pattern and separated from its nontoxic mimic snakes: "Red on yellow, kill a fellow, red on black, venom lack" differentiates the coral snake from its nontoxic mimics such as the king snake Figure 23 .

Assessment

First and foremost, you need to make certain that the scene is safe and that the snake is not a threat to the EMS team or the patient. Confirm that the snake is dead, trapped, or gone. Note the time at which the bite occurred. Due to the serious damage

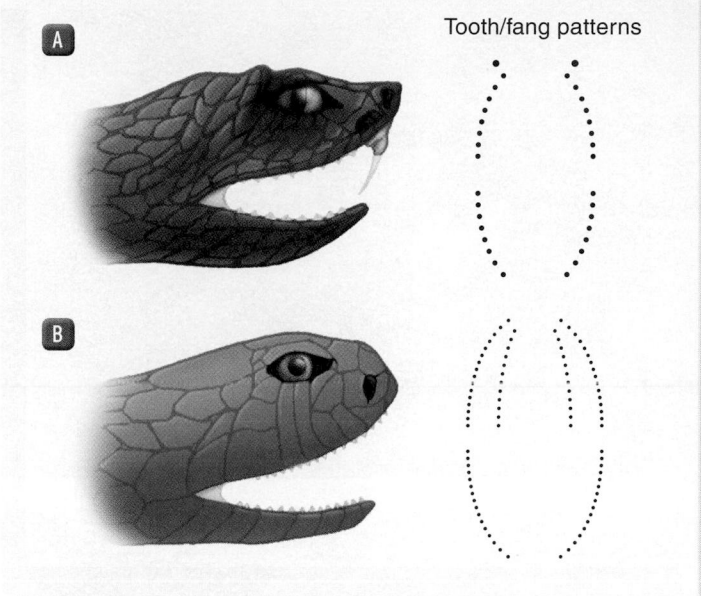

Tooth/fang patterns

Figure 22 Characteristics of pit vipers and nonpoisonous snakes. **A.** Pit vipers have vertical pupils, a pit between the eye and the nostril, a single row of teeth, and two erectile fangs. **B.** Nonpoisonous snakes have round pupils and often a double row of upper teeth; they do not leave fang marks.

that venom can cause, the amount of time that passes from the bite to the time of care is important. Determine the type of snake, if possible. This needs to be done without endangering yourself or others—dead snakes can still bite.

Venoms Crotalid venom is a mixture of enzymes that promote tissue destruction through proteolysis, hemolysis, thrombogenesis, and some degree of neurologic and cardiac toxicity in higher doses. These venom components cause the signs and symptoms of toxicity. Severity is determined by how much venom is injected as well as the location. Upwards of 25% of bites are actually "dry bites," in which no venom was injected. The ultimate severity of a bite is difficult to determine immediately after the bite, and therefore all patients should be transported. Elapid venom is primarily a neurotoxin, the injection of which leads to respiratory failure and death. The Mojave rattlesnake is an exception to the typical separation of crotalids and elapids. It is a crotalid, but it also has a potent neurotoxin in its venom, and thus its bites are a varied combination of crotalid and elapid envenomation.

Crotalid Bite Symptoms Crotalid bites cause swelling and pain at the bite site Figure 24 . In all cases of envenomation there will be bleeding from the site. Fang marks with no bleeding means that a "dry bite" has occurred. These patients should still be evaluated at the emergency department to ensure that no further signs of envenomation develop.

Bites with envenomation will usually be painful and bleed from the wound site and, as severity increases, swelling progresses up the affected extremity. Systemic symptoms also occur. Initial symptoms include an abnormal taste in the mouth, often described as metallic. Weakness, dizziness, altered mental status, and unconsciousness can occur. Diaphoresis and tachycardia

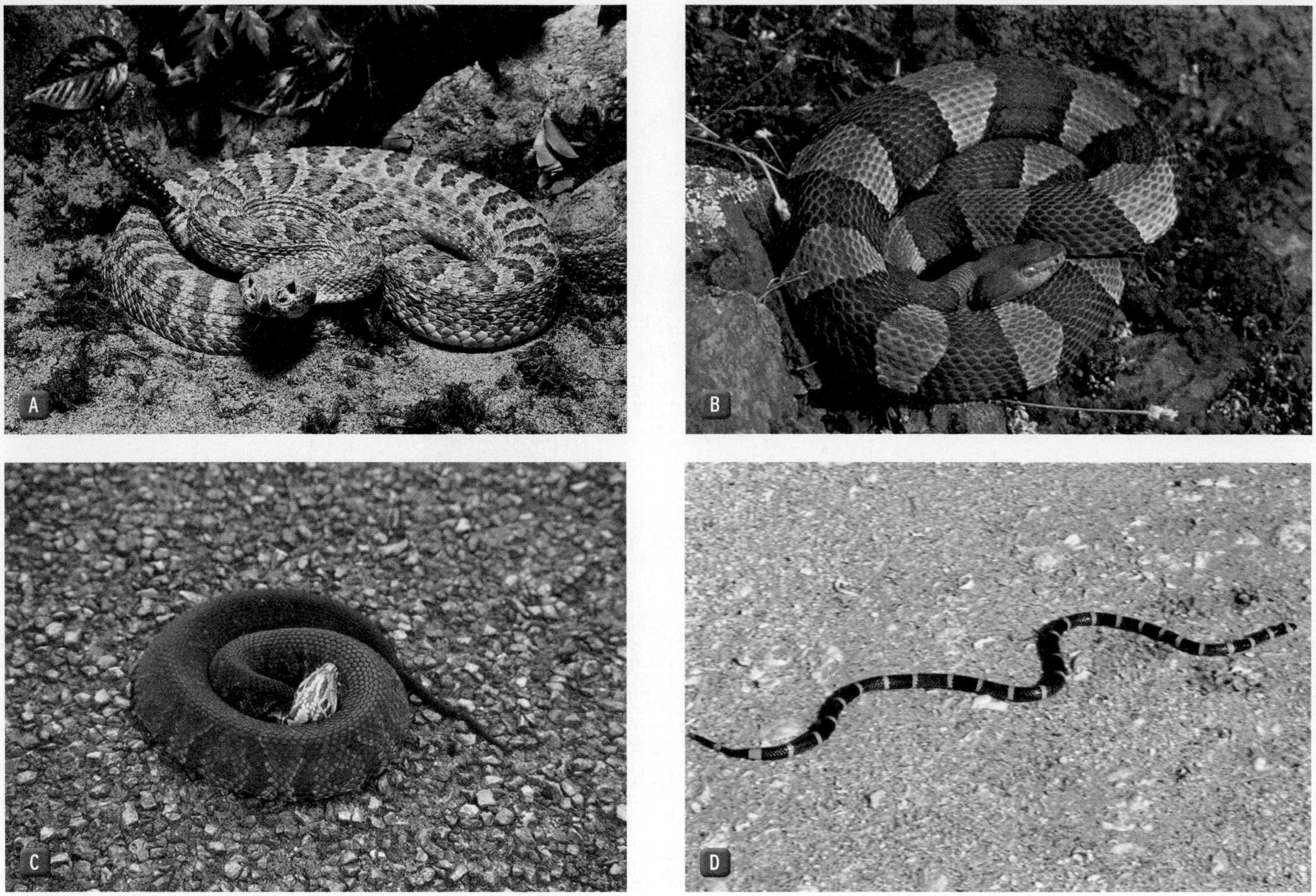

Figure 23 **A.** Rattlesnake. **B.** Copperhead. **C.** Cottonmouth. **D.** Coral snake.

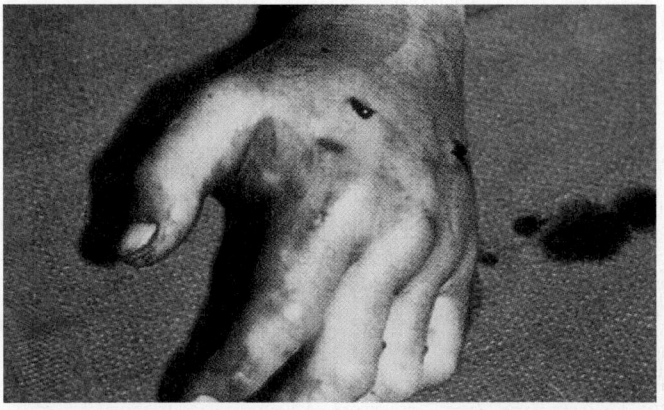

Figure 24 A snake bite wound from a poisonous snake has characteristic markings: two small puncture wounds about 1/2 inch apart, discoloration, and swelling.

can occur. Nausea and vomiting are common. As coagulopathies develop, spontaneous bleeding is seen, which may be followed by shock and cardiovascular collapse.

The degree of envenomation of a crotalid bite is determined by the degree of swelling of the affected extremity as well as the presence of any systemic symptoms.

- A mild envenomation has minimal local swelling only with no systemic symptoms.
- Moderate envenomation has swelling extending up the extremity and the presence of systemic symptoms. Coagulation abnormalities, if they occur, are minimal and no significant bleeding is seen.
- Severe envenomation has extensive soft-tissue swelling and severe systemic effects and bleeding up to and including disseminated intravascular coagulation and shock. Coagulation abnormalities are prominent.

Management

The treatment for any significant snake envenomation is the provision of antivenin. EMS systems that encounter envenomations should have protocols in place for appropriate triage to facilities with antivenin.

Monitor the ABCs in a standard fashion. An IV line should be placed and oxygen provided. Keep the patient calm, supine, and motionless to decrease venom spread and absorption. Quickly clean the wound with available antimicrobials. If local protocols allow, blood should be drawn for hospital use because coagulation studies may be unreliable in blood obtained later in the patient's course. Immobilize the involved extremity in a neutral position below the level of the heart, without applying excessive constriction. Rings and any other constricting jewelry should be removed because swelling occurs rapidly in a crotalid envenomation. Finally, begin immediate transport to a facility where the patient can receive antivenin.

Table 11 outlines lay treatments for snake bites that are not beneficial and may be outright dangerous.

Spider Bites

Pathophysiology

There are an estimated 34,000 species of spiders worldwide. Most spiders are carnivores and can bite; they normally use their venom to subdue their prey. There are three important spider species that cause envenomation in the United States. They are the black widow, brown recluse, and the hobo spiders.

Table 11 Snake Bites: Treatments to Avoid

Do not ice bites. Ice has no benefit and can increase tissue damage.

Do not incise and suction. Incision markedly increases tissue damage because a coagulopathy may have developed. The rapidity of absorption of the toxin and angle of the fangs in injecting the venom also precludes incision and suction from being of any benefit other than to increase tissue damage. Commercial suction devices without incision have been shown to be of limited benefit only if used within the first 3 minutes of the bite. If used after this time, they are of no benefit.

Do not provide electric shock to the bite. Electric shock has been touted as a method of decreasing the toxicity of venom by denaturing the venom proteins. This does not work; the amount of electricity that would be required to actually denature the snake venom would be such that it would cause third-degree burns and massive tissue destruction.

Do not use tourniquets. Tourniquets will localize the venom and in crotalid envenomation will increase the local tissue damage. This is as opposed to a constriction dressing that is designed only to limit lymphatic flow. In elapid bites, which contain a neurotoxin and little-to-no toxin that causes local tissue damage, there is a benefit to the use of constriction dressings. By inhibiting lymphatic flow, the constriction bandage slows the absorption of the neurotoxin. Constriction dressings have been used for years in the treatment of elapid bites outside of the US. Previously somewhat controversial, constriction dressings are now recommended for elapid bites in the US. A constriction bandage is made by wrapping an elastic compressive bandage tightly and proximally up the bitten extremity starting just over the site of the bite. The wrap is extended up above the next major joint and then wrapped back down the extremity to the bite site. The extremity is then immobilized.

Only the female of the black widow species poses a danger to humans. Her name derives from her disagreeable practice of devouring her mate. This spider is glossy black with a ½-inch oval body, a leg span of about 1.5 inch, and a characteristic orange or reddish hourglass mark on the abdomen **Figure 25**.

The black widow spider is found throughout the United States, but especially in the Southeast. Most of the 500 or 1,000 or so black widow spider bites that occur each year in the United States happen between the months of April and October. This spider makes its home in sheds, basements, garages, woodpiles, and similar areas. Because it likes to live in outhouses, bites may occur in some rather unusual and sensitive areas of the anatomy. However, most wounds involve the hands or forearms.

The brown recluse spider, also known as the fiddleback spider due to its unique violin-like back marking, is found from the southern Midwest of the United States to Texas and across the Southeast **Figure 26**. It is not found in the far West unless accidently transported to the region from a native state. There are species of loxoceles found in every other state, but these are not known for causing envenomation. The Northwest, however, is home to the hobo spider—a member of *Tegenara* species whose bite may be similar clinically to the brown recluse, and thus is grouped with it for clinical approach. The brown recluse is not aggressive and bites only when accidently pressed against the skin—for example, when a person puts on clothes that

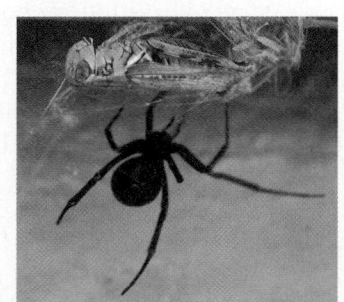

Figure 25 Black widow spiders are distinguished by their glossy black body and bright red-orange hourglass marking on the abdomen.

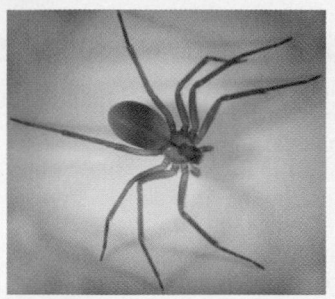

Figure 26 Brown recluse spiders are dull brown and have a dark, violin-shaped mark on the back.

the spider has crawled into. The hobo spider, while described as an "aggressive house spider," is considered to be only slightly more aggressive than the brown recluse spider.

Assessment

A history of a spider bite is not often confirmed. Instead, the patient may report a sudden, sharp prick followed by a cramping or numbing pain that begins at the bite area and gradually spreads. Extreme restlessness is the classic sign of the reaction to a black widow spider bite.

Special Populations

In children, a black widow spider bite can be fatal.

The black widow is one of the most venomous of North American spiders. Its venom is predominantly a neurotoxin (which triggers multiple neurotransmitters from presynaptic nerves) that causes local pain and swelling followed by muscle spasm and paralysis. The local pain is rapid in onset, occurring within 30 to 60 minutes of the bite. Local muscle spasm and localized diaphoresis can occur. Diffuse and more pronounced muscular spasms may then follow. These typically involve the thigh and shoulder girdle and later the abdomen. The abdominal spasm can cause a "boardlike" appearance and can be confused with an acute abdomen. Systemic symptoms of nausea and vomiting also occur. Respiratory difficulty may develop as the diaphragm becomes affected by the venom.

Brown recluse spider bites are typically painless, and most people go on to have little or no subsequent symptoms, local or systemic. In a small percentage of people bitten, local and/or systemic symptoms may develop. There is a small subset of patients who, for unknown reasons, will have more pronounced symptoms and will develop <u>loxoscelism</u> **Figure 27** . Loxoscelism is a potentially fatal condition resulting from a brown recluse spider bite that begins with a painful, inflamed vesicle that may progress to a gangrenous sloughing of the skin. Most commonly this condition presents cutaneously with pruritus and pain developing 2 to 8 hours after the bite. These symptoms worsen over the next day to day and a half, followed by the development of a necrotic lesion that can take a month or more to heal and may require skin grafting. Systemic symptoms are much rarer and include nausea, vomiting, and fever. In rare cases it has been reported that hemolysis and coagulopathies have led to death.

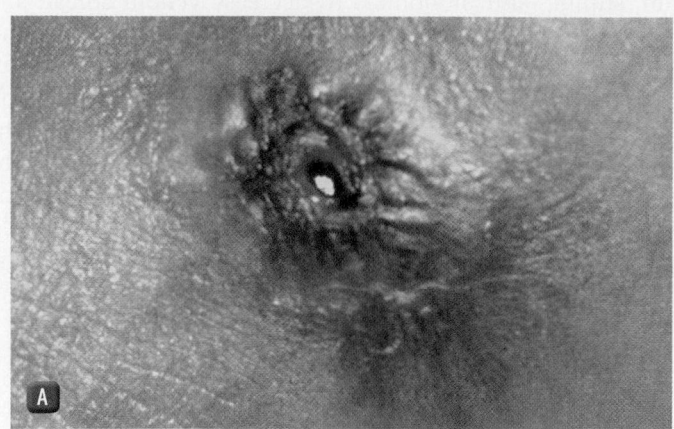

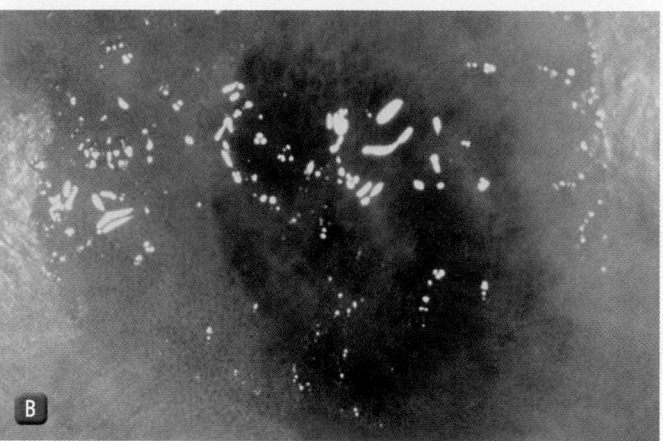

Figure 27 Brown recluse spider bite in early stage (**A**) and late stage (**B**).

Management

Treatment for a black widow spider bite includes intermittent use of ice and antimicrobial cleansing of wound, as well as providing pain and muscle spasm relief, and prompt transport. ABCs and monitoring are standard. IV access should be obtained and oxygen applied. Narcotics and muscle relaxants/sedatives are the other prehospital mainstays of therapy. Severe muscle spasms may be treated with the benzodiazepines diazepam or lorazepam. Narcotics should be used for pain relief. An antivenin is available for treatment of black widow spider bites, but its use is typically reserved for the young and old who have severe envenomation. This antivenin has a high incidence of allergic reactions inherent in all equine-derived antivenin.

Treatment for both brown recluse and hobo spider bites is supportive. Antivenin is not routinely available. Dapsone had previously been recommended for brown recluse envenomation but has recently shown to be of no benefit in the treatment of confirmed brown recluse bites. Likewise, electric shock, steroids, hyperbaric oxygen, colchicine, antihistamines, and early excision have also not been shown to be of any benefit.

Controversies

Calcium gluconate given intravenously was previously recommended for treatment of the muscle spasms and pain associated with black widow spider bites but is no longer recommended because it has been shown to be no better than placebo in symptom relief. There is an antivenin available in the United States. Contact your poison control center.

Scorpion Stings

Pathophysiology

There are approximately 90 scorpion species in the continental United States, only one of which, the *Centruroides* species (bark scorpion), is of any potential threat to humans 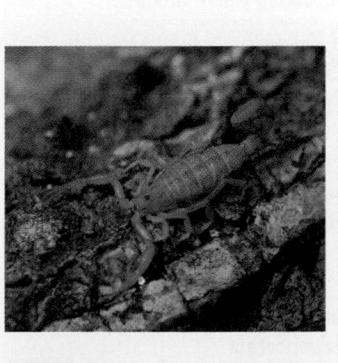. The vast majority of the 15,000 scorpion stings seen in the United States are from other species and result only in a painful local reaction. The bark scorpion is found living along the Mexican border of Arizona and California, though its habitat extends up to parts of Nevada, New Mexico, and Utah. It is not aggressive, but is nocturnal and can crawl into places such as shoes or other personal items. The bark scorpion can also climb walls, where it can be accidently encountered.

A scorpion's venom is located in the glands of the stinger with which the scorpion will stab its prey after grasping it with its claws. Scorpion venom is made up of a mixture of many toxins that affect virtually every body system.

Assessment

Local scorpion sting symptoms are similar to hymenoptera stings, with development of erythema, pruritis, urticaria, and a sharp burning pain or paresthesia. The paresthesias have been described as feeling like a strong electric shock. Local effects begin within minutes of a sting, and last for several hours. Local tissue necrosis is not common. These local symptoms are all that occur in the vast majority of scorpion stings. In contrast, a sting from the more neurotoxic bark scorpion causes minimal local symptoms. Systemic symptoms typically begin within minutes and peak by 4 to 6 hours, with resolution in 24 to 72 hours if treated symptomatically only (without the use of antivenin).

The most predominant effect of the bark scorpion venom is a neurotoxic one that causes an autonomic excitation. The toxin causes nerve sodium channels to remain open, allowing continuous activation of nerves of the sympathetic, parasympathetic, and somatic nerve systems. The symptoms seen are due to this diffuse neuronal excitation. These symptoms are

Figure 28 The bark scorpion.

myriad and depend to a great extent on which portion of the nervous system is most in overdrive, the sympathetic or parasympathetic. If the sympathetic is predominant, then tachycardia, palpitations, tachypnea, hypertension, dry mouth, and elevated temperature are seen. Sympathetically-induced pulmonary edema also may be seen. If the parasympathetic stimulation predominates, then bradycardia, hypotension, lacrimation, salivation, urination, priapisim, and defecation are seen. Cranial nerve findings are common and include nystagmus or wandering eye movements as well as tongue fasciculations and dysphagia. Muscle contractions, myoclonic jerking, and fasciculations are signs of somatic nervous system involvement. The typical bark scorpion victim has nystagmus, hypersalivation, dysphagia, mydriasis, and restlessness.

Management

Prehospital treatment primarily involves maintenance of ABCs, monitoring of the patient, and transport to the hospital. Intubation, if required for airway maintenance, should be performed. An IV line should be initiated and volume given as required for the maintenance of blood pressure. Ice packs may be applied to areas of local pain and swelling. There is no role for suction or extraction devices. The extremity should be immobilized. Application of a constricting band just above the wound site (but not tight enough to occlude the pulse) may reduce lymph flow and the subsequent spread of venom; follow your local protocol. In the unlikely event of seizures, treat with benzodiazepines per local protocol and transport the patient to an appropriate facility.

For a bark scorpion sting in which the patient shows signs of severe toxicity, a reasonable treatment is now available. Anascorp, a Mexican-manufactured scorpion antivenin, was FDA approved in 2011. This ovine-derived antivenin can rapidly decrease morbidity in those with more severe toxicity.

In-hospital treatment is protection of the ABCs through supportive care. This may include the use of alpha and beta blockers as well as atropine to control the excessive nervous system symptoms. Vasoactive drugs are used as required to control the neurologic overstimulation. If available, bark scorpion antivenin is given.

Tick Bites

Pathophysiology

Ticks are blood-sucking arthropods found around the world, often in rural, wooded areas 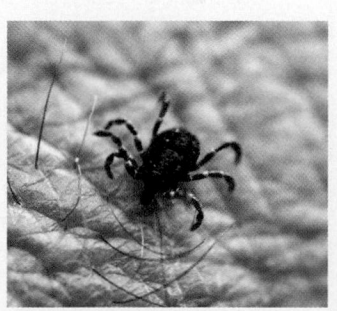. Ordinarily, tick bites are not a medical emergency, but they are of concern because ticks serve as disease vectors. Bacteria, viruses, and protozoa can be transmitted via a tick bite, and they are linked to a variety of serious

Figure 29 Ticks typically attach themselves directly to the skin.

illnesses, including febrile illness, Lyme disease (associated with a bull's-eye rash around the location of the bite), Rocky Mountain spotted fever, and tularemia.

In rare cases, a tick bite on the back of the head, neck, or spine may produce potentially life-threatening "Tick Paralysis" that cannot be reversed unless the tick is removed. The clinical presentation mirrors that of Guillain-Barré syndrome. Although this is a rare occurrence, consider this possibility in unexplained weakness or paralysis after a person (especially a child) has recently been out in a wooded area.

Assessment and Management

The principal treatment of a tick bite is careful removal of the tick. Ticks attach themselves tenaciously to their victims using their mouth parts and a cementlike adhesive. If you try to pull the tick away from the skin, the mouth parts may remain embedded. To remove the tick, after putting on gloves, use a curved forceps to grasp the tick by the head, as close to the skin as possible, and pull straight upward using steady gentle traction. Use even pressure as you pull, and avoid twisting or jerking the tick. Do not squeeze or crush the tick's body. Dispose of the tick in a container of alcohol.

Once you have removed the tick, wash the area around the bite with soap and water. Depending on your local protocol, there may be no reason to transport the patient if he or she remains asymptomatic, but do advise your patient to see a physician. If you suspect tick paralysis or Lyme disease (with its cardiac or neurologic manifestations), transport the patient.

YOU are the Medic — SUMMARY

1. What are your assessment and treatment priorities?

Assessment priorities include assessing for trauma injuries. The patient is feeling sleepy and weak and has a rapid radial pulse. Therefore, treatment priorities will focus on treatment of occult trauma injuries as well as passive rewarming. In addition, treatment priorities include spinal precautions (because he fell through the ice) and supporting airway and breathing. Assessment and treatment for cold-related injuries (frostbite) are also important.

2. What other information would you obtain about the patient and the incident?

It is important to identify any trauma injuries, especially head and spine trauma. What does the patient recall regarding the event? Were alcohol or drugs involved? Or, can any information be revealed from the patient's medical history or recent health complaints?

3. What are your early communication and transport plans?

Effective early communication with the receiving facility and transport to a trauma center will improve this patient's outcome. Depending on your location, you may consider transport by air.

4. What do these physical findings indicate to you?

His pale, cold, and moist skin could be a result of peripheral vasoconstriction as a result of frostbite. The fact that his peripheral-vascular and motor assessment is abnormal can be attributed to his frostbite. This is also evidenced by his weak and uncoordinated lower extremity movements. His fingers and toes are soft to the touch so they most likely sustained superficial frostbite. If they were firm, you should suspect deep frostbite.

5. Why is his shivering significant?

The shivering means that his core body temperature (CBT) is still probably above 91°F (32.7°C) because shivering usually ceases when the CBT drops below 91°F (32.7°C). It also means that his body is compensating for the hypothermia and trying to generate heat through movement of skeletal muscle. The implication of this action is that he will burn energy at a faster rate than if he were resting. Therefore, checking his blood glucose level is important.

6. What can you conclude from the patient's vital signs?

The patient's blood pressure and pulse rate are low. His pulse is irregular and indicates some type of dysrhythmia. He will need a 12-lead ECG and continuous cardiac monitoring for lethal dysrhythmias. In addition, you should obtain a CBT.

7. Why is the blood glucose reading of 48 mg/dL significant?

According to the American Diabetic Association, a normal random glucose level should be between 70 and 125 mg/dL. Therefore, his blood glucose level is too low. This would explain his feeling of being sleepy and weak. It is possible that the hypoglycemia was a contributing factor to the snowmobile accident, but unlikely because he is healthy otherwise and has no history of diabetes.

8. Would you support the patient drinking warm fluids?

Drinking warm fluids would have to be limited in this patient. The patient should not have caffeinated beverages because they have a diuretic effect and hypovolemia is often associated with hypothermia. Because the patient is immobilized and he is still shivering, he may be at risk for aspiration.

9. What is the significance of his dysrhythmia?

The patient is shivering and has a CBT of 91°F (32.7°C). Atrial flutter may be observed in such patients until their CBT increases. The patient remains at risk for lethal dysrhythmias, so continuous cardiac monitoring is important.

YOU *are the Medic* | **SUMMARY,** *continued*

10. What are your reassessment priorities?

It is important to reassess his vital signs and CBT for hemodynamic changes because active external rewarming can cause *afterdrop*–the continued lowering of the CBT even after the patient is removed from the cold. Because he is still at risk for dysrhythmias, cardiac monitoring remains important. Continue to reassess his frostbitten extremities for peripheral-vascular, motor, and sensory changes.

11. Why is it important to treat the patient's pain?

It is important to make the patient comfortable and treat his pain because pain causes unfavorable physiologic changes in perception and vital signs. However, careful monitoring is required when narcotic analgesics are given. Remember that side effects of narcotic analgesics include respiratory depression, bradycardia, and hypotension.

EMS Patient Care Report (PCR)

Date: 01-10-11	Incident No.: 130	Nature of Call: Hypothermia		Location: 1090 County Aire Dr	
Dispatched: 1400	En Route: 1405	At Scene: 1415	Transport: 1445	At Hospital: 1525	In Service: 1555

Patient Information

Age: 20	Allergies: No known drug allergies
Sex: M	Medications: None
Weight (in kg [lb]): 100 kg (220 lb)	Past Medical History: None
	Chief Complaint: Upper & lower extremity pain/hypothermia

Vital Signs

Time: 1425	BP: 80/40	Pulse: 104	Respirations: 10	Spo$_2$: 95%
Time: 1435	BP: 89/54	Pulse: 104	Respirations: 12	Spo$_2$: 98%
Time: 1445	BP: 110/64	Pulse: 104	Respirations: 14	Spo$_2$: 98%

EMS Treatment
(circle all that apply)

Oxygen @ __4__ L/min via (circle one): (NC) NRM Bag-mask device	Assisted Ventilation	Airway Adjunct	CPR
Defibrillation	**Bleeding Control**	**Bandaging**	**Splinting:** Spinal immobilization	**Other:** IV NS Lock #18 GA left AC, heat packs, blankets

Narrative

Pt 20-year-old male who fell through the ice while riding his snowmobile about 1300 today. Pt then walked about ½ mile home unassisted. Upon arrival found pt sitting on kitchen floor A & O X 3, but slow to answer questions. Skin is pale, cold, and moist. Shivering noted. Extremities cold with absent distal pulses, absent sensation, and unable to move fingers and toes upon command. Wet clothes removed and pt dried and blankets applied. Physical exam otherwise unremarkable. Pt recalls entire event and denies LOC, neck pain, numbness/tingling in extremities, headache, N/V, abdominal pain, chest pain, or dyspnea. Reports bilateral hand, foot, finger/toe pain and "aching all over." Pain an "8" on "0–10" scale. Fitted pt with c-collar and immobilized to long backboard. Heat packs applied to groin, neck, and axillae. En route fingers and toes remain soft and now pt can move fingers/toes, but sensation remains absent. Bulky dressings applied to hands, feet, fingers, and toes. Blood glucose 48 mg/dL. Medical direction is called and spoke to Dr. Patterson who advised a 500-mL warm NS IV bolus PRN and gave orders for morphine sulfate 2 mg IVP PRN and as vital signs permit titrated to effect and D$_{50}$ 25 grams IVP. Meds given as ordered and IV bolus X 2 given. Pain now a "4" on "0–10" scale and blood glucose is 149 mg/dL. Transported pt to St. Anthony's Hospital room # 14 and report given to Julia, RN. No pt belongings transported. Paramedic Fred #12211. **End of report**

Prep Kit

- Environmental emergencies are medical conditions caused or worsened by the weather, terrain, or unique atmospheric conditions such as high altitude or being underwater.

- Risk factors that predispose people to environmental emergencies include being very young, being elderly, being in a poor state of health, and taking certain medications.

- Thermoregulation is the body's ability to ensure a balance between heat production and release. The hypothalamus is the organ involved in regulating this balance. The skin also has a major role.

- The body produces heat through metabolism. The basal metabolic rate (BMR) is the heat energy produced at rest from normal metabolic reactions. Metabolism can be increased through exertion, which also creates body heat. Absorption of heat from the environment can also occur.

- Thermolysis is the release of heat and energy from the body. Thermogenesis is the production of heat and energy for the body.

- The body has four main means of cooling itself: radiation—transfer of heat to the environment; conduction—transfer of heat to a cooler object through direct contact; convection—loss of heat to air moving across the skin; and evaporation—conversion of liquid to a gas (sweating).

- Heat illness is the increase in core body temperature (CBT) due to inadequate thermolysis; the body cannot get rid of a heat buildup.

- Heat cramps are acute, involuntary muscle pains in the abdomen or lower extremities resulting from profuse sweating and sodium loss. The patient's pulse rate is usually rapid, the skin pale and moist, and the temperature normal. Treatment includes moving the patient to a cool environment, providing a salt-containing solution if the patient is not nauseated, or administering IV normal saline.

- Heat syncope can occur when an overheated patient suddenly changes position. Treatment includes placing the patient supine and replacing fluids.

- Heat exhaustion can result from dehydration and heat stress. Symptoms include headache, fatigue, dizziness, nausea, vomiting, and abdominal cramping. Skin is usually pale and clammy, and the pulse rate and respirations are rapid. Treatment consists of removing the patient from heat and providing fluids through sports drinks or an IV line.

- Heatstroke is defined as a core temperature above 104°F (40°C) and altered mental status. Signs include changes in behavior, nervous system disturbances (such as tremors), elevated temperature, tachycardia, hyperventilation, and skin that is dry and red or pale and sweaty. Treatment is to remove the patient from the heat, perform cooling measures, administer normal saline, and monitor the cardiac rhythm.

- Fever can mimic heatstroke. Obtain a thorough history, and treat for heatstroke if in doubt.

- To prevent heat illness, dress appropriately, stay hydrated, and stay in the shade or air conditioning. Community-based programs aimed at high-risk populations can provide valuable education.

- Frostbite is local freezing of a body part; it is classified as superficial or deep. Frostnip is a mild form of frostbite.

- Superficial frostbite is characterized by numbness, tingling, or burning. The skin is white, waxy, and firm to palpation. When thawed, the skin turns cyanotic and the patient feels a hot, stinging sensation. Treatment consists of getting the patient out of the cold; rewarming the injured part with body heat; covering with a warm, sterile dressing; and transporting the patient.

- In deep frostbite, the injured body part looks white, yellow-white, or mottled blue-white and is hard, cold, and without sensation. Major tissue damage can occur when the part thaws. Gangrene (permanent cell death) can result in the need for amputation. Treatment includes leaving the part frozen if it is found frozen, or rewarming the part if it is partially thawed.

- Trench foot is similar to frostbite but results from prolonged exposure to cool, wet conditions. Prevention is the best treatment.

- Hypothermia is a decrease in core body temperature. It can be mild, moderate, or severe.

- Mild hypothermia is a core body temperature of greater than 93°F (33.9°C). The patient shivers and may be confused, have slurred speech, or have impaired coordination. Treatment is passive rewarming such as removing wet clothing or drying the patient's skin and possibly providing warm fluids.

- Moderate hypothermia is a core body temperature in the range of 86°F to 93°F (30°C to 33.9°C). Treatment is passive rewarming, active external rewarming of truncal areas, administering warmed IV fluids, and potentially using special rewarming devices.

- Severe hypothermia is a core body temperature of less than 86°F (30°C). Treatment is active internal rewarming, such as administering warm IV fluids, and in-hospital measures.

- Hypothermic patients who are not breathing or who do not have a pulse need resuscitation. Patients in cardiac arrest require high-quality CPR and possibly a single shock depending on the heart rhythm; follow local guidelines. Attempt to insert an advanced airway; deliver ventilation with warm, humidified oxygen; and provide IV fluids.

- Hypothermic patients with obvious lethal traumatic injuries or patients who are so frozen as to block the airway or chest compression efforts generally are dead. If the patient appears dead after prolonged exposure, hypothermia may protect the brain and organs. Resuscitation can be attempted in cases of cardiac arrest and hypothermia.

- Drowning is the process of experiencing respiratory impairment from submersion or immersion in liquid. Drowning progresses from breath holding, to laryngospasm, to respiratory and cardiac arrest.

- Caring for a patient who drowned starts with reaching the patient, a task that should be undertaken by specially trained rescuers. Treatment includes caring for the ABCs and taking cervical spine precautions. Positive end-expiratory pressure may be used to keep the alveoli open and drive fluid out. A nasogastric tube may be inserted to decompress the stomach if the patient is intubated. Submersion patients may develop bronchospasm and may require administration of a beta-2 adrenergic drug.

- In diving injuries, obtain as many details as possible about the patient, including the type of diving, type of tank, number of dives in the past 72 hours, and pre-dive and post-dive activities.

- Barotrauma can result during dive descent, owing to a pressure imbalance between the inside of the body and the outside atmosphere. It may result in ear pain. Treatment is a loose dressing for ear bleeding, and possibly IV antiemetics or sedatives.

- Nitrogen narcosis is a state of altered mental status caused by breathing compressed air at depth. Signs and symptoms include feeling euphoric; exhibiting inappropriate, foolish behavior; and tingling of the lips, gums, and legs.

- When a diver ascends too quickly, pulmonary overpressurization syndrome (POPS, also known as burst lung) can occur. Signs and symptoms include mediastinal and subcutaneous emphysema, a sense of fullness in the throat, pain on swallowing, dyspnea, and substernal chest pain.

- Arterial gas embolism is a dangerous consequence of pulmonary overpressurization syndrome. Air bubbles may travel to the coronary arteries, causing cardiac arrest. Symptoms include weakness or paralysis of the extremities, seizure activity, unresponsiveness, and other neurologic symptoms.

- Treatment of barotrauma depends on whether an air embolism is present. A pneumothorax may require needle decompression. With an air embolism, the patient must receive treatment in a hyperbaric chamber.

- Decompression sickness encompasses a broad range of signs and symptoms caused by nitrogen bubbles in blood and tissues coming out of solution on dive ascent. Symptoms include itchy skin, subcutaneous emphysema, swelling, rashes, joint and muscle pain, sensory and motor disturbances, incoordination, paralysis, chest pain, and dyspnea. Treatment is 100% oxygen, IV normal saline, and transport to a hyperbaric facility.

- Shallow water blackout occurs when a person hyperventilates just before diving underwater and passes out before resurfacing. Treatment is the same as for any other submersion.

- The Divers Alert Network is a valuable resource for diving-related injuries. Callers are immediately connected to a physician experienced in diving medicine who can provide advice regarding specific management.

- Altitude illness occurs when unacclimatized people ascend to altitude. Types of altitude illness include acute mountain sickness (AMS), high-altitude cerebral edema (HACE), and high-altitude pulmonary edema (HAPE).

- Symptoms of acute mountain sickness include headache plus fatigue, weakness, gastrointestinal symptoms, dizziness, light-headedness, and difficulty sleeping.

- Symptoms of high-altitude cerebral edema include a change in mental status and/or ataxia in a person with acute mountain sickness or the presence of both in a person without acute mountain sickness.

- Symptoms of high-altitude pulmonary edema include at least two of the following: dyspnea at rest, cough, weakness, or chest tightness or congestion and at least two of the following: central cyanosis, audible rales, wheezing, tachypnea, or tachycardia.

- Treatment of altitude illnesses includes descending or using a portable hyperbaric chamber, providing oxygen, and administering certain IV medications.

- Cardiopulmonary resuscitation should be started promptly for lightning strike victims.

- Lightning strike victims should be evaluated using "reverse triage," meaning that those people who appear to be dead should be treated first.

- Anaphylactic reaction is the most frequent cause of mortality from all insect bites and envenomations.

- Prompt removal of hymenoptera stingers or venom sacs can decrease toxin exposure.

- Fire ant stings often result in infection.

- Pit vipers (crotalids) are responsible for the greatest number of snake bites in the United States.

- With a crotalid bite, if there are visible fang marks with no bleeding, this indicates that a "dry bite" (with no venom) has occurred.

- In terms of scene safety, it is important to make sure the snake is dead, gone, or trapped in cases of envenomation.

- All significant snake envenomations require treatment with antivenin; transport promptly. The time between the occurrence of the bite and the time of treatment is crucial.

- The female black widow, the brown recluse, and the hobo spider produce the most concerning spider bites.

- A small subset of patients with brown recluse spider bites may develop loxoscelism.

- Scorpion stings produce a neurotoxic reaction that causes autonomic excitation.

- Treatment of scorpion stings is largely supportive, with protection of the airway.

- Tick bites can transmit a variety of serious illnesses, and in rare cases, can cause life-threatening paralysis. Principal treatment is careful removal of the tick, and washing the area around the bite. Transport all patients with any neurologic symptoms.

Prep Kit, continued

■ Vital Vocabulary

acute lung injury A condition in which lung tissue is damaged, characterized by hypoxemia, low lung volume, and pulmonary edema.

acute mountain sickness (AMS) An altitude illness characterized by headache plus at least one of the following: fatigue or weakness, gastrointestinal symptoms (nausea, vomiting or anorexia), dizziness or light-headedness, or difficulty sleeping.

afterdrop Continued fall in core temperature after a victim of hypothermia has been removed from a cold environment, due at least in part to the return of cold blood from the body surface to the body core.

altitude illnesses Conditions caused by the effects from hypobaric (low atmospheric pressure) hypoxia on the central nervous system and pulmonary systems as a result of unacclimatized people ascending to altitude; range from acute mountain sickness (AMS) to high-altitude cerebral edema (HACE) and high-altitude pulmonary edema (HAPE).

arterial gas embolism (AGE) The resultant gaseous emboli from the forcing of gas into the vasculature from barotrauma.

ataxia Inability to coordinate the muscles properly; often used to describe a staggering gait.

atmosphere absolute (ATA) A measurement of ambient pressure; the weight of air at sea level, equivalent in pressure to 33 feet of seawater (fsw).

barotrauma Injury resulting from pressure disequilibrium across body surfaces.

basal metabolic rate (BMR) The heat energy produced at rest from normal body metabolic reactions, determined mostly by the liver and skeletal muscles.

Boyle's law At a constant temperature, the volume of a gas is inversely proportional to its pressure (if you double the pressure on a gas, you halve its volume); written as PV = K, where P = pressure, V = volume, and K = a constant.

breath-hold diving Also called free diving, this type of diving does not require any equipment, except sometimes a snorkel.

chilblains Itchy reddish and purple swollen lesions that occur primarily on the extremities, due to longer exposure to temperatures just above freezing or sudden rewarming after exposure to cold.

classic heatstroke Also called passive heatstroke, this is a serious heat illness that usually occurs during heat waves and is most likely to strike very old, very young, or bedridden people.

cold diuresis Secretion of large amounts of urine in response to cold exposure and the consequent shunting of blood volume to the body core.

conduction Transfer of heat to a solid object or a liquid by direct contact.

convection Mechanism by which body heat is picked up and carried away by moving air currents.

core body temperature (CBT) The temperature in the part of the body comprising the heart, lungs, brain, and abdominal viscera.

Dalton's law Each gas in a mixture exerts the same partial pressure that it would exert if it were alone in the same volume, and the total pressure of a mixture of gases is the sum of the partial pressures of all the gases in a mixture.

decompression illness (DCI) A term for decompression sickness (DCS) and air gas embolism (AGE).

decompression sickness (DCS) A broad range of signs and symptoms caused by nitrogen bubbles in blood and tissues coming out of solution on ascent.

deep frostbite A type of frostbite in which the affected part looks white, yellow-white, or mottled blue-white and is hard, cold, and without sensation.

drowning The process of experiencing respiratory impairment from submersion or immersion in liquid.

envenomation The injecting of venom via a bite or sting.

environmental emergencies Medical conditions caused or exacerbated by the weather, terrain, or unique atmospheric conditions such as high altitude or underwater.

evaporation The conversion of a liquid to a gas.

exercise-associated hyponatremia A condition due to prolonged exertion in hot environments coupled with excessive hypotonic fluid intake that leads to nausea, vomiting, and, in severe cases, mental status changes and seizures (also known as exertional hyponatremia).

exertional heatstroke A serious type of heatstroke usually affecting young and fit people exercising in hot and humid conditions.

feet of seawater (fsw) An indirect measure of pressure under water, equal to one atmosphere absolute (ATA).

frostbite Localized damage to tissues resulting from prolonged exposure to extreme cold.

frostnip Early frostbite, characterized by numbness and pallor without significant tissue damage.

gangrene Permanent cell death.

heat cramps Acute and involuntary muscle pains, usually in the lower extremities, the abdomen, or both, that occur because of profuse sweating and subsequent sodium losses in sweat.

heat exhaustion A clinical syndrome characterized by volume depletion and heat stress that is thought to be a milder form of heat illness and on a continuum leading to heatstroke.

heat illness The increase in core body temperature due to inadequate thermolysis.

heatstroke The least common and most deadly heat illness, caused by a severe disturbance in thermoregulation, usually characterized by a core temperature of more than 104°F (40°C) and altered mental status.

heat syncope An orthostatic or near-syncopal episode that typically occurs in nonacclimated people who may be under heat stress.

Henry's law The amount of gas dissolved in a liquid is directly proportional to the partial pressure of the gas above the liquid.

high-altitude cerebral edema (HACE) An altitude illness in which there is a change in mental status and/or ataxia in a person with acute mountain sickness or the presence of mental status changes and ataxia in a person without acute mountain sickness.

high-altitude pulmonary edema (HAPE) An altitude illness characterized by at least two of the following: dyspnea at rest, cough, weakness or decreased exercise performance, or chest tightness or congestion. Also, at least two of the following signs: central cyanosis, audible rales or wheezing in at least one lung field, tachypnea, or tachycardia.

homeostasis Body processes that balance the supply and demand of the body's needs.

hyperthermia Unusually elevated body temperature.

hypothalamus Portion of the brain that regulates a multitude of body functions, including core temperature.

hypothermia Condition in which the core body temperature is significantly below normal.

laryngospasm Severe constriction of the larynx in response to allergy, noxious stimuli, or illness.

loxoscelism A potentially fatal condition resulting from a brown recluse spider bite that begins with a painful, inflamed vesicle that may progress to a gangrenous sloughing of the skin.

malignant hyperthermia A condition that can result from common anesthesia medications (notably succinylcholine) and present with hyperthermia, muscular rigidity, altered mental status, and a hyperdynamic state.

neuroleptic malignant syndrome (NMS) A condition caused by antipsychotic and even common antiemetic medications that presents with hyperthermia, muscular rigidity, altered mental status, and a hyperdynamic state.

nitrogen narcosis A state resembling alcohol intoxication produced by nitrogen gas dissolved in the blood at high ambient pressure; also called rapture of the deep.

odynophagia Painful swallowing.

orthostatic hypotension A fall in blood pressure that occurs when moving from a recumbent to a sitting or standing position.

partial pressure The amount of the total pressure contributed by various gases in solution.

pulmonary overpressurization syndrome (POPS) Also called "burst lung," this diving emergency can occur during rapid ascent and can cause pneumothorax, mediastinal and subcutaneous emphysema, alveolar hemorrhage, and the lethal arterial gas embolism (AGE).

radiation Emission of heat from an object into surrounding, colder air.

saturation diving A type of diving in which the diver remains at depth for prolonged periods.

self-contained underwater breathing apparatus The expansion of the acronym (SCUBA) for specialized underwater breathing equipment.

shallow water blackout A diving emergency that occurs when a person hyperventilates just before submerging underwater and loses consciousness before resurfacing due to hypoxemia and cerebral vasoconstriction.

superficial frostbite A type of frostbite characterized by altered sensation (numbness, tingling, or burning) and white, waxy skin that is firm to palpation, but the underlying tissues remain soft.

surface-tended diving A type of diving in which air is piped to the diver through a tube from the surface.

thermogenesis The production of heat in the body.

thermolysis The liberation of heat from the body.

thermoregulation The process by which the body compensates for environmental extremes, for example, balancing between heat production and heat release.

trench foot A process similar to frostbite but caused by prolonged exposure to cool, wet conditions.

wind chill factor The factor that takes into account the temperature and wind velocity in calculating the effect of a given ambient temperature on living organisms.

Assessment in Action

It is a hot, humid summer day (98°F ambient air temperature/80% humidity) and you are dispatched to the scene of a local grocery store for a 2-year-old girl who is unresponsive. According to law enforcement personnel at the scene, the child was left in the car "with the windows cracked" while her mother went in the store "for just a minute." When you arrive, you find the child with the police who now have her in their air-conditioned patrol car; she is lying supine on some towels in the back seat. A police officer is fanning the child as he sits next to her in the squad car. The child is extremely flushed and her skin is hot, dry, and red. Her extremities are mottled and her lips are gray. She is unresponsive to voice and pain (no motor response), and without eye opening. Her airway is open with dried secretions around the mouth.

Her vital signs are: respirations, 70 breaths/min with retractions; carotid pulse, 180 beats/min, weak and regular; blood pressure cannot be measured; and pulse oximetry, 88% on room air; rectal thermometer reads 106°F; capillary refill time is 5 seconds. Lung sounds are diminished, but clear and equal bilaterally. Her weight is estimated at 16 kg using a length-based resuscitation tape. There are no signs of trauma injuries. The patient's clothes are removed as she is placed on the stretcher and bag-mask ventilations are initiated with 100% oxygen. While en route to the closest pediatric specialty center, IV access is attempted twice without success. Intraosseous access in the left tibia is obtained. Cold packs are applied to the patient's neck, groin, and axillae, and the air conditioner in the back of the ambulance is turned to its lowest setting. Medical direction is consulted and a rapid infusion of a 10 mL/kg NS bolus is ordered PRN. Her blood glucose level is 38 mg/dL. D_{25} 12.5 grams IVP is given per protocol. En route a complete trauma assessment is performed and found to be unremarkable.

1. The body reacts to hot environmental conditions by releasing stored heat and energy by a process called:
   A. thermolysis.
   B. hemolysis.
   C. thermogenesis.
   D. shivering.

2. Normally, body temperature is controlled by an internal thermostat called the:
   A. thymus.
   B. pituitary gland.
   C. hypothalamus.
   D. adrenal glands.

3. All of the following are ways the body compensates for an increased core body temperature EXCEPT:
   A. increased cardiac output.
   B. opening of sweat glands.
   C. increased basal metabolic rate.
   D. cutaneous vasoconstriction.

4. The only way the body can dissipate heat when the ambient temperature approaches body temperature is through:
   A. perspiration (sweat).
   B. decreasing respirations.
   C. shivering.
   D. increased basal metabolic rate.

5. A severe heat-related disturbance in the body's thermoregulation system characterized by a core temperature more than 104°F is called:
   A. heat exhaustion.
   B. heatstroke.
   C. heat syncope.
   D. heat cramps.

6. When you are treating a patient for heatstroke, cooling efforts should continue until the rectal temperature has fallen below:
   A. 98.6°F (37°C).
   B. 100°F (38°C).
   C. 102°F (39°C).
   D. 104°F (40°C).

7. When you are treating a patient for heatstroke, cooling should:
   A. occur in such a way as to not allow the core body temperature to drop more than 1 degree per hour.
   B. occur as slowly as possible.
   C. not be considered a priority.
   D. occur as rapidly as possible.

8. Patients with heatstroke are at risk for the development of:
   A. metabolic alkalosis.
   B. seizures.
   C. hyperglycemia.
   D. exertional hypernatremia.

9. All of the following are effective means of cooling a patient with heatstroke EXCEPT:
   A. cold water or ice immersion.
   B. spraying the patient with tepid water while fanning constantly.
   C. covering the patient with wet sheets.
   D. applying ice packs to the patient's groin, neck, and axillae.

Additional Questions

10. How can a paramedic differentiate from a patient experiencing heatstroke, a febrile illness, or sepsis?

11. Why are the elderly more at risk for cold-related emergencies than younger adults?

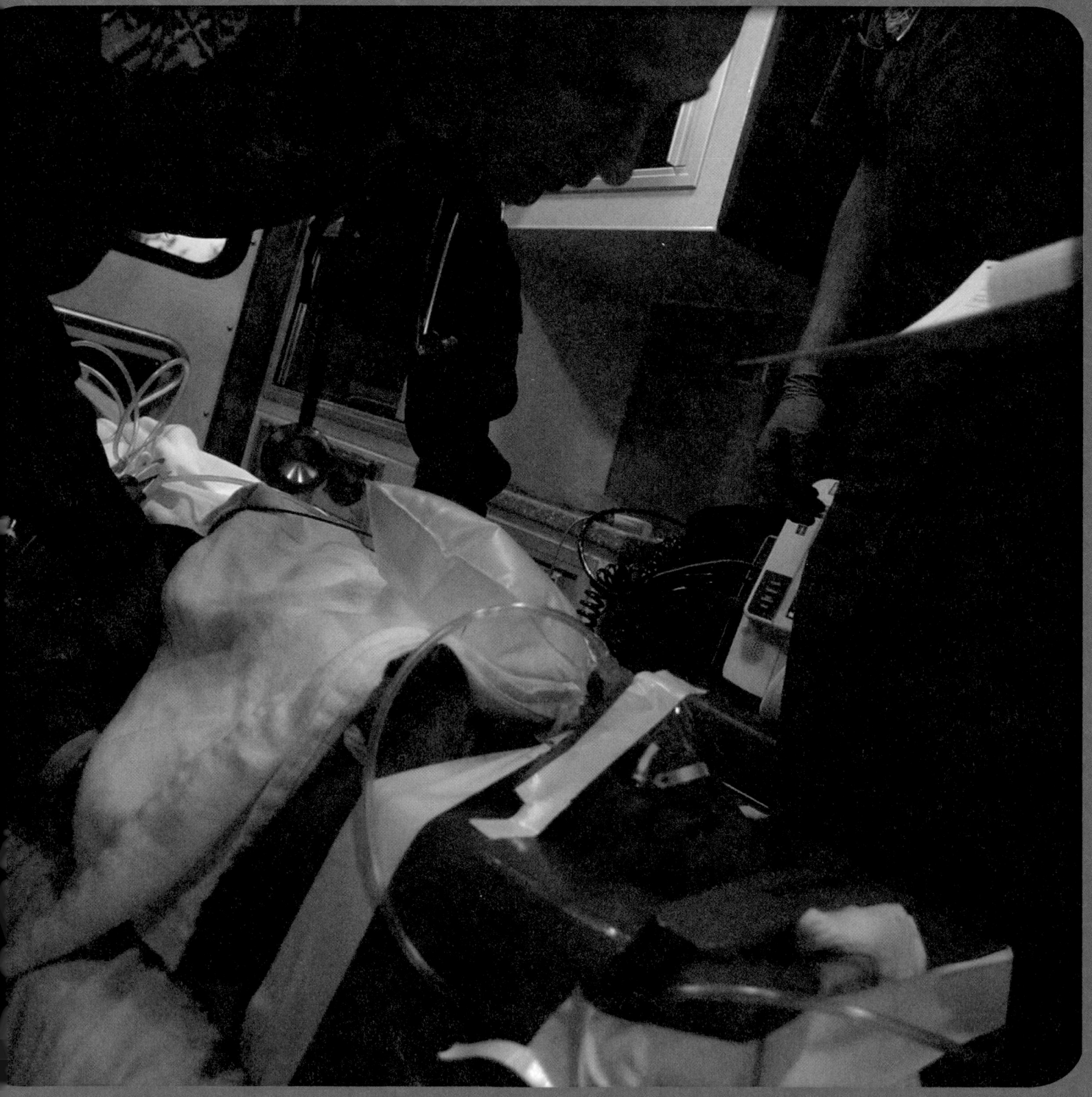

Responding to the Field Code

National EMS Education Standard Competencies

Shock and Resuscitation

- Integrates comprehensive knowledge of causes and pathophysiology into the management of cardiac arrest and pre-arrest states.

Knowledge Objectives

1. Discuss the importance of the American Heart Association's five links of the Chain of Survival to a successful code. (pp 1851-1852)
2. Describe the management acronym SMART and each of its objectives. (p 1852)
3. Describe how progressive communities can improve survival of prehospital cardiac arrest patients. (p 1852)
4. Discuss the use of simulation in CPR training. (pp 1852-1853)
5. Discuss some of the revisions made by the American Heart Association (AHA) and International Liaison Committee on Resuscitation (ILCOR) to the Emergency Cardiovascular Care (ECC) and CPR guidelines. (pp 1853-1854)
6. Describe how you, your crew, and your agency can incorporate the latest guidelines into the management of field codes. (pp 1852-1854)
7. Discuss some of the theories that have shifted the focus of certain CPR techniques. (p 1854)
8. Summarize the steps of the BLS healthcare provider algorithm and identify the key to a successful outcome in patients with cardiac arrest. (pp 1854-1855)
9. Explain how two-rescuer CPR can benefit the paramedic and the patient. (p 1856)
10. Explain the steps in providing two-rescuer adult CPR, including the method for switching positions during the process. (p 1856)
11. Identify the various age groups of infants and children for the purposes of resuscitation procedures and equipment. (p 1856)
12. Explain the steps in providing child and infant CPR, including the method for switching positions during the process. (pp 1858-1860)
13. Discuss guidelines for circumstances that require the use of an automated external defibrillator (AED) on both adult and pediatric patients experiencing cardiac arrest. (pp 1861-1862)
14. Describe situations in which manual or automated defibrillation would be appropriate. (p 1862)
15. Summarize how to perform manual defibrillation on an adult and child/infant. (p 1862)
16. Summarize how to use an automated external defibrillator. (pp 1864-1865)
17. Describe how to manage a witnessed arrest versus a nonwitnessed arrest. (p 1865)
18. Explain special situations related to the use of automated external defibrillation. (pp 1865-1866)
19. Review the management of a cardiac arrest based on analysis of the electrocardiogram (ECG) as either a shockable (ventricular fibrillation or ventricular tachycardia) or a nonshockable (pulseless electrical activity or asystole) rhythm. (pp 1866, 1868)
20. List the "Hs and Ts" and how they can be managed in the field. (p 1869)
21. Describe the different mechanical devices that are available to assist in delivering improved circulatory efforts during CPR. (pp 1870-1872)
22. Describe the general steps of postresuscitative care. (p 1872)
23. Describe the ethical issues related to patient resuscitation, providing examples of when not to start CPR on a patient. (pp 1872-1873)
24. Explain the various factors involved in the decision to stop CPR once it has been started on a patient. (p 1873)
25. Discuss the value of scene choreography at a field code. (pp 1873-1874)
26. Describe the typical roles of the code team leader and code team members at a field code. (p 1874)
27. Plan for a code by reviewing a sample script for a typical prehospital cardiac arrest resuscitation. (p 1875)

Skills Objectives

1. Demonstrate how to perform one- and two-rescuer adult CPR. (p 1857, Skill Drill 1)
2. Demonstrate how to perform CPR in a child who is between age 1 year and the onset of puberty. (p 1859, Skill Drill 2)
3. Demonstrate how to perform CPR in an infant who is between ages 1 month and 1 year. (p 1860, Skill Drill 3)
4. Demonstrate how to perform manual defibrillation in an adult patient. (p 1863, Skill Drill 4)
5. Demonstrate how to perform manual defibrillation in an infant or child. (pp 1863-1864)
6. Demonstrate how to manage a patient in ventricular fibrillation or ventricular tachycardia. (pp 1864-1865, 1868-1869)
7. Demonstrate how to manage a patient in asystole or pulseless electrical activity. (pp 1869-1870)
8. Demonstrate the steps of postresuscitative care. (p 1872)
9. Demonstrate how to be committed to the success of the team. (pp 1873-1874)
10. Demonstrate the roles of the code team member and the code team leader. (p 1874)

Introduction

In the early 1970s, when the first edition of this text was written, the technique of cardiopulmonary resuscitation (CPR) was only in its second decade. A prehospital sudden cardiac arrest was a terminal event and there were few survivors. In the mid 1970s, stories about the success of programs such as the Seattle and King County Medic One CPR training began to circulate. These programs brought CPR training to the public through schools, firehouses, and mailings. The training programs brought about a paradigm shift from the expectations of the 1970s that most cardiac arrests would result in death to the post 2010 expectation for a return of spontaneous circulation (ROSC).

Today, EMS systems have taken the time to train the public in CPR and place automated external defibrillators (AEDs) in public places and thus are achieving tremendous success in the ROSC. It is not unusual to find communities with a ROSC rate as high as 40%. Crews are no longer surprised when they achieve getting a patient's pulse back; they expect it to come back! This is especially true of those communities that have worked hard to implement each of the details in the current Emergency Cardiovascular Care (ECC) guidelines. It is clear that treating a sudden cardiac arrest is a discipline that requires attention to all the details as well as involvement of the entire community.

This chapter explores ways that practice and planning can help increase your resuscitation success. You will learn about planning for the resuscitation or "field code," and what actions are performed by the code team leader and code team members. As a wise person once said, "Failure to plan is planning to fail," and this expression is never more apparent than in the resuscitation of the patient who has experienced sudden cardiac arrest. The American Heart Association (AHA), in concert with the International Liaison Committee on Resuscitation (ILCOR), come together to revise the guidelines for ECC and CPR every 5 years. This chapter describes how you, your crew, and your agency can incorporate the latest guidelines into the management of adult, child, and infant field codes. The care of newly born and neonate patients is discussed in the chapter, *Neonatal Care*.

Improving the Response to Cardiac Arrest

The Chain of Survival

For success to be achieved in the assessment and management of a cardiac arrest patient in the field, all the links in the Chain of Survival must be solidly in place Figure 1. There needs to be recognition of a cardiac emergency, early access to 9-1-1, early high-quality CPR by the public or responders, early defibrillation, early advanced life support care, and transport to a hospital that can provide state-of-the-art postresuscitative care (ie, hypothermia, continuous electroencephalogram [EEG] or brain wave monitoring, coronary catheterization, and seizure control). It takes a team of skilled providers, beginning

YOU are the Medic · PART 1

At 4:15 PM you are dispatched to a golf course located in a gated island community. Local volunteer emergency responders have also been dispatched. You are advised that you are responding to a 54-year-old man who has collapsed while golfing. He is reported to be pulseless and apneic with hands-only CPR in progress. You have requested that the field supervisor respond to the call with you. On arrival you find CPR being performed on a man lying on the ground. An AED is attached to the patient. You are met by a man who tells you that his friend was complaining of "indigestion" after lunch when they began playing. Thanks to a recent community CPR course, compressions were initiated immediately. The bystander is not aware of any medical history or medications taken regularly by his friend. He explains that the patient's wife is being driven to the scene from their home within the community.

Local responders arrive to assist you and your paramedic partner as you begin two-rescuer CPR and ventilating the patient with a bag-mask device. You are told CPR has been in progress approximately 6 minutes. The AED was retrieved and one shock was delivered prior to your arrival. You connect your cardiac monitor and analyze the ECG. The patient's rhythm is ventricular fibrillation. You are aware that this is a lethal, but shockable, rhythm and prepare to defibrillate as the responders continue high-quality compressions at 100 per minute and your partner provides ventilations using high-concentration oxygen. You assume the role of team leader.

1. What links of the Chain of Survival are present that would make you optimistic about the potential for return of spontaneous circulation (ROSC)?

2. On the basis of the events occurring prior to your arrival and your own ECG analysis, what are your next steps as team leader?

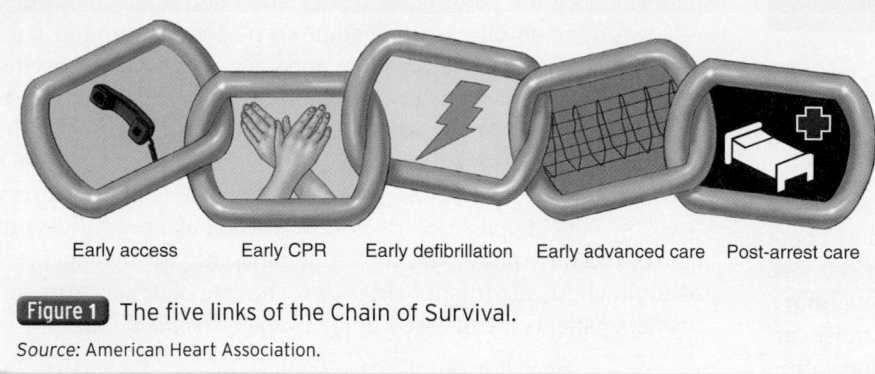

Early access   Early CPR   Early defibrillation   Early advanced care   Post-arrest care

Figure 1 The five links of the Chain of Survival.

Source: American Heart Association.

with community members who are trained in CPR, to the first responders who show up with an automated external defibrillator (AED), to the EMTs and paramedics who have been well trained in high-quality CPR and frequently practice simulated codes. The prehospital team should practice so they are able to work together in tandem, with their moves choreographed by a code team leader.

Developing Prehospital Program Objectives: The SMART Way

When you are undertaking a community-based program to improve the survival of prehospital cardiac arrest patients, consider adopting the management acronym **SMART** to describe the program's objectives: Specific, Measurable, Attainable and Achievable, Realistic and Relevant, and Timely. The following are a few questions that progressive communities must ask themselves in order to improve their response:

- Is there a universal access number (ie, 9-1-1), and do all members of the public know how and when to use it?
- Are all the dispatchers/communicators trained to provide hands-only CPR telephone instruction? Does the medical director for the communications center review 100% of the cardiac arrests to analyze the times and listen to the tapes for compliance with medical dispatch protocols?
- Is a community CPR training program readily available at all times of the day and days of the week at little to no cost for the citizens? If so, does the public know it is available? Have 10% to 20% of the population been trained? (Part of attaining this objective can be addressed by convincing the public to take the self-help approach to CPR training as provided by the 30-minute CPR Anytime program.)
- Is learning how to perform CPR a requirement to graduate high school? If not, how can you change this?
- Are 100% of the responders to emergencies (police, fire, EMS) currently trained in CPR and use of the AED? Do all response vehicles have an AED?
- Are AEDs and qualified personnel who are trained in their use available in all locations of public assembly for more than 500 people or in high-risk locations (ie, golf courses, sports arenas, concert halls, nursing homes)?

- Do all schools have AEDs readily available, and is the AED available at all sporting events?
- Do fitness centers have personnel trained in CPR and AEDs readily available?
- How long does it take for the first emergency responder to arrive on the scene? How long does it take for the paramedics to arrive? Is this data published on a regular basis? If it does not get "measured" it is difficult to improve.
- Is the EMS agency's medical director actively involved in reviewing all cardiac arrests and making quality improvements to the EMS system's response on a regular basis?
- Are the cardiac arrest events reported using the Recommended Guidelines for Uniform Reporting of Data from Out-of-Hospital Cardiac Arrest, "The Utstein Style" (approved by AHA and European Resuscitation Council in 1991), so your community's data can be compared with the data of other progressive communities?
- Do all hospitals you transport to participate in the AHA's Get With The Guidelines® quality improvement suite (previously called the National Registry of Cardiopulmonary Resuscitation [NRCPR] data system)? This is the only national registry of in-hospital resuscitation events.
- Do the prehospital and in-hospital code teams practice their response with simulated patients on a regular basis? These code drills should focus on teamwork, following the current guidelines, and ensuring a minimal amount of interruptions in high-quality CPR.

If you answered no to some of the questions above, there is more work to be done in your community! If you answered yes to all of the questions, share your best practices with neighboring communities to help them improve!

Simulation Training, or "Mock Code" Training

In the past, simulation training, or "mock" code training, in medicine typically involved using "simulated patients" in a classroom setting; the students assessed people who were instructed to mimic having symptoms of different ailments. However, technology today has helped to streamline this method by creating simulation modules. Regardless of the type of industry or training, one question always comes up: "How do I train my personnel for the 'low-frequency, high-risk' situation?" For example, How do I train the EMT to recognize a dangerous intersection? How do I train the paramedic to recognize and manage a serious medical condition (eg, lethal dysrhythmia, cardiac arrest, multisystem trauma)?

Today's simulation technology allows you to gain knowledge about real-life scenarios, performed in a virtual world where no one is injured if you make a mistake. Using "high-fidelity" manikins and videotaping to mock the code for review and analysis, this type of training is invaluable because your actions and results are tracked and available for critique, to review, and to learn from. High-fidelity manikins integrate with a computer simulator and have the ability to play out preprogrammed scenarios involving alterations in the vital signs, electrocardiogram (ECG), Spo_2, end-tidal carbon dioxide ($ETCO_2$), and other parameters.

Many services spend time in simulation centers to practice their codes and team leadership. This helps to fill the void of lack of actual skill performance with actual patients.

Development of New CPR Guidelines

Reemphasis on Quality CPR

During the 1990s the emphasis on performing quality CPR seemed to slip as providers became more focused on intubation, drug administration, defibrillation, and other aspects of field code management. Studies published in medical journals, which prompted the development of the 2005 ECC guidelines, showed that the quality of CPR was poor in both in-hospital and prehospital settings: The depth of compressions was inadequate, the rate of compressions was too slow, almost half the time no compressions were being provided, the ventilations were too fast, and the chest was rarely allowed to fully recoil. Studies investigating the value of intubation and the use of resuscitation drugs were inconclusive at best, but it was determined that performing CPR is clearly important both before and immediately after defibrillation. In addition, it was determined that immediate CPR can double or triple the rate of survival in a patient who is experiencing ventricular fibrillation (V-fib) or sudden cardiac arrest.

Both the 2005 and 2010 CPR guidelines emphasize the importance of providing high-quality CPR beginning with compressions (push hard and fast, and allow full chest recoil). In fact, the "resuscitation pyramid" is built on a strong base of high-quality CPR beginning with compressions as illustrated in **Figure 2**. When you arrive at the scene of a patient in cardiac arrest, you need to understand that the success of the resuscitation does not rely on an IV line, an endotracheal (ET) tube, a circulatory adjunct, or drugs you have in your drug box. Your best chance of succeeding at resuscitation hinges on providing continuous, uninterrupted high-quality CPR compressions.

Airway Management

If you were to compare the first edition of this textbook to this current edition on the management of cardiac arrest, an obvious difference would be the change in the emphasis of "securing" the patient's airway with the "gold standard" technique of endotracheal intubation. Clearly, the airway is no less important today than it was three decades ago. However, with research showing that high-quality compressions can double if not triple the chance of survival if administered promptly, the focus

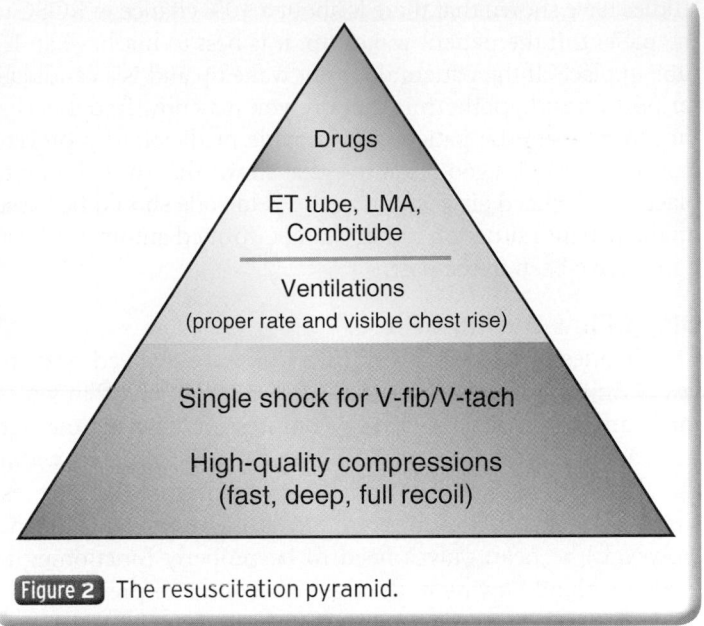

Figure 2 The resuscitation pyramid.

has shifted to interventions that make a measurable difference in survival (ie, defibrillation). If the airway can be opened and ventilation is successful using basic adjuncts such as an oropharyngeal or nasopharyngeal airway and bag-mask ventilation, it is not a priority for you to ensure that an ET tube is inserted. Today, paramedics are taught to consider use of advanced airways during the field code if a basic airway is not adequate or the airway needs to be better protected, such as in a patient who is vomiting. Paramedics should be trained to place advanced airways with a minimum interruption in chest compressions (less than 10 seconds). If this cannot be accomplished, a rescue airway such as the King LT or Combitube may be an acceptable alternative.

Another consideration with airway maintenance and adjunct placement is control of the ventilation volume and rate. During a field code, ventilations should be administered, each 1 second in duration, and only with sufficient volume for you to see visible chest rise. Do not overventilate the patient because this can cause gastric distention or regurgitation. It is just as important not to hyperventilate the patient because excessive gas in the chest has been shown to significantly reduce coronary artery perfusion. Some EMS medical directors have encouraged paramedics to use an impedance threshold device (ResQPOD), which is placed in the ventilation circuit between the mask and the bag-mask device or automated transport ventilator (ATV). The device is designed to enhance compressions by creating a vacuum in the chest that allows more blood to flow to the heart and brain. The device also has a prompt that helps the person providing ventilations to keep track of the rate of ventilations so as to not exceed the recommended ventilation rate (2 ventilations every 30 compressions OR 1 ventilation every 6 to 8 seconds when an advanced airway is inserted).

Another consideration you should take into account when you are using advanced airways early in the treatment of the field code is that if the links of the Chain of Survival are all "in place," studies have shown that there is about a 40% chance of ROSC in the patient. If the patient wakes up, it is best to not have an ET tube in place. If the patient does not wake up and is a candidate for post-arrest hypothermia therapy, you may now find it necessary to intubate the patient and provide medication to prevent shivering. This is a good example that shows that the decision to place an advanced airway during the field code should be based on the patient's situation rather than performed automatically as it may have been in the past.

Blood Flow During CPR

The theories on blood flow during CPR have evolved over the years. An early thought was the "heart pump theory," in which the heart is directly squeezed by compression between the sternum and the spinal column. The pressure is increased within the chambers of the heart and blood flows from higher pressured chambers to the lowered pressured vessels and organs. However, the heart valves need to be properly functioning to keep the blood flowing in the right direction and prevent retrograde flow of blood.

The next thought on how blood flows during CPR was the "thoracic pump theory," in which compression of the sternum raises the pressure in the entire chest cavity. With the pressure in the extrathoracic spaces remaining low, the pressure gradient is established in which venous collapse prevents the backflow of blood and open arteries allow for the forward flow of blood out of the chest. Administration of epinephrine and other vasopressors is thought to be a benefit in helping to keep those essential arteries open. Building on the concepts of both these theories, researchers have found success in promoting the use of harder and faster compressions that can increase the pressure to a greater degree. However, all of this blood movement ceases when there are interruptions in the chest compressions; thus the current emphasis is for the provision of continuous chest compressions with minimum, if any, interruptions.

Finally, the current theories on blood flow during CPR consider the importance of negative intrathoracic pressure. Because patients in cardiac arrest are not breathing on their own, they do not produce negative inspiratory pressure to assist in circulatory system blood flow, most specifically the coronary arteries. During CPR, some negative pressure develops in the chest as the sternum and ribs rebound to their normal position during the decompression or relaxation phase. In fact, researchers have noted that in the studies on pigs, using Thumper-type devices to actually perform the CPR chest compressions, it is essential to ensure that the pad of the compressor releases complete pressure on the chest wall or there is little to no coronary blood flow. Thus the emphasis on "full chest recoil" was introduced in the 2005 guidelines. When a greater amount of negative pressure can be achieved in the chest (push hard and fast and allow full chest recoil), a greater amount of blood is returned to the heart. Then on the next compression, a greater amount of blood is forced to circulate to the heart's coronary arteries and the rest of the body's vital organs. You can see how the concept of a device, such as the impedance

threshold device or ResQPOD could be effective in enhancing this negative pressure gradient. As the theories of how to best resuscitate a patient in cardiac arrest continue to evolve through ongoing research, it is apparent that providing the highest quality of CPR in a timely manner, with little to no interruptions, is the patient's best chance for ROSC.

Words of Wisdom

When the heart stops contracting, the blood stops flowing and blood, oxygen, and essential substrates cannot be delivered or removed from the cells of the body. The body cannot survive when the heart stops because organ damage begins quickly after the blood stops circulating. Of all the organs, the brain is the most sensitive to lack of blood flow and oxygen. Brain damage begins within 4 to 6 minutes after the patient experiences a cardiac arrest. The arrest is considered irreversible within 8 to 10 minutes. Reperfusion of the brain with oxygenated blood is essential to ROSC.

The heart can stop beating for many reasons but the primary reasons are sudden death due to a life-threatening dysrhythmia (ie, ventricular fibrillation [V-fib] or ventricular tachycardia [V-tach]), heart disease, electrolyte imbalances, and severe trauma. Medical emergencies such as asthma, anaphylaxis, and being struck in the chest at the wrong time in the cardiac cycle (ie, commotio cordis) can also lead to cardiac arrest. The downward spiral from respiratory distress to respiratory failure, respiratory arrest, and finally, cardiac arrest commonly occurs in infants and children.

■ Adult CPR

The initial steps for managing the adult patient in cardiac arrest follow the adult *BLS healthcare provider algorithm* **Figure 3**. These steps are discussed in detail in the chapter, *Cardiovascular Emergencies*, and are summarized here. As previously discussed, research findings showed that the key to a successful outcome in patients with cardiac arrest is the speed at which compressions are initiated. As per the guidelines, after establishing unresponsiveness and the lack of "normal" breathing, (ie, agonal gasps or absent breathing), you should spend no more than 10 seconds determining pulselessness. If there is no pulse, begin CPR and continue for 2 minutes or five cycles of 30 compressions and 2 ventilations. You should always bring your AED or defibrillator/monitor to the patient on any potential cardiac arrest call. In all patients, begin CPR and attach the AED as soon as it is available. In some instances, CPR may have been started prior to your arrival.

To help make CPR easier to learn, remember, and perform, the general public or "lay rescuers" are taught to provide hands-only or compression-only CPR. In some cases, bystanders may have taken a traditional CPR course, which taught the compression to ventilation ratio of 30:2. The public is generally not taught to take a pulse, to perform rescue breathing, or to perform two-person CPR. Unfortunately, studies have

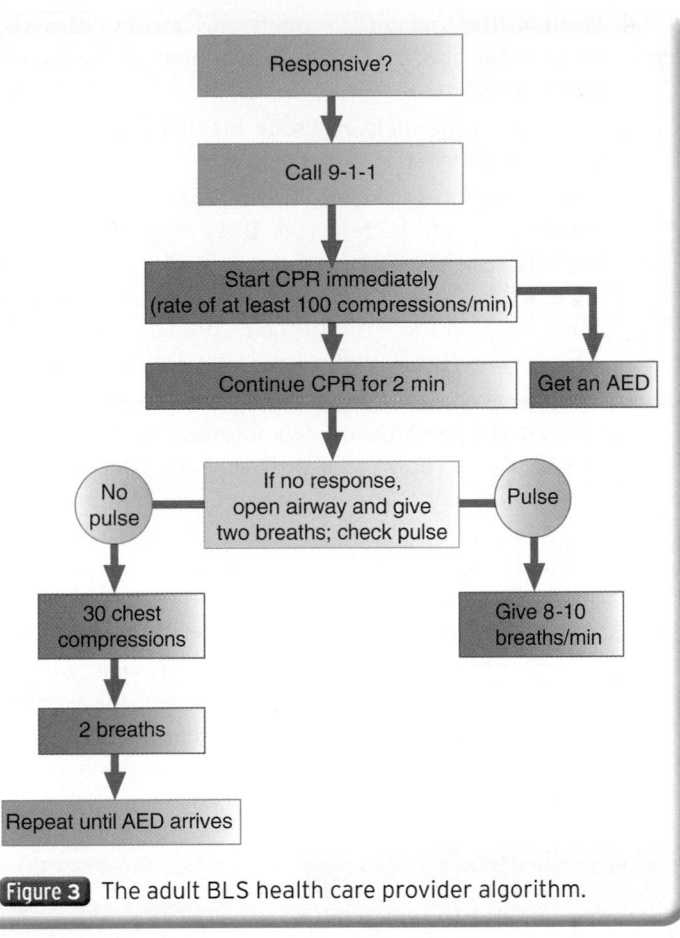

Figure 3 The adult BLS health care provider algorithm.

shown that bystander CPR is performed in only one third or fewer of witnessed cardiac arrests and is often poorly performed. Bystanders who have been trained previously in CPR are often reluctant to begin this procedure for the following reasons:

- CPR steps may have been too complicated and included too many steps to remember. However, the new guidelines have made a significant effort to simplify the steps taught to the public with the emphasis on hands-only CPR with the focus on compressions.
- Training methods may have been inadequate, and skill retention typically declines rapidly after a course. This issue is being studied to try to determine which methods of training will produce the greatest skill retention. A video-based watch-and-do method, as opposed to watch-then-do, was incorporated into most courses.
- Some members of the public may be afraid of transmitted diseases and therefore may be reluctant to perform mouth-to-mouth resuscitation. Although the guidelines strongly emphasize that the risk of transmission of infection is low, those people who are concerned about disease are encouraged to use barrier devices. In addition, the technique of hands-only/compression-only CPR is encouraged for those people who are reluctant to perform ventilations and for dispatcher-assisted CPR instruction.
- Finally, many bystanders who were trained but did not help when confronted with a cardiac arrest stated that they were afraid they might do the wrong thing.

YOU are the Medic   PART 2

Your field supervisor arrives as you prepare to defibrillate. Once the defibrillator has charged, you announce that everyone should "Clear the patient!" Once you have confirmed that the patient is clear and the bag-mask device has been removed from the patient, you deliver a 200 J biphasic shock. CPR is resumed immediately and your field supervisor prepares to gain venous access. After delegating medication preparation, she has 40 units of vasopressin ready to administer via the IV line while responders complete their five cycles of compressions. You check the patient's rhythm and find ventricular tachycardia on the monitor. You confirm that the patient has no pulse and complete the assessment in less than 10 seconds. The vasopressin has been administered so you prepare to defibrillate again. As responders complete their fifth cycle, you announce that everyone should "Clear the patient" and after verifying that the patient is clear, deliver another shock of 200 J. Your field supervisor has now prepared 1.5 mg/kg of lidocaine for IV administration. Once this has been administered, she prepares the intubation equipment for your partner, who is continuing to ventilate the patient using a bag-mask device.

Recording Time: 1 Minute	
Appearance	Pale and mottled
Level of consciousness	Unresponsive
Airway	Patent
Breathing	Apneic, ventilations provided at a rate of 10 breaths/min via bag-mask device
Circulation	Pulseless with CPR in progress, skin is cool

4. What other alternative medications are indicated for ventricular fibrillation/ventricular tachycardia and at what dosages?

5. If the rhythm had been analyzed as torsades de pointes, what medication might be beneficial and at what dosage?

■ Two or More Rescuer CPR

Two-rescuer CPR is always preferable because it is less tiring and facilitates effective chest compressions. In fact, a team approach to CPR and AED use is far superior to the one-rescuer approach. Once one-rescuer CPR is in progress, additional rescuers can be added easily. Prior to assisting with CPR, a second rescuer should apply the AED and then set up airway adjuncts including a bag-mask device and suction, and should insert an oral airway. If CPR is in progress, the second rescuer should enter the procedure after a cycle of 30 compressions and two ventilations.

When you are using two or more rescuers, rotate the compressor every 2 minutes. To do so, position a third rescuer so he or she is kneeling on the other side of the patient's chest from the rescuer actually performing chest compressions. Now, you can have an "active compressor" and an "on-deck compressor" who is ready to take over after the five cycles or 2-minute intervals. Studies of rescuer fatigue show that the compressor tires after 2 to 5 minutes and that the quality of compressions will suffer if the compressor is not replaced.

To perform two-rescuer adult CPR, follow the steps in Skill Drill 1 :

Skill Drill 1

1. While moving to the patient's head, establish unresponsiveness as your partner moves to the patient's side to prepare to deliver chest compressions Step 1 .

2. If the patient is unresponsive, determine pulselessness by checking the carotid pulse (a maximum of 10 seconds). If the patient has no pulse and an AED is available, apply it now Step 2 .

3. If no AED is available or the elapsed time from collapse is greater than 4 to 5 minutes, begin chest compressions at a ratio of 30:2. Once an advanced airway is inserted, rescuers should switch from cycles of CPR to continuously delivered compressions at a rate of at least 100/min Step 3 .

4. Position the patient to open the airway Step 4 . If breathing is adequate, place the patient in the recovery position and monitor.

5. If not breathing, deliver rescue breaths at a rate of 8 to 10 breaths/min Step 5 .

6. After 2 minutes of CPR, the rescuer providing compressions should be replaced. If there is a third rescuer available, position him or her at the chest opposite the compressor. Make the switch when both rescuers are ready, keeping the switch time as brief as possible (5 to 10 seconds). If only two rescuers are available, make the switch mid-cycle during compressions.

7. Reassess the patient every few minutes. Each assessment should last no more than 10 seconds. Depending on the patient's condition, continue CPR, continue rescue breathing only, or place the patient in the recovery position and monitor breathing and pulse.

Note: Once an advanced airway has been inserted, the compressions and ventilations are no longer in cycles. Instead, they are asynchronous with the compressor providing at least 100 per minute without pauses for breaths and the ventilator giving 8 to 10 breaths/min (every 6 to 8 seconds). Because the compressor will inevitably get tired, switch compressors every 2 minutes with no more than 10-second pauses, if any.

■ CPR for Infants and Children

A question often asked is "For the purposes of resuscitation, what age defines a child?" Many pediatricians say, "If the patient looks like a child, then he or she is a child; if the patient looks like an adult, then he or she is an adult." The guidelines use the following definitions of age groups for the purposes of resuscitation:

- Newly born—an infant within the first few hours after birth
- Neonate—an infant within the first month after birth
- Infant—1 month to 1 year
- Child—age 1 year to adolescence (signs of puberty or secondary sexual characteristic development)
- Adult—adolescent and older

Skill Drill | 1

Performing Two-Rescuer Adult CPR

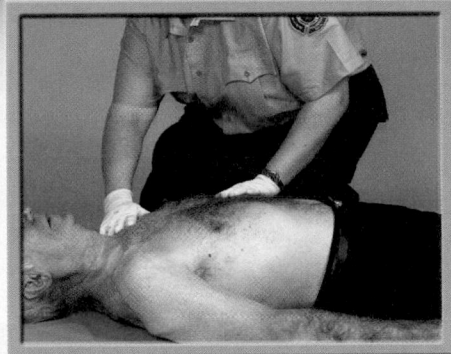

Step 1 Determine unresponsiveness and take positions.

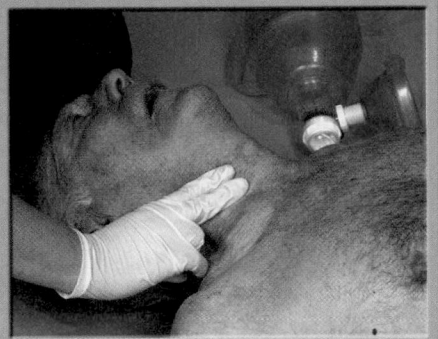

Step 2 Check for a carotid pulse (maximum of 10 seconds). If there is no pulse but an AED is available, apply it now.

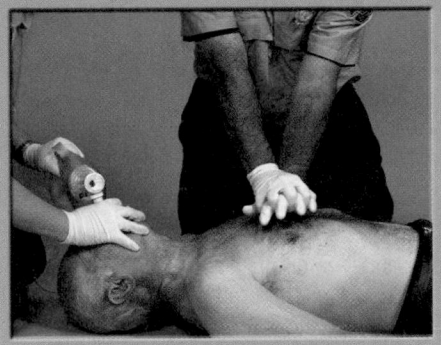

Step 3 If there is no pulse and an AED is not available or the elapsed time from collapse is greater than 4 to 5 minutes, begin chest compressions at a ratio of 30:2. Once an advanced airway is inserted, rescuers should switch from cycles of CPR to continuously delivered compressions at a rate of at least 100/min.

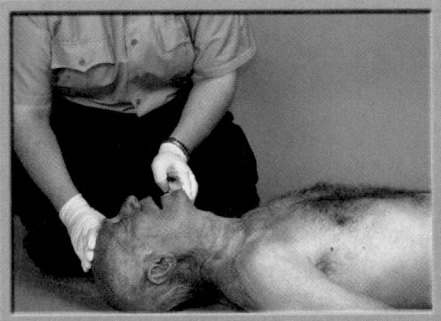

Step 4 Open the airway. Check for breathing. If breathing is adequate, place the patient in the recovery position and monitor.

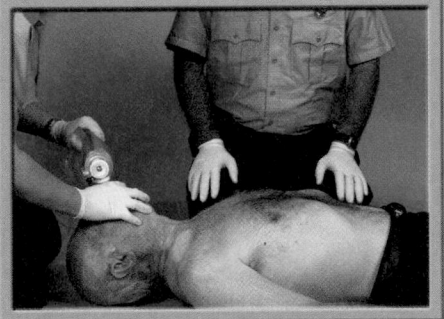

Step 5 If not breathing, give two breaths of 1 second each. After 2 minutes, switch rescuer positions to minimize fatigue. Keep switch time to 5 to 10 seconds. Depending on patient condition, continue CPR, continue ventilations only, or place in recovery position and monitor breathing and pulse.

In most cases, cardiac arrest in infants and children follows respiratory arrest, which triggers hypoxia and ischemia of the heart. Children consume oxygen two to three times as rapidly as adults. Therefore, you must open the airway and provide artificial ventilation. Often, this will be enough to allow the child to resume spontaneous breathing and, thus, prevent cardiac arrest. Therefore, airway and breathing are a focus of pediatric BLS Table 1 .

Respiratory problems leading to cardiopulmonary arrest in children can have a number of different causes, including the following:

- Injury, both blunt and penetrating
- Infections of the respiratory tract or another organ system
- A foreign body in the airway
- Submersion
- Electrocution

Table 1   Review of Pediatric BLS Procedures

Procedure	Infants (between age 1 month and 1 year[a])	Children (1 year to onset of puberty[b])
Circulation		
Pulse check	Brachial artery	Carotid or femoral artery
Compression area	Just below the nipple line	In the center of the chest, in between the nipples
Compression width	2 fingers or 2 thumb-encircling-hands technique	Heel of one or both hands
Compression depth	At least one third anterior-posterior diameter (about 1½ inches)	At least one third anterior-posterior diameter (about 2 inches)
Compression rate	At least 100/min	At least 100/min
Compression-to-ventilation ratio (until advanced airway is inserted)	30:2 (one rescuer); 15:2 (two rescuers)[c]	30:2 (one rescuer); 15:2 (two rescuers)[c]
Foreign body obstruction	Responsive: Back slaps and chest thrusts Unresponsive: CPR	Responsive: Abdominal thrusts Unresponsive: CPR
Airway		
	Head tilt–chin lift; jaw thrust if spinal injury is suspected	Head tilt–chin lift; jaw thrust if spinal injury is suspected
Breathing		
Ventilations with advanced airway	1 breath every 6 to 8 seconds (8 to 10 breaths/min) Asynchronous with chest compressions. About 1 second per breath. Visible chest rise.	1 breath every 6 to 8 seconds (8 to 10 breaths/min) Asynchronous with chest compressions. About 1 second per breath. Visible chest rise.

[a]The American Heart Association defines neonatal patients as birth to age 1 month, and infants as age 1 month to 1 year. Neonatal resuscitation is covered in the chapter, *Neonatal Care*.

[b]Onset of puberty is approximately 12 to 14 years of age, as defined by secondary characteristics (eg, breast development in girls and axillary hair in boys).

[c]Pause compressions to deliver ventilations.

- Poisoning or drug overdose
- Sudden infant death syndrome

Pediatric BLS can be divided into four steps:

1. Determining responsiveness
2. Circulation
3. Airway
4. Breathing

Note that neonatal patients are defined as birth to age 1 month, and infants as age 1 month to 1 year. Neonatal resuscitation is covered in the chapter, *Neonatal Care*.

■ Technique for Children

The technique of CPR has a few slight variations for children as opposed to the adult technique Skill Drill 2 :

Skill Drill   2

1. Place the child on a firm surface.
2. Prepare to place the heel of one or two hands in the center of the chest, in between the nipples. Avoid compression over the lower tip of the sternum, which is called the xiphoid process Step 1 .

3. Compress the chest at least one third the anterior-posterior diameter of the chest (approximately 2 inches in most children) at a rate of at least 100/min Step 2 . With pauses for ventilation, the actual number of compressions delivered will be about 80 per minute. In between compressions, allow the chest to fully recoil. Compression and relaxation time should be the same duration. Use smooth movements. Hold your fingers off the child's ribs, and keep the heel of your hand(s) on the sternum.

4. Coordinate rapid compressions and ventilations in a 30:2 ratio for one rescuer and 15:2 for two rescuers, making sure the chest rises with each ventilation. At the end of each cycle, pause briefly for two ventilations Step 3 .

5. Continue cycles of compressions and ventilations until an AED becomes available or the patient shows signs of spontaneous breathing.

6. If the child resumes effective breathing, place him or her in a position that allows for frequent reassessment of the airway and vital signs during transport Step 4 .

Switching rescuer positions is the same for children as it is for adults—every 2 minutes of CPR. Remember, if the child is past the onset of puberty, use the adult CPR sequence, including the use of the AED.

Skill Drill   2

Performing CPR on a Child

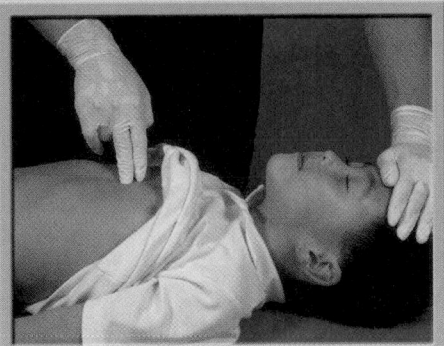

Step 1 Place the child on a firm surface. Prepare to place the heel of one or both hands in the center of the chest, in between the nipples, avoiding the xiphoid process.

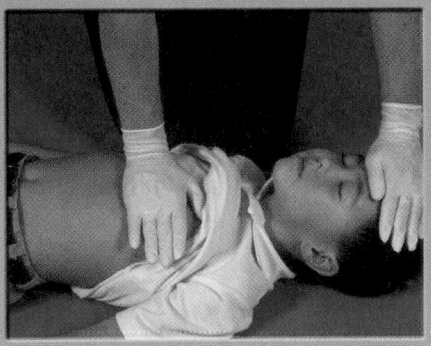

Step 2 Compress the chest one third the anterior-posterior diameter of the chest at a rate of 100/min.

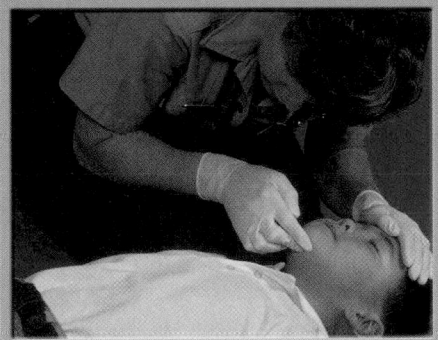

Step 3 Coordinate compressions with ventilations in a 30:2 ratio (one rescuer) or 15:2 (two rescuers). At the end of each cycle, pause for two ventilations.

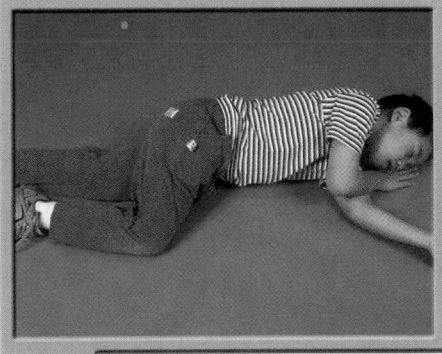

Step 4 Continue cycles of compressions and ventilations until an AED becomes available or the patient shows signs of spontaneous breathing. If the child resumes effective breathing, place him or her in a position that allows for frequent reassessment of the airway and vital signs during transport.

Note: Once an advanced airway has been inserted, the compressions and ventilations are no longer in cycles. Instead, they are asynchronous with the compressor providing at least 100 per minute without pauses for breaths and the ventilator giving 8 to 10 breaths/min (every 6 to 8 seconds). Because the compressor will inevitably get tired, switch compressors every 2 minutes with no more than 10-second pauses, if any.

■ Technique for Infants

The technique of CPR for an infant has a few slight variations from the adult and child technique, as shown in **Skill Drill 3**:

Skill Drill   3

1. Place the infant on a firm surface, using one hand to keep the head in an open airway position. You can also use a pad or wedge under the shoulders and upper body to keep the head from tilting forward **Step 1**.

2. Imagine a line drawn between the nipples. Place two fingers in the middle of the sternum, about ½ inch below the level of the imaginary line (one finger-width).

3. Using two fingers, compress the sternum at least one third the anterior-posterior diameter of the chest

Skill Drill 3

Infant CPR

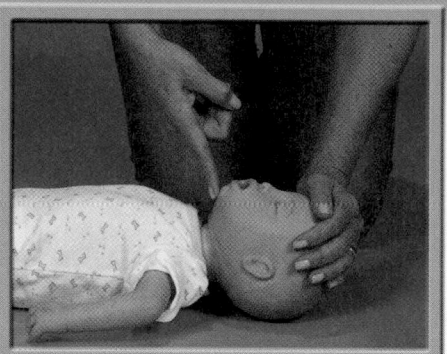

Step 1 Position the infant on a firm surface while maintaining the airway.

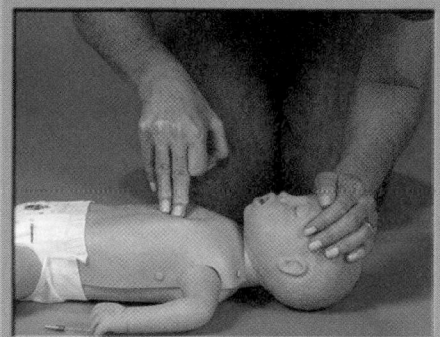

Step 2 Place two fingers in the middle of the sternum just below a line between the nipples. Use two fingers to compress the chest one third the anterior-posterior diameter of the chest at a rate of at least 100/min. Allow the sternum to return to its normal position between compressions.

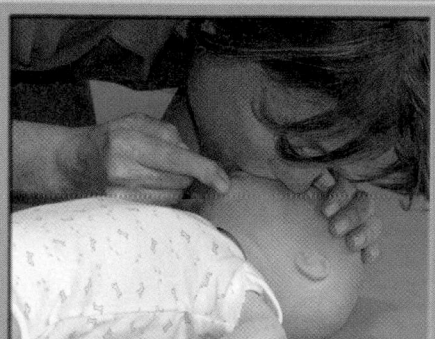

Step 3 Coordinate compressions with ventilations in a 30:2 ratio (one rescuer) or 15:2 (two rescuers), pausing for two ventilations at the end of each cycle. Continue cycles of compressions and ventilations until an AED becomes available or the infant shows signs of spontaneous breathing.

(approximately 1½ inches in most infants). Compress the chest at a rate of at least 100/min.

4. After each compression, allow the sternum to return briefly to its normal position. Allow equal time for compression and relaxation of the chest. Do not remove your fingers from the sternum, and avoid jerky movements Step 2.

5. Coordinate rapid compressions and ventilations in a 30:2 ratio for one rescuer and 15:2 for two rescuers, making sure the chest rises with each ventilation. At the end of each cycle, pause for two ventilations.

6. Continue cycles of compressions and ventilations until an AED becomes available or the infant shows signs of spontaneous breathing Step 3.

7. If the infant resumes effective breathing, place him or her in a position that allows for frequent reassessment of the airway and vital signs during transport.

If two rescuers are present, compressions can also be performed using the two thumb-encircling-hands technique Figure 4. If the chest does not rise, or rises only a little, use a head tilt–chin lift to open the airway. Reassess the infant for signs of spontaneous breathing after five cycles (about 2 minutes) of CPR.

Controversies

The use of advanced airway devices seems to be deemphasized in the current guidelines–particularly the use of the endotracheal (ET) tube, which previously was considered the "gold standard." When used by skilled providers, bag-mask ventilation with supplementary oxygen can be as effective as an ET tube in terms of oxygenation, ventilation, and protection from aspiration for short transportation times.

Many service medical directors have been reluctant to train their EMTs in the optional endotracheal intubation skill because of the marginal results when the skill is not practiced frequently. In the past, unrecognized, uncorrected esophageal intubations or tube dislodgements occurred with unacceptable frequency. One study of paramedics providing pediatric field intubations revealed that 8% of patients arriving at the emergency department had a tube in their esophagus. Another study in a large adult group of cardiac arrests found that 25% of the tubes were incorrectly placed by paramedics. As a consequence, the advanced airway option now favors the use of easier-to-insert devices (eg, LMA, Combitube, or King LT).

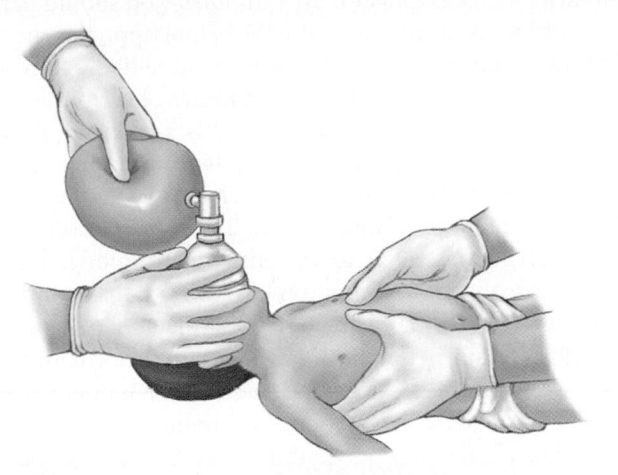

Figure 4 The two thumb-encircling-hands technique for infant chest compressions can be used when two rescuers are present.

■ Defibrillation

When an unresponsive patient is receiving CPR, the AED is probably one of the first pieces of equipment you will obtain from the ambulance. **Defibrillation** is the process by which a surge of electric energy is delivered to the heart. As a paramedic you are likely to administer electricity to a patient in one of three different ways: defibrillation, cardioversion, or transcutaneous pacing (TCP). In the context of a patient who is in cardiac arrest, defibrillation is appropriate when the patient is in V-fib or pulseless V-tach. Cardioversion and TCP are reserved for patients who are not yet in cardiac arrest and are further discussed in the chapter, *Cardiovascular Emergencies*. Occasionally you may actually be the "first responder," as in the case of a cardiac arrest in a public place such as a school where you are playing in a community basketball league or a health club. In those situations, you are likely to use an AED as opposed to the manual defibrillator you would carry in your paramedic unit. Many communities

YOU *are the Medic* | PART 3

After 2 minutes of compressions, you check the patient's rhythm. The patient continues to be in ventricular tachycardia. While responders continue CPR and the field supervisor assists your partner with intubation, you remind them that this action should delay compressions no longer than 10 seconds. The intubation is completed and while tube placement is confirmed by cord visualization, auscultation, and using end-tidal carbon dioxide ($ETCO_2$) monitoring, you prepare to administer epinephrine 1 mg to the patient. The supervisor prepares the second dose of lidocaine 1.5 mg/kg for the patient as you note that the $ETCO_2$ is 37 mm Hg and appropriate waveforms are present. Responders complete another five cycles of CPR and you identify that the patient remains in ventricular tachycardia. You prepare to deliver the third shock by charging to 200 J. You again announce and verify the patient should be cleared and then defibrillate. Compressions resume as the second dose of lidocaine is administered.

The patient's wife arrives and you take this opportunity to obtain a SAMPLE history. She advises you her husband has complained of occasional indigestion for the last week and finally contacted his physician this morning. He was scheduled for a stress test tomorrow. Current medications are limited to over-the-counter products such as acid-reducers and pain relievers. She is aware of no allergies. She tells you that until now she believed her husband to be healthy because he regularly exercised and watched his diet. She thinks he ate lunch with friends immediately prior to beginning this round of golf. You advise her that her husband's condition is extremely critical but that you are providing him with the best care possible.

Recording Time: 6 Minutes	
Respirations	10 breaths/min via ET tube ventilations
Pulse	Pulseless with CPR in progress at 100 compressions/min
Skin	Pale and cool
Blood pressure	Not obtainable
Oxygen saturation (SpO_2)	Not obtainable
Pupils	Equal, round, and unresponsive to light
End-tidal carbon dioxide ($ETCO_2$)	37 mm Hg

5. Why is intubation not an early intervention consideration in the cardiac arrest patient?

6. What is the importance of $ETCO_2$ monitoring in the cardiac arrest patient?

7. If resuscitative efforts are eventually successful, what is the significance of transporting the cardiac arrest patient to a facility capable of advanced cardiac care?

have placed AEDs in public places such as health clubs, public pools, concert halls, sports venues, airports, schools, and government buildings. The AED has been shown to be an effective lifesaving treatment for adults, children, and infants. The following guidelines should be used for AED use:

- Adults: use a standard adult AED unit.
- Children (age 1 year to the onset of puberty): Use an AED with pediatric dose-attenuation if available **Figure 5**. If no pediatric dose-attenuator system is available, use a standard adult AED.
- Infants (ages 1 month to 1 year): A manual defibrillator should be used if available. If a manual defibrillator is not available, use a pediatric dose-attenuator. If neither is available, use a standard adult AED with the pads in the A/P position.
- Newborns (birth to age 1 month): Focus attention on CPR with emphasis on ventilation.

Defibrillation needs to be carried out as soon as possible in two rhythms—V-fib and pulseless V-tach—because the likelihood of its success declines rapidly with time. If you witness a patient's cardiac arrest, begin CPR starting with chest compressions and attach the AED as soon as it is available. However, if the patient's cardiac arrest was not witnessed, especially if the call-to-arrival time is longer than 4 minutes, you should perform five cycles (about 2 minutes) of CPR before applying the AED. The rationale for this is that the heart is more likely to respond to defibrillation within the first few minutes of the onset of ventricular fibrillation. If the arrest interval is prolonged, however, metabolic waste products accumulate within the heart, energy stores are rapidly depleted, and the chance of successful defibrillation is reduced. Therefore, a 2-minute period of CPR before applying the AED to patients with prolonged cardiac arrest (greater than 4 to 5 minutes) can "prime the pump," thus restoring oxygen to the heart, removing metabolic waste products, and increasing the chance of successful defibrillation.

If the cardiac arrest is not witnessed and CPR is not in progress, immediately start CPR and continue for 2 minutes before delivering the first shock. If the patient's rhythm converts to V-fib or pulseless V-tach and the defibrillator is already attached, perform CPR only long enough to charge the defibrillator and then defibrillate. Defibrillation is *not* useful in asystole because there is no evidence that the myocardial cells are spontaneously depolarizing. Defibrillation of asystole is unlikely to be beneficial and is harmful (due to the unnecessary interruption of compressions). Thus, if you are unsure about asystole after checking more than one lead, resume CPR and follow the asystole pathway in the pulseless arrest algorithm until the next pulse and rhythm check.

■ Manual Defibrillation

Some defibrillators are combination units that can perform either manual or automated defibrillation. In **manual defibrillation**, you interpret the cardiac rhythm and determine if defibrillation is needed. Manual defibrillator units require you to select the appropriate dose. A default setting of 200 J is usually used; however, settings may range from 120 J to 200 J, depending on the specifications of the manufacturer. For simplicity, we will use the default setting of 200 J. After delivering a shock it is important for you to immediately begin chest compressions for a 2-minute cycle and then reassess the patient for pulse return and rhythm change. If your unit has both manual and AED mode, it is faster to use the unit in the manual mode because you can interpret the rhythm quicker than the time it takes the AED to interpret the rhythm or a rhythm change.

Skill Drill 4 summarizes the procedures for manual defibrillation in an adult:

Skill Drill 4

1. Take standard precautions.
2. Prepare the skin for placement of the defibrillation pads if needed. Attach the adhesive defibrillation pads to the patient's chest as instructed on the package **Step 1**. If using paddles, lubricate them with a conductive gel.
3. Turn on the main power switch.
4. Set the energy level to 200 J (for biphasic devices), or follow the defibrillator manufacturer's recommendations regarding the appropriate energy level **Step 2**. Monophasic defibrillators should be set to 360 J for the first and all successive shocks.
5. Charge the defibrillator.

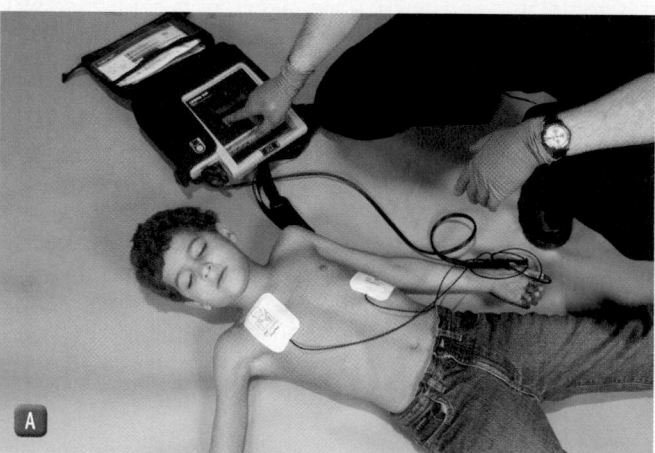

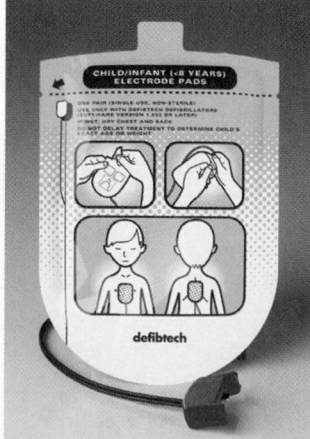

Figure 5 The pediatric dose-attenuator system. **A.** Attenuator pads in use. **B.** Attenuator pads in packaging.

Skill Drill | 4

Performing Manual Defibrillation in an Adult

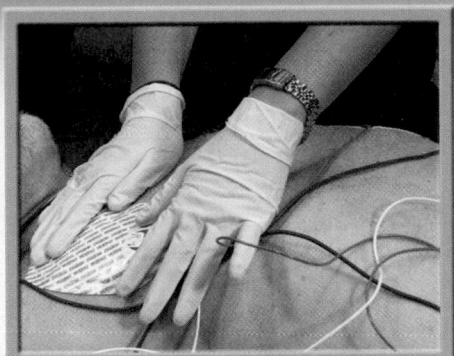

Step 1 Take standard precautions. Prepare the skin. Attach the adhesive defibrillation pads to the patient's chest as instructed on the package. If using paddles, lubricate them with a conductive gel.

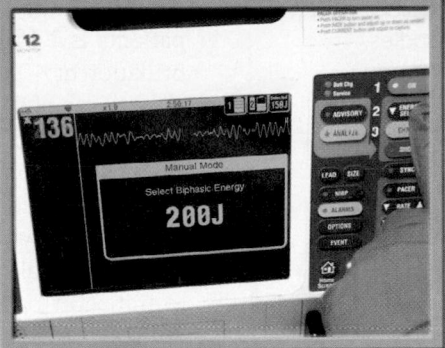

Step 2 Turn on the main power switch. Set the defibrillator to the proper energy setting. Charge the defibrillator. If using paddles, exert firm pressure to make good skin contact. Ensure that no one is touching the patient.

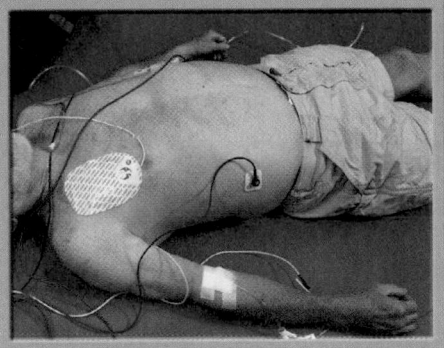

Step 3 Clear the area. Announce, "All clear!" Press the button on the machine if using a hands-free system; if not, discharge the defibrillator by pressing the button on each handle simultaneously. Observe for contraction of the patient's chest muscles. Resume CPR immediately. Continue CPR for 2 minutes or five cycles, and then pause to check for a pulse and reevaluate the rhythm. If at any point you see an organized rhythm on the monitor, check for a pulse (maximum of 10 seconds).

6. If using paddles, exert firm pressure (20 to 25 lb) on each paddle to make good skin contact.

7. Ensure that no one is touching the patient. Remember not to defibrillate a patient who is in pooled water. Ensure that the patient is not touching metal.

8. Clear the area. Announce, "All clear!"

9. Press the button on the machine if using a hands-free system; if not, discharge the defibrillator by pressing the button on each handle simultaneously **Step 3**.

10. Observe for contraction of the patient's chest muscles. If you do not see contraction, check the defibrillator to be certain the synchronizing switch is off and the battery is charged.

11. Resume CPR immediately. Continue CPR for 2 minutes or five cycles, and then pause to check for a pulse and reevaluate the rhythm. If at any point you see an organized rhythm on the monitor, check for a pulse (maximum of 10 seconds).

Follow these steps to perform manual defibrillation in an infant or a child:

1. Take standard precautions. Confirm unresponsiveness, pulselessness, and apnea.

2. Begin CPR if a defibrillator is not immediately available.

3. Use defibrillation pads for hands-free system (or select the proper paddle size if using paddles) **Table 2**. If using paddles, apply conductive gel to the paddles.

4. Place one pad on the anterior chest wall to the right of the sternum, inferior to the clavicle; place the other pad on the left midclavicular line at the level of the xiphoid process. Apply firm pressure **Figure 6**.

5. For children who are younger than 1 year or who weigh less than 22 lb (10 kg), you may use anterior-posterior placement **Figure 7**.

6. Assess the cardiac rhythm to confirm the presence of V-fib or pulseless V-tach.

7. Select the appropriate energy setting, and charge the defibrillator.

8. Verbally and visually ensure that no one is in contact with the patient; stop CPR if it is in progress.

9. Deliver the shock at the appropriate energy setting.

10. Give five cycles of CPR (approximately 2 minutes).

11. Reassess the rhythm.

12. If a shockable rhythm persists, give an additional shock at an increased or the same energy, and immediately resume CPR.

13. Establish IV/IO access, and begin medication therapy as indicated. Consider an advanced airway. Repeat the defibrillation after five cycles of CPR (approximately 2 minutes) if refractory V-fib or pulseless V-tach persists.

Table 2 Pediatric Defibrillation Paddle Size	
Age/Weight	**Paddle Size**
Older than 1 year or > 22 lb (10 kg)	8-cm (adult) paddles
Up to 1 year or < 22 lb (10 kg)	4.5-cm (pediatric) paddles

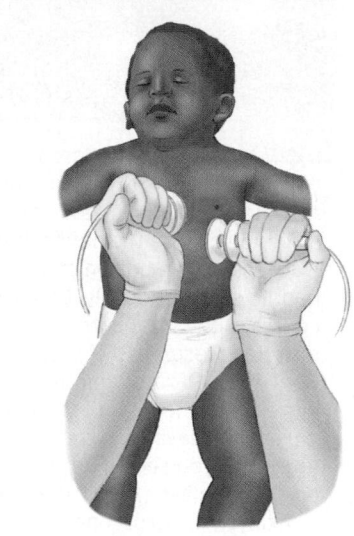

Figure 6   Anterior chest wall position in infants.

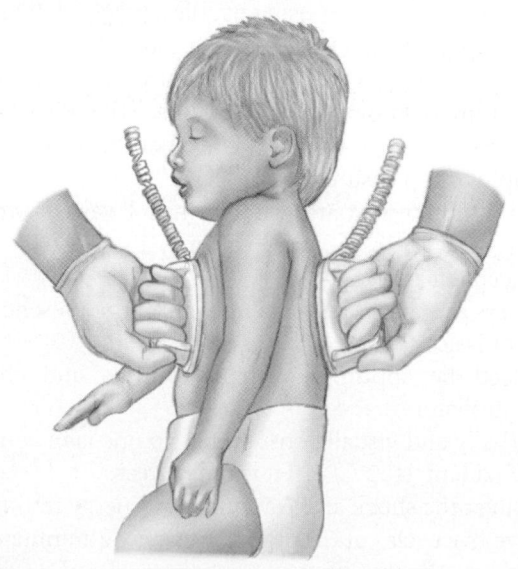

Figure 7   Anterior-posterior position for children who are younger than 1 year or who weigh less than 10 kg.

Most EMS systems use pre-gelled defibrillator pads instead of paddles. In fact it is difficult to find a defibrillator used in the field that still has paddles. If your system uses defibrillator pads, place them in the same location as you would when you are using an AED. When you are applying the pads, ensure that there are no air pockets in the pad-skin interface because they may result in skin burns and decreased defibrillation effectiveness.

The initial energy setting for defibrillation of pediatric patients is 2 J/kg. If this level is not successful, repeat the defibrillation at 4 J/kg. Further defibrillation should occur at 4 J/kg after cycles of CPR, as needed. With ongoing CPR, remember to search for and treat any underlying reversible causes (the Hs and Ts). Give epinephrine only after you have delivered two shocks, doubling the dose for the second attempt.

Consult with your medical director, medical control physician, or local protocols for the decision on when and where to transport patients who are in cardiopulmonary arrest. Early ROSC (less than 5 min) and V-fib or V-tach as a presenting rhythm are associated with improved neurologic outcome for survivors of pediatric cardiopulmonary arrest.

Automated External Defibrillation

As discussed, paramedics usually perform manual defibrillation, but as a paramedic you may encounter AEDs when you are responding to a scene where law enforcement personnel or other EMS providers have already attached an AED to the patient; therefore, you must know how to use AEDs.

An **automated external defibrillator (AED)** interprets the cardiac rhythm and determines if defibrillation is needed. AED units are used by personnel who are not trained in ECG rhythm interpretation. AEDs can assess the patient's rhythm and—if V-fib or V-tach is present—charge the pads and prompt the rescuer to deliver a countershock, without any intervention by the rescuer. AEDs can also be preprogrammed so that the user does not have to select a dose. Some AEDs may be fully automated, though these are now rare. A semiautomated AED detects V-fib and rapid V-tach, and a voice prompt may say, "Shock advised. Press to shock." The rescuer must then depress the shock button to defibrillate the patient.

Remember to observe safety measures. Distance yourself from the patient. Do not defibrillate a patient who is in pooled water. Do not defibrillate a patient who is touching metal. Remove a nitroglycerin patch from a patient's chest and wipe the area with a dry towel before defibrillation to prevent ignition of the patch. To review the steps for using an AED, see the chapter, *Cardiovascular Emergencies*.

The care of the patient after the AED delivers a shock depends on your location and EMS system; therefore, you should follow your local protocols. After the AED protocol is completed, one of the following outcomes is likely:

- Pulse is regained.
- No pulse is regained, and the AED indicates that no shock is advised.
- No pulse is regained, and the AED indicates that a shock is advised.

For each of these scenarios, the sequence of compressions and defibrillation is the same as described in the earlier section on manual defibrillation, with the only difference being that the AED determines whether the cardiac rhythm is shockable.

Shockable ECG Rhythms

The two shockable ECG rhythms are V-fib and pulseless V-tach. When a patient is in a shockable rhythm, the heart is quivering but blood is not pumping. Defibrillation stuns the heart muscle momentarily and allows the patient's normal conduction system to resume control. If the patient is not defibrillated, the V-fib will ultimately deteriorate to asystole or flatline.

In the first moments of a cardiac arrest, when the patient is in V-fib or V-tach, the heart is oxygenated and "ready" to receive a shock. This explains why the rescuer should begin the steps of CPR and get the AED attached as quickly as possible. If a shock is recommended in this circumstance, administer it immediately—the chances of a successful defibrillation drop 7% to 10% for every minute that passes.

When the V-fib or V-tach is not "fresh," however, a rapid shock is not always the best initial treatment. When a patient is in cardiac arrest for an interval of 4 to 5 minutes or longer, even if the initial ECG showed a shockable rhythm, the success rate is poor because the heart is no longer "ready" for a shock. Instead, perfusion and oxygenation are needed first. The guidelines state that it would be more appropriate to begin the steps of CPR, proceeding with five cycles or approximately 2 minutes of 30 compressions to two ventilations, and then analyze the patient's ECG. If the patient is still in V-fib or V-tach at this point, he or she is ready for a dose of electricity.

Words of Wisdom

Nonarrest rhythms include bradycardia and tachycardia. See the chapter, *Cardiovascular Emergencies*, for management of these conditions.

Shock First or Compressions First?

The decision to deliver a shock first versus provide CPR first is a local medical control policy decision. Many medical directors implement a policy similar to the following:

- If the EMS provider witnesses the cardiac arrest, begin CPR with chest compressions and attach an AED as soon as it is available.
- If the cardiac arrest is not witnessed by the EMS provider, then five cycles (2 minutes) of CPR should be performed prior applying the AED.
- The decision of whether to count bystander CPR as the first 2 minutes is a judgment call. If you enter the room and observe high-quality compressions being performed (at the proper rate and depth, and with full chest recoil), it probably makes the most sense to allow the bystander to finish out the 2 minutes, unless he or she is tiring, and apply the electrodes around the compressor. Then, at the 2-minute point, you will be ready to analyze and shock, if recommended.

The success rate for a biphasic dose is excellent (better than 93%) if the heart is ready to receive the shock. The three-shock series of defibrillation that was taught prior to 2005 is no longer used; it would mean delaying compressions for the sake of providing two additional shocks that may not benefit the patient at this point. If the shock does not work, the patient needs 2 minutes of high-quality CPR. You can then quickly reanalyze the rhythm and shock as recommended by the device.

Effective Shocks and Special Circumstances

When a shock is effective, occasionally the patient wakes up. However, the majority of the effective defibrillations take a minute or so to produce an effective return of circulation. The defibrillation actually stuns the heart, allowing the pacemaker to begin to beat. This may not be enough of a heartbeat to generate a pulse just yet. For this reason, as soon as the patient is defibrillated, you should immediately begin compressions. Do not be surprised if the patient begins to move after a minute or so. After a cycle of 2 minutes of CPR, it is then acceptable to take 10 seconds to check for a pulse and review the rhythm. If there is ROSC, you can then cease the compressions and check for a pulse, respirations, and blood pressure.

Because defibrillator pads or electrodes are safer, paddles are rarely used today. Instead, the patient's ECG is monitored and displayed throughout the arrest—not just when you are taking a "quick look" or when asking the AED to analyze the rhythm. Thus it is possible to observe V-fib or V-tach while compressions are being done and begin to charge up the unit. Once the AED is fully charged, the operator should clear all rescuers and deliver the shock. With this approach, compressions can be delivered while the unit is charging, which minimizes the interruption.

The code team member who delivers the shock *must* always first clear the patient! It is also recommended that the ventilation device be removed from the patient or detached from the advanced airway to prevent oxygen from flowing across

Controversies

In some settings, the LMA, Combitube, or King LT are thought to be superior to bag-mask ventilation and oxygenation. Surprisingly, research shows that these devices are equivalent to the ET tube in the adult patient. In addition, the Combitube and King LT offer protection from aspiration of the stomach contents into the lungs. The LMA, Combitube, and King LT are similar in several ways:
- They are advanced airway devices that are inserted blindly.
- They are placed orally and inserted past the hypopharyngeal space.
- They are easy to use and do not require extensive training in laryngoscopy.

By training selected EMS providers on the use of these devices, your service may expand the number of patients who have access to an advanced airway. The specifics on how to use these devices are included in the airway chapter, *Airway Management and Ventilation*.

the patient's chest while a shock is being delivered, because the simultaneous delivery poses a fire hazard.

You should review the following special circumstances for defibrillation and understand the solutions or modifications to the procedure should they arise:

- **The patient is an infant.** Use the appropriate pediatric pads and an attenuator if available.
- **The patient has a hairy chest and the electrodes will not stick.** Quickly shave the patient just as you would to obtain a 12-lead ECG.
- **The patient is submersed in water or is soaking wet.** Get out of the rain, quickly moving the patient to your ambulance,

or remove the patient from the pool and dry him or her off prior to applying the electrodes or providing a shock.

- **The patient has an implantable cardioverter defibrillator (AICD) or pacemaker.** Avoid these devices by a few inches when you are placing the electrodes.
- **The patient has a transdermal medication patch on the chest.** Quickly remove the patch and wipe the chest dry. You should wear disposable gloves while removing the patch to avoid absorbing the nitroglycerin into your skin.

A comparison of the key elements of adult, child, and infant CPR is shown in **Table 3**.

Table 3 Key Elements of CPR for Adults, Children, and Infants, 2010 Guidelines

Procedure	Age 9 to Adult	Age 1 to 8 Years	Younger Than 1 Year[a]
Circulation			
Recognition	Unresponsive with no breathing, or only agonal (gasping) respirations		
Pulse check	Carotid artery	Carotid artery	Brachial artery
Compression location	In the center of the chest, in between the nipples	In the center of the chest, in between the nipples	Just below the nipple line
Compression area	Heel of both hands	Heel of one or both hands	Two fingers or two-thumb encircling-hands technique
Compression depth	At least 2 inches	At least one third of chest depth Approximately 2 inches	At least one third of chest depth Approximately 1½ inches
Compression rate	At least 100/min		
Chest wall recoil	Allow full chest recoil in between compressions Rotate professional rescuers delivering compressions every 2 minutes		
Interruptions	Limit interruptions in delivery of chest compressions to less than 10 seconds		
Ratio of compressions to ventilations (until an advanced airway is inserted)	30:2 (one or two rescuers)	30:2 (one rescuer); 15:2 (two professional rescuers)	
Airway			
	Head tilt–chin lift maneuver; jaw-thrust maneuver if spinal injury is suspected		
Breathing			
Untrained rescuer	Compressions only		
Ventilations without advanced airway	2 breaths with a duration of 1 second each, with enough volume to produce chest rise[b]		
Ventilations with advanced airway	1 breath every 6 to 8 seconds (8 to 10/min) Asynchronous with chest compressions. Duration of 1 second each with enough volume to produce chest rise		
Rescue breaths	1 breath every 5 seconds (12 breaths/min)	1 breath every 3 seconds (20 breaths/min)	1 breath every 3 seconds (20 breaths/min)
Defibrillation			
Device	Adult AED	Use pediatric dose-attenuator unit if available; if not available, use adult unit	Use manual defibrillator if available; if not, use unit with pediatric dose-attenuator; if neither is available, use adult unit

Continues

Table 3   Key Elements of CPR for Adults, Children, and Infants, 2010 Guidelines, continued

Procedure	Age 9 to Adult	Age 1 to 8 Years	Younger Than 1 Year[a]
Procedure	Attach AED as soon as it is available. If two rescuers are available, one should immediately begin CPR while the second retrieves and applies the AED. Minimize CPR interruptions. Resume CPR immediately after shock, beginning with chest compressions.		
Airway Obstruction			
Foreign body obstruction	Conscious: abdominal thrusts	Conscious: abdominal thrusts	Conscious: back slaps and chest thrusts
	Unconscious: CPR[c]		

[a]Excluding newborns, in whom arrest is usually the result of asphyxiation and requires the rescue ventilations.
[b]Pause compressions to deliver ventilations.
[c]Look in the mouth for objects before delivering breaths in a patient with a known airway obstruction.

YOU are the Medic   PART 4

You reassess your patient to find that his skin appears to have more color and you quickly check for a pulse. A carotid pulse rate of 68 beats/min is detected. The compression device has been paused and you analyze the patient's rhythm. You detect clear ST-segment elevation and begin to obtain a 12-lead ECG. You identify the presence of the ST elevation myocardial infarction (STEMI) and your partner transmits the ECG to the hospital. You prepare to call in your report to the receiving facility while your partner obtains vital signs. Although the patient has not shown signs of regaining consciousness, you are pleased to have an ROSC. After completing your radio report, the hospital advises you they have received your ECG transmission and your patient should be taken to the cardiac procedure lab on arrival without stopping in the emergency department.

You and your team move to the back of the ambulance with the patient loaded and secured to a backboard. Your partner has also applied a cervical collar to help secure the endotracheal tube. Your partner continues to deliver ventilations while the field supervisor prepares the automated transport ventilator. The patient is connected and the supervisor advises she will drive you to the hospital. Transport time is estimated to be approximately 10 minutes.

You obtain another set of vital signs prior to reaching the hospital. On arrival, you unload the patient with the assistance of your partner and supervisor. Your supervisor goes to locate your patient's wife to update her on her husband's location in the hospital. As you transfer your patient to the staff in the lab, you provide a bedside report and your updated assessment findings to the receiving nurse and cardiologist. You return to the EMS workroom in the emergency department to complete your patient care report. You are aware of the importance of accurate and specific documentation of this field resuscitation for data collection and reporting for cardiac arrests.

Recording Time: 16 Minutes	
Respirations	10 breaths/min via ET tube using an automated transport ventilator
Pulse	68 beats/min
Skin	Pink, cool, and dry
Blood pressure	88/54 mm Hg
Oxygen saturation (Spo$_2$)	99% on 100% F$_{IO_2}$
Pupils	Equal, round, and sluggish but reactive to light
End-tidal carbon dioxide (ETCO$_2$)	38 mm Hg

8. What is the significance of completing advanced life support care prior to transport?

9. What is the significance of good documentation for improvement of survival in prehospital cardiac arrests?

The Advanced Cardiac Life Support Algorithm

The *Advanced Cardiac Life Support (ACLS) Algorithm* used to manage an adult in cardiac arrest builds on the *BLS Healthcare Provider Algorithm* discussed earlier in this chapter **Figure 8**. After making sure the patient has been placed on supplementary oxygen, the monitor or defibrillator is used to determine whether the patient is still in a shockable rhythm. The ACLS algorithm separates the treatment approach into two basic pathways: shockable rhythms (V-fib or V-tach) or nonshockable rhythms (asystole or pulseless electrical activity).

The key difference in management from the past approaches is that some preplanning is done so that the medications are

drawn up and ready to administer prior to the rhythm checks. The medications are administered during CPR, and compressions need not stop for this treatment.

As long as the patient has an effective BLS airway and is being adequately ventilated, placement of an advanced airway (LMA, Combitube, King LT, or ET tube)—although helpful—should never take priority over delivery of high-quality compressions or a shock when needed. Practice your intubation techniques so you are able to insert the advanced airway device with no more than a 10-second interruption in chest compressions. Refer to the chapter, *Airway Management and Ventilation*, for more information about advanced airway devices.

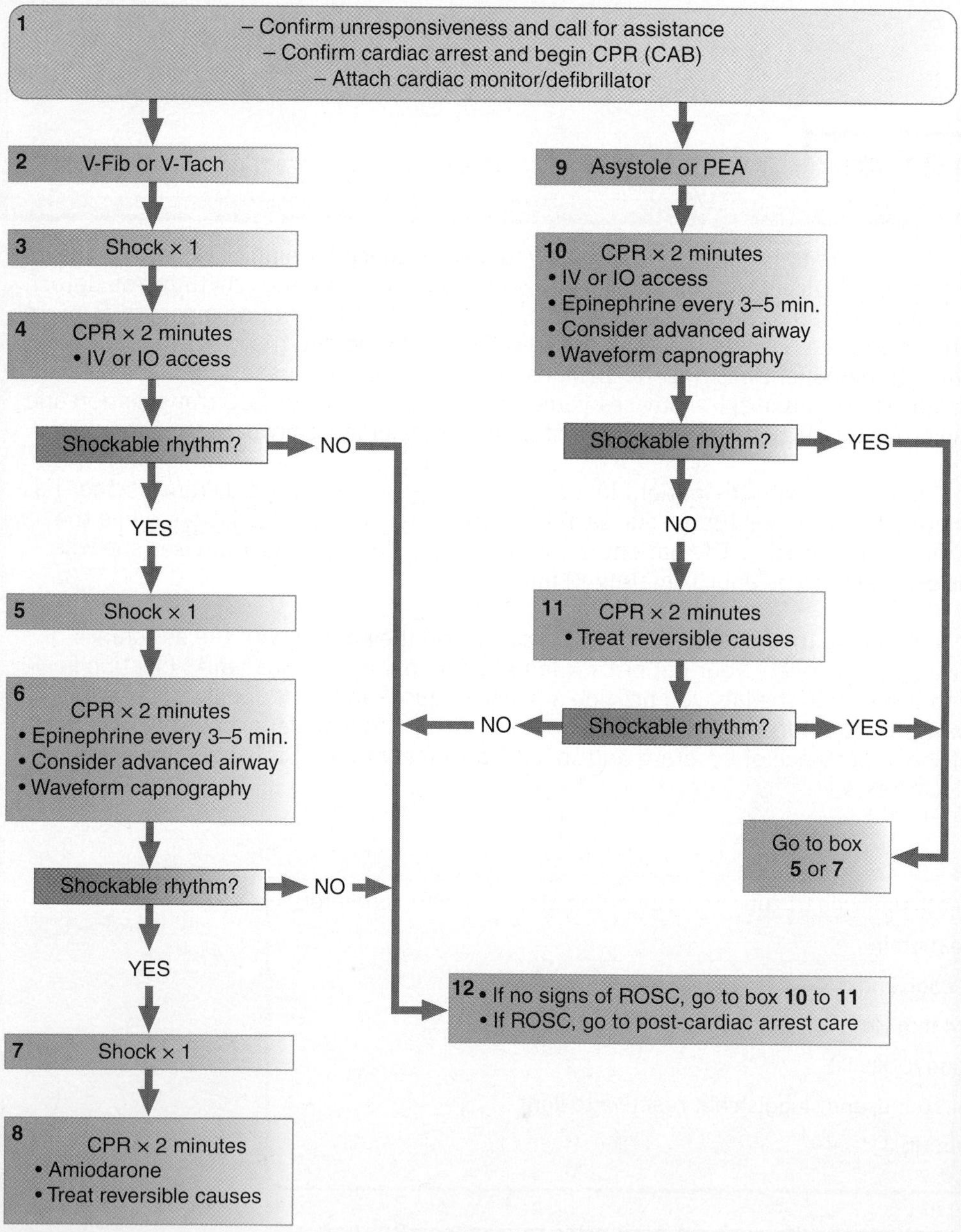

Managing Patients in Ventricular Fibrillation or Ventricular Tachycardia

Patients with V-fib or pulseless V-tach are the most likely to be resuscitated—if they receive timely and appropriate treatment. Per the ACLS algorithm, you should continue to perform high-quality CPR and do a rhythm check at each 2-minute point. If the patient is in a shockable rhythm, administer a single shock and immediately begin compressions. If three rescuers are performing CPR (ventilator, active compressor, and on-deck compressor) and an advanced airway has been placed, the compressions and ventilations can be asynchronous. Medications should be prepared and administered while performing CPR. A timekeeper can remind the code team leader what should be coming up in the next 30 seconds, in the next 15 seconds, and so on.

Drug therapy for V-fib or V-tach includes a vasopressor (epinephrine or vasopressin). Epinephrine (1:10,000) is given as a 1-mg IV push; this dose should be repeated every 3 to 5 minutes as long as the pulse is absent. Vasopressin is given as 40 units IV push, one time only. A single dose of vasopressin 40 U IV or IO may be substituted for either the first or second epinephrine dose (but not both).

After the third shock, you may decide to administer an antidysrhythmic such as amiodarone, which is given as a 300-mg bolus during CPR. Amiodarone may be repeated once at 150 mg in 3 to 5 minutes after the initial dose. If amiodarone is unavailable, you may administer lidocaine (1 to 1.5 mg/kg IV push, then 0.5

Figure 8 Advanced Cardiac Life Support (ACLS) Algorithm for cardiac arrest (adult or pediatric).

Words of Wisdom

The American Heart Association has defined ACLS for a patient in cardiac arrest (or a patient at immediate risk of cardiac arrest) as consisting of the following elements:

- Effective and minimally interrupted chest compression (for cardiac arrest)
- Use of adjunctive equipment for ventilation and circulation
- Cardiac monitoring for dysrhythmia recognition and control
- Establishment and maintenance of an IV infusion line
- Use of definitive therapy, including defibrillation and drug administration, to:
  1. Prevent cardiac arrest
  2. Aid in establishing an effective cardiac rhythm and circulation when cardiac arrest occurs
  3. Stabilize the patient's condition
- Administration of hypothermia therapy for patients who are in a coma after ROSC
- Transport to an appropriate facility—one that is prepared to provide successful resuscitation treatment
- Transport with continuous monitoring

to 0.75 mg/kg, up to a maximum of 3 doses, or 3 mg/kg). Do not combine these two antidysrhythmics and always follow local protocol.

If the patient has torsades de pointes, consider administering magnesium (loading dose 1 to 2 g IV or IO). After each drug has been administered, allow it to circulate and then reanalyze the patient at the next 2-minute point. If the patient remains in a shockable rhythm, administer another shock and consider other treatable causes (ie, the Hs and Ts) **Table 4**. Refer to the chapter, *Cardiovascular Emergencies*, for more detailed information about the specific steps in managing V-fib and pulseless V-tach.

Words of Wisdom

Whenever you administer a medication through a peripheral IV line during CPR, follow it immediately with a 20- to 30-mL bolus of IV fluids and then elevate the extremity to facilitate delivery of the medication to the central circulation (which may take 1 to 2 minutes). Note that IO administration has the same effect on central circulation.

■ Managing Patients in Pulseless Electrical Activity or Asystole

The term pulseless electrical activity (PEA) refers to an organized cardiac rhythm (other than ventricular tachycardia) on the monitor that is not accompanied by any detectable pulse. You should continue to provide high-quality CPR and do a rhythm check at each 2-minute point. If the patient is in a nonshockable rhythm, such as asystole or PEA, the potential cause must be taken into consideration (the "Hs and Ts"). Some of these issues can be managed in the field; others will require intervention in the emergency department.

Table 4 Possible Causes and Treatment of Cardiac Arrest Rhythms

Possible Cause of PEA to Consider During Arrest	Clues to Cause	Treatment (Beyond Managing the Cardiac Arrest)
Hypovolemia	Patient history	Volume infusion
Hypoxemia	Cyanosis, airway problem	Intubation and ventilation with 100% oxygen
Hypoglycemia	Blood glucose level < 60 mg/dL	Dextrose 50% in water, 25 g
Hypothermia	History of exposure to cold	See hypothermia algorithm in the chapter, *Environmental Emergencies*.
Hyperkalemia, hypokalemia, hydrogen ions (acidosis)	History, ECG changes	Immediate transport. Consider sodium bicarbonate if certain of acidosis.
Tension pneumothorax	History, no pulse with CPR, unequal breath sounds with hyperresonance to percussion on affected side	Needle decompression of the affected side of the chest
Cardiac tamponade	History, no pulse with CPR, jugular venous distention	Pericardiocentesis (immediate transport)
Others: Drug overdose, trauma, massive MI, pulmonary embolism	History	Consider need for immediate transport. Naloxone (Narcan) for opioid or narcotic overdose.

If three rescuers are performing CPR (ventilator, active compressor, and on-deck compressor) and an advanced airway has been placed, the compressions and ventilations can be asynchronous. Medications should be prepared and administered while doing CPR. A timekeeper can remind the code team leader what should be coming up in the next 30 seconds, in the next 15 seconds, and so on.

Drug therapy for PEA or asystole includes a vasopressor (epinephrine or vasopressin). Epinephrine (1:10,000) is given as a 1-mg IV push; this dose should be repeated every 3 to 5 minutes as long as the pulse is absent. Vasopressin is given as 40 units IV push, one time only. A single dose of vasopressin of 40 units IV or IO may be substituted for either the first or second epinephrine dose (but not both).

Consider the reversible causes and manage them (Hs and Ts). If the patient changes to V-fib or V-tach at any point or when the rhythm is checked every five cycles of CPR (approximately

2 minutes), move back to the shockable side of the algorithm. After each drug has been administered, allow it to circulate and then reanalyze the patient at the next 2-minute point. Refer to the chapter, *Cardiovascular Emergencies*, for more detailed information about the specific steps in managing PEA and asystole.

Paramedics are trained to follow the current algorithms and use good medical judgment. To be successful you need to practice. Simulation can be helpful because today's high-fidelity simulators can provide excellent learning opportunities for those low-frequency, high-risk, or high-impact calls such as the patient in cardiac arrest.

The following information is NOT an algorithm; rather these are the key points when you are managing a patient in cardiac arrest:

- Perform high-quality CPR beginning with compressions and minimizing interruptions from start to completion of the code. Organize the code around 2-minute cycles of 30:2 (compressions to ventilations) and then switch compressors and analyze the rhythm. If an advanced airway is inserted, you should switch to **asynchronous** compressions of at least 100 per minute and ventilate every 6 to 8 seconds (that is a rate of 8 to 10 per minute).
- If a shockable rhythm is identified, continue compressions until the defibrillator is charged to the appropriate dose and then stop, clear, deliver the shock, and immediately begin compressions unless the patient wakes up.
- Without interrupting CPR, obtain IV/IO access and administer epinephrine every 3 to 5 minutes for the duration of the code (provided the patient is not hypothermic). After a cycle of CPR and shock, if necessary, administer an antidysrhythmic drug for V-fib/V-tach (amiodarone 300 mg which may be repeated at 150 mg).
- For asystole or PEA, do not deliver shocks.
- For all arrests, regardless of the rhythm, consider the reversible causes and treat them appropriately.
- If you decide to insert an advanced airway (supraglottic or ET tube), confirm and monitor with waveform capnography and switch to asynchronous compressions/ventilations. Never overventilate the patient because this causes a deadly restriction on coronary perfusion.
- If the patient experiences ROSC, the capnography readings might show a sustained increase in ETCO$_2$ (typically greater than or equal to 40 mm Hg). Turn your attention to monitoring vital signs, obtain a 12-lead ECG, and prepare to transport the patient to the most appropriate facility that can perform postresuscitative care (ie, hypothermia, EEG monitoring, coronary catheterization lab).

Mechanical Adjuncts to Circulation

Several devices are available to provide immediate feedback to rescuers on the quality of their compressions (rate, depth, and chest recoil). There is currently no research to support the use of these devices, however four devices hold considerable promise in improving the quality and consistency of compressions as well as improving the blood flow during CPR: the impedance

threshold device (ITD) and three mechanical compression adjuncts (AutoPulse, Thumper, Lucas 2).

Impedance Threshold Device

The impedance threshold device (ITD) is marketed as the ResQPOD in the United States **Figure 9**. It has been shown to enhance the vacuum in an adult's chest, which forms during the chest recoil phase of CPR. Imagine a bellows fanning a fireplace. As the bellows opens to its full size, it sucks in air. A similar process occurs when the chest wall re-expands—the vacuum that results pulls air into the lungs and blood back into the heart. An ITD selectively prevents that unnecessary air from rushing into the chest, maximizing the vacuum during the recoil phase of the compression. This results in enhanced return of blood that increases cardiac output, blood pressure, and perfusion to vital organs, and ultimately improves survival rates. Use of the ITD may therefore improve circulation during CPR and increase the ROSC in cardiac arrest patients. This device was given a strong recommendation (a Class IIa rating) by the AHA in its 2005 guidelines due to the strength of the available data on this point. As the patient's pulse returns, however, the ITD should be removed from the ventilation system because it is designed to be used in conjunction with compressions.

Load-Distributing Band CPR or Vest CPR Device

The AutoPulse device is designed to deliver consistent, uninterrupted adult chest compressions and therefore improve hemodynamics during cardiac arrest **Figure 10**. This automated,

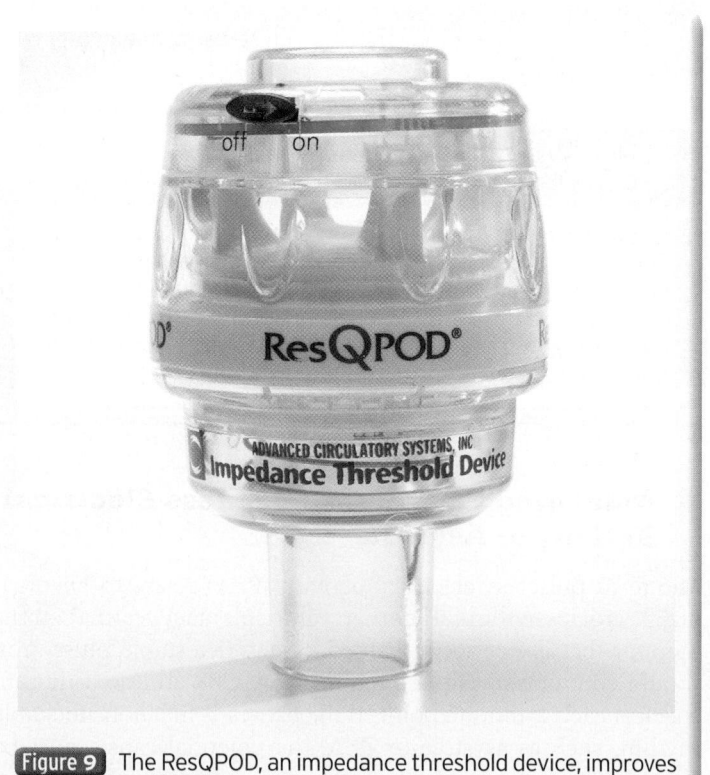

Figure 9 The ResQPOD, an impedance threshold device, improves perfusion during CPR.

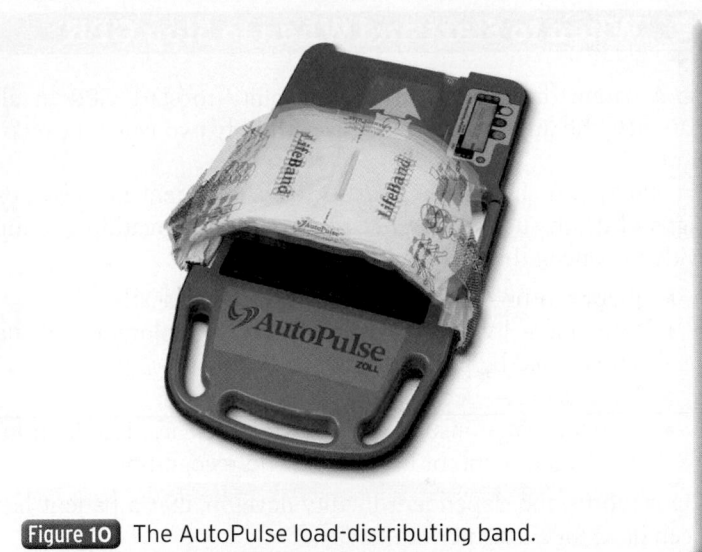

Figure 10 The AutoPulse load-distributing band.

portable device offers an easy-to-use, load-distributing LifeBand that squeezes the entire chest, thereby improving blood flow to the heart and brain during cardiac arrest. Its use can also free up rescuers to focus on other lifesaving interventions and eliminate fatigue from the performance of CPR chest compressions.

The AutoPulse can be integrated into a code as follows:

1. Ensure that CPR is in progress and that effective, high-quality compressions are being provided.
2. Align the patient on the AutoPulse platform.
3. Close the LifeBand chest band over the patient's chest.
4. Press the start button (AutoPulse performs the compressions automatically).
5. Provide bag-mask ventilation at a rate of two ventilations for every 30 compressions. Each ventilation should be given over 1 second to provide visible chest rise.
6. If an advanced airway is in place (LMA, Combitube, King LT, or ET tube), there are no longer cycles of compressions to ventilations. The compression rate is continuous (at least 100/min) and the ventilation rate is 8 to 10 per minute.
7. After 2 minutes of CPR, reassess for pulse and/or shockable rhythm (maximum interruption of 10 seconds).

Thumper CPR Device

The Thumper is an adjunct to adult CPR that provides both continuous chest compressions (at least 100 per minute) and ventilations Figure 11 . It can be used with a pocket mask or an advanced airway. Because this device is powered by oxygen and delivers oxygen when it ventilates, it does go through a large volume of oxygen. If you use the Thumper, plan to carry additional portable oxygen tanks equipped with high-pressure hose adapters to facilitate rapid transfer of the gas. Use these high-pressure adapters in the ambulance and keep them available for use in the emergency department if the Thumper is used to transport the patient to the emergency department. The Thumper has been particularly useful in lengthy arrests (eg, hypothermic arrest), because it can produce excellent CPR compressions for a long time.

In the past, some services have reserved the use of the Thumper for transport to the hospital. Given that high-quality compressions are important to the success of the resuscitation, it makes more sense for the code team to practice simulated codes to ensure they can apply the Thumper as early as possible without any interruptions in manual CPR.

Mechanical Piston Device

A mechanical piston device is a device that depresses the adult sternum via a compressed gas-powered plunger mounted on a backboard. A more recent device to become available is the Lucas 2 mechanical piston device Figure 12 . This device is similar to the Thumper with a piston that compresses the chest, yet it is not designed to offer the ventilation component because many services use an ATV for this purpose. The device is portable and easy to deploy; a small back plate fits behind the patient and allows the piston to snap down directly into the back plate. The Lucas 2 is powered by a small battery at the top of the piston, eliminating all the air hoses of the Thumper and the prior version of the Lucas device.

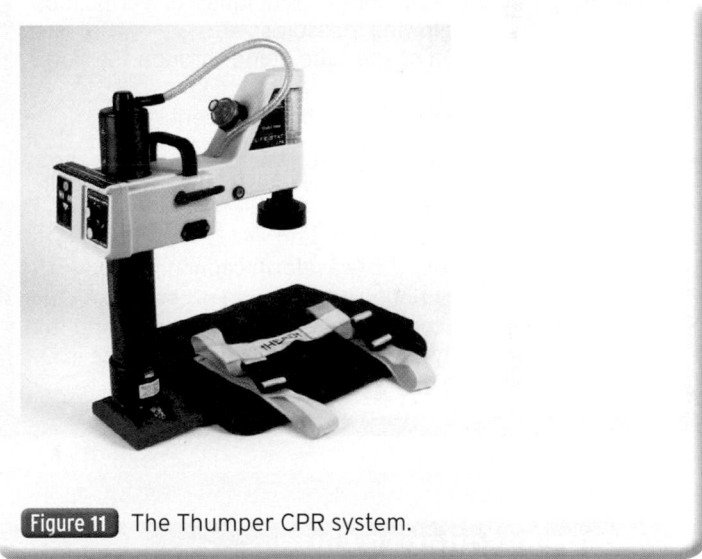

Figure 11 The Thumper CPR system.

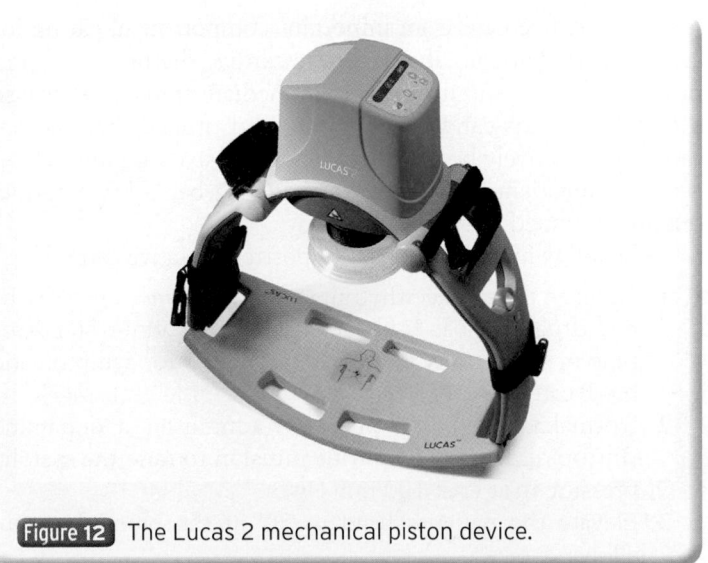

Figure 12 The Lucas 2 mechanical piston device.

When you are using any of the adjuncts to circulation, it is important that they are easy to deploy without interrupting high-quality manual CPR compressions. If they are not easy to deploy, they will not be used early in the field code. If your agency purchases an adjunct to circulation, practice with the device so all members of your service can deploy it and make sure it arrives on the scene as early as possible in the field code.

Words of Wisdom

The ECC guidelines include recommendations on tube placement confirmation and continuous monitoring of the tube's position to avoid its dislodgement. To ensure that the tube is inserted in the correct location, after the tube is seen to pass through the vocal cords and the tube position is verified by chest expansion and auscultation during positive-pressure ventilation, you should obtain additional confirmation of placement using continuous waveform $ETCO_2$ (capnography). No single confirmation technique, including clinical signs or the presence of water vapor in the tube, is completely reliable. Your initial techniques of verification should include the following measures:

- Direct visualization of the tube going through the vocal cords
- Physical examination of the tube placement
- Bilateral chest expansion
- Five-point auscultation (two in each lung and epigastrium)
- Tube condensation
- Initial monitoring of $ETCO_2$ (waveform capnography)

Be sure to provide continuous monitoring of the $ETCO_2$ throughout the field code and closely note and respond to any changes. Not only will the $ETCO_2$ tell you if the tube is misplaced, it will also give you an indication of ROSC.

Postresuscitative Care

Postresuscitative care is an important component of caring for cardiac arrest patients. If an effective cardiac rhythm is restored in the field, you should provide immediate transport because the patient needs careful monitoring and titrated therapy that can most effectively be provided in an intensive care unit. However, if the patient is comatose after ROSC, begin hypothermia treatment immediately.

The following is a summary of postresuscitative care:

1. Stabilize the cardiac rhythm (administer an antidysrhythmic drug for post–V-fib or post–V-tach; administer atropine or use a transcutaneous pacemaker for symptomatic bradycardia).
2. Normalize the blood pressure (administer a dopamine [Intropin] or norepinephrine infusion to raise the systolic pressure to at least 100 mm Hg).
3. Elevate the patient's head to 30° if the blood pressure allows.

When to Start and When to Stop CPR

As a paramedic, it is your responsibility to start CPR in all patients who are in cardiac arrest, with only two general exceptions.

First, you should not start CPR if the patient has obvious signs of death such as absence of a pulse and breathing, along with any one of the following findings:

- Rigor mortis—stiffening of the body after death
- Dependent lividity (livor mortis)—a discoloration of the skin caused by pooling of blood
- Putrefaction—decomposition of the body
- Evidence of nonsurvivable injury such as decapitation, dismemberment, or burned beyond recognition

Rigor mortis and dependent lividity develop after a patient has been dead for a long period.

Second, you should not start CPR if the patient and his or her physician have previously agreed not to resuscitate. This may apply only to situations in which the patient is known to be in the terminal stage of an incurable disease. In this situation, CPR serves only to prolong the patient's death. However, this can be a complicated issue. Do not resuscitate (DNR) orders, Medical Orders for Life-Sustaining Treatment (MOLST) forms, and advance directives such as living wills may express the patient's wishes; however, these documents may not be readily producible by the patient's family or caregiver. In such cases, the safest course is to assume that an emergency exists and begin CPR under the rule of implied consent and contact medical control for further guidance. Conversely, if a valid DNR, MOLST form, or living will is produced, resuscitative efforts may be withheld. Learn your state laws and local protocols as well as the standards in your system for treating terminally ill patients, and refer to the chapter, *Medical, Legal, and Ethical Issues*, for further discussion on advance health care directives. Some EMS systems have computer notes on patients who are preregistered with the system, specifying the amount and extent of treatment desired. Other states have specific EMS DNR forms that allow EMS providers to withhold care when the patient, family, and physician have agreed in advance that such a course is most appropriate. It is critical that you understand your local protocols and are aware of the specific restrictions these advance directives imply.

In all other cases, you should begin CPR on anyone who is in cardiac arrest. It is usually impossible to know how long the patient has been without oxygen to the brain and vital organs unless you were there to witness the cardiac arrest. Factors such as air temperature and the basic health of the patient's tissues and organs can affect their ability to survive. Therefore, most legal advisers recommend that, when in doubt, always give too much care rather than too little. You should always start CPR if any doubt exists.

Once you begin CPR in the field, you should not stop until one of the following events occurs:

- The patient starts breathing and has a pulse (ROSC).
- The patient is transferred to another health care provider of equal or more advanced training.

- You are completely out of strength and energy and are no longer physically able to perform CPR.
- A physician who is present or providing online medical direction assumes responsibility for the patient and gives direction to terminate the resuscitative efforts.

In short, CPR should always be continued until the patient's care is transferred to a physician or higher medical authority in the field. In some cases, your medical director or a designated medical control physician may order you to stop CPR on the basis of the patient's condition. Every EMS system should have clear standing orders or protocols that provide guidelines for starting and stopping CPR. Your medical director and your system's legal adviser should agree on these protocols, which should be closely administered and reviewed by your medical director.

Terminating Resuscitative Efforts

The 2010 AHA guidelines say the following about lengthy resuscitative efforts and transporting cardiac arrest patients:

- There are few instances that require transporting a nontraumatic cardiac arrest patient who has failed a successfully executed prehospital ACLS resuscitation effort to an emergency department to continue the resuscitation attempt.
- In the absence of mitigating factors, prolonged resuscitative efforts are unlikely to be successful. If ROSC of any duration occurs, however, it may be appropriate to consider extending the resuscitative effort.
- Rare exceptions may include severe prehospital hypothermia (eg, submersion in icy water) and drug overdose. A successfully executed prehospital resuscitation includes an "adequate trial" of BLS and ALS.

Transporting a deceased patient who is refractory to proper BLS and ALS is usually not appropriate. Protocols for pronouncement of death and appropriate transport of the body by non-EMS vehicles should be established.

Termination Rules

According to the 2010 AHA guidelines, the quality of CPR is compromised during transport and survival is linked to optimizing scene care, rather than simply rushing to the hospital. Specifically, for a patient who is receiving only BLS, the BLS termination of resuscitation rule was established to consider terminating BLS support before ambulance transport if all of the following criteria are met:

1. The arrest was not witnessed by anyone.
2. No ROSC after three full rounds of CPR and AED analysis.
3. No AED shocks were delivered.

For situations where ALS personnel are present to provide care for an adult with prehospital cardiac arrest, the ALS termination of resuscitation rule was established to consider terminating resuscitative efforts before ambulance transport if all of the following criteria are met:

1. The arrest was not witnessed by anyone.
2. Bystander CPR was not provided.
3. No ROSC after complete ALS care in the field.
4. No AED shocks were delivered.

Of course, the local decision on transportation should involve preplanning by the regional and service medical directors.

Scene Choreography and Teamwork

During resuscitation, many tasks need to be performed. This is where teamwork comes in. Teamwork divides the task while multiplying the chances for a successful resuscitation. There is a role for each health care provider who is committed to fulfilling his or her part. Teams who practice together regularly are more successful in their resuscitation attempts.

Consider the following analogy from the world of sports. From 1999 to 2005, Lance Armstrong and his international team of cyclists set an unprecedented record by winning the Tour de France seven consecutive times **Figure 13**. The Tour is

Controversies

Rescuers who begin BLS are taught to continue until one of the following events occurs:
- Effective spontaneous circulation and ventilation are restored.
- Care is transferred to a higher level of care provider, who in turn may determine whether the patient is not responsive to the resuscitative attempt.
- Reliable criteria indicating irreversible death are present.
- The rescuer is unable to continue because of exhaustion or the presence of dangerous environmental hazards or because continuation of the resuscitation effort places other lives in jeopardy.
- A valid DNR order or MOLST form is presented to the rescuers.

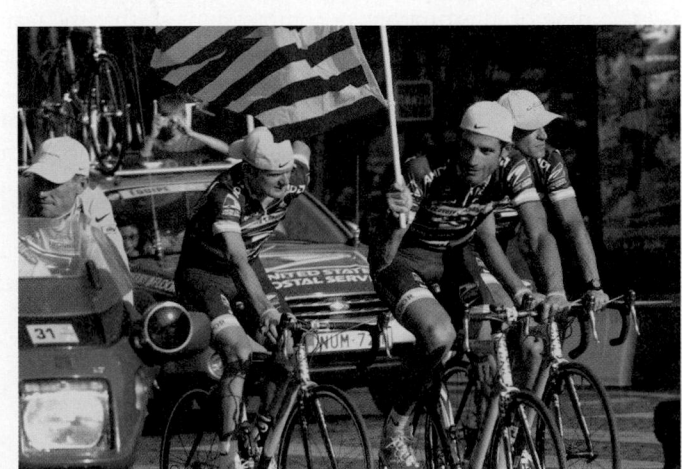

Figure 13 Even though Lance Armstrong (yellow jersey) is the only household name on this team, cycling is a team sport.

a grueling 21-stage bike race traveling 3,607 km through the tallest mountains and smallest towns into Paris. Cycling is a *team sport*. Each member of the team has a specific role in maintaining the pace, blocking the wind, collecting water bottles and food bags, and helping the team succeed. All team members must be totally committed to the success of the team rather than to their own personal achievements.

The intense preparation and teamwork that characterize any type of high-level sports team hold a few pertinent lessons for code team members:

- Athletes do not only excel on their own. They need the support of their team and coach.
- The coach helps the team members understand the rules of the game and prepare for its challenges.
- The coach drills the athletes with routines or plays and provides constant feedback and plenty of practice opportunities to measure their progress.
- The team trains with the best equipment, eats nutritious meals, develops a positive mental attitude about winning, and gets plenty of rest after enduring rigorous demanding physical and mental exercise.
- When it is time to compete, team members are well prepared, on time, and ready to go. The coach can support them from the sidelines and may offer signals and guidance or "plays" in some sports, but he or she cannot compete for the team.

Code team members who are rested, fit, and well nourished, and who bring a positive attitude to their work, practice their skills, know the "plays," and work together as a team, are on top of their game. They are ready to resuscitate patients. To be successful, your team needs to take the following steps:

- Know the plays expertly and automatically. This takes much practice. When there are questions, use posters and pocket cards to explain and prepare.
- Listen to your "coaches." They have the best interests of the patients in mind—and your best interests, too.
- Have a "practice ethic." Pull out the manikins and run mock codes or simulations frequently. Collect data on the cumulative time of interruptions of compressions so that the team has feedback and can work to improve its performance. How long does it take you to do each procedure? If you measure it and provide feedback you can improve performance.
- Remember that success equals practice, a positive mental attitude, well-designed plays (ie, the algorithms), and excellent coaching.
- Recognize that the effectiveness of the team is not about you. It is about succeeding as a group. Patients and their families are counting on you to get this right so come prepared!

Code Team Member and Code Team Leader Roles

Whether you are a code team member or a code team leader, you should know both your own role and the roles of the other members of your code team during the resuscitation attempt. This will help you anticipate what steps are coming next and see how your role is an essential part of the resuscitation attempt. Whatever skills you are trained and appropriately authorized to perform, it is essential to the success of the resuscitation that you are prepared, have practiced regularly, have mastered the algorithms, and are committed to success.

Code Team Member Roles

A code team member may be called on to perform all of the following roles (and more):

- **Ventilator**—managing the airway. This team member's duties include suctioning the patient, ventilating the patient with a bag-mask device or ATV, inserting an advanced airway device (ie, LMA, Combitube, King LT, or ET tube), and maintaining manual in-line immobilization of the head and neck.
- **Active compressor**—providing high-quality chest compressions. The responsibility of this team member is to compress for 2 minutes and be the on-deck compressor for 2 minutes.
- **On-deck compressor**—At the 2-minute point, this team member needs to be ready to relieve the compressor without any interruption in compressions. Other functions include assisting with application of a mechanical CPR adjunct device (if available), checking on vital signs, and preparing the patient for transport.
- **Other support personnel**—responsible for analyzing the ECG and delivering shocks, gaining venous (IV or IO) access, providing documentation for the patient care report (PCR), and supporting family members.

Code Team Leader Roles

Every resuscitation team needs a leader to organize the efforts of the group. Clearly the code team leader must know all of the specific skills and be able to perform each skill expertly—occasionally the code team leader will serve as the backup for a team member who may be having difficulty inserting a tube or gaining IV/IO access. The code team leader is often responsible for making sure everything gets done at the right time in the right way.

The roles of the code team leader may include all of the following:

- Obtaining the patient's history and performing the physical exam.
- Interpreting the ECG.
- Keeping track of the time.
- Making a medication decision following the algorithm.
- Clearly delegating tasks to code team members.
- Completing documentation after the resuscitation attempt.
- Talking with medical control.
- Controlling the resuscitation scene.

Code team leaders must also model excellent behavior and leadership skills for their team and all others who may be involved in the resuscitation. The code team leader should help train future team leaders, seek to improve the effectiveness of the entire team through continuous quality improvement, and practice after the resuscitation to help prepare for the next code.

Plan for a Code

The following plan is merely an example and is not the "only way"; obviously, different communities have different resources that arrive at different times in different ways. The point is that you need a plan and you need to practice this plan diligently.

This example focuses on a prehospital EMS agency response to a cardiac arrest in a private home, assuming a five-person team that could arrive on different units (eg, EMT unit, paramedic unit, EMS field supervisor with a Thumper or other mechanical CPR-type device) at different times in the first few minutes. Roles for the adult scenario include Compressor 1, Compressor 2, Ventilator, Code Team Leader, and the EMS Field Supervisor:

- **Compressor 1.** Responsible for performing high-quality chest compressions (at least 100/min, press hard and fast, and full chest recoil), stays in position and compresses for 2 minutes and then rests for 2 minutes (for the duration of the time the patient is pulseless), may assist with application of the Thumper or other adjunct to circulation (provided Compressor 2 is continuing uninterrupted compressions).

- **Compressor 2.** Responsible for performing high-quality chest compressions (at least 100/min, press hard and fast, and full chest recoil), stays in position and compresses for 2 minutes and then rests for 2 minutes (for the duration of the time the patient is pulseless), may assist with application of the Thumper or other adjunct to circulation (provided Compressor 1 is continuing uninterrupted compressions).

- **Ventilator.** Responsible for providing ventilations (bag mask, oropharyngeal airway, oxygen) at a ratio of 30:2, ensuring visible chest rise with each ventilation (1 second in duration). May need to briefly suction the patient as necessary, and then as appropriate will switch over to the ATV. Will assist with the transition from BLS airway to advanced airway (not a high priority). Once an advanced airway is placed, ventilate 8 to 10 times/min to achieve visible chest rise over a 1-second duration for each ventilation.

- **Code team leader.** Responsible for initial ECG analysis and defibrillation with a single shock (200 J). Responsible for overall timing of the code and reassessment after 2 minutes of cycles of CPR with the interruption not to exceed 10 seconds. After the initial shock (or ascertaining "no shock" rhythm), proceeds to establish IV or IO access (no medications down the tube), then begins administration of a vasopressor every 3 to 5 minutes (1 mg epinephrine 1:10,000, with vasopressin as an acceptable substitute for the first or second—but not both—doses of epinephrine), helps to transition the airway from BLS to an advanced airway (ET tube, Combitube, King LT, or LMA), and continues with single shocks every 2 minutes if patient is still in V-tach or V-fib. Makes the decision with input from the code team and medical control that the resuscitation should be terminated if there is no ROSC in the first 15 minutes. If there is ROSC, administers the appropriate antidysrrhythmic (eg, amiodarone, lidocaine), ensures appropriate ventilations, and assists the team in preparing for transport.

- **EMS field supervisor.** Brings in the Thumper or other adjunct to circulation and works with one of the compressors to transition the patient to mechanical CPR compressions with minimal interruption. Assists the medic with IV or IO, advanced airway placement, and preparation of medications, and contacts medical control, per local protocols.

Managing the field code is complex, but not impossible. Have confidence and expect patients to survive if you come on the scene and someone is already performing CPR. Remember, the paradigm has changed since the early years of EMS and this textbook's first edition. Today, with all of the links of the Chain of Survival in place, you should expect patients to survive more than 40% of the time!

YOU are the Medic   SUMMARY

1. What links of the Chain of Survival are present that would make you optimistic about the potential for ROSC?

Early access to 9-1-1 following a witnessed arrest contributed to immediate response of an advanced life support unit. Early CPR was provided at the scene by a layperson who had recently completed CPR training. Early defibrillation was available due to the close proximity of an automated external defibrillator (AED) at the golf course.

2. On the basis of the events occurring prior to your arrival and your own ECG analysis, what are your next steps as team leader?

Based on finding CPR in progress, you are aware that at least five cycles or 2 minutes of compressions have been performed since the AED delivered a shock to the patient. You have found the patient to be in a shockable rhythm so delivering another shock is appropriate. Once additional advanced life support resources are available, you can delegate preparation of medications for administration. You should also be tracking times throughout the incident, interventions performed, and assessment findings.

3. What other alternative medications are indicated for ventricular fibrillation/ventricular tachycardia and at what dosages?

Amiodarone 300 mg IV bolus in 20 to 30 mL of normal saline may be used instead of lidocaine as an antidysrhythmic medication. Epinephrine 1 mg of 1:10,000 concentration may be used instead of vasopressin as the vasopressor during an arrest. Vasopressin may only be administered once.

YOU *are the Medic*   **SUMMARY,** *continued*

4. **If the rhythm had been analyzed as torsades de pointes, what medication might be beneficial and at what dosage?**

For a patient with torsades de pointes, magnesium 1-2 g IV over 1 to 2 minutes might be helpful. It is indicated in refractory ventricular fibrillation and pulseless ventricular tachycardia, especially torsades de pointes. Hypomagnesemia may cause these types of cardiac dysrhythmias.

5. **Why is intubation not an early intervention consideration in the cardiac arrest patient?**

Studies that assess the value of intubation are inconclusive. Quality compressions with minimal disruption should be the primary focus during resuscitation. Oxygen can be administered effectively using a bag-mask device. Skill degradation affects the ability of the paramedic to intubate correctly and rapidly. Multiple or extended attempts to intubate can disrupt effective compressions, thereby decreasing the potential for successful ROSC. Alternative advanced airway options should be considered if successful, rapid intubation is questionable.

6. **What is the importance of ETCO$_2$ monitoring in the cardiac arrest patient?**

Carbon dioxide levels rise in cardiac arrest due to anaerobic metabolism. As effective CPR is delivered, these levels can begin to normalize and assist you in monitoring the effectiveness of CPR. In the prehospital environment, potential for dislodgement of an ET tube is high with movement and transferring of the patient. Monitoring ETCO$_2$ levels and waveform capnography can provide for early detection of proper and improper tube placement, as well as potential obstructions in the ET tube such as secretions or disconnection from automated transport ventilator devices.

7. **If resuscitative efforts are eventually successful, what is the significance of transporting the cardiac arrest patient to a facility capable of advanced cardiac care?**

Considering the links in the Chain of Survival, your goal is to continue to seek an optimal outcome for the patient. Based on a patient's recent medical history, there may be a cardiac event that resulted in the arrest. Assuming you are successful in achieving resuscitation with ROSC, a facility capable of interventional cardiac procedures may offer more definitive treatment if this is the case.

8. **What is the significance of completing advanced life support care prior to transport?**

Survival of cardiac arrest is linked to optimizing on-scene care. Preparation for transport and moving of patients to the ambulance can significantly compromise the quality of the CPR being delivered. By providing full ALS care at the scene, you are ensuring high-quality compressions can be delivered with minimal disruption during the heart's most receptive period to resuscitation. You are also better able to secure your airway, obtain IV access, and prepare and deliver front-line medications as indicated. Most of these interventions are more difficult to perform in the confines of the ambulance and there is often less room for additional personnel to assist in carrying out the resuscitative efforts safely.

9. **What is the significance of good documentation for improvement of survival in prehospital cardiac arrests?**

Data collection for the purposes of research and providing quality improvement in cardiac arrest patients includes information you document on your patient care report. The receiving hospital may participate in the AHA's Get With The Guidelines program (previously called the National Registry of Cardiopulmonary Resuscitation [NRCPR] data system). There are recommended guidelines for reporting of data for the prehospital cardiac arrest. By participating, your community can compare its data with other progressive communities. Quality improvement and medical review allow for the ability to optimize your system's performance in managing these patients. By considering the SMART management acronym, you are providing data that are specific and measurable to allow your system and community to develop programs that have attainable and achievable goals. These goals must also be realistic and relevant based on the limitations and potential for your community and emergency response system. Timely data collection and review increase the likelihood of establishing programs that have the potential to make a difference in the lives of your patients.

YOU *are the Medic*   **SUMMARY,** *continued*

EMS Patient Care Report (PCR)

Date: 06-28-10	Incident No.: 201032591	Nature of Call: Cardiac arrest	Location: 1 Golf Club Drive		
Dispatched: 1415	En Route: 1416	At Scene: 1420	Transport: 1448	At Hospital: 1458	In Service: 1525

Patient Information

Age: 54 Sex: M Weight (in kg [lb]): 78.2 kg (172 lb)	Allergies: No known drug allergies Medications: OTC acid-reducers and pain relievers Past Medical History: Indigestion per wife Chief Complaint: Cardiac arrest

Vital Signs

Time: 1426	BP: Not obtainable	Pulse: 0	Respirations: 0	Spo$_2$: Not obtainable
Time: 1432	BP: Not obtainable	Pulse: 0	Respirations:	Spo$_2$: Not obtainable
Time: 1436	BP:	Pulse:	Respirations:	Spo$_2$: Not obtainable
Time: 1441	BP: 86/60	Pulse: 80	Respirations: 10 via bag-mask	Spo$_2$: Not obtainable
Time: 1447	BP: 88/54	Pulse: 68	Respirations: 10 via bag-mask	Spo$_2$: 98%
Time: 1453	BP: 100/68	Pulse: 72	Respirations: 10, ventilator assisted	Spo$_2$: 99%

EMS Treatment
(circle all that apply)

Oxygen @ __15__ L/min via (circle one): NC NRM (Bag-mask device)	(Assisted Ventilation)	(Airway Adjunct)	(CPR)
(Defibrillation)	Bleeding Control	Bandaging	Splinting	(Other:) Vasopressin, epinephrine, and lidocaine

Narrative

EMS requested to above location for a man not breathing and without a pulse. On arrival, pt found lying supine on the ground with CPR in progress. Several bystanders and emergency responders on scene with AED attached to the pt. Pt confirmed to be in V-fib. CPR continued with bag-mask assisted ventilations using high concentration oxygen at 10/min. Defibrillated pt with 200 J at 1423. IV established 16 gauge in left AC. Vasopressin 40 U administered IV at 1427. Confirmed rhythm to be V-tach and defibrillated pt with 200 J at 1427. Lidocaine 1.5 mg/kg (117 mg) administered IV at 1429. Confirmed rhythm to be V-tach and defibrillated with 200 J at 1431. Pt intubated with size 7.5 ET tube orally in first attempt at 1433. Placement confirmed via cord visualization, auscultation, and ETCO$_2$ with waveforms. Tube secured at 27 cm mark with tube holder device. Epinephrine 1 mg IV administered at 1433. Confirmed rhythm to be V-tach and defibrillated with 200 J at 1434. Lidocaine 1.5 mg/kg (117 mg) administered IV at 1439. Pt had ROSC at 1440. Ventilations continued via ATV at 1441. EMS advised pt's wife of receiving facility. Pt will be transported to for evaluation and treatment. Pt reassessed en route with changes. Report called to emergency department prior to arrival which included pt's current condition and ETA. ECG transmission of 12-lead showing STEMI. Medical control advises to transport pt directly to cardiac procedure lab. On arrival, pt was transferred to the cardiac procedure table and report given to RN and cardiologist. Physician signature obtained for medications delivered under ACLS protocol. **End of report**

Prep Kit

- Use the links in the Chain of Survival as a guide to manage cardiac arrest: recognition of a cardiac emergency, early access to 9-1-1, early high-quality CPR by the public or responders, early defibrillation, early advanced life support care, and transport to a hospital that can provide state-of-the-art postresuscitative care.
- Both the 2005 and 2010 CPR guidelines emphasize the importance of providing high-quality CPR beginning with compressions (push hard and fast, and allow full chest recoil).
- Advanced airways are only considered during the field code if a basic airway is not adequate or the airway needs to be better protected due to a patient who is vomiting. The focus of care should be CPR with high-quality compressions.
- The basic principles of BLS are the same for infants, children, and adults. According to the American Heart Association (AHA), anyone between the ages of 1 month and 1 year is considered an infant. A child is between age 1 year and puberty. Adulthood is from onset of puberty and older.
- You must first assess the patient's circulation. If the patient has no pulse, you must provide artificial circulation by beginning with chest compressions at the rate and depth appropriate for the patient's age.
- CPR can be performed with one or two rescuers. Two-rescuer CPR or a team approach is always the first choice. When a rescuer is performing adult CPR alone or with another rescuer, the ratio of compressions to ventilations is 30:2.
- Defibrillation needs to be carried out as soon as possible in the presence of two rhythms—ventricular fibrillation and pulseless ventricular tachycardia—because the likelihood of its success declines rapidly with time.
- When you use a manual defibrillator, you interpret the cardiac rhythm and determine if defibrillation is needed. An automated external defibrillator interprets the cardiac rhythm for you and determines if defibrillation is indicated.
- Defibrillation is indicated for patients in nontraumatic cardiac arrest who are older than 1 month. If you are using an automated external defibrillator on a child between age 1 year and the onset of puberty, if available, you should use pediatric-sized pads and a dose-attenuating system (energy reducer).
- The ACLS algorithm separates the treatment approach into two basic pathways: shockable rhythms (ventricular fibrillation or ventricular tachycardia) or nonshockable rhythms (asystole or pulseless electrical activity).

- For all arrests, regardless of the rhythm, you should consider the reversible causes and treat them as appropriate.
- For asystole or pulseless electrical activity, do not deliver shocks.
- Certain devices may be used as adjuncts to circulation to help improve the quality of compressions when you are providing CPR. These devices include the impedance threshold device, the mechanical piston device, and the load-distributing band.
- For postresuscitative care, if an effective cardiac rhythm is restored in the field, transport immediately. However, if the patient is comatose after ROSC, consider hypothermia treatment depending on protocol.
- Terminating resuscitative efforts in an adult with a prehospital cardiac arrest should follow the ALS termination of resuscitation rule.
- Teamwork divides tasks while multiplying the chances for a successful resuscitation.
- Whether you are a code team member or a code team leader, you should know both your own role and the roles of the other members of your code team during the resuscitation attempt.

asynchronous In CPR, when two rescuers perform ventilations and compressions individually and not timed or waiting for the other rescuer to pause.

automated external defibrillator (AED) A "smart" defibrillator that can analyze the patient's ECG rhythm and determine whether a defibrillating shock is needed.

code team leader The code team member who has the responsibility for managing the rescuers or team members during a cardiac arrest, as well as choreographing the effort of the group.

code team member A member of the resuscitation team trying to revive the patient.

defibrillation The use of an unsynchronized direct current electric shock to terminate ventricular fibrillation or ventricular tachycardia.

manual defibrillation A mode available on automated external defibrillators, allowing the paramedic to interpret the cardiac rhythm and determine whether defibrillation is indicated (rather than the monitor making the determination).

return of spontaneous circulation (ROSC) The return of spontaneous heart beat and blood pressure during the resuscitation of a patient in cardiac arrest.

SMART An acronym used to describe a prehospital program's objectives: Specific, Measurable, Attainable and Achievable, Realistic and Relevant, and Timely.

Assessment in Action

At 3:10 AM you are dispatched to a single-family residence. Dispatch information indicates you are responding to an 82-year-old woman who is not breathing and has no pulse. Dispatch has also requested the assistance of the local fire engine as well as the field supervisor. Emergency responders are estimated to be on scene within 6 minutes and are capable of BLS treatment while your ALS unit's response time will be approximately 8 minutes. You begin to consider the potential outcome for this patient. Dispatch advises you that they are providing hands-only CPR instructions by phone to bystanders. On arrival you note that the engine company is on scene as the field supervisor pulls in behind you. You are met at the door by a woman who states she is the patient's daughter. She advises you that when she arrived home at approximately 3:00 AM, she found her mother on the couch not breathing. She quickly called 9-1-1 but would not provide CPR as dispatch requested because she said "I was afraid I might hurt my mother." You assess the scene and find the two responders performing high-quality CPR on an older woman who has been placed on the floor in the living room. There is an AED attached. As a code team leader who has practiced this type of scenario, you begin delegating tasks to ensure all efforts are coordinated and compression disruption is minimized. Your partner, also a paramedic, is instructed to take over the role of ventilator while your field supervisor moves to connect your cardiac monitor. You ask that the responders continue their compressions while you obtain a patient history and begin tracking times. The patient's daughter tells you that her mother had hip surgery 1 week ago and takes aspirin 81 mg daily, hydrocodone/acetaminophen (Lorcet) 10 mg every 4 hours for pain, and levothyroxine (Synthroid) 0.5 mg every day. Your supervisor notes that the patient's rhythm is asystole and that the responders have reported the AED advised "No Shock Indicated" when the rhythm was analyzed.

1. Which of the following is not a component of high-quality CPR?
   - A. Intubate early
   - B. Allow complete chest recoil after each compression
   - C. Compression depth of at least 2 inches (5 cm)
   - D. Compression rate of at least 100 per minute

2. It is important to rotate the compressor every 2 minutes or after five cycles of compressions.
   - A. True
   - B. False

3. Which factor would influence the rescuer to shock first before initiating compressions?
   - A. Bystander tells you the patient just "stopped breathing" as you arrived.
   - B. Dispatch advised CPR was in progress while you were responding.
   - C. You witness the patient arrest after connecting the cardiac monitor/defibrillator.
   - D. The patient has an automatic implantable cardioverter defibrillator.

4. Which of the following is a contraindication for defibrillation in the cardiac arrest patient?
   - A. Patient is submerged in water or wet
   - B. Patient has a pacemaker or automatic implantable cardioverter defibrillator
   - C. Patient is an infant or child
   - D. None of the above

5. The patient's rhythm should be analyzed and a pulse check performed immediately following defibrillation.
   - A. True
   - B. False

6. Which of the following interventions is not appropriate for the patient in asystole or pulseless electrical activity?
   - A. Vasopressor administration
   - B. High-quality CPR
   - C. Defibrillation
   - D. Consideration of potential causes

7. On the basis of this patient's recent medical history and considering the "Hs and Ts", what may have been a potential cause of her cardiac arrest?
   - A. Hyperkalemia
   - B. Tension pneumothorax
   - C. Pulmonary embolism
   - D. Hypothermia

Additional Questions

8. During resuscitation, how does scene choreography and teamwork improve chances of a successful resuscitation?

9. Current guidelines offer both a "BLS Termination Rule" and an "ALS Termination Rule." Considering these rules and your findings for this patient, what next steps and decisions should be considered?

Management and Resuscitation of the Critical Patient

National EMS Education Standard Competencies

Shock and Resuscitation

- Integrates a comprehensive knowledge of the causes and pathophysiology into the management of shock, respiratory failure or arrest with an emphasis on early intervention to prevent arrest.

Knowledge Objectives

1. List examples of peri-arrest conditions that critical patients can present with in the field. (p 1882)
2. Describe the process of determining a differential diagnosis in the field assessment of a critical patient. (pp 1882-1883)
3. Discuss the rapid decision making involved in the assessment and management of a critical patient. (p 1883)
4. List examples of bias that can affect your critical decision making. (pp 1883-1884)
5. Describe the body's physiologic response to changes in perfusion. (pp 1886-1889)
6. Discuss the pathophysiology of shock and peri-arrest situations. (pp 1889-1895)
7. Describe the effects of decreased perfusion at the capillary level. (pp 1892-1893)
8. Define shock based on aerobic and anaerobic metabolism. (pp 1890-1892)
9. Relate pulse pressure changes to perfusion status. (pp 1886-1889, 1896)
10. Relate orthostatic vital sign changes to perfusion status. (p 1896)
11. Predict shock based on mechanism of injury. (p 1895)
12. Discuss the progression of shock. (pp 1895-1897)
13. Discuss the pathophysiologic changes associated with compensated shock. (p 1896)
14. Discuss the assessment findings associated with compensated shock. (pp 1897-1899)
15. Identify the need for intervention and transport of the patient with compensated shock. (p 1898)
16. Discuss the treatment plan and management of compensated shock. (pp 1900-1903)
17. Discuss the pathophysiologic changes associated with decompensated shock. (p 1896)
18. Discuss the assessment findings associated with decompensated shock. (pp 1897-1899)
19. Identify the need for intervention and transport of the patient with decompensated shock. (p 1898)
20. Discuss the treatment plan and management of the patient with decompensated shock. (pp 1900-1903)
21. Differentiate between compensated and decompensated shock. (pp 1895-1897)
22. Discuss the assessment findings associated with shock and the peri-arrest situations. (pp 1897-1899)
23. Identify the need for intervention and transport of the patient with shock or other peri-arrest situations. (pp 1903-1911)
24. Discuss the treatment plan and management of shock and other peri-arrest situations. (pp 1903-1911)
25. Describe the pathophysiology, assessment, and management of specific types of shock, including cardiogenic, obstructive, distributive, and hypovolemic shock. (pp 1903-1911)

Skills Objectives

1. Defend the importance of teamwork, experience, and practice in preparation to manage the critical patient. (p 1881)
2. Demonstrate rapid decision making based on differential field diagnosis of the critical patient with a peri-arrest condition. (pp 1884-1885)
3. Demonstrate the management of shock. (pp 1901-1902, Skill Drill 1)

Introduction

Expertise in critical thinking and decision making are essential tools to use when you are confronted with a critical patient. This process involves conducting a rapid assessment, providing life-saving treatment, and developing a <u>differential field diagnosis</u>, a short list of the potential causes of the patient's presenting condition. If you use this process consistently, it will become routine when you need it most. It takes plenty of practice to make the "right" decisions for each unique situation; eventually, however, making decisions quickly and working as part of a team will become an integral part of who you are.

When the patient's condition is critical, it is essential that you are well trained to make the right decisions, take the right amount of time to do the right assessment, and provide the right care to the patient. In addition, on the basis of the patient's condition, he or she will need to be transported to the right hospital for the most appropriate definitive care. This approach also involves having the right equipment, using the right resources, crew management, leadership skills, prioritization, and compliance with protocols, as well as working with other public safety personnel and family members. A critical patient's survival should be a function of all of these rights coming into alignment.

This chapter discusses the approach that you should take when you are confronted with a critical patient. Managing critical patients often involves confronting pre-morbid or peri-arrest conditions. This chapter also takes a close-up look at perfusion, the function that fails in patients who are in shock. Next it looks at the physiologic causes of shock and describes each of its major forms. Finally, it discusses the assessment and emergency treatment of shock in general and of each particular type of shock.

Developing Critical Thinking and Decision-Making Abilities

EMS educators tell their students that excellent decision-making abilities come with experience. This is true, provided that the student acquires the right "entry level" knowledge and skills, followed by the appropriate guided experience. According to the paramedic curriculum design, the training is developed to prepare a competent "entry level" paramedic. The internship experience is a good first step to help you pull together the didactic, lab skills, and clinical experiences in order to function as a paramedic in the field. An excellent internship experience guided by an experienced mentor (preceptor) will bring you to the competent "entry level" milestone. State and national

Words of Wisdom

Leadership is something you need to see in order to emulate; therefore, it is important to spend time with exceptional leaders. Having no "vision" of quality leadership, critical thinking, and decision making is like bowling with a blindfold on. You can hear the pins falling but you don't know how many you knocked down!

YOU are the Medic   PART 1

At 9:15 AM, you are the paramedic on an advanced life support unit dispatched to an apartment at a senior residence complex. The dispatcher advises you that a home health aide found an unresponsive 77-year-old man in bed this morning. You are told he is breathing and has a pulse. When you arrive at the apartment complex, you are escorted by the security officer to the elevator to get to the fifth floor. The security officer tells you he has not seen Mr. Oliver for his last two shifts. Because you are responding to an upstairs unit and due to the nature of the call, you are bringing your ECG monitor/defibrillator, rapid response (ABCs) bag, and IV/medication kit with you.

You are met at the apartment by the home health aide. She tells you she routinely visits Mr. Oliver twice a week to help with cleaning and cooking. This morning when she arrived, security personnel were needed to gain access to his apartment because he did not open the door when she knocked. She explains that she found Mr. Oliver in bed and unresponsive. She says he was sick the last time she saw him 3 days ago and encouraged him to see his physician. She follows you to his bedroom. As you move through the apartment you conduct a scene size-up. The apartment appears relatively neat and clean. No dirty dishes are seen and no evidence of a recent meal is visible. All furniture is upright and no evidence of a disturbance is noted. When you reach the bedside, your general impression is of a thin, older male who appears to be asleep. He has audible respirations that sound congested, and his skin appears pale and mottled. Your partner prepares oxygen while you assess his level of consciousness. He is unresponsive except to painful stimuli. You request additional assistance by having the field supervisor dispatched to your location.

1. **What should your next course of action be for this patient?**

2. **Discuss the role of intuition in forming a field diagnosis as well as the potential for bias.**

certification/registration/licensure follows, and from there, the paramedic has a license to practice and learn from continued experiences.

Critical Patients

When caring for <u>critical patients</u> that require your critical thinking skills, you will be confronting premorbid conditions, major trauma, or patients who are in the peri-arrest period. The <u>peri-arrest period</u> is the period either just before or just after cardiac arrest, when the patient is critical and care must be taken to prevent progression or regression into cardiac arrest. Examples of peri-arrest conditions include unstable dysrhythmias (bradycardia, tachycardia, ventricular tachycardia, and complete heart block), shock, syncope, myocardial ischemia, or heart failure. <u>Premorbid conditions</u> are conditions that precede the onset of a disease. In the context of emergency medicine, the "disease" is life-threatening trauma or medical conditions that need to be rapidly identified and managed. Typically, premorbid conditions are sorted into those occurring in presumed to be healthy adults and more frequently occuring in unhealthy adults as shown in Table 1.

Many adult patients have other preexisting conditions that can make them fit into the critical patient category. This is especially true if a patient experiences trauma such as a full-thickness burn over 15% to 20% of the total body surface area or when the head, chest, or abdomen are involved with significant hemorrhage leading to shock. Other examples of conditions that would fit into the critical patient category include acute coronary syndrome (ACS), congestive heart failure (CHF), renal failure, uncontrolled hypertension, uncontrolled diabetes, obesity, electrolyte imbalance, electrocution, drowning or submersion, hypothermia, drug toxicity, stroke, near-fatal asthma, anaphylaxis, and pulmonary embolus Figure 1. The epidemiology and

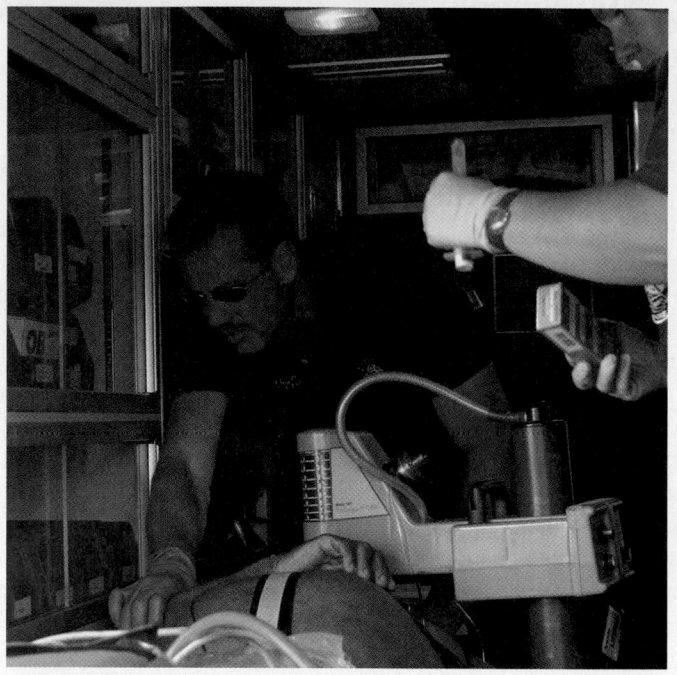

Figure 1 A critical patient being managed in the field.

pathophysiology of these conditions are discussed in detail in other chapters of this text.

The EMS Approach to Diagnosis

Common complaints of critical patients may include altered mental status, difficulty breathing, severe pain, and chest pain. The EMS approach to determining a field diagnosis involves following the standard approach emphasized in this text and as illustrated in Figure 2. To arrive at a field diagnosis, after considering the most serious life threats and managing them, your approach involves considering or ruling out various conditions. This leaves you with the differential diagnosis.

For example, you have a patient who has a chief complaint of altered mental status and you need to consider the differential diagnosis. To start this process you will need to consider each of the potential causes. There are many ways to do this; you may choose to consider using the "M-T SHIP" acronym:

M: Medication overdose/noncompliance (ie, barbiturates, narcotics, alcohol), metabolic causes (ie, B_{12} or thiamine deficiency)

T: Tumor, trauma, toxins (ie, lead, mercury, carbon monoxide, toxidromes)

S: Seizures (ie, status epilepticus, postictal state), stroke

H: Hypoxia (ie, pulmonary, cardiac, anemia, or carbon dioxide retention), hyperthermia/hypothermia, hyperglycemia/hypoglycemia, hypertensive crisis, hypovolemia, hyperkalemia/hypokalemia (and other electrolyte imbalances)

I: Infection and uremia (ie, renal or hepatic dysfunction)

P: Psychiatric or behavioral disorders

By determining whether trauma was involved, whether or not the patient has a diabetic history, or whether there is fever or

Table 1 Adult Premorbid Conditions Directly Affecting EMS

Condition	Healthy Adult	Unhealthy Adult
Congestive heart failure	Unlikely	X
Coronary Artery Disease	Unlikely	X
Drug toxicity	X	X
Electrolyte imbalance	X	X
Obesity	Unlikely	X
Pulmonary embolus	X	X
Renal failure	Unlikely	X
Stroke	Unlikely	X
Uncontrolled hypertension	Unlikely	X
Uncontrolled diabetes	Unlikely	X

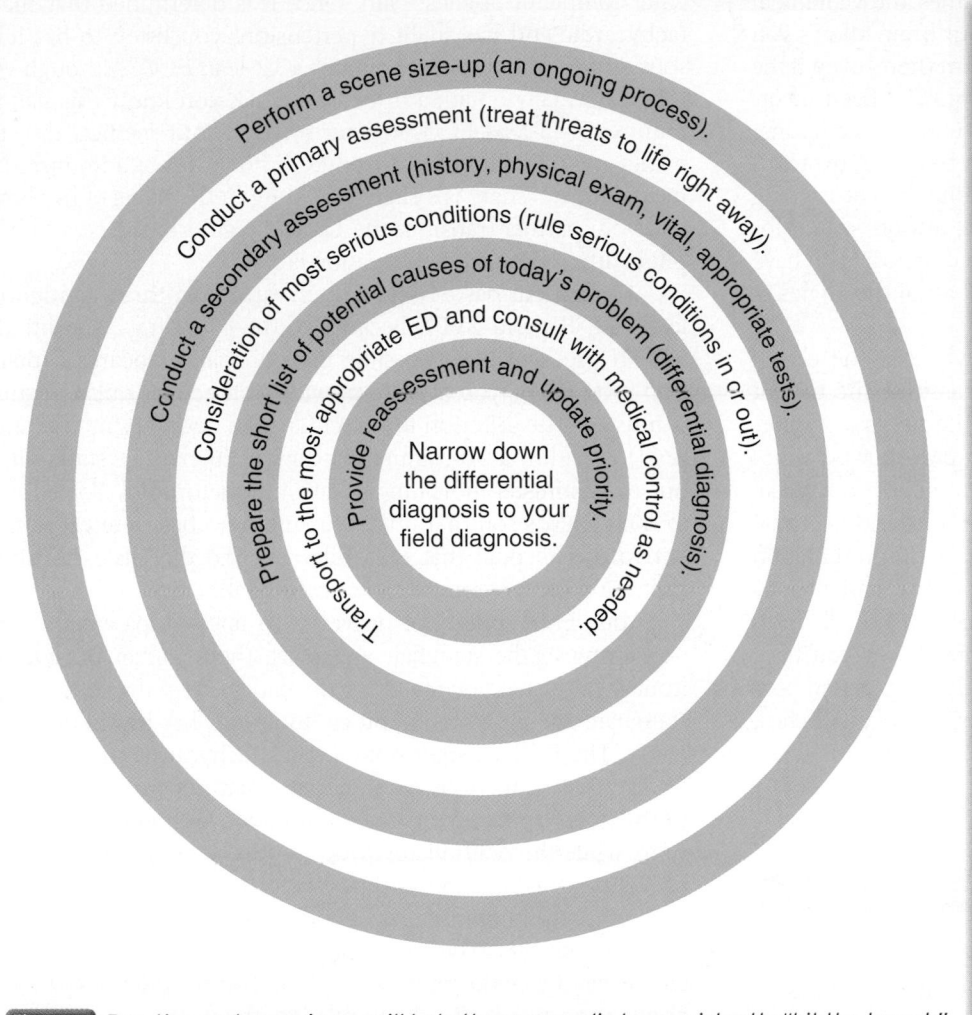

Perform a scene size-up (an ongoing process).

Conduct a primary assessment (treat threats to life right away).

Conduct a secondary assessment (history, physical exam, vital, appropriate tests).

Consideration of most serious conditions (rule serious conditions in or out).

Prepare the short list of potential causes of today's problem (differential diagnosis).

Transport to the most appropriate ED and consult with medical control as needed.

Provide reassessment and update priority.

Narrow down the differential diagnosis to your field diagnosis.

Figure 2 Practice and experience will help the paramedic to consistently "hit the target."

infection, this list can be narrowed down considerably. Further questioning will also narrow down the differential diagnosis.

Suppose your patient has a chief complaint of chest pain and you need to consider the differential diagnosis. The patient could have ischemic chest pain indicating a possible cardiac condition such as acute myocardial infarction (AMI), angina, aortic dissection, coronary spasm, pericarditis, myocarditis, or hypertropic cardiomyopathy. Gastrointestinal (GI) system causes of the chest pain may be heartburn, esophageal spasm, hiatal hernia, and gallbladder or pancreas problems. Or, the patient could be experiencing musculoskeletal problems such as costochondritis, sore muscles, injured ribs, or a pinched nerve. There are also a number of respiratory causes of chest pain such as pulmonary embolism, pleurisy, pneumothorax, and asthma. Finally, the chest pain may be due to a panic attack, shingles, or cancer in the chest.

Experience will guide you to the most serious problems that could lead to the cause of the chest pain, and help you to narrow down the list and arrive at the differential diagnosis.

The Role of Intuition in Critical Decision Making

Some paramedics describe a sense they get when the situation is much worse than it initially appears from reviewing the patient's vital signs. Others describe having a gut feeling when they first look at a patient who gives a poor general impression, such as a patient who is so diaphoretic that an ECG electrode will not stick to his or her skin.

The intuition that comes with experience is hard to teach. Intuition can be described as pattern recognition and pattern matching, based on your own past experiences. Intuition can keep you out of trouble by forewarning you or get you in trouble and lead you to make treatment decisions based on the wrong assumptions. In medicine, intuition may be used to "up-triage" the patient rather than "down-triage" the patient. For example, if your instinct tells you the patient is more serious than he or she seems, treat the patient as such; however, if your instinct tells you otherwise, you will need to investigate the complaint thoroughly before downgrading the response.

How can your intuition lead you astray? Researchers explain that just because you are good at pattern recognition in one field, or level of training, does not mean you are automatically good at pattern recognition in another field, or level of training, that you have less experience in. Be cautious not to misuse analogies and make a decision based on intuition that draws on incorrect experiences. It has been shown that in highly complex, ambiguous situations, complexities can obscure pattern-recognition ability.

When decisions are being made based on intuition, it is often difficult for the team leader to communicate to the other team members his or her thought process. Therefore, it may be difficult for the team members to stay onboard with the line of thinking (or treatment plan in this case). The organizational scholar Karl Weick has proposed a simple five-step process for communicating intuitive decisions and obtaining feedback from team members to ensure a clear understanding of all involved:

1. Here is what I think we are dealing with.
2. Here is what I think we should do.
3. Here is why.
4. Here is what we should keep our eyes on.
5. Now talk to me. Are there any other concerns?

Bias to Decision Making

There are a number of biases that can lead to faulty decision making. One of the most prevalent biases that you will face is confirmation bias. A **confirmation bias** is a tendency to gather and rely on information that confirms your existing views and avoids or downplays information that does not confirm your preexisting hypothesis or field differential. Another bias is anchoring bias. In this case, you may sometimes allow an initial reference point to distort your estimates. Your brain allows you to begin at that reference point and adjust from there, even if the initial reference point was arbitrary and may have been incorrect. This is often seen in financial negotiations and price setting.

Be careful about making a misjudgment based on overconfidence. This occurs when you assume you know what is going on with the patient. To avoid this situation, always search for information that would refute the differential diagnosis you have arrived at and make sure you have looked at all of the angles of the problem. Never assume anything.

Last, when you are treating a patient who has the classic presentation of a specific condition, do not assume the patient has that condition without obtaining all of the necessary information and data. The same holds true for a patient who is not presenting with the classic signs and symptoms; do not make the mistake of not considering the spectrum of the differential diagnosis. One of the best examples is the classic presentation of a male patient with symptoms of an AMI. The patient may have crushing substernal chest pain radiating down the left arm accompanied by nausea and shortness of breath. As you have learned in your training, many women, elderly people, and people with diabetes experiencing an AMI do not complain of chest pain. Be careful not to prematurely jump to conclusions when you are assessing a critical patient.

■ A Snapshot of Critical Decision Making

It is 5:00 AM and you have been dispatched to the home of a 62-year-old woman whose son called 9-1-1. The son states he woke up and found his mother sitting in the living room complaining of pressure in the center of her chest. Because of the complaint of chest pain and the patient's age, this is a priority dispatch and your medic unit, a backup unit, and the supervisor are quickly en route. The traffic is light and your equipment is ready. As you pull up in front of the home, you are met at the doorway by the son, who quickly leads you to his mother.

The scene appears to be safe, but you realize you will need to pay attention to the environment you are entering and all potential hazards. The police, who respond on most of your calls, are just pulling up outside the residence. You introduce yourselves to the patient and ask about the chief complaint. The woman, Judith, explains that she has been to her private physician twice, who determined that her chest pain was caused by stress and acid reflux. She has been taking antacids, but they have not alleviated the crushing sensation beneath her breastbone, accompanied by nausea and tingling in her right arm. The pain is a 7 out of 10 and it began around 4:30 AM today. You explain to Judith that you have a few more questions to ask her while your partner places her on oxygen using a nonrebreathing mask and obtains her vital signs. You know that oxygen is helpful and she is breathing well on her own, but you need to know if her blood pressure is where it should be and if her pulse rate is regular. Once you have determined that she has no cardiac history and no allergies, and she is not taking an anticoagulant, you give her four baby aspirin to chew, not swallow, per your protocols. You quickly go through the OPQRST mnemonic which helps to elaborate on the

chief complaint of chest pain. Once it is determined that she is tachycardic and has slight hypertension, you listen to her lung sounds while your partner obtains a 12-lead ECG. Although you might normally obtain a three-lead ECG, you know this patient requires a 12-lead ECG. In your system, your medical director wants you to obtain the 12-lead ECG just prior to administering nitroglycerin. There is a slight crackling in the bases of her lungs and your partner transmits the 12-lead results to the nearest hospital with a coronary catherization lab.

The patient has ST-segment elevations in three contiguous leads (II, III, and AVF). Because of these findings, she fits the STEMI protocol for a possible inferior wall myocardial infarction (MI). Thus, you need to provide immediate transport; time is muscle! The criterion for percutaneous coronary intervention (PCI) is within a 90-minute window. Your partner starts an IV line to administer morphine sulfate and metoprolol. You explain to the patient's son that it is in his mother's best interest to take her to the hospital that is 2 miles beyond the closest hospital because it has a coronary catherization lab.

Your EMS supervisor arrives with another paramedic, and they bring in the stairchair and place the stretcher outside the front door. Just as you are lifting the patient from the couch to the stairchair, she passes out. You try to arouse her by shouting her name. The ECG changes from a sinus tachycardia to ventricular fibrillation. Instinctively, you and your partner move the patient to the floor. In the absence of a pulse, you begin chest compressions while the defibrillator pads are placed on the patient. The EMT from the backup unit kneels at the patient's head, removes the nonrebreathing mask, sizes and inserts an oropharyngeal airway, and prepares to begin bag-mask ventilations with supplemental oxygen. Once the pads are in place, compressions are stopped briefly to ensure ventricular fibrillation, the defibrillator is charged up to 200 joules, the patient is cleared, and the first shock is delivered. Immediately thereafter, CPR compressions resume.

At this point, all EMS personnel have a specific task because there will be five cycles of CPR (30:2) taking 2 minutes. You need to make sure each task occurs at the right time. This includes the following steps:

1. Get the mechanical CPR device (Thumper, Auto-Pulse, Lucas-2) ready to deploy with no interruption in manual chest compressions for more than 10 seconds.
2. Ensure the BLS ventilations are effective, producing visible chest rise (and not too often) and switching over to the automatic transport ventilator with the impedance threshold device.
3. Start an IV line. If this is not going to be easy, switch to plan B, and prepare for intraosseous (IO) infusion with the EZ-IO bone drill. IV access is needed because you are going to administer 1 mg of epinephrine 1:10,000 every 3 minutes until her pulse returns.
4. Ensure there will be a fresh person to supply compressions for the second 2 minutes in case there is a delay in applying the mechanical CPR device. The quality of the compressions is crucial to the success of this resuscitation.
5. Draw up 300 mg of amiodarone because an antidysrhythmic will need to be administered soon.
6. Reanalyze and reshock the patient again at the 2-minute point.

After the third shock, the patient appeared to have a rhythm but now remains pulseless. CPR continues and an antidysrhythmic is administered IO in her right tibia. A medic considers placing an ET tube and readies the equipment while ventilations continue. Necessary actions are taking place so you take a moment to consider the causes of cardiac arrest. You know that you need to consider the reversible causes of cardiac arrest because they are your differential field diagnoses in the case of a patient who is in cardiac arrest Table 2 .

Patient history reveals that Judith did not sustain any trauma or report symptoms of GI bleeding (ie, diarrhea; dark, tarry, smelly stool). Her systolic blood pressure was initially slightly high so it is not likely that she is hemorrhaging. She is not a diabetic and was initially alert, so low levels of blood glucose are unlikely. She did not have respiratory distress and was not cold to the touch, so pulmonary embolus and hypothermia are not likely. She did have ST elevation MI (STEMI), and with the vague presentation that elderly women often have, it is likely she is experiencing a massive AMI or coronary thrombosis.

Just after the fourth shock, the patient wakes up. She is anxious and scared. You ask the EMT managing the airway to switch back to the nonrebreathing mask. You tell Judith that she is sick and her condition warrants going to the hospital right away. You assure her that all of her needs are being taken care of and that her son is nearby and will be coming along. In the meantime, crew members are assigned to package and carry the patient on the long backboard out to your stretcher. One medic sets up an amiodarone drip and prepares to administer a mild sedative to calm the patient without affecting her respirations.

Once you are en route, you contact the emergency department (ED) to update the staff and another 12-lead ECG is transmitted. Because the patient is alert on return of spontaneous circulation, she does not fit your system's field hypothermia protocol. You proceed to reassess the vital signs, document the incident, and discuss the situation with the patient. On arrival, because you have already transmitted the 12-lead ECG to the ED, the patient is admitted directly to the catheterization lab. Two arteries, each 90% blocked, are cleared and stents are inserted by the interventional cardiologist.

■ Shock: The Critical Patient Evolving In Front of You

Shock is a state of collapse and failure of the cardiovascular system in which blood circulation slows and eventually ceases, leading to insufficient perfusion of organs and tissues. Shock is a normal compensatory mechanism used by the body to maintain systolic blood pressure and brain perfusion during times of distress. This response can accompany a broad spectrum of events, ranging from heart attacks, to falls, to allergic reactions, to motor vehicle crashes. If not treated promptly, shock will injure the body's vital organs and ultimately lead to death.

Table 2 The "H and T" Questions of Cardiac Arrest

Reversible Causes of Cardiac Arrest	Ask your team...
Hypovolemia	Does this patient have any evidence of internal or external bleeding or fluid loss?
Hypoxia	How well is the patient oxygenating? Could there have been a respiratory event that led to this cardiac arrest?
Hydrogen ion (acidosis)	Is there any reason for metabolic or respiratory acidosis in this patient?
Hypokalemia/hyperkalemia	Does this patient undergo renal dialysis? Might the electrolytes be altered (ie, is the patient on a liquid diet)?
Hypothermia	Does the patient feel cold to touch? If so, obtain the core body temperature.
Hypoglycemic/hyperglycemic	Is the patient a diabetic? What is the blood glucose level?
Tension pneumothorax	Does the patient have bilateral lung sounds? Is the patient becoming difficult to ventilate? Consider the need for chest decompression.
Tamponade (cardiac)	Is there penetrating trauma to the patient's heart? Consider the need for pericardiocentesis (in the ED).
Toxins	Consider substance abuse (ie, narcotics or opiates). Consider naloxone (Narcan).
Thrombosis (pulmonary)	Does the patient have a history of blood clots? Is the patient a smoker and/or take birth control? Has the patient had a recent long bone immobilization?
Thrombosis (coronary)	Does the patient have a large AMI developing? Is this patient a candidate for PCI?
Trauma	Is there a mechanism of injury for life-threatening trauma?

Anatomy and Physiology of Perfusion

<u>Perfusion</u> is the circulation of blood within an organ or tissue in adequate amounts to meet the cells' current needs for oxygen, nutrients, and waste removal. Perfusion requires having a working cardiovascular system. It also requires adequate gas exchange in the lungs, adequate nutrients in the form of glucose in the blood, and adequate waste removal, primarily through the lungs. Because tissue perfusion is primarily a function of the cardiovascular system, an examination of that system is important in understanding shock, or <u>hypoperfusion</u>.

To keep the blood moving continuously through the body, the cardiovascular system requires three intact components Figure 3 :

- A functioning pump: the heart
- Adequate fluid volume: the blood and body fluids
- An intact system of tubing capable of reflex adjustments (constriction and dilation) in response to changes in pump output and fluid volume: the blood vessels

The heart's contractility allows it to increase or decrease the volume of blood it pumps with each contraction, also known as the <u>stroke volume (SV)</u>. The heart can also vary the speed at which it contracts by raising or lowering the pulse rate. <u>Cardiac output (CO)</u> is the volume of blood that the heart can pump per minute, and it is dependent on several factors. First, the heart must have adequate strength, which is largely determined by the ability of the heart muscle to contract. This ability to contract is referred to as <u>myocardial contractility</u>. Second, the heart must receive adequate blood to pump. As the volume of blood flowing to the heart increases, the precontraction pressure in the heart builds up. This precontraction pressure is known as preload. The <u>preload</u> is the initial stretching of the cardiac muscles prior to contraction. It is related to the chamber volume of blood just prior to contraction. As preload increases, the volume of blood within the ventricles increases, which causes the heart muscle to stretch. When the muscle is stretched, myocardial contractility increases, leading to greater force of contraction and increased cardiac output. Lastly, the resistance to flow in the peripheral

YOU are the Medic | PART 2

Your partner attempts to open the patient's airway with a head tilt–chin lift maneuver. On the basis of your scene assessment, there is no indication that Mr. Oliver has fallen or sustained trauma that would necessitate taking spinal precautions. You suction the airway and remove loose but thick, light brown secretions. You note this stimulates his gag reflex and induces coughing. You assess your patient's breathing, and it is slightly labored with a respiratory rate of 24 breaths/min. Chest rise is equal bilaterally. Auscultation reveals scattered rales and rhonchi in all lung fields. You assess for a radial pulse and detect one that is weak with a rate of 120 beats/min. Your impression of his skin is that it is pale, mottled, cool, and clammy to touch. The patient appears to be critical, and a rapid assessment is indicated before initiating transport. Because the patient is nonverbal and unable to respond to your questions, you look to his home health aide for assistance. Your paramedic partner is assisting the patient's ventilations with a bag-mask device and supplemental oxygen at 15 L/min.

You obtain a limited SAMPLE history from his aide. She tells you that Mr. Oliver had a terrible cough 3 days ago and a temperature of 101°F. She said he also reported pain when he took a deep breath. She told him she was concerned he may have pneumonia and should call his doctor. She knows he has an allergy to shellfish. His medications are in the kitchen, and she tells you he took them regularly as far as she knows. She hands you her information sheet on Mr. Oliver's medical history. You note he has a history of hypertension, chronic bronchitis, and had a myocardial infarction approximately 5 years ago. The aide is unsure as to when he last ate but tells you he refused lunch during her last visit when he said he had no appetite. She is not sure how long he has been like this or when his condition changed, but he normally walked daily around 8:00 AM. You recall the security officer telling you he did not see Mr. Oliver for his last two shifts.

Recording Time: 6 Minutes	
Appearance	Poor
Level of consciousness	Unresponsive
Airway	Partially obstructed by secretions, then patent after suctioning
Breathing	24 breaths/min, shallow and slightly labored, assisted with bag-mask device
Circulation	120 beats/min and weak, skin is pale, mottled, and cool

3. Describe what contributing factors would lead you to label this patient as critical.

4. Discuss pathophysiologic changes associated with septic shock.

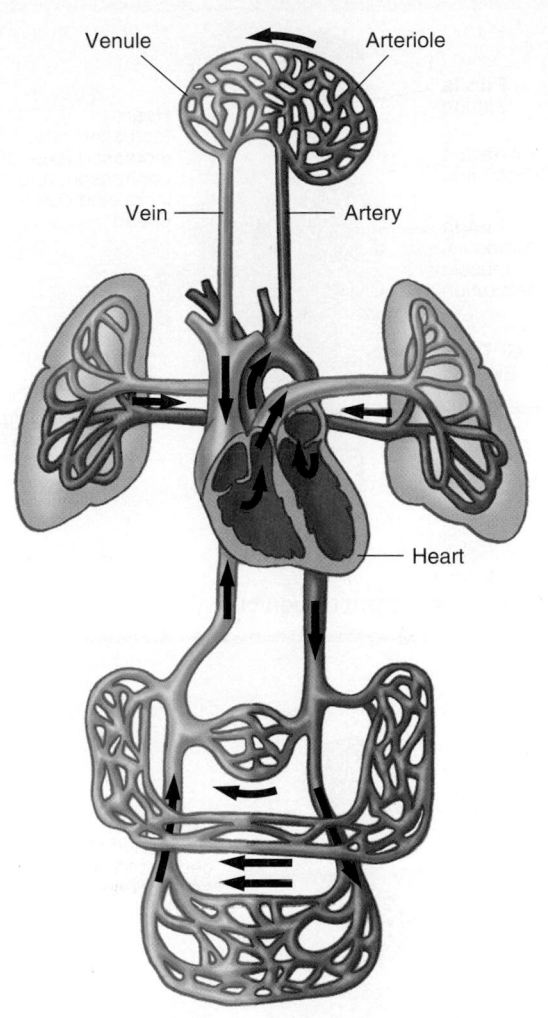

Figure 3 The cardiovascular system requires continuous operation of its three components: the heart (or pump), the blood vessels (or container), and the blood and body fluids (or contents).

maintained within the arteries while the heart rests between heartbeats.

Perfusion depends on cardiac output, SVR, and transport of oxygen.

$$CO = HR \times SV$$
Cardiac Output = Heart Rate × Stroke Volume

$$BP = CO \times SVR$$
Blood Pressure = Cardiac Output × Systemic Vascular Resistance

<u>**Mean arterial pressure (MAP)**</u> is generally considered to be the patient's blood pressure and takes into consideration the systolic blood pressure (SBP) as well as the diastolic blood pressure (DBP). However, MAP is ultimately the blood pressure required to sustain organ perfusion and is roughly 60 mm Hg in the average person. If the MAP falls significantly below 60 mm Hg for an appreciable amount of time, the result will be ischemia of the organ(s) from lack of perfusion. Thus, the MAP needs to be greater than 60 mm Hg to ensure that the brain, coronary arteries, and kidneys remain perfused. MAP is determined with this formula:

$$MAP = DBP + \frac{1}{3}(SBP - DBP)$$

Using the example of a patient who has a blood pressure of 120/60 mm Hg, the <u>**pulse pressure**</u> (difference between the systolic and diastolic pressures) would equal 60 mm Hg (120 mm Hg – 60 mm Hg = 60 mm Hg). To calculate the MAP, take one third of the pulse pressure and add the diastolic pressure to it (20 + 60 = 80 mm Hg). **Table 3** shows an example of how this data affects the field provider.

The body is perfused via the cardiovascular system. Control of the cardiovascular system is a function of the autonomic nervous system, which is composed of competing subsystems circulation must be appropriate. The force or resistance against which the heart pumps is known as <u>afterload</u>.

Blood pressure (BP), the pressure that is generated by the contractions of the heart and the dilation and constriction of the blood vessels, is usually carefully controlled by the body so that there is always sufficient circulation in the various tissues and organs; it is also considered a rough measure of perfusion. Because the heart cannot pump out what is not in its holding chambers, blood pressure varies directly with cardiac output, systemic vascular resistance, and blood volume. <u>**Systemic vascular resistance (SVR)**</u> is the resistance to blood flow within all of the blood vessels except the pulmonary vessels. Remember that blood pressure is the pressure of blood within the vessels at any one time. The systolic pressure is the peak arterial pressure, or pressure generated every time the heart contracts; the diastolic pressure is the pressure

Table 3 Mean Arterial Pressure (MAP)

Formula: $\frac{1}{3}$ (pulse pressure) + diastolic pressure = MAP
Example: 120/60 mm Hg (20 + 60 = MAP 80 mm Hg)

	Systolic								
	120	116	112	96	92	86	82	78	74
80	93	92	91	85	84	82	-	-	-
76	91	89	88	84	83	79	-	-	-
72	88	87	85	80	76	77	75	-	-
68	85	84	83	77	76	74	73	71	-
64	83	81	80	75	73	71	70	69	-
60	80	79	77	72	71	69	67	66	65
56	77	76	75	69	68	66	65	63	62

(Diastolic — left column labels)

Table 4 . One of the subsystems, the sympathetic nervous system, which is sometimes known as the "fight or flight" system, prepares the body for physical activity during a stressful situation. This preparation includes increasing the pulse rate, blood pressure, and respiratory rate while dilating blood vessels in areas required for physical activity and constricting those in areas primarily involved with reproduction and restoration.

The autonomic nervous system is primarily housed in the upper part of the medulla oblongata of the brain. Nerve signals caused by stimulation of the sympathetic nervous system travel between the brain and the body by way of nerves travelling through the spinal cord. These nerves leave the spinal cord between each pair of vertebrae and spread out to affect the tissues in those areas Figure 4 . Another mechanism used by the sympathetic nervous system is the chemical release of epinephrine and norepinephrine from the adrenal glands into the bloodstream. These chemicals travel through the bloodstream to all parts of the body to activate a sympathetic response in those areas.

The other subsystem of the autonomic nervous system is the parasympathetic nervous system, which is primarily responsible for rest and regeneration Figure 5 . The parasympathetic nervous system opposes every action of the sympathetic nervous system. Where the sympathetic system increases the pulse rate, blood pressure, and respiratory rate, the parasympathetic system decreases these. The parasympathetic system also constricts blood vessels in muscular tissue and dilates those in the digestive system.

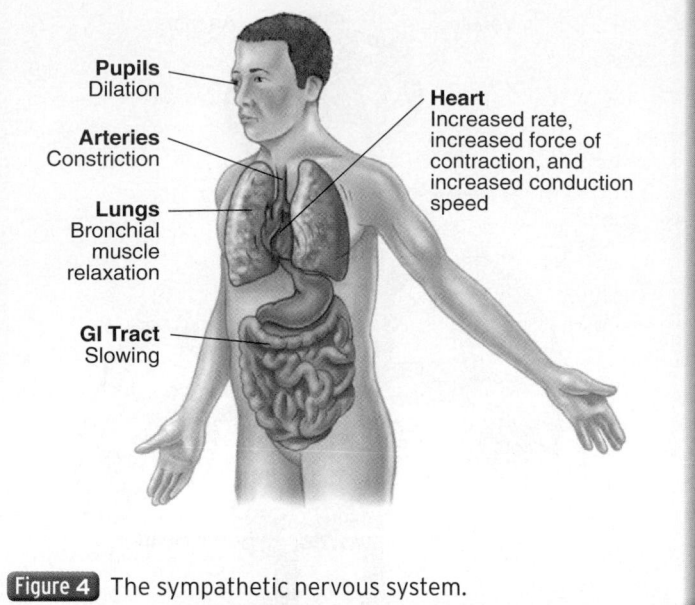

Figure 4 The sympathetic nervous system.

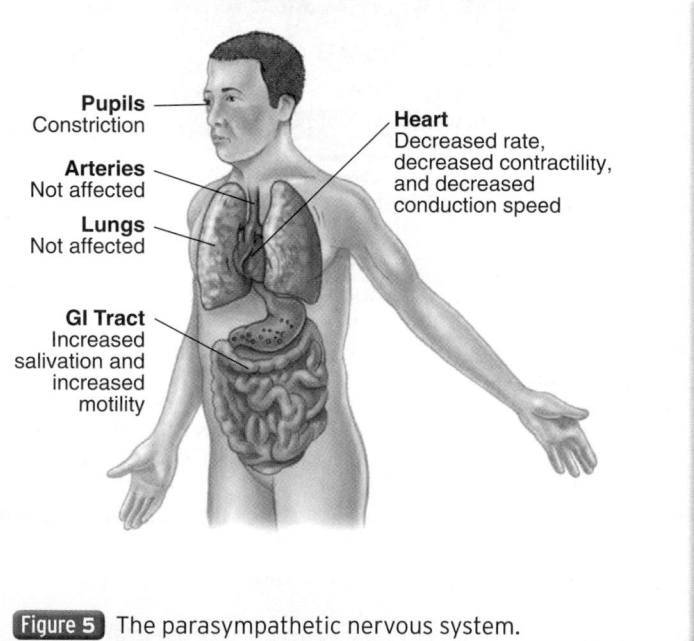

Figure 5 The parasympathetic nervous system.

Table 4 Comparison of Sympathetic and Parasympathetic Nervous Systems

Features	Parasympathetic	Sympathetic
Other name for system	Cholinergic, "rest and digest"	Adrenergic, "fight or flight"
Natural chemical mediator	Acetylcholine	Norepinephrine, epinephrine
Primary nerve(s)	Vagus	Nerves from the thoracic and lumbar ganglia of the spinal cord
Effect of stimulation	Decreases contractility (negative inotropic effect) Slows conduction velocity (negative dromotropic effect) Slows the heart* (negative chronotropic effect) Constricts pupils Increases salivation Increases gut motility	Increases contractility (positive inotropic effect) Speeds conduction velocity (positive dromotropic effect) Speeds the heart* (positive chronotropic effect) Dilates pupils Slows the gut Dilates the bronchi

*Slowing occurs (mostly in the atria).

Words of Wisdom

The following elements are collectively known as the **Fick principle**, which states that the movement and use of oxygen in the body is dependent on:

1. Adequate concentration of inspired oxygen (F_{IO_2} [fraction of inspired oxygen])
2. Appropriate movement of oxygen across the alveolar-capillary membrane into the arterial bloodstream
3. Adequate number of red blood cells to carry the oxygen
4. Proper tissue perfusion
5. Efficient off-loading of oxygen at the tissue level

Respiration and Oxygenation

Each time you take a breath, the alveoli (microscopic, thin-walled air sacs) receive a supply of oxygen-rich air. The oxygen then dissolves in the blood plasma and attaches to the blood's hemoglobin. The oxygen gas molecules from the oxygenated blood pass through the alveolar wall into the walls of a fine network of pulmonary capillaries that are in close contact with the alveoli. If the oxygenated blood is not properly circulated, some of the cells and organs will not receive proper nutrients, possibly resulting in cellular death.

Oxygen and carbon dioxide pass rapidly across these thin tissue layers through diffusion. <u>Diffusion</u> is a passive process in which molecules move from an area with a higher concentration of molecules to an area of lower concentration. There are more oxygen molecules in the alveoli than in the blood. Therefore, the oxygen molecules move from the alveoli into the blood. Because there are more carbon dioxide molecules in the blood than in the inhaled air, carbon dioxide moves from the blood into the alveoli.

Just like oxygen, carbon dioxide is dissolved in the plasma and attaches to the blood's hemoglobin. The body takes the carbon dioxide, combines it with water, and creates carbonic acid. Carbonic acid concentrations become high just as the blood is moving toward the lungs. Once it reaches the lungs, the carbonic acid breaks down and the carbon dioxide is exhaled. All of this action takes place to maintain the delicate balance between the gases and maintain the pH of the body.

Regulation of Blood Flow

Blood flow through the capillary beds is regulated by the capillary sphincters, circular muscular walls that constrict and dilate, acting as a gate to increase or decrease flow. These <u>sphincters</u> are under the control of the autonomic nervous system, which regulates involuntary functions such as sweating and digestion. Capillary sphincters also respond to other stimuli such as heat, cold, the need for oxygen, and the need for waste removal. Under normal circumstances, not all cells have the same needs at the same time. For example, the stomach and intestines have a high need for blood flow during and shortly after eating, when digestion is at a peak. Between meals, blood flow is lessened, and blood is diverted to other areas. The brain, by contrast, needs a constant and consistent supply of blood to function.

Regulation of blood flow is determined by cellular need and is accomplished by vessel constriction or dilation, together with sphincter constriction or dilation. Maintenance of blood flow, or perfusion, is accomplished by the heart, blood vessels, and blood working together.

Pathophysiology of Shock

Shock can result from inadequate cardiac output, decreased SVR, or the inability of red blood cells (RBCs) to deliver oxygen to tissues. If there is a disturbance in the transportation of oxygen and removal of carbon dioxide, dangerous waste products will build up leading to cellular death and eventually death of the entire organ. Because the body is built in a framework where every cell ultimately relates to the body, conditions such as inadequate perfusion will cause damage to the cells as well as the body **Figure 6**. If the shock state persists, it will ultimately lead to death. As mentioned, shock is a state of failure and ultimate collapse of the cardiovascular system that causes inadequate cellular oxygenation and hypoperfusion. To protect vital organs, the body attempts to compensate by shunting (directing) blood flow from organs that are more tolerant of low flow (such as the skin and intestines) to vital organs that cannot tolerate hypoperfusion (such as the heart, brain, and lungs). If the cause of shock is not promptly addressed, the patient will most likely die.

The cardiovascular system consists of three parts: the heart, the blood vessels or arteries, and the fluid or blood. These three parts can be referred to as the "perfusion triangle" **Figure 7**. When a patient is in shock, one or more of the three parts is not working properly.

Blood is the vehicle for carrying oxygen and nutrients through the vessels to the capillary beds to tissue cells, where these supplies are exchanged for waste products created during metabolism. For this process to happen, the vessels (container) must be intact. Blood contains RBCs, white blood cells, platelets, and plasma. As discussed in the chapter, *Anatomy and*

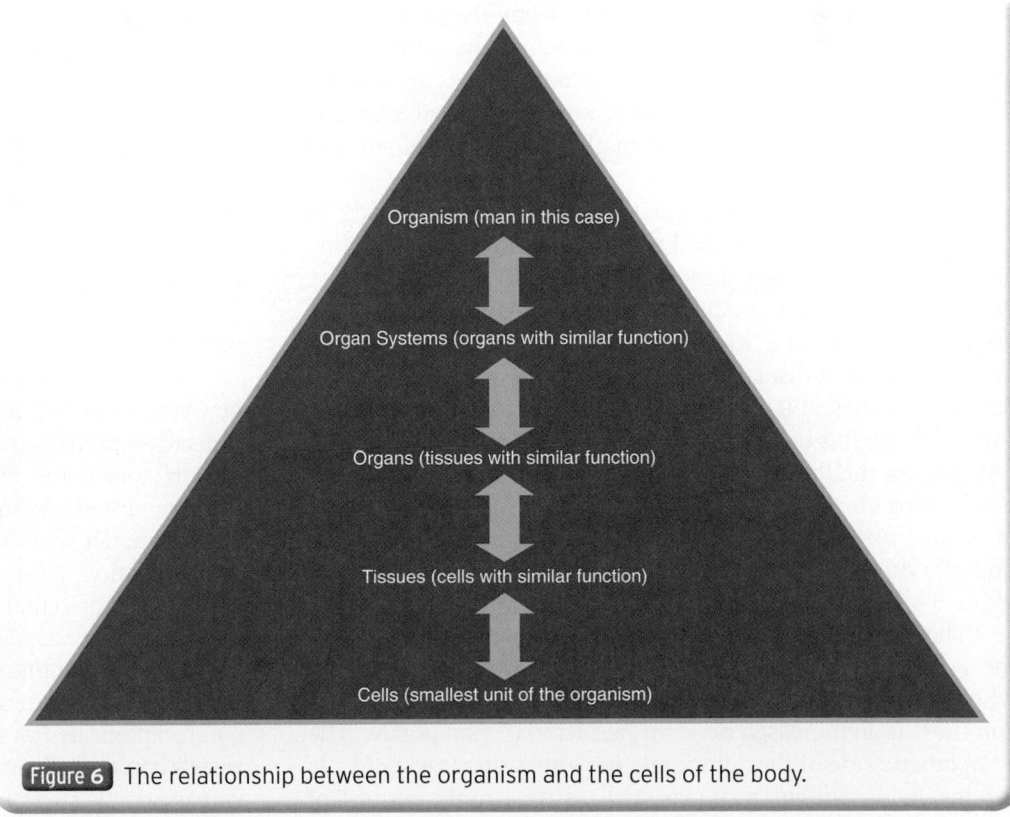

Figure 6 The relationship between the organism and the cells of the body.

- Organism (man in this case)
- Organ Systems (organs with similar function)
- Organs (tissues with similar function)
- Tissues (cells with similar function)
- Cells (smallest unit of the organism)

Perfusion Triangle

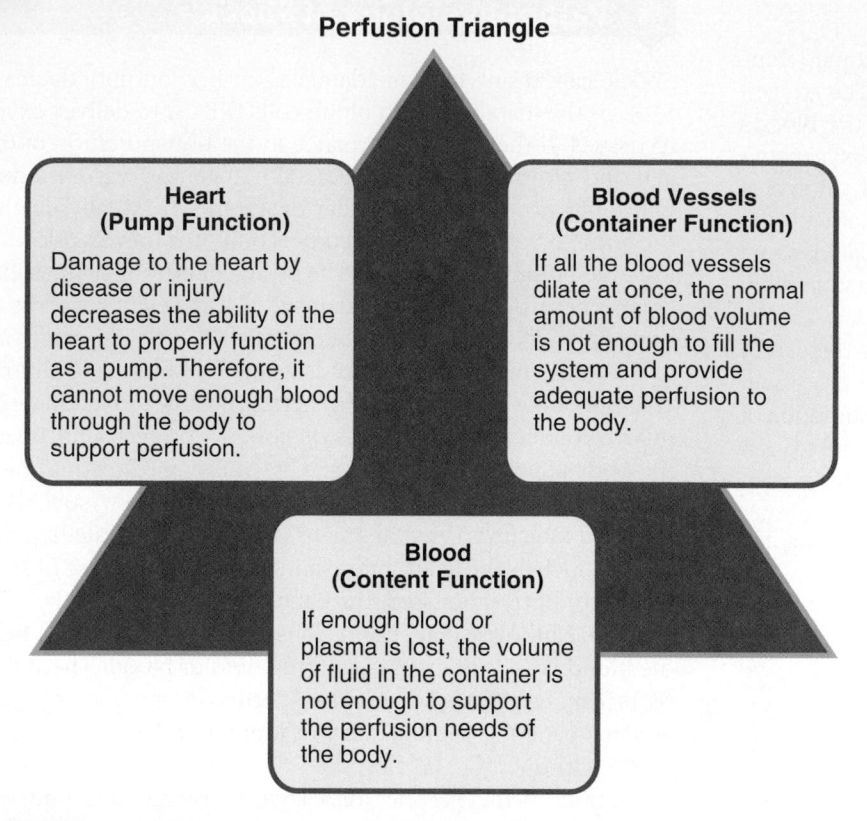

**Heart
(Pump Function)**

Damage to the heart by disease or injury decreases the ability of the heart to properly function as a pump. Therefore, it cannot move enough blood through the body to support perfusion.

**Blood Vessels
(Container Function)**

If all the blood vessels dilate at once, the normal amount of blood volume is not enough to fill the system and provide adequate perfusion to the body.

**Blood
(Content Function)**

If enough blood or plasma is lost, the volume of fluid in the container is not enough to support the perfusion needs of the body.

Figure 7 The heart, the blood vessels, and the blood and body fluids represent the perfusion triangle.

Physiology, RBCs are responsible for the transportation of oxygen to the cells and for transporting carbon dioxide (a waste product of cellular metabolism) away from the cells to the lungs where it is exhaled and removed from the body. White blood cells help the body to fight infection. Platelets are responsible for forming blood clots. There are also formed elements and the plasma, also discussed in the chapter, *Anatomy and Physiology*.

Blood clots are an important response from the body to control blood loss. In the body, a blood clot forms depending on one of the following principles: retention of blood because of blockage in blood circulation (blood stasis), changes in the vessel wall (such as a wound), and the blood's ability to clot (as the result of a disease process or medication). When injury occurs to tissues in the body, platelets begin to aggregate at the site of injury; this causes the RBCs to become sticky and clump together. As the RBCs begin to clump, another substance in the body called fibrinogen reinforces the RBCs. This is the final step in the formation of a blood clot. However, clots are unstable and prone to rupture because blood is continually moving as a result of the blood pressure.

The body's neural and hormonal mechanisms, including the autonomic nervous system and hormones, are triggered when the body senses that the pressure in the system is falling and there is an increased need for perfusion of vital organs. The sympathetic side of the autonomic nervous system, responsible for the fight-or-flight response, will assume more control of

the body's functions during a state of shock. The parasympathetic nervous system controls involuntary functions by sending signals to the cardiac, smooth, and glandular muscles. When the autonomic nervous system releases epinephrine and norepinephrine, these hormones cause changes in certain body functions such as an increase in the pulse rate, an increase in the strength of cardiac contractions, and vasoconstriction in nonessential areas, primarily in the skin, muscles, and GI tract (peripheral vasoconstriction). Together, these actions are designed to maintain pressure in the system and, as a result, sustain perfusion of the vital organs (ie, brain, heart, lungs, kidneys, and liver).

Eventually, there is also a shifting of body fluids to help maintain pressure within the system. However, the response of the autonomic nervous system and hormones comes within seconds. It is this response that causes all the signs and symptoms of shock in a patient.

Compensation for Decreased Perfusion

Central among the homeostatic mechanisms that regulate cardiovascular dynamics are those that maintain blood pressure. When any event results in decreased perfusion (such as in blood loss, MI, loss of vasomotor tone, or tension pneumothorax), the body must respond immediately to preserve the vital organs. <u>Baroreceptors</u> located in the aortic arch and carotid sinuses (as well as in most of the large arteries of the neck and thorax) sense the decreased blood flow and activate the vasomotor center in the medulla oblongata, which oversees changes in the diameter of blood vessels, to begin constriction of the vessels and, therefore, increase blood presssure. Along with baroreceptors are <u>chemoreceptors</u>, which measure subtle shifts in the amounts of carbon dioxide in the arterial blood. In the chapter, *Anatomy and Physiology*, you learned that this has an effect on the regulation of the respiratory rate as well as control of the acid/base balance in the body.

Normally, stimulation occurs when the systolic pressure is between 60 and 80 mm Hg in adults or even lower in children. A decrease in the systolic pressure to less than 80 mm Hg stimulates the vasomotor center to increase the arterial pressure by constricting vessels. As the arterial pressure drops, the walls of the arteries are not stretched as much, thereby decreasing baroreceptor stimulation. Normally, baroreceptor stimulation prevents the vasoconstrictor center of the medulla from constricting the vessels, leading to vasodilation in the peripheral circulatory system and a decrease in pulse rate and contractility, causing a concomitant decrease in arterial pressure. With dropping pressure, the baroreceptors are not stimulated to allow for vasodilation, so the vessels constrict to raise the blood pressure. The sympathetic nervous system is also stimulated as the body recognizes a potential catastrophic event. This message is sent to the adrenal glands to release epinephrine and norepinephrine into the bloodstream. These two naturally occurring "medications" will cause tachycardia and increase the contractility of the heart. Additionally, they will cause venous and arteriolar constriction resulting in a decrease in blood flow to the skin, muscles, the GI tract, and often the kidneys. This allows for a relative redistribution of blood to the brain and heart. Capillary hydrostatic pressure decreases in the compensated phase of shock, allowing fluid from the interstitial compartment to flow into the vessels.

Also, in response to hypoperfusion, the renin-angiotensin-aldosterone system in the kidneys is activated and antidiuretic hormone is released from the pituitary gland. Together, these mechanisms trigger salt and water retention and peripheral vasoconstriction. The result is an increase in the patient's blood pressure and maintenance of cardiac output. Depending on the severity of the insult, variable amounts of fluid will shift from the interstitial tissues into the vascular compartment. The spleen also releases some RBCs that are normally sequestered there to augment the blood's oxygen-carrying capacity. The overall response of the initial compensatory mechanisms is to increase the preload, stroke volume, and pulse rate, which usually results in an increase in cardiac output. This "autotransfusion" effect, along with the subtle effects in other response systems of the body (ie, osmosis, insulin and glucagon production in the pancreas, as well as the effects of the hormones arginine vasopressin, adrenocorticotropic hormone cortisol system, and somatotropin), allows the body to compensate adequately for a volume loss of up to 25%. Remember that shock is a normal compensatory response of the body, and disease can occur or become exacerbated when normal response systems are activated under abnormal conditions.

As hypoperfusion persists, the myocardial oxygen demand continues to increase. Eventually, the accelerated compensatory mechanisms are no longer able to keep up with the body's demand. Myocardial function then worsens, with decreased cardiac output and ejection fraction. Tissue perfusion decreases, leading to impaired cell metabolism. Often, the systolic blood pressure decreases, especially in progressive hypoperfusion or "decompensated" shock. Fluid may leak from the blood vessels, as in the case of a severe allergic reaction, causing systemic and pulmonary edema. As the patient decompensates, perfusion to the brain and coronary arteries decreases. Cells switch to anaerobic metabolism when they do not have enough oxygen available to them. The switch from **aerobic metabolism** (or all of the cells' processes occurring with adequate oxygen supply) to **anaerobic metabolism** (cellular processes occurring in the absence of oxygen) is a critical point that begins to produce lactic acidosis from this inefficient form of metabolism. This will shift the oxygen-hemoglobin dissociation curve to the right to increase tissue oxygen delivery. This shift in the curve also decreases cardiac function and makes the heart more susceptible to the effect of the circulating catecholamines (ie, causing dysrhythmias). Other signs of hypoperfusion may also be present, such as dusky skin color, oliguria, and impaired mentation.

The body produces its own "medicines," epinephrine and norepinephrine, in the adrenal glands in response to hypoperfusion. These substances are released by the body as part of the global compensatory state. Epinephrine is also administered by caregivers in cases of anaphylaxis, severe airway disease, and cardiac arrest.

Release of epinephrine improves cardiac output by increasing the pulse rate and strength. The alpha-1 response to its release includes vasoconstriction, increased peripheral vascular resistance, and increased afterload from the arteriolar constriction. Alpha-2 effects ensure a regulated release of alpha-1. Beta responses from the release of epinephrine primarily affect the heart and lungs. Increases in pulse rate, contractility, conductivity, and automaticity occur in tandem with bronchodilation.

Effects of norepinephrine are primarily alpha-1 and alpha-2 in nature and center on vasoconstriction and increasing peripheral vascular resistance. Table 5 lists the alpha and beta effects of epinephrine and norepinephrine. This vasoconstriction allows the body to shunt blood from areas of lesser need to areas of greater need, serving to keep the brain and other vital organs perfused in the early phases of shock. In an effort to maintain circulation to the brain, the body will shunt blood away from the following tissues, in this order: placenta, skin, muscles, gut, kidneys, liver, heart, lungs. This planned shunting of blood is often referred to as the "pecking order." The skin and muscles can survive with minimal blood flow from vasoconstriction for a much longer period than can major organs such as the kidneys, liver, heart, and lungs. If the blood supply is inadequate to the major organs for more than 60 minutes, they often develop complications that will lead to death, such as renal failure and shock lung. This concept has been traditionally referred to as the "Golden Period", and it explains why it is so important for you to address the cause of the shock immediately.

Table 5	Effects of Epinephrine and Norepinephrine
Epinephrine	
Alpha-1	Vasoconstriction Increase in peripheral vascular resistance Increased afterload from arteriolar constriction
Alpha-2	Inhibit insulin release Relax gastrointestinal smooth muscle
Beta-1	Positive **chronotropic effects** (increase in the heart's rate of contraction) Positive **inotropic effects** (increase in the contractility of the heart muscle) Positive **dromotropic effects** (increase in the heart's velocity of conduction)
Beta-2	Bronchodilation Gastrointestinal smooth muscle dilation
Norepinephrine	
Alpha-1 and alpha-2	Vasoconstriction Increase in peripheral vascular resistance Increased afterload from arteriolar constriction

Failure of compensatory mechanisms to preserve perfusion leads to decreases in preload and cardiac output. Myocardial blood supply and oxygenation decrease, reducing myocardial perfusion. As cardiac output further decreases, coronary artery perfusion also decreases, leading to myocardial ischemia. As all of these changes are occurring, other organ systems are affected too. The normal functions of the liver and pancreas are impacted by the low perfusion state inhibiting insulin release. This is why patients in shock have been described as being in a diabetic-like state. Gastrointestinal motility is decreased causing stress ulcers to develop. When kidney perfusion is diminished, so is urine production; this leads to kidney failure if not reperfused within 45 minutes to 1 hour. Normal urine output is roughly 30 to 40 mL/h. When the patient has an output of less than 500 mL per day, this is considered oliguria and can lead to acute kidney insufficiency, an indicator of the severity of acute underlying illness, also associated with mortality in sepsis and pneumonia.

Shock-Related Events at the Capillary and Microcirculatory Levels

As perfusion decreases, cellular ischemia occurs. Minimal blood flow passes through the capillaries, causing the cells to switch

Words of Wisdom

The Frank-Starling mechanism states that the length of the fibers constituting the heart's muscular wall determines the force of the heartbeat. In other words, an increase in diastolic filling increases the force of the contraction, whereas a decrease in diastolic filling decreases the force of the contraction. Decreased perfusion in shock is partially the result of decreased cardiac contractility, which may be the result of loss of fluid, increased container size, or a damaged pump.

from aerobic metabolism to anaerobic metabolism or all the cells' processes occurring in the absence of oxygen, which can quickly lead to metabolic acidosis. With less circulation, the blood stagnates in the capillaries. The precapillary sphincter relaxes in response to the buildup of lactic acid, vasomotor center failure, and increased amounts of carbon dioxide. The postcapillary sphincters remain constricted, causing the capillaries to become engorged with fluid.

The capillary sphincters—circular muscular walls that constrict and dilate—regulate blood flow through the capillary beds. These sphincters are under the control of the autonomic nervous system, which regulates involuntary functions such as sweating and digestion. Capillary sphincters also respond to other stimuli

YOU are the Medic   PART 3

Your supervisor arrives and obtains vital signs while you establish intravenous access. After initiating access, you provide an infusion of normal saline. The patient's blood pressure is 68 mm Hg by palpation so you administer a fluid bolus of normal saline at 20 mL/kg. You attach the cardiac monitor and identify the rhythm as a sinus tachycardia at a rate of 118 beats/min and without ectopy. Your partner and supervisor prepare the patient for transport while the home health aide gathers his medication at your request so that you can evaluate them and turn them over to hospital personnel. She also gathers pertinent identification for you to take with you. The security officer assists you to the elevator and helps you remove your equipment from the scene. Once you have loaded your patient into the ambulance, your supervisor advises he will drive you to the closest appropriate facility so your partner can continue assisting ventilations while you provide care and assessment during transport. You evaluate the patient's medications once transport has begun. His medications include lisinopril 10 mg daily, aspirin 81 mg daily, albuterol metered dose inhaler two puffs three times daily and PRN, and furosemide 20 mg daily. After a quick count, you notice that it appears there are two more tablets of lisinopril than there should be if Mr. Oliver had been compliant with his medications. This supports your concerns that he has been in bed for at least 24 hours. You reevaluate his vital signs as transport continues.

Recording Time: 10 Minutes	
Skin	Pale, cool, moist
Pulse	118 beats/min and weak
Blood pressure	68 mm Hg by palpation
Respirations	20 breaths/min, assisted with bag-mask device
Oxygen saturation (Spo$_2$)	Not obtainable secondary to poor perfusion
Pupils	Equal, round, and responsive to light
Temperature	96°F

5. Discuss the potential phase of shock this patient may be in.

6. Describe how you should manage this patient with suspected shock.

such as heat, cold, increased demand for oxygen, and the need for waste removal. Thus, regulation of blood flow is determined by cellular need and is accomplished by vessel constriction or dilation, working in tandem with sphincter constriction or dilation.

The body can tolerate anaerobic metabolism for only a limited time. Anaerobic metabolism is much less efficient than aerobic metabolism and leads to systemic acidosis and depletion of the body's normally high energy reserves (adenosine triphosphate [ATP]). Although hypoxia decreases the rate of ATP synthesis in the cells, it will not damage the mitochondria unless it is sustained and severe.

During anaerobic metabolism, incomplete glucose breakdown leads to an accumulation of pyruvic acid. Pyruvic acid cannot be converted to acetyl coenzyme A without oxygen, however, so it is transformed in greater amounts to lactate and other acid by-products. Acidosis develops because ATP is hydrolyzed to adenosine diphosphate and phosphate with the release of a proton. Hydrogen ions accumulate, decreasing the pool of bicarbonate buffer. Lactate also buffers protons, and lactic acid accumulates in the body.

At the same time, ischemia stimulates increased carbon dioxide production by the tissues. The higher the body's metabolic rate, the higher the carbon dioxide level in hypoperfused states. The excess carbon dioxide combines with intracellular water to produce carbonic acid. Increased tissue acids will, in turn, react with other buffers to form more intracellular acidic substances. Thus, acidosis serves as an indirect measure of tissue perfusion. The acidic condition of the blood inhibits hemoglobin in the RBCs from binding with and carrying oxygen. This adds to the cellular oxygen debt, shifting the oxyhemoglobin dissociation curve to the right.

Meanwhile, sodium, which is usually more abundant outside the cells than inside them, is naturally inclined to diffuse into the cells. Normally the sodium-potassium pump acts like a "bouncer" at the cell membrane, sending the sodium back out against the concentration gradient. This mechanism involves active transport and requires an ample supply of ATP to fuel the bouncer. Reduced levels of ATP, however, result in a dysfunctional sodium-potassium pump and alter the cell membrane function. Excessive sodium begins to diffuse into the cells, along with water, which ultimately depletes the interstitial compartment.

The intracellular enzymes that usually help digest and neutralize bacteria introduced into a cell are bound in a relatively impermeable membrane. Cellular flooding explodes that membrane and releases these lysosomal enzymes, which then autodigest the cell. If enough cells are destroyed in this way, organ failure will become evident. The release of the lysosomes opens the floodgates for the onset of the last phase of shock, called irreversible or terminal shock.

To compound these problems, accumulating acids and waste products act as potent vasodilators, further decreasing venous return and diminishing blood flow to the vital organs and tissues. The arterial pressure falls to the point at which even the "protected organs" such as the brain and heart are no longer being perfused. When aortic pressures fall below a MAP of 60 mm Hg, the coronary arteries no longer fill, the heart is

weakened, and the cardiac output falls. Myocardial depressant factor is released from an ischemic pancreas, further decreasing the pumping action of the heart and slowing the cardiac output.

Eventually, the reduced blood supply to the vasomotor center in the brain results in slowing and then stopping of sympathetic nervous system activity. The metabolic wastes are released into the slower-flowing blood. The blood's sluggish flow, coupled with its acidity, leads to platelet agglutination and formation of microthrombi. Because the capillary walls are stretched, they lose their ability to retain large molecules, allowing them to leak into the surrounding interstitial spaces. Hydrostatic pressure forces plasma into the interstitial spaces, further increasing the distance from the capillaries to the cells. In turn, oxygen transport decreases, increasing cellular hypoxia.

The continuing buildup of lactic acid and carbon dioxide acts as a potent vasodilator, leading to relaxation of the postcapillary sphincters. The accumulated hydrogen, potassium, carbon dioxide, and thrombosed (clotted) RBCs wash out into the venous circulation, increasing the metabolic acidosis. This has been referred to as the capillary "washout phase." The result is an even greater drop in cardiac output. Ischemia and necrosis ultimately lead to multiple-organ dysfunction syndrome, in which the various organ systems fail in succession.

> ### Words of Wisdom
>
> Capillary hydrostatic pressure tends to force fluids through capillary walls, whereas interstitial fluid hydrostatic pressure pushes fluid back into the cells.
>
> Oncotic pressure pulls fluids from the surrounding tissue into the capillaries as a result of a difference in the concentration of solutes in the fluid inside the capillaries. Fluid leaves the capillaries as a result of hydrostatic pressure, while albumin and other large proteins remain inside, resulting in a greater concentration of solutes inside the capillaries. The oncotic pressure rises, pulling more water into the capillaries in order to balance the solute concentration. If capillary hydrostatic pressure is greater, fluid will leave the capillaries. If capillary oncotic pressure is greater, fluid will be pulled into the capillaries.

In conjunction with all this injury going on, the white blood cells and blood clotting system are impaired. There is a decreased resistance to infection and disseminated intravascular coagulation (DIC) may occur. DIC is a serious disorder whereby the proteins that normally control clotting become active. Once again, a normal function becomes activated under abnormal circumstances. Research shows that 97% of patients who die from hemorrhagic shock have evidence of coagulation defects prior to fluid or blood administration. This occurs most often in patients with head trauma and suggests preexisting DIC. The most frequent abnormality was elevated prothrombin (97%), followed by depressed platelet counts (72%), and elevated partial thromboplastin time (70%). DIC has also been found to complicate septic shock.

Multiple-Organ Dysfunction Syndrome

Multiple-organ dysfunction syndrome (MODS) is a progressive condition characterized by combined failure of two or more organs or organ systems that were initially unharmed by the acute disorder or injury that caused the patient's initial illness. Six organ systems are surveyed when you are diagnosing MODS: the respiratory, hepatic, renal, hematologic, neurologic, and cardiovascular systems. Each system is assigned a score to determine the patient's overall risk. For example, the Glasgow Coma Scale score is used to score the patient's neurologic system function.

Consider this; if each type of tissue has its warm ischemic time—that is, the time it can be deprived of oxygenated blood before it starts to die—then different tissue types (ie, nervous, muscle, epithelial tissue) will begin to exhibit the effects of poor perfusion, depending on how much time has transpired prior to adequate reperfusion by the surgeon in the operating suite. As previously discussed, the warm ischemic time of the brain and central nervous system tissue is approximately 4 to 6 minutes, and the warm ischemic time for the skin and muscles is almost 2 hours. The Golden Period corresponds to the warm ischemic time of the rest of the vital organs (ie, liver, kidneys, heart and lungs). When a patient has poor perfusion in the field and it is not adequately restored within the first hour, blood is diverted, in order, from the skin and muscles, gut, liver, kidneys, and the heart and lungs in an effort to keep the brain well perfused. This is often the cause of the development of serious, often life-threatening complications of organ damage to the liver (liver failure), the kidneys (renal failure), the lungs (acute respiratory distress syndrome), and the heart (massive MI). Thus, what was initially a single injury causing the patient to lose significant amounts of blood or fluids can have a devastating impact on multiple organs and organ systems. It is all directly related from the single cell to the organism.

First described in 1975, patients with MODS have an overall mortality rate of 60% to 90%. Previously called multisystem organ failure, today MODS is considered the major cause of death following septic, traumatic, and burn injuries. MODS is classified as primary or secondary. Primary MODS is a direct result of an insult, such as a pulmonary contusion from striking the chest on the steering wheel during a crash. Secondary MODS encompasses the organ dysfunction that occurs as an integral component to the patient's response (ie, renal failure following trauma).

MODS occurs when injury or infection (sepsis) triggers a massive systemic immune, inflammatory, and coagulation response, resulting in the release of numerous inflammatory mediators and activation of the following systems:

- **Activation of the complement system.** Normally, this group of plasma proteins functions to eliminate invading bacteria—that is, these components are part of the immune response. In MODS, an overactive complement system activates phagocytes and induces further inflammation and damage to cells.
- **Activation of the coagulation system.** Endothelial damage and coagulation, especially in the microscopic venules and arterioles, become uncontrolled in MODS, which results in microvascular thrombus formation and tissue ischemia.
- **Activation of the kallikrein-kinin system.** The release of bradykinin, a potent vasodilator, leads to tissue hypoperfusion and may contribute to hypotension.

The net outcome of overactivity in these systems is maldistribution of systemic and organ blood flow. Often the body attempts to compensate by accelerating tissue metabolism. The result is an oxygen supply-demand imbalance that leads to tissue hypoxia, tissue hypoperfusion, exhaustion of the cells' fuel supply (ATP), metabolic failure, lysosome breakdown, anaerobic metabolism, acidosis, and impaired cellular function. As MODS progresses, various organs begin to malfunction as a result of the cell and tissue hypoxia.

MODS typically develops within hours to days following resuscitation. The signs and symtoms include hypotension, insufficient tissue perfusion, uncontrollable bleeding (coagulopathy), and multisystem organ failure. A low-grade fever may develop from the inflammatory response, tachycardia, and dyspnea. It also may be difficult to oxygenate patients because of acute lung injury and acute respiratory distress syndrome.

In a 14- to 21-day period, renal and liver failure can develop, along with collapse of the GI and immune systems. If the patient does not respond to treatment of the underlying condition, cardiovascular collapse and death typically occur within days to weeks of the initial insult.

MODS affects specific organs and organ systems in the following ways:

- **Heart.** Hypoperfusion may stun a healthy heart and result in dysrhythmias, muscle ischemia, infarction, and pump failure with ejection fractions falling far below 40%. Peripheral pulses are weak or absent. Extremities become cyanotic and cold.
- **Lungs.** Failure is evidenced by adult respiratory distress syndrome or noncardiogenic pulmonary edema. Hypoxic vasoconstriction of pulmonary beds increases pulmonary arterial pressures and produces pulmonary hypertension, putting a strain on the right ventricle. Pulmonary capillary blood flow reduction results in impaired gas exchange, a reduced Pao_2 level, and an increased $Paco_2$ level. Alveolar cells become ischemic and slow their production of surfactant, resulting in massive atelectasis and a reduction in pulmonary compliance. At the same time, pulmonary capillaries become permeable to water, resulting in interstitial and intra-alveolar edema at low wedge pressures (< 18 mm Hg). The net results are respiratory failure, severe hypoxemia, and respiratory acidosis.
- **Central nervous system.** Decreased cerebral perfusion pressure and cerebral blood flow result in confusion, reduced responses to verbal and painful stimuli, and, ultimately, unresponsiveness.
- **Kidneys.** A reduction in renal blood flow produces acute tubular necrosis, which in turn leads to oliguria (urine output of less than 20 mL/h). Toxic waste products cannot be excreted, so they are retained in the blood. Metabolic acidosis worsens as the kidneys become unable to excrete acids or retain bicarbonate.

- **Liver.** Impaired metabolic function and alterations in clotting factors produce coagulopathies such as disseminated intravascular coagulation, in which clotting and bleeding occur at the same time. The liver fails to filter bacteria, leaving the patient vulnerable to infections. Failure to metabolize waste products, such as ammonia and lactate, causes markedly increased blood levels of these toxins. Cell death is evidenced by an increase in enzyme levels (including lactate dehydrogenase, aspartate aminotransferase, and alanine aminotransferase) in the blood. The net result is ischemic hepatitis, hypoxic hepatitis, or shock liver.
- **GI tract.** Hypoperfusion results in ischemic gut syndrome. Release of vasodilating endotoxins into the gut causes the gut to leak, which further contributes to the progression of shock.

Causes of Shock

Recall that normal tissue perfusion requires three intact mechanisms: a pump (heart), fluid volume (blood and body fluids), and tubing capable of reflex adjustments (constriction and dilation) in response to changes in pump output and fluid volume (blood vessels). If any one of those mechanisms is damaged, tissue perfusion may be disrupted, and shock will ensue.

Shock can result from many conditions, including bleeding, respiratory failure, acute allergic reactions, and overwhelming infection. In all cases, however, the damage occurs because of insufficient perfusion of organs and tissues. As soon as perfusion stops or becomes impaired, tissues start to die, affecting all local body processes. If the conditions causing shock are not promptly arrested and reversed, death soon follows.

You should have a high index of suspicion for shock in many emergency medical situations. For example, you would expect hemorrhagic shock to accompany massive external or internal bleeding. You should also expect shock if a patient has any one of the following conditions:

- Multiple severe fractures
- Abdominal or chest injury
- Spinal injury
- Severe infection
- Major heart attack
- Anaphylaxis

Understanding the basic physiologic causes of shock will better prepare you to treat it. There are three basic causes of shock (Figure 8).

Words of Wisdom

Shock is a complex physiologic process that gives subtle signs to its presence before it becomes severe. These early signs relate closely to the events that lead to more severe shock, so it is important for you to know the underlying processes thoroughly. If you understand what causes shock, you will be able to recognize it in many patients before it becomes out of control.

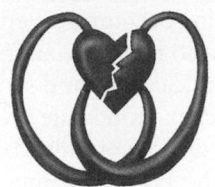 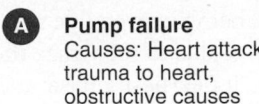
A   Pump failure
Causes: Heart attack, trauma to heart, obstructive causes

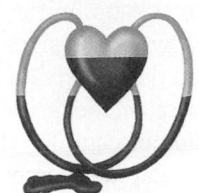
B   Low fluid volume
Causes: Trauma to vessels or tissues, fluid loss from GI tract (vomiting/diarrhea can also lower the fluid component of blood)

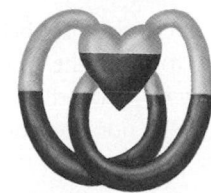
C   Poor vessel function
Causes: Infection, drug overdose (narcotic), spinal cord injury, anaphylaxis

Figure 8 There are three basic causes of shock and impaired tissue perfusion. **A.** Pump failure occurs when the heart is damaged by disease, injury, or obstructive causes. The heart may not generate enough energy to move the blood through the system. **B.** Low fluid volume, often a result of bleeding, leads to inadequate perfusion. **C.** Poor vessel function—if blood vessels dilate excessively, the blood within them, even though it is of normal volume, is inadequate to fill the system and provide efficient perfusion.

Certain categories of patients are at high risk to develop shock. They include patients known to have had trauma or bleeding; patients with massive MI; pregnant women; and patients with a possible source for septic shock (such as burned patients and people with diabetes or cancer). The elderly are particularly at risk for shock, especially elderly men with urinary tract infections. Increased age works against patients in that they normally have a decreased resting cardiac output, decreased cardiac reserves (as much as 50%), and atherosclerosis that affects vasoconstriction.

Words of Wisdom

More than one type of shock may be present at one time. Consider the patient who was in a motor vehicle crash who presents with hypovolemic shock from a ruptured spleen and other internal injuries as well as spinal shock from a severed spine. Or, consider the burn patient who is losing body fluid and has cells that are leaking and swelling tremendously.

The Progression of Shock

Shock occurs in three successive phases (compensated, decompensated, and irreversible). This is also referred to as the four grades of hemorrhage or four classes of shock, with class I and II being compensated shock, class III being decompensated shock, and class IV being irreversible shock, also referred to as terminal shock. Your goal is to recognize the clinical signs and symptoms of shock in its earliest phase and begin immediate treatment before permanent damage occurs. To do so, you must be aware of the subtle signs exhibited while the body is compensating effectively and treat the patient aggressively **Table 6**. Anticipate the potential for shock from the scene size-up and evaluation of the mechanism of injury (MOI). Recognize the signs of poor perfusion that precede hypotension, and do not rely on any one sign or symptom to determine the phase of shock the patient is going through. Always err on the side of caution when you are treating a potential shock patient. Rapid assessment and immediate transportation are essential to preserve any chance of survival.

Altered mental status changes are late indicators because a key purpose of the shock syndrome is to keep the brain well perfused. Sometimes "alert" patients may be agitated or anxious during the compensated phase but this is not considered an altered mental status.

Compensated Shock

The earliest stage of shock, in which the body can still compensate for blood loss, is called compensated shock. In this phase, the patient's level of responsiveness is a better indicator of tissue perfusion than most other vital signs. Release of chemical mediators by the autonomic nervous system as it recognizes a potential catastrophic event causes the arterial blood pressure to remain normal or slightly elevated. There is an increase in the rate and depth of respirations as the body attempts to bring in more oxygen and remove more carbon dioxide. This effort helps to maintain the acid-base balance by creating respiratory alkalosis to offset the metabolic acidosis.

During the compensated phase of shock, blood pressure is maintained. Blood loss in hemorrhagic shock can be estimated

Table 6 Compensated Versus Decompensated Shock

Compensated Shock	Decompensated Shock
■ Agitation, anxiety, restlessness	■ Altered mental status (verbal to unresponsive)*
■ Sense of impending doom	■ Hypotension
■ Weak, rapid (thready) pulse	■ Labored or irregular breathing
■ Clammy (cool, moist) skin	■ Thready or absent peripheral pulses
■ Pallor with cyanotic lips	■ Ashen, mottled, or cyanotic skin
■ Shortness of breath	
■ Nausea, vomiting	■ Dilated pupils
■ Delayed capillary refill in infants and children	■ Diminished urine output (oliguria)
■ Thirst	■ Impending cardiac arrest
■ Normal blood pressure	

*Mental status changes are late indicators.

to be at 15% to 30% at this point. A narrowing of the pulse pressure (the difference between the systolic and diastolic pressures) also occurs. The pulse pressure reflects the tone of the arterial system and is more sensitive to changes in perfusion than the systolic or diastolic blood pressure alone. Patients in the compensated phase will also have a positive orthostatic tilt test result.

Words of Wisdom

The term orthostatic has to do with positioning. Orthostatic hypotension, for example, is a drop in systolic blood pressure when a person is moved from a sitting to a standing position. An orthostatic tilt test is used to determine dehydration or hypovolemia. Blood pressure and pulse rate are measured as patients are lying, seated, and standing. A positive tilt test result occurs if a patient becomes dizzy, has a pulse rate increase of at least 20 beats/min, or has a systolic blood pressure decrease of at least 20 mm Hg. Remember, if patients are dizzy in the supine position, they will most likely pass out if asked to stand up; lift them to the stretcher!

Decompensated Shock

The next stage of shock, when blood pressure is falling, is decompensated shock (also called uncompensated shock or progressive shock). It occurs when blood volume drops by more than 30%. The compensatory mechanisms begin to fail, and signs and symptoms become much more obvious. The cardiac output falls dramatically, leading to further reductions in blood pressure and cardiac function. The signs and symptoms become more obvious as blood is shunted to the brain, heart, and kidneys. At this point, vasoconstriction can have a disastrous effect if allowed to continue. Cells in the nonperfused tissues become hypoxic, leading to anaerobic metabolism. Treatment at this stage will sometimes result in recovery.

Blood pressure may be the last measurable factor to change in shock. The body has several automatic mechanisms to compensate for initial blood loss and to help maintain blood pressure. Thus, by the time you detect a drop in blood pressure, shock is well developed. This is particularly true in infants and children, whose blood pressure may be maintained until they have lost more than 35% to 40% of their blood volume. In all patients where you suspect shock and they are already hypotensive, consider this an emergency and start transport in less than 10 minutes, providing fluid resuscitation en route to the most appropriate ED.

Irreversible (Terminal) Shock

The last phase of shock, when this condition has progressed to a terminal stage, is irreversible shock. Arterial blood pressure is abnormally low (typically in hemorrhagic shock there is a 40% or greater blood volume loss). A rapid deterioration of the cardiovascular system occurs that cannot be reversed by compensatory mechanisms or medical interventions.

Life-threatening reductions in cardiac output, blood pressure, and tissue perfusion are observed. Blood is shunted away from the liver, kidneys, and lungs to keep the heart and brain perfused. Cells begin to die. Even if the cause of shock is treated and reversed, vital organ damage cannot be repaired, and the patient may eventually die. Providing aggressive treatment at this stage does not usually result in recovery; however, because it is difficult to determine who will or will not survive, you should provide aggressive treatment en route to the trauma center!

Patient Assessment of Shock

Scene Size-up

The general assessment plan of a patient who is suspected of having hypoperfusion or shock follows the plan reinforced throughout this text. Size up the scene for hazards, follow standard precautions, and determine the number of patients and the need for additional or specialized resources.

The size-up also includes a quick assessment of the MOI or nature of illness (NOI). For a patient with suspected shock, this information can give you clues about the causes of non-hemorrhagic shock or the extent of any bleeding (whether internal or external). For example, a patient lying unconscious at the base of a building where a third-floor window is open suggests the possibility that the person fell or was pushed out.

Primary Assessment

Form a General Impression

Start the primary assessment by forming a general impression. How does the patient look to you? Some patients simply do not pass the "look test" and will need to be fast tracked based on the MOI/NOI and the poor impression you have. A patient who is blue or has a sweaty pale look will need your immediate attention. If patients do not greet you as you approach, it may be because they are concentrating on breathing, their injuries, or they are in severe pain. Next, assess the patient's mental status (using AVPU). Introduce yourself and ask if they know their name, where they are, and the day of the week.

Words of Wisdom

If you suspect a cardiac arrest, use a CAB (circulation/compressions, airway, breathing) approach during the primary assessment.

Airway and Breathing

Next, you will need to quickly assess the patient for any threats to airway and breathing. If you suspect cardiac arrest, use the CAB (circulation/compressions, airway, breathing) approach. Otherwise, assess the ABCs (airway, breathing, circulation). If the patient is conscious, listen to the patient speak. Patients with

---

YOU are the Medic: PART 4

You become concerned that peripheral perfusion has become too diminished. You consult medical direction for orders to initiate a vasopressor to increase cardiac output. You receive orders for dopamine (Intropin) with an initial dose of 5 µg/kg/min. You will monitor and titrate as needed to increase cardiac output and systolic blood pressure. Your partner notes the patient's decreasing respirations and indicates he is prepared to intubate. Based on the history of chronic bronchitis, you also consider that your patient has end-stage chronic obstructive pulmonary disease and a hypoxic drive that is failing due to the high concentrations of oxygen. Securing his airway and providing positive-pressure ventilations should allow for controlling his breathing and ensuring adequate oxygenation in the presence of decreased peripheral perfusion. You obtain another set of vital signs prior to initiating intubation.

Recording Time: 15 Minutes	
Skin	Pink, cool, and dry
Pulse	100 beats/min
Blood pressure	72 mm Hg by palpation
Respirations	8 breaths/min and shallow without assistance via bag-mask device
Oxygen saturation (Spo$_2$)	Not obtainable due to poor perfusion
Pupils	Equal, round, and sluggish but reactive to light

7. Why should a patient's hypoxic drive not be a consideration when treating shock?

8. What are the anticipated benefits of dopamine administration for this patient?

life-threatening airway problems cannot speak or they speak in short one- or two-word sentences. If there are any immediate threats to the patient's airway or breathing, manage them immediately. This may involve positioning the unconscious patient's airway (ie, head tilt–chin lift or jaw thrust); clearing the airway of secretions, blood, or vomitus; and administering oxygen. If you suspect there is difficulty breathing, examine the chest for flail segments, impaled objects that need to be stabilized, and holes that need to be sealed with an occlusive dressing. Assess the adequacy of the patient's ventilation in respect to volume and rate, and make a decision if it will be necessary for you to assist the patient with bag-mask ventilation and high-concentration oxygen. Once the airway is open, secure, and breathing is adequate, move on to assess circulation.

Circulation

If you suspect the patient does not have a pulse, you would take the CAB approach and perform chest compressions at this time. With a patient who has a pulse, your approach should be to determine whether the pulse is adequate to sustain life, for now, and then perform a rapid exam to check for external blood loss that you can control.

In conscious patients, you will usually assess the pulse at the radius; in unconscious patients, you will typically check the carotid pulse in the neck. The radial pulse can give you clues about the phase of shock and the patient's ability to compensate for shock. Ask yourself, "Is the radial pulse strong and regular, or weak and thready, or irregular?" If the radial pulse is barely palpable, and yet the patient is sitting up and talking to you with a bullet hole in the abdomen, remember that the purpose of the shock syndrome is to keep the brain perfused—but the reduction in the radial pulse is an indicator to you that the systolic blood pressure is dropping fast. In such a case, you may then decide that you cannot take the time to measure the patient's blood pressure because you already know the patient is hypotensive (indicating decompensated shock) and instead, make the decision to provide immediate transport to the ED.

The rapid exam to determine locations of uncontrolled external bleeding is designed to help you detect an injury that is life threatening and needs to be dealt with immediately. Otherwise, note the patient's skin color, temperature, and condition as you move on to determine the priorities for the patient's condition.

Transport Decision

At this point, all patients need to be prioritized. Patients who are in shock will usually be prioritized as "high." If the shock originates from a medical problem, the patient should be fast-tracked through your elaboration of the chief complaint using OPQRST to an assessment based on the body systems involved. In the more likely case—the patient has experienced some sort of trauma. In the trauma patient, the MOI should guide your assessment of the major body cavities and regions. For example, the patient was standing on a corner at a busy intersection when a truck cut the corner too tight and ran over both her legs. She may have stable vital signs and no immediate life threats, but beware: Given the

typical bleeding from a broken bone—and in this case, there are multiple fractures in both the upper and lower legs—you should suspect significant blood loss for this patient.

History Taking

In a high-priority patient, history taking can be done en route to the ED along with the secondary assessment and the reassessment. Time is of the essence in shock patients; focus on getting to the ED and keep the on-scene care to the essential items that must be done before moving the patient (ie, ABCs and spinal immobilization). Unless the patient is pinned and there may be a delay in extrication, delay establishing IV/IO access until you are en route. Keep in mind that the interventions that add time to the scene time must be justified by the benefits they will produce for the patient.

Secondary Assessment

Shock is considered hypovolemic or hemorrhagic until proven otherwise. **Table 7** summarizes the hemodynamic parameters in the differentiation of shock. The phase of shock in hypovolemic or hemorrhagic shock (compensated, decompensated, or terminal/irreversible) relates to the percentage of blood loss. In the other types of shock, the best indicator that the body is no longer able to compensate is a drop in the systolic blood pressure or altered mental status.

Other indicators you need to pay attention to (in addition to mental status and vital signs) include the end-tidal carbon dioxide ($ETCO_2$) (which is lowered in hypoperfused states) and lactic acid buildup. Lactate is a sign of metabolic distress and is an early indicator of severe sepsis (ie, lactate levels above 4 mmol/dL). Portable lactate monitors are tools traditionally used by elite athletes **Figure 9**. This tool is similar to a glucometer and has been incorporated into sepsis alert programs in cities such as Denver, Colorado. Sepsis alert programs use specific criteria for early sepsis recognition, allowing caregivers to provide more effective care.

Reassessment

This portion of patient assessment is important in patient care. The rule of thumb is to assess, intervene, then reassess. In this portion of the assessment, you revisit the primary assessment, the vital signs, the chief complaint, and any treatment performed on the patient, including oxygen administration. You must reassess the patient to determine whether the interventions you performed are having any effect on the patient. This step prepares you to present the patient at the hospital with a complete, concise account of the patient encounter and care.

You must determine what interventions are needed for your patient at this point based on the findings of your assessment. You should focus on supporting the cardiovascular system. Treating for shock early and aggressively will help to prevent inadequate perfusion from harming your patient. Provide oxygen and put

Table 7   Differentiation of Shock

Characteristics

Origin	Etiology	BP	Pulse	Skin	Lungs	EMS Treatment
↓ Pump performance	Cardiogenic	↓	↓ → ↑	Pale, cool, moist	Crackles	Low-dose dopamine
↓ Fluid volume	Hypovolemic, hemorrhagic	↓	↑	Pale, cool, moist	Clear	IV fluids
Vessels or container dilates: maldistribution of blood; low peripheral resistance	Neurogenic	↓	↓	Flushed, dry, warm	Clear	IV fluids, atropine, high-dose dopamine
	Septic	↓	↑	Flushed or pale, hot or cool, moist	Crackles if pulmonary origin	IV fluids, high-dose dopamine
	Anaphylactic	↓	↑	Flushed, warm, moist	May have wheezes; may be ↓ with no sounds	Epinephrine Diphenhydramine, albuterol, ipratropium, corticosteroids

Hemodynamic Parameters

Parameter	Hypovolemic	Cardiac	Neurogenic	Septic
Mean arterial pressure	↓	↓	↓	↓
Pulse rate	↑	↑ or ↓	↓	↑
Central venous pressure	↓	Variable	↓	↑
Cardiac output	↓	↓	↓	↑ then ↓
Peripheral vascular resistance	↑	↑	↓	↑
pH	↓	↓	↓	↓
Pao_2	↓	↓	↓	↓
$Paco_2$	↓	↓	Increase and decrease the rate	↓

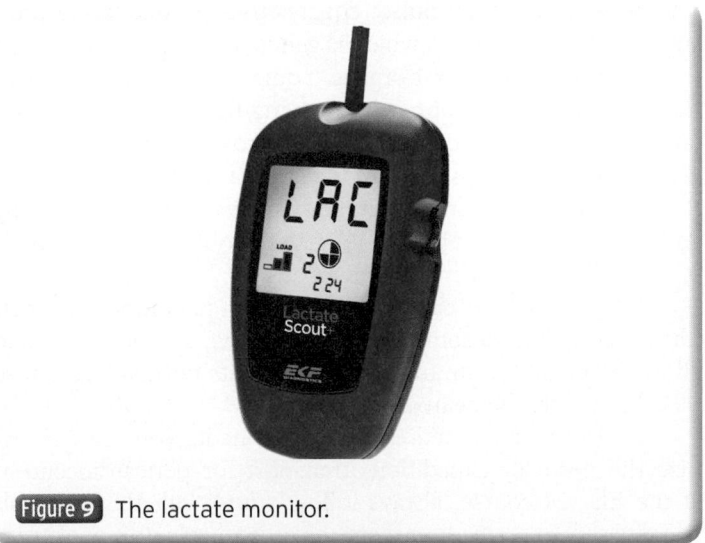

Figure 9 The lactate monitor.

the patient in the position dictated by local protocol for shock patients. Provide warmth, gain IV access, and administer fluid as needed based on patient presentation. Specific interventions

are discussed in the emergency medical care section later in this chapter.

Patients who are in decompensated shock will need rapid interventions to restore adequate perfusion. The hospital may or may not have suggestions on how best to support a patient's failing cardiovascular system. Most of the interventions used to treat shock do not require a specific physician's order; however, some do. Determine, based on the signs and symptoms found in your assessment, whether your patient is in compensated or decompensated shock. Document these findings after you have treated for shock.

■ Special Considerations for Assessing Shock

Healthy, fit, young adults usually are well prepared to combat a situation of life-threatening blood loss. When young adults stay fit through aerobic exercise, their cardiovascular system is resilent and their heart's stroke volume is usually larger than the average patient. In addition, keeping their weight within the normal range for their height and consuming a diet low in salt, fats, and cholesterol help prepare the body to handle the effects of the epinephrine and norepinephrine released during compensated shock. Their blood vessels can handle the vasoconstriction of the body's pecking order without developing clots, and arteries are generally free of obstructions such as plaque. Being a nonsmoker also contributes to better oxygenation when extra cardiac output is needed to combat the challenges of shock. If you want to be best prepared to deal with life-threatening blood loss, review the Simple 7 material covered in the chapter, *Workforce Safety and Wellness*.

Pediatric Considerations

When you are managing pediatric patients, remember that their bodies can compensate well until they have lost about 30% to 35% of their blood volume; then their condition declines rapidly. In pediatric patients, their ability to compensate relies on increasing their pulse rate and systemic vascular resistance. However, this causes the body to burn glucose rapidly, and pediatric patients have little glucose in storage. Pediatric patients are able to compensate through vasoconstriction and are able to increase their pulmonary vascular resistance (PVR) up to the point where not enough blood is perfused to the brain, heart, and lungs to keep them alive. Treat pediatric patients aggressively and early if there is a significant MOI or any indication of developing shock. You should never wait to see a drop in the systolic blood pressure to be aggressive in the management of a child you suspect may be in the early phase of shock. You should provide oxygen, manage the body temperature, place the patient in the appropriate position, and initiate IV access en route to the appropriate facility. See the chapter, *Pediatric Emergencies*, for more information on pediatric patients and shock.

Geriatric Considerations

When you are treating elderly patients, remember that their ability to manage a loss of blood volume is diminished. Vasoconstriction is less effective and their renal and vascular systems cannot effectively handle infusion of large volumes of fluid. Thermoregulation is less effective in the elderly and many of these patients have a history of smoking, leading to chronic obstructive pulmonary disease (COPD). When elderly patients receive significant burns, their survival is about half that of a younger adult because their bodies cannot handle the calories needed to heal a burn injury as well as the tremendous fluid volumes needed for resuscitation. Fluid therapy should be carefully managed by administering fluid boluses and reassessing the patient, including the lung sounds. Be aware that the anemic patient starts off at a disadvantage for managing shock. Older patients may also have cardiovascular disorders or diabetes, affecting their body's ability to compensate when confronted with shock (ie, warafin). Finally, these patients may be on blood-thinning medications (warfarin) that prevent them from forming clots to major injuries (a fractured leg can bleed significantly). Minor bleeding (ie, nosebleed) can also be a serious issue when a patient is on a blood-thinning medication.

■ Emergency Medical Care of a Patient With Suspected Shock

As with any patient, airway and ventilatory support take top priority when you are treating a patient with suspected shock. Maintain an open airway, and suction as needed. Administer high-flow supplemental oxygen via a nonrebreathing mask or assist ventilation with a bag-mask device. Consider early definitive management in patients who are unable to maintain their own airway. Control any external hemorrhage, and try to estimate the amount of blood lost. Look for signs of internal hemorrhage, and consider the potential for loss in the area of suspected hemorrhage. For example, a patient may lose as much as a liter of blood in the tissues of the thigh in a closed, uncomplicated femur fracture. Consider the MOI, and maintain a high index of suspicion for occult injuries, especially when the patient has signs of shock (ie, tachycardia, dizziness, pallor, thirst) with no obvious cause.

IV fluid therapy can be helpful in supplementing the initial therapies; however, this should be done en route to the ED so as to not prolong the time at the scene, especially when you are managing a patient who is actively bleeding. While en route, establish IV access with two large-bore catheters (14 or 16 gauge) and administer IV volume expanders to replace blood loss. Isotonic crystalloids, such as normal saline or lactated Ringer's, should be used (synthetic solutions may also be used). If the patient is trapped or the extrication will be delayed, it is reasonable to begin IV fluid resuscitation at the scene. Solutions of dextrose in water are not effective for resuscitation of trauma patients and as such, most EMS systems have removed them from their protocols. The goal of volume replacement is to maintain perfusion without increasing internal or uncontrollable external hemorrhage. For this reason, most protocols advise administration of IV fluid in boluses of 20 mL/kg until radial pulses return. The presence of radial pulses equates to a systolic blood pressure of 80 to 90 mm Hg, which is generally sufficient to perfuse the brain and other vital organs. Some studies suggest a permissive hypotensive approach involving fluid therapy to maintain the systolic blood pressure at approximately 80 mm Hg. This is thought to be safer for the patient than to attempt restoration of normotension, which may aggravate ongoing bleeding and also release clots that would cause problems in other parts of the circulatory system or vital organs.

If the patient exhibits signs of a tension pneumothorax, perform needle chest decompression to improve cardiac output and allow the mediastinum to shift back into its normal location so blood can enter the heart.

In cases of suspected cardiac tamponade, you must recognize the need for expeditious transport for pericardiocentesis at the ED. Of course, always follow your local ALS protocols because some paramedic systems have received additional training to provide these skills. Both of these conditions further impair circulation by compressing the heart and decreasing cardiac output.

Nonpharmacologic interventions for shock include proper positioning of the patient, prevention of hypothermia, and rapid transport. Apply the cardiac monitor, and be alert for possible dysrhythmias. When you are making your transport decision, consider the need for a regional trauma center. If travel time is lengthy, air medical transportation may be the best option. Provide psychological support en route; even unresponsive patients can sometimes hear and understand. Speak calmly and reassuringly to the patient throughout assessment, care, and transport.

Skill Drill 1 provides a basic review of shock management:

Skill Drill   1

1. Follow standard precautions. Make sure the patient has an open airway, maintain manual stabilization if necessary, and check breathing and pulse rate. In general, keep the patient in a supine position Step 1 . Patients who have experienced a severe heart attack or who have lung disease may find it easier to breathe in the Fowler's or semi-Fowler's position. Never allow the patient to eat or drink anything prior to being evaluated in the ED.

2. Control all obvious external bleeding Step 2 . Refer to the chapter, *Bleeding*, for more information.

3. Splint bone or joint injuries to minimize pain, bleeding, and discomfort, all of which can aggravate shock Step 3 . Splinting also prevents the ends of the broken bone from further damaging adjacent soft tissue and, in general, makes it easier to move the patient. To minimize time spent on the scene, you may use a long backboard as a temporary splint until you are headed to the ED. Handle the patient gently and no more than is necessary.

4. Always provide supplemental oxygen, assist with ventilation as needed, and use airway control adjuncts as needed. Continue to monitor the patient's breathing. To prevent the loss of body heat, place blankets under and over the patient Step 4 . Do not overload the patient with covers or attempt to warm the body too much, however; the goal is to maintain a normal body temperature. Do not use external heat sources, such as hot water bottles or heating pads because they may cause vasodilation and decrease blood pressure even more.

5. Once you have positioned the patient on a backboard or a stretcher, consider placing him or her in the Trendelenburg position if your local protocols allow. This position is easily accomplished by raising the foot of the backboard or stretcher about 6 in to 12 in. Raising the lower extremities any higher may aggravate a patient's breathing because the abdominal organs push against the diaphragm. If the patient is not on a backboard and no lower extremity fractures are suspected, place the patient in the position dictated by local protocol for shock patients. Do not use the Trendelenburg or shock position for patients who have associated chest injury or intra-abdominal injury, which may be aggravated by causing the abdominal contents to push against the diaphragm and further impair breathing. These positions may help to return blood from the extremities back to the core of the body, where it is needed most.

6. En route to the ED, insert at least one, and preferably two, large-bore peripheral IV lines (14 to 16 gauge), using an over-the-needle catheter. Obtain IV access at the scene only if transport of the patient is delayed (such as if the patient is pinned).

7. If allowed by protocol, draw blood (two red-top blood collection [Vacutainer] tubes and one purple-top tube) so that ED personnel may obtain a hematocrit, type- and cross-match, and other tests immediately on your arrival Step 5 .

8. Unless local protocol favors a different resuscitation fluid, administer isotonic crystalloids of normal saline or lactated Ringer's solution in 250- to 500-mL increments to maintain systolic blood pressure in low normal ranges. Many trauma surgeons prefer lactated Ringer's over normal saline because lactated Ringer's may help decrease the acidosis in patients with severe hemorrhagic hypovolemia. However, this belief remains controversial and either solution will benefit the patient. The use of hypertonic saline, 5 mL/kg of 7.5% sodium chloride, in 250-mL increments may also be effective in treating hypovolemic shock caused by hemorrhage. Studies have shown that hypertonic solutions may optimize blood pressure, cardiac output, intracranial pressure, and microvascular flow without increasing bleeding or causing volume overload. However, there has been no change in survival rates compared with standard fluid resuscitation. More research in this area may change the face of fluid therapy, but for now, most disciplines in the United States continue to use isotonic crystalloid therapy.

In addition to the basic treatment of suspected shock, you will provide fluid therapy, airway management, and pharmacologic interventions (ie, antiemetics, pain relief, volume expanders, sympathomimetics) as guided by your local protocols.

■ IV Therapy

Intravenous lines are inserted for one of three purposes: (1) to provide a route for *immediate replacement* of fluid in patients who have already lost significant volumes of fluid or blood, (2) to provide a route for *potential replacement* in patients who are at risk of losing significant volumes of fluid or blood, and (3) to provide a route for the administration of medication. The IV fluid of choice will be normal saline or lactated Ringer's.

Specifically, all patients in hypovolemic shock need IV fluid replacement. In addition, IV access should be obtained in patients who are likely to develop hypovolemic shock because they have one or more of the following conditions: profuse external bleeding, internal bleeding, ulcer (vomiting blood or blood in the stool), vaginal bleeding, blunt trauma to the abdomen, fracture of the pelvis or femur, severe or widespread burns, heat exhaustion, intractable vomiting or diarrhea, and neurogenic shock or septic shock.

In case of need for emergency administration of drugs, IV lines should also be inserted to keep a vein open. When a

Skill Drill | 1

Basic Treatment of Suspected Shock

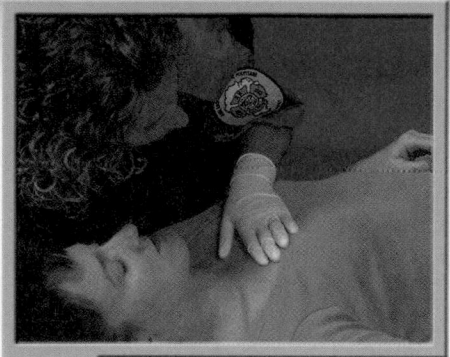

Step 1 Keep the patient supine, open the airway, and check breathing and pulse.

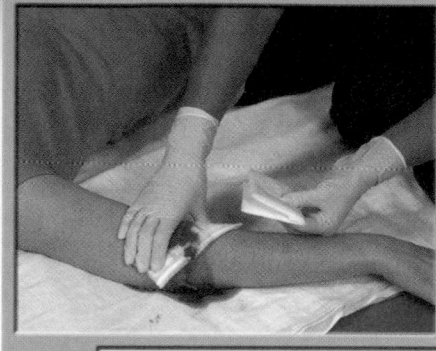

Step 2 Control obvious external bleeding.

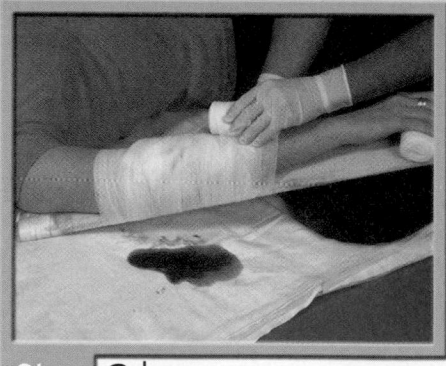

Step 3 Splint broken bones and joint injuries.

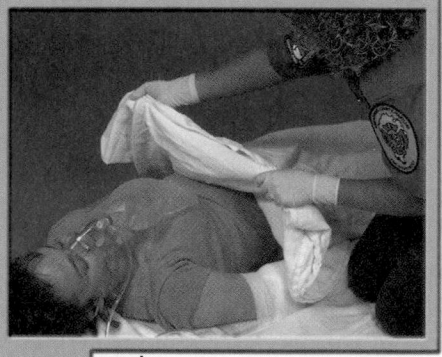

Step 4 Administer high-flow supplemental oxygen, and assist ventilations as needed. Place blankets under and over the patient.

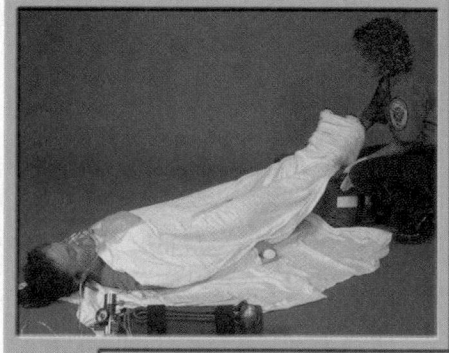

Step 5 If no fractures are suspected and local protocol allows, consider Trendelenburg positioning by elevating the foot of the backboard or stretcher 6 in to 12 in. Obtain IV or IO access, and administer warm fluid en route to the ED. If allowed by protocol, draw blood.

patient has poor cardiac output (as in shock), blood is shunted away from the skin and skeletal muscles. Thus, drugs administered subcutaneously or intramuscularly are absorbed at a low and unpredictable rate. Giving a drug directly into the vein ensures that the desired dose of the drug reaches the circulation. The IV fluid that had traditionally been used to keep the vein open was D_5W. However, most EMS services have stopped carrying D_5W, and carry only normal saline. Patients who need a vein kept open include those at risk of cardiac arrest (it is easier to start the IV line before the arrest) and patients who may need

parenteral medication (such as patients with seizures, diabetes, congestive heart failure, or coma).

The IV flow rate is typically determined by local protocol. The decision on flow rates usually reflects the patient's presumptive diagnosis and the condition of his or her lungs (wet or dry), and takes into account whether the IV line was inserted to keep the vein open for future medication administration. **Table 8** shows the blood pressure indicators that are often referenced when determining IV flow rates for patients with dry lungs (not pulmonary edema).

Table 8 IV Fluid Therapy

Adult Systolic BP (mm Hg)	Fluid Volume (presumes dry lungs)*
Normotensive (100 to 130; higher end depends on age)	Fluid challenge not needed unless signs/symptoms suggestive of shock
Hypotensive (80 to 90)	Fluid challenge of 20 mL/kg normal saline, and reevaluate patient for further infusion
Severe hypotension (50 to 80)	Fluid challenge of 1 L normal saline, then titrate additional fluid boluses of 20 mL/kg to achieve low end or normotensive state

*Fluid therapy for burn patients should follow the Parkland formula (see the chapter, *Burns*).

Volume Expanders and Plasma Substitutes

Hypovolemic shock should be treated with volume expanders to replace what has been lost or to "fill the container" in relative hypovolemia. For cardiogenic shock, cautious use of volume expanders may increase preload and, subsequently, cardiac output. Positive cardiac inotropic drugs may be administered to increase the strength of contractions, along with rate-altering medications to further enhance perfusion. An example is epinephrine, which serves both purposes with its beta-1 effects.

The vasodilation that accompanies distributive shock creates relative hypovolemia. Treatment involves volume expanders and positive cardiac inotropic drugs. Volume expanders are also indicated for obstructive shock and spinal shock.

A variety of macromolecular solutions have colloidal and osmotic properties similar to those of plasma and are used to maintain circulatory volume in the emergency treatment of shock. Although such solutions cannot replace the RBCs, platelets, or plasma proteins lost in hemorrhage, they are more readily available than whole blood or plasma in an emergency because they do not require typing and can be carried in the ambulance. Furthermore, during multiple-casualty incidents, the supply of blood and blood products may not be adequate, and substitutes must be used. Plasma substitutes do not carry the risk of hepatitis or acquired immunodeficiency syndrome. Available plasma substitutes and volume expanders include dextran (Gentran), plasma protein fractions, and polygeline.

Dextran is a high-molecular-weight glucose polymer that stays in the vascular space because of its large size. Because it tends to coat RBCs, this substance may cause clotting problems if given in large quantities, and it can also interfere with the cross-matching of blood. For that reason, blood for type- and cross-matching should be drawn *before* administration of dextran. Dextran also interferes with platelet function, so it may increase bleeding. Given that virtually no prehospital research shows dextran to be superior to crystalloid solution administration, medical directors are not likely to approve its use in the field at this time.

Plasma protein fraction (Plasmanate) contains mainly albumin plus a small amount of serum globulin. It is an excellent plasma substitute but is expensive and has been reported to produce hypotensive reactions in some patients.

Polygeline (Haemaccel), hetastarch (Hespan), and other starch solutions are constituted to resemble the osmotic and electrolyte composition of the plasma and do not interfere with clotting or blood typing. Many of these products have long shelf lives and may be ideally suited for prehospital use once research proves them effective in improving patient outcomes.

Crystalloids

Crystalloids are solutions that do not contain proteins or other large molecules; that is, they are noncolloids. Their effects in restoring volume in shock are usually quite transitory because the fluid rapidly equilibrates across the capillary walls into the tissues. For example, approximately 60% of infused normal saline, when given as a bolus, diffuses out of the intravascular space within 20 minutes of administration. Thus, when noncolloid solutions are used in the treatment of hemorrhagic shock, you need to administer two to three times the volume of blood lost.

Crystalloids are clearly the fluids of choice when only salt and water have been lost, such as in dehydration. Debate continues, however, about the role of crystalloids versus colloids in the treatment of shock. Despite a great deal of research on the subject, no overwhelming evidence supports one therapeutic approach over the other. Until such evidence is forthcoming, practical considerations will continue to favor the use of crystalloids for initial fluid resuscitation in the field.

The crystalloids most commonly used for that purpose are normal saline and lactated Ringer's solution. Normal saline is simply sodium chloride (0.9% NaCl) in water at a concentration isotonic with the extracellular fluid. Lactated Ringer's solution is similarly constituted but includes small amounts of potassium and calcium. Lactated Ringer's solution contains 28 mEq of lactate as well, which is added as a buffer (the liver breaks lactate down into bicarbonate). Many trauma surgeons prefer lactated Ringer's over normal saline because lactated Ringer's may help decrease the acidosis in patients with severe hemorrhagic hypovolemia. However, this belief remains controversial and either solution will benefit the patient.

There is a limit on the usefulness of crystalloids because they do not carry oxygen, change the viscosity of the blood by thinning it, and dissolve the clotting factors. Thus, most ALS protocols limit the number of liters administered to the patient (two or three) and then will switch to blood products administered in the ED.

■ Pathophysiology, Assessment, and Management of Specific Types of Shock

The three primary classifications of shock coincide with the conditions that cause them: cardiogenic, distributive, and hypovolemic.

Cardiogenic shock results from a weakening pumping action of the heart. Distributive shock, which is characterized as a relative hypovolemia, can be further broken down into chemical and neural causes. Septic shock results from fluid shifts associated with massive infections and poisons resulting in vasodilation. Neurogenic shock results from blood vessel dilation caused by a brain or spinal/nerve injury, also causing vasodilation. There are also other conditions that decrease tissue perfusion, indirectly affecting the cardiovascular system. Among these are the conditions that obstruct the flow of oxygen into the bloodstream and into the starving tissue, leading to obstructive shock. Conditions that produce obstructive shock include tension pnuemothorax, cardiac tamponade, pulmonary embolism, airway obstruction, and carbon monoxide poisoning. Whereas hypovolemic shock reduces the total fluid in the body, hemorrhagic shock, a form of hypovolemic shock, is a direct result of blood loss. Refer to the chapter, *Bleeding*, for more information on hemorrhagic shock. The non-hemorrhagic causes of hypovolemic shock (eg, severe burns, heatstroke, gastroenteritis), discussed in this chapter, are commonly grouped by how they reduce perfusion. These types of shock involve either a weakening of the pump, an increase in the size of the container, or a direct mechanical interference with the circulation. The initial management is the same for each type of shock and includes the following steps:

1. Manage the airway.
2. Administer supplemental oxygen.

3. Put the patient in a position of comfort (some regions still use Trendelenburg).
4. Obtain vital signs, Spo$_2$, lung sounds, and a 12-lead ECG.
5. Obtain IV access for medication or fluid bolus.
6. Maintain body heat.

Additional management may be necessary Table 9 :

Words of Wisdom

The Weil-Shubin classification considers shock from a mechanistic point of view. From this perspective, two types of shock are distinguished: <u>central shock</u>, which consists of cardiogenic shock and obstructive shock, and <u>peripheral shock</u>, which includes hypovolemic shock and distributive shock.

Cardiogenic Shock

<u>Cardiogenic shock</u> occurs when the heart is unable to circulate sufficient blood to maintain adequate peripheral oxygen delivery. Circulation of blood throughout the vascular system requires the constant pumping action of a normal and vigorous heart muscle. Many diseases can cause destruction or inflammation of this muscle. Within certain limits, the heart can adapt to

YOU *are the Medic*   PART 5

You prepare to intubate your patient nasally due to the presence of spontaneous respirations and a positive gag reflex. The patient is intubated with lubrication without difficulty using the Beck Airway Airflow Monitor (BAAM) device on the tube. You confirm tube placement by auscultation and initiation of end-tidal carbon dioxide monitoring. The tube is secured and connected to the automated transport ventilator. You reassess all vital signs including cardiac rhythm and decide to obtain a 12-lead ECG to see if the patient may have also had a myocardial infarction. Your patient continues to be in a sinus tachycardia. You are aware that dopamine is a sympathomimetic and may precipitate ventricular dysrhythmias so you continue to monitor your patient closely. Once you have completed your reassessment, you contact the receiving facility to report on your patient. On arrival you carefully transfer your patient to the ED stretcher in the assigned room. You provide a bedside report as the patient is transitioned to the hospital's equipment and monitors. You complete your patient care report while your partner prepares the ambulance for the next call.

Recording Time: 20 Minutes	
Skin	Pale and cool
Pulse	104 beats/min
Blood pressure	76/48 mm Hg
Respirations	12 breaths/min via ETT using an ATV
Oxygen saturation (Spo$_2$)	99% on 100% oxygen
End-tidal carbon dioxide	42 mm Hg

9. What is the benefit of assessing lung compliance in the ventilated shock patient?

10. Discuss how your assessment findings for this patient led you to a differential field diagnosis of septic shock.

Table 9 Types of Shock

Type of Shock	Examples of Potential Causes	Signs and Symptoms	Assessment and Treatment (beyond initial 6 steps presented above)
Cardiogenic	Inadequate heart function Disease of muscle tissue Impaired electrical system Disease or injury	Chest pain Irregular pulse Weak pulse Low blood pressure Cyanosis (lips, under nails) Cool, clammy skin Anxiety Rales Pulmonary edema	If lungs are clear and protocols allow, administer a fluid challenge of 200 mL (to increase preload) Consider CPAP/BiPAP

Obstructive	Mechanical obstruction of the cardiac muscle causing a decrease in cardiac output
	1. Tension pneumothorax
	2. Cardiac tamponade
		Dependent on cause:
		■ Dyspnea
		■ Rapid, weak pulse
		■ Rapid, shallow breaths
		■ Decreased lung compliance
		■ Unilateral, decreased, or absent breath sounds
		■ Decreased blood pressure
		■ Jugular vein distention
		■ Subcutaneous emphysema
		■ Cyanosis
		■ Tracheal deviation toward affected side
		■ Beck triad (cardiac tamponade):
		  – Jugular vein distention
		  – Narrowing pulse pressure
		  – Muffled heart tones
			Dependent on cause:
			■ Administer fluid at a KVO rate
			■ Consider chest decompression (injured side for suspected tension pneumothorax)
			■ Consider pericardiocentesis for cardiac tamponade if appropriately trained and authorized by protocol

Septic	Severe bacterial infection	Warm skin Tachycardia Low blood pressure	Administer fluid boluses to maintain radial pulses Consider sepsis alert program if protocol exists in your region. Consider medications depending on the existence of warm versus cold shock
Neurogenic	Cervical or thoracic spinal card injury, which causes widespread blood vessel dilation	Bradycardia (slow pulse) or normal pulse Low blood pressure Signs of neck injury	Administer warmed IV fluids to maintain radial pulses Consider vasopressors, steroids, or vagal blocker per local protocols
Anaphylactic	Extreme life-threatening allergic reaction	Can develop within seconds Mild itching or rash Burning skin Vascular dilation Generalized edema Coma Rapid death	Determine cause of anaphylaxis Administer epinephrine IM or a vasopressor Administer fluid at a KVO rate Consider bronchodilator or antihistamine
Psychogenic (fainting)	Temporary, generalized vascular dilation Anxiety, bad news, sight of injury or blood, prospect of medical treatment, severe pain, illness, tiredness	Rapid pulse Normal or low blood pressure	Determine duration of unresponsiveness Suspect head injury if patient is confused or slow to respond

Continues

Table 9 Types of Shock, *continued*

Type of Shock	Examples of Potential Causes	Signs and Symptoms	Assessment and Treatment (beyond initial 6 steps presented above)
Hypovolemic	Loss of blood or fluid	Rapid, weak pulse Low blood pressure Change in mental status Cyanosis (lips, under nails) Cool, clammy skin Increased respiratory rate	Control external bleeding Provide fluid resuscitation en route Consider use of vasopressors to maintain the blood pressure
Respiratory insufficiency	Severe chest injury, airway obstruction	Rapid, weak pulse Low blood pressure Change in mental status Cyanosis (lips, under nails) Cool, clammy skin Increased respiratory rate	Seal hole in chest Stabilize flail segments/impaled objects Administer fluid at a KVO rate

these problems. If too much muscular damage occurs, however, the heart no longer functions effectively. Filling is impaired because of a lack of pressure to return blood to the heart (preload), or outflow is obstructed by a lack of pumping function. In either case, direct pump failure is the cause of shock. In the case of ischemic heart disease, pump failure is generally due to a loss of 40% or more of the functioning myocardium.

The most common cause of cardiogenic shock is an AMI accompanied by 40% dysfunction of the left ventricle. Anterior infarcts more commonly lead to cardiogenic shock than do inferior ones. Studies show that 50% of the patients who develop cardiogenic shock as a complication of AMI do so within the first 24 hours. Other causes of cardiogenic shock may be right ventricular failure, valvular disorders, cardiomyopathies, ventricular septal defects, papillary muscle rupture, myocardial insufficiency, and sustained dysrhythmias. Some experts consider ventricular fibrillation as the ultimate form of cardiogenic shock. The causes may be classified as intrinsic or extrinsic, with the aforementioned examples being intrinsic causes. These conditions manifest with poor contractility, decreased cardiac output, or impaired ventricular filling. Extrinsic causes of cardiogenic shock include pericardial tamponade, effusion, pulmonary emboli, and tension pneumothorax. Cardiogenic shock may occur in approximately 5% to 8% of patients admitted to the hospital following an AMI. Populations at the greatest risk of developing cardiogenic shock are elderly patients, patients with a history of diabetes mellitus, and patients with a history of AMI with an ejection fraction of less than 35%. Ejection fraction is the portion of the blood ejected from the ventricle during systole. Normal ejection fraction is 55% to 70% of the blood in your heart leaving the left ventricle. This is measured with an echocardiogram, MRI, or CT of the heart, or during cardiac catherization.

The diagnosis of cardiogenic shock may be difficult to make in the field. Once the diagnosis has been made in a definitive setting, newer treatment modalities (ie, medications such as super aspirins, blood thinners, inotropic agents, fibrinolytics, surgical procedures such as angioplasty and stenting, coronary artery bypass, and insertion of a ventricular assist device) have greatly improved the long-term prognosis.

Prolonged efforts to stabilize the condition of a patient in cardiogenic shock in the field are not recommended. Because this is a time-sensitive patient, you should expedite transport as quickly as possible. Place the patient in a position of comfort, secure the airway, monitor the SpO_2, and administer supplemental oxygen via a nonrebreathing mask at 12 to 15 L/min. Consider CPAP/BiPAP. Apply ECG electrodes, document the initial rhythm, and obtain a 12-lead ECG. IV access should consist of administration of a crystalloid solution. Auscultate the lungs; if they are clear and protocols allow, try a fluid challenge of 200 mL to increase the preload and evaluate the effects on the blood pressure and lung sounds.

Some EMS systems advocate the use of dopamine (Intropin) at low doses in the beta range (5 μg/kg/min) if the patient has a MAP of less than 60 mm Hg. Elevating the blood pressure by using high-dose dopamine in the alpha range may be temporarily ordered by medical control at the expense of other target organs. In such a case, anticipate rapid tachycardia that could adversely impact ventricular filling. Combination drug therapy is often needed at the hospital (eg, dopamine plus dobutamine, or norepinephrine) while awaiting cardiac catheterization, hemodynamic monitoring catheters, and insertion of an intra-aortic balloon pump.

Obstructive Shock

Obstructive causes of shock are those not directly associated with loss of fluid, pump failure, or vessel dilation. <u>Obstructive shock</u> occurs when blood flow in the heart or great vessels becomes blocked. Two of the most common examples of obstructive shock causes in trauma are tension pneumothorax and cardiac tamponade. Others include a pulmonary embolus, which can block the oxygen from entering the bloodstream through the alveoli, or carbon monoxide poisoning, which can block the oxygen from loading into the RBCs as they pass through the lungs.

Tension Pneumothorax

Tension pneumothorax is caused by damage to the lung tissue. This damage allows air normally held within the lung to escape into the chest cavity. If a pneumothorax is allowed to continue untreated, a sufficient amount of air will accumulate within the chest cavity and begin applying pressure to the structures of the mediastinum. When the trapped air begins to shift the chest organs toward the uninjured side, a pneumothorax becomes known as a tension pneumothorax. A pneumothorax is a respiratory problem but a tension pneumothorax is a serious and life-threatening condition because the kinking of the vena cava that occurs as the mediastinum shifts can precede cardiac arrest. Usually the only action that can prevent eventual death from a tension pneumothorax is decompression of the injured side of the chest, relieving the pressure in the chest cavity and allowing the heart to expand fully again. Fortunately, needle chest decompression is a skill many providers are allowed to perform. The decision to decompress the chest should always be based on good evidence that a tension pneumothorax exists with decreased perfusion. See the chapter, *Chest Trauma*, for more information on this procedure.

Cardiac Tamponade

Cardiac tamponade is another traumatic condition that leads to obstructive shock. It is caused by blunt or penetrating trauma, tumors, or pericarditis and can progress quickly. Cardiac tamponade occurs when blood leaks into the tough fibrous membrane known as the pericardium, causing an accumulation of blood within the pericardial sac.

Blood accumulates quickly within the pericardium. This accumulation of leaked blood leads to compression of the heart. Because the pericardium has minimal ability to stretch, each contraction of the heart allows more blood accumulation betweeen the heart and the sac. This accumulated blood prevents the heart from opening up to allow complete refilling. Continued pressure within the pericardial sac obstructs the flow of blood into the heart, resulting in decreased outflow from the heart. You may note electrical alternans and a small QRS on the ECG as this condition is developing.

The ultimate treatment for cardiac tamponade is pericardiocentesis, which involves inserting a needle attached to a syringe into the chest far enough to penetrate the pericardium and then withdrawing fluid. This technique is risky, however, and medical control rarely allows it to be performed by paramedics. Early recognition along with rapid transport is the key treatment available to providers. As always, follow your local ALS protocols. Vital clues that a cardiac tamponade is present include muffled heart sounds and systolic and diastolic blood pressures starting to merge (ie, the systolic drops and the distolic rises). This is a serious and life-threatening condition.

◼ Distributive Shock

Distributive shock occurs when there is widespread dilation of the resistance vessels (small arterioles), the capacitance vessels (small venules), or both. As a result, the circulating blood volume pools in the expanded vascular beds and tissue perfusion decreases. The four most common types of distributive shock are septic shock, neurogenic shock, anaphylactic shock, and psychogenic shock.

Septic Shock

Sepsis comes from the Greek word *sepein* meaning "to putrefy." Septic shock is defined as the presence of sepsis syndrome plus a systolic blood pressure of less than 90 mm Hg or a decrease from the baseline blood pressure of more than 40 mm Hg.

Sepsis occurs as a result of widespread infection, usually due to gram-negative bacterial organisms; gram-positive bacteria, fungi, viruses, and rickettsia can also be causative agents. Complex interactions occur between the pathogen and the body's defense systems. Initially, the body's defense mechanisms may keep the infection under control. The infection activates the inflammatory-immune response, which invokes humoral, cellular, and biochemical pathways. This response results in increased microvascular permeability (leaky capillaries), vasodilation, third-space fluid shifts, and microthrombi formation. In some patients, an uncontrolled and unregulated inflammatory-immune response occurs, resulting in hypoperfusion to the cells owing to opening of arteriovenous shunts, tissue destruction, and organ death. Left untreated, the result is multiple-organ dysfunction syndrome and, often, death.

Septic shock is a complex problem. First, there is an insufficient volume of fluid in the container, because much of the blood has leaked out of the vascular system (hypovolemia). Second, the fluid that leaks out often collects in the respiratory system, interfering with ventilation. Third, a larger-than-normal vascular bed is asked to contain the smaller-than-normal volume of intravascular fluid.

Septic shock presents similarly to hemorrhagic shock in that the patient will have a weak, thready pulse; shallow, rapid respirations; and altered mental status. One major difference is that patients with septic shock usually present with warm or hot skin due to the elevated core body temperature associated with the infection.

The proper treatment of septic shock requires complex hospital management, including antibiotics. If you suspect that a patient has septic shock, you must use appropriate standard precautions and transport as promptly as possible. Use high-flow oxygen during transport. Ventilatory support may be necessary to maintain adequate tidal volume. If the patient is normotensive after initial fluid therapy, dopamine (Intropin) is used to maintain the blood pressure and renal perfusion. If the patient remains hypotensive and vasodilated in "warm" shock, norepinephrine is the appropriate intervention. If the patient remains hypotensive and vasoconstricted in "cold" shock, epinephrine is the most appropriate course of action. Consider medications depending on the existence of warm versus cold shock. Use blankets to conserve body heat. Gain IV or IO access en route and administer fluid boluses to maintain radial pulses.

Neurogenic Shock

Neurogenic shock usually results from spinal cord injury. Less commonly, it may derive from medical causes such as brain conditions, tumors, or pressure on the spinal cord.

The effect of these conditions is loss of normal sympathetic nervous system tone and vasodilation.

In neurogenic shock, the muscles in the walls of the blood vessels are cut off from the nerve impulses that cause them to contract. As a consequence, all vessels below the level of the spinal injury dilate widely, increasing the size and capacity of the vascular system and causing blood to pool. There may actually be visible lines of demarcation on the skin found in the patient with spinal shock. The available 5 to 6 L of blood in the body can no longer fill this enlarged vascular system. Perfusion of organs and tissues becomes inadequate, even though no blood or fluid has been lost, and shock occurs. The patient experiences relative hypovolemia, which leads to hypotension (systolic blood pressure usually between 80 and 100 mm Hg). In addition, relative bradycardia occurs because the sympathetic nervous system is not stimulated to release catecholamines. The skin is pink, warm, and dry because of cutaneous vasodilation. There is no release of epinephrine and norepinephrine, which would otherwise produce the classic sign of pale, cool, diaphoretic skin. Instead, a characteristic sign of neurogenic shock is the absence of sweating below the level of injury.

The term **spinal shock** refers to the local neurologic condition that occurs after a spinal injury produces motor and sensory losses (which may not be permanent). Damage to the spinal cord, particularly at the upper cervical levels, may cause significant injury to the autonomic nervous system, which controls the size and muscular tone of the blood vessels. Swelling and edema of the cord begin within 30 minutes after an insult, creating a "physiologic" transaction with nerve conduction disruption. Secondary cord injury, aside from the initial lesions, often develops over the first few days due to the ischemic spinal cord tissue. Severe pain may be present just above the level of injury owing to a zone of heightened sensitivity. Spinal shock is characterized by flaccid paralysis, flaccid sphincters, and absent reflexes. There is an absence of all pain, temperature, touch, proprioception, and pressure below the level of the lesion; absent or impaired thermoregulation; absent somatic and visceral sensations below the lesion; bowel distention; and loss of peristalsis. The level of the injury to the cord is related to the severity of neurogenic shock development. Injury above the T-1 level can disrupt all the spinal tracts that control the entire sympathetic system. Injuries from T-1 to L-3 may only partially interrupt sympathetic outflow. The higher the level of the injury, the more severe and the more likely the patient will develop spinal shock.

The care of a patient with suspected neurogenic shock is similar to the general management approach for any patient with shock. In addition, the patient should be immobilized to minimize further movement and injury to the spine. Specific concerns relate to keeping the patient warm because a spinal injury can disrupt the thermoregulatory mechanisms and leave the patient vulnerable to hypothermia.

Another specific concern relates to the issue of fluid therapy. You should determine the necessity for IV fluids based on the patient's hemodynamic status. Maintain adequate hydration and volume status to keep the systolic blood pressure at 90 mm Hg or higher. General hemodynamic resuscitation includes volume loading with normal saline IV fluid boluses in 20-mL/kg increments up to 2 L through a large-bore IV catheter. If possible, use warm fluid to prevent hypothermia.

In pure neurogenic shock not associated with hypovolemic shock or still present after concomitant injuries have been stabilized, vagal blockers—such as atropine, 0.5 mg, by rapid IV push (up to a maximum of 3 mg) if the pulse remains severely bradycardic—and vasopressor agents—such as a dopamine drip beginning at 10 µg/kg/min and titrating to 20 µg/kg/min—may be used to better advantage than overhydrating the patient. Monitor the patient's response to vasopressors because it may be less than expected owing to the compromise of the sympathetic nervous system.

Anaphylactic Shock

Anaphylaxis occurs when a person reacts violently to a substance to which he or she has been sensitized. **Sensitization** means developing a heightened reaction to a substance. An allergic reaction typically does not occur, or occurs in a milder form, during sensitization. Do not be misled by a patient who reports no history of allergic reaction to a substance following a first or second exposure: Each subsequent exposure after sensitization tends to produce a more severe reaction.

In **anaphylactic shock**, there is no loss of blood, no vascular damage, and only a slight possibility of direct cardiac muscular injury. Instead, the patient experiences widespread vascular dilation, resulting in relative hypovolemia. In other words, relative to the now larger container, the normal blood volume is less. The combination of poor oxygenation and poor perfusion, however, may easily prove fatal.

In anaphylaxis, immune system chemicals, such as histamine and other vasodilator proteins, are released when exposed to an allergen. Their release causes the severe bronchoconstriction that accounts for wheezing if the patient is actually moving enough air. Anaphylaxis is also accompanied by urticaria (hives). The results are widespread vasodilation, which causes distributive shock, and blood vessels that continue to leak. Fluid leaks out of the blood vessels and into the interstitial space, resulting in hypovolemia and potentially causing significant swelling. In some cases, this swelling may occlude the upper airway, resulting in a life-threatening condition **Figure 10**.

Recurrent large areas of subcutaneous edema of sudden onset, usually disappearing within 24 hours and mainly seen in young women (frequently as a result of allergy to food or drugs), are called **angioedema**.

When a patient experiences shock due to a severe allergic reaction, you need to act fast. Remove the inciting cause if possible. Resolve any immediate life threats to the ABCs, which may require aggressive airway management (ie, intubation and/or rapid sequence intubation) and supplemental oxygen administration. Evaluate the patient's ventilatory status and the need for bag-mask ventilation.

Provide cardiovascular support with IV fluid challenges of crystalloid solution. Reverse the target-organ effect by administering epinephrine or a vasopressor such as dopamine (Intropin) in high doses. Consider the need for a bronchodilator such as albuterol (Proventil) or ipratropium (Atrovent). Impede further mediator release with an antihistamine such as

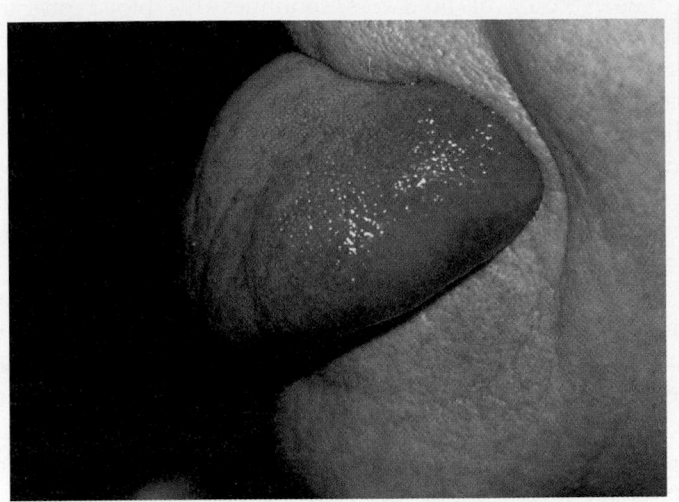

Figure 10 In anaphylaxis, interstitial fluid may cause significant swelling. In some cases, this swelling may occlude the upper airway, resulting in a life-threatening condition.

diphenhydramine (Benadryl). If the patient has an epinephrine injector, take it to the hospital. All paramedics carry epinephrine in their drug box, and you should administer epinephrine IM as early as possible (prior to intubation).

Psychogenic Shock

A patient who is experiencing **psychogenic shock** has had a sudden reaction of the nervous system that produces a temporary, generalized vascular dilation, resulting in syncope (vasovagal syncope). Blood pools in the dilated vessels, reducing the blood supply to the brain; as a result, the brain ceases to function normally, and the patient faints. Whereas there are many causes of syncope, it is important to realize that some are of a serious nature but others are not. Causes of syncope that are potentially life threatening result from events such as an irregular heartbeat or a brain aneurysm. You should always consider all the potential causes of syncope before deciding it was just a simple vasovagal syncope. Syncope is discussed in detail in the chapter, *Neurologic Emergencies*. Other non–life-threatening events that cause syncope may be the receipt of bad news or experiencing fear or unpleasant sights (such as the sight of blood).

In an uncomplicated case of fainting, once the patient collapses and becomes supine, circulation to the brain is usually restored and with it, a normal state of functioning. Remember that psychogenic shock can significantly worsen other types of shock. If the attack has caused the patient to fall, you must check for injuries, especially in older patients. However, you should also assess the patient thoroughly for any other abnormality. If, after regaining consciousness, the patient is unable to walk without weakness, dizziness, or pain, you should suspect another problem, such as head injury. You should transport this patient promptly.

Be sure to record your initial observations of vital signs (including orthostatic) and level of consciousness. Obtain an ECG. In addition, try to learn from bystanders whether the patient complained of anything before fainting and how long he or she was unresponsive.

Hypovolemic Shock

As discussed in the chapter, *Bleeding*, when shock comes about because of inadequate blood volume, it is termed **hypovolemic shock** (*hypo* = deficient + *vol* = volume + *emia* = in the blood). There are hemorrhagic and non-hemorrhagic causes of hypovolemic shock. Volume can be lost as blood (internal or external hemorrhagic shock), plasma (burns), or electrolyte solution (vomiting, diarrhea, sweating) (non-hemorrhagic shock).

Non-hemorrhagic hypovolemic shock will be discussed in this chapter. See the chapter, *Bleeding*, for information about hemorrhagic shock.

Non-hemorrhagic shock occurs when the fluid loss is contained within the body, as in dehydration, burn injury, crush injury, and anaphylaxis. With severe thermal burns, for example, intravascular plasma leaks from the circulatory system into the burned tissues that lie adjacent to the injury. By comparison, crushing injuries may result in the loss of blood and plasma from damaged (crushed) vessels into injured tissues.

Abnormal losses of fluids and electrolytes (dehydration) may occur through a variety of mechanisms listed as follows:

- GI losses, especially through vomiting and diarrhea
- Increased loss as a consequence of fever, hyperventilation, or high environmental temperatures (through the lungs)
- Increased and excessive sweating
- Internal losses ("third-space" losses), as in peritonitis, pancreatitis, and ileus
- Plasma losses from burns, drains, and granulating wounds

Other causes of body fluid deficits include ascites, diabetes insipidus, acute renal failure, and osmotic diuresis secondary to hyperosmolar states (ie, diabetic ketoacidosis).

Most of the typical symptoms and signs of shock result from inadequate tissue oxygenation and the body's attempts to compensate for volume loss. The earliest signs of shock are restlessness and anxiety: The patient looks scared! The decline in tissue perfusion may not be enough to produce obvious asphyxia, but it *is* setting off alarms all over the body, to which the patient responds with a feeling of apprehension—a "gut" feeling that something is not right. If conscious, the patient may report being thirsty, reflecting the deficit of fluids in the body; at the same time, the patient may feel nauseated and even vomit. The diversion of blood flow away from low-priority peripheral tissues causes the skin to become pale, cold, and clammy; sometimes it has a mottled appearance. Meanwhile, the heart speeds up to circulate the remaining RBCs more rapidly, producing a rapid, weak pulse—rapid because the heart is beating faster, weak because the blood vessels are now narrow and the volume moving through them is decreased.

In each case, the fluid lost has a unique electrolyte composition, and long-term therapy aims to restore the deficient body chemicals. For treatment in the field, however, all excessive fluid losses can be considered to lead to dehydration.

Symptoms of dehydration include loss of appetite (anorexia), nausea, vomiting, and sometimes fainting when standing up (postural syncope). Physical examination of a dehydrated patient reveals poor skin turgor (the skin over the forehead or sternum will "tent" when pinched); a shrunken, furrowed tongue; and sunken eyes. The pulse will be weak and rapid, rising more than 15 beats/min when the patient is raised from a recumbent to a sitting position (a maneuver that may cause the patient to feel faint). When fluid and electrolyte depletion are severe, shock and coma may be present.

A dehydrated patient needs replacement of fluid and electrolytes and should be given an IV infusion of normal saline or lactated Ringer's solution at a rate of 20 mL/kg for an adult, depending on the circumstances. Keep the patient flat or in the Trendelenburg position (depending on local protocol) to optimize circulation to the brain.

The priorities in treating a patient in hypovolemic shock are the same as in treating any other patient—namely, the ABCs. Establish and maintain an open airway. Keep suction at hand to clear the mouth and pharynx if the patient should vomit. Administer supplemental oxygen, and assist ventilation as needed. Keep the patient warm.

En route to the ED, establish at least one, and preferably two, large-bore peripheral IV lines (14 to 16 gauge), using an over-the-needle catheter. If required by protocol, draw blood (two red-top blood collection [Vacutainer] tubes and one purple-top tube) so that ED personnel may obtain a hematocrit, type- and cross-match, and other tests immediately on your arrival. Unless local medical policy favors a different resuscitation fluid, administer normal saline or lactated Ringer's solution. For guidance, refer to the IV fluid flow rates table and to your local protocol. Run in the first 500-mL "fluid challenge" as fast as it will flow, and then reassess the patient to see the impact of the intervention. If warmed fluids are available, consider their use as well.

Do not give the patient anything by mouth because he or she is likely to vomit. If this occurs, administration of an antiemetic should be appropriate, especially if you have a long bumpy ride to the ED. Keep the patient at normal temperature, covering the patient with a blanket and warming the patient compartment of the ambulance—patients in hypovolemic shock are often unable to conserve body heat effectively and are easily chilled. Place the patient in a position with the head elevated 15° to 30° and the legs elevated 30° on pillows (injuries permitting).

Monitor the ECG rhythm because any critically ill or injured patient is like to have dysrhythmias. Also monitor the patient's mental status, pulse rate, blood pressure, SpO_2, and $ETCO_2$. In a patient with substantial vasoconstriction, the blood pressure sounds may be difficult to hear, especially under field conditions. If you can feel a pulse over the femoral artery, but not over the radial artery, the systolic blood pressure is most likely between 70 and 80 mm Hg. The pulse oximetry and $ETCO_2$ findings will help you assess perfusion status and the need for ventilation intervention. Depending on local practice, medical control may order sodium bicarbonate to treat acidosis or a vasopressor (such as dopamine [Inotropin], metaraminol, or norepinephrine) to enhance vasoconstriction.

As bleeding or fluid loss continues, the blood pressure finally falls in the shock patient. Do not wait until the blood pressure falls before you suspect shock and begin treatment! Falling blood pressure is a *late* sign in shock (decompensated shock), signaling the collapse of all compensatory mechanisms and the fact that the patient may have already lost 30% or more fluid volume. Furthermore, the blood pressure measured at the arm provides you with little information about perfusion of vital organs; it tells only about perfusion of the arms.

The goal in treating shock is to save the brain, lungs, and kidneys; these organs must remain perfused if the patient is to survive and return to a healthy life. The best indication of brain perfusion is the patient's state of consciousness. If the patient is conscious and alert, the brain is being perfused adequately despite what the blood pressure findings show. If the patient has an altered mental status, perfusion of the brain is inadequate. Kidney perfusion can be gauged by urine output in a catheterized patient. Adequately perfused kidneys put out at least 30 mL to 50 mL of urine per hour; poorly perfused kidneys shut down and stop putting out any urine.

In the field—where patients will not ordinarily have urinary catheters—you can estimate the patient's peripheral perfusion by testing for capillary refill, although this is not the most reliable indicator. To do so, press on one of the patient's fingernails until it blanches, then release the pressure. If the skin under the nail does not "pink up" within 2 seconds, peripheral perfusion is compromised. To determine how well the *vital* organs are being perfused, you must rely on the patient's state of consciousness.

■ Respiratory Insufficiency

A patient with a severe chest injury such as flail chest, or obstruction of the airway, may be unable to breathe in an adequate amount of oxygen. This affects the ventilation process of respiration; enough oxygen cannot be inspired to meet the metabolic demand.

An insufficient concentration of oxygen in the blood can produce shock as rapidly as vascular causes, even if the volume of blood, the volume of the vessels, and the action of the heart are all normal. Without oxygen, the organs in the body cannot survive, and their cells promptly start to deteriorate.

Certain types of poisoning may affect the ability of cells to metabolize or carry oxygen. Carbon monoxide has a 200 to 250 times greater affinity for hemoglobin than oxygen. If a patient is in an environment where he or she inhales carbon monoxide, it will bind to the hemoglobin, forming carboxyhemoglobin, rather than allowing oxygen to bind. This results in a hypoxic state if not corrected. Cyanide impairs the ability of cells to metabolize oxygen within the cell and cellular asphyxia may occur.

Anemia occurs when there is an abnormally low number of RBCs. RBCs contain hemoglobin, an iron-containing pigment. Hemoglobin transports oxygen from the lungs to the tissues. Each hemoglobin molecule is able to carry four molecules of oxygen. Anemia may be the result of either chronic or acute bleeding, a deficiency in certain vitamins or minerals, or an underlying disease process. If anemia is present, tissues may be hypoxic because the blood may not be able to carry adequate oxygen, even though the hemoglobin is fully saturated. In this situation, a pulse oximeter may indicate that there is adequate saturation, even though the tissues are hypoxic. This type of hypoxia is known as hypoxemic hypoxia.

When you are treating a patient who is in shock as a result of inadequate respiration, you must immediately seal the hole in the chest, stabilize impaled objects in the chest, and secure and maintain the airway. Clear the mouth and throat of anything obstructing the air passages, including mucus, vomitus, and foreign material. Assess the SpO_2 and $ETCO_2$ as well as vital signs, and determine the need to assist ventilations with a bag-mask device and supplemental oxygen. Determine the most appropriate transportation destination based on the patient's condition and local protocols.

Transportation of Shock Patients

If you suspect that a patient is in shock, transport is inevitable; the questions you should be asking yourself are when, where, and how. Remember that scene time should be limited to 10 minutes or less; preplanning will help determine where the patient should be taken as well as how to get the patient to the ED. Know how to access aeromedical transportation in your community. Consideration for the priority of the patient and the availability of a regional trauma center should be your concerns, and local transport protocols may specifically deal with these issues. Patients who are suspected to be in shock, whether compensated or decompensated, may benefit from early surgical intervention and should be transported to a facility with appropriate capabilities. Patients with cardiogenic shock may need to go to a hospital with comprehensive cardiac care capabilities such as an interventional catheterization lab or a heart surgery program. If a facility of this type is not readily available, medical control should help you make the transport decision. In some communities, this will involve transport to a local facility and transfer (often aeromedical) to a tertiary care facility with the appropriate facilities and staff to handle the patient's complex needs.

Prevention Strategies

Prevention of shock and its deadly effects begins with your immediate assessment of the MOI, primary assessment findings, and the patient's clinical picture. Be alert, and search for early signs of shock. Do not rationalize irregularities away because the irregularities may soon become much more obvious if the patient truly is in shock—by then it may be too late. For example, at the scene of what appears to be a minor motor vehicle crash, do not assume the patient has tachycardia because he is upset. Instead, consider the MOI and manage the suspected shock aggressively and immediately.

YOU are the Medic   SUMMARY

1. What should your next course of action be for this patient?

After conducting a scene size-up and forming a general impression of this patient, you recognize that you are dealing with a critical patient. There was no sign of trauma, and indications lead you to believe that this patient has been sick for several days. His altered mental status is a possible indication of the critical nature of his condition. It is important to conduct a primary assessment so that you can identify and treat immediate life threats. A secondary assessment performed as a rapid scan will also provide clues to assist you in determining the field diagnosis and initiate appropriate treatment. Consider all the potential causes of an altered mental status, as discussed in this chapter, to help you reach the most accurate working field diagnosis.

2. Discuss the role of intuition in forming a field diagnosis as well as the potential for bias.

Every patient assessed and treated by the paramedic contributes to the bank of experience and knowledge that shapes future decisions. Intuition is not a skill that can be taught and is essentially based on recognition of patterns then matched to previous experiences. Intuition is safest to use in making treatment decisions that heighten your index of suspicion and result in increased care as opposed to downgrading your response to the patient's condition. However it is important to remember that the more complex the patient, the greater the risk of obscuring patterns and matching them incorrectly. There are three forms of bias that lead the paramedic astray when making decisions: confirmation bias (ignoring information that does not conform to a preexisting field diagnosis), anchoring bias (making decisions based on an arbitrary initial reference point), and a bias of representativeness (failure to obtain all information or data because a patient has a classic presentation). If the paramedic remains aware of the potential biases, then it is easier to avoid being trapped by them.

3. Describe the contributing factors that would lead you to label this patient as critical.

Critical patients require that the paramedic employ critical thinking skills. Patients identified as critical usually present as being in a peri-arrest period and may have any of the premorbid conditions listed in Table 1. The peri-arrest period is prior to and following cardiac arrest. Shock, especially in its decompensation phase, is one of the conditions that can progress to cardiac arrest. While you are assessing this patient, you have determined he has a history of acute coronary syndrome, as well as chronic obstructive pulmonary disease. He takes medication that supports these findings.

4. Discuss pathophysiologic changes associated with septic shock.

Shock is a systemic state of collapse and failure of the cardiovascular system. Under normal compensatory mechanisms, the body is able to maintain system blood pressure and brain perfusion when the body is stressed. In prolonged shock, the vital organs suffer and death results. When the body is stressed, the autonomic nervous system redirects blood flow toward the vital organs, which include the heart, brain, lungs, and kidneys. Inadequate circulatory support to other areas of the body will lead to inadequate tissue perfusion or hypoperfusion. This means the areas affected have inadequate supplies of oxygen, nutrients, and waste removal. Pale or mottled skin discoloration is a good indicator of hypoperfusion. As shock progresses due to a failure to correct the precipitating cause, the vital organs become hypo-perfused. This may become evident through an altered mental status before changes in other vital signs occur. As systemic vascular resistance begins to fall, cardiac output drops. This eventually leads to system-wide collapse of perfusion including that to the myocardium, which further worsens the ability of the body to compensate. In septic shock, the initial changes are due to widespread vasodilation due to infection that has activated the inflammatory-immune response. Septic shock can be complex because of the multi-system involvement. Fluid shifts and micro-vascular permeability decreases the available volume of fluid for circulation. Leakage in the pulmonary system creates congestion that reduces the ability for adequate gas exchange. Inadequate volume leads to decreased preload, which further compromises adequate cardiac output and perfusion status.

5. Discuss the potential phase of shock this patient may be in.

Based on assessment findings, this patient may be in decompensated shock. It is characterized by a drop in blood volume of greater than 30%. Compensatory mechanisms have begun to fail as indicated by a reduction in blood pres-sure and cardiac function. This means that cardiac output is decreasing. System vasoconstriction is occurring as noted by the pale, cool, and mottled skin. These nonperfused tissues are becoming hypoxic. Because there is clear indication that reduc-tions in cardiac output, blood pressure, and tissue perfusion are occurring, consideration should be given to the potential that this patient is entering the irreversible phase of shock. Efforts should be focused on aggressive treatment to increase tissue perfusion and circulation until definitive care for the underlying cause can be provided.

6. Describe how you should manage this patient with suspected shock.

Airway and ventilatory support are always a high priority in the shock patient. After establishing a patent airway and suctioning as needed, high-flow supplemental oxygen should be provided. In the patient who is unable to maintain his or her own airway, assisted ventilations via a bag-mask device or placement of an advanced airway is preferred. Gaining IV access and supporting circulation through administration of

isotonic fluids such as normal saline can improve blood pressure and tissue perfusion. Establishing an available IV access port allows for rapid medication administration when it is indicated. Consider administering vasopressors appropriate to the patient's condition. Nonpharmacologic interventions such as body positioning and prevention of hypothermia should also be employed. Cardiac monitoring allows for early identification of possible dysrhythmias and changes in cardiac function.

7. Why should a patient's hypoxic drive not be a consideration when treating shock?

Hypoxic drive is an alternative mechanism for the central nervous system to determine whether respirations should be increased or decreased. In healthy people, peripheral chemoreceptors detect levels of carbon dioxide in the blood ($Paco_2$) and respond by increasing the respiratory rate when there is too much. In some patients with chronic bronchitis or emphysema, the patient maintains a higher than normal level chronically. The chemoreceptors no longer are sensitive to this, and the central nervous system does not respond to these higher levels. The amount of oxygen in the blood (Pao_2) becomes the new mechanism for determining the need to alter respiratory rates. As levels rise with the administration of high concentrations of oxygen, the central nervous system may slow or cease respirations. Although this is possible, the acutely ill patient, such as those in shock, should still receive high concentrations of oxygen in response to hypoxia due to diminished perfusion. If respiratory efforts cease, the paramedic should take control of the patient's airway and initiate ventilations to ensure oxygenation is continued and the patient's condition is not worsened by further hypoxia.

8. What are the anticipated benefits of dopamine administration for this patient?

Dopamine (Intropin) is a sympathetic agonist that acts on alpha, beta-1, and dopaminergic adrenergic receptors. Its action on alpha and beta-1 adrenergic receptors can result in increased blood pressure and specific to beta-1 receptors may have a posi-tive inotropic effect on the heart. Cardiac output, stroke volume, and myocardial contractility should increase without excessive increases in myocardial oxygen demands. It also has less chrono-tropic effects than other sympathetic agonists such as isoproter-enol and epinephrine. At mid-range dosages there is less effect on systemic vascular resistance with increases to renal blood flow. It also has less potential for causing tachydysrhythmias. The body's response to the medication is affected by the dosages being delivered.

9. What is the benefit of assessing lung compliance in the ventilated shock patient?

Lung compliance refers to the amount of resistance for the lungs to expand. Normal compliance indicates that the lungs expand with minimal resistance and lower pressures are required to ventilate your patient. Decreased lung compli-ance indicates that the lung tissue is stiff and difficult to

YOU are the Medic   SUMMARY, continued

ventilate. You may notice increased resistance and greater effort required to ventilate using a manual resuscitation bag. If the patient is being artificially ventilated using a mechanical ventilator, high pressure alarms will sound and greater pressures are required to achieve the desired tidal volume. Decreased compliance can be seen in patients with traumatic chest injuries such as chest wall trauma or in the presence of a tension pneumothorax due to increased pressures in the chest. Patients with acute respiratory distress syndrome (ARDS) may also have decreased compliance due to the formation of interstitial fluid accumulation in the lungs. Surfactant is lost and alveolar sacs collapse creating impaired gas exchange. ARDS may be seen in the acute sepsis or shock patient, so assessment for lung compliance is beneficial to aid in identification of the presence of ARDS.

10. Discuss how your assessment findings for this patient led you to a differential field diagnosis of septic shock.

Assessment of this patient revealed an older man (77 years old) with a recent history of cough and fever. He had comorbid factors that included chronic bronchitis. Complaints on deep breathing lead you to suspect there was a potential for pneumonia. He had not been seen for at least 24 hours, indicating less mobility than usual and a possible decrease in appetite based on his refusal of lunch at least 3 days ago. His clinical presentation of shock signs and symptoms in conjunction with your review of potential causes leads you to conclude infection as the underlying condition. You are aware that an untreated infection in the older patient in addition to comorbid conditions increases the likelihood of progression to sepsis.

EMS Patient Care Report (PCR)

Date: 11-03-10	**Incident No.:** 201064376	**Nature of Call:** Unresponsive patient	**Location:** 4950 Waters Way, Apartment 512		
Dispatched: 0915	**En Route:** 0916	**At Scene:** 0924	**Transport:** 0933	**At Hospital:** 0946	**In Service:** 1510

Patient Information

Age: 77 **Sex:** M **Weight (in kg [lb]):** 64.5 kg (142 lb)	**Allergies:** Shellfish **Medications:** Lisinopril 10 mg daily, aspirin 81 mg daily, albuterol MDI 2 puffs TID and PRN, furosemide 20 mg daily **Past Medical History:** HTN, MI × 5 years ago, chronic bronchitis **Chief Complaint:** Altered mental status

Vital Signs

Time: 0934	**BP:** 68 by palpation	**Pulse:** 118	**Respirations:** assisted	**Spo$_2$:** Not obtainable
Time: 0939	**BP:** 72 by palpation	**Pulse:** 100	**Respirations:** 8 spont.	**Spo$_2$:** Not obtainable
Time: 0944	**BP:** 76/48	**Pulse:** 104	**Respirations:** 12 ATV	**Spo$_2$:** 99%

EMS Treatment
(circle all that apply)

Oxygen @ __15__ L/min via (circle one): NC NRM Bag-mask device	**Assisted Ventilation:** 12 breaths/min	**Airway Adjunct:** Oral ETT	**CPR**
Defibrillation	**Bleeding Control**	**Bandaging**	**Splinting**	**Other:** Dopamine 5 µg/kg/min drip; airway suction; saline IV

Narrative

EMS requested to above location for a man who is unresponsive. On arrival, pt found lying supine in his bed. Home health aide is on scene. Pt confirmed to be responsive to painful stimuli only. No signs of trauma noted on scene. Building security notes pt has not been seen outside of his apartment for at least 24 hours. Pt's airway noted to be partially obstructed by secretions. Bag-mask assisted ventilations with high concentrations of oxygen initiated after opening and suctioning airway. Pt found with audible respirations and suctioning reveals thick, light brown sputum. Medications assessed and patient identification as well as medications gathered for transport. SAMPLE history obtained from aide on scene. Cardiac monitor reveals sinus tachycardia without ectopy. IV established with an 18 gauge to the right AC. Fluid bolus of NS initiated at 20 mL/kg (1,200 mL). Pt transferred to unit for transport. Once en route, pt noted to have decreased respiratory effort and perfusion. Medical control contacted for orders for administration of a vasopressor. Dopamine drip initiated using pre-mix bag at rate of 12 drops per minute. Pt intubated with 7.0 ETT nasally and secured at 28-cm mark. Placement confirmed via auscultation and ETCO$_2$ monitoring and waveforms. Pt transport continued without further incident and report called to receiving facility. No changes noted to cardiac rhythm during transport. On arrival at the ED, pt transferred to stretcher in Room 6 and report given to RN at bedside. Pt placed in stretcher with all rails up and placed on ventilator by respiratory therapist. Signature for medication order obtained from Dr. Jackson. **End of report**

Prep Kit

- The paramedic needs to develop expertise in rapidly developing a differential field diagnosis of the critical patient found in a peri-arrest condition or during a peri-arrest period.
- The novice paramedic can benefit from working with an experienced paramedic to help develop skills in intuition and becoming comfortable in making critical decisions when they are needed most.
- Hypoperfusion occurs when the level of tissue perfusion decreases below normal.
  - Early decreased tissue perfusion may result in subtle changes, such as aberrant mental status, long before a patient's vital signs appear abnormal.
  - Shock refers to a state of collapse and failure of the cardiovascular system that leads to inadequate circulation, creating inadequate tissue perfusion.
- The body is perfused via the cardiovascular system. Control of the cardiovascular system is a function of the autonomic nervous system, which is composed of competing subsystems.
- Tissue perfusion requires three intact mechanisms: a pump (heart), fluid volume (blood and body fluids), and tubing capable of reflex adjustments (constriction and dilation) in response to changes in pump output and fluid volume (blood vessels). If any one of those mechanisms is damaged, tissue perfusion may be disrupted, and shock will ensue.
- Shock occurs in three successive phases (compensated, decompensated, and irreversible). This is also referred to as the four grades of hemorrhage or four classes of shock, with class I and II being compensated shock, class III being decompensated shock, and class IV being irreversible shock, also referred to as terminal shock.
- As with any patient, airway and ventilatory support take top priority when you are treating a patient with suspected shock.
- If a patient is suspected to be in shock, transport is inevitable; the questions to be asked are when, where, and how.
  - The priority of the patient and the availability of a regional trauma center should be your concerns. Local transport protocols may specifically deal with these issues.
  - Patients who have suspected shock, whether compensated or decompensated, will benefit from early medical or surgical intervention and should be transported to a facility with those capabilities.
- Never wait for the blood pressure to drop; always treat shock aggressively in its compensated phase.

- The non-hemorrhagic causes of hypovolemic shock are commonly grouped by how they reduce perfusion. These types of shock involve either a weakening of the pump, an increase in the size of the container, or a direct mechanical interference with the circulation.
- Prevention of shock and its deadly effects begins with your immediate assessment of the MOI, primary assessment findings, and the patient's clinical picture. Be alert, and search for early signs of shock.

aerobic metabolism Metabolism that can proceed only in the presence of oxygen.

afterload The pressure in the aorta against which the left ventricle must pump blood.

anaerobic metabolism Metabolism that takes place in the absence of oxygen.

anaphylactic shock A severe hypersensitivity reaction that involves bronchoconstriction and cardiovascular collapse.

anchoring bias Occurs when an initial reference point distorts your estimates.

angioedema Recurrent large areas of subcutaneous edema of sudden onset, usually disappearing within 24 hours, which is seen mainly in young women, frequently as a result of allergy to food or drugs.

baroreceptors Receptors in the blood vessels, kidneys, brain, and heart that respond to changes in pressure in the heart or main arteries to help maintain homeostasis.

capacitance vessels The smallest venules.

cardiac output (CO) The volume of blood pumped through the circulatory system in 1 minute.

cardiogenic shock A condition caused by loss of 40% or more of the functioning myocardium; the heart is no longer able to circulate sufficient blood to maintain adequate oxygen delivery.

cardiovascular collapse Failure of the heart and blood vessels; shock.

central shock A condition that consists of cardiogenic shock and obstructive shock (Weil-Shubin classification).

chemoreceptors Sense organs that monitor the levels of oxygen and carbon dioxide and the pH of cerebrospinal fluid and blood and provide feedback to the respiratory centers to modify the rate and depth of breathing based on the body's needs at any given time.

chronotropic effect The rate of contraction of the heart.

compensated shock The early stage of shock, in which the body can still compensate for blood loss. The systolic blood pressure and brain perfusion are maintained.

confirmation bias Occurs with the tendency to gather and rely on information that confirms your existing views and to avoid or downplay information that does not conform to your preexisting hypothesis or field differential.

critical patients Patients in either pre-morbid conditions, with major trauma, or in the peri-arrest period.

decompensated shock The late stage of shock, when blood pressure is falling.

differential field diagnosis The short list of the potential causes of the patient's presenting condition.

diffusion A process in which molecules move from an area of higher concentration to an area of lower concentration.

distributive shock A condition that occurs when there is widespread dilation of the resistance vessels, the capacitance vessels, or both.

dromotropic effect The effect on the velocity of conduction.

Fick principle A principle that states the movement and use of oxygen in the body is dependent on an adequate concentration of inspired oxygen, appropriate movement of oxygen across the alveolar-capillary membrane into the arterial bloodstream, adequate number of red blood cells to carry the oxygen, proper tissue perfusion, and efficient off-loading of oxygen at the tissue level.

hypoperfusion A condition that occurs when the level of tissue perfusion decreases below that needed to maintain normal cellular functions; also called shock.

hypovolemic shock A condition that occurs when the circulating blood volume is inadequate to deliver adequate oxygen and nutrients to the body.

inotropic effect Affecting the contractility of muscle tissue, especially cardiac muscle.

irreversible shock The final stage of shock, resulting in death.

mean arterial pressure (MAP) The blood pressure required to sustain organ perfusion; roughly 60 mm Hg in the average person.

multiple-organ dysfunction syndrome (MODS) A progressive condition usually characterized by combined failure of several organs, such as the lungs, liver, and kidneys, along with some clotting mechanisms, which occurs after severe illness or injury.

myocardial contractility The ability of the heart to contract.

neurogenic shock Circulatory failure caused by paralysis of the nerves that control the size of the blood vessels, leading to widespread dilation; seen in patients with spinal cord injuries.

non-hemorrhagic shock Shock that occurs as a result of fluid loss contained within the body, such as in dehydration, burn injury, crush injury, and anaphylaxis.

obstructive shock Shock that occurs when there is a block to blood flow in the heart or great vessels, causing an insufficient blood supply to the body's tissues.

orthostatic hypotension A drop in systolic blood pressure when moving a patient from a sitting to a standing position.

perfusion The delivery of oxygen and nutrients to the cells, organs, and tissues of the body.

peri-arrest period The period either just before or just after cardiac arrest when the patient is critical and care must be taken to prevent progression or regression into cardiac arrest.

peripheral shock A condition that consists of hypovolemic shock and distributive shock (Weil-Shubin classification).

preload The initial stretching of the cardiac muscles prior to contraction. It is related to the chamber volume of blood just prior to the contraction.

premorbid condition A condition preceding the onset of disease.

psychogenic shock A sudden reaction of the nervous system that produces a temporary, generalized vascular dilation, resulting in syncope (vasovagal syncope).

pulse pressure The difference between the systolic and diastolic pressures.

resistance vessels The smallest arterioles.

sensitization Developing sensitivity to a substance that initially caused no allergic reaction.

septic shock Shock caused by severe infection, usually a bacterial infection.

shock An abnormal state associated with inadequate oxygen and nutrient delivery to the metabolic apparatus of the cell; also called hypoperfusion.

sphincters Circular muscular walls of capillaries that constrict and dilate, acting as a gate to increase or decrease blood flow.

spinal shock The local neurologic condition that occurs after a spinal injury produces motor and sensory losses (which may not be permanent).

stroke volume (SV) The amount of blood that the left ventricle ejects into the aorta per contraction.

systemic vascular resistance (SVR) The resistance to blood flow within all of the blood vessels except the pulmonary vessels.

Assessment in Action

At 5:30 PM you are the paramedic on an advanced life support unit responding to a patient who has collapsed. Dispatch advises that the scene is safe. An engine crew is also being sent. On arrival, you are directed to an area of a field where a small group of people has gathered. You note the ambient temperature today has been hot and there is no shaded area near the field. You are aware that environmental exposure to this temperature for extended periods may result in heat-related emergencies. The initial general impression of your patient as you approach is a petite young woman who is pale and silent with her eyes closed. You are approached by a woman who advises you she is the coach of the ladies track team and they have been practicing for the last few days. Your patient, Jennifer, was running but then stopped, vomited, and collapsed to the ground. Your assessment of the scene does not reveal any structures or objects that she may have hit during her collapse, but you do note a small amount of green vomitus near the patient. You move to the patient's side to continue your primary assessment, and the patient opens her eyes when you call her name. You ask her age and she tells you she is 18 years old. Assessment of her breathing reveals a respiratory rate of 28 breaths/min and they are slightly labored. She has a radial pulse rate that is tachycardic at 120 beats/min and her skin is mottled, cool, and dry. Your rapid scan confirms that there are no obvious signs of trauma but there are positive signs and symptoms of dehydration, including sunken eyes and poor skin turgor, as well as syncope, nausea, and vomiting. These findings indicate an immediate life threat, and you begin delegating care by assuming the role of team leader. She is a high-priority patient, and a short scene time and rapid transport to definitive care is appropriate.

While your partner applies a nonrebreathing mask with high-concentration oxygen at 15 L/min, emergency responders begin to prepare the patient for transport. You obtain a SAMPLE history and continue with a secondary assessment. The patient tells you she has been running all day trying to improve her times for an upcoming competition. This morning she felt nauseated so she did not eat or drink much during lunch. Her last full meal and fluid intake was at approximately 8:00 AM. She is allergic to penicillin and takes 10 units of insulin at 7:30 AM daily for her diabetes. You remind your partner to check her blood glucose level when obtaining vital signs. Her vital signs are a pulse rate of 120 beats/min and weak; respirations, 22 breaths/min and slightly labored; blood pressure, 108/64 mm Hg; oxygen saturation, 98% on high concentrations of oxygen; and a blood glucose level of 66 mg/dL.

1. Which form of shock is this patient experiencing?
   A. Septic shock
   B. Neurogenic shock
   C. Cardiogenic shock
   D. Hypovolemic shock

2. Total blood volume in the adult is approximately how many liters?
   A. 3
   B. 6
   C. 8
   D. 10

3. Which phase of shock does this patient appear to be in?
   A. Compensated
   B. Decompensated
   C. Irreversible
   D. Terminal

4. Which of the following are signs and symptoms of hypovolemic shock?
   A. Feelings of anxiety and restlessness
   B. Thirst
   C. Pale, cool, and moist skin
   D. All of the above

5. Which of the following is a concern for IV fluid therapy in patients with hypovolemic shock?
   A. Congestive heart failure
   B. Hypertension
   C. Increased external hemorrhage
   D. Extravasation

6. Which of the following is not a component of the body's initial compensatory mechanisms for shock?
   A. Increase preload and cardiac output
   B. Maintain brain perfusion
   C. Increase available oxygen
   D. Increase urine output

7. Which of the following is typically the last factor to change in shock?
   A. Mental status
   B. Blood pressure
   C. Skin condition
   D. Pulse rate

Additional Questions

8. Why is it important to consider the preexisting medical conditions of the critical patient?

9. What physiologic changes associated with shock place the patient at risk for multiple-organ dysfunction syndrome (MODS)?

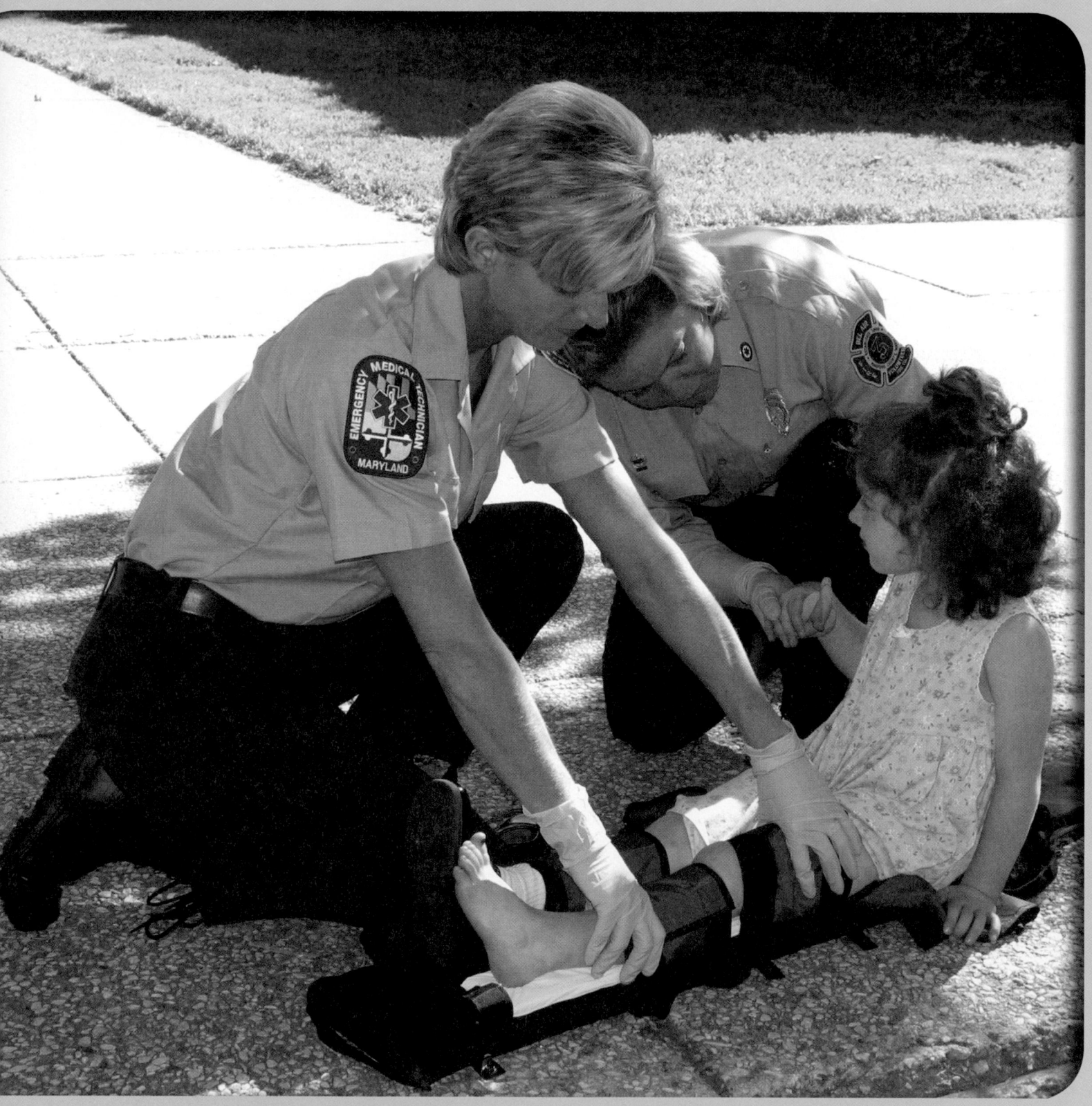

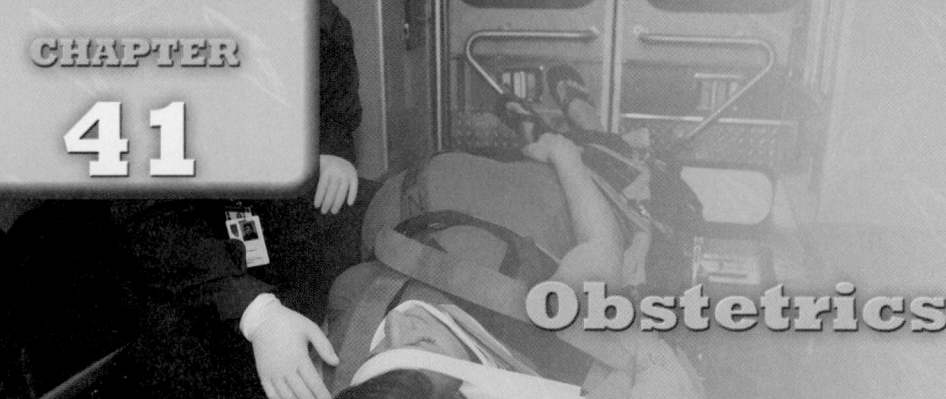

Obstetrics

National EMS Education Standard Competencies

Special Patient Populations

Integrates assessment findings with principles of pathophysiology and knowledge of psychosocial needs to formulate a field impression and implement a comprehensive treatment/disposition plan for patients with special needs.

Obstetrics

- Recognition and management of
  - Normal delivery (pp 1938–1944)
  - Vaginal bleeding in the pregnant patient (pp 1936–1938)
- Anatomy and physiology of normal pregnancy (pp 1922–1923)
- Pathophysiology of complications of pregnancy (pp 1931–1935)
- Assessment of the pregnant patient (pp 1927–1931)
- Psychosocial impact, presentations, prognosis, and management of
  - Normal delivery (pp 1938–1944)
  - Abnormal delivery
    - Nuchal cord (pp 1949–1950)
    - Prolapsed cord (p 1950)
    - Breech delivery (pp 1948–1949)
  - Third-trimester bleeding
    - Placenta previa (pp 1937–1938)
    - Abruptio placenta (pp 1937–1938)
  - Spontaneous abortion/miscarriage (pp 1936–1937)
  - Ectopic pregnancy (p 1937)
  - Preeclampsia/eclampsia (pp 1931–1932)
  - Antepartum hemorrhage (p 1937)
  - Pregnancy induced hypertension (pp 1931–1932)

Trauma

Integrates assessment findings with principles of epidemiology and pathophysiology to formulate a field impression to implement a comprehensive treatment/disposition plan for an acutely injured patient.

Special Considerations in Trauma

Recognition and management of trauma in

- Pregnant patient (p 1951–1954)
- Pediatric patient (see chapter, *Pediatric Emergencies*)
- Geriatric patient (see chapter, *Geriatric Emergencies*)

Pathophysiology, assessment, and management of trauma in the

- Pregnant patient (pp 1952, 1953–1954)
- Pediatric patient (see chapter, *Pediatric Emergencies*)
- Geriatric patient (see chapter, *Geriatric Emergencies*)
- Cognitively impaired patient (see chapter, *Patients With Special Challenges*)

Knowledge Objectives

1. Discuss the anatomy and physiology of the female reproductive system, including the female hormones. (pp 1922-1923)

2. Understand the normal changes that occur in the various body systems during pregnancy. (pp 1925-1927)

3. Describe the process of conception and fetal development, from ovulation to the fetal stage. (pp 1923-1924)

4. Discuss the various functions of the placenta. (pp 1923-1924)

5. Be aware of special considerations involving pregnancy in different cultures and with teenage patients. (p 1927)

6. Describe commonly used obstetric terminology. (p 1927)

7. Discuss the process of assessing a patient who is experiencing an emergency related to pregnancy, or who is in labor. (pp 1927-1931)

8. Discuss complications related to pregnancy, including abuse, substance abuse, supine hypotensive disorder, diabetes mellitus, heart disease, hyperemesis gravidarum, hypertensive disorders, Rh sensitization, and infections, including sexually transmitted diseases. (pp 1931-1935)

9. Discuss bleeding during pregnancy, including third-trimester bleeding and its potential causes and management. (pp 1936-1938)

10. Differentiate between the three stages of labor. (p 1939)

11. Describe the indications of an imminent delivery. (p 1930)

12. Explain the steps involved in normal delivery management. (p 1942-1943)

13. Explain the necessary care of the baby as the head appears. (p 1942-1943)

14. Describe the procedure followed to cut and tie the umbilical cord. (p 1943)

15. Describe delivery of the placenta. (pp 1943-1944)

16. Discuss management of complications of labor, including cephalic presentation, breech presentation, shoulder dystocia, nuchal cord, and prolapsed cord. (pp 1948-1950)

17. Discuss management of high-risk pregnancy considerations, including precipitous labor and birth, post-term pregnancy, meconium staining, fetal macrosomia, multiple gestation, intrauterine fetal death, amniotic fluid embolism, hydramnios, and cephalopelvic disproportion. (pp 1946-1948)

18. Discuss management of complications of delivery, including premature rupture of membranes, preterm labor, uterine rupture, and fetal distress. (pp 1945-1946)

19. Discuss management of postpartum complications, including uterine inversion, postpartum hemorrhage, pulmonary embolism, and postpartum depression. (pp 1950-1951)

20. Discuss concerns related to trauma in the pregnant patient, including assessment and management of the woman and the unborn fetus. (pp 1951-1954)

Skills Objectives

1. Demonstrate how to listen to fetal heart sounds. (p 1930)

2. Demonstrate the procedure to assist in a normal cephalic delivery. (pp 1942-1943)

3. Demonstrate care procedures of the infant as the head appears. (pp 1942-1943)

4. Demonstrate the steps to follow in postdelivery care of the infant. (pp 1942-1943)

5. Demonstrate how to cut and tie the umbilical cord. (p 1943)

6. Demonstrate how to assist in delivery of the placenta. (pp 1943-1944)

7. Demonstrate the postdelivery care of the mother. (p 1944)

8. Describe how to assist with a breech delivery in the field. (pp 1948-1949)

9. Describe how to assist with a limb presentation in the field. (pp 1948-1949)

■ Introduction

When you are responding to an obstetric (OB) or maternity call, keep several key issues in mind. First, pregnancy itself is not a disease that needs treatment; it is the natural continuation of the human species. Women have been having children without the benefit of emergency departments, epidurals, painkillers, and enhanced 9-1-1 since time began. For the most part, childbirth is a happy event for all involved. Emotions can be out of control—ranging from extreme excitement to panicked distress; therefore, your role is to bring professional calm and control to the scene. Second, the number of patients increases to a minimum of two—the pregnant woman and the fetus—or perhaps even more if more than one fetus is expected.

Whereas childbirth and pregnancy are both naturally occurring states, they are not without potential complications, including maternal death and fetal death. With the advent of modern medicine, maternal and infant mortality rates have been significantly reduced, and close medical monitoring usually discovers problems well before childbirth.

■ Anatomy and Physiology of the Female Reproductive System

The female reproductive organs include the mammary glands (breasts), vagina, uterus (womb), and ovaries and fallopian tubes. The ovaries are the beginning point for reproduction. These paired glands are found next to the uterus, one ovary on each side. They are about the size and shape of an unshelled almond and are similar to the testes in the male. The ovaries are positioned in the upper pelvic cavity but typically descend to the brim of the pelvis during the third month of fetal development.

Each ovary contains about 200,000 follicles, and each follicle contains an **oocyte** (egg). The human female is born with all the eggs she will ever release (approximately 400,000). Each month, during the menstrual cycle, about 20 of these follicles begin the process of maturation, but only a single follicle ultimately matures and releases an ovum; the other follicles die off and are reabsorbed by the body. (The chapter, *Gynecologic Emergencies* covers the menstrual cycle in detail.)

The oocyte matures when the follicular cells respond to **follicle-stimulating hormone (FSH)** released by the anterior pituitary gland, which is first stimulated by the release of gonadotropin-releasing factor (GnRF) from the hypothalamus. As the preovulatory phase of the menstrual cycle progresses, the anterior pituitary gland releases **luteinizing hormone (LH)**, which stimulates the process of **ovulation**—that is, the release of the egg (or at this point, the **ovum**). LH continues to be excreted throughout the ovarian cycle and subsequent pregnancy, should it occur, stimulating the ovarian cells to produce the hormones relaxin, progesterone, and various estrogens. At the end of the pregnancy, the uterus and placenta produce prostaglandins that, along with oxytocin, will signal the uterus to contract and labor will begin.

What is left of the follicle after the egg has been released becomes the **corpus luteum**, which in turn secretes another female hormone, **progesterone**. Under the influence of progesterone, the second phase of the menstrual cycle takes place. The glands of the endometrium increase in size and secrete the materials on which the fertilized egg will implant and grow. There it will develop into an **embryo** and then a **fetus** Figure 1. If the ovum is *not* fertilized, it dies and degenerates 36 to 48 hours after being released. The endometrium then breaks down and is shed as menstrual flow on about the 28th day of the cycle (ie, about 14 days after ovulation).

The ovum passes from the ovaries to the uterus through the **fallopian tubes**. These paired structures measure about 4 inches long. Each tube extends out laterally from the uterus, terminating just short of an ovary. The proximal end of each fallopian tube is very thick and narrow and connects to the uterus itself. Each fallopian tube is composed of three layers of tissue. The outer layer consists of a serous membrane that protects the tubes. The middle layer is made of smooth muscle that contracts to help move the ovum through the tube and into the uterus. The innermost layer contains secretory cells and cilia which also move the ovum along and may also play a part in providing nutrition to the ovum. In summary, when an ovary releases an egg, the ciliary motion sweeps the egg into the fallopian tube. Smooth muscle contractions and the inner mucosa move the ovum through the tube to the uterus. If the egg encounters a sperm cell along the way, it may become fertilized. Fertilization can occur at any time within about a 24-hour window following ovulation.

YOU are the Medic   PART 1

Your unit is dispatched as a second unit for a motor vehicle crash. The first unit on scene advises you they have a critical trauma patient and you are responding for a woman who is 20 weeks' pregnant who was the driver of one of the vehicles. When you arrive on scene, you find a rear-end type collision. You are directed to your patient who is sitting in the vehicle that struck the rear of the first car. You don your safety equipment and approach the patient.

1. What is your primary concern after scene safety is established?
2. What questions are in your mind given knowledge that the patient is pregnant?

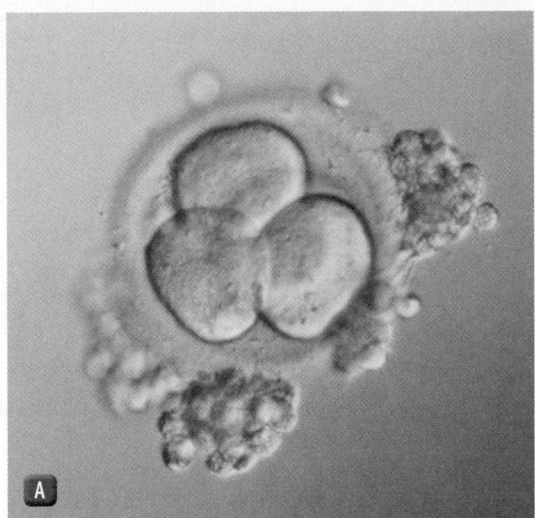 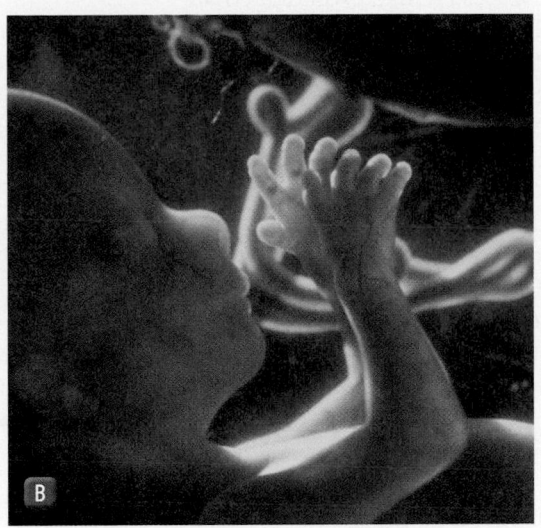

Figure 1 A. Embryo. B. Fetus.

The <u>uterus</u> is a muscular, inverted pear-shaped organ that lies between the urinary bladder and the rectum. The dome-shaped top of the uterus is called the <u>fundus</u>. Below the dome, the uterus begins to taper and narrow, forming the body. The narrowest portion of the uterus, called the <u>cervix</u>, opens into the vagina. The interior of the body of the uterus is the <u>uterine cavity</u>, and the interior of the cervix is the <u>cervical canal</u>.

The uterus is where the fertilized ovum will implant, where the fetus will develop, and where the act of labor takes place. It consists of three layers of tissue: the <u>perimetrium</u> (outer protective layer), the <u>myometrium</u> (middle layer), and the <u>endometrium</u> (inner lining). The myometrium is composed of three layers of muscle fibers; the contractions of these muscles help expel the fetus during childbirth. The endometrium is a mucous membrane composed of two layers; the layer innermost to the uterine cavity, is shed during menstruation. As the follicle starts developing and pumping out estrogen, the endometrium is stimulated to increase its thickness in preparation for the reception and future growth of a fertilized egg.

The <u>vagina</u> is a highly muscular, tubular organ lined with mucous membranes. Functions include the receptacle for the penis during sexual intercourse, the passage for exit of the menstrual flow, and the passage for childbirth. The interior of the vagina is acidic owing to the breakdown of glycogen (found in large amounts in the vaginal mucosa), which creates a low-pH environment that inhibits bacterial growth. This acidity, while beneficial, is injurious to sperm cells. Semen is alkaline in nature and likewise has antibacterial properties. The alkalinity of seminal fluid neutralizes the acidity of the vagina, allowing the sperm cells to survive and fertilize the ovum.

The vagina is the lower portion of the birth canal and can stretch widely to accommodate the delivery of a fetus. If the vagina is unable to stretch far enough, the tissues in and around the perineum may tear, causing significant pain and bleeding. In the hospital setting, the physician may make an incision in the perineal skin called an <u>episiotomy</u>. In the prehospital setting, you are limited to providing gentle pressure against the newborn's head to prevent an explosive birth and give the tissues time to expand.

The mammary glands (breasts) are modified sweat glands that are mainly composed of adipose tissue. Their primary purpose is lactation, or milk secretion, to provide nourishment to the newborn. Milk is carried to the surface of each breast through lactiferous ducts that terminate in a nipple. The nipple of the breast is surrounded by a darker pigmented area called the areola. Breast enlargement, tenderness, and milk excretion are all signs that a woman is most likely pregnant. Unilateral enlargement, discolored or foul fluid excretion, or pain and tenderness in the breasts may indicate a more serious underlying condition.

◼ Conception and Fetal Development

Once the egg has been fertilized and implanted in the endometrium of the uterus, both the egg and the pregnant woman begin to undergo major physiologic, hormonal, and chemical changes. The egg, on entering the uterus, begins absorbing uterine fluid through the cell membrane. As the fluid fills the interior of the egg, cell division increases rapidly, and the cells multiply on the outside of the egg surface, forming layers that will eventually generate the fetal membrane, <u>placenta</u>, and embryo. The egg, now called a <u>blastocyst</u>, will migrate to the endometrial wall and become implanted there approximately 1 week after conception. On implantation, the egg will adhere to the endometrium, and enzymatic activity from the egg will dissolve endometrial tissue and provide nourishment for its development. Occasionally, the mechanism of implantation may result in vaginal bleeding that is spotty and painless, but of concern to the patient who does not yet realize that she is pregnant.

The implantation and subsequent actions of the blastocyst trigger the development of placental tissues, whose formation stimulates the release of human chorionic gonadotropin hormone, which in turn sends signals to the corpus luteum that pregnancy has begun. The corpus luteum then begins to produce hormones designed to support the pregnancy until the placenta has developed. By the second week after conception, the blastocyst has evolved into an embryonic disc, and the amniotic sac and placenta are starting to differentiate into their specialized duties. The developing placenta produces projections that tap into the external tissue layer tissue of the blastocyst, where spaces called *lacunae* have been formed. These spaces are filled with maternal blood, and the connection allows both the embryo to draw on the maternal circulation for oxygenation and nutrition and embryonic waste products to be shunted safely away. This connection serves as the beginning of the umbilical cord.

In the third week after conception, the egg, now officially the *embryo* is ready to begin the process of forming specialized body systems. The rudiments of the central nervous system, cardiovascular system, spine, and portions of the skeletal anatomy begin to appear. At the end of this week, an S-shaped tubular heart begins to beat, and blood cells produced in the yolk sac begin to circulate. The pregnant woman, by this point, may notice that she has missed her period and begin to suspect that she is pregnant.

Around the fourth week of pregnancy, the placenta begins to develop. Essentially an enlarged endocrine gland, the placenta carries out a number of crucial functions during pregnancy. The placenta serves as an early liver, taking care of the synthesis of glycogen and cholesterol, metabolizes fatty acid, and produces antibodies that protect the fetus. It also provides the following functions:

- **Respiratory gas exchange.** The placenta functions as the fetal lungs, enabling the fetus to exchange its carbon dioxide–laden blood for oxygen-rich blood.
- **Transport of nutrients** from maternal to fetal circulation.
- **Excretion of wastes,** some of which pass into the maternal circulation and others of which are excreted into the amniotic fluid.
- **Transfer of heat** from the woman to the fetus.
- **Hormone production.** The placenta produces chorionic gonadotropin, a hormone that maintains the pregnancy and stimulates changes in the woman's breasts, vagina, and cervix that prepare her for delivery and motherhood.
- **Formation of a barrier** against harmful substances in the pregnant woman's circulation, such as chemicals or microorganisms. When the placenta blocks a drug from reaching the fetal bloodstream, this means that the drug "does not cross the placenta." The placenta is not able to exclude every harmful substance, so you need to be very careful about which drugs are administered to women during pregnancy.

The **umbilical cord** connects the placenta to the fetus via the fetal umbilicus (navel) **Figure 2**. The cord is gray, easily compressed, and soft and pliant though structurally tough. The interior of the cord contains a mucous material (Wharton jelly—it keeps the umbilical cord from becoming knotted) and a supportive framework of loose connective tissue. The umbilical cord also contains two arteries and one vein. Occasionally, a child will be born with only a single umbilical artery (SUA). SUA may be normal genetically in some children, but may also indicate a congenital abnormality, such as heart or kidney malformations.

Fetal circulation differs from that of the pregnant woman. The umbilical *vein* carries oxygenated blood from the placenta to the fetus, while the umbilical *arteries* carry arteriovenous blood to the placenta. Because the fetus obtains its oxygen via

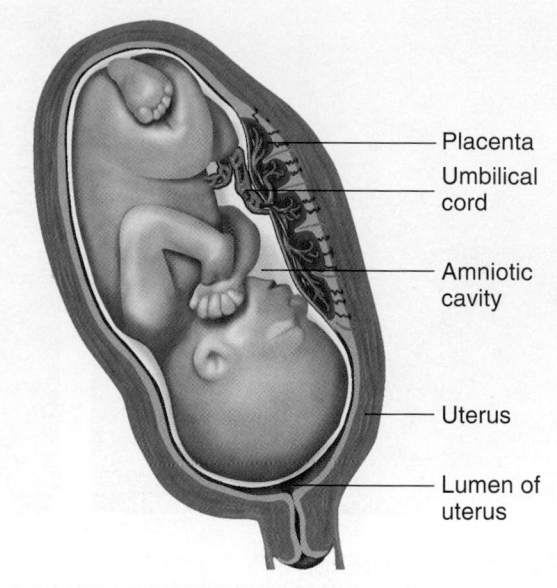

Figure 2 The umbilical cord and other structures of the pregnant uterus.

Labels: Placenta; Umbilical cord; Amniotic cavity; Uterus; Lumen of uterus

the placenta, the fetal circulation bypasses the lungs until birth. A duct connects the umbilical vein and the inferior vena cava, another duct connects the pulmonary artery and the aorta, and an opening separates the right and left atria of the fetal heart. At birth, the neonate's lungs begin to function, and the arteriovenous shunts close.

The **amniotic sac** is a membranous bag that encloses the fetus in a watery fluid called **amniotic fluid**. The amniotic fluid, whose volume reaches about 1 L by the end of pregnancy, provides the fetus with a weightless environment in which to develop. In the latter stages of pregnancy, the fetus swallows amniotic fluid and passes wastes out into the fluid. In this way amniotic fluid assists in fetal excretory function.

The 4th through the 8th weeks of embryonic development are critical for normal development. During this period, the major organs and other body systems are forming and are most susceptible to damage. Some prescription drugs and even over-the-counter medications may have side effects that harm the fetus. Women who use illicit drugs, smoke tobacco, drink alcohol, or are exposed to other toxic substances during their pregnancy also run the risk of creating birth defects in the fetus.

The **gestational period** is the time that it takes for the fetus to develop in utero. It normally takes 38 weeks, with significant developmental progress occurring each week. The time of pregnancy is calculated from the first day of the pregnant woman's last menstrual period. Because the placental tissues normally start sending hormonal signals to the corpus luteum to start changing the internal environment in the second week after conception, this dating method adds 2 weeks to the entire calculation, leading to 40 total weeks of pregnancy from conception to birth (prenatal period).

Physiologic Maternal Changes During Pregnancy

When a woman conceives, carries a fetus to term, and then gives birth, several physiologic changes occur within her body. Many of these changes can alter the normal response to trauma or exacerbate or create medical conditions that can threaten the health of both the woman and fetus. In particular, hormonal changes precipitate physiologic changes, and the rapidly changing internal environment puts stress on the woman. Metabolic demands increase during pregnancy, and the enlarging uterus with its significant vascularity creates mechanical changes as well.

The most significant physiologic changes occur in the uterus. Before a woman's first pregnancy, the uterus measures about 3 inches long by 2 inches wide and is approximately 1 inches thick. After pregnancy has stretched the uterus, it will rarely return to its previous dimensions. In the nonpregnant patient, the uterus weighs only about 0.07 oz (2 g) and has a fluid capacity of about 10 mL. By the end of pregnancy, the uterus may weigh as much as 2.2 lb (1 kg) and have a capacity of about 5,000 mL.

The measurement of the fundus of the uterus (the top portion, opposite the cervix) can indicate possible developmental problems. The fundus is measured in centimeters by running a measuring tape vertically from the top of the pubic bone to the top of the fundus **Figure 3**. The length in centimeters roughly corresponds to length of gestation. For example, if the patient is 32 weeks' pregnant, the measurement would be 32 cm. If the length is longer or shorter than expected, it could indicate uterine growth problems or breech position (if shorter) or the possibility of twins (if longer).

As the pregnancy continues, the uterus enlarges and increases in weight. This weight places pressure on the lower end of the intestine and the woman's rectum and often results

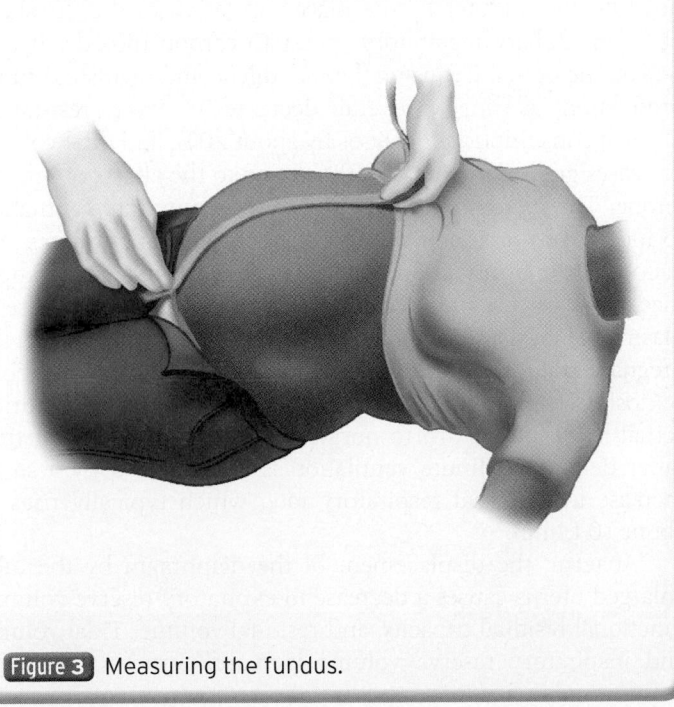

Figure 3 Measuring the fundus.

in constipation. The smooth muscle in the gastrointestinal (GI) tract relaxes due to increased progesterone levels, which causes a decrease in GI motility (decrease in moving stomach contents to duodenum). This decreased motility sometimes can also cause heartburn and burping.

Physiologic changes also occur to the urinary system as the kidneys increase in size and volume. Kidney volume can increase up to 30%. The ureters also have an increase in diameter, with the right side being more dilated than the left in most cases. These changes result in increased urinary frequency for the pregnant woman and an increased chance of urinary tract infection if she does not empty her bladder frequently. Increased pressure on the urinary bladder from the enlarging uterus also causes increased urinary frequency.

Most women also experience changes to their skin, hair, and eyes from the hormones in pregnancy. Increased hair and nail growth and changes in texture are common. It is also common for women to have a "pregnancy mask"—brown and yellowish color changes to the face (around eyes, cheeks, and nose). The skin may darken around the areola, axilla, and genitalia. A dark line of pigment down the midline of the abdomen, which is called *linea nigra*, also develops in many women.

Pregnancy has an impact on a woman's circulatory system in several ways. The average woman has about 4 to 5 L of blood available as total circulating volume. Blood volume in a pregnant woman increases gradually throughout the pregnancy to as much as a 40% to 50% overall increase at term. The increase in the level of blood volume depends on such factors as patient size, if she is carrying multiples, and the number of times **gravid** (total number of times pregnant, including current pregnancy) and **para** (number of live births). This increase in blood volume is necessary to meet the metabolic needs of the developing fetus, to adequately perfuse maternal organs—especially the uterus and kidneys—and to help compensate for blood loss during delivery. At term, the uterus normally contains 15% to 16% of the woman's total circulating blood volume. During vaginal delivery, a woman may lose as much as 500 mL of blood (1,000 mL in case of cesarean section). The uterus, as it contracts, tends to shunt blood back into maternal circulation (autotransfusion), thereby preserving maternal circulatory hemostasis.

As blood volume increases, so does the number of red blood cells (RBCs), which increases by as much as 33% over the normal count. The increase in RBCs heightens the pregnant woman's need for iron, which is why most women take **prenatal** vitamins. If the woman does not take iron supplements, the fetus will rob maternal stores for its needs, resulting in anemia for the woman—and often leading to preterm labor and spontaneous abortion. Women who live in socioeconomically deprived areas and lack access to prenatal health care are the most likely to experience pregnancy-related anemia.

A woman's white blood cell (WBC) count also increases during pregnancy, with an average of 4,300 to 4,500 mL before pregnancy to as high as 12,000 mL or more in the third trimester of pregnancy. Clotting factors are similarly increased, while fibrinolytic factors are depressed. These issues are important considerations if the paramedic has to deal with obstetric hemorrhage or thromboembolic disease.

As blood volume increases, so does the size of the pregnant woman's heart, by an average of 10% to 15% from prepregnancy levels, with a collateral capacity increase of 70 mL to 80 mL. Cardiac output increases to about 40% more than before pregnancy, reaching its maximum capacity at about 22 weeks' gestation and then maintaining this level until term. As the uterus enlarges and the diaphragm becomes elevated, internal maternal organs begin to shift to make room. The myocardium is displaced upward and to the left with a slight rotation in its long axis, which causes the apex of the heart to shift laterally (remember this point when you are auscultating the S_3 and S_4 heart sounds). In addition, the intensity of the "lub-dub" S_1 heart sound increases, while the S_2 heart sound generally remains normal. Increased cardiac output can also cause a benign systolic flow murmur, which results from hypertrophy of the heart and dilation across the tricuspid valve.

A pregnant woman's heart rate gradually increases during pregnancy, by an average of 15 to 20 beats/min by term. ECG changes that can occur during pregnancy include ectopic beats and supraventricular tachycardia, which is often considered normal. Other changes include a slight left axis deviation and lead III changes such as low-voltage QRS, T-wave inversion or flattening, or even occasional Q waves.

As gestation increases, a woman's sensitivity to body positioning increases as well. Resting or lying supine can cause the weight of the uterus to compress the inferior vena cava, thereby decreasing venous return to the heart. Pressure by the fetus on the common iliac vein creates this problem as well. Over time, if pressure is not relieved, cardiac output is decreased, blood pressure drops, and lower extremity edema will result. In about the 12th week of gestation, systolic pressure may drop slightly, but diastolic pressure usually declines by 5 to 10 mm Hg. Diastolic pressure usually returns to normal prepregnancy levels at about 36 weeks' gestation.

The pressures exerted on the circulatory system and the increased blood volume combine to produce venous distention of about 150% of prepregnancy levels. Blood return to the heart is reduced as the venous ends of the capillaries become dilated. Pregnant women who are bedridden or who spend a great deal of time lying down are in particular danger of experiencing deep venous thrombosis, which can lead to pulmonary embolism. This slow blood return to the heart also causes delayed absorption of subcutaneously or intramuscularly injected medications.

When the patient goes into labor, the birthing position she is in may also stress the cardiovascular system. In the United States, the standard position is the lithotomy position, in which the woman is supine (on her back) with her knees spread apart, or her feet in stirrups **Figure 4** .

The workload of the heart increases significantly during both gestation and labor. For a healthy woman, this presents no undue complications. For a woman with heart disease or other forms of cardiac compromise, however, the increased work can result in ventricular failure or pulmonary edema, culminating in congestive heart failure. The pain and pressures of labor can further stress the heart, resulting in cardiac arrest.

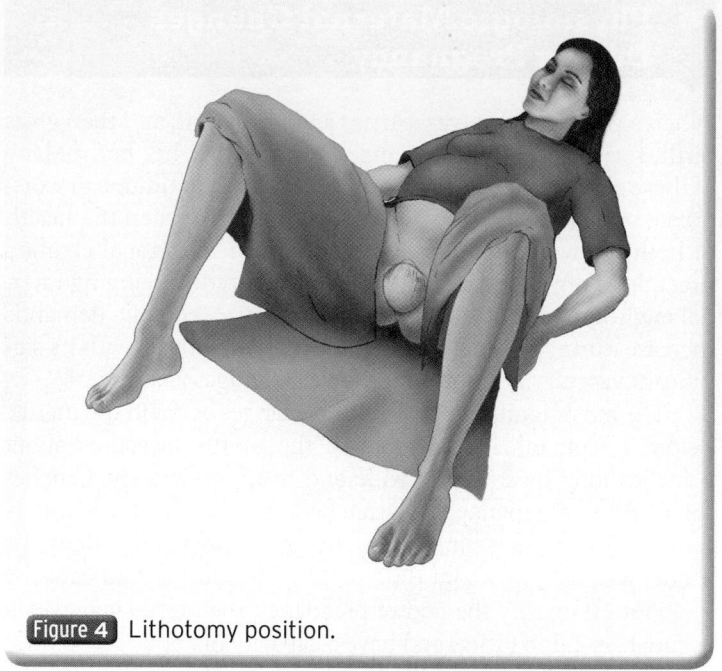

Figure 4 Lithotomy position.

During pregnancy, the respiratory system undergoes stresses as well. The uterus pushes the diaphragm up toward the abdominal cavity, resulting in about a 1½-inches (4-cm) displacement of the diaphragm. To compensate for this change, the rib margins flare outward, increasing the lower thoracic diameter and the total thoracic circumference by as much as 2½ inches (6 cm). This allows the respiratory system to maintain intrathoracic volume. The abdominal muscles tend to lose their tone during pregnancy, which allows respiration to be more diaphragmatic.

As maternal oxygen demand increases, the respiratory physiology changes to accommodate this need. The hormone progesterone, which is produced early in pregnancy by the corpus luteum and later by the placenta, decreases the threshold of the medullary respiratory center to carbon dioxide. It also acts on the bronchi, causing them to dilate, and regulates mucus production, causing an overall decrease in airway resistance. Oxygen consumption increases by about 20%, and tidal volume increases gradually to about 40% owing to the effects of progesterone. The increase in tidal volume causes minute ventilation to increase by as much as 50% over prepregnancy values and Pa_{CO_2} to drop by about 5 mm Hg. The latter change is accompanied by a decrease in blood bicarbonate and a slight increase in plasma pH levels, which in turn affects acid-base balance. In the pregnant state, respiratory alkalosis is balanced by a metabolic acidosis. The acid-base changes become quite marked during actual labor, but return to normal about 3 weeks __postpartum__ (after delivery). Minute ventilation is also affected by a slight increase in maternal respiratory rate, which typically rises to about 10 L/min.

At term, the displacement of the diaphragm by the fully enlarged uterus causes a decrease in expiratory reserve volume, functional residual capacity, and residual volume. Tidal volume and inspiratory reserve volume increase. Structural changes within the respiratory mucous membrane result in increased vascularity and edema.

As the pregnancy progresses, the maternal metabolism undergoes phenomenal changes—most obviously, weight gain and alterations in physical structure. Weight gain is partly due to increased blood volume and increases in intracellular and extracellular fluid (6 to 7 lb), uterine growth (3 lb), placental growth (2 lb), fetal growth (7 lb), and increased breast tissue (2 to 3 lb). Some weight gain is also attributable to increased proteins and fat deposits, with the average weight gain in pregnancy being 27 lb (12.3 kg).

The hormone relaxin, which is released during pregnancy, causes collagenous tissues to soften and produces a generalized relaxing of the ligamentous system, especially along the spine; this effect contributes to the characteristic lordosis of latter pregnancy and the increased flexion of the neck, both of which help the pregnant patient compensate for balance. Animal studies have shown that relaxin also appears to enhance mammary gland enlargement, soften the cervix, and loosen the pelvic joints.

Pregnancy increases the demand for carbohydrates, which seems to be based on fetal demand for glucose. Because the insulin molecule is too large to pass through the placental barrier, several hormones are used to compensate for the increased carbohydrate requirement. Women who are predisposed to a diabetic state may become chemical diabetics during pregnancy, but return to a normal carbohydrate metabolism postpartum. During pregnancy, the pancreas secretes insulin in greater amounts and at a faster pace, while cellular sensitivity to insulin declines. The increased production of insulin is the result of increased levels of free cortisol and progesterone. Estrogen has the effect of blunting the action of insulin, whereas progesterone decreases the utilization of insulin by the cells. The net effect is to make glucose available to the fetus from increased energy production from fat. In a healthy woman, these systems work a very fine balancing act to maintain homeostasis. In obese women or women who have been diagnosed with or are predisposed to diabetes, this balance is much harder to achieve.

Cultural Value Considerations

The United States is among the most culturally diverse nations in the world. This diversity may be a factor when you are assessing and treating an obstetric patient from a culture different than yours. Women of some cultures may have a value system that will affect their pregnancy, the choice of how they care for themselves during pregnancy, and how they have planned the childbirth process. Some cultures may not permit a male health care provider, especially in the prehospital setting, to assess or examine a pregnant patient. Different cultures may view pregnancy different than you do, socially, psychologically, and emotionally. Some may see pregnancy as a means of achieving status and recognition within the family unit where others may experience a drop in self-esteem. Your responsibility is to the patient and is limited to providing care and transport. You should

respect these differences and honor requests from these patients. A competent, rational adult has the right to refuse all or any part of your assessment or care.

Adolescent Pregnancy

The United States has one of the highest teenage pregnancy rates compared with other developed countries. It is likely during your career that you will respond to a pregnant teen who may or may not be in labor. Adolescents present their own challenges to the EMS community in physical and psychological development, even when there is not the contributing factor of the female teenager being pregnant.

Pregnant teens may or may not know that they are pregnant or can be in denial of their situation. As you begin to assess all female teenagers, you should remember that pregnancy is a possibility. The pregnancy itself may or may not be related to the nature of the call, but you should consider it when you are assessing the patient, talking to the patient, obtaining a history, and providing treatment. Respect the teenager's privacy and need for independence. If possible, question all teenagers and perform your assessment away from parents.

Patient Assessment

Special terminology is used when referring to a pregnant patient. As mentioned, **gravidity** refers to the number of times a woman has been pregnant, regardless of the outcome (abortion, stillborn, or live birth). **Parity** refers to delivery of an infant who is alive. The following are some other commonly encountered obstetric terms:

- Primigravida—a woman who is pregnant for the first time.
- Primipara —a woman who has had only one delivery.
- Multigravida—a woman who has had two or more pregnancies, irrespective of the outcome.
- Multipara—a woman who has had two or more deliveries. A woman who has had more than five deliveries is referred to as a "grand multipara."
- Nullipara—a woman who has never delivered.

For example, a woman who has had four pregnancies but carried only one of them to term—the three others ended in miscarriage—would be classified as gravida 4, para 1. The medical shorthand annotation would be G4P1. You could also write the preceding case history as G4A3P1, showing abortive history.

Scene Size-up

Perform a scene size-up as with any other call. As with every emergency call, your safety is a priority. Take standard precautions—gloves and eye protection are a minimum if delivery has already begun or is complete. If the call is going to result in a field delivery and if time allows, a mask and gown should also be used. Consider calling for additional or specialized resources. You will encounter pregnant patients who are not in labor, so it is important to determine the mechanism of injury or nature of illness in a pregnant patient. Because a pregnant woman's balance may be altered by the weight and size of the fetus and hormones that relax the musculature, falls and spinal immobilization must be considered.

■ Primary Assessment

The primary assessment is the same as with any patient—airway, breathing, and circulation.

Form a General Impression

The general impression is a good across-the-room assessment that should tell you whether the patient is in active labor or if you have time to assess for imminent delivery and address other possible life threats. Perform a rapid scan of the patient to determine whether there are airway, breathing, or circulation problems. The chief complaint may be, "The baby is coming!" Take a moment to confirm whether the fetus will be delivered in the next few minutes or, again, whether you have time to continue to evaluate the situation. When trauma or other medical problems such as vaginal bleeding or seizures are the presenting complaint, evaluate these first and then assess the impact of these problems on the fetus. Use the AVPU (*Alert* to person, place, and day; responsive to *Verbal* stimuli; responsive to *Pain*; or *Unresponsive*) scale to determine the patient's level of consciousness.

Airway and Breathing

During an uncomplicated birth, life-threatening conditions with the mother's airway and breathing usually are not an issue. However, a motor vehicle crash, an assault, or any number of medical conditions in a pregnant woman may cause a life threat to exist and, sometimes, result in a complicated delivery. In these situations, assess the airway and breathing to ensure they are adequate. If needed, provide airway management and high-flow oxygen.

Circulation

External and internal bleeding are potential life threats to the patient and should be assessed early on. Blood loss after delivery is expected, but significant bleeding is not. Recall that normal changes in pregnancy result in increased overall blood volume, increased heart rate, and changes in blood clotting. These changes can have a significant impact on a pregnant patient who is bleeding, regardless of the cause. Quickly assess for any potential life-threatening bleeding, and begin treatment immediately. Assess the skin for color, temperature, and moisture, and check the pulse rate to determine whether it is too fast or too slow. If there are signs of shock, control the bleeding, give oxygen, and keep the patient warm.

Transport Decision

If delivery is imminent, you must prepare to deliver at the scene. The ideal place for the delivery is in the security of your ambulance or the privacy of the woman's home. The area should be warm and private with plenty of room to move around.

If the delivery is not imminent, prepare the patient for transport and perform the remainder of the assessment en route to the emergency department. Administer oxygen.

Pregnant women in the last two trimesters of pregnancy should be transported lying on the left side when possible. If spinal immobilization is indicated, secure the woman to the backboard and elevate the right side of the board with rolled towels or blankets to prevent supine hypotensive syndrome. Provide rapid transport for pregnant patients who have significant bleeding and pain, are hypertensive, are having a seizure, or have an altered mental status.

Special Populations

Blood pressure is an unreliable indicator of perfusion in any patient, but it is even less reliable in the pregnant patient because a greater volume of blood can be lost before hypotension develops.

■ History Taking

Proper medical history and physical assessment are an important part in treating the obstetric patient. Determine the patient's chief complaint, investigate the chief complaint using OPQRST, and obtain the SAMPLE history. Specifically, you want to know if the patient is pregnant, how many times she has been pregnant (gravida), and how many times she has had a live birth (para). The first question can generally be bypassed if the patiently is obviously pregnant. Asking a woman who is near term if she is pregnant (the unspoken implication is that she is obese) is not a good way to develop trust, but if in doubt, ask. The number of times pregnant may also need to be clarified, because many women do not count abortions or miscarriages as pregnancies, and tend to think only of actual deliveries. Also ask about the length of gestation and her estimated due date or date of confinement.

Has the woman had a baby before? Labor in a first time mother is usually slower and longer (averages 16 hours) than in subsequent pregnancies, allowing more time for transport.

Ask the patient whether she has experienced complications with any of her pregnancies, or whether she has had any obstetric or gynecologic complications. Has she ever had a cesarean section? If so, is a cesarean delivery planned for the current pregnancy or does the patient intend to have a vaginal birth after cesarean (VBAC)? Complications of VBAC can include uterine rupture. Is the patient currently under a physician's care? Has she been taking prenatal vitamins? When was her last visit to her physician? Has her physician indicated any concerns about this pregnancy?

Has the patient had a recent ultrasound? What were the findings? Did the ultrasound reveal more than one fetus or any abnormal presentations? Is the patient taking any current medications? Any over-the-counter drugs, recreational drugs, or herbals? Does the patient have any allergies?

What is your general impression of the patient's overall health? Has she been smoking, consuming alcohol, or used any illicit drugs during the pregnancy? If yes, how recently? Is the patient currently experiencing pain? If yes, what is the quality and duration? Where is it located and does it radiate? Was the onset gradual or sudden? When did the pain start, and does anything relieve it? Has the patient experienced this type of pain before? When? Is the pain occurring regularly? Is it sporadic or constant?

Has the patient noticed any vaginal bleeding or spotting? If so, what was the amount of bleeding? How long did the bleeding last? What color was the blood? What was the patient doing prior to the bleeding? Did she use sanitary pads to absorb the bleeding? How many pads? Did the bleeding stop? Has the patient passed any clots or tissue? If so, try to obtain samples to give to the emergency department. Has the patient experienced any other type of vaginal discharge? What was the amount, color, and duration of that discharge? Was any identifiable or disagreeable odor associated with the discharge?

If the patient is in active labor, has her water broken? Does she need to move her bowels or push? That sensation occurring during labor is caused by the fetus's head in the woman's vagina pressing against the rectum; it indicates that delivery is imminent. If the woman reports an urge to move her bowels, *do not allow her to go to the toilet.*

What are the contractions like? Some women experience Braxton-Hicks contractions throughout the pregnancy, so it is important to distinguish false labor from the real thing. The pains of true labor are regularly spaced and increase in intensity over time. **Table 1** distinguishes false labor from true labor.

How frequent are the contractions? If they are more than 5 minutes apart, you generally have enough time to get the woman to a nearby hospital. Contractions that are less than 2 minutes apart signal impending delivery, especially in a multipara.

The answers to those questions should give you a good idea of whether there will be time to transport the woman to the hospital. To double-check, *inspect* the woman for **crowning**—crowning indicates that the fetus will be born within the next few minutes.

Table 1 **False Labor Versus True Labor**

Parameter	True Labor	False Labor
Contractions	Regularly spaced	Irregularly spaced
Interval between contractions	Gradually shortens	Remains long
Intensity of contractions	Gradually increases	Stays the same
Effects of analgesics	Do not abolish the pain	Often abolish the pain
Cervical changes	Progressive effacement and dilation	No changes

■ Secondary Assessment

Your physical exam should be based on the patient's chief complaint. Just because a woman is pregnant, you should not rule out the possibility of asthma, heart attack, or allergic reactions, for example. No matter what the chief complaint, the full-body exam should also include fetal heart tones and heart rate. By feeling the abdomen, you can roughly palpate the fetal position. Ask her when was the last time she felt the baby move or if there has been any change to how much the baby has been moving. Pay close attention to the vital signs of both patients—the woman and the fetus. If the patient tells you she has abdominal pain, ask her to describe the pain; this information will help determine whether she is having contractions.

Inspect the vaginal area for crowning or vaginal bleeding or discharge. Crowning indicates that you will need to deliver the fetus on scene. If there is no crowning, ask the woman

YOU are the Medic   PART 2

Your patient is sitting in the driver's seat of the vehicle. She is still wearing her seat belt, which is across the widest part of her abdomen. The airbag has deployed from the steering wheel. The patient is responsive, alert, and oriented. She reports a cramping-type pain in her pelvis.

Recording Time: 1 Minute	
Appearance	Awake
Level of consciousness	Alert, oriented
Airway	Open
Breathing	Adequate
Circulation	Adequate

3. Is the location of the seat belt concerning to you?

4. What steps will you take in your further assessment of this patient?

Special Populations

If you note a scar above a woman's pubic hair line **Figure 5**, it may mean she has delivered once before by cesarean. Ask whether she knows of any reason why she would not be able to delivery vaginally, and report her response to medical control. Women who have previously delivered by cesarean are not precluded from having a normal, vaginal delivery, but doing so may increase the risk for uterine rupture.

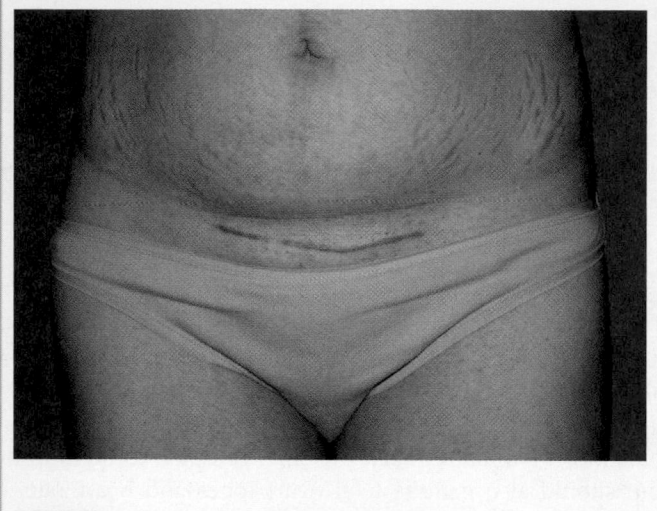

Figure 5 A scar from a cesarean section.

how far apart the contractions are, and then time them. Ask the patient if her water has broken, and, if so, how long ago. First-time pregnant women typically take more time to deliver.

If you see bleeding or discharge, determine when it started and check the abdomen for tenderness and rigidity. Normal abdomens are not rigid during pregnancy. Assessment of the serial vital signs will tell you if the woman or fetus is in distress.

If the patient's water has broken, ask about the color of the fluid and whether it had an odor. If it is brown or black or has a strong odor, it may be an indication of meconium staining, discussed later in this chapter. Meconium can be aspirated into the fetus's lungs, resulting in potentially life-threatening sepsis. Its presence requires special techniques discussed later in this chapter.

Some women may experience Braxton-Hicks contractions, or intermittent uterine contractions that may occur every 10 to 20 minutes. Usually seen in the third trimester of the pregnancy, this condition is also known as false labor. Because you have no way of telling in the field if a patient's contractions are from a miscarriage or another complication of pregnancy, the patient needs to be transported.

Imminent Delivery

If delivery is imminent, you will not have time to conduct an extensive physical examination, but you should attempt to do the following:

- **Assess the woman's vital signs.** If the woman's blood pressure is elevated or her hands and face look puffy, test the deep tendon reflexes at the knees ("knee jerks") for hyperactivity. Any of those signs—elevated blood pressure, facial edema, or hyperactive reflexes—strongly suggest that the woman has preeclampsia, and you must be prepared to deal with seizures before, during, or after delivery.
- **Try to estimate the gestational age.** Palpate the abdomen to estimate the height of the uterus. If the top of the uterus (the fundus) is palpable just above the symphysis pubis, the gestational age is 12 to 16 weeks; if the fundus is palpable at the level of the woman's umbilicus, the gestational age is 22 weeks; if the fundus reaches all the way to the xiphoid, the fetus is at or near term.
- **Listen for fetal heart tones.** Anything lower than 120 beats/min suggests fetal distress. To measure the fetal heart rate, listen with the bell of the stethoscope over the pregnant woman's abdomen at the 4 o'clock position, about 2 inches from the woman's umbilicus. You may have to move the stethoscope around the abdomen until you can hear the fetal heart tones. Palpate the woman's pulse at the same time as you count the fetal heart rate. If the fetal heart rate is identical to the maternal pulse, you are probably listening to an echo of the maternal heartbeat and not the fetal heart, so change the position of your stethoscope and try again. It takes a lot of practice to hear fetal heart tones and requires quiet surroundings. Some modern ambulances may be equipped with Doppler stethoscopes, which make assessment of fetal heart sounds much easier.

If the history and physical assessment indicate that there is ample time to reach the hospital, place the woman in the lateral recumbent position, remove any of her underclothing that might obstruct delivery in the event delivery suddenly appears to be imminent en route to the hospital, and begin transport.

If you reach the conclusion that there is *not* enough time to get to the hospital, prepare to assist in delivery of the fetus at the scene. In a crowded or public place, try to find an area of maximum privacy and cleanliness in which to work. In the patient's home, deploy nervous bystanders in such a way as to keep them occupied, preferably elsewhere. The pregnant woman may find it reassuring to have another woman (eg, a friend, sister, mother, or neighbor) or her husband present. But your own behavior, if calm and reassuring, will be the most effective sedative for patient and bystanders alike.

Reassessment

Ongoing examination should include an assessment of the woman's serial vital signs and the fetal heart rate and heart tones. Also, time the contractions and perform a full-body exam of the woman (if you have not already done so) to avoid missing other possible injuries and complications. Check any interventions and transport to an appropriate facility.

If your assessment determines that delivery is imminent, notify staff at the receiving hospital. Provide an update on the status of the mother and newborn after delivery. On the rare occasion that the delivery does not occur within 30 minutes or you determine that a complication is occurring that cannot be treated in the field, notify the hospital staff of your findings and provide rapid transport. For a pregnant patient with complaints unrelated to childbirth (such as trauma or difficulty breathing), be sure to include the pregnancy status of your patient in your radio report.

Pathophysiology, Assessment, and Management of Complications Related to Pregnancy

Several medical conditions and situations may adversely affect the health of both the woman and the developing fetus. Pregnancy has the tendency to aggravate preexisting medical conditions and give rise to new ones.

Substance Abuse

When a pregnant woman is a drug addict, the illicit drugs she uses pass through the placenta barrier and enter into the fetal circulation. The fetus may then develop birth defects and also becomes an addict. When you are delivering the fetus of a woman with a history of drug abuse, be aware that the newborn may have signs of withdrawal after it is born—for example, respiratory depression, bradycardia, tachycardia, seizures, and cardiac arrest. Treatment should revolve around cardiorespiratory support.

Supine Hypotensive Syndrome

When the pregnant uterus compresses the inferior vena cava, venous blood return to the heart is diminished or, in some cases, occluded. This problem occurs mainly when a pregnant patient is in the supine position (hence the term supine hypotensive syndrome) but can also occur when the woman is sitting. This condition is usually seen in the third trimester, when the uterus is at its largest, and patient mobility is significantly impaired. It also occurs more commonly in women who have venous variscosities. The woman is most prone to this syndrome during labor, but may also experience difficulties in sleep states, particularly if she falls asleep on her back. Left uncorrected, supine hypotensive syndrome can result in significant maternal hypotension and potentially lead to fetal distress because the maternal hypotension translates into placental hypoperfusion. It generally takes 3 to 7 minutes of compression before signs and symptoms manifest. Nausea, dizziness, tachycardia, and claustrophobia are early signs, progressing to breathing difficulty and syncopal episodes. Precipitating factors may include hypovolemia, from either blood loss or dehydration.

Management includes placing the patient in the left lateral recumbent position (tilting your backboard if needed) and treating underlying causes (ie, IV fluids, if hypovolemic). In addition, you must monitor the blood pressure and other vital signs and obtain an ECG.

Cardiac Conditions

Heart disease is of major concern when you are dealing with a pregnant patient. When you are obtaining the patient's medical history, find out the nature and treatment of any heart conditions. Which cardiac medications has the patient been taking? Has she previously been diagnosed with dysrhythmias or heart murmurs? Has she had a history of rheumatic fever, or was she born with a congenital heart defect? Such heart defects may be benign under normal conditions, but the added stresses of pregnancy could create major problems. Has the patient experienced any episodes of dizziness, light-headedness, or syncopal episodes with the pregnancy? Such episodes can be indicative of dysrhythmias that can become critical during the stresses of labor.

Hypertensive Disorders

A major cause of mortality and morbidity in the pregnant woman is hypertension. Blood pressure is generally lower during the gestational period than at prepregnancy levels, but women who are hypertensive or borderline hypertensive may have their hypertension exacerbated by pregnancy.

Chronic hypertension is a blood pressure that is equal to or greater than 140/90 mm Hg, which exists prior to pregnancy, occurs before the 20th week of pregnancy, or continues to persist postpartum. Diastolic pressures higher than 110 mm Hg place the patient in an increased risk category for stroke and other cardiovascular dangers.

Pregnancy-induced hypertension develops after the 20th week of pregnancy in women with previously normal blood pressures and resolves spontaneously in the postpartum period. It is more commonly experienced by women who are obese or glucose intolerant. Pregnancy-induced hypertension may be an early sign of preeclampsia.

Preeclampsia occurs in about 8% of all pregnancies and, along with the other hypertensive disorders, accounts for about 76,000 deaths annually in the United States. Women younger than 20 years who are experiencing their first pregnancy are at highest risk, followed by women with advanced maternal age, histories of multiple pregnancies, and risk factors of chronic hypertension, renal disease, and diabetes. Race also tends to play a factor, with African-American women being most susceptible. The disorder manifests after the 20th week of pregnancy, with the onset of a triad of symptoms: edema, usually of the face, ankles, and hands; gradual onset of hypertension; and protein in the urine. Other symptoms include severe headache, nausea and vomiting, agitation, rapid weight gain, and visual disturbances. Chronic hypertension can retard growth and development of the fetus, impair liver and renal function, cause pulmonary edema, or progress to life-threatening grand mal seizures. Eclampsia exists when the patient experiences a seizure as a result of the severe hypertension. Other risk factors that may accompany preeclampsia include liver or renal failure, cerebral hemorrhage, placental abruption, and HELLP syndrome (Hemolysis, Elevated Liver enzymes, Low Platelets), the presence of which necessitates immediate delivery of the fetus to save the woman's life. A systolic pressure exceeding 160 to 180 mm Hg and a diastolic pressure exceeding 105 mm Hg, in the presence of these other risk factors, may require administration of emergency hypertensive medications, such as labetalol (Normodyne, Trandate) or hydralazine (Alazine, Apresoline). Preeclampsia normally resolves with delivery, but can still be present postpartum.

Seizures

When a seizure occurs in pregnancy, two patients are involved—the pregnant woman and the fetus. Seizures can be caused by hypertension, toxemia, preeclampsia, or a preexisting seizure disorder. Treatment for a pregnant patient is especially difficult because diazepam (Valium) and phenobarbital—the drugs commonly used to treat seizures—can cross the placental barrier, causing fetal distress. In pregnant patients, magnesium sulfate is the recommended treatment, especially in the patient with eclampsia. In addition, high-flow supplemental oxygen is needed for both patients to counteract the hypoxia that occurs in seizures. Potential complications in such cases may include abruptio placenta, hemorrhage, disseminated intravascular coagulation, and death.

Diabetes

Gestational diabetes mellitus (GDM) is the inability to process carbohydrates during the pregnancy. Increased maternal insulin production may lead to an imbalance between the supply of the woman's insulin and glucose production. The patient may be asymptomatic or may exhibit the same signs observed in patients with diabetes mellitus: polyuria, polydipsia, and polyphagia. Treatment consists of diet control and oral hypoglycemic medications. As GDM may occur early in the pregnancy, it is recommended that patients undergo a fasting glucose test as part of routine prenatal testing.

Diabetes may be markedly affected by pregnancy. As the hormones of pregnancy alter the insulin-regulating mechanisms, diabetics may experience wildly fluctuating blood glucose levels, manifested as hyperglycemic or hypoglycemic episodes. Unfortunately, oral hypoglycemic agents can cross the placental barrier and affect the fetus, so insulin-dependent diabetics may have to adjust their daily dosing during pregnancy.

Pregnant patients with a history of diabetes or who present with an altered mental status or seizures should have their blood glucose level checked with a glucometer. Prehospital management should include high-flow oxygen, IV fluids, and administration of $D_{50}W$ if indicated by a low blood glucose reading. Patients who are hyperglycemic should receive oxygen and IV fluid therapy per local protocol.

Respiratory Disorders

One of the most common complaints of pregnant patients is shortness of breath or general dyspnea. This is often precipitated by hormone-related anatomic changes to the respiratory system and is generally only of minor concern and discomfort to the patient. Careful patient assessment and a thorough SAMPLE history may reveal an underlying condition that is being aggravated by the pregnancy.

Asthma is one of the most common conditions that can complicate pregnancy. It can either be aggravated as a preexisting illness or occur for the first time during pregnancy, triggered by the effects of stress or respiratory irritants on an already-sensitized respiratory system. Acute asthma attacks render the fetus and woman vulnerable to progressive hypoxia. Maternal complications of an asthma attack may include premature labor, preeclampsia, respiratory failure, vaginal hemorrhage, or eclampsia. Fetal complications may include premature birth, low birth weight, growth retardation, and quite possibly fetal death.

Pneumonia is one of the leading indirect causes of maternal death in the United States. This illness of the respiratory system and lungs results in alveolar inflammation and edema. Pneumonia can be caused by fungal, viral, or bacterial infection; parasitic infestation; or traumatic or chemical insult to the lungs (eg, aspiration of vomitus). Pneumonia can be especially virulent during pregnancy because of the pregnant woman's already depressed immune system. In conjunction with other medical conditions, it can have a significant impact on maternal mortality and morbidity. Low birth weight and premature labor are common complications, with preterm delivery occurring in as many as 43% of patients and before 36 weeks' gestation.

Hyperemesis Gravidarum

Hyperemesis gravidarum is a condition of persistent nausea and vomiting during pregnancy. Nearly all women experience the infamous—but normal—"morning sickness," especially during the first several weeks of pregnancy. Hyperemesis gravidarum is a much more serious condition, sending more than 50,000 women to US hospitals each year. Prolonged vomiting leads to dehydration and malnutrition, which have negative effects on the woman and fetus. The exact cause of the condition is unknown, but suspects include increased hormone levels (especially estrogen and human chorionic gonadotropin), stress, and changes to the gastrointestinal system. Hyperemesis gravidarum is most common in first-time pregnancies, with multiple gestations, and in women who are obese. Symptoms include severe and persistent vomiting, in excess of three or four times daily. Vomiting is usually projectile and generally consists of bile and possibly blood. Severe nausea, pallor, and possibly jaundice may also be seen.

Prehospital treatment of hyperemesis gravidarum includes the following steps:

1. Provide 100% supplemental oxygen via nonrebreathing mask.
2. Start an IV line of normal saline and administer the first 250 mL of fluid.
3. If protocols allow, administer diphenhydramine, 10 to 50 mg IV or deep IM. This drug has both sedative and antiemetic effects and is contraindicated if the patient is taking MAO inhibitors.
4. Check blood glucose level.
5. Check orthostatic vital signs, and obtain an ECG.
6. Transport. Severe cases will ultimately require hospitalization.

Renal Disorders

As pregnancy progresses, a woman's kidneys increase in length by 1 cm to 1.5 cm (0.4 inches to 0.6 inches), and her ureters get longer, wider, and more curved. Although these changes increase the capacity of the ureters, they can also lead to urinary stasis, resulting in urinary tract infections. These infections can be mild, but they may also progress to states that result in low fetal birth weight and retarded fetal development, premature labor, or even intrauterine fetal death.

Pressure on the bladder as the uterus enlarges can also result in increased urinary frequency. The renal plasma flow rate increases by as much as 25% to 50%, and the glomerular filtration rate increases by about 50%. Patients with preexisting renal disease are likely to experience compounding of associated problems, and those without a diagnosis of renal disease may experience renal malfunctions or failure due to hypertensive disorders or conditions such as hyperemesis gravidarum.

Rh Sensitization

Rh factor is a protein found on the RBCs of most people. When this factor is absent, the person is said to be Rh negative. When a woman who is Rh negative becomes pregnant by a man who has the Rh factor (Rh positive) and the fetus inherits this factor, the fetal blood can pass into the woman's circulation and produce maternal antibody (isoimmunization) to the factor. Rh disease is normally not a problem in first pregnancies, but in subsequent pregnancies the antibody will aggressively cross the placental barrier to attack the fetal RBCs, which the woman's body identifies as foreign proteins. This attack can result in death of the fetus or cause hemolytic disease (erythroblastosis fetalis) in a newborn. Newborns with hemolytic disease may present with jaundice, anemia, and hepatomegaly.

Infections

Viral and parasitic infections in pregnancy can cause significant problems for the pregnant woman and the fetus. Infections early in pregnancy can affect the formation of the organ systems of the fetus; infections later in pregnancy can result in neurologic impairments, growth disturbances, and heart and respiratory conditions. The most commonly encountered infections include varicella zoster virus, human parvovirus B19 (fifth disease), toxoplasmosis, and cytomegalovirus.

Urinary Tract Infections

Group B streptococcus (GBS) is the leading cause of life-threatening infections in newborns, yet remains one of the conditions for which pregnant women are not routinely screened. This infection is caused by *Streptococcus agalactiae*, bacteria that live in the genitourinary and GI tracts of healthy people, generally without causing any ill effects. In pregnancy, the bacteria can proliferate, resulting in urinary tract infection, infection of the uterus, and stillbirth. If the infection is passed on to the newborn, it can cause respiratory problems, pneumonia, septic shock, and meningitis. Infant illness generally manifests within the first 7 days after birth, but can occur several months later.

Human Immunodeficiency Virus (HIV)

Human immunodeficiency virus (HIV) causes acquired immune deficiency syndrome (AIDS), which leads to some types of cancers, severe infections, and other life-threatening conditions. HIV is most often spread by unprotected sex with a person who is HIV positive. It is also transmitted by contact with infected blood, so IV drug users and health care providers who sustain a dirty needlestick are at risk of acquiring this infection. Pregnant women may infect their fetus during pregnancy, during delivery, or from breastfeeding. Many pregnant women are asymptomatic and do not know that they are infected with HIV.

There are medications that an HIV-positive woman may take to control the infection. If the pregnant patient's HIV status is known, these medications may significantly decrease the chance of transmitting the HIV infection to the infant. HIV-infected women are instructed not to breastfeed their newborns.

Cholestasis

Cholestasis is a disease of the liver that can occur during pregnancy. Hormones affect the gallbladder by slowing down or blocking the normal bile flow from the liver. Bile, which aids the process of digestion by breaking down fats, is produced in the liver and stored in the gallbladder. When its normal flow is altered, bile acids build up in the liver and then spill out into the bloodstream. The most common symptom of this condition is profuse, painful itching, particularly of the hands and feet. Patients may also report fatigue or depression, nausea, and right upper quadrant pain. They may also notice color changes in waste elimination—dark urine and abnormally colored stools (light gray, yellow, light brown, or white). Women who are carrying multiple fetuses are at a higher risk for the development of cholestasis, as are women who have a familial history of cholestasis or who have had previous liver damage.

Cholestasis is relatively benign and transitory for the pregnant woman, but can have serious effects on the fetus. Because the fetus relies on the woman's liver to remove bile acids from the blood, any impediment to this process puts stress on the developing fetal liver. Preterm birth and stillbirth are potential complications of untreated cholestasis.

Sexually Transmitted Infections

Bacterial Vaginosis   Bacterial vaginosis is one of the most common conditions to afflict women. In this infection, normal bacteria in the vagina are replaced by an overgrowth of other bacterial forms. Symptoms may include itching, burning, or pain and may be accompanied by a "fishy," foul-smelling discharge. Left untreated, bacterial vaginosis can lead to premature birth or low birth weight babies and may result in pelvic inflammatory disease (PID) for the woman. It is treated with an antibiotic called metronidazole which, if the patient consumes alcohol while taking, will result in severe nausea and vomiting.

Candidiasis   Vaginal infections are common in pregnancy, and candidiasis or *thrush* can develop after having sex with someone who is also infected. It is not technically defined as a sexually transmitted infection. More commonly known as a yeast infection, candidiasis occurs in pregnant and nonpregnant females, although it seems to be more common during pregnancy due to the chemical changes in the vagina (increased glycogen facilitates growth). Risk factors include poorly controlled diabetes and gestational diabetes, taking antibiotics, wearing tight-fitting clothing (increases warmth and decreases air flow), and other activities as insignificant as a bubble bath that can cause an irritation that leads to an infection.

Treatment involves the use of prescription creams and over-the-counter medications. The fetus will not be affected by this infection while in utero. There is a chance the infant may develop thrush in the mouth after delivery if the infection is active during a vaginal delivery or if the woman breastfeeds.

Chlamydia <u>Chlamydia</u> is a common sexually transmitted disease (STD); reported annual diagnoses in the United States exceed 1.2 million every year. Symptoms are usually mild or absent, although some women may report lower abdominal pain, low back pain, nausea, fever, painful intercourse, and bleeding between menstrual periods. A chlamydial infection of the cervix can spread to the rectum, leading to rectal pain, discharge, and bleeding. Left untreated, the disease can progress to pelvic inflammatory disease (PID).

Gonorrhea <u>Gonorrhea</u> is a bacterial infection that grows and multiplies rapidly in the warm, moist areas of the reproductive tract, including the cervix, uterus, and fallopian tubes in women and in the urethra. The bacterium can also grow in the mouth, throat, eyes, and anus. Symptoms, which are generally more severe in men than in women, appear approximately 2 to 10 days after exposure. Women may be infected with gonorrhea for months but be asymptomatic until the infection spreads to other parts of the reproductive system. Symptoms, when they occur, are dysuria with associated burning or itching, a yellowish or bloody vaginal discharge (can be a foul odor), and bleeding associated with vaginal intercourse. More severe infections may present with cramping and abdominal pain, nausea and vomiting, and bleeding between periods. Rectal infections generally present with anal discharge and itching, plus occasional painful bowel movements with fecal blood spotting.

Human Papilloma Virus (HPV) Genital warts are caused by the <u>human papilloma virus (HPV)</u>. There are more than 100 types of HPV (most types are harmless) with about 30 types that can be spread through sexual contact. HPV is the most common STD, with millions of new cases being reported every year. Some infected people have no symptoms. In others, multiple growths develop in the genital areas. HPV has been identified as a causative agent in cervical, vulvar, and anal cancers. In pregnant women, warts may develop that become large enough to affect urination or obstruct the birth canal. If the virus is passed to the fetus, the newborn may develop *laryngeal papillomatosis* (throat warts that block the airway), a potentially life-threatening condition.

Syphilis Approximately 40,000 cases of <u>syphilis</u> are reported each year in the United States, mostly in the 20- to 40-year-old group. Many of the signs and symptoms of syphilis mimic other diseases. Syphilis presents in three stages: primary, secondary,

and late. Transmission occurs through direct contact with open sores, which may arise anywhere on the body, but tend to appear on the genitals, anus, rectum, lips, or mouth. A person with syphilis may remain asymptomatic for years, not realizing that the sores are manifestations of a disease.

The primary stage of syphilis is usually marked by the appearance of a single sore, although in some people, multiple sores develop. The sore is usually painless and is small, firm, and round. It usually goes away after 3 to 6 weeks, marking the second stage of the disease.

The secondary stage of syphilis is characterized by the development of mucous membrane lesions and a skin rash. The characteristic rash may manifest on the palms of the hands and the bottoms of the feet as rough, red or reddish brown spots. Alternatively, it may be barely discernible or resemble rashes from other diseases. The rash generally does not itch. Symptoms of secondary syphilis may include fever, swollen lymph glands, sore throat, patchy hair loss, headaches, weight loss, muscle aches, and fatigue. The symptoms will resolve without treatment. Left untreated, the secondary stage invariably leads to late-stage syphilis.

In the late stage, syphilis has no signs or symptoms, but internal damage is occurring as it attacks the brain, nerves, eyes, heart, blood vessels, liver, bones, and joints. Paralysis, numbness, dementia, gradual blindness, and difficulty coordinating muscle movements are possible and may cause death. Pregnant women with syphilis may have stillborn babies, babies who are born blind, developmentally delayed babies, or babies who die shortly after birth.

Trichomoniasis <u>Trichomoniasis</u> is caused by a single cell parasite that is transmitted through sexual contact, with the vagina being the most common site of infection. Approximately 7 million cases are reported in the United States each year. The infected person may be asymptomatic or may experience signs and symptoms including a frothy, yellow-green vaginal discharge with a strong odor. The infection may also cause irritation and itching of the female genital area, discomfort during intercourse, dysuria, and lower abdominal pain. When present, symptoms usually appear in women within 5 to 28 days of exposure. If the pregnant patient does not get treated for this condition, there is an increased chance for a low birth weight newborn or premature birth and an increased susceptibility to HIV infection.

Finally, cytomegalovirus and herpes are also sexually transmitted infections, but will be discussed within the next section on TORCH syndrome.

TORCH Syndrome

The acronym TORCH stands for toxoplasmosis, other agents, rubella, cytomegalovirus, and herpes simplex. TORCH syndrome refers to infections that occur in neonates as a result of organisms passing through the placenta from the woman to the fetus. While the woman may show no symptoms, neonates show similar symptoms regardless of which of the five infections they have.

Toxoplasmosis <u>Toxoplasmosis</u> is an infection caused by a parasite that pregnant women may get from handling or eating contaminated food or exposure from handling cat litter (cat ingests contaminated food and then passes the infection on in the feces). Depending on when the infection occurs, early versus late pregnancy, there is a chance of the fetus becoming infected. Persons with this infection may not have any signs and symptoms and not know they have the infection. Pregnant women are encouraged not to change cat litter boxes and to only eat meat that has been thoroughly cooked. Some women may have their physician perform a blood test to detect the condition if they have risk factors.

It has been estimated that only about 50% of infected pregnant women will transmit the infection to the fetus. If the pregnant woman becomes infected early in the pregnancy, there is a decreased chance of spread to the fetus, although signs and symptoms are usually more severe for the fetus if the transmission occurs early in the pregnancy.

Newborns usually do not show any signs of the infection but may develop learning, visual, and hearing disabilities as they grow older.

Rubella "German measles" or <u>rubella</u> is a viral infection that some women may become infected with during their pregnancy if they are not immune. Infections that occur in early pregnancy, less than 20 weeks, have a significant chance of causing developmental issues with the fetus, depending on where fetal development is at the time of infection. Rubella infection after 20 weeks rarely causes these issues. Adverse effects on the developing fetus may result in the infant being born blind or deaf, and there is the possibility of significant cardiac and respiratory abnormalities.

Cytomegalovirus <u>Cytomegalovirus (CMV)</u> is a member of the herpesvirus family. This common viral infection has no known cure, and the virus can remain dormant in the body for years. An estimated 80% of the US population has been exposed to CMV. In its active stages, CMV may produce symptoms including prolonged high fever, chills, headache, malaise, extreme fatigue, and an enlarged spleen. Pregnant women are among those with an increased risk for developing an active infection and more serious complications. Newborns who acquire CMV are susceptible to lung problems, blood problems, liver problems, swollen glands, rash, and poor weight gain.

Herpes Genital <u>herpes</u> is an infection of the genitals, buttocks, or anal area caused by herpes simplex virus, type 1 or type 2. The most common is type 1, which infects the mouth and lips, causing cold sores or "fever" blisters. Genital sores may also be present. Type 2, the more serious infection, can affect the mouth as well, but is more commonly known as the primary cause of genital herpes. Genital herpes infection is more prevalent in women. While over one in five Americans has genital herpes, one in four women in the United States are infected with type 2 herpes.

In an active herpes infection, symptoms generally appear within 2 weeks of primary infection and can last for several weeks. Symptoms may include tingling or sores near the area where the virus has entered the body, such as on the genital or rectal area, on the buttocks or thighs, or on other parts of the body where the virus has entered through broken skin. In women, the sores may be inside the vagina, on the cervix, or in the urinary tract. Other symptoms that may accompany the first outbreak, and possibly subsequent outbreaks, include fever, muscle aches and pains, headache, dysuria, vaginal discharge, and swollen glands in the groin area.

YOU are the Medic   PART 3

Your patient confirms she is 20 weeks' pregnant and has been being followed by her doctor throughout the pregnancy. She is expecting no complications. This is her second child; the first child is not in the vehicle with her. She states that her child is being cared for by her grandmother.

Recording Time: 5 Minutes	
Respirations	20 breaths/min
Pulse	100 beats/min
Skin	Pink, warm, dry
Blood pressure	130/72 mm Hg
Oxygen saturation (Spo$_2$)	98% on room air
Pupils	Equal and reactive

5. What trimester is this patient in?

6. Do you have any additional concerns because this is the patient's second pregnancy?

Pathophysiology, Assessment, and Management of Bleeding Related to Pregnancy

Pathophysiology

Abortion

Abortion is defined as expulsion of the fetus, from any cause, before the 20th week of gestation (some sources consider any loss of the pregnancy up to the 28th week of gestation to be an abortion). Most abortions occur during the first trimester, before the placenta is fully mature.

Abortions can be broadly classified as spontaneous or elective (induced). A spontaneous abortion (miscarriage) occurs naturally, affecting about 1 of every 5 pregnancies. Causes may include acute or chronic illness in the pregnant woman, maternal exposure to toxic substances (illicit drugs), abnormalities in the fetus, or abnormal attachment of the placenta. In many cases, the cause of a spontaneous abortion cannot be found.

An elective abortion is brought about intentionally. When you are obtaining a medical history that includes an abortive history, you must be dispassionate and professional regardless of your personal convictions. You may encounter a patient who is experiencing complications following an elective abortion, such as vaginal bleeding or sepsis from having parts of the fetus remaining in the uterus. You may also encounter a patient who has "self-medicated" in an attempt to induce an abortion and is experiencing toxic effects of the herbal remedy as well as a threatened or progressing abortion. Herbal preparations work by making the uterus and bloodstream too toxic for the fetus to survive, which in turn may be too toxic for the woman to survive.

You will most likely find yourself attempting to manage an abortion that is occurring spontaneously. The specific management of such a case depends to some extent on the stage of the abortion when the patient presents for treatment. All pregnant patients presenting with vaginal bleeding or abdominal pain should be transported and evaluated by a physician.

Some women experience recurrent miscarriages or habitual abortions, which is defined as three or more consecutive pregnancies that end in miscarriage. Habitual abortion is seen in less than 1% of patients. Causes include chromosomal and endocrine disorders, ovarian issues, uterine malformations, cervical conditions (incompetence), infections, and lifestyle factors.

A threatened abortion is an abortion that is attempting to take place. It is generally characterized by vaginal bleeding during the first half of pregnancy—usually in the first trimester. The patient may present with abdominal discomfort or report menstrual cramps. Severe pain is rarely a presenting complaint because uterine contractions are not rhythmic. The cervix remains closed. A threatened abortion can progress to an incomplete abortion, or it may subside, allowing the pregnancy to go to term. The treatment for a threatened abortion is usually complete bed rest, often in a hospital environment, so that the woman's condition can be monitored. Your role in this case is usually transport and emotional support.

An imminent abortion is a spontaneous abortion that cannot be prevented. The patient will generally present with severe abdominal pain caused by strong uterine contractions. Vaginal bleeding, often massive, will be present, as well as cervical dilation because the uterus is preparing to expel the products of conception. When you are treating a patient who is experiencing a spontaneous abortion, your goals are to maintain blood pressure and prevent hypovolemia. Treatment consists of establishing an IV line of normal saline to maintain blood pressure, 100% supplemental oxygen via a nonrebreathing mask at 15 L/min, obtaining an ECG, and providing emotional support with rapid transport. Be alert for signs of shock.

An incomplete abortion occurs when part of the products of conception are expelled but some remain in the uterus. (For example, the fetus is expelled but the placenta remains, or only part of the fetus is expelled.) Because the cervix has dilated to expel the fetus, vaginal bleeding will be present, which may be slight or profuse, but will be continuous. Be alert for signs and symptoms of shock, and start an IV line of normal saline. If products of conception are protruding from the vagina, consult medical control for instructions; gentle removal of protruding tissues may prevent or relieve signs of shock. You will most often encounter this situation when you find the patient on the toilet, having attempted a bowel movement, with the fetus in the toilet still attached to the umbilical cord hanging from the vagina. The fetus should be gently collected, and emotional support provided to the patient. Fundal massage may be beneficial in stimulating the placenta to deliver. All products of conception need to be collected and presented to the receiving facility. Do not deter the patient from viewing the fetus if she wishes, but be prepared for a strong emotional reaction. A complete abortion has occurred when all the products of conception have been expelled.

In a missed abortion, the fetus dies during the first 20 weeks of gestation but remains in utero. There is no field management of a missed abortion other than providing transport and emotional support. Management at the hospital will consist of a dilation and curettage (D&C), in which the cervix will be manually dilated and the endometrial lining scraped and suctioned. You should suspect a missed abortion when the patient presents with a history of threatened abortion. The typical history will be a cessation of vaginal bleeding followed by a gradual diminishing of the signs of pregnancy, such as uterine and breast enlargement. The woman may also report having had a brownish vaginal discharge, possibly accompanied by a rank smell. On examination, the uterus may feel like a hard mass in the abdomen, and fetal heart sounds cannot be heard. Missed abortion is generally caused by maternal disease or abnormalities with the embryo, uterus, placental, or fetal chromosomes. It almost always occurs because of a problem with the fetus, but occasionally a healthy fetus can be expelled by a diseased or damaged uterus. A missed abortion generally precedes a spontaneous abortion.

Septic abortion was once the leading cause of maternal death worldwide. In medical literature, a common complication of childbirth was puerperal fever, which was caused by

Words of Wisdom

Any vaginal bleeding during the third trimester of pregnancy must be regarded as a dire medical emergency until proved otherwise.

a streptococcal infection of the genital tract. The incidence of puerperal fever declined significantly in the early 20th century when physicians began routinely washing their hands between patients **Figure 6** . Septic abortion occurs when the uterus becomes infected—often by common vaginal bacterial flora—following any type of abortion. The patient will generally give a history of fever and bad-smelling vaginal discharge, usually starting within a few hours after abortion. Physical examination will generally reveal fever and abdominal tenderness.

In severe cases, the infection will have progressed to septicemia, resulting in septic shock. For this life-threatening emergency, prehospital management consists of establishing an IV line of normal saline, administering 100% supplemental oxygen via a nonrebreathing mask, ECG monitoring, and rapid transport. The fluid administration rate should maintain the patient's blood pressure at an acceptable level.

Third-Trimester Bleeding

Abortion accounts for the majority of vaginal bleeding that results in an emergency call. Any detachment of the ovum or embryo from the uterine wall will result in bleeding. The patient may report light or heavy bleeding, normally accompanied by cramping abdominal pain. She may also report the passage of tissue or clots. Vaginal bleeding is a serious sign at any stage of pregnancy, but the complications of bleeding increase as the gestation time lengthens.

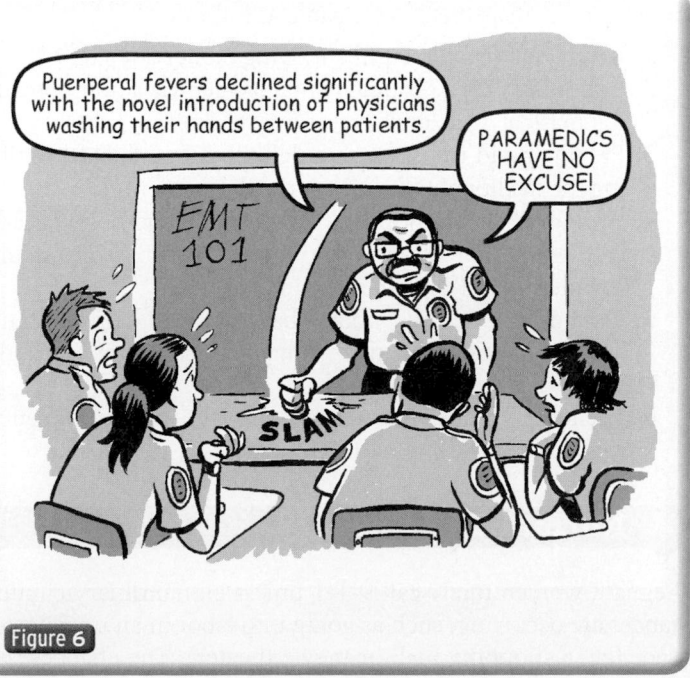

Figure 6

Third-trimester bleeding presents the greatest danger of hemorrhage, which becomes more acute as the woman approaches term. A complicating factor of third-trimester bleeding is the large volume of blood present within the pregnant woman's body and the compensatory mechanisms that are functioning as a result of pregnancy. A pregnant woman can lose a full 40% of her circulating volume before significant signs and symptoms of hypovolemia become apparent.

Ectopic Pregnancy

Ectopic pregnancy is a life-threatening condition. In an ectopic pregnancy, a fertilized ovum becomes implanted somewhere other than in the uterus, usually in one of the fallopian tubes. The fetus will not develop to term. All the normal signs and symptoms of pregnancy are usually present. You are typically dispatched to a patient with abdominal pain. The patient is in severe pain (from the threatened rupture of the tube), and may be in hypovolemic shock. It is important for you to be understanding, empathetic, and supportive. All female patients of child-bearing age with severe, lower abdominal pain should be considered as experiencing an ectopic pregnancy. Treatment for shock and rapid transport are your priorities. Ectopic pregnancy is discussed in detail in the chapter, *Gynecologic Emergencies*.

Special Populations

A pregnant woman may lose a large amount of blood before she shows signs of shock. Do not wait for signs and symptoms. Suspect shock from the mechanisms of injury.

Bleeding and the Placenta

Major causes of significant hemorrhage before delivery are abruptio placenta and placenta previa.

Abruptio placenta refers to a premature separation of a normally implanted placenta from the wall of the uterus **Figure 7** . It most commonly occurs during the last trimester of pregnancy, but can take place in the second trimester as well. Abruptio placenta affects about 1 of every 100 pregnancies that go to term. Maternal hypertension is the most common cause of abruption (44%), followed by trauma (eg, motor vehicle crash), assault, falls, and infection. Drug abuse, alcohol use, and smoking are also contributing factors. Incidence is greater among multiparous women and those who have previously experienced abruptio placenta.

The patient with abruptio placenta will usually report vaginal bleeding, with bright red blood, although in some cases the blood does not emerge through the cervix and the bleeding may remain concealed within the endometrium. In any case, the woman will experience the sudden onset of severe abdominal pain, and she may report that she no longer feels the fetus moving inside her. Physical examination may reveal signs of shock, often out of proportion to the apparent volume of blood loss. The abdomen will be tender and the uterus rigid to palpation. Fetal heart sounds are often absent because the fetus, being

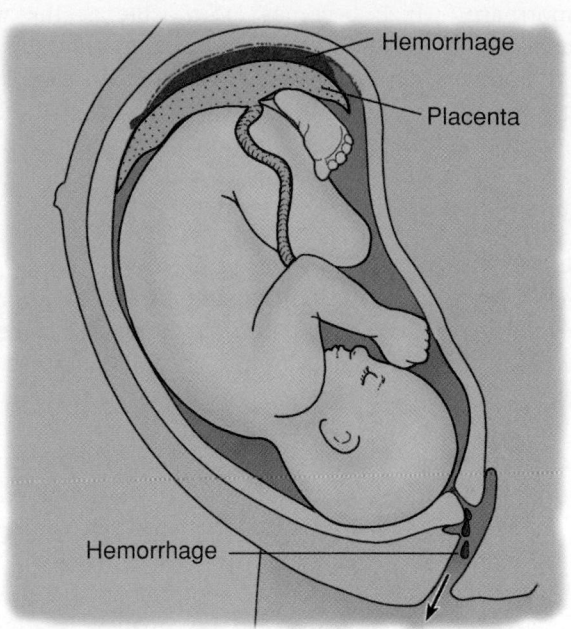

Figure 7 In abruptio placenta, the placenta separates prematurely from the wall of the uterus.

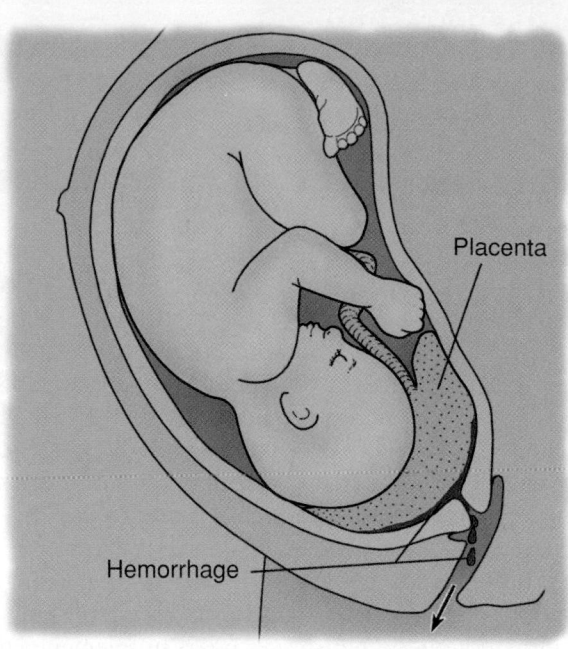

Figure 8 In placenta previa, the placenta develops over and covers the cervix.

partly or completely cut off from its blood supply, is likely to die. Other complications include severe hemorrhaging. If the hemorrhaging cannot be controlled after delivery, a hysterectomy may be necessary.

In <u>placenta previa</u>, the placenta is implanted low in the uterus and, as it grows, it partially or fully obscures the cervical canal **Figure 8**. This condition is the leading cause of vaginal bleeding in the second and third trimesters of pregnancy, with the majority of problems occurring near term because the cervix begins to dilate in preparation for delivery. Maternal age and multiparity are risk factors. Placenta previa occurs in about 5 of every 1,000 births, with a maternal mortality rate of 0.03%. Complications include disseminated intravascular coagulation, hemorrhage, and low fetal birth weight.

The chief complaint of a woman with placenta previa is usually painless vaginal bleeding, with the loss of bright red blood. Because the blood supply to the fetus is not immediately jeopardized, fetal movements continue and fetal heart sounds remain audible. On gentle palpation, the uterus is soft and nontender. (Do *not* try to palpate the abdomen deeply in any woman with third-trimester bleeding; if she does have placenta previa, deep palpation may induce heavy bleeding.)

■ Assessment and Management

When the patient presents with the chief complaint of vaginal bleeding, try to determine as much as possible about the nature of the bleeding. When did it start? What activity was the woman engaged in at the onset? Was she active or at rest? How much blood has been lost? Is the patient experiencing abdominal pain? What is the nature of the pain? Sharp? Cramping? Dull?

Achy? Use OPQRST to elaborate on the chief complaint of labor pain. Rate its severity on a scale of 1 to 10. During the physical examination, identify any changes in orthostatic vital signs. Orthostatic changes indicate a significant blood loss, which may be contrary to the physical evidence of bleeding, which may be slight. Look for a positive Grey Turner sign or Cullen sign, which can help correlate the presence of internal bleeding.

You do not need to identify the underlying cause of the bleeding to treat it. Regardless of the source of hemorrhaging, prehospital management is the same as follows:

1. Keep the woman recumbent, lying on her left side.
2. Administer 100% supplemental oxygen via a nonrebreathing mask at 15 L/min.
3. Provide rapid transport to a definitive care facility, notifying the facility of the patient's condition en route.
4. Start an IV line of normal saline with a large-bore IV catheter. Infuse at a rate necessary to maintain blood pressure. An additional IV line may be indicated.
5. Obtain an ECG and obtain baseline vital signs. Do not attempt to examine the woman internally or pack the vagina with trauma pads.
6. Use loosely placed trauma pads over the vagina in an effort to stop the flow of blood.

■ Normal Childbirth

Pregnant women rarely call 9-1-1 unless extraordinary circumstances are occurring, such as going into labor in an unexpected place (eg, a shopping mall or movie theater). The chances that complications will occur increase significantly when delivery occurs unplanned outside of the hospital. You will usually be working in an uncontrolled, nonsterile environment, so having a good working knowledge of potential complications and strategies to resolve them is mandatory.

Stages of Labor

The following information discusses the stages of normal labor. Labor refers to the mechanism by which the products of conception—that is, the fetus and the placenta—are expelled from the pregnant woman's uterus. It is called labor because it is *hard work*.

Labor progresses through several well-defined stages. The time for each stage depends, in part, on whether the woman is going through her first pregnancy or has had previous deliveries. The premonitory signs of labor, which often are unnoticed, include the woman beginning to feel a relief of pressure in her upper abdomen (lightening) and a simultaneous increase of pressure in her pelvis as the fetus starts its descent toward the birth canal. A plug of mucus, sometimes mixed with blood (called the bloody show) is expelled from the dilating cervix and discharged from the vagina.

The first stage of labor begins with the onset of labor pains—crampy abdominal pains that may radiate into the small of the back and reflect the contractions of the uterus. Those early contractions come at 5- to 15-minute intervals, and they serve to maneuver the fetus into position and prepare the cervical opening for the delivery of the fetus. The latent phase is when the cervix begins to dilate and efface. As the uterus contracts, its less muscular lower segment is pulled upward over the presenting part, resulting in effacement (thinning and shortening) of the cervix. Effacement is accompanied by progressive cervical dilation—that is, stretching of the cervical opening until it is wide enough to accommodate passage of the fetus. The first stage of labor lasts until the cervix is fully dilated, an average of about 12 hours in a nullipara and anywhere up to 8 hours in a multipara. During the active phase, there is a noticeable increase in intensity and the contractions are more painful. Contractions occur more regularly, last longer, and are closer together. Cervical dilation occurs to about 7 centimeters in this phase. The transition phase begins when the cervix is fully dilated to 10 centimeters and the woman may feel an urge to bear down, push, or have a bowel movement. Toward the end of this first stage of labor, the amniotic sac often ruptures, with a gush of fluid pouring out of the vagina.

The second stage of labor begins as the head of the fetus descends and flexes (chin to chest) to enter the birth canal. The fetus must go through several positional changes in order to pass through the pelvic ring and completely through the birth canal. The next position is internal rotation, in which the head is rotated so that the face is toward the woman's rectum. Extension occurs next, as the head of the fetus tilts to a position such that the crown of the head can be seen at the vaginal opening. The baby's head then rotates to the side (restitution) to align the head again with the shoulders. The final external rotation occurs with the movement of the shoulders that results in expulsion of the body of the fetus.

The woman's contractions in this stage are more intense and more frequent, occurring 2 to 3 minutes apart. Her pulse rate increases, and sweat appears on her face. She tends to bear down with each contraction and, because of the pressure of the fetus' head against her rectum, she may feel as if she has to move her bowels. The cervix meanwhile becomes fully dilated and effaced, and the presenting part of the fetus (the part that emerges from the woman first—normally the head) begins bulging out of the vaginal opening (crowning). When crowning occurs, delivery is imminent. The second stage of labor concludes when the newborn is fully delivered. Altogether, the second stage of labor takes 1 to 2 hours in a nullipara and about 30 minutes in a multipara.

The third stage of labor (placental stage) is the period that involves separation of the placenta from the uterine wall. It lasts from the delivery of the newborn until the placenta has been fully expelled and the uterus has contracted. Uterine contraction is necessary to squeeze shut all of the tiny blood vessels left exposed when the placenta separates from the uterine wall. Table 2 summarizes the stages of labor.

Maternal and Fetal Response to Labor

The body systems of the pregnant woman and the fetus respond differently during the strenuous stages of labor. Almost all of the responses are the direct result of the intense physical stressors the woman is going through with each contraction. Contractions and the positional changes of the fetus through the birth canal are the primary causes of the fetal responses seen.

The woman experiences an increased workload on the heart during labor. Blood pressure, pulse, and cardiac output are all increased to ramp up the necessary energy for childbirth. It is

Table 2 The Stages of Labor: Nullipara Versus Multipara

Stage of Labor	Nullipara	Multipara
First stage	8 to 12 hours	6 to 8 hours
Second stage	1 to 2 hours	30 minutes
Third stage	5 to 60 minutes	5 to 60 minutes

common to see an increase in systolic blood pressure as much as 15 points during a contraction. The respiratory system responds by increasing the breathing rate to accommodate the increased demand for oxygen. During the second stage of labor, the woman's need for and consumption or use of oxygen approaches 100%. Pain from contractions and perineal stretching will also cause an increase in respiratory rate during labor.

Typically, the woman's immune system responds to the stress and exertion of labor with an increase in WBC production. The renal system (kidneys) will preserve fluids and electrolytes. The significant muscle exertion results in protein breakdown, which is shown by finding protein in the woman's urine. The increase in physical exertion also increases the woman's body temperature; diaphoresis is common in laboring patients in an attempt to regulate their body temperature. The woman's body diverts blood flow to areas most needed during labor so the gastrointestinal system is essentially inactive, resulting in delayed stomach emptying and loose bowel movements. Nausea, vomiting, and diarrhea are common.

Most of the responses to labor seen in the fetus are the result of the powerful uterine contractions on the body of the fetus. During a contraction, blood flow is greatly reduced, which can affect the hemodynamic status of the fetus. This results in a decrease in the amount of oxygen and nutrients reaching the fetus, as well as insufficient removal of waste from the fetus, and a decreased fetal heart rate during a contraction. Fetal acidosis is the acid-base response from hypoxia and the buildup of lactic acid and can be caused by a nuchal cord, multiple births, abnormal fetal position, respiratory conditions, shoulder dystocia, and other complications of childbirth.

◼ Preparing for Delivery

When you have to assist in childbirth outside the hospital, it means that birth is imminent and you may not have enough time to reach the hospital. Consequently, you generally do not have much time to make a lot of preparations. You may have only a minute or two to get the woman into position, open the OB kit, and deliver the newborn. Thus the sequence of actions in emergency childbirth needs to be well planned and well rehearsed before you use it in the field.

Position the pregnant woman. If childbirth is to take place in the patient's home, the fetus is usually delivered with the woman

lying supine in her bed or at least on a flat surface. While placing the woman in the supine position makes things much easier for you assisting delivery, it makes things harder for the woman because she has to push against gravity. Some women therefore prefer to sit at the edge of a chair or to squat for delivery—positions that enable the woman to take advantage of gravity.

Delivery modalities have changed dramatically in recent years. More women are opting for home deliveries versus in-hospital care, and the phenomenon of natural childbirth is becoming more popular. The use of nurse midwives, lay midwives, professional birth assistants, chiropractors, and doulas (an assistant who "mothers" the woman) are gradually gaining acceptance within the medical community. With the advent of these professions, alternative "pushing" positions are also becoming more popular.

Birthing Positions

Standing Birth Birthing from a standing position is an ancient practice, and one that is used in several areas of the world Figure 9. This position is sometimes used in the active birth model, in which the woman is allowed total freedom to move around and be active up to the point of delivery. Standing birth allows the woman to take advantage of gravity and allows the pelvis to open to a maximal position. The fetal head is moved away from the sacral area as the woman arches her back, a movement that is not easily accomplished while supine.

Semi-Fowler's Position The semi-Fowler's position is basically the supine lithotomy position, with the woman's torso propped up to a high Fowler's or Fowler's position Figure 10. Sitting up seems to help some women with pushing because they can lie back to rest in between contractions.

Kneeling Birth In the kneeling birth position, the woman kneels with her buttocks in the air and usually rests on her elbows Figure 11. This position provides some of the same advantages as squatting: It enables the woman to arch her back to assist delivery, which allows the fetal head to move away from the sacrum, thereby facilitating the birth. Some women may use this method in a bathtub full of water (water birth), which is reputed to ease delivery. Unintentional submersion (of the woman and newborn) is a possible downside to this method, but is technically a low risk. The newborn continues to be oxygenated through the umbilical cord until the face breaks water, or the newborn is stimulated.

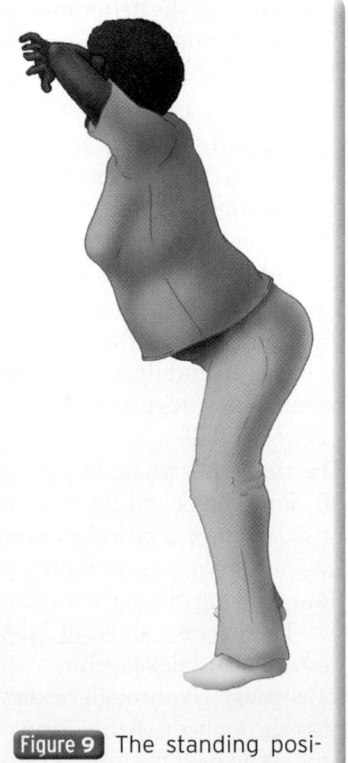

Figure 9 The standing position.

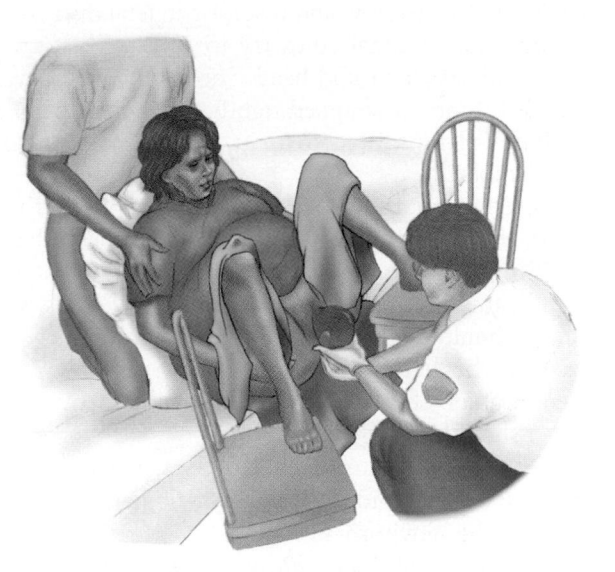

Figure 10 Semi Fowler's position.

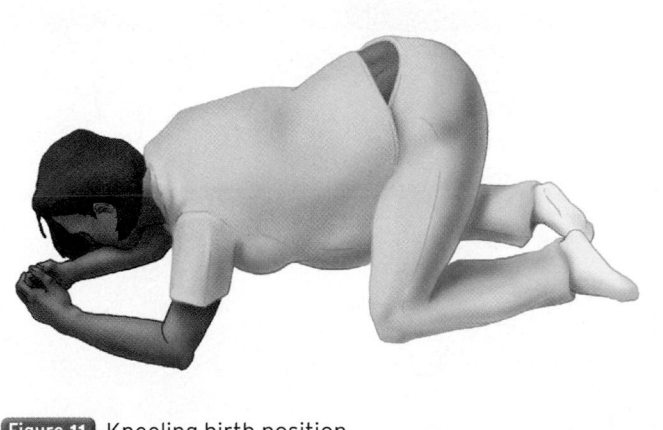

Figure 11 Kneeling birth position.

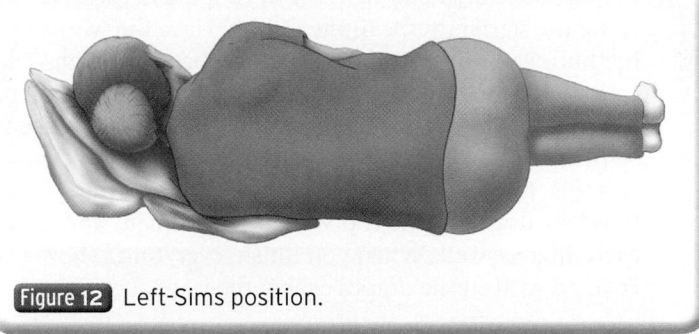

Figure 12 Left-Sims position.

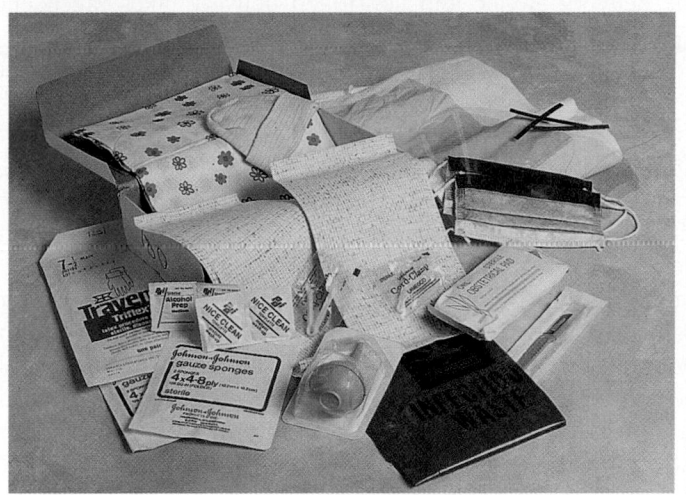

Figure 13 Your unit should contain a sterile OB kit. Items usually found in this kit are listed in Table 3.

Table 3 Sterile Obstetrics Kit for Ambulances

Quantity	Item	Quantity	Item
1	Pair surgical scissors	1 to 2	Surgical masks
4	Cord clamps	12	4-in × 4-in gauze sponges
4 to 6	12-in lengths of umbilical tape	1	Bulb syringe
4 to 6	Towels	1	Baby blanket
2 to 3	Pairs surgical gloves	2	Large plastic bags
1	Surgical gown	3	Povidone-iodine scrub brushes

Side-Lying Position This position is essentially a left-Sims position, with the upper torso possibly supported with pillows **Figure 12**. This position ensures that the uterus and the fetus are moved away from the inferior aorta. Some midwives report a significantly reduced incidence of perineal tears using this method. While some women may prefer to have their legs widely spread during birth, the side-lying position allows the knees to be held together, which also purportedly reduces tearing, especially during the crowning stage.

If the woman prefers to be in one of these positions, you need to adapt to the circumstances and let her use whatever position she is most comfortable with as long as the alternative method does not endanger the woman.

The OB Kit and Preparation

Take the following steps to prepare for the delivery:

- Open the sterile OB kit, making sure to maintain sterility by touching only the outside **Figure 13** (see **Table 3** for kit contents).
- Wash your hands thoroughly with a povidone-iodine or chlorhexidine scrub solution, if available.
- Put on sterile gloves, using a sterile donning technique.
- Maintain standard precautions. Deliveries are often messy, and the chance of contamination from body fluid exposure is high. Put on a sterile gown and surgical mask, and wear eye protection.

- Prepare the woman for delivery by draping her with towels using the sterile towels in the OB kit. Have the woman lift her buttocks, and place the first towel beneath them. Take care not to touch her or the sheet she has been sitting on so that you do not break your sterile field. Lay a second sterile towel flat on the bed or stretcher between the woman's legs, just below the vaginal opening. Lay a third sterile towel or drape across the woman's abdomen, and drape each thigh as well. When you finish, everything should be covered with sterile drapes except the vaginal opening.

If the delivery of the fetus is imminent and you do not have time to place the sterile drapes, just concentrate on controlling the delivery. A safe and controlled delivery takes precedence over draping procedures.

Do not forget to attend to the emotional needs of the patient and family members who are bystanders. This job should be managed by your partner while you are getting prepared. Emotions tend to run high during deliveries, and additional stress may be experienced if the delivery is occurring in a crowded area. Your partner should take a position at the woman's head to help keep her calm and should administer oxygen to her if indicated (a high-risk pregnancy, hypotension or hypertension, or pain). Your partner should also ensure that an emesis basin and portable suction are at hand. If there is time, an IV line should be established (especially if your protocols call for oxytocin administration after delivery), and apply the ECG monitor. Consideration should be given to IV fluid boluses if the woman is hypotensive. Although not common, some protocols will direct you to administer analgesic pain medication. As always, follow your local protocol.

Encourage the woman to rest between contractions and to resist bearing down until you are ready to assist with the delivery. This may be challenging, because once your patient is ready to push, she is *going* to push. If she finds it difficult not to bear down, instruct her to "pant like a dog" during each contraction. Panting makes it nearly impossible to push because bearing down requires a closed glottis.

Assisting Delivery

Follow these steps to assist with the delivery:

1. Control the delivery. When crowning occurs, place *gentle* pressure on the newborn's head with the palm of your gloved hand to prevent the head from delivering too quickly and tearing the woman's vagina.
2. As the newborn's head begins to emerge from the vagina, it will start to turn. Support the head as it turns. Do *not* attempt to pull the newborn from the vagina! If the membranes cover the head after it emerges, tear the amniotic sac with your fingers or forceps to permit escape of amniotic fluid and enable the newborn to breathe.
3. Slip your middle finger alongside the newborn's head to check for a nuchal cord. In such a case, the umbilical cord becomes wrapped around part of the infant's body, generally the neck and as a single loop. In most cases, a nuchal cord is not a significant problem, but as the fetus descends

during labor, cord compression may occur, causing the fetal heart rate to slow and resulting in fetal distress.

4. If you find a nuchal cord, try to slip it gently over the newborn's shoulder and head. Should this maneuver fail, and if the cord is wrapped tightly around the neck, place umbilical clamps 2 inches apart and cut the cord between the clamps.
5. With the newborn's head cradled and supported in your hand, clear the airway by suctioning with the bulb syringe **Figure 14**.
6. Gently guide the head downward to allow delivery of the upper shoulder **Figure 15**. Do not pull on the newborn to facilitate the delivery.
7. Gently guide the head upward to allow delivery of the lower shoulder **Figure 16**.
8. Once the shoulders are delivered, the newborn's trunk and legs will follow rapidly **Figure 17**. Be prepared to grasp and support the newborn as it emerges, keeping in mind an important fact: *Newborns are wet and slippery.*

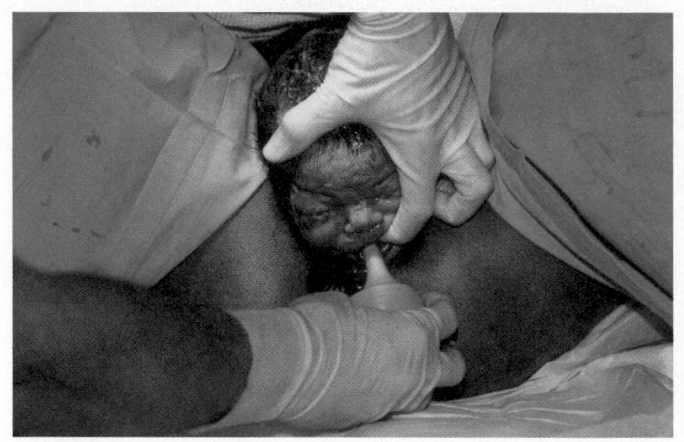

Figure 14 Clear the newborn's airway.

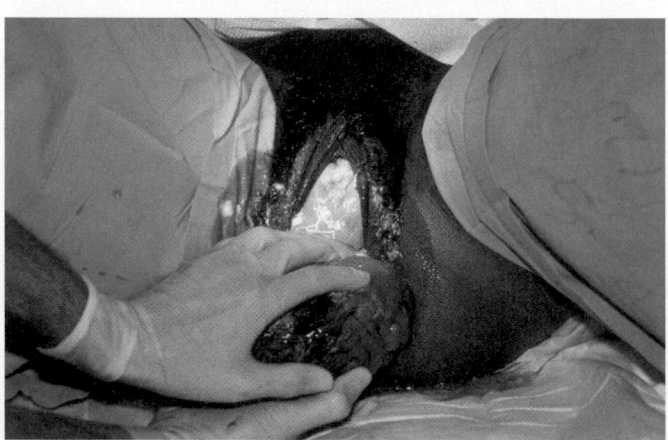

Figure 15 Gently guide the newborn's head downward to allow delivery of the upper shoulder.

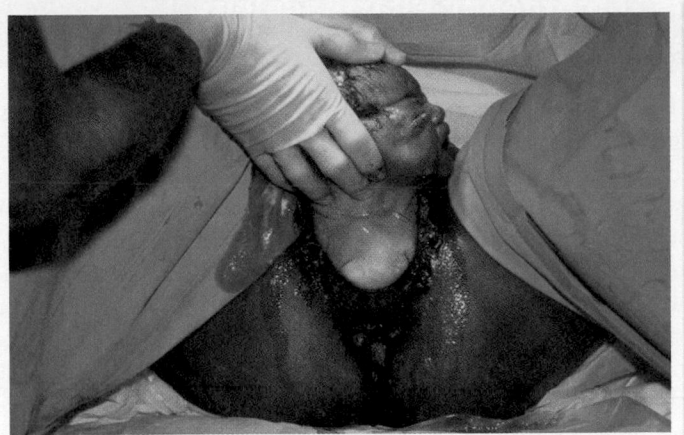

Figure 16 Gently guide the head upward to allow delivery of the lower shoulder.

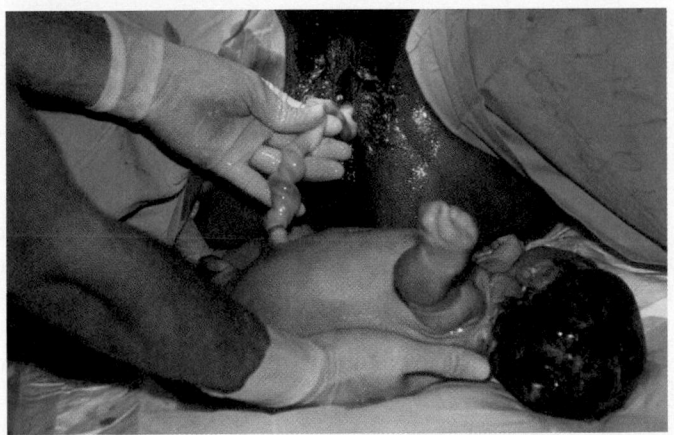

Figure 17 Once the shoulders are delivered, the newborn's trunk and legs will follow rapidly.

9. Once the newborn is delivered, maintain its body position at the same level as the vagina to prevent blood drainage from the umbilical cord.
10. Wipe any blood or mucus from the newborn's nose and mouth with a sterile gauze. Use the bulb syringe to suction the mouth and nostrils. Be sure to squeeze the bulb *before* inserting the tip, and only *then* place the tip in the newborn's mouth or nostril and release the bulb slowly. Withdraw the bulb, expel its contents into a waste container, and repeat suctioning as needed.
11. Dry the newborn with sterile towels (wet newborns lose heat faster than dry ones), and wrap with a dry blanket.
12. Record the time of birth for your PCR.

In a normal delivery, the newborn will usually be breathing on his or her own, if not crying, by the time you finish suctioning the airway. Newborns are usually born blue, but after taking several breaths or crying they should turn a pink color, although their extremities may remain dusky.

Apgar Scoring

The <u>Apgar scoring system</u> (devised by Virginia Apgar, MD) is a useful means of evaluating the adequacy of a newborn's vital functions immediately after birth; such information will prove useful to those who take over the care of the newborn after your delivery. In this system, five parameters—heart rate, respiratory effort, muscle tone, reflex irritability, and color—are each given a score from 0 to 2 both 60 seconds and then 5 minutes after birth. Most newborns are vigorous and have a total score of 7 to 10; they cough or cry within seconds of delivery and require no further resuscitation. Newborns with a score in the 4 to 6 range are moderately depressed; they may be pale or blue 1 minute after delivery, with poorly sustained respirations and flaccid muscle tone. These newborns will require resuscitation. Neonatal resuscitation is discussed in the chapter, *Neonatal Care*.

Cutting the Umbilical Cord

Once the newborn has been delivered and is breathing well, the umbilical cord can be clamped and cut because it is no longer necessary for the newborn's survival. The steps are as follows:

1. Handle the umbilical cord with care. It tears easily.
2. Tie or clamp the cord about 8 inches from the newborn's navel, with two ties (or clamps) placed 2 inches apart. Cut the cord between the two ties or clamps.
3. Examine the cut ends of the cord to be certain there is no bleeding. If the cut end attached to the newborn is bleeding, tie or clamp the cord *proximal* to the previous clamp, and examine it again (do *not* remove the first clamp). There should not be any oozing from the newborn's end of the cord.
4. Once the cord is clamped and cut, wrap the newborn in a dry blanket. If the mother's condition is stable, you may give the newborn to her. This will give her a chance to bond and she may want to begin breastfeeding the newborn. The suckling reflex triggers the uterus to contract, which will speed the delivery of the placenta and reduce bleeding.

Delivery of the Placenta

With the delivery of the newborn, the second stage of labor is complete, and the third stage—delivery of the placenta—begins. The placenta is usually delivered within 20 minutes of the newborn's arrival. During this time, you should reassess the mother and wait for the placenta to begin to separate spontaneously. *Do not* attempt to speed delivery of the placenta by pulling on the umbilical cord.

The first sign that the placenta is separating from the uterine wall is usually the patient reporting that her contractions are starting again. The uterus rises in the abdomen and feels hard to palpation. The end of the umbilical cord protruding from the vagina lengthens, and there is usually a gush of blood from the vagina. When these signs occur, you should instruct the patient to bear down to expel the placenta.

One side of the placenta (fetal side) should be gray, shiny, and smooth; the other side (maternal side) should be dark maroon with a rough texture **Figure 18**. Place the placenta in a plastic bag from the OB kit and transport it with you to the hospital.

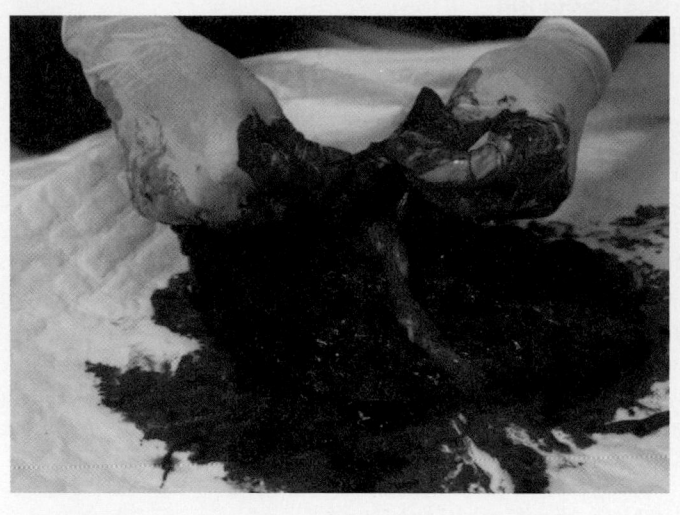

Figure 18   A whole placenta.

Words of Wisdom

Never pull on the umbilical cord to try to hasten delivery of the placenta.

Examine the perineum for lacerations and apply pressure to any bleeding tears. Clean up and place a sanitary pad over the woman's vaginal opening, lower her legs, and prepare for transport. If the placenta has not delivered after 15 minutes, do not wait; begin your transport.

Some women may request to keep the placenta. This is standard practice in some parts of the world, where consumption of the placenta is considered a means for the mother to quickly regain her strength. Women from some cultures may want to keep the placenta to bury it and plant a tree over the spot, so that the tree and the child grow together. If possible, you should respect such requests.

Postpartum Care

After delivery of the newborn, obtain the mother's vital signs. Place a sanitary napkin in front of the vagina to collect any discharge after the birth. Monitor the mother's condition closely for postpartum hemorrhage and shock, seizure activity, or respiratory difficulty. Assess the fundus (you should easily be able to palpate it around the mother's umbilicus—it should be firm). Massaging the fundus (after placenta delivery) will help control excessive postpartum hemorrhage (more than 500 mL). Note the vaginal discharge following delivery—lochia is the expected normal vaginal discharge of blood and mucus. This discharge is usually red in the first few days and will decrease in amount and change to a brownish color for several weeks after delivery. Finally, cover the mother with blankets to prevent mild hypothermia.

Emergency Pharmacology in Pregnancy

There is always some concern in pregnancy of pharmacologic agents having dangerous effects on the fetus. However, these concerns are secondary when the life of the pregnant woman is at stake. As noted earlier, maternal physiology is altered in pregnancy, and these changes have an impact on pharmacologic therapies. Hepatic metabolism increases, as does renal excretion, which may cause IV-administered medications to pass quickly through the maternal system. Volume changes may affect distribution, resulting in higher doses needed to gain appreciable systemic affects. Gastric absorption is slowed, meaning oral drugs may require a longer period than normal to achieve the desired effect.

Drugs given in the field for pregnancy-related problems constitute a very short list.

Magnesium Sulfate

Magnesium sulfate is classified as an electrolyte. Magnesium sulfate acts as a central nervous system depressant; in pregnancy, it is principally used in the management of eclampsia. Some physicians may order a magnesium sulfate infusion in patients with preeclampsia to prevent seizures from occurring.

Magnesium sulfate can cause respiratory depression, hypotension, and, potentially, circulatory collapse. This drug needs to be administered slowly because rapid infusion can potentiate these effects.

Magnesium sulfate may also be considered as a slow IV push in the presence of seizures during or immediately following labor (eclampsia). (Hydralazine or labetalol can also be used to control blood pressure once seizures have stopped, if the patient is still hypertensive.) IM injection can also be used, but the total dose should be placed in two separate syringes, with an equal dose in each syringe, and administered at different sites.

Calcium Chloride

Classified as a supplement, calcium chloride is mainly used in the field for managing cases of hypocalcemia. When magnesium sulfate has been given in patients with eclampsia and respiratory depression has developed, calcium chloride (or calcium gluconate) acts as an antidote to counter the effects of magnesium sulfate.

Side effects of calcium chloride include nausea and vomiting, syncope, bradycardia, and dysrhythmias, and the drug may precipitate cardiac arrest. This agent is typically administered as an IV push with repeat doses per state or regional protocol. This may be repeated in 10-minute intervals as a buffer to magnesium toxicity.

Terbutaline

Terbutaline is a tocolytic and sympathetic agonist. In pregnancy, this drug can be administered to suppress preterm labor through the action of uterine relaxation, a step that becomes necessary in the field in case of cord prolapse. Terbutaline can also be used to treat pregnancy-induced asthma because it has immediate bronchodilatory effects.

Side effects of terbutaline administration may include hypertension, nausea and dizziness, vomiting, chest pain, and cardiac dysrhythmias. The standard dosage is 0.25 mg SC; a repeat dose can be administered after 30 minutes. A terbutaline drip can also be administered and should begin with a starting infusion of 30 mL/h. Administration of 10 mg in 1,000 mL of normal saline, or 5 mg in 500 mL, will produce 5 μg/min infused at 30 mL/h. This rate can be slowly titrated to effect, but should not exceed 80 μg/min.

Valium

Diazepam (Valium) is a benzodiazepine that is classified as a sedative/anticonvulsant. It is used principally in EMS as a seizure medication. Its use is indicated in eclampsia when the patient's seizures do not respond to magnesium sulfate. Valium may also be ordered to treat anxiety in cases of hypertensive crisis, such as in preeclampsia.

The principal side effects of diazepam administration include nausea and vomiting, respiratory depression, and hypotension. Ancillary side effects include headache and amnesia. The dosage is 5 to 10 mg slow IV push for management of seizure states. The dosage for anxiety management is 2 to 5 mg. The anxiety dosage should be given IM if conditions permit, or by IV if anxiety is high and is accompanied by significant hypertension and dependent or facial edema is present.

Diphenhydramine

Diphenhydramine (Benadryl) is an antihistamine used principally to treat allergic reactions. Because of its sedative and antiemetic properties, it is also useful in treating hyperemesis gravidarum.

Side effects include drowsiness, headache, tachycardia, and hypotension. The dosage for emesis is 25 to 50 mg IV.

Oxytocin

Oxytocin (Pitocin) is a naturally occurring hormone that causes uterine contractions by acting on smooth muscle. This uterine stimulant can be used to induce labor, but is commonly used to control postpartum hemorrhage. In the prehospital setting, oxytocin should be used only to manage severe postpartum bleeding, and only after *all* products of conception have been expelled from the uterus (including additional fetuses).

Side effects include nausea and vomiting, tachycardia, seizures, and cardiac dysrhythmias. Oxytocin can also induce coma or result in uterine rupture and hypertension if administered in excess. The dosage is 3 to 10 units IM, or 10 to 20 units in 500 or 1,000 mL normal saline, slowly titrated to effect.

Words of Wisdom

Any fetus who is not delivering headfirst or buttocks-first must be managed at the hospital.

Pathophysiology, Assessment, and Management of Complications of Labor

Premature Rupture of Membranes

When the amniotic sac ruptures or "opens" more than an hour before labor, it is called *premature rupture of the membranes*. In some instances, the sac will self-seal and heal itself, but more

---

YOU are the Medic   PART 4

You and your partner place the patient in full spinal precautions and move her to the back of your ambulance for further assessment. The patient still reports cramping pain that is staying constant. The patient has no signs of bleeding. You see a seat belt burn on the patient's abdomen but the skin is not broken.

Recording Time: 10 Minutes	
Respirations	18 breaths/min
Pulse	98 beats/min
Skin	Pink, warm, dry
Blood pressure	130/72 mm Hg
Oxygen saturation (Spo$_2$)	99% at 4 L/min via nasal cannula
Pupils	Equal and reactive

7. Because the patient is in spinal precautions, what should you do to the backboard to make this patient more comfortable?

8. Should you administer a pain medication to reduce the cramping pain the patient is experiencing?

commonly, labor will begin within 48 hours. If the pregnancy is term or near term, there is usually no concern. However, if the pregnancy is not yet term, there is a risk of infection. In this situation, you should provide emotional support to the patient and provide transport to the hospital.

Preterm Labor

Labor (uterine contractions that are regular, intense, and accompanied by effacement) that begins after the 20th week but before the 37th week of gestation is considered preterm. The threat to the unborn fetus is a premature birth. Signs and symptoms are the same as normal childbirth labor. If the pregnancy is not near term, the patient's physician may admit her to the hospital for medications, bed rest, and close monitoring.

Fetal Distress

There are many conditions that may cause fetal distress including hypoxia, nuchal cord, trauma, abruptio placenta, fetal developmental disabilities, and a prolapsed cord. It will be difficult for you to assess for fetal distress in the field. Most pregnant women will be acutely aware of how much or how decreased the fetus is moving. You should rely on the information the woman tells you if the fetus is not moving or if she tells you the movement is markedly decreased. Remember that the best care for the fetus is quality care for the woman. Provide support to the woman and rapid transport.

Uterine Rupture

Uterine rupture occurs during labor. Patients at greatest risk are women who have had many children and those with a scar on the uterus (eg, from a previous cesarean section). Typically, you will find a woman in active labor who is reporting weakness, dizziness, and thirst. She may tell you that she initially had very strong and painful contractions, but then the contractions slackened off. Physical examination will reveal signs of shock—sweating, tachycardia, and falling blood pressure. Significant vaginal bleeding may or may not be obvious. Treat the patient for shock and provide rapid transport.

Pathophysiology, Assessment, and Management of High-Risk Pregnancy Considerations

Precipitous Labor and Birth

When EMS receives a call for a precipitous labor and birth, the newborn has usually been delivered prior to your arrival. This condition means that the entire labor time and actual birth of the newborn occurred in less than 3 hours. These types of births are not common in women pregnant for the first time but the chances increase as the woman has more children. You should be prepared for this situation if the woman tells you that a prior delivery was precipitous. Contractions are usually more intense and thus effective. Assess the woman post delivery for

tears and bleeding. Newborns normally do not have any adverse effects but there is a chance of infant facial bruising or a more than usual misshaped head.

Post-Term Pregnancy

A pregnancy is considered "post term" if the fetus has not been born after 42 weeks (normal pregnancy is 40 weeks). The cause of this condition is unknown. This type of pregnancy is considered high risk because of the potential effects on the fetus, which may become malnourished because the placenta may no longer function as it should to provide nourishment to the fetus. There is also an increased chance for meconium aspiration. There is little to no effect on the woman.

Risk factors include previous post-term pregnancy and irregular menstrual cycles that increase the chance of a miscalculation of the due date. Because these fetuses may be larger than normal, there is a risk for a longer labor and a complicated delivery (see section on cephalopelvic disproportion and shoulder dystocia). Generally, these deliveries should be performed by cesarean section.

Meconium Staining

While in utero, the fetus passively ingests several elements—for example, lanugo (fine, downy hair), mucus, and amniotic fluid. This material is stored in the intestines and constitutes the first stool the fetus passes. This first stool, which is called **meconium**, is odorless, greenish-black, and has a tar-like consistency. Unlike later feces, it is also sterile. In cases of fetal distress, or with the stresses of labor and delivery, the fetus may void the meconium into the amniotic fluid. If this occurs in utero, it may result in chemical pneumonia in the newborn. Umbilical cord prolapse is one condition that can cause such fetal distress, if compression of the cord has occurred.

There is no way for you to ascertain whether meconium is in the amniotic fluid until the bag of waters breaks. Normally, the waters should be clear. A yellow tint to the amniotic fluid suggests the meconium has been in the amniotic fluid for a while. A greenish black color, especially with the presence of particulate matter, indicates recent passage of meconium and is a sign of danger.

You need to be vigilant regarding the need for suctioning if meconium staining is present and the newborn is not responding normally. The viscosity of meconium can cause the newborn's airway to become partially or completely blocked, and meconium trapped in the airways will irritate the respiratory tract, further hampering the newborn's efforts to breathe.

If the newborn is depressed, you should perform tracheal suctioning through an endotracheal tube if you observe meconium in the airway. If the newborn is vigorously moving and is not presenting with indications of needing ventilation assistance, suctioning is not recommended.

Fetal Macrosomia

Fetal macrosomia, also known as "big baby syndrome," refers to a large fetus—usually defined as weighing more than

4,500 grams or almost 9 pounds. Another term used for this condition is "large for gestational age."

Risk factors for this condition include gestational diabetes or the woman having diabetes that is not properly controlled. Other factors include excessive weight gain (woman), male fetus, post-term pregnancy, number of pregnancies, obesity (woman), and some genetic conditions (fetus).

Potential complications that you may face in the prehospital setting have to do with the size of the fetus in relation to the woman's anatomy such as cephalopelvic disproportion and shoulder dystocia. Your treatment should be focused on supporting the woman and providing rapid transport because most fetuses are delivered by cesarean section. If a field delivery should occur, encourage the woman to breastfeed the newborn, and check the newborn's blood glucose level because there is an increased risk of hypoglycemia.

Multiple Gestation

The incidence of women carrying multiple infants has been on the increase in the United States. Twins occur about once in every 80 births. Sometimes, there is a family history of twins or the woman may suspect that she is having twins due to an unusually large abdomen. Usually, however, multiples are diagnosed early in pregnancy with modern ultrasound techniques. With twins or multiples, always be prepared for more than one resuscitation, and call for assistance.

Twins are smaller than single newborns, and delivery is typically not difficult. Consider the possibility that you are dealing with twins any time the first newborn is small or the woman's abdomen remains fairly large after the birth. You should also ask the woman about the possibility of multiples. If twins are present, the second one usually will be born within 45 minutes of the first. About 10 minutes after the first birth, contractions will begin again, and the birth process will repeat itself.

The procedure for delivering twins is the same as that for single newborns. Clamp and cut the cord of the first newborn as soon as it has been born and before the second newborn is delivered. The second newborn may deliver before or after the first placenta. There may be only one placenta, or there may be two. When the placenta has been delivered, check whether there is one umbilical cord or two. If two cords are coming out of one placenta, the twins are called identical. If only one cord is coming out of the placenta, then the twins are called fraternal, and there will be two placentas. Remember, if you see only one umbilical cord coming out of the first placenta, there is still another placenta to be delivered. If both cords are attached to one placenta, the delivery is over. Identical twins are of the same sex; fraternal twins may be of different sexes, or they may be the same.

Record the time of birth of each twin separately. Twins may be so small that they look premature; handle them very carefully, and keep them warm. In the case of twins, you should identify the first newborn delivered as "Baby A" by loosely tying an extra length of tape around a foot. With the delivery of more than two newborns, you can indicate the order of delivery by writing on a piece of tape and placing it on the blanket or towel that is wrapped around each newborn.

Intrauterine Fetal Death

Unfortunately, you may find yourself delivering a fetus who died in the woman's uterus before labor. This will be a true test of your medical, emotional, and social abilities. Grieving parents will be emotionally distraught and will require all your professionalism and support skills.

Intrauterine fetal death is when a fetus dies in a normal pregnancy; it occurs in approximately 1% of all pregnancies. Definitions vary by state and source but, in general, it is considered death of the fetus after the 20th week of gestation or when the weight of the fetus is 500 grams or more. Fetal deaths that occur at less than 20 weeks' gestation or with lower weights are considered miscarriages. Regardless of the definition, your treatment and care will focus on the woman.

The actual cause of intrauterine fetal death is usually difficult to determine, with many of the causes of death unknown. If a cause is determined, it is usually attributed to a complication with the fetus, placenta, or the woman. Risk factors for this condition include infections, genetic disorders, poorly controlled diabetes in the woman, hypertension, preeclampsia, eclampsia, Rh factor conditions, and multiple gestations.

The onset of labor can occur up to 2 weeks or longer after fetal death. Some women may already know that the fetus has died; others may not. In most cases, labor will progress normally. If an intrauterine infection has caused the demise, you may note an extremely foul odor. The delivered fetus may have skin blisters, skin sloughing, and a dark discoloration, depending on the stage of decomposition. The head will be soft and perhaps grossly deformed.

Do not attempt to resuscitate an obviously dead fetus. However, do not confuse such a newborn with those who have had a cardiopulmonary arrest as a complication of the birthing process. You should attempt to resuscitate normal-appearing newborns.

Amniotic Fluid Embolism

Amniotic fluid embolism is a life-threatening condition that is extremely rare and is hardly ever seen in the hospital setting. Factors for this high-risk pregnancy include women older than 35 years, eclampsia, abruptio placenta, placenta previa, uterine rupture, and fetal distress. Amniotic fluid embolism occurs when amniotic fluid and fetal cells enter the woman's pulmonary and circulatory system through the placenta via the umbilical veins. This may be from ruptured membranes and ruptured cervical or uterine veins. Regardless of the cause, the result is an exaggerated response from the pregnant woman's body (allergic reaction) that causes coagulopathies, cardiac and respiratory collapse, and eventually death.

Signs and symptoms include a sudden onset of respiratory distress and hypotension. Many of these patients are very cyanotic and may have seizures. They eventually go into cardiogenic shock, become unresponsive, and may experience cardiac arrest. If these patients survive this initial reaction, they typically develop coagulopathies (their blood loses the ability to clot). Your treatment is aimed at supporting the vital systems (respiratory and circulatory) and providing rapid transport. Treatment for the fetus is aimed at successful resuscitation of the woman and probable cesarean section delivery in the hospital.

Hydramnios

Hydramnios (also known as polyhydramnios) is a condition in which there is too much amniotic fluid. On average, most pregnancies will have about 500 mL of amniotic fluid. Carrying multiples (twins), fetal anemia, diabetic pregnant patients, and fetal conditions that cause the fetus to stop swallowing the fluid are all potential causes of hydramnios. This condition is usually detected on ultrasound and these patients will be closely followed by their obstetrician.

If you encounter a patient with this condition, you should be prepared for the possibility of a prolapsed cord and abruptio placenta due to the increased size of the uterus from the extra fluid. These patients also have an increased risk of postpartum hemorrhage (an overstretched uterus may not contract as efficiently to stop bleeding).

Cephalopelvic Disproportion

In cephalopelvic disproportion, the head of the fetus is larger than the pelvis. Cephalopelvimetry (a radiographic measurement) is performed to obtain the dimensions of the fetal head. In most cases, a cesarean section will be required to prevent maternal and fetal distress. You should ask the patient about this complication before you attempt delivery in the field. Cephalopelvic disproportion may cause massive hemorrhage, along with other postpartum complications.

Pathophysiology, Assessment, and Management of Complications of Delivery

Most deliveries are normal. The fetus arrives headfirst, followed shortly by the placenta. Occasionally, however, complications arise. For you to successfully deal with obstetric complications, you must know when to anticipate them, how to recognize them when they do occur, and what action to take to ensure that everyone makes it through the event successfully.

Cephalic Presentation

With most deliveries, newborns present in the vertex or top of the head position. This occurs over 95% of the time. Variations in the exact position of the newborn's head as it is exiting the birth canal can vary and define the different types of cephalic presentations. If the newborn's head is overly extended, you may encounter a face presentation. Face presentations are rare but can occur with premature fetuses, fetal macrosomia, and cephalopelvic disproportion. In a brow presentation, the head

is extended, but only slightly. Occiput-posterior presentations (face up) can stall out and result in prolonged labor times. A military presentation occurs when the head is in a more neutral position—not flexed or only partially flexed—similar to a soldier in the military standing at attention. This head position causes a wider diameter of the head to attempt to exit through the birth canal, which can make for a more painful and difficult delivery. If you are faced with one of these presentations and the newborn's head does not externally rotate into position or you are unable to complete the delivery, support the woman and the newborn and provide rapid transport.

Breech Presentations

Most term newborns enter the world headfirst. The head serves to open a path through the cervix for the more narrow shoulders and hips. In a breech presentation, however, another part of the body leads the way, usually the buttocks (the word *breech* means "buttocks") **Figure 19**, but sometimes one of the feet comes first. Breech presentations occur in 4% of all deliveries and are more common with premature births. There are different types of breech presentations:

- Frank: Hips flexed and knees extended with the buttocks as the presenting part
- Incomplete: One or both hips and knees may be extended with one or both feet as the presenting part
- Complete: Hips and knees both flexed with the buttocks as the presenting part

The best place for a breech presentation to be delivered is in the hospital. However, there will be times when you will not realize that you are dealing with a breech delivery until the woman is crowning and you notice that the head is not the presenting part. At this point, it is usually too late to get the woman to the hospital.

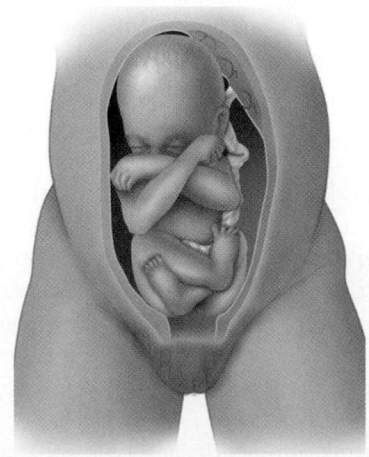

Figure 19 In a breech presentation, the buttocks are delivered first. These deliveries are usually slow, so you will often have time to transport the woman to the hospital.

If you have determined that the buttocks are the presenting part and that delivery is imminent, proceed as follows:

- Position the woman with her buttocks at the edge of the bed or stretcher and her legs flexed.
- Allow the buttocks and trunk of the newborn to deliver spontaneously. *Do not pull on the newborn.*
- Once the newborn's legs are clear, support the newborn's body.
- Lower the newborn slightly so that it very nearly hangs by its own weight downward; that will help the head pass through the pelvic outlet. You can tell when the head is in the vaginal canal because you will be able to see the newborn's hairline at the nape of the neck just below the woman's symphysis pubis.
- When you can see the hairline, grasp the newborn by the ankles and lift him or her upward in the direction of the woman's abdomen. The head should then deliver without difficulty.
- If the head does not deliver within 3 minutes, the newborn is in danger of suffocation, and immediate action is indicated. Suffocation may occur when the newborn's umbilical cord is compressed by his or her head against the birth canal, which cuts off the supply of oxygenated blood from the placenta, and the face is pressed against the vaginal wall, which prevents the newborn from breathing on his or her own. Place your gloved hand in the vagina, with your palm toward the newborn's face. Form a V with your fingers on either side of the newborn's nose, and push the vaginal wall away from the face until the head is delivered.
- Remember: *This is a delivery, not an extrication.* Do not attempt to forcibly pull the newborn out or allow an explosive delivery. If the head does not deliver within 3 minutes of establishing the airway, provide rapid transport to the hospital, with the woman's buttocks elevated on pillows. Try to maintain the newborn's airway throughout transport. En route, alert the hospital so they can prepare for your arrival.

There are a variety of other abnormal ways in which the fetus may present for delivery; fortunately, most of them are quite rare. In a footling breech, one or both feet will dangle down through the vaginal opening **Figure 20**. In a <u>transverse presentation</u> (transverse lie), the fetus lies crosswise in the uterus and one hand may protrude through the vagina. Even the fetus who is coming headfirst may deflex the head and present with the face or brow instead of the top of the head (vertex). With all of those abnormal presentations, the most important point for you to remember is *not to attempt delivery in the field.* Nearly all of these abnormal presentations will require delivery by cesarean section, so prehospital management is to provide rapid transport.

Shoulder Dystocia

Another complication of delivery is <u>shoulder dystocia</u> or difficulty in delivering the shoulders. A diabetic woman, large fetuses, and fetuses that are post term are at increased risk for

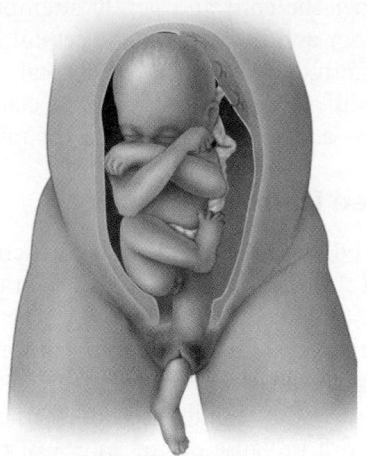

Figure 20 In very rare instances, a fetus' limb—usually a single arm or leg—presents first. This is a serious situation, and you must provide prompt transport for hospital delivery.

this complication. Shoulder dystocia occurs after the head has been delivered and the shoulder cannot get past the woman's symphysis pubis; there is either difficulty in getting it to pass or it gets "stuck" behind the pelvic bones and the fetus is unable to be delivered. This unexpected complication is a threat is to the life of the fetus if it is not delivered due to the increased chance of cord compression. As time passes and the shoulders are not clearing, the fetus cannot breathe (lungs are still inside the birth canal) and/or the cord is compressed between the fetus and the woman's tissue. The delivery needs to be completed in order for the fetus to breathe. The major concern for the newborn once it is born is damage to the brachial nerve plexus.

There are several maneuvers that may be attempted in an effort to widen the woman's pelvis or reposition the fetus to allow for a successful delivery. The McRoberts maneuver is one of the safest (for woman and fetus) maneuvers to use in the case of shoulder dystocia and is reported to be over 40% effective. To widen the woman's pelvis and flatten the lower back, hyperflex her legs tightly to her abdomen. It may be necessary to apply suprapubic pressure (woman's lower abdomen) and to *gently* pull on the fetus's head.

Nuchal Cord

There is a chance that during delivery the umbilical cord may become wrapped around the newborn's neck; this is termed a <u>nuchal cord</u>. Most sources report that nuchal cords occur in about 2 out of 10 births (20%), with an approximate 5% possibility of the cord being wrapped around the neck twice. As the fetus descends during labor, cord compression may occur, causing the fetal heart rate to slow and resulting in fetal distress. Nuchal cords rarely result in death of the fetus, but it is one of the first things you should assess for when the fetus' head is delivered.

If the umbilical cord is found around the fetus' neck, slip your finger under the cord and gently attempt to slip it over the fetus' shoulder and head. If not successful or if the cord is wrapped too tightly, carefully place umbilical clamps 2 inches apart and carefully cut the cord between the clamps in a motion that is away from, as opposed to towards, the infant.

Prolapsed Umbilical Cord

With a __prolapsed umbilical cord__, the cord emerges from the uterus ahead of the fetus **Figure 21**. With each uterine contraction, the cord is then compressed between the presenting part and the bony pelvis, shutting off the fetus' supply of oxygenated blood from the placenta. Fetal asphyxia may ensue if circulation through the cord is not rapidly reestablished and maintained until delivery. Cord prolapse occurs in 3% of deliveries and is more likely when the presenting part does not completely fill the pelvic brim, such as in abnormal presentations or with small fetuses (premature births, multiple births).

Treatment of cord prolapse is clearly urgent. Take the following steps:

1. Position the woman supine with her hips elevated as much as possible on pillows.
2. Administer 100% supplemental oxygen via a nonrebreathing mask.
3. Instruct the woman to pant with each contraction, which will prevent her from bearing down.
4. With two fingers of your gloved hand, gently push the presenting part (not the cord) back up into the vagina until it no longer presses on the cord.
5. While you maintain pressure on the presenting part, have your partner cover the exposed portion of the cord with dressings moistened in normal saline.
6. You must then try to maintain that position, with a gloved hand pushing the presenting part away from the cord, throughout *urgent transport* to the hospital.

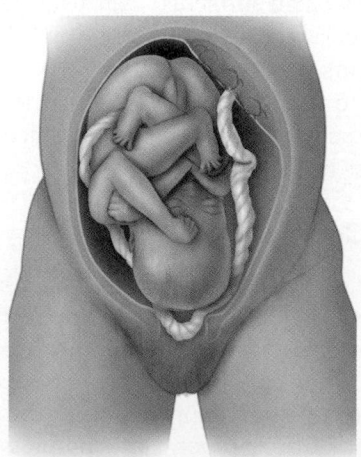

Figure 21 A prolapsed umbilical cord, another rare situation, is very dangerous and must be cared for at the hospital.

Pathophysiology, Assessment, and Management of Postpartum Complications

Uterine Inversion

__Uterine inversion__ is a rare but potentially fatal complication of childbirth, occurring in 1 of every 3,000 pregnancies. In this condition, the placenta fails to detach properly and adheres to the uterine wall when it is expelled. As a result, the uterus literally turns inside out. Uterine inversion usually occurs as a result of mismanaging the third stage of labor, such as placing excessive pressure on the uterus during fundal massage or by exerting strong traction on the umbilical cord in an attempt to hasten delivery of the placenta.

The severity of inversion is graded by how much the uterus has reversed itself and ranges from incomplete inversion, to complete inversion, to prolapsed inversion, and finally to total inversion. With incomplete and complete inversions, the uterus does not protrude externally. You will most likely encounter a prolapsed or a total inversion. (The other forms are not readily identifiable in the field.) In a prolapsed inversion, the fundus of the uterus can be seen protruding from the vagina. In a total inversion, both the uterus and the vagina protrude inside out. This is a very painful condition, and hypovolemic shock may develop rapidly.

Management of uterine inversion is as follows:

1. Keep the patient recumbent.
2. Administer 100% supplemental oxygen via a nonrebreathing mask.
3. Start two IV lines with normal saline, and titrate to vital signs.
4. If the placenta is still attached to the uterus, do *not* attempt to remove it.
5. Carefully monitor vital signs, and treat for shock.
6. Consider giving oxytocin (Pitocin), 10 units IM, to help control exsanguinating hemorrhage, if your local protocol permits it.

Make *one* attempt to replace the uterus. Push the uterine fundus up and through the vaginal canal by applying pressure with the fingertips and the palm of your gloved hand. If this procedure fails, cover all protruding tissues with moist sterile dressings and provide rapid transport.

Postpartum Hemorrhage

Postpartum hemorrhage can either be defined as early or late hemorrhage. Early postpartum hemorrhage is bleeding within 24 hours of delivery and is the most common type of postpartum hemorrhage seen. Only a very small percentage of late postpartum hemorrhage occurs, and it is defined as bleeding that occurs from 24 hours to 6 weeks after delivery. The average blood loss during the third stage of labor is normally about 150 mL. When blood loss exceeds 500 mL during the first 24 hours after giving birth, it is considered postpartum hemorrhage (bleeding after birth). Anything that interferes with the contractions of the interlacing uterine muscle fibers after delivery of the placenta will promote postpartum hemorrhage. The following are possible causes:

- **Lacerations.** The mother may have tears or lacerations around the vaginal opening and in the perineum.
- **Prolonged labor or delivery of multiple babies.** They may lead to a "tired" uterus.
- **Retained products of conception.** Retained pieces or fragments of the placenta may cause bleeding, and the uterus cannot contract fully until it is empty.
- **Uterine atony.** The uterus loses the ability to contract after childbirth.
- **Grand multiparity.** After many pregnancies, the muscle tissue in the uterus is gradually replaced with fibrous tissue, which does not contract.
- **Multiple pregnancy.** The placental site is larger, and the overstretched uterine muscles do not contract as well.
- **Placenta previa.** Muscles in the lower segment of the uterus, where the placenta is implanted, do not contract efficiently.
- **A full bladder.** It may prevent proper placental separation and uterine contraction.

The only measures feasible in the field to manage postpartum hemorrhage are those that encourage uterine contraction and help restore circulating volume. Follow these guidelines when you encounter this type of situation:

1. Continue uterine massage (gently but firmly knead and massage the uterus in a circular motion).
2. Encourage the woman to breastfeed.
3. If allowed by protocol, add 10 units of oxytocin to the IV bag (1,000 mL), and infuse at a rate of 20 to 30 mL/min.
4. Notify the receiving hospital of the woman's status and your estimated time of arrival.
5. Transport without delay.
6. Start another large-bore IV line en route, and infuse normal saline wide open.
7. Do not attempt internal examination of the vagina.
8. Do not attempt to pack the vagina with any form of dressing.
9. Manage *external* bleeding from perineal tears with firm pressure. It may be necessary to open the labia and place ice packs at the bleeding site.

Pulmonary Embolism

One of the most common causes of maternal death during childbirth or postpartum is pulmonary embolism. An embolism may form from a number of sources, but a blood clot arising in the pelvic circulation is a frequent cause. Leakage of amniotic fluid into the maternal circulation (amniotic embolism), a clot arising from deep venous thrombosis (pregnancy-related venous thromboembolism), and water or air entering the vagina after a water birth (water embolism) are examples of potential embolic processes. Should the woman experience sudden dyspnea, tachycardia, atrial fibrillation, or hypotension in the postpartum state, you should suspect pulmonary embolism. The patient may report sudden, sharp chest or abdominal pain, or may experience syncope. Physical examination may reveal nothing unusual except for an increased pulse rate, tachypnea, and hypotension—signs that may be mistaken for shock. Management of a postpartum embolism is the same as management of a pulmonary embolism occurring in nonpregnant states: awareness/recognition, high-flow oxygen, and rapid transport.

Postpartum Depression

Experts estimate that one out of eight women experience postpartum depression, or the "baby blues," and some would say that it is the most common pregnancy complication. Symptoms of this disorder can appear any time during the pregnancy and up to 1 year after birth. Adolescent mothers and those in lower income levels have an increased chance of having this condition.

There are several factors that have been identified that, if present, increase the risk for the woman to experience postpartum depression. Some of these risk factors include a previous history of depression or family history; financial or marital/relationship issues; diabetes; a complicated pregnancy or delivery; major life-changing events such as job loss, divorce, or death of a family member; infertility issues; and multiples.

You should be aware of the signs and symptoms of this type of depression in order to provide the best care to your patient. Women with postpartum depression exhibit signs similar to those of other depressed people including a lack of interest to care for themselves, insomnia to sleeping all the time, overwhelming sadness and crying, and lack of an appetite. However, some women may also have strong feelings of anger that may be directed toward their infant, may not have an interest in the infant, may have strong feelings of guilt, and may even have thoughts of harming themselves or the infant. This is a serious condition that requires definitive treatment you will not be able to provide in the prehospital setting.

Your assessment and management of the woman in this situation may be a critical step in getting her the help she needs. Be aware of the signs and symptoms of postpartum depression so you may recognize the condition in your patients. Maintain a professional approach and be a patient advocate. If at all possible, provide transport for the patient so she may seek and obtain the medical care she needs.

Words of Wisdom

What is good for the pregnant woman is good for the fetus.

Trauma and Pregnancy

Trauma is a serious complicating factor in pregnancy, partly because of the many physiologic changes that occur during pregnancy, but mostly because of the involvement of two patients—the woman and her fetus. Both patients are particularly vulnerable to trauma because of the unique features of pregnancy.

Special Populations

Throughout pregnancy, seat belts should be used with both the lap belt and the shoulder harness in place. The lap belt portion should be placed under the abdomen and over the iliac crests and the pubic symphysis. The shoulder harness should be positioned between the breasts.

Trauma is the leading cause of maternal death in the United States, with an estimated 5% of all pregnant women experiencing some type of trauma during the pregnancy, usually in the last trimester. The major causes of injury to pregnant women are motor vehicle crashes, falls, domestic abuse, and penetrating injuries such as gunshot wounds. Motor vehicle trauma accounts for a large percentage of trauma in pregnancy. Homicides and motor vehicle trauma are the two largest causes of maternal death. Domestic abuse statistics indicate that more than 324,000 women are abused each year by an intimate partner during their pregnancy. Approximately 70% of all penetrating abdominal wounds (such as gunshot wounds, stabbings) result in injury to the fetus.

■ Pathophysiology and Assessment Considerations

In general, abdominal trauma occurs from the same mechanisms in pregnant women as in nonpregnant women. However, because the likelihood of domestic abuse increases greatly during a woman's pregnancy, you should be suspicious for evidence of this crime. Sexual assault is also a form of trauma that can occur during pregnancy, and is covered in the chapter, *Gynecologic Emergencies*.

The anatomic changes during pregnancy have important implications for trauma. As the woman approaches term, her abdominal contents are compressed into the upper abdomen. The diaphragm is elevated by about 1½ inches (4 cm), so there is a higher incidence of abdominal injuries in association with chest trauma. Meanwhile, because the peritoneum is maximally stretched, significant abdominal trauma may occur without peritoneal signs.

In the first trimester of pregnancy, the uterus is well protected in the woman's bony pelvis and is rarely damaged from abdominal trauma. In the second and third trimesters of pregnancy, the uterus grows out from the pelvis and extends into the abdomen, making it more vulnerable to blunt and penetrating trauma. In motor vehicle crashes, for example, the use of a lap belt increases the likelihood of uterine damage because the lap belt compresses the uterus. Shoulder restraints, by contrast, decrease the chance of uterine injury. In penetrating injuries, the large uterus protects the other organs from injury. Because the uterus shields the other organs, pregnant women with penetrating wounds may have a better outcome, although the fetus is often injured by the trauma. In addition to abdominal tenderness, the examination of an injured pregnant woman may reveal an abnormal fetal position, an easily palpated fetus, inability to palpate the top of the uterus, or vaginal bleeding.

As early as the second trimester of pregnancy, the bladder is displaced upward (superior) and forward (anterior) so that it lies outside the pelvic cavity. It is therefore at increased risk of injury, particularly from a deceleration injury caused by a lap seat belt. Should you encounter a restrained pregnant patient in a motor vehicle crash, make a note of belt placement. If the patient is found with the belt placed over the abdomen or on top of the uterine dome, this positioning should dramatically increase your index of suspicion for internal injuries to the woman and the fetus. The uterus also becomes more vulnerable to injury as it increases in size, and deceleration forces, such as those produced by vehicular trauma, may bring about abruptio placenta or uterine rupture.

A pregnant patient will show different signs and responses to trauma due to the physiologic changes to her body from being pregnant. As noted earlier, pregnancy is accompanied by a significant increase in vascular volume. Normal vascular volume increases by nearly 50% during the first 6 months of pregnancy as a result of the pregnant woman having to perfuse her own circulation and that of the fetus. To meet this demand, normal cardiac output increases by about 40% as a result of the increasing pulse rate and stroke volume. The resting pulse rate increases by 15 to 20 beats/min over the rate in a nonpregnant patient, so the resting pulse may be as high as 100 beats/min by the end of the second trimester of pregnancy. This physiologic change makes it much more difficult to interpret tachycardia. Furthermore, because of the pregnant woman's vastly expanded blood volume, other signs of hypovolemia, such as a falling blood pressure, may not be evident until she has lost as much as 40% of her blood volume. Therefore you need to be aggressive in managing a pregnant woman with a mechanism of injury that indicates shock.

A relative redistribution of blood volume also occurs during pregnancy, with blood flow to the pelvic region increasing tenfold. If a pregnant woman sustains a pelvic fracture, her chances of bleeding to death are therefore significantly higher than those of a nonpregnant woman. A large amount of blood volume can be lost before signs and symptoms of shock develop because other mechanisms are compensating for the loss.

Regarding respiration, the pregnant woman has a higher basal metabolism and therefore an increased need for oxygen. At the same time, she has more carbon dioxide to eliminate—hers and that produced by fetal metabolism. Her body responds by increasing her tidal volume and, therefore, her minute volume. In general, a respiratory rate that is less than 20 breaths/min is not considered adequate ventilation in the pregnant trauma patient. If she should need artificial ventilation, you will have to administer supplemental oxygen at a higher minute volume than usual.

During pregnancy, digestion slows and bowel motility decreases, resulting in the stomach staying full longer. With the gravid uterus placing pressure on the stomach, the chances of aspiration are dramatically increased.

Special Populations

A fetal heart rate below 100 to 120 beats/min likely means fetal distress. Other factors related to fetal distress include the length of time that a decreased fetal heart rate is sustained.

Considerations for the Fetus and Trauma

The muscular wall of the uterus acts as a cushion for the fetus against the direct effects of blunt trauma, but fetal injury can occur as a result of rapid deceleration or may be secondary to impaired fetal circulation. The most common cause of fetal death from trauma is maternal death, but a woman will often survive an incident that proves fatal for the fetus. Blunt trauma resulting in abruptio placenta, for instance, provides a good statistical outcome for the pregnant woman but often results in the death of the fetus.

If the pregnant woman has sustained trauma and is bleeding massively, the maternal circulation will shunt blood away from fetal circulation to maintain maternal homeostasis—maternal circulation takes precedence over the requirements of the fetus. Therefore, any injury that involves significant maternal bleeding will threaten the life of the fetus. The woman's increased heart rate is not an early sign of hypovolemic shock. By the time the woman shows clinical signs of shock, fetal circulation will be so compromised that you can expect a fetal mortality of 70% to 80%.

The best indication of the status of the fetus after trauma is the fetal heart rate. A normal fetal heart rate is between 120 and 160 beats/min. A rate slower than 120 beats/min means fetal distress and signals a dire emergency. The earlier section, *Imminent Delivery* within the section, *Patient Assessment*, discusses how to measure the fetal heart rate.

Special Populations

Every pregnant woman who has been in a crash must be evaluated at the hospital, even if her own injuries appear trivial.

Management of the Pregnant Trauma Patient

Although trauma in a pregnant woman involves at least *two* patients, you can treat only one of them directly: the woman. During your assessment, determine the gestational age of the fetus if possible and relay this information to the receiving facility staff so they can better prepare to care for the newborn if needed. In general, what is good for the woman will be good for the fetus. For example, any effort to improve maternal perfusion will have a collateral effect of improving fetal circulation. Potential for injury to the fetus cannot be adequately assessed in the field, however, only presumed or suspected. Whereas a decreased fetal heart rate signals an emergency

situation, a normal fetal heart rate does not guarantee that all is well. Even minor deceleration forces can cause significant injury to the fetus.

In general, the prehospital management of pregnant women with abdominal trauma is the same as for nonpregnant patients. Airway, breathing, and circulation remain the highest priorities. However, because the large uterus can compress the vena cava (decreasing right atrial preload), a pregnant woman should be transported on her left side unless a spinal injury is suspected Figure 22. If you must transport a patient in the supine position, elevate her right hip about 6 inches to minimize the pressure of the vena cava. Be aware that because of the physiologic changes that occur in a woman's body during pregnancy, the fetus may lack appropriate circulation even if the woman's vital signs appear normal. The fetus may be in shock before signs appear in the mother, so initiate early, aggressive fluid resuscitation.

Field treatment of a pregnant trauma patient is as follows:

1. **Ensure an adequate airway.** Regurgitation and aspiration are much more likely in a pregnant woman than in a patient who is not pregnant, so if the patient is unresponsive, provide early endotracheal intubation to isolate the airway. Provide cricoid pressure until the airway is secured.
2. **Administer oxygen.** A pregnant woman's oxygen needs are 10% to 20% higher than normal, so provide 100% supplemental oxygen via a nonrebreathing mask if the patient is responsive.
3. **Assist ventilations as needed, and provide a higher minute volume than usual.** Because the uterus of a pregnant woman presses up against the diaphragm, ventilation will be more difficult. Once the patient is intubated, therefore, you may want to use a positive-pressure ventilator periodically to ensure visible chest rise (representing an adequate tidal volume).

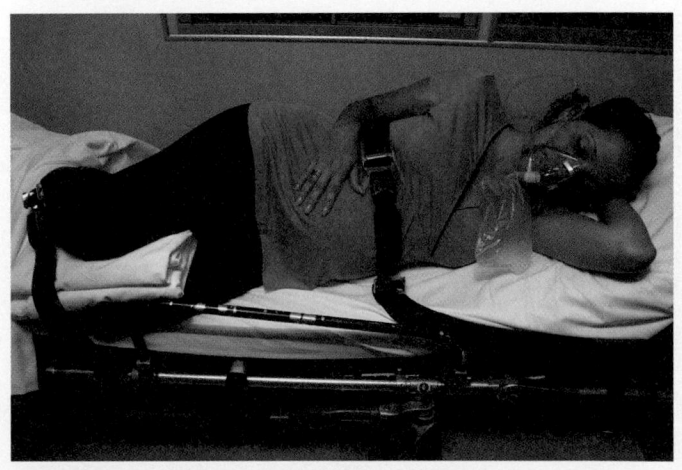

Figure 22 Whenever possible, transport a pregnant patient lying on her left side to allow for sufficient circulation through the vena cava.

4. **Control external bleeding promptly.** Splint any fractures.

5. **Start one or two IV lines of normal saline.** Use large-bore catheters and macrodrip sets. Administer a bolus if signs and symptoms of hemodynamic compromise are present, with the goal of maintaining blood pressure. Remember that a larger volume of fluid is necessary for the pregnant patient.

6. **Notify the receiving hospital of the patient's status.** Also indicate your estimated time of arrival.

7. **Transport the woman in the lateral recumbent position.** If she is on a backboard, tilt the backboard 30° to the left by wedging pillows beneath it. This will cause the uterus to shift, taking the weight off the inferior vena cava and improving venous return to the heart.

Maternal Cardiac Arrest

If cardiac arrest occurs, provide CPR and ALS as you would for any trauma patient. The normal landmarks you would use for chest compressions may not be obvious in a third trimester pregnant patient—use the sternal notch as a guideline for hand placement (about 5 to 7 inches below the angle of Louis).

Once the patient arrives at the hospital, an emergency cesarean section may be performed. A cesarean section may be the only chance a term or near-term fetus has to survive. A pregnant trauma patient in cardiac arrest requires rapid transport and early notification to the hospital. Even if the woman is *obviously* dead (eg, in case of decapitation), good CPR and ventilatory support may keep the fetus viable until a cesarean section can be performed.

YOU *are the Medic* — SUMMARY

1. What is your primary concern after scene safety is established?

Your immediate concern is the overall presentation of the patient. Does your rapid exam reveal any obvious life threats? Is she responsive? Does she have obvious breathing difficulty or evidence of injury? Does she appear pale, cyanotic, red, or gray? Is she alert and oriented or confused?

2. What questions are in your mind given knowledge that the patient is pregnant?

Focus on the patient's chief complaint. If the chief complaint is abdominal pain, you need to find out more about the pain itself. The OPQRST method (Onset; Provoking factors; Quality of pain; Region of pain and whether it radiates or refers; Severity; and Time) discussed in previous chapters works well for this purpose. How many weeks pregnant is the patient? Is the patient receiving prenatal care from a physician or nurse practitioner? These are important questions to answer in the care of this patient.

3. Is the location of the seat belt concerning to you?

As a general rule, all people, including pregnant women, should wear seat belts with the lap belt low on the hips. Because the seat belt is located visibly high on the patient, you would be wise to suspect a potential fetal injury. Relatively minor trauma to the abdomen can cause injury to the placenta and uterus.

4. What steps will you take in your further assessment of this patient?

As mentioned earlier, you need to establish the status of the patient's pregnancy with more specific information such as the term and whether the patient expects any problems with her pregnancy. You should also perform all the steps in proper patient care as you would for any patient. Spinal precautions need to be applied, vital signs need to be assessed, and a secondary assessment including palpation of abdominal quadrants should be performed.

5. What trimester is this patient in?

Pregnancy is assumed to be a 9-month process. The 9-month period is divided into three equal trimesters. The first 3 months or 12 weeks are the first trimester; the period between months 4 through 6 or weeks 13 through 24 are the second trimester; and the third trimester covers months 7 through 9 or from week 25 through week 36. This patient states that she is 20 weeks' pregnant, which indicates her pregnancy is in the second trimester.

6. Do you have any additional concerns because this is the patient's second pregnancy?

Generally, a pregnancy that is the woman's second pregnancy or greater delivers more easily than a first pregnancy. This may be a concern with the patient in this scenario. Additionally, the patient should be able to tell you if something feels different or wrong because she has already delivered a child. If the patient has given birth previously, ask how the child was delivered. Was it natural or did the birth occur by cesarean section?

7. Because the patient is in spinal precautions, what should you do to the backboard to make this patient more comfortable?

You should consider raising the right edge of the backboard approximately 15% so the patient is lying in a left lateral position. This is especially important with patients who are 24 weeks' apostrophe pregnant or greater, due to the possibility of supine hypotension syndrome. You can accomplish this by using pillows, rolled linen, or low-rise equipment that you will not need in the care of the patient. Remember that the backboard and patient still need to be secured to the stretcher.

8. Should you administer a pain medication to reduce the cramping pain the patient is experiencing?

At this point you should avoid analgesia because whatever you administer will also be administered to the fetus that may or may not be in distress. It is best to wait until an assessment can be made in a hospital setting to determine the cause of the cramping.

YOU *are the Medic* | **SUMMARY,** *continued*

EMS Patient Care Report (PCR)

Date: 05-15-11	Incident No.: 9745	Nature of Call: MVC		Location: Mason/3rd Ave	
Dispatched: 1012	En Route: 1012	At Scene: 1015	Transport: 1030	At Hospital: 1042	In Service: 1100

Patient Information

Age: 28 Sex: F Weight (in kg [lb]): 98 kg (215 lb)	Allergies: No known drug allergies Medications: Prenatal vitamins Past Medical History: Denies Chief Complaint: Abdominal pain

Vital Signs

Time: 1020	BP: 130/72	Pulse: 100	Respirations: 20	Spo$_2$: 98% room air
Time: 1030	BP: 130/72	Pulse: 98	Respirations: 18	Spo$_2$: 99% at 4 L/min
Time: 1040	BP: 130/70	Pulse: 100	Respirations: 18	Spo$_2$: 99% at 4 L/min

EMS Treatment
(circle all that apply)

Oxygen @ __4__ L/min via (circle one): (NC) NRM Bag-mask device	Assisted Ventilation	Airway Adjunct	CPR
Defibrillation	Bleeding Control	Bandaging	Splinting	(Other) Spinal immobilization

Narrative

Arrived to find 28-year-old, 20-week pregnant female sitting in driver's seat of a midsize passenger car that struck another vehicle from behind. Moderate damage is noted to the front of this vehicle. Air bags have deployed in this vehicle. This pt was still restrained by her 3-point seat belt, the lap belt portion of the restraint was found high on the abdomen. There is a corresponding seat belt abrasion across the pt's abdomen. Pt is complaining of a cramping-like pain in her pelvis. The pt states the pain is constant. Pt removed from vehicle using full spinal precautions. Backboard raised approx 15 degrees so pt is left lateral. Backboard and pt secured to stretcher and secured in ambulance. O$_2$ 4 L/min NC established. IV lock established in right forearm 18 ga. No change in pt condition during transport to trauma center at Regional Hospital. Report to RN Julia on arrival in the ED. **End of report**

Prep Kit

- The ovaries are the beginning point for reproduction. During the menstrual cycle, one follicle releases an ovum. If the ovum becomes fertilized, it develops into an embryo, and then into a fetus.
- The fallopian tubes are the structures that transport the ovum from the ovary to the uterus (a muscular, inverted pear-shaped organ). Once an egg is fertilized, it implants in the endometrium (the inner lining of the uterus).
- The fetus is enclosed in the amniotic sac, which contains amniotic fluid, allowing the fetus to develop in a weightless environment.
- The gestational period (the time that it takes for the infant to develop in utero) normally lasts 38 weeks.
- In the first trimester of pregnancy, the placenta, umbilical cord, specialized body systems, and limbs form. In the second trimester of pregnancy, the fetus gains weight and body systems become more specialized. In the last trimester of pregnancy, the fetus primarily puts on weight.
- Pregnancy is considered at term by week 37. Newborns born before 37 weeks of gestation are considered premature, and newborns born after 42 weeks of gestation are considered postmature.
- Physiologic changes during pregnancy can alter a woman's normal response to trauma or exacerbate or create medical conditions that can threaten the health of the woman and the fetus.
- When you are assessing a patient with an obstetric emergency, identify the length of gestation, estimated due date, any complications with this pregnancy or others, and the presence of any vaginal bleeding.
- There are many potential complications related to pregnancy, including abuse of the pregnant woman, substance abuse by the pregnant woman, and disorders that can develop during pregnancy or be exacerbated by pregnancy. Specific disorders include diabetes mellitus, heart disease, supine hypotensive syndrome, hyperemesis gravidarum, seizures, renal disorders, respiratory disorders, vaginal bleeding, placental problems, hypertensive disorders, Rh sensitization, and infections, including sexually transmitted diseases.
- Preeclampsia is the most serious hypertensive disorder, manifesting after the 20th week of pregnancy. Symptoms include edema, gradual onset of hypertension, protein in the urine, severe headache, nausea and vomiting, agitation, rapid weight gain, and visual disturbances. Preeclampsia may lead to seizures and eclampsia.
- Abortion can cause bleeding during pregnancy. Abortion is expulsion of the fetus, from any cause, before the 20th week of gestation.
- An incomplete abortion occurs when only some of the products of conception are expelled. In such patients, be alert for signs and symptoms of shock.
- Causes of bleeding during pregnancy include ectopic pregnancy or bleeding related to the placenta (abruptio placenta or placenta previa).
- Vaginal bleeding may cause shock. Keep the woman lying on her left side, administer supplemental oxygen, provide rapid transport, IV fluids and ECG monitoring, and place sanitary pads over the vagina.
- Labor may begin with a bloody show, or release of mucus (sometimes with blood) from the vagina.

- The first stage of labor begins with the onset of contractions—crampy abdominal pains that may radiate into the lower back. The amniotic sac may also rupture.
- The second stage of labor begins when the fetus's head enters the birth canal. The woman's contractions become more intense and more frequent. When the head becomes visible at the vaginal opening (crowning), delivery is imminent.
- The third stage of labor occurs when the placenta is expelled.
- When you are assessing a pregnant patient, determine whether there is time to provide transport to the hospital.
- If delivery is imminent, quickly prepare a private clean area. Behave in a calm and reassuring way. Control the delivery. Clear the newborn's airway.
- Never pull on the umbilical cord to deliver the placenta. Gently massage the abdomen to aid in delivery of the placenta.
- Pharmacology during pregnancy may include magnesium sulfate for eclampsia, calcium chloride to reverse respiratory depression following magnesium sulfate administration; terbutaline for asthma and as a uterine relaxant and occasionally for cord prolapse, diphenhydramine for treating hyperemesis gravidarum, and oxytocin for treatment of postpartum hemorrhage.
- Complications related to high-risk pregnancy include precipitous labor and birth, post-term pregnancy, meconium staining, fetal macrosomia, multiple gestation, intrauterine fetal death, amniotic fluid embolism, hydramnios, and cephalopelvic disproportion.
- Meconium is the fetus's first stool. A yellow or greenish black tint to the amniotic fluid indicates the presence of meconium. Vigilantly suction the newborn if meconium staining is present and the newborn is depressed (not vigorous).
- Complications of labor include premature rupture of membranes, preterm labor, uterine rupture, and fetal distress.
- Complications of delivery include cephalic presentation, breech presentation, shoulder dystocia, nuchal cord, and prolapsed cord.
- Postpartum complications include uterine inversion, postpartum hemorrhage, pulmonary embolism, and postpartum depression.
- In the case of postpartum hemorrhage, massage the abdomen, provide IV fluid resuscitation, and transport urgently.
- Pulmonary embolism can cause maternal death during childbirth or postpartum. Suspect this complication if the patient experiences sudden dyspnea, tachycardia, atrial fibrillation, or postpartum hypotension.
- The major causes of injury to pregnant women are motor vehicle crashes, falls, domestic abuse, and penetrating injuries such as gunshot wounds. Treatment of trauma in a pregnant woman is the same as treatment of a nonpregnant woman, except that the pregnant patient should be transported on her left side unless spinal injury is suspected.

Prep Kit, continued

■ Vital Vocabulary

abortion Expulsion of the fetus, from any cause, before the 20th week of gestation.

abruptio placenta A premature separation of the placenta from the wall of the uterus.

amniotic fluid A watery fluid that provides the fetus with a weightless environment in which to develop.

amniotic fluid embolism An extremely rare, life-threatening condition that occurs when amniotic fluid and fetal cells enter the pregnant woman's pulmonary and circulatory system through the placenta via the umbilical veins, causing an exaggerated allergic response from the woman's body.

amniotic sac The fluid-filled, baglike membrane in which the fetus develops.

Apgar scoring system A scoring system for assessing the status of a newborn that assigns a number value to each of five areas of assessment.

bacterial vaginosis An overgrowth of bacteria in the vagina, characterized by itching, burning, or pain, and possibly a "fishy" smelling discharge.

blastocyst The term for an oocyte once it has been fertilized and multiplies into cells.

bloody show A plug of mucus, sometimes mixed with blood, that is expelled from the dilating cervix and discharged from the vagina.

breech presentation A delivery in which the buttocks come out first.

candidiasis A vaginal infection that is not technically a sexually transmitted infection, and which can occur in a pregnant or nonpregnant female, but which is more common in pregnancy; also called thrush or a yeast infection.

cephalopelvic disproportion A situation in which the head of the fetus is larger than the woman's pelvis; in most cases, cesarean section is required for such a delivery.

cervical canal The interior of the cervix.

cervix The narrowest portion of the uterus that opens into the vagina.

chlamydia A sexually transmitted disease (STD) caused by the bacterium *Chlamydia trachomatis*; has the highest incidence in sexually transmitted diseases; signs and symptoms include inflammation of the urethra, epididymis, cervix, and fallopian tubes, and discharge from the urethra.

cholestasis A disease of the liver that occurs only during pregnancy, in which hormones affect the gallbladder by slowing down or blocking the normal bile flow from the liver; the most common symptom is profuse, painful itching, particularly of the hands and feet.

chronic hypertension A blood pressure that is equal to or greater than 140/90 mm Hg, which exists prior to pregnancy, occurs before the 20th week of pregnancy, or continues to persist postpartum.

complete abortion Expulsion of all products of conception from the uterus.

corpus luteum The remains of a follicle after an oocyte has been released, and which secretes progesterone.

crowning The appearance of the newborn's body part (usually the head) at the vaginal opening at the beginning of labor.

cytomegalovirus (CMV) A herpesvirus that can produce the symptoms of prolonged high fever, chills, headache, malaise, extreme fatigue, and an enlarged spleen.

eclampsia Seizures that result from severe hypertension in a pregnant woman.

ectopic pregnancy An egg that attaches outside the uterus, typically in a fallopian tube.

effacement Thinning and shortening of the cervix; this is a normal process that occurs as the uterus contracts.

elective abortion Intentional expulsion of the fetus.

embryo The fetus in the earliest stages after fertilization.

endometrium The innermost layer of tissue in the uterus.

episiotomy An incision in the perineal skin made to prevent tearing during childbirth.

fallopian tubes The vehicles of transportation of the ova from the ovaries to the uterus; also called oviducts.

fetal macrosomia A situation in which a fetus is large, usually defined as weighing more than 4,500 grams or almost 9 pounds; also known as "large for gestational age."

fetus The developing, unborn infant inside the uterus.

first stage of labor The stage of labor that begins with the onset of regular labor pains, crampy abdominal pains, during which the uterus contracts and the cervix effaces.

follicle-stimulating hormone (FSH) A hormone produced by the anterior pituitary gland that is important in the menstrual cycle.

fundus The dome-shaped top of the uterus.

gestational period The time that it takes for the fetus to develop in utero, normally 38 weeks.

gonorrhea A sexually transmitted disease (STD) that results in infection caused by the gonococcal bacteria, *Neisseria gonorrhoeae*; signs and symptoms include pus-containing discharge from the urethra and painful urination in men and signs and symptoms of an acute abdomen in women.

gravid The total number of times pregnant, including the current pregnancy.

gravidity A term used to refer to the number of times a woman has been pregnant, regardless of the outcome.

habitual abortion Three or more consecutive pregnancies that end in miscarriage.

herpes An infection of the genitals, buttocks, or anal area caused by herpes simplex virus, type 1 or type 2.

human immunodeficiency virus (HIV) An infection that causes acquired immune deficiency syndrome or AIDS.

human papilloma virus (HPV) The most common sexually transmitted disease that can cause genital warts and some types of cancer.

hydramnios A condition in which there is too much amniotic fluid; also known as polyhydramnios.

hyperemesis gravidarum A condition of persistent nausea and vomiting during pregnancy.

imminent abortion A spontaneous abortion that cannot be prevented.

incomplete abortion Expulsion of the fetus that results in some products of conception remaining in the uterus.

labor The mechanism by which the fetus and the placenta are expelled from the uterus.

lightening In pregnancy, a feeling of relief of pressure in the upper abdomen; a premonitory sign of labor.

lochia The vaginal discharge of blood and mucus that occurs following delivery of a newborn; usually lasts several days and then gradually decreases over the weeks following delivery.

luteinizing hormone (LH) A hormone released by the anterior pituitary gland that stimulates the process of ovulation.

meconium A dark greenish black material in the amniotic fluid that indicates fetal distress; can be aspirated into the fetus' lungs during delivery; the fetus's first bowel movement.

missed abortion A situation in which a fetus has died during the first 20 weeks of gestation, but has remained in utero.

myometrium The middle layer of tissue in the uterus.

nuchal cord A situation in which the umbilical cord is wrapped around the fetus's neck; cord compression may occur during labor, causing the fetal heart rate to slow and resulting in fetal distress.

oocyte An egg produced from the female ovary.

ovulation A process in which an ovum is released from a follicle.

ovum A mature oocyte.

para The number of live births.

parity Number of live births a woman has had.

perimetrium The outer protective layer of tissue in the uterus.

placenta The tissue attached to the uterine wall that nourishes the fetus through the umbilical cord.

placenta previa A condition in which the placenta develops over and covers the cervix.

postpartum The period of time after a woman has given birth.

preeclampsia A condition of late pregnancy that involves gradual onset of hypertension, headache, visual changes, and swelling of the hands and feet; also called pregnancy-induced hypertension or toxemia of pregnancy.

pregnancy-induced hypertension High blood pressure that develops after the 20th week of pregnancy, in women with previously normal blood pressures, and resolves spontaneously in the postpartum period.

prenatal The state of the pregnant woman before birth.

progesterone A hormone that influences the second phase of the menstrual cycle, when the oocyte is either fertilized or dies.

prolapsed umbilical cord A situation in which the umbilical cord comes out of the vagina before the newborn.

Rh factor A protein found on the red blood cells of most people; when a woman without this protein is impregnated by a man with this protein, the woman's body can create antibodies against the protein and attack future pregnancies.

rubella A viral disease similar to measles, best known by the distinctive red rash on the skin; not nearly as infectious or severe as measles.

second stage of labor The stage of labor in which the newborn's head enters the birth canal, during which contractions become more intense and more frequent.

septic abortion A life-threatening emergency in which the uterus becomes infected following any type of abortion.

shoulder dystocia A complication of delivery in which there is difficulty delivering the shoulders of a newborn; the shoulder cannot get past the woman's symphysis pubis.

spontaneous abortion Expulsion of the fetus that occurs naturally; also called miscarriage.

supine hypotensive syndrome Low blood pressure resulting from compression of the inferior vena cava by the weight of the pregnant uterus when the woman is supine.

syphilis A sexually transmitted disease caused by the bacterium *Treponema pallidum*, which manifests in three stages—primary, secondary, and late—and is transmitted through direct contact with open sores; characterized by an ulcerative lesion or chancre of the skin or mucous membrane at the site of infection, commonly in the genital region.

third stage of labor The stage of labor in which the placenta is expelled.

threatened abortion Expulsion of the fetus that is attempting to take place but has not occurred yet; usually occurs in the first trimester.

toxoplasmosis An infection caused by a parasite that pregnant women may get from handling or eating contaminated food or exposure from handling cat litter; the fetus can become infected.

transverse presentation A delivery in which the fetus lies crosswise in the uterus; one hand may protrude through the vagina.

trichomoniasis A parasitic infection caused by a single-cell parasite that is transmitted through sexual contact, with the vagina being the most common site of infection; infected person may be asymptomatic or may experience frothy, yellow-green vaginal discharge with a strong odor, irritation, and itching of the female genital area, discomfort during intercourse, dysuria, and lower abdominal pain.

umbilical cord The conduit connecting the pregnant woman to the fetus via the placenta; contains two arteries and one vein.

uterine cavity The interior of the body of the uterus.

uterine inversion A potentially fatal complication of childbirth in which the placenta fails to detach properly and results in the uterus turning inside out.

uterus A muscular inverted pear-shaped organ that lies situated between the urinary bladder and the rectum.

vagina A tubular organ lined with mucous membranes, that is the lower portion of the birth canal.

Assessment in Action

You are dispatched to a local residence for a patient with a severe headache. The dispatcher tells you this patient is 8 months' pregnant and has a severe headache and dizziness. When you arrive at the residence, you find a 30-year-old woman who appears to be extremely overweight. The patient tells you her hands and feet have swollen a lot over the past day and she is dizzy.

1. Increasing hypertension in a third trimester pregnancy may indicate:
   A. preeclampsia.
   B. eclampsia.
   C. oliguria.
   D. hypertensive crisis.

2. A normal blood pressure for a patient in the third trimester should be:
   A. much higher than normal.
   B. much lower than normal.
   C. normal or slightly lower than normal.
   D. normal or slightly higher than normal.

3. What is the difference between preeclampsia and eclampsia?
   A. In eclampsia, the patient is primigravid.
   B. In eclampsia, the patient has had a seizure.
   C. In eclampsia, the patient has liver damage.
   D. In eclampsia, the patient has placenta previa.

4. What medication is indicated for seizures in eclampsia?
   A. Amiodarone
   B. Calcium chloride
   C. Etomidate
   D. Magnesium sulfate

5. What is the correct dosing for magnesium sulfate in a patient with eclampsia?
   A. Loading dose of 1 to 2 g in 50 to 100 mL of D_5W over 5 to 60 minutes IV
   B. 25 to 50 mg/kg IV/IO of a 10% solution over 15 to 30 minutes to a maximum dose of 2 grams
   C. 1 to 2 g of a 10% solution IV/IO over 5 to 20 minutes
   D. 1 to 4 g of a 10% solution IV/IO over 3 minutes; maximum dose of 30 to 40 g/day

6. What medication is indicated as an antagonist to magnesium sulfate?
   A. Amiodarone
   B. Calcium chloride
   C. Etomidate
   D. Diphenhydramine

Additional Questions

7. What is false labor?

8. What are the three stages of labor, and during which stage is the fetus delivered?

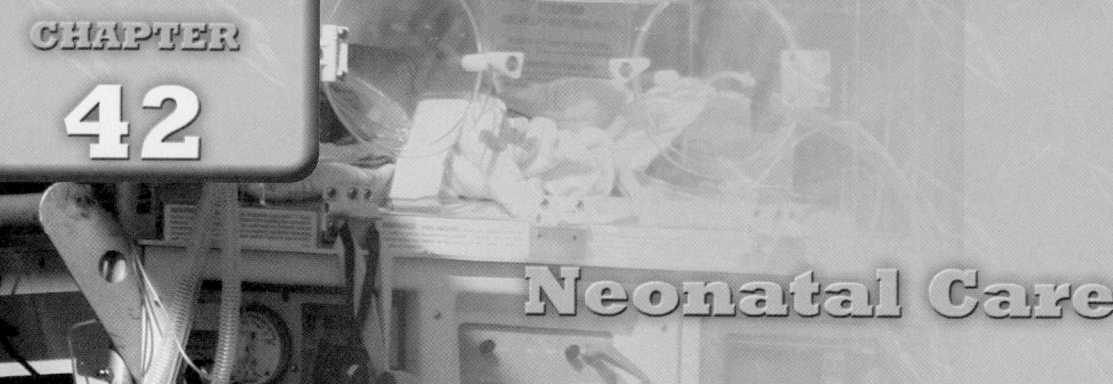

National EMS Education Standard Competencies

Special Patient Populations

Integrates assessment findings with principles of pathophysiology and knowledge of psychosocial needs to formulate a field impression and implement a comprehensive treatment/disposition plan for patients with special needs.

Neonatal Care

Anatomy and physiology of neonatal circulation (pp 1963-1968)

Assessment of the newborn (pp 1963-1970)

Presentation and management

- Newborn (pp 1964-1967)
- Neonatal resuscitation (pp 1970-1977)

Knowledge Objectives

1. Explain terminology associated with infants, including newborn versus neonate. (p 1963)
2. List antepartum and intrapartum risk factors that can lead to a need for neonatal resuscitation. (pp 1963-1964)
3. Discuss the process of transitioning from a fetus to a newborn. (p 1964)
4. List causes of delayed transition in newborns. (p 1964)
5. Discuss measures to take to prepare for neonatal resuscitation. (pp 1964-1966)
6. List equipment for neonatal resuscitation. (pp 1964-1967)
7. Discuss the initial steps of assessment for neonates, including drying and warming, positioning, suctioning, and stimulation. (pp 1963-1970)
8. Explain how to measure essential parameters including pulse rate, color, and respiratory effort. (pp 1964-1967)
9. Discuss Apgar scores, including how and when to obtain them. (pp 1967; 1968)
10. Discuss how to determine whether a neonate requires resuscitation. (pp 1968-1970)
11. Discuss methods used to improve oxygenation during neonatal resuscitation, including the use of positive end-expiratory pressure, free-flow oxygen, oral airways, and bag-mask devices. (pp 1970-1975)
12. Describe the technique for using a bag-mask device on a neonate. (pp 1971-1972)
13. Discuss when endotracheal intubation is required in a neonate. (pp 1972-1973)
14. Describe vascular access considerations in the neonate. (p 1977)
15. Discuss pharmacologic interventions used to treat specific emergencies in a neonate, including bradycardia, low blood volume, acidosis, respiratory depression secondary to narcotics, and hypoglycemia. (pp 1977-1979)
16. Describe family and transport considerations that apply to neonatal emergencies. (p 1979)
17. Discuss the pathophysiology, assessment, management of specific emergencies including pneumothorax, meconium-stained amniotic fluid, diaphragmatic hernia, and apnea or inadequate respiratory effort. (pp 1979; 1980-1982)
18. Discuss the pathophysiology, assessment, and management of hypoglycemia in a neonate. (p 1986)
19. Discuss the pathophysiology, assessment, and management of premature or low birth weight infants. (pp 1983-1984)
20. Discuss the pathophysiology, assessment, and management of seizures in neonates. (pp 1984-1986)
21. Discuss the pathophysiology, assessment, and management of emergencies related to thermoregulation, including fever and hypothermia. (pp 1988-1989)
22. Discuss the pathophysiology, assessment, and management of vomiting in a neonate. (pp 1986-1987)
23. Discuss the pathophysiology, assessment, and management of diarrhea in a neonate. (pp 1987-1988)

Skills Objectives

1. List the steps of neonatal resuscitation. (pp 1968-1977)
2. Describe the technique for performing endotracheal intubation in a neonate. (pp 1972-1975, Skill Drill 1)
3. Describe the technique for inserting an orogastric tube in a newborn. (pp 1975-1976, Skill Drill 2)
4. Explain how to perform chest compressions on a neonate. (pp 1975-1976)
5. Describe the technique for cannulating the umbilical vein in a newborn. (p 1977)

Introduction

The care of a newborn or neonate must be tailored to meet the unique needs of this population. A **newborn** refers to an infant within the first few hours after birth; a **neonate** refers to an infant within the first month after birth. A healthy neonate is completely dependent on others for nourishment, warmth, and protection from the environment. Most parents recognize this need and instinctively wish to fulfill the role of nurturer and caregiver. However, when a newborn needs special support that necessitates intervention by trained caregivers, the parents may feel isolated and inadequate. It is important for you to support the needs of both the newborn and the parents or other caregivers by allowing them to be physically close as much as possible, explaining what is being done, and providing details of the plan for transport to the next level of care.

This chapter reviews the physiologic changes that occur in a newborn during birth, the care that should be provided during and immediately after birth, and the special needs of premature births or births complicated by other factors. It also reviews the steps involved in neonatal resuscitation and outlines the process of transporting an infant to a hospital or between hospitals.

General Pathophysiology and Assessment

Additional skilled care intervention is needed for approximately 10% of newborn deliveries. The rate of birth complications, as well as mortality and morbidity, increase as the newborn's birth weight and gestational age decrease. In the United States, approximately 34,000 (8%) newborns delivered each year weigh less than 3 lb (1,500 g), with the majority requiring resuscitation. **Table 1** and **Table 2** outline risk factors for complications before and during birth.

Initial steps of neonatal resuscitation include:

- Airway (position and clear)
- Breathing (stimulate to breathe)
- Circulation (assess heart rate and oxygenation)

In newborns, unlike adults, the resuscitation efforts are focused on establishing the airway and ensuring adequate ventilation.

The initial stabilization of a newborn includes the following specific steps:

- Warming the newborn to prevent hypothermia
- Positioning the newborn
- Clearing the airway if necessary
- Drying and stimulating breathing

The newborn can be kept warm by placing him or her on prewarmed towels or blankets, drying, and then replacing the wet towels with dry, prewarmed towels. Once resuscitation is complete, the newborn can stay warm if placed on the mother's chest, or abdomen, on another heat source, or under a radiant warmer.

The newborn should be positioned on the back or side. The neck should be placed in the sniffing position (slightly extended) to open up the airway. A small shoulder roll may be required to keep the head in this position given the relatively large head size.

YOU are the Medic   PART 1

You are called to the home of a 29-year-old woman who is 41 weeks' pregnant. She was doing housework when her amniotic sac ruptured. She contacted her obstetrician who instructed her to call 9-1-1. On entering the residence, you find the patient sitting on the edge of her bed clutching her abdomen in pain. You observe a large green puddle of fluid on the floor. The patient tells you her water broke approximately 45 minutes ago, was green in color, and had a foul smell.

Maternal Assessment Recording Time: 1 Minute	
Appearance	Anxious, in pain
Level of consciousness	Alert (oriented to person, place, and day)
Airway	Patent
Breathing	Respirations, increased; adequate tidal volume
Circulation	Radial pulses present, increased and regular; no gross bleeding

1. What is the significance of the green amniotic fluid?

2. What further information would you like to obtain from the patient?

Table 1 Antepartum (Before Birth) Risk Factors

▪ Multiple gestation	▪ Inadequate or no prenatal care
▪ Pregnant woman's age < 16 y or > 35 y	▪ Prior history of perinatal morbidity or mortality
▪ Post-term (> 42 weeks) gestation	▪ Maternal use of drugs/ medications
▪ Hypertension, preeclampsia	▪ Fetal anemia
▪ Diabetes	▪ Oligohydramnios (decreased volume of amniotic fluid during a pregnancy)
▪ Polyhydramnios (excessive amount of amniotic fluid)	
▪ Premature rupture of the membrane	▪ Maternal infections
▪ Fetal malformation	▪ Known malformations (high-risk OB patient)
▪ Decreased fetal movement	▪ Bleeding during pregnancy (abruptio)

Table 2 Intrapartum (During Birth) Risk Factors

▪ Premature labor	▪ Meconium-stained amniotic fluid
▪ Rupture of membranes > 18 hours before delivery	▪ Use of narcotics within 4 hours of delivery
▪ Breech or abnormal presentation	▪ Prolonged labor (> 24 hours) or precipitous delivery
▪ Prolapsed cord	▪ Significant bleeding
▪ Chorioamnionitis	▪ Placenta previa

If there are significant oral secretions, the airway can be cleared using a bulb syringe or suction catheter. Turn the newborn's head to the side; suction the mouth before the nose to prevent aspiration. Do not suction vigorously or deeply, as this can induce a vagal response and bradycardia. Once the airway is cleared, return the newborn to the sniffing position.

Drying the newborn's head and body with towels provides adequate stimulation in most cases. If the newborn does not appear vigorous with adequate respirations, additional safe tactile stimulation methods include:

- Slapping/flicking the soles of the feet
- Rubbing the back or trunk gently

Maintain a patent airway while performing all the resuscitation steps by appropriate positioning of the head.

In some cases, additional resuscitation steps may be required. These include the following:

- Providing supplemental oxygen
- Assisting in ventilation by providing positive pressure
- Intubating
- Providing chest compressions
- Administering medications

Because both short- and long-term outcomes in newborns have been linked to initial stabilization efforts, it is imperative that you anticipate complications during resuscitation, have the appropriate resuscitation equipment readily available and the skills to use this equipment, and, lastly, carefully consider the newborn's ultimate transport destination.

Transition from Fetus to Newborn

In utero (ie, in the pregnant woman's womb), a fetus receives its oxygen from the placenta Figure 1 . The fetal lung is collapsed and filled with fluid, receiving only 10% of the total blood supply. As the fetus is delivered, a rapid series of events needs to occur to enable the newborn to breathe. This process is called fetal transition. The first breath is triggered by mild hypoxia and hypercapnia related to partial occlusion of the umbilical cord during normal delivery. Tactile stimulation and cold stress also promote early breathing. As the newborn's lungs become filled with air, the pulmonary vascular resistance drops, causing more blood to flow to the lungs, picking up oxygen to supply to the body. Any event that delays this decline in pulmonary pressure can lead to delayed transition, hypoxia, brain injury, and, ultimately, death Table 3 .

A newborn delivered at less than 37 completed weeks of gestation is considered preterm; a newborn born at 38 to 42 weeks of gestation is described as term; and a newborn born at more than 42 weeks of gestation is described as post-term (or post-dates).

Arrival of the Newborn

Use any time available before the fetus arrives to obtain a patient history and prepare the environment and equipment that may be necessary. Key questions you need to ask when you are at a scene involving a pregnant woman or a recent home birth include the woman's age; length of the pregnancy (preferably expressed in weeks); the presence and frequency of contractions; the presence or absence of fetal movement; whether there have been any pregnancy complications (eg, diabetes, hypertension, fever); whether membranes have ruptured, including the timing and the makeup of the fluid (clear, meconium stained, or bloody); and the medications being taken (see the list of

Table 3 Causes of Delayed Transition in Newborns

- Hypoxia
- Meconium or blood aspiration
- Acidosis
- Hypothermia
- Pneumonia
- Hypotension
- Sepsis
- Birth asphyxia
- Pulmonary hypoplasia
- Respiratory distress syndrome

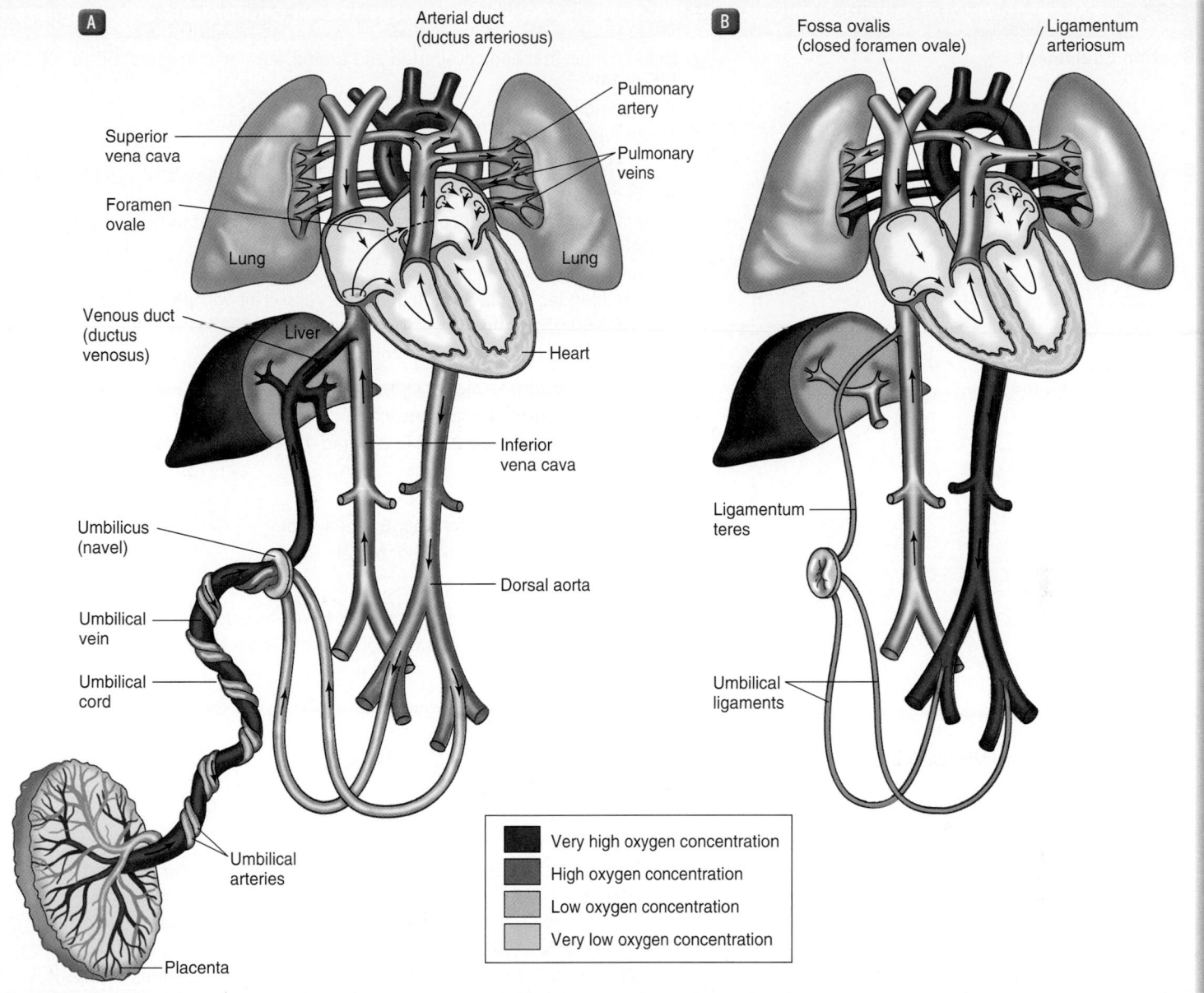

Figure 1 Fetal circulation. **A.** Oxygenated blood from the placenta reaches the fetus through the umbilical vein. Blood returns to the placenta via two umbilical arteries. Right-to-left shunts occur at the ductus venosus, foramen ovale, and the ductus arteriosus. **B.** Fetal circulation following transition.

risk factors in Tables 1 and Table 2). All of these questions will help you determine what resuscitation and equipment may be needed.

Nearly 90% of newborns are born vigorous and at term. These newborns transition well, often with minimal, basic intervention. At a minimum, you will need warm, dry blankets, a bulb syringe, two small clamps or ties, and a pair of clean scissors to cut the umbilical cord. However, any complications need prompt management. Even if a piece of equipment is in a sealed sterile wrap, having it near at hand will expedite its use once the newborn is delivered. Table 4 lists additional equipment that may be needed if more extensive resuscitation becomes necessary.

If the newborn is delivered in the ambulance, the foot of the stretcher, covered with clean, warm blankets, can be used for

Words of Wisdom

Steps to improve fetal circulation:
- Roll the pregnant woman onto her side to take the weight of her uterus off the great vessels.
- Administer 100% oxygen by mask to the pregnant woman.

the initial stabilization steps. The newborn can then be placed on mother's chest after you confirm adequate patency of the airway, breathing, and pulse rate. If more extensive resuscitation is needed, this area can be used as needed initially, optimally transitioning to a second ambulance equipped with a neonatal

Table 4 Preparation of Area for Newborn Resuscitation, Including Resuscitation Equipment and Supplies

Suction Equipment	■ Bulb syringe, mechanical suction and tubing, suction catheters, 5F, 6F, 8F, 10F, 12F, or 14F ■ 8F feeding tube and 20-mL syringe ■ Meconium aspirator
Bag-Mask Equipment	■ Device for delivering positive-pressure ventilation, capable of delivering up to 100% oxygen ■ Face masks, newborn and premature infant size (cushioned-rim masks preferred) ■ Compressed air source ■ Oxygen blender to mix oxygen and compressed air with flowmeter (flow rate up to 10 L/min) and tubing ■ Pulse oximeter and oximeter probe
Intubation Equipment	■ Laryngoscope with straight blades, size 0 (preterm) and 1 (term) ■ Extra bulb, batteries for laryngoscope ■ Endotracheal tubes size 2.5, 3.0, 3.5, and 4.0 internal diameter ■ Stylet (optional) ■ Scissors ■ Tape or securing device for endotracheal tube ■ Capnograph or carbon dioxide detector ■ Laryngeal mask airway
Medications	■ Epinephrine 1:10,000 (0.1 mg/mL), 3- or 10-mL ampules ■ Isotonic crystalloid (normal saline or lactated Ringer's solution), 100- or 250-mL bag ■ Normal saline for flushes ■ Dextrose, 10%, 250 mL
Umbilical Vessel Catheterization Equipment	■ Sterile gloves ■ Scalpel or scissors ■ Antiseptic prep solution ■ Umbilical tape ■ Umbilical catheters, 3.5F, 5F (a sterile 3.5F feeding tube can be used in an emergency) ■ Three-way stopcocks for each catheter ■ Syringes: 1, 3, 5, 10, 20, and 50 mL ■ Needles: 25, 22, and 18 gauge or puncture device for needleless system
Miscellaneous	■ Gloves and appropriate standard precautions ■ Radiant warmer or other heat source ■ Firm, padded resuscitation surface ■ Clock with second hand, timer optional ■ Warmed towels ■ Stethoscope, neonatal head ■ Tape, 1/2 or 3/4 inch ■ Cardiac monitor and electrodes or pulse oximeter and probe (optional for delivery room) ■ Oropharyngeal airways (0, 00, and 000 sizes or 30-, 40-, and 50-mm lengths)
For Very Preterm Newborns	■ Size 00 laryngoscope blade (optional) ■ Reclosable, food-grade plastic bag (1-gallon size) or plastic wrap ■ Chemically activated warming pad (optional) ■ Transport incubator to maintain newborn's temperature during move to the nursery

Adapted from: American Academy of Pediatrics Neonatal Resuscitation Program.

transport incubator to allow maintenance of a thermoneutral environment and observation of the newborn's color and tone.

Do not milk the umbilical cord **Figure 3** .

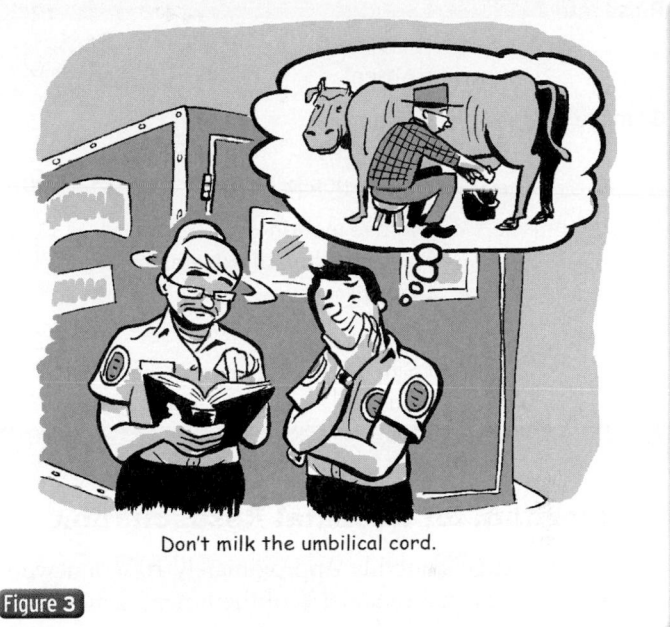

Don't milk the umbilical cord.

Figure 3

Special Populations

A delay in clamping the umbilical cord and keeping the newborn below the level of the placenta may cause more blood to flow into the newborn, which can in turn lead to <u>polycythemia</u> (an abnormally high red blood cell count). If the newborn is kept above the level of the placenta, reverse blood flow occurs and may cause anemia in the newborn.

When the newborn's head is delivered, suction the mouth and then the nose with a bulb syringe. Nasal suctioning helps clear the secretions and provides a stimulus to breathe. After delivery, keep the newborn at the level of the mother, with the head slightly lower than the body, while you clamp the umbilical cord in two places and then cut between the clamps **Figure 2** .

If the umbilical cord comes out ahead of the newborn (more common with polyhydramnios, a condition characterized by extra amniotic fluid), the blood supply through the umbilical cord to the fetus may be cut off. In this case, relieving pressure on the cord (by gently moving the presenting part of the newborn's body off the cord and pushing the cord back) can be lifesaving.

Your initial rapid assessment of the newborn may be done simultaneously with any treatment interventions. Note the time of delivery, and monitor the ABCs. In particular, assess patency of the airway, respiratory rate, respiratory effort, tone, pulse rate, and color.

The newborn is at risk for hypothermia because of significant heat loss through evaporation, a large surface area to volume ratio, limited ability to generate heat, and poor insulation from the environment. Ensure <u>thermoregulation</u> by placing the newborn on prewarmed towels or a radiant warmer, drying the head and the body thoroughly, discarding the wet towels, and then covering the newborn with a dry towel. Cover the head with a cap to minimize heat loss. Position the newborn to ensure a patent airway, clear the airway of secretions as needed, and assess the newborn's respiratory effort. All newborns are cyanotic immediately after birth. If the newborn remains vigorous and begins to become pink in the first 5 minutes of life, ongoing observation and continued thermoregulation with direct skin-to-skin contact with the mother should be maintained while on the way to a local hospital. Bonding with the mother should be encouraged in a stable newborn.

The Apgar Score

The <u>Apgar score</u>, named after Dr. Virginia Apgar, who developed the measure in 1953, and helps record the condition of the newborn in the first few minutes after birth based on five signs **Table 5** . This score can help paramedics determine the need for specific resuscitation measures and the effectiveness of their resuscitation efforts to facilitate the transition from fetus to newborn. Each sign is assigned a value of 0, 1, or 2. The Apgar score is the sum total of these values and is typically recorded at 1 and 5 minutes after birth. If the 5-minute Apgar score is less than 7, the newborn's condition should be reassessed and an additional score assigned every 5 minutes until 20 minutes after birth. If resuscitation is necessary, the Apgar score is completed by determining the result of the resuscitation.

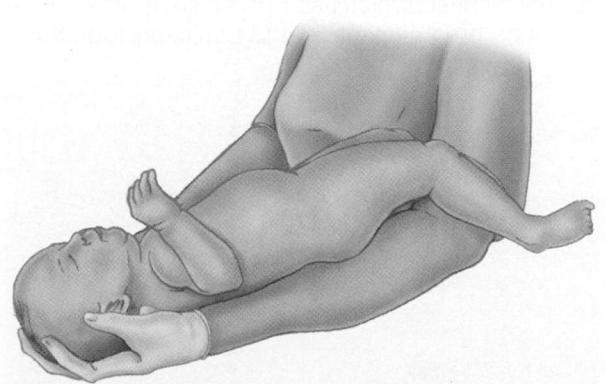

Figure 2 Positioning. Immediately after delivery, hold the newborn with the head slightly lower than the body to facilitate drainage of secretions.

Table 5 The Apgar Score

Condition	Description	Score
Appearance–skin color	Completely pink Body pink, extremities blue Centrally blue, pale	2 1 0
Pulse rate	>100 <100, >0 Absent	2 1 0
Grimace–irritability	Cries Grimaces No response	2 1 0
Activity–muscle tone	Active motion Some flexion of extremities Limp	2 1 0
Respiratory–effort	Strong cry Slow and irregular Absent	2 1 0

Algorithm for Neonatal Resuscitation

Not all deliveries go smoothly. Approximately 10% of newborns need additional assistance and 1% of them need major resuscitation to survive. If a problem arises, it is important for you to follow the clearly defined algorithm developed by the American Academy of Pediatrics and the American Heart Association to optimize the outcome **Figure 4** . In this algorithm, interventions, assessment, and determination of need to progress to the next level of resuscitation are delineated in 30-second intervals.

Following delivery of the newborn, the initial steps of bulb suctioning of the mouth and nose, drying, and stimulating the newborn are followed for 30 seconds. If the newborn does not respond to these actions, further intervention is indicated. Assess the newborn's respiratory rate, respiratory effort, pulse rate, and color. Count the respiratory rate and pulse rate for 6 seconds and then multiply by 10 to quickly determine the rate per minute. The pulse rate can be determined either by auscultation or by feeling the base of the umbilical cord at the baby's abdomen because the umbilical artery should still have pulsatile flow **Figure 5** . Be sure to communicate the heart rate to other members of your resuscitation team. Many newborns become centrally pink but have blue hands and feet (**acrocyanosis**). This is considered normal. If the newborn has a normal breathing pattern and a pulse rate of greater than 100 beats/min but maintains **central cyanosis** of the trunk or of the mucous membranes, provide supplemental **free-flow oxygen**. If there is no other warming source available, keep the newborn on the mother's chest and continue to manage the airway.

If the baby is apneic (ie, has a 20-second or longer respiratory pause) or has a pulse rate of less than 100 beats/min after 30 seconds of drying and stimulation and supplemental free-flow (blow-by) oxygen, begin **positive-pressure ventilation (PPV)** by bag-mask device, being sure to use a newborn-sized bag-mask device. You should use caution when you are squeezing the bag in order to avoid inadvertently delivering too much volume, potentially resulting in a pneumothorax. The size of breath provided should result in a physiologic chest rise.

YOU are the Medic   PART 2

Your patient tells you that this is her fifth pregnancy and she has been receiving regular prenatal care. Her doctor had her scheduled to induce labor 2 days from now. She has not experienced any complications during her pregnancy. The only medication she takes is a daily prenatal vitamin.

As you apply appropriate standard precautions and perform a visual inspection of the patient's vaginal area, your partner obtains a baseline set of vital signs. Your exam reveals crowning of the newborn's head, which has a green stain. You call for additional assistance, anticipating a second patient. You apply oxygen via a nonrebreathing mask at 12 L/min, position the patient for delivery, and have your partner open the OB kit.

Maternal Assessment Recording Time: 2 Minutes	
Respirations	24 breaths/min; adequate tidal volume
Pulse	104 beats/min; strong and regular
Skin	Pink, warm, and moist
Blood pressure	128/74 mm Hg
Oxygen saturation (Spo$_2$)	97% on room air

3. Besides the OB kit, what additional equipment should you have available?

4. Should you stimulate the newborn immediately after birth?

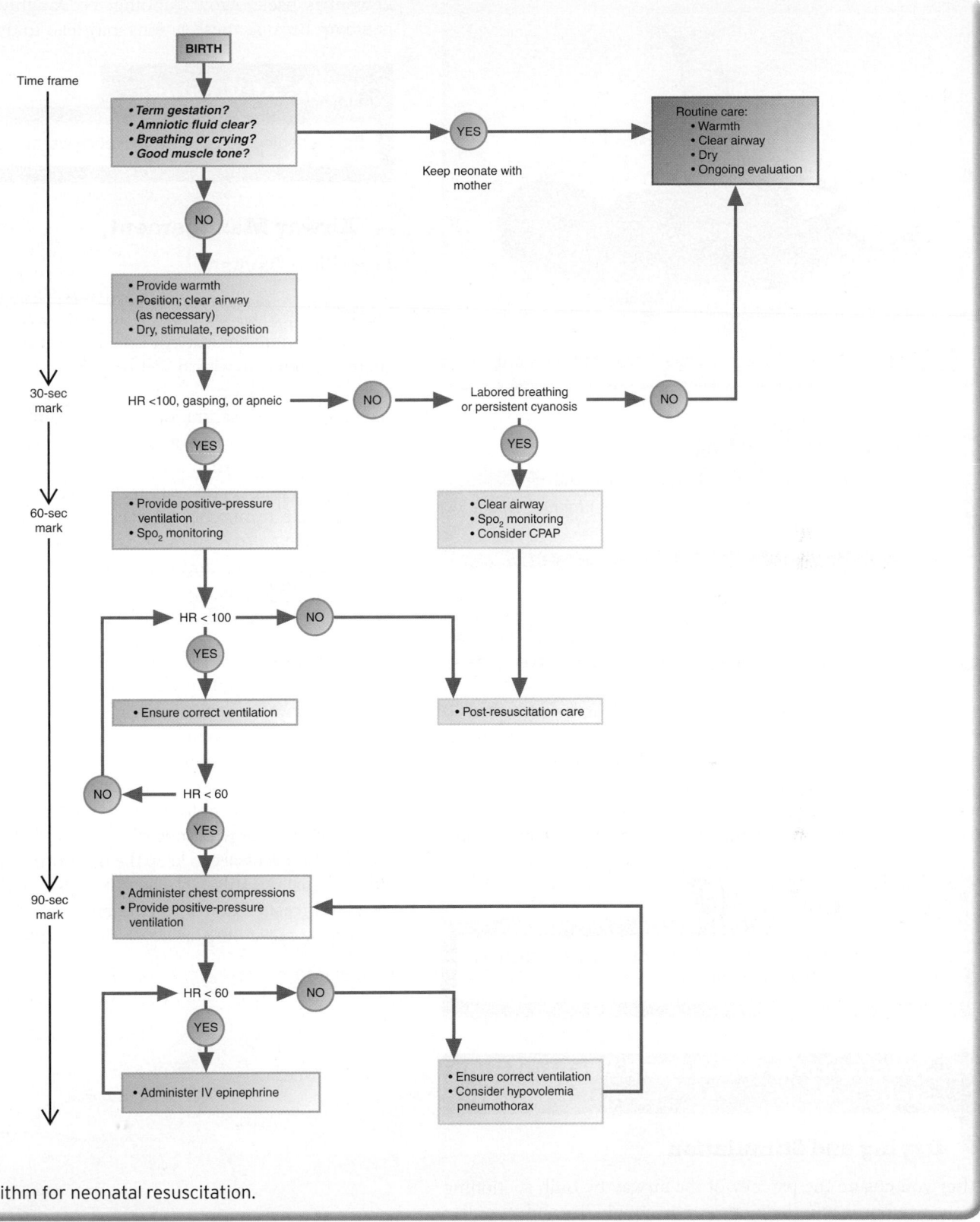

Figure 4 Algorithm for neonatal resuscitation.

Commonly used peak inspiratory pressure (PIP) and peak end-expiratory pressure (PEEP) are 25 and 5. After 30 seconds of adequate ventilation by PPV via a bag-mask device. If blended oxygen is not available, start with room air and then switch to 100% oxygen if needed per Neonatal Resuscitation Program (NRP) guidelines. If the newborn's pulse rate is less than 60 beats/min, begin chest compressions in addition to PPV. Effective chest compressions should result in palpable pulses.

Fewer than 1% of deliveries involve <u>bradycardia</u> that requires treatment with chest compressions. The most common etiology for bradycardia in a newborn is hypoxia, which is readily reversed by effective PPV. Profound hypoxia or shock is also

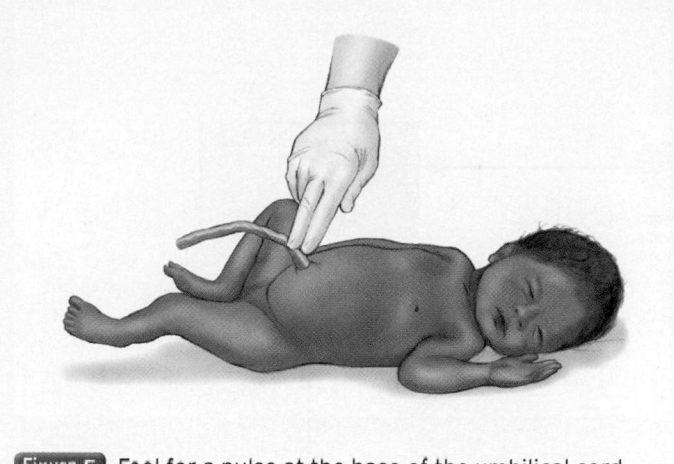

Figure 5   Feel for a pulse at the base of the umbilical cord.

Words of Wisdom

Do not wait until you have measured the 1-minute Apgar score before you start resuscitation.

the cause of cardiac arrest, which is almost always a secondary event after respiratory failure in these patients. Another less common etiology—but one that requires prompt intervention—is tension pneumothorax, which needs to be recognized and treated with needle decompression if resuscitation is to be successful. If ventilation and chest compressions do not improve the bradycardia, you should administer epinephrine via intravenous (IV) line or endotracheal (ET) intubation. Even newborns who have been resuscitated for 20 minutes can have positive long-term outcomes. Newborns are resilient, and most respond readily to interventions.

Words of Wisdom

Do not suction deep into the oropharynx. Do not suction for more than 10 seconds at a time.

Specific Intervention and Resuscitation Steps

Drying and Stimulation

After you ensure the patency of the airway by bulb suctioning of the newborn's mouth and nose, you should dry and stimulate the newborn (in the absence of meconium-stained fluid, see specific resuscitation steps below). Nasal suctioning is a stimulus for the newborn to breathe. The newborn should be positioned on his or her back or side, with the neck in the sniffing position. If the airway is not clear, suction using a bulb syringe or suction catheter, with the head turned to the side. Remember to suction the mouth before the nose to prevent aspiration. Finally, flick the soles of the newborn's feet and gently rub the

newborn's back. Avoid rubbing too roughly or slapping the newborn because these actions may lead to traumatic injury.

Words of Wisdom

Do not neglect to keep the newborn warm.

Airway Management

Free-Flow Oxygen

If a newborn is cyanotic or pale, you should provide supplemental oxygen. Given that 5 g/dL of deoxygenated hemoglobin is needed before clinical cyanosis becomes apparent, a severely anemic hypoxic newborn will be pale, but not cyanotic. Therefore, you should provide oxygen to a pale newborn until an accurate oxygen saturation reading can be obtained using a pulse oximeter. Warm and humidify the oxygen if it will be provided for more than a few minutes. If PPV is not indicated (ie, the pulse rate is greater than 100 beats/min and the newborn has adequate respiratory effort), oxygen can initially be delivered through an oxygen mask or via oxygen tubing within your hand that is cupped and held close to the newborn's nose and mouth **Figure 6** . The oxygen flow rate should be set at 5 L/min. Do not blow oxygen directly into the newborn's eyes.

Oral Airways

Oral airways are rarely used for newborns, but they can be lifesaving if airway obstruction leads to respiratory failure. Some conditions that may require an oral airway are bilateral choanal atresia, Pierre Robin sequence, <u>macroglossia</u> (large tongue size), and other craniofacial defects that may affect the airway. In all the above cases, except for bilateral choanal atresia, an (ET) tube can be inserted down a nostril to a level below the base of the tongue. It is necessary to keep the newborn's mouth open to provide adequate ventilation when these conditions exist. Bilateral <u>choanal atresia</u> (bony or membranous obstruction of the back of the nose preventing air flow) can be rapidly fatal, but usually

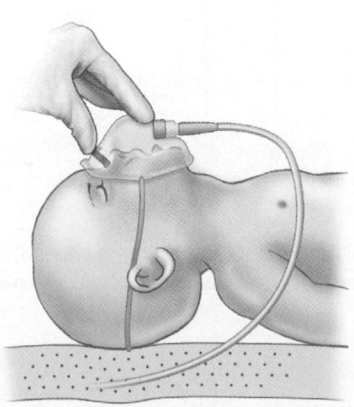

Figure 6   Free-flow oxygen can be delivered through an oxygen mask.

Table 6	Common Causes of Respiratory Distress	
- Lung or heart disease - Central nervous system disorders - Pneumothorax - Meconium aspiration - Lung immaturity/ respiratory distress syndrome - Shock and sepsis - Diaphragmatic hernia	- **Persistent pulmonary hypertension** - Mucous obstruction of nasal passages - Choanal atresia - Amniotic fluid aspiration - Pneumonia - Metabolic acidosis	

responds to placement of an oral airway (or a gloved finger until an adequate oral airway is located). The **Pierre Robin sequence** is a series of developmental anomalies including a small chin and posteriorly positioned tongue that frequently lead to airway obstruction. Positioning the patient prone (chest down) may relieve the obstruction. If not, you should insert an oral airway. As with infants and small children, use a tongue blade to depress the tongue and insert the oral airway without rotating it.

Bag-Mask Ventilation

Bag-mask ventilation is indicated when a newborn is apneic, has inadequate respiratory effort, or has a pulse rate of less than 100 beats/min (bradycardia) after you clear the airway of secretions, relieve obstruction from the tongue, and dry and stimulate the newborn. Signs of respiratory distress that suggest a need for bag-mask ventilation include periodic breathing, **intercostal retractions** (sucking in between the ribs), **nasal flaring**, and **grunting** on expiration. Respiratory distress occurs in approximately 8 of every 1,000 live births and accounts for approximately 15% of neonatal deaths. Table 6 summarizes the most common conditions leading to respiratory distress.

Three devices may be used to deliver bag-mask ventilation to a newborn. First, you may use a self-inflating bag with an oxygen reservoir (an oxygen source is not necessary to provide PPV but is necessary to provide supplementary oxygen). Second, you may use a flow-inflating bag, though it needs a gas source to provide PPV; this technique is therefore more common in the operating room. Third, you may apply a T-piece resuscitator (also needs a gas source, mostly found in neonatal intensive care units).

In the field, you will most likely use a self-inflating bag for bag-mask ventilation. If available, always use the infant size (240 mL). Given that the breath size (tidal volume) of a newborn is only 3 to 6 mL/kg, only one tenth of the bag's volume will be used for each breath—which explains why a larger bag can easily create problems. If a neonatal bag is not available and the newborn is in severe respiratory distress, has apnea, or has bradycardia, you can use a bag designed for adults or older children (750 mL or greater volume) as long as you carefully keep the delivered breath size appropriately small and monitor chest rise to avoid excessive volumes of delivered breaths.

When you are administering bag-mask ventilation with 100% oxygen, the face mask needs to provide an airtight seal, fitting over the newborn's mouth and nose, and extending down to the chin but not over the eyes Figure 7 . Pressure on the eyes, like deep suctioning, can lead to a vagal response and bradycardia. The newborn needs to have a patent airway, cleared of secretions, with his or her neck slightly extended in the sniffing position Figure 8 . The first

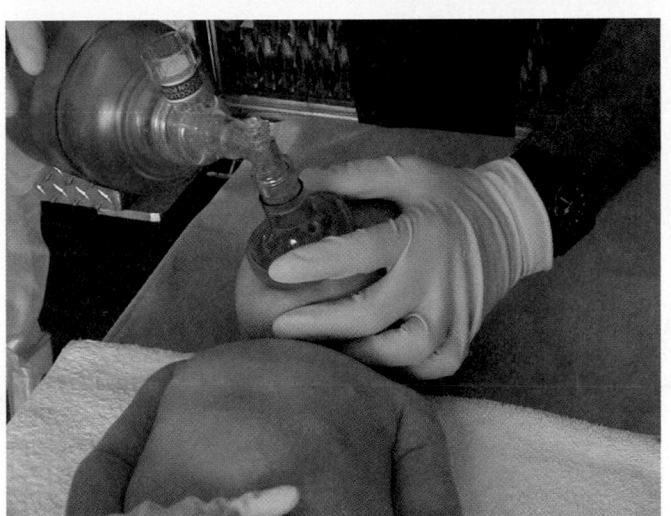

Figure 7 Bag-mask ventilation of the newborn. Hold the mask securely to the face with your thumb and index finger. Apply countertraction under the bony part of the chin with your middle finger.

few breaths after birth will frequently require higher pressures (possibly around 30 mm Hg) because the lungs are not yet expanded and are still full of fluid. To deliver these initial breaths, you may need to manually (cover with your finger) disable the spring-loaded pop-off valve (it is usually set by the manufacturer at 30 to 40 cm H_2O). Subsequent breaths should be delivered with sufficient pressure to result in visible but not excessive chest rise, with the pop-off valve on.

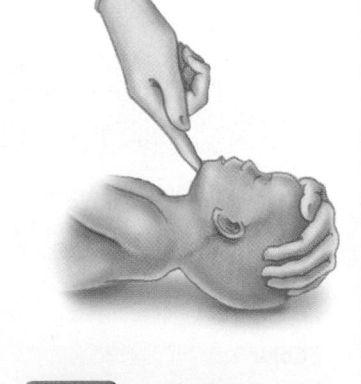

Figure 8 The sniffing position.

In a newborn, it is important for you to provide the correct timing for ventilation at a rate of 40 to 60 breaths/min because breaths delivered at a higher rate can lead to hypocapnia, air trapping, or pneumothorax. To help with the timing, count "breath–two–three, breath–two–three" as you ventilate: Give a breath on "breath," and release on "two–three." Continue PPV as long as the pulse rate remains at less than 100 beats/min or the newborn's respiratory effort is ineffective. If prolonged PPV is needed (more than 1 minute), hook the system to a pressure manometer to aid in monitoring and minimizing excessive pressures (target peak inspiratory pressure less than 25 mm Hg in full-term newborns, less in preterm newborns).

The most common reasons for ineffective bag-mask ventilation are inadequate seal of the mask on the face and incorrect head position. Other causes such as copious secretions, pneumothorax, or equipment malfunction need to be considered as well.

Words of Wisdom

When treating a newborn with <u>cleft lip</u> and/or <u>cleft palate</u>, airway resuscitation is not needed, but you may need to apply some cricoid pressure if intubation becomes necessary. Consider delivering PPV via a bag-mask device. You may need to use a little extra positive pressure in a newborn with a cleft palate. Owing to the risk of aspiration and regurgitation, do not feed the newborn with a cleft lip and palate in the field.

Controversies

Whereas resuscitation with 100% oxygen has been the norm in the United States, a growing body of evidence shows that routine exposure to 100% oxygen is unnecessary and possibly harmful for the term newborn. Doing newborn resuscitation with room air is a safe alternative. If there is need for oxygen, full-term and preterm infants can be stabilized with less than 100% oxygen. Regardless of the amount of oxygen initiated, the American Academy of Pediatrics recommends using a pulse oximeter to titrate the amount of oxygen delivered. Bag-mask ventilation can be initiated with room air while an oxygen source is being secured.

- Meconium-stained fluid is present and the newborn is not vigorous (ie, poor muscle tone, bradycardia, inadequate ventilation, no respiratory effort), a condition for which tracheal suctioning is indicated.
- Congenital **diaphragmatic hernia** (a congenital defect in which abdominal organs herniate through an opening in the diaphragm into the chest cavity) is known or suspected and respiratory support is indicated.
- The newborn does not respond to bag-mask ventilation and chest compressions, necessitating ET administration of epinephrine (ie, no umbilical venous line or intraosseous (IO) site has been established).
- Prolonged PPV is needed.
- Craniofacial defects impede the ability to maintain an adequate airway.

Before you begin ventilation, make sure that you have the following equipment available:

- Suction equipment (10F tubing, with 5F to 8F being available, suction set to 100 mm Hg)
- Laryngoscope (check the light to ensure that the bulb is bright and screwed in tightly)

Intubation

Bag-mask ventilation provides successful resuscitation of most newborns. Intubation, however, may be necessary if the newborn requires resuscitation beyond simple interventions **Figure 9**. Intubation is indicated in the following situations:

YOU *are the Medic*   PART 3

As the newborn's head delivers, you carefully suction the mouth and nose. The newborn continues to deliver without difficulty. Immediately following delivery, because the newborn's respirations are weak and muscle tone is low, you do not begin to dry and stimulate the infant. Instead, you cut and clamp the umbilical cord, intubate the trachea, use a meconium aspirator attached to the end of the endotracheal tube, and a suction catheter to clear the airway of any meconium. After suctioning dark green material from the airway, you resume with drying and stimulating the newborn, then perform a newborn assessment.

Newborn Assessment Recording Time: 11 Minutes	
Respiratory effort	Weak and irregular; no cry
Pulse rate	85 beats/min, regular
Color	Cyanosis to the trunk and extremities

5. What treatment is indicated for this newborn?
6. When is endotracheal intubation indicated in the newborn?

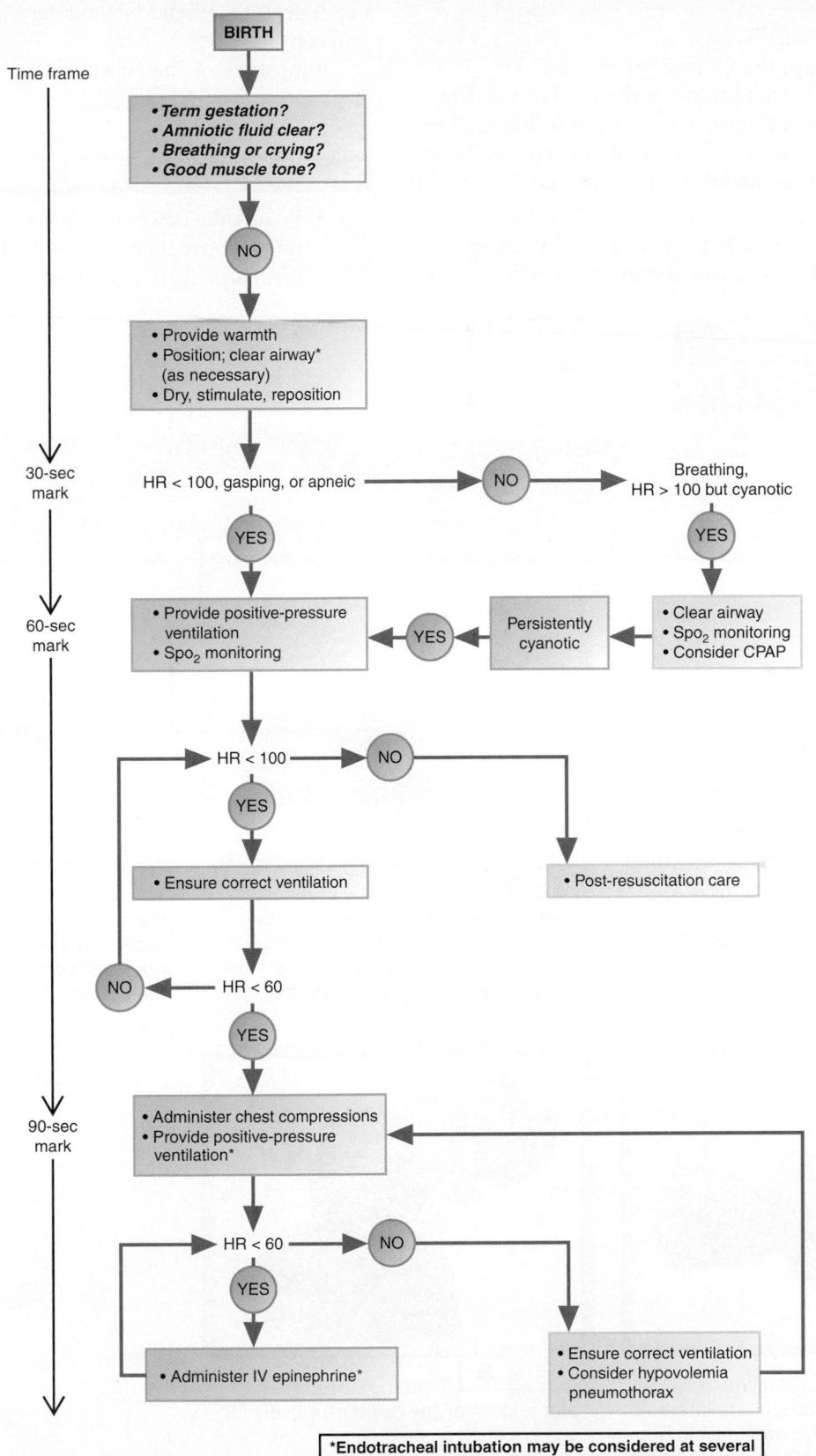

Figure 9 Resuscitation algorithm for the distressed newborn.

- Blades—straight: No. 1 for full-term newborns, No. 0 for preterm newborns
- Shoulder roll
- Adhesive tape, to tape the ET tube
- ET tube: 2.5 to 4.0 mm (2.5 mm if the newborn is delivered before 28 weeks of gestation, 3.0 mm if delivered at 28 to 34 weeks of gestation, 3.5 mm if delivered at 34 to 38 weeks of gestation, and 4.0 mm if delivered after 38 weeks of gestation)

Some paramedics use a stylet to provide rigidity to the ET tube. In such a case, you must secure the stylet (bending it over at the top of the ET tube so it cannot advance) and make sure that it does not extend beyond the ET tube, or tracheal perforation may occur.

Intubation of the newborn is discussed in the following steps and shown in Skill Drill 1:

Skill Drill   1

1. Be sure the newborn is preoxygenated to an oxygen saturation above 95% by bag-mask ventilation using supplemental oxygen prior to making an intubation attempt

Skill Drill   1

Intubating a Newborn

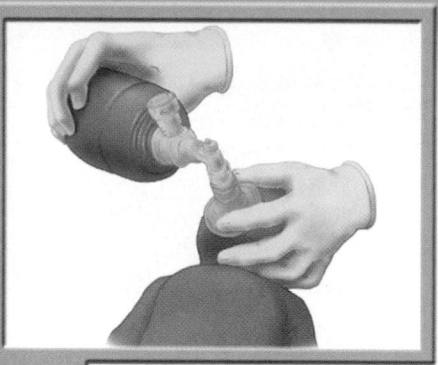

Step 1 Preoxygenate the newborn by bag-mask ventilation to an oxygen saturation greater than 95%.

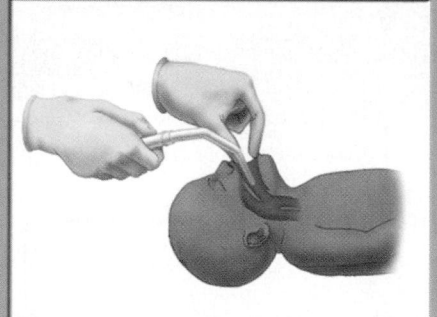

Step 2 Suction the oropharynx if there are copious secretions that prevent adequate ventilation. Avoid deep suctioning and provide bag-mask ventilation if bradycardia results.

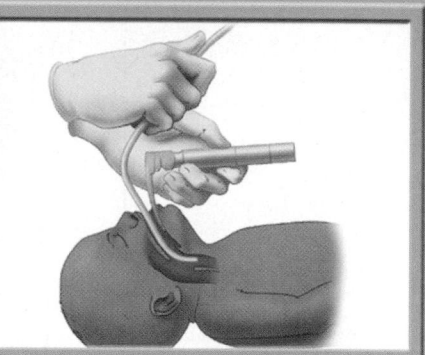

Step 3 Place the laryngoscope blade in the oropharynx. Visualize the vocal cords. Place the ET tube between the vocal cords until the black line on the ET tube is at the level of the cords.

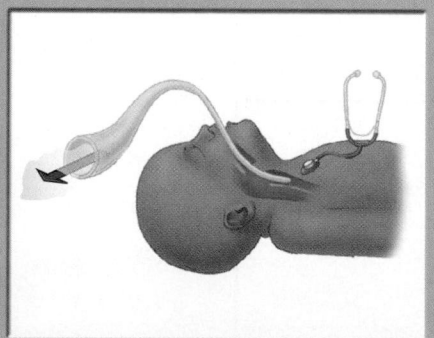

Step 4 Confirm placement. Observe chest rise, auscultate laterally and high on the chest, note mist in the ET tube, note equal breath sounds on both sides, and observe for clinical improvement. Monitor ETCO$_2$ via waveform capnography and consider using pulse oximetry.

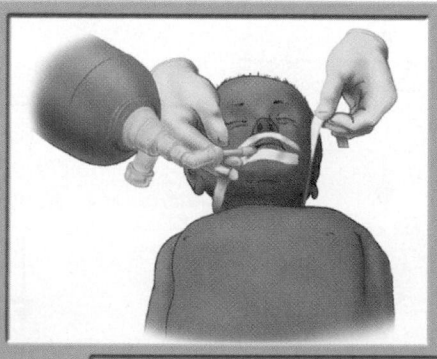

Step 5 Tape the ET tube in place. Monitor the newborn closely for complications.

Step 1. Use of 100% oxygen is not needed and can have deleterious effects in preterm infants.

2. If the infant appears to have copious secretions that hinder adequate ventilation, suction the oropharynx to remove any secretions. This can be a vagal stimulus, so pay close attention to the pulse rate and avoid repeated or vigorous suctioning. Bag-mask ventilation may be needed if the newborn develops bradycardia at this point Step 2.

3. Place the laryngoscope blade in the oropharynx and then visualize the vocal cords. Avoid applying torque to the blade because it increases the risk of trauma. Place the ET tube between the vocal cords until the black line on the tube is at the level of the cords Step 3. For full-term newborns, the ET tube is usually advanced until it is at 9 cm at the lip. A premature newborn may need to have the ET tube advanced to only 6½ to 7 cm at the lip. Limit the intubation attempt to 20 seconds, and initiate bag-mask ventilation if it is unsuccessful or if significant bradycardia develops.

4. Confirm placement by observing chest rise when applying positive pressure through the ET tube, auscultating laterally in the epigastric region and high on the chest, noting mist in the ET tube (seen when the patient exhales through the tube from condensation of humidified air leaving the lungs), noting equal breath sounds on both sides, and observing for clinical improvement. As with adult and pediatric intubation, all tubes inserted into a newborn must be checked initially and monitored continuously with a waveform capnography device to measure the $ETCO_2$ level Step 4. This is also often the earliest indicator of return of spontaneous circulation (ROSC). In addition, pulse oximetry monitoring provides the peripheral oxygen saturation and reflects the response to adequate oxygenation and ventilation.

5. Tape the ET tube in place on the face to minimize the risk of the tube dislodging . Monitor the newborn closely for complications such as tube dislodgement, tube occlusion by mucous plug or meconium, or pneumothorax Step 5.

Complications of ET tube placement include oropharyngeal or tracheal perforation, esophageal intubation with subsequent persistent hypoxia, and right mainstem intubation that can lead to atelectasis, persistent hypoxia, and pneumothorax. You can minimize these risks by ensuring optimal placement of the laryngoscope blade and carefully noting how far the ET tube is advanced.

Gastric Decompression

Gastric decompression using an orogastric tube is indicated when you are providing prolonged bag-mask ventilation (more than 5 to 10 minutes), if abdominal distention is impeding ventilation, and in the presence of a diaphragmatic hernia or a gastrointestinal congenital anomaly such as pyloric stenosis. Many diaphragmatic hernias are diagnosed prenatally by routine ultrasound; postnatally they are suspected clinically if there are decreased breath sounds on the left side (90% of diaphragmatic hernias are on the left), a scaphoid or concave abdomen (many of the abdominal contents are in the chest), and increased work of breathing. Skill Drill 2 shows gastric decompression in a newborn.

Skill Drill 2

1. To determine the length of tube to insert, use an 8F feeding tube and measure the length from the bottom of the earlobe to the tip of the nose to halfway between the xiphoid process (lower tip of sternum) and the umbilicus Step 1.

2. Insert the tube through the mouth to the appropriate depth. Leave the nose open to allow for ventilation Step 2.

3. Attach a 10-mL syringe and suction the stomach contents. Tape the tube to the newborn's cheek. Remove the syringe from the feeding tube to allow venting of air from the stomach, and intermittently suction the feeding tube Step 3.

Words of Wisdom

Indications for endotracheal intubation of the newborn:
- Inability to ventilate effectively by bag-mask device
- Necessity to perform tracheal suctioning, especially if meconium is present and newborn is depressed at birth
- When prolonged ventilation will be necessary

Circulation

Chest Compressions

Chest compressions are indicated if the pulse rate remains at less than 60 beats/min despite positioning, clearing the airway, drying and stimulation, and 30 seconds of effective PPV. Two people are needed to deliver effective chest compressions while continuing ventilation. Two different techniques are used Figure 10.

1. **Thumb technique:** This is the preferred technique because it appears to generate superior peak systolic and coronary arterial perfusion pressure, while causing less fatigue in the rescuer. Encircle the torso with both hands, with fingers under the newborn's back, supporting the spine. Place your two thumbs side by side, or one over the other in a small preterm baby, over the lower third of the sternum. This area is between the xiphoid process and a line drawn between the nipples. Once the newborn's airway is secure or you have intubated, the chest compressions using this technique can be delivered from the head of the bed, allowing your colleague easier access to the umbilicus for insertion of an umbilical catheter.

2. **Two-finger technique:** The tips of your index and middle fingers of one hand are placed over the lower third of the sternum. This area is between the xiphoid process and a line drawn between the nipples. The second hand is placed behind the newborn's back to support the spine.

Skill Drill 2

Inserting an Orogastric Tube in the Newborn

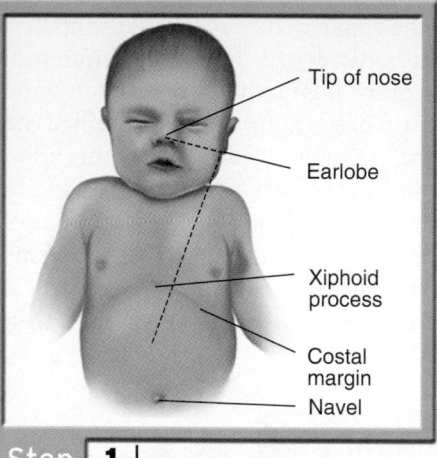

Tip of nose
Earlobe
Xiphoid process
Costal margin
Navel

Step 1 Measure for correct depth—from the bottom of the earlobe to the tip of the nose to halfway between the xiphoid process (lower tip of sternum) and the umbilicus.

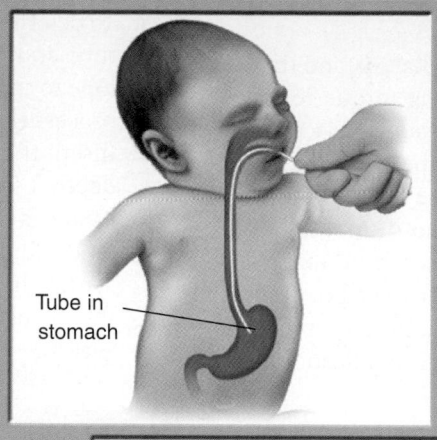

Tube in stomach

Step 2 Insert the tube to the appropriate depth. Leave the nose open to allow for ventilations.

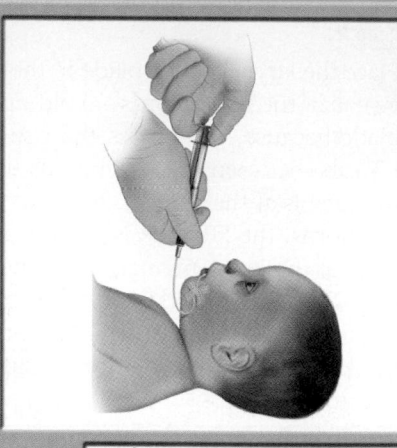

Step 3 Remove the gastric contents with a 10-mL syringe. Tape the tube to the newborn's cheek. Remove the syringe and leave the tip of the tube open to allow air to vent from the stomach.

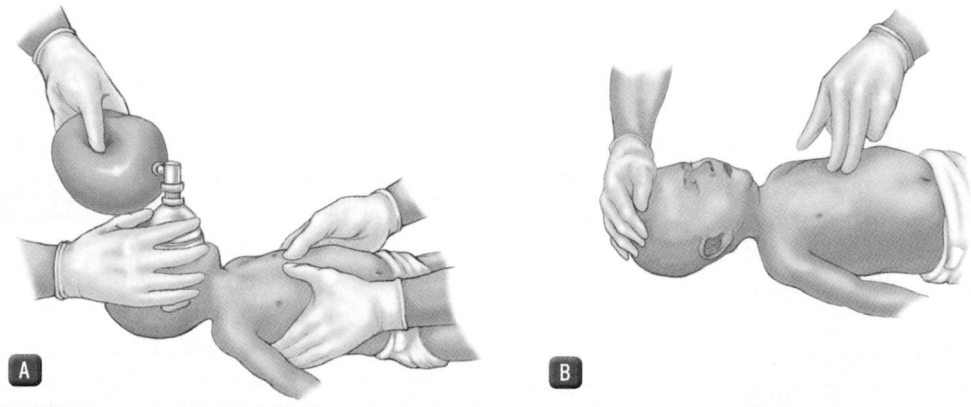

Figure 10 Chest compressions in the newborn. **A.** When using the thumb technique, use your thumbs side by side, placed between the xiphoid and an imaginary line drawn between the two nipples. Support the spine by encircling your fingers around the torso. **B.** When the newborn is large, use two fingers placed between the xiphoid and an imaginary line drawn between the nipples. Use the other hand to support the newborn's head.

In newborns, the chest compressions and artificial ventilation should not be delivered simultaneously; rather, they should be coordinated to result in 90 compressions and 30 breaths/min. This equals a rate of 120 events per minute, meaning that each event should occur every half second. The person doing the compressions takes over the counting out loud. The compressor counts "one-and-two-and-three-and-breathe-and." The person ventilating squeezes the bag or occludes the T-piece cap during "breathe-and" and releases during "one-and."

The depth of compression is one third of the anteroposterior diameter of the chest. Your thumbs or fingers should remain in contact with the chest at all times. It is important for you to allow the chest to completely recoil after giving a compression. Liver laceration and rib fractures are possible risks when you are delivering chest compressions to a newborn. Refer to the chapter, *Responding to the Field Code* for coverage of infant CPR.

In the past, pulse rate was assessed every 30 seconds. However, studies suggest that return of spontaneous circulation may take up to a minute after chest compressions are started. Any interruption of chest compressions required to assess the pulse may result in decrease of perfusion to the coronary arteries. Therefore, it is recommended that you wait at least 45 to 60 seconds after establishing well-coordinated ventilation and chest compressions before pausing to check the pulse rate. If the pulse rate is above 60 beats/min, chest compressions may be stopped. Effective ventilation should be continued at the higher rate of 40 to 60 breaths/min after stopping the chest compressions. Recheck the pulse rate after 30 seconds. Once the pulse rate rises above 100 beats/min, gradually slow the rate and decrease the pressure of PPV.

Vascular Access

Emergent access becomes necessary when fluid administration is needed to support circulation, and when resuscitation medications (eg, epinephrine, sodium bicarbonate) and therapeutic drugs (eg, IV dextrose, antibiotics) must be administered intravenously. However, establishing peripheral access in a newborn can prove difficult.

The **umbilical vein** can be catheterized using an umbilical vein line in a newborn using the following steps:

1. Clean the umbilical cord with alcohol or another antiseptic such as povidone-iodine (Betadine). Drape the area with sterile towels, keeping the umbilical stump exposed. Place a sterile tie firmly, but not too tightly, around the base of the cord to control bleeding. Although the line must be placed quickly in a code situation, maintain sterile technique as much as possible.

2. Attach a 3-mL syringe and a stop-cock to a sterile 3.5F to 5F umbilical vein line catheter (a comparable-size sterile feeding tube can be used in an emergency) and prefill the catheter. Turn the stop-cock to off toward the patient.

3. Cut the cord with a scalpel between the clamp placed on the cord and the cord tie, keeping about 1 to 2 cm from the skin.

4. Insert a "low-UV line": The umbilical vein is a large, thin-walled vessel usually found at the 12 o'clock position, as compared with the two thick-walled, smaller umbilical arteries usually found at 4 and 8 o'clock **Figure 11**. Insert the catheter into this vein for a distance of 2 to 4 cm (less in preterm newborns) until blood can be aspirated. If the catheter is advanced too deep and into the liver, the infusion of hypertonic solutions may lead to irreversible damage **Figure 12**. If the catheter is advanced into the heart, dysrhythmias may develop.

5. Flush the catheter with 0.5 mL of normal saline and tape it in place.

A peripheral IV or IO line can also be placed. Placement of an IO line is discussed in the chapter, *Medication Administration*. Whereas the technique for placing an IO line is similar to that used with older children or adults, a smaller needle should be used in newborns to avoid exiting the far side of the bone.

Pharmacologic Interventions

Medications are rarely needed in newborn resuscitation because most newborns can be resuscitated with effective ventilatory support. Medications in newborns are based on weight, so you may need to estimate the newborn's weight for dosing.

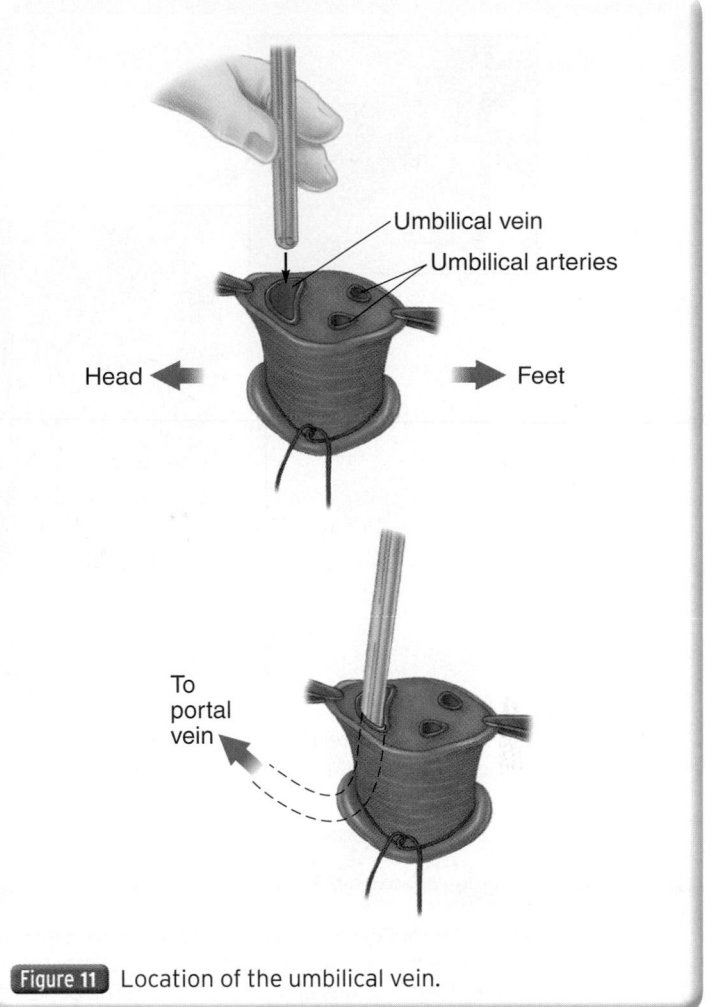

Figure 11 Location of the umbilical vein.

A full-term newborn usually weighs 6½ to 9 lb (3 to 4 kg) and is 20 inches (50 cm) long; a newborn born at 28 weeks of gestation, on average, weighs 2½ lb (1 kg) and is approximately 14¾ inches (37.5 cm) long. A weight of 3 kg is often used for dose calculations in a full-term newborn.

Bradycardia

Bradycardia in a newborn is often a result of inadequate ventilation and usually responds to effective PPV. If hypoxia continues, there could be persistent bradycardia. Administration of epinephrine is indicated when the newborn has a pulse rate of less than 60 beats/min after 30 seconds of effective ventilation and 30 seconds of effective chest compressions coordinated with ventilation. The recommended concentration for newborns is 1:10,000. The recommended dose is 0.1 to 0.3 mL/kg of 1:10,000 epinephrine IV, equal to 0.01 to 0.03 mg/kg, administered rapidly, and followed by a 0.5- to 1-mL normal saline flush to clear the line. A low umbilical vein catheter is the preferred access to administer medications during resuscitation.

Administration of epinephrine via ET tube may be considered while IV access is being established. The dose via ET tube is much higher, 0.5 to 1 mL/kg of 1:10,000 epinephrine.

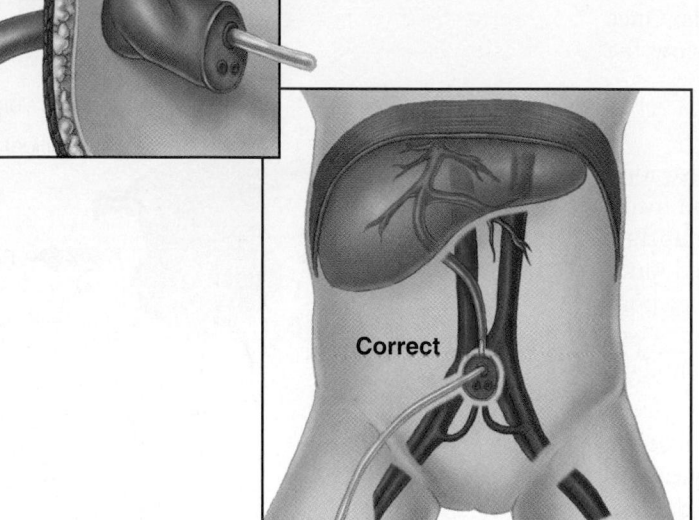
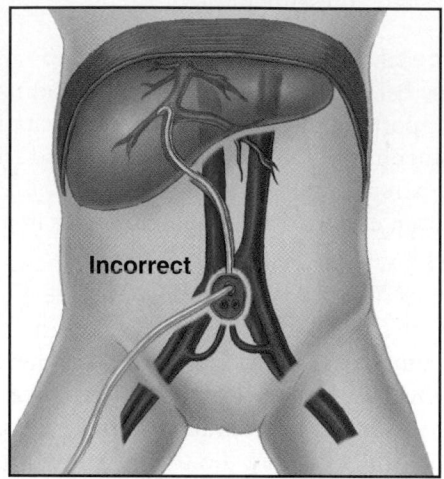

Figure 12 Umbilical vein catheterization. Inset shows cross section through abdominal wall.

Words of Wisdom

Special consideration for IV access: You may encounter newborns with exposed abdominal contents. A developmental defect may lead to the intestines appearing outside the abdomen. There are two types of abdominal wall defects seen.

1. Gastroschisis occurs when there is a skin defect and the uncovered intestines herniate outside the abdomen. An intact omphalocele occurs when abdominal contents that routinely herniated into the umbilical cord during early development fail to return into the abdominal cavity.
2. Omphalocele: A nonintact omphalocele occurs if there is rupture of the umbilical cord and the intestine is no longer protected by being within the cord.

In these situations, while providing standard resuscitation, place the newborn from the waist down into a sterile, clear plastic bag immediately to keep the bowel clean and minimize heat/fluid loss. Intubate and secure the airway of the newborn to prevent distention and kinking of the intestinal loops. Monitor the color of the intestines through the clear bag (pink is an abnormal finding, blue/black is a normal finding) and position the newborn on his or her side to maintain the blood supply to the intestines. Place a peripheral IV or IO in these infants. Keep the intestines moist, using sterile saline as needed.

Check the pulse rate about 1 minute after administering epinephrine (longer if administered via ET tube). Dosing may be repeated every 3 to 5 minutes when there is persistent bradycardia. In addition, ensure that ventilation is adequate and effective, that the ET tube is not dislodged, and that chest compressions are being given to adequate depth of one third the anteroposterior diameter.

Low Blood Volume

If the newborn has significant intravascular volume depletion owing to conditions such as placenta abruptio (separation of the placenta from the uterus, which leads to excessive bleeding), twin-to-twin transfusion, placenta previa, or septic shock, fluid resuscitation may be needed. Signs of hypovolemia include pallor, persistently low pulse rate, weak pulses, or no improvement in circulatory status despite adequate resuscitation efforts. In a newborn, you should place a low umbilical vein line as outlined earlier. In a newborn who is more than a few days old, place a peripheral IV or IO line. A fluid bolus in a newborn consists of 10 mL/kg of normal saline, lactated Ringer's, or O Rh-negative blood IV given over 5 to 10 minutes. Multiple boluses may be administered if the patient remains clinically hypovolemic.

Acidosis

If bradycardia persists after adequate ventilation, chest compressions, and volume expansion, suspect metabolic acidosis. A 10-mL/kg normal saline bolus may aide in improved perfusion and clearance of acid. Administration of sodium bicarbonate has been associated with increased morbidity and should be avoided.

Respiratory Depression Secondary to Narcotics

In the case of a drug-addicted mother, administration of naloxone (Narcan) to the newborn to reverse the narcotic effect may precipitate seizures that can potentially cause death, so this intervention is no longer recommended as a first-line drug in resuscitation. In the case of a newborn experiencing respiratory suppression from the mother's chronic use of narcotics, you should provide ventilatory support and transport immediately. If respiratory depression is the result of the mother being treated acutely with narcotics, and there is no chronic narcotic exposure, naloxone, 0.1 mg/kg, may be administered to the newborn via the IV (preferred) or intramuscular route to reverse the narcotic effect.

Hypoglycemia

Hypoglycemia is most frequently seen in newborns who are small for their gestational age, those who are large for their gestational age, and those whose mothers were diabetic during pregnancy. Neurologic symptoms consist of jitteriness, decreased response to stimuli, hypotonia (floppy), apnea, poor feeding, and seizures. In these cases, blood glucose measurement and administration of dextrose may be lifesaving in the field. Obtain the newborn's baseline vital signs and oxygen saturation readings and provide additional oxygen, assisted ventilation, blood pressure support, and IV access as necessary. A 10% dextrose solution may be given as an IV bolus (2 mL/kg) if the newborn's blood glucose level is less than 40 mg/dL, with a recheck of the blood glucose level in about 30 minutes. IV administration of dextrose often needs to be followed by a 10% dextrose infusion run at 60 to 100 mL/kg/d.

Family and Transport Considerations

Once you have stabilized the newborn as much as possible in the field, transport the patient to the nearest facility that can provide the next level of care. This facility will not necessarily be a tertiary hospital. A nearby community hospital, if it is located much closer, may be able to perform additional stabilization procedures for an ill newborn, such as placement of a chest tube for a clinically significant pneumothorax. Ideally, the paramedic will contact this facility to discuss the situation and obtain advice regarding care and disposition. Throughout the care process, you should provide ongoing communication with the family regarding what is being done for the newborn and what care is planned to help allay their fears. Do not be specific about survival statistics. Many factors play into mortality and morbidity, and you do not want to be misleading. If family members have questions you cannot answer, be straightforward. Tell them that you do not have a definite answer, but you will help put them in touch with the people who do (ie, the center to which the newborn is being transferred).

During transport, you should continuously observe the newborn and perform frequent reassessments to ensure timely intervention should the newborn's status change. Attention to thermoregulation, respiratory effort, patency of airway, skin color, and pulse rate is vital. If the newborn is being transferred between facilities after the initial stabilization, continue to provide close observation and assessment of these factors to facilitate initiation of interventions should the newborn's condition change.

The development of new and more sophisticated techniques for the care of newborns, especially premature newborns, together with round-the-clock care by expert medical personnel, has significantly reduced the mortality among high-risk newborns in hospitals where such capabilities are available. Because the average community hospital cannot provide the specially trained doctors and nurses or the specialized equipment needed for such care, it sometimes becomes necessary to transfer the critically ill newborn to a regional center, where the newborn may benefit from highly skilled personnel and sophisticated equipment. In the well-organized regional referral system, transport of a high-risk newborn proceeds through the following several steps:

1. A physician at the referring hospital initiates a request for transport. A physician in the regional control center decides which intensive care nursery can accommodate the patient and gives the referring physician advice on management of the patient until the transport team arrives.
2. A mode of transportation is chosen—ground transportation, helicopter, or fixed-wing aircraft, depending on the distance, availability of services, and weather conditions.
3. The transport team is mobilized, and equipment is assembled. The ideal team consists of a nurse with special training in neonatal intensive care, a respiratory therapist with similar special training, and a paramedic who has undertaken a period of apprenticeship in a neonatal intensive care unit. For particularly critical patients, a physician may also attend. The equipment is highly specialized, requiring appropriately designed ventilation and oxygenation units and an incubator meeting stringent criteria.
4. On arriving at the referring hospital, the transport team continues to stabilize the newborn before embarking on transport. Conditions such as hypoxemia, acidosis, hypoglycemia, and hypovolemia should be treated before leaving the referring hospital.
5. While stabilizing the newborn, the team collects information and materials including a copy of the mother's and newborn's charts and any radiographic studies taken of the newborn.

Words of Wisdom

Transport of a distressed newborn should be expedited to allow initiation of additional support not available in the field.

Pathophysiology, Assessment, and Management of Specific Conditions

The remaining sections in this chapter discuss specific neonatal emergencies and their assessment and management.

Apnea

Apnea is common in newborns delivered before 32 weeks of gestation, but is rarely seen in the first 24 hours after delivery, even in premature newborns. Apnea is defined as a respiratory pause of greater than 20 seconds. If it does not respond to stimulation and further steps are not taken such as PPV, apnea can lead to hypoxemia and bradycardia. Apnea often follows a period of hypoxia or hypothermia. Other causes include maternal or infant narcotic exposure, airway or respiratory muscle weakness, septicemia, prolonged or difficult labor and delivery, gastroesophageal reflux, central nervous system abnormalities including seizures, and metabolic disorders.

The pathophysiology of apnea depends on the underlying etiology. Apnea of prematurity is due to an underdeveloped central nervous system. Gastroesophageal reflux can trigger a vagal response, leading to apnea. Drug-induced apnea frequently results from direct central nervous system depression. Regardless of the cause, a newborn with apnea needs respiratory support to minimize hypoxic brain damage and other organ damage.

Assessment and Management

Assessment of an apneic newborn includes obtaining a careful history to elicit possible etiologic risk factors and performing a physical exam that focuses on neurologic signs and symptoms or signs of infection. At birth it is important to differentiate between **primary apnea** and **secondary apnea**. If the newborn has experienced a relatively short period of hypoxia, he or she will have a period of rapid breathing, followed by apnea and bradycardia. At this point, the use of drying and stimulation may cause a resumption of breathing and improvement in the pulse rate. If hypoxia continues during primary apnea, the newborn will gasp and enter secondary apnea. At this point, stimulation alone will not restart the newborn's breathing. Instead, PPV by bag-mask device is required. Follow the steps for neonatal resuscitation discussed earlier in the chapter.

■ Bradycardia

Bradycardia occurs in about 1% of newborns. Bradycardia in a newborn is most frequently a result of inadequate ventilation and often responds to effective PPV. If hypoxia continues, there could be persistent bradycardia. Other causes of bradycardia include hypothyroidism, acidosis, and congenital atrioventricular block in infants whose mothers have lupus. While increased intracranial pressure in older children can result in bradycardia, neonates have open fontanelles so they rarely present with increased intracranial pressure. Interventions can result in bradycardia as well. Prolonged suctioning or attempts at intubation, or vagal stimulation from an inadequately secured ET tube or orogastric tube, often result in bradycardia. The morbidity and mortality of bradycardia are determined by the underlying cause and how quickly it can be corrected.

Assessment and Management

Heart rate in a newborn is assessed via auscultation or by palpating the base of the umbilical cord. NRP guidelines outline the management of bradycardia in a newborn. Bradycardia in a neonate is often a result of inadequate ventilation and often responds to effective PPV (initially using room air per the 2010 NRP guidelines, increasing to 100% oxygen per clinical response) if heart rate is less than 100 beats/min. Assess the patency of the airway. If hypoxia continues, there could be persistent bradycardia. Begin chest compressions per NRP guidelines for a heart rate that is less than 60 beats/min in spite of effective bag-mask ventilation. Administration of epinephrine is indicated when the newborn has a pulse rate of less than 60 beats/min after 30 seconds of effective ventilation and 30 seconds of chest compressions. The recommended concentration of epinephrine for newborns is 1:10,000. The recommended dose is 0.1 to 0.3 mL/kg of 1:10,000 epinephrine IV, equal to 0.01 to 0.03 mg/kg, administered rapidly, followed by a 0.5- to 1-mL normal saline flush to clear the line. If IV access is not yet established, consider starting with the higher dose of 0.3 up to 1 mL/kg of 1:10,000 epinephrine given via the ET tube. Dosing may be repeated every 3 to 5 minutes in case of persistent bradycardia. Focus on maintaining normothermia. Transport the patient to a facility that is able to handle high-risk neonates.

■ Pneumothorax Evacuation

A pneumothorax can occur if an infant inhales meconium at birth, if the lung is weakened by infection, or if PPV is needed. If a newborn has signs of a significant pneumothorax—severe respiratory distress unresponsive to PPV with unilateral decreased breath sounds and (if the pneumothorax is on the left side) shift of heart sounds—a needle evacuation of the pneumothorax may be necessary.

Assessment and Management

On the side of the suspected pneumothorax, clean the area around the second intercostal space, midclavicular line (usually just above the nipple), with alcohol. Prepare the equipment needed: a 22-g butterfly needle attached to extension tubing, a three-way stopcock, and a 20-mL syringe. Palpate the upper edge of the second rib and insert the needle above that rib as a second provider pulls back on the syringe (which is open to the patient). The nerves and blood vessels run below the ribs, so avoid piercing this area. Continue to slowly advance the needle until air is recovered. The butterfly needle is rigid, so be gentle so as to avoid further tearing the lung. If the 20-mL syringe becomes filled with air, turn the stopcock off to the newborn, push out the air from the syringe, open the stopcock to the newborn, and continue withdrawing air. Once no more air can be withdrawn, remove the needle.

> ### Words of Wisdom
>
> Before you resort to the use of a syringe, recheck the effectiveness of assisted ventilation.

If there is a symptomatic ongoing air leak, a 22-g angiocatheter can be inserted in a similar location, the introducer needle removed, and the angiocatheter attached to the extension tubing. Note that the angiocatheter may further tear the lung during its initial placement and is more likely to kink than the butterfly needle.

Remove as much air as possible with the syringe. At this point, the tubing may be taped to the chest and briefly occluded while you place the end of the tubing that had been attached to the syringe in a small bottle of sterile water and release the tubing occlusion.

This can relieve the pressure buildup from the pneumothorax until the patient can be transferred to a facility for placement of a chest tube. During transport, you should monitor the newborn closely for signs of a reaccumulation of the pneumothorax.

Words of Wisdom

Whereas positive-pressure ventilation and chest compressions can be performed in a moving emergency vehicle, you should pull the vehicle over to the side of the road while placing and securing an advanced airway.

While you are performing the pneumothorax evacuation, continue your reassessment—use proper positioning to maintain the airway and avoid aspiration, take steps to maintain thermoregulation, and ensure adequate communication with the family and with the medical team receiving the newborn. If the newborn is distressed, transport as rapidly as possible.

Meconium-Stained Amniotic Fluid

Meconium-stained amniotic fluid, which is present in 10% to 15% of deliveries, carries a high risk of morbidity. Passage of meconium may occur either before or during delivery. It is more common in post-term newborns and in those who are small for their gestational age (weighing less than the 10th percentile for their age), and in newborns who are stressed before or during delivery. Newborns do not normally pass stool before birth, but if they do and then inhale the meconium-stained amniotic fluid either in utero or at delivery, their airways may become plugged and hypoxia may ensue. This, in turn, can lead to atelectasis, persistent pulmonary hypertension (delayed transition from fetal to neonatal circulation), hypoxemia, and aspiration pneumonitis. Partial plugging of airways with meconium can lead to ball-valve effects, increasing the risk of pneumothorax, which may require needle aspiration. Any condition that leads to a delayed drop in pulmonary vascular resistance after birth, such as meconium aspiration, can result in right-to-left shunting across the foramen ovale or the patent ductus arteriosus, a condition referred to as persistent pulmonary hypertension of the newborn. Ensuring a clear airway, keeping the newborn warm, minimizing stimulation, and providing supplemental oxygen when needed decrease the risk of the development of persistent pulmonary hypertension.

Once meconium aspiration has occurred, the newborn should be followed closely for signs of deterioration, including progressive hypoxia, hypercapnia, acidosis, and development of a pneumothorax.

Assessment and Management

When a newborn is delivered through meconium-stained amniotic fluid, determine whether the fluid is thin and green stained versus thick and particulate. Assess the newborn's activity level. If the newborn is crying and vigorous, employ standard interventions. If the newborn is depressed (poor muscle tone, bradycardia of less than 100 beats/min, inadequate ventilation, no respiratory effort), *do not* dry or stimulate the newborn.

Clear the airway of meconium, intubate the trachea, attach a meconium aspirator and suction catheter to the end of the ET tube, and suction the ET tube while withdrawing the tube from the trachea. Be sure to cover the hole of the meconium aspirator with your finger while you are suctioning **Figure 13**.

After you have performed tracheal suctioning under direct visualization, drying and stimulation are often enough to establish adequate breathing and pulse rate in the newborn; in many cases, however, oxygen and PPV are needed. If intubation for direct tracheal suctioning is unsuccessful and the newborn has bradycardia, continue with standard resuscitation per Neonatal Resuscitation Program (NRP) guidelines, recognizing that the newborn will be at high risk of meconium aspiration. The 2010 NRP guidelines recommend starting resuscitation with room air, and if hypoxia persists more than a few minutes providing blended oxygen or 100% oxygen if blended gas is not available, to reverse hypoxia. Keep in mind that a healthy newborn's preductal oxygen saturation, measured in the right upper extremity, is typically about 60% within a minute of birth, and takes on average 10 minutes to reach 90%. If the newborn is not breathing effectively on his or her own, begin bag-mask ventilation. If the infant remains bradycardic (heart rate less than 60 beats/min) after effective PPV, initiate chest compressions and further interventions per NRP guidelines. If the newborn is not responding well to resuscitation, airway occlusion or pneumothorax should be suspected. Steps should be taken to minimize hypothermia by avoiding cold environments, covering the newborn with warm blankets when possible, and placing the newborn, once stabilized, skin-to-skin on the mother, again covered with a blanket. Frequent reassessment of the newborn is indicated to ensure that his or her condition has not changed. If the newborn has prolonged hypoxia after significantly delayed resuscitation, the outcome will likely be poor. When you are transporting a newborn with these respiratory symptoms, stay in communication with a facility skilled at managing high-risk newborns to help with management and identification of an appropriate transport destination. To help support the family, explain what is being done for the newborn but do not discuss "chance of survival."

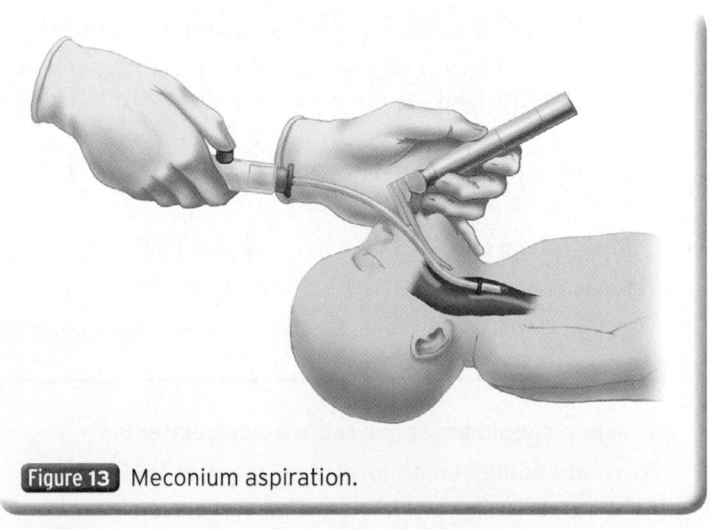

Figure 13 Meconium aspiration.

Diaphragmatic Hernia

Diaphragmatic hernia—that is, an abnormal opening in the diaphragm, most commonly on the left side causing the abdominal contents to herniate into the chest cavity and the heart and mediastinum to be shifted to the contralateral side of the hernia—has an incidence of 1 in 2,200 live births. This diagnosis is often made on prenatal ultrasound before birth. Postnatally, the diagnosis is suspected clinically in a newborn with respiratory distress, heart sounds shifted to the right, decreased breath sounds on the left side (which can also be signs of a pneumothorax), bowel sounds heard in the chest (most commonly on the left side; 90% of these hernias are left-sided), and scaphoid abdomen (ie, the abdomen, rather than being round, is sunken due to the abdominal contents being in the chest cavity). Mortality may be as high as 50% for this condition.

Assessment and Management

A newborn with a congenital diaphragmatic hernia may demonstrate few or no symptoms, or may present with severe hypoxia and increased work of breathing, depending on the size of the hernia, the degree of lung hypoplasia, and associated anomalies such as cardiac disease. If there is significant mediastinal shift, the contralateral side can also have significant pulmonary hypoplasia. Although the NRP currently advocates initiating resuscitation using room air in full-term newborns, an exception to this rule is the newborn with a severe congenital diaphragmatic hernia who should be resuscitated on 100% oxygen. If a newborn has a diaphragmatic hernia, bag-mask ventilation will introduce air that distends the intestines in the chest cavity, further compromising the newborn's ability to ventilate. If PPV is needed in such a newborn, place an ET tube and deliver a peak ventilatory pressure of 25 mm Hg or less to minimize barotrauma—these newborns have poorly developed lungs and are at high risk of a pneumothorax developing even at fairly low peak inspiratory pressures. These infants are at increased risk of persistent pulmonary hypertension in addition to lung hypoplasia and

may remain hypoxic in spite of supplemental oxygen. Put an orogastric tube in place and provide intermittent suctioning to minimize intestinal distention. The patient's heart rate should be monitored continuously throughout transport. Ultimately, a newborn with a diaphragmatic hernia will require surgical correction, so transport the newborn to a facility with a neonatal intensive care unit and a pediatric surgical team.

Respiratory Distress and Cyanosis

Prematurity is the single most common cause of respiratory distress and cyanosis in the neonate. These conditions occur more frequently in newborns younger than 30 weeks of gestation or weighing less than 1,200 g. Women with multiple gestations and pregnancy complications increase the risk as well.

There are many etiologies of respiratory distress and cyanosis in the neonate. Respiratory causes include airway obstruction, aspiration (meconium, amniotic fluid, maternal blood at delivery, gastroesophageal reflux, foreign body), pneumonia, pneumothorax, tracheoesophageal fistula, congenital diaphragmatic hernia, or immature lungs. Any process that results in a delay in drop of pulmonary vascular resistance after birth (including all of the previously described conditions as well as acidosis, stress, and hypoxia) can lead to shunting of blood across the patent ductus arteriosus and patent foramen ovale, resulting in persistent pulmonary hypertension and cyanosis. Central nervous system depression can lead to ineffective respirations and subsequent cyanosis. Septic shock and severe metabolic acidosis often present with increased work of breathing and cyanosis. Cardiac anomalies typically result in cyanosis without increased work of breathing.

Assessment and Management

Remember your ABCs—ensure the airway is patent, breathing is adequate, and a pulse is present. Assess respiratory rate, respiratory effort (including periodic breathing, intracostal retractions, nasal flaring, grunting, choking, or gagging) and breath sounds. Ask the parents if they have noted increased symptoms with

---

YOU are the Medic   PART 4

You provide positive-pressure ventilation for 30 seconds and then reassess the newborn. The assessment reveals a strong respiratory effort with adequate tidal volume and a strong rapid pulse rate palpated at the umbilical cord.

Newborn Assessment Recording Time: 14 Minutes	
Respiratory effort	Strong, rapid, and regular; good cry
Pulse rate	156 beats/min; regular
Color	Pink trunk but cyanosis to the extremities

7. When should an Apgar score be calculated?

8. What should you do for the newborn at this time?

feeding attempts. Is the newborn cyanotic or pale? (Remember that a hypoxic newborn who is severely anemic will look pale, not cyanotic.)

Treatment focuses on establishing a patent airway (suction mouth, oropharynx as needed), ensuring adequate oxygen delivery by providing supplemental oxygen if needed, establishing effective ventilation, including providing PPV as needed, and ensuring adequate circulation, including chest compressions if bradycardia of less than 60 beats/min persists once supplemental oxygen and adequate ventilation have been established. Keep in mind that occasionally resuscitative efforts do not result in improvement in cyanosis or bradycardia due to an underlying pneumothorax. In this situation, needle thoracentesis can be a lifesaving intervention. Remember to keep the family updated regarding the newborn's condition and what is being done to help him or her, and maintain communication with the receiving hospital for advice and to allow them to prepare for your arrival.

Premature and Low Birth Weight Infants

Newborns delivered before 37 completed weeks of gestation are considered <u>**premature**</u> Figure 14 . While prematurity is often idiopathic, there are maternal conditions associated with preterm labor and delivery. These include maternal infection, including urinary tract infection, chorioamnionitis, maternal illness leading to dehydration, placental insufficiency, polyhydramnios, preeclampsia/eclampsia, and pregnancy-induced hypertension. In addition to the increased overall mortality when a fetus is delivered prematurely, there are a number of morbidities associated with prematurity. These include respiratory distress syndrome, respiratory suppression and apnea, hypothermia, sepsis, and central nervous system compromise, including intraventricular hemorrhage and periventricular leucomalacia (increased in newborns with hypoxemia and fluctuations in blood pressure and serum osmolarity).

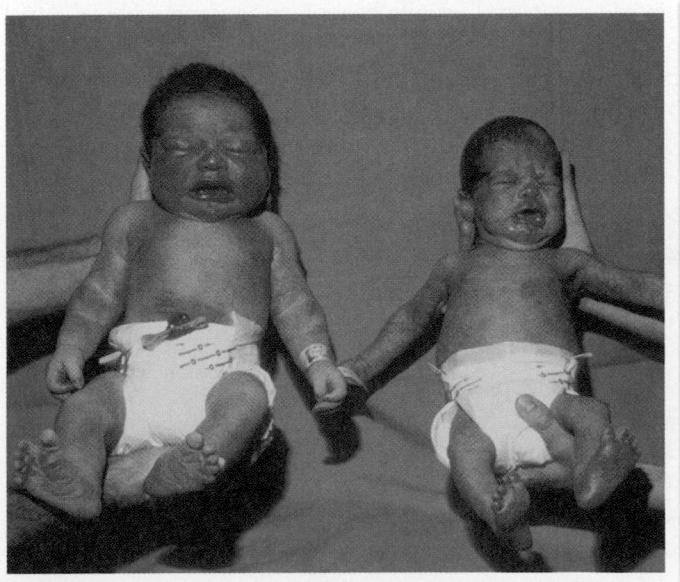

Figure 14 Premature newborns (right) are smaller and thinner than full-term newborns (left).

Newborns weighing less than 5½ lb (2,500 g) are considered low birth weight. The most common etiology for low birth weight is prematurity. A number of factors can predispose a woman to deliver prematurely, including genetic factors, infection, cervical incompetence (early opening of cervix), abruption (blood under the placenta), multiple gestations (eg, twins, triplets), previous delivery of a premature infant, drug use, and trauma. Other factors that may contribute to low birth weight include chronic maternal hypertension, smoking, placental anomalies, and chromosomal abnormalities. If a newborn is delivered prior to 24 weeks of gestation or weighs less than 1 lb (500 g) and is born outside of a center that is equipped to manage such deliveries, the newborn is unlikely to survive. If a premature infant is born after 32 weeks of gestation or weighs at least 3 lb (1,500 g) and is provided warmth and cardiorespiratory support as needed until transfer to a center with a neonatal intensive care unit, survival is close to that of an infant born at term. The degree of immaturity can be estimated by physical characteristics such as skin appearance (more thin and translucent in more premature newborns). If you observe signs of life, you should attempt resuscitation until the newborn can be transported to an appropriate facility.

Approximately 12% of births in the United States are preterm (less than 37 weeks of gestation). Morbidity and mortality in this population are, in large part, related to the degree of prematurity. Most newborns delivered after 28 weeks of gestation who receive needed cardiovascular support after birth survive and do well over the long term. Newborns delivered at 24 weeks of gestation have a high morbidity and mortality. Approximately one third die and one third experience significant long-term problems—typically respiratory issues, related to the need for long-term ventilation and oxygen treatment, and neurologic issues, related to recurrent hypoxia and bleeding into the brain.

Assessment and Management

The degree of prematurity is the most predictive indicator of significant morbidity and mortality. Significant respiratory distress occurs most frequently at less than 32 weeks gestation, and newborns with lower birth weights will become hypothermic more quickly than full-term newborn. In addition to physical features of prematurity (maturity of skin, size of infant, degree of respiratory distress), the family can give additional information related to dating (last menstrual period, estimated date of confinement assigned by the obstetrician, ultrasound dating) and information related to other maternal or fetal complications.

If a newborn is delivered prematurely in the field, providing cardiorespiratory support and a thermoneutral environment will optimize his or her survival and long-term outcome. Premature newborns are at higher risk for respiratory distress owing to <u>**surfactant**</u> deficiency. Their thermoregulation can be improved with careful environmental control (eg, warm blankets, plastic wrap or plastic bag up to neck). The lungs of a premature newborn are weak, so use only the minimum pressure necessary to move the chest when you are providing PPV. Brain injury can result from hypoxemia, rapid changes in blood pressure, or infusion of hyperosmolar solutions, leading to intraventricular hemorrhage. Premature newborns are also at risk of <u>**retinopathy of prematurity**</u> (abnormal vascular development of the retina), which may be worsened by long-term oxygen exposure.

Because hypoxia causes irreparable brain damage, however, do not withhold oxygen from a cyanotic premature newborn.

The management of premature newborns focuses on clearing the airway, providing gentle stimulation, and providing supplemental oxygen if needed based on oxygen saturation and PPV if needed for ineffective or absent respiratory effort. Peak inspiratory pressures should be provided to maintain physiological chest rise because excessive pressures increase the risk of pneumothorax. Finally, chest compressions should be initiated if effective ventilation does not result in adequate heart rate. As always, maintaining a warm environment for the newborn is critical.

Because it can be difficult to assess gestational age or predicted morbidity or mortality in the field, if there are signs of life, maintain resuscitative efforts until you can transfer the patient to a facility that can continue support.

Seizures in the Newborn

Seizures are the most distinctive sign of neurologic disease in the newborn. A seizure is defined clinically as a paroxysmal alteration in neurologic function (ie, behavioral and/or autonomic function). The degree of myelination will affect the manner of seizure presentation and observed clinical signs. Seizures are more common in premature newborns. The incidence in this population can be as high as 57.5 per 1,000 infants who weigh less than 3 lb (1,500 g) at birth, compared with 2.8 per 1,000 infants who weigh between 5½ lb and 9 lb (2,500 g and 3,999 g) at birth. In the field, seizures are identified by direct observation; in the hospital, an electroencephalogram (EEC) is used to confirm the diagnosis of seizures.

Newborns may exhibit normal motor activity that can sometimes be mistaken for seizures. These myoclonic, dysconjugate eye movements or sucking movements are often seen when the newborn is drowsy or asleep. In addition, jitteriness is often confused with a seizure Table 7 . Jitteriness is characteristically a disorder of the newborn and is rarely seen at a later age. Jitteriness is most commonly seen with hypoxic-ischemic encephalopathy, hypocalcemia, hypoglycemia, and drug withdrawal. Clinically, gastroesophageal reflux and choking episodes can also mimic seizures.

Seizures, by contrast, represent a relative medical emergency. They are usually related to a significant underlying abnormality—one that often requires specific therapy. Seizures may also interfere with cardiopulmonary function, feeding, and metabolic function. Finally, prolonged seizures may even cause brain injury.

Types of Seizures   Four major types of seizures are distinguished as follows:

- **Subtle seizure.** A seizure characterized by eye deviation, blinking, sucking, pedaling movements of the legs, and apnea.
- **Tonic seizure.** A seizure characterized by tonic extension of the limbs. Less commonly, flexion of the arms and extension of the legs may also occur. This type of seizure is more common in premature infants, especially in those with intraventricular hemorrhage.
- **Focal clonic seizure.** A seizure characterized by clonic localized jerking. This type of seizure can occur in both full-term and premature infants.

Table 7   Jitteriness Versus Seizures in the Newborn

Characteristic	Jitteriness	Seizures
Ocular phenomenon (deviation or fixation of the eyes)	Not seen	Commonly associated
Stimulus sensitive (may be triggered by a stimulus)	Yes	No
Dominant movement	Tremor	Clonic jerking
Application of gentle pressure to limb	Stops jitteriness	Does not stop seizures
Autonomic phenomenon	Not associated	Common association

- **Myoclonic seizure.** A seizure characterized by flexion jerks of the upper or lower extremities. This type of seizure may occur singly or in a series of repetitive jerks.

When describing seizures, a multifocal seizure refers to clonic activity that involves more than one site, is asynchronous, and is usually migratory. A generalized seizure refers to activity that is bilateral, synchronous, and nonmigratory.

Causes of Seizures   Table 8 lists the most common (and important) causes of neonatal seizures. The time of onset for hypoxic ischemic encephalopathy, hypoglycemia, and other metabolic disturbances is up to 3 days after delivery. With all other causes listed in Table 8, seizures may begin 3 days or longer after birth.

Hypoxic ischemic encephalopathy, usually secondary to perinatal asphyxia (lack of oxygen to tissues), is the single most common cause of seizures in both term and preterm newborns. Seizures characteristically occur 12 to 24 hours after a hypoxic event, and usually become more severe over the first 2 to 3 days of life. Metabolic abnormalities include disturbances in the levels of glucose, calcium, magnesium, or other electrolytes. Other metabolic disturbances include abnormalities of amino acids, organic acids, blood ammonia, and certain toxins.

Table 8   Causes of Neonatal Seizures

- **Hypoxic ischemic encephalopathy**
- Intracranial infections (meningitis)
- Hypoglycemia
- Other metabolic disturbances
- Epileptic syndromes
- Intracranial hemorrhage
- Development defects
- Hypocalcemia
- Meningitis
- Encephalopathy
- Drug withdrawal

Hypoglycemia is most frequently seen in newborns who are small for their gestational age, those who are large for their gestational age, and those whose mothers were diabetic during pregnancy. Neurologic symptoms consist of jitteriness, stupor, hypotonia (floppy), apnea, poor feeding, and seizures.

Hypocalcemia has two major peaks of incidence. The first peak occurs at 2 to 3 days after delivery and is most commonly seen in low birth weight newborns and in newborns of diabetic mothers. Late-onset hypocalcemia is rare in the United States but may be seen in infants who consume cow's milk or synthetic formulas high in phosphorus.

Other metabolic disturbances are uncommon in newborns, although hyponatremia, hyperammonemia, other amino acid and organic acid abnormalities, or seizures from drug withdrawal (eg, narcotic analgesics, sedative hypnotics, tricyclic antidepressants, cocaine, or alcohol) may be seen.

Assessment and Management

When you evaluate a newborn with seizures, you must include a quick evaluation of prenatal and birth history and perform a careful physical exam. You may observe a quiet, often hypotonic infant. The newborn may be lethargic or apneic. Hypoglycemia must be recognized quickly and treated promptly. In these patients, blood glucose measurement and administration of dextrose may be lifesaving in the field. Obtain the newborn's baseline vital signs and oxygen saturation readings, and provide additional oxygen, assisted ventilation, blood pressure evaluation, and IV access as necessary. A 10% dextrose solution may be given as an IV bolus (2 mL/kg) if the newborn's blood glucose level is less than 40 mg/dL, with a recheck of the blood glucose level in about 30 minutes. IV administration of dextrose often needs to be followed by a 10% dextrose infusion.

Consult with medical control if you are considering giving the newborn anticonvulsant medication. Phenobarbitol (Luminal) and phenytoin (Dilantin)—the drugs most commonly used in such cases—require care in administration and may interfere with respiratory and cardiac function. Lorazepam (Ativan) is a benzodiazepine that may be administered IV or rectally.

Monitor the newborn's respiratory status and oxygen saturations carefully. Maintain the newborn's normal body temperature

YOU are the Medic   PART 5

You and your partner prepare the newborn and mother for transport, when a second paramedic unit arrives on scene. You load the mother into your ambulance, and depart for the hospital which is 12 miles away; the second paramedic unit transports the newborn. En route you start an IV line of normal saline in the mother and check for delivery of the placenta. The mother remains in stable condition throughout transport. The placenta is delivered without difficulty as you are turning into the hospital parking lot.

You bring the mother to the labor and delivery department. The second paramedic unit arrives a moment later, and brings the newborn to the neonatal team that is awaiting their arrival.

Mother Recording Time: 23 Minutes	
Respirations	18 breaths/min; adequate tidal volume
Pulse	94 beats/min; strong and regular
Skin	Pink, warm, and moist
Blood pressure	124/70 mm Hg
Oxygen saturation (Spo$_2$)	99% on 100% via NRM at 12 L/min

Newborn Recording Time: 23 Minutes	
Respirations	46 breaths/min; adequate tidal volume
Pulse	154 beats/min; strong and regular
Skin	Pink, warm, and moist
Blood pressure	Not obtained
Oxygen saturation (Spo$_2$)	99% on 5 L/min blow-by

9. What are the five components that make up the Apgar score?

and keep the family informed about the care you are providing as transport gets under way.

Hypoglycemia

In full-term or preterm newborns, <u>hypoglycemia</u> is a blood glucose level of less than 45 mg/dL. This condition represents an imbalance between glucose supply and utilization. Glucose levels may be low due to inadequate intake or storage or increased utilization of glucose. Most newborns remain asymptomatic until the glucose level falls below 20 mg/dL for a significant period of time. Because the brain relies on glucose as its primary fuel, hypoglycemia may result in seizures and severe, permanent brain damage. Table 9 lists risk factors for hypoglycemia in the newborn.

The fetus receives glucose from the mother and deposits glycogen in the liver, lung, heart, and skeletal muscle in utero. The newborn then begins to use those glycogen stores to meet glucose needs after birth; most full-term newborns will have sufficient glycogen stores to meet their glucose needs for 8 to 12 hours. Disorders related to decreased glycogen stores (small for gestational age, prematurity, postmaturity) or to increased use of glucose (newborn of a diabetic mother, large for gestational age, hypoxia, hypothermia, sepsis) place the newborn at increased risk for hypoglycemia. Metabolic adaptations to maintain normal glucose levels are regulated by counterregulatory hormones such as glucagon, epinephrine, cortisol, and growth hormone. Frequently, stressed newborns will become hypoglycemic.

Table 9 Risk Factors for Hypoglycemia in the Newborn

Risk Factor	Specific Indicators
Disorders of fetal growth and maturity	<ul><li>Small for gestational age</li><li>Smaller of discordant twins (weight difference > 25%)</li><li>Large for gestational age</li><li>Low birth weight infant (birth weight < 2,500 g)</li></ul>
Prematurity	<ul><li>Less than 37 weeks of gestation or less than 5.5 pounds (2.5 kg)</li></ul>
Disorders of maternal glucose regulation	<ul><li>Insulin-dependent diabetic mother</li><li>Gestational diabetic mother</li><li>Morbid obesity in mother</li></ul>
Neonatal conditions with disturbed oxidative metabolism	<ul><li>Perinatal distress (eg, 5-minute Apgar score < 5)</li><li>Hypoxemia due to cardiac or lung disease</li><li>Shock, hypoperfusion, sepsis, cold stress</li></ul>
Severe anemia	<ul><li>Pallor (in the absence of hypovolemia)</li></ul>
Congenital anomalies and genetic disorders	<ul><li>Visible anatomic deformities/abnormalities</li></ul>

Assessment and Management

Symptoms of hypoglycemia can be quite nonspecific. They may include cyanosis, apnea, irritability, poor sucking or feeding, limpness, irregular respirations, eye rolling, and hypothermia. These symptoms may also be associated with lethargy, tremors, twitching or seizures, and coma. Newborns may also have tachycardia, tachypnea, or vomiting.

Check the blood glucose level in all sick newborns (by heel stick), and evaluate the newborn's vital signs. After you establish good oxygenation, ventilation, and circulation (ABCs), manage the hypoglycemia. Medical control personnel may order the administration of a 10% dextrose solution as a bolus at 2 mL/kg via IV access if the newborn's blood glucose level is less than 45 mg/dL. This intervention may be followed by an IV infusion of 10% dextrose based on the newborn's gestational age (60 mL/kg/d for a full-term newborn; adjust upward based on the recommendations of the referring hospital for premature newborns). As always, maintain normal body temperature—hypothermia places additional stress on glucose demand.

Vomiting

Vomiting is common in newborns. Approximately 85% of infants vomit during the first week of life, and another 10% have vomited by age 6 weeks. Vomiting ranges from "spitting up" to severe, bloody or bilious, projectile vomiting. Most episodes of vomiting are benign and do not result in weight loss, dehydration, or other ill effects. Bilious and/or bloody emesis (vomiting) indicates a pathologic condition that needs medical attention. Persistent vomiting is a warning sign and can cause excessive loss of fluid, dehydration, and changes in electrolyte levels (ie, sodium, potassium, and glucose).

Vomiting mucus, occasionally blood streaked, in the first few hours of life is not uncommon. Persistent vomiting in the first 24 hours of life suggests obstruction in the upper digestive tract or increased intracranial pressure. Vomitus containing dark blood is often a sign of a life-threatening illness; it indicates bleeding in the gut. Sometimes, vomitus may be accompanied by bloody or tarry stool, another worrisome sign. Aspiration of vomitus can cause respiratory insufficiencies or obstruction of the airway.

Causes of Vomiting A newborn's presenting symptoms may give a clue to the site of obstruction or other problem that is causing the vomiting. One possible cause is esophageal atresia (a failure to develop the distal lumen) with or without a congenital tracheoesophageal fistula. Its incidence is 1 case per 2,000 to 4,000 births. Newborns are seen with excessive frothing soon after birth and may choke when attempting to feed because the swallowed milk is returned promptly.

Another possible cause of vomiting, <u>pathogenic gastroesophageal reflux (GER)</u>, is common in infants, with a reported prevalence of 2% to 20% based on the age. GER is most commonly seen in infancy, with its incidence peaking in the 1- to 4-month age group. The infant may vomit either immediately or a few hours after a feeding. The vomiting may not be forceful. In uncomplicated GER, the vomitus is not bile stained or bloody. GER in infants and young children can present as typical or atypical crying and/or irritability, apnea and/or bradycardia, poor appetite, apparent life-threatening event, vomiting, wheezing, stridor, weight loss or poor growth (failure to thrive), hoarseness, and/or laryngitis.

In infantile hypertrophic pyloric stenosis (IHPS), marked hypertrophy and hyperplasia of the two (circular and longitudinal) muscular layers of the pylorus occur. As a consequence, the pylorus becomes thickened and obstructs the end of the stomach. The incidence of IHPS is 2 to 4 cases per 1,000 live births, with a male-to-female predominance of 4:1; 30% of patients with IHPS are first-born males. The usual age of presentation is approximately age 3 weeks (range, 1 to 18 weeks). In IHPS, the stomach muscles contract forcibly to overcome the obstruction. Affected infants usually present with projectile vomiting, dehydration, malnutrition, and electrolyte changes. The vomitus in this case is not bile stained, but it can be brown or coffee colored due to blood, resulting from gastritis or a Mallory Weiss tear at the gastroesophageal junction.

Malrotation is a congenital anomaly of rotation of the midgut. In this condition, the small bowel is found predominantly on the right side of the abdomen; the cecum is found in the epigastrium–right hypochondrium. Malrotation predisposes the infant to midgut volvulus and secondary obstruction of the blood supply to the intestines. In cases of malrotation with midgut volvulus, the vomitus is bile stained and may be feculent (like feces/stool) if the obstruction is distal in the intestines. With symptomatic malrotation, 75% to 90% of cases occur in infants younger than age 1 year, 50% to 64% of cases occur in infants younger than age 1 month, and 25% to 40% of cases occur in the first week of life. During the first week of life, the ratio of male-to-female presentation is 2:1. Early mortality rate ranged from 23% to 33%, with most deaths resulting from bowel dysfunction and malnutrition. With the advent of new corrective surgical procedures, the morbidity and mortality have decreased significantly.

Intestinal atresia or intestinal stenosis include congenital conditions where parts of the bowel may not have developed well (atresia) or may be narrow (stenosis). Conditions that affect the upper bowel—ie, duodenum, jejunum, and upper small bowel—may present with bilious vomiting within the first day or two after birth. Obstruction to the lower bowel (distal small intestine and large intestine) often presents as feeding intolerance and abdominal distention.

Another cause of vomiting, meconium plug, is seen in Hirschsprung disease. In this disease, the last segment of colon fails to relax and it causes mechanical obstruction. The infant usually has a history of not passing meconium in the first 24 hours of life.

Vomiting may also happen in conjunction with asphyxia, meningitis (infection of the layers covering the brain and spine), and hydrocephalus (large head size is a clue). It is often sudden, unexpected, and forceful in such cases, and it may be accompanied by persistent irritability. Meningitis and hydrocephalus may also be associated with increased intracranial pressure (ICP).

Use of drugs during pregnancy can lead to several withdrawal symptoms in newborns, including vomiting. The drugs that most commonly cause vomiting in newborns are barbiturates.

Assessment and Management

On physical exam, you may note a distended stomach that has been caused by vomiting. You should suspect an infection if the newborn has a fever or hypothermia, or a history of contact with people who are ill. You may also note temperature instability, apnea/bradycardia, abdominal tenderness/guarding, and minimal or absent bowel sounds.

Initial management steps for a newborn with vomiting start with the ABCs. Maintain a patent airway, while staying aware that a vomiting newborn can aspirate the vomitus and compromise the airway. Keep the newborn's face turned to one side to prevent further aspiration. Suction or clear the vomitus from the airway with the help of a suction catheter or suction bulb. Ensure adequate oxygenation, providing either free-flow supplemental oxygen or bag-mask ventilation as necessary. Bradycardia may be caused by vagal stimulus and is usually transient; it may resolve with stimulation and free-flow oxygen. Consider using a nasogastric or orogastric tube to decompress the stomach and reduce emesis or vagal effects of distention.

Antiemetics should not be administered in the field. The newborn may be dehydrated, however, and need fluid resuscitation. Dry mucous membranes, tachycardia, or a sunken fontanelle are clues that the patient needs hydration. Normal saline (10 mL/kg per bolus) may be required in that case.

On transport, place the newborn on his or her side, identify a facility capable of managing a high-risk newborn, and explain what is being done for the newborn to the family.

◼ Diarrhea

A normal number of stools per day for an infant is five to six, especially if the infant is breastfeeding, when infants often produce stool after every feeding. Diarrhea is an excessive loss of electrolytes and fluid in the stool. In the United States, infants younger than 3 years have 1.3 to 2.3 episodes of diarrhea each year. The prevalence is higher in infants attending daycare centers. Nine percent of all hospitalizations of children younger than age 5 years are for diarrhea.

The most common cause of acute diarrhea in children is viral infection (especially rotavirus infection during the winter months). Less frequently encountered causes include poisoning due to insecticides, organophosphates, and carbamates. Diarrhea related to these agents is accompanied by profuse sweating, lacrimation, hypersalivation, and abdominal cramps, or more serious conditions such as intussusception, malrotation, increased ICP, and metabolic acidosis. Other causes of diarrhea include gastroenteritis, lactose intolerance, neonatal abstinence syndrome, thyrotoxicosis, and cystic fibrosis.

Severe cases of diarrhea can cause dehydration and subsequent electrolyte imbalance. Combinations of physical signs—such as ill general appearance, poor vital signs, capillary refill of greater than 2 seconds, dry mucous membranes, absent tears, weight loss, and low urine output—are good objective predictors of the degree of dehydration.

Assessment and Management

Assessment includes estimating the number and volume of loose stools, decreased urinary output, and degree of dehydration based on skin turgor, mucous membranes, presence of sunken eyes, and other signs. Patient management, as always, begins with the ABCs. The newborn's airway and ventilation may be compromised if he or she is severely dehydrated and is obtunded, so ensure adequate oxygenation and ventilation.

Perform chest compressions in addition to PPV in a newborn if the pulse rate is less than 60 beats/min.

Fluid therapy may be indicated when a newborn has diarrhea. Normal saline (10-mL/kg boluses) may be needed immediately to provide fluid resuscitation to the newborn.

Neonatal Jaundice

Jaundice in the newborn results from the immaturity of the liver to conjugate bilirubin in the first week of life. This transient hyperbilirubinemia has therefore been called "physiologic jaundice." Neonatal jaundice is considered pathologic when:

- Jaundice is clinically visible in the first 24 hours after birth
- Total serum bilirubin increases by more than 5 mg/dL /d
- Total bilirubin exceeds 12 mg/dL in full-term infants
- Conjugated bilirubin exceeds 15 to 20 mg/dL
- Clinical jaundice persisits for more than 1 week in full-term infants or for more than 2 weeks in preterm infants

Jaundice can result from hemolysis (ABO incompatibility, Rh incompatibility), various types of red blood cell deficiencies, polycythemia, or bowel obstruction, among other causes.

Additionally, cholestasis can present after the first 2 weeks of life. Causes of cholestasis in the neonate include hepatitis, metabolic disorders, and prolonged total parenteral nutrition, among other causes.

Assessment and Management

It is clinically difficult to determine the extent of the problem just based on the distribution of the yellow color. Initial evaluation includes total and direct bilirubin measurement at the hospital; therefore, transport is essential. Additional assessment includes blood type and Rh of both mother and infant, antiglobulin (Coombs) test on the infant, hematocrit value, and reticulocyte count. These tests are not available in the field. A neonate with significant clinical jaundice can be started on IV fluids in the field to help decrease the level of bilirubin and minimize the longer term neurologic effects. Any newborn with jaundice must be specifically communicated to medical control. Phototherapy and other modes of treatment will be available at the medical center. Treatment will need to be started early in sick neonates and preterm infants as bilirubin-induced encephalopathy may develop at lower bilirubin levels than in healthy term infants.

For newborns with potential cholestasis, because it is not toxic, management includes diagnostic testing and then treatment of the cause; therefore, transport the patient to a facility where this can occur.

Pathophysiology, Assessment, and Management of Conditions Related to Thermoregulation

Thermoregulation is the body's ability to balance heat production and heat loss so as to maintain a normal body temperature. This ability is limited in the newborn. The average normal temperature of a newborn is 37.5°C (99.5°F). For the neonate, the thermoneutral temperature range is 36.6° to 37.2°C (97.9°F to 99°F).

Nonshivering thermogenesis, the production of heat by metabolism, is the primary source of heat production in the newborn. Brown fat (deposited in the fetus after 28 weeks of gestation, and principally stored around the scapula, kidneys, adrenal glands, neck, and axilla) is a thermogenic tissue unique to the newborn.

Heat loss occurs when heat is lost to the environment, through any of the following four mechanisms. In evaporation, heat is lost when water evaporates from the skin and respiratory tract. In convection, heat is lost to cooler surrounding air; the extent of heat loss depends on the air temperature and air movement. In conduction, heat is lost to cooler solid objects in direct contact with the body. In radiation, heat is lost to cooler surrounding objects not in direct contact with the body.

Fever

Fever is defined as a rectal temperature of greater than 38°C (100.4°F). Oral and axillary temperatures are, respectively, 0.6°C (1°F) and 1.1°C (2°F) lower than the rectal temperature on average.

A newborn's temperature regulation system is relatively immature, so fever may not always be a presenting feature with infection or illness. In fact, newborns may become hypothermic with infection. Neonates may also become hypoglycemic during a fever because their enteral intake decreases and may even develop lactic acidosis because of anaerobic metabolism. Also, hypoglycemia may be a symptom of septicemia. No matter what the presenting symptoms are, it is important to identify newborns with serious bacterial infection (eg, bacteremia, urinary tract infection, meningitis, bacterial gastroenteritis, and pneumonia) or serious viral infection (eg, herpes simplex) for which treatment is available. Approximately 13% of infants younger than age 28 days with a temperature of more than 38.1°C (100.6°F) will have a serious bacterial infection.

Fever may also be caused by overheating. Infants can easily become too hot when dressed in many layers of clothing, overbundled in a heated car, or placed in direct sunlight, even through a window, or near heating vents at home. Fever related to dehydration is an important consideration in breastfeeding infants, especially in the first week after birth. These infants have often lost more than 10% of their weight and may have a history of difficulty in initiating breastfeeding.

Newborns have limited ability to control their temperature. They do not sweat when they are hot to allow cooling, and they do not shiver to raise their temperature when they are cold. Term infants may produce sweat over their brow but not the rest of their body. Premature infants do not produce sweat. Moreover, many newborns with serious life-threatening infections may actually see their core temperature drop; these newborns are at a higher risk for hypoglycemia and metabolic acidosis. A careful examination will reveal irritability, somnolence, and decreased feeding. The newborn may feel warm to touch. Some newborns with fever, however, may be initially asymptomatic.

Assessment and Management

When fever is suspected, you should examine the newborn for the presence of rashes, especially petechiae or pinpoint pink or red skin lesions **Figure 15**. Obtain a careful history regarding

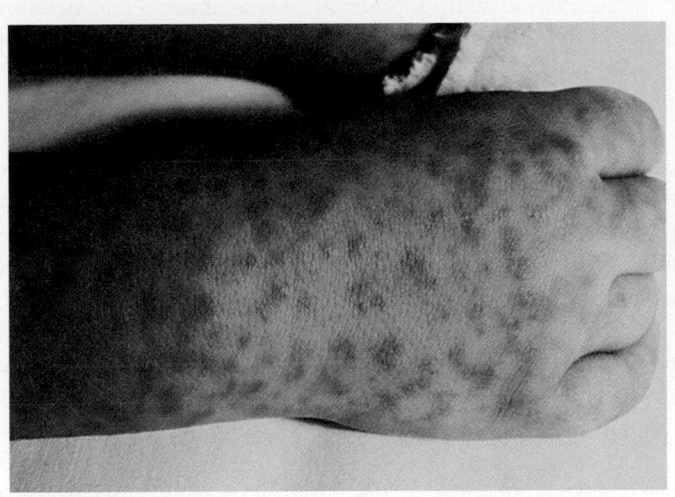

Figure 15 A newborn with a fever may also have petechiae or pinpoint pink or red skin lesions.

Table 10 Risk Factors for Hypothermia
■ All newborns in the first 8 to 12 hours after birth
■ Home delivery
■ Prolonged resuscitation
■ **Small for gestational age** infant
■ Infant with central nervous system problems
■ Prematurity
■ Sepsis
■ Inadequate measures to keep the infant warm during transport

general activity, feeding, voiding, and stooling. Note increased respiratory rate, along with increased work of breathing. Obtain the newborn's vital signs and ensure adequate oxygenation and ventilation, providing free-flow supplemental oxygen if necessary. Perform chest compressions, if indicated. Administration of antipyretic agents such as acetaminophen or ibuprofen is controversial in the prehospital setting; do not give ibuprofen to a newborn. To cool the newborn, remove additional layers of clothing and improve ventilation in the environment.

■ Hypothermia

<u>Hypothermia</u> is a drop in body temperature to less than 35°C (95°F). Hypothermia in the newborn occurs in all climates, but is more common during the winter months. It has been linked to impaired growth and may make the newborn vulnerable to infections. Moderate hypothermia is associated with an increased risk of death in low birth weight newborns. Sick or low birth weight infants admitted to a hospital with hypothermia are more likely to die than those admitted with normal temperature. Infants may die of cold exposure at temperatures adults find comfortable. Table 10 lists risk factors for hypothermia.

Newborns have increased surface area-to-volume ratio, making them extremely sensitive to environmental conditions, especially when wet after delivery. An increase in metabolic function in an attempt to overcome the heat loss can cause hypoglycemia, metabolic acidosis, <u>pulmonary hypertension</u>, and hypoxemia. Every hypothermic newborn should also be investigated for infection.

Assessment and Management

Hypothermic newborns are cool to the touch, initially in the extremities; as their temperature drops, however, the skin becomes cool all over. The newborn may also be pale and have acrocyanosis. The hypothermic newborn may present with decreased respiratory effort, apnea, bradycardia, cyanosis, irritability, and a weak cry. As a newborn's temperature drops, he or she may become lethargic and obtunded. In severely hypothermic newborns, the face and extremities may appear bright red. Sclerema—hardening of the skin associated with reddening and edema—may be seen on the back, limbs, or all over the body. Thermal shock, disseminated intravascular coagulopathy, and death may occur in more serious cases.

Preventive measures include warming your hands before touching the newborn. Dry the newborn thoroughly after birth and remove any wet blankets. Place a cap on the newborn's head because the head is the largest source of heat loss. Place the newborn "skin to skin" with the mother, if possible, using warm blankets over the newborn. This serves two purposes: The mother keeps the newborn warm, and mother and newborn can more readily bond. Ensure adequate oxygenation and ventilation, and perform chest compressions if necessary. If the newborn is hypoglycemic, you may administer $D_{10}W$. Warm IV fluids can assist in rewarming the newborn. The critically ill newborn, once stabilized, should be placed in a prewarmed incubator or, if none is available, covered with warm blankets and kept on mother's chest.

At home, skin-to-skin contact is the best method to rewarm a newborn with mild hypothermia. Ideally, the room should be warm (24°C to 26.5°C), and the newborn should be covered with a warm blanket and wear a prewarmed cap. Continue the rewarming process until the newborn's temperature reaches the normal range or his or her feet are no longer cold. Do not use hot water bottles—they may cause burns because blood circulation is poor in the cold skin of newborns.

Recent studies in newborns with hypoxic-ischemic injury indicate improved outcomes when the newborn is provided mild therapeutic hypothermia within 6 hours of birth. This approach is not recommended in the field, although it is prudent to prevent hyperthermia. Maintain the newborn at the lower margin of normal temperature (axillary temperature no higher than 36.5°C (97.7°F)).

■ Pathophysiology, Assessment, and Management of Common Birth Injuries in the Newborn

Birth trauma includes both avoidable and unavoidable injuries to the newborn resulting from mechanical forces (ie, compression, traction) during the delivery process. Such trauma is estimated to occur in 2 to 7 of every 1,000 live births. Most birth injuries are self-limiting and have a favorable outcome. Nearly half are potentially avoidable with recognition and anticipation of obstetric risk factors.

Birth injuries account for 2% to 3% of all infant deaths, with 5 to 8 of every 100,000 newborns dying of birth trauma and 25 of every 100,000 newborns dying of anoxic injury. Separating the effects of a hypoxic ischemic insult from the effects of a traumatic birth injury may prove difficult.

A difficult birth or injury to the newborn can occur because of the newborn's size or position during labor and delivery. Conditions associated with a difficult birth include **primigravida** (first pregnancy), prolonged labor, cephalopelvic disproportion (the size and shape of the maternal pelvis are not adequate for the vaginal delivery of the newborn), prolonged or rapid labor, abnormal presentation (eg, breech), large size (birth weight exceeding 9 lb, or 4,000 g), shoulder dystocia, prematurity, or low birth weight.

Birth trauma includes a variety of injuries. For example, abrasions, lacerations, bruises, and subcutaneous fat necrosis can occur with deliveries that involve instruments (eg, a vacuum or forceps). Molding of the head and overriding parietal bones are part of the normal process of labor, but occasionally excessive molding may be seen.

Caput succedaneum is swelling of the soft tissue of the newborn's scalp as it presses against the dilating cervix. This type of cranial injury is common. The swelling usually disappears in the first day or two after birth.

A cephalhematoma is an area of bleeding between the parietal bone and its covering periosteum. It often appears several hours after birth as a raised lump on the newborn's head, is limited by the boundaries of the bone, and may take 2 weeks to 3 months to resolve. If the bleeding is severe, jaundice may be seen as the red blood cells break down. Newborns born by instrumental vaginal delivery are more likely to have a cephalhematoma. Do not try to drain a rapidly expanding scalp hematoma because this may worsen or prolong the bleeding. Subperiosteal hemorrhage and intracranial hemorrhage may occur.

Linear skull fractures are occasionally seen with difficult births (spontaneous vaginal deliveries or deliveries using instruments). Nondisplaced fractures can be managed conservatively. Care should be observed to avoid pressure to the involved area. Displaced fractures warrant neurosurgical evaluation.

Brachial plexus injuries typically occur in large newborns and have an incidence of 0.5 to 2.0 cases per 1,000 live births. The most common brachial plexus injury is **Erb palsy** (involvement of C5, C6). **Klumpke paralysis** (involvement of C7–C8, T1) is rare and results in the weakness of the intrinsic muscles of the hand.

Although branches of the facial nerve may be injured in forceps delivery, most facial nerve palsy is unrelated to trauma. Physical findings include asymmetric faces with crying (lack of movement on the affected side makes the face appear to be "pulled" to the opposite side). Full resolution of cranial nerve injuries may take several weeks. Additionally, subconjunctival and retinal hemorrhage are possible results of birth trauma.

Diaphragmatic paralysis may occur as an isolated finding when the cervical roots supplying the phrenic nerve are injured or in association with a brachial plexus injury. The newborn may experience respiratory distress with hypoxemia, hypercapnea, and acidosis. Approximately 80% of the lesions are on the right side, and 10% are bilateral.

Laryngeal nerve injury appears to result from an intrauterine posture in which the head is rotated and flexed laterally. The newborn presents with stridor or a hoarse cry. Bilateral injury may be associated with severe respiratory distress needing respiratory support. The paralysis often resolves in 4 to 6 weeks, but may occasionally take as long as 6 to 12 months to clear up.

Spinal cord injury may result from excessive traction (in a breech delivery) or rotation and torsion (in a vertex delivery). The clinical presentation is stillbirth or rapid neonatal death with failure to establish an adequate airway.

The clavicle is the most frequently fractured bone in the newborn; such a bone injury is most often an unpredictable, unavoidable complication of normal birth. Risk factors may include large size, mid-forceps delivery, and shoulder dystocia (ie, the newborn's shoulders get stuck in the birth canal). The newborn may present with pseudoparalysis as he or she tries not to move the affected extremity to minimize pain. Examination will show crepitus and palpable bony irregularity. There may be lack of movement of the arm freely on the side of the fractured clavicle.

Loss of spontaneous arm or leg movement is an early sign of long bone fracture. The femur and humerus are the most commonly affected long bones. The fractures are treated by splinting. Look for signs of radial nerve injury with a humerus fracture.

Intra-abdominal injury is uncommon and may be overlooked as a cause of death in a newborn. Possible intra-abdominal injuries include liver contusion or fracture, rupture of the spleen, or adrenal hemorrhage. Hemorrhage is the most serious complication, and the liver is the organ most commonly injured. The bleeding may be catastrophic or insidious, and the patient presents with circulatory collapse. Consider intra-abdominal bleeding in every newborn presenting with shock, or unexplained pallor, plus abdominal distention. Finally, hypoxia and shock could be caused by birth trauma.

■ Pathophysiology, Assessment, and Management of Cardiac Conditions in Newborns

Various congenital heart diseases or malformations of the heart may cause cardiac emergencies in newborns; therefore, it is useful for you to be familiar with them. **Figure 16** shows the locations of pulmonary stenosis, atrial septal defect, and ventricular septal defect, which will be discussed next.

■ Pathophysiology

Congenital Heart Disease
Congenital heart disease (CHD) is the most common birth defect and occurs in 8 per 1,000 live births. Approximately one third of these conditions are considered critical—forms of CHD that are usually associated with hypoxia in the newborn period and require intervention during the first months of life.

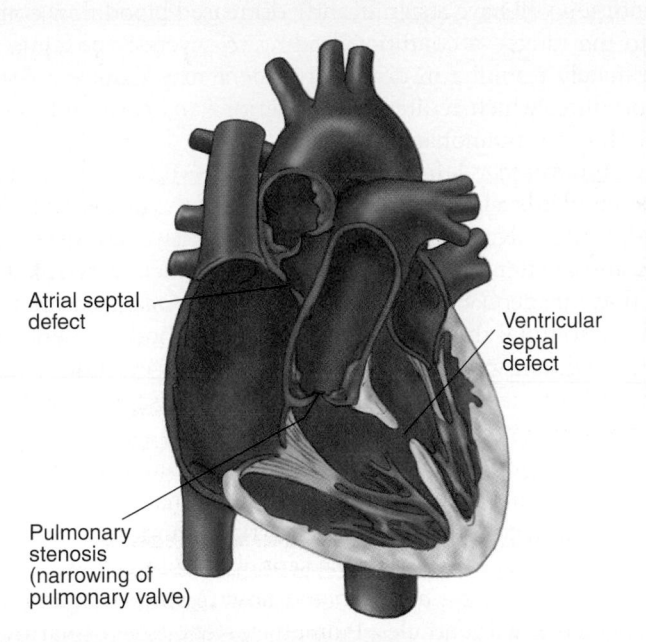

Figure 16 Locations of various congenital heart malformations.

This important cause of morbidity and mortality accounts for approximately 40% of deaths caused by congenital anomalies, the majority of which occur in the first year of life. Ten percent of neonates who died of CHD before 1 year of age were diagnosed at autopsy. Although there have been great improvements in surgical care of these infants, there remains much room for improvement in early detection of CHD.

It is well recognized that visual detection of cyanosis is difficult. A painless, noninvasive way to detect cyanosis is to measure oxygen saturation of hemoglobin in arterial blood. Pulse oximetry has been found to be a noninvasive and accurate method to detect oxygenated versus nonoxygenated blood.

Monitoring oxygen saturation has been shown to have the highest sensitivity and highest specificity with the right hand and one foot, using cutoff values of less than 95% or a greater than 3% difference between the two. The best outcomes are found when a physical examination is paired with pulse oximetry screening.

In 2011, the Department of Health and Human Services and the American Academy of Pediatrics recommended pulse oximetry screening for full-term healthy newborns in an effort to diagnose CHD early in the neonatal period. Because some disorders may present with significant cardiopulmonary compromise without apparent cyanosis, the recommended term is critical CHD rather than term cyanotic heart disease, which is sometimes used.

Pulmonary stenosis is a disease in which the pulmonic valve located near the right ventricle of the heart becomes damaged. When this exists, the patient will have a decrease in blood flow to the lungs and will present with jugular vein distention, cyanosis, or right ventricular hypertrophy. Pulmonary stenosis is typically associated with CHD but can also be a result from rheumatic heart disease.

Septal defects can exist in the atrias or the ventricles within the heart. When an **atrial septal defect (ASD)** is present,

deoxygenated blood is able to shift from the right atrium or left atrium to the other atria and mix with oxygen-rich blood. The failure of the **foramen ovale** to close after birth allows for this process to take place. The foramen ovale exists in utero, during which time it enables the fetus to receive oxygen-rich blood from the placenta—essential because the fetus's lungs are nonfunctioning. After the fetus has been born, a drop in circulatory pulmonary pressure occurs, allowing the foramen ovale to close. In a patient with an open foramen ovale, hemodynamic status can be dependent on how much blood flow is being shunted. In a **ventricular septal defect (VSD)**, the left ventricle contracts, forcing some of the blood flow back into the right ventricle. This causes an increase in the right ventricle pressure, which subsequently results in pulmonary hypertension developing in the patient.

Patent ductus arteriosus (PDA) exists when the ductus arteriosus fails to close after birth. In the fetus, an open ductus arteriosus allows blood flow to bypass the right ventricle and lungs due to the fetus's lungs being filled with fluid. The ductus arteriosus connects the pulmonary artery and the aorta; after birth, it is supposed to evolve into the ligamentum arteriosum **Figure 17**. An untreated PDA may cause the patient to subsequently develop congestive heart failure.

Coarctation of the aorta (CoA) is a narrowing of the aorta, the largest oxygen-carrying artery in the human body. When CoA is present, the heart must push harder to force blood flow past the narrowed portion of the aorta. These patients may experience shortness of breath, chest pain, hypertension, headaches, and muscle weakness. Treatment is usually heart surgery.

In a normal circulatory system, the pulmonary artery and the aorta are two separate vessels. In **truncus arteriosus**, these vessels are combined into one **Figure 18**. This merger greatly increases the blood flow coming into the lungs, ultimately

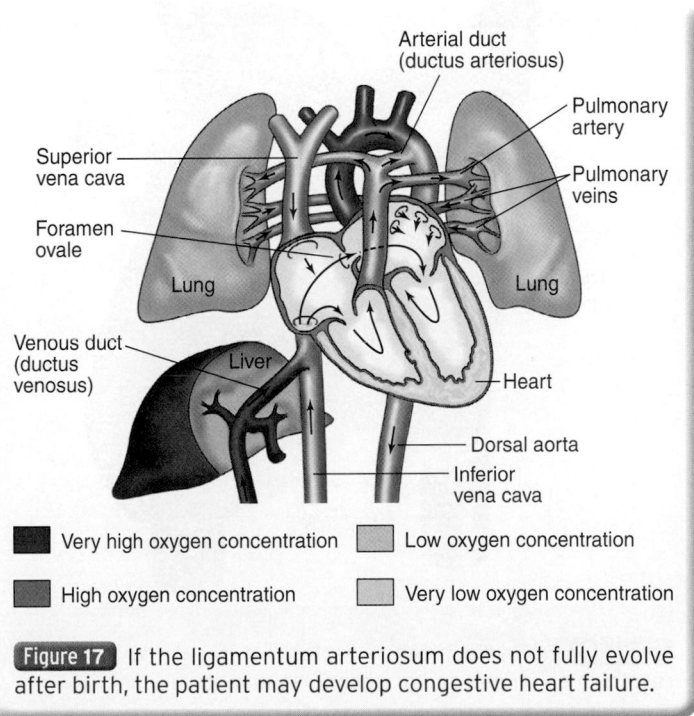

Figure 17 If the ligamentum arteriosum does not fully evolve after birth, the patient may develop congestive heart failure.

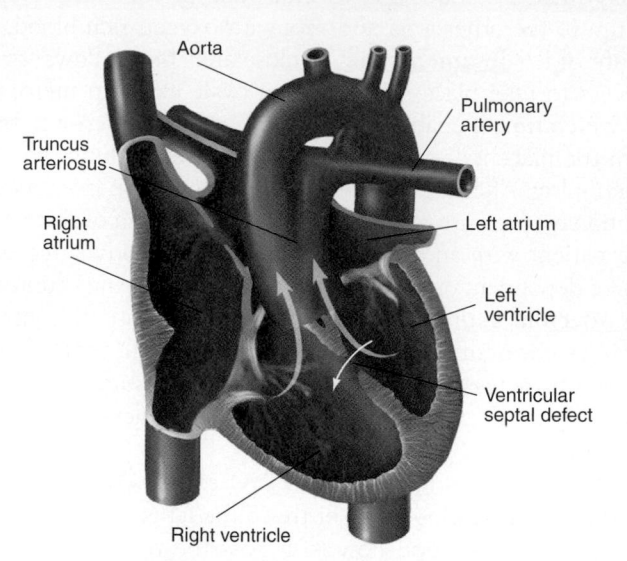

Figure 18 In truncus arteriosus, the pulmonary artery and the aorta are combined into one vessel.

causing these patients to have congestive heart failure. Early in life, the patient will demonstrate slightly lower oxygen levels, which eventually result in cyanosis. Affected patients will require surgical intervention.

In **tricuspid atresia**, the patient lacks the tricuspid valve, which normally separates the right atrium and the right ventricle. The lack of the tricuspid valve results in an undersized or absent right ventricle **Figure 19**. Patients who present with this

condition will have a significantly decreased blood flow coming into the lungs—a condition leading to severe hypoxemia and ultimately resulting in death. Treatment may require a Fontan procedure, which redirects the inferior vena cava and hepatic vein into the pulmonary circulation.

Hypoplastic left heart syndrome (HLHS) is the complete underdevelopment of the left side of the heart. The mitral and aortic valves may be closed or severely underdeveloped, the aorta extremely small, and the left ventricle very small. All of these inadequacies result in the left side of the heart being unable to fulfill the circulation needs of the body. Patients with this condition will present with a murmur or cyanosis. A heart transplant is necessary to resolve the cardiovascular insufficiencies resulting from HLHS.

Tetralogy of Fallot (ToF) is a combination of four heart defects: a ventricular septal defect, pulmonary stenosis, right ventricular hypertrophy, and an overriding aorta. The ventricular septal defect is a hole in the septum that separates the right and left ventricles; it allows blood flow to shift back and forth between the two ventricles. Pulmonary stenosis is the narrowing of the pulmonary valve that causes the heart to have to pump harder due to the lack of blood flow to the lungs. Right ventricular hypertrophy is a thickening of the right ventricle that occurs so that the body can efficiently pump blood to the lungs. In a normal circulatory system, the aorta is connected to the left ventricle. In ToF, the aorta is connected between the left and right ventricles over the ventricular septal defect. All of these defects result in poor oxygenation; open heart surgery is required to correct ToF.

In **transposition of the great arteries (TGA)**, blood goes to the lungs to become oxygenated. Instead of then going to the body, however, the blood returns back to the lungs **Figure 20**. Blood that comes from the body to the heart ends up going right back to the body without ever becoming oxygenated. Patients present with

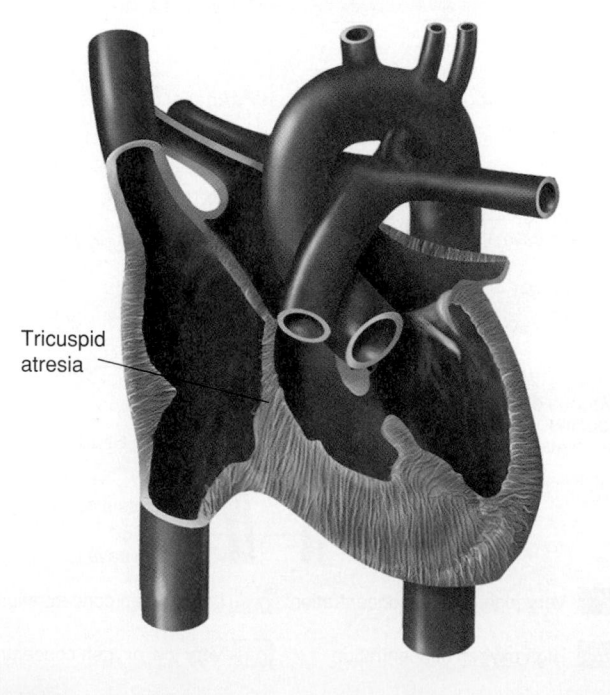

Figure 19 Tricuspid atresia, or lack of the tricuspid valve, results in an undersized or absent right ventricle.

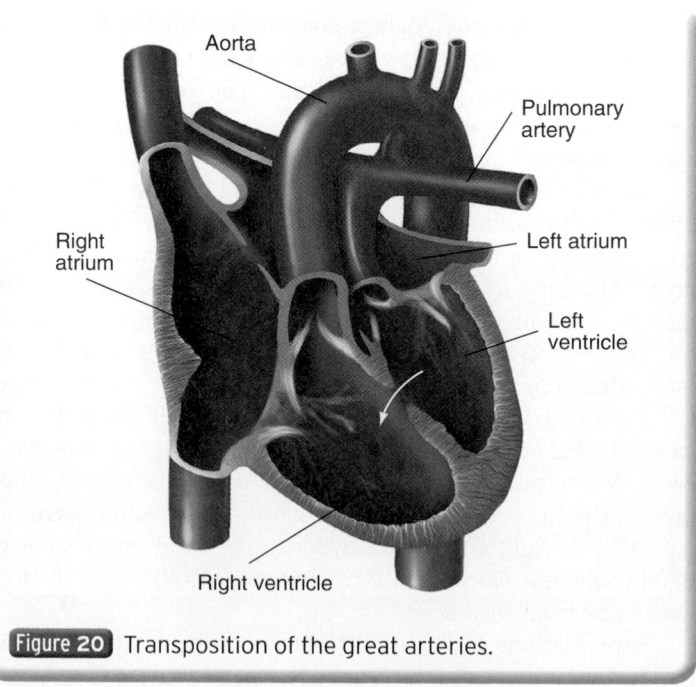

Figure 20 Transposition of the great arteries.

shortness of breath, clubbing of fingers and toes, and cyanosis. They may require surgical intervention to correct the defect.

Total anomalous pulmonary venous return (TAPVR) is a rare congenital defect in which the four pulmonary veins do not connect to the left atrium. Instead, the pulmonary veins connect to the right atrium, resulting in diminished oxygen and an increased load on the right ventricle. These patients will present with signs and symptoms shortly after birth.

■ Assessment and Management

Critical CHD commonly presents in the neonatal period. Rapid detection and transport are mandatory because the conditions of patients can become unstable very quickly. Communication with medical control is critical to having adequate services available for diagnosis and treatment upon arrival at the emergency facility.

YOU *are the Medic* | SUMMARY

1. What is the significance of the green amniotic fluid?

Amniotic fluid should be clear and odorless. The presence of a green or greenish-black staining indicates that the fetus has passed fetal stool or meconium. This occurs because of fetal, distress. If the fetus inhales the meconium into his or her lungs it can cause a severe pneumonia leading to respiratory distress, respiratory failure, or death.

2. What further information would you like to obtain from the patient?

At this point in time you should obtain information to answer two important questions. The first one is "are you going to be delivering at the house or do you have time to transport to the hospital?" Ask the woman whether she feels the need to push or have a bowel movement. If she answers "yes" to either question, check for crowning because an urge to push signifies that the fetus will likely deliver soon. The second question that you need to ask is "are there any other risk factors, other than four prior pregnancies and deliveries, present that might require resuscitation of the newborn once it is born?" Key information includes the use of drugs (including prescription drugs, illicit drugs, and alcohol) within the past 4 hours and knowledge of any other complications she had throughout the pregnancy.

3. Besides the OB kit, what additional equipment should you have available?

Because you already detected the presence of meconium, you must have your resuscitation equipment available and ready to go. At a minimum, make sure that your intubation equipment is functioning properly, that you have a meconium aspirator to attach between the end of the ET tube and the suction tubing, and ensure that the suction unit is working. Most importantly, you need help. Call for additional assistance!

4. Should you stimulate the newborn immediately after birth?

No. If the newborn is depressed on delivery, do not dry or stimulate him or her. This is the time to intubate the trachea and attempt to remove any meconium that may be blocking the airway.

5. What treatment is indicated for this newborn?

Because the newborn has a pulse rate below 100 beats/min and has a weak respiratory effort after drying and stimulation, positive-pressure ventilation via a bag-mask device is necessary. Make sure that you ventilate at a rate of 40 to 60 breaths/min and use only enough pressure to cause chest rise.

6. When is endotracheal intubation indicated in the newborn?

Endotracheal intubation is not routinely required during the resuscitation of a newborn. However, there are certain circumstances when intubation is necessary. These include: 1) meconium-stained fluid is present and the newborn is not vigorous; 2) a congenital diaphragmatic hernia is suspected and respiratory support is needed; 3) the newborn does not respond to bag-mask ventilation and chest compressions, requiring the administration of endotracheal epinephrine; and 4) prolonged positive-pressure ventilation is required. Epinephrine is best administered IV, but the endotracheal route may be used if there is no IV access.

7. When should an Apgar score be calculated?

The Apgar score is a tool that is used to help you determine the need for and effectiveness of resuscitation. Usually the Apgar score is calculated at 1 and 5 minutes after birth if the newborn does not require immediate interventions. DO NOT delay resuscitation efforts to calculate an Apgar score! You can obtain an Apgar score once the newborn is stabilized.

8. What should you do for the newborn at this time?

Because the newborn now has a good respiratory rate and pulse rate, and you have already cut and clamped the cord after your last reassessment, you should now make sure that the newborn stays warm. Wrap the newborn in clean, dry towels or the swaddler that is contained in the OB kit, and place the hat on the newborn's head. In this scenario, do not give the newborn to the mother, as the risk of ET tube dislodgment is too high.

9. What are the five components that make up the Apgar score?

When you assess the newborn to calculate an Apgar score, there are five key parameters to evaluate. The first parameter, "A", stands for appearance. Appearance is determined by looking at the newborn's color. As always, pink is good and blue is bad. A newborn may have a pink body but blue hands and feet. This is normal in the newborn and will gradually disappear over the next several hours as the new blood vessels open up and increase

YOU *are the Medic* | SUMMARY, *continued*

perfusion to those areas. The second parameter "P," stands for pulse rate. The pulse rate can be determined by palpating the base of the umbilical cord or listening to the chest. The pulse rate should be greater than 100 beats/min. If the pulse rate remains less than 60 beats/min after 30 seconds of effective positive-pressure ventilation, you must immediately begin cardiac compressions. The third parameter, "G," stands for grimace or irritability. Simply

put, how does the newborn act when you rub his or her back or flick the sole of the foot? The fourth parameter, activity, is the second "A". How is newborn moving his or her extremities? Is the newborn kicking and screaming or just lying there? Finally, the last parameter, "R," stands for respirations. What kind of effort is the newborn making to breathe? Is the newborn screaming at you full force, barely moving the chest, or not breathing at all?

YOU *are the Medic* | SUMMARY, *continued*

Maternal Patient Care Report

EMS Patient Care Report (PCR)

Date: 07-06-12	Incident No.: 187444	Nature of Call: Possible childbirth		Location: 8901 NW Pembroke Road	
Dispatched: 0910	En Route: 0911	At Scene: 0917	Transport: 0952	At Hospital: 1012	In Service: 1020

Patient Information

Age: 29 years Sex: F Weight (in kg [lb]): 78 kg (172 lb)	Allergies: None Medications: Prenatal vitamins Past Medical History: None Chief Complaint: Water broke

Vital Signs

Time: 0919	BP: 128/74	Pulse: 104	Respirations: 24	Spo$_2$: 97%
Time: 0940	BP: 124/70	Pulse: 94	Respirations: 18	Spo$_2$: 99%
Time: 1000	BP: 122/74	Pulse: 86	Respirations: 18	Spo$_2$: 99%

EMS Treatment
(circle all that apply)

Oxygen @ __12__ L/min via (circle one): NC (NRM) Bag-mask device		(Assisted Ventilation)	Airway Adjunct	CPR
Defibrillation	Bleeding Control	Bandaging	Splinting	(Other:)OB kit, IV

Narrative

Dispatched to the home of a 29-year-old female for possible childbirth. Arrived on scene to find the pt sitting on the edge of her bed, clutching her abdomen and grimacing in pain. Pt states that her "water broke about 45 minutes ago and when she saw that it was green she called her OB who told her to call 9-1-1." There is a large puddle of green fluid on the floor beside the bed. Pt states that she is 41-weeks' pregnant with her fifth child. Pt denies other PMH. Pt states that she was scheduled to be induced two days from now. Pt states that she has had routine prenatal care with no known complications. Pt takes prenatal vitamins and denies any medication allergies. Additional assistance requested from dispatch. Pt placed on O$_2$ 12 L/min via nonrebreathing mask. Pt placed in supine position with legs flexed towards the abdomen to facilitate inspection of the vaginal area. Crowning is noted upon inspection at 0920. OB kit and neonatal resuscitation equipment are prepared. Following delivery and stabilization of the baby, mother and baby were placed on stretchers and secured with straps. Separate PCR filed by second paramedic unit that transported newborn. En route to Grand View Hospital an 18-gauge IV was placed in the mother's left AC and a 1,000 mL bag of normal saline was hung at a rate of 200 mL/h. Physical assessment findings: Pt AAO x 4. PEARRL. No JVD or tracheal deviation noted. Chest symmetrical with bilateral chest rise and clear lung sounds. Abdomen soft and non-tender following delivery. PMS x 4. Hospital contacted and report given to labor and delivery. No further orders were given. Mother remained stable through transport. The placenta was delivered as rescue was entering the parking lot of the hospital. Mother was brought to labor and delivery. Report given to Dr. Aarons and Judy ARNP. Cleared for service at 1020. **End of report**

YOU *are the Medic* | **SUMMARY,** *continued* |

Newborn Patient Care Report

EMS Patient Care Report (PCR)

Date: 07-06-12	**Incident No.:** 596833	**Nature of Call:** Possible childbirth		**Location:** 8901 NW Pembroke Road
Dispatched: 0910	**En Route:** 0932	**At Scene:** 0940	**Transport:** 0952	**At Hospital:** 1012 **In Service:** 1020

Patient Information

Age: Newborn **Sex:** F **Weight (in kg [lb]):** Approx. 4 kg (8 lb)	**Allergies:** None **Medications:** None **Past Medical History:** None **Chief Complaint:** Childbirth

Vital Signs

Time	BP	Pulse	Respirations	O₂ / SpO₂
Time: 0927	**BP:** N/A	**Pulse:** 85	**Respirations:** N/A	**O$_2$:** N/A
Time: 0931	**BP:** N/A	**Pulse:** 156	**Respirations:** N/A	**O$_2$:** N/A
Time: 0940	**BP:** N/A	**Pulse:** 154	**Respirations:** 46	**Spo$_2$:** 99%
Time: 1000	**BP:** N/A	**Pulse:** 154	**Respirations:** 46	**Spo$_2$:** 99%

EMS Treatment
(circle all that apply)

Oxygen @ __5__ L/min via (circle one): (NC) NRM Bag-mask device	(**Assisted Ventilation**) Newborn	(**Airway Adjunct**) Intubation, ET tube	**CPR**
Defibrillation	**Bleeding Control**	**Bandaging**	**Splinting**	(**Other:**) Suction, warming

Narrative

See separate narrative filed by first paramedic unit for information regarding the mother. Called to a private residence for possible childbirth. Arrived to find newborn had been born and was stabilized. The following notes were obtained from the first paramedic unit:

   Upon physical examination of the mother at 0920 crowning was noted. OB kit and neonatal resuscitation equipment are prepared. At approximately 0929 the baby's head was delivered and the mouth and nose were suctioned with a bulb syringe. Moderate amounts of thick green meconium was removed from the oral cavity. Upon delivery the baby was noted to have a weak respiratory effort and cyanosis to the trunk and extremities. Umbilical cord was clamped and cut. A 3.5 ETT with a meconium aspirator was attached to suction and the vocal cords were visualized using a Miller 1 blade. The ETT was passed below the level of the vocal cords and removed as suction was applied. Moderate amount of thick green meconium was removed. A new ETT was placed and the procedure was repeated and baby was ventilated at a rate of 60 breaths/min for 30 seconds with enough pressure to produce visible chest rise. After 30 seconds of positive-pressure ventilation, the baby was noted to have a good cry, pink trunk with blue hands and feet, and a pulse rate of 156 beats/min. Breath sounds are clear and equal. The baby was dried with a towel and wrapped in the silver swaddler.

   Mother was transported by first medic unit. Baby placed on stretcher and secured with straps. Hospital contacted and report given to labor and delivery. No further orders were given. Baby remained stable through transport. Baby was brought to labor and delivery. Report given to Dr. Aarons and Judy ARNP. Cleared for service at 1020. **End of report**

Prep Kit

- The care of a newborn or neonate must be tailored to meet the unique needs of this population. The rate of complications increases as birth weight and gestational age decrease. Approximately 10% of newborns need additional assistance to survive.

- Initial steps of neonatal resuscitation include positioning and clearing the airway, stimulating the newborn to breathe, and assessing heart rate and oxygenation. In a newborn, resuscitation efforts are focused on establishing the airway and ensuring adequate ventilation.

- Both short- and long-term outcomes have been linked to initial stabilization efforts, which include warming the newborn; positioning; clearing the airway if necessary; drying the newborn's head, face, and body; and stimulating the newborn. Additional steps that may be required include providing supplemental oxygen, assisting ventilation by providing positive pressure, intubating, providing chest compressions, and administering medications as needed.

- At birth, a fetus must transition from receiving oxygen from the placenta to receiving oxygen via breathing. A rapid series of events must occur to enable the newborn to breathe. Anything that delays this decline in pulmonary pressure can lead to delayed transition, hypoxia, brain damage, and, ultimately, death.

- While a delivery is occurring, use any time available to obtain a patient history and prepare the environment and equipment that may be necessary for neonatal resuscitation.

- Your initial rapid assessment of the newborn may be done simultaneously with any treatment interventions. Note the patency of the airway, respiratory rate, respiratory effort, pulse rate, color, and capillary refill.

- The Apgar score is used to determine the need for and the effectiveness of resuscitation. It includes a score for appearance, pulse rate, grimace or irritability, muscle activity, and respiratory effort. This score is obtained at 1 and 5 minutes after birth.

- It is important to follow the neonatal resuscitation algorithm developed by the American Academy of Pediatrics and the American Heart Association.

- Thermoregulation is limited in the newborn; therefore, you must take an active role in keeping the newborn's body temperature in the normal range. Place the newborn directly on the mother's chest. Dry the head and the body with towels. Cover the newborn with a dry towel; cover the head with a cap. Position the newborn to ensure a patent airway.

- If the newborn does not respond by 30 seconds after initial stabilization efforts (bulb suctioning mouth and nose, drying and stimulating), further intervention is indicated.
  - If the newborn has a normal breathing pattern and a pulse rate of greater than 100 beats/min but maintains central cyanosis of the trunk or of the mucous membranes, provide supplemental free-flow oxygen.
  - If the newborn remains apneic or has a pulse rate of less than 100 beats/min, begin positive-pressure ventilation by bag-mask device.
  - If the newborn's pulse rate is less than 60 beats/min after 30 seconds of adequate ventilation by positive-pressure ventilation with 100% oxygen via a bag-mask device, begin chest compressions.

- Airway management in the newborn follows these steps. If a newborn is cyanotic or pale, administer warmed, humidified free-flow oxygen. If the newborn has an airway obstruction, for example from a congenital malformation, insert an oral airway. If these measures are not effective and the newborn is apneic, has inadequate respiratory effort, or is bradycardic, perform bag-mask ventilation. If this is not effective, endotracheal intubation is required.

- Gastric decompression using an orogastric tube is indicated for prolonged bag-mask ventilation (more than 5 to 10 minutes), if abdominal distention is impeding ventilation, and in the presence of diaphragmatic hernia or a gastrointestinal congenital anomaly like a tracheoesophageal fistula.

- Chest compressions are indicated if the pulse rate remains less than 60 beats/min despite positioning, clearing the airway, drying and stimulation, and 30 seconds of effective positive-pressure ventilation.

- Emergent vascular access becomes necessary when fluid administration is needed to support circulation, when resuscitation medications must be administered IV, and when therapeutic drugs must be given IV. Vascular access in a newborn occurs via the umbilical vein.

- Most newborns can be resuscitated with effective ventilatory support. Medications may be needed in patients with bradycardia, low blood volume, acidosis, respiratory depression secondary to narcotics, and hypoglycemia. Remember that neonatal medication doses are based on weight.

- Once the newborn is stabilized as much as possible in the field, you should provide transport to the nearest facility that can provide the next level of care.

- Ongoing communication with the family is a must. Do not be specific about survival statistics. If you do not have an answer, put the family in touch with the people who do.

- Bradycardia in a newborn is usually caused by hypoxia, which is readily reversed by effective positive-pressure ventilation. Another cause is a tension pneumothorax that requires needle decompression. If ventilation and chest compressions do not improve the bradycardia, administer epinephrine via an IV line or ET tube.

- When a newborn is delivered through meconium-stained amniotic fluid, there is a high risk of morbidity. If the newborn is depressed, *do not* dry or stimulate the newborn. Clear the airway of meconium, intubate the trachea, attach a meconium aspirator and suction catheter to the end of the endotracheal tube, and suction the ET tube while withdrawing the tube from the trachea.

- Diaphragmatic hernia is an abnormal opening in the diaphragm. If positive-pressure ventilation is needed in a newborn with this condition, endotracheal intubation will be necessary, along with an orogastric tube to minimize intestinal distention. Surgical correction is required for this condition.

- Newborns born before 37 weeks of gestation are considered premature. You should provide cardiorespiratory support and a thermoneutral environment to optimize their survival and long-term outcome.

- Seizures are a very distinctive sign of neurologic disease in the newborn. Quickly evaluate prenatal and birth history, and perform a careful physical exam. Consult with medical control if you are considering administering anticonvulsant medication.

- Non-bilious vomiting is common in newborns. Keep the newborn's face turned to one side to prevent further aspiration. Suction or clear the vomitus from the airway with the help of a suction catheter or suction bulb. Ensure adequate oxygenation. Consider fluid resuscitation. Transport the newborn on his or her side.

- In an infant with diarrhea, estimate the number and volume of loose stools, decreased urinary output, and degree of dehydration. Ensure adequate oxygenation and ventilation. Perform chest compressions in addition to positive-pressure ventilation in a newborn if the pulse rate is less than 60 beats/min. Administer fluid therapy.

- If fever is suspected, observe the newborn for the presence of rashes. Obtain a careful history and vital signs. Ensure adequate oxygenation and ventilation. Remove additional layers of clothing and improve ventilation in the environment. Perform chest compressions, if indicated. Do not administer antipyretic agents.

- Birth trauma includes both avoidable and unavoidable injuries to the newborn resulting from mechanical forces during the delivery process. A difficult birth or injury to the newborn can occur because of the newborn's size or position during labor or delivery.

- Various congenital heart diseases or malformations of the heart may cause cardiac emergencies in newborns.

Prep Kit, continued

■ Vital Vocabulary

<u>acrocyanosis</u> A decrease in the amount of oxygen delivered to the extremities. The hands and feet turn blue because of narrowing (constriction) of small arterioles (tiny arteries) toward the end of the arms and legs.

<u>amniotic fluid</u> A clear, slightly yellowish liquid that surrounds the fetus during pregnancy; contained in the amniotic sac.

<u>Apgar score</u> Scale used to assess the status of a newborn 1 and 5 minutes after birth (range, 0 to 10).

<u>apnea</u> Respiratory pause greater than or equal to 20 seconds.

<u>asphyxia</u> Condition of severely deficient supply of oxygen to the body leading to end organ damage.

<u>atrial septal defect (ASD)</u> A hole in the atrial septal wall that allows oxygenated and deoxygenated blood to mix; patients with this hole have a higher incidence of stroke.

<u>bradycardia</u> A pulse rate of less than 100 beats/min in the newborn.

<u>central cyanosis</u> Bluish coloration of the skin due to the presence of deoxygenated hemoglobin in blood vessels near the skin surface.

<u>choanal atresia</u> A narrowing or blockage of the nasal airway by membranous or bony tissue; a congenital condition, meaning it is present at birth.

<u>cleft lip</u> An abnormal defect or fissure in the upper lip that failed to close during development. It is often associated with cleft palate.

<u>cleft palate</u> A fissure or hole in the palate (roof of the mouth) that forms a communicating pathway between the mouth and nasal cavities.

<u>coarctation of the aorta (CoA)</u> Pinching or narrowing of the aorta that obstructs blood flow from the heart to the systemic circulation.

<u>congenital heart disease (CHD)</u> The most common birth defect; associated with hypoxia in the newborn period requiring intervention during the first months of life.

<u>diaphragmatic hernia</u> Passage of loops of bowel with or without other abdominal organs, through a developmental defect in the diaphragm muscle; occurs as the bowel from the abdomen "herniates" upward through the diaphragm into the chest (thoracic) cavity.

<u>Erb palsy</u> Lack of movement at the shoulder due to nerve injury resulting from the stretching of the cervical nerve roots (C5 and C6 most commonly) during delivery of the newborn's head during birth. The effect is usually transient, but can be permanent.

<u>fetal transition</u> The process through which the fluid in the fetal lungs is replaced with air, the ductus arteriosus constricts, and the newborn begins adequate oxygenation of its own blood.

<u>foramen ovale</u> An opening in the septum of the heart that closes after birth.

<u>free-flow oxygen</u> Oxygen administered via oxygen tube and a cupped hand on patient's face.

<u>generalized seizure</u> Seizure activity that is bilateral, synchronous, and nonmigratory.

<u>gestation</u> Period of time from conception to birth. For humans, the full period is normally 9 months (or 40 weeks).

<u>grunting</u> Noises heard when an infant is having difficulty breathing; short inarticulate guttural sounds as effort is expended.

<u>hypoglycemia</u> A deficiency of glucose in the blood caused by too much insulin or too little glucose; in the newborn it is a level of less than 40 mg/dL, and in older neonates it is a level of less than 60 mg/dL.

<u>hypoplastic left heart syndrome (HLHS)</u> Underdevelopment of the aorta, aortic valve, left ventricle, and mitral valve; this defect involves the entire left side of the heart.

<u>hypothermia</u> A condition in which the core body temperature is significantly below normal (less than 35°C [95°F]).

<u>hypotonia</u> Low or poor muscle tone (floppy).

<u>hypoxic ischemic encephalopathy</u> Damage to cells in the central nervous system (the brain and spinal cord) from inadequate oxygen.

infantile hypertrophic pyloric stenosis (IHPS) Marked hypertrophy and hyperplasia of the two (circular and longitudinal) muscular layers of the pylorus, resulting in the pylorus becoming thick and obstructing the end of the stomach.

intercostal retractions Skin sucking in between the ribs, seen when a patient creates increased negative intrathoracic pressure to breathe.

intestinal atresia A congenital condition in which part of the bowel does not develop.

intestinal stenosis A congenital condition in which part of the bowel is narrow.

intussusception An event where one part of the intestine folds into another part of the intestines leading to a blockage.

Klumpke paralysis An injury of childbirth affecting the spinal nerves C7, C8, and T1 of the brachial plexus. It can be contrasted to Erb palsy, which affects C5 and C6.

macroglossia Large tongue size.

malrotation A congenital anomaly of rotation of the midgut, the small bowel is found predominantly on the right side of the abdomen. Results in increased incidence of intestinal volvulus.

meconium A dark green fecal material that accumulates in the fetal intestines and is discharged around the time of birth.

multifocal seizure Seizure activity that involves more than one site, is asynchronous, and is usually migratory.

nasal flaring Intermittent outward movements of the nostrils with each inspiration; indicates an increase in the work needed to breathe.

neonate Infant during the first month after birth.

newborn Infant within the first few hours after birth.

oligohydramnios Decreased volume of amniotic fluid during a pregnancy; a risk factor associated with abnormalities of the urinary tract, postmaturity (birth after a prolonged pregnancy), and intrauterine growth retardation.

patent ductus arteriosus (PDA) A situation in which the ductus arteriosus, which assists in fetal circulation, does not transition as it should after birth to become the ligamentum arteriosum; the result is that the connection between the pulmonary artery and the aorta remains, allowing some oxygenated blood to move back into the heart rather than all of it moving out of the aorta and into the systemic circulation.

pathogenic gastroesophageal reflux (GER) A condition in which stomach acid rises into the esophagus on a regular or frequent basis, potentially causing irritation and damage; a common cause of vomiting.

persistent pulmonary hypertension Delayed transition from fetal to neonatal circulation.

Pierre Robin sequence A condition present at birth marked by a small lower jaw (micrognathia). The tongue tends to fall back and downward (glossoptosis), and there is a cleft soft palate.

placenta previa Abnormal location of the placenta in the lower part of the uterus, near or over the cervix.

polycythemia Abnormally high red blood cell count.

polyhydramnios An excessive amount of amniotic fluid. May cause preterm labor.

positive-pressure ventilation (PPV) Method for assisting ventilation (bag-mask or intubated) with high-flow air or supplemental oxygen.

post-term Any pregnancy that lasts more than 42 weeks.

premature Underdeveloped; the condition of an infant born too soon. Refers to infants delivered before 37 weeks from the first day of the last menstrual period.

preterm Used to describe an infant delivered at less than 37 completed weeks.

primary apnea Apnea caused by oxygen deprivation; usually corrected with stimulation, such as drying or slapping the newborn's feet. Primary apnea is typically preceded by an initial period of rapid breathing.

primigravida First pregnancy.

prolapsed cord When the umbilical cord presents itself outside of the uterus while the fetus is still inside; an obstetric emergency during pregnancy or labor that acutely endangers the life of the fetus; can happen when the amniotic sac breaks and with the gush of amniotic fluid the cord comes along.

pulmonary hypertension Elevated blood pressure in the pulmonary arteries from constriction; causes problems with the blood flow in the lungs, and makes the heart work harder.

pulmonary stenosis Narrowing of the pulmonary valve.

retinopathy of prematurity A disease of the eye that affects prematurely born infants, thought to be caused by disorganized growth of retinal blood vessels resulting in scarring and retinal detachment; can lead to blindness in serious cases.

secondary apnea When asphyxia continues after primary apnea, infant responds with a period of gasping respirations, falling pulse rate, and falling blood pressure. Positive-pressure ventilation is indicated to reverse secondary apnea.

seizure A paroxysmal alteration in neurologic function—ie, behavioral and/or autonomic function.

small for gestational age An infant whose size and weight are considerably less than the average for infants of the same age.

surfactant A substance formed in the lungs that helps keep the small air sacs or alveoli from collapsing and sticking together; a low level in a premature infant contributes to respiratory distress syndrome.

term Used to describe a newborn delivered at 38 to 42 weeks of gestation.

tetralogy of Fallot (ToF) A cardiac anomaly that consists of four defects: a ventricular septal defect, pulmonary stenosis, right ventricular hypertrophy, and an overriding aorta.

thermoregulation The process by which the body maintains temperature through a combination of heat gain by metabolic processes and muscular movement and heat loss through respiration, evaporation, conduction, convection, and perspiration.

total anomalous pulmonary venous return (TAPVR) A rare congenital defect in which the four pulmonary veins do not connect to the left atrium; instead, the pulmonary veins connect to the right atrium, resulting in diminished oxygen and an increased load on the right ventricle.

transposition of the great arteries (TGA) A defect in which the great vessels are reversed; the aorta is connected to the right ventricle, and the pulmonary artery is connected to the left ventricle.

tricuspid atresia The absence of a tricuspid valve, which normally separates the right atrium and the right ventricle.

truncus arteriosus A condition in which the pulmonary artery and the aorta are combined into one.

umbilical vein The blood vessel in the umbilical cord used to administer emergency medications.

ventricular septal defect (VSD) A hole in the septum separating the ventricles, allowing blood from the left ventricle to flow into the right ventricle.

Assessment in Action

You and your partner just delivered a newborn who is premature at 27 weeks' gestation. During your newborn assessment you observe a slow, weak respiratory effort, slow pulse rate, and cyanosis of the trunk and extremities. An additional rescue unit arrives and assumes care of the mother, allowing you and your partner to treat the newborn. After 30 seconds of drying and stimulation there is no change in your assessment.

1. What intervention should be performed immediately?
   A. Chest compressions
   B. Endotracheal intubation
   C. Administration of epinephrine
   D. Positive-pressure ventilation

2. Which of the following is the correct ventilation rate for a newborn requiring positive-pressure ventilation?
   A. 10 to 20 breaths/min
   B. 20 to 40 breaths/min
   C. 40 to 60 breaths/min
   D. 60 to 80 breaths/min

3. At what point during resuscitation should chest compressions be started?
   A. If the newborn's pulse rate remains below 60 beats/min following 30 seconds of positive-pressure ventilation via a bag-mask device
   B. If the newborn's pulse rate remains below 60 beats/min following 30 seconds of positive-pressure ventilation via an endotracheal tube
   C. If the newborn's pulse rate remains below 60 beats/min following 30 seconds of drug administration
   D. If the newborn's pulse rate remains below 60 beats/min following 30 seconds of free-flow oxygen at 5 L/min

4. How deep should you compress the chest when performing cardiopulmonary resuscitation on a newborn?
   A. Two thirds the anteroposterior diameter of the chest
   B. One half the anteroposterior diameter of the chest
   C. One third the anteroposterior diameter of the chest
   D. One quarter the anteroposterior diameter of the chest

5. What is the compression-to-ventilation ratio for neonatal cardiopulmonary resuscitation?
   A. 15:2
   B. 30:2
   C. 3:1
   D. 5:1

6. What is the recommended dose and concentration of epinephrine for neonates?
   A. 0.1 to 0.3 mg/kg; 1:10,000
   B. 0.1 to 0.3 mL/kg; 1:10,000
   C. 0.01 to 0.03 mg/kg; 1:1,000
   D. 0.01 to 0.03 mL/kg; 1:1,000

7. Most newborns can be resuscitated with:
   A. ventilatory support.
   B. chest compressions.
   C. fluid replacement.
   D. medication administration.

Additional Question

8. What are some of the factors that can cause a woman to deliver prematurely?

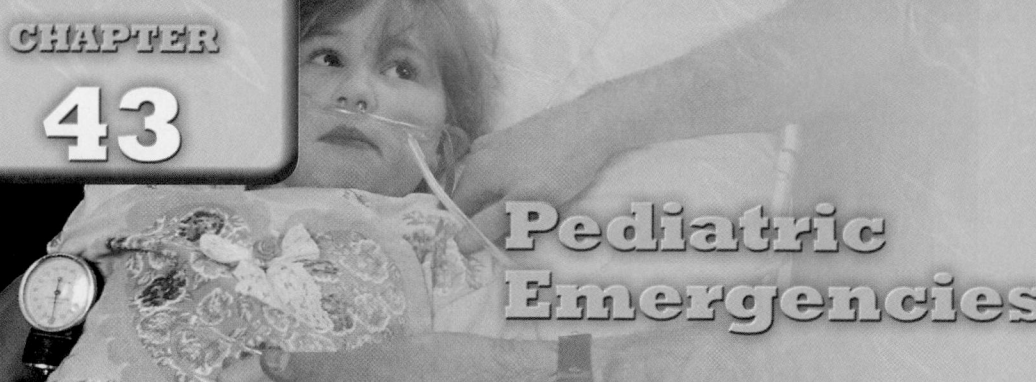

National EMS Education Standard Competencies

Special Patient Populations

Integrates assessment findings with principles of pathophysiology and knowledge of psychosocial needs to formulate a field impression and implement a comprehensive treatment/disposition plan for patients with special needs.

Pediatric Emergencies

Age-related assessment findings, and age-related and developmental-stage-related assessment and treatment modifications for pediatric-specific major or common diseases and/or emergencies:

- Foreign body (upper and lower) airway obstruction (pp 2021-2022)
- Lower airway reactive disease (pp 2024-2025)
- Respiratory arrest distress/failure (pp 2019-2020)
- Shock (pp 2035-2040)
- Seizures (pp 2046-2048)
- Sudden infant death syndrome (SIDS) (p 2062)
- Gastrointestinal disease (pp 2049-2051)
- Bacterial tracheitis (p 2023)
- Asthma (p 2024)
- Bronchiolitis (pp 2024-2025)
  - Respiratory Synctial Virus (RSV) (pp 2024-2025)
- Pneumonia (p 2025)
- Croup (pp 2022-2023)
- Epiglottitis (p 2023)
- Hyperglycemia (pp 2051-2052)
- Hypoglycemia (p 2053)
- Pertussis (p 2025)
- Cystic fibrosis (p 2025)
- Bronchopulmonary dysplasia (pp 2025-2026)
- Congenital heart disease (pp 2043-2044)
- Hydrocephalus and ventricular shunts (pp 2048-2049)

Patients With Special Challenges

- Recognizing and reporting abuse and neglect (pp 2060-2062 and see chapter, *Geriatric Emergencies*)

Health care implications of

- Abuse (pp 2060-2062 and see chapters, *Geriatric Emergencies* and *Patients With Special Challenges*)
- Neglect (pp 2060-2062 and see chapters, *Geriatric Emergencies* and *Patients With Special Challenges*)
- Homelessness (see chapter, *Patients With Special Challenges*)
- Poverty (see chapter, *Patients With Special Challenges*)
- Bariatrics (see chapter, *Patients With Special Challenges*)

- Technology dependent (see chapter, *Patients With Special Challenges*)
- Hospice/terminally ill (see chapter, *Patients With Special Challenges*)
- Tracheostomy care/dysfunction (see chapter, *Patients With Special Challenges*)
- Home care (see chapter, *Patients With Special Challenges*)
- Sensory deficit/loss (see chapter, *Patients With Special Challenges*)
- Developmental disability (see chapter, *Patients With Special Challenges*)

Trauma

Integrates assessment findings with principles of epidemiology and pathophysiology to formulate a field impression to implement a comprehensive treatment/disposition plan for an acutely injured patient.

Special Considerations in Trauma

Recognition and management of trauma in

- Pregnant patient (see chapter, *Obstetrics*)
- Pediatric patient (pp 2063-2068)
- Geriatric patient (see chapter, *Geriatric Emergencies*)

Pathophysiology, assessment, and management of trauma in the

- Pregnant patient (see chapter, *Obstetrics*)
- Pediatric patient (pp 2063-2068)
- Geriatric patient (see chapter, *Geriatric Emergencies*)
- Cognitively impaired patient (see chapter, *Patients With Special Challenges*)

Knowledge Objectives

1. Explain some of the challenges inherent in providing emergency care to pediatric patients and why effective communication with both the patient and his or her family members is critical to a successful outcome. (p 2004)
2. Describe the developmental stages of children, including examples of each stage. (pp 2005-2007)
3. Describe differences in the anatomy, physiology, and pathophysiology of the pediatric patient as compared with the adult patient and their implications for the health care provider. (pp 2007-2010)
4. Describe the challenges in dealing with the stressed parents or caregivers of ill and injured children. (pp 2010-2011)
5. Describe the steps in the primary assessment for providing emergency care to a pediatric patient, including the elements of the pediatric assessment triangle (PAT), hands-on ABCs, and transport decision considerations. (pp 2011-2017)
6. Describe the steps in the secondary assessment, including the systematic assessment, which may include a full-body examination or a focused assessment on the body part or body system specifically involved. (pp 2017-2018)
7. Describe the different causes of pediatric respiratory emergencies; the signs and symptoms of increased work of breathing; the difference between respiratory distress, respiratory arrest, and respiratory failure;

and the emergency medical care strategies used in the management of each. (pp 2019-2035)

8. Describe upper airway emergencies in a pediatric patient, including anaphylaxis, croup, epiglottitis, and bacterial tracheitis; their possible causes, signs and symptoms; and steps in the management of a child who is experiencing these conditions. (pp 2021-2023)

9. List the steps in the management of foreign body airway obstruction of an infant and child. (pp 2021-2022)

10. Describe lower airway emergencies in a pediatric patient, including asthma, bronchiolitis, pneumonia, and pertussis; their possible causes, signs and symptoms; and steps in the management of a child who is experiencing these conditions. (pp 2024-2025)

11. Discuss other respiratory conditions, including cystic fibrosis and bronchopulmonary dysplasia; their possible causes, signs, and symptoms; and steps in the management of a child who is experiencing these conditions. (pp 2025-2026)

12. Discuss the most common causes of shock (hypoperfusion) in a pediatric patient, its signs and symptoms, and emergency medical management in the field. (pp 2035-2040)

13. Describe the procedure for establishing IV access in the pediatric patient. (pp 2036-2039)

14. Discuss the steps to establish an IO infusion in pediatric patients. (pp 2036-2039)

15. Describe common pediatric heart rhythm disturbances and how to manage each dysrhythmia. (pp 2040-2043)

16. Discuss the most common causes of altered mental status (AMS) in a pediatric patient, its signs and symptoms, and emergency medical management in the field. (pp 2045-2046)

17. List the common causes of seizures in a pediatric patient, the different types of seizures, and their emergency medical management in the field. (pp 2046-2048)

18. List the common causes of meningitis, patient groups who are at the highest risk for contracting it, its signs and symptoms, special precautions, and emergency medical management in the field. (p 2048)

19. Discuss the types of gastrointestinal emergencies that might affect pediatric patients, including intussusception, Meckel diverticulum, and pyloric stenosis. (pp 2049-2051)

20. Discuss the pathophysiology, assessment, and management of endocrine emergencies, including hyperglycemia, hypoglycemia, and congenital adrenal hyperplasia. (pp 2051-2054)

21. Describe conditions in which the pituitary produces inadequate amounts of some or all of its hormones. (pp 2053-2054)

22. Describe special considerations in patients with childhood immunodeficiencies. (pp 2054-2056)

23. Discuss hematologic disorders, including sickle cell disease, hemophilia, and thrombocytopenia; signs and symptoms; special precautions; and emergency medical management in the field. (pp 2054-2056)

24. Discuss toxicologic emergencies in pediatric patients, including common sources, assessment findings, and techniques for emergency medical management including decontamination and antidotes. (pp 2056-2058)

25. Describe special considerations during the management of a pediatric behavioral or psychiatric emergency, including safety precautions and assessment and management techniques. (pp 2058-2059)

26. Discuss the common causes of a fever emergency in a pediatric patient and management techniques. (pp 2059-2060)

27. Describe child abuse and neglect and its possible indicators, and then describe the medical and legal responsibilities when caring for a pediatric patient who is a possible victim of child abuse. (pp 2060-2062)

28. Discuss sudden infant death syndrome (SIDS), including its risk factors, patient assessment, and special management considerations related to the death of an infant patient. (p 2062)

29. Discuss the common causes of pediatric trauma emergencies, and differentiate between injury patterns in adults, infants, and children. (p 2063)

30. Describe the procedure for performing needle decompression in the pediatric patient. (pp 2063-2065)

31. List the steps to immobilize an infant and a child. (pp 2065-2067)

32. Describe the indications for fluid and pain management for a pediatric trauma patient. (pp 2067-2068)

33. Discuss the significance of burns in pediatric patients, common causes, and general assessment and management techniques. (pp 2068-2069)

34. Describe the needs of technology-assisted children, including the various types of medical technology used. (pp 2069-2070)

35. Describe injury patterns and identify potential areas for intervention and prevention. (p 2071)

Skills Objectives

1. Demonstrate the steps for removal of an upper airway obstruction with Magill forceps. (p 2022)

2. Demonstrate the steps for inserting an oropharyngeal airway in a child. (pp 2026-2027, Skill Drill 1)

3. Demonstrate the steps for inserting a nasopharyngeal airway in a child. (pp 2027-2028, Skill Drill 2)

4. Demonstrate how to perform bag-mask ventilation for an infant or child. (pp 2029-2031, Skill Drill 3)

5. Demonstrate the steps to perform endotracheal intubation in an infant or a child. (pp 2031-2034, Skill Drill 4)

6. Describe how to insert an orogastric and nasogastric tube in a pediatric patient, including how to prepare the patient, the equipment, and assess the placement of the tubes. (pp 2034-2035)

7. Demonstrate how to establish intraosseous access in pediatric patients. (pp 2036-2039, Skill Drill 5)

8. Demonstrate how to perform needle decompression in a child. (pp 2063-2065, Skill Drill 6)

9. Demonstrate how to immobilize a child who has been involved in a trauma emergency. (pp 2065-2066, Skill Drill 7)

10. Demonstrate how to immobilize an infant who has been involved in a trauma emergency. (pp 2065-2067, Skill Drill 8)

Introduction

Children differ anatomically, physiologically, and emotionally from adults. In addition, the types of illnesses and injuries they sustain and their responses to them vary across the pediatric age span. Sick or injured children present unique challenges in evaluation and management. Their perceptions of their illness or injury, their world, and you differ from the perceptions of adults. Depending on their age, they may not be able to report what is bothering them. Fear or pain may make children difficult to assess as well. In addition, you will have to work with concerned parents and caregivers who may be stressed or frightened and acting irrationally. In the midst of this chaos, you are expected to be an island of calm and authority, carrying out your job systematically, carefully, and confidently Figure 1 .

The manner in which you approach a sick or injured child will depend on the child's age and developmental level. Childhood extends from the neonatal period, just after birth, until age 18 years. An enormous amount of physical and psychological development occurs in these 18 years. A child's anatomy, physiology, and psychosocial development will all influence your assessment and treatment. For these reasons, you must tailor your approach to accommodate the developmental and social issues unique to pediatric patients.

This chapter addresses some of the special considerations that will enhance your effectiveness in caring for an ill or injured child. It begins by discussing the approach to pediatric patients, with an eye toward their developmental level and the anatomic or physiologic differences unique to the age group. This information is used to outline an approach to pediatric assessment, review specific pediatric emergencies, and address their prehospital management. Finally, the chapter details the skills needed to care efficiently and effectively for pediatric patients, regardless of the diagnosis.

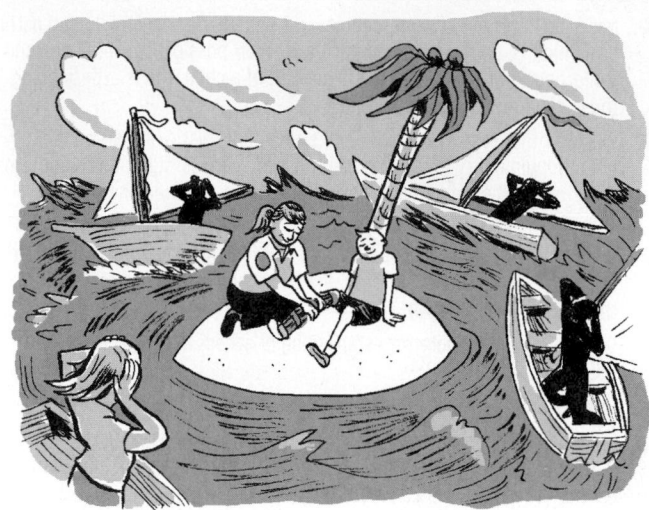

The paramedic is asked to be an island of calm and authority.

Figure 1

YOU are the Medic   PART 1

You and your partner are sitting down for lunch when dispatch sends you to an apartment for a sick child. You are met at the door by a 14-year-old girl. She is crying and saying she can't wake up her brother. She brings you into the living room where you see a 3-year-old boy lying supine on the couch. The girl tells you that she and her brother were watching television and fell asleep. She woke up and found that she could not wake her brother. She became scared and called 9-1-1.

Recording Time: 1 Minute	
Appearance	Toddler lying on the couch who appears to be asleep
Level of consciousness	U (unresponsive to verbal or painful stimuli)
Airway	Open
Breathing	Adequate rate and volume; no retractions or audible sounds
Circulation	Pale, cold, dry skin, with some mottling noted to the extremities; absent radial pulses and weak central pulses

1. Using the Pediatric Assessment Triangle as a guide, what is your general impression of the child?

2. What information would you like to get from the sister?

Developmental Stages

The growth and development of infants, toddlers, preschoolers, school-age children, and adolescents are discussed in the chapter, *Life Span Development*. Refer to that chapter to familiarize yourself with pediatric physical and psychosocial stages of development. Infancy and toddlerhood have their own specific phases that are discussed in detail in the next section.

Neonate and Infant

The first month of life is called the neonatal period, whereas infancy refers to the first 12 months of life. Neonates do not do much, other than eat, sleep for up to 16 hours per day, and cry in order to communicate. This can be a particularly difficult time for new parents, adjusting to a demanding schedule. See the chapter, *Neonatal Care*, for more information about infants that are younger than age 1 month. As infants reach the 2- to 6-month threshold, they begin to hold their heads up and seek attention. At 6 to 12 months, infants begin to crawl and babble. A great deal of development occurs in this interval Table 1.

Because infants cannot communicate their feelings or needs verbally, it is especially important to respect a caregiver's perception that "something is wrong." Persistent crying, irritability, and lack of eye contact may be a symptom of a serious problem such as a bacterial infection, a cardiac problem, depressed mental status, or an electrolyte disturbance. Nonspecific concerns about a young infant's behavior, feeding, sleep pattern, or arousability may be tip-offs to a serious underlying illness or injury.

You should also pay particular attention to the child's stage of development because increased mobility in an infant or toddler can often lead to injury. Any behaviors out of line with development (ie, a 2-month-old infant that reportedly sustained injuries from rolling off of a couch) should increase your suspicion for the possibility of abuse; the history should match the child's developmental stage.

Consider the best location for performing your assessment and keep the child warm to avoid hypothermia. Support the head and neck of young infants. Although separating a 2-week-old infant from a parent will not cause distress, an older infant in stable condition will be calmest in a parent's arms. Make sure that your hands and stethoscope are warm—a startled, crying infant will be difficult to examine. Be opportunistic with your exam, use a soft voice, and smile. If the child is quiet, listen to the heart and lungs first. If a young infant starts crying, letting the infant suck on a pacifier or gloved finger may quiet the child enough to allow you to complete your assessment. Jingling keys or shining a penlight may distract an older infant long enough for you to finish an exam. Do not provide small objects that pose a risk of aspiration.

Toddler

The toddler period includes the ages from 1 to 3 years. It includes the "terrible twos," a behavioral manifestation of the child's struggle between continued dependence on caregivers for food, shelter, and love and his or her emerging drive for independence Table 2. Children in this age group are not capable of reasoning, and they have a poorly developed sense of cause and effect. Language development is occurring rapidly, along with the ability to explore the world by crawling, walking, running, and climbing. Many toddlers will develop associations—possibly negative—with health care providers. Painful procedures may make lasting impressions.

Your assessment of a toddler begins with observation of the child's interactions with the caregiver, vocalizations, and mobility, measured through the Pediatric Assessment Triangle (PAT), which is described in detail later. Examine a toddler in stable condition on the parent's lap in order to avoid separation anxiety. Get down to the child's level, sitting or squatting for the exam. Talk to the child throughout the assessment. You may need to be creative to perform a good exam on a toddler with stranger anxiety: Use a parent to lift the shirt so that you can count the respiratory rate, or have the parent press on the abdomen to see if that appears painful. Use play and distraction techniques whenever possible—listening to a doll's chest first may buy you a few minutes of cooperation. Offer toddlers limited choices when possible because they like to be in control. If you ask yes or no questions, the answer is likely to be "No!" Consider saving the more upsetting parts of

Table 1	Infant Development		
	Birth–2 months	**2–6 months**	**6–12 months**
Physical Development	■ Controls gaze ■ Turns head	■ Can recognize caregivers ■ Makes eye contact ■ Uses both hands ■ Rolls over ■ Most sleep through the night	■ Sits without support ■ Crawls ■ Puts things in mouth ■ Teething begins ■ Eats soft foods
Cognitive Development	■ Begins crying to communicate needs ■ Crying peaks at 6 weeks	■ Increased awareness ■ Explores their own body	■ Babbles (learns first word by 12 months) ■ Remembers objects ■ Curious about what objects do
Emotional Development	■ Trust develops in parents	■ Uses expressions of joy, anger, fear, surprise ■ Seeks attention	■ Separation anxiety develops ■ Start of tantrums ■ Self-determination while eating

Table 2 Toddler Development

	12–18 months	18–24 months	24–36 months
Physical Development	▪ Crawls ▪ Walks ▪ Front teeth emerge ahead of molars ▪ Sensory development	▪ Improved gait and balance ▪ Runs ▪ Climbs ▪ Head grows more slowly than body	▪ Develops fine motor skills ▪ Toilet training ▪ Goes up and down stairs with help ▪ Jumps with both feet ▪ Can draw a circle
Cognitive Development	▪ Imitates others ▪ Makes believe ▪ Understands more than expressed ▪ Knows major body parts ▪ Knows 4–6 words	▪ Begins to understand cause/effect ▪ Labels objects ▪ Speech picks up to ~100 words by 24 months	▪ Follows 2-step commands ▪ Names at least 1 color ▪ Knows 250–500 Words
Emotional Development	▪ Basic reasoning ▪ Understands object permanence ▪ Separation anxiety	▪ Attachment to certain objects, such as a pacifier, doll, or blanket	▪ Can name a friend ▪ Separates fairly easily from parents

the exam, such as palpating a tender abdomen or examining an injured extremity, for last. Be flexible in your approach—some toddlers will not let you complete an orderly head-to-toe exam.

■ Preschool-Age Child

During the preschool years (3 to 5 years), the child is becoming rapidly verbal and active. He or she can understand directions and be engaged with an activity or set of goals. Generally, a preschooler will be able to tell you what hurts and may have a story to share about the illness or injury. Preschoolers will understand as you explain what you are going to do, but choose your words carefully because preschoolers are literal. Saying "I'm going take your pulse" may lead preschoolers to believe that you are taking something from them and wonder if you plan to give it back! Speak to them in plain language about what you are going to do and provide lots of reassurance—this is the stage of monsters under the bed and many other fears. At this age, they often believe that their thoughts or wishes can cause injury or harm to themselves or to others. They may believe that an injury is the result of a bad deed they did earlier in the day.

Words of Wisdom

Keep infants and young children close to their parents during your assessment to help them feel safe and to improve your ability to perform the assessment.

By age 4 years, the child develops 20/20 vision and performs normal running and walking, in addition to throwing, catching, and kicking as a school-age child would. Right or left handedness is also discovered.

As you perform your assessment, take advantage of the child's curiosity, rich fantasy life, and desire to cooperate. Respect their modesty by keeping them covered. If the child is in medically stable condition, offer to take turns in listening to the heart and lungs. Let the preschooler play with or hold equipment that

is safe. To help give the child some sense of control, offer simple choices and avoid procedures on the dominant hand or arm. Tantrums may occur when preschool-age children feel they cannot control the situation or its outcomes. Avoid yes or no questions. Set limits on behavior if the child acts out. Children at this age know what acceptable behavior is. Appeal to their thinking, and you should be able to talk a preschooler through an orderly exam.

■ School-Age Child (Middle Childhood)

As a child enters the school-age period (6 to 12 years), he or she becomes much more analytic and capable of abstract thought. School is important at this stage and concerns about popularity and peer pressure occupy a great deal of time and energy. At this age, the child can understand cause and effect. Children with chronic illness or disabilities can become self-conscious because of concerns about fitting in with their peers. At this stage, children begin to understand that death is final, which may increase their anxieties about illness or injury. School-age children will have their own stories to tell about the illness or injury and may have their own ideas about the care to be given. By age 8 years, the child's anatomy and physiology are similar to those of adults. Girls develop breasts between ages 8 and 13 years, and their menstrual period begins between ages 9 and 16 years. Boys experience an increase in the size of their testicles around age 10 years. Children at this age may be self-conscious about their body image.

During assessment of a school-age child, ask the child about the history leading to calling 9-1-1 and let the child describe the symptoms, rather than focusing on the caregiver. Explain what you plan to do in simple language, and answer the child's questions. Give the child appropriate choices and control whenever possible, and provide ongoing reassurance and encouragement.

School-age children can understand the difference between emotional and physical pain. They also have concerns about the meaning of pain. Give them simple explanations about what is causing their pain and what will be done about it. Respect the patient's modesty and keep them covered as much as possible during your examination. Games and conversation may distract them. Asking about school will often allow them to warm up to you. Ask them to describe their favorite place, their pets, or their toys. Ask the caregiver's advice in choosing the right distraction.

Rewarding the school-age child after a procedure can be helpful in his or her recovery, but only reward a child for completing the procedure.

Adolescence

The adolescent years, from 13 to 17 years, can be difficult. Adolescents are struggling with issues of independence, body image, sexuality, and peer pressure. Friends are key support figures, and this is a time of experimentation and risk-taking behaviors. Adolescents begin to understand who they are, and develop morals and the ability to reason. Relationships may shift from same sex to those with the opposite sex. With respect to CPR and foreign body airway obstruction procedures, once secondary sexual characteristics have developed (breasts or facial/axillary hair), the child should be treated as an adult. During the assessment, you must address and reassure the patient. Failure to do so can result in the adolescent feeling left out of his or her own care, which can alienate the patient, making it difficult for you to get an accurate assessment or give appropriate treatment. Encourage the patient's questions and involvement. Address all concerns and fears. Also, provide accurate information—a teen may become alienated and uncooperative if you are suspected of being misleading. When you perform the physical exam, respect the patient's privacy. If possible, address the adolescent without a caregiver present, especially about sensitive topics such as sexuality or drug use. If the adolescent's friends are on scene, he or she may want them to remain during the assessment. Let the patient have as much control over the situation as appropriate. Of course, do not let down your guard regarding scene safety.

Pediatric Anatomy, Physiology, and Pathophysiology

Anatomic and physiologic differences can create difficulties with your assessment of the child if you do not understand them. This section provides an overview of the anatomic and physiologic differences of children.

Special Populations

Children have more head injuries than adults because of their large heads.

The Head

When you are looking at an infant or young child, you will note that children have heads that are large relative to the rest of their bodies. In fact, an infant's head is already two thirds the size it will be in adulthood. The large surface area means more mass relative to the rest of the body—an important factor in the incidence of head injuries in young patients, who tend to lead with

their head in a fall. Traumatic brain injury is the leading cause of death and significant disability in pediatric trauma patients.

Because of the proportionally larger occiput, special care must be taken when you are positioning the child's airway. In seriously injured children younger than 3 years, place a thin layer of padding under the back to obtain a neutral position. In seriously ill children younger than 3 years, place a folded sheet under the occiput to obtain a sniffing position. The large head also means more surface area for heat loss. Always keep the child's head covered to provide warmth.

During infancy, the anterior and posterior fontanelles are open. The fontanelles are areas where the infant's skull bones have not fused together, thus allowing compression of the head during the birthing process and for rapid growth of the brain. By the time the child reaches 4 months, the posterior fontanelles close; by the time the child reaches 1 year, the anterior fontanelles close.

The fontanelles are an important anatomic landmark when you are assessing a sick or injured infant. Bulging of the fontanelles suggests increased intracranial pressure; sunken fontanelles suggest dehydration. These conditions will be discussed later in this chapter.

The Neck and Airway

Children have short, stubby necks, which can make it difficult for you to feel a carotid pulse or see jugular veins. Not surprisingly, the airway of a young child is also much smaller than an adult airway. That smaller diameter makes the airway more prone to obstruction, either by foreign body inhalation, inflammation with infection, or the child's disproportionately large tongue. During the first few months of life, infants are obligate nose breathers, and nasal obstruction with mucus can result in significant respiratory distress. Their epiglottis is long, floppy, U-shaped, and narrow, extending at a 45° angle into the airway, making it difficult to visualize the vocal cords during intubation. Finally, the narrowest part of a young child's airway occurs at the level of the cricoid cartilage below the vocal cords, rather than at the vocal cords as in adults; this issue should influence your choice of endotracheal (ET) tubes.

You must have a thorough understanding of the anatomic and physiologic differences in the child's airway to provide appropriate management. With the aforementioned anatomic differences, it is important for you to remember the following:

- Keep the nares clear with suctioning in infants younger than 6 months.
- The tracheal cartilage is softer and more collapsible as compared with an adult; avoid hyperextension of the child's neck. Hyperextension may result in reverse hyperflexion and kinking of the trachea and may also displace the tongue posteriorly, creating an airway obstruction.
- Keep the airway clear of all secretions; even a small amount of particulate matter may result in an airway obstruction.
- Use care when you are managing the child's airway, such as when you are inserting airway adjuncts; the jaw is smaller than an adult's jaw and the soft tissues are delicate and prone to swelling. In many cases, the child's airway can be maintained by correct positioning, thereby negating the use of airway adjuncts (that is, oral or nasal airways).

The Respiratory System

Proportionally, tidal volume in children is slightly smaller than in adults. However, the metabolic oxygen demand of children is doubled. In addition, their functional residual capacity is smaller, resulting in proportionally smaller oxygen reserves. Functional residual capacity is the volume of air remaining in the lungs following exhalation, also referred to as oxygen reserve.

An infant breathes faster than an older child. The child's lungs will grow and develop better abilities to handle the exchange of oxygen as the child ages. A respiratory rate of 30 to 60 breaths/min is normal for newborns, whereas teenagers are expected to have rates closer to the adult range Table 3.

The higher respiratory rate and oxygen demand needed to meet the higher metabolic rate of infants and children puts them at higher risk for effects from inhaled toxins. Children typically inhale a proportionately larger amount of toxic fumes than adults and become symptomatic sooner.

Infants have little use of their chest muscles to make their chests expand during inspiration; they use the diaphragm (belly breathers). Anything that puts pressure on the abdomen of an infant or young child can block the movement of the diaphragm and cause respiratory compromise. Young children also experience muscle fatigue much more quickly than older children, which can lead to respiratory failure if a child has had to breathe hard for long periods.

You must be aware that infants and children, especially during respiratory distress, are highly susceptible to hypoxia because of their decreased functional residual capacity, increased oxygen demand, and easily fatigued respiratory muscles. Infants and children will develop hypoxia rapidly with apnea and ineffective bagging and can spiral into cardiovascular collapse. Use a larger bag if needed to ventilate a pediatric patient, but use only enough pressure to achieve visible chest rise in order to avoid pneumothorax. The bag's volume should have no less than 450–500 mL.

The Cardiovascular System

It is important for you to know the normal pulse rate ranges when you are evaluating children because this is the primary method for the child's body to compensate for decreased oxygenation Table 4. Children rely mainly on their pulse rate to maintain adequate cardiac output. An infant's pulse rate can be 200 beats/min or more if the body needs to compensate for injury or illness.

Children have limited but vigorous cardiac reserves. Proportionally, they have a larger circulating blood volume compared with adults; however, their absolute blood volume is less, approximately 70 mL/kg. The ability of a child to constrict blood vessels (vasoconstriction) provides the ability to keep vital organs well perfused.

Because a child's circulating blood volume is large compared with an adult's, injured children can maintain their blood pressure for longer periods than adults, even though they are still in shock (hypoperfusion). In other words, a proportionally larger volume of blood loss must occur in the child before hypotension develops.

Suspect shock when an infant or child presents with tachycardia. Bradycardia, however, usually indicates severe hypoxia and must be managed aggressively. Remember that hypotension, when it occurs in a child, is an ominous sign and often indicates impending cardiopulmonary arrest.

Constriction of the blood vessels can be so profound that blood flow to the periphery of the body diminishes. Signs of vasoconstriction can include weak peripheral (for example, radial) pulses, delayed capillary refill (in children younger than 6 years), and pale, cool extremities.

Special Populations

When you are assessing a sick or injured child, be aware that bradycardia is most often the result of hypoxia; therefore, treatment is aimed at ensuring adequate oxygenation and ventilation. In addition, despite the presence of a normal blood pressure, a child, even more so than an adult, may still be in shock.

The Heart

Circulation in the fetus is much different from that in the newborn, and large right-sided forces on the electrocardiogram (ECG) are normal in young infants. During the first year

Table 3 Pediatric Respiratory Rates	
Age	Respirations (breaths/min)
Neonate: 0 to 1 month	30 to 60
Infant: 1 month to 1 year	25 to 50
Toddler: 1 to 3 years	20 to 30
Preschool-age: 3 to 5 years	20 to 25
School-age: 6 to 12 years	15 to 20
Adolescent: 13 to 17 years	12 to 20
Adult: Older than 18 years	12 to 20

Table 4 Pediatric Pulse Rates	
Age	Pulse Rate (beats/min)
Neonate: 0 to 1 month	100 to 180
Infant: 1 month to 1 year	100 to 160
Toddler: 1 to 3 years	90 to 150
Preschool-age: 3 to 5 years	80 to 140
School-age: 6 to 12 years	70 to 120
Adolescent: 13 to 17 years	60 to 100
Adult: Older than 18 years	60 to 100

of life, the ECG axis and voltages shift to reflect left ventricular dominance. Cardiac output is rate-dependent in infants and young children. They have relatively poor ability to increase stroke volume, which is reflected in their normal pulse rates (higher in newborns than in older children and adults) and in rate response to physiologic stress and hypovolemia.

The mediastinum of pediatric patients is more mobile than adults. This is important to remember when you are dealing with pediatric trauma or abuse cases because these patients are at a high risk of injury to mediastinal organs that may not be immediately evident on exam. Cardiac tamponade can present with muffled heart tones, whereas cardiac contusions can cause dysrhythmias.

The Nervous System

The nervous system continually develops throughout childhood. Until the nervous system is fully developed, the neural tissue and vasculature are fragile, easily damaged, and prone to bleeding from injury. The brain and spinal cord are not as well protected by the developing skull and spinal vertebrae.

Because the brain and spinal cord are less well protected, it takes less force to cause brain and spinal cord injuries in children than in adults. Brain injuries in young children, when they occur, are frequently more devastating.

The subarachnoid space in a child is relatively smaller than that of an adult, providing less cushioning effect for the brain. Bruising and damage to the brain may be the result of head momentum such as seen with "shaken baby syndrome." The pediatric brain also requires nearly twice the cerebral blood flow as an adult's brain, making even minor injuries significant. This requirement increases the risk of hypoxia. Head injuries are greatly exacerbated by hypoxia and hypotension, causing ongoing damage.

The brain continues to develop after birth. As the brain matures, the infant's responses to the environment, outside stimuli, and even pain become more organized and purposeful. The rapidity of brain development can be appreciated by comparing the abilities and interactions of a 4-day-old infant, whose repertoire is limited to eating, sleeping, and defecating, with those of a 4-month-old infant, who smiles socially, rolls over, and plays with a rattle, and with those of a 12-month-old infant, who walks, is beginning to talk, and expresses preferences for people and activities.

The Spinal Column

The vertebral column develops along with the child. When the child is younger, the cervical spine fulcrum (or bending point) is higher, closer to C1-C2, because the head is heavier. As the child grows, the fulcrum descends to "adult level," around C5 through C7. An infant who sustains blunt head trauma involving acceleration-deceleration forces is at high risk for a fatal, high cervical spinal injury. By comparison, a school-age child who experiences the same injury will likely sustain a lower cervical spinal injury and may be paralyzed.

Fortunately, vertebral fractures and spinal cord injuries in young children are uncommon. Spinal ligaments and joint capsules are more lax in children than in adults, leading to increased mobility and the phenomenon of cord injury in the absence of identifiable vertebral bony fracture or dislocation. Vertebral bodies are also aligned anteriorly and can slide forward, potentially causing cord damage with significant forward flexion.

Words of Wisdom

Spinal cord injuries with normal-appearing radiographs are referred to as SCIWORA (spinal cord injury without radiographic abnormalities).

Thoracic and lumbar spinal injuries are also encountered relatively infrequently until a child is pursuing adult activities, such as driving and diving. Nevertheless, these injuries are seen in children in association with specific mechanisms—for example, seat belt-associated lumbar spine injuries (often associated with abdominal injury) and compression fracture due to axial loading in a fall. When you are confronted with a significant mechanism of injury (MOI), the safest course is to assume that the child has a cervical spine injury and transport with spinal immobilization precautions.

The Abdomen and Pelvis

Abdominal injuries are the second leading cause of serious trauma in children (after head injuries). Abdominal organs are situated more anteriorly. As a result, they are less protected by the ribs and are closer together as compared with an adult. In addition, organs such as the liver and spleen are relatively large, making them vulnerable to blunt trauma. The appearance of abdominal distention in a healthy infant is due to two factors: the weak abdominal wall muscles and the larger size of the solid organs.

The liver and the spleen extend below the rib cage in young children and, therefore, do not have as much bony protection as they do in adults. These organs have a rich blood supply, so injuries to them can result in large blood losses. The kidneys are also more vulnerable to injury in children because they are more mobile and less well supported than in adults. Finally, the duodenum and pancreas are likely to be damaged in handlebar injuries. As the child grows, the organs become more proportionate and better protected. In the meantime, remember that even seemingly insignificant forces can cause serious internal injury and that multiple organ injuries are common.

Pelvic fractures are relatively rare in young children and are generally seen only with high-energy MOIs. The risk for pelvic fracture increases in adolescence, when the skeleton and MOIs become more like those of adults.

Special Populations

Because of children's shorter rib cages and less well-developed abdominal musculature, you should expect more intra-abdominal injuries in pediatric patients than in adults.

The Musculoskeletal System

Reaching adult height requires active bone growth. The growth plates (<u>ossification centers</u>) of a child's bones are made of cartilage, are relatively weak, and are easily fractured. As a consequence, the bones of growing children are weaker than their ligaments and tendons, making fractures more common than sprains. Joint dislocations without associated fractures are not common. Bones finish growing at differing times, but most growth plates will be closed by late adolescence.

Growth plate fractures can be seen with low-energy MOIs, and they may be lacking the degree of tenderness, swelling, and bruising usually associated with a broken bone. Immobilize all sprains or strains and suspect fractures; growth plate injuries may result in poor bone growth.

The Chest and Lungs

Chest trauma is the third leading cause of serious injury in pediatric trauma. A child's chest wall is quite thin, with less musculature and less subcutaneous fat to protect ribs and organs. A child's ribs, however, are more pliable and flexible than those of an adult. This increased laxity and flexibility can lead to significant intrathoracic injury with minimal external findings. Children often have fewer rib fractures and flail chest events, but injuries to the thoracic organs may be more severe because the pliable rib cage and fragile lung tissue are more easily compressed during blunt trauma. As a consequence, children are more vulnerable than adults to pulmonary contusions, cardiac tamponade, and diaphragmatic rupture. The lungs are also prone to pneumothorax from excessive pressures during bag-mask ventilation.

The thin chest wall makes it easy to hear heart and lung sounds; however, pneumothoraces and esophageal intubations are often missed due to sounds readily transmitted throughout the chest. The rib cage is more compliant, making retractions easy to see.

Be sure to look for signs of chest injuries in a child with suspected chest trauma, but note that the signs of pneumothorax or hemothorax in children are often subtle. You may not see signs such as jugular vein distention, and it may be difficult to determine tracheal deviation.

The Integumentary System

In comparison with adults, infants and children have thinner and more elastic skin, a larger body surface area (BSA)/weight ratio, and less subcutaneous (fatty) tissue.

The above factors contribute to the following:

- Increased risk of injury following exposure to temperature extremes
- Increased risk of hypothermia (can complicate resuscitative efforts) and dehydration
- Increased severity of burns
  - Many burns that would ordinarily be classified as minor or moderate in adults are classified as severe in children.

Infants and young children also have a relatively large surface area that predisposes them to hypothermia.

Metabolic Differences

Infants and children have limited stores of glycogen and glucose that are rapidly depleted as a result of injury or illness. You should maintain a high index of suspicion for hypoglycemia and check blood glucose levels in any patient with lethargy, seizures, or decreased activity. Because it takes glucose to produce energy and energy is required to maintain body temperature, children are highly susceptible to hypothermia. The risk of hypothermia is further increased because of the child's large BSA/weight ratio. When you are assessing and treating a newborn (neonate), you must remain aware that these young infants lack the ability to shiver—one of the body's ways of producing heat. Hypothermia is a serious risk and may predispose the newborn to spontaneous bleeding in the head.

Significant hypovolemia and electrolyte derangements are also more common in children as a result of severe vomiting and diarrhea.

It is critical to keep the child warm during transport and take measures to prevent the loss of body heat. To conserve body heat, be sure to cover the child's head, which because of its proportionally large size, is a source of significant heat loss. Newborns requiring aggressive resuscitation after delivery should not be overly warmed because this can worsen their neurologic outcome.

Parents of Ill or Injured Children

The majority of children you will treat will have at least one parent or caregiver present. Thus, in many pediatric calls, you will be dealing with more than one patient—even if only the child is ill or injured. Serious illness or injury to a child is one of the most stressful situations caregivers can face. Some may react to this stress by becoming angry—at the fact that their child is sick, at the person or situation that caused the injury, or at you simply because they need someone to blame! Other parents will be frightened or guilty about the circumstances that led to the illness or injury. Establishing a rapport with caregivers is vital, however, because they will be a source of important information and assistance. Children look to their parents when they are frightened and often mimic their response, so helping calm a parent may also help the patient cope.

Approach stressed caregivers in a calm, quiet, and professional manner. Enlist their help in caring for the child. Along the way, explain what you are doing and provide honest reassurance and support. Above all, do not blame the parent for what has happened. Finally, transport at least one caregiver with the child.

If the parent is extremely emotional, provide support, but remember that your first priority is the child. Do not let a distraught or aggressive parent interfere with your care. If necessary, enlist the help of other family members or law enforcement personnel.

Pediatric Patient Assessment

Just as your general approach to a pediatric patient differs somewhat from your approach to an adult patient, so, too, will your assessment. In particular, you may need to adapt your assessment skills. Ensure you have age-appropriate equipment and review age-appropriate vital signs in anticipation of potential developments.

Scene Size-up

On the way to the scene, prepare for a pediatric scene size-up, the use of pediatric equipment, and an age-appropriate physical assessment. If possible, collect information from dispatch on the age and gender of the child, the location of the scene, and the NOI or MOI.

As with any call, the scene size-up begins with ensuring that you and your partner have taken the appropriate standard precautions. On arriving at the scene, observe for any hazards or potential hazards that may pose a threat to you, your partner, or the patient. Resist the temptation to hastily access the patient because you know the patient is a child. Personal safety must always remain your priority.

As you enter the scene, note the position in which the child is found. Observe the area for clues to the MOI or NOI; these observations will help guide your assessment and management priorities. By looking and listening as you enter the scene, you should be able to determine the severity of the patient's illness or injury.

At a traumatic scene when the child is unable to communicate because of his or her developmental age or is unresponsive, assume that the MOI was significant enough to cause head or neck injuries. Spinal immobilization with a cervical collar should be performed if you suspect the MOI to be severe. Remember the need to pad under the pediatric patient's head and/or shoulders to facilitate a neutral position for airway management.

Note the presence of any pills, medicine bottles, alcohol, drug paraphernalia, or household chemicals that would suggest toxic exposure or possible ingestion by the child. If the child has been injured—a motor vehicle crash, fall, or pedestrian incident—carefully observe the scene or vehicle (if involved) for clues to the potential severity of the child's injuries.

You must not discount the possibility of child abuse. Conflicting information from the parents or caregivers, bruises or other injuries that are not consistent with the MOI described, or injuries that are not consistent with the child's age and developmental abilities should increase your index of suspicion for abuse. Observe and note the parents' or caregivers' interaction with the child. Do they appear to be appropriately concerned, angry, or indifferent? Does the child seem comforted by their presence or scared by them? Child abuse will be discussed in greater detail later in this chapter.

Primary Assessment

Using the Pediatric Assessment Triangle to Form a General Impression

After ensuring scene safety, the first step in the primary assessment of any patient begins with your general impression of how the patient looks (the "sick–not sick" classification). An assessment tool called the Pediatric Assessment Triangle (PAT) Figure 2 has been developed to help EMS providers form a "from-the-doorway" general impression of pediatric patients. Providers with experience in treating ill and injured children intuitively use some version of the PAT to make the important distinction between sick and not-sick patients. The PAT standardizes this approach by including three elements—the child's appearance, work of breathing, and circulation—that collectively paint an accurate clinical picture of the patient's cardiopulmonary status and level of consciousness. This 15- to 30-second assessment is conducted prior to assessing the ABCs and does not require touching the patient. It applies a rapid, hands-off systematic approach to observing an ill or injured child and helps establish urgency for treatment or transport.

Special Populations

Use the PAT to help with your hands-off, from-the-doorway general impression of pediatric patients.

Appearance

The first element of the PAT is the child's appearance. In many cases, this is the most important factor in determining the severity of illness, the need for treatment, and the response to therapy. Appearance reflects the adequacy of ventilation, oxygenation, brain perfusion, body homeostasis, and central nervous system (CNS) function. The TICLS (tickles) mnemonic highlights the most important features of a child's appearance:

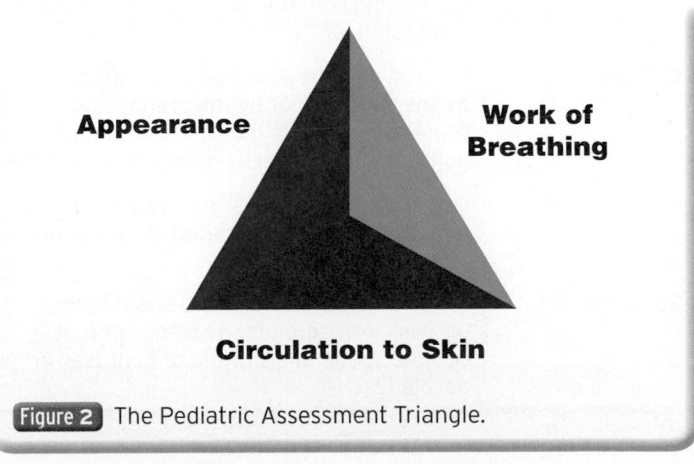

Figure 2 The Pediatric Assessment Triangle.

Tone, Interactiveness, Consolability, Look or gaze, and Speech or cry Table 5. In addition, you can evaluate the child's level of consciousness by using the AVPU scale, modified as necessary for the child's age.

To assess appearance, observe the child from a distance, allowing the child to interact with the caregiver as he or she chooses. Walk through the characteristics of the TICLS mnemonic while observing the child from the doorway. Delay touching the patient until you have developed your general impression because the child may become agitated by your touch. Unless a child is unconscious or critically ill, take your time in assessing his or her general appearance by observation before you begin the hands-on assessment and obtain vital signs. Figure 3 and Figure 4 demonstrate examples of an infant with a normal appearance and one with an abnormal appearance.

An abnormal appearance may result from numerous underlying physiologic abnormalities. A child may show evidence of inadequate oxygenation or ventilation, as in respiratory emergencies; inadequate brain perfusion, as from cardiovascular emergencies; systemic abnormalities or metabolic derangements, such as with poisoning, infection, or hypoglycemia; or acute or chronic brain injury. In any event, a child with a grossly abnormal appearance is seriously ill and requires immediate life-support interventions and transportation. The remainder of the PAT—work of breathing and circulation—plus the hands-on portion of the primary assessment (assessment of the ABCs) may help you identify the cause of the abnormal appearance and

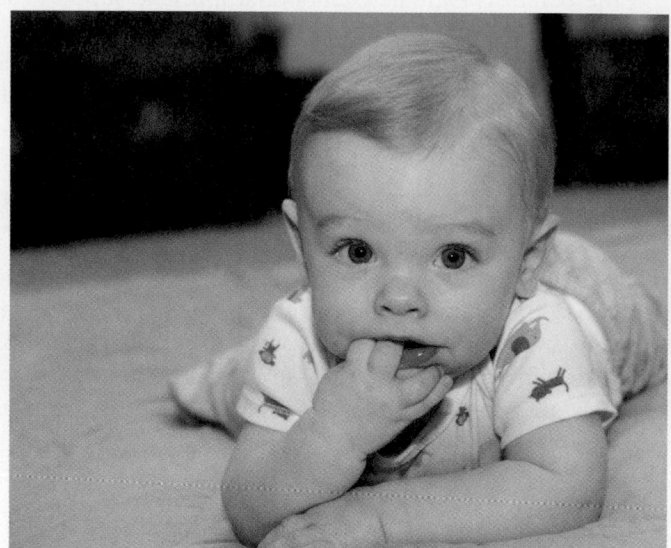

Figure 3 A child with a normal appearance. An infant or child who is not very sick will make good eye contact.

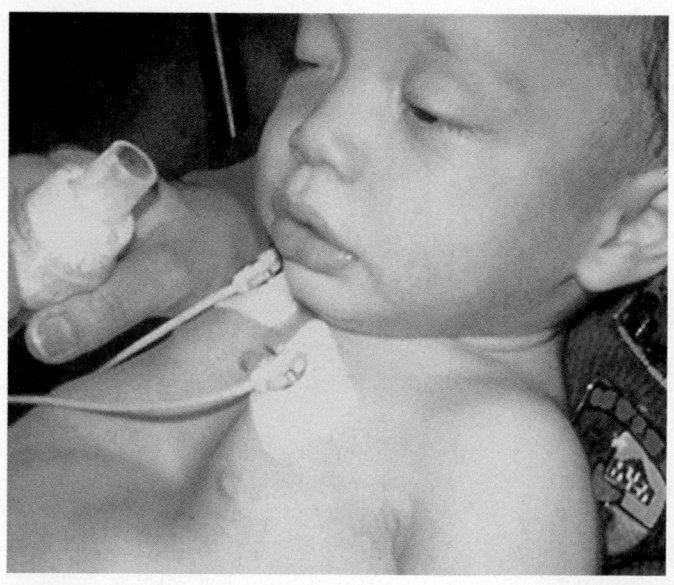

Figure 4 A child with an abnormal appearance. A limp child unable to maintain eye contact may be critically ill or injured.

determine the severity of a child's illness and the need for treatment and transportation.

Work of Breathing

A child's work of breathing is often a better assessment of his or her oxygenation and ventilation status than the auscultation or respiratory rate. The work of breathing reflects the child's attempt to compensate for abnormalities in oxygenation and ventilation, and, therefore, it is a proxy for effectiveness of gas exchange. The hands-off assessment of work of breathing includes listening for abnormal airway sounds and looking for signs of increased breathing effort Table 6.

Table 5	Characteristics of Appearance: The TICLS Mnemonic
Characteristic	**Features to Look For**
Tone	Is the child moving or resisting examination vigorously? Does the child have good muscle tone? Or is the child limp, listless, or flaccid?
Interactiveness	How alert is the child? How readily does a person, object, or sound distract the child or draw the child's attention? Will the child reach for, grasp, and play with a toy or exam instrument, like a penlight or tongue blade? Or is the child uninterested in playing or interacting with the caregiver or prehospital professional?
Consolability	Can the child be consoled or comforted by the caregiver or by the prehospital professional? Or is the child's crying or agitation unrelieved by gentle reassurance?
Look or gaze	Does the child fix his or her gaze on a face, or is there a "nobody home," glassy-eyed stare?
Speech or cry	Is the child's cry strong and spontaneous or weak or high-pitched? Is the content of speech age-appropriate or confused or garbled?

Table 6 Characteristics of Work of Breathing

Characteristic	Features to Look For
Abnormal airway sounds	Snoring, muffled or hoarse speech, stridor, grunting, or wheezing
Abnormal posturing	Sniffing position, tripod position, refusing to lie down
Retractions	Supraclavicular, intercostal, or substernal retractions of the chest wall; head bobbing in infants
Flaring	Flaring of the nares on inspiration

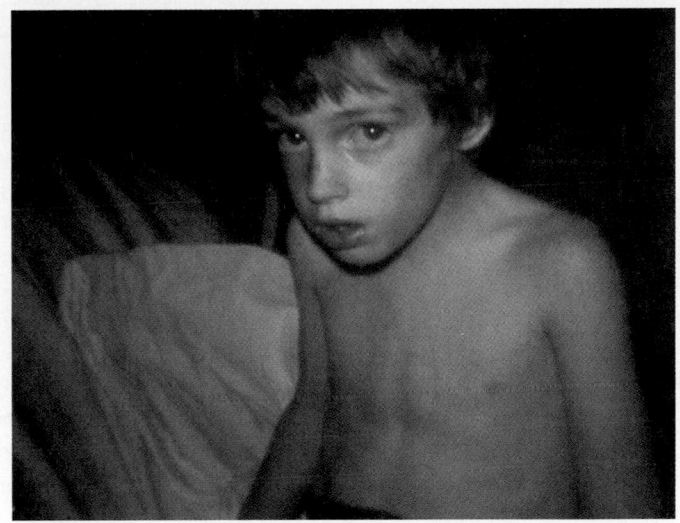

Figure 5 A child in the sniffing position is trying to align the airway to increase patency and improve airflow.

Some abnormal airway sounds can be heard without a stethoscope and can indicate the likely physiology and anatomic location of the breathing problem. For example, snoring, muffled or hoarse voice, or stridor (a harsh sound during inspiration, high-pitched due to partial upper airway obstruction) can indicate obstruction at the level of the oropharynx, glottis or supraglottic structures, or glottis or subglottic structures, respectively. Such an upper airway obstruction may result from croup, bacterial upper airway infections, bleeding, or edema.

Lower airway obstruction is suggested by abnormal grunting or wheezing. Grunting is a form of auto-PEEP (positive end-expiratory pressure), a way to distend the lower respiratory air sacs or alveoli to promote maximum gas exchange. **Grunting** involves exhaling against a partially closed glottis. This short, low-pitched sound is best heard at the end of exhalation and is often mistaken for whimpering. Grunting suggests moderate to severe hypoxia and is seen with lower airway conditions such as pneumonia and pulmonary edema. It reflects poor gas exchange because of fluid in the lower airways and air sacs. Wheezing is a musical tone caused by air being forced through constricted or partially blocked small airways. It often occurs during exhalation only but can occur during inspiration and expiration during severe asthma attacks. Although this sound is often heard only by auscultation, severe obstruction may result in wheezing that is audible even without a stethoscope.

Abnormal positioning and retractions are physical signs of increased work of breathing that can easily be assessed without touching the patient. A child who is in the **sniffing position** is trying to align the axes of the airways to improve patency and increase air flow **Figure 5**; such a position often reflects a severe upper airway obstruction. The child who refuses to lie down or who leans forward on outstretched arms (**tripoding**) is creating the optimal mechanical advantage to use accessory muscles of respiration **Figure 6**.

Retractions represent the recruitment of accessory muscles of respiration to provide more "muscle power" to move air into the lungs in the face of airway or lung disease or injury. To optimally observe retractions, expose the child's chest. Retractions are a more useful measure of work of breathing in children than in adults because a child's chest wall is less muscular, so the inward excursion of skin and soft tissue between the ribs is more apparent. Retractions may be evident in the supraclavicular area

(above the clavicle), the intercostal area (between the ribs), or the substernal area (under the sternum) **Figure 7**. Another form of retractions that is seen only in infants is head bobbing, the use of neck muscles to help breathing during severe hypoxia. The infant extends the neck as he or she inhales, then allows the head to fall forward during exhalation. Nasal flaring is the exaggerated opening of the nostrils during labored inspiration and indicates moderate to severe hypoxia.

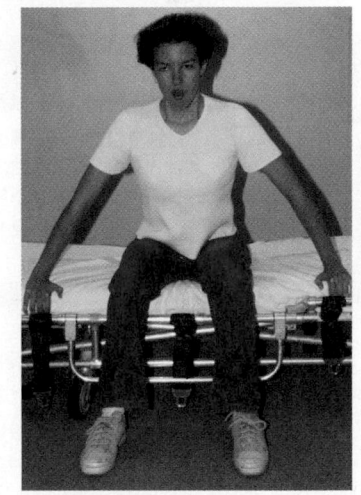

Figure 6 A child in the tripod position is maximizing his or her accessory muscles of respiration.

Combine the characteristics of work of breathing—abnormal airway sounds, abnormal positioning, retractions, and nasal flaring—to make your general assessment of the child's oxygenation and ventilation status. Together with the child's appearance, the child's work of breathing suggests the severity of the illness and the likelihood that the cause is in the airway or is a respiratory process.

Circulation to Skin

The goal of rapid circulatory assessment is to determine the adequacy of cardiac output and core perfusion. When cardiac output diminishes, the body responds by shunting circulation from nonessential areas (eg, skin) toward vital organs. Therefore, circulation to the skin reflects the overall

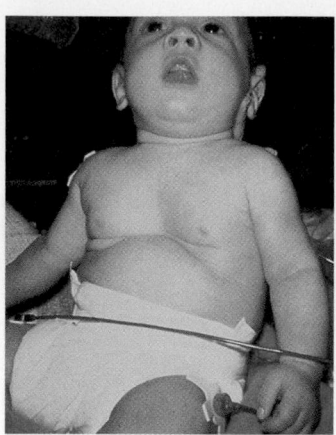

Figure 7 Retractions can occur in the suprasternal, intercostal, and substernal areas and indicate increased work of breathing.

status of core circulation. The three characteristics considered when you are assessing the circulation are pallor, mottling, and cyanosis **Table 7**.

Pallor or paleness may be the initial sign of poor circulation or even the only visual sign in a child with compensated shock. It indicates reflex peripheral vasoconstriction that is shunting blood toward the core. Pallor may also indicate anemia or hypoxia.

Mottling reflects vasomotor instability in the capillary beds demonstrated by patchy areas of vasoconstriction and vasodilation. It may also be a child's physiologic response to a cold environment.

Words of Wisdom

Note the line of demarcation of any mottling or pallor on the child's limbs during your assessment. An increase in mottling or pallor with movement toward the core of the body indicates a worsening "shell to core" shunt from peripheral vasoconstriction.

Cyanosis, a bluish discoloration of the skin and mucous membranes, is the most extreme visual indicator of poor perfusion or poor oxygenation. **Acrocyanosis**, blue hands or feet in an infant younger than 2 months, is distinct from cyanosis; it is a normal finding when a young infant is cold. True cyanosis is seen in the skin and mucous membranes and is a late finding of respiratory failure or shock.

After assessing the child's appearance and work of breathing, visually scan the child's skin and mucous membranes looking for pallor, mottling, and cyanosis. You can then combine the

three pieces of the PAT to estimate the severity of illness and the likely underlying pathologic cause. For example, a child with an abnormal appearance with poor circulation may be in shock from a cardiovascular cause.

Stay or Go

On the basis of the findings from the PAT, you will determine whether the pediatric patient is in stable condition or requires urgent care. If the pediatric patient is in unstable condition, assess the ABCs, treating any life threats, and transport the pediatric patient immediately to an appropriate facility. If the pediatric patient is in stable condition, then you have time to perform the entire patient assessment process.

Hands-on ABCs

After using the PAT to form a general impression of the patient, you will need to complete the rest of the primary assessment—that is, you must assess the child's ABCs and mental status and prioritize the care and need for transport. Threats to the ABCs are managed as they are found, providing a prioritized sequence of life-support interventions to reverse critical physiologic abnormalities. The steps are the same as with adults, albeit with differences related to the child's anatomy, physiology, and signs of distress. If you suspect this is cardiac arrest, which is rare, the order is CAB because chest compressions would be the priority. You will also assess disability and exposure.

Early in your assessment of a young child, you will need to estimate the child's weight, because much of your care will depend on the child's size. The best way to estimate a child's weight is with a pediatric resuscitation tape measure (Broselow tape, also called a length-based resuscitation tape), which will also provide appropriate medication doses and equipment sizes **Figure 8**. The pediatric resuscitation tape measure can estimate weight and height in pediatric patients weighing up to 75 lb (34 kg).

To use the pediatric resuscitation tape measure, follow these steps:

1. Measure the child's length, from head to heel, with the tape (with the red portion at the head).
2. Note the weight in kilograms that corresponds to the child's measured length at the heel.

Table 7	Characteristics of Circulation to Skin
Characteristic	**Features to Look For**
Pallor	White or pale skin or mucous membranes from inadequate blood flow
Mottling	Patchy skin discoloration due to vasoconstriction or vasodilation
Cyanosis	Bluish discoloration of skin and mucous membranes

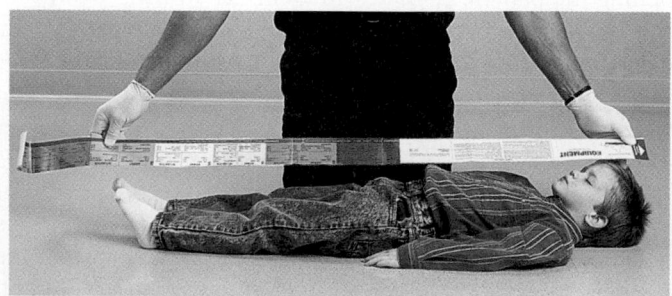

Figure 8 Use of a pediatric resuscitation tape measure is one way to estimate a child's weight and identify the correct size for pediatric equipment and medication doses.

3. If the child is longer than the tape, use adult equipment and medication doses.
4. From the tape, identify appropriate equipment sizes.
5. From the tape, identify appropriate medication doses.

Airway

The PAT may suggest the presence of an airway obstruction based on abnormal airway sounds and increased work of breathing. As with adults, determine whether the airway is open and the patient has adequate chest rise with breathing. Check for mucus, blood, or a foreign body in the mouth or airway. If there is potential obstruction from the tongue or soft tissues, position the airway and suction as necessary. Determine whether the airway is open and patent, partially obstructed, or totally obstructed. Do not keep the suction tip or catheter in the back of a child's throat too long because young patients are extremely sensitive to vagal stimuli and the pulse rate may plummet.

Breathing

The breathing component of the primary assessment involves calculating the respiratory rate, auscultating breath sounds, and checking pulse oximetry for oxygen saturation. Verify the respiratory rate per minute by counting the number of chest rises in 30 seconds and then doubling that number. Healthy infants may show periodic breathing, or variable respiratory rates with short periods of apnea (< 20 s). As a consequence, counting for only 10 to 15 seconds may give a falsely low respiratory rate. Interpreting the respiratory rate requires knowing the normal values for the child's age and putting the respiratory rate in context with the rest of the primary assessment. Rapid respiratory rates may simply reflect high fever, anxiety, pain, or excitement. Normal rates, by contrast, may occur in a child who has been breathing rapidly with increased work of breathing and is becoming fatigued. Serial assessment of respiratory rates may be especially useful because the trend may be more accurate than any single value.

Words of Wisdom

Consider pulse oximetry readings in terms of the environmental context and the physiologic status of the child. Peripheral vasoconstriction from hypothermia or poor perfusion may alter these readings. Always correlate the pulse oximetry waveform with the patient's pulse rate and ECG reading.

Auscultate the breath sounds with a stethoscope over the midaxillary line to hear abnormal lung sounds during inhalation and exhalation. Listen for extra breath sounds such as inspiratory crackles, wheezes, or rhonchi; rhonchi often indicate harsh breath sounds or sounds that may be transmitted from the upper airways. If you cannot determine whether the sounds are being generated in the lungs or the upper airway, hold the stethoscope over the nose or trachea and listen. Also, listen to the breath sounds for adequacy of air movement. Diminished breath sounds may signal severe respiratory distress. Auscultation over the trachea may also help distinguish stridor from other sounds.

Check the pulse oximetry reading to determine the oxygen saturation level while the child breathes ambient air. You can place the pulse oximetry probe on a young child's finger just as you would with an adult. In infants or young children who try to remove the probe, it may be helpful to place the probe on a toe, possibly with a sock covering it. A pulse oximetry reading of greater than 94% saturation while breathing room air indicates good oxygenation.

As with the respiratory rate, evaluate the pulse oximetry reading in the context of the PAT and remainder of the primary assessment. A child with a normal pulse oximetry reading, for example, may be expending increasing amounts of energy and increasing the work of breathing to maintain his or her oxygen saturation. The primary assessment would identify the respiratory distress and point to the need for immediate intervention despite the normal oxygen saturation level.

Circulation

The information obtained from the PAT about circulation to the skin directs the next step of the primary assessment. Integrate this assessment of circulation with the pulse rate and quality, and skin CTC (color, temperature, and condition plus capillary refill time) to obtain an overall assessment of the child's circulatory status.

Obtain the child's pulse rate by listening to the heart or feeling the pulse for 30 seconds and doubling the number. As with respiratory rates in pediatric patients, it is important to know normal pulse rates based on age. Interpret the pulse rate within the context of the overall history and primary assessment. Tachycardia may indicate early hypoxia or shock or a less serious condition such as fever, anxiety, pain, or excitement.

Feel for the pulse to ascertain the rate and quality of pulsations. If you cannot find a peripheral (distal) pulse (that is, radial or brachial), feel for a central pulse (that is, femoral or carotid). Check the femoral pulse in infants and young children and the carotid pulse in older children and adolescents. As with adults, if there is no pulse, start CPR.

After checking the pulse rate, do a hands-on evaluation of skin CTC. Check whether the hands and feet are warm or cool to the touch. Check capillary refill time in the fingertip, toe, heel, or pads of the fingertips; a normal refill time is 2 seconds or less. These two pieces of information need to be placed in context with the PAT and remainder of the primary assessment because cool extremities and delayed capillary refill are commonly seen in a child in a cool environment.

Disability

The assessment of the pediatric patient's level of consciousness can be done using the AVPU scale **Table 8** or the Pediatric Glasgow Coma Scale **Table 9**.

After evaluating the patient's response with the AVPU scale, assess the pupillary response to a beam of light to assess brainstem response. Note if the pupils are dilated, constricted, reactive, or fixed. Next, evaluate motor activity, looking for symmetric movement of the extremities, seizures, posturing, or flaccidity. Combine this information with the PAT results to determine the child's neurologic status.

Table 8 AVPU Scale

Category	Stimulus	Response Type	Reaction
Alert	Normal environment	Appropriate	Normal interactiveness for age
Verbal	Simple command or sound stimulus	Appropriate Inappropriate	Responds to name Nonspecific or confused
Painful	Pain	Appropriate Inappropriate Pathologic	Withdraws from pain Makes sound or moves without purpose or localization of pain Posturing
Unresponsive			No perceptible response to any stimulus

Table 9 Pediatric Glasgow Coma Scale (GCS)

Activity	Score	Infant	Score	Child
Eye opening	4	Open spontaneously	4	Open spontaneously
	3	Open to speech or sound	3	Open to speech
	2	Open to painful stimuli	2	Open to painful stimuli
	1	No response	1	No response
Verbal	5	Coos, babbles	5	Oriented conversation
	4	Irritable cry	4	Confused conversation
	3	Cries to pain	3	Cries
				Inappropriate words
	2	Moans to pain	2	Moans
				Incomprehensible words/sounds
	1	No response	1	No response
Motor	6	Normal spontaneous movement	6	Obeys verbal commands
	5	Localizes pain	5	Localizes pain
	4	Withdraws to pain	4	Withdraws to pain
	3	Abnormal flexion (decorticate)	3	Abnormal flexion (decorticate)
	2	Abnormal extension (decerebrate)	2	Abnormal extension (decerebrate)
	1	No response (flaccid)	1	No response (flaccid)

Numerous studies have found that children are much less likely than adults to receive effective pain medications. Inadequate treatment of pain has many adverse effects on the child and family. Pain causes morbidity and misery for the child and caregivers, and it interferes with your ability to accurately assess physiologic abnormalities. Children who do not receive appropriate analgesia may be more likely to have exaggerated pain responses to subsequent painful procedures. Also, posttraumatic stress may be more common among children who experience pain during an illness or injury.

Assessment of pain must consider developmental age. The ability to identify pain improves with the age of the child. In infants and preverbal children, it may be difficult to distinguish crying and agitation due to hypoxia, hunger, or pain. Further assessment and discussion with caregivers about their perceptions of the child's pain are essential to identify pain in this age group. Pain scales using pictures of facial expressions, such as the Wong-Baker FACES scale, may prove helpful **Figure 9** .

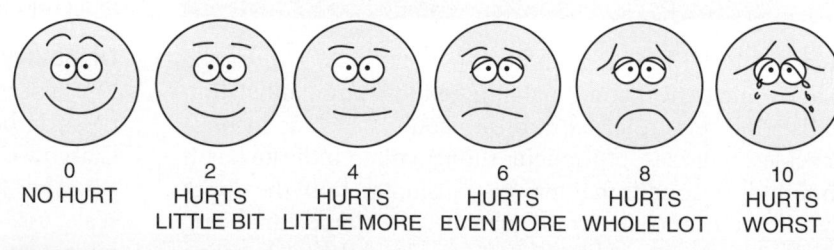

0	2	4	6	8	10
NO HURT	HURTS LITTLE BIT	HURTS LITTLE MORE	HURTS EVEN MORE	HURTS WHOLE LOT	HURTS WORST

Figure 9 The Wong-Baker FACES scale.

From Hockenberry MJ, Wilson D, Wikelstein ML: *Wong's Essentials of Pediatric Nursing*, 8th ed, St. Louis, 2009, p. 1259. Used with permission. © Mosby.

Remaining calm and providing quiet, professional reassurance to parents and child is critical for managing pediatric pain and anxiety. A calm parent will help keep the child calm and more at ease. Distraction techniques with toys or stories may prove helpful in reducing pain, as may visual imagery techniques and music. Sucrose pacifiers may reduce pain in neonates. Pharmacologic methods for reducing pain—such as acetaminophen, opiates, benzodiazepines, and nitrous oxide—are available to paramedics in a number of EMS systems. The benefit of such analgesic or anxiolytic medication must be weighed against the risks of its administration (respiratory depression, bradycardia, hypoxemia, and hypotension are potential side effects of sedatives), including the potential route of administration. Medications that are given intravenously are often most effective at reducing pain, but they require establishing intravenous (IV) access, which itself is a painful procedure.

Special Populations

Consider pain to be a vital sign in pediatric patients. Assess and reassess pain along with the other vital signs. Treat pain accordingly.

Today, assessment of pain is recognized as part of vital sign assessment, and management of pediatric pain and anxiety should be a routine part of field care. This effort requires a thorough understanding of nonpharmacologic techniques, drugs, potential drug contraindications and complications, and management of the complications.

Exposure

Proper exposure of the child is necessary to complete the primary assessment. The child will need to be at least partially undressed to assess the work of breathing and circulation. However, it is also important to perform a rapid exam of the entire body to look for unsuspected injuries and anatomic abnormalities. Be careful to avoid heat loss, especially in infants, by covering the child as soon as possible. Keep the temperature in the ambulance high, and use blankets when necessary.

Transport Decision

After completing the primary assessment and beginning resuscitation when necessary, you must make a crucial decision: whether to immediately transport the child to the emergency department (ED) or continue the additional assessment and treatment on scene. Immediate transport is imperative if the emergency call is for trauma and the child has a serious MOI, a physiologic abnormality, or a potentially significant anatomic abnormality or if the scene is unsafe. In these cases, manage all life threats, and begin transport. Attempt vascular access on the way to the ED. If the emergency call is for an illness, the decision to stay or go is less clear-cut and depends on the following factors: expected benefits of treatment, EMS system regulations, comfort level, and transport time.

History Taking

If the child seems to be in physiologically unstable condition based on the primary assessment, you may decide to begin transport immediately and conduct history taking and the secondary assessment in the ambulance en route to the ED. The goal of history taking is to elaborate on the chief complaint (ie, OPQRST) and obtain a patient history (ie, SAMPLE) Table 10.

Secondary Assessment

Whereas the primary assessment addresses immediately life-threatening pathologic problems, the secondary assessment includes a systematic assessment of the patient that may include a full-body examination or a focused assessment on the body part or body system specifically involved. A complete set of baseline vital signs, using monitoring devices as appropriate, should also be obtained at this time.

For a full-body examination, infants, toddlers, and preschool-age children should be assessed starting at the feet and ending at the head; older children can be assessed using the head-to-toe approach, as with adults. Tailor the exam to the child's age and developmental stage. The extent of the examination will depend on the situation and may include the following:

- **Head.** The younger the infant or child, the larger the head is in proportion to the rest of the body, increasing the risk for head injury with deceleration (such as in

Table 10 Pediatric SAMPLE History Components

Component	Explanation
Signs and symptoms	Onset and nature of symptoms of pain or fever Age-appropriate signs of distress
Allergies	Known drug reactions or other allergies
Medications	Exact names and doses of ongoing drugs (including over-the-counter, prescribed, herbal, and recreational drugs) Timing and amount of last dose Time and dose of analgesics or antipyretics
Past medical history	Previous illnesses or injuries Immunizations History of pregnancy, labor, delivery (infants and toddlers)
Last oral intake	Timing of the child's last food or drink, including bottle or breastfeeding
Events leading to illness or injury	Key events leading to the current incident Fever history

motor vehicle crashes). Look for bruising, swelling, and hematomas. Significant blood can be lost between the skull and scalp of a small infant. Assessment of the bulging fontanelle suggests elevated intracranial pressure caused by meningitis, encephalitis, or intracranial bleeding. A sunken fontanelle suggests dehydration.

- **Pupils.** Note the size, equality, and reactivity of the pupils to light. The response of the pupils is a good indication of how well the brain is functioning, particularly when trauma has occurred.
- **Nose.** Young infants prefer to breathe through their nose, so nasal congestion with mucus can cause respiratory distress. Gentle bulb or catheter suction of the nostrils may bring relief.
- **Ears.** Look for any drainage from the ear canals. Leaking blood suggests a skull fracture. Check for bruises behind the ear or Battle sign, a late sign of skull fracture. The presence of pus may indicate an ear infection or perforation of the eardrum.
- **Mouth.** In the trauma patient, look for active bleeding and loose teeth. Note the smell of the breath. Some ingestions are associated with identifiable odors, such as hydrocarbons. Acidosis, as in diabetic ketoacidosis, may impart an acetone-like smell to the breath.
- **Neck.** Examine the trachea for swelling or bruising. Note if the pediatric patient cannot move his or her neck and has a high fever. This may indicate that the pediatric patient has bacterial or viral meningitis.
- **Chest.** Examine the chest for penetrating injuries, lacerations, bruises, or rashes. If the pediatric patient is injured, feel the clavicles and every rib for tenderness and/or deformity.
- **Back.** Inspect the back for lacerations, penetrating injuries, bruises, or rashes.
- **Abdomen.** Inspect the abdomen for distention. Gently palpate the abdomen and watch closely for guarding or tensing of the abdominal muscles, which may suggest infection, obstruction, or intra-abdominal injury. Note any tenderness or masses. Look for any seat belt abrasions or bruising.
- **Extremities.** Assess for symmetry. Compare both sides for color, warmth, size of joints, swelling, and tenderness. Put each joint through full range of motion while watching the eyes of the pediatric patient for signs of pain, unless there is obvious deformity of the extremity suggesting a fracture.
- **Capillary refill (in children younger than 6 years).** Normal capillary refill time should be 2 seconds or less. As discussed earlier, assess capillary refill time by blanching the finger or toenail beds; the soles of the feet may also be used. Cold temperatures will increase capillary refill time, making it a less reliable sign.
- **Level of hydration.** Assess skin turgor, noting the presence of **tenting**, a condition in which the skin slowly retracts after being pinched and pulled away slightly from the body. In infants, note whether the fontanelles are sunken or flat. Ask the parent or caregiver how many diapers the infant has soiled over the last 24 hours. Determine whether the child is producing tears when crying; note the condition of the mouth. Is the oral mucosa moist or dry?

Words of Wisdom

Blood pressure is just one component of the overall assessment of pediatric patients. Determination of physiologic stability should be based on all data collected from the PAT, physical exam, and initial vital signs.

It may be difficult to obtain an accurate measurement of blood pressure in a young child or infant because of a lack of cooperation and need for proper cuff size. Nevertheless, you should attempt to measure the blood pressure on the upper arm or thigh, making sure the cuff has a width two thirds the length of the upper arm or thigh. One formula for determining the lower limit of acceptable blood pressure in children ages 1 to 10 years is this: minimal systolic blood pressure = 80 + (2 × age in years). For example, a 2-year-old toddler should have a minimal systolic blood pressure of 84; a lower rate indicates decompensated shock. (**Table 11** shows normal minimal systolic blood pressure values for different ages.) Given the technical difficulty of trying to measure the blood pressure in a pediatric patient, make one attempt in the field; if unsuccessful, move on to the rest of the assessment.

Special Populations

For children 1 to 10 years, calculate the lower limit of acceptable blood pressure for age with the following formula:
Minimal systolic blood pressure = 80 + (2 × age in years)

Reassessment

The elements in the reassessment include the PAT, patient priority, vital signs (every 5 minutes if the patient is in unstable condition and every 15 minutes if in stable condition), assessment of the effectiveness of interventions (eg, medications

Table 11 Normal Blood Pressure for Age

Age	Minimal Systolic Blood Pressure (mm Hg)
Infant	> 70
Toddler	> 80
Preschool-age child	> 80
School-age child	> 80
Adolescent	> 90

administered, splints applied, bleeding controlled), and reassessment of the focused exam areas. Perform the reassessment on all patients to observe their response to treatment, to guide ongoing treatments, and to track the progression of identified pathologic and anatomic problems. New problems may also be identified on reassessment. The reassessment may also guide the choice of an appropriate transport destination and your radio or telephone communications with medical oversight or ED staff.

Documentation and Communication

Perform frequent reassessment of serial vital signs, and record them on your patient care report. By recording each set of vital signs, you can visualize trends and transfer important information to the accepting physicians.

◼ Pathophysiology, Assessment, and Management of Respiratory Emergencies

Respiratory problems are among the medical emergencies that you will most frequently encounter in children. Pediatric patients with a respiratory chief complaint will span the spectrum from mildly ill to near death. In pediatrics, respiratory failure and arrest precede the majority of cardiopulmonary arrests; by contrast, a primary cardiac event is the usual cause of sudden death in adults. Early identification and intervention can stop the progression from respiratory distress to cardiopulmonary failure and help to avert much pediatric morbidity and mortality.

◼ Respiratory Arrest, Distress, and Failure

When you are faced with a respiratory emergency, the first step is to determine the severity of the disease: Is the patient in respiratory distress, respiratory failure, or respiratory arrest? Keep the anatomic and physiologic respiratory differences in mind as you approach the child.

Respiratory distress entails increased work of breathing to maintain oxygenation and/or ventilation; that is, it is a compensated state in which increased work of breathing results in adequate pulmonary gas exchange. The hallmarks of respiratory distress—which is classified as mild, moderate, or severe—are retractions (suprasternal, intercostal, subcostal), abdominal breathing, nasal flaring, and grunting.

A patient in respiratory failure can no longer compensate for the underlying pathologic or anatomic problem by increased work of breathing, so hypoxia and/or carbon dioxide retention occur. Signs of respiratory failure may include decreased or absent retractions owing to fatigue of the chest wall muscles, altered mental status owing to inadequate oxygenation and ventilation of the brain, and an abnormally low respiratory rate Table 12 . Respiratory failure is a decompensated state, requiring urgent intervention to ensure adequate oxygenation and ventilation and prevent respiratory arrest. Do not be afraid to assist ventilations at this point if you judge the tidal volume or respiratory effort to be inadequate.

YOU are the Medic   PART 2

Using the Pediatric Assessment Triangle, you classify the child as sick. His abnormal appearance, abnormal circulation, and normal work of breathing leads you to believe that the child may be in shock. Your partner applies 100% oxygen via a nonrebreathing mask and places him on the cardiac monitor, which shows a narrow complex tachycardia. On questioning the sister, you learn that the child has had a stomachache with vomiting and diarrhea for the past few days and has not eaten or drank anything since the night before. She says that he never gets sick.

Recording Time: 5 Minutes	
Respirations	22 breaths/min unlabored; clear breath sounds
Pulse	180 beats/min, regular; absent distally and weak centrally
Skin	Pale, cool, and dry; some mottling to the extremities
Blood pressure	68/42 mm Hg
Oxygen saturation (Spo$_2$)	99% at 12 L/min of oxygen on nonrebreathing mask
Capillary refill	5 seconds

3. What is the significance of the child's blood pressure?

4. What should your treatment consist of at this point?

Table 12 Signs of Impending Respiratory Failure

Assess	Sign
Mental status	Agitation, restlessness, confusion, lethargy (VPU of AVPU)
Skin color	Cyanosis, pallor
Respiratory rate	Tachypnea → bradypnea → apnea
Respiratory effort	Severe retractions, nasal flaring, grunting, paradoxical abdominal motion, tripod positioning
Auscultation	Stridor, wheezing, rales, or diminished air movement
Blood oxygen saturation	< 90% with supplemental oxygen
Pulse rate	Tachycardia, bradycardia, or cardiac arrest

Special Populations

Initiate aggressive airway management and ventilatory support with a bag-mask device and supplemental oxygen as soon as possible for a child with respiratory failure.

Respiratory arrest means that the patient is not breathing spontaneously. Administer immediate bag-mask ventilation with supplemental oxygen to prevent progression to cardiopulmonary arrest. Resuscitation of a child from respiratory arrest is often successful, whereas resuscitation of a child in cardiopulmonary arrest usually fails.

By combining the three components of the PAT, you can determine the severity of disease before you even touch the patient. The child's appearance will give you clues about the adequacy of CNS oxygenation and ventilation. If a child with trouble breathing is sleepy, assume the child is hypoxic. Assess the work of breathing by noting the patient's position of comfort, presence or absence of retractions, and grunting or flaring. A patient who prefers to sit upright, in the sniffing position, or to use his or her arms for support is trying to optimize breathing mechanics. Deep retractions herald the use of accessory muscles of respiration to move air. Assessment of circulation for the presence of pallor or cyanosis will give you further information on the adequacy of oxygenation.

For respiratory emergencies, focus on the child's airway and breathing. Assess the airway by listening for stridor in awake patients or checking for obstruction in **obtunded** patients. Assess breathing by determining the child's respiratory rate, listening to the lungs for adequacy of air entry and abnormal breath sounds, and checking pulse oximetry readings. A respiratory rate that is too low may be more worrisome than a rate that is too high for the child's age. The presence of abnormal breath sounds may identify the anatomic or pathologic abnormality and suggest a likely diagnosis. For example, symmetric,

diffuse wheezing implies bronchospasm and possibly asthma, whereas diffuse rhonchi, rales, and wheezing in an infant or toddler are typical signs of lower airway inflammation associated with bronchiolitis. The presence of stridor in the context of clear lung fields is consistent with upper airway obstruction, often due to croup. Poor air entry with decreased breath sounds is an ominous sign that must be addressed immediately. Determine oxygen saturation by assessing pulse oximetry via a finger or toe or, in a small infant, around the foot.

Your determination of whether the patient is in respiratory distress, respiratory failure, or respiratory arrest will drive your next steps, by indicating the urgency for treatment and transport. You can obtain the SAMPLE history at the scene or during transport, depending on the patient's stability. Table 13 lists key questions to ask during a respiratory emergency.

Most pediatric patients with a primary respiratory complaint will have respiratory distress and require only generic treatment. Allow the child to assume a position of comfort, and provide supplemental oxygen. The choice of oxygen delivery method will depend on the severity of illness and the child's developmental level. Young children may become agitated by a nasal cannula or face mask. Because crying and thrashing increase metabolic demands and oxygen consumption, you must weigh the benefits of this therapy against the potential cost. Allowing a caregiver to deliver blow-by oxygen to a calm toddler may be your best choice, if the child does not show signs of respiratory failure.

As a child becomes fatigued, respiratory distress may progress to respiratory failure. As part of your reassessment, electronically monitor the patient's pulse rate, respiratory rate, and oxygen saturation level. A significant change or trend in any of these variables requires prompt attention. You should also perform frequent reassessment to evaluate the effects of your treatment.

Table 13 Key Questions in Respiratory Emergencies

Component	Key Questions
Signs and symptoms	Shortness of breath? Hoarseness? Stridor? Wheezing? Cough? Chest pain? Choking? Rash/Hives? Cyanosis?
Allergies	Known drug or food allergies; smoke exposure
Medications	Names and doses of ongoing medications; recent use of corticosteroids
Past medical history	History of asthma, chronic lung disease, heart problems, prematurity; prior hospitalizations and intubation for breathing problems; history of choking or anaphylaxis; immunizations
Last oral intake	Timing of last food, including bottle or breastfeeding
Events leading to illness or injury	Fever history or recent illness; history of injury to chest; history of choking on food or object

Upper Airway Emergencies

Foreign Body Aspiration or Obstruction

Infants and toddlers explore their environment by putting objects into their mouths, resulting in a high risk of foreign body aspiration. Any small object or food item has the potential to obstruct a young child's narrow trachea. Peanuts, hot dogs, grapes, balloons, and small toys or pieces of toys are frequent offenders. Swallowed foreign bodies can also cause respiratory distress in infants and young children because a rigid esophageal foreign body can compress the relatively pliable trachea. In addition, the tongue, owing to its large size relatively to the upper airway, frequently causes mild upper airway obstruction in a child with a decreased level of consciousness (LOC) and diminished muscle tone.

Suspect foreign body aspiration when you encounter signs of mild or severe airway obstruction during the primary assessment. An awake patient with stridor, increased work of breathing, and good color on the PAT has mild upper airway obstruction. Auscultation may reveal fair to good air entry, and the presence of unilateral wheezing may tip you off to a foreign body lodged in a mainstem bronchus. In contrast, a patient with severe airway obstruction is likely to be cyanotic and unconscious when you arrive, owing to profound hypoxia. If the child has spontaneous respiratory effort, you will hear poor air entry, but you may *not* hear stridor owing to minimal air flow through the trachea. A typical SAMPLE history for foreign body aspiration reveals a previously healthy child with sudden onset of coughing, choking, or gagging while eating or playing.

Initial management of mild airway obstruction involves allowing the patient to assume a position of comfort, providing supplemental oxygen as tolerated, and transporting the child to an appropriate treating facility. Avoid agitating the child because this stimulus could worsen the situation. Continuous monitoring and frequent reassessments are needed to ensure that the problem does not progress to severe airway obstruction.

Removing a Foreign Body Airway Obstruction in Responsive Infants

For a responsive infant, deliver five back slaps and five chest thrusts **Figure 10** :

1. Hold the infant face down, with the body resting on your forearm. Support the infant's head and face with your hand, and keep the head lower than the rest of the body.
2. Deliver five back blows between the shoulder blades using the heel of your hand.
3. Place your free hand behind the infant's head and back, and bring the infant upright on your thigh, sandwiching the infant's body between your two hands and arms. The infant's head should remain below the level of the body.

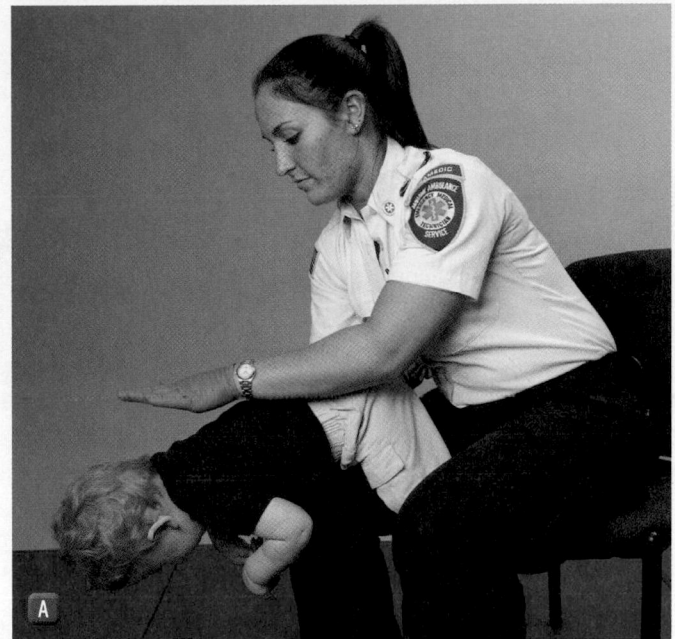

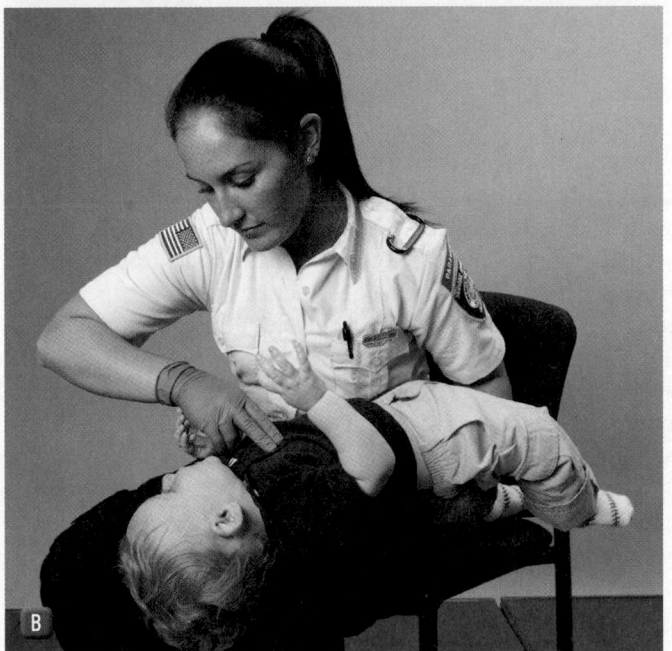

Figure 10 Perform back slaps and chest thrusts to clear a foreign body airway obstruction in a responsive infant. **A.** Deliver five quick back blows between the shoulder blades, using the heel of your hand. **B.** Give five quick chest thrusts, using two fingers placed on the lower half of the sternum.

4. Give five quick chest thrusts in the same location and manner as for chest compressions, using two fingers placed on the lower half of the sternum. For larger infants, or if you have small hands, you can place the infant in your lap and turn the infant's whole body as a unit between back blows and chest thrusts.
5. Check the airway. If you can see the foreign body now, remove it. If not, repeat the cycle as often as necessary. Do not stick your fingers in the infant's mouth to

remove an object unless you can actually visualize the object.

6. If the infant becomes unresponsive, begin CPR with compressions, remembering to look in the airway before ventilations each time.

Words of Wisdom

According to 2010 guidelines for CPR and emergency cardiovascular care, a child is a person from about age 1 year until the onset of puberty (age 12 to 14 years).

Removing a Foreign Body Airway Obstruction in Unresponsive Infants As with the adult and child, if the infant loses consciousness, look inside the mouth. If you see the object, remove it. If not, start CPR beginning with 30 chest compressions (15 compressions if two rescuers are present and the patient is an infant or child). Also, if there is no pulse, or the pulse rate is less than 60 beats/min, begin CPR. Continue the process of compressions, always looking in the mouth, and attempting ventilations until the obstruction is relieved. Then, assess for a pulse.

Removing a Foreign Body Airway Obstruction in Children The abdominal thrust manueuver (also called the Heimlich maneuver) is the most effective method of dislodging and forcing an object out of the airway of a responsive adult or child. This method aims to increase the pressure in the chest, creating an artificial cough that may force a foreign body from the airway. Use this manueuver until the obstructing object is expelled or the child becomes unresponsive. If the child becomes unresponsive, carefully position him or her supine and perform 30 chest compressions (15 compressions if two rescuers are present and the patient is an infant or child), and then open the airway and look in the mouth. You should attempt to remove the foreign body only if you can see it. After looking in the mouth, attempt to ventilate the patient. If the first breath does not produce visible chest rise, reopen the airway and reattempt to ventilate. If both breaths fail to produce visible chest rise, continue chest compressions. If you are unable to relieve a severe airway obstruction in an unresponsive patient with the basic techniques previously discussed, you should proceed with direct laryngoscopy (visualization of the airway with a laryngoscope) for the removal of the foreign body. Insert the laryngoscope blade into the patient's mouth. If you see the foreign body, carefully remove it from the upper airway with Magill forceps, a special type of curved forceps.

The steps for removal of an upper airway obstruction with Magill forceps are listed here:

1. With the patient's head in the sniffing position, open the patient's mouth and insert the laryngoscope blade.
2. Visualize the obstruction, and retrieve the object with the Magill forceps.
3. Remove the object with the Magill forceps.
4. Attempt to ventilate the patient.

Refer to the chapter, *Airway Management and Ventilation*, for more information on this procedure.

Anaphylaxis

Anaphylaxis is a potentially life-threatening allergic reaction, triggered by exposure to an antigen (foreign protein). Food—especially nuts, shellfish, eggs, and milk—and bee stings are among the most common causes, although anaphylaxis to antibiotics and other medications can occur as well. Exposure to the antigen stimulates the release of histamine and other vasoactive chemical mediators from white blood cells, leading to multiple organ system involvement. Onset of symptoms generally occurs immediately after the exposure and may include hives, respiratory distress, circulatory compromise, and gastrointestinal symptoms (vomiting, diarrhea, abdominal pain). See the chapter, *Immunologic Emergencies* for more information about the sequence of events in anaphylaxis.

Although a child with mild anaphylaxis may experience only hives and some wheezing, a child with severe anaphylaxis may be in respiratory failure and shock when you arrive. The PAT may reveal an anxious child (many adults describe a sense of impending doom at the onset of anaphylaxis). With severe anaphylaxis, the child may be unresponsive due to respiratory failure and shock. He or she may have increased work of breathing due to upper airway edema or bronchospasm and poor circulation. The primary assessment will usually reveal hives, with other findings potentially including swelling of the lips and oral mucosa, stridor and/or wheezing, and diminished pulses. If the child has a known allergy, the SAMPLE history may reveal recent contact with or ingestion of the potentially offending agent (including consumption of prepared foods containing traces of eggs, nuts, and milk at daycare or school).

The "gold standard" treatment for anaphylaxis is epinephrine. Epinephrine's alpha-agonist effect decreases airway edema by **vasoconstriction** and improves circulation by increasing peripheral vascular resistance. Its beta-agonist effect causes bronchodilation, resulting in improved oxygenation and ventilation. Epinephrine should be given by the intramuscular (IM) route at a dose of 0.01 mg/kg of the 1:1,000 solution, to a maximum dose of 0.3 mg. This dose may be repeated as necessary every 5 minutes. If several doses are needed, the child may require a continuous IV epinephrine drip. In addition to epinephrine, treatment of anaphylaxis should include supplemental oxygen, fluid resuscitation for shock, diphenhydramine (Benadryl) for its antihistamine effect (dose: 1 to 2 mg/kg IV to a maximum of 50 mg), and bronchodilators for wheezing.

Many children with a history of anaphylaxis will have been treated with IM epinephrine by a caregiver before EMS activation. Given the short half-life of this drug, the child should be transported, even if asymptomatic on your arrival.

Croup

Croup (laryngotracheobronchitis) is a viral infection of the upper airway and the most common cause of upper airway emergencies in young children. The parainfluenza virus is the pathogen most commonly responsible for croup, but respiratory syncytial virus (RSV), influenza, and adenovirus have also been implicated. The virus is transmitted by respiratory secretions. Croup primarily affects children age 5 years and younger, with most cases occurring in the fall and winter months. The virus has an affinity for the <u>subglottic space</u>—the narrowest part of the pediatric airway—and causes edema and progressive airway obstruction. Turbulent air flow through the narrowed subglottic airway causes the hallmark sign of croup—stridor.

Most cases of croup are mild. EMS may be called when the symptoms come on abruptly, often in the middle of the night, or if symptoms cause moderate to severe respiratory distress. The PAT for a child with croup will typically reveal an alert infant or toddler who has audible stridor with activity or agitation, a barky cough, some increased work of breathing, and normal skin color. If a child with a history compatible with croup is sleepy or obtunded or has significant respiratory distress or cyanosis, be concerned about critical airway obstruction. On your primary assessment, breath sounds will likely be clear over the lung fields, although you may hear stridor (originating at the level of the subglottic space). Because the pathophysiology of croup largely involves the upper airway, hypoxia is uncommon, and its presence should alert you to critical obstruction and the need for immediate treatment. The SAMPLE history usually reveals several days of cold symptoms and low-grade fever, followed by the onset of a barky cough, stridor, and trouble breathing. The cough and respiratory distress are often worse at night.

The initial management of croup is the same as for most respiratory emergencies. Allow the child to assume a position of comfort, and avoid agitating him or her. The use of cool mist or nebulized saline is controversial. For patients with stridor at rest, moderate to severe respiratory distress, poor air exchange, hypoxia, or altered appearance, nebulized epinephrine is the treatment of choice. It works by causing vasoconstriction and decreasing upper airway edema. Nebulized epinephrine is available in two formulations: racemic epinephrine and L-epinephrine. The dose for racemic epinephrine (2.25%) is 0.5 mL mixed in 3 mL of normal saline. The dose for L-epinephrine is 0.25 to 0.5 mg/kg of the 1:1,000 solution (maximum, 5 mg per dose); this form can be diluted with normal saline to bring the volume to 3 mL. Although only a small amount of epinephrine is absorbed via the nebulized route, side effects may include tachycardia, agitation, tremor, and vomiting.

Special Populations

The presence of hypoxia in a child with croup is a potentially ominous finding, indicating significant subglottic edema. Assess and transport quickly.

In the case of croup and respiratory failure, nebulized epinephrine alone may not be adequate and assisted ventilation may be necessary. Assisted ventilation with bag-mask ventilation will often succeed in overcoming the upper airway obstruction. Advanced airway placement is rarely needed in croup. If performed, choose an ET tube one-half to one size smaller than normal for age or size to accommodate the subglottic edema. Children requiring nebulized epinephrine or assisted ventilation need to be transported immediately to an appropriate treatment facility.

Words of Wisdom

Bag-mask ventilation is the mainstay of treatment for most upper airway emergencies.

Epiglottitis

<u>Epiglottitis</u>, a once-dreaded inflammation of the supraglottic structures, usually due to bacterial infection, is now rare in children. With the introduction of a childhood vaccine against *Haemophilus influenzae*, type B, the incidence of this life-threatening condition has decreased dramatically. Nevertheless, sporadic cases have been reported among adolescents, adults, and unimmunized children.

The classic presentation of epiglottitis is easily distinguishable using the PAT. A child with epiglottitis looks sick and will be anxious, will sit upright in the sniffing position with the chin thrust forward to allow for maximal air entry, and may be drooling because of an inability to swallow secretions. The work of breathing is increased, and pallor or cyanosis may be evident. Stridor heard on auscultation over the neck, a muffled voice, decreased or absent breath sounds, and hypoxia are all signs of a significant airway obstruction. The SAMPLE history will reveal a sudden onset of high fever and sore throat in preschool- or school-age children. Because symptoms progress rapidly, children with epiglottitis are generally sick for only a few hours before they come to medical attention. Remember to ask about immunizations as part of the pertinent medical history for patients suspected of having epiglottitis.

Your goal is to get the child with epiglottitis to an appropriate hospital with a maintainable airway. Because rapidly progressive disease carries a risk for acute airway obstruction and respiratory arrest, you should minimize your scene time and not attempt procedures that might agitate the child. Allow the patient to assume a position of comfort, and provide supplemental oxygen only if tolerated by the patient. Do not attempt to look in the mouth because this can precipitate complete airway obstruction, and do not insert an IV line. Be prepared with a bag-mask device and an ET tube one to two sizes smaller than anticipated for the child's age and length in the event of complete obstruction during transport and the need for assisted ventilation. ET intubation of a child with epiglottitis is difficult because of the extreme distortion of the airway anatomy. Alert personnel at the receiving facility to the suspected diagnosis and the patient's condition because they will need to mobilize a team for the management of this difficult airway.

Some uncommon conditions can also cause upper airway obstruction, including retropharyngeal abscess, peritonsillar abscess, tracheitis, and diphtheria. Presentation may include fever, stridor, difficulty handling secretions, and respiratory distress. Regardless of the underlying diagnosis, assessment and management will be the same as for croup.

Bacterial Tracheitis

<u>Bacterial tracheitis</u> is an invasive exudative bacterial infection of the soft tissues of the trachea. Children typically present with

cough, stridor, and respiratory distress of varying degree with a history of a preceding viral infection. Toddlers are at increased risk of complications due to their relatively narrow airway diameter and may present in extremis. Patients are often febrile, and may prefer the sniffing position to increase airway diameter.

Allow the patient to assume a position of comfort, and provide supplemental oxygen as tolerated by the patient. Do not attempt to look in the mouth because this can precipitate complete airway obstruction, and do not insert an IV line. Try to keep the patient as calm and comfortable as possible. You should be prepared with a bag-mask device and an ET tube one to two sizes smaller than anticipated for the child's age and length in the event of complete obstruction during transport and the need for assisted ventilation. Alert the receiving facility of the potential need for intubation of a difficult airway.

■ Lower Airway Emergencies

The underlying pathophysiology in upper airway emergencies involves restriction of air flow *into* the lungs (inhalation). By contrast, the pathophysiology of lower airway respiratory emergencies involves restriction of air flow *out* of the lungs (exhalation).

Asthma

Asthma is the most common chronic illness of childhood and the most common respiratory complaint encountered by prehospital providers. An estimated 5% to 10% of children are affected by asthma, many of whom will be treated in the ED. Recent studies indicate that the incidence and mortality of this disease are increasing.

In this disease of the small airways, three main components lead to obstruction and poor gas exchange: bronchospasm, mucus production, and airway inflammation. Lower airway inflammation in asthma results in hypoxia because of **ventilation-perfusion mismatch**, a situation in which blood flowing to parts of the lung is poorly oxygenated. Triggers for asthma attacks include upper respiratory infections, environmental allergies, exposure to cold, changes in the weather, and secondhand smoke. Clinical signs include frequent cough, wheezing, and more general signs of respiratory distress.

The primary assessment of a child with an acute exacerbation of asthma will vary based on the degree of obstruction and the presence or absence of respiratory fatigue. A child with mild to moderate respiratory distress will be awake and alert, sometimes preferring a seated posture. Although increased work of breathing may be evident by retractions and nasal flaring, circulation will seem normal. Decreasing alertness, assumption of the tripod position, deep retractions, and cyanosis are signs of severe respiratory distress and impending respiratory failure. The primary assessment will reveal shortness of breath as evidenced by inability to speak in full sentences, increased respiratory rate, prolonged expiration phase, and wheezes noted on auscultation. Expiratory wheezing alone may be heard in patients with mild to moderate asthma attacks, but wheezing may be heard on inspiration and expiration in patients with moderate to severe disease. Decreased air movement and the absence of wheezes in a person with asthma who has activated the EMS system suggest severe lower airway obstruction and respiratory fatigue and signal the need for immediate treatment to prevent respiratory arrest.

The SAMPLE history for a patient suspected of having asthma should reveal the frequency and severity of previous asthma attacks, as reflected by ED visits and hospitalizations. A patient who has previously been admitted to an intensive care unit or intubated for asthma is at increased risk for severe—even possibly fatal—attacks. The medication history should identify any preventive treatment (controller medications) and any rescue medications administered by the caregiver before your arrival. Inhaled steroids are the most common controller medications used in pediatrics, whereas inhaled albuterol is the most common beta-2 agonist drug used as a rescue medication.

The initial management of an asthma exacerbation remains basic respiratory care: Allow the patient to remain in a position of comfort, and administer supplemental oxygen. The gold standard treatment consists of bronchodilators, beta-agonists that act to relax smooth muscles in the bronchioles, thereby decreasing bronchospasm and improving air movement and oxygenation. Bronchodilators may be delivered by nebulizer or metered-dose inhaler (MDI) with a spacer-mask device. Unit doses of 2.5 mg of albuterol premixed with 3 mL of normal saline are often used for nebulization and represent an acceptable starting dose for most young children. For a larger child or a child of any age who is in severe distress, consider administering 5 mg of albuterol as the initial dose. If nebulized albuterol is used, four puffs are equivalent to 2.5 mg administered by nebulizer. Children with moderate to severe respiratory distress can be given treatments as often as needed during transport, including back-to-back nebulizer treatments.

Although albuterol is a relatively safe medication, its potential side effects include tachycardia, tremor, and mild hyperactivity. An isomer of albuterol, levalbuterol, reportedly has fewer side effects. It has not been studied in the prehospital setting but is likely an acceptable alternative to albuterol.

Children with moderate to severe respiratory distress may also benefit from treatment with inhaled ipratropium (Atrovent), an anticholinergic bronchodilator. Studies have shown that the combination of albuterol and ipratropium (which may be mixed and delivered together by nebulizer) is more effective than albuterol given alone. The dose of ipratropium given is based on the patient's weight: a 0.25 mg unit dose nebulized or one puff by MDI for children weighing less than 10 kg; a 0.5 mg unit dose nebulized or two puffs by MDI for children weighing more than 10 kg.

If a child is in severe respiratory distress, is obtunded, or has markedly diminished air movement on auscultation, a dose of epinephrine may be required. Epinephrine will cause immediate relaxation of bronchial smooth muscles, opening the airways to allow bronchodilators to work. The dose is 0.01 mg/kg of 1:1,000 epinephrine injected IM; single doses should not exceed 0.3 mg. Initiate bronchodilator therapy immediately after administering the epinephrine.

Assisted ventilation is problematic for patients with an asthma exacerbation. High inspiratory pressures force air into the lungs, but exhalation is compromised by bronchospasm, mucus production, and inflammation, leading to air trapping and a high risk of pneumothorax and pneumomediastinum. Assisted ventilation should be undertaken only if the patient has respiratory failure and has failed to respond to IM epinephrine and high-dose bronchodilators. If this therapy is performed, use slow rates to allow time for adequate exhalation: Your goal is adequate oxygenation.

Bronchiolitis

Bronchiolitis is an inflammation or swelling of the small airways (bronchioles) in the lower respiratory tract due to viral infection. The most common source of this disease is respiratory syncytial virus (RSV), although a newer virus, metapneumovirus, has also been found to cause this illness. These viruses occur with highest frequency during the winter months, and they primarily affect infants and children younger than 2 years. A highly contagious disease, the severity ranges from mild to moderate respiratory distress with hypoxia and respiratory failure. Younger infants are at particularly high risk for episodes of apnea associated with RSV infection, which may not be associated with severe respiratory distress.

The signs and symptoms of bronchiolitis can be difficult to distinguish from those of asthma. One clue is the child's age: Asthma is rare in children younger than 1 year. An infant with a first-time wheezing episode occurring in late fall or winter likely has bronchiolitis. Mild to moderate retractions, tachypnea, diffuse wheezing, diffuse crackles, and mild hypoxia are characteristic findings during the primary assessment. As with asthma, a sleepy or obtunded patient or one with severe retractions, diminished breath sounds, or moderate to severe hypoxia (oxygen saturation less than 90%) is in danger of respiratory failure and requires immediate transport. Infants in the first months of life or who have a history of prematurity, underlying lung disease, congenital heart disease, or immunodeficiency are at greatest risk for respiratory failure and arrest.

The management of infants and young children with bronchiolitis is entirely supportive. Leave the patient in a position of comfort (eg, in the caregiver's arms, if the child does not seem to be in respiratory failure), and provide supplemental oxygen. Although bronchodilator therapy has not proved effective in the majority of cases, inhaled albuterol or nebulized racemic epinephrine (0.5 mL of a 2.25% solution for inhalation) may be given as a therapeutic trial in children with moderate to severe respiratory distress. Be prepared to assist ventilation with bag-mask ventilation or ET intubation if needed.

Pneumonia

Pneumonia is a common disease process that infects the lower airway and the lung. Although it can occur at any age, in pediatric patients it is commonly seen in infants, toddlers, and preschoolers. In infants and toddlers, pneumonia is often caused by a virus. As children get older, however, the incidence of bacterial pneumonia increases. Children with pneumonia typically have a recent history of a cough or cold, or a lower airway infection (ie, bronchiolitis).

Often pediatric patients will present with unusually rapid breathing, or will breathe with grunting or wheezing sounds. Additional signs and symptoms include nasal flaring, tachypnea, crackles, chest pain, and hypothermia or fever. The patient may also exhibit unilateral diminished breath sounds. Assess the work of breathing by observing for signs of accessory muscle usage. Pneumonia in the infant population may not be tolerated as well as in the older child or adult populations because infants have an increased oxygen demand and less reserve amounts.

For a pediatric patient with suspected pneumonia, your primary treatment will be supportive, consisting of monitoring the patient's airway and breathing status, and administering supplemental oxygen if required. Follow standard precautions and consider placing a mask on the child if tolerated. Vascular access is generally not indicated for children with pneumonia; however, if the child's condition warrants medication therapy, establish IV or intraosseous (IO) access en route to the hospital.

Pertussis

Pertussis, also known as whooping cough, is a highly contagious disease caused by a bacterium that is spread through respiratory droplets. As the result of vaccinations, this potentially deadly disease is less common in the United States. Unfortunately, immunization rates have fallen because of apathy, lack of access to medical care, and the growing fear of some parents that immunization has negative consequences. The typical signs and symptoms are similar to a common cold: coughing, sneezing, and a runny nose. As the disease progresses, the coughing becomes more severe and is characterized by the distinctive whoop sound heard during the inspiratory phase. The cough can be so severe that it can cause postcough vomiting, conjunctival hemorrhage, and cyanotic hypoxia. To treat these pediatric patients, keep the airway patent and transport to the ED. Because pertussis is a contagious disease, follow standard precautions, including wearing a mask and eye protection.

■ Other Respiratory Conditions

Cystic Fibrosis

Cystic fibrosis (CF) is a genetic disease that primarily affects the respiratory and digestive systems. It is the most common life-shortening hereditary disease among people of European descent. People with CF chronically produce copious amounts of thick mucus in their respiratory and digestive tracts, which makes them susceptible to recurrent respiratory infections and requires them to maintain a relatively strict regimen of aerosol treatments, mucus management, and pulmonary exercise. People with CF have frequent respiratory illnesses that require hospitalization.

Pediatric patients may present with tachypnea, chest pain, and crackles, though it may be difficult to separate acute exam findings from chronic disease. Assess the work of breathing by observing for signs of accessory muscle usage, tachypnea, and nasal flaring. Apply supplemental oxygen as needed. Vascular access is generally not needed.

Bronchopulmonary Dysplasia

Bronchopulmonary dysplasia is a spectrum of lung conditions found in premature neonates who required long periods of high-concentration oxygen and ventilator support, ranging from mild reactive airways to debilitating chronic lung disease. Whereas efforts to save premature infants during the past several decades have resulted in the ability to save smaller and smaller infants, some are left with severely damaged lungs, occasionally requiring long-term ventilator support. Researchers in this area initially thought that barotrauma from ventilators was the primary cause, but studies have increasingly pointed to the role of high-concentration oxygen in damaging the lungs. Children with bronchopulmonary dysplasia may use home ventilators, have tracheostomies, or have chronic lung disease. These patients are at high risk for recurrent pulmonary infections including pneumonias, bronchiolitis, and tracheitis. Many patients will be on home oxygen, thus it is important to ask caregivers about baseline oxygen requirements, tracheostomy secretions, and ventilator settings and note any acute changes that have occurred with illness.

Like all pediatric patients with respiratory symptoms, upper airway obstruction can cause distress, so remembering the ABCs of airway management is important. Positioning the airway with a head tilt–chin lift or jaw-thrust maneuver, or with a nasopharyngeal or oropharyngeal airway, may help overcome the obstruction and distress. Bag-mask ventilation and positive airway pressure should also be considered. Continuous positive airway pressure (CPAP) or bilevel positive airway pressure (BiPAP) may be beneficial, but ultimately patients with bronchopulmonary dysplasia may require intubation for severe distress or respiratory failure. When intubating, consider the patient's size and weight when choosing an ET tube; the size needed may be smaller than you would typically pick if you considered only the chronological age. A weight-based system such as the pediatric resuscitation tape measure may be helpful.

Though oxygen may lead to lung damage in premature infants causing bronchopulmonary dysplasia, children with desaturations require oxygen therapy. If bronchospasm is present, bronchodilators such as albuterol may be tried, though improvement may not be seen since the mechanism could be related to the underlying lung disease. Ipratropium may be beneficial in some patients with bronchopulmonary dysplasia and should be considered. Oral and IM steroids such as prednisone or dexamethasone can be considered acutely, but they should be avoided if there is a concern for overwhelming infection.

General Assessment and Management of Respiratory Emergencies

Infants and young children with severe tachypnea and retractions, in association with hypoxia, bradycardia, or altered mental status, are in respiratory failure and need immediate intervention to prevent respiratory arrest. A respiratory rate too slow for age in a child with a history of respiratory distress should also raise concerns for respiratory fatigue and failure.

Airway Management
The first step in managing any respiratory emergency is to start with the airway. Check for obstruction, and position the airway using the head tilt–chin lift or jaw-thrust maneuver **Figure 11** . In a young infant, place a small roll under the shoulders to align the airway **Figure 12** .

An airway adjunct may be helpful if the patient is unresponsive and cannot maintain a patent airway. The use of a nasal or oral airway will help to maintain an open airway, improve bag-mask ventilation, and may avert the need for an advanced airway (such as an ET tube, laryngeal mask airway, King LT airway, or Combitube). When you are placing the adjunct, make sure to start by choosing the appropriately sized equipment.

Oropharyngeal Airway
An oropharyngeal (oral) airway is designed to keep the tongue from blocking the airway, and it makes suctioning the airway easier. This kind of airway should be used for pediatric patients who are unresponsive and cannot maintain their own airway

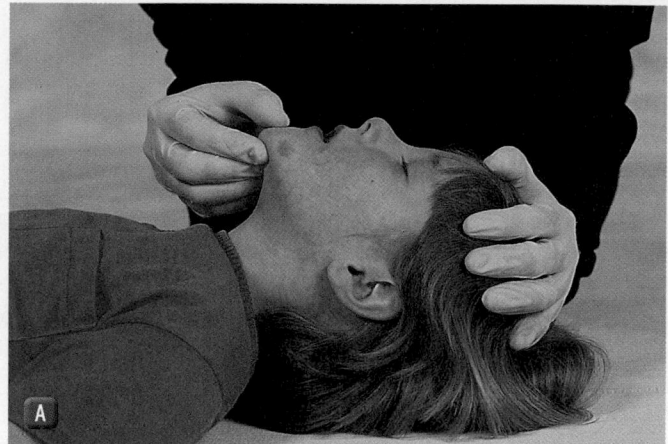

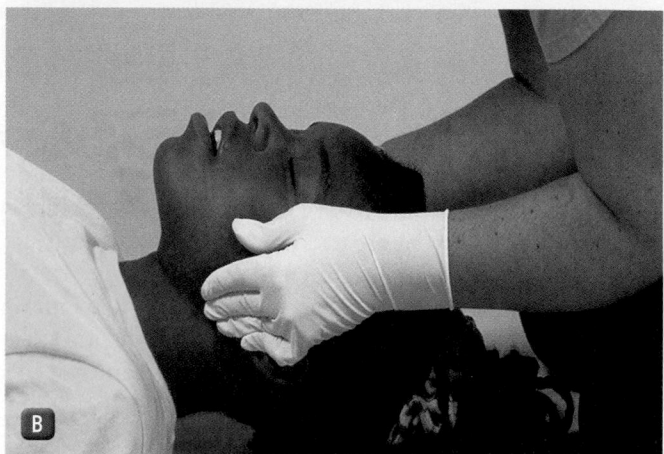

Figure 11 **A.** Use the head tilt-chin lift maneuver to open the airway of a child without trauma. **B.** For a child with suspected spinal injury, use the jaw-thrust manueuver to open the airway.

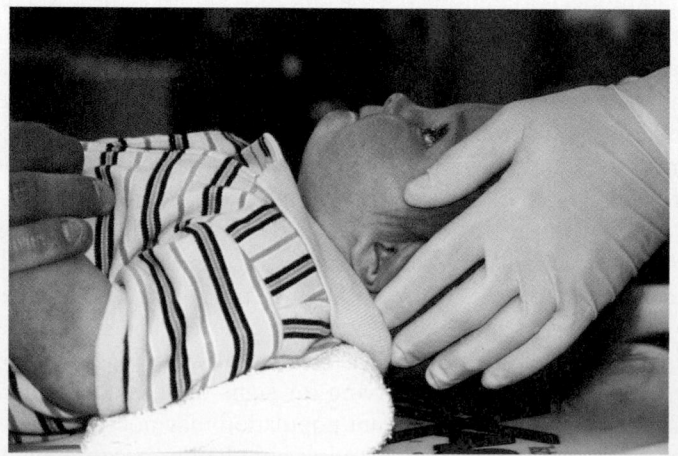

Figure 12 Use a shoulder roll in an infant without trauma to position the airway in a neutral position.

spontaneously. It should *not* be used for conscious patients or patients with a gag reflex—an oropharyngeal airway may stimulate vomiting, thereby increasing the risk of aspiration. In addition, this adjunct should *not* be used for children who have ingested a caustic (corrosive) or petroleum-based product.

Skill Drill 1 shows the preferred technique for inserting an oropharyngeal airway in a child.

Skill Drill 1

1. Determine the appropriately sized airway by measuring from the corner of the mouth to the earlobe or by using the length-based resuscitation tape to measure the patient.
2. Place the airway next to the face, with the flange at the level of the central incisors and the bite block segment parallel to the hard palate. The tip of the airway should reach the angle of the jaw Step 1.
3. Position the patient's airway. For medical patients, use the head tilt–chin lift maneuver, avoiding hyperextension; you may place a towel under the patient's shoulders. If the patient has a traumatic injury, use the jaw-thrust maneuver and provide in-line spinal stabilization Step 2.
4. Open the mouth by applying pressure on the chin with your thumb.
5. Insert the airway by depressing the tongue with a tongue blade on the base of the tongue and inserting the airway directly over the tongue blade. If a tongue blade is not available, point the airway tip toward the roof of the mouth to depress the tongue. Gently rotate the airway

into position as it passes through the mouth toward the curve of the tongue. Insert the airway until the flange rests against the lips.
6. Reassess the airway after insertion Step 3.

Take care to avoid injuring the hard palate as you insert the airway. Rough insertion can cause bleeding that may aggravate airway problems and cause vomiting. If the oropharyngeal airway is too small, the tongue may be pushed back into the pharynx, obstructing the airway. If it is too large, it may obstruct the larynx.

Nasopharyngeal Airway

A nasopharyngeal (nasal) airway is usually well tolerated and is not as likely as the oropharyngeal airway to cause vomiting. The nasopharyngeal airway is used for conscious patients and patients with altered levels of consciousness. In pediatric patients, it is typically used in association with respiratory failure. It is also a good choice for maintaining an airway in patients who are experiencing a seizure or who are in a postictal state. This type of airway is rarely used for children younger than 1 year because of the small diameter of their nares, which tend to become easily obstructed by secretions.

Follow the steps in Skill Drill 2 to insert a nasopharyngeal airway in a child:

Skill Drill 2

1. Determine the appropriately sized airway. The external diameter of the airway should not be larger than the diameter of the naris, and there should be no blanching (turning white) of the naris after insertion.

Skill Drill 1

Inserting an Oropharyngeal Airway

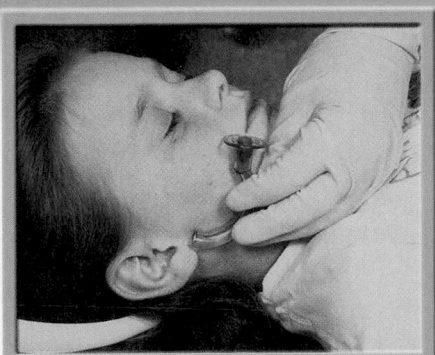

Step 1 Determine the appropriately sized airway by measuring from the corner of the mouth to the earlobe.

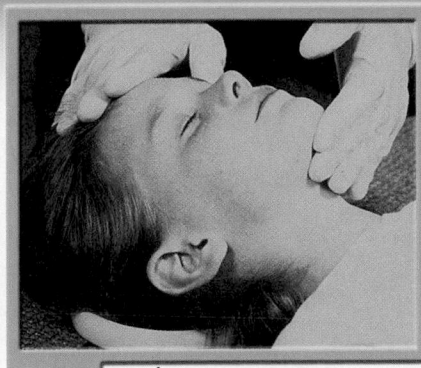

Step 2 Position the child's airway with the appropriate method.

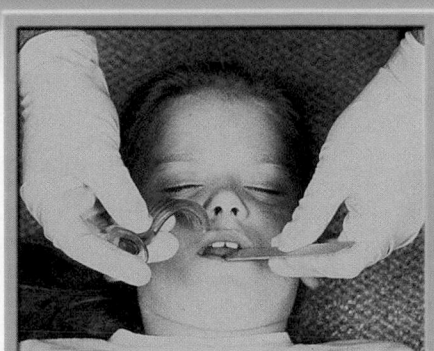

Step 3 Open the mouth. Insert the airway until the flange rests against the lips. Reassess the airway.

2. Place the airway next to the patient's face to make sure the length is correct. The airway should extend from the tip of the nose to the tragus of the ear (that is, the small cartilaginous projection in front of the opening of the ear).

3. Position the patient's airway, using the techniques described for the oropharyngeal airway (Step 1).

4. Lubricate the airway with a water-soluble lubricant.

5. Insert the tip into the right naris with the bevel pointing toward the septum, or central divider of the nose (Step 2).

6. Carefully move the tip forward, following the curvature of the nose, until the flange rests against the outside of the nostril. If you are inserting the airway on the left side, insert the tip into the left naris upside down, with the bevel pointing toward the septum. Move the airway forward slowly until you feel a slight resistance, and then rotate the airway 180°.

7. Reassess the airway after insertion (Step 3).

Several problems are possible with the nasopharyngeal airway. A diameter that is too small may become obstructed by mucus, blood, vomitus, or the soft tissues of the pharynx. If the airway is too long, it may stimulate the vagus nerve and slow the pulse rate; it may also enter the esophagus, causing gastric distention. Inserting the airway in responsive patients may cause spasm of the larynx and result in vomiting. A nasopharyngeal airway should not be used when the patient has facial trauma because the airway may tear soft tissues and cause bleeding into the airway. Similarly, a nasopharyngeal airway should not be used for a patient with moderate to severe head trauma because it could increase intracranial pressure (ICP).

Oxygenation

As part of your breathing assessment, you will assess the patient's ventilatory and oxygenation status. All patients with respiratory emergencies should receive supplemental oxygen. The two most common ways to deliver oxygen to pediatric patients are the blow-by technique and the nonrebreathing mask.

The **blow-by technique** does not deliver high concentrations of oxygen to the patient, so it is best used when only a small amount of supplemental oxygen is needed or when the patient cannot tolerate wearing the mask needed for higher oxygen delivery. You can use oxygen tubing, a mask, a cup, or a similar device to deliver blow-by oxygen (Figure 13). The child or caregiver can hold the device near the patient's face. Do not use a Styrofoam cup because it may blow fluorocarbons into the child's airway. The idea is to increase the oxygen concentration immediately around the patient's mouth and nose.

For children in significant respiratory distress or respiratory failure or for older children, a nonrebreathing mask is the preferred method of oxygen delivery. With this technique, the patient does not "rebreathe" exhaled air (which has a lower oxygen concentration); as a result, a nonrebreathing mask can deliver up to 90% oxygen to the patient. You must fit the mask appropriately onto the patient's face and use high flow rates (10 to 15 L/min) to achieve the maximum oxygen concentration (Figure 14).

Skill Drill 2

Inserting a Nasopharyngeal Airway

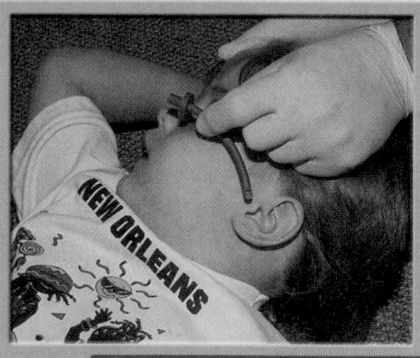

Step 1 Determine the correct airway size by comparing its diameter with the opening of the naris. Place the airway next to the patient's face to confirm correct length. Position the airway appropriately.

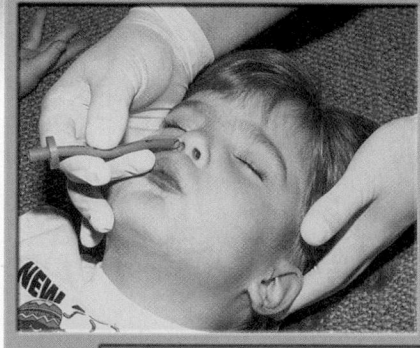

Step 2 Lubricate the airway. Insert the tip into the right naris with the bevel pointing toward the septum.

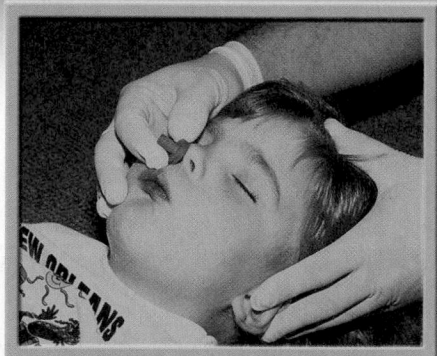

Step 3 Carefully move the tip forward until the flange rests against the outside of the naris. Reassess the airway.

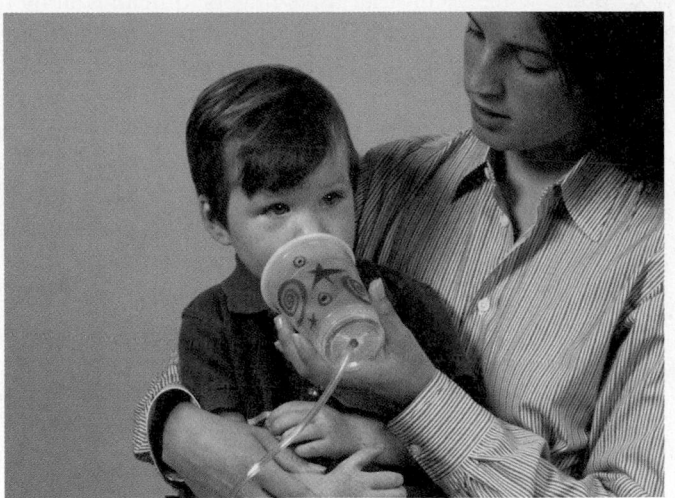

Figure 13 Blow-by oxygen technique can be used for a child with mild respiratory distress who will not tolerate a facial mask. Make a small hole in the base of a 6- to 8-oz cup. Connect the oxygen tubing to an oxygen source, and hold the cup about 1 to 2 inches from the child's mouth.

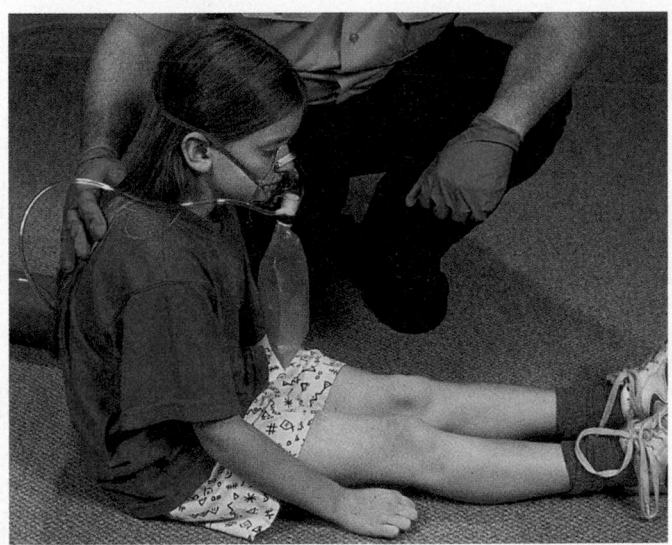

Figure 14 A pediatric nonrebreathing mask is the oxygen delivery method of choice for children who can tolerate it.

Bag-Mask Ventilation

If the patient's respiratory effort is not improved with airway positioning or insertion of an airway adjunct, you should start assisted ventilation using a bag-mask device. Bag-mask ventilation is always the first step in assisted ventilation, and it represents definitive airway management for many patients. Proficiency in bag-mask ventilation is a critical skill for all EMS providers and may avert the need for ET intubation, a procedure with a much higher complication rate. You may need to try a variety of mask sizes to find the one that gives the optimal seal. Do not hesitate to change providers, hand position, or technique if difficulty with ventilation continues.

Words of Wisdom

Limit ventilation volume to just that necessary to cause the chest to rise.

Avoid excessive tidal volumes and rate to minimize gastric distention, vomiting, and aspiration. Deliver breaths at a rate of 12 to 20 breaths/min for infants and children (one breath every 3 to 5 seconds), squeezing the bag only until you see the chest rise. Do not overdistend the chest.

Assist the ventilation of an infant or child using a bag-mask device in the following way:

1. Ensure that you have the appropriate equipment in the right size. The mask should extend from the bridge of the nose to the cleft of the chin, avoiding compression of the eyes **Figure 15**. The mask is transparent, so you can observe for cyanosis and vomiting. The mask volume should be small to decrease dead space and avoid rebreathing; however, the bag should contain at least 450 mL of air. Use an infant bag rather than a neonatal bag for children older than 1 year. Older children and adolescents may need an adult-size bag. Make sure that there is no pop-off valve on the bag; if there is one, make sure that you can hold it shut as necessary to achieve adequate chest rise.

2. Maintain a good seal with the mask on the face. An inadequate mask-to-face seal will result in inadequate tidal volume delivery and a decreased concentration of delivered oxygen. Consider the use of airway adjuncts (nasal and oral pharyngeal airways) in tandem with bag-mask ventilation.

3. Ventilate at the appropriate rate and volume using a slow, gentle squeeze (1 second per breath), until the chest visibly rises. Do not hyperventilate.

Errors in technique, including providing too much volume with each breath, squeezing the bag too forcefully, and ventilating at too fast a rate, can result in gastric distention or

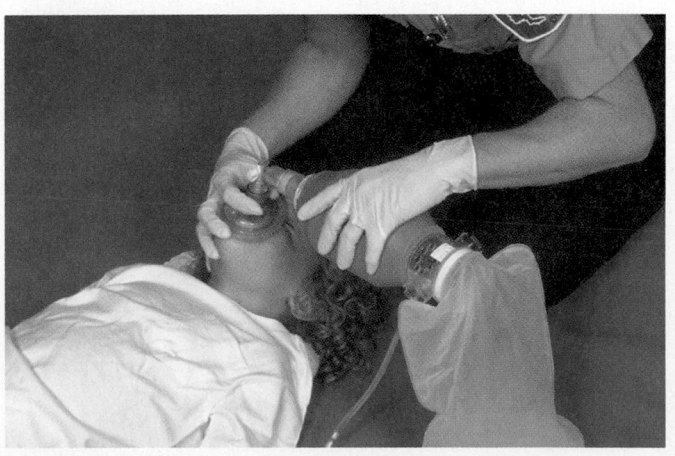

Figure 15 Proper mask size for bag-mask ventilation.

a pneumothorax. Even with the best technique, however, the patient may regurgitate and aspirate the stomach contents. An inadequate mask-to-face seal or improper head position can lead to inadequately delivered tidal volume and hypoxia.

One-Person Bag-Mask Ventilation Perform one-person bag-mask ventilation for an infant or child by following the steps in Skill Drill 3:

Skill Drill   3

1. Open the airway, and insert the appropriate airway adjunct Step 1.
2. Hold the mask on the patient's face by using the one-handed head tilt–chin lift technique (E-C grip) method: Form a C with your thumb and index finger along the

mask, while your other three fingers form an E along the mandible. With infants and toddlers, support the jaw with only your third finger. Do not compress the area under the chin because you may push the tongue into the back of the mouth and block the airway. Keep your fingers on the mandible.
3. Make sure the mask forms an airtight seal on the face. Maintain the seal while checking that the airway is open Step 2.
4. Squeeze the bag, using the correct ventilation rate: 12 to 20 breaths/min for infants and children (one breath every 3 to 5 seconds).
5. Allow 1 second per ventilation, providing adequate time for exhalation Step 3.
6. Assess the effectiveness of ventilation by watching for adequate bilateral rise and fall of the chest Step 4.

Skill Drill   3

One-Person Bag-Mask Ventilation for a Child

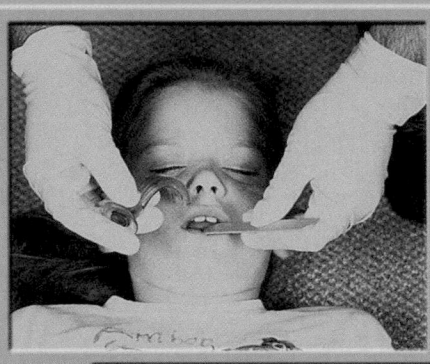

Step 1 Open the airway and insert the appropriate airway adjunct.

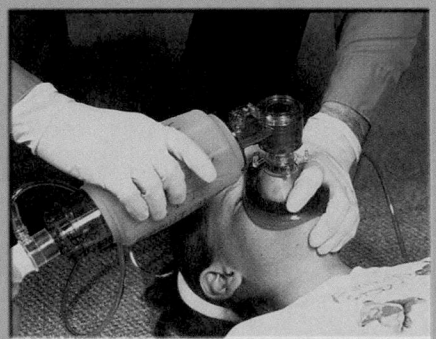

Step 2 Hold the mask on the patient's face with a one-handed head tilt–chin lift technique (E-C clamp). Ensure a good mask-to-face seal while maintaining the airway.

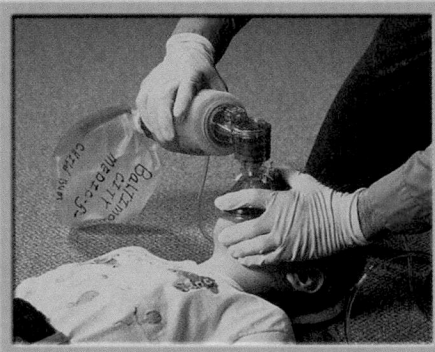

Step 3 Squeeze the bag using the correct ventilation rate of 12 to 20 breaths/min. Allow adequate time for exhalation.

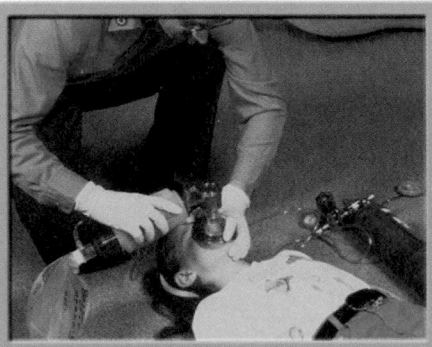

Step 4 Assess effectiveness of ventilation by watching the bilateral rise and fall of the chest.

Two-Person Bag-Mask Ventilation This procedure requires two rescuers—one to maintain an adequate mask-to-face seal and maintain the patient's head position and one to ventilate the patient. This technique is usually more effective at maintaining a tight seal and delivering adequate tidal volume. Because it is not possible to perform a one-handed jaw-thrust manueuver and also maintain spinal immobilization, ventilating the trauma patient is a two-person skill.

Endotracheal Intubation

ET intubation is defined as passing an ET tube through the glottic opening and sealing the tube with a cuff inflated against the tracheal wall. Consider ET intubation only if adequate oxygenation and ventilation cannot be achieved with good bag-mask technique or if transport times are long. Intubation has the advantage of providing a definitive airway and carrying a decreased risk of aspiration, but studies have shown significant failure and complication rates when using this technique in the prehospital setting. Potential complications include damage to teeth and oral structures, aspiration of gastric contents, bradycardia due to a vagal response, bradycardia due to hypoxemia from prolonged attempts, increased ICP, and incorrect placement. Incorrect placement of the ET tube into the right mainstem bronchus may result in hypoxia and inadequate ventilation. A potentially catastrophic complication is an unrecognized esophageal intubation. Indications for ET intubation in pediatric patients are the same as those in adults:

- Cardiopulmonary arrest
- Respiratory failure or arrest
- Traumatic brain injury
- Unresponsiveness
- Inability to maintain a patent airway
- Need for prolonged ventilation
- Need for ET administration of resuscitative medications (if no IV or IO access available)

When you are preparing to intubate an infant or a young child, remember the differences between the adult and pediatric airways Table 14.

Equipment for Endotracheal Intubation Access to pediatric-specific equipment is mandatory, including a range of laryngoscope blades in sizes 0 to 3 and ET tubes in sizes 2.5 (for field deliveries of premature infants) to 6.0. ET tube size selection is based on the child's age. Any size of laryngoscope handle can be used, although many paramedics prefer the thinner pediatric handles. Straight (Miller or Wis-Hipple) blades make it easy to lift the floppy epiglottis to provide a direct view of the vocal cords. If a curved (Macintosh) blade is used, the tip of the blade is positioned in the vallecula to lift the jaw and epiglottis to visualize the vocal cords.

The appropriately sized blade extends from the patient's mouth to the tragus of the ear. Acceptable means of measuring include using the length-based resuscitation tape measure or following these general guidelines:

- Premature newborn: size 0 straight blade
- Full-term newborn to 1 year: size 1 straight blade
- 2 years to adolescent: size 2 straight blade
- Adolescent or older: size 3 straight or curved blade

Table 14	**Differences in the Pediatric Airway**

Infants and small children (up to age 5 or 6 years) have a larger, rounder occiput, which causes the head of an infant or small child who lies supine to be in a flexed position.

In children, the tongue is proportionately larger and the mandible is proportionately smaller—differences that increase children's propensity for airway obstruction.

The epiglottis in a child is more floppy and omega-shaped, so it must be lifted, or positioned, out of the way to visualize the vocal cords.

The trachea in a child is smaller, shorter, and narrower than an adult's, and it is positioned more anteriorly and superiorly.

The narrowest portion of the child's airway is the cricoid ring, which is below the vocal cords (subglottic), and the anatomy below the vocal cords is funnel-shaped. This difference makes a cuff less necessary for occluding the trachea; the developing cartilage of the cricoid ring could be injured by inflation of a cuffed ET tube.

Use a length-based resuscitation tape measure to choose the appropriate ET tube size or, for children older than 1 year, use this formula for uncuffed ET tubes:

$$[\text{Age (in years)} + 16] \div 4 = \text{Size of tube (in mm)}$$

If using a cuffed ET tube, size down half a size. For example, a 4-year-old child would need a 5.0-mm uncuffed ET tube:

$$[(4+16) \div 4 = 5.0] \text{ or a 4.5 cuffed ET tube}$$

Always have a tube that is one size smaller and one that is one size larger than expected available for situations in which there is variability in upper airway diameter.

For patients who are younger than 8 to 10 years, you may choose to use uncuffed ET tubes, although a non-inflated cuffed tube is acceptable. A cuff at the cricoid ring may be unnecessary to obtain a seal in young children. Furthermore, there is the possibility of ischemia and damage to the mucosa of the trachea at this location when cuffs are inflated at high pressures.

The appropriate depth for insertion is 2 to 3 cm beyond the vocal cords. This depth should be recorded as the mark at the corner of the child's mouth. For uncuffed tubes, there is often a black glottic marker at the tube's distal end to use as a guide. When you see this line go through the vocal cord, stop. For cuffed tubes, when the cuff is just below the vocal cords, stop. Another guideline is to insert the tube to a depth that is equal to three times the inside diameter of the ET tube. The depth of insertion is important in order to avoid right mainstem intubation or unplanned extubation.

Pediatric stylets will fit into tubes sized 3.0 to 6.0 mm, whereas adult stylets are used for tubes 6.0 mm or larger. The use of a stylet is based on personal preference. If you use a stylet, insert it into the ET tube, stopping at least 1 cm from the end of the tube; a stylet that protrudes beyond the end of the tube can damage the oral mucosa and vocal cords. With the stylet in place, bend the ET tube into a gentle upward curve. In some cases, bending the tube into the shape of a hockey stick is beneficial.

Preparing for and Performing Endotracheal Intubation Pediatric patients should be preoxygenated (but not hyperventilated) with a bag-mask device and 100% supplemental oxygen for at least 2 to 3 minutes before you attempt intubation using the "squeeze, release, release" technique. Adequate preoxygenation cannot be overemphasized because respiratory failure or arrest is the most common cause of cardiopulmonary arrest in the pediatric population. During this time, you must also ensure that the child's head is in the proper position—the neutral position for patients with suspected spinal trauma or the sniffing position for patients without trauma. Insert an airway adjunct if one is needed to ensure adequate ventilation.

Because stimulation of the parasympathetic nervous system and bradycardia can occur during intubation, you should apply a cardiac monitor if one is available. Use a pulse oximeter before, during, and after the intubation attempt to monitor the patient's pulse rate and oxygen saturation. Have suction handy.

To perform endotracheal intubation in an infant or a child, follow the steps listed in Skill Drill 4 :

Skill Drill ⎯⎯ 4 ⎯⎯

1. Take standard precautions (gloves and face shield) Step 1 .
2. Check, prepare, and assemble your equipment Step 2 .
3. Measure an adjunct if needed Step 3 .
4. Manually open the child's airway, and insert an adjunct, if needed Step 4 .

5. Preoxygenate the child with a bag-mask device and 100% oxygen for at least 2 to 3 minutes Step 5 .
6. Measure the length of the child using a length-based resuscitation tape Step 6 .
7. Remove the airway adjunct if one was placed. Insert the laryngoscope in the right side of the mouth, and sweep the tongue to the left. Lift the tongue with firm, gentle pressure. Avoid using the teeth or gums as a fulcrum Step 7 .
8. Identify the vocal cords. If the cords are not yet visible, instruct your partner to perform the BURP maneuver, if possible Step 8 .
9. Introduce the ET tube in the right corner of the child's mouth Step 9 .
10. Pass the ET tube through the vocal cords to approximately 2 to 3 cm below the vocal cords. Inflate the cuff if a cuffed tube is used Step 10 .
11. Attach an ETCO$_2$ detector (waveform capnography preferred).
12. Attach the bag-mask device, and auscultate for equal breath sounds over each lateral chest wall high in the axillae. Ensure absence of breath sounds over the epigastrium Step 11 .
13. Secure the ET tube, noting the placement of the distance marker at the child's teeth or gums, and reconfirm tube placement Step 12 .

If an intubated child deteriorates, use the DOPE mnemonic (**D**isplacement, **O**bstruction, **P**neumothorax, **E**quipment failure) to identify the potential problem, and institute an appropriate intervention Table 15 .

Skill Drill ⎯ 4 ⎯

Performing Pediatric Endotracheal Intubation

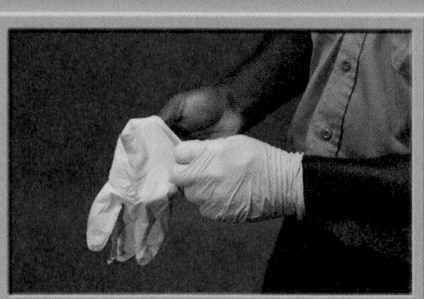

Step 1 Take standard precautions (gloves and face shield).

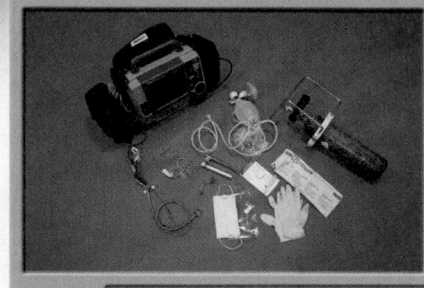

Step 2 Check, prepare, and assemble your equipment.

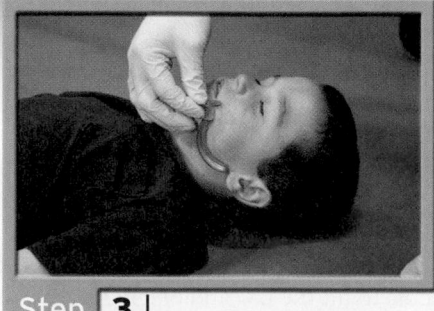

Step 3 Measure an adjunct if needed.

Continues

Skill Drill 4

Performing Pediatric Endotracheal Intubation, continued

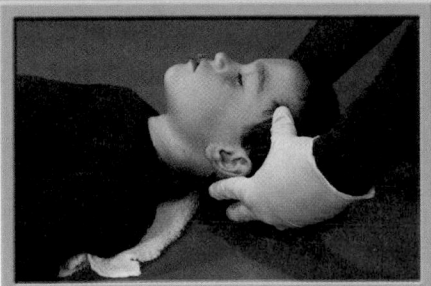

Step **4** Manually open the child's airway and insert an adjunct if needed.

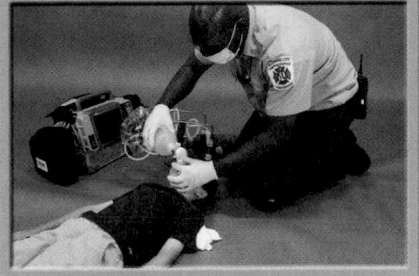

Step **5** Preoxygenate the child with a bag-mask device and 100% oxygen for at least 2 to 3 minutes.

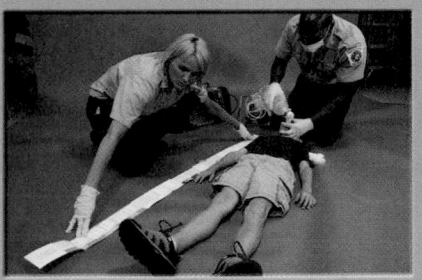

Step **6** Measure the length of the child using a length-based resuscitation tape.

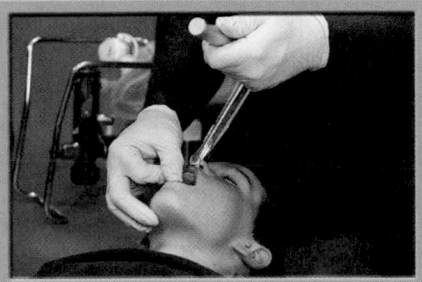

Step **7** Remove the airway adjunct if one was placed. Insert the laryngoscope in the right side of the mouth, and sweep the tongue to the left. Lift the tongue with firm, gentle pressure. Avoid using the teeth or gums as a fulcrum.

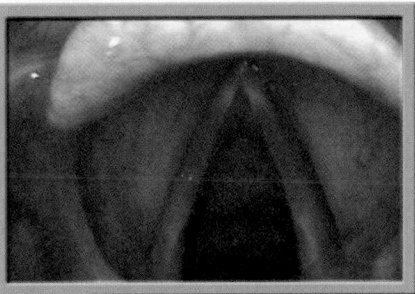

Step **8** Identify the vocal cords. If the cords are not yet visible, instruct your partner to perform the BURP maneuver, if possible.

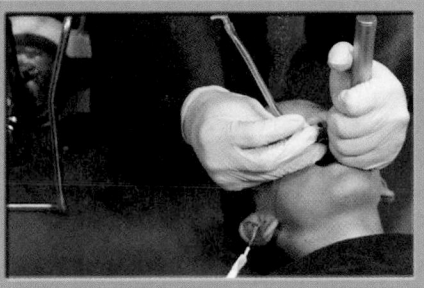

Step **9** Introduce the ET tube in the right corner of the child's mouth.

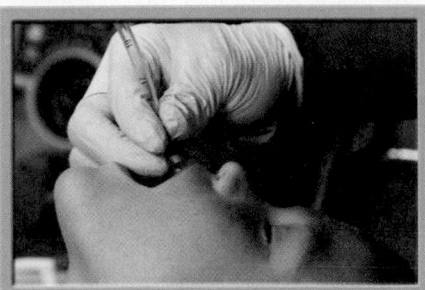

Step **10** Pass the ET tube through the vocal cords to approximately 2 to 3 cm below the vocal cords. Inflate the cuff if a cuffed tube is used.

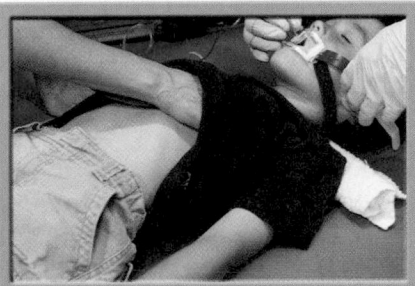

Step **11** Attach an ETCO$_2$ detector. Attach the bag-mask device, and auscultate for equal breath sounds over each lateral chest wall high in the axillae. Ensure absence of breath sounds over the epigastrium. Ensure proper tube placement with waveform capnography.

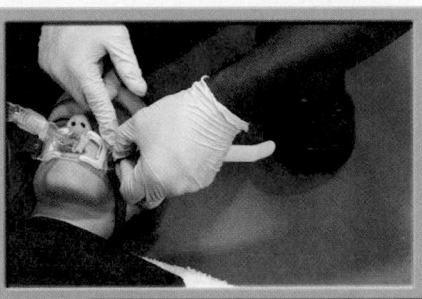

Step **12** Secure the ET tube.

Table 15 **DOPE: Troubleshooting Acute Deterioration With the DOPE Mnemonic in an Intubated Child**

Displacement	■ Reauscultate breath sounds and any sounds over the epigastrium. ■ If breath sounds are stronger on the right, slowly withdraw the tube until they are equal bilaterally. ■ If breath sounds are absent and you hear epigastric gurgling, immediately remove the endotracheal tube, suction as needed, and ventilate with a bag-mask device and 100% oxygen.
Obstruction	■ If thick pulmonary secretions are interfering with your ability to effectively ventilate an intubated child, perform tracheobronchial suctioning. ■ Consider tube obstruction if ventilation compliance is decreased (that is, it is difficult to squeeze the bag).
Pneumothorax	■ Suspect a pneumothorax if breath sounds are stronger on the *left* side and decreased or absent on the right; such findings are not consistent with right mainstem bronchus intubation. ■ Ventilation compliance may also be decreased in a child with a pneumothorax. ■ Prepare to perform needle decompression.
Equipment failure	■ Ensure that you are giving 100% oxygen. ■ Check the reservoir bag on the bag-mask device for tears, ensure that the device is attached to a 100% oxygen source, and check the bag itself for tears. ■ Immediately replace defective or damaged equipment.

Complications of Endotracheal Intubation Complications associated with ET intubation in pediatric patients are essentially the same as those for adult patients:

- Unrecognized esophageal intubation. *Frequently* monitor the position of the tube, especially after *any* major patient move. Use continuous waveform capnography.
- Induction of emesis and possible aspiration. *Always* have a suctioning device immediately available.
- Hypoxia resulting from prolonged intubation attempts. Limit pediatric intubation attempts to *20 seconds*. Monitor the child's cardiac rhythm and oxygen saturation during intubation.
- Damage to teeth, soft tissues, and intraoral structures. Technique, technique, technique!

Documentation and Communication

Vital signs, especially pulse rate and oxygen saturation, should be recorded before and after each intubation attempt. Record the size of the ET tube and the depth of insertion as measured at the patient's lip.

Orogastric and Nasogastric Tube Insertion

During positive-pressure ventilation, it is common to inflate the stomach, as well as the lungs, with air and liquid. Gastric distention slows downward movement of the diaphragm and decreases tidal volume, making ventilation more difficult and necessitating higher inspiratory pressures. It also increases the risk that the patient will vomit and aspirate stomach contents into the lungs. Invasive gastric decompression involves placement of a nasogastric (NG) tube or an orogastric (OG) tube to decompress the stomach by removing the contents with suction, making assisting ventilation easier. Gastric decompression with an NG or OG tube is contraindicated in unresponsive children

with a poor or absent gag reflex and an unsecured airway. Instead, you should perform ET intubation first to decrease the risk of vomiting and aspiration.

Special Populations

A single intubation attempt should be limited to 20 seconds. If the attempt is not successful after 20 seconds, resume bag-mask ventilation and preoxygenate the child for the next attempt.

Preparation of Equipment To perform NG or OG tube insertion, you will need an appropriately sized NG or OG tube; a 30- to 60-mL syringe with a funnel-tipped adapter for manual removal of stomach contents through the tube; mechanical suction; adhesive tape; and a water-soluble lubricant. To prepare the patient and the equipment for NG or OG tube placement, take the following steps:

1. Select the proper size of tube. Use a pediatric resuscitation tape measure to determine the proper size, or use a tube size twice the uncuffed ET tube size that the child would need. For example, a child who needs a 5.0-mm uncuffed ET tube requires a 10F OG or NG tube.
2. Measure the tube on the patient. The length of the tube should be the same as the distance from the lips or tip of the nose (depending on whether the OG or NG route is used) to the earlobe *plus* the distance from the earlobe to the xiphoid process **Figure 16**.
3. Mark this length on the tube with a piece of tape. When the tip of the tube is in the stomach, the tape should be at the lips or nostril.
4. Place the patient in a supine position.
5. Assess the gag reflex. If the patient is unresponsive and has a poor or absent gag reflex, perform ET intubation before gastric tube placement.

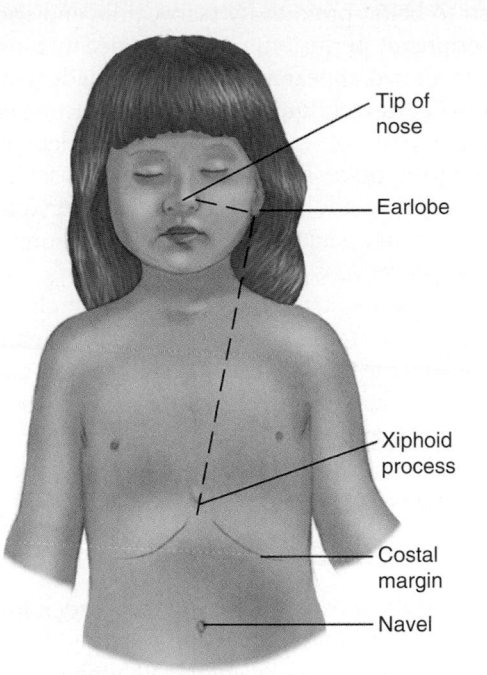

Figure 16 Technique for measuring the distance to insert an NG or OG tube.

6. In a trauma patient, maintain in-line stabilization of the cervical spine if a neck injury is possible. Choose the OG route of insertion if the patient has a severe head or midfacial injury.

7. Lubricate the end of the tube.

OG Tube Insertion Follow these steps to insert an OG tube in an infant or child:

1. Insert the tube over the tongue, using a tongue blade if necessary to facilitate insertion.

2. Advance the tube into the hypopharynx, then insert it rapidly into the stomach.

3. If the child begins coughing or choking or has a change in voice, immediately remove the tube; it may be in the trachea.

NG Tube Insertion Follow these steps to insert an NG tube in an infant or child:

1. Insert the tube gently through the naris, directing the tube straight back along the nasal floor. Do not angle the tube superiorly. If the tube does not pass easily, try the opposite naris or a smaller tube. Never force the tube.

2. Advance the tube into the stomach.

3. If NG passage is unsuccessful, use the OG approach.

Assessing Placement of OG and NG Tubes Follow these steps to confirm successful placement of an NG or OG tube:

1. Check tube placement by aspirating stomach contents. Use a syringe with an appropriate adapter to quickly instill 10 to 20 mL of air through the tube while auscultating over the left upper quadrant. If you hear a rush of air (or gurgling) over the stomach, the placement is correct.

2. If correct placement cannot be confirmed, remove the tube.

3. Secure the tube to the bridge of the nose or to the cheek, using adhesive tape.

4. Aspirate air from the stomach, using a 30- to 60-mL catheter-tipped syringe, or connect the tube to mechanical suction at a low, continuous suction of 20 to 40 mm Hg or to the intermittent setting.

Complications of OG or NG Tube Insertion As with ET intubation, you must be aware of the potential complications associated with the placement of an NG or OG tube—namely, placement of the tube into the trachea, resulting in hypoxia; vomiting and aspiration of stomach contents; airway bleeding or obstruction; and passage of the tube into the cranium. The last complication can occur if you insert an NG tube into a patient with severe head or midfacial trauma because the tube may be passed through the fracture and into the brain.

■ Cardiopulmonary Arrest

Cardiopulmonary arrest in infants and children is most often associated with respiratory failure and respiratory arrest. Children are affected differently than adults when it comes to decreasing oxygen concentrations. An adult becomes hypoxic and the heart gets irritable, and sudden cardiac death occurs from a dysrhythmia. This is often in the form of ventricular fibrillation, and is the reason why defibrillation is the treatment of choice. A child, on the other hand, becomes hypoxic and the heart slows down, becoming more and more bradycardic. The heart will beat slower and become weaker with each beat until no pulse is felt. The survival rate from cardiac arrest in the prehospital setting is poor and clearly improved by strengthening the links in the chain of survival. However, the survival rate from respiratory arrest is 75%. Therefore, a child who is breathing poorly with a slowing pulse rate must be ventilated with high concentrations of oxygen early to try to oxygenate the heart and avoid the development of cardiac arrest. The chapter, *Responding to the Field Code* covers providing CPR to pediatric patients in detail.

The signs, symptoms, and treatment of cardiopulmonary arrest are discussed in other chapters. The following section will address methods of maintaining and improving circulation in the infant or child, including vascular access IV and IO, and IV fluid resuscitation.

■ Pathophysiology, Assessment, and Management of Shock

Shock is defined as inadequate delivery of oxygen and nutrients to tissues to meet metabolic demand. The types of shock that you may encounter are the same in adults and children: hypovolemic, distributive, and cardiogenic.

Besides determining the cause of shock, you must quickly determine whether the child is in a compensated or decompensated state. In compensated shock, although the child has critical abnormalities of perfusion, his or her body is (for the moment) able to mount a physiologic response to maintain adequate perfusion to vital organs by shunting blood from the periphery, increasing the pulse rate, and increasing the vascular tone. A child in compensated shock will have a normal appearance, tachycardia, and signs of decreased peripheral perfusion, such as cool extremities with prolonged capillary refill. Timely intervention is needed to prevent a child in compensated shock from decompensating.

Decompensated shock is a state of inadequate perfusion in which the body's own mechanisms to improve perfusion are no longer sufficient to maintain a normal blood pressure. Remember that decompensated shock includes hypotension. Hypotension is relative to the age of the child, as illustrated in Table 16 .

Table 16	Lower Limits of Normal Systolic Blood Pressure by Age	
Age	**Minimal Systolic Blood Pressure**	
Infant (1 month to 1 year)	> 70 mm Hg	
1-year-old child	> 80 mm Hg	
Child (1 to 10 years)	80 + (2 × age in years)	
Child or adolescent > 10 years	> 90 mm Hg	

In addition to being profoundly tachycardic and showing signs of poor peripheral perfusion, a child in decompensated shock may have an altered appearance, reflecting inadequate perfusion of the brain. Because children typically have strong cardiovascular systems, they are able to compensate for inadequate perfusion by increasing the pulse rate and peripheral vascular resistance more efficiently than adults. Hypotension is, therefore, a late and ominous sign in an infant or a young child, and urgent intervention is needed to prevent cardiac arrest.

Initial management involves allowing the child to assume a position of comfort and administering supplemental oxygen. After completing the primary assessment, make a transport decision based on the severity of the problem. Start resuscitation on scene for any child who shows signs of decompensated shock. Whereas rapid transport is imperative, the risk of deterioration to cardiac arrest is too high to permit a "load-and-go" approach.

■ Hypovolemic Shock

Hypovolemia is the most common cause of shock in infants and young children, with loss of volume occurring due to illness or trauma. Because of their small blood volume (80 mL/kg body weight), a combination of excessive fluid losses and poor intake in an infant or a young child with gastroenteritis ("stomach flu") can result in shock relatively quickly. The same vulnerability exists with hemorrhage from trauma.

A patient with hypovolemic shock will often appear listless or lethargic and may have compensatory tachypnea. The child may appear pale, mottled, or cyanotic. In medical shock, further assessment may identify signs of dehydration such as sunken

YOU are the Medic — PART 3

You ask your partner to obtain a blood glucose level while you prepare to start an IV line. A quick look for a peripheral vein yields nothing, so you choose to insert an intraosseous needle into the proximal tibia. You successfully insert the intraosseous needle and confirm placement by aspirating bone marrow and observing free flow of fluids into the bone without swelling behind the insertion site. According to the pediatric resuscitation tape measure, the child weighs approximately 14 kg and requires 280 mL of normal saline for a fluid bolus. As you start administering the initial fluid bolus, your partner tells you the blood glucose level is 28 mg/dL.

Recording Time: 9 Minutes	
Respirations	22 breaths/min; adequate depth and volume
Pulse	180 beats/min, regular; absent peripheral pulses and weak central pulses
ECG	Narrow complex tachycardia
Skin	Pale, cool, and dry; some mottling of the extremities
Blood pressure	74/50 mm Hg
Oxygen saturation (Spo$_2$)	98% at 12 L/min on nonrebreathing mask
Pupils	Equal and reactive to light

5. What are the potential complications of intraosseous needle insertion?

6. How should you manage the blood glucose level?

eyes, dry mucous membranes, poor skin turgor, or delayed capillary refill with cool extremities. In an injured child, the site of bleeding may be identified.

Allow the child to remain in a position of comfort, administer supplemental oxygen, and keep the child warm. Apply direct pressure to stop any external bleeding. Volume replacement is the mainstay of treatment for hypovolemic shock, whether medical or traumatic in origin.

If the child is in compensated shock, you can attempt to establish IV or IO access en route to the hospital. As with all procedures, gather all the equipment necessary before beginning this step. Catheters—preferably an over-the-needle catheter—are available in pediatric sizes of 20, 22, and 24 gauge. A butterfly needle is a temporary alternative if an over-the-needle catheter is unavailable; this stainless steel needle stays in the vein, predisposing it to infiltration.

Many of the sites used for IV access in adults are the same for children. The most commonly used sites are the dorsum of the hand and the antecubital fossa. In children, veins in the foot may also be used Figure 17 . Scalp veins and the external jugular veins are used less commonly.

The procedure for establishing IV access in the pediatric patient is as follows:

1. Choose the appropriate fluid, and examine the bag for clarity and expiration date. Make sure that no particles are floating in the fluid and that the fluid is appropriate for the child's condition and not expired.
2. Choose the appropriate drip set, and attach it to the fluid. A macrodrip set (eg, 10 gtt/mL) should be used for a child who needs volume replacement; a microdrip set (eg, 60 gtt/mL) should be used for a child who needs a medication infusion.
3. Fill the drip chamber by squeezing it.
4. Flush or "bleed" the tubing to remove any air bubbles by opening the roller clamp. Make sure no errant bubbles are floating in the tubing.

5. Tear the tape before venipuncture, or have a commercial device available.
6. Apply gloves before making contact with the patient. Secure the appropriate limb to minimize movement during the procedure (ie, use of an arm board). Palpate a suitable vein. Veins should be "springy" when palpated. Stay away from areas that are hard when palpated.
7. Apply the constricting band above the intended IV site. It should be placed approximately 4 inches to 8 inches above the intended site.
8. Clean the area using aseptic technique. Use an alcohol pad to cleanse in a circular motion from the inside out. Use a second alcohol pad to wipe straight down the center.
9. Choose the appropriately sized catheter and twist the catheter to break the seal. Do not advance the catheter upward because this may cause the needle to shear the catheter. Examine the catheter and discard it if you discover any imperfections. Occasionally you will find "burrs" on the edge of the catheter.
10. Insert the catheter at an angle of approximately 45° with the bevel up while applying distal traction with your other hand. This traction will stabilize the vein and help to keep it from "rolling" as you insert the catheter.
11. Observe for "flashback" as blood enters the catheter. The clear chamber at the top of the catheter should fill with blood when the catheter enters the vein. If you note only a drop or two, you should gently advance the catheter farther into the vein.
12. Occlude the catheter to prevent blood leaking while removing the stylet. Hold the hub while withdrawing the needle so as not to pull the catheter out of the vein.
13. Immediately dispose of all sharps in the proper container.
14. Attach the prepared IV line. Hold the hub of the catheter while connecting the IV line.
15. Remove the constricting band.
16. Open the IV line to ensure fluid is flowing and the IV is patent. Observe for any swelling or infiltration around the IV site. If the fluid does not flow, check whether the constriction band has been released. If infiltration is noted, immediately stop the infusion and remove the catheter while holding pressure over the site with a piece of gauze to prevent bleeding.
17. Secure the catheter with tape or a commercial device. Wrap the IV tubing with extra gauze to prevent the child from pulling out the IV catheter.

Once IV access is established, fluid resuscitation should begin with isotonic fluids *only*, such as normal saline or lactated Ringer's. Begin with 20 mL/kg of isotonic fluid, and then reassess the patient's status. The use of warm IV fluids (when possible) can counteract the effects of systemic hypothermia from environmental exposure, blood loss, or open wounds. Multiple fluid boluses may be necessary during transport.

Volume resuscitation should be addressed separately from treatment of hypoglycemia. In a child with shock due to medical illness, perform a bedside glucose check; treat with dextrose-containing fluid only for a documented low blood glucose level. Hypoglycemia is unlikely in shock due to acute injury.

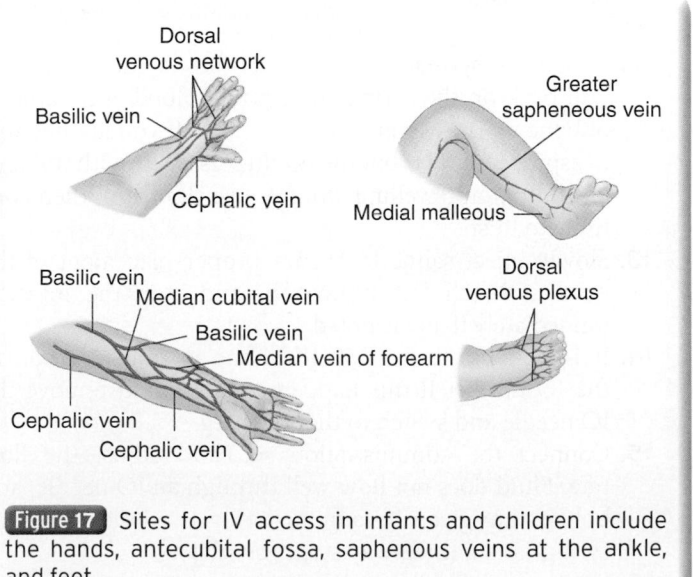

Figure 17 Sites for IV access in infants and children include the hands, antecubital fossa, saphenous veins at the ankle, and feet.

If a child is in decompensated shock with hypotension, begin initial fluid resuscitation at the scene. Evaluate sites for IV access. If this is unsuccessful, begin IO infusion. When an IO needle is placed correctly, it will rest in the medullary canal, the space within the bone that contains bone marrow. An IO infusion is contraindicated if a secure IV line is available or if a fracture (or possible fracture) exists in the same bone in which you plan to insert the IO needle. Anything that can be administered through an IV line can be administered through an IO line (such as isotonic fluids, medications).

The IO needles are usually double needles, consisting of a solid-bore needle inside a sharpened hollow needle **Figure 18**. This double needle is pushed into the bone (usually the proximal tibia) with a screwing, twisting action away from the joint to avoid disruption of the growth plate. Once the needle pops through the bone, the solid needle is removed, leaving the hollow steel needle in place. The EZ-IO uses a drill mechanism for quick and safe IO insertion, and can be used on any age patient, including adults. The EZ-IO comes with two standard needle sizes: pink pediatric (13 to 39 kg weight) and blue adult (greater than 40 kg weight). Standard IV tubing is attached to this catheter.

Words of Wisdom

If the patient "fits" on a length-based resuscitation tape measure (Broselow tape), "think pink" for pediatric EZ-IO needle color. If the patient is too big for the length-based resuscitation tape measure, use the adult EZ-IO needle.

The IO lines require full and careful immobilization because they rest at a 90° angle to the bone and are easily dislodged. Stabilize the IO needle, thereby ensuring adequate flow, in the same manner that you would any impaled object. As with any invasive procedure, several complications may be associated with IO infusion: compartment syndrome, failed infusion, growth plate injury, bone inflammation caused by infection

(osteomyelitis), skin infection, and bony fracture. Proper technique will help to minimize these complications.

Follow the steps in **Skill Drill 5** to establish an IO infusion in pediatric patients:

Skill Drill   5

1. Check the IV fluid for proper fluid, clarity, and expiration date. Look for any discoloration or particles floating in the fluid. If any are found, discard and choose another bag of fluid.

2. Select the appropriate equipment, including an IO needle, syringe, saline, and extension set **Step 1**. A three-way stopcock may also be used to facilitate easier fluid administration.

3. Select the proper administration set. Connect the administration set to the bag. Prepare the administration set. Fill the drip chamber, and flush the tubing. Make sure no air bubbles remain in the tubing.

4. Prepare the syringe and extension tubing **Step 2**.

5. Cut or tear the tape and prepare bulky dressings. This can be done at any time before the IO puncture.

6. Take standard precautions. This must be done before the IO puncture.

7. Identify the proper anatomic site for IO puncture **Step 3**. To miss the epiphyseal (growth) plate, you should measure two fingerbreadths below the knee on the medial side of the leg.

8. Cleanse the site using aseptic technique (that is, in a circular manner from the inside out).

9. Stabilize the tibia. Place a folded towel under the knee, and hold it so that you keep your fingers away from the puncture site.

10. Insert the needle at a 90° angle to the leg. Advance the needle with a twisting motion until you feel a "pop" **Step 4**. Unscrew the cap, and remove the stylet from the needle **Step 5**.

11. Remove the stylet from the catheter.

12. Attach the syringe and extension set to the IO needle. Pull back on the syringe to aspirate blood and particles of bone marrow to ensure placement. If you are not able to aspirate marrow but the IO flushes easily with no signs of infiltration (swelling around insertion site), then continue to flush.

13. Slowly inject saline to ensure proper placement of the needle. Watch for infiltration, and stop the infusion immediately if any is noted.

14. It is possible to fracture the bone during insertion of the IO needle. If this happens, you should remove the IO needle and switch to the other leg.

15. Connect the administration set, and adjust the flow rate. Fluid does not flow well through an IO needle, and boluses are given by administering the fluid using the syringe and a three-way stopcock **Step 6**.

16. Secure the needle with tape, and support it with a bulky dressing. Be careful not to tape around the entire

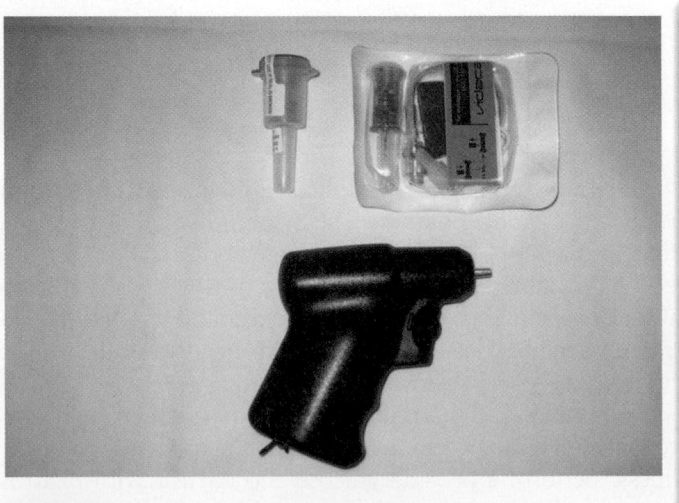

Figure 18   Standard pediatric intraosseous needle.

Skill Drill 5

Pediatric IO Infusion

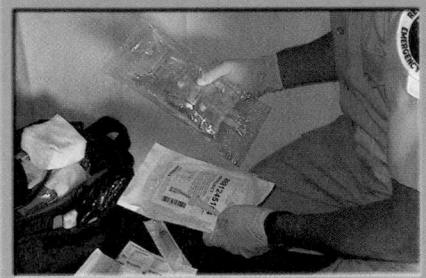

Step 1 Check selected IV fluid for proper fluid, clarity, and expiration date. Select the appropriate equipment, including an IO needle, syringe, saline, and extension set.

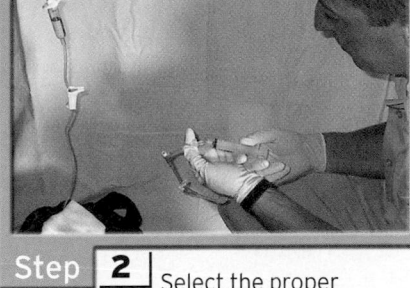

Step 2 Select the proper administration set. Connect the administration set to the bag. Prepare the administration set. Prepare the syringe and extension tubing.

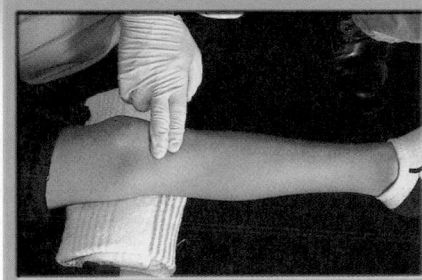

Step 3 Cut or tear the tape. Take standard precautions. Identify the proper anatomic site for IO puncture.

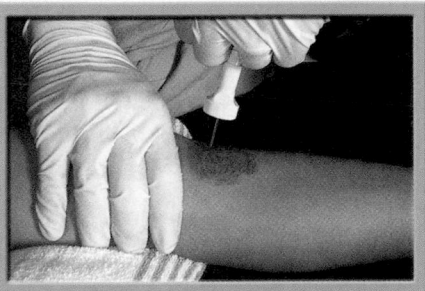

Step 4 Cleanse the site appropriately. Stabilize the tibia. Insert the needle at a 90° angle to the leg. Advance the needle with a twisting motion until you feel a "pop".

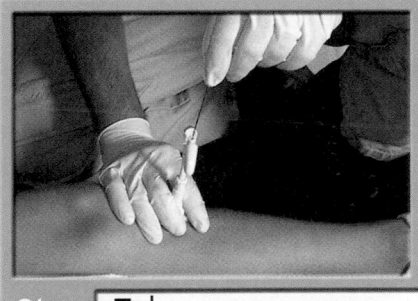

Step 5 Unscrew the cap, and remove the stylet from the needle.

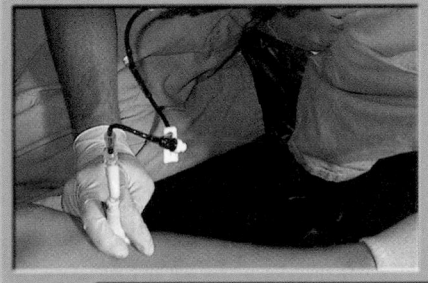

Step 6 Attach the syringe and extension set to the IO needle. Pull back on the syringe to aspirate blood and particles of bone marrow to ensure placement. Slowly inject saline to ensure proper placement of the needle. Watch for infiltration, and stop the infusion immediately if any noted. Connect the administration set, and adjust the flow rate as appropriate.

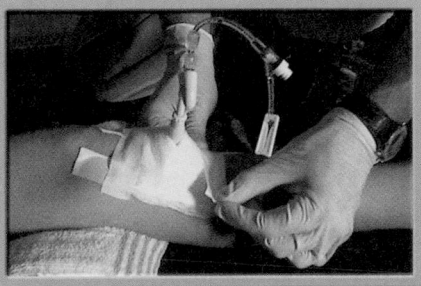

Step 7 Secure the needle with tape, and support it with a bulky dressing. Dispose of the needle in the proper container.

circumference of the leg because this could impair circulation and create compartment syndrome.

17. Dispose of the needle in the proper container (**Step 7**).

As with IV administration, administer 20 mL/kg boluses of isotonic fluid via IO infusion to treat hypovolemia, reassessing after each bolus and repeating as needed based on physiologic response. As much as 60 mL/kg may be needed during transport to improve the child's blood pressure, pulse rate, mental status, and peripheral perfusion. Rapidly transport the patient to an appropriate treatment facility.

Distributive Shock

In distributive shock, decreased vascular tone develops, resulting in vasodilation and third spacing of fluids due to increased vascular permeability (leakage of plasma out of the blood vessels and into the surrounding tissues). This results in a drop in effective blood volume and functional hypovolemia. Distributive shock may be due to sepsis, anaphylaxis, and spinal cord injury; sepsis accounts for the bulk of pediatric cases.

Early in distributive shock, the child may have warm, flushed skin and bounding pulses as a result of peripheral vasodilation. In contrast, the symptoms and signs of *late* distributive shock will look much like hypovolemic shock on primary assessment. Fever is a key finding in septic shock, whereas urticarial rash and wheezing may be noted in anaphylaxis, and neurologic deficits are apparent in shock due to spinal cord injury.

Front-line treatment of pediatric patients in distributive shock is volume resuscitation because the child is in a state of relative hypovolemia. In a child with apparent sepsis who remains persistently hypotensive despite administration of a total of 60 mL/kg of isotonic fluid, vasopressor support to improve vascular tone may be considered.

Anaphylactic shock should be treated immediately with IM epinephrine, 0.01 mg/kg of 1:1,000 solution (maximum dose, 0.3 mg). This dose should be repeated as necessary every 5 minutes. If several doses are needed, the child may require a low-dose, continuous epinephrine IV drip. The decision about timing of IV access and transport for patients in distributive shock considers the same factors as for patients in hypovolemic shock. Additional therapies for anaphylactic shock include diphenhydramine 0.5 to 1 mg/kg IV (max of 50 mg) and methylprednisone 0.5 mg IV (max of 60 mg) or dexamethasone 0.15 mg/kg (max of 16 mg) to decrease ongoing exacerbation.

Cardiogenic Shock

Cardiogenic shock is the result of pump failure: intravascular volume is normal, but myocardial function is poor. This type of shock is uncommon in the pediatric population but may be present in children with underlying congenital heart disease, myocarditis, or rhythm disturbances. It is important to recognize cardiogenic shock by the child's history or from the primary assessment because the treatment for this type of shock is different from that for hypovolemic or distributive shock.

A child in cardiogenic shock will appear listless or lethargic (like children in hypovolemic or distributive shock) but is likely to show signs of increased work of breathing owing to congestive heart failure and pulmonary edema. Circulation will be impaired, and the skin will look pale, mottled, or cyanotic. Your primary assessment may reveal an abnormal pulse rate or rhythm or findings of a murmur or gallop. The child's skin may feel clammy, and you may feel an enlarged liver. The caregiver may describe the infant sweating with feeding and, in many cases, will recount a history of congenital heart disease.

Special Populations

Shock in children is most likely due to hypovolemia. Fluid resuscitation with isotonic fluid is the mainstay of treatment.

If you suspect cardiogenic shock, allow the child to remain in a position of comfort (often sitting upright), administer supplemental oxygen, and transport. The transport destination is a critical decision because the facility needs to be capable of providing pediatric critical care. Supplemental oxygen may not increase the SpO_2 in children with particular types of congenital heart disease, and parents will often alert you to this fact. Consider establishing IV access en route to the receiving facility. Unless you are sure of the diagnosis of cardiogenic shock (the child has a history of congenital heart disease, is afebrile, and has no history of volume loss), err on the side of fluid resuscitation. If you suspect cardiac dysfunction, administer a single isotonic fluid bolus slowly, and monitor the patient carefully to assess its effect. Increased work of breathing, a drop in oxygen saturation, or worsening perfusion after a fluid bolus will confirm your suspicion of cardiogenic shock. Although inotropic agents may be needed to improve cardiac contractility and improve perfusion, they are rarely administered in the field. See the chapter, *Management and Resuscitation of the Critical Patient*, for more information on cardiogenic shock.

Special Populations

A child with decompensated shock from hypovolemia needs fluid resuscitation. Do not waste time with multiple IV insertion attempts. Insert an IO needle, and begin fluid therapy.

Pathophysiology, Assessment, and Management of Cardiovascular Emergencies

Cardiovascular emergencies are relatively rare in children. When such problems arise, they are often related to volume or infection rather than a primary cardiac cause, unless the child has congenital heart disease. Through the primary assessment, you can quickly identify a cardiovascular emergency, understand the likely cause, and institute potentially lifesaving treatment.

Dysrhythmias

Rhythm disturbances can be classified based on whether the pulse rate is too slow (bradydysrhythmias), too fast (tachydysrhythmias), or absent (pulseless). The signs and symptoms associated with a rhythm disturbance are often nonspecific—for example, the patient or caregiver may report fatigue, irritability, vomiting, chest or abdominal pain, palpitations, and shortness of breath.

If you suspect a rhythm disturbance, quickly move through the primary assessment, supporting the airway and breathing as necessary. An ECG or rhythm strip will help you to identify the underlying rhythm, thus allowing you to decide which specific management steps should be initiated. Address reversible causes of dysrhythmias such as hypoxemia. The decision to stay on scene to obtain additional history and perform a secondary assessment will be dictated by the child's overall physiologic status.

Bradydysrhythmias

Bradydysrhythmias, a condition in which the pulse rate is lower than normal for age, most often occurs secondary to hypoxia in children, rather than as a result of a primary cardiac problem (such as heart block). Airway management, supplemental oxygen, and assisted ventilation as needed are always first-line treatment. Also, treat any underlying respiratory problem. Less common causes of bradycardia include congenital or acquired heart block and toxic ingestion of beta blockers, calcium channel blockers, or digoxin. Elevated ICP can also cause bradycardia and should be considered in children with ventricular shunts, a history of head injury, or suspected child abuse without a consistent injury history.

Initiate electronic cardiac monitoring as part of your primary assessment. If the child is asymptomatic, no further treatment is indicated in the field. Healthy, athletic adolescents may have sinus bradycardia as an incidental finding and should be transported to a hospital for further evaluation if they are symptomatic (ie, chest pain, dizziness, syncope).

If the child's pulse rate is lower than normal for age despite oxygenation and ventilation and perfusion is poor, begin chest compressions and attempt IV or IO access. For chest compressions to be effective, the patient should be placed on a firm, flat surface with the head at the same level as the body. If you need to carry an infant while providing CPR, your forearm and hand can serve as the flat surface. See the chapter, *Responding to the Field Code* for more information about infant and child CPR.

Heart block can be congenital or acquired in varying degrees. First-degree block is an asymptomatic, often incidental finding seen on ECG or cardiorespiratory monitoring with slight prolongation of the PR interval. No intervention is needed. Second-degree heart block may involve a progressive prolongation of the PR interval with a subsequent drop of the QRS complex (type I) or a random drop of the QRS complex (type II). Type II second-degree blocks may progress to third-degree heart blocks in which the atrial and ventricular rates are totally uncoordinated. These rhythms can lead to poor perfusion and cardiovascular compromise.

Transcutaneous pacing may be used in patients with symptomatic bradycardia or third-degree heart block to provide the patient with adequate circulation until they can be evaluated by a cardiologist.

Tachydysrhythmias

Sinus tachycardia, a pulse rate higher than normal for age, is common in children. Although it may be a sign of serious underlying illness or injury, it may also be due to fever, pain, or anxiety. Interpret the presence of tachycardia in the context of the remainder of the PAT and the primary assessment. For example, if a child appears well but has a fever, sinus tachycardia is likely and treatment with antipyretics is all that is necessary. If a child with tachycardia has a history of copious vomiting or diarrhea, fluid resuscitation is the appropriate treatment.

Special Populations

The preferred agent for pediatric bradycardia is epinephrine unless the bradycardia is suspected to be from increased vagal tone.

If a child with tachycardia appears ill and has poor perfusion with no history of fever, trauma, or excessive volume loss, continue your assessment for a primary cardiac cause while initiating resuscitation. Your assessment should include determination of the pulse rate along with interpretation of an ECG or rhythm strip.

Tachydysrhythmias are subdivided into two types based on the width of the QRS complex. A narrow complex tachycardia exists when the QRS complex is 0.09 second or less (less than two standard boxes on the rhythm strip); a wide complex tachycardia exists when the QRS complex is greater than 0.08 second (more than two standard boxes on the rhythm strip).

Narrow Complex Tachycardia Although sinus tachycardia is the most common dysrhythmia in children, supraventricular tachycardia (SVT) is the most frequent tachydysrhythmia requiring antidysrhythmic treatment. **Table 17** compares sinus tachycardia, reentry SVT, and ventricular tachycardia (V-tach). You may identify sinus tachycardia based on the presence or absence of P waves, pulse rate, and history of preceding illness or injury. Its treatment is geared toward the underlying cause and may include oxygen, fluids, splinting, and analgesia.

SVT, which involves abnormal conduction pathways, can be identified by a narrow QRS complex, absence of P waves, and an unvarying pulse rate of more than 220 beats/min in an infant or more than 180 beats/min in a child. The child may have a history of SVT or exhibit nonspecific signs and symptoms, including irritability, vomiting, and chest or abdominal pain. Parents of young infants may report poor feeding for several days. The treatment of SVT depends on the patient's perfusion and overall stability. If the child is in stable condition, consider attempting vagal maneuvers while obtaining IV access: Have an older child hold his or her breath, blow into a straw with the end crimped over, or bear down as if having a bowel movement; in a younger child, place an exam glove filled with ice firmly over the midface, being careful not to obstruct the nose and mouth. Attempt these techniques only once, while continually monitoring the child's rhythm.

If the child has adequate perfusion and vagal maneuvers do not succeed in converting SVT to a sinus rhythm, consider administering adenosine. Adenosine has a short half-life and must be injected quickly into a vein near the heart, usually an antecubital vein. It can be given IO, however, the higher 0.2 mg/kg dose is frequently needed for SVT when it is administered IO, since it

Table 17 Features of Sinus Tachycardia, Supraventricular Tachycardia, and Ventricular Tachycardia

	History	Pulse Rate	Respiratory Rate	QRS Interval	Assessment	Treatment
Sinus tachycardia	Fever Volume loss Hypoxia Pain Increased activity or exercise	< 220 beats/min (infant) < 180 beats/min (child)	Variable	Narrow: < 0.09 s	Hypovolemia Hypoxia Painful injury	Fluids Oxygen Splinting Analgesia or sedation
Supraventricular tachycardia	Congenital heart disease Known SVT Nonspecific symptoms (such as poor feeding, fussiness)	> 220 beats/min (infants) > 180 beats/min (child)	Constant	Narrow: < 0.09 s	CHF* may be present Adenosine	Vagal maneuvers (ice to face) Synchronized electrical cardioversion
Ventricular tachycardia	Serious systemic illness	> 150 beats/min	Variable	Wide: > 0.09 s	CHF may be present	Synchronized electrical cardioversion Amiodarone Procainamide

*CHF indicates congestive heart failure.

takes longer to reach the heart and because of the short half-life of adenosine. Its administration will be followed by a brief run of bradycardia, ventricular tachycardia, ventricular fibrillation, or asystole, which will convert spontaneously to sinus rhythm. Persistence of any of these rhythms is rare, but be prepared to switch dysrhythmia algorithms if necessary.

For a child with SVT who has poor perfusion, **synchronized cardioversion** is recommended. Synchronized cardioversion is the timed administration of electrical energy to the heart to correct a dysrhythmia. If the child is generating a regular but ineffective rhythm, it is important to time the jolt of electricity with the appropriate phase of the electrical activity (corresponds with the R wave on an ECG). A burst of electricity to the myocardium during the relative refractory period (the downward slope of the T wave) can precipitate ventricular fibrillation (V-fib)—a potentially lethal effect. Follow the same steps with synchronized cardioversion as with defibrillation, except that you must press the "sync" button on the defibrillator to alert the machine to time the electrical jolt. The dose of the initial synchronized cardioversion attempt is 0.5 to 1.0 joules per kilogram of body weight (J/kg). If the first dose is unsuccessful, a repeated dose of 2 J/kg can be given. In the hospital setting, sedation is provided before cardioversion, but its administration must not delay the procedure in a child in unstable condition.

An alternative approach to treating the child in SVT with poor perfusion is to give a dose of IV adenosine if vascular access is readily available. Do not delay synchronized cardioversion if vascular access is not already established, however. If the child remains in SVT and is in unstable condition or shock or is unconscious, you may give additional antidysrhythmic medications in conjunction with cardiology consultation.

Wide Complex Tachycardia A child with a wide QRS complex tachycardia with a palpable pulse is likely in V-tach, a rare, but potentially life-threatening rhythm in children. Its presence may reflect underlying cardiac pathology. SVT may sometimes manifest as a wide complex rhythm, and distinguishing between the two can be challenging.

If a child with suspected V-tach is in hemodynamically stable condition and IV access is available, consider administering antidysrhythmic medication. Amiodarone is the drug of choice for V-tach with a pulse, although procainamide is an acceptable alternative. Do not give amiodarone *and* procainamide because both prolong the QT interval. If a child with V-tach is in an unstable condition or shock or is unconscious, the treatment is synchronized cardioversion. Prior sedation is ideal, but do not delay cardioversion for this reason. The same dose of synchronized cardioversion is used for SVT and V-tach.

Special Populations

The most common cause of tachycardia in an infant or a young child is sinus tachycardia from fever, dehydration, or pain.

If a child with a tachydysrhythmia is or becomes pulseless, begin CPR and follow the pulseless arrest treatment guidelines. Prepare to immediately transport any child with a dysrhythmia to an appropriate receiving facility. Copies of rhythm strips or ECG tracings will be helpful to hospital personnel for diagnostic and therapeutic purposes.

Pulseless Arrest Cardiopulmonary arrest exists when the child is unresponsive, apneic, and pulseless. In children, this type of dysrhythmia is usually a secondary event—that is, the end result of profound hypoxemia and acidosis owing to respiratory failure. Asystole is the most common arrest rhythm. Pulseless electrical activity (PEA), V-tach, and V-fib are seen with lower frequency in children than in adults. The survival rate for children with asystolic arrest in the prehospital setting is poor, and few survivors have good neurologic outcomes. The survival rate for children with V-fib arrest is slightly better and, as in adults, depends on early defibrillation.

When you are confronted with a pediatric patient in cardiopulmonary arrest, the most important consideration is to provide high-quality BLS skills. You should also attempt IV or IO access. Attach a monitor or defibrillator to determine the underlying cardiac rhythm. If it is asystole or PEA, defibrillation is not indicated, and additional treatment is limited to epinephrine or a single dose of vasopressin. After administering the medication, perform five cycles of CPR (approximately 2 minutes) before rechecking the rhythm and assessing for the presence of a pulse. If asystole or PEA persists, continue with CPR and epinephrine. High-dose epinephrine is not routinely recommended, however. Consider the "Hs and Ts" as the potential causes—for example, Hypoxia, Hypothermia, Hypovolemia, Tamponade (cardiac), Tension pneumothorax, Toxins, and Trauma.

Defibrillation is performed before administration of medication in the treatment of V-fib or pulseless V-tach. See the chapter, *Responding to the Field Code* for more information on pediatric defibrillation.

Special Populations

Approximately half of all prehospital calls for pediatric patients are trauma-related; the other half are medical. Medical calls may include respiratory complaints (as previously discussed in this chapter), fever, seizures, and altered level of consciousness.

Congenital Heart Disease

Congenital heart disease is the most common congenital disorder in newborns. Neonates and infants can present with varying degrees of cardiorespiratory compromise depending on the particular cardiac lesion. With the advent of prenatal ultrasonography, many congenital heart problems are diagnosed in utero and preparations made for treatment well in advance, but patients may lack prenatal care or decompensate while waiting for evaluation and repair.

Cyanotic Disease

Cyanotic lesions comprise approximately one third of potentially fatal forms of congenital heart disease. These lesions are typically ductal dependent, requiring a patent ductus arteriosus for adequate pulmonary or systemic vascular flow. Examples of cyanotic disease include hypoplastic left heart syndrome (HLHS), tricuspid atresia, transposition of the great arteries (TGA), Tetralogy of Fallot (TOF), total anomalous pulmonary vasculary return (TAPVR), and truncus arteriosus. Patients with these congenital defects typically present in the neonatal period with increasing respiratory distress, poor perfusion, cyanosis, and eventual cardiovascular collapse if left unrecognized. Early recognition, emergent stabilization, and transport to an appropriate cardiac care center are critically important in the outcome of newborns with these lesions.

Initial management includes cardiorespiratory support and monitoring to ensure sufficient organ/tissue perfusion and oxygenation. If there is respiratory compromise, an adequate airway should be established immediately and supportive therapy (eg, supplemental oxygen and/or mechanical ventilation) instituted as needed. Patients with hypotension or poor perfusion require cardiopulmonary resuscitation. Vital signs should be monitored and vascular access established for sampling of blood and administration of medications.

In infants who have a clinical suspicion for a ductal-dependent congenital heart defect, prostaglandin E_1 should be administered until a definitive diagnosis or treatment is established. The initial dose is dependent on the clinical setting because the risk of apnea, one of the major complications of prostaglandin E_1 infusion, is dose dependent. The dose should be managed in conjunction with a pediatric cardiologist, starting at an initial dose of 0.01 µg/kg per minute with a maximum dose of 0.1 µg/kg per minute.

Noncyanotic Disease

Noncyanotic congenital heart disease, including atrial septal defects (ASDs), ventricular septal defects (VSDs), and patent ductus arteriosus (PDA) constitute the most common forms of congenital heart disease. The clinical presentation varies depending on the size of the defect and may range from an isolated murmur that is detected incidentally at a health supervision visit to severe heart failure. Coarctation of the aorta, also typically a noncyanotic lesion, can mimic cyanotic lesions in severe cases and will be discussed later.

Isolated ASDs, as well as most small ASDs of any type, do not cause symptoms in infancy and childhood. The diagnosis is usually made because of a murmur detected incidentally on physical examination. Larger lesions can lead to failure to thrive, frequent respiratory infections, or heart failure.

Infants with small, restrictive VSDs usually remain asymptomatic while those with moderate to large VSDs can manifest signs of heart failure by age 3 to 4 weeks. Common signs and symptoms include tachypnea, poor feeding or sweating with feeds, poor weight gain, tachycardia, and hepatomegaly.

The ductus arteriosus (DA) is a fetal vascular connection between the main pulmonary artery and the aorta that diverts blood away from the pulmonary bed in utero. After birth, the DA constricts and closes because pulmonary flow begins to oxygenate the newborn. A PDA occurs when the DA fails to completely close postnatally.

A murmur is often the only sign of a PDA. The respiratory and cardiac exams are often normal and there is no cyanosis. Larger lesions may lead to symptoms of heart failure, including failure to thrive, poor feeding, and respiratory distress. The older child may present with shortness of breath or easy fatigability.

Coarctation of the aorta (CoA) is typically a discrete narrowing of the thoracic aorta just distal to the left subclavian artery near the DA. The major clinical finding in infants and children with coarctation of the aorta is a difference in systolic blood pressure between the upper and lower extremities. The classic findings are hypertension in the upper extremities with diminished or delayed femoral pulses. Critical lesions can be ductal dependent and significant hemodynamic compromise can occur if the DA closes prior to recognition of this defect, leading to poor systemic circulation. Most older infants and children remain asymptomatic, resulting in delayed diagnosis. They may report chest pain with exercise, cold extremities, and claudication with physical activities. Heart failure rarely occurs beyond the neonatal period.

Words of Wisdom

Keep a laminated copy of the pediatric algorithms with you at all times for your reference during a cardiovascular emergency.

Congestive Heart Failure

Congestive heart failure (CHF) occurs when the heart can no longer meet the metabolic demands of the body at normal physiologic venous pressures. Infants will typically present with tachypnea, respiratory distress (retractions), grunting, and difficulty with feeding. Often, children with CHF have profuse sweating and increased work of breathing during feedings. Older children may have tachycardia, tachypnea, crackles or rales on exam, or an enlarged liver.

Initial management involves assessment of the patient's airway, breathing, and circulation to determine cardiovascular stability. The patient should be supported with oxygen and diuretics may be given in consultation with a cardiologist. IV fluids should be used judiciously because these patients are prone to worsening symptoms from fluid overload.

Neonates with symptoms suggestive of or a history of a ductal dependent lesion who present with symptoms of CHF may require a prostaglandin infusion to preserve systemic circulation until definitive care. This decision should be made in conjunction with a pediatric cardiologist.

Myocarditis

Myocarditis is a condition resulting from inflammation of the heart muscle that results in myocardial dysfunction and can lead to heart failure. In contrast to adults, the majority of children with myocarditis present with acute or fulminant disease. Viral infections are the most common cause of myocarditis in children but autoimmune disorders and toxins should be considered.

Infants and children often present with signs and symptoms of CHF including dyspnea at rest, exercise intolerance (sweating during feeding), syncope, tachypnea, tachycardia, and hepatomegaly. A gallop or new murmur may be heard on cardiac auscultation. However, nonspecific signs and symptoms such as respiratory distress or gastrointestinal symptoms may be the most prominent features early in the illness and can make diagnosis difficult.

Patients may present with fulminant disease with signs of decreased cardiac output, including hypotension, poor pulses, and decreased perfusion, that may progress to cardiovascular collapse. Malignant dysrhythmias can occur leading to sudden cardiac death.

Because of the high risk of dysrhythmias and hemodynamic compromise, the patient with suspected myocarditis should be transported on cardiorespiratory monitors with close attention to the pulse rate, blood pressure, and perfusion. Obtain vascular access but use IV fluids judiciously because these patients are prone to fluid overload from inefficient heart function. Patients will often need inotropic support with dopamine or dobutamine. Oxygen should be applied to all patients during transport.

Cardiomyopathy

In dilated cardiomyopathy (DCM), the heart becomes weakened and enlarged, making it less efficient and causing a negative impact to the pulmonary, hepatic, and other systems. The weakening of the heart is typically due to viral infection or medication toxicity in the pediatric patient. In hypertrophic cardiomyopathy (HCM), the heart muscle is unusually thick, which means that the heart has to pump harder to get blood to leave the heart. Patients with HCM can present with chest pain, hypertension, fatigue, heart failure, syncope, difficulty breathing, and/or cardiac arrest. It is critical for you to thoroughly investigate reports of unexplained syncope in all patients, but especially in the younger population and athletes.

General Assessment and Management of Cardiovascular Emergencies

As with all pediatric emergencies, when you are called to a scene for a suspected cardiac complaint, begin the hands-off assessment by using the PAT and then move to the hands-on assessment of the ABCs. The child's appearance gives an overview of perfusion, oxygenation, ventilation, and neurologic status. For a suspected cardiovascular problem, an abnormal appearance may indicate inadequate brain perfusion and the need for rapid intervention. Tachypnea, without retractions or abnormal airway sounds, is common in an infant or child with a primary cardiac problem; it is a mechanism for blowing off carbon dioxide to compensate for metabolic acidosis related to poor perfusion. In contrast, when cardiac compromise progresses to CHF, pulmonary edema leads to increased work of breathing and a fast respiratory rate. The presence of pallor, cyanosis, or mottling may give you clues to this problem.

For suspected cardiovascular compromise, start with airway and breathing, and provide supportive care as needed. Ensure adequate oxygenation and ventilation, and then assess the circulation by checking the pulse rate, pulse quality, skin CTC, and blood pressure when possible. Combine information from the primary assessment to make a decision about the likely underlying cause, the patient's priority, and the need for immediate treatment or transport.

If you determine that the patient's condition is stable enough for you to continue the assessment on site, continue the assessment. (Table 18 reviews key elements of a cardiovascular SAMPLE history.) Repeat the PAT and ABCs after each intervention, and monitor trends over time.

Table 18 SAMPLE Components for a Child With Cardiovascular Problems

Components	Features
Signs and symptoms	Presence of vomiting or diarrhea Number of episodes of vomiting or diarrhea Vomiting blood or bile; blood in stool External hemorrhage Presence or absence of fever Rash Respiratory distress or shortness of breath
Allergies	Known allergies History of anaphylaxis
Medications	Exact names and dosages of ongoing medications Use of laxative or antidiarrheal medications Long-term diuretic therapy Potential exposure to other medications or drugs Timing and dosages of analgesics or antipyretics
Past medical problems	History of heart problems History of prematurity Prior hospitalizations for cardiovascular problems
Last oral intake	Timing of the child's last food or drink, including bottle or breastfeeding
Events leading to injury or illness	Travel Trauma Fever history Symptoms in family members Potential toxic exposure

Special Populations

A large number of emergencies requiring cardiopulmonary resuscitation in children are preventable.

Pathophysiology, Assessment, and Management of Neurologic Emergencies

Neurologic emergencies can be benign (eg, febrile seizure) or life threatening (eg, ventricular shunt failure). When such problems arise, it is important for you to obtain a thorough past medical history, including previous seizures, shunts, cerebral palsy, or any recent trauma or ingestions. Infants and children are particularly difficult to assess neurologically because they can often be uncooperative with your exam due to a lack of understanding or fear. Assess the child's general appearance and seek the parent's impression of changes in behavior because they will be in tune to more subtle changes in their child's demeanor and activity level.

Altered LOC and Mental Status

An altered LOC or mental status is an abnormal neurologic state in which a child is less alert and interactive with the environment than normal. Table 19 uses the mnemonic AEIOU-TIPPS to highlight some common causes of altered LOC. Without a good history, it may be difficult to determine the underlying cause, and you may find yourself simply identifying and treating concerning symptoms.

Run through the PAT and ABCs quickly to determine possible points of intervention. Assess the need to protect the airway. Pay special attention to possible disability and dextrose issues. Use the AVPU scale (Alert, responsive to Voice, responsive to Pain, Unresponsive) to identify the level of disability. In addition, check the patient's glucose level because hypoglycemia (defined as a serum glucose concentration of less than 40 mg/dL in a newborn and of less than 60 mg/dL in all other infants and children) is easily treatable.

History taking and the secondary assessment, whether performed at the scene or en route to the hospital, may also provide clues about the underlying cause. For example, a child with a history of epilepsy may be in a postictal state after an unwitnessed seizure; a child with diabetes may be hypoglycemic or in diabetic ketoacidosis. A history of toxic ingestion, recent illness, or injury may also reveal the cause of the altered mental status.

Regardless of the cause, the management of altered mental status is the same. Support the ABCs by carefully assessing the patient's airway and breathing. Provide assisted ventilation or airway support as needed. If the child is hypoglycemic, give glucose at a targeted dose of 0.5 g/kg. Depending on which glucose solution is available, this dose can be given as 5 mL/kg of D_{10} solution, 2 mL/kg of D_{25} solution, or 1 mL/kg of D_{50} solution. Always recheck the blood glucose level after giving IV glucose.

Table 19 AEIOU-TIPPS: Possible Causes of Altered Level of Consciousness and Mental Status

A	Alcohol
E	Epilepsy, endocrine, electrolytes
I	Insulin
O	Opiates and other drugs
U	Uremia
T	Trauma, temperature
I	Infection
P	Psychogenic
P	Poison
S	Shock, stroke, space-occupying lesion, subarachnoid hemorrhage

The goal is to maintain a *normal* glucose level: Hyperglycemia is associated with worse neurologic outcomes in patients with cerebral ischemia. For children with altered mental status and signs or symptoms suggestive of an opiate toxidrome Table 20, consider giving naloxone. All patients with altered mental status should be transported expeditiously to an appropriate medical facility. Assess for increased ICP and intervene as appropriate.

When you are intubating a pediatric patient with an altered mental status, atropine 0.02 mg/kg (minimal dose 0.1mg) is given. Etomidate is a common induction agent if septic shock is not suspected. The dose is 0.3 mg/kg, and it is considered a good agent if the patient is hypotensive because it has less effect on blood pressure than other choices. Midazolam 0.1 mg/kg or ketamine 2 mg/kg are other options. Ketamine is a bronchodilator, so it is a good choice for patients with respiratory problems such as asthma, though it can cause increased bronchorrhea and may cause a transient drop in the blood pressure. Muscle relaxants such as succinylcholine 1 to 2 mg/kg or rocuronium 1 mg/kg can be used in the pediatric population. You should be cautious about using succinylcholine in patients who may have hyperkalemia because of medications such as thiazide diuretics or ACE inhibitors, crush injuries, severe burns, renal diseases, Addison disease, or adrenal disease.

In patients for whom increased ICP is suggested, the addition of lidocaine 1 mg/kg prior to intubation may blunt the increase in ICP associated with intubation. Signs of increased ICP include Cushing triad: bradycardia, irregular respirations, and hypertension (with or without a widened pulse pressure). If you suspect increased ICP, elevation of the head can help decease the pressure using the force of gravity. Barbiturates may also help, and mannitol 0.5 to 1 g/kg push or hypertonic saline (3% NS) will cause diuresis and lower ICP until definitive management can be obtained with a neurosurgeon.

■ Seizures

Seizures result from abnormal electrical discharges in the brain. Although many types of seizures exist, generalized seizures manifest as abnormal motor activity and an altered LOC. Some children are predisposed to seizures because of underlying brain abnormalities, whereas others experience seizures as a result of trauma, metabolic disturbances, ingestion, or infection. Seizures associated with fever (febrile seizures) are unique to young children and are typically benign, though frightening to the parents.

The physical manifestation of a seizure will depend on the area of the brain firing the electrical discharges and the age of the child. Infants have immature brains, so seizures in this age group may be subtle. Repetitive movements such as lip smacking, chewing, and "bicycling" suggest seizure activity. Apnea and cyanosis can also be signs of underlying seizure activity.

Words of Wisdom

Always check the glucose level for a patient with an altered mental status.

The prognosis following a seizure is closely linked to the underlying cause. For example, a child with a febrile seizure will not have brain damage as a consequence of the event, whereas a child who has a seizure as a complication of a head injury or meningitis may have long-term neurologic abnormalities. All types of seizures (but especially first-time seizures) are frightening to caregivers, and they often result in 9-1-1 calls.

Types of Seizures

The classification system for seizures is the same for children and adults (see the chapter, *Neurologic Emergencies*, for an in-depth discussion of seizures). Briefly, seizures that involve the entire brain are considered **generalized seizures**, whereas those that involve only one part of the brain are called **partial seizures**. The most common type of seizures are generalized **tonic-clonic seizures** (grand mal), that involve jerking of both arms and/or legs. **Absence seizures** (petit mal) are generalized seizures that involve a brief loss of attention without abnormal body movements. Partial seizures can be further subclassified

Table 20 Common Toxidromes

Toxidrome	Agent	Signs and Symptoms
Anticholinergic	Antihistamines, tricyclic antidepressants	"Hot as a hare, red as a beet (hot, dry skin; hyperthermia), blind as a bat (dilated pupils), mad as a hatter (delirium, hallucinations)"
Cholinergic	Organophosphates	DUMBELS: Diarrhea/diaphoresis, Urination, Miosis, Bradycardia/bronchoconstriction, Emesis, Lacrimation, Salivation
Narcotic	Morphine, methadone	Bradycardia, hypoventilation, miosis, hypotension
Sympathomimetic	Cocaine, amphetamines	Tachycardia, hypertension, hyperthermia, mydriasis (dilated pupils), diaphoresis (sweating)
Opiate	Opiates such as morphine, fentanyl, oxycodone Reversal agent: Naloxone	Pinpoint pupils, decreased respiratory drive or apnea, decreased LOC, coma. Note that with meperidine (Demerol), you will see dilated pupils.

into <u>simple partial seizures</u>, that involve focal motor jerking without loss of consciousness, and <u>complex partial seizures</u>, that feature focal motor jerking with loss of consciousness.

Febrile Seizures

Febrile seizures occur in about 25% of young children. To make this diagnosis, the child must be between age 6 months and 6 years, have a fever, and have no identifiable precipitating cause (such as head injury, ingestion, or meningitis). Most febrile seizures occur in children between the ages of 6 months and 3 years. The strongest predictor for having a febrile seizure is a history of this diagnosis in a first-degree relative.

Simple febrile seizures are brief, generalized tonic-clonic seizures (lasting less than 15 minutes) that occur in a child without underlying neurologic abnormalities. <u>Complex febrile seizures</u> are longer (lasting more than 15 minutes), are focal, or occur in a child with baseline developmental or neurologic abnormality. They may also be associated with serious illness.

The majority of your calls for fever and seizures will involve simple febrile seizures. The postictal phase after a brief seizure tends to be short, so the child will often be waking up or back to baseline by the time you arrive at the scene. Depending on your agency's policy, a well-appearing child who has a history consistent with a simple febrile seizure may be transported by EMS or by parents but always needs urgent physician evaluation.

The prognosis for children with simple febrile seizures is excellent. Although one third of children who have one simple febrile seizure will have another such seizure, their prognosis does not change. There is no relationship between simple febrile seizures and brain damage or future developmental or learning disabilities, and children with this diagnosis have only a slightly increased risk for subsequent development of epilepsy.

Special Populations

Febrile seizures are unique to children. Reassure the parents that febrile seizures are extremely common and that children who experience them typically recover completely.

Assessment of Seizures

When you are conducting the primary assessment of a child with a history of seizures, you should give special attention to compromised oxygenation and ventilation and signs of ongoing seizure activity. Seizures place a child at risk for respiratory distress or failure because of airway obstruction (often from the tongue), aspiration, or depressed respiratory drive. Given the typical EMS response time, any child who is still having a seizure when you arrive has likely been having seizure activity for at least 10 minutes and should be considered to be in status epilepticus; therefore, you need to initiate treatment to stop the seizure in such cases. <u>Status epilepticus</u> has historically been defined as any seizure lasting more than 20 minutes or two or more seizures without return to neurologic baseline between seizures. In recent years, however, neurologists have begun urging treatment for any seizure lasting more than 5 minutes. As part of history

taking, ask about prior seizures; anticonvulsant medications; recent illness, injury, or suspected ingestion; duration of the seizure activity; and the character of the seizure.

Management of Seizures

Treatment of seizures at the scene will be limited to supportive care if the seizure has stopped by your arrival, but status epilepticus requires more extensive intervention. For a child with ongoing seizure activity, open the airway using the chin-lift or jaw-thrust maneuver. Proximal airway obstruction is common during a seizure or postictal state because the tongue and jaw fall backward because of the decreased muscle tone associated with altered mental status. If the airway is not maintainable with positioning, consider inserting a nasopharyngeal airway. Suction for secretions or vomitus, and consider the lateral decubitus position in case of ongoing vomiting. Do not attempt to intubate during an active seizure because endotracheal intubation in this setting is associated with serious complications and is rarely successful. More appropriate care should include using BLS airway management, stopping the seizure, and then considering the child's need for ALS airway support.

Provide 100% supplemental oxygen to the patient, and start bag-mask ventilation as indicated for hypoventilation. Consider placing an NG tube to decompress the stomach if the patient requires assisted ventilation.

Assess the child for IV sites. Measure the serum glucose level, and treat any documented hypoglycemia.

Consider your options for anticonvulsant administration. Insertion of an IV line can be difficult in a child having a seizure, and alternative routes for medication delivery may be needed. The goal of medical therapy is to stop the seizure while minimizing anticonvulsant side effects.

First-line anticonvulsant treatment consists of a benzodiazepine—lorazepam, diazepam, or midazolam. All benzodiazepines can cause respiratory depression, so you should monitor oxygenation and ventilation carefully, especially when you give repeated doses or combinations of anticonvulsants. Lorazepam is an excellent choice for seizure management because of its rapid onset, lower risk of respiratory depression, and relatively long half-life. Its usefulness in the field is limited because it must be refrigerated. Diazepam is frequently used in the prehospital setting, given by the IV or rectal route. The advantages of rectal administration include ease of access and a lower rate of respiratory depression, although onset of action is longer (approximately 5 minutes). The half-life of diazepam is relatively short, however, and breakthrough seizures may occur with longer transport times. Midazolam may be administered by the IV, IM, and intranasal (using an atomizer) routes. Although it has excellent anticonvulsant effects, it has the shortest duration of action of the three benzodiazepines mentioned. Be prepared to repeat dosing for recurrent seizures.

If the seizures do not stop after two or three doses of a benzodiazepine, a second-line agent is necessary. Phenobarbital is the second-line agent of choice for neonates. Phenobarbital, phenytoin, and fosphenytoin are acceptable second-line agents for infants and children outside of the neonatal age group. Phenobarbital has sedative effects and causes respiratory depression, so be vigilant if you administer it after a benzodiazepine. Although phenytoin has the advantage of not compromising the respiratory system or causing sedation, it is difficult to administer and can cause hypotension and bradycardia. Fosphenytoin, a drug that is metabolized to phenytoin, allows for more rapid infusion with fewer side effects; it may be administered by the IV or IM route.

Any child with a history suggestive of seizures requires physician evaluation to look for the cause. Although treatment at the scene is appropriate for a child in status epilepticus, detailed assessment should be performed during transport. Monitor cardiorespiratory status in any postictal child, and reassess frequently for recurrent seizure activity.

Meningitis

Meningitis entails inflammation or infection of the meninges, the covering of the brain and spinal cord. It is most often caused by a viral or bacterial infection. Although children may look and feel quite ill, viral meningitis is rarely a life-threatening infection. By contrast, bacterial meningitis is potentially fatal. Children with bacterial meningitis can progress rapidly from mildly ill-appearing to coma and even death. In the early stages of illness, it is difficult to tell which type of infection is present, so take the safe route: Always proceed as if the child may have bacterial meningitis.

The symptoms of meningitis vary depending on the age of the child and the agent causing the infection. In general, the younger the child, the more vague the symptoms. A newborn with early bacterial meningitis may have a fever as the only symptom. Young infants will often have a fever and perhaps localizing signs such as lethargy, irritability, poor feeding, and a bulging fontanelle. Young children rarely show typical "meningeal signs" such as nuchal rigidity (neck stiffness with movement of the neck) until they are older. Verbal children will often report headaches and neck pain. An altered LOC and seizures are ominous symptoms at any age. Projectile vomiting and photosensitivity are also common findings. Other signs may include Kernig sign (the patient cannot extend his or her leg at the knee when the thigh is flexed because of stiffness in the hamstrings) and Brudzinski sign (passive flexion of the leg on one side causes a similar movement in the opposite leg).

Neonates most often contract meningitis-causing bacteria during the birthing process: The bacteria that are a normal part of the mother's vaginal tract—*Escherichia coli*, group B *Streptococcus*, and *Listeria monocytogenes*—can produce serious infections in newborns. Older infants and young children are at risk for contracting viral meningitis from enteroviruses, which are widespread during the summer and fall. Bacterial meningitis in this age group most often involves *Streptococcus pneumoniae* (also known as pneumococcus) and *Neisseria meningitidis* (also known as meningococcus), although pneumococcus infection is becoming less frequent because more young children are vaccinated against this bacterium. Meningitis from *H influenzae* is rare because a vaccine against this pathogen was introduced several years ago.

Neisseria meningitidis may also cause sepsis (an overwhelming bacterial infection in the bloodstream). Meningococcal meningitis with sepsis is typically characterized by a petechial (small, pinpoint red spots) or purpuric (larger purple or black spots) rash in addition to the other symptoms of meningitis Figure 19 .

Infection control is an important part of managing a child who may have meningitis. Meningococcus, in particular, is quite contagious. Protect yourself and others from contracting this illness by being vigilant about using standard and respiratory precautions. Wear a gown, gloves, and a mask if meningitis is a possibility and remember to place a mask on the patient.

Children with meningococcal sepsis and meningitis quickly become extremely sick, so you need to move quickly through your assessment. Form your general impression, and perform the primary assessment as usual, while recognizing that the initial presentation of a child with meningitis can be highly variable. Look for fever, altered mental status, bulging fontanelle, photophobia, nuchal rigidity, irritability, petechiae, purpura, and signs of shock. Perform a bedside glucose check because hypoglycemia may result from the hypermetabolic state. Helpful components of a SAMPLE history are shown in Table 21 .

For children in physiologically unstable condition, provide lifesaving interventions as needed and transport them quickly, ideally to a facility with a pediatric intensive care unit. En route, perform frequent reassessments—one of the hallmarks of this disease is rapid deterioration. Monitor vital signs and changes in physical exam findings closely to anticipate a child's needs and intervene early. Patient needs may include oxygen, airway management, and ventilation support. Medical control may order IV fluids based on patient signs and symptoms, and medications may be ordered en route if seizures occur or the patient shows signs of shock. See the chapter, *Infectious Diseases* for more information about meningitis.

Hydrocephalus

Hydrocephalus is a condition resulting from impaired circulation and absorption of cerebrospinal fluid (CSF), leading to increased size of the ventricles (fluid-filled spaces in

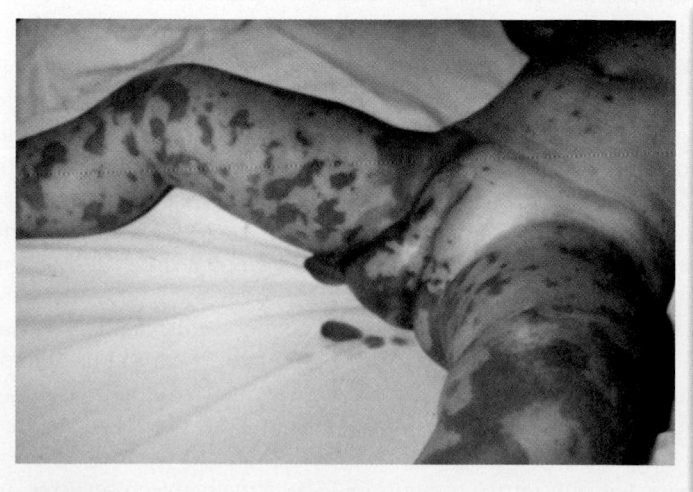

Figure 19 Purpura in a child with meningococcal sepsis.

Table 21   SAMPLE History for a Child With Suspected Meningitis

Component	Explanation
Signs and symptoms	Onset and duration of illness, including "cold symptoms"–runny nose, cough Onset and duration of fever Rash? Headache? Neck pain? Photophobia? Irritability?
Allergies	Known drug reactions or other allergies
Medications	Exact names and doses of ongoing drugs Timing and amount of last dose Time and dose of analgesics and antipyretics
Past medical history	Previous illnesses or injuries Immunizations Perinatal history for young infants
Last oral intake	Timing of the child's last food or drink, including bottle or breastfeeding
Events leading to illness or injury	Any known exposures to children with illnesses and what kind of illnesses

the brain) and increased ICP. Hydrocephalus may be congenital or acquired; it is most commonly seen in children born with brain malformations, as a complication of prematurity, or following surgery for a brain tumor. To decrease the increased ICP, patients will often have a cerebral shunt placed; ventriculoperitoneal (VP), or less commonly, a ventriculoatrial (VA) shunts are surgically inserted into the ventricles of the brain by neurosurgeons. VP shunts drain excess fluid from the ventricular system of the brain into the peritoneal cavity through a tube that exits the skull at a valve. VA shunts are similar, except the tubing terminates in the right atrium of the heart. The tubing can often be felt in the lateral portion of the neck. In thin or young children, coils of tubing may also be palpable in the abdomen. Draining off the extra CSF prevents herniation of the brain.

Complications of cerebral shunts include infections, blockages, and overdrainage. Signs of a cerebral shunt malfunction include vomiting, headache, altered LOC, visual changes, and with infection, fever, redness, or tenderness over the shunt itself. In patients with VP shunts, peritonitis can also accompany VP shunt infections. For any of these conditions, management of increased ICP and immediate transport to a medical center with pediatric neurosurgical capabilities is required.

Closed Head Injuries

Head trauma is common in childhood. Most head trauma in children is minor and not associated with brain injury or long-term sequelae. However, a small number of children who appear to be at low risk may have an intracranial injury. A number of states have laws requiring medical evaluation prior to allowing children who have been concussed in a sporting event

back into play. The goal of the evaluation of children with head trauma is to identify those with traumatic brain injury (TBI) and prevent deterioration and secondary injury. Any child who presents with head injury should also be evaluated for signs of potential abuse.

An epidural hematoma is a hemorrhage into the space between the dura and the overlying skull. It is almost exclusively caused by trauma. Morbidity and mortality result from mass effect on the brain as the hematoma grows and strips the dura away from the skull. Prompt diagnosis is critical to successful management and improved neurologic outcome. Epidural hematomas are more likely to occur with trauma to the temporal bone that can damage the middle meningeal artery. Patients often present with loss of consciousness or altered mental status. Patients also often report a severe headache accompanied by persistent vomiting, or ataxia. Infants may be difficult to console and have a cephalohematoma on exam. Older patients may have a lucid interval with minimal symptoms after head trauma, followed several hours later by rapid clinical deterioration.

By contrast, a subdural hematoma forms when there is hemorrhage into the potential space between the dura and the arachnoid membranes. In children, this bleeding differs significantly from those in adults because inflicted head injury from abuse is a common etiology, especially in pediatric patients younger than 2 years. The bleeding may or may not be associated with skull fractures. Any infant or toddler with a subdural hematoma should be suspected of having been abused until proven otherwise.

Management includes stabilization of airway, breathing, and circulation during the primary assessment. Vascular access is often indicated in patients with epidural hematomas but is often not needed for patients with subdural bleeding. The patient should be kept comfortable on cardiorespiratory monitors, and you should perform frequent neurologic checks to assess for any developing deficits or changes in responsiveness.

Pathophysiology, Assessment, and Management of Gastrointestinal Emergencies

Complaints of gastrointestinal origin are common in the pediatric population. In fact, gastrointestinal-related complaints are the 5th most common pediatric complaint seen in the ED. The gut embryonically develops external to the body, then regresses into the abdominal cavity. Features of maldevelopment are responsible for certain pediatric gastrointestinal diseases such as Meckel diverticulum or malrotation with volvulus. Organs like the liver mature over the first few months of life.

Neonatal Jaundice

Neonatal jaundice (hyperbilirubinemia) is due to the immature liver's inability to conjugate and excrete bilirubin from red blood cell breakdown. Severe hyperbilirubinemia can lead to kernicterus, a form of developmental delay from the deposition of bilirubin in neuronal tissues. The treatment for most cases of neonatal hyperbilirubinemia is phototherapy. Light helps break down the unconjugated bilirubin and aids in its excretion. In extreme cases, patients may require exchange transfusion.

Biliary Atresia

Children with severe liver disease, though rare, can also present with jaundice. Biliary atresia can present in the newborn period. In this disease, the biliary tract is malformed such that bilirubin cannot be excreted. This leads to liver disease and failure. Some rare genetic disorders can also present as liver failure. These children may have esophageal varices which can bleed profusely. Transport children with massive gastrointestinal bleeds to the nearest ED, obtain IV access, and administer fluid boluses with isotonic saline or lactated Ringer's solution.

Viral Gastroenteritis

A common source of gastrointestinal upset is acute viral gastroenteritis, an infection caused by a variety of viruses, or the ingestion of certain foods, such as milk or ice cream (lactose intolerance), or unknown substances. In most cases, you will be faced with a pediatric patient who is experiencing abdominal discomfort with nausea, vomiting, and/or diarrhea. Many patients also have a fever. These findings can become a concern because both vomiting and diarrhea can quickly cause dehydration in children. If you suspect dehydration, an IV line should be placed and 20 mL/kg of an isotonic fluid such as normal saline should be administered. Do not administer a bolus with one half normal saline or fluids containing dextrose or potassium.

Appendicitis

Appendicitis is common in pediatric patients and if untreated can lead to peritonitis (inflammation of the peritoneum, which lines the abdominal cavity) or shock. Patients with appendicitis will typically present with a fever and pain on palpation of the right lower abdominal quadrant. Patients often describe the pain as having started in the periumbilical region and migrating to the right lower quadrant over time, usually hours. Some patients have a fever or vomiting when they have appendicitis. Rebound tenderness is a common sign associated with appendicitis. Remember that constipation also can be a cause of severe abdominal pain in children. The pain often follows a meal, is intermittent, and a history of constipation is often lacking. These patients have diffuse abdominal pain, but do not have guarding or rebound tenderness on examination. The severity can often mimic appendicitis. Never assume that you can distinguish between appendicitis and constipation based on history and physical examination in the field alone. Immediately transport the pediatric patient to the ED for further evaluation.

Ingestion of Foreign Bodies

The ingestion of foreign bodies is a common cause of gastrointestinal complaints in pediatric patients. Though most foreign bodies pass without trouble, if a foreign object gets lodged in the esophagus, patients will often present with gagging, vomiting, and difficulty swallowing. Worsening pain raises the concern for perforation of a viscus, and difficulty breathing or choking raises the possibility of a foreign body airway obstruction. In this situation, keep the child in a calm, comfortable position, often on the parent's lap, and transport the child to the ED immediately.

Gastrointestinal Bleeding

Gastrointestinal bleeds are rare in the pediatric population. The causes are often different compared to adults. An important difference to note is that because of the rapid transport times in the pediatric gastrointestinal tract, ingested, upper, and lower bleeding may all present with hematochezia or bright red rectal bleeding. In adults, upper bleeding may present as melena or dark black, tar-like stools because of the digestion of the blood in the gastrointestinal tract.

In newborns, blood ingested during birth can present as rectal bleeding. This is seen in the first few days of life and is harmless. Infants may have blood in their stool if there is maternal bleeding from the nipples during breastfeeding. Maternal mastitis, an infection of the breast, is a common cause. Children may have rectal bleeding from ingested blood from epistaxis (nosebleeds), after surgery such as tonsillectomy, or after multiple episodes of forceful vomiting. Children with gastroenteritis and repetitive vomiting can get small tears of the esophagus called Mallory-Weiss tears. These mucosal tears can present as blood streaking of the emesis or blood in the stool. They are usually small, harmless, and self-limited. Finally, children with constipation can have small anal fissures that present as rectal bleeding. The blood from fissures presents as blood-streaking on the surface of the stool. They can be painful but are also self-limiting. Abusive trauma should always be on the differential diagnosis of rectal bleeding in the pediatric population.

Intussusception

Intussusception is a disease that most commonly occurs in children between ages 6 months and 6 years. It involves the telescoping of the bowel into itself, commonly the small intestine into the large intestine at the cecum. Patients present with intermittent severe abdominal pain and lethargy and there can be bloody stools (or currant jelly-like stools). This is considered a surgical emergency and patients should be transported to the ED for immediate evaluation.

Meckel Diverticulum

Meckel diverticulum is one of the most common congenital malformations of the small intestines, and patients present with painless rectal bleeding or hematochezia. The condition presents with the "rule of 2s": 2% of the population, symptomatic by age 2 years, and usually presents by the second decade of life. Classically it is seen in young boys. Meckel diverticulum can cause concern because of the large volume of blood loss. If you suspect Meckel diverticulum, transport the patient to the ED for further evaluation.

Pyloric Stenosis and Malrotation With Volvulus

In infants younger than 2 months, pyloric stenosis and malrotation with volvulus are two diseases that cause vomiting that need prompt attention. <u>Pyloric stenosis</u> occurs when the pylorus, the muscle that serves as a one-way valve for contents leaving the stomach, becomes hypertrophied. Infants with this condition classically present with projectile vomiting occurring after feedings. Poor weight gain or weight loss, dehydration, and electrolyte abnormalities can be seen due to the amount of vomiting. Surgery is curative in these children. <u>Malrotation with volvulus</u> occurs when there is a twisting of the bowel around its mesenteric attachment to the abdominal wall. Patients present with bilious emesis (dark green), pain, and a distended, rigid abdomen. They may have blood in the vomitus or stool, and this condition is considered a surgical emergency. Infants who are vomiting should be transported immediately to an ED with pediatric capabilities.

General Assessment and Management of Gastrointestinal Emergencies

When obtaining a history for a child with gastrointestinal complaints, it is important to consider the patient's age, the patient's sex, and whether the child was born premature. Ask about current medication use, as well as a history of similar complaints in the past. For example, severe abdominal pain is a common complaint with a large differential diagnosis list; however, recurrent abdominal pain that can mimic the pain of appendicitis can be seen with constipation or gastroenteritis. Patients on polyethylene glycol may have pain from constipation, whereas patients on H2-blockers such as ranitidine may have gastritis or ulcer disease.

Physical examination findings of patients with gastrointestinal complaints include looking for pallor or jaundice. Scleral jaundice may also be present. These may be signs of hepatic disease or blood breakdown or loss. Tachycardia is seen before hypotension in pediatric patients with significant dehydration or blood loss. Tachycardia should be treated with an intravenous fluid bolus of 20 mL/kg. Location and severity of abdominal pain should be assessed and reassessed at regular intervals for change in severity or location. The pain of appendicitis, for example, commonly starts periumbilically then migrates to the right lower quadrant. Premature infants and those with symptoms in the first weeks of life require further evaluation at a center with pediatric capabilities.

Special consideration should be paid to patients with gastrostomy tubes (G-tubes) since these patients may require continuous feeds to maintain hydration. G-tubes can become dislodged by the child playing or pulling them, or when the balloon that secures the tube deflates. Many parents have been trained in replacing G-tubes. If a replacement tube is not available, insertion of a sterile urinary catheter or other similar catheter into the stoma is important. Stomas can become narrow quickly and completely close off after the tube is removed. Reinsertion of the original tube into the stoma can also help

prevent this. When replacing a G-tube or inserting another catheter through the abdominal wall stoma, consider the time since the tube was originally inserted and therefore the age of the tract the G-tube follows. Mature tracts, or those over six months old, can safely be replaced. Immature G-tube tract tubes should not be replaced in the field because of the risk of tract perforation and insertion of the G-tube into the abdominal cavity rather than the stomach. To replace a G-tube, use a lubricant on the end of the tube being inserted through the stoma. Gentle pressure should allow the tube to slide into the stoma. If significant resistance is felt or if there is pain or bleeding, then the attempt should be aborted. Tape the replacement into place and transport the child to the ED for definitive replacement.

Because the pediatric population is sensitive to fluid loss, obtain a thorough history from the primary caregiver. In particular, ask questions such as:

- How many wet diapers has the child had today?
- Is your child tolerating liquids and is he or she able to keep them down?
- How many times has your child had diarrhea and for how long?
- When he or she cries, are there tears present?

These questions can help you determine just how dehydrated the pediatric patient may be.

When transporting a patient with a suspected gastrointestinal emergency, the patient should be given nothing to eat or drink until a thorough assessment can be completed. Vascular access is often indicated in patients who show signs of clinical dehydration and need IV fluids. The patient should be kept comfortable on cardiorespiratory monitors with frequent assessment for change in hemodynamic status.

Pathophysiology, Assessment, and Management of Endocrine Emergencies

When you are caring for pediatric patients with endocrine-related emergencies, it is important to remember that children are not just "small adults." Children and young adults are much more commonly diagnosed with type 1 diabetes; therefore, they are susceptible to DKA, a life-threatening event. Events of hypoglycemia can be particularly damaging to the developing brain. Children are at varying stages of cognitive development, depending on age and maturity; therefore, consistent maintenance of blood glucose levels within the normal range can be challenging.

Hyperglycemia

Hyperglycemia is an abnormally high blood glucose level. It can either be the presenting problem in a child with new-onset diabetes mellitus or it may occur as a complication in a child with a known history of diabetes. If not recognized or promptly treated, hyperglycemia can result in severe dehydration and diabetic ketoacidosis (DKA), both of which are potentially life-threatening. In DKA, the deficiency of insulin prevents cells from taking up the extra glucose. The cells are starving, and a distress signal goes out over the sympathetic nervous system, causing the release of various stress hormones. Because the body cannot use glucose, it turns instead to other sources of energy—principally, fat. The metabolism of fat generates *acids* and *ketones* as waste products. (The ketones give the characteristic fruity odor to the breath of a patient in DKA, but not all providers are able to smell this.) Because glucose must be excreted in the urine in solution, the body loses excessive amounts of water and electrolytes (sodium and potassium). This may lead to disturbances in water balance and acid–base balance.

During your assessment of the child with suspected hyperglycemia, you will typically find that a dose of insulin was missed, a greater proportion of food was eaten compared with the dose of insulin, or the insulin pump malfunctioned.

Like hypoglycemia, the signs and symptoms of hyperglycemia depend on how high the level of blood glucose is. During your assessment, ask about insulin administration; functioning of an insulin pump, including when the site of insertion was last changed; changes in urine output; changes in mental status, patterns on recent glucose checks, the presence of urine ketones (if they check these); and any other symptoms, including headache, visual changes, seizures, abnormal speech, or the presence of vomiting and abdominal pain.

Management of hyperglycemia begins by administering 100% oxygen or assisted ventilation if needed. Monitor vital signs closely. Obtain IV access and administer isotonic fluids such as normal saline or lactated Ringer's. A 10-mL/kg bolus may be administered if the patient is in shock; this may be repeated as needed to maintain adequate perfusion.

There is a risk of cerebral edema with rapid IV fluid administration to a patient in DKA; therefore, if needed, IV fluids should be run slowly during transport to a hospital (such as 20 mL/kg over an hour). Cerebral edema associated with DKA increases mortality by 20% to 90%. Patients who survive have a 20% to 40% risk of neurologic impairment. Signs and symptoms include an altered mental status, headache, nausea, vomiting, bradycardia, and hypertension. Seizures, changes in pupils, incontinence, and respiratory arrest signal rapid deterioration. These conditions usually present clinically 4 to 12 hours after treatment has been initiated; however, they may occur even prior to treatment. Successful management includes IV administration of 5 to 10 mL/kg of 3% NaCl over 30 minutes or 0.25 to 1 g/kg of mannitol over 20 minutes. Intubation and ventilation may be necessary; however, hyperventilation should be used with caution or avoided. Neurologic improvement is rapid.

Children with hyperglycemia and DKA are often severely dehydrated, but because the process of becoming dehydrated is usually slow, patients will usually tolerate slower rehydration with a decreased risk of cerebral edema and herniation. Bicarbonate therapy should not be administered to correct the acidosis of DKA because this greatly increases the risk of cerebral edema and herniation. If patients report worsening of a headache or their mental status deteriorates during fluid administration, fluids should be discontinued and the patient assessed and treated for increased ICP from cerebral edema and impending herniation.

Closely monitor the patient's ABCs and be prepared to adjust your treatment accordingly. The patient in DKA desperately needs insulin; however, this is not a drug that is administered in the prehospital setting. If an insulin pump is working, however, do not discontinue the use of it in the field. Immediate transport of the patient to the closest appropriate facility is critical.

YOU *are the Medic*   PART 4

Prior to packaging the patient for transport, you administer 28 mL of D$_{25}$ solution. The child begins to move around as he is placed on the stretcher and is opening his eyes by the time you are ready to leave. Law enforcement personnel arrive to care for the sister as you are loading the child into the back of the ambulance.

Recording Time: 15 Minutes	
Respirations	20 breaths/min; adequate depth and volume
Pulse	160 beats/min, regular; weak peripheral pulses and strong central pulses
Skin	Pale, warm, and dry; decreased mottling of the extremities
Blood pressure	80/54 mm Hg
Oxygen saturation (Spo$_2$)	98% at 12 L/min on nonrebreathing mask
Pupils	Equal and reactive to light

7. What do you think was the cause for shock in this patient?

8. What additional treatment should be performed en route to the hospital?

Hypoglycemia

Hypoglycemia is defined as an abnormally low blood glucose level. Infants and children have limited stores of glucose that can be quickly depleted in times of illness, injury, or stress. You must recognize that hypoglycemia is a life-threatening emergency that requires immediate treatment. If hypoglycemia is unrecognized or treatment is delayed, permanent brain damage or death can result.

Special Populations

Although hypoglycemia is more common in children with diabetes, physical exertion, illness (particularly severe gastroenteritis), or injury can result in hypoglycemia in children without diabetes. Alcohol ingestion can also lead to hypoglycemia in young children. Remember to assess blood glucose levels in all ill or injured children with an altered mental status or bizarre behavior.

General signs and symptoms of hypoglycemia include hunger, malaise, tachycardia, tachypnea, diaphoresis, tremors, decreased LOC, confusion, and coma. The severity of the patient's clinical presentation depends on how low the blood glucose level has dropped. You should obtain a blood glucose reading in any infant or child who you suspect is hypoglycemic. Normal blood glucose levels range from 80 to 120 mg/dL. In children with a known history of diabetes, ask the pertinent questions.

Management of hypoglycemia begins by administering 100% oxygen or assisted ventilation if needed. Monitor vital signs closely. Treat the symptomatic child with glucose if the blood glucose reading is less than 80 mg/dL.

If the child is responsive and alert enough to swallow, administer oral glucose as allowed by local protocol. However, if the child has an altered mental status or is otherwise incapable of swallowing, administer IV glucose in the following dosages:

- Younger than 2 years: 25% dextrose (D_{25}), 2 to 4 mL/kg. Dilute 50% dextrose (D_{50}) 1:1 with normal saline to make D_{25}.
- Older than 2 years: 50% dextrose (D_{50}), 1 to 2 mL/kg.

If an IV line cannot be established, insert an IO needle. If vascular access (IV or IO) is not available, medical control may order the administration of 1 mg of glucagon via IM injection.

Repeat a blood glucose reading 10 to 15 minutes following the administration of glucose. If the patient is still symptomatic and the blood glucose reading remains below 80 mg/dL, repeat the glucose as needed.

Congenital Adrenal Hyperplasia

Congenital adrenal hyperplasia (CAH) is an autosomal-recessive disorder of an enzyme responsible for the metabolism of cortisol (steroidogenesis) and aldosterone in the adrenal glands. The most common form is due to 21-hydroxylase deficiency. Males born with this disorder appear normal, but females may be masculinized, with an enlarged clitoris that may resemble a penis. Patients sometimes undergo early pubertal development with pubic hair growth, early growth acceleration, and the development of facial hair.

When children with CAH become sick, their bodies may not be able to compensate because of the lack of cortisol. This lack can lead to salt wasting from decreased aldosterone (decreased levels of mineralocorticoids). Though this condition is screened for in newborn screenings, it can sometimes be missed. Infants who present with salt-wasting crisis because of loss of urinary sodium may present with metabolic acidosis and hyperkalemia.

Clinically, infants with this condition may have vomiting, poor weight gain, dehydration, and may progress to shock in the first few weeks of life. Hypoglycemia may also be present. If this condition is suspected, hydrocortisone and IV boluses of normal saline (and glucose if hypoglycemic) are needed. Stress-dose steroids should be considered for patients with suspected CAH. Contact medical control before administration. For children on chronic steroid replacement, ask the parents if they have a stress-dose steroid regimen. Parents usually know the appropriate dose to give if their child becomes ill. If the parents do not know the appropriate dose, it is reasonable to give an extra dose of the child's home steroid dose, which is often tripled (or given three times a day rather than once a day) during acute illnesses. Consult with medical control. For children who appear in shock, IV hydrocortisone or methylprednisone may be considered in consultation with medical control.

Panhypopituitarism

Located at the base of the brain, the pituitary produces eight hormones. Examples include growth hormone, adrenocorticotropic hormone (ACTH), follicle-stimulating hormone (FSH), thyroid-stimulating hormone (TSH), and antidiuretic hormone (ADH). Hypopituitarism, a condition in which the pituitary gland does not produce normal amounts of some or all of its hormones, can be congenital; secondary to tumors, infection or strokes, or develop after trauma or radiation therapy. When there is hyposecretion of any of these hormones, patients require replacement therapy.

Because several pituitary hormones affect the production of secretions of the adrenal glands, patients with panhypopituitarism can be at risk for adrenal crisis. Panhypopituitarism is the inadequate production or absence of the pituitary hormones, including ACTH, cortisol, thyroxine (T_4), luteinizing hormone (LH), FSH, estrogen, testosterone, growth hormone, and ADH. When stressed or sick, these patients can present with symptoms similar to CAH, including hypoglycemia, dehydration, poor weight gain or weight loss, vomiting, muscle cramping, weakness, dizziness, hypotension, and if gradual in onset, tanning of the skin. These patients require IV fluid boluses with normal saline, glucose replacement, and replacement of steroids with IV hydrocortisone.

It is important for a pediatric endocrinologist to manage children diagnosed with panhypopituitarism. Often these conditions are a result of the hypothalamus, rather than the pituitary gland, functioning abnormally. These hormones control growth and sexual maturation, and once hormone therapy is initiated, children can generally live a normal life. Hormone replacement therapy will need to be continually monitored throughout the patient's life.

Inborn Errors of Metabolism

Inborn errors of metabolism (IEM) are a group of congenital conditions that cause either accumulation of toxins or disorders of energy metabolism in the neonate. These conditions are characterized by an infant's failure to thrive and by vague signs such as poor feeding. Because they are inherited, there may be a family history of the disorder; however, many are recessive, so a family history may not be obvious. Examples of these disorders are included in Table 22.

All IEMs present in early childhood, though the presenting symptoms can vary significantly, from poor weight gain and failure to thrive, to loss of milestones in development, to recurring vomiting and diarrhea, skin problems, dental deformities, deafness, blindness, and various cancers. Dietary restrictions and replacements can control many of these disorders. For example, diet soda labels contain the following information to prevent people with phenylketonuria (PKU) from consuming it: "Warning, contains phenylketone". Some patients with IEM become hypoglycemic, particularly when they are sick or vomiting. They may also be hypermetabolic when ill, so the administration of boluses of glucose and the use of D_{10} fluids may be necessary to maintain normoglycemia. Consider IEM in patients with severe hypoglycemia who are resistant to initial therapy. If the patient has been diagnosed with an IEM, many geneticists give families specific care plans with instructions on emergent treatment.

Table 22	Examples of Inborn Errors of Metabolism Disorders
Disorders of:	**Examples**
Carbohydrate metabolism	Glycogen storage diseases such as Pompe disease and von Gierke disease
Amino acid metabolism	Phenylketonuria (PKU) and maple syrup urine disease (MSUD)
Fatty acid oxidation and mitochondrial metabolism	Medium-chain acyl-coenzyme A dehydrogenase deficiency (MCADD)
Porphyrin metabolism	Porphyria
Purine or pyrimidine metabolism	Lesch-Nyhan syndrome
Steroid metabolism and function	Congenital adrenal hyperplasia
Peroxisomal function	Zellweger syndrome
Lysosomal storage	Gaucher disease and Niemann-Pick disease

Pathophysiology, Assessment, and Management of Hematologic, Oncologic, and Immunologic Emergencies

Hematologic, oncologic, and immunologic diseases are common in pediatrics, ranging from cancers to bleeding disorders to immune deficiencies. Children may be immunosuppressed for several reasons, including cancer, congenital diseases of the immune system, chronic steroid use, chemotherapy, immunosuppressive medications after transplant, and infections like human immunodeficiency virus (HIV). Because of the altered immunity, children may present with severe illness and even shock. Early recognition of shock and initiation of IV fluids can be extremely important for a positive long-term outcome.

Children have a great capacity for compensation when in shock due to their ability to increase cardiac output by greatly increasing heart rate; hypotension is a late finding. Tachycardia associated with a fever or hypothermia should indicate the possibility of sepsis. When these patients are ill, the oxygen-carrying capacity of hemoglobin is altered, resulting in decreased oxygen-carrying capacity. Oxygen supplementation is an important early intervention if a patient is suspected of being potentially septic. Special considerations besides sepsis for you to remember in patients with childhood immunodeficiencies and cancer include acute chest syndrome associated with sickle cell crisis, stroke with sickle cell crisis, tumor lysis syndrome in chemotherapy patients, and an increased overall risk of infection, including bacterial infections, viral infections (varicella or shingles, herpes, and viremia), and fungal infections.

Patients with abnormal hematologic systems, including bleeding disorders or blood cancers, may also have either increased or decreased tendencies to clot. Because of these alterations, your primary assessment of these patients needs to include evaluation of the ABCs, pain and location, shortness of breath, weakness or neurologic symptoms, bleeding or swelling, fever, or other concerns. Remember that hypoglycemia can cause altered mental status, particularly in young children because of low glucose stores (as compared to adults). Decreases in blood glucose can occur quickly, so bedside glucose checks should be considered in these patients.

Patients with congenital or acquired immunodeficiencies are at high risk for recurrent infections and invasive disease. Bacterial, viral, and fungal organisms can quickly lead to severe morbidity and mortality. Patients should be quickly assessed for signs of sepsis and decompensation.

Examination of these patients should include a thorough lung, circulatory, and neurologic examination, and evaluation of the extremities for swollen joints that could be a sign of infection, hemarthrosis (bleeding into the joint), or a pain crisis. Delay in the capillary refill and diminished peripheral pulses can be an indicator of early sepsis and should be treated with aggressive boluses of isotonic fluids. Because some patients with hematologic, oncologic, and immunologic problems have indwelling catheters such as peripherally inserted central catheter (PICC) lines, Broviacs, and Port-A-Caths, evaluation of the catheter site for erythema, swelling, and tenderness is imperative. These can be signs of central line infections and warrant early initiation of antibiotics after blood cultures are obtained.

Sickle Cell Disease

Sickle cell disease (SCD) is a genetically inherited autosomal-recessive disorder of red blood cells. It usually presents in childhood in people of African American descent. Up to 1 out of every 500 African Americans will have the disorder that results in abnormal sickling of the red blood cells in the microvasculature resulting in occlusion, leading to ischemia and painful crises.

Sickle cell vaso-occlusive episodes can be precipitated by hypoxia, infection, fever, dehydration, cold environment, and acidosis. An infant experiencing a vaso-occlusive crisis may present with fussiness, irritability, crying, poor feeding, and other nonspecific findings because young children are nonverbal. Older children may report pain in specific locations of the body, including joints, the back, and the chest. Pain reported in the chest is particularly worrisome because acute chest syndrome can develop. Acute chest syndrome is a vaso-occlusive crisis of the vasculature of the chest. It can result in inflammation of the lung, infiltrates seen on chest radiographs, decreased oxygen saturations, fever, and respiratory failure.

Splenic sequestration occurs in younger children before children become functionally asplenic. Red blood cells become trapped in the spleen, leading to enlargement of the spleen, a swollen and painful abdomen, and profound anemia with hypotension progressing to circulatory collapse. The crises can be transient, but must be treated aggressively, oftentimes with blood transfusions.

Priapism is an uncommon side effect of SCD caused by sickling of cells within the vasculature of the penis. Blood flow out of the penis is blocked, which results in an erection that is sustained. The condition is painful and can lead to damage of the penile tissues if not treated in an ED quickly. Fluids and pain medications should be started en route to the nearest hospital.

Strokes can result from sickling of red blood cells within the vasculature of the brain. The result is ischemia and symptoms similar to a patient experiencing a stroke. Because the mechanism is sickled blood cells rather than thromboembolic events, thrombolytics do not help patients who are having a stroke because of SCD. These patients should be placed on oxygen, given IV fluids, and transported to a hospital where an exchange transfusion can take place. During an exchange transfusion, the patient's sickled blood is removed and replaced with normal red blood cells. Strokes are the second leading cause of death in young sickle cell patients, after acute chest syndrome.

Treatment of patients who are having a sickle cell crisis includes gentle hydration rather than fast boluses of fluids. A 20-mL/kg bolus can be given over 1 hour. Oxygen saturations of less than 90% should be treated with supplemental oxygen. Pain control may be obtained with anti-inflammatory medications and narcotics. In pediatric patients, the concern for addiction is minimal, so medications should be given until pain is relieved.

Bleeding Disorders

A bleeding or clotting disorder is a condition in which there is an abnormality in clotting of the blood. The development of a blood clot, called thrombosis, can occur in either arterial or venous blood vessels. The patient's symptoms depend on which part of the vascular system the clot occurs in, how large the clot is, and whether the clot becomes dislodged and travels to another part of the body.

Most bleeding is the result of trauma, but when a patient has a bleeding disorder, bleeding may be more severe or spontaneous. For all bleeding patients, the first thing for you to consider is how to best control the bleeding, if possible. Local pressure, elevation, packing, and the judicious use of tourniquets may be necessary. As with all patients, significant blood loss can lead to shock, so fluid replacement with boluses of isotonic fluids such as saline or lactated Ringer's solution is necessary until the patient is at a hospital for definitive care and blood transfusions.

Bleeding may be drug-induced, inherited, or acquired. Drugs such as aspirin and the NSAID class (ibuprofen) can cause a decrease in platelet adhesion, making patients more prone to bleeding. Drugs such as aspirin, warfarin (Coumadin), and heparin interfere with the clotting cascade and decrease the tendency to form a clot. Over-the-counter medications (ginkgo biloba, ginger, vitamin E, ginseng, and garlic) and some antibiotics can also increase bleeding tendencies. Though rare in young children, ethanol use or diseases that affect the liver can lead to bleeding by decreasing the liver's capacity to synthesize the factors needed in the clotting cascade.

Thrombocytopenia

Thrombocytopenia is when the body has an abnormally low number of platelets in the blood. The normal platelet count is between 150,000 and 450,000 platelets per microliter of blood; when the platelet count falls below this level, thrombocytopenia is present. The risk of bleeding is proportional to the degree of thrombocytopenia. Platelet counts below 100,000 are associated with impaired ability for the blood to form clots, and platelet counts below 20,000 can lead to spontaneous bleeding. Thrombocytopenia can have many causes, including infections, cancers such as leukemia, rheumatologic diseases such as lupus, and splenic sequestration. Some inherited conditions may also cause low platelet counts. In addition, many medications (including valproic acid used to treat seizures) and chemotherapy drugs can reduce the platelet count.

Besides spontaneous bleeding or prolonged bleeding with injury, patients with low levels of platelets may exhibit petechiae or purpura. Large bruises may develop from minimal injuries or with no history of injury. Physical abuse should always be considered in children with unexplained bruising until proven otherwise.

Treatment of patients with bleeding secondary to thrombocytopenia includes treating the underlying cause if present (treating infections, stopping offending medications) and transfusing platelets if bleeding cannot be controlled with local measures. Consultation with a hematologist is required for these patients, so transport to a hospital with these capabilities should not be delayed.

Hemophilia

Hemophilia is a genetic disorder usually inherited from the mother. People with hemophilia have a significant decrease in one of their clotting factors, or proteins in the blood that work with platelets to help blood to clot. Without the clotting factor, it is more difficult for bleeding to stop. This condition occurs predominantly in males and is seen in approximately 1 in every 5,000 to 10,000 births. The disease is classified into two primary types, hemophilia A and hemophilia B.

Hemophilia A involves a deficiency of factor VIII and is responsible for approximately 80% of the disease. Hemophilia B is due to a deficiency of factor IX and makes up the majority of the other 20% of hemophiliacs. Type A and type B have the same signs and symptoms. Though not curable, hemophilia is treated with replacement of the missing factor. When injuries occur, extra factor is often needed. Most families have factor available, that must be delivered intravenously, and local blood banks also have factor available.

von Willebrand Disease

von Willebrand disease is the most common heritable disorder of coagulation, and its presentation can mimic hemophilia A. Though the prevalence is roughly 1/100, only about 1 person in 10,000 has significant disease. Most people with von Willebrand disease are undiagnosed. von Willebrand disease is due to a decreased amount or abnormal production of von Willebrand factor, a protein that is required for platelet adhesion and subsequent clot formation. There are several types of von Willebrand disease that can range in severity from mild (presenting with nosebleeds) to severe with uncontrolled bleeding tendencies. In the field, treatment is aimed at controlling bleeding and transporting the patient to a hospital with hematology services.

◼ Leukemia/Lymphoma

Approximately 10,000 children under the age of 15 years are diagnosed with cancer each year, the most common type being acute leukemia. Patients with childhood cancers, including leukemia and lymphoma, are often immunocompromised because of their treatment regimens. Chemotherapeutic agents cause significant immunosuppression in these patients, and this is compounded by the use of steroids and radiation therapy. Because of this, the patients are particularly prone to severe infections, even though they may not present with fevers (in fact, hypothermia may be present in septic children).

In patients with leukemia, the immunosuppressed state is often secondary to the leukemic cells overtaking the bone marrow or the treatments they are receiving. These patients are susceptible to bacteremia, sepsis, and shock. Illness progression can be fast because of the poor innate immunity these patients have. Neutropenia, or a low white blood cell count, is classified as mild if the absolute neutrophil count (ANC) is between 1,000 and 1,500. If the ANC is between 500 and 1,000, patients have moderate neutropenia, and an ANC of less than 500 is classified as severe. Severe patients are at an extreme risk and need to be started on antibiotics at the first sign of illness, including fever.

Patients who are being treated for cancer, patients with a history of immunosuppression, or patients who are on drugs that can alter immunity should have blood cultures drawn and isotonic fluids started. Fluid therapy should be aggressive in pediatric patients who are tachycardic because this can be the first sign of sepsis. Hypotension is a late sign of sepsis in the pediatric population. In consultation with a physician, early antibiotic therapy may be indicated for immunosuppressed patients.

One special condition to consider with oncology patients is tumor lysis syndrome (TLS). TLS is a condition that can occur after treatment of certain cancers, particularly leukemias and lymphomas. It is caused by the rapid increase of breakdown of the cancer cells after treatment (it can sometimes occur without treatment) and may result in hyperkalemia, hypocalcemia, hyperphosphatemia, and hyperuricemia. TLS can lead to acute renal injury and failure if not treated quickly. Besides renal injury and failure, patients can present with cardiac dysrhythmias because of the high potassium levels, and seizures, tetany, myopathy, and emotional lability can result from the hypocalcemia.

If TLS is suspected, rapid fluid therapy should be instituted as soon as IV access is obtained. The IV use of isotonic sodium bicarbonate to promote alkaline diuresis has potential benefits of solubilizing and thus minimizing intratubular (renal) precipitation of uric acid during TLS. The goal is to increase urinary pH to 7.0 to maximize uric acid solubility and excretion. A drawback to systemic alkaline therapy is worsening of clinical hypocalcemia, and routine use of alkalinization is controversial. Ultimately, hemodialysis may be necessary if the renal injury is severe.

◼ Pathophysiology, Assessment, and Management of Toxicologic Emergencies

Toxic exposures account for a significant number of pediatric emergencies. In 2009, almost 2.5 million poisoning cases were reported to Poison Centers. More than half of these poisonings occurred in children younger than 6 years, and 65% (more than 1.5 million cases) occurred in patients younger than 20 years.

Toxic exposures can take the form of ingestion, inhalation, injection, or application of a substance (see the chapter, *Toxicology*, for more information on specific exposures). A toddler or preschool-age child is most likely to have an unintentional exposure, the result of developmentally normal exploration. In this age group, ingestion tends to involve small quantities of a single cleaning product, cosmetic product, or plant, or a few pills. In contrast, toxic exposures in adolescents are typically the result of recreational drug use or suicide attempts and often involve multiple agents. Although intentional exposures among adolescents lead to greater morbidity and mortality, in small children, the toxic effects of some medications are such that "one pill can kill" Table 23.

Table 23 One Pill Can Kill: Potentially Lethal Toddler Ingestion

Medicine	Lethal Dose
Camphor	One teaspoon of oil
Chloroquine	One 500-mg tablet
Clonidine	One 0.3-mg tablet
Diphenoxylate/atropine	Two 2.5-mg tablets
Glyburide	Two 5-mg tablets
Imipramine	One 150-mg tablet
Lindane	Two teaspoons of 1% lotion
Oil of wintergreen	One teaspoon of oil
Propranolol	One or two 160-mg tablets
Theophylline	One 500-mg tablet
Verapamil	One or two 240-mg tablets

Table 24 SAMPLE History for a Child With Toxic Exposure

Components	Features
Signs and symptoms	Time of suspected exposure Behavior changes in child Emesis and content of vomit
Allergies	Known drug reactions or other allergies
Medications	Identity of suspected toxin Amount of toxin exposure (count pills or measure volume) Pill or chemical containers on scene Exact names and doses of prescribed medications
Past medical problems	Previous illnesses or injuries
Last oral intake	Timing of the child's last food or drink Type and time of home treatment
Events leading to injury or illness	Key events leading to the exposure Type of exposure (inhaled, injected, ingested, or absorbed through the skin) Poison Center contact

Assessment of Toxicologic Emergencies

The evaluation of a child who has experienced a potentially toxic exposure follows the standard assessment sequence. Identify the agents to which the child was exposed, the quantity, and the route and time of exposure. Findings of physical assessment will vary widely based on these factors. Make special note of vital signs, pupillary changes, skin temperature and moisture, and any unusual odors. Putting together these pieces of the puzzle may allow you to identify a toxidrome—a pattern of symptoms and signs typical of a particular poisoning.

When you are performing the primary assessment, attend to the ABCs as indicated. A dextrose (glucose) check is an important test because ingestion of some common substances can lead to hypoglycemia—namely, ethanol and other alcohols, insulin, oral hypoglycemic agents, and beta blockers. Treat documented hypoglycemia as part of your resuscitation.

If the child is in stable condition without physiologic abnormalities and without a serious toxic exposure, stay on scene to obtain additional history and perform a secondary assessment. See Table 24 for the SAMPLE history for a pediatric patient with a potential toxic exposure. During the secondary assessment, look for toxidromes by assessing the patient's mental status, pupillary changes, skin CTC, gastrointestinal activity (bowel sounds, emesis, or diarrhea), and abnormal odors. Perform frequent reassessments because the child's condition may change.

Words of Wisdom

Have the national Poison Center number (1-800-222-1222) in your clipboard for suspected poisonings.

Children with potentially life-threatening toxic exposures may be asymptomatic on your arrival, and the dose of drug in an accidental toddler ingestion may be high. Always attempt to collect any pill containers or bottles and transport them with the patient to the hospital to assist the ED staff in making treatment decisions.

Management of Toxicologic Emergencies

The management of any potential toxic exposure begins with supportive care and attention to the ABCs. Other management options include reducing the absorption of the substance by decontamination, enhancing elimination of the substance, and/or providing an antidote. Give special attention to the risks of environmental exposures for the EMS crew, who may also require decontamination measures.

If you are not sure if an exposure is dangerous or potentially toxic to a child, the national Poison Center hotline is available 24 hours a day at 1-800-222-1222. This nationwide number puts you in contact with experts who can help manage the care of ingestions, exposures, inhalations, and other toxicologic emergencies.

Decontamination

If a toxic substance has been applied to the skin, reducing absorption involves removal of all clothing and a thorough washing of the skin. With ocular exposure, immediately wash out the eyes. For ingested toxins, options to reduce gastric absorption include dilution, gastric lavage, and activated charcoal.

Depending on the substance ingested, it may be useful to dilute the substance by having the child drink a glass of milk or water. This decision should be made in conjunction with a Poison Center consultant or your medical control physician or nurse, depending on your protocols. If the child has any airway or breathing concerns, do not allow the child to drink.

Although parents were once encouraged to keep syrup of ipecac available to induce vomiting in young children, this treatment is no longer recommended by the American Academy of Pediatrics. Ipecac does not remove significant amounts of ingested toxins and can cause prolonged emesis; it should not be used in the prehospital management of pediatric toxic ingestion.

The most common method currently used for gastrointestinal decontamination in the ED setting is the administration of activated charcoal. Activated charcoal absorbs many ingested toxins in the gut, making less of the toxin available for systemic absorption if it is administered within the first hour after exposure. However, some common toxins do not bind to charcoal—for example, heavy metals, alcohols, hydrocarbons, acids, and alkalis. Activated charcoal is messy to administer and is rarely readily accepted by pediatric patients. For these reasons, as well as the risk of severe chemical pneumonia if a child with altered mental status or vomiting aspirates the charcoal, this treatment may be best given in the hospital setting. If activated charcoal is given in the field, the ideal dose is 10 times the mass of the ingested substance. The amount of drug ingested is often not known, so the typical dose is 1 to 2 g/kg.

For substances that are renally excreted, diuresis may be beneficial. IV fluid administration can increase diuresis, as can mannitol. Care must be taken with mannitol administration for this purpose as it can lead to hypotension. Some substances have enhanced excretion in an alkali environment, such as salicylates and methyl alcohol (antifreeze or wood alcohol). For these substances, the use of sodium bicarbonate to alkalinize the urinary pH can be beneficial. Dialysis is required for some overdoses and overdoses that do not improve with other therapies such as alkalization of the urine. Examples of ingestions or overdoses that dialysis is helpful for include salicylates, lithium, methyl alcohol, ethylene glycol, and barbiturates such as phenobarbital.

If the substance is inhaled, special consideration should be given to the respiratory status of the patient. Bronchodilators may be needed for bronchial irritation and bronchospasm. Monitoring of oxygen saturations and intubation may be necessary, particularly with inhalational injuries associated with house fires. If there is the presence of soot in the upper airway, if the patient has stridor, or if there is any swelling of the upper airway, early intubation is indicated. Carbon monoxide inhalation injuries may be difficult to diagnose because the patient's oxygen saturation level will be near 100%. This is because the oximeter may misinterpret carboxyhemoglobin as oxyhemoglobin. These patients should be placed on a nonrebreathing mask until blood carboxyhemoglobin levels can be checked at the hospital.

Enhanced Elimination

Cathartics such as sorbitol or magnesium citrate are sometimes combined with activated charcoal. They work by speeding up elimination. In general, cathartics are not recommended for young children because they have been known to cause significant diarrhea with serious—sometimes life-threatening—electrolyte abnormalities. Hospital providers have additional options for enhancing elimination, such as whole bowel irrigation, urinary alkalinization for salicylate overdoses, dialysis, and hemoperfusion.

Antidotes

Antidotes can be lifesaving but are available for only a few poisonings. They work by reversing or blocking the effects of the ingested toxin. Table 25 lists some of the more commonly available antidotes; indications for their use are the same for young children as for adults. The dose depends on the weight of the child.

Table 25 Common Antidotes

Poison	Antidote
Carbon monoxide	Oxygen
Organophosphate	Atropine/pralidoxime
Tricyclic antidepressants	Bicarbonate
Opiates	Naloxone
Beta blockers	Glucagon
Calcium channel blockers	Calcium
Benzodiazepine	Flumazenil
Acetaminophen	N-acetylcysteine (NAC)

Pathophysiology, Assessment, and Management of Psychiatric and Behavioral Emergencies

As a paramedic, you will encounter children with behavioral and psychiatric problems. The call may be for out-of-control behavior or for a suicide attempt. Unfortunately, EMS calls for behavioral emergencies are increasing, reflecting in part the limited community resources available for children with mental health problems. A recent study of one pediatric ED found that 5% of all pediatric ED visits were for mental health concerns.

Safety

When you are called to a home for a behavioral or psychiatric emergency, safety should be your first priority. Assess the scene for your own safety and for the safety of your patient. If weapons are involved or you cannot determine the degree of risk, call for law enforcement backup.

Approach the child calmly, letting him or her know you are there to help. Address the patient directly when you are obtaining the history, and explain clearly what you are doing and why. Some children are flight risks, so determine how best to deploy your squad so that they do not leave the scene. As always, answer questions as honestly as possible.

A small percentage of children cannot be safely talked down for transport and must be mechanically restrained for their own protection and the protection of the EMS crew. Applying these restraints may be a task for EMS or for law enforcement personnel. If you decide to apply restraints, carefully document the reason and keep the restraints in place until arrival at the ED. Try to avoid using chemical restraint (that is, tranquilizing drugs) in the prehospital setting.

Assessment and Management of Psychiatric and Behavioral Emergencies

The PAT will give you a general impression of the child's mental status and cardiovascular stability. A child who has attempted suicide by ingestion may have life-threatening medical complications that take precedence over his or her psychiatric concerns. In the absence of acute medical issues, the bulk of your assessment will be based on observation and history. In cases involving an agitated child, your hands-on assessment may be limited. **Table 26** lists specific SAMPLE questions for behavioral emergencies. As always, treat any existing medical problems or injuries by using standard protocols.

Table 26 SAMPLE History for a Child With Behavioral Problems

Component	Features
Signs and symptoms	Out-of-control behavior? Suicidal or homicidal thoughts or actions? Harm to self, others, or pets? Recent change in behavior? Recent change in medication? Auditory or visual hallucinations?
Allergies	Known food or drug allergies and their reactions
Medications	List of all patient's medications and vitamins, prescribed and over-the-counter
Past medical history	History of any behavior or psychiatric problems? Therapist, counselor, or psychiatrist contact information? Prior psychiatric or behavioral hospitalizations? Any medical illnesses?
Last oral intake	Timing and identification of last food and drink
Events leading to behavioral problems	Ongoing or new stressors? Argument or fight with boyfriend, girlfriend, or family members?

Special Populations

Any child with unexplained hyperpnea should be suspected to have salicylate poisoning.

Pathophysiology, Assessment, and Management of Fever Emergencies

Fever is a common pediatric complaint but often not a true medical emergency. A symptom of an underlying infectious or inflammatory process, fever can have multiple causes. Most pediatric fevers are caused by viral infections that are often mild and self-limiting. In other cases, fever is a symptom of a more serious bacterial infection.

Your general impression and primary assessment will help you determine the severity of illness. Remember that young children with a fever can look quite ill because increased body temperature causes increased metabolism, tachycardia, and tachypnea. Record temperature as part of the vital signs, but recognize that the height of the fever does not reflect the severity of the illness. If the patient is a young infant, a rectal temperature is most accurate, but recognition that fever is present is more important than the exact temperature. As you move through the primary assessment, look for signs of respiratory distress, shock, seizures, stiff neck, petechial or purpuric rash, or a bulging fontanelle in an infant. These signs may tip you off to the presence of pneumonia, sepsis, or meningitis, all of which can be life threatening and require prompt transport to an appropriate facility.

Young infants (younger than 2 months) should always be considered at risk for serious infection. Young infants have few ways of interacting with the world, and a fever (defined as body temperature greater than 100.4°F [greater than 38°C]) may be the only sign of a potentially life-threatening illness. Regardless of how well a child in this age group looks, he or she should be assessed and transported quickly to an ED for a full sepsis workup, including blood, urine, and CSF analysis. All children younger than 28 days with a fever, and most children younger than 2 months of age will require admission to the ED.

History taking and the secondary assessment will help you to determine the underlying cause of the fever and the severity of illness. Perform this assessment on scene if the child is in stable condition or en route to the ED if the child appears seriously ill. Ask about the presence of vomiting, diarrhea, poor feeding, headache, neck pain or stiffness, and rash. A history of infectious exposure may provide clues to the likely cause of the child's current illness. History taking may also identify a child at high risk for serious bacterial illness. For example, sickle cell disease, HIV infection, and childhood cancers may all lead to an immunocompromised state.

A child with a fever may require little intervention in the field. You should simply support the ABCs as needed. Although fever by itself is not dangerous, temperature control will make the child with a minor acute illness look and feel better. Consider treating with acetaminophen or ibuprofen, but avoid aspirin in children. Use of aspirin in children has been linked with a rare illness called Reye syndrome, which can result in cerebral edema and liver failure. Other cooling measures should be limited to undressing the child. Transport the patient to an appropriate medical facility with ongoing reassessment for clinical deterioration.

Special Populations

Fever itself is generally not an emergency, but rather a symptom of an underlying process. Use your assessment skills to determine the child's severity of illness.

■ Child Abuse and Neglect

Sadly, child abuse is prevalent in our society. <u>Child abuse</u> is any improper or excessive action that injures or otherwise harms a child or infant; it includes physical abuse, sexual abuse, neglect, and emotional abuse. In 2009, national child protective services reported more than 800,000 confirmed cases of child abuse in the United States. Approximately 2,000 of these patients died as a result of maltreatment.

Physical abuse involves the infliction of injury to a child. Sexual abuse occurs when an adult engages in sexual activity with a child; it can range from inappropriate touching to intercourse. Emotional abuse and child neglect are often difficult to identify and may go unreported. Neglect is refusal or failure on the part of the caregiver to provide life necessities, whereas emotional abuse may be described as lack of emotional support by the caregiver.

Words of Wisdom

EMS providers are mandated reporters of suspected child abuse and neglect in all states.

Keep the possibility of child abuse in mind when you are called to assist with an injured child. The information you gather from the scene size-up and interviews may prove invaluable. If you suspect child abuse, you should act on your suspicions because child abuse involves a pattern of behavior. A child who is abused once is likely to be abused again—and next time, it may be more serious or even fatal.

■ Risk Factors for Abuse

No child asks to be abused, but certain risk factors make abuse more likely. Younger children are more often abused than older children, perhaps a function of their helplessness and limited ability to communicate their needs. Children who require extra attention, such as children with handicaps, chronic illnesses, or other developmental problems, are also more likely to be abused.

Child abuse occurs across all socioeconomic levels, although it is more prevalent in lower socioeconomic families. Divorce, financial problems, and illness can contribute to the overall stress level of parents, placing them at higher risk to abuse their children. Drug and alcohol abuse can also interfere with a caregiver's ability to parent, and both are associated with higher rates of abusive behavior. Domestic violence in the home places a child at a much higher risk for child abuse.

Special Populations

Autism can vary in severity and falls under a broader category known as pervasive developmental disorders (PDDs). PDDs cause delays in many areas of childhood development, such as the development of skills to communicate and interact socially, and the effects can be lifelong. See the chapter, *Patients With Special Challenges*, for more information on this condition.

■ Suspecting Abuse or Neglect

When you are called to the home of an injured child and suspect abuse, trust your instincts. Look for "red flags" that could suggest child maltreatment (summarized in the mnemonic CHILD ABUSE; Table 27):

- A history inconsistent with the type of injury sustained—for example, a child who fell from a tree but whose bruises are only on the buttocks
- An account of the injury that is inconsistent with the developmental abilities of the child—for example, a 2-month-old infant rolling off a bed
- An old injury that went unreported
- Inappropriate actions or language from the caregiver

Table 27   CHILD ABUSE Mnemonic for Suspicion of Child Abuse

C	Consistency of the injury with the child's developmental age
H	History inconsistent with injury
I	Inappropriate parental concerns
L	Lack of supervision
D	Delay in seeking care
A	Affect (of the parent or caregiver and the child in relation to the caregiver)
B	Bruises of varying ages
U	Unusual injury patterns
S	Suspicious circumstances
E	Environmental clues

Assessment and Management of Abuse and Neglect

To recognize abuse, you first have to suspect it. Once you begin to question whether abuse is involved, it becomes important to carefully document what you see. Although it may be difficult to remain impartial when child abuse is suspected, it is an important part of professionalism. Record what you see and hear, but do not editorialize. Be detailed in your incident report about the child's environment, noting the condition of the home and the interactions among the caregivers, the child, and the EMS crew. Record concerning comments verbatim, as well as the name of the person who made the comments and when. In all states, prehospital personnel are mandated reporters, meaning you have an independent obligation under the law to report a suspicion of child abuse to child protective services and law enforcement. Failure to make a report may be a crime. Review the specific law in your state. Reporting is done in conjunction with emergency physicians, social workers, and child protection teams at the ED. Involving police early is important to secure the crime scene and collect evidence that may be destroyed or lost. In cases where death occurs, the medical examiner will investigate the cause of death. The medical examiner should be notified of any death if the child is not being transported to the ED.

Documentation and Communication

If you suspect child abuse, take extra care with your documentation. Record conversations verbatim (in quotes) and document on your patient care report what you see and hear.

Do not approach the caregiver with your concerns, but make sure that you pass these concerns on to staff at the ED. In all states, EMS providers are mandatory reporters of suspected child abuse. Be aware of local regulations; you may have a legal—and an ethical—obligation to ensure that a report is made to the local **child protection services (CPS)**. The primary objective of CPS is to ensure the safety of children and keep children safe within their own families.

Although child abuse can generate an emotional response from the EMS crew, remember that your primary focus should be on trauma assessment and management and on ensuring the safety of the child. Base your general impression on the PAT, which may range from normal in a child with minor inflicted injuries to grossly abnormal in a child with severe internal or central nervous system injuries. In shaken baby syndrome, you may encounter a child with an abnormal appearance but no external signs of injury. In such a case, the child receives a severe brain injury when a caregiver violently shakes the infant, often when the child is crying inconsolably. Given that few caregivers will admit to having hurt the child, be alert for a history that is inconsistent with the clinical picture.

Pay special attention to the child's skin while looking for bruises, especially in different stages of healing or in concerning locations. Active toddlers often have bruises on their shins from

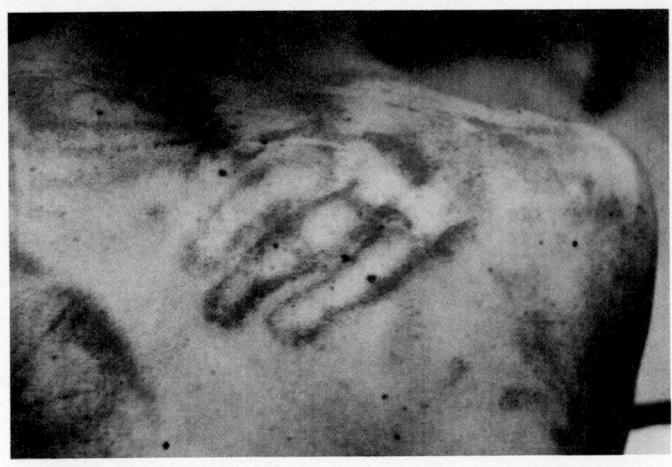

Figure 20 Bruises from child abuse. Look for bruises that look like finger or hand marks.

falls and active playing but rarely on their backs or buttocks. Bruises in identifiable patterns such as belt buckles, looped cords, or straight lines are rarely incurred accidentally. **Figure 20** and **Figure 21** are examples of bruises that are suggestive of physical abuse.

Use the CHILD ABUSE mnemonic when you obtain additional history. Ask yourself, "Does the caregiver's explanation make sense? Could this child produce this bruise or injury through his or her normal activities?"

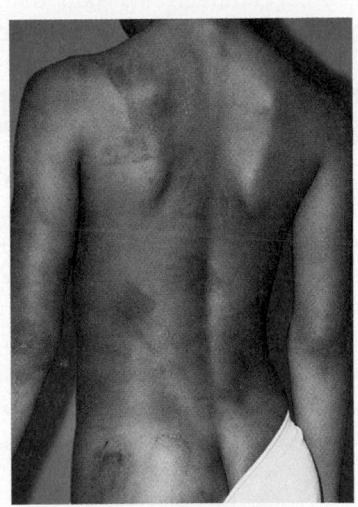

Figure 21 Multiple bruises or injuries that are in different stages of healing are concerns for abuse.

Mimics of Abuse

It can be difficult to distinguish some normal skin findings from inflicted injuries. For example, Mongolian spots **Figure 22** can mimic bruises. These birthmarks are generally found on the lower back and buttocks of children of Asian or African American descent; they may be mistaken for bruises because of their unique bluish coloring. Other medical conditions can mimic bruises, such as the purpura of meningitis and Henoch-Schönlein purpura, or the petechiae of idiopathic thrombocytopenic purpura and leukemia. Exposure to the sun can cause reactions with certain medications or fruits (limes, mangos), causing reddish-purple discolorations of the skin called phytophotodermatitis.

Certain cultural customs also produce skin markings that can mimic child abuse. Coining **Figure 23** and cupping **Figure 24** are traditional Asian healing practices, often used in the treatment

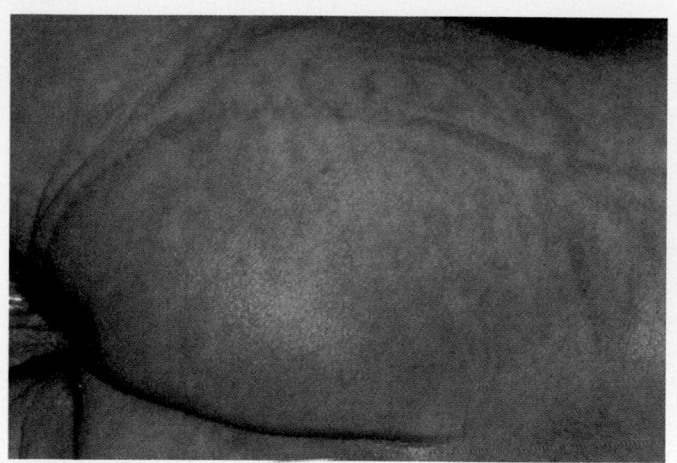

Figure 22 A Mongolian spot is a birthmark that can mimic a bruise. It may be on the back, buttocks, or extremities.

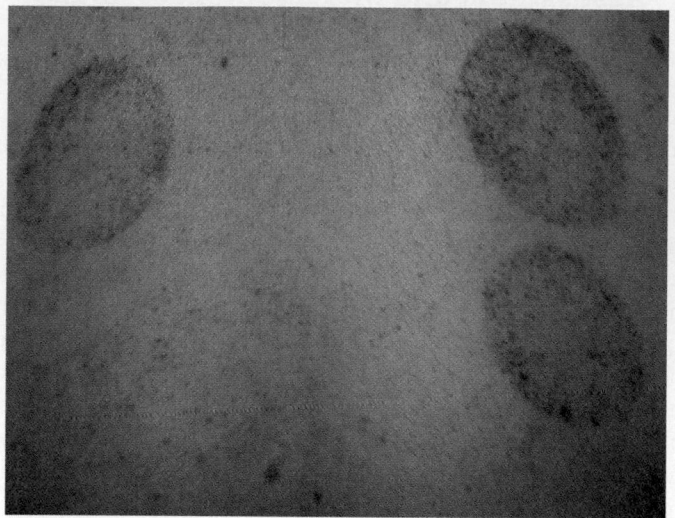

Figure 24 Round, flat, red circles on a child's back may be from the practice of cupping—placing warm cups on the skin to draw out illness from the body.

of fever. Although the skin markings can be impressive, the practice is not harmful and does not represent abuse.

Sudden Infant Death Syndrome

Sudden infant death syndrome (SIDS), formerly known as crib death, is the sudden and unexpected death of an infant younger than 1 year for whom a thorough postmortem examination (autopsy) fails to demonstrate an adequate cause of death. Whatever the cause, the sudden death of an apparently healthy infant is devastating to families and to the EMS crew that responds to the call. Risk factors associated with SIDS include male sex; prematurity; low birth weight; young maternal age; sleeping in the prone position; sleeping with soft, bulky blankets or soft objects; sleeping on soft surfaces; and exposure to tobacco smoke.

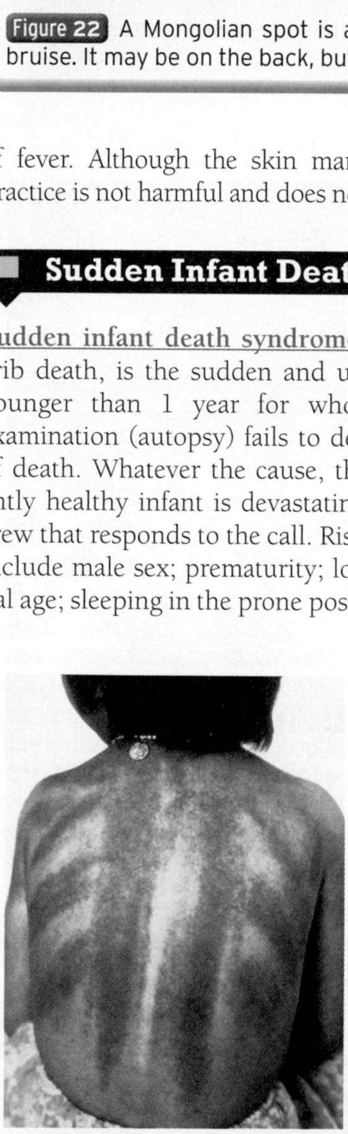

SIDS is the leading cause of death in infants ages 1 month to 1 year, with a peak incidence between 2 and 4 months. Approximately 250,000 SIDS deaths occur each year in the United States.

Assessment and Management of SIDS

The typical scenario for a SIDS call is that of a healthy infant who was put down for a nap and later found dead in bed. On arrival of EMS, the baby will be lifeless and, depending on discovery time, may have rigor mortis and dependent lividity (pooling of blood on the underside of the body). The presence of frothy or blood-tinged fluid in the mouth or nose or on the bedding is typical of SIDS. Be alert for clues to other potential causes of death, such as trauma, suffocation, or maltreatment.

Your decision to start resuscitative efforts, or to stop CPR that was started by first responders or family members, can be difficult in cases of suspected SIDS. Your actions will be guided by local protocols on declaring death in the field and by your assessment of the patient and the needs of the family. Although a victim of SIDS cannot be resuscitated, failure to initiate care may not be acceptable to the shocked family. Likewise, ED care will not change the outcome for the infant, but hospital-based social services for the family may be an important resource. In cases that meet the criteria for declaring death at the scene and nontransport, notify the coroner, medical examiner, or law enforcement personnel, as dictated by local protocol, so that appropriate scene investigation can be undertaken. You also have an important role in mobilizing support for the survivors—for example, a chaplain or minister, SIDS team, social worker, or other family members.

Despite the emotionally charged atmosphere, doing a thorough scene size-up and obtaining the pertinent history is important. A history of recent illnesses, chronic conditions, medications, or trauma may decrease the likelihood of SIDS as the cause of death. The presence of pillows, stuffed toys, window blind cords, or sheepskin in the baby's crib may make suffocation a possibility.

Figure 23 Coining, the practice of rubbing hot coins on the back as a treatment of medical illnesses, can leave impressive markings that can mimic child abuse.

Apparent Life-Threatening Event

An apparent life-threatening event (ALTE) is an episode during which an infant becomes pale or cyanotic; chokes, gags, or has an apneic spell; or loses muscle tone. These changes are sufficiently dramatic that the caregiver becomes frightened and may think that the baby is dying. ALTEs frequently prompt 9-1-1 calls. Their causes may include benign diagnoses, such as a brief episode of laryngospasm during feedings or gastroesophageal reflux, and serious diagnoses, such as sepsis, congenital heart disease, and seizures.

ALTEs were once thought of as existing along a spectrum with SIDS; hence they were called near-miss or aborted SIDS. More recent evidence demonstrates that although both events occur in early infancy, the two are not related. It is common to find a distraught caregiver and a well-appearing baby on arrival at the scene of an ALTE call. Provide life support if the infant shows signs of cardiorespiratory compromise or altered mental status, and transport all infants with a history of an ALTE to an appropriate medical facility for evaluation. This is a challenging age group to assess, and overtriage is the safest path. Because ALTEs may be associated with serious underlying illness, failure to transport may be associated with grave consequences for the child.

Pathophysiology, Assessment, and Management of Pediatric Trauma Emergencies

Pediatric trauma is the leading cause of death among children older than 1 year. Motor vehicle crashes cause the most deaths in this age group, followed by falls and submersions. Among adolescents, homicide and suicide are also common causes of death.

Children's age-related anatomy and physiology make their injury patterns and responses to trauma different from those seen in adults. In addition, a child's developmental stage will affect his or her response to injury. For a young child, being strapped to a backboard may be as traumatic as the injury leading to the EMS call! Refer to the beginning of this chapter for a review of age-related anatomy and physiology and a discussion on how trauma impacts children as a result of their anatomic and physiologic differences.

Pathophysiology of Traumatic Injuries

Blunt trauma is the MOI in more than 90% of pediatric injury cases. Because children have less muscle and fat mass than adults, they have less protection against the forces transmitted in blunt trauma.

Falls are common in pediatric patients, and the injuries sustained will reflect the anatomy of the child and the height of the fall. For example, a 6-year-old child playing on the monkey bars is most likely to sustain an upper extremity fracture when falling onto an outstretched arm. Internal or head injuries would be uncommon with this mechanism. Conversely, an infant, with a big head and no protective reflexes, who falls out of a shopping cart will commonly have a skull fracture and could have an intracranial hemorrhage. Falls from a standing position usually result in isolated long bone injuries, whereas high-energy falls (such as from a window, ejection from a motor vehicle, car-versus-pedestrian collision) may result in multisystem trauma.

Injuries from bicycle handlebars typically produce compression injuries to the intra-abdominal organs. Duodenal hematomas and/or pancreatic injuries are common with this MOI, as are upper extremity injuries. You must also consider a head injury if the patient went over the handlebars, especially if not wearing a helmet.

Motor vehicle crashes can result in a variety of injury patterns depending on whether the child was properly restrained and where the child was seated in the car. For unrestrained passengers, assume multisystem trauma. Restrained passengers may sustain chest and abdominal injuries associated with seat belt use. If you see chest or abdominal bruising in a seat belt pattern, you should have a high suspicion for spinal fractures. Air bags pose a particular threat for head and neck injuries in young children.

A child who is the victim of a car-versus-pedestrian collision is likely to sustain multisystem trauma. Depending on the child's height and the height of the vehicle's bumper, a child may receive chest, abdominal, and lower extremity injuries at impact. Head and neck injuries may result from the fall when the child is thrown.

Assessment and Management of Traumatic Injuries

The first steps in managing pediatric trauma are the same as for medical emergencies. Begin with a thorough scene size-up addressing safety concerns, determining the MOI or NOI as you approach the scene, noting the number of patients, and following standard precautions before coming into contact with the patient. Also determine whether or not additional resources are needed.

Use the PAT to form a general impression. If the PAT findings are grossly abnormal, quickly move on to the management of the ABCs to prevent death or disability. An abnormal appearance should make you think immediately of a head injury. With an isolated closed head injury, the child's breathing and circulation may be normal. Of course, abnormal appearance may also reflect inadequate oxygenation of the brain owing to shock or respiratory failure. Abnormalities in work of breathing will tip you off to chest or airway injury and abnormal circulation to a hemorrhage problem. If multisystem injuries are present, all three sides of the PAT may be abnormal.

Initiate life support interventions as you identify problems. Assess the airway for obstruction with teeth, blood, vomit, or edema. Suction as needed. For cervical spinal injury, open the airway using the jaw-thrust maneuver. If the child cannot maintain the airway, consider placement of an NG or oropharyngeal airway. If you attempt ET intubation, maintain cervical spinal precautions. Establishment of an emergency surgical airway in a child is fraught with complications, and the failure rate is high; for these reasons, tracheotomy should be reserved for the most expert surgeons in a controlled setting. The chances of needing to perform a needle cricothyrotomy in a child are remote. In younger children, identification of the cricothyroid membrane is difficult. Needle cricothyrotomy is described in the chapter, *Airway Management and Ventilation.*

Breathing assessment includes evaluation for symmetric chest rise and equal breath sounds. Provide 100% supplemental oxygen, give bag-mask ventilation as needed, and place an NG or OG tube for stomach decompression.

Pneumothorax is not common in pediatric blunt chest injury, but it may be present when there is penetrating trauma of the chest or upper abdomen. Remember that you are less likely to see jugular venous distention and tracheal deviation in a child. If the mechanism suggests a possible tension pneumothorax and the child is in significant respiratory distress, perform needle decompression. The signs and symptoms of tension pneumothorax include the following:

- Tachycardia
- Difficult ventilation despite an open airway
- Absent or decreased breath sounds on the affected side
- Jugular vein distention (may not be present with associated hemorrhage)
- Hyperresonance to percussion on the affected side
- Tracheal deviation away from the affected side (this late sign is not always present)
- Pulsus paradoxus

Trachial deviation, hyperresonance, pulsus paradoxus, and even decreased breath sounds can be difficult to assess in a young child.

Follow the steps in **Skill Drill 6** to perform needle decompression in a child:

Skill Drill 6

1. Assess the child to ensure that the presentation is due to a tension pneumothorax.
2. Prepare and assemble the necessary equipment: large-bore IV catheter, preferably 14 to 16 gauge, alcohol or povidone iodine preps, and adhesive tape.
3. Obtain orders from medical control.
4. Locate the appropriate site. Find the second or third intercostal space in the midclavicular line on the affected side **Step 1**.

Skill Drill 6

Pediatric Needle Decompression (Thoracentesis) of a Tension Pneumothorax

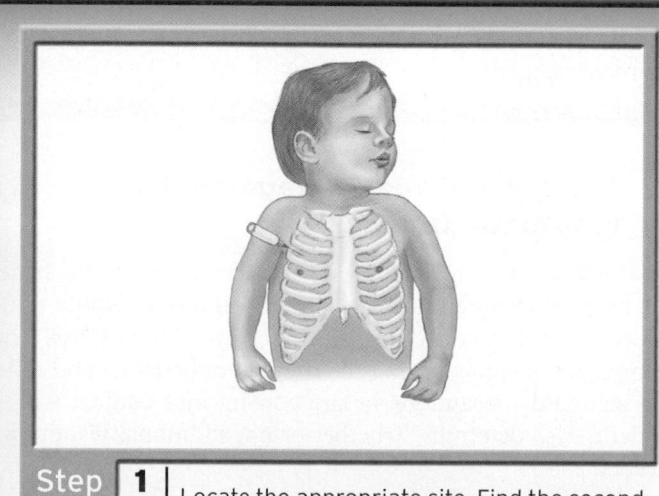

Step 1 Locate the appropriate site. Find the second or third intercostal space at the midclavicular line on the affected side.

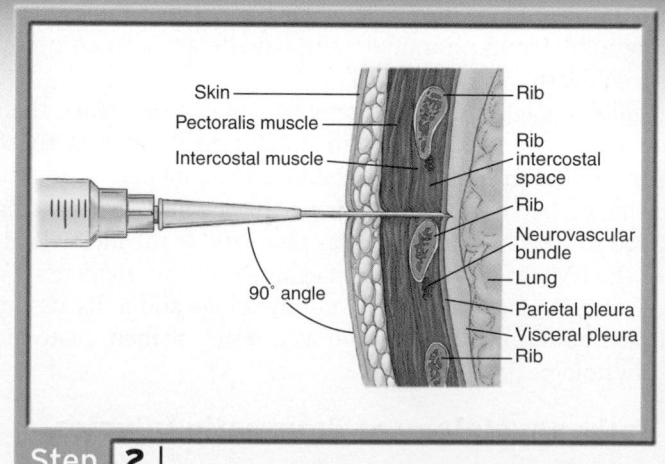

Step 2 Cleanse the appropriate area using aseptic technique. Insert the needle at a 90° angle and listen for the release of air.

5. Cleanse the appropriate area using aseptic technique.

6. Insert the needle at a 90° angle, just superior to the third rib (nerves, arteries, and veins run along the inferior borders of each rib), and listen for the release of air **Step 2**.

7. Advance the catheter over the needle, and place the needle in the sharps container.

8. Secure the catheter in place the same way you would secure an impaled object.

9. Monitor the child closely for recurrence of the tension pneumothorax.

Any trauma patient should be considered to be at risk for developing shock from visible external bleeding or internal bleeding. Assess the child's circulation by checking the pulse rate and quality, capillary refill, skin temperature, and blood pressure. In pediatric patients, the only sign of compensated shock might be an elevated pulse rate—children have a remarkable capacity for peripheral vasoconstriction and can maintain their blood pressure despite significant blood loss. If the MOI is concerning and the child is tachycardic, assume the presence of compensated shock and initiate volume resuscitation with 20 mL/kg of isotonic fluid (normal saline or lactated Ringer's). Ideally, you will insert two peripheral IV lines, but an IO line may be best in a child with hemorrhagic shock. Control external bleeding as you would in any trauma patient. Once the ABCs are stabilized, continue your assessment of disability with the AVPU scale. Your assessment of appearance in the PAT will already have identified an altered LOC. Check the child's pupils and motor function. Place a cervical collar, and immobilize the child on a long backboard as indicated.

If increased ICP is a concern, keep the head midline to facilitate jugular venous return to the heart. If the child is not in shock, elevate the backboard or head of the stretcher to 30°. Perform shock resuscitation with IV fluids—brain hypoperfusion will worsen the situation. If the child has acute signs of herniation such as a "blown" pupil or the Cushing triad (elevated blood pressure, bradycardia, abnormal respiratory pattern), consider mild hyperventilation guided to an $ETCO_2$ of 32 to 35 mm Hg and administer mannitol.

Assess "exposure"—that is, perform a rapid exam to identify all injuries. Log roll the child, and examine the back and buttocks. Once you have completed this exam, cover the child with blankets. Do not forget to cover the head, especially in infants and young children, and avoid drafts from heating or air conditioning units. Children have a relatively large skin surface area–body mass ratio, increasing their risk for heat loss and hypothermia. Consider the use of warm IV fluids, warm oxygen, and a warm patient transport environment, and keep the patient covered. Also be sure to remove any wet clothing that could conduct heat away from the patient.

Treat any fractures—open or closed—as you would in an adult. Check out your equipment ahead of time to ensure that you have splints appropriate for pediatric patients.

■ Transport Considerations

After stabilization of the child, you are faced with the transport decision. Some traumas are load-and-go situations because

of the severity of injuries and the child's unstable condition. Examples include trauma involving an ominous MOI regardless of how the child looks on scene, a child with an unstable or compromised airway, a child in shock, a child with difficulty breathing, and a child with a severe neurologic disability. For these situations, perform lifesaving procedures on scene or en route, and quickly transfer them to an appropriate trauma center according to local trauma triage protocols.

All trauma victims for whom spinal injury is suspected require appropriate spinal stabilization. The indications are the same for children and adults. You may have difficulty finding an appropriately sized cervical collar for infants or young children. Do not attempt to place a collar that is too big on a small child—use towel rolls and tape to immobilize the head. Apply the tape across the temples and forehead, but avoid tape over the chin or throat because it may impair ventilation. Choose a pediatric immobilizer with a recess for the child's large occiput, or place a towel or small blanket under the shoulders and back to prevent neck flexion in infants and toddlers **Figure 25**.

Immobilize a child with the following steps **Skill Drill 7**:

Skill Drill   7

1. Maintain a child's head in a neutral position by placing a towel under the shoulders **Step 1**.

2. Place an appropriately sized cervical collar on the child **Step 2**.

3. Carefully log roll the child onto the immobilization device **Step 3**.

4. Secure the child's torso to the immobilization device first **Step 4**.

5. Secure the child's head to the immobilization device **Step 5**.

6. Complete immobilization by ensuring that the child is strapped in properly **Step 6**.

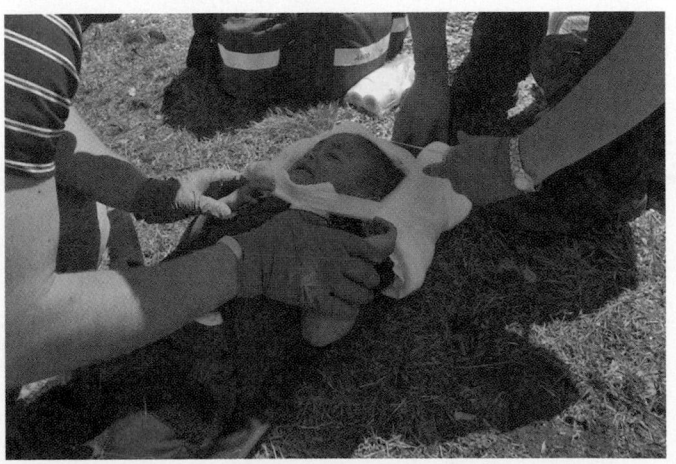

Figure 25 Cervical spinal stabilization with towels and tape for a young infant.

Skill Drill 7

Immobilizing a Child

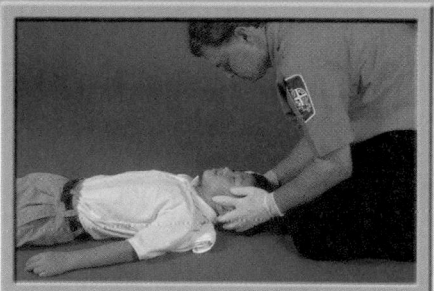

Step 1 Use a towel under the shoulders of a child to maintain the head in a neutral position.

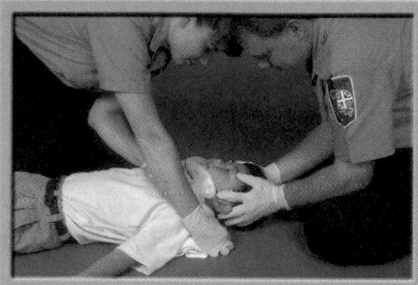

Step 2 Apply an appropriately sized cervical collar.

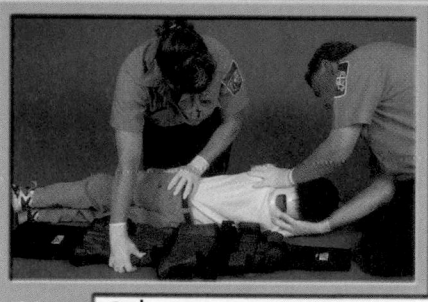

Step 3 Log roll the child onto the immobilization device.

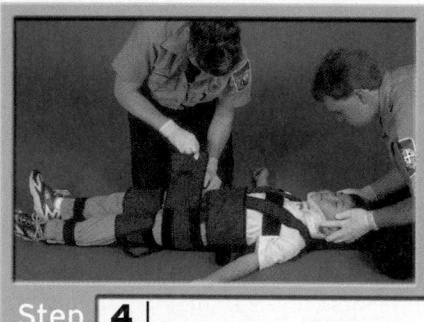

Step 4 Secure the torso first.

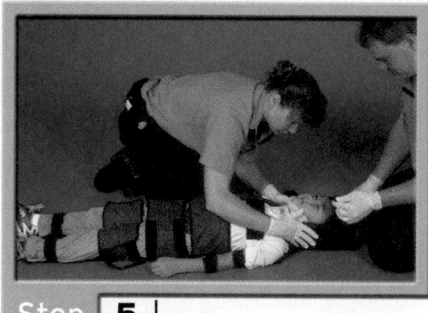

Step 5 Secure the head next.

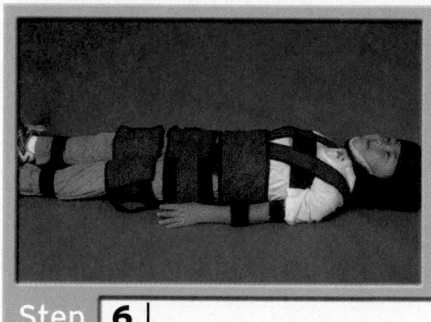

Step 6 Ensure that the child is strapped in properly.

Secure the child firmly onto the backboard but leave room for adequate chest expansion. Being immobilized is a frightening experience, especially for a young child who cannot understand your intent. Use developmentally appropriate language to explain what you are doing and why, and keep a parent close by when possible.

Follow the steps in **Skill Drill 8** to immobilize an infant:

Skill Drill 8

1. Carefully stabilize the infant's head in a neutral position and lay the seat down into a reclined position on a hard surface **Step 1**.
2. Position a pediatric board or other similar device between the infant and the surface on which the infant is resting **Step 2**.
3. Carefully slide the infant into position on the board **Step 3**.
4. Make sure the infant's head is in a neutral position by placing a towel under the infant's shoulders **Step 4**.
5. Secure the torso first, and place padding to fill any voids **Step 5**.

6. Secure the infant's head to the backboard **Step 6**.

The identification of the nearest appropriate facility depends on local protocols and the capabilities of local EDs. In some areas of the country, you may be directed to take the patient directly to a pediatric trauma center or to arrange for air transport to a pediatric trauma center. In other areas of the country, children are evaluated primarily at local EDs and then transferred to a pediatric trauma center.

▌ History Taking and Secondary Assessment

If the patient is in stable condition and does not meet the load-and-go criteria, obtain additional history as outlined in **Table 28** and perform a more thorough physical exam. A full-body, back-to-front detailed physical examination should be performed on all trauma patients with significant MOI en route to the ED. For infants, this will include checking the anterior fontanelle for bulging (a sign of increased ICP). Look for bruises, abrasions, or other subtle signs of injury that may have been missed during the primary assessment. Be sure to revisit the primary assessment during your reassessment on the way to the ED because the patient's condition can change quickly.

Skill Drill   8

Immobilizing an Infant

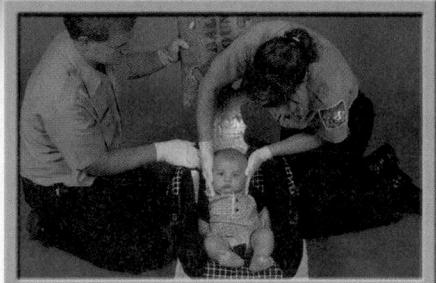

Step 1 Stabilize the infant's head in a neutral position.

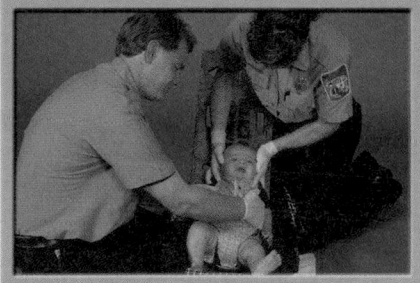

Step 2 Place an immobilization device between the infant and the surface on which he or she is resting.

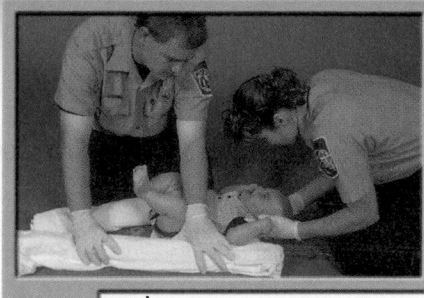

Step 3 Slide the infant onto the board.

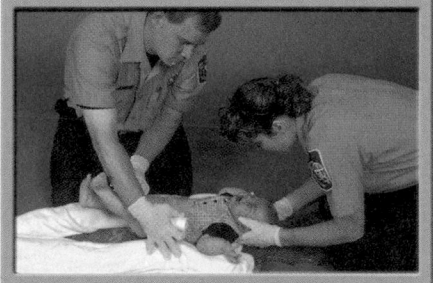

Step 4 Place a towel under the shoulders to ensure neutral head position.

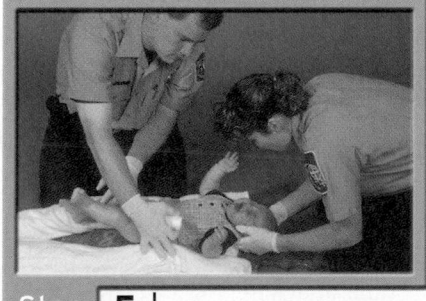

Step 5 Secure the torso first; pad any voids.

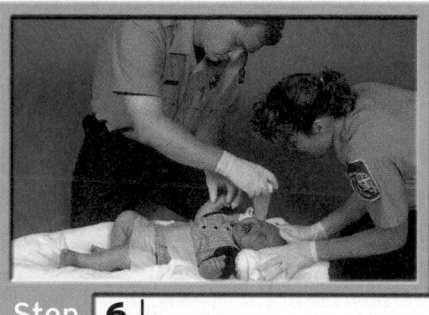

Step 6 Secure the head.

Table 28 SAMPLE History in Pediatric Trauma

Component	Explanation
Signs and symptoms	Time of event Nature of symptoms or pain Age-appropriate signs of distress
Allergies	Known drug reactions or other allergies
Medications	Timing and last dose of long-term medications Timing and dose of analgesics or antipyretics
Past medical history	Prior surgeries Immunizations, especially last tetanus
Last oral intake	Time of child's last food and drink, including bottle or breastfeeding
Events leading to the injury	Key events leading to the current incident MOI Hazards at the scene

Fluid Management

Circulatory compromise is less common in children than in adults as the result of trauma; therefore, airway management and ventilatory support take priority over management of circulation. Tachycardia is usually the first sign of circulatory compromise in a child, but tachycardia can also be caused by agitation, being scared, or being restrained. Children are able to compensate for blood loss from any cause, including trauma, so hypotension is a late finding in pediatric trauma. Once a pediatric patient is hypotensive, they are already in severe trouble. Recognizing circulatory compromise and treating early are even more important in the pediatric population. Consider the following when you are establishing vascular access in the injured child:

- Large-bore IV catheters should be inserted into a large peripheral vein whenever possible. In infants and young children, 20 or 22 gauge IV needles may be considered "large bore."
- Because definitive care can only be provided at the ED, never delay transport for the purpose of starting an IV line; this procedure should be performed en route.

- To maintain perfusion in a child, administer an initial bolus of 20 mL/kg using an isotonic crystalloid solution (ie, normal saline, lactated Ringer's).

  - Frequently reassess the child's vital signs and provide additional IV fluid boluses of 20 mL/kg if no improvement is noted following the initial bolus. Up to 60 mL/kg can be given for resuscitation of a pediatric patient. If the patient is over 50 kg, adult resuscitation fluid volumes should be used.

  - If the child's condition does not improve following two boluses of an isotonic crystalloid, blood loss is likely severe and the patient may need surgical intervention. Provide rapid transport with continuous monitoring of the child en route.

If the child is hypotensive and IV access cannot be obtained within 90 seconds, consider inserting an IO needle to gain access to the vascular system.

■ Pain Management

Pain is often undertreated in young children. Whether or not a child can communicate with you verbally, do not overlook signs of pain in pediatric trauma patients. Consider pain assessment as important as the vital signs, and use one of the many tools available to elicit the child's self-report of pain level. Tachycardia and inconsolability may be the only way a child has to express pain, and findings may be similar to those of early shock or plain old fear.

Pain treatment includes use of a calm, reassuring voice, distraction techniques, and, when appropriate, medications. Commonly used pain medications include morphine and fentanyl. Patients who are intubated should receive pain medication and sedation (such as diazepam and midazolam) if they are in hemodynamically stable condition. These medications, which may need to be redosed depending on transport time, can also be used in conjunction with narcotics for patients in stable condition. Side effects of narcotics and benzodiazepines include respiratory depression, hypoxemia, bradycardia, and hypotension.

You must weigh the risks and benefits when deciding to administer these medications. Children who are in shock and hemodynamically unstable condition are not good candidates for narcotics or sedatives; these medications may worsen their already precarious status. All children receiving such medications should be carefully monitored in terms of their pulse rate, respiratory rate, pulse oximetry, and blood pressure.

■ Pathophysiology, Assessment, and Management of Burns

The initial assessment and management of pediatric burn victims is similar to that of adults, with a few key differences. The larger skin surface–body mass ratio of children makes them more susceptible to heat and fluid loss. Worrisome patterns of injury or suspicious circumstances should also raise concerns of child abuse.

■ Assessment and Management of Burns

The assessment of scene safety is an important element in a burn call. Check for ongoing dangers such as fire, chemicals, or other hazardous materials. Your from-the-doorway assessment may identify signs of smoke inhalation, such as abnormal airway sounds and respiratory distress, or soot around the nose. Quickly move the patient and crew to a well-ventilated area.

An estimation of the percentage of BSA burned may affect your decision to start fluid resuscitation in the field and influence the transport destination. For adolescents, use the same rule of nines that you use for adult burn victims. For younger children, this rule of nines is modified to account for a child's disproportionately larger head size. For infants, the head and trunk each account for 18% of BSA, the arms each count as 9%, and the legs each count as 14%. The size of a child's palm (not including fingers) represents about 1% total BSA. You can also use this rule of palm to assess the extent of the burn **Figure 26**.

Burns suggestive of abuse include those in which the mechanism or pattern observed does not match the history or the child's developmental capabilities. For example, a child who cannot stand independently is unlikely to pull a hot cup of coffee off a table. Splash burns—as from tipping over a pot of boiling water—should have an irregular configuration because the hot liquid runs down the child's body. Be suspicious if a burn has clear demarcation lines or is on the buttocks.

Initial management begins with removal of burning clothing and support of the ABCs. If you observe signs of smoke inhalation, consider early intubation. Make sure that you have a range of tubes available because airway edema and sloughing may mandate use of a smaller tube than originally estimated.

All burn victims should be provided 100% supplemental oxygen, regardless of the presence or absence of signs of respiratory distress. Smoke inhalation may cause bronchospasm

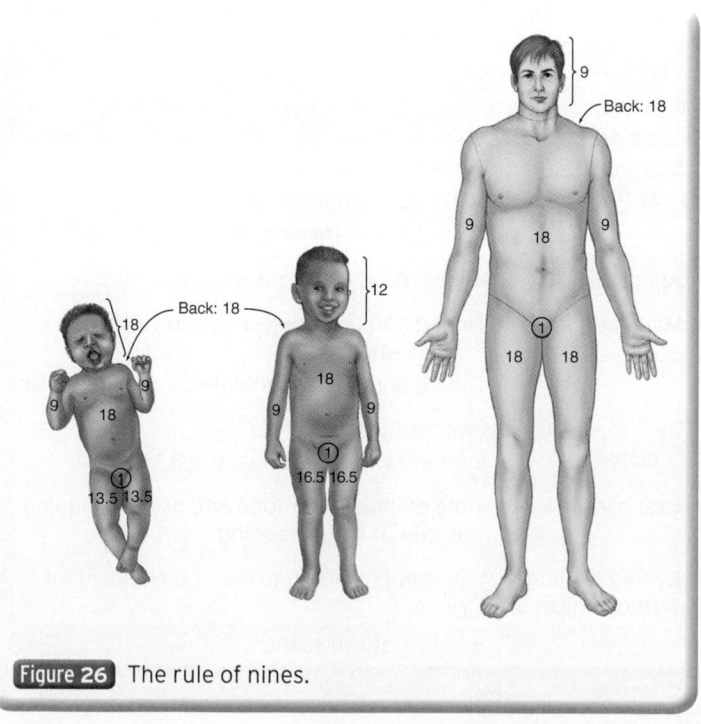

Figure 26 The rule of nines.

resulting in wheezing and mild respiratory distress. Consider using a bronchodilator such as albuterol or epinephrine IM.

If possible, insert an IV line and initiate fluid resuscitation in transport for patients with more than 5% of burned BSA. Start with 20 mL/kg of isotonic fluid, and reassess the need for additional boluses because large burns can lead to huge fluid shifts.

Clean burned areas minimally to avoid hypothermia, and cover them with clean, dry cloth. Avoid putting lotions or ointments on burned skin because they can trap heat and bacteria. Avoid heat loss by covering the burn and the patient as needed.

Analgesia is a critical part of the early management of burns; these injuries can be incredibly painful. Assess and treat pain and anxiety as discussed previously. Carefully monitor any child given narcotics or benzodiazepines for signs of respiratory or hemodynamic compromise.

Once the patient's condition is stabilized, begin transport to an appropriate medical facility. Larger burns, full-thickness burns, and burns involving the face and neck are best treated at a regional burn center.

Special Populations

Use the rule of palm to estimate the percentage of body surface area burned in a young child or infant: A child's palm is equal to 1% of body surface area.

Children With Special Health Care Needs

Children with special health care needs include those with physical, developmental, and learning disabilities. The disabilities have a broad range of causes, including premature birth, traumatic brain injury, congenital anatomic anomalies, and acquired illnesses. Advances in technology and drugs have enabled an increasing number of children with disabilities to receive care in the community, leading to a corresponding increase in the number of EMS calls for this medically complex population.

Technology-Assisted Children

Technology-assisted children constitute a subset of children with special health care needs that may require your assistance. It is important to familiarize yourself with the various types of medical technology that you may encounter and have to troubleshoot.

Tracheostomy Tubes and Artificial Ventilators

Tracheostomy is a surgical procedure, involving creation of a stoma—in this case, a permanent connection between the skin of the throat and trachea—through which a tracheostomy tube can be placed for long-term ventilatory needs Figure 27. A child might need a tracheostomy for a variety of reasons, including long-term ventilator support for chronic lung disease, inability to protect the airway because of neurologic impairment, or a congenital airway anomaly leading to airway obstruction. Caregivers have been trained in the use and care of their child's

tracheostomy and are a source of valuable information. In general, they will have a spare tracheostomy tube available.

A child with a tracheostomy tube may breathe spontaneously with room air, if the function of the tube is simply to bypass mechanical upper airway obstruction. Alternatively, the child may be dependent on a home ventilator and supplemental oxygen if he or she has severe lung disease or problems with respiratory drive.

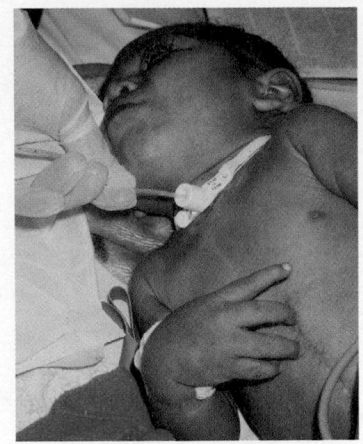

Figure 27 A tracheostomy is a surgical opening in the neck into the trachea, creating an artificial airway.

Although a tracheostomy tube is intended to provide a secure, permanent airway, problems can arise, as with any mechanical device. The most common problem is obstruction of the tracheostomy tube with secretions, resulting in respiratory distress or respiratory failure. Displacement of the tube is another potential problem. If you are faced with a child with a tracheostomy tube and respiratory distress, start by assessing tube position and suctioning the tube. If the child is using a home ventilator, disconnect the circuit and provide bag-mask ventilation. If these measures fail to lead to improvement or if the child is cyanotic or in severe distress, you may need to remove and replace the tracheostomy tube, preferably using a tube of the same diameter and length. Confirmation of tube position is done in the same manner as for an ET tube. See the chapter, *Airway Management and Ventilation* for more information on tracheostomy tubes.

Gastrostomy Tubes

Gastrostomy tubes (G-tubes) are surgically placed directly into the patient's stomach through the skin Figure 28. They provide nutrition or medications directly into the stomach, bypassing the oropharynx and esophagus. Some children are unable to take food or medication by mouth and depend on a G-tube for all of their nutrition; for other patients, the tube is used to supplement intake and ensure adequate nutrition.

Problems such as obstruction, dislodgment, or leakage of a G-tube are not uncommon but rarely represent an emergency. Most of these calls can be managed by supportive care and transport. Urgent physician evaluation is needed if a G-tube has been pulled out because the opening on the abdominal wall tends to constrict quickly, making replacement difficult.

Central Venous Catheters

A central venous catheter may be inserted when a child needs long-term IV access for medications or nutrition. Such a device is placed surgically or by interventional radiologists into large central veins, such as the subclavian. Completely implanted central lines, with a port or reservoir accessible under the skin, may be left in place for months to years. For example, they are

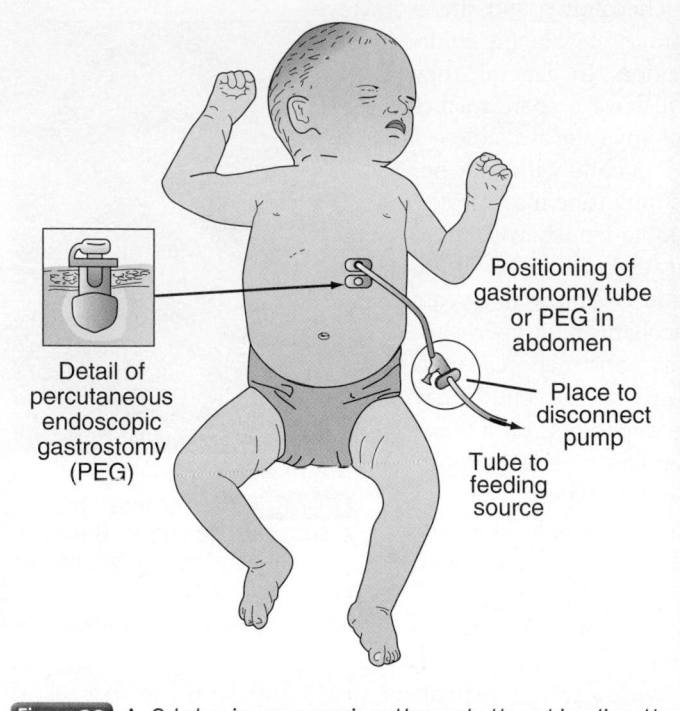

Figure 28 A G-tube is an opening through the skin directly into the stomach.

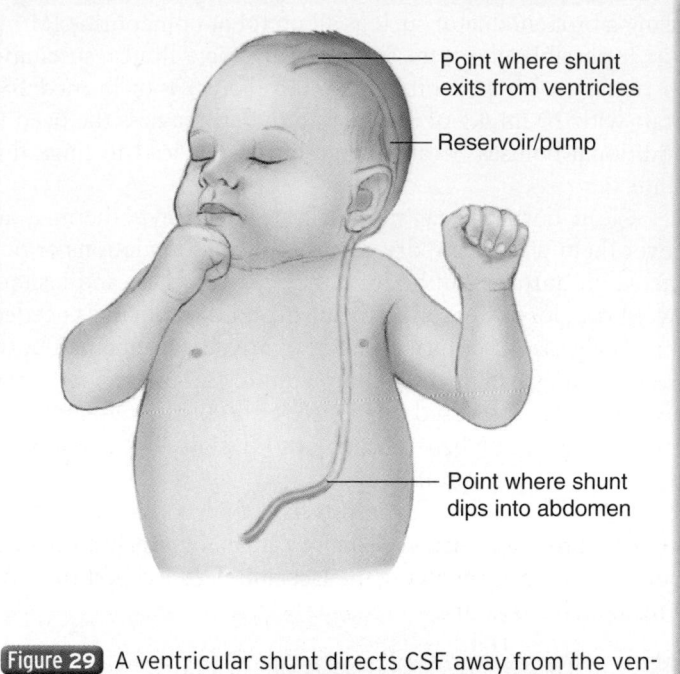

Figure 29 A ventricular shunt directs CSF away from the ventricles in the brain to the abdomen to relieve pressure.

commonly placed in children with cancer who are undergoing long courses of chemotherapy. Partially implanted central lines have tubing external to the skin.

Complications associated with central venous catheters include infections, obstruction, and dislodged or broken catheters. Children with an infection of the central line may have redness, swelling, tenderness, or pus at the skin site of insertion; they may also have systemic signs of infection (such as fever) or signs of septic shock. Central line obstruction may be a medical emergency, depending on what is infusing through the line. If the child is not in urgent need of the infusion, simply assess the child and provide transport to the ED. Dislodged or broken catheters may result in leakage of fluid or blood. In such a case, use sterile technique to clamp off the broken line to minimize risk of infection or air embolus.

On rare occasions, you will be confronted with a child who has a functioning central line but requires emergency IV access for field treatment. Because these permanent lines carry a high risk for infection, look for peripheral access and avoid using the central line whenever possible.

Ventricular Shunts

Ventricular shunts are inserted to drain excessive fluid from the brain, thereby normalizing ICP **Figure 29**. A neurosurgeon places the tube and connects it to a one-way, pressure-sensitive valve that runs from the enlarged ventricle subcutaneously into the abdominal peritoneal space. When pressure builds up in the ventricle, the one-way valve opens, and CSF drains into the peritoneum, where it is reabsorbed.

A ventricular shunt obstruction occurs when the drainage of fluid from the brain through the shunt tubing becomes blocked—perhaps due to a break in the tubing, problems with

the valve, or buildup of debris in the tubing. Without adequate fluid drainage, the CSF fluid continues to accumulate, resulting in hydrocephalus. A child with a shunt obstruction will show signs of increased ICP, which may range from subtle changes in behavior to impending brain herniation. Typical symptoms include headache, fatigue, vomiting, and even coma.

A ventricular shunt infection results from bacterial contamination during the surgery to place the shunt or from bacteria in the blood adhering to and infecting the hardware. Infections are encountered most frequently within months of shunt surgery. Children with shunt infections are generally extremely sick and have fever and signs of shunt obstruction.

Shunt obstructions and shunt infections are true medical emergencies. The patient should be transported to appropriate treatment facilities where neurosurgical evaluation is available. The child's condition can deteriorate rapidly, so maintain continuous cardiopulmonary monitoring during transport. Shunt obstruction may be recognized by signs and symptoms of increased ICP, including Cushing triad (hypertension, bradycardia, and widened pulse pressure or irregular respirations).

Assessment and Management of Children With Special Health Care Needs

Follow the standard pediatric assessment sequence when you are approaching children with special health care needs. Ask questions of the parent or caregiver to establish the child's baseline level of neurologic function and baseline physiologic status. Meet every child at his or her unique developmental level. An otherwise healthy 10-year-old child with a perinatal brain injury may have the developmental skills of a toddler. Conversely, a 6-year-old child with severe cardiopulmonary compromise may be ventilator-dependent and have an oxygen saturation level in the 80s but be cognitively intact.

Your treatment goal is to restore a child to his or her own physiologic baseline, which will require collaboration with caregivers to determine what is normal for the child and management strategies that have been successful in the past.

Special Populations

> Caregivers will be key resources when you are managing a child with special health care needs. Draw on their expertise to assist you in assessing and managing the child.

Transport of Children With Special Health Care Needs

Most children with special health care needs will have a medical home—that is, a hospital, clinic, or private practice where they receive their care. Transporting the child to a facility where the clinical team is familiar with the patient's history and needs will streamline their care. If this is not possible, take along any medical records available to assist the team at the receiving facility to sort out the potentially complex issues faced by the patient. Take any assistive devices as well, including home ventilators and feeding pumps. Most important, take the parent or caregiver of the child! Children with special health care needs rely on their caregivers for much—if not all—of their caretaking needs, so it can be emotionally difficult for the child to be separated from the caretaker.

An Ounce of Prevention

Emergency care for children involves a team approach by health care professionals in the community and in the ED. Paramedics are a critical part of the community responsible for caring for sick and injured children, but their role in prevention is not always highlighted, even though this is an area in which they can have a greater public health impact than possible by running a code or controlling an airway. To be an effective child safety advocate, you must be knowledgeable about local and national prevention programs, such as those conducted through the Emergency Medical Services for Children (EMSC) initiative.

Emergency Medical Services for Children

EMSC is a federally funded program that was created more than 25 years ago in an effort to reduce child disability and death due to severe illness and injury. EMSC works with local communities and hospitals to improve care for children in and out of the ED. It also works with existing EMS systems to improve the quality of children's emergency care, such as by creating pediatric-specific protocols and procedures. For example, EMSC has helped provide ambulances and EDs with child-appropriate equipment. The program also supports training EMTs, paramedics, and other emergency care providers in pediatric-specific emergency care.

Prevention of Injuries

Most injuries are not accidents, but rather are predictable and preventable events. When injury patterns are tracked and tabulated, this knowledge helps emergency care providers target potential areas for intervention and prevention. For example, childhood poisonings can be prevented by effective storage of medications and chemicals. Toddler drowning and submersion can be virtually eliminated by installation of four-sided pool fencing. The risk of serious injury from a bike crash is lessened by use of a helmet. The morbidity and mortality from motor vehicle crashes is dramatically decreased by the appropriate use of child restraint devices.

As you care for children, you may be frustrated by the illnesses and injuries that you encounter, especially when they are preventable. Take this frustration as a call to action. Get involved in your community. Participate in existing prevention programs or start your own program. Numerous types of pediatric injury can be targeted Table 29 ; choose something that interests you, and take a leadership role.

Table 29 Examples of Common Injuries and Possible Prevention Strategies

Injury	Preventive Measures
Vehicle trauma	Infant and child restraint seats Seat belts and air bags Pedestrian safety programs Motorcycle helmets
Cycling	Bicycle helmets Bicycle paths separate from vehicle traffic
Recreation	Appropriate safety padding and apparel Cyclist, skateboard, and skater safety programs Soft, energy-absorbent playground surfaces
Drowning and submersion	Four-sided locked pool enclosures Pool alarms Immediate adult supervision Caretaker CPR training Swimming lessons Pool and beach safety instruction Personal flotation devices
Poisoning and household injuries	Proper storage of chemicals and medications Child safety packaging
Burns	Proper maintenance and monitoring of electrical appliances and cords Fire and smoke detectors Proper placement of cookware on stove top
Other	Discouragement of infant walker use Gated stairways Babysitter first-aid training Child care worker first-aid training

YOU *are the Medic* | SUMMARY |

1. Using the Pediatric Assessment Triangle as a guide, what is your general impression of the child?

By using the Pediatric Assessment Triangle, you should be able to determine that the child is sick and requires immediate attention. Further application will help you figure out what may be wrong with him. His initial appearance is abnormal. His work of breathing is normal because he has an adequate respiratory rate and tidal volume and there are no retractions or audible sounds. Circulation is definitely abnormal with pale skin and some mottling seen on the extremities. The combination of an abnormal appearance, normal respiratory status, and abnormal circulation should guide you toward looking for a circulatory problem.

2. What information would you like to get from the sister?

It is important to get as much information as possible to help you figure out what the problem might be and the best approach for treatment. Information that could provide you with clues would be how long the child has been sick, what he has been complaining of, the last time he ate or drank, if he has been urinating regularly, and the last time he was awake and talking with his sister.

3. What is the significance of the child's blood pressure?

The child's blood pressure is extremely low. The minimal acceptable systolic blood pressure for a 3-year-old child is 86 mm Hg – 80 + (2 × age in years). This blood pressure should be grabbing your attention; you need to take action before the child deteriorates further!

4. What should your treatment consist of at this point?

You have the child on high-flow oxygen and identified the cardiac rhythm as sinus tachycardia. Because the child is in decompensated shock, the focus of your treatment should be fluid replacement and checking the glucose level to prevent missing hypoglycemia. Insertion of an IO needle is the ideal way to gain vascular access due to the child's poor hemodynamic status.

5. What are the potential complications of IO needle insertion?

Caution should be taken when you are inserting the intraosseous needle to help minimize the chance for complications. Several complications such as compartment syndrome, failed infusion, injury to the growth plate, infection, and fracture have all occurred as a result of IO needle insertion.

6. How should you manage the blood glucose level?

This child is hypoglycemic! Glucose should be administered at a dose of 0.5 g/kg to bring the glucose level back to a normal level. Depending on the concentration you have available, you can give 5 mL/kg of D_{10} solution, 2 mL/kg of D_{25} solution, or 1 mL/kg of D_{50} solution. Always remember to recheck a blood glucose level after you have administered IV glucose to ensure the child is not hyperglycemic.

7. What do you think was the cause for shock in this patient?

Hypovolemia and dehydration secondary to prolonged vomiting and diarrhea were the conditions that caused the development of shock in this child.

8. What additional treatment should be performed en route to the hospital?

Now that the child is beginning to respond to treatment and improve, it is your job to keep him warm and perform frequent reassessments. Remember that children lose body heat quickly, so you need to keep the child warm.

YOU are the Medic   SUMMARY, continued

EMS Patient Care Report (PCR)

Date: 07-06-11	Incident No.: 05839	Nature of Call: Altered mental status		Location: 3920 E. 152 Ave.	
Dispatched: 1325	En Route: 1327	At Scene: 1333	Transport: 1350	At Hospital: 1359	In Service: 1431

Patient Information

Age: 3 Y Sex: M Weight (in kg [lb]): 14 kg (30 lb)	Allergies: None known Medications: None known Past Medical History: None known Chief Complaint: Altered mental status

Vital Signs

Time: 1338	BP: 68/42	Pulse: 180	Respirations: 22	Spo$_2$: 99%
Time: 1342	BP: 74/50	Pulse: 180	Respirations: 22	Spo$_2$: 98%
Time: 1348	BP: 80/54	Pulse: 160	Respirations: 20	Spo$_2$: 98%
Time: 1353	BP: 80/54	Pulse: 160	Respirations: 20	Spo$_2$: 98%

EMS Treatment
(circle all that apply)

Oxygen @ __12__ L/min via (circle one): NC (NRM) Bag-mask device	Assisted Ventilation	Airway Adjunct:	CPR
Defibrillation	Bleeding Control	Bandaging	Splinting	Other: IO insertion

Narrative

Dispatched to an apartment for a 3-year-old boy with altered mental status. Upon arrival met at door by 14-year-old sister, who is the only other person on-scene. Brought to living room where the child is observed lying on the couch appearing to be asleep. Pt is unresponsive to painful stimuli. Skin is noted to be pale, cool, and dry, with some mottling of the extremities. Unable to palpate radial pulse. Carotid pulse is weak. Capillary refill is 5 seconds. Pt placed on O$_2$ at 12 LPM via nonrebreathing mask. Cardiac monitor applied showing a narrow complex tachycardia. Lung sounds are clear and equal. Unable to locate peripheral vein for IV access. IO inserted into left tibia. Placement confirmation; Needle stands upright on its own, small amount marrow aspirated, fluids flowing easily, and no signs of infiltration. 1,000 mL bag of normal saline hung and initial fluid bolus of 280 mL ran. Blood glucose 28 mg/dL. Administered 28 mL of D$_{25}$. Reassessment prior to transport shows improving mental status and circulation. Child is waking up as we leave. En route pt becomes fully awake and alert and radial pulses are able to be palpated. Contacted Northwest Regional Medical Center who advised to continue fluid administration. Pt remained stable during transport. Arrived at the ED and care was transferred to Jocelyn RN. Rescue 20 available for transport at 1431. **End of report**

Prep Kit

- Children differ anatomically, physiologically, and emotionally from adults.

- Sick or injured children present unique challenges in evaluation and management. Their perceptions of their illness or injury, of their world, and of paramedics differ from the perceptions of adults.

- The majority of children you treat will come with at least one parent or caregiver. Thus, in many pediatric calls, you will be dealing with more than one patient—even if only the child is ill or injured.

- Serious illness or injury to a child is one of the most stressful situations caregivers can face.

- An assessment tool called the Pediatric Assessment Triangle (PAT) has been developed to help EMS providers form a from-the-doorway general impression of pediatric patients.

- Respiratory problems are among the medical emergencies that you will most frequently encounter in children. Pediatric patients with a respiratory chief complaint will span the spectrum from mildly ill to near death.

- In pediatrics, respiratory failure and arrest precede the majority of cardiopulmonary arrests.

- The types of shock that you may encounter are the same in adults and children. Because children typically have strong cardiovascular systems, they are able to compensate for inadequate perfusion more efficiently than adults.

- Cardiovascular emergencies are relatively rare in children. When such problems arise, they are often related to volume or infection rather than to a primary cardiac cause, unless the child has congenital heart disease.

- Through the PAT and primary assessment, you can quickly identify a cardiovascular emergency, understand the likely pathologic cause, and institute potentially lifesaving treatment.

- Children are particularly difficult to assess neurologically because they can often be uncooperative during the assessment.

- The ingestion of foreign bodies is a common cause of gastrointestinal complaints in pediatrics.

- Children and young adults are much more commonly diagnosed with type 1 diabetes; therefore, they are susceptible to diabetic ketoacidosis (DKA), a life-threatening event.

- Hematologic and immunologic diseases are common in pediatric patients, and because of the altered immunity of many of these children, often result in severe presentations of illness and even shock.

- Toxic exposures account for a significant number of pediatric emergencies. Toxic exposures can take the form of ingestion, inhalation, injection, or application of a substance.

- Behavioral and psychiatric problems relating to pediatric patients may range from out-of-control behavior to a suicide attempt.

- Most pediatric fevers are caused by viral infections that are often mild and self-limiting. In other cases, fever is a symptom of a more serious bacterial infection.

- Child abuse or maltreatment comes in many forms: physical abuse, sexual abuse, emotional abuse, and child neglect.

- The sudden death of an apparently healthy baby is devastating to families and the EMS crew that responds to the call.

- An apparent life-threatening event (ALTE) is an episode during which an infant becomes pale or cyanotic; chokes, gags, or has an apneic spell; or loses muscle tone.

- Pediatric trauma is the leading cause of death among children older than 1 year.
  - Motor vehicle crashes cause the most deaths in this age group, followed by falls and submersions.
  - Among adolescents, homicide and suicide are major causes of death.

- The initial assessment and management of pediatric burn victims is similar to that of adults, with a few key differences.
  - The larger skin surface–body mass ratio of children makes them more susceptible to heat and fluid loss.
  - Worrisome patterns of injury or suspicious circumstances should raise concerns of child abuse.

- Children with special health care needs include children with physical, developmental, and learning disabilities.
  - These disabilities have a broad range of causes, including premature birth, traumatic brain injury, congenital anatomic anomalies, and acquired illnesses.
  - Advances in technology and drugs have enabled an increasing number of children with disabilities to receive care in the community, leading to a corresponding increase in the number of EMS calls for this medically complex population.

- Emergency care for children involves a team approach by health care professionals in the community and in the hospital.

Vital Vocabulary

absence seizures The type of seizures characterized by a brief lapse of attention in which the patient may stare and not respond; formerly known as petit mal seizures.

acrocyanosis Cyanosis of the extremities.

apparent life-threatening event (ALTE) An unexpected sudden episode of color change, tone change, or apnea that requires mouth-to-mouth resuscitation or vigorous stimulation.

bacterial tracheitis An invasive exudative bacterial infection of the soft tissues of the trachea.

blow-by technique A method of delivering oxygen by holding a face mask or similar device near an infant's or a child's face; used when a nonrebreathing mask is not tolerated.

bronchiolitis A condition seen in children younger than 2 years, characterized by dyspnea and wheezing.

bronchopulmonary dysplasia A spectrum of lung conditions found in premature neonates who require long periods of high-concentration oxygen and ventilator support, ranging from mild reactive airways to debilitating chronic lung disease.

central venous catheter A catheter inserted into the vena cava to permit intermittent or continuous monitoring of central venous pressure and to facilitate obtaining blood samples for chemical analysis.

child abuse Any improper or excessive action that injures or otherwise harms a child or infant; it includes physical abuse, sexual abuse, neglect, and emotional abuse.

child protective services (CPS) An agency that is the community legal organization responsible for protection, rehabilitation, and prevention of child maltreatment and neglect; it has the legal authority to temporarily remove children from homes if there is reason to believe they are at risk for injury or neglect and to secure foster placement.

complex febrile seizures An unusual form of seizure that occurs in association with a rapid increase in body temperature.

complex partial seizures Seizures characterized by alteration of consciousness with or without complex focal motor activity.

congenital adrenal hyperplasia (CAH) Inadequate production of cortisol and aldosterone by the adrenal gland.

congenital heart disease Abnormalities of the heart during development, many of which lead to cyanosis.

croup A common disease of childhood due to upper airway obstruction and characterized by stridor, hoarseness, and a barking cough.

cystic fibrosis (CF) A genetic disease that primarily affects the respiratory and digestive systems.

dilated cardiomyopathy (DCM) A condition in which the heart becomes weakened and enlarged, making it less efficient and causing a negative impact to the pulmonary, hepatic, and other systems.

epiglottitis Inflammation of the epiglottis.

gastrostomy tube (G-tube) A tube that is surgically placed directly into the patient's stomach through the skin in order to provide nutrition or medications.

generalized seizures The seizures characterized by manifestations that indicate involvement of both cerebral hemispheres.

grunting A short, low-pitched sound at the end of exhalation, present in children with moderate to severe hypoxia; reflects poor gas exchange because of fluid in the lower airways and air sacs.

hemophilia A bleeding disorder that is primarily hereditary, in which clotting does not occur or occurs insufficiently.

hydrocephalus The increased accumulation of cerebrospinal fluid within the ventricles of the brain.

hypertrophic cardiomyopathy (HCM) A condition in which the heart muscle is unusually thick, which means that the heart has to pump harder to get blood to leave.

hypopituitarism A condition in which the pituitary gland does not produce normal amounts of some or all of its hormones, can be congenital; secondary to tumors, infection, strokes, or develop after trauma or radiation therapy.

inborn errors of metabolism (IEM) A group of congenital conditions that cause either accumulation of toxins or disorders of energy metabolism in the neonate. These conditions are characterized by an infant's failure to thrive and by vague signs such as poor feeding.

intussusception Telescoping of the intestines into themselves.

malrotation with volvulus A condition that occurs when there is a twisting of the bowel around its mesenteric attachment to the abdominal wall.

Meckel diverticulum One of the most common congenital malformations of the small intestines, which presents with painless rectal bleeding.

meningitis Inflammation of the meningeal coverings of the brain and spinal cord; usually caused by a virus or bacterium; the viral type is less severe than the bacterial; the bacterial type can result in brain damage, hearing loss, learning disability, or death.

mottling A condition of abnormal skin circulation, caused by vasoconstriction or inadequate perfusoin.

myocarditis Inflammation of the myocardium.

nuchal rigidity A stiff or painful neck; commonly associated with meningitis.

obtunded A condition when the patient is dulled to pain and sensation.

ossification centers Areas where cartilage is transformed through calcification into a new area of bone.

panhypopituitarism The inadequate production or absence of the pituitary hormones, including adrenocorticotropic hormone (ACTH), cortisol, thyroxine, luteinizing hormone (LH), follicle-stimulating hormone (FSH), estrogen, testosterone, growth hormone, and antidiuretic hormone (ADH).

partial seizures Seizures that involve only one part of the brain

Pediatric Assessment Triangle (PAT) An assessment tool that allows rapid formation of a general impression of the type and level of illness or injury in an infant or child without touching him or her; consists of assessing appearance, work of breathing, and circulation to the skin.

pertussis An acute infectious disease characterized by catarrhal stage, followed by a paroxysmal cough that ends in a whooping inspiration; also called whooping cough.

petechial Characterized by small purplish, nonblanching spots on the skin.

pneumonia An inflammation of the lungs caused by bacterial, viral, or fungal infections or infections with other microorganisms.

purpuric Pertaining to bruising of the skin.

pyloric stenosis Hypertrophy (enlargement) of the pyloric sphincter of the stomach; ultimately leads to intestinal obstruction, often in infants.

respiratory arrest The absence of respirations with detectable cardiac activity.

respiratory distress A clinical state characterized by increased respiratory rate, effort, and work of breathing.

respiratory failure A clinical state of inadequate oxygenation, ventilation, or both.

respiratory syncytial virus (RSV) A virus that affects the upper and lower respiratory tracts, but disease, namely pneumonia and bronchiolitis, is more prevalent in the lower respiratory tract.

retractions Skin pulling between and around the ribs and clavicles during inhalation; a sign of respiratory distress.

sepsis A pathologic state, usually in a febrile patient, resulting from the presence of invading microorganisms or their poisonous products in the bloodstream.

sickle cell disease (SCD) A disease that causes red blood cells to be misshapen, resulting in a poor oxygen-carrying capability and potentially resulting in lodging of the red blood cells in blood vessels or the spleen.

simple febrile seizures A brief, self-limited, generalized seizure in a previously healthy child between ages 6 months and 6 years that is associated with the onset of or sudden increase in fever.

simple partial seizures Focal seizures that involve a motor or sensory abnormality in a patient who remains conscious.

sniffing position An upright position in which the patient's head and chin are thrust slightly forward to keep the airway open; appears to be sniffing.

status epilepticus A condition in which seizures recur every few minutes, or in which seizure activity lasts more than 30 minutes.

stoma In the context of the airway, the resultant orifice of a tracheostomy that connects the trachea to the outside air; located in the midline of the anterior part of the neck.

subglottic space The narrowest part of the pediatric airway.

sudden infant death syndrome (SIDS) The abrupt and unexplained death of an apparently healthy child younger than 1 year.

synchronized cardioversion The use of synchronized direct current (DC) electric shock to convert tachydysrhythmias (such as atrial fibrillation) to normal sinus rhythm.

tenting A condition in which the skin slowly retracts after being pinched and pulled away slightly from the body; a sign of dehydration.

thrombocytopenia A reduction in the number of platelets in the blood.

thrombosis The development of a blood clot.

tonic-clonic seizures Seizures that feature rhythmic back-and-forth motion of an extremity and body stiffness.

tripoding An abnormal position to keep the airway open; involves leaning forward onto two arms stretched forward.

vasoconstriction Narrowing of the diameter of the blood vessels.

ventilation-perfusion mismatch A pathologic state in which there is an imperfect match between the areas of the lung being ventilated and the areas being perfused.

ventricular shunt A surgically inserted tube draining cerebrospinal fluid from the cerebral ventricles into a body cavity, often the peritoneal cavity or the right atrium.

von Willebrand disease The most common heritable disorder of coagulation. Its presentation can mimic hemophilia A.

Assessment in Action

You and your partner are dispatched to an elementary school for a 7-year-old child experiencing a seizure. On arrival you are met by the school principal who escorts you to the playground. As you enter the area you observe a young girl next to the swings exhibiting tonic-clonic movement. A teacher approaches and tells you that the girl was playing tag with her friends when she stated that she "felt funny" and collapsed. According to the teacher the girl has a history of seizures and has been actively seizing for approximately 15 minutes.

1. Which of the following types of seizures is your patient most likely having?
   A. Absence
   B. Febrile
   C. Grand mal
   D. Simple partial

2. What type of seizure is unique to children?
   A. Grand mal
   B. Complex partial
   C. Simple partial
   D. Febrile

3. How should you manage the airway of a child who is actively seizing?
   A. Endotracheal intubation
   B. Head tilt-chin lift or jaw-thrust
   C. Oropharyngeal airway
   D. LMA

4. Which of the following medications may be used as first-line anticonvulsant therapy?
   A. Diazepam
   B. Morphine
   C. Phenobarbital
   D. Phenytoin

5. What is a major side effect associated with the administration of benzodiazepines?
   A. Hypertension
   B. Tachycardia
   C. Respiratory depression
   D. Vomiting

6. Which benzodiazepine can be administered intranasally?
   A. Midazolam
   B. Diazepam
   C. Lorazepam
   D. Alprazolam

Additional Question

7. When can you use the mnemonic DOPE?

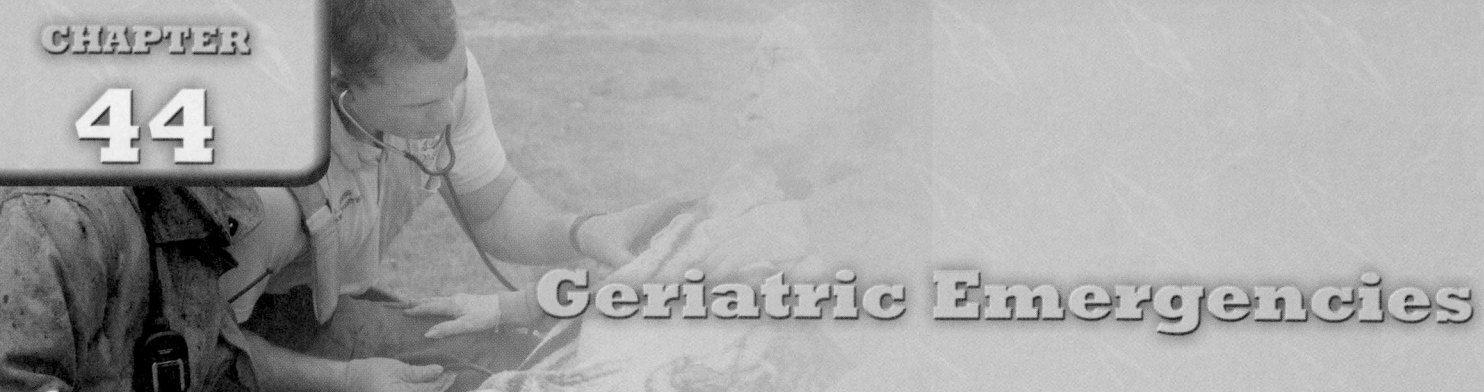

Geriatric Emergencies

National EMS Education Standard Competencies

Special Patient Populations

Integrates assessment findings with principles of pathophysiology and knowledge of psychosocial needs to formulate a field impression and implement a comprehensive treatment/disposition plan for patients with special needs.

Geriatrics

Impact of age-related changes on assessment and care (pp 2088-2092)

Changes associated with aging, psychosocial aspects of aging, and age-related assessment and treatment modifications for the major or common geriatric diseases and/or emergencies

- Cardiovascular diseases (pp 2082-2083)
- Respiratory diseases (p 2082)
- Neurologic diseases (pp 2083-2084)
- Endocrine diseases (p 2085)
- Alzheimer disease (pp 2097-2098)
- Dementia (p 2097)
- Fluid resuscitation in the elderly (pp 2085, 2103)

Normal and abnormal changes associated with aging, pharmacokinetic changes, psychosocial and economic aspects of aging, polypharmacy, and age-related assessment and treatment modifications for the major or common geriatric diseases and/or emergencies

- Cardiovascular diseases (pp 2093-2096)
- Respiratory diseases (pp 2092-2093)
- Neurologic diseases (pp 2096-2098)
- Endocrine diseases (pp 2102-2103)
- Alzheimer disease (pp 2097-2098)
- Dementia (p 2097)
  - Acute confusional state (pp 2096-2097)
- Fluid resuscitation in the elderly (pp 2085, 2103)
- Herpes zoster (p 2107)
- Inflammatory arthritis (p 2108)

Patients With Special Challenges

- Recognizing and reporting abuse and neglect (pp 2112-2113 and see chapter, *Pediatric Emergencies*)

Health care implications of

- Abuse (pp 2112-2113 and see chapter, *Pediatric Emergencies*)
- Neglect (pp 2112-2113 and see chapter, *Pediatric Emergencies*)
- Homelessness (see chapter, *Patients With Special Challenges*)
- Poverty (see chapter, *Patients With Special Challenges*)
- Bariatrics (see chapter, *Patients With Special Challenges*)
- Technology dependent (see chapter, *Patients With Special Challenges*)
- Hospice/terminally ill (see chapter, *Patients With Special Challenges*)
- Tracheostomy care/dysfunction (see chapter, *Patients With Special Challenges*)
- Home care (see chapter, *Patients With Special Challenges*)
- Sensory deficit/loss (see chapter, *Patients With Special Challenges*)
- Developmental disability (see chapter, *Patients With Special Challenges*)

Trauma

Integrates assessment findings with principles of epidemiology and pathophysiology to formulate a field impression to implement a comprehensive treatment/disposition plan for an acutely injured patient.

Special Considerations in Trauma

Recognition and management of trauma in

- Pregnant patient (see chapter, *Obstetrics*)
- Pediatric patient (see chapter, *Pediatric Emergencies*)
- Geriatric patient (pp 2108, 2110-2112)

Pathophysiology, assessment, and management of trauma in the

- Pregnant patient (see chapter, *Obstetrics*)
- Pediatric patient (see chapter, *Pediatric Emergencies*)
- Geriatric patient (pp 2108, 2110-2112)
- Cognitively impaired patient (see chapter, *Patients With Special Challenges*)

Knowledge Objectives

1. Describe the old-age dependency ratio. (p 2080)
2. Describe the phenomenon "the greying of America." (p 2080)
3. Discuss the social, economic, and psychosocial factors affecting the older population. (pp 2080-2081)
4. Discuss the physiologic changes that occur in the various body systems as people age. (pp 2081-2086)
5. Describe the steps in the primary assessment for providing emergency care to a geriatric patient, including the elements of the GEMS diamond. (pp 2088-2089)
6. Discuss special considerations when performing the patient assessment process on a geriatric patient. (pp 2087-2088)
7. Describe the pathophysiology of geriatric respiratory conditions, the signs and symptoms, and the emergency medical care strategies used in the management of each condition. (pp 2092-2093)
8. Describe the pathophysiology of geriatric cardiovascular conditions, the signs and symptoms, and the emergency medical care strategies used in the management of each condition. (pp 2093-2096)
9. Describe the pathophysiology of geriatric nervous system conditions, the signs and symptoms, and the emergency medical care strategies used in the management of each condition. (pp 2096-2098)
10. Describe the pathophysiology of geriatric gastrointestinal conditions, the signs and symptoms, and the emergency medical care strategies used in the management of each condition. (pp 2098-2100)
11. Describe the pathophysiology of geriatric renal conditions, the signs and symptoms, and the emergency medical care strategies used in the management of each condition. (pp 2100-2102)
12. Describe the pathophysiology of geriatric endocrine conditions, the signs and symptoms, and the emergency medical care strategies used in the management of each condition. (pp 2102-2103)
13. Describe the pathophysiology of sepsis, the signs and symptoms, and the emergency medical care strategies used in the management of sepsis. (p 2103)
14. Describe the pathophysiology of geriatric toxicology, the signs and symptoms, and the emergency medical care strategies used in the management of adverse drug reactions. (p 2104)
15. Discuss polypharmacy and medication non-compliance and their effects on patient assessment and management. (p 2104)
16. Describe the pathophysiology of geriatric depression, the signs and symptoms, and the emergency medical care strategies used in the management of depression. (p 2106)
17. Describe the pathophysiology of geriatric integumentary conditions, the signs and symptoms, and the emergency medical care strategies used in the management of each condition. (p 2107)
18. Describe the pathophysiology of geriatric musculoskeletal conditions, the signs and symptoms, and the emergency medical care strategies used in the management of each condition. (pp 2107-2108)
19. Describe special considerations for a geriatric patient who has experienced trauma, including performing the patient assessment process on a geriatric patient with a traumatic injury. (pp 2108, 2110-2112)
20. Discuss elder abuse and neglect, and its implications in assessment and management of the patient. (pp 2112-2113)

Skills Objectives

There are no skills objectives for this chapter.

■ Introduction

Geriatrics is the assessment and treatment of disease in someone 65 years or older. According to the 2010 census, there are 40,267,984 Americans who are age 65 and older. This is a 15.1% increase from the 2000 census. Whereas the elderly population represents 15% of emergency department (ED) visits, they are four times more likely to use EMS for transportation to the ED.

Elderly people constitute an ever-increasing proportion of patients in the health care system, particularly the emergency care sector. People who are 65 years and older account for 36% of all hospital stays in the United States. People are receiving more of their care out of hospitals, and because of efforts by insurance companies and public health assistance programs to reduce costs, along with potential changes from health care legislation, this trend will most likely continue in the future. This population also has more contacts with doctors than people younger than 65 years. As a result, as the number of older Americans increases, the need for physician services will also likely increase because 80% of seniors have at least one chronic medical condition and 50% of this population have two or more.

The old-age dependency ratio is used to determine the number of older people in a society as compared with the number of potential workers who are theoretically capable of providing resources to sustain the whole population. The old-age dependency ratio is the number of older people (65 years and older) for every 100 adults (potential caregivers) between the ages 18 and 64 years. It is used by social scientists and researchers to compare the differences in age structure between time periods in a single society or to compare age structures between two different societies. It can be used as an indicator of the aging of a population, as a whole.

Many social scientists refer to a phenomenon as "the greying of America," which is a term used to describe the increasing number of older Americans. In 1990, there were 20 older people for every 100 working-age persons. By 2025, it is projected that there will be 32 older people for every 100 working-age "caregivers." In other words, the supply of people capable of providing resources for the older population is not keeping pace

with the growth of the older population. The need for caregivers is going to increase, and society may have difficulty keeping up with the demand for services as the population continues to age. As the older population grows, EMS personnel will be required to offer services that are cost-effective and efficient. Insurance regulations, costs associated with providing care, and facility issues will make cost a continuing concern.

Most of your geriatric patients will not reside in nursing homes. According to the 2004 Centers for Disease Control and Prevention (CDC) National Nursing Home Survey (NNHS), there are 16,100 nursing homes with 1.7 million beds across the United States. The average nursing home stay was 835 days. Although nursing home admissions are increasing because of the larger number of older persons in the United States, a countertrend is for elderly people to maintain independent lives. In 2003, for example, 96% of older people lived in the same residence that they had lived in during the previous year, and half of those who moved stayed in the same county. Many older adults continue to live at home with support from a spouse or family member and a visiting nurse; others live in a more dependent care environment such as a senior center facility. Still others may seek an assisted-living facility or a total care nursing home, which is known as a skilled nursing facility.

Determining how and where older adults will spend their retirement years is a difficult and complex process involving numerous social and economic issues such as the person's marital status, financial resources, religious beliefs, ethnicity, gender, and general health. Because such decisions may place a burden on grown children and other family members, their wishes must be considered by health care providers when making care decisions. Older adults and their families can also seek advice from medical social workers, professional care managers, discharge planners at health care facilities, and a large number of private and public resources. The range of services available includes delivered meals, personal care, housekeeping, adult day care, transportation, caregiver support, respite care, and emergency response systems, including EMS services and lifelines **Figure 1**.

One factor that frequently affects decisions regarding living conditions and services used by older adults is their unique financial situation. Older Americans are more likely than those younger than them to have wealth (which includes the sum

YOU *are the Medic* | PART 1

The first day after you have successfully completed a paramedic training program you head to the EMS service where you work with a paramedic partner. As soon as you enter the building, you are dispatched to a local bowling alley at 982 Stover Street for an elderly person who fell. Two minutes later you are en route after storing your belongings.

1. What type of injuries might you suspect on the basis of the dispatch information?

2. What dictates the type of skills that a paramedic may perform?

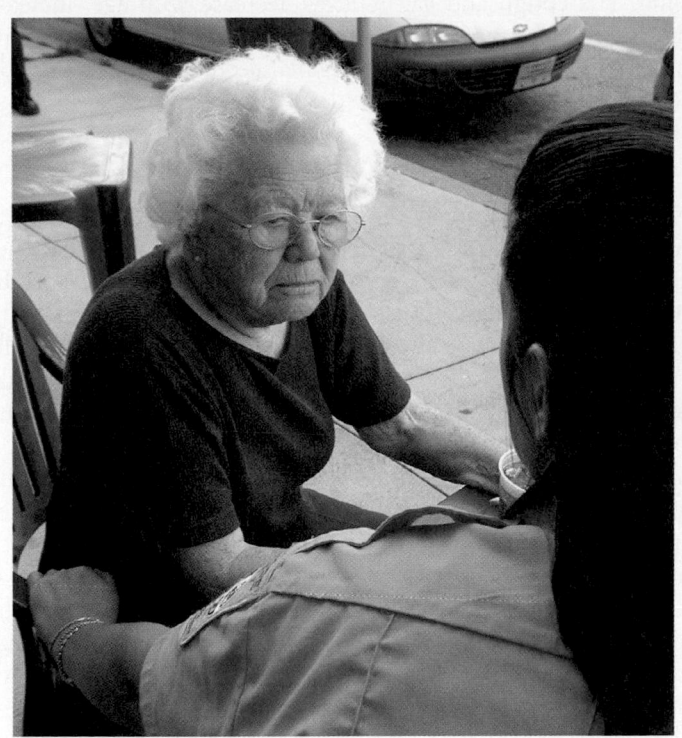

Figure 1 EMS professionals should be familiar with available resources.

of a person's assets, such as residential and business properties, retirement accounts, savings, and stocks). Many elders have also delayed retirement. They are also more likely to have health insurance coverage, although it is likely that health care reforms will decrease the number of uninsured people in all age categories.

You cannot assume, however, that all retired people live comfortably. Recent research has revealed that more than 10% of seniors have been uncertain about whether they would have enough food to eat each day, and older people who report "food insecurity" generally have poorer nutrition, poorer self-reported health, and more limitations in their abilities to care for themselves. Not surprisingly, older people who live in poverty are less likely to feel confident that they will have enough food. They may also have difficulty paying for medical expenses and housing costs, and may attempt to save money by skipping doses of medication or using a kerosene heater rather than the central heating unit; these actions may pose serious risks to their health.

Psychosocial factors may influence successful aging. For example, at retirement, people may no longer feel useful or productive in society and may experience diminished self-esteem. They may also feel frustrated at their inability to do things as easily as they once did, or they may mourn the loss of activities in which they can no longer participate because of complications from medical conditions. Conversely, some people experience feelings of freedom on retirement and accomplishment when looking back on their lives. The psychologist Erik Erikson refers to this as the crisis of integrity versus despair; at this particular point in life, a person can either experience integrity because

of his or her accomplishments, or despair at the idea that he or she may not have enough time to accomplish all of their goals. When people are unable to view their lives with integrity, they are significantly more likely to feel depressed, useless, or as though they are a burden on others.

Age may also bring **bereavement**—sadness over the loss of friends and loved ones. Notably, the likelihood of death increases during the year following the death of one's spouse. As friends and family die, elderly persons tend to experience increasing loneliness and isolation—factors shown to have negative effects on health. The death of a spouse, in particular, may also increase financial concerns, especially in lower-income families who may not have adequate retirement resources or life insurance coverage. Those people who were previously reliant on their spouse for daily assistance may no longer be able to meet basic needs on their own, requiring more help from their children or from other sources.

The social situations and health problems of older people are quantitatively and qualitatively different from the problems of younger people. You cannot simply transfer the principles of caring for and interacting with the younger population without modification. The special problems of older people require special approaches.

■ Geriatric Anatomy and Physiology

Human growth and development peaks in the late 20s and early 30s, at which point the aging process sets in. Aging is a linear process; that is, the rate at which a person loses functions does not increase with age. A 35-year-old person is aging just as fast as an 85-year-old person, but the older person exhibits the cumulative results of a longer process. Organ and tissue aging may be accelerated by a variety of factors including genetic qualities, preexisting diseases, diet, exposure to toxins, activity levels, and psychosocial characteristics. It is difficult to generalize the rate of aging for any person, and this process can vary dramatically from one person to another. You can most likely recall meeting 60-year-old people who look frail and 80-year-old people who are healthy enough to run a marathon Figure 2 .

The aging process is inevitably accompanied by changes in physiologic function, such as a decline in the function of the liver and kidneys. All tissues in the body undergo aging, albeit not at the same rate. The decrease in the functional capacity of various organ systems is normal but can affect the way in which a patient responds to

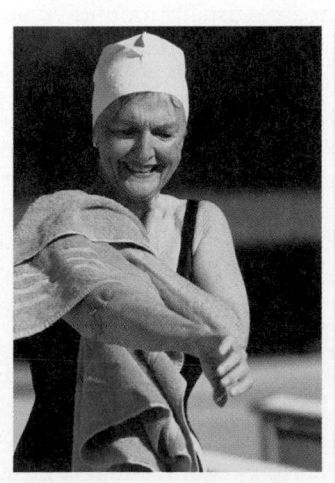

Figure 2 Many older people, especially those who have hobbies and activities, are healthy and vital.

illness. Older patients may report signs and symptoms different than those generally experienced by younger people, even when both are experiencing the same disease or disorder. In addition, diseases that may generally be short-lived and without detrimental effect can have a much longer course and cause significantly worse effects in older patients.

The aging process and its associated changes can also affect the way health professionals respond to a patient's illness. It is important to differentiate between normal physiologic changes of aging and acute changes that indicate pathologic processes. For example, a health care provider who is unaware of the normal changes of aging may mistake the changes for signs of illness and be tempted to provide treatment when none is necessary. At the other end of the spectrum, the health care provider may attribute genuine disease symptoms to "just getting old" and fail to provide proper treatment. Because of this, it is particularly important for you to determine the patient's baseline level of function when you are caring for older patients.

Changes in the Respiratory System

A person's respiratory capacity undergoes significant reductions with age, largely due to decreases in the elasticity of the lungs and in the size and strength of the respiratory muscles. In addition, calcification of costochondral cartilage tends to make the chest wall stiffer. As a result of these changes, the vital capacity (the amount of air that can be exhaled following a maximal inhalation) decreases, and the residual volume (the amount of air left in the lungs at the end of a maximal exhalation) increases. Thus, although the total amount of air in the lungs does not change with age, the proportion of that air usefully used in gas exchange progressively declines. Air flow, which depends largely on airway size and resistance, also deteriorates somewhat with age.

Meanwhile, changes in the distribution of blood flow within the lungs result in declining partial pressure of oxygen (Pao_2). The Pao_2 is a measurement of the amount of oxygen in the blood. At 30 years, the Pao_2 of a healthy person breathing ambient air is usually around 90 mm Hg; at 80 years, the Pao_2 under the same conditions is around 75 mm Hg ($Pao_2 = 100 - age/3$). Furthermore, the respiratory drive becomes dulled as a person ages because of decreased sensitivity to changes in arterial blood gases or decreased central nervous system (CNS) response to such changes. The number of alveoli also decreases, which makes the exchange of gases more difficult. As a consequence of these changes, elderly people have a slower reaction to hypoxemia and hypercarbia.

Musculoskeletal changes, such as kyphosis (outward curvature of the thoracic spine), may also affect pulmonary function by limiting lung volume and maximal inspiratory pressure. Chest expansion is also limited by decreased pulmonary muscle strength and mass. The decreased mass and strength requires an elderly person to exert a greater amount of energy to perform ventilations.

The respiratory system is physically limited by these changes in its ability to modify either the respiratory rate or tidal volume as a compensatory mechanism. In addition, the lung's defense mechanisms become less effective as a natural consequence of

aging. The cough and gag reflexes decrease with age, increasing the risk of aspiration. Furthermore, the ciliary mechanisms that normally help remove bronchial secretions are markedly slowed.

Changes in the Cardiovascular System

As with the respiratory system, a variety of changes occur in the cardiovascular system as a person grows older, with their net effect being to decrease the efficiency of this system. Specifically, the heart hypertrophies (enlarges) with age, most likely in response to the chronically increased afterload imposed by stiffened blood vessels. Over time, cardiac output declines, mostly as a result of a decreasing stroke volume. <u>Arteriosclerosis</u>—the stiffening of vessel walls—contributes to systolic hypertension in many older patients, which places an extra burden on the heart. This phenomenon may be a consequence of disease states such as diabetes, <u>atherosclerosis</u> **Figure 3**, and renal compromise, and it is associated with an increased risk of cardiovascular disease, dementia, and death. Compliance of the vascular walls depends on the production of collagen and elastin, proteins that are the primary components of muscle and connective tissue. An increase in blood pressure (normal hypertension seen in aging) leads to overproduction of abnormal collagen and decreased quantities of elastin, both of which contribute to vascular stiffening. The result is a widening pulse pressure, decreased coronary artery perfusion, and changes in cardiac ejection efficiency.

<u>Aortic sclerosis</u> occurs when the aortic valve thickens due to fibrosis and calcification. The thickening of the aortic valve obstructs blood flow from the left ventricle. Aortic sclerosis ultimately leads to <u>aortic stenosis</u>, a condition in which the aortic valve does not open fully, decreasing blood flow from

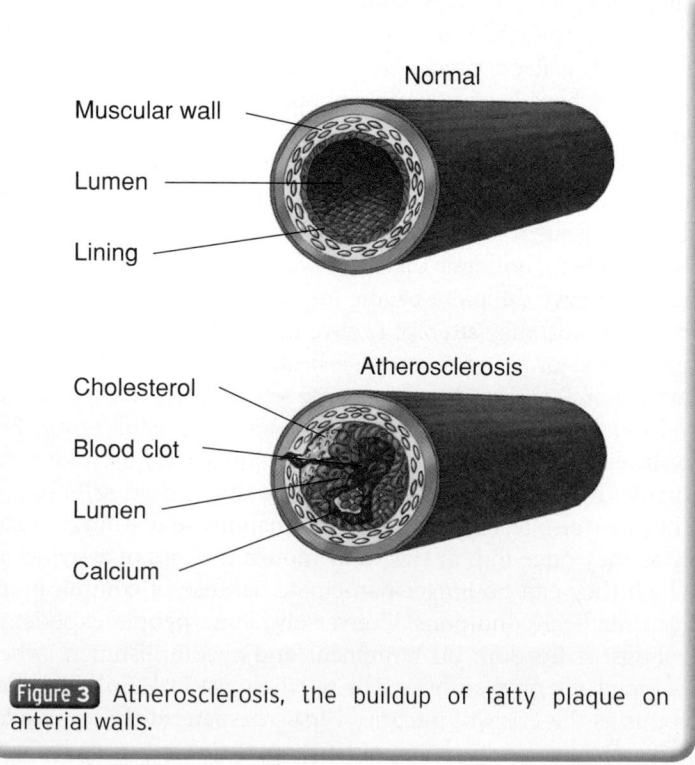

Figure 3 Atherosclerosis, the buildup of fatty plaque on arterial walls.

the heart. The walls of peripheral vessels also lose elasticity with age, which can result in a higher blood pressure due to less flexibility. The older patient is at a higher risk for the development of peripheral vascular disease, dependent venous pooling, and stasis ulcers.

At the same time, the electrical conduction system of the heart deteriorates over time. For example, the number of pacemaker cells in the sinoatrial node decreases dramatically as a person ages. In many cases, the changes in the conduction system lead to bradycardia that can in turn contribute to the decline in cardiac output. Other possible changes include the failure of the primary pacemaker and the development of alternate pacemakers within the atria, which must function as the primary pacemaker. This often leads to atrial dysrhythmias, such as atrial fibrillation, that causes irregular heartbeats and may cause clots to be distributed within the body. Additionally, it is much more difficult for the aging conduction system to produce a faster heart rate as a compensatory mechanism for decreased circulatory volume or increased cellular demand.

Some changes in cardiovascular performance are probably not a direct consequence of aging, but rather reflect the deconditioning effect of a sedentary lifestyle. Whether because of other disabilities (such as arthritis) or for social, financial, or psychological reasons, many people tend to decrease their physical activity as they grow older. The bodybuilder's slogan, "Use it or lose it," applies just as much to the cardiac muscle as to the biceps.

The sum of these changes leaves the cardiovascular system much more vulnerable to any dysfunction. Because the aging heart is less efficient at its baseline, when acute circulatory changes occur, the effects may be much worse than would be expected for younger populations. This means that all potential cardiac compromise should be recognized and treated quickly, and you should always be alert for presenting or potential cardiac concerns.

■ Changes in the Nervous System

Aging produces changes in the nervous system that are reflected in the neurologic examination. Changes in thinking (cognitive) speed, memory, and postural stability are the most common normal findings in older people. Studies have documented age-associated declines in mental function, especially slower central processing of sensory stimuli and language, and longer retrieval times for short- and long-term memory. Collectively, these changes affect performance on the mental status portion of the neurologic examination, with common findings including slow responses to questioning or requests to repeat a question.

The brain decreases in terms of weight (5% to 10%) and volume (atrophy) as a person ages. The functional significance of these changes is not clear, however. The human brain has an enormous reserve capacity, and having a smaller and lighter brain does not interfere with the mental capabilities of productive elderly people.

Because the brain is responsible for coordinating the other systems of the body, as mental function declines, the specific functions of other body systems may decline, as well. Regulation of respiratory rate and depth, pulse rate, blood pressure, hunger, and thirst may all be affected by changes to the CNS. Reflexes often slow, resulting in older people not being able to protect themselves in normal ways. For example, older patients with slowed responses to pain may sustain a serious burn if it takes them longer to remove their hand from a hot surface. Changes in both temperature regulation and temperature perception also occur, meaning that older people are less capable of recovering from exposure to extreme temperatures and less likely to recognize these exposures.

Sensory Changes

Undeniably, the performance of most of the sense organs declines with increasing age. Decreases in the ability to see and hear are the most common sensory impairments among the elderly, along with a decreased ability to discern tastes and decreased tactile sensation. Although these senses are not as sharp as they once may have been, this does not mean you should assume that all older people are blind or deaf. Use the same communication techniques that you would use with other age groups when you are caring for an older patient. If you sense an inability to communicate effectively, gradually modify your technique until you are able to speak with the patient in a comfortable manner.

Visual changes may begin as early as 40 years, such that as many as 50% of patients older than 65 years have vision problems. Tear production decreases with age, which can lead to sensations of dry or itchy eyes and increase the chances of mild eye injury (such as corneal abrasion) and infection. Causes of visual impairment in elderly people may include diabetes, age-related macular degeneration, and retinal detachment, which may also be associated with diabetes.

The two most common causes of visual disturbances in elderly people, however, are cataracts and glaucoma. **Cataracts** are a result of hardening of the lenses over time. The lenses eventually become opaque, preventing light and images from being transmitted to the rear of the eye. Patients with cataracts may report blurred vision, double vision, spots, and/or ghost images. Surgical treatment may be required to improve vision. By contrast, **glaucoma** is caused by an increase in intraocular pressure severe enough to damage the optic nerve, potentially resulting in permanent loss of peripheral and central vision. Treatment of glaucoma consists of oral medications and eye drops.

Decreases in visual acuity are common in older people, even without disease processes such as cataracts. Night vision becomes impaired, as does the ability to adjust to rapid changes in lighting conditions, depth perception, and perception of color. Presbyopia, or "far-sightedness," is caused by a loss of elasticity in the lens of the eye, and it is much more common in middle and older age adults. Difficulty differentiating among colors is also more common in older age. Changes in a patient's vision can affect independence, the ability to read, and the ability to drive a vehicle. All of these factors again increase the risk of injury from a vehicle crash or an unintentional overdose of medications.

Although not all older people experience hearing loss, some gradual loss of hearing is not uncommon as people age. A common cause of hearing impairment in geriatric patients is

<u>presbycusis</u>, a progressive hearing loss, particularly in the high frequencies, along with a lessened ability to discriminate between a particular sound and background noise. Patients who lose the ability to interpret most speech experience a decreased ability to communicate, which may lead to isolation and depression. Even when hearing loss is not severe enough to consistently interfere with conversation, certain activities, like going to the movies or listening to music, may be less enjoyable. Hearing loss may also threaten safety because many warnings, such as smoke detectors and car horns, are auditory.

Hearing aids are among the most commonly used assistive devices in the United States, and most people who use hearing aids are older **Figure 4**. They generally consist of a microphone and an amplifier, and some models are so small that they fit entirely into the ear canal. Hearing aids are almost always battery-operated. If inspection of the ear canal is necessary, hearing aids will most likely need to be removed. If the patient is conscious and able to remove them, you should ask the patient to do so because manipulation of hearing aids may cause loud feedback or a squealing noise. These devices are expensive and not always covered by insurance, so be certain that they are not lost during transport or transfer of patient care.

Another hearing-related impairment noted in the elderly population is <u>Meniere disease</u> (prevalence, 2 people per 1,000 population). Onset of symptoms usually occurs in early middle age, with symptoms presenting in cycles that last several months at a time. The typical symptoms include vertigo (a sudden loss of normal balance or equilibrium), hearing loss, tinnitus, and pressure in the ear.

Special Populations

With patients who have some degree of hearing loss, do not yell! Lean closer and speak into the patient's ear using a somewhat low pitch. Remember that patients with limited vision are not necessarily hard of hearing.

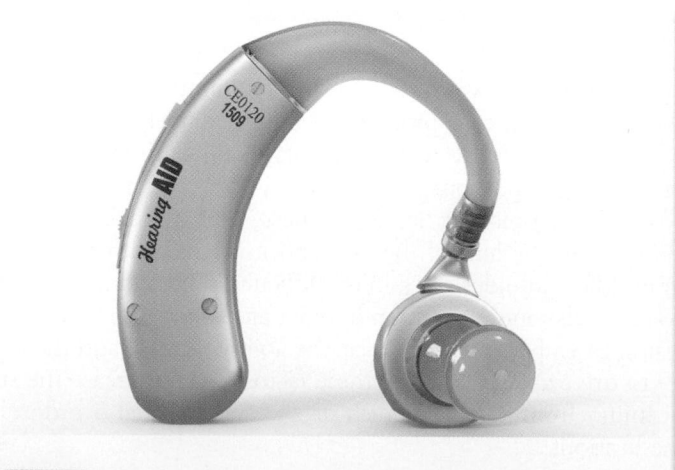

Figure 4 Hearing aids are among the most commonly used assistive devices in the United States.

Changes in appetite may occur because of a decrease in the number of taste buds. By 70 years, the number of taste buds a person has is reduced by one third. Although these changes are gradual, the salty and sweet sensation appears to be among the first to diminish.

The sense of touch decreases from loss of the end nerve fibers. This loss, in conjunction with the slowing of the peripheral nervous system, can result in a delayed reflex reaction.

The sense of smell is among the last to diminish in older patients. However, factors such as upper respiratory infections (ie, the common cold), to which older persons are more prone, can affect the sense of smell.

For many older people, physiologic changes make it difficult to produce speech that is loud enough, clear, and well-spaced. Weakness, paralysis, poor hearing, or brain damage can damage the delicate functions that make these abilities possible. Changes in cognition may also impact speech and conversation because the person may not be able to recall specific information fast enough to carry on a normal conversation. This may be frustrating to patients, as well, so do not rush them for answers to your questions or interrupt them; give them time to put their thoughts together.

Sense of body position (<u>proprioception</u>) also becomes impaired with age. Proprioception enables a person to maintain postural stability by using a variety of receptors in the joints and information provided by the eyes. As these mechanisms fail with age, people become less steady on their feet, and the tendency to fall increases markedly. This may be exacerbated by many of the previously described changes in sensory perception, as well.

Changes in the Digestive System

The process of digestion begins in the mouth, which is also where aging-related changes in the digestive system may first be noted. As discussed previously, a decrease in the number of taste buds and changes in olfactory receptors may diminish an older person's senses of taste and smell, which may, in turn, interfere with the enjoyment of food. The consequent decrease in appetite may lead to malnutrition. Other changes in the mouth include a reduction in the volume of saliva, with a resulting dryness of the mouth. Dental loss is not a normal result of the aging process, but rather the result of disease of the teeth and gums; nevertheless, dental loss is widespread in the elderly population and contributes to nutritional and digestive problems. Even when dentures are present, ill-fitting dentures may result in pain or discomfort when eating, or they may not allow the wearer to chew effectively, increasing the likelihood of choking, heartburn, and abdominal pain.

Like oral secretions, gastric secretions are reduced as a person ages—although enough acid is still present to produce ulcers under certain conditions. Because of the esophageal sphincter's weakening and decreased ability to hold back stomach contents, the acid present in the stomach may also cause heartburn, indigestion, or acid reflux. Whereas these symptoms tend to be related to diet and eating practices, the possibility exists that the patient may ignore symptoms of cardiac compromise, thinking of them simply as the after-effects of a spicy or greasy meal. Changes in gastric motility also occur that may lead to slower gastric emptying—a factor of some importance when you are assessing the risk of aspiration, and a contributing factor to uncomfortable (but not life-threatening) heartburn and acid reflux.

Function of the small and large bowel changes little as a consequence of aging, although the incidence of certain diseases involving the bowel (such as diverticulosis) increases as a person grows older. As with other sphincters within the body, rectal sphincter muscles may decrease in size and strength causing the possibility of unintentional bowel release, or fecal incontinence.

Slowing of peristalsis can lead to constipation. Constipation may also be caused or worsened by certain medications, changes in diet, and decreased physical activity. This may lead to difficult bowel movements with straining that can cause hemorrhoids. Forceful straining or retching (vagus nerve stimulation) may also lead to syncope or bradycardia. The patient may attempt to treat constipation without the assistance of a physician, often with diet techniques or medications that may or may not be intended to treat constipation. When treated too aggressively, diarrhea may result, sometimes leading to dehydration. For constipation that cannot be resolved with diet and medications, manual removal of stool by a physician or nurse may be necessary.

In the liver, there are changes in hepatic enzyme systems, with some systems declining in activity and others increasing. Notably, the activity of the enzyme systems concerned with the detoxification of drugs declines as a person ages. The decrease in hepatic function can complicate drug absorption, resulting in drug toxicity. When patients are prescribed numerous medications, the risk for hepatic damage or drug toxicity increases.

Changes in the Renal System

The kidneys are responsible for maintaining the body's fluid and electrolyte balance and have important roles in maintaining the body's long-term acid-base balance and eliminating drugs from the body. In a young adult, the kidneys weigh between 250 and 270 g; in a healthy 70-year-old person, they weigh between 180 and 200 g. This decline in weight results from a loss of functioning nephron units that translate into a smaller effective filtering surface. At the same time, renal blood flow decreases by as much as 50% as a person ages.

Acute illness in elderly patients is often accompanied by derangements in fluid and electrolyte balance. Aging kidneys, for example, respond sluggishly to sodium deficiency. An elderly patient may lose a large amount of sodium before the kidneys halt urinary sodium excretion, a problem that is exacerbated by the markedly decreased thirst mechanism in elderly people. The net result may be a rapid development of severe dehydration.

Conversely, elderly patients are at considerable risk of overhydration if they are exposed to large sodium loads (such as from intravenous [IV] saline solutions or heavily salted foods). Because of its lower glomerular filtration rate, the aging kidney is less able to excrete a large sodium load, making the patient vulnerable to acute volume overload.

The same factors that reduce an older person's ability to handle sodium also affect the body's ability to handle potassium. Thus, elderly patients are prone to hyperkalemia that can reach serious—even lethal—levels if the patient becomes acidotic or if the potassium load is increased from any source.

Changes in the Endocrine System

According to the Centers for Disease Control and Prevention, 26.9% of US residents, or 10.9 million people, aged 65 years and older had diabetes in 2010. This does not include the approximate 50% of geriatric patients who, according to fasting glucose tests, were classified in the prediabetic category. The reason older patients are at greater risk for developing type 2 diabetes is multifaceted. As patients age, the metabolism of carbohydrates becomes more difficult. Furthermore, older patients who are diagnosed with diabetes may have a multitude of comorbid disorders and may be prescribed various medications that may affect glucose metabolism.

As patients age, an increase in the production of antidiuretic hormone (ADH) can occur. This can cause various electrolyte imbalances, particularly hyponatremia, as well as fluid balance issues. Patients may present with pedal or other peripheral edema, although peripheral edema may also be the result of cardiovascular compromise. Again, it is important for you to determine a baseline for edema; worsening of edema is much more significant than its presence alone.

In women, menopause (or cessation of the reproductive cycles of menstruation and ovulation) results in decreased secretion of hormones, specifically estrogen. Because estrogen plays an important role in the preservation of bone mass, the decline in estrogen levels may lead to decreased bone density and osteoporosis. Changes in both estrogen and progesterone levels also cause symptoms of menopause, such as "hot flashes" and mood disturbances.

Changes in the Immunologic System

Because nearly every function of the immune system is affected by aging, older persons are more prone to infection and secondary complications than younger people. Chronic conditions such as diabetes, dementia, malnutrition, and cardiovascular disease place older people at greater risk of serious infection.

Older persons manifest infections differently. Although fever is often present with minor illness in young people, fever in older persons usually indicates a serious infection. However, as many as 30% of older persons with a serious infection may not have a fever. This is due to the inability of the aging immune system to initiate a fever. Pneumonia is the leading cause of death from infection in Americans older than 65 years.

Changes in the Integumentary System

Wrinkling and loss of resiliency of the skin are the most visible signs of aging. Wrinkling occurs because the skin becomes thinner, drier, less elastic, and more fragile. As subcutaneous fat becomes thinner, bruising becomes more common because subcutaneous fat normally cushions blood vessels from mild blunt forces. Elastin (the substance that makes the skin pliable) and collagen (the substance that makes the skin strong) decrease with age. Thinner skin tears much more easily, and the loss of elasticity allows for more bleeding before hemostasis occurs. Because of the decreased resiliency of the skin, it may also be more prone to tenting when skin turgor is checked, even when dehydration is not present.

As a person ages, the sebaceous glands produce less oil and the skin becomes drier. Sweat gland activity also decreases, hindering the ability to sweat and to regulate heat. Hair follicles produce thinner hair or may stop producing hair. Follicles produce less melanin (the pigment that gives hair color), making the hair color revert to gray or white. The number of melanocytes in the epidermis decrease, making the skin appear paler than in younger years and increasing sensitivity to sun exposure. As the number of melanocytes decreases, existing melanocytes grow larger. This may lead to benign pigmentation changes in sun-exposed areas, such as age spots or "liver spots."

The blood vessels that supply the skin also are affected by atherosclerosis and provide less oxygenated blood at the cellular level. As a consequence of the skin's lower metabolism, epidermal cells develop more slowly and do not replace outgoing cells as quickly as with younger skin. Fingernails and toenails may change, as well, generally becoming thinner and more brittle. These changes are more profound when combined with inadequate nutrition from any of a number of causes. Fingernails that are poorly cared for can be a source of infection, particularly for patients with significantly decreased cognitive abilities. Inadequate or incorrect self-care of toenails can result in infection of the soft tissue of the toes, and when combined with peripheral vascular disease or diabetes, the complications from poor toenail care can lead to amputation.

Homeostatic and Other Changes

Homeostasis is the process by which the body maintains a constant internal environment. Many homeostatic mechanisms work on a feedback principle, much like the thermostat in a house—that is, a change in the internal environment feeds back to the control system to induce a corrective response. For example, when the body temperature starts to rise, temperature sensors are activated, which in turn activate compensatory responses: Cutaneous blood vessels dilate, and excess heat is transferred from the body to the environment. Similarly, when the concentration of glucose in the blood rises, the pancreas is stimulated to secrete insulin, which leads to uptake of glucose by cells and reduction of the blood glucose level back toward normal.

With aging, there is a progressive loss of these homeostatic capabilities. For that reason, a specific illness or injury in elderly people is more likely to result in generalized deterioration. For example, the thirst mechanism that ordinarily protects a person from dehydration becomes depressed in elderly patients. Likewise, temperature-regulating mechanisms tend to become disordered, which when combined with integumentary changes makes elderly patients much more vulnerable to environmental stresses such as heat exhaustion and accidental hypothermia after relatively minor exposures. A defect in temperature regulation also may account for the absence of a febrile response to illness in many elderly people. As discussed previously, infections that would ordinarily produce high fever, such as pneumococcal pneumonia, may produce only a low-grade or no fever in elderly people. Likewise, an elderly patient may have warm, flushed skin even though the patient may be hypothermic.

Words of Wisdom

A specific illness or injury in the elderly is more likely to result in generalized deterioration.

The regulatory system that manages the blood glucose level similarly becomes impaired with increasing age, such that an elevated blood glucose level occurs quite commonly in older patients. Ordinarily, moderate hyperglycemia does no harm, but overly aggressive treatment of this problem may produce damaging hypoglycemia.

Changes in the Musculoskeletal System

Aging brings a widespread decrease in bone mass in men and women, but especially among postmenopausal women. Bones become more brittle and tend to break more easily. Tendons and ligaments begin to lose elasticity, synovial fluids in joints thicken, and cartilage that cushions joints decreases. Narrowing of the intervertebral disks and compression fractures of the vertebrae contribute to a decrease in height as a person ages, along with changes in posture. Joints lose their flexibility and may be further immobilized by arthritic changes. In fact, more than half of all elderly people have some form of arthritis. Muscle mass decreases throughout the body, with an accompanying decrease in muscle strength. Atrophy, or wasting of muscles, occurs when mobility is limited for a prolonged period of time, such as during bed confinement after surgery or illness.

From your perspective, the changes in the musculoskeletal system most often translate into fractures incurred as the result of falls. The aging musculoskeletal system not only makes the person more susceptible to fractures when falls occur, but also increases the likelihood of falling because joint stiffness, loss of elasticity in tendons and ligaments, and weakening of muscles may impair mobility. Changes may cause patients to have difficulty caring for themselves; this is especially true regarding tasks that require fine motor coordination and strength in the hands and fingers. Because of this, patients may have difficulty taking medications, self-administering medication, or caring for wounds.

Loss of bone density and muscle mass may be slowed by remaining physically active. People who enter older adulthood with larger muscles and a history of performing physical labor or participating in regular strenuous exercise are the least susceptible to musculoskeletal decline. Elderly people may also experience less pain from arthritis when they consistently and gently use arthritic joints.

Special Populations

Growing old does not naturally or normally include confusion, dementia, delirium, depression, falls, weakness, syncope, and other conditions related to disease processes.

Special Populations

When an elderly person calls for an ambulance, there is usually a good reason, even if it is not the reason the patient tells you.

■ Geriatric Patient Assessment

Although illness is common among elderly people, it is not an inevitable part of aging. Complaints of elderly people cannot be ascribed simply to "getting old." Aging is a continuous process and a normal development sequence that affects people in multiple ways. The normal wear-and-tear concept and genetic makeup are two theories that have been suggested to explain the biologic effects of aging.

Special Populations

Getting old is not a disease, and it does not by itself produce symptoms of disease.

Along the same lines, there is a widespread misconception that elderly people tend to be hypochondriacs, with many imaginary or minor complaints. In reality, hypochondria is far less common among elderly patients than among younger patients. Indeed, older patients tend not to complain, even when they have legitimate symptoms. When an elderly person calls for an ambulance, he or she usually has a real problem.

Knowing what is and what is not part of the aging process constitutes the first challenge when you are assessing elderly patients. A second challenge is that signs and symptoms of disease may be altered from their presentation in younger patients as a consequence of the aging process. A myocardial infarction (MI) may present without chest pain; fever may be minimal in pneumonia; uncontrolled diabetes is more likely to present as hyperosmolar nonketotic coma (HONK)/hyperosmolar hyperglycemic nonketotic coma (HHNC) than as diabetic ketoacidosis. A variety of acute illnesses—from congestive heart failure to an acute abdomen—may present simply as delirium.

Another challenge relates to the fact that the older the patient, the more likely there are multiple problems—medical, psychological, and social. Interestingly, the proportion of older people with a disability has decreased; however, the total number of older people with a chronic disability has increased simply because there are more elderly people. Debilitating health conditions often found in this population include hypertension, arthritic symptoms, heart disease, cancer, diabetes, stroke, and chronic obstructive pulmonary disease (COPD). The incidence of depression also increases with age, with 15% to 20% of people older than 85 years having some form of depression. With the baby boomers moving into this age group, this is likely to be a very significant issue in the next decade.

The co-occurrence of multiple pathologic conditions has several consequences for patients and health care providers alike. The symptoms of one disease or disability may alter or hide the symptoms of another condition. The patient with severe leg pain from arthritis, for example, may not pay much attention to new pain caused by thrombophlebitis. In addition, when several organ

YOU are the Medic   PART 2

On arrival you are directed by the manager to an area in front of an alley where a 72-year-old woman is sitting with her right leg propped up on a chair. Several bystanders tell you that she twisted her right ankle and they heard a "pop." She fell forward onto her knees and they assisted her back to the chair.

Recording Time: 1 Minute	
Appearance	No significant distress
Level of consciousness	Alert
Airway	Open and clear
Breathing	Normal
Circulation	Strong radial pulses

3. Is safety an issue here?

4. What are your primary responsibilities at this point during the call?

systems are in borderline condition, a disturbance in function in only one of the systems may have repercussions throughout the body, leading to failure of multiple organs in a domino-like manner. The presence of multiple underlying illnesses also makes it much more difficult for you to sort out which problem is causing which symptom. Furthermore, chronic comorbidities may make it much more difficult to treat the patient's acute problem. For example, the medication a patient needs for a cardiac problem may be contraindicated because of a renal or hepatic problem or, at the least, may require a major modification in the dosage.

Scene Size-up

Begin the patient assessment process by ensuring scene safety, and take standard precautions. Be mindful of clues that may help you to determine the mechanism of injury or the nature of illness. Immediately determine the number of patients that require your assistance, and consider any additional or specialized resources that may need to be called. You also need to be aware of the numerous factors that affect the assessment process in geriatric patients: sensory alterations, verbal communication skills, and mental and physical capabilities. You need to be able to accommodate and comprehend these conditions.

Words of Wisdom

Always assume that an elderly patient's mental status is normal until you have evidence to the contrary.

Primary Assessment

Using the GEMS Diamond to Form a General Impression

As you approach the patient, you will want to form a general impression that may prove relevant to the case and help you to address life threats. You will look for potential clues such as general living conditions; availability of social and family support; activity level; medications; overall appearance with respect to nutrition, general health, cleanliness, personal hygiene, and attitude and mental well-being.

There are many acronyms in the prehospital setting to help you remember steps in your assessment and treatment. The GEMS diamond was created to help providers recall key themes when caring for geriatric patients **Table 1**. It was designed to assist the prehospital professional in the assessment and treatment of elderly patients.

"G" of the GEMS diamond is to recognize that the patient is a geriatric patient. Your thought process needs to be geared to the possible problems of an aging patient. When you are responding to an emergency involving an older patient, you should consider that older patients are different from younger patients and may present atypically.

Table 1 The GEMS Diamond

G—Geriatric Patients

- Present atypically.
- Deserve respect.
- Experience normal changes with age.

E—Environmental Assessment

- Check the physical condition of the patient's home: Is the exterior of the home in need of repair? Is the home secure?
- Check for hazardous conditions that may be present (for example, poor wiring, rotted floors, unventilated gas heaters, broken window glass, clutter that prevents adequate egress).
- Are smoke detectors present and working?
- Is the home too hot or too cold?
- Is there an odor of feces or urine in the home? Is bedding soiled or urine-soaked?
- Is food present in the home? Is it adequate and unspoiled?
- Are liquor bottles present? If so, are they lying empty?
- If the patient has a disability, are appropriate assistive devices (for example, a wheelchair or walker) present?
- Does the patient have access to a telephone?
- If living with others, is the patient confined to one part of the home?
- If the patient is residing in a nursing facility, does the care appear to be adequate to meet the patient's needs?

M—Medical Assessment

- Older patients tend to have a variety of medical problems, making assessment complex. Keep this in mind in all cases—both trauma and medical. A trauma patient may have an underlying medical condition that could have caused or may be exacerbated by the injury.
- Obtaining a medical history is important in older patients, regardless of the chief complaint.
- Are medications out of date or unmarked, or are prescriptions for the same or similar medications from many physicians?
- Primary assessment
- Reassessment

S—Social Assessment

- Assess activities of daily living (eating, dressing, bathing, toileting).
- Are these activities being provided for the patient? If so, by whom?
- Are there delays in obtaining food, medication, or other necessary items? The patient may complain of this, or the environment may suggest this.
- If in an institutional setting, is the patient able to feed himself or herself? If not, is food still sitting on the food tray? Has the patient been lying in his or her own urine or feces for prolonged periods?
- Does the patient have a social network? Does the patient have a mechanism to interact socially with others on a daily basis?

"E" of the GEMS diamond stands for an environmental assessment. Assessment of the environment can help give clues to the patient's condition or the cause of the emergency. Is the home too hot or cold? Is the home well kept and secure? Are there hazardous conditions? Preventive care is also important for a geriatric patient, who may not carefully study the environment or may not realize where risks exist.

"M" of the GEMS diamond stands for medical assessment. Older patients tend to have a variety of medical problems and may be taking numerous prescription, over-the-counter, and herbal medications. Obtaining a thorough history is important in older patients. Keep this in mind throughout the assessment process.

"S" stands for social assessment. Older people may have less of a social network because of the death of a spouse, family members, or friends. Older people may also need assistance with activities of daily living (ADL), such as dressing and eating. There are numerous social agencies that are readily available to help geriatric patients, and these agencies can share with you and your patients a listing of the services they provide.

The GEMS diamond provides a concise way for you to remember the important issues for older patients. Using this concept will help you make appropriate referrals, and as a result, you will help older patients maintain their quality of life.

Words of Wisdom

Cover the patient with a blanket to protect privacy and keep the patient warm. This action shows respect for the patient and will improve your exam.

Airway and Breathing

Anatomic changes occur as a person ages, predisposing geriatric patients to airway problems. Aging and disease can compromise a patient's ability to protect his or her airway with loss of a gag reflex and normal swallowing mechanisms. Changes in level of consciousness, dementia, and poststroke weakness or paralysis can cause airway obstruction or aspiration. Ensure that the patient's airway is open and is not obstructed by dentures, vomitus, fluids, or blood. Suction may be necessary.

Anatomic changes with aging also affect a person's ability to breathe effectively. Increased chest wall stiffness, brittle bones, weakening of the airway musculature, and decreased muscle mass contribute to breathing problems. Loss of mechanisms that protect the upper airway, like cough and gag reflexes, cause a decreased ability to clear secretions. A decrease in the number of cilia that line the bronchial tree results in the inability of the patient to remove material from the lung, which can cause infection. In some patients, the alveoli are damaged, and a lack of elasticity results in a decreased ability to exchange oxygen and carbon dioxide. Superimposed on the physiologic changes are the chronic respiratory diseases common in elderly people that affect the ability of the patient to breathe effectively. Airway and breathing issues should be treated with oxygen as soon as possible.

Circulation

People who normally live with compromised circulation have little in the way of reserves during a circulatory crisis. Physiologic changes may negatively affect circulation. Less responsive nerve stimulation may lower the rate and strength of the heart's contractions, so lower heart rates and weaker and irregular pulses are common in elderly patients. Vascular changes and circulatory compromise might make it difficult to feel a radial pulse on an older patient. If choosing an alternative pulse point like the carotid, press gently. Another option is to listen to the apical pulse right over the heart. The pulse may be irregular because of common heart rhythm problems. Circulation problems in older adults should be treated with oxygen as soon as possible.

Documentation and Communication

Be patient when you are interviewing older people, recognizing that physical, intellectual, and psychological barriers may slow or interfere with effective communication.

Transport Decision

Your most important task during the primary assessment is to determine conditions that are life threatening, treat them to the best of your ability, and provide transport to priority patients. Priority patients include patients who have a poor general impression, airway or breathing problems, acute altered level of consciousness, shock, any severe pain, or uncontrolled hemorrhage. Elderly people do not have the reserves that younger people do, and they will easily decompensate. Even a general complaint of weakness and dizziness can be an indication of something more serious like a heart problem. Consider early on in your call if advanced life support (ALS) treatment and immediate transport is appropriate and available. If possible, try to take the patient to a facility where the patient has been treated before and his or her medical records reside.

History Taking

Good communication skills will help you gather the information you need during your assessment. Without good communication skills, you could frighten, alienate, insult, anger, or even harm your patients. Your first words should focus on gaining the patient's trust. Introduce yourself. Use respect when you are addressing the patient; use his or her name, if you know it; and avoid terms such as "buddy," "honey," "dear," and "grandma" when addressing an older patient. Speak slowly, distinctly, and respectfully. Do not raise your voice excessively. Attempt to get the patient history from the patient, rather than family and bystanders, whenever possible. The ability to elicit a thorough patient history reflects education and experience. For example, a thorough knowledge of prescription medications will help in understanding the patient's diagnoses as well as medication compliance.

Communication is not just talking; it is also listening. When you are asking questions of older patients, wait for their answers. Older people may need more time to process your questions, and they may speak slowly when responding. Active listening also involves paying attention to the patient's tone, especially if it conveys fear or confusion.

Nonverbal communication is just as important as verbal communication. Eye contact, hand gestures, body position, facial expressions, and touch communicate a message. When you are speaking with patients, get face to face with them and make sure there is plenty of light. Have patients put in hearing aids (ensure they are turned on) or wear glasses to facilitate better communication, and be sure to take these aids with the patients to the hospital so other health care providers can communicate as well.

Explain everything you plan to do, especially if the patient seems confused. Part of your task in the assessment is to determine whether this confused state is normal, a new manifestation of a preexisting medical problem, or a result of the patient's lack of understanding. Preserve the patient's dignity during exposure and when you are discussing his or her history around others.

A comprehensive patient history includes many elements to investigate—the patient's chief complaint, present illness or injury, pertinent medical history, and current health care status and needs. Keep in mind that pertinent past medical history would include current cardiovascular health (such as palpitations or flutters), exercise tolerance, diet history, medications, smoking and drinking habits, sleep patterns, and other intrinsic and extrinsic factors. Obtaining the chief complaint would seem to be a straightforward procedure, but it may not be simple with some elderly patients. Older patients tend not to report significant symptoms for several reasons. Many share the misconception that illness and assorted aches and pains are simply part of aging. Other older people may not mention even legitimate symptoms to avoid being identified as old and a hypochondriac. Some older patients fear that mentioning a symptom will lead to a diagnosis or treatment that will jeopardize their independence. "If I mention those pains in my stomach," the person may reason, "they'll put me in the hospital, and I may never come out of that place again."

Whereas elderly patients tend to underreport serious symptoms, the symptoms they do report are often vague and may appear trivial. It may be difficult for older patients to report symptoms, particularly in front of their spouse or other family members. Furthermore, elderly patients are likely to have several chief complaints, each of which may have a different source.

When a patient's chief complaint seems trivial, it may be necessary to go through a standard list of screening questions to confirm that you are not missing important pieces of information. In such a review of systems, questions are designed to evaluate the functions of the body's major organ systems. In the field, you do not have sufficient time to conduct a complete review of all systems, but a few well-chosen questions can provide you with a great deal of information about the function of the patient's more important systems:

- Cardiovascular
  - Have you had any pain or discomfort in your chest? When?
  - Have you had any pain in your left arm or jaw?
  - Have you noticed any fluttering in your chest or fast heartbeats?
- Respiratory
  - Do you ever get short of breath? When?
  - Have you had a cough lately? Is it painful?
- Neurologic
  - Can you explain the reason for calling 9-1-1?
  - Have you had any dizzy spells? Have you fainted?
  - Have you had any trouble speaking?
  - Have you had headaches recently?
  - Have you noticed any unusual weakness or odd sensations in your arms or legs?
- Gastrointestinal
  - Have there been any changes in your appetite lately?
  - Have you gained or lost any weight?
  - Have there been any changes in your bowel movements?
  - Have you had any nausea or vomiting?
- Genitourinary
  - Do you have any pain or difficulty urinating?
  - Have you noticed any change in the color of your urine?
  - Have you noticed any changes in the frequency of urination?

Documentation and Communication

Interviewing techniques:
- Introduce yourself.
- Speak to the patient first rather than family or bystanders.
- Be aware of your body language.
- Look directly at the patient.
- Speak slowly and distinctly.
- Explain what you are doing.
- Allow time for the patient to answer.
- Show the patient respect, and preserve dignity.
- Do not talk about the patient with others in front of the patient.
- Be patient.
- Locate hearing aids or eyeglasses if needed.
- Turn on lights.

If any of these screening questions yields a positive answer, follow up with further questions. For example, if the patient states that he has been coughing lately, find out whether he is bringing up sputum and, if so, what the sputum looks like (for example, is there blood in the sputum?).

Once you have elicited what you believe to be the chief complaint, go through the usual process of assembling the history of the present illness. This history may be complicated if other chronic problems are affecting the acute problem. To sort out which symptoms relate to the current chief complaint and which are chronic difficulties, try asking questions such as "How does this problem differ from what it was like last week?" or "What happened today to make you decide to get help?"

Just as it is not practical to go through a comprehensive review of systems in the field, it is not usually feasible to obtain a complete medical history in the prehospital setting. Nevertheless, you should obtain a SAMPLE history to inquire about recent hospitalizations and allergies **Table 2**.

Most important, you should obtain the most detailed history possible of the patient's medications because medications account for a significant percentage of medical problems in elderly people. A medication history should include all medications, not just prescription drugs, because many people do not think to mention common over-the-counter preparations such as aspirin, antacid tablets, and herbal medicines. Ask the patient to list the medications by name, and determine the dosing and frequency for each one. Also, inquire about medications that are prescribed but not taken (such as because of cost issues or side effects) and medications that may have been provided by other sources (such as a spouse's medication). Obtain the patient's permission to take medications to the hospital, and then collect them all—prescription and nonprescription drugs. If the patient cannot tell you where the medicines are stored, check the bathroom medicine cabinet, the bedside table, the kitchen table and counters, and the refrigerator.

Obtaining a history from an elderly patient requires patience. You must be prepared to listen, often for an extended period. But your listening will be rewarded—not only by helping you discover the patient's problem, but also by allowing you to provide part of the solution to the problem. Listening is a demonstration of caring, and your caring can mean a great deal to a lonely or frightened older person.

Secondary Assessment

During the secondary assessment of an elderly patient, you may have to adjust your usual methods. Poor cooperation and easy fatigability on the part of the patient may require that you keep manipulations to a minimum. In addition, older people are more prone to hypothermia, so be sure to keep the patient warm and maintain body temperature. Inspection and palpation can be hampered by multiple layers of clothing, so remove only the clothing that is necessary to perform an accurate examination. Be sure to cover the patient when you are finished.

Whereas the primary assessment addresses immediately life-threatening pathologic problems, the secondary assessment includes a systematic assessment of the patient that may include a full-body examination or a focused assessment on the body part or body system specifically involved. A complete set of baseline vital signs, using monitoring devices as appropriate, should also be obtained at this time.

Postural changes in blood pressure vary among elderly people, but changes increase with increasing frailty and heighten the person's risk for falls. Marked postural changes in blood pressure and pulse rate may indicate hypovolemia or overmedication. As you obtain the vital signs, bear in mind that blood pressure tends to be higher in elderly people. An elderly patient who has a blood pressure in a normal adult range could be hypotensive. If possible, determine the patient's baseline blood pressure. When you are obtaining a patient's blood pressure, be aware of the possibility of significant hypertension and orthostatic changes. Consider obtaining vital signs in both arms and checking pulses proximally and distally in all extremities. This process will allow you to gather information and observe for signs of dependent edema, dehydration, and the patient's circulatory status without raising his or her anxiety level.

Pay attention to the respiratory rate. Tachypnea can be a sensitive indicator of acute illness in elderly people—especially pulmonary infection—even when patients show few, if any, other signs. When you are assessing the patient's respirations, listen to lung sounds in all fields, noting adventitious sounds that might aid in the development of a treatment plan. You can also use the stethoscope to listen for carotid bruits; note jugular vein distention.

Table 2 Geriatric SAMPLE History Components	
Component	**Explanation**
Signs and symptoms	Onset and nature of symptoms of pain or fever
Allergies	Known drug reactions or other allergies
Medications	Exact names and doses of ongoing drugs (including over-the-counter, prescribed, herbal, and recreational drugs) Timing and amount of last dose Time and dose of analgesics or antipyretics
Past medical history	Previous illnesses or injuries Immunizations Important family history
Last oral intake	Timing of the last food or drink What was ingested and when
Events leading to illness or injury	Key events leading up to the current injury or illness

Special Populations

Consider the possibility of hypovolemia in any elderly person whose systolic blood pressure is less than 120 mm Hg.

When you are examining the mouth, make a note of any upper or lower dentures. In the chest examination, keep in mind that elderly people may have pulmonary crackles without apparent pathology. Similarly, edema in the legs may be the result of chronic venous insufficiency and not right-sided heart failure.

Reassessment

Reassess the geriatric patient often because the condition of an older adult may deteriorate quickly. Repeat the primary assessment. Reassess the vital signs. Reassess the patient's complaint.

Recheck interventions. Identify and treat changes in the patient's condition.

Pathophysiology, Assessment, and Management of Respiratory Conditions

Chronic lower respiratory disease, influenza, and pneumonia remain in the top five causes of geriatric deaths. In fact, one of the most common causes of death in older patients is infection with *Pneumococcus* bacteria.

Pneumonia

Pneumonia involves an inflammation of the lung, secondary to infection by bacteria, viruses, or other organisms. Although it can affect people at any age, this disease has its biggest impact on very young and elderly people, typically during the colder seasons (winter and early spring). People considered at risk include elderly people; people with underlying health problems such as COPD, diabetes mellitus, and vascular diseases; and any person with a depressed immune system because of acquired immunodeficiency syndrome, cancer therapy, or organ transplantation. General immobility, bed confinement (ie, rehabilitation from a fractured hip), and conditions that limit the ability to breathe deeply, such as rib fractures, also increase the risk for pneumonia.

An older patient with pneumonia often does not have the classic presentation of chills, fever, and productive cough. Instead, these symptoms are often supplanted by acute confusion (delirium), normal temperature, and a minimal to absent cough. Some patients may report abdominal pain, as well. Rhonchi may be auscultated in the affected lobes, and inflammation of the bronchi may result in wheezing.

Treatment is primarily supportive, consisting of fluids, oxygen therapy via a nasal cannula or mask to relieve dyspnea, and analgesics to reduce fever. Preventive measures include a *Pneumococcus* vaccine given once, with booster doses after 3 to 5 years (although this will not prevent infection from other bacterial species), along with smoking cessation and respiratory exercises during bed confinement. The receiving facility will determine whether antibiotics are necessary.

Chronic Obstructive Pulmonary Disease

Chronic obstructive pulmonary disease (COPD) is the name given to a set of diseases, including chronic bronchitis and emphysema, along with asthma, all of which are characterized by the presence of bronchial obstruction and airway inflammation. Distinguishing among these diseases can be difficult, so the problem may not be diagnosed or treated correctly. COPD affects approximately 10% of the older population, and tobacco use is strongly correlated with this diagnosis. Its effects reflect the age-related loss of elastic tissue in the lungs (senile emphysema) and a decreased ability to defend against infection. These factors may increase the baseline disability of COPD and set up older patients for an increased risk of acute exacerbation, often caused by infection. Patients with COPD may experience dyspnea upon exertion, and when the disease is in its later stages, even minor physical activities like position changes and walking may become difficult for the patient.

Preventive measures for COPD include smoking cessation, avoidance of certain environmental pollutants, and immunization for influenza and pneumococcal pneumonia. Long-term oxygen therapy has proven helpful in hypoxemic patients. In addition, pulmonary rehabilitation may improve functional status and the quality of life for some patients. Patients with COPD frequently use inhaled beta-adrenergic agents and inhaled or oral steroids. In a patient of any age, treatment goals for COPD are to reduce the symptoms and complications. Along with shortness of breath, presenting symptoms may include fatigue and a decreased activity level. Treatment consists of immediate assessment and correction of respiratory difficulties with the application of supplemental oxygen. Use of CPAP for COPD patients has proven to decrease the morbidity and mortality of patients. The patient may also receive bronchodilators to decrease the shortness of breath, inhaled or oral steroids to decrease inflammation, and antibiotics to treat infection.

Asthma

Approximately 1 in 20 elderly people has a history of asthma or is affected by it. Onset can occur in old age with presenting symptoms of shortness of breath (especially with effort), chronic or nocturnal cough, and wheezing. Patients with asthma that is worsened by exertion may find that they are more susceptible to asthma attacks as they age. Management of asthma in the elderly population is similar to management in other age groups, although when asthma and cardiac disease coexist, the administration of preferred beta-adrenergic agents for asthma may exacerbate cardiac symptoms. Asthma clinical practice guidelines are the same for younger and older patients **Figure 5**. On rare occasions, epinephrine may be indicated for a life-threatening asthma exacerbation. See the chapter, *Respiratory Emergencies* for more information about asthma.

Pulmonary Embolism

Another condition that can cause respiratory distress is pulmonary embolism. Pulmonary embolism occurs when a blood vessel supplying the lung becomes blocked by a clot. Just as is true with the heart, any obstruction in blood flow to the lung can result in irreversible damage or infarction. An embolus is often released from a vein in a lower extremity, the pelvis, or the abdomen but could also result from a damaged heart. Deep venous thrombosis (DVT) is a common cause of pulmonary embolus in which an embolus may become displaced from the vein in which it formed (generally one of the larger veins in the leg).

Prevention of embolism is based on the patient's risk level—high, moderate, or low. Surgical patients are in the highest risk category for potential emboli, and prophylaxis is generally recommended, including warfarin (Coumadin) and/or heparin and compression stockings. The risk of pulmonary embolus increases with age because of increasing immobility

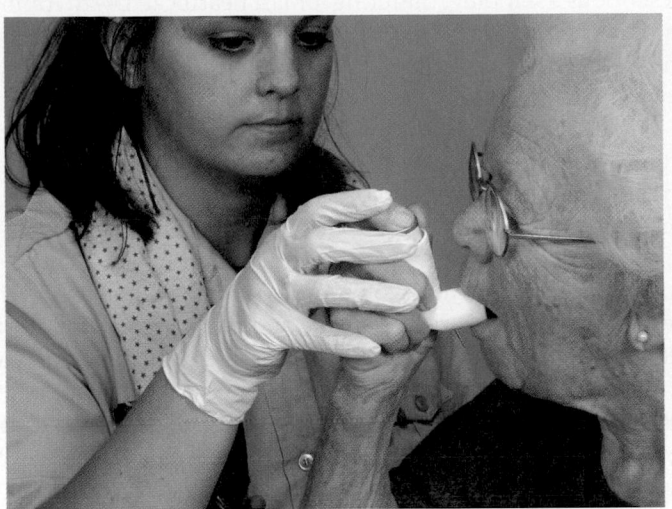

Figure 5 A patient having an asthma attack may have a bronchodilator medication in a metered-dose inhaler. Older patients often do not use an inhaler correctly, so you may need to help with its use.

and increased vascular stasis in the lower extremities. Bed confinement during illness or after surgery will further decrease blood flow in the legs and feet, increasing the chance of DVT and/or pulmonary embolism. Finally, elderly patients have an increased incidence of diseases associated with a higher risk of pulmonary embolus, such as cancer, heart attack, cardiac dysrhythmias, and clotting disorders.

Many pulmonary emboli are silent or present with tachypnea alone—that is, the classic triad of dyspnea, chest pain, and hemoptysis is often altered or absent. If you suspect a pulmonary embolus, check for swelling, erythema, and warmth or tenderness of the lower leg; all of these are signs of a DVT. If DVT might be present, handle the leg gently and monitor the patient for respiratory changes. Prehospital treatment is largely supportive after ensuring that airway and ventilation are adequate. Lysing the thrombus and use of anticoagulation therapies may be considered after a risk assessment is performed, with these measures being followed by rapid transport.

Pathophysiology, Assessment, and Management of Cardiovascular Conditions

The human heart beats 2.5 billion times and moves 200 million liters of blood in an average lifetime. Not surprisingly, this workload affects the cardiovascular system throughout the entire body over the lifespan. Diseases of the heart remain the leading cause of death among older adults in the United States, and coronary artery disease (CAD) is the number one culprit. Heart attack or myocardial infarction is the major cause of morbidity and mortality in people older than 65 years, and

its potential for mortality increases significantly after a person reaches 70 years **Figure 6** .

Myocardial Infarction

Myocardial infarction (MI) or heart attack is the death of part of the heart muscle due to the blockage of one of the coronary arteries. Although chest pain is a common presentation for acute myocardial infarction in older patients, it may be decreased in intensity or atypical. In fact, it may even be absent, with the patient reporting dyspnea, syncope, weakness, confusion, nausea, vomiting, or fatigue. Major risk factors for MI include tobacco use, hypertension, diabetes, obesity, psychosocial factors, genetic predisposition, lack of physical activity, high cholesterol, and alcohol consumption. Preventive strategies include measures to prevent the first MI, avoidance of recurring MIs, and lifestyle interventions. Lifestyle changes include the cessation of tobacco use, eating a healthy diet, control of blood glucose (in diabetics), exercise, weight control, and control of hypertension. A physician may also order aspirin to help reduce the risk of heart attack.

Congestive Heart Failure

People 65 years and older are a high-risk group for congestive heart failure (CHF). In fact, this problem is the most common reason for hospitalization in the geriatric population. CHF is on the rise in this group for two paradoxical reasons: better care of the diseases that might otherwise result in failure (such as CAD and hypertension), which enables patients to live long enough to develop heart failure, and more effective management of heart failure once it develops. Risk factors include gender, ethnicity, family history and genetics, long-term alcohol abuse, and multiple medical conditions—CAD, emphysema, hyperthyroidism,

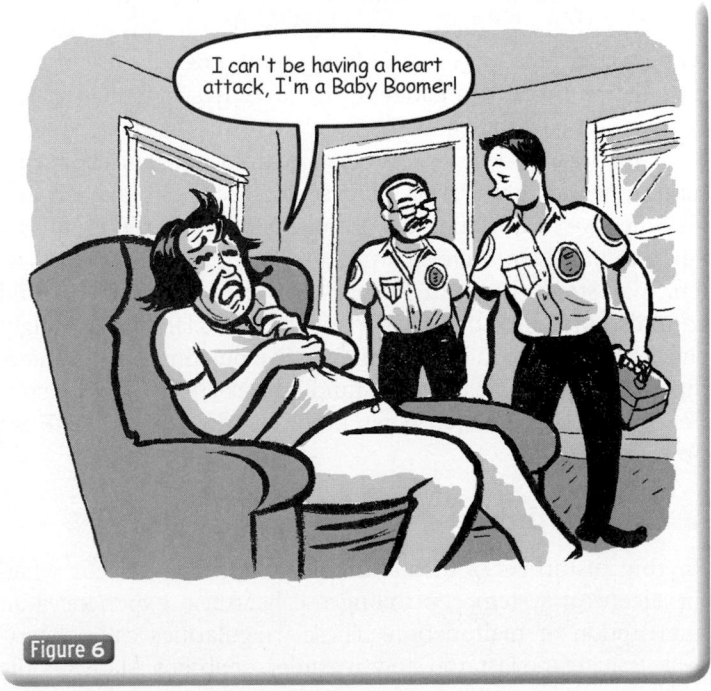

Figure 6

thiamine (vitamin B) deficiency, and human immunodeficiency virus infection, among others. As with MI, prevention is aimed at lifestyle changes: cessation of tobacco use, eating a healthy diet, control of blood glucose (in diabetics), exercise, weight control, and control of hypertension.

Acute exacerbation of CHF results in pulmonary edema that decreases the ability of the lungs to exchange gases. It may present with dyspnea or orthopnea. Because of the decreased oxygenation of all of the organ systems, including the brain, mental status changes may also be seen in acute exacerbation of CHF, including a sensation of air hunger, or the perception that the person cannot take deep enough breaths to get enough air. Peripheral edema may also indicate worsening CHF, although in the absence of other more serious symptoms, it may also be the result of any number of other circulatory, integumentary, or infectious conditions.

The presentation of CHF in an older person can be confused by symptoms and signs symbolic of old age and shared by a number of chronic diseases—for example, dyspnea on exertion, easy fatigability (especially with left-sided heart failure), confusion, crackles on lung exam, orthopnea, dry cough progressing to productive cough, and dependent peripheral edema in right-sided heart failure. Acute exacerbations of CHF are often related to poor diet, medication noncompliance, onset of dysrhythmias such as atrial fibrillation, or acute myocardial ischemia.

Prehospital treatment is unchanged from that of younger patients, although greater consideration is given to becoming familiar with the patient's medications and their implications for your proposed treatment. Evaluation of end-tidal carbon dioxide ($ETCO_2$) should be done immediately and be monitored throughout the transport. For example, the patient taking long-term furosemide (Lasix) may not respond to the usual dose of the same drug that you administer as an acute therapy. Additional treatments by prehospital providers should include close monitoring of fluids and avoidance of excessive fluid overload, use of CPAP, use of digoxin or diltiazem (Cardizem) in patients with atrial fibrillation or atrial flutter, and, possibly, use of anti-coagulation therapy in patients with atrial dysrhythmias to prevent thromboembolism.

CHF may also be exacerbated by fluid imbalances, particularly when overhydration occurs. Because the weakened and less-effective heart is not able to adequately pump normal vascular volumes, an increase in volume within the vascular system may stress the heart further. It is important that IV fluid administration be judicious in patients with CHF because slight changes can result in significant negative outcomes, and achieving an appropriate balance of fluid and electrolyte administration may be complicated when both dehydration and CHF are present.

Dysrhythmias

Rhythm disturbances (dysrhythmias) of the heart occur when the electrical system controlling the heartbeat experiences an interruption or malfunction. These irregularities cause heartbeats that are too fast, too slow, irregular, or absent. Many people experience an occasional or harmless dysrhythmia that they may

describe as a skipping, fluttering, or fast heartbeat. Dysrhythmias in older people are generally a result of age-related changes in the heart, existing cardiac disease, adverse drug effects, or a combination of these factors.

Cardiac dysrhythmias are classified by the part of the heart from which they originate. Unlike tachydysrhythmias or brady-dysrhythmias that speed up or slow down the heart, premature beats signify no change in speed but rather alter the regularity of the heartbeat. In contrast, atrial fibrillation (coming from the atria), which is the most common dysrhythmia among elderly people, increases the risk of stroke and heart failure. The fibrillating atria allow stasis of the blood, thereby encouraging clot formation and increasing the chances that a clot fragment might travel to the brain and cause a stroke. Most of the blood in the atria enters the ventricles when the valves open, with about 20% being kicked in by contraction of the atria. The aging heart may function adequately when preload provided by the atria ends up in the ventricles; however, when that 20% remains in the atria, new signs or symptoms of heart failure may develop or stable heart failure may decompensate.

Bradycardias are also more common in elderly people. The aging conduction system may produce sinus abnormalities such as sick sinus syndrome. CAD may produce high-degree blocks, whereas medications such as beta blockers or calcium channel blockers can slow the heart too much. Even seemingly benign conditions, such as constipation, can result in bradycardia, particularly when the patient strains to have a bowel movement. Nonperfusing rhythms receive the same treatment as given to younger adults. Survival depends on the prearrest health of the patient and the early deployment of the links in the chain of survival (early recognition, early CPR, early defibrillation, early ALS and post-resuscitative measures).

Hypertension

More than half of all older persons are hypertensive. The majority have isolated systolic hypertension resulting from a loss of arterial elasticity. Controlling systolic and/or diastolic hypertension in elderly people helps prevent strokes and MIs. Geriatric hypertensive emergencies require a controlled decline in blood pressure that often cannot be achieved in the field, and the use of nitroglycerin for treatment of hypertensive emergencies is heavily debated. In case of rapid onset of symptomatic systolic hypertension, treatment aims to reduce the systolic pressure with antihypertensive therapy that can minimize cardiovascular and cerebrovascular morbidity and mortality.

Aneurysms

The incidence of aneurysm increases with age. An aneurysm is a weakness in any artery that produces a balloon defect, weakening the arterial wall. This weakness may be congenital (present at birth) or acquired. In the latter case, hypertension, atherosclerotic disease, and obesity are contributing factors to development of this defect. For example, a blood pressure reading of greater than 160/95 mm Hg doubles the mortality risk in men and can lead to kidney loss and blindness by damaging the blood vessels that supply the kidney and eyes. Life-threatening aneurysms can develop in the brain, chest, or abdomen. A new headache or a change in chronic headache patterns, for example, may signal early cerebral bleeding from an aneurysm; all too often, the first manifestation is a sudden and devastating stroke. Use of anticoagulants for the management of cardiac disease increases the negative effects of an aneurysm by increasing the amount of time necessary for bleeding to stop. Preventive measures—proper diet, exercise, smoking cessation, and cholesterol control—aim to control the risk factors associated with hypertension and atherosclerotic diseases.

Thoracic aneurysms generally remain asymptomatic until they become large or rupture. Early symptoms may be related to compression by the aneurysm, such as difficulty swallowing or hoarseness from laryngeal nerve pressure. Abdominal aortic aneurysms present typically with abdominal pain or possibly only with back pain. Asymptomatic thoracic and abdominal aneurysms that do not exceed a certain size and are not expanding are generally treated without surgery but are reassessed on a regular schedule. In an older patient with back pain, examine the chest and abdomen carefully. The treatment of abdominal emergencies is surgical, so early recognition, assessment, stabilization, and rapid transport to an appropriate medical facility are essential.

Traumatic Aortic Disruption

Traumatic aortic disruption or aortic dissection occurs when the inside wall of the artery becomes torn and allows blood to collect between the arterial wall layers. It may occur with trauma or sustained hypertension, particularly when an abdominal aortic aneurysm (AAA) is present. Dissection weakens the arterial wall, making it prone to rupture. A thoracic dissection, for example, can produce chest pain that is difficult to differentiate from cardiac ischemia. Therefore, it is helpful to obtain blood pressure readings in both arms in all patients with chest pain. A systolic blood pressure difference of 15 mm Hg or higher suggests a thoracic dissection.

Stroke

Stroke is a significant cause of death and disability in elderly people. More than 80% of all stroke deaths occur in persons older than 65 years, and stroke is the leading cause of long-term disability at any age. Strokes, which are mainly caused by atherosclerosis, are responsible for 1 of every 15 deaths in the United States. The risk of stroke doubles each decade after 35 years, mirroring the increase in risk factors such as hypertension and atrial fibrillation. Hypertension is the primary risk factor for stroke, but age, family history, smoking, diabetes, high cholesterol, and heart disease also contribute. Normal changes of aging, such as loss of vascular elasticity, also place the older patient at an increased risk of hemorrhagic stroke. Prevention is aimed at reduction of risk factors, improving diet, exercise, and lowering cholesterol. Because time is crucial in stroke treatment, many communities are also encouraging early recognition of stroke symptoms through public media campaigns.

Effective prehospital acute stroke care includes early recognition, discovery of conditions that mimic strokes (such as hypoglycemia or hypoxia), and timely transport to the most appropriate facility. Use a stroke assessment tool as appropriate, taking the patient's history into account when you are assessing the components of the scale. An older person with severe arthritis may not move as well on one side, or damage from a previous stroke may make his or her speech difficult to assess. Always ask family or caregivers for information that may help you identify deviations from the patient's normal pattern of behavior or activity.

Family members or caregivers can provide valuable input into the patient's baseline cognitive status, personality, and ADL. When you are evaluating the patient's cognitive level, evaluate the patient's ability to perform basic cognitive functions such as recalling events, learning, and remembering (such as the provider's name) and the ability to follow commands. Caregivers will also have an insight into the patient's normal responses. They will be able to inform the providers if the patient is normally agitated, irritable, or depressed, if the personality change is a new onset or if the personality change is a symptom of an underlying disorder, or if the change is caused by the presence of unfamiliar people. ADLs are the skills required for daily self-care. These skills include the ability to walk, the ability to dress appropriately for the environment, the ability to maintain reasonable standards for home cleanliness, and the ability to care for basic hygiene needs. Caregivers will be aware of the patient's ability to perform ADLs and if this ability has decreased.

Documentation and Communication

A stroke is a traumatic and emotional event for the patient, and a sensitive and compassionate approach is essential. Even though the patients may not be able to communicate with you, they can often understand. Communicate with them as you would any other patient—in a calm and reassuring manner.

Transient Ischemic Attack

Transient ischemic attacks (also called TIAs and ministrokes) entail a temporary disturbance of blood supply to the brain that results in a sudden, temporary decrease in brain function. The symptoms are the same as those for a stroke but generally last less than 24 hours; they are warning signs of a future stroke. Although a TIA results in no lasting damage to the brain, the gravity of this condition should not be minimized in the field. Because of the short amount of time that you often have with your patient, you most likely will not be able to make a determination of whether the patient is experiencing a stroke or a TIA, and for this reason, any patient experiencing stroke-like symptoms should be treated as though he or she is having a stroke. Furthermore, patients who report a history of previous TIAs should be considered at a much higher risk of having a stroke instead of another TIA.

Words of Wisdom

Prehospital treatment for chest pain remains essentially unchanged in elderly patients, albeit with extra cautions because of the increased potential for medication side effects. As in all prehospital emergencies, health care providers must prioritize the patient's airway, breathing, and circulatory status. Nitroglycerin and morphine may produce more hypotension or respiratory compromise than in younger patients or may react adversely with long-term medications. Ensure that patients are not taking erectile dysfunction medications prior to nitroglycerin administration. Aspirin may increase bleeding in a patient who is already taking anticoagulants. For patients 75 years or older with ST-segment elevation infarcts, angioplasty offers a better outcome than peripheral fibrinolysis.

■ Pathophysiology, Assessment, and Management of Neurologic Conditions

Normal age-related cognitive changes have two major features: (1) They are relatively isolated (that is, they are not associated with multiple abnormal neurologic findings that suggest specific disease states), and (2) the onset and progression of these findings are "in time" with the person's aging process (that is, the findings are not sudden or extreme, and they do not extend to other abnormalities).

■ Delirium

Delirium (also known as acute brain syndrome or acute confusional state) is a symptom, not a disease. This temporary state is generally a reflection of an underlying disturbance to a person's well-being (usually a treatable physical or mental illness) and is usually reversible.

Delirium is characterized by disorganized thoughts, inattention, memory loss, disorientation, striking changes in personality and affect, hallucinations, delusions, or a decreased level of consciousness. The confusion and disorientation fluctuate with time, and hallucinations may lead to bizarre, uncharacteristic, or confusing behavior. The patient experiences a rapid alteration between mental states, such as lethargy and agitation, serious attention disruption, disorganized thinking, and changes in perception and sensation. Symptoms of delirium may mimic intoxication, drug abuse, or severe psychological disorders, such as schizophrenia.

The assessment and subsequent management of its numerous causes is complicated. In patients with delirium, assess for recent changes in the patient's level of consciousness or orientation. Specifically, look for an acute onset of anxiety, an inability to think logically or maintain attention, and an inability to focus. Also assess for changes in vital signs, temperature (indicating infection), glucose level, and medications—all frequent causes of delirium.

In elderly people, delirium often replaces or confounds the typical presentation caused by a medical problem, an adverse medication effect, or drug or alcohol withdrawal. Causes of delirium may include medications; poisons; electrolyte imbalances; nutritional deficiencies; respiratory, cardiovascular, or nervous system disorders; hyperglycemia or hypoglycemia, environmental emergencies; trauma; and infections such as urinary tract infections and pneumonia. Most important, prehospital providers need to consider neurologic causes (such as Alzheimer disease and Parkinson disease) and endocrine changes (such as diabetes).

YOU are the Medic   PART 3

As you perform your assessment, the patient tells you that she has pain only at the site of the injury. Examination reveals swelling and discoloration of the right ankle. She has good pedal pulses in her right foot. The rest of the assessment findings are unremarkable, and she states that her pain is minimal as long as there is no movement.

Recording Time: 4 Minutes	
Respirations	18 breaths/min
Pulse	98 beats/min, regular and strong
Skin	Warm and dry
Blood pressure	148/86 mm Hg
Spo$_2$	99% on room air
Pupils	Equal and reactive to light

5. Does this patient need ALS care? Why or why not?

6. How would you care for this patient?

Use the mnemonic "DELIRIUMS" to identify other causes of delirium:

D Drugs or toxins (including intoxication or withdrawal)

E Emotional (psychiatric)

L Low Pao_2 (carbon monoxide poisoning, COPD, CHF, acute myocardial infarction, pneumonia)

I Infection (pneumonia, urinary tract infection, sepsis)

R Retention of stool or urine

I Ictal (seizures)

U Undernutrition (including vitamin deficiencies) or underhydration

M Metabolism (thyroid or endocrine, electrolytes, kidneys)

S Subdural hematoma

With delirium, the onset of confusion or disorientation is abrupt (occurring within hours to days) and generally resolves with treatment of the underlying problem. Because of this, treatment of delirium is focused on resolution of the causative disease or disorder, but this may be complicated by the patient's inability to provide an accurate medical history and uncooperative behavior while obtaining diagnostic information.

◼ Dementia

Unlike delirium, <u>dementia</u> produces irreversible brain failure. Dementia signs and symptoms take months to years to become apparent and may include short-term memory loss or shortened attention span, jargon aphasia (talking nonsense), hallucinations, confusion, disorientation, difficulty in learning and retaining new information, and personality changes such as social withdrawal or inappropriate behavior. Dementia is not synonymous with delirium, however, and a patient with dementia can also have delirium.

Disorders that cause dementia include conditions that impair vascular and neurologic structures within the brain, such as infections, strokes, head injuries, poor nutrition, and medications. The two most common degenerative types of dementia in older people are Alzheimer disease (one of the fastest-growing health care problems in the United States) and multi-infarct or vascular dementia, both of which cause structural damage to the brain. Dementia may also be the result of tumors within the brain, emotional disorders, Parkinson disease, or Huntington chorea.

An estimated 6% to 10% of elderly people will eventually have dementia, although this percentage increases with advancing age. Risk factors that may predispose a patient to dementia include a low level of education, female gender, and African American ethnicity, although these are more accurately described as correlating factors rather than causes of dementia.

Dementia may be diagnosed when two or more brain functions are impaired. These cognitive and psychomotor functions consist of language, memory, visual perception, emotional behavior and/or personality, and cognitive skills. Patients with dementia have progressive loss of cognitive function; impairments in long-term or short-term memory, or both; loss of communication skills; inability to perform daily activities; an increased ability to become lost, even in familiar places; and changes in temperment and affect, specifically increasing anger.

Because dementia is a chronic condition, most requests for emergency care will be related to new presentation of dementia-related symptoms or inability to manage behavioral disruptions, such as angry outbursts. There is no treatment for dementia, but acute change in mental status may be related to underlying medical problems that can be treated. It is important to ascertain from caregivers the patient's baseline behaviors and abilities and to ask specifically about the changes that led them to request emergency services at the point that services are provided. Patients may provide inaccurate or conflicting information about their own conditions, and information provided by patients with advancing dementia should be checked against information provided by caregivers. Although most cases of dementia cannot be prevented, some experts suggest that low-fat diets and exercise may help ward off vascular dementia.

Despite the weakened physical condition of patients with dementia, you should be cautious when you are caring for patients with dementia-related complaints because these patients may not be able to rationally evaluate the impact of their behaviors and may attempt to harm you because of confusion or anxiety. Patients with dementia are also at an increased risk of victimization at the hands of caregivers because they are unable to report injury or neglect accurately. Caregiver stress is an additional concern when caring for patients with dementia; referrals to home health agencies, respite care programs, and other community services may be helpful.

◼ Alzheimer Disease

The most common type of dementia in the United States is <u>Alzheimer disease</u>. This progressive loss of function begins with subtle symptoms, such as frequently losing items or difficulty recalling the names of people. With time, patients lose their ability to think, reason clearly, solve problems, and concentrate. They may forget the identities of close family members, including their spouses and children, and they may also forget their own past experiences. In Alzheimer disease, symptoms may present as confusion (lack of familiarity with surroundings), changes in personality or judgment, and extreme difficulty with daily activities, such as feeding, bathing, and bowel and bladder control. As of 2011, this progressive disease cannot be cured or reversed by any known treatment or intervention.

There are approximately 4 million people diagnosed with Alzheimer disease, which is costing the United States over 100 billion dollars annually. It is projected that there will be over 15 million diagnosed patients by the year 2050. There are demonstrated genetic links, including a 40% likelihood that a twin will develop the disease if their twin sibling has it. African Americans are more likely to develop Alzheimer disease, and Latinos are more likely to develop Alzheimer disease earlier. There is also a correlation between decreased education (< 12 years) and Alzheimer disease.

Progression of Alzheimer disease is classified into stages. The earliest stage, mild cognitive impairment (MCI), is more accurately described as a pre-Alzheimer stage because not all patients who develop MCI will progress to Alzheimer disease. It is characterized by forgetfulness, especially forgetting earlier conversations or recent events, difficulty when attempting to perform more than one task at once, diminished problem-solving skills, and increases in the amount of time required to perform more difficult tasks.

Early-stage Alzheimer disease, which involves more cognitive impairment than MCI, involves language problems, misplacing items, getting lost on familiar routes, personality changes and loss of social skills, loss of interest in previously enjoyed activities, and difficulty performing moderately complex tasks that were once easy, such as balancing a checkbook or preparing food using a recipe.

As Alzheimer disease progresses, symptoms become more profound, and include forgetting details about current events and components of a person's life history; changes in sleep patterns, sometimes called "sundowners"; difficulty reading and writing; impairment in assessment of danger and risk; disorganized language use and construction of nonsensical sentences; hallucinations and delusions; dangerous or violent behaviors and agitation; and difficulty performing basic tasks, like preparing simple foods, choosing proper clothing, and driving.

Severe or end-stage Alzheimer disease is seen when people forget things learned in the first 2 or 3 years of life. These patients can no longer understand language, recognize even close family members, or perform basic self-care tasks, such as eating, dressing, and bathing. Patients with end-stage Alzheimer may no longer interact verbally with family members or caregivers. They may also have medical devices, such as gastric tubes and urinary catheters, placed to facilitate the tasks that they can no longer perform, like eating and voiding.

Alzheimer disease is not diagnosed by specific tests, but rather the exclusion of other causes of dementia. The only way to truly diagnose Alzheimer disease is after death by evaluating the brain tissue. When thickened neurofilaments encircle and obscure the nuclei of nerve cells, it is referred to as neurofibrilliary tangles. Neurotic plaques are developed when neurons die and accumulate into clusters. When dying neurons accumulate around proteins, they develop a product known as senile plaque.

Treatment of Alzheimer disease in the prehospital and interfacility setting will generally revolve around supportive care and treating the symptoms. Communicate slowly with these patients and consider other illnesses. Antipsychotics or benzodiazipines may be used for combative patients who are a danger to themselves or others. However, the use of chemical restraints should only be considered after other means of verbal containment have proven ineffective. Daily treatment regimens that Alzheimer patients may be prescribed include the use of antidepressants to assist with depression and cholinesterase inhibitors to help prevent further deterioration and further cognitive decline associated with Alzheimer disease. Examples of cholinesterase inhibitors include donepezil, rivastigmine, and rivastigmine transdermal. Newer medications that have been introduced include memantine, which is an NMDA inhibitor, and galantamine, which is an acetylcholinesterase inhibitor.

Experts have not identified a single cause for Alzheimer disease, but most believe it is not a normal part of the aging process. Although age is a significant risk factor for this disease

(Alzheimer disease typically affects patients older than 60 years), age alone is not the cause.

Parkinson Disease

Patients with Parkinson disease—another age-related neurologic disorder—have two or more of the following symptoms: resting tremor of an extremity, slowness of movement (bradykinesia), rigidity or stiffness of the extremities or trunk, and poor balance. Parkinson disease is caused by degeneration of the substantia nigra, an area of the brain that controls voluntary movement by producing the neurotransmitter dopamine. Cells use dopamine to transmit impulses, so a loss of dopamine results in the loss of muscle function. Parkinson disease can affect one or both sides of the body and produces a wide range of functional loss. Parkinson disease may present as dyskinesia (involuntary movements or tremors affecting one or both sides of the body), dementia, depression, autonomic dysfunction (bladder and GI problems), and postural instability (loss of reflexes or inability to "right oneself").

Seizures

The incidence of seizures (including status epilepticus) is also increased in elderly people, partly because of the increase in risk factors such as stroke, dementia, primary or metastatic brain tumors, and acute metabolic disorders (such as hyperglycemia, hyponatremia, alcohol withdrawal). Prehospital treatment for seizures is the same for younger and older patients.

Pathophysiology, Assessment, and Management of Gastrointestinal Conditions

Constipation is a frequent and significant problem in elderly people. Although it can cause acute abdominal pain, it should not be the initial suspect when a patient experiences such discomfort. Instead, causes with high mortality, such as bleeding from an acute abdominal aneurysm or dead bowel from mesenteric ischemia, should be investigated first. In your assessment of a gastric emergency, ask the patient about food and fluid intake, history of abdominal complaints, current bowel and bladder habits, and medications and supplements before proceeding with a physical exam. Symptoms are often vague and manifest only as diffuse abdominal pain with no particular point of origin. Abdominal and gastric complaints often require surgical treatment, so early recognition and rapid transport for definitive hospital care are the best practice.

Bowel Obstruction

Large bowel obstructions in elderly people are likely to be caused by cancer, impacted stool, or sigmoid volvulus. In addition, small bowel obstruction secondary to gallstones increases significantly with age. One third to one half of all elderly people have cholelithiasis (gallstones), although most remain asymptomatic for life. With one or more episodes of cholecystitis (inflammation of the gallbladder), the gallbladder adheres to the small bowel and, over time, creates an opening, or fistula. The stone(s) drop into the bowel and produce the obstruction. Such a gallstone ileus may account for as many as 25% of geriatric small bowel obstructions. The large and small intestines are at risk for obstruction from adhesions due to previous surgery or infection or when a segment of bowel is forced into a fascial defect (hernia) in the abdominal wall.

Biliary Diseases

Along with implications for small bowel obstructions, biliary diseases, including cirrhosis, hepatitis, and cholecystitis, may also present independently in older patients. Signs and symptoms of biliary disease include jaundice, fever, right upper quadrant pain with possible radiation to the upper back or shoulder, and vomiting or nausea. Jaundice may be more profound in paler patients because less melanin is present to interfere with visibility of bilirubin. Although these diseases cause fever, this response may be repressed in older patients. Pain sensation may be altered, as well, resulting in unusual referral paths or the absence of abdominal pain. Pain management may be indicated for patients with acute cholecystitis; be cautious in administering opiates to older patients, however, because of their decreased ability to compensate for cardiovascular and respiratory changes that may accompany these medications.

Peptic Ulcer Disease

Older patients are more likely than younger ones to have stomach or duodenal ulcers (peptic ulcer disease). The main risk factors for peptic ulcers are regular use of NSAIDs and infection with *Helicobacter pylori* (an ulcer-associated bacterium of the stomach), both of which are more common in older patients. Other medications have also been implicated in ulcer formation. Social factors, such as high-stress professions, and certain personality types have also been associated with ulcer formation. The main symptom of peptic ulcer disease is dyspepsia (gnawing, burning pain in the upper abdomen), which usually improves immediately after eating but returns several hours later. Other causes of dyspepsia include acid reflux, gastritis, and gastric cancer.

Gastrointestinal Bleeding

Gastrointestinal bleeding also becomes more common with age, and it is almost always the result of either physiologic changes that lead to an increased likelihood of bleeding systemically or pathologic processes that specifically impact the digestive system. A number of normal changes of aging increase the time necessary to obtain hemostasis, including decreased vascular tone and thinning of various epithelial tissues. Decreased rates of peristalsis also increase the likelihood that irritating substances will damage the gastric lining. Older patients are also more likely to take medications that alter coagulation, including warfarin, aspirin, and heparin. Pathologic processes within the gastrointestinal system that are sometimes responsible for bleeding include ulcers and varices; cancers of the stomach, esophagus, colon, and rectum; diverticulitis; cirrhosis; and bowel obstructions.

Although the source of gastrointestinal bleeding may vary, the signs and symptoms vary more by the location of the bleeding than the origin. Bleeding from the esophagus is most commonly associated with varices and alcohol abuse; the patient will present with violent vomiting of emesis that contains almost no food and a large quantity of bright red, uncoagulated blood. Bleeding from the stomach may produce either red or darker coffee-ground emesis, and it is most commonly associated with peptic ulcer disease. Bloody stool is usually indicative of bleeding from the lower gastrointestinal system, although blood from the stomach may be digested and appear as dark, tarry stool. Bright red blood in the stool usually comes from the large intestine or rectum, and may be caused by diverticulitis, large bowel obstructions, anal fissures, or hemorrhoids. In general, the darker the blood, the longer it has been in the body, and therefore, the further the distance between the site of bleeding and the portal of exit.

Upper GI hemorrhage occurs when there is bleeding from the esophagus, stomach, or duodenum **Figure 7** . When severe, this condition is a true medical emergency that must be recognized and assessed quickly. Not only are older people more prone to upper GI bleeding, they are in need of urgent surgery and also at a greater risk of complications and death.

It is not possible to determine the cause of upper GI bleeding without an endoscopic examination (inspection of the inside of a hollow organ or body cavity) of the esophagus, stomach, and duodenum. However, obtaining a thorough history can

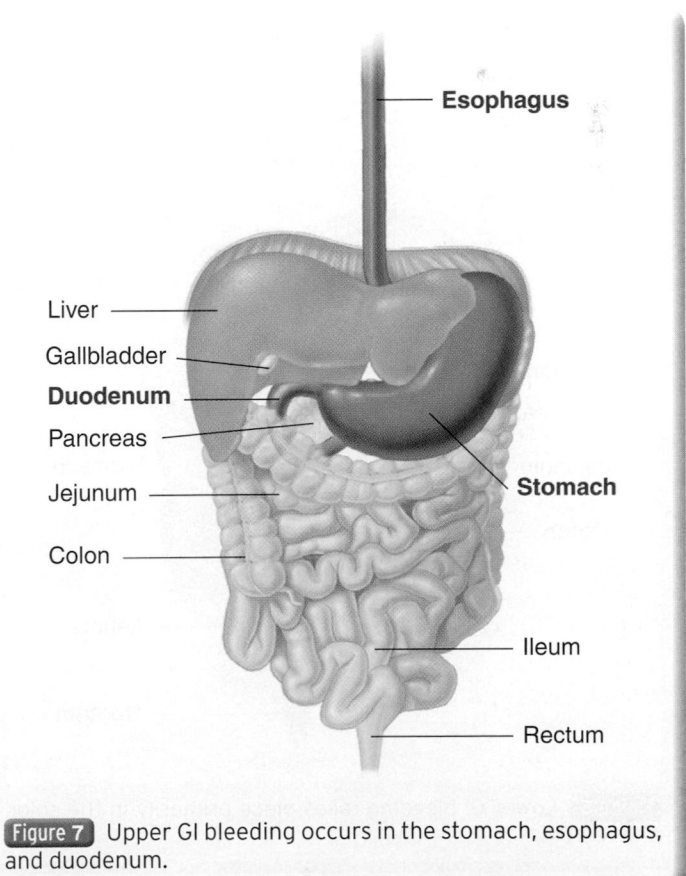

Figure 7 Upper GI bleeding occurs in the stomach, esophagus, and duodenum.

provide you with clues to the cause. Regular use of NSAIDs or alcohol may result in bleeding from irritation of the lining of the stomach or from ulcers (a hollowing out or disintegration of tissue) in the stomach or duodenum. Forceful vomiting can cause tears in the esophagus that may bleed. Cirrhosis of the liver from long-term alcohol use or chronic infectious hepatitis may cause enlargement of the veins (varices) in the esophagus. These varices can rupture and result in massive bleeding. Stomach cancer or esophageal cancer can also produce upper GI bleeding. Recent weight loss or difficulty swallowing would raise the suspicion of cancer as the source of bleeding.

Lower GI hemorrhage primarily describes bleeding from the colon and rectum and should never simply be attributed to hemorrhoids **Figure 8**. Colon polyps and colon cancer are also possible causes, among others. Minor lower GI bleeding is characterized by small amounts of red blood covering formed brown stools or scant amounts of red blood noticed on the toilet paper. Severe lower GI bleeding is characterized by passing significant amounts of red blood or maroon-colored stools.

Assessment should begin with identifying risk factors such as a history of previous lower GI bleeding, symptoms or signs suggestive of colon cancer, recent constipation or diarrhea, and use of medications such as blood thinners. Treat for shock. Blood administration may be necessary during interfacility transport if the patient's hematocrit and hemoglobin decrease significantly. Severe lower GI bleeding requires immediate transportation to the nearest emergency department.

Some signs and symptoms of gastrointestinal bleeding are associated with hypovolemia that occurs from the blood loss. These include agitation, dizziness, syncope, hypotension, and changes in mental status. Others may be associated with the disease processes that caused the bleeding, including jaundice, hepatomegaly, constipation or diarrhea, pain with voiding, nausea, and abdominal pain.

When you arrive at the scene, it is more important for you to be able to assess the severity of the bleeding than to determine the cause of bleeding. Slower bleeding is characterized by emesis with coffee-grounds appearance. With minor bleeding, the pulse rate and systolic blood pressure are normal. Brisk bleeding presents with hematemesis (vomiting red blood) or melena (black, tarlike stools). It is important to note that melena, not pain, is the most common presenting symptom of GI bleeding. Prehospital treatment is supportive, including adequate pain control.

Regardless of the cause of gastrointestinal bleeding, treatment should be focused on recognition and management of hypovolemic shock and transport to a facility capable of providing definitive care because many patients with gastrointestinal bleeding may require surgery to repair the site of injury or disease. Again, be cautious in fluid resuscitation and bear in mind that the older adult's compensatory mechanisms may be altered because of normal aging processes. Finally, keep in mind that these patients may be on blood-thinning medications (warfarin) that prevent them from forming clots to major injuries.

Pathophysiology, Assessment, and Management of Renal Conditions

Although the kidneys of an elderly person may be capable of dealing with day-to-day demands, they may not be able to meet unusual challenges, such as those imposed by illness.

Urinary Tract Infections

The most common hospital-associated infection to cause sepsis in the United States is urinary tract infections (UTI). UTIs usually develop in the lower urinary tract (urethra and bladder) when normal flora (bacteria that naturally populate the skin) enter the urethra and grow. Although UTIs are usually more common in women due to the relatively short urethra and its close proximity to the vagina and rectum, after age 50 years, there is an increase in UTIs in men because of obstruction of the urethra by the prostrate. Common risk factors include diabetes, prostatitis, cystocele (prolapse of the bladder into the vagina), urethrocele (prolapse of the urethra into the vagina), kidney obstruction, and indwelling urinary catheters. While you are performing a physical assessment, you may notice a fever, shortness of breath, gastrointestinal symptoms, neurologic symptoms, poor urinary output, increased urinary frequency, and hematuria. These patients will report painful urination, frequent urges to urinate, and difficulty urinating. You should evaluate the patient's indwelling catheter, if applicable, for sediment, opacity, color, or presence of blood. A strong odor may be present. Later signs and

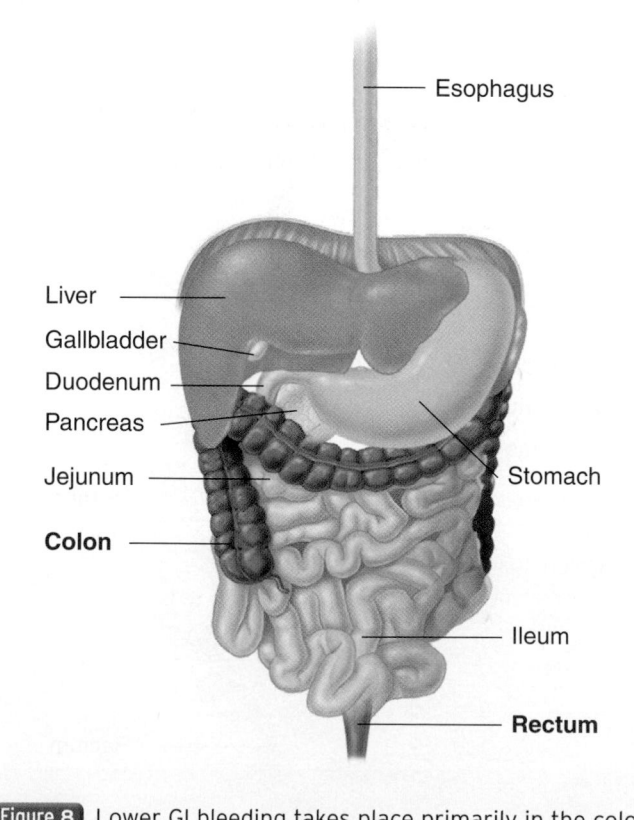

- Esophagus
- Liver
- Gallbladder
- Duodenum
- Pancreas
- Jejunum
- **Colon**
- Stomach
- Ileum
- **Rectum**

Figure 8 Lower GI bleeding takes place primarily in the colon and rectum.

symptoms may include hypotension, tachycardia, diaphoresis, and pale skin.

Renal Failure

Renal failure is the sudden decrease in the rate of filtration through the glomeruli, causing toxins to accumulate in the blood. If the kidneys are no longer able to excrete waste, concentrate urine, and control electrolytes, pH, or blood pressure, then renal failure develops. Approximately 11.5% of US adults older than 20 years have chronic renal failure. Risk factors for chronic renal failure include diabetes, cardiac disease, pyelonephritis, hypertension, autoimmune disorders, glomerulonephritis, and polypharmacy. Chronic renal failure may require lifelong hemodialysis or a kidney transplant. Hemodialysis is a process where patients are attached to a hemodialysis machine for a period of 3 to 4 hours three times a week so that the patient's blood can be filtered through the machine and waste can be removed.

Whereas dialysis treatments are generally considered a BLS nonemergency transport, if a patient misses a treatment, the situation can become an ALS emergency. Signs and symptoms include hypertension, headache, anxiety, fatigue, anorexia, vomiting, increased dark urination, altered mental status, and seizures. A thorough assessment will include obtaining a 12-lead ECG. Electrolyte changes may be present on the ECG. All vital signs should be monitored regularly; however, you should not take blood pressures on the same arm that has a fistula. ETCO$_2$ should be monitored throughout the transport. Breath sounds and bowel sounds should also be monitored. The patient should be transported to a hospital that has hemodialysis capabilities. IV fluids should be administered to assist circulation as necessary. If dysrhythmias are present, they should be treated according to current American Heart Association ACLS guidelines.

Incontinence

Bowel and bladder continence require anatomically correct gastrointestinal and genitourinary tracts, functioning and intact sphincters, and properly working cognitive and physical functions. Urinary incontinence (involuntary loss of urine) can have a significant social and emotional impact, but relatively few people admit to the problem and even fewer seek treatment. Incontinence can lead to skin irritation, skin breakdown, and UTIs. As people age, the capacity of the bladder and the strength of the sphincter muscles decrease. Because pressure on the urinary sphincter is responsible for triggering recognition of the need to urinate, a decrease in sphincter tone may keep older people from realizing that their bladder is full until they can no longer wait to urinate. As a consequence, older people may find it difficult to postpone voiding or may have involuntary bladder contractions. Nighttime incontinence may also be problematic for older people because the weakened sensations of the need to urinate are less likely to wake them from sleep. Additionally,

---

YOU are the Medic   PART 4

You use a pillow to splint her ankle, taking care to mark pedal pulses and check them before and after splinting. An ice pack is also applied. She is loaded onto the stretcher and placed in the ambulance. She tells you that she is not allergic to any medications and that she takes lisinopril for high blood pressure and metformin for diabetes. You establish a 20-gauge IV line in her left antecubital fossa and run normal saline at a keep-vein-open rate. She is transported to Randolph Medical Center for evaluation. On arrival, you give your report to the receiving nurse, restock the truck, and call to report that you are back in service. As part of continuous quality improvement, the run is reviewed by peers.

Recording Time: 18 Minutes	
Respirations	18 breaths/min
Pulse	94 beats/min, regular and strong
Skin	Warm and dry
Blood pressure	146/78 mm Hg
Spo$_2$	100% on room air
Pupils	Equal and reactive to light

7. Is IV therapy within your scope of practice?

8. Does this patient need care that could only be provided by a paramedic-level provider?

9. What type of community service can a paramedic become involved in to become a patient advocate and increase safety?

incontinence sometimes occurs when elderly people recognize the need to urinate and have adequate sphincter control to prevent accidental bladder release, but their physical ability to move to the restroom is limited. In this case, simple modifications, like placing a toilet chair in the person's bedroom, may eliminate incontinence.

Two major types of incontinence are distinguished: stress and urge. Stress incontinence occurs during activities such as coughing, laughing, sneezing, lifting, and exercise. Urge incontinence is triggered by hot or cold fluids, running water, and sometimes simply thinking about going to the bathroom.

Treatment of incontinence consists of bladder training programs, medications, physical therapy, and, depending on the cause, surgery. Because incontinence can be embarrassing, always be discreet and nonjudgmental when you are addressing the topic with patients. If you have enough time and the patient's condition allows you to do so, you may want to help the patient gather his or her own incontinence supplies before being transported to the hospital. If your patient experiences a loss of bladder control, you should cover the patient until his or her clothing can be changed. During long transports, you should make an effort to reduce the amount of time that the patient wears urine-soaked clothing or absorbent undergarments; beyond the temporary discomfort and shame associated with incontinence, a patient who must sit in urine for a long period of time may experience new or worsening skin breakdown.

The opposite of incontinence is urinary retention or difficulty urinating. Patients may have difficulty voiding or absence of voiding as a result of many medical causes. In men, benign enlargement of the prostate, also known as benign prostatic hypertrophy, can place pressure on the urethra, making voiding difficult and frequent. Patients with this condition may experience difficulty sleeping because of the frequent need to urinate with little production. Bladder and urinary tract infections can also cause inflammation that results in retention of urine; the pain associated with urination during such infections may lead patients to intentionally avoid urination, as well. The placement and subsequent removal of a urinary catheter can also lead to retention. Because of the loss of elasticity of the bladder wall, some patients are able to urinate and empty most of the bladder's contents while retaining a small amount of urine. This residual retention can lead to an increased risk of UTIs.

Temporary urinary retention may lead to pain and abdominal distention, and in severe or prolonged cases of urinary retention, patients may have acute or chronic renal failure.

Pathophysiology, Assessment, and Management of Endocrine Conditions

Many endocrine changes may have occurred earlier in life and been diagnosed before intervention by prehospital providers became necessary. Geriatric patients may have diseases such as Grave disease (hyperthyroidism), Addison disease (hypoadrenalism), Cushing syndrome (hyperadrenalism), osteoporosis, or diabetes.

Special Populations

Acute delirium in the elderly is always a sign of physical illness or drug intoxication and is always an emergency.

Diabetic Disorders

Diabetes is the result of the body's inability to oxidize complex carbohydrates (sugars) due to impaired pancreatic activity—namely, production of insulin. Insulin moves carbohydrates out of the bloodstream, through the cellular walls, and into the cells to be metabolized. With diabetes, more glucose is present in the blood than the body can handle. In people older than 65 years, one of every five people in the United States has diabetes—primarily type 2 diabetes (formerly called adult-onset, or non–insulin-dependent diabetes mellitus [NIDDM]). Type 1 diabetes has historically been referred to as insulin-dependent diabetes mellitus (IDDM) or juvenile diabetes, because it generally affects children. Many normal changes of aging contribute to the development of diabetes. The most common risk factor for this disease is having more than one chronic disease, and many elderly people with diabetes also have hypertension, heart disease, and stroke. Other risk factors for diabetes include a family history of diabetes, genetics, age, diet, obesity, and a sedentary lifestyle. Management of diabetes is complicated when other acute diseases are present, particularly infections, and because the elderly are more likely to have several comorbid disorders, this is especially true for them.

In the emergency setting, diabetes can result in two life-threatening conditions: hypoglycemia and hyperglycemia. Normal blood glucose levels range from approximately 70 to 120 mg/dL. Hypoglycemia occurs when blood glucose levels drop to 45 mg/dL or less, and hyperglycemia occurs when the levels of glucose in the blood exceed the normal range of 70 to 120 mg/dL.

Geriatric patients with diabetes are at increased risk for hypoglycemia for several reasons: confusion about medication doses or usage, inadequate or irregular dietary intake, inability to recognize the warning signs due to cognitive problems, and/or blunted warning signs. Delirium may be the only indication of hypoglycemia in an elderly patient. Other symptoms include mental status changes and confusion, diaphoresis, and decreased respiratory effort.

Symptoms of an elevated blood glucose level (hyperglycemia) include fatigue, poor wound healing, blurred vision, and frequent infections. Other symptoms of chronic hyperglycemia include the three Ps: polyuria (excessive urine output), polydipsia (excessive thirst), and polyphagia (excessive eating). New-onset diabetes in geriatric patients is often a mild progression that produces no symptoms.

Older people with diabetes and consistently high blood glucose levels are more prone to hyperosmolar nonketotic coma (HONK), also called hyperosmolar hyperglycemic nonketotic coma (HHNC), than diabetic ketoacidosis (DKA). DKA is a life-threatening condition that is associated predominantly with type 1 diabetes (patients who have this condition tend to be young—teenagers and young adults). See the chapter, *Endocrine Emergencies*, for more information on this condition.

The most frequent cause for HONK/HHNC is infection. Other potential risk factors include hypothermia, hyperthermia, cardiac disease, pancreatitis, and stroke. The patient is likely to present with hyperglycemia that is generally greater than 500 mg/dL and has acute confusion with dehydration, although signs of dehydration may be altered in elderly patients Table 3. With HONK/HHNC, hyperglycemia and hyperosmolarity lead to osmotic diuresis and an osmotic shift of fluid to the intravascular space, resulting in further intracellular dehydration. Signs and symptoms include dizziness, confusion, altered mental status, and polydipsia. Prehospital treatment remains the same as for younger patients, albeit with a cautious approach to fluid resuscitation.

Assessment of hyperglycemia and hypoglycemia are complicated by many of the changes associated with aging. Changes in peripheral vascular function, in particular, make assessment of skin condition for key signs of hypoglycemia much more difficult because many older patients may be paler and cooler at baseline. Diaphoresis may also be less prominent due to changes in regulatory mechanisms and secretory functions of the skin. Baseline alterations of mentation may also be confused with acute mental status changes that are related to either hyperglycemia or hypoglycemia.

You should ensure that all vital signs, including blood pressure, blood glucose levels, temperature, and distal pulses, are assessed every 15 minutes and monitored for changes. A 12-lead ECG should also be obtained to help evaluate for other possible causes. Capnography should be used throughout the transport to monitor ETCO$_2$ as well as ventilatory status. Whereas SpO$_2$ is a valuable tool, poor perfusion may make it difficult to obtain an SpO$_2$ reading.

Treatment of diabetic emergencies in the elderly patient is no different than treatment in other populations, although care with fluid resuscitation and electrolyte balance is of particular importance. Recognition of return to baseline levels of function is also more important because this may not be as universal in older populations as it is in younger groups.

Prevention of type 2 diabetes is aimed at changes in lifestyle that include dietary restrictions, exercise, and controlling obesity. Long-term management may include limiting of carbohydrate intake and the use of insulin and oral antihyperglycemic agents. Diabetes management also focuses on preventing many of the devastating systemic effects of the disease, including aggressive wound management, frequent screening for impaired renal function, and management of pain associated with neuropathy.

Thyroid Disorders

Thyroid abnormalities also increase with aging. Many older patients remain asymptomatic, and the disease is diagnosed only when a routine blood test reveals a thyroid problem. Adult hypothyroidism is sometimes called *myxedema*. The condition is manifested by a general slowing of the body's metabolic processes due to the reduction or absence of thyroid hormone. With hypothyroidism, the signs and symptoms may match those seen with normal aging: cold intolerance, constipation, dry skin, weakness, and weight gain. Prior thyroidectomy is also more common in elderly patients, and most of them will take synthetic thyroid hormones.

For acute-onset hyperthyroidism (thyrotoxicosis), the presentation can be blunted; although tachycardia is generally present, older patients may experience less tremor, anxiety, or hyperactive reflexes than younger patients. Atrial fibrillation is more likely to be induced by an overactive thyroid gland in a geriatric patient. A smaller percentage of elderly patients with hyperthyroidism present with symptoms opposite of those expected: weakness, lethargy, and depression. Patients with hyperthyroidism or hypothyroidism are likely to require supplemental oxygen. Hypoglycemia may need correction with 50% dextrose (D$_{50}$). Hypothyroid conditions may lead to diminished respiratory effort that may require positive-pressure ventilation.

Continued decrease of hormone levels may lead to myxedema coma, an extreme manifestation of hypothyroidism that is accompanied by physiologic decompensation. Myxedema coma is four to eight times more likely in women than men and occurs primarily in the elderly population. See the chapter, *Endocrine Emergencies*, for more information on these conditions.

Pathophysiology, Assessment, and Management of Immunologic Conditions

Infections in older persons can be severe and dangerous. Sepsis occurs as the result of an infection and is a disease state that results from the presence of microorganisms or their toxic products in the bloodstream. This is a serious problem that you should know how to recognize and treat. Think of sepsis whenever you see a hot, flushed patient who is also tachycardic and tachypneic. Other signs of sepsis include an oral temperature of greater than 100.4°F (38°C) or less than 96.8°F (36°C), a respiratory rate of more than 20 breaths/min or a partial pressure of carbon dioxide in the blood (PaCO$_2$) of less than 32 mm Hg, and a pulse rate of greater than 90 beats/min. If available, consider measuring lactate levels with a point of care device. Sepsis can be caused by bacteria, fungi, and viruses.

Table 3 Signs of Dehydration in Elderly People

- Dry tongue
- Longitudinal furrows in the tongue
- Dry mucous membranes
- Weak upper body musculature
- Confusion
- Difficulty in speech
- Sunken eyes

Pathophysiology, Assessment, and Management of Toxicologic Conditions

As the number of uses for medications increases, there is a proportional increase in the likelihood of adverse drug reactions and interactions. Elderly people are particularly prone to adverse reactions, even when they take drugs at doses that would be safe in younger people. This increased incidence of adverse drug reactions among elderly people seems to reflect changes in drug metabolism because of diminished hepatic function; in drug elimination because of diminished renal function; in body composition, including increased body fat and decreased body water, altering the distribution of drugs through the various body compartments; and in the responsiveness to drugs that affect the CNS. A change in any one of these processes can lead to toxic effects in elderly people.

Other body changes may affect medication use by geriatric patients in a more general way. As vision declines with age, reading small print becomes more difficult. Night vision becomes less acute, so reading labels in dim light can lead to errors. Short-term memory loss may lead to forgetfulness about whether medications have been taken. An inability to distinguish flavors may cause patients to take multiple doses of medications before they detect problems.

Polypharmacy and Medication Noncompliance

Elderly people consume more than 25% of all prescribed and over-the-counter drugs sold in the United States. Community-dwelling older persons take an average of three to five medications per day. Nursing home patients take an average of six to seven routinely scheduled medications daily (polymedicine) and two to three additional medications on an as-needed basis. This kind of **polypharmacy** may be therapeutic when multiple drugs are needed to manage different medical problems, but it may prove harmful when these medications interact because they have not been adjusted for the multiple medications or multiple organs that are affected. Elderly patients are particularly prone to having multiple chronic diseases, which may lead to a vicious cycle: The presence of multiple disease states leads to the use of multiple medications, which increases the likelihood of adverse reactions, which in turn leads to treatment with more medications. In turn, a person's chance of ending up in the hospital because of an adverse reaction to a medication increases with the number of drugs taken and should be considered when you are assessing the patient's chief complaint. Ultimately, the best dosage of a drug for an elderly patient is the lowest dosage that will achieve a therapeutic effect.

Another compounding issue that may arise is that the patients may not be receiving their medication due to caregiver theft. This is not isolated to home caregivers, but can also occur in long-term care facilities. This should be suspected if patients report immense pain with corresponding vital signs.

Medication noncompliance in older patients is also associated with negative effects on health. Many patients—not just older patients—do not follow instructions or advice on the use of their medications. Because elderly people use more medications than the rest of the population, noncompliance issues are more likely. Noncompliance issues include failure to fill a prescription (for example, the patient does not have the money to pay for the drug or does not see the benefits of it), improper administration of medication (for example, the patient decreases the dosage to make the prescription last longer), discontinuation of medication (for example, the patient feels better and decides not to take the medication), and taking inappropriate medications (for example, the patient had medication left over from a previous prescription or shares the medicine with family or friends). Patients may be taking medications prescribed by more than one physician, each dispensing prescriptions without knowledge of the others' orders. Patients may also take over-the-counter medications or medications prescribed for a family member or friend. Compliance can become complicated because of difficult drug regimens that may change based on physician evaluation. Difficult drug regimens may be forgotten by the patient, especially if it has changed recently. Furthermore, patients may not understand the prescribed drug regimen or may have some difficulty opening the medication containers.

Special Populations

The best dosage of a drug for an elderly patient is the lowest dose that will achieve a therapeutic effect.

Pharmacokinetics

Another factor contributing to the toxic effects of drugs in elderly people is aging-related alterations in pharmacokinetics (that is, the absorption, distribution, metabolism, and excretion of drugs). Geriatric patients are predisposed to medicine-related reactions owing to the previously mentioned age-related physiologic changes that occur in body systems and body composition. For example, an increase in the proportion of adipose tissue can prolong the half-life of a drug. In particular, medications that affect the CNS are the most common source of adverse or unexpected reactions, and barbiturates and benzodiazepines are the drugs most often associated with toxic effects. For this reason, you should consider reducing the dosage of medications that affect the CNS. For example, consider administering 25 μg instead of 50 μg of fentanyl. A reduction in the nervous system response—especially the decrease in parasympathetic activity typically seen with the aging process—increases the risk that adverse anticholinergic effects will occur. Reduced beta-adrenergic receptor sensitivity (which is responsible for bronchodilation) makes most bronchodilator medications less effective. The use of diuretics and antihypertensive medications by geriatric patients can cause hypotension and orthostatic changes due to reduced cardiac output and a decrease in total body water. Finally, decreased glucose tolerance may cause medications such as diuretics and corticosteroids to have hyperglycemic effects.

Pharmacokinetics may also be influenced by diet, smoking, alcohol consumption, and use of other drugs. Drugs such as digoxin that depend on the liver and kidney for metabolism and excretion are particularly likely to accumulate to toxic levels in older patients. With most drugs, little is known about the optimal dosage for elderly people because nearly all clinical trials to establish the safe dosages of drugs are performed in young populations. For the most part, dosages for elderly people need to be reduced compared with those for younger patients ("start low, go slow").

Although almost any drug can produce toxic effects in an older person, certain drugs and classes of drugs are implicated more often than others; Table 4 lists the "dirty dozen." Typically toxic effects present with psychiatric symptoms (such as hallucinations, paranoia, delusions, agitation, and psychosis) and cognitive impairment (such as delirium, confusion, disorientation, amnesia, stupor, and coma) Figure 9 .

Table 4 Drugs Most Commonly Causing Toxic Reactions in Elderly People

Medication	Symptoms
Anti-inflammatory agents (NSAIDs, steroids)	Drowsiness, dizziness, confusion, anxiety, bradypnea, tachypnea, GI bleeding
Antibiotics	GI signs, altered mental status, seizures, coma
Anticholinergics and antihistamines	Urination difficulty, constipation, drowsiness, restlessness, irritability, hypertension
Anticoagulants (warfarin)	Ecchymosis, epistaxis, hematuria, abdominal pain, vomiting, fecal blood
Antidysrhythmics (amiodarone, lidocaine)	Restlessness, hypotension, bradycardia, tachycardia, palpitations, angina
Antidepressants (tricyclics, long-acting selective serotonin reuptake inhibitors)	Confusion, delirium, disorientation, memory impairment
Antihypertensives (diuretics, alpha blockers, beta blockers; angiotensin-converting enzyme inhibitors)	Hypotension, palpitations, angina, fluid retention, headache
Antipsychotics (phenothiazines, atypicals)	Drowsiness, tachycardia, dizziness, restlessness
Digoxin	Headache, fatigue, malaise, drowsiness, depression
Insulin and oral antidiabetic medications	Hypoglycemia presenting as confusion
Narcotics	Delirium, respiratory depression, apnea, involuntary muscle movements
Sedative-hypnotics (benzodiazepines, barbiturates)	Incoordination, dizziness, disturbances in cognitive function

Words of Wisdom

Bring all of the patient's medications—prescription and non-prescription—to the hospital.

Drug and Alcohol Abuse

Alcohol is the preferred substance of abuse among older persons, in whom its use is on the rise. A much smaller but increasing segment of the geriatric population uses illicit drugs. Another common form of abuse includes prescription drug abuse. Many geriatric patients see multiple physicians for various disorders that may include pain management and/or require sedation. Some states have instituted a statewide system to control and monitor scheduled medication distribution, and it is used by all pharmacies in the participating states. These measures help prevent the same medications being prescribed by multiple physicians. Most users are men, and more than half carry their addiction into old age. About one third develop an abuse problem after reaching 65 years, often in response to a life-changing event such as the loss of a spouse, declining health, or low self-esteem.

The prevalence of alcohol and drug misuse among older people is also attributable to the multiplicity of medications that are prescribed for them and their heightened vulnerability to abuse owing to the effects of aging. Decreased body mass and total body water means higher concentrations of blood alcohol; at the same time, the combination of digestive, renal, and hepatic system changes means slower elimination of alcohol from the body.

As the geriatric population continues to grow and experiences even more chronic disabilities, the likelihood of substance

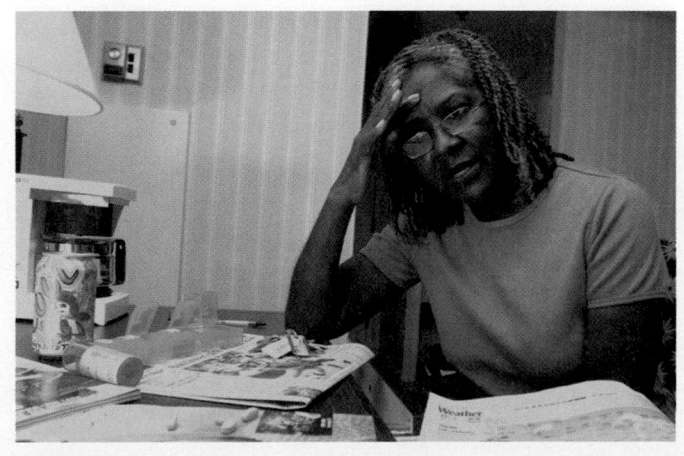

Figure 9 The toxic effects of drugs may initially manifest in the form of confusion.

abuse–related problems in this group will increase. Recognizing substance abuse in older people can be difficult. If they have engaged in this behavior for a long time, it may be well hidden from—or even accepted by—family and friends. Because substance abuse can complicate your field assessment and treatment, it is important to ask about this issue.

Pathophysiology, Assessment, and Management of Psychological Conditions

Depression is not part of normal aging, but rather a medical disease that occurs in about 6% of the population older than 65 years. Depression can be a normal, short-term reaction to a particular event. When sadness, restlessness, fatigue, and hopelessness persist for weeks, however, it becomes a larger concern. Depression in the geriatric population is a major health problem with an incidence growing in tandem with the progressive aging of the population. This trend can be attributed to increases in polypathology, psychosocial stress, and aging-related changes in the brain that collectively lead to greater cognitive impairment, increased medical illness, dependency on health care services, and more suicide attempts Figure 10 . Depression may also occur when a patient takes a variety of medications; such polypharmacy is more likely when the person has multiple medical conditions that result in more vulnerability to toxic effects.

The good news is that depression is treatable with medication and therapy. The bad news is that if depression goes unrecognized or untreated, it is associated with a higher suicide rate in the elderly population than in any other age group. Depression in elderly patients can mimic the effects of many other medical problems (such as dementia). Risk factors for depression in older people include a history of depression, chronic disease, and loss (function, independence, or significant others). This condition may be difficult to recognize in older people because many do not want to complain about feeling sad, worthless, or unwanted.

Disturbingly, the majority of elder suicides occur in people who have recently been diagnosed with depression. In addition, the majority of suicide victims have seen their primary care physician within the month before the event. Unlike younger people, geriatric patients typically do not make suicidal gestures or attempt to get help. Instead, the rate of completed suicide is disproportionately high in the geriatric population. Many geriatric patients see no other way out when they have a terminal illness or debilitating cardiac or neurologic condition (such as severe heart disease or stroke). At highest risk are Caucasian men 85 years and older who use firearms as their suicide method of choice.

When you are dealing with psychological emergencies with geriatric patients, you need to determine whether the situation is a true behavioral emergency or a behavioral crisis. A behavioral emergency implies a significant risk of serious harm to self or others unless intervention is undertaken immediately. Examples include serious suicidal states, potential violence, and impaired judgment that could leave a person at risk of injury or death. In a behavioral crisis, the patient's ability to cope is insufficient and he or she becomes overwhelmed, sending the patient in search of alternative methods of coping Figure 11 .

When you are dealing with a patient's mental illness or psychotic episodes, always remember that a person who is psychotic is out of touch with reality. Many forms of psychotic behavior are possible, including schizophrenic and paranoid behaviors. All symptoms associated with psychotic conditions may not be present when a patient is having an episode, however. Clues to psychotic behavior might include the patient becoming excited or angry for no apparent reason, engaging in antisocial activity or being a loner, and sleeping during the day and staying awake at night. You should consider underlying medical conditions as possible causes of altered behavior. Information about changes in the patient's normal routine may be obtained from family, friends, or caregivers.

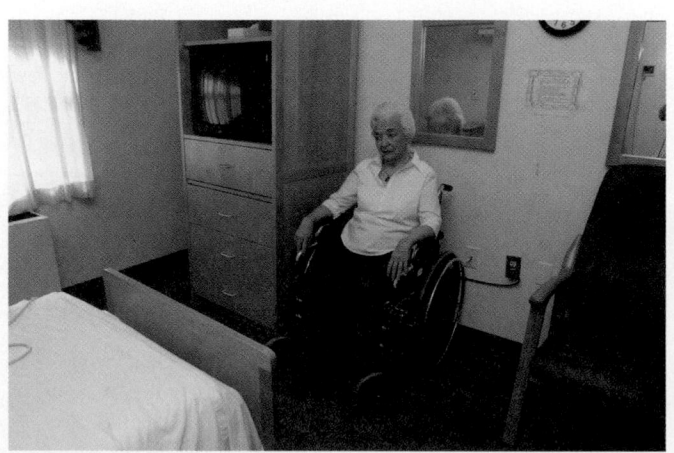

Figure 10 Isolation and chronic medical problems are among the factors that contribute to depression in older adults.

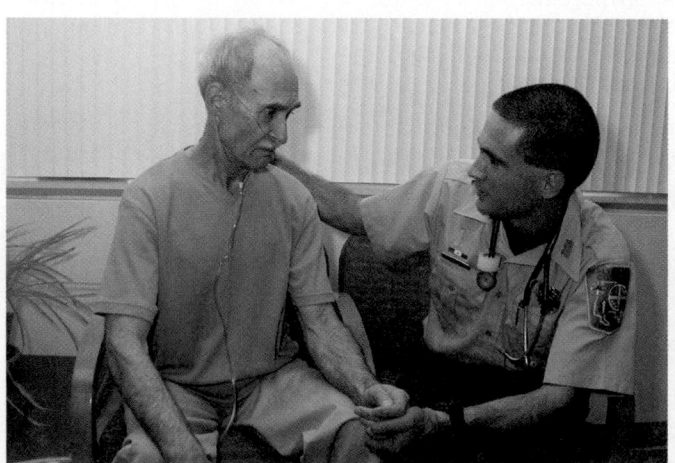

Figure 11 A patient in a behavioral crisis may be searching for alternative methods of coping.

Pathophysiology, Assessment, and Management of Integumentary Conditions

Elderly patients are at higher risk for secondary infection after the skin breaks, skin tumors, and fungal or viral infections of the skin. Many wounds that heal quickly in younger patients take much longer to heal in older patients. Cumulative sun and toxin exposure also increase the likelihood of developing cancerous skin lesions.

Herpes Zoster

Herpes zoster (shingles) is caused by the reactivation of the varicella virus on nerve roots. This condition is more common in the older population, especially if they had chicken pox during the first year of life. Most people with herpes zoster are in good health, but people with cancer or immunosuppression are at higher risk. This condition affects any nerve in the body, but the thoracic nerves and the ophthalmic division of the trigeminal nerve are most common. The disease usually starts with pain in the affected area. Subsequently, a cluster of tiny blisters (vesicles) erupts on reddened skin in the same area. The rash is typically unilateral; it rarely crosses the midline.

One of the most common complications of herpes zoster is pain, or postherpetic neuralgia. During the acute phase of the infection, the person may have severe pain and require narcotic pain relievers. Antiviral medications such as acyclovir and famciclovir can be used, preferably within 48 hours of the activation of the disease. These medications decrease healing time, new lesion formation, and pain.

Cellulitis

Cellulitis is an acute inflammation in the skin caused by a bacterial infection Figure 12 . This condition usually affects the lower extremities. Symptoms include fever, chills, and general malaise. Cellulitis can cause warmth, swelling, redness, tenderness,

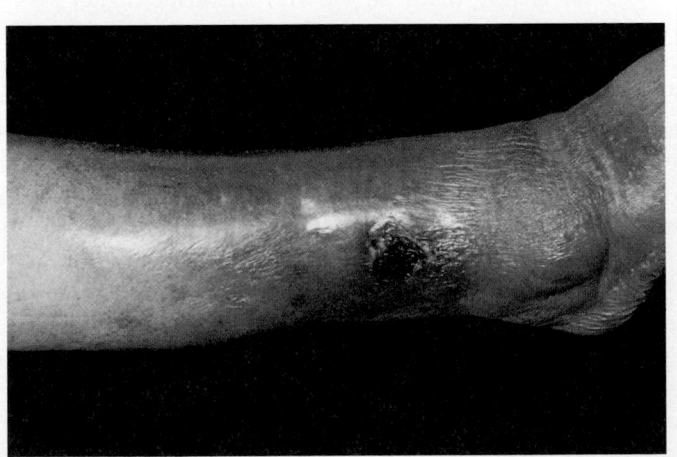

Figure 12 Cellulitis is a diffuse, acute inflammation in the skin caused by bacterial infection.

and enlarged nodes in the affected area. Blood tests may show elevation of the white blood cell count and the presence of bacteria. Treatments include antibiotic therapy, ensuring adequate fluid intake, and local dressings if there is an open sore.

Pressure Ulcers

Pressure ulcers are a major concern of elderly patients, particularly those who are bedridden. They occur when pressure is applied to body tissue, resulting in a lack of perfusion and ultimately necrosis. Possible risk factors include brain or spinal cord injury, neuromuscular disorders, and nutritional problems. These ulcers are exacerbated by fecal and urinary incontinence, particularly when the patient is exposed to saturated materials for a prolonged period of time. You should be particularly aware of pressure sores during spinal immobilization and ensure that padding is adequate throughout the posterior to prevent sores. Sores are most commonly located on the lower legs, sacrum, greater trochanter, and the glutes.

According to the CDC, pressure ulcers can be classified as follows:

- **Stage 1:** A persistent area of skin redness (without a break in the skin) that does not disappear when pressure is relieved.
- **Stage 2:** A partial thickness is lost and may appear as an abrasion, blister, or shallow crater.
- **Stage 3:** A full thickness of skin is lost, exposing the subcutaneous tissues; presents as a deep crater with or without undermining adjacent tissue.
- **Stage 4:** A full thickness of skin and subcutaneous tissues are lost, exposing muscle or bone.

Over 10% of US nursing home patients have some stage of pressure ulcer. Half of these patients have stage 2 ulcers, the most common type of pressure ulcer. The least common type of pressure ulcer is stage 3, encompassing 1% of the nursing home population. Of the patients who have a stage 3 ulcer or higher, 35% of them receive specialty wound care.

Prehospital treatment for pressure ulcers is mostly BLS. However, ulcers that remain untreated can go on to be a source of significant infection and potentially lead to sepsis. You should monitor the patient's body temperature and vital signs, administer oxygen, establish an IV line, and consider administration of a fluid bolus.

Pathophysiology, Assessment, and Management of Musculoskeletal Conditions

Changes in physical abilities can affect older adults' confidence in their mobility. Many older adults choose to limit their physical activity due to a fear of falling and sustaining injuries. The muscle system atrophies and weakens with age. Muscle fibers become smaller and fewer, motor neurons decline in number, and strength declines. The ligaments and cartilage of the joints lose their elasticity. Cartilage also goes through degenerative changes with aging, contributing to arthritis.

The stooped posture of older people comes from atrophy of the supporting structures of the body. Two of every three older patients will show some degree of kyphosis (outward curvature of thoracic spine). Lost height in older adults generally results from compression in the spinal column, first in the disks and then from the process of osteoporosis in the vertebral bodies.

Osteoporosis

Osteoporosis is characterized by a decrease in bone mass leading to reduction in bone strength and greater susceptibility to fracture. The extent of bone loss that a person experiences is influenced by numerous factors, including genetics, smoking, level of activity, diet, hormonal factors, and body weight and structure. Use of anticonvulsant medications, steroids, and alcohol also increase the likelihood of development of osteoporosis. Generally speaking, women are more likely to develop osteoporosis than men, and Caucasian and Asian women are more likely to develop osteoporosis than African American or Hispanic women.

Osteoporosis is classified into two categories. The most rapid loss of bone occurring in women during the years following menopause is identified as type I osteoporosis. The most common fractures that occur from type I osteoporosis are radius and hip fractures. Type II osteoporosis is seen in both men and women, generally older than 50 years. The most common fractures associated with type II include hip and vertebral fractures. The vertebral fractures may cause the patient to develop dorsal kyphosis.

Although hormone replacement therapy (HRT) was the preferred treatment to prevent or slow osteoporosis in the past, newer medications that specifically target the bones are now available. These medications, classified as bisphosphonates, include alendronate (Fosamax) and ibandronate (Boniva), and they generally have lower risks than HRT. These are also useful in the treatment of bone loss in men, which is generally not true of HRT. Calcium and vitamin D supplementation is another treatment for the condition, and many other medications are available to improve bone strength. Older people should remain active and perform low-impact exercises to maintain bone and muscle strength.

Arthritis

Osteoarthritis is a progressive disease of the joints that destroys cartilage, promotes the formation of bone spurs in joints, and leads to joint stiffness. This type of arthritis is thought to result from "wear and tear" and, in some cases, from repetitive trauma to the joints. It affects 35% to 45% of the population older than 65 years. Typically, osteoarthritis affects several joints of the body, most commonly those in the hands, knees, hips, and spine. Patients report pain and stiffness that gets worse with exertion; some patients report increasing pain with changes in outside temperature or humidity levels. The end result is often substantial disability and disfigurement. Patients are typically treated with anti-inflammatory medications and physical therapy to improve the range of motion. Some patients may use topical lidocaine patches or opiates to manage pain, as well, along with herbal supplements that claim to improve cartilage health. Although arthritis is not life threatening, patients may seek emergency care for pain management.

Rheumatoid arthritis (RA) is a long-term autoimmune disorder that is classified by inflammation of the joints and the surrounding tissues. Symptoms are usually bilateral and most commonly affect the hands, feet, wrists, ankles, and knees. Patients may note pain and stiffness at the joints, and smaller joints in the fingers and toes are usually affected long before larger joints, like the elbows, shoulders, knees, or hips. You may observe deformities that are baseline for the patient as well as a poor range of motion. Care for RA is strictly supportive in the prehospital setting. If RA causes chest pain associated with pleurisy, this should be treated according to pain management protocols.

Management of Medical Emergencies in Elderly People

With the exception of patients who require immediate interventions to maintain a patent airway, adequate and supportive breathing, or circulatory status, most prehospital care is supportive and focuses on pain relief and palliative interventions. Additional steps in the patient treatment plan will depend on the patient's specific medical emergency and chief complaint. **Table 5** reviews common medical complications encountered with geriatric patients and their management strategies.

Pathophysiology, Assessment, and Management of Geriatric Trauma Emergencies

Deaths from injury in people older than 65 years account for one fourth of all trauma deaths in the United States, and injury is the seventh leading cause of death in the older population.

Several factors place an elderly person at higher risk of trauma than a younger person—namely, slower reflexes, visual and hearing deficits, equilibrium disorders, and an overall reduction in agility. In particular, changes in the body's homeostatic compensatory mechanisms combined with the effects of aging on body systems and any preexisting conditions usually add up to less favorable outcomes in trauma situations. Compensation in trauma is successful when an increased pulse rate, increased respirations, and adequate vasoconstriction make up for trauma-related blood loss. Reduced cardiac reserve, decreased respiratory function, impaired renal activity, and ineffective vasoconstriction, by contrast, may lead to unsuccessful recovery from traumatic situations. Furthermore, an elderly person is more likely to sustain serious injury in a trauma situation because stiffened blood vessels and fragile tissues tear more readily, and brittle, demineralized bone is more vulnerable to fracture.

Table 5 Common Medical Complications in Elderly People and Their Management

Medical Complication	Management
Incontinence	Some cases are managed surgically. Other considerations include absorptive devices for fecal and urinary incontinence, placement of catheters, and awareness of the patient's self-esteem and social issues.
COPD	Nebulizer treatment with a bronchial dilator could include metaproterenol (Alupent), racemic epinephrine, isoetharine (Bronkosol), ipratropium (Atrovent), and albuterol (Ventolin) or an IV dose of methylprednisolone (Solu-Medrol). Inhaled or oral steroids to decrease inflammation, and antibiotics to treat infection. CPAP.
Pulmonary emboli	Lysing the thrombus and anticoagulation therapies are indicated. Once all risk factors for bleeding have been reviewed, anticoagulants such as heparin or enoxaparin (Lovenox) can be considered.
Heart failure	Heart failure that produces signs and symptoms of pulmonary edema can be managed with sublingual nitroglycerin, IV furosemide (Lasix), and IV morphine. Providers can also consider a vasoactive medication such as dopamine (Intropin) for patients with hemodynamically unstable hypotension.
Dysrhythmias	Unless a patient is in unstable condition, dysrhythmias are handled with supportive care only. Unstable dysrhythmias are treated following current CPR and electrocardiographic (ECG) guidelines.
Aneurysm	Treatment is handled surgically, and prehospital interventions focus on supportive care.
Hypertension	Hypertensive emergencies require a controlled decline in blood pressure, which is not often feasible in prehospital care. A hypertensive crisis or urgency may be addressed by using labetalol (Normodyne) or sodium nitroprusside (Nipride).
Cerebral vascular disease	Prehospital management targets recognition and support. Definitive treatment is surgery.
Delirium	Recognize and treat the underlying cause, and provide supportive interventions.
Dementia, Alzheimer disease, Parkinson disease	Provide supportive care.
Diabetes	In hypoglycemia, treatments address the elevation of the blood glucose level with intramuscular or IV injections when not contraindicated. In hyperglycemia, treatment aims to eliminate additional glucose by using fluid boluses for patients with adequate renal function.
GI problems	Few treatments using medications for GI problems are possible in the prehospital environment, other than antiemetics. For nausea and vomiting, consider promethazine (Phenergan), zofran (Ondansetron), dimenhydrinate (Dramamine; especially for narcotic-induced nausea and vomiting), or prochlorperazine (Compazine; for severe nausea and vomiting or acute psychosis).
Drugs' toxic effects	■ Lidocaine: CNS depression may occur, so be alert for respiratory changes. No antidote is used in prehospital care to reverse its effects. ■ Beta blockers: Provide supportive care; give activated charcoal; and consider the use of atropine, epinephrine, and glucagon in symptomatic patients. ■ Antihypertensives: Provide supportive care. No antidote is used in prehospital care to reverse the drugs' effects. ■ Diuretics: Provide supportive care. Consider treatments aimed at restoring volume depletion and electrolyte imbalance. No antidote is used in prehospital care to reverse the drugs' effects. ■ Digitalis: Provide supportive care. Consider fluid replacement, vasoactive medications such as dopamine, and activated charcoal. ■ Psychotropics: Provide supportive care. Consider aggressive fluid replacement. ■ Antidepressants: Provide supportive care. Give fluid therapy for hypotension and sodium bicarbonate.
Alcohol abuse	Provide supportive care. Later care includes identification of abuse potential and referral to an appropriate treatment facility.
Behavioral disorders	Use psychological support and communication strategies. Consider haloperidol (Haldol), droperidol (Inapsine), or chlorpromazine (Thorazine).
Depression, suicide	Provide supportive care. Later care includes identification of the potential condition and referral to an appropriate treatment facility.

Most geriatric trauma cases involve falls or motor vehicle crashes. The incidence of falls, for example, increases with increasing age. Although most falls do not produce serious injury, in 2006, more than 20,800 patients died from fall-related injuries, with 17,700 of these patients older than 65 years. This increased mortality in geriatric patients is directly related to the patient's age, preexisting disease processes, and complications related to the trauma. Falls are associated with a higher incidence of anxiety and depression, a loss of confidence, and post-fall syndrome. With this syndrome, geriatric patients develop a lack of confidence and anxiety about potential falls. Ultimately, they may become immobile, risk incontinence, and develop pneumonia or pressure ulcers from lack of movement.

Falls among elderly people are divided between those resulting from extrinsic (external) causes, such as tripping on a loose rug or slipping on ice, and those resulting from intrinsic (internal) causes, such as a dizzy spell or a syncopal attack Table 6. The risk of falls increases in people with preexisting gait abnormalities (such as from neurologic or musculoskeletal impairment) and cognitive impairment. Older patients with osteoporosis have lower-density bones, so even a sudden, awkward turn may

Table 6 Causes of Falls in the Elderly

Cause	Clues to Suggest This Cause
Extrinsic (accidental)	Obvious environmental hazard at the scene, such as poor lighting, scatter rugs, uneven sidewalk, ice or other slippery surface
Intrinsic drop attacks	Sudden fall; patient found on the ground somewhat confused, often temporarily paralyzed and unable to get up; no premonitory symptoms
Postural hypotension	Fall when getting up from a recumbent or sitting position (Check medications the patient is taking, and ask about occult blood loss, such as presence of black stools. Measure blood pressure in recumbent and sitting positions.)
Dizziness or syncope	Marked bradycardia or tachydysrhythmias
Stroke	Other characteristic signs of stroke, such as hemiparesis, hemiplegia, or aphasia
Fracture	Patient felt something snap before falling.

fracture a bone. When you are treating a patient who has fallen, you need to obtain a careful history. Although the patient often attributes the fall to an accidental cause ("I must have tripped over the rug."), meticulous questioning often reveals a period of dizziness or palpitations just before the fall, suggesting a different cause. Home safety assessments by EMS—during a routine visit or as part of an outreach program—may reduce fall incidence. Components of this assessment should include clear pathways to and from the bathroom, handrails in bathtubs and on steps, no loose rugs or other objects on the floor, wheelchair ramps with grip tape, and caregivers who are trained to lift and move patients.

After falls, motor vehicle crashes are the second leading cause of accidental death among elderly people. An older patient is five times more likely than a younger patient to be fatally injured in a motor vehicle crash, even though excessive speed is rarely a causative factor in the older age group. Impaired vision, errors in judgment, and underlying medical conditions contribute to the higher risk. Impairments in vision and hearing, along with diminished agility, also contribute to pedestrian deaths involving elderly people.

■ Pathophysiology

Changes associated with normal aging and with diseases of aging make elderly people particularly vulnerable to certain types of injuries. In particular, head trauma or injury is a serious problem. The increased fragility of cerebral blood vessels, enlargement of the subdural space, and a decrease in the supportive tissue of the meninges all contribute to make an elderly person more vulnerable than a younger person to intracranial bleeding, particularly subdural hematoma. In many cases, the hematoma develops slowly, over a period of days or weeks. By the time the patient becomes symptomatic, the person or his or her caretakers may not remember the incident, or the family or caretakers may feel guilty about their own negligence in the incident. As a result, it may be difficult to obtain an accurate history of the initial trauma. The most important early symptom of a subdural hematoma is a headache that may be worse at night. Sometimes the headache occurs on the same side of the head as the blood clot. With increasing intracranial pressure, the state of consciousness becomes depressed, and the patient becomes increasingly drowsy.

Elderly people are also more vulnerable than their younger counterparts to cervical spinal cord injury and cord compression, even after apparently minor trauma. Degenerative changes in the cervical spine (cervical **spondylosis**) cause arthritic "spurs" and narrowing of the vertebral canal; the nerve roots exiting from the cervical spine gradually become compressed, and pressure on the spinal cord increases. Any injury to the cervical spine, therefore, is much more likely to injure the already compromised spinal cord. Even a sudden movement of the neck may result in spinal cord injury.

Injuries to the chest in elderly people are much more likely to produce rib fracture and flail chest, owing to the brittleness of the ribs and overall stiffening of the chest wall as the costochondral cartilage becomes calcified. Abdominal trauma often produces liver injury, perhaps because the liver is less protected by the abdominal musculature.

Orthopaedic injuries are a common result of falls in geriatric patients, with hip fractures the most common acute orthopaedic injury, followed, in severity and frequency, by fractures of the femur, pelvis, tibia, and upper extremities. Hip fracture may occasionally (this is rare) occur without trauma, simply because of vigorous contracture of the hip musculature. The most important risk factor for hip fracture is osteoporosis: Approximately half of older women and one of eight older men will sustain an osteoporosis-related fracture (hip or other).

Burns are a significant risk of morbidity and mortality in elderly people because of physiologic and pathophysiologic changes. The risk of mortality is increased when preexisting medical conditions exist, defense mechanisms to protect against infection are weakened, and fluid replacement is complicated by renal compromise. When you are assessing a burn patient, you need to monitor the patient's hydration status by assessing current vital signs, mucous membranes, and urine output, which is typically 50 to 60 mL/h or 0.5 to 1.0 mL/kg/h.

Internal temperature regulation is slowed in elderly people and gets slower with increasing age. The body's ability to recognize fluctuations in temperature becomes delayed owing to a slowed endocrine system. Heat gain or loss in response to environmental changes is delayed by atherosclerotic vessels, slowed circulation, and decreased sweat production in the skin. In addition, thermoregulation can be adversely affected by chronic disease, medications, and alcohol use, all of which are more frequent in elderly people.

Not surprisingly, about half of all deaths from hypothermia occur in elderly people, and most indoor hypothermia deaths involve geriatric patients. Although living where harsh winters occur is a risk factor, hypothermia can develop at temperatures above freezing when an older person is exposed for a prolonged period.

The death rates from hyperthermia are more than doubled in elderly people compared with younger persons; people older than 85 years are at highest risk. Arizona has more heat-related deaths than all other states combined, reflecting its long, hot summers and large geriatric population.

Providers should be aware of environmental emergencies during extreme heat and cold, particularly in lower socioeconomic areas that may not have sufficient heat or air conditioning. This may require public awareness and preplanning. You may have to keep the patient compartment at a temperature that is higher than normal, and perhaps uncomfortable, in order to adequately maintain the patient's temperature.

■ Assessment and Management of Trauma

Begin the assessment by looking at the mechanism of injury. Falls account for the largest number of injuries in elderly people, followed by injuries related to motor vehicles (including passenger and pedestrian trauma) and then burns and other injuries. Always look for signs or symptoms that the patient may have experienced a medical problem before the trauma. A syncopal event while driving, for example, may result in a crash.

The initial management of an injured elderly patient follows the basic ABC pattern of trauma care with some special concerns.

When you are securing the airway, check for dentures. If they are intact and in place, leave them where they are; if the dentures are broken or loose in the mouth, remove them and place them in a safe container. Aggressive suctioning of blood or secretions is required because of the older patient's lessened airway and gag reflexes Figure 13 .

When you are assessing breathing, check for rib fracture. If assisted ventilation is required, use a bag-mask gently, exerting just enough pressure to inflate the lungs so as to lessen the

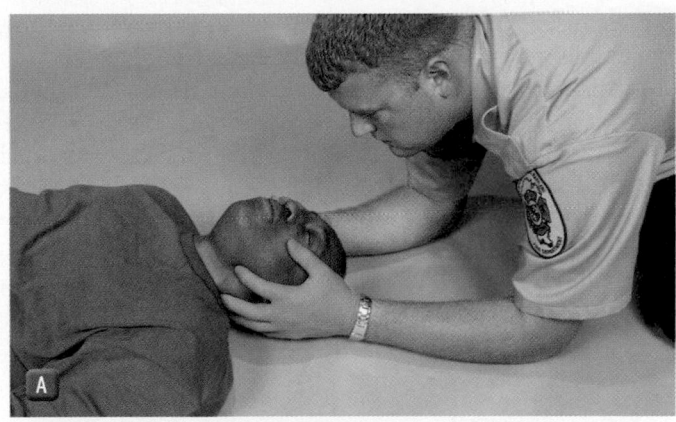

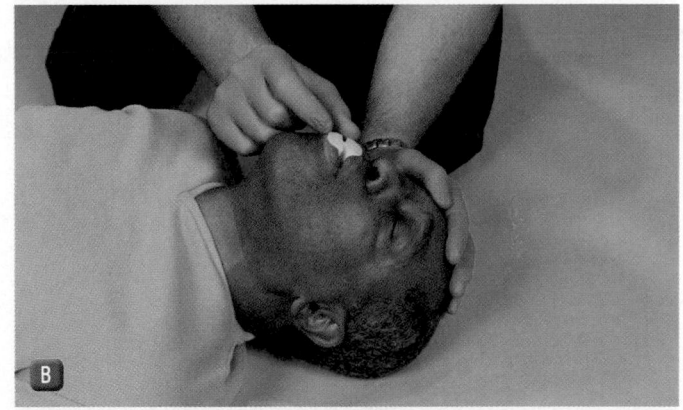

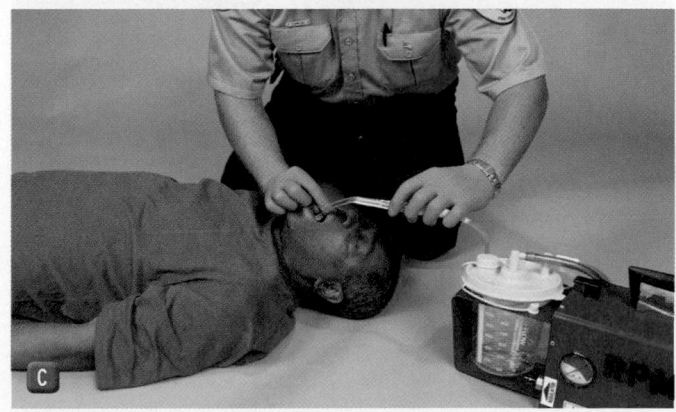

Figure 13 The airway should initially be addressed using simple techniques, such as (A) the jaw-thrust, (B) placement of an oropharyngeal or nasopharyngeal airway, and (C) suctioning.

chance of creating a pneumothorax. Administer supplemental oxygen early to assist the body in compensating for early states of trauma.

When you are evaluating circulation, remember that what is a normal blood pressure in a younger person may mean hypotension in an older person. If possible, try to determine the patient's normal baseline blood pressure and circulatory status.

The assessment of disability (neurologic status) should include an evaluation of the pupils and the level of consciousness, according to the AVPU scale. Finally, be sure to expose the entire injured area, even if it means peeling away many layers of clothing.

Once the primary assessment is complete, try to obtain a complete history of the trauma event from the patient and from anyone who may have witnessed the event **Figure 14**. Be aware that the patient may have sustained the trauma several hours or days prior to the ambulance call but symptoms may have developed due to the patient's medication regimens. If the patient fell, from what height? Did the patient have any symptoms beforehand, such as dizziness? If the patient was struck by a car, how fast was the car moving? If the patient was the driver of a car involved in a crash, did he or she feel dizzy or black out before the crash? Did the patient have chest pain? Did witnesses notice the car moving erratically before it crashed?

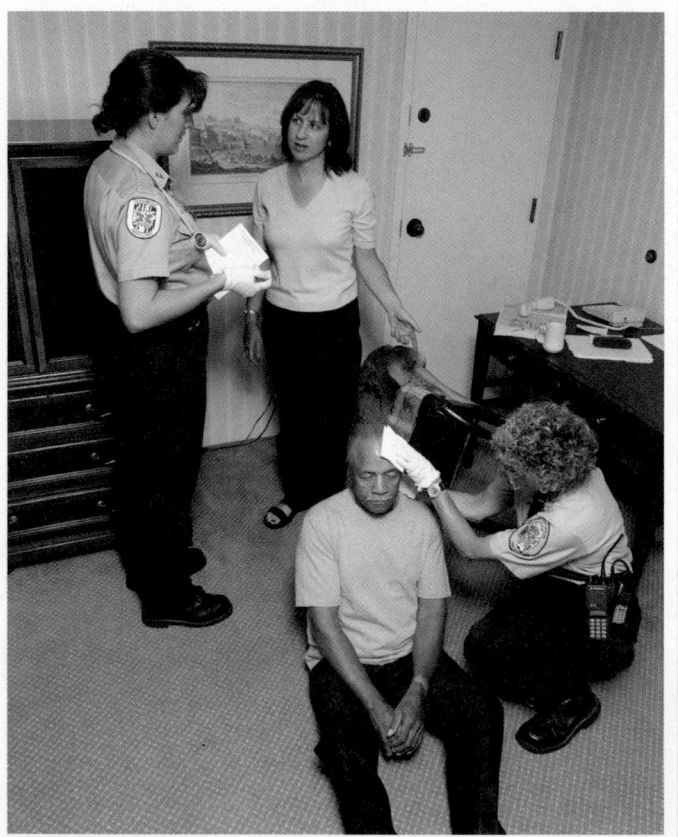

Figure 14 History is especially important in older patients who have lost consciousness.

Obtain a complete list of all medications the patient takes regularly. Inquire in particular about beta blockers, antihypertensives, and medications for diabetes because they may affect the patient's response to resuscitation measures and to anesthesia.

Conduct the secondary assessment as usual, staying particularly alert for signs of injuries to the head, cervical spine, ribs, abdomen, and long bones. Pain from fractures or peripheral injury may be difficult to assess if the patient has decreased pain perception.

Additional treatment will depend on the patient's specific injuries, although there are a few general principles to keep in mind:

- Use caution inserting IV catheters and administering isotonic solutions. It is very easy to overload an elderly person with sodium, and you must balance that with the need to maintain adequate perfusion pressure. Use small boluses, and reassess the patient frequently, especially for signs of pulmonary edema.
- Monitor cardiac rhythm throughout care of the patient, and be alert for changes. Previous or continuing cardiac disease predisposes a person to ECG changes.
- Take steps to preserve temperature in elderly trauma patients. Regulation of temperature is slowed in elderly people, and the blood in cold patients does not clot as well.
- Frail elderly patients may not do well with a traction splint for a femoral fracture. If possible, place the patient on a well-padded backboard and buttress him or her well with pillows secured firmly in place.
- Consider the use of pain medication. Remember that elderly patients require a lower dosage of pain medications to reach therapeutic levels.
- Immobilize the cervical spine before transporting the patient. Pad the backboard generously, because the skin of an older person may be damaged by the direct trauma of the pressure and the decrease in blood flow. Target areas where the bone is near the surface, from top to bottom: occiput, scapula, spinous processes, elbows, sacrum, and heels. A pressure ulcer can develop in as little as 45 minutes and can complicate the original injury.

Elder Abuse

One category of geriatric trauma that deserves special mention is elder abuse—that is, any form of mistreatment that results in harm or loss to an older person. Five types of abuse are distinguished: physical, sexual, emotional, neglect, and financial. The first four are similar to the forms found in child abuse. Financial abuse involves improper use of an older person's funds, property, or assets. The average victim of elder abuse is 80 years old, is female, and has multiple chronic conditions. These conditions make patients unable to function on their own, leaving them dependent on others for at least part of their care. The abuser is almost always known to the abused and is often a family member (such as adult children or a spouse). Whereas elder abuse does occur in long-term care facilities, abuse is more likely to occur at the patient's home or the home of a caregiver.

One clue to elder abuse is unexplained injuries that do not fit the stated cause. Assessment of elder abuse must include not only the physical exam, but also the environmental and social clues. Look at the patient's overall hygiene, and review how he or she interacts with caregivers. Take adequate time to listen patiently to any concerns expressed by older patients about their care (or lack of it) **Figure 15** . If the patient is in stable condition but the situation is unsafe, see if the patient will accept transportation to the hospital. If the patient refuses transport, see if he or she will accept help from the local **adult protective services (APS)**. In some cases, patients may be hesitant to go with EMS personnel because of fear of caregiver retaliation. If the situation is immediately unsafe, notify law enforcement personnel and remain with the patient only if the scene remains safe to do so.

Many states have elder abuse statutes, and the reporting of suspected abuse is mandatory in some jurisdictions. Nevertheless, only one of five cases of elder abuse is ever reported. The way elder abuse is defined varies considerably from state to state, so it is advisable to become familiar with the legislation that applies to your own area. However, regardless of the legislation, if you have any reason to suspect elder abuse in a given case of geriatric injury—for example, if you found evidence of gross patient neglect in the patient's residence—objectively document your observations and report your findings and suspicions to the receiving facility. APS could use these observations as an indicator of whether assistance is required.

End-of-Life Care

You will inevitably be involved with end-of-life care for many patients. Of course, "do not resuscitate" (DNR) does not mean "do not respond to the needs of a terminal patient." You can treat various disorders, administer various medications, and perform other various treatments as long as they do not include providing artificial ventilations or cardiovascular assistance. There is much you can do, beginning with demonstrating a caring and concerned attitude and approach. Many of your visits may be "no transport" decisions and may not be perceived as valuable by those who decide on reimbursement, but they prove no less valuable to the patient than more aggressive measures. Many communities have a local **hospice**, an organization that provides terminal care for patients and support for their families. If one exists in your community, consider how you or your service might collaborate on providing quality care for a person at the end of life **Figure 16** .

Controversies

Is a DNR order from a state other than yours valid? It depends on your state's law. About a dozen states recognize out-of-state DNR orders.

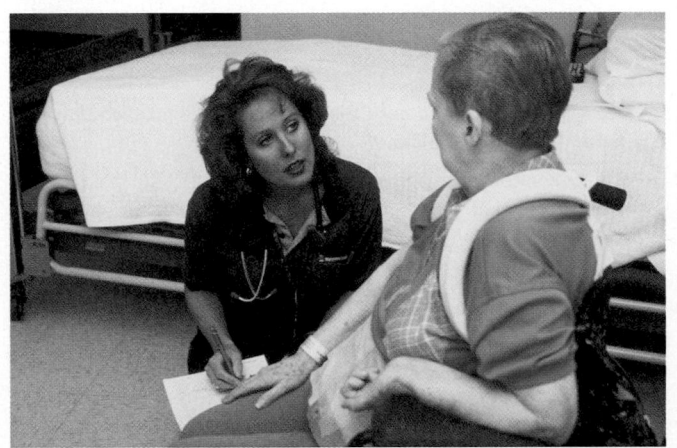

Figure 15 Take time to listen patiently to older patients.

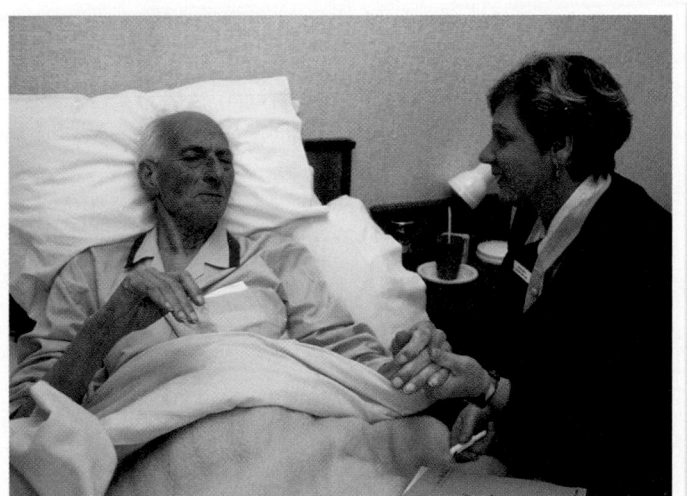

Figure 16 Hospice care allows people with terminal illnesses to receive palliative care in their own homes.

YOU are the Medic | SUMMARY

1. What type of injuries might you suspect on the basis of the dispatch information?

Because this person is elderly, her bones may be brittle, making fractures of the hip more common. Also, depending on whether she landed on an outstretched arm or other extremity, the potential for fractures in those areas may be greater. Neck or back injuries may be possible as well. Consider the cause of the fall. Did the patient become dizzy, have a syncopal episode, or just step onto a slippery surface? Research has shown that being barefooted, wearing only socks, and wearing slippers increase the incidence of falls in the elderly. In this situation, slippery soles on bowling shoes may have contributed to the fall.

2. What dictates the type of skills that a paramedic may perform?

Your EMS service has a physician medical director who authorizes providers to perform specific duties in the field in accordance with their level of training. Along with online medical control, physicians also provide authorization through the use of standing orders and protocols.

3. Is safety an issue here?

Safety is a concern on every call. Fortunately, the hazards are minimal in this situation. This scene involves a controlled environment, and dispatch information did not indicate any hazards, such as a large crowd or a violent situation that led to the injury. As you approach a scene, you should always look for anything that poses a threat to the safety of you, your partner, bystanders, or the patient. If a scene that initially appeared safe becomes potentially unsafe, remove yourself immediately and call for law enforcement assistance.

4. What are your primary responsibilities at this point during the call?

You have already prepared yourself to respond to the call. The next responsibility is scene management. Make sure the scene is safe before you enter and as you approach the patient.

Once you establish that the scene is safe, patient assessment and care begin. You must perform a primary assessment, including obtaining a thorough history that investigates the chief complaint and obtain a SAMPLE history. Prioritize the needs of the patient based on the patient's illness or injury and provide care accordingly.

Patient treatment also involves determining the most appropriate mode of transport and destination. Follow protocols for treatment and, if necessary, contact medical control for direction. Choose a receiving facility that can provide the appropriate care for your patient's condition. The closest facility may not be the most appropriate for the situation.

Patient transfer may begin this early in the call, depending on the emergency. On arrival at the receiving facility, give a brief, pertinent report to the receiving staff. Be sure to explain the patient's signs and symptoms, assessment findings, the care given, and the patient's response to treatment.

A paramedic is also responsible for writing a patient care report and preparing and restocking the ambulance unit as quickly as possible in order to return to service.

5. Does this patient need ALS care? Why or why not?

This patient does not need ALS care. She is not in any apparent distress and her vital signs are within normal limits. If her pain level increases, she may need an analgesic. A paramedic may administer narcotic analgesics such as morphine or meperidine (Demerol).

6. How would you care for this patient?

Perform a thorough patient assessment. Check for pedal pulses prior to moving the ankle. Mark pulses with an "x" to indicate where the pulse was found; this is useful in the event that pulses are lost with movement. Have another provider carefully lift the leg and ankle as a unit and place a pillow underneath to use as a splint. Because there is no need for spinal immobilization, the patient may be transported in a position of comfort. Establish IV access and administer normal saline at a keep-vein-open rate. Reassess the patient after interventions and every 15 minutes because her condition is stable.

7. Is IV therapy within your scope of practice?

Yes, a paramedic can establish IV access and administer fluid. Monitor vital signs, including breath sounds, carefully so you do not overload the patient with fluid.

8. Does this patient need care that could only be provided by a paramedic-level provider?

Cardiac monitoring or administration of analgesics for pain are the only skills that are strictly paramedic level that this patient may require. Level of care should be dictated by the patient's presentation and direction by online medical control if needed.

9. What type of community service can a paramedic become involved in to become a patient advocate and increase safety?

Providing safety inspections at the bowling alley and other establishments may help prevent future problems before they arise. You can have a role in this simply by looking around your environment as you are surveying the scene to see if there are any potential hazards such as spills or loose rugs. A suggestion should also be made to examine the bottom of rental shoes for slippery materials. Discuss the importance of other safety issues such as using bike helmets, safety belts, and child car seats whenever you can. As a professional, it is your job to be a patient advocate. Showing concern for your patients, their families, and others is part of being a paramedic.

YOU *are the Medic*   SUMMARY, *continued*

EMS Patient Care Report (PCR)

Date: 01-11-12	Incident No.: 572819	Nature of Call: Fall		Location: 982 Stover Street	
Dispatched: 1813	En Route: 1815	At Scene: 1822	Transport: 1842	At Hospital: 1854	In Service: 1902

Patient Information

Age: 72 **Sex:** F **Weight (in kg [lb]):** 78 kg (172 lb)	**Allergies:** No known drug allergies **Medications:** Lisinopril, Metformin **Past Medical History:** Non-insulin-dependent diabetes mellitus, hypertension **Chief Complaint:** Ⓡ ankle pain

Vital Signs

Time: 1826	BP: 148/86	Pulse: 98/regular	Respirations: 18	Spo$_2$: 99% on room air
Time: 1840	BP: 146/78	Pulse: 94/regular	Respirations: 18	Spo$_2$: 100% on room air
Time:	BP:	Pulse:	Respirations:	Spo$_2$:

EMS Treatment
(circle all that apply)

Oxygen @ _____ L/min via (circle one): NC NRM Bag-mask device	Assisted Ventilation	Airway Adjunct	CPR
Defibrillation	**Bleeding Control**	**(Bandaging)**	**(Splinting)**	**Other**

Narrative

Dispatched for a "fall." On arrival found a 72-year-old woman sitting in a chair reporting Ⓡ ankle pain after twisting her ankle while bowling. Bystanders report hearing a "pop" as she fell to her knees. Pt denies having any other complaint. Vital signs are within normal limits, no apparent distress, skin warm and dry. Presents with pain, swelling, and discoloration to Ⓡ ankle, but good pedal pulses. No other abnormal findings during assessment. Ⓡ ankle is splinted with a pillow for comfort and an ice pack applied to reduce swelling. Pulses present and marked before and after splinting. Pt is transported in position of comfort. Established 20-g IV Ⓛ antecubital fossa with normal saline at a keep-vein-open rate. Transport uneventful—no changes en route. **End of report**

Prep Kit

Ready for Review

- Elderly people constitute an ever-increasing proportion of patients presenting to the health care system, particularly to the emergency care sector.

- The health problems of older people are quantitatively and qualitatively different from those of younger people. The special problems of older people require special approaches.

- The aging process is accompanied by changes in physiologic function. The decrease in the functional capacity of various organ systems can affect the way in which the patient responds to illness.

- A person's respiratory capacity undergoes significant reductions with age due to decreases in the elasticity of the lungs and in the size and strength of the respiratory muscles, calcification of costochrondral cartilage in the chest wall, and musculoskeletal changes.

- A variety of changes occur in the cardiovascular system as a person ages. The heart hypertrophies (enlarges), arteriosclerosis (the stiffening of vessel walls) develops, and the electric conduction system of the heart deteriorates.

- Changes in the nervous system lead to a decrease in the performance of sense organs, as evidenced by visual changes (glaucoma and cataracts are common) and hearing loss.

- Digestive system changes include a decrease in taste buds and a reduction in saliva and gastric secretions. These changes may interfere with the enjoyment of food, leading to malnutrition in elderly people.

- Geriatric patients may experience renal system changes. Although the kidneys of an elderly person may be capable of handling day-to-day demands, they may not be able to meet unusual challenges, such as those imposed by illness. Therefore, acute illness in elderly patients is often accompanied by derangements in fluid and electrolyte balance.

- Changes in the endocrine system may lead to diabetes and thyroid abnormalities in older patients.

- Nearly every function of the immune system is affected by aging. Older persons are therefore more prone to infection and secondary complications than younger people.

- Changes in the integumentary system include thinner skin and loss of elasticity, allowing skin to be torn easily and more bleeding to occur.

- Aging is accompanied by a progressive loss of homeostatic capabilities. A specific illness or injury in elderly people is more likely to result in generalized deterioration.

- Aging brings a widespread decrease in bone mass in men and women, but especially among postmenopausal women. Bones become more brittle and tend to break more easily.

- Knowing what is and what is not part of the aging process constitutes the first challenge when you are assessing elderly patients. A second challenge is that signs and symptoms of disease may be altered from their presentation in younger patients as a consequence of aging.

- The GEMS diamond was designed to assist the prehospital professional in the assessment and treatment of elderly patients. It can be integrated into the patient assessment process and it will help you to form a general impression of your patient.

- Whereas the primary assessment addresses immediately life-threatening pathologic problems, the secondary assessment includes a systematic assessment of the patient that may include a full-body examination or a focused assessment on the body part or body system specifically involved.

- The physical exam of older patients can be difficult. Poor cooperation and easy fatigability may require that you keep manipulations of the patient to a minimum.

- Stroke is a significant cause of death and disability in elderly people. More than 80% of all stroke deaths occur in persons older than 65 years, and stroke is the leading cause of long-term disability at any age.

- Diseases of the heart remain the leading cause of death among older adults in the United States. Heart attack is the major cause of morbidity and mortality in people older than 65 years, and its potential for mortality increases significantly in people older than 70 years.

- In elderly people, delirium often replaces or confounds the typical presentation caused by a medical problem, an adverse medication effect, or drug withdrawal. Disorders that cause delirium may also include poisons, electrolyte imbalances, nutritional deficiencies, and infections such as urinary tract infections and pneumonia.

- Unlike delirium, dementia is a disease that produces irreversible brain failure. Disorders that cause dementia include conditions that impair vascular and neurologic structures within the brain, such as infections, stroke, head injuries, poor nutrition, and medications.

- The two most common degenerative types of dementia in older people are Alzheimer disease and multi-infarct or vascular dementia, both of which cause structural damage to the brain.

- Gastrointestinal problems in elderly people include peptic ulcer disease, small bowel obstruction due to gallstones, and stomach or duodenal ulcers (peptic ulcer disease).

- The most common hospital-associated infection to cause sepsis in the United States is urinary tract infections (UTIs).

- A geriatric patient with diabetes is at increased risk for hypoglycemia for several reasons: medications, inadequate or irregular dietary intake, inability to recognize the warning signs due to cognitive problems, and/or blunted warning signs. Delirium may be the only indication of hypoglycemia in an elderly patient.

- Older patients with diabetes whose blood glucose levels tend to be high are prone to hyperosmolar nonketotic coma (HONK), also called hyperosmolar hyperglycemic nonketotic coma (HHNC). The most frequent cause for HONK/HHNC is infection. Presentation is likely to be acute confusion with dehydration.

- Elderly people are particularly prone to adverse drug reactions because of changes in the following: drug metabolism because of diminished hepatic function; drug elimination because of diminished renal function; body composition, including increased body fat and decreased body water, altering the distribution of drugs through the various body compartments; and the responsiveness to drugs of the central nervous system.

- Alcohol is the preferred substance of abuse among older persons, in whom its use is on the rise. A much smaller but increasing segment of the geriatric population uses illicit drugs.

- Depression in elderly patients can mimic the effects of many other medical problems (such as dementia). Risk factors for depression in an older person include a history of depression, chronic disease, and loss (function, independence, or significant others).

- Osteoporosis is characterized by a decrease in bone mass leading to reduction in bone strength and greater susceptibility to fracture. Osteoarthritis is a progressive disease process of the joints that destroys cartilage, promotes the formation of bone spurs in joints, and leads to joint stiffness.

- Several factors place an elderly person at higher risk of trauma than a younger person: slower reflexes, visual and hearing deficits, equilibrium disorders, and an overall reduction in agility.

- Most geriatric trauma cases involve falls or motor vehicle crashes. Falls among elderly people are evenly divided between those resulting from extrinsic (external) causes, such as tripping on a loose rug or slipping on ice, and those resulting from intrinsic (internal) causes, such as a dizzy spell or a syncopal attack.

- Elder abuse is any form of mistreatment that results in harm or loss to an older person. Five types of abuse are distinguished: physical, sexual, emotional, neglect, and financial.

- Hospice care allows people with terminal illnesses to receive palliative care in their own homes. You will be involved with end-of-life care for many patients.

■ Vital Vocabulary

adult protective services (APS) Organizations that investigate cases involving abuse and neglect and provide case management services in some cases.

Alzheimer disease A progressive organic condition in which neurons die, causing dementia.

aortic sclerosis A condition in which the aortic valve thickens due to fibrosis and calcification, obstructing blood flow from the left ventricle.

aortic stenosis A condition in which the aortic valve does not open fully, decreasing blood flow from the heart.

arteriosclerosis A pathologic condition in which the arterial walls become thickened and inelastic.

atherosclerosis A disorder in which cholesterol and calcium build up inside the walls of the blood vessels, forming plaque, which eventually leads to partial or complete blockage of blood flow.

bereavement Sadness from loss; grieving.

cataracts A clouding of the lens of the eye or its surrounding transparent membrane; normally a result of aging.

cellulitis An acute inflammation in the skin caused by a bacterial infection.

delirium An acute confusional state characterized by global impairment of thinking, perception, judgment, and memory.

dementia A chronic deterioration of mental functions.

geriatrics The assessment and treatment of disease in someone 65 years or older.

glaucoma A disease of the eye caused by an increase in intraocular pressure; when severe enough, this may damage the optic nerve and potentially cause permanent loss of vision.

herpes zoster Shingles; a contagious condition caused by the reactivation of the varicella virus on nerve roots.

homeostasis A tendency to constancy or stability in the body's internal milieu.

hospice An organization that provides end-of-life care to patients with terminal illnesses and their families.

Meniere disease An inner ear disorder in which endolymphatic rupture creates increased pressure in the cochlear duct, which then leads to damage to the organ of Corti and the semicircular canal; symptoms include severe vertigo, tinnitus, and sensorineuronal hearing loss.

old-age dependency ratio A formula used to determine the number of older people in a society as compared with the number of potential workers who are theoretically capable of providing resources to sustain the whole population. It is the number of older people (65 years and older) for every 100 adults (potential caregivers) between the ages of 18 and 64 years.

osteoarthritis The degeneration of a joint surface caused by wear and tear that leads to pain and stiffness.

osteoporosis A decrease in bone mass and density.

Parkinson disease A neurologic condition in which the portion of the brain responsible for production of dopamine has been damaged or overused, resulting in tremors.

polypharmacy The use of multiple medications.

presbycusis Progressive hearing loss, particularly in the high frequencies, along with lessened ability to discriminate between a particular sound and background noise.

pressure ulcers Ulcers that occur when pressure is applied to body tissue, resulting in a lack of perfusion and ultimately necrosis.

proprioception The ability to perceive the position and movement of one's body or limbs.

rheumatoid arthritis An inflammatory disorder that affects the entire body and leads to degeneration and deformation of joints.

sepsis A disease state that results from the presence of microorganisms or their toxic products in the bloodstream.

spondylosis Degenerative condition resulting in decreased mobility of vertebral joints and compression of neural elements.

Assessment in Action

It is just after 10:00 AM when you are dispatched to a residence for a fall. On arrival a man meets you at the door and tells you that his mother is "not acting right." He also tells you that she lives alone and apparently fell sometime during the night. He says that she has been confused lately and that the doctor ran tests but found nothing significant. She takes medication for hypertension, and has had a stroke and a myocardial infarction in the past. He says that the doctor thinks she may have mild dementia. She also takes "many medications." He has not seen or talked to her since yesterday morning and came over to check on her just prior to calling 9-1-1.

You enter the kitchen to find an elderly woman sitting at the kitchen table looking at you in a bewildered fashion. She has dried blood matted in the back of her white hair, and her son tells you the blood is from her fall. You also note blood on the edge of the countertop that she apparently struck on the way down. She says that she does not remember what happened and cannot tell you her age or what day of the week it is. You note several loose throw rugs on the floor, and her clothes are disheveled and buttoned inappropriately. Her vital signs are within normal limits, pupils are equal and reactive to light, and the blood glucose level is normal. She says she is fine and does not want to go to the hospital.

1. The loose rugs may have contributed to the patient's fall. What part of the GEMS diamond does this represent?
   A. Geriatric assessment
   B. Environmental assessment
   C. Medical assessment
   D. Social assessment

2. If the rugs are the cause of the fall, this would be considered:
   A. an extrinsic factor.
   B. an intrinsic factor.
   C. proprioception.
   D. a result of spondylosis.

3. The state of the patient's clothing offers important information during what portion of the GEMS diamond assessment?
   A. Geriatric assessment
   B. Environmental assessment
   C. Medical assessment
   D. Social assessment

4. Changes in the patient's neurologic system due to the aging process and her history of a stroke may indicate which condition as the cause of her confusion?
   A. Delirium
   B. Presbycusis
   C. Dementia
   D. Organic brain syndrome

5. Her confusion and instability may be the result of a toxicologic impairment as a result of:
   A. polypharmacy.
   B. alcohol.
   C. noncompliance.
   D. psychiatric conditions.

6. The patient's fall may have resulted from a cardiac dysrhythmia as a result of her aging cardiovascular system. What is the most common dysrhythmia among elderly people?
   A. Sinus tachycardia
   B. Sinus bradycardia
   C. Ventricular fibrillation
   D. Atrial fibrillation

7. Confusion in any patient may be the result of endocrine disorders. Older patients, and particularly those with a known history of diabetes, are more likely to present with which condition as a result of elevated glucose levels?
   A. Diabetic ketoacidosis (DKA)
   B. Hyperosmolar hyperglycemic nonketotic coma (HHNC)
   C. Hyperthyroidism
   D. Thyrotoxicosis

Additional Questions

8. It is important for you to assess any elderly patient for signs of abuse. What should you look for and how should you proceed if abuse is suspected?

9. Explain what is meant by a *review of systems*, and why this is important when you are assessing an elderly patient.

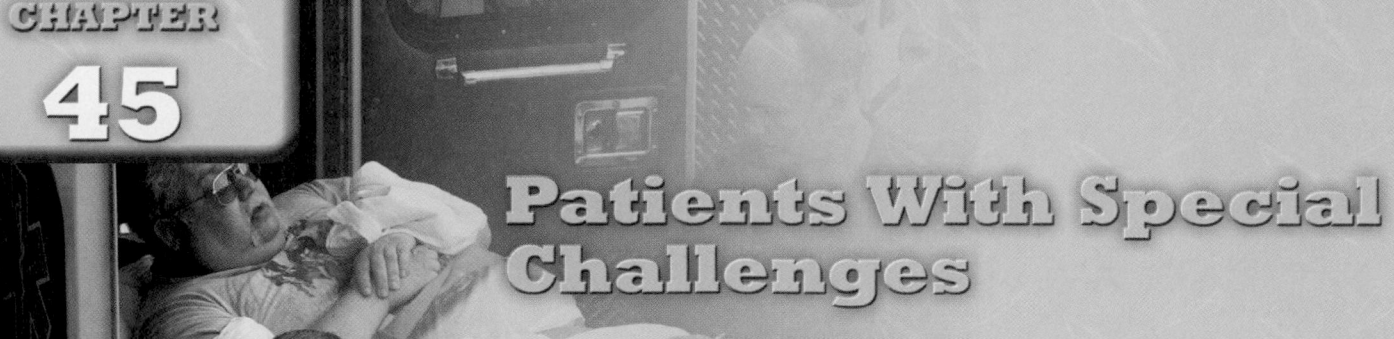

Patients With Special Challenges

National EMS Education Standard Competencies

Special Patient Populations

Integrates assessment findings with principles of pathophysiology and knowledge of psychosocial needs to formulate a field impression and implement a comprehensive treatment/disposition plan for patients with special needs.

Patients With Special Challenges

Recognizing and reporting abuse and neglect (pp 2123-2129)

Health care implications of:

- Abuse (see chapter, *Pediatric Emergencies*, and see chapter, *Geriatric Emergencies*)
- Neglect (see chapter, *Pediatric Emergencies*, and see chapter, *Geriatric Emergencies*)
- Homelessness (pp 2122-2123)
- Poverty (pp 2122-2123)
- Bariatrics (pp 2130-2131)
- Technology dependent (pp 2132-2147)
- Hospice/terminally ill (pp 2129-2130)
- Tracheostomy care/dysfunction (pp 2132-2135)
- Home care (pp 2129-2130)
- Sensory deficit/loss (pp 2153-2156)
- Developmental disability (p 2151)

Trauma

Integrates assessment findings with principles of epidemiology and pathophysiology to formulate a field impression to implement a comprehensive treatment/disposition plan for an acutely injured patient.

Special Considerations in Trauma

Pathophysiology, assessment, and management of trauma in the

- Pregnant patient (see chapter, *Obstetrics*)
- Pediatric patient (see chapter, *Pediatric Emergencies*)
- Geriatric patient (see chapter, *Geriatric Emergencies*)
- Cognitively impaired patient (pp 2156-2157)

Knowledge Objectives

1. Discuss how poverty and homelessness adversely impact patient health and EMS system performance. (pp 2122-2123)
2. Identify ways to advocate for patients' rights to health care services. (pp 2122-2123)
3. Recognize signs and symptoms of neglect and various forms of abuse, including physical abuse, neglect, sexual abuse, and emotional abuse. (pp 2123-2129)
4. Identify benign physical findings that may be confused with signs of abuse. (pp 2125-2127)

5. Discuss the unique management and documentation concerns related to suspected cases of abuse or neglect. (pp 2127-2129)
6. Describe mandatory reporting and how it relates to cases of suspected abuse. (p 2129)
7. Describe specific concerns related to patients with a terminal illness, including situations in which hospice may be involved. (pp 2129-2130)
8. Discuss situations in which advance directives and do not resuscitate (DNR) orders may exist, and how the paramedic should proceed in situations where the validity of such a document is in question. (p 2130)
9. Describe specific clinical and management concerns related to bariatric patients. (pp 2130-2131)
10. Discuss operational concerns related to emergency management of bariatric patients. (p 2131)
11. Describe specific concerns related to patients with a communicable disease. (pp 2131-2132)
12. Discuss medical technology and adaptive devices used in the prehospital setting, including long-term ventilators, apnea monitors, long-term vascular access devices, medication infusion pumps, insulin pumps, gastric tubes, colostomies, urinary diversion devices, dialysis shunts, surgical drains and devices, and cerebrospinal fluid shunts. (pp 2132-2147)
13. Discuss the purpose of tracheostomy tubes, and how to troubleshoot problems that may occur in a patient with a tracheostomy. (pp 2132-2135)
14. Discuss the types of medical technology that may be used during interfacility transports, including hemodynamic monitoring, intra-aortic balloon pumps, and intracranial pressure monitoring. (pp 2147-2150)
15. Identify strategies for providing care to patients with cognitive impairment, including patients with development delay, Down syndrome, mental retardation, and autism. (pp 2150-2152)
16. Identify strategies for providing care to patients with communication impairment, including hearing, vision, and speech impairments. (pp 2153-2156)
17. Identify strategies for providing care to patients with sensory impairment, including paralysis, paraplegia, and quadriplegia. (p 2156)
18. Discuss concerns related to managing a cognitively impaired patient who experiences trauma. (pp 2156-2157)
19. Identify chronic medical conditions likely to be encountered by paramedics, including arthritis, cancer, cerebral palsy, cystic fibrosis, multiple sclerosis muscular dystrophy, myasthenia gravis, spina bifida, postpolio syndrome, systemic lupus erythematosus, and traumatic brain injury. (pp 2157-2162)
20. Discuss treatment and transportation concerns for patients with a chronic illness. (pp 2157-2162)

Skills Objectives

1. Demonstrate how to suction and clean a tracheostomy. (pp 2132-2135, Skill Drill 1)
2. Demonstrate how to access an implantable venous access device. (pp 2137-2139, Skill Drill 2)
3. Demonstrate how to replace an ostomy device. (pp 2140-2141; 2142, Skill Drill 3)
4. Demonstrate how to catheterize an adult male patient. (pp 2143-2144, Skill Drill 4)
5. Demonstrate how to catheterize an adult female patient. (pp 2143-2145, Skill Drill 5)

■ Introduction

As a paramedic, you will encounter patients with a wide variety of special challenges. It is often necessary to modify how you communicate with, assess, treat, or transport a patient when that person has a chronic medical condition, sensory impairment, cognitive or emotional disorder, or other anomaly. An understanding of many of the special challenges highlighted in this chapter will help you provide optimal care when EMS assistance is required for these patients.

The combined incidence of cognitive, sensory, and communication impairments in the US population is staggering. One to three percent of the population has mental retardation, making it the cognitive impairment that you are most likely to encounter. Slightly less than 1% of children have autism or a related condition. Overall, 13% of children have some form of developmental disability.

Patients with complicated illnesses and those who require invasive medical devices are no longer confined to acute health care settings **Table 1**. Many life-sustaining therapies such as mechanical ventilation and intravenous (IV) medication administration are continued outside the hospital, often performed by members of the patient's family or by the patients themselves. You should expect to provide care to these patients during EMS response in the community and when these patients require transportation between various health care facilities.

Many social and economic factors adversely impact the health of people. Paramedics are frequently requested as a last resort when a patient cannot otherwise access health care services

| Table 1 | Home Care Patients in the United States, 2000 and 2007 | | | | |

Year	Number of Persons Receiving Home Care	>65 Years Old	<65 Years Old	Female	Male
2000	1,355,290	29.5%	70.5%	64.8%	35.2%
2007	1,459,900	68.7%	31.3%	64.0	36.0

Source: www.cdc.gov/nchs/fastats/homehealthcare.htm. Accessed March 17, 2012.

or when attempts to manage an illness, injury, or chronic medical condition without assistance have suddenly failed. This situation can overwhelm EMS and emergency department resources, placing a heavy burden on paramedics in many EMS systems.

Patient care is further complicated when caregivers abuse or neglect people who are dependent on them. You must learn to recognize signs and cues suggestive of abuse or neglect. Abuse and neglect recognition and reporting become essential when children, incapacitated elderly, and many patients with the special challenges outlined in this chapter are victimized.

■ General Strategies for Patients With Special Challenges

You should not feel overwhelmed when you are confronted by a patient with special challenges. In many instances, the patient

YOU are the Medic   PART 1

You and your partner are called to the health department for a child in respiratory distress. On arrival a nurse meets you at the registration desk and brings you back to an examination room where you find a 15-year-old girl seated on the examination table leaning forward in the tripod position with noted accessory muscle use, increased respiratory rate, and faint audible expiratory wheezes. The patient's mother explains that her daughter, Amanda, has been having increased shortness of breath for the past 2 days. Amanda has been out of her breathing medication for the past week due to the inability to pay.

Recording Time: 1 Minute	
Appearance	Teenager small for stated age, in respiratory distress
Level of consciousness	Alert (oriented to person, place, and day)
Airway	Open
Breathing	Increased work of breathing with accessory muscle use and faint expiratory wheezes
Circulation	Strong radial pulse, slightly increased; clubbing noted

1. Using the pediatric assessment triangle as a guide, what is your general impression of the child?
2. What information would you like to get from the mother?

Special Populations

Chronic conditions necessitating home care occur across all age groups. Different conditions are more prevalent in certain age groups. In addition, the age of the person affects his or her response to the chronic condition.

In childhood, chronic conditions may impede the attainment of normal developmental milestones and affect trust and autonomy. In adolescence, body image and peer acceptance become primary concerns, and normal teenage rebellion may interfere with treatment plans. The development of intimate relationships and achievement of vocational goals may be impaired when chronic illness strikes in early adulthood. Chronic illness in middle age may hinder professional or career growth, resulting in early retirement and the need to use retirement income for medical expenses. Spouses of older patients may become the primary caregiver even though they are experiencing a similar decline in health.

and his or her caregivers have already become experts on a particular condition or impairment. An open mind and willingness to listen are often your greatest assets. You should demonstrate confidence while enlisting the expertise of the patient or other caregiver when you are determining the optimal method to communicate with, assess, treat, and transport a patient. This alliance will help you provide optimal patient care while minimizing the risk of mistakes, complications, or injuries to the patient or others. The collaboration may be as simple as the patient showing you the best place to start an IV line or as complicated as helping you troubleshoot a malfunctioning ventilator or infusion pump.

Patients and caregivers have often received large amounts of education related to a particular condition, device, or technique. It is a mistake for you to claim to have more familiarity with the situation than you actually have. The patient or caregivers are likely to immediately recognize any disparity, and their trust in you will be undermined. Conversely, a well-educated paramedic may be able to explain some important nuance related to the situation, greatly enhancing the understanding by the patient or his or her caregiver.

Resources such as online medical control, electronic medical reference materials, and the experience of coworkers will also prove extremely valuable when you encounter unfamiliar conditions, technology, or situations. A dedicated paramedic will learn from these encounters and become better prepared for similar challenges in the future.

EMS, Health Care, and Poverty

Paramedics, other EMS providers, and emergency departments are on the frontlines of the economic and health care crisis facing the United States. Over the last 5 years, the number of people without health insurance has increased. In 2010, almost 50 million people did not have health insurance in the US. For people fortunate enough to have any health insurance, a greater number are forced to rely on government health programs. According to the US Census Bureau report *Income, Poverty, and Health Insurance in the United States: 2010*, 46.2 million people were in poverty in the US in 2010. The definition of poverty depends on a calculation that factors how many people are in a household, their ages, and the household's combined total income. For example, two people under the age of 65 who have one child would be in poverty if their combined annual income were less than $15,030. These trends profoundly impact EMS.

Poverty and the lack of health insurance impact a person's health habits in a variety of ways. As people lose the ability to pay for health care, they stop seeking or receiving many preventive health services. Without preventive measures, the incidence and severity of a disease process can increase significantly. Health care is often delayed until an emergent situation develops.

Chronic medical conditions such as diabetes, hypertension, reactive airway disease, mental disorders, and certain infectious diseases such as tuberculosis and acquired immune deficiency syndrome (AIDS) require ongoing medication to control the disease process. Poverty and the lack of health insurance may prevent patients from receiving needed medications. People may be forced to choose between paying for medications and paying for such necessities as food, clothing, or shelter. Interruption of needed medications can lead to catastrophic complications. Exacerbation of chronic illness due to lack of medication may lead to expensive hospitalization and worsening financial woes. Loss of a job or depletion of personal savings during periods of economic hardship can cause a patient to lose access to basic health care services.

Homelessness is a complicated economic and social problem. Homeless people are typically prone to numerous chronic medical conditions, frequently accompanied by mental illness and substance abuse. Medical care for homeless people is made more difficult by problems associated with environmental exposure, crime/violence, malnutrition, and lack of hygiene. Rates of pregnancy, infectious diseases, and mental illness in homeless people far exceed rates in the general population. People who are homeless have difficulty accessing preventive health care services and are subject to the same financial barriers to health maintenance as other people who live in poverty.

Patients frequently seek EMS and emergency department assistance when a chronic medical condition becomes severe or when health care is needed and no other options are available. Federal laws require emergency departments to stabilize patients experiencing an emergency or active labor, regardless of the patient's ability to pay. This protection allows people with no means to pay for health care services to access health care providers without demand for upfront payment. The stress that this practice places on emergency departments is significant.

An alarming number of emergency departments have closed in recent years because of financial pressures and changes within the health care industry. Many of the emergency departments that remain are becoming overcrowded. You may be forced to transport patients greater distances to an available emergency department or experience longer delays when turning patients over to emergency department staff due to overcrowding.

The situation is further complicated by seemingly frivolous requests for EMS assistance and transportation. Paramedics and other EMS providers are often placed in a precarious position because they may recognize that a patient does not need transportation to an emergency department, but they still feel obligated to transport the patient because of a fear of legal liability or regulations prohibiting patient abandonment. Depending on the nature of a particular EMS system, people may request EMS assistance simply as a method to obtain a "free ride" to the hospital or in an attempt to bypass overcrowded emergency department waiting rooms. Although other health care settings may be more appropriate for the needs of a particular patient, paramedics must be extremely careful to avoid legal liability or charges of patient abandonment. The distinction between an informed patient refusal and abandonment by EMS providers becomes problematic in many situations. Paramedics are in the unique position to assist people in the community by advocating for patient rights and suggesting safe alternatives so patients can receive appropriate medical care. Remember, when patients call for assistance, even when you do not believe such assistance is necessary, the safest thing to do is to provide that assistance. Never refuse to transport a patient if requested unless your EMS system and medical director specifically authorize you to do so.

Various health care organizations and communities have taken creative approaches to providing health care services outside the emergency department to people without health insurance or those who have limited financial resources. Whereas emergency departments are well suited to handle a patient in crisis, management of chronic medical conditions is often less than optimal. Such issues as medication monitoring, prescription refills, diagnostic testing, referrals, and coordination among specialists, as well as assistance with social needs, lifestyle modification, or long-term care, are best coordinated by primary health care providers. You may see changes in education and scope of practice as practices in the health care industry place increasing stress on emergency departments and EMS systems. Creative ideas include having EMS providers offer more primary care services or allowing EMS providers to transport 9-1-1 patients to health care settings other than emergency departments.

Health care resources are available for patients with financial need **Figure 1**. Government agencies and private organizations provide health care services to at-risk groups through a variety of community-based health care facilities. These may be targeted at homeless people, children, families, or any person with financial need. Many immunizations are provided at little or no cost by the government in the interest of public health. Hospitals are frequently able to provide financial assistance, payment plans, low-cost health care services, or help enrolling eligible people in government health insurance programs. EMS treatment or transportation should never be discouraged because of a person's perceived financial difficulty.

■ Care of Patients With Suspected Abuse and Neglect

You are likely to provide care to victims of **abuse** and **neglect**. However, you will most likely find that caring for these patients is made difficult by a host of emotional, legal, and regulatory concerns. In addition, the care you are trying to provide is frequently complicated by your interactions with the possible perpetrator(s). You must continue to provide effective care to these patients while taking affirmative steps to protect the potential victim from future harm **Figure 2**.

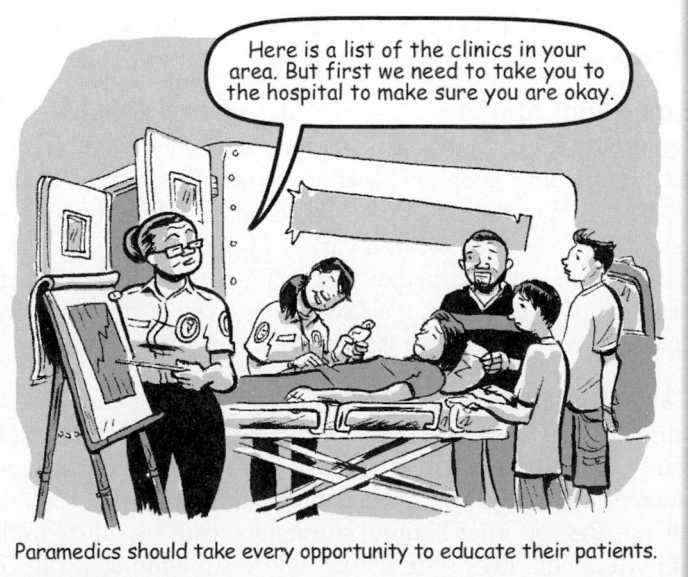

Paramedics should take every opportunity to educate their patients.

Figure 1

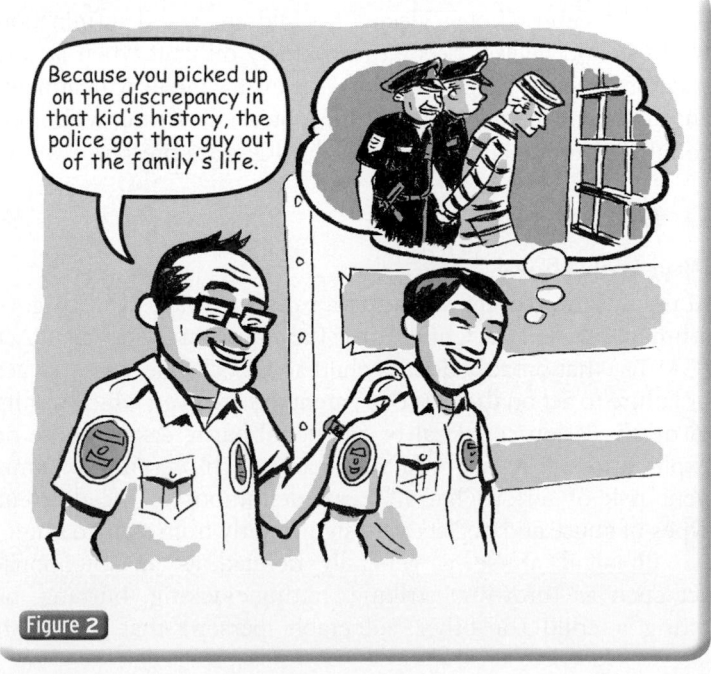

Figure 2

Several groups of people are particularly susceptible to abuse or neglect by caregivers. Children and dependent elderly are at high risk for abuse and neglect. Adults with medical, cognitive, or emotional impairments may also be subject to abuse or neglect by caregivers. Many adult patients with specific challenges discussed later in this chapter are potential victims of abuse and neglect by family members or caregivers.

Epidemiology

Millions of children and vulnerable adults are abused or neglected each year in the United States. Six million children and up to 2 million elderly adults are victimized each year, though the actual incidence is widely believed to be much higher than the number of reported cases. An average of five children die every day from abuse or neglect. Over three quarters of the children that die from abuse or neglect are killed by one or both parents.

Infants and young children are more likely to be victims of abuse or neglect than older children. Approximately 80% of abused or neglected children who die are younger than 4 years; more than 45% are younger than 1 year. Boys and girls are abused or neglected at roughly equal rates. Approximately 70% of all child abuse or neglect cases involve substance abuse by the perpetrator. Children with a disability or chronic medical condition have twice the likelihood of being abused or neglected as healthy children.

Abuse and neglect occur with varied frequency across the spectrum of race and socioeconomic status. Child maltreatment can be committed by any person who has care, custody, or control of the child, including parents, step-parents, foster parents, babysitters, and relatives. Abusive parents frequently receive little enjoyment from parenting and are more isolated from the community than are nonabusive parents. They have unrealistic expectations of their child and try to control the child through negative and authoritarian means. Abusive parents are often afraid of asking for help from sources of support in their community, or are emotionally unable to ask for help. Most were themselves abused or neglected as children. The determination of abuse and neglect becomes extremely difficult when factors such as poverty, religious beliefs regarding medical treatment, autonomy of mature minors, and potential victims with concomitant emotional or behavioral disorders are present.

Definitions

Physical Abuse

Abuse and neglect may occur in a variety of ways. The US government enacted the Child Abuse Prevention and Treatment Act (CAPTA) that broadly defines child abuse or neglect as: ". . . act or failure to act on the part of a parent or caregiver, which results in death, serious physical or emotional harm, sexual abuse or exploitation, or an act or failure to act which presents an imminent risk of serious harm." Legal definitions of the different types of abuse and neglect vary significantly from state to state.

Physical abuse is generally defined as an intentional act such as throwing, striking, hitting, kicking, burning, or biting a child (or other vulnerable person) that results in physical impairment or injury. Approximately 650,000 children are victims of physical abuse each year. You may encounter victims of physical abuse when you are requested to respond for a dramatic injury, or suspected abuse may be discovered while you are treating and transporting patients with a seemingly unrelated complaint. Physical abuse also occurs if a caregiver places the child or other susceptible person in circumstances that create a substantial risk of harm. When a child is injured because of inadequate supervision or the caregiver's failure to use seat belts or other safety devices, it may or may not be considered physical abuse depending on the specific circumstances or the particular state where the injury occurred.

Neglect

Neglect of vulnerable people is roughly four times more common than physical abuse. Children, certain vulnerable or impaired adults, and the dependent elderly require the assistance of caregivers to provide basic necessities such as food, shelter, medical care, supervision, and possibly financial guidance. When caregivers fail to provide such protection and the health or well-being of the vulnerable person is impacted, neglect occurs. Signs of neglect are often subtle, requiring greater awareness on the part of paramedics and other health care providers.

Sexual Abuse and Sexual Exploitation

Vulnerable people may become victims of **sexual abuse** or **sexual exploitation**. This may range from outright sexual contact, to forced prostitution, inappropriate undressing, sexually suggestive photography, or simply forcing the victim to watch sexual acts or pornography. Almost 10% of reported child abuse or neglect cases involve sexual abuse or exploitation, though the actual incidence is unfortunately underreported. Elder sexual abuse statistics are not readily available, although one study revealed that 81% of elderly female sexual abuse incidents were committed by the patient's primary caregiver. Certain behavioral cues, genital trauma, and the presence of a sexually transmitted disease are highly suggestive of sexual abuse. In extreme cases, comatose women have become pregnant, leading to criminal charges for caregivers.

Emotional Abuse

Emotional abuse impacts children, dependent elderly, and other vulnerable people. This abuse causes a substantial change in the victim's behavior, emotional response, or cognitive function, or it may manifest as a variety of mental illnesses. Emotional abuse may be verbal in the form of ridicule, threats, blaming, or humiliation. It also occurs nonverbally when a caregiver ignores the victim or isolates the victim from others.

Caregiver Substance Abuse

Various states have enacted laws that specifically address substance abuse by the parents or other caregiver. It may be considered abuse or neglect when pregnant women use alcohol, illicit drugs, or other harmful substances, causing injury to the unborn child. Other state statutes address providing alcohol or drugs to a child, manufacturing or selling drugs in the presence of a child, or when a caregiver becomes impaired by alcohol or drugs while caring for a child or other vulnerable person. States may prosecute adults for child abuse when they drive while intoxicated with a child in the car or allow an underage child to become the designated driver for an intoxicated caregiver.

Abandonment

Caregivers may be prosecuted for abandonment in certain states. Abandonment occurs when a child or vulnerable adult suffers harm because the identified caregiver has failed to maintain adequate contact. Leaving a young child home alone and/or allowing the child to wander the streets unsupervised are two possible examples of abandonment.

Recognizing Abuse or Neglect

Paramedics and other health care providers have a duty to recognize and report suspected abuse or neglect in children and vulnerable adults. A variety of behavioral cues and physical findings will prompt suspicion of abuse or neglect in these patients.

The demeanor, behaviors, and history provided by the caregiver are often the first clues that abuse or neglect may be present. You should become immediately suspicious if the designated caregiver appears to be under the influence of alcohol or other intoxicating substance. Agitation, slurred speech, bloodshot eyes, speech alteration, unsteady gait, or other unexplained abnormality is suggestive of intoxication.

Caregivers in abuse or neglect situations may interfere with the physical examination of the child or vulnerable adult. Behaviors such as refusing to allow a physical examination, looming over the health care provider during the physical examination, preventing paramedics from removing clothing during the physical examination, or offering unsolicited explanations for abnormal physical findings during the examination may all be suggestive of abuse or neglect. The caregiver may also interrupt or otherwise prevent the patient from answering questions related to the particular illness or injury. Remember, do not confront a suspected perpetrator; rather, simply report to the "hot-line" and ED physician. These behaviors should raise your suspicion of abuse or neglect.

You should pay particular attention when a caregiver provides the history of present illness/injury (HPI) or describes the events that prompted the call for EMS involvement. In many instances, the story provided by the caregiver simply does not make sense in relation to the age, capability, or medical condition of the patient. In other situations, the story provided by the caregiver will frequently change with each subsequent discussion or the explanations provided by the patient and various caregivers will be significantly different.

A caregiver may occasionally self-report facts that are highly suggestive of abuse or neglect. Statements such as "I lost my temper," "I couldn't get her to stop crying," or "I did it to teach him a lesson" should raise immediate concerns regarding abuse or neglect. Other situations such as a child being injured due to obviously careless actions of an intoxicated caregiver should trigger your concerns regarding abuse or neglect.

The child or vulnerable adult may demonstrate a wide range of behaviors, symptoms, or physical signs that are suggestive of abuse or neglect. When you are assessing a potential child abuse case, be attuned to suspicious behavioral traits. A child who does not become agitated when a parent leaves the room or who does not look to a parent for reassurance may be abused. Children who are abused may also cry excessively or not at all, may be wary of physical contact, or may appear apprehensive.

In many instances there is a legitimate reason for the findings that is related to normal growth and development or a particular medical or mental health condition, not resulting from any maltreatment. You should discuss abnormal behavioral cues or other findings with receiving health care providers when you observe unusual findings during patient assessment.

A variety of physical signs are highly suggestive of the possibility of nonaccidental trauma, particularly in young children and infants. Physical abuse is commonly associated with fractures, burns, and bruises **Figure 3**. Bruises on the torso, ears, proximal arms, abdomen, and buttocks are suggestive of abuse **Figure 4**. Closed head injury in the absence of a realistic mechanism is also suggestive of abuse. One author reports 80% of head injuries in patients younger than 2 years are a result of physical abuse. Burns, particularly symmetric burns or those without splash marks and ligature marks suggest abuse **Figure 5**. Bruises in patterns resembling finger marks, shoes, or other common items are also extremely concerning for physical abuse. Seizure activity without a prior history in an afebrile child should raise suspicion for the possibility of physical abuse.

Table 2 outlines a variety of signs, symptoms, and behaviors that may be a manifestation of abuse or neglect. Multiple types of abuse or neglect may be present in the same patient, and there may be considerable variability among the signs, symptoms, and behaviors outlined in Table 2.

Benign Physical Findings

Paramedics and other EMS providers should be aware of notable physical findings that appear to mimic signs of physical abuse.

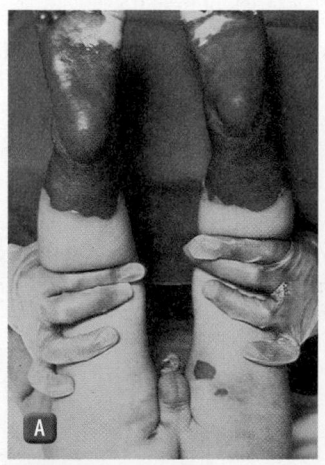
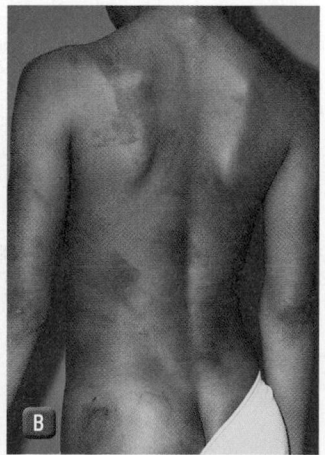

Figure 3 Signs of child abuse. **A.** Scald. **B.** Multiple injuries at different stages of healing.

At first glance these findings may appear highly suggestive of nonaccidental trauma, but on further investigation maltreatment is often ruled out.

Ambulatory toddlers are prone to bruising or minor injuries as psychomotor skills develop through early childhood. Bruises in various locations and various stages of healing are often present on the arms, legs, and faces of normal, healthy, and well cared-for toddlers and young children. As children grow older, a wide assortment of injuries may occur from bicycling, contact sports, and a vast array of horseplay and recreational activities. Scald burns from a toddler grabbing an unguarded pot off the stove will appear different from submersion injuries associated with intentional physical abuse. It is possible that toddlers and young children will sustain bites or scratches from young playmates rather than the malice of a parent or other caregiver. When odd injuries are present on a toddler or child, you should keep an open mind when you are assessing for the possibility of physical abuse.

Mongolian spots are lesions that resemble bruises, typically on the buttocks or back, that are present at birth on many infants of Asian or African origin **Figure 6** . Mongolian spots occur

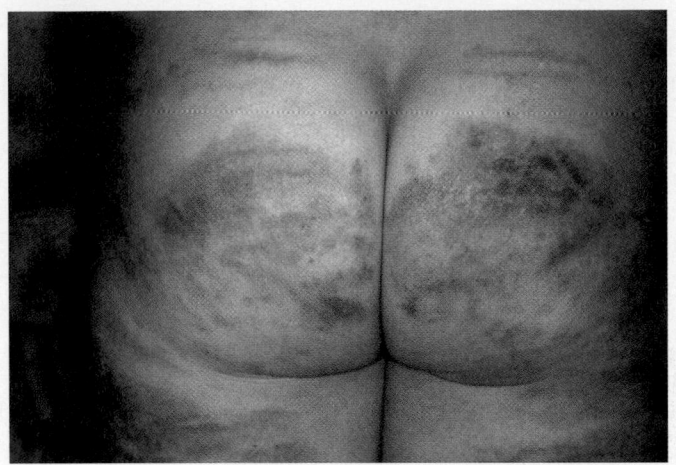

Figure 4 Bruises on the buttocks are usually inflicted injuries.

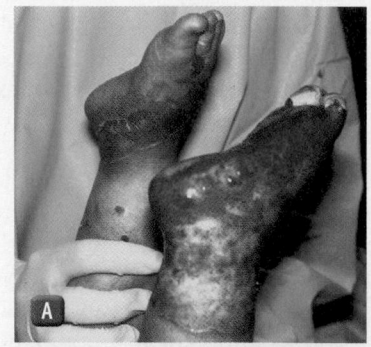
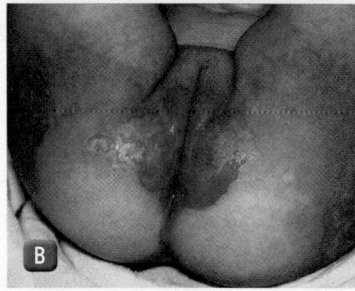

Figure 5 **A.** Stocking/glove burns of the feet or hands in an infant or a toddler are almost always inflicted injuries. **B.** A doughnut burn occurs when a child is held in a hot bath and the area in contact with the cooler porcelain is spared.

Table 2 General Signs and Symptoms of Abuse and Neglect

General	Physical Abuse	Neglect	Sexual Abuse	Emotional Abuse
Sudden change in behavior or school performance	Unexplained (or poorly explained) bruises, bites, burns, fractures	Frequent absences from school	Difficulty walking or sitting	Extremes in behavior (passive, aggressive, labile, demanding)
Hypervigilant behavior	Numerous injuries in various stages of healing	Appears malnourished	Nightmares, bedwetting, or sleep disturbances	Developmental delays
Learning difficulties	Injuries inconsistent with reported mechanism	Dirty clothes, inappropriate clothes for weather	Unusual sexual behaviors or knowledge in young children	Acting inappropriately adult or inappropriately infantile
Suicide attempts or self-harm	Injuries inconsistent with age, developmental stage, or ability	Obvious inadequate medical or dental care	Sexually transmitted diseases	Wide variety of emotional or behavioral disorders
Demonstrates lack of attachment to parent or caregiver	Injury patterns suggestive of nonaccidental trauma	Poor hygiene	Injuries or bleeding from anus or genitalia	
Unusual attachment or comfort with strangers		Pressure ulcers in people who are nonambulatory	Suspicious pregnancy	
		Soiled bedding, unsanitary living conditions, unsafe living conditions		

Original table by A. Bartkus, adapted from the Child Welfare Information Gateway at www.childwelfare.gov/pubs/factsheets/signs.cfm.

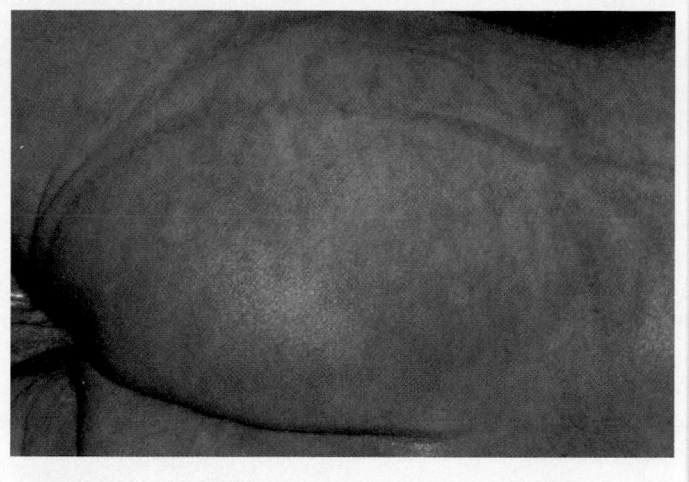

Figure 6 Mongolian spots can be mistaken for bruises.

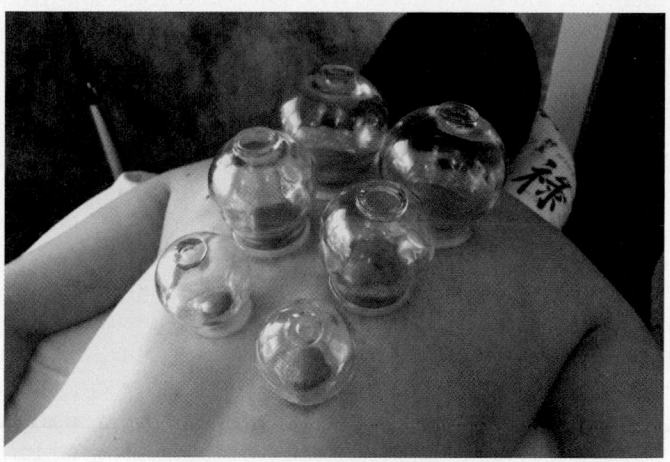

Figure 8 Cupping is the cultural practice of placing warm cups on the skin to pull out illness from the body. The red, flat, rounded skin lesions are often more intensely red at the borders.

less frequently in other locations throughout the body surface. These lesions generally fade over time and are not associated with other signs of soft-tissue trauma.

Certain Asian cultures practice two techniques known as **coining** (*cao gio*) and **cupping** (*baguanfa, dijiufa,* or *shanhuofa*). These techniques are practiced in Eastern medicine to relieve a wide variety of symptoms or conditions. In coining, a coin with warm oil is rubbed vigorously across the torso, causing superficial skin trauma in a linear pattern that could be easily mistaken for physical abuse Figure 7 . Cupping is performed by heating the inside of a small glass vessel (cup), then applying it to the patient's skin. A vacuum is created as the vessel cools, creating round red marks or bruising, usually on the patient's torso Figure 8 . Marks from these techniques appear highly suggestive of physical abuse; however, they are actually healing techniques practiced for many centuries and are not associated with any malice or maltreatment.

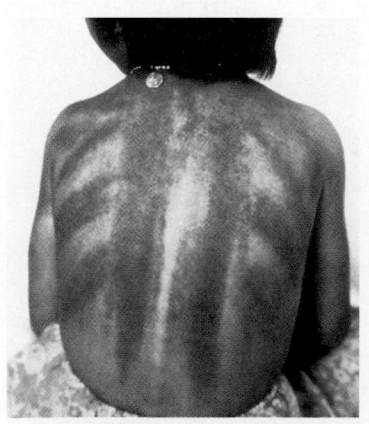

Figure 7 Rubbing hot coins, often on the back, produces rounded and oblong red, patchy, flat skin lesions.

Health care providers in certain cultures apply citrus or vegetable juices to the patient's skin for healing purposes. As the juices get exposed to sunlight, redness of the skin, known as **phytophotodermatitis**, may develop. These patterns may resemble splash burns or similar injury, prompting suspicion of physical abuse.

You may also encounter benign physical findings that are suggestive of sexual abuse. Poor hygiene, masturbating, skin irritation from cleansing products, marks from poorly fitting undergarments, and various infections can all cause physical findings that are suggestive of sexual abuse. You should use caution before labeling manifestations of many of these benign conditions as sexual abuse.

Words of Wisdom

It is a good idea to establish a "code" between you and your partner indicating that the provider should discreetly call for police. This signal can be as simple as "Could you go to the ambulance and get the extra set of latex-free gloves?" This way, you will not aggravate or "tip off" the abuser to your request for police, further riling him or her.

■ Management of Suspected Abuse or Neglect

Care of patients who are victims of abuse or neglect may present a considerable challenge for paramedics. Innocent victims suffer devastating injuries at the hands of people who are supposed to be responsible for that patient's well-being. When innocent children, vulnerable adults, or frail elderly patients are victimized, it is likely to evoke powerful emotions in you and other health care providers. These emotions have the potential to undermine patient care and ultimately worsen the situation for the patient.

Assessment Process

You should focus on several key priorities when you are caring for a patient with suspected abuse or neglect. The first priority is the safety of emergency responders. Other forms of domestic violence accompany 30% to 50% of child abuse incidents. Domestic violence incidents are notorious for placing police, emergency responders, and even innocent bystanders at considerable risk of harm. Law enforcement assistance should be requested whenever the threat of continued violence is present. Scene safety is discussed in greater depth in other areas of this text.

The second priority is for you to provide optimal clinical care to any patient with suspected abuse or neglect. This includes a patient assessment that is appropriate for the clinical situation. You should not waste large amounts of time conducting a meticulous head-to-toe examination when immediate threats to a patient's life are present. Life-sustaining interventions and prompt transport are the most appropriate treatment for any patient with a critical illness or injury. Immediate threats to life must be treated aggressively, regardless of whether abuse or neglect is present or suspected. As time permits, you should conduct a thorough patient assessment that includes a history of present illness, head-to-toe exam, and any relevant medical and psychosocial history. The value of full patient exposure must be balanced against privacy needs of the patient and the risks of further traumatizing a victim of suspected abuse or neglect.

It is likely that all the facts of a particular situation will not be fully disclosed when you initially interact with the patient and any caregivers present. You should not make any hasty assumptions regarding the identity of an alleged perpetrator or circumstances surrounding a particular event. It is possible that the caregiver present with the patient is also a victim of abuse, neglect, or violence.

You must use careful judgment when you are deciding whether to allow a particular parent or caregiver to remain or travel with the patient. Separating an ill or injured child from a trusted caregiver may cause additional stress, especially if this caregiver turns out not to be a perpetrator or in situations when no abuse or neglect has actually occurred. Conversely, the presence of a violent perpetrator may continue to threaten the patient and place you at risk of injury.

You should make every attempt to remain nonjudgmental when you are providing patient care. This is often not easy when powerful emotions are present. You need to remain professional and provide the patient with the best treatment possible. Comments and hostility directed toward the patient's caregiver are unlikely to do anything except complicate the situation, and are unprofessional.

Documentation

Careful documentation is essential whenever abuse or neglect is present or suspected. Paramedics should expect that any patient care reports (PCRs) and related documentation are going to be reviewed by law enforcement officers, by social service agencies, and in court. Simple documentation errors such as incorrect spelling or grammar and inconsistent times will undermine both the credibility of the documentation and the paramedic responsible for the documentation. Use accurate quotations whenever possible, identifying the source of the information. Carefully document any physical findings or indicate whether assessment of a particular body area was accomplished or deferred. Avoid inaccurate terms such as "normal" or "within normal limits," if a particular area has not been adequately evaluated. Use objective descriptions and measurements whenever possible when

YOU *are the Medic*   **PART 2**

Using the pediatric assessment triangle, you classify Amanda as sick. Her normal appearance, normal circulation, and abnormal work of breathing lead you to believe that she is in respiratory distress. You have your partner apply a nebulizer with 2.5 mg albuterol/3 mL normal saline and attach the cardiac monitor. The mother tells you that Amanda was born with cystic fibrosis. She is supposed to take breathing treatments with albuterol four times a day followed by chest physical therapy, digestive enzymes before each meal, and vitamins.

Recording Time: 3 Minutes	
Respirations	24 breaths/min; labored, faint expiratory wheezes, and rhonchi bilaterally
Pulse	110 beats/min, regular; strong radial pulses
Skin	Pink, warm, and dry
Blood pressure	116/72 mm Hg
Oxygen saturation (Spo$_2$)	92% on nebulizer at 8 L/min of oxygen
Pupils	2 seconds

3. What is cystic fibrosis?
4. Which body systems are most affected by cystic fibrosis?

you are documenting findings on the physical examination. You should carefully document the timing or time frame of a particular injury or event. Subsequent changes in the reported timing of an event may disclose or substantiate suspicions of abuse or neglect. Avoid labeling a person as a victim or perpetrator. Cite a specific source when you are charting a history of present illness. Avoid photography unless there is a formal policy at the EMS agency that outlines appropriate consent, technique, storage, security, and release of any patient photographs. Special training is often required for forensic photography. It is quite easy for an otherwise well-intentioned paramedic to violate HIPAA or other patient privacy rules by taking and sharing patient photographs.

Words of Wisdom

If you and your partner can safely get the patient and the person suspected of abuse away from each other, by all means do so. This separation will help make the scene safer; it also gives you a chance to compare current histories.

Mandatory Reporting and Legal Involvement

Paramedics, EMS providers, and other health professionals are **mandatory reporters** of suspected child abuse and neglect. If you have a reasonable suspicion that child abuse or neglect has occurred, you must report the circumstances to the appropriate child welfare agency for a particular jurisdiction. If you fail to report suspected child abuse or neglect, you may be subject to a variety of civil, criminal, or regulatory penalties. Many states have enacted statutes specifically addressing mandatory reporting of abuse to elderly and incapacitated adults, though the scope of these statutes may vary significantly from state to state. You should consult your applicable state laws and EMS regulations regarding mandatory reporting of suspected abuse and neglect of the elderly and other vulnerable adults.

Suspected abuse and neglect are reported to the state or government social services agency of a particular jurisdiction. Agency titles vary by location, but are usually called something similar to **Adult Protective Services (APS)**, Department of Youth Services, or Children Youth and Family Division. In most states, central hotline telephone numbers are available for abuse or neglect reports involving children or vulnerable adults. These agencies evaluate the circumstances of a particular report and determine whether an investigation is indicated. Unfortunately, not every report of abuse or neglect will automatically trigger an investigation. Rates of investigations of abuse and neglect reports vary significantly from state to state. Circumstances of the case and the severity of the alleged abuse or neglect will determine whether an investigation is initiated or how urgently the social services agency intervenes. Intervention may range from providing support to an at-risk family all the way to immediate removal of the victim from the home or facility.

Law enforcement personnel frequently become involved in cases of suspected abuse or neglect. Law enforcement officers may respond simultaneously with EMS, may discover abuse or neglect while engaged in other law enforcement activities, or may be requested by health care providers, EMS responders, or an investigator from the social services agency. Law enforcement officers have two primary roles when abuse or neglect is suspected. They may intervene when there is an immediate threat to the health or safety of a child or vulnerable adult. Officers are typically empowered to take custody of a child or vulnerable adult for a short duration until the appropriate social services agency can intervene or the immediate threat resolves. In addition, law enforcement officers conduct a simultaneous investigation into potential criminal activity associated with the suspected abuse or neglect. When suspected abuse or neglect results in death, these cases are referred to the medical examiner for autopsy.

Paramedics and other emergency responders may benefit from emotional support following their response to dramatic or heart-wrenching cases of abuse or neglect. Many areas have specially trained crisis intervention personnel who are familiar with the difficult role of EMS and other emergency responders. These personnel can help paramedics and other emergency responders recognize and manage the enormous emotional stress associated with these extremely challenging situations.

■ Care of Patients With Terminal Illness

Death is inevitable. Despite advances in the science and technology of modern health care, many disease processes simply cannot be reversed. As patients confront the reality of failing health, many choose to forego uncomfortable, invasive, and often marginally effective medical treatment of a particular condition or disease. Paramedics and other EMS providers will encounter patients with a wide variety of terminal illnesses as well as those who decline aggressive medical intervention for otherwise potentially treatable conditions.

Most sources define **terminal illness** as a disease process that is expected to cause death within 6 months, verified by a physician. Other medical conditions will ultimately cause death because of a lack of effective medical treatment options or simply the devastating impact of the disease process itself. These conditions may persist for years as the health of the patient either fluctuates or steadily declines. Common terminal conditions include cancer, heart failure, pulmonary disease, liver failure, AIDS, Alzheimer disease, and amyotrophic lateral sclerosis (ALS; Lou Gehrig disease). When you are treating these patients, you must be prepared to alter or forego the aggressive, lifesaving interventions that have historically defined the paramedic profession. If you are called to a scene in which death is imminent, the actions you take will have a lasting impact on the family. This is a time when compassion, understanding, and sensitivity are most needed.

Patients with a terminal illness often receive continued medical care. Some continue aggressive medical treatment, hoping for a statistically improbable recovery or attempting to prolong life as much as possible. This approach is known as **curative care**.

Other patients may pursue curative care, but refrain from treatment options that are risky, minimally effective, or cause significant discomfort. As the disease process worsens and hopes for recovery fade, patients may transition from curative care to **comfort care**, also known as **palliative care**. When a patient is receiving comfort or palliative care, the focus changes from prolonging life to improving the quality of the time that the patient has left. Medical care continues, but aggressive, invasive, and uncomfortable interventions cease. Patients undergoing comfort care frequently continue to receive analgesic medications, oxygen, IV fluids, treatment of fevers, and possibly antibiotic medications.

Terminally ill patients seen by EMS usually need only supportive care. Therapy is usually aimed at making the patient as comfortable as possible. The patient may have a displaced urinary catheter, need assistance in returning to bed, or need intervention in a pain crisis.

Patients with a terminal illness and their caregivers will often know the best way to manage sudden increases in discomfort. Pain assessment and management are often primary tasks for paramedics treating patients with a terminal illness. Patients should be assessed for pain using a variety of techniques depending on the patient's age, ability to communicate, and cognitive function. You should obtain a history that includes the patient's use of, effectiveness of, and adverse reactions to particular pain medications, especially if you have limited pharmacologic options for pain management. Terminally ill patients may use a complex array of pain medications, transdermal patches, or self-administered pain management devices. You should perform a patient assessment that includes the patient's level of consciousness, vital signs, past medical history, and pain medication history, and then either follow standing protocols or contact medical control in order to administer analgesic or sedative medications for patient comfort.

Many patients with a verified terminal illness choose to enter hospice treatment. **Hospice** is a program and philosophy that attempts to help the patient maximize the quality of remaining life. Hospice programs provide social and emotional support, treat discomfort with pharmacologic and nonpharmacologic approaches, and help patients and families cope with the prospect of impending death. Patients may receive hospice treatment at home, in hospitals, or while living at long-term care facilities.

■ Advance Directives

Large numbers of patients and people in the community have advance directives in place. These forms are either signed by the patient or **surrogate decision-maker**. A surrogate decision-maker is somebody who is legally authorized to make health care decisions for that patient when the patient is not capable of making or communicating the decision himself or herself. The forms instruct health care providers how medical decisions for the patient are to be made when the patient is unable to comprehend or communicate such a decision due to incapacity. Advance directives can specify which medical interventions are authorized in particular situations or who is authorized

to make these decisions on behalf of the patient. Patients with decision-making capacity may revoke a prior advance directive. You should contact online medical control when there is any confusion regarding the documentation or in situations when a patient's surrogate decision-maker is contradicting a written advance directive.

Hospice patients, along with many hospital patients and those living at home or in long-term care facilities, have do not resuscitate (DNR) orders in place. These forms are physician orders that instruct other health care providers to withhold some or all resuscitation efforts in the event that a patient experiences respiratory or cardiovascular collapse. These orders may be generic or may specifically discuss whether resuscitation procedures such as external cardiac compressions, vasopressor medications, endotracheal intubation, and bag-mask ventilation are indicated or withheld.

EMS providers can be placed in a precarious situation when they are encountering a patient in cardiac or respiratory arrest. State EMS agencies may require a specific DNR form for prehospital providers in the event of a prehospital cardiac or respiratory arrest. These forms may not be readily available when a prehospital resuscitation decision must be made. Other indicators of DNR status include wristbands and bracelets. EMS regulations will specify whether a symbolic indication of DNR status is sufficient for EMS providers to withhold resuscitation efforts. The situation becomes further complicated when conflict exists between DNR paperwork and the stated wishes of a family member or surrogate decision-maker for the patient. Paramedics should consult the EMS regulations for a particular state for specific requirements related to DNR orders and advance directives. Additional information regarding EMS patient consent and refusal can be found in the chapter, *Medical, Legal, and Ethical Issues*.

■ Care of Bariatric Patients

Obese patients create great difficulties for health care providers. Paramedics and other EMS responders must overcome many significant clinical and logistical hurdles when they are treating and transporting profoundly obese patients. As the obesity epidemic worsens, EMS systems may require additional resources to provide optimal care to this at-risk patient population.

The medical specialty of **bariatrics** has emerged in response to the widespread and profound incidence of adult and childhood obesity. Over one third of American adults are considered obese, defined by a body mass index (BMI) of greater than 30 kilograms per meters squared (kg/m^2). People with a BMI of between 40 and 49.9 kg/m^2 are considered to be morbidly obese. A BMI above 50 kg/m^2 is considered extreme obesity. Approximately 12.5 million (17%) children and adolescents are obese. Obesity adds from 80 to 168 billion dollars, depending on the source, to annual US health care costs. Several studies have found that EMS personnel and fire fighters have obesity rates that exceed the general population; one such study demonstrated that 75% of firefighter and paramedic recruits in a particular state were either overweight or obese.

A wide variety of lifestyle, genetic, metabolic, and environmental causes are responsible for obesity Table 3 .

Obesity causes or worsens a number of serious medical conditions. Heart disease, cerebrovascular accident, diabetes, hypertension, some cancers, and asthma are only some of the diseases linked to obesity. These patients are also prone to physical injury and a variety of musculoskeletal problems. Patients who are more than 40% overweight have double the likelihood of premature death.

Clinical Concerns for the Bariatric Patient

Routine procedures for obese patients can become extremely complicated. Airway procedures are made more difficult by a larger tongue, larger patient head size, and limited neck mobility associated with obesity. Bag-mask ventilation may be ineffective with patients in a supine position. Airway and ventilation procedures may need to occur with the patient in a semi-Fowler or reverse Trendelenburg position to facilitate optimal chest expansion. Obese patients will have a diminished respiratory reserve, decreasing the window to perform airway procedures before the patient becomes hypoxic. These patients often require bag-mask ventilations with positive end-expiratory pressure (PEEP), continuous positive airway pressure (CPAP), or bilevel positive airway pressure (BiPAP or BPAP) as a way to avoid endotracheal intubation or as a bridge until successful intubation can occur. Even bag-mask ventilation can become difficult because of poor mask seal or increased resistance due to excess body tissue on the chest wall and abdomen.

Peripheral IV access is often problematic in obese patients. A large neck mass may obscure landmarks for external jugular IV line placement or surgical cricothyrotomy. Many conventional intramuscular (IM) needles will not be able to actually reach the IM space through excess adipose tissue. Absorption and distribution will be altered for many lipophilic medications, potentially causing dramatic patient response at a given dose. (See the chapter, *Principles of Pharmacology* for further discussion of obesity and medication distribution.) Auscultation of

heart, lung, or bowel sounds may be more difficult through extra abdominal and chest wall mass.

Words of Wisdom

When you are transporting an obese or bariatric patient, be sure to alert the receiving facility in advance if special accommodations, equipment, or other resources may be needed.

Operational Concerns for the Bariatric Patient

EMS treatment and transportation of obese patients can quickly become complicated. Obese patients are often too heavy for traditional two-person EMS crews to package and transport safely or effectively. Additional lifting assistance is frequently necessary, although small rooms and narrow staircases limit the utility of additional lifting personnel. As patient weights become extreme, the capacity of EMS equipment such as stretchers, backboards, and stair chairs is quickly exceeded. EMS providers have attempted novel solutions such as using doors, tarps, or plywood for transporting extremely obese patients. These improvised devices are not designed to be carried safely and typically have no reliable way to secure the patient. There are reports of emergency responders needing to remove house walls or bay windows in order to extricate obese patients for transportation to a hospital. All of these operations put EMS providers at high risk for serious injury. Careful planning and proper body mechanics are essential to avoid injury to emergency responders or the patient. Whereas the creative solutions above may have been effective at the moment, both the patient and emergency responders were placed at considerable risk during the process.

Paramedics need to advocate for EMS equipment that is capable of safely transporting obese patients. Some EMS systems use ambulances with special winches, stretchers, and ramps that allow safe loading of bariatric patients. Even simple items such as larger blood pressure cuffs, longer injection or intraosseous (IO) needles, or special cervical collars may dramatically improve the paramedic's ability to provide patient care.

The reality is that the obesity epidemic will continue to grow. You should be prepared to encounter these patients with a vast array of illnesses and injuries in any conceivable scene location. Careful planning, a thorough understanding of the challenges involved, and the proper equipment will help you provide the best care possible to this extremely high-risk group.

Care of Patients With Communicable Diseases

Communicable diseases (also known as contagious diseases) are medical conditions that can be passed from one person to another by a variety of modes. The severity of these diseases ranges from almost completely undetectable to causing death

Table 3   Causes of Obesity

Primary Causes	Poor dietary choices
	Excessive food intake
	Lack of exercise
Secondary Causes	Hormonal changes
	Inadequate sleep
	Low basal metabolic rate
	Environmental toxins
	Genetic predisposition
	Declining smoking
	Widespread dependence on air conditioning

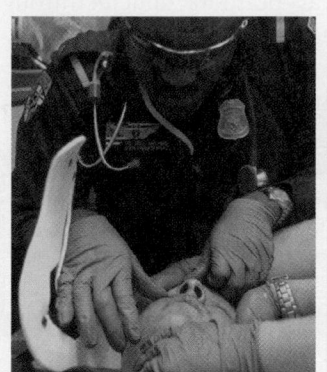

Figure 9 Always wear gloves and eye protection as a bare minimum.

within several days or weeks. Many patients live for years with a particular communicable disease and the continuous potential to transmit this disease to others. You should expect to encounter patients with communicable disease in every segment of the population and every geographic region. Therefore, safety protocols should always be followed. Gloves and eye protection should be considered mandatory attire. Gowns, masks, and other protective measures should be deployed if the situation warrants **Figure 9**. Safety for yourself, your crew, and your patient is paramount. (The chapters, *Workforce Safety and Wellness* and *Infectious and Communicable Diseases* discuss specific infectious diseases and infection control precautions in greater depth.)

Many communicable diseases have significant psychosocial implications. Having a communicable disease can take an emotional toll on the patient, his or her family, and loved ones. Also, certain communicable diseases are commonly associated with particular lifestyle choices that may not be well accepted by others. Communicable diseases often prompt paranoia in people who lack an understanding of the actual risk and mode(s) of transmission. People suspected of having a communicable disease may face discrimination, stigmatization, threats, or hostile treatment in the community. For these reasons, respect and privacy by paramedics is essential.

Patient assessment and communication should be conducted with as much privacy as possible. Bystanders, other emergency responders, and even personnel at a receiving facility may have an indirect relationship with the patient. Any unnecessary release of private information could adversely affect the patient. Violation of patient privacy rules can ultimately have harsh legal consequences for the paramedic as well.

You should endeavor to treat patients who have a communicable disease with all the respect and dignity afforded other patients. Patients may acquire a communicable disease through occupational exposure, sexual assault, blood transfusion, close family contact, or other method, without ever participating in any high-risk behaviors. Assumptions based on stereotypes of a particular communicable disease are unlikely to accomplish anything except to undermine patient care efforts.

Medical Technology in the Prehospital Setting

Patients with complex medical needs are no longer confined to acute health care settings. Many invasive, unusual, or life-sustaining therapies, once reserved for hospitals, are now widely used in patient homes and long-term care facilities. Chronically ill patients are cared for at home by a wide range of caregivers who may include family members, unlicensed caregivers, licensed nonprofessional caregivers, licensed professionals, or a combination of these. As mentioned, many family members who care for chronically ill patients are medically knowledgeable and are often your best source for information and care guidelines. In addition to frail or chronically ill elderly patients in the home care setting, you may encounter patients, for example, who have recently had a hospital stay, surgery, or a high-risk pregnancy, or a newborn with medical complications. When you encounter medical technology and adaptive devices during an EMS response or an interfacility patient transport, this technology may simplify, complicate, or have no impact whatsoever on your patient care. You may need to troubleshoot these devices when they malfunction or incorporate this technology into traditional prehospital patient care.

■ Tracheostomy Tubes

Tracheostomy (trach) tubes **Figure 10** function as a long-term replacement for endotracheal tubes. These devices are used for patients requiring long-term ventilator support, frequent tracheal suctioning, or airway protection resulting from a long list of possible medical conditions. If a patient experiences an unexpected loss of a tracheostomy tube due to occlusion or an accidental removal, it may or may not create an emergency. Many patients, even those on long-term ventilators, may tolerate interruptions in ventilator support for a period of time. Other patients, including those with cervical spinal cord injuries or serious neuromuscular disease are completely dependent on the ventilator. Loss of a tracheostomy tube may become an immediate threat to life.

Tracheostomy tubes can be placed emergently by health care providers when a profound upper airway obstruction occurs. They may also be placed electively in patients already receiving mechanical ventilation via endotracheal tubes or in patients with a slowly evolving upper airway obstruction or tumor. Tracheostomy tubes may be used by patients in the community, with or without an attached ventilator.

The tracheostomy tube passes directly from an opening in the anterior neck, below the thyroid cartilage, into the trachea. Speech is not possible unless expired air is allowed to pass around the tracheostomy tube and through the larynx (vocal cords). A tracheostomy tube bypasses the nasal passages that filter, warm, and humidify inspired air. Patients with a tracheostomy tube in place will need humidification and

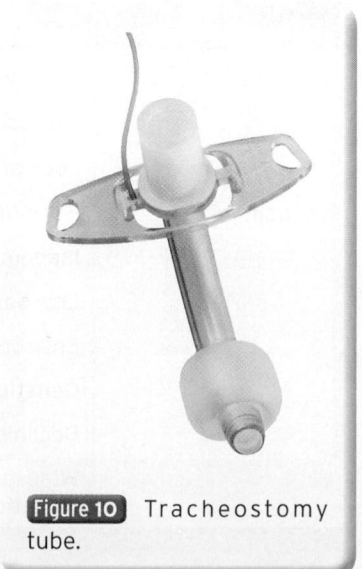

Figure 10 Tracheostomy tube.

heating of inspired air whenever possible. These patients also need frequent deep suctioning with an appropriate size suction catheter. In health care settings, deep tracheal suctioning is performed with sterile technique. Secretions may accumulate above the tracheostomy tube, requiring oral suctioning in addition to deep tracheal suctioning.

Tracheostomy tubes consist of three main parts with several notable additional features **Figure 11**. The **outer cannula** is the larger tube that passes from the anterior neck surface, inferior to the thyroid cartilage, into the trachea. Part of the outer cannula is a **flange** that helps stabilize the tracheostomy tube on the skin of the patient's neck and gets secured with ties or a strap around the patient's neck. The outer cannula may or may not have a cuff, similar to an endotracheal tube cuff. If a cuff is present, a short length of tubing with a cuff port (pilot balloon) and Luer valve will be visible. In adults, tracheostomy tube cuffs are necessary for bag-mask or ventilator assistance. Children may or may not require a tracheostomy tube cuff for assisted ventilation.

The second part of the tracheostomy tube is the **inner cannula**. The inner cannula is a tube that runs inside the outer cannula and can typically be removed for cleaning, although not all inner cannulas are capable of being removed. The inner cannula has a 15-mm port that can be attached to a bag-mask or ventilator circuit.

Words of Wisdom

If a tracheostomy tube becomes plugged, the patient may be ventilated by deflating the cuff, covering the nose and mouth with a mask, and using a bag-mask device. If you are unable to ventilate the patient through the tracheostomy, tube, plug the tracheostomy stoma and attempt to ventilate the patient in the traditional manner with a bag-mask device.

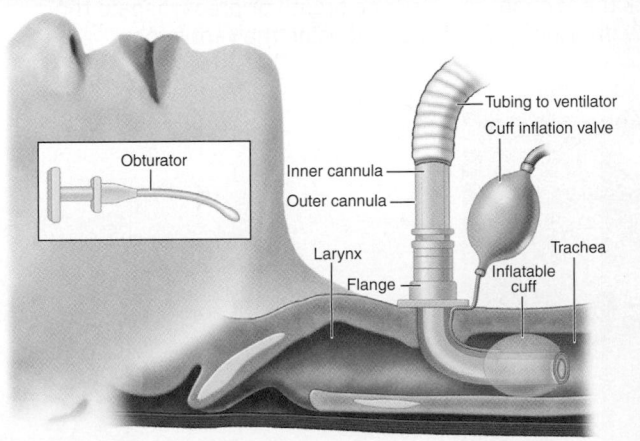

Figure 11 A tracheostomy is a surgical procedure in which an opening is placed in the trachea below the cricoid ring. A tracheostomy tube can be inserted into the opening to maintain it. It can also be attached to a ventilator or bag-mask device to assist with ventilations.

Special Populations

If you are transporting a child with a tracheostomy tube in a standard car seat, avoid using seats with a tray or shield. The tray or shield could come into contact with the tracheostomy tube and injure the child or block the airway.

The third part of the tracheostomy tube is the removable **obturator**, which is a solid plug with a rounded tip that extends out the bottom (inside) end of the trachea. The obturator is only used for reinserting the tracheostomy tube (outer cannula) if it becomes dislodged. In the unlikely event that traditional mask-to-mouth ventilations must be performed on a patient with tracheostomy tube in place, such as cuff failure in a ventilator-dependent patient with no backup outer cannula, the obturator may be inserted to keep air from escaping out the tracheostomy tube.

Tracheostomy tubes may be **fenestrated**, which means that holes or openings are present in the outer cannula or both the inner and the outer cannula. These holes allow the patients to speak, breathe, or clear secretions from the upper airway. Not every tracheostomy tube has fenestrations. These may be used for patients who are being evaluated for tracheostomy tube removal or for patients who only require intermittent ventilator support. It is essential that any cuff is deflated before a fenestrated tube is capped for speaking or clearing of secretions.

Patients and their family members or caregivers are likely to be thoroughly familiar with tracheostomy tube problems. You should not be afraid to accept assistance when you are evaluating, using, or troubleshooting a tracheostomy tube. Any needed equipment is likely to be close by if the patient is at home or in a long-term care facility. Many health care facilities have a policy to keep an extra correctly sized tracheostomy tube at the patient's bedside at all times. Routine care for tracheostomy tubes includes keeping the stoma clean and dry. The outer cannula should be changed as needed. Patients may also require periodic suctioning, depending on their ability to keep the airway clear of secretions or sputum.

Troubleshooting tracheostomy tube problems is similar to troubleshooting endotracheal tube problems. You should follow the DOPE acronym (Dislodged/displaced/disconnected, Obstruction, Pneumothorax, Equipment). First, check for a dislodged, displaced, or disconnected tracheostomy tube. It is possible for a tracheostomy tube to end up in a **false lumen**, outside the trachea, following removal and reinsertion or partial removal. A false lumen can be detected by placing an endotracheal suction catheter into the tracheostomy tube. If the suction catheter meets resistance immediately beyond the expected end of the tracheostomy tube, placement into a false lumen should be considered. If this happens, the tracheostomy outer cannula will need to be removed and then reinserted. Continuous end-tidal capnography monitoring will alert you of any unexpected dislodging, displacement, or disconnect of the tracheostomy tube during transport.

You also need to evaluate for tracheostomy (or ventilator circuit) obstruction. Obstruction of a tracheostomy tube may be cleared by removing the inner cannula, and then using a suction catheter to push the mucous plug out. Alternatively, an obstruction may be removed by using a combination of tracheostomy tube suctioning and mechanical ventilation through the tracheostomy tube to loosen and remove a mucous plug.

If the patient's only available tracheostomy tube becomes lost or unusable, you can carefully insert an appropriately sized endotracheal tube into the tracheostomy tube opening (called a **stoma**). Care must be taken to ensure that the endotracheal tube enters the trachea, not a false lumen under the skin but outside the trachea. Various techniques such as bougie, gloved finger, or hemostat guidance can be used to ensure correct placement. A correctly placed endotracheal tube will appear unusually shallow when placed directly into the trachea. Correct placement is confirmed using a combination of end-tidal CO_2, breath sounds, ventilation compliance, chest rise, and clinical improvement. Finally, pneumothorax and equipment (ventilator or ventilator tubing) failure should be evaluated when you are attempting to troubleshoot a malfunctioning tracheostomy tube.

To suction and clean a tracheostomy tube, follow the steps given here and in [Skill Drill 1]:

Skill Drill 1

1. Wash your hands and apply a mask, goggles, and clean nonlatex gloves. Suctioning a home care patient is a clean procedure, not a sterile one.

2. Open supplies may be used. For cost reasons, home care patients often reuse their suction catheters. If the catheters do not have visible contamination and have been stored in a clean manner, they are acceptable for use.

Skill Drill   1

Cleaning a Tracheostomy Tube

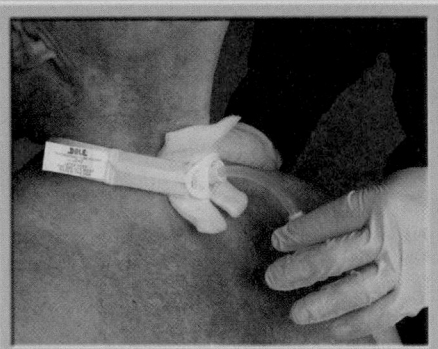

Step 1 Remove the inner cannula and place the device to soak in the proper solution.

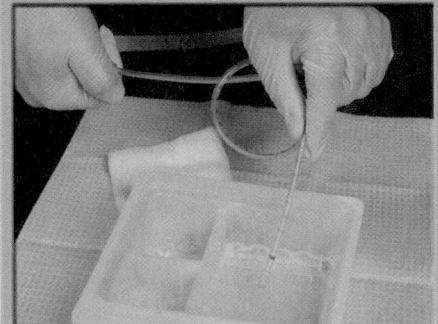

Step 2 Attach the catheter to negative pressure. Check the suction and clear the catheter by drawing up a small amount of saline.

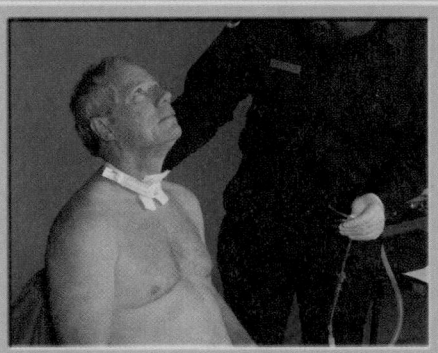

Step 3 Have the patient take a deep breath or preoxygenate the patient using the ventilator.

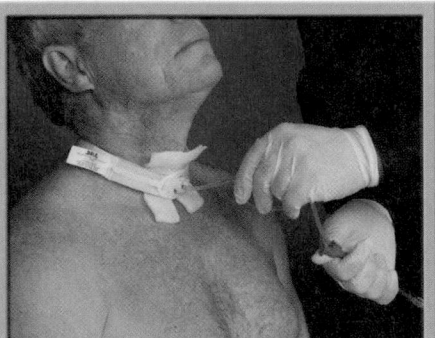

Step 4 Insert the catheter into the trachea without suction. Apply intermittent suction while removing the catheter. Repeat as necessary.

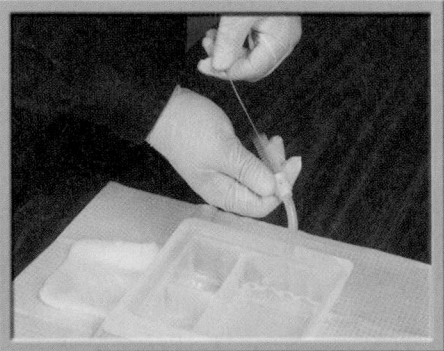

Step 5 Clean the inner cannula with the tracheostomy brush, rinse, and replace and lock into place.

3. Remove the inner cannula. Check with your patient's caregiver, if available, and place the device to soak in the appropriate recommended solution. If the caregiver is not available, use a mixture of hydrogen peroxide and water. Placing the cannula in plain water is acceptable in short-term situations. With one-piece tracheostomy tubes, this step is unnecessary. If the patient is dependent on a ventilator, have a replacement cannula immediately available Step 1.

4. Attach the catheter to negative pressure. Check the suction and clear the catheter by drawing up a small amount of saline Step 2.

5. Have the patient take a deep breath or preoxygenate the patient Step 3.

6. Insert the catheter into the trachea without suction. Apply intermittent suction while removing the catheter. Repeat as necessary. Keep the patient well oxygenated during the procedure Step 4.

7. Clean the inner cannula with the tracheostomy brush, rinse, and replace and lock into place. Omit this step for a one-piece tracheostomy tube Step 5.

8. Remove your gloves and wash your hands.

9. Document the procedure and assessment on your PCR.

Long-Term Ventilators

Patients may be on long-term ventilators at home for a variety of reasons Figure 12. Spinal cord injury, neuromuscular disease, and lung injury are all conditions associated with long-term ventilator use. It is possible that ventilator use will have nothing at all to do with the reason that EMS was requested for a particular patient.

The primary assessment for any patient on a long-term ventilator should include determining whether the ventilator is working effectively for the patient. Patients with a chronic lung disease may have oxygen levels well below what is considered normal for healthy people. You should inquire whether unusual findings such as an elevated respiratory rate or decreased oxygen saturation level are "normal" for this particular patient. Certain serious medical conditions can be made worse by overly aggressive oxygenation and ventilation. If the ventilator appears to be adequate for the particular patient, it is typically best to leave

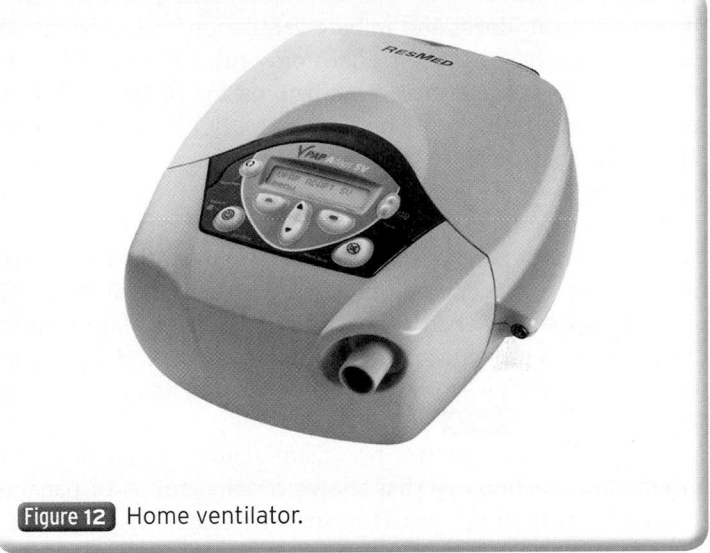

Figure 12 Home ventilator.

YOU are the Medic PART 3

You establish a 20-gauge IV line in the patient's left antecubital space and hang a 500-mL bag of saline running at a KVO rate and prepare for transport. Reassessment of lung sounds after the nebulizer treatment reveals no change. Amanda tells you that she is still struggling to breathe and asks you if there is anything else you can do. You contact medical control and receive orders to administer methylprednisolone (Solu-Medrol) and a second nebulizer with 2.5 mg albuterol and 0.5 mg ipratropium (Atrovent).

Recording Time: 7 Minutes	
Respirations	24 breaths/min; labored with accessory muscle use; faint expiratory wheezes and rhonchi bilaterally
Pulse	115 beats/min, regular; strong radial pulses
Skin	Pink, warm, and dry
Blood pressure	118/74 mm Hg
Oxygen saturation (Spo$_2$)	93% on nebulizer at 8 L/min of oxygen
Pupils	Equal and reactive to light

5. Your patient weighs 43 kg. How much methylprednisolone (Solu-Medrol) should you administer?

the ventilator settings unchanged and leave it connected to the patient.

If the ventilator does not appear to be working effectively for the patient, you have two possible options. It is possible to work with the patient or caregiver to adjust ventilator settings. You should be familiar with the clinical impact of various ventilator changes before attempting to adjust the patient's ventilator. It is possible to severely injure a patient by improperly adjusting his or her ventilator. Additional discussion of ventilator management is in the chapter, *Airway Management and Ventilation*.

You always have the option of disconnecting the ventilator completely if the patient is in unstable condition or there is a ventilator malfunction that you are unable to correct. You may choose to disconnect the ventilator during cardiac arrest or other critical illness and initiate ventilation with a bag-mask device or via the patient's tracheostomy tube. PEEP is likely to be needed during bag-mask ventilations for patients who are receiving long-term ventilator support. PEEP valves can be attached to many disposable bag-mask devices.

Patients often have CPAP and BPAP or BiPAP devices in homes and long-term care facilities. These devices offer a noninvasive option for patients who require oxygenation and ventilation support. A plastic mask is typically connected to the CPAP or BPAP device and then attached over a patient's face or nose using straps. A growing number of people with sleep apnea are using CPAP machines for improved ventilation and oxygenation while sleeping **Figure 13**.

Diaphragm and phrenic nerve stimulators (pacemakers) are an emerging technology that allows certain groups of patients to breathe without the assistance of a ventilator. External electrical impulses cause the diaphragm to contract and then passively relax. This movement creates enough tidal volume for effective respiration, eliminating the need and risks associated with ventilator support. In the event of failure of these devices, you can support ventilation using conventional bag-mask technique. It is possible that **asynchrony** may occur between patient breathing and mechanical ventilations if the nerve stimulator

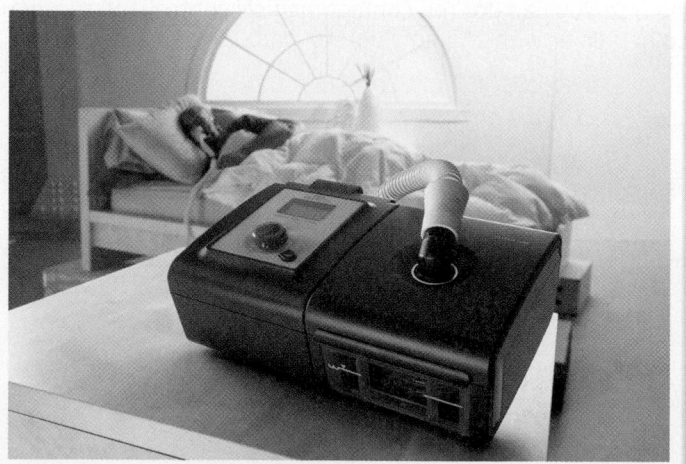

Figure 13 Continuous positive airway pressure machine.

device is activated while patients are receiving bag-mask or ventilator assistance. These devices typically consist of a small box connected to wires that are inserted into the anterior lower chest/upper abdominal wall.

Words of Wisdom

Both CPAP and BiPAP can be administered in the home by nasal or facemask without endotracheal intubation. This technique is referred to as "noninvasive ventilation."

Ventricular Assist Devices

Ventricular assist devices (VADs) provide a life-saving bridge for patients with severe heart failure. In the hospital setting, VADs are temporarily placed into a patient's chest cavity during or after heart surgery to augment the performance of a failing heart. Advances in medical technology have allowed these devices to become portable for use by persons with heart failure in the community.

Patients receive VADs while awaiting a heart transplant or as a long-term treatment for patients who are not candidates for heart transplantation. A patient undergoes surgery to have the pump connected to the left, right, or both heart ventricles. Blood exits the heart ventricle into large diameter tubing. The tubing is connected to a pump that propels blood into either the aorta or pulmonary artery. Occasionally, VADs are placed into the right atrium, completely bypassing the right ventricle and propelling blood into the pulmonary artery. The VAD pump or pumps are connected to a wire that exits through the abdominal wall and is connected to an external power supply or battery pack.

Complications of VAD placement include bleeding, infection, and device failure, among others. Other than correcting problems with the battery or power supply, there are very few interventions that you can perform on VADs in the prehospital setting. In the event of VAD failure, provide supportive treatment and immediate transport to a facility capable of definitive intervention.

Apnea Monitors

You may occasionally encounter patients using an apnea monitor. Infants who are identified as having a high risk for sudden infant death syndrome or other causes of apnea are provided with apnea monitors along with infant CPR instruction for parents and caregivers. Adults and children may be using apnea monitors for diagnosis and evaluation of sleep apnea.

Sleep apnea monitors will vary depending on purpose. Infant apnea monitors typically record an electrocardiogram (ECG) tracing and record respirations based on transthoracic electrical impedance. Central apnea (usually from neurogenic causes) will be detected, but apnea caused all or partially by airway obstruction may or may not be detected until cardiac arrest occurs.

Many home apnea models do not display numeric values or ECG and respiratory waveforms. It is essential that you use ALS resuscitation equipment rather than home apnea monitors for any patient requiring EMS assistance. You may or may not need to remove apnea monitor leads and electrodes in order to perform ALS monitoring or procedures.

Words of Wisdom

False alarms are common with apnea monitors and may be caused by movement, loose lead wires, or improperly placed electrodes. When you are in doubt, follow your local EMS protocols and have the family contact the manufacturer of the device.

Long-Term Vascular Access Devices

Many patients in the community use a variety of long-term vascular access devices 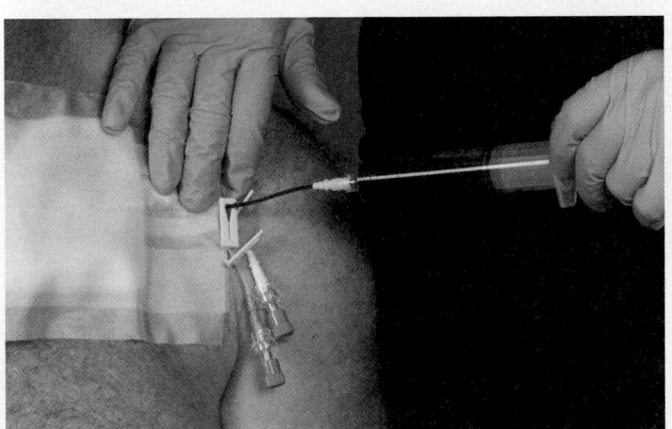. Patients may also present with central venous access devices during interfacility transport. Central and long-term vascular access devices are placed for a variety of reasons including inadequate or impossible peripheral IV access, administration of medications that are irritating to smaller blood vessels, vasopressor medication infusion, chemotherapy, frequent blood draws, long-term antibiotic therapy, or dialysis.

Extreme caution is required when you are considering whether to use a long-term vascular access device. Many of these devices are maintained with the anticoagulant heparin, some in dangerously high concentrations. You should obtain additional training and medical director authorization prior to using any long-term vascular access devices.

In emergency situations, this may be the only IV access available. You should contact online medical control for guidance in these situations. As a general rule, in order to remove any heparin, these catheters require up to 10 mL of blood to be removed and discarded before any flush, medication push,

Figure 14 Paramedics may encounter patients with long-term vascular access devices.

or infusion is given. Contamination of these catheters can lead to serious bloodstream infections. Meticulous sterile technique or port cleaning should be used when you are accessing these devices. Below are common long-term vascular access devices that you may encounter.

- **Peripherally inserted central catheter (PICC):** A long intravenous catheter that is usually placed in either arm and follows peripheral veins into the superior vena cava. It may be in place up to 1 year. The smaller diameter and longer catheter length may increase resistance during rapid infusion. These may or may not be flushed with heparin after use.
- **Midline catheter:** A catheter placed into an upper extremity that is not as long as the PICC catheter above and does not reach central circulation. Midline catheters are longer than traditional peripheral IV catheters and are better suited for many irritating medications. These catheters typically contain heparin.
- **Double or triple lumen central catheter:** Traditional central lines are placed through the skin in relatively close proximity to a large central vein. The femoral, internal jugular, and subclavian veins are the most common sites. These catheters are placed in an acute care setting, but still may be in place for a short time following discharge or transfer to another health care facility. These also contain heparin when not being used for an ongoing infusion.
- **Hickman, Broviac, and Groshong catheters:** These three similar brands of catheters are "tunneled" under the skin and placed into the superior vena cava. These catheters typically contain heparin and look similar to a dialysis catheter, described below. The ports of these catheters may be colored red, blue, or green. Contrary to many other uses in medicine, red does not indicated that this port enters an artery. Do not use any clamps or hemostats on the catheter itself. These catheters contain heparin when not in use.
- **Implanted ports (Port-a-Cath or similar):** These catheters are placed completely under the patient's skin and are tunneled into a central vein, typically the superior vena cava. The ports are similar in size and shape to one or two large hazelnuts under the skin. The top of the implanted ports have a flat or slightly rounded top with a clearly palpable edge. In hospital settings, these ports are accessed with a needle bent 90° that has plastic wings for the health care provider to hold while inserting. There is a metal plate in the base of the port that keeps the needle from piercing the bottom. Implanted ports contain heparin when not in use.
- **Dialysis catheter (Vas-Cath/Permcath):** These devices are thick-walled, high-volume catheters, usually placed into a patient's neck or groin for dialysis. Many hospitals require that only dialysis nurses or specially trained RNs access or use dialysis catheters. These devices are stored with high-dose heparin that can become problematic if adequate blood is not discarded before the catheter is used. The large catheter diameter may allow significant bleeding if the caps and clamps are not used properly.

To access an implantable venous access device, follow the steps in **Skill Drill 2**:

Skill Drill   2

1. Wash your hands and apply a mask, goggles, and nonlatex gloves.
2. Open needed supplies, including the port access kit.
3. Palpate the skin over the device **Step 1**.

4. Cleanse the skin over the device using a cleansing solution (eg, Betadine) **Step 2**. Draw up a small amount of saline.
5. Prime the needle tubing and needle with saline. Use a special access needle, called an unbeveled or noncutting needle, to avoid slicing the silicone reservoir wall **Step 3**.
6. While you are stabilizing the device, insert the needle at a 90° angle to the skin until the needle tip reaches the back of the device **Step 4**.
7. Aspirate 5 mL of blood **Step 5**.

Skill Drill   2

Accessing an Implantable Venous Access Device

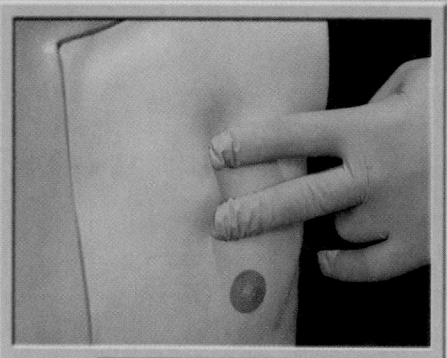

Step 1 Palpate the skin over the device.

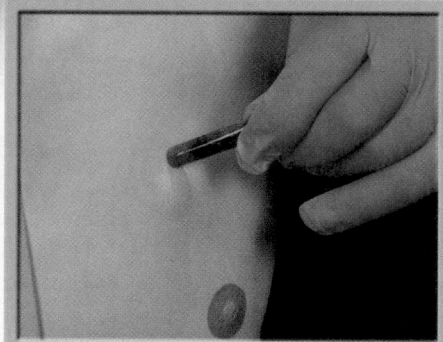

Step 2 Cleanse the skin over the device (betadine solution). Draw up a small amount of saline.

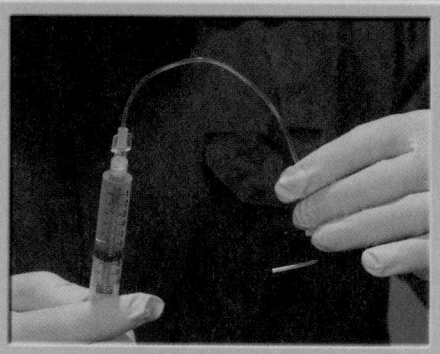

Step 3 Prime the needle tubing and needle with saline.

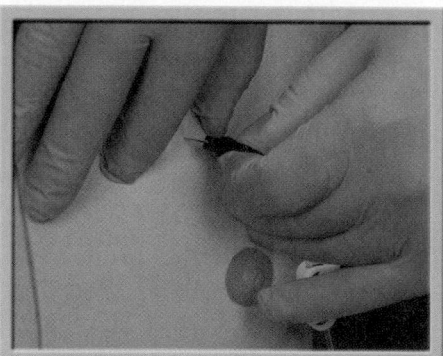

Step 4 While you are stabilizing the device, insert the needle at a 90° angle to the skin until the needle tip reaches the back of the device.

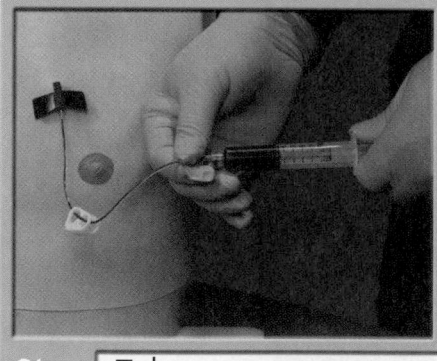

Step 5 Aspirate 5 mL of blood.

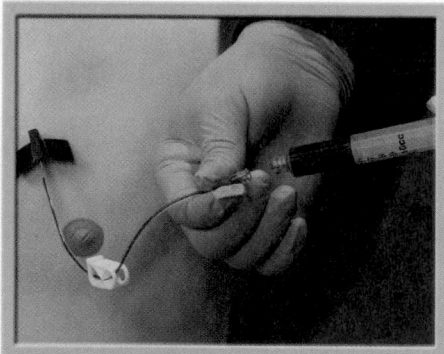

Step 6 Block the flow in the line using the crimping device, and then discard the initial aspirate. Obtain additional blood samples as necessary. To avoid air aspiration into the line, never remove the syringe without blocking the flow in the line.

Continues

Skill Drill   2

Accessing an Implantable Venous Access Device (continued)

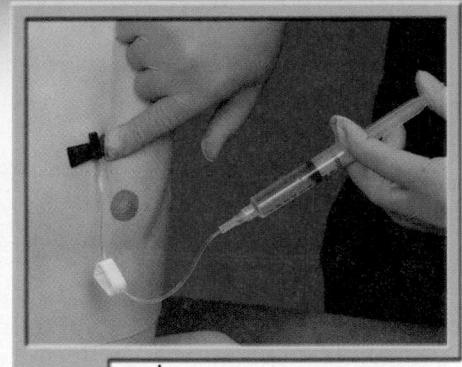

Step 7 Flush the line with normal saline.

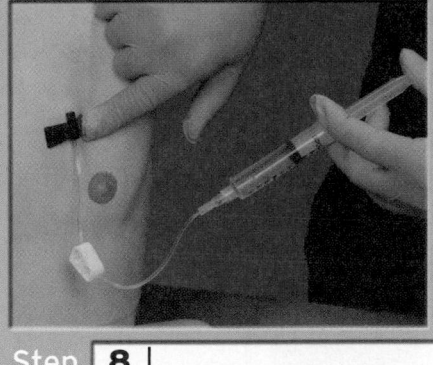

Step 8 Administer medications or fluids as directed.

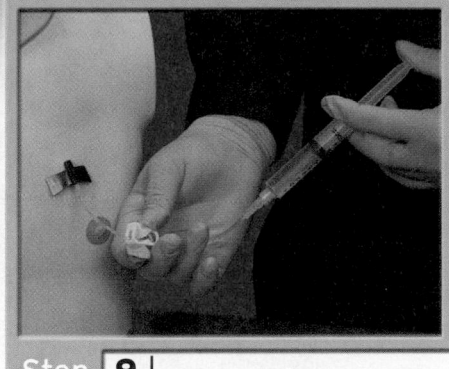

Step 9 Flush the device. Block the flow in the device.

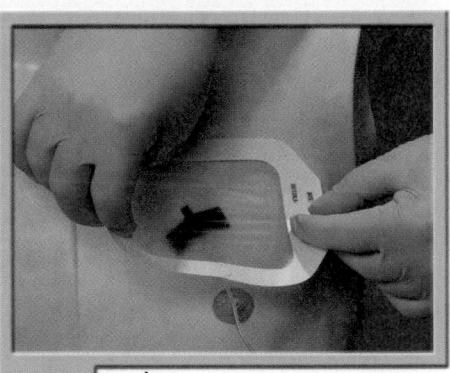

Step 10 Secure the needle with a sterile dressing.

8. Block the flow in the line using the crimping device, and then discard the initial aspirate. Obtain additional blood samples as necessary. To avoid air aspiration into the line, never remove the syringe without blocking the flow in the line **Step 6**.

9. Flush the line with normal saline **Step 7**. Block the flow in the device.

10. Administer medications or fluids as directed **Step 8**.

11. Flush the device **Step 9**.

12. Secure the needle with a sterile dressing or remove by pulling straight out of the device **Step 10**.

13. Apply a dressing to the skin over the device if the needle was removed.

14. Identify the tubes of blood by writing the date and time drawn and your name on the side of the tube, and ready them for transport by securing them in a leak-proof protected container. Transport tubes to the patient's physician,

hospital personnel, or usual lab. Do not shake blood collection tubes because this may cause the blood to hemolyze.

15. Document the procedure and assessment on the PCR.

16. Dispose of contaminated equipment.

Medication Infusion Pumps

Patients receive a wide assortment of IV medications in their homes. Medication categories include inotropic medications for heart failure, IV nutrition, chemotherapy, IV antibiotics, and a variety of other substances. Many of these medications will be administered with infusion pumps **Figure 15**. If infusion pumps fail while the patient is receiving certain vasoactive medications, a life-threatening emergency may result.

Several problems related to medication infusion pumps will trigger requests for EMS assistance. The underlying medical condition may become exacerbated, despite a properly functioning medication infusion system. In these situations, it is often

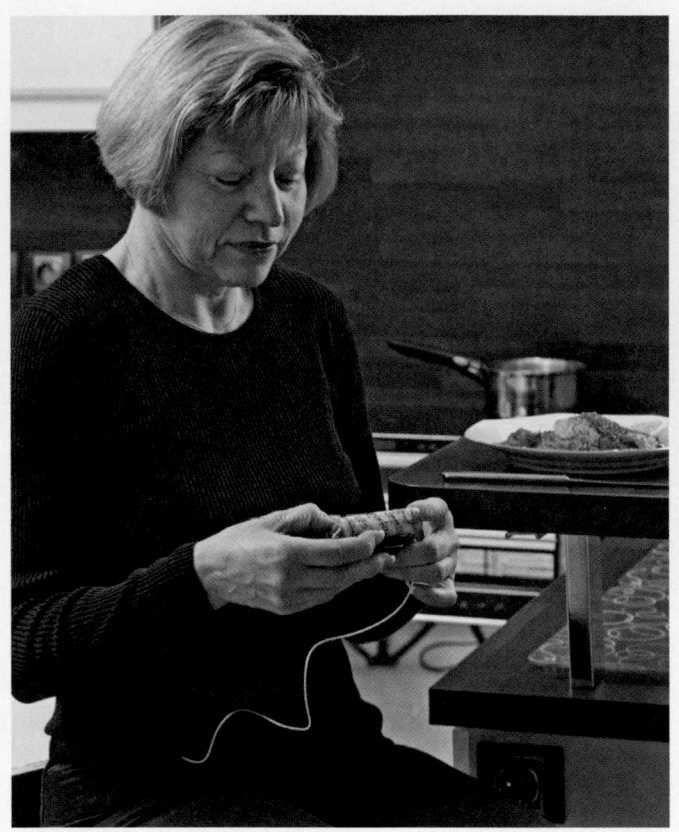

Figure 15 Patients may receive IV medication at home via a medication infusion pump.

advisable for you to continue the current medication infusion while contacting medical control for guidance, especially with unfamiliar medications or medical conditions. Most situations will not require titration or manipulation of a patient's medication infusion pump.

It is also possible that problems will occur with a long-term vascular access device. Each device outlined above has a limited life span. These devices can become clogged with blood clots and can harbor infections, and all are subject to either potential mechanical failure or accidental removal. You may need to emergently reestablish alternative vascular access such as a peripheral IV line or IO needle.

You may need to troubleshoot a medication infusion system. Medication infusion pumps require either a battery or a continuous power supply. An electrical outage or battery depletion has the potential to become a life-threatening emergency for the patient. Device malfunction is also a continuous possibility. Sudden, unexpected loss of a medication infusion pump may present you with a considerable challenge.

Simple solutions such as using an ambulance inverter to provide external power after a device battery failure may prove lifesaving. In other instances, another suitable backup device may be available in the patient's home or facility. You should not overlook the timeless practice of calculating the drip rate of IV tubing when a malfunctioning infusion pump cannot be immediately repaired or replaced. Collaboration with the patient or caregivers and creative solutions for infusion pump malfunction have the potential to save the patient's life.

Insulin Pumps

Insulin pumps are electronic devices that allow diabetic patients to carefully titrate exogenous insulin needs to activity, body stress, and dietary intake. A small needle is inserted into subcutaneous tissue and connected by a short length of tubing to the insulin pump. Insulin pumps are similar in size to a pager or cellular telephone. Patients can make careful adjustments on the insulin pump to effectively control glucose levels throughout the day.

Insulin pumps have the potential to complicate EMS treatment of patients with insulin-dependent diabetes who develop hypoglycemia. Insulin pumps may continue to infuse insulin even after a patient has become profoundly hypoglycemic. Unless you disconnect the insulin pump or turn it off, insulin will continue to be delivered. Steps for deactivation of insulin pumps will differ among various models and brands. Care must be taken to avoid accidental needle sticks if the needle is removed from the patient. With increasing use of insulin pumps, you should get in the habit of searching for insulin pumps as part of the physical examination of diabetic patients with hypoglycemia.

Tube Feeding

Patients in homes and long-term care facilities may receive some or all nourishment from tube feeding. Flexible catheters can be placed through the mouth or nose, or directly through the skin into the patient's stomach or small intestine. These tubes allow nourishment and water to enter the digestive system directly without the need for chewing or swallowing. These tubes can decrease the risk of aspiration in patients who lack the ability to swallow effectively or protect his or her airway. It is still possible for aspiration of tube feeding to occur, especially when feeding tubes are placed into the stomach rather than intestine.

Nasogastric and orogastric feeding tubes are placed from the nose and mouth, respectively, into the patient's stomach. Nasoduodenal and nasojejunal feeding tubes are inserted through the nose and end in the duodenum and jejunum of the small intestine, respectively. Gastrostomy (G) tubes are surgically inserted through the skin into the patient's stomach. Jejunostomy (J) tubes are placed through the patient's skin directly into the jejunum of the small intestine. Percutaneous endoscopic gastrostomy (PEG) and percutaneous endoscopic jejunostomy (PEJ) tubes are placed into the stomach and jejunum respectively, using endoscopic surgical technique.

It is unlikely that you will need to troubleshoot or otherwise manipulate feeding tubes during an EMS response. Unless a nasogastric or orogastric tube interferes with bag-mask seal on a patient's face and cannot be adequately displaced to the side, you will likely not need to remove a feeding tube.

You may need to monitor continuous tube feeding during interfacility transports. An infusion pump is typically used at a rate specific for a particular patient. You should monitor for malfunction of the infusion pump and any signs of the patient vomiting or aspirating tube feeding. The patient's head should remain elevated during and after completion of tube feeding.

Words of Wisdom

Be careful not to cut an ostomy appliance when you are using trauma shears to cut away clothing. The drainage can contaminate wounds and damage intact skin.

If any complications develop, you should simply stop the tube feeding infusion and possibly flush the catheter with tap water to prevent the tube feed solution from clogging the catheter.

To replace an ostomy device, follow the steps in Skill Drill 3:

Skill Drill   3

1. Help position the patient in a comfortable area in which to change the appliance and easily dispose of the contaminated articles.

2. Wash your hands and apply a mask, goggles, and clean nonlatex gloves.

3. Open supplies. Ostomy equipment includes a skin barrier called a wafer and one of several styles of drainage bags. Some bags can be opened along the bottom and emptied at regular intervals; others are sealed around a system similar to a urine drainage bag.

4. Empty/remove the current appliance and dispose of it appropriately Step 1.

5. Wash the area around the stoma with soap and water. Cleanse the stoma with water only, being careful not to rub or irritate the area Step 2.

6. Place a clean gauze pad over the stoma to prevent contamination of the clean skin with stool or urine Step 3.

7. Cut the wafer to the correct size using the patient's measurement or tracing. Home care patients usually have the stoma already sized or have a tracing to cut a hole in the wafer large enough for the stoma but keeping exposed skin to a minimum Step 4.

8. Attach the appliance to the wafer. Be sure the distal end is closed Step 5.

9. Remove the gauze Step 6.

10. Remove the paper backing from the wafer Step 7.

11. Apply the appliance with the stoma centered in the wafer cutout Step 8.

12. Remove your gloves and wash your hands.

13. Document the procedure and assessment on the PCR.

Colostomy

Patients may receive a colostomy following intestinal trauma or surgery. A colostomy is a surgical procedure that directs the large intestine (colon) out through an opening in the anterior abdominal wall called a stoma. The stoma has a raised, circular mass of tissue that appears moist and vascular. A colostomy bag is a plastic bag with a hard, circular opening that is attached around the stoma by an adhesive ring Figure 16. Stool and intestinal liquid is collected in this plastic bag for disposal.

You generally do not need to do much in the way of care for a colostomy or colostomy bag. Occasionally the bag will separate from the abdominal wall, requiring replacement or temporary reinforcement with tape. If the colostomy bag becomes full, you may need to assist the patient in emptying the bag. A clamp is located at the bottom of the bag. The clamp is opened and any contents are drained into a suitable collection device. Care should be taken to avoid spilling or splashing the contents of the bag. Abdominal gas may accumulate in the colostomy bag, requiring periodic release during longer transports.

Urostomy/Urinary Diversion

Patients occasionally require urinary diversion for certain medical conditions. Bladder cancer, congenital anomalies, and massive urinary tract obstructions are possible indications for urinary diversion.

Part of the urinary system is diverted through an opening in the anterior abdominal wall, also called a stoma. This procedure is called a urostomy. Urine is collected in a plastic bag, similar to the colostomy bag discussed earlier Figure 17. Interventions by paramedics are similar to those for a colostomy. Occasional emptying and reinforcement or reattachment are likely to be all that you will be required to perform in most EMS settings.

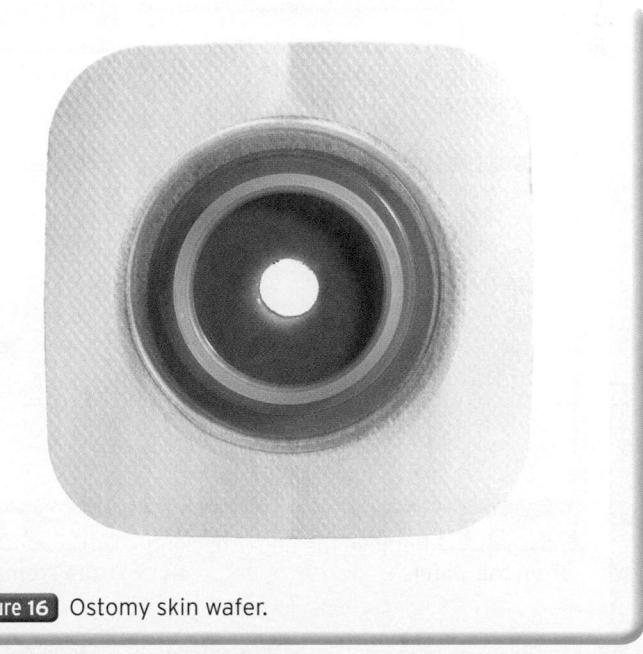

Figure 16 Ostomy skin wafer.

Skill Drill | 3

Replacing an Ostomy Device

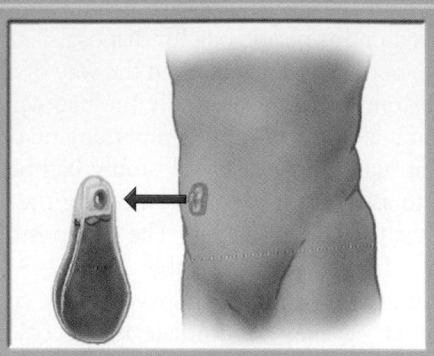

Step 1 Empty/remove the current appliance and dispose of it appropriately.

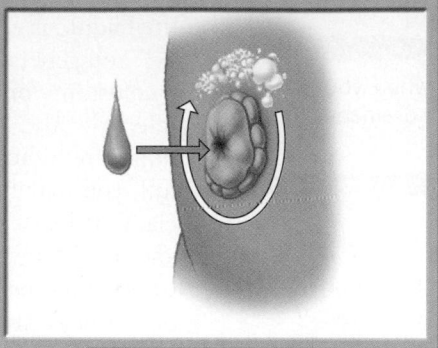

Step 2 Wash the area around the stoma with soap and water. Cleanse the stoma with water only.

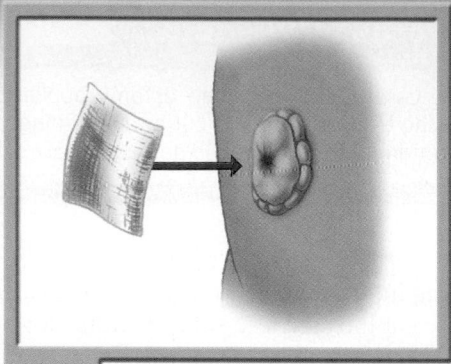

Step 3 Place a clean gauze pad over the stoma.

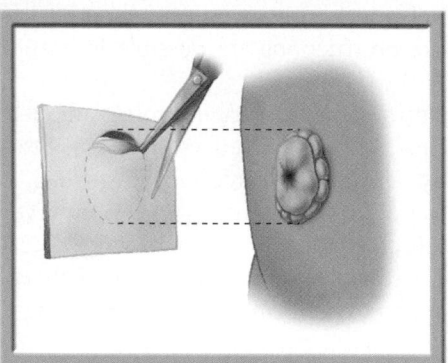

Step 4 Cut the wafer to the correct size using the patient's measurement or tracing.

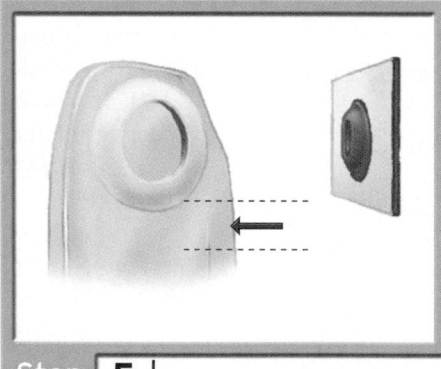

Step 5 Attach the appliance to the wafer.

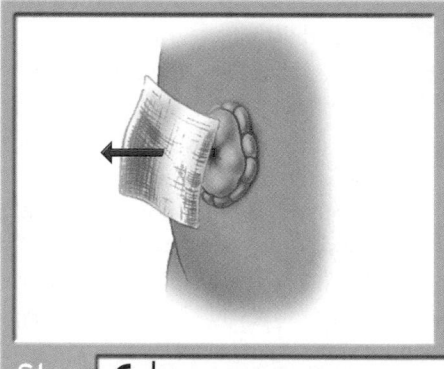

Step 6 Remove the gauze.

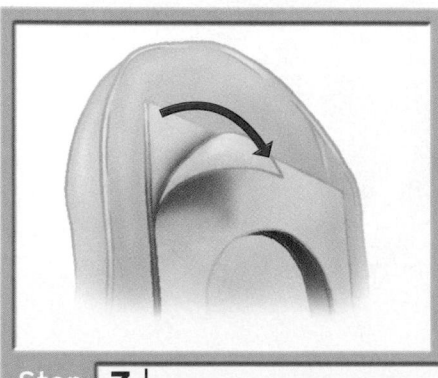

Step 7 Remove the paper backing from the wafer.

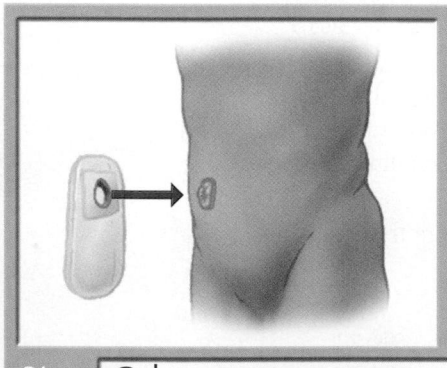

Step 8 Apply the appliance with the stoma centered in the wafer cutout.

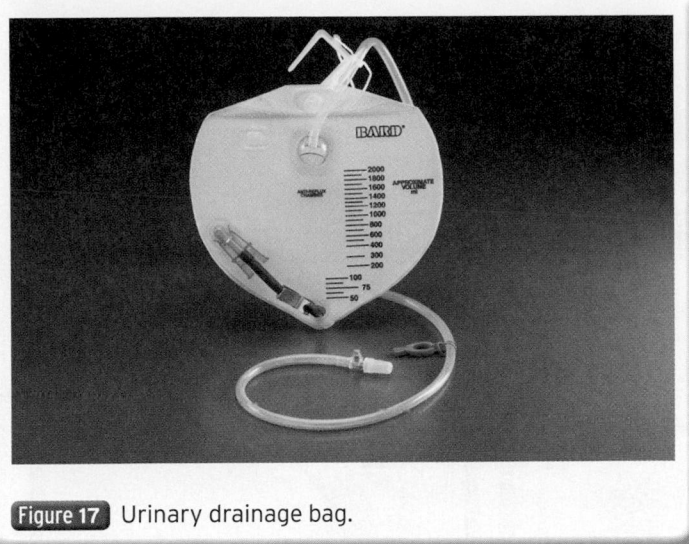

Figure 17 Urinary drainage bag.

Urinary Catheterization

Patients who are not able to void (urinate) on their own may need to be catheterized. Catheters may remain in place (ie, indwelling catheters such as Foley catheters) or may be used intermittently (straight catheters). Whereas the principles for catheterization remain the same for either gender, anatomy differences change the process.

To catheterize adult male patients, follow steps in **Skill Drill 4**:

Skill Drill — 4

1. Help position the patient supine with the legs slightly spread apart. Maintain privacy as much as possible.

2. Wash your hands and apply a mask, goggles, and sterile nonlatex gloves.

3. Open supplies including the urinary catheter and placement kit. Home care patients may reuse their catheters provided that they have been stored in a clean manner. Place necessary supplies onto a clean area within reach. If placing an indwelling catheter, use sterile technique throughout. Do not allow the catheter to be inserted to come into contact with anything that is not also sterile. If you are inserting an indwelling catheter, connect a syringe filled with saline to the balloon port. Also connect the indwelling catheter to the drainage system. There are no connecting ports for either a balloon or a drainage bag on a straight catheter.

4. Wash the penis with chlorhexidine solution, betadine solution, or another antiseptic depending on local protocols. Make sure that the foreskin has been retracted. Use great caution throughout to avoid breaks in sterile technique.

5. Coat the end of the catheter with a water-soluble gel. An anesthetic gel is preferred for patients with sensation in the penile area.

6. Hold the penis at a 90° angle to the body and insert the catheter (Step 1).

7. When urine is evident in the tubing, insert the catheter until the Y between the drainage port and the balloon port is at the tip of the penis. For a straight catheter, insert approximately 1 inch more (Step 2).

8. Inflate the balloon and gently pull back on the catheter until you feel resistance, which indicates that the balloon is snug against the neck of the bladder. This step is unnecessary for a straight catheter. Never inflate the balloon if you do not see any urine in the tubing or if you meet resistance to inflation, as this may indicate that the balloon is in the urethra instead of the bladder and inflation would therefore cause urethral injury.

9. Allow urine to drain. Note the amount and color (Step 3).

10. To remove a catheter, remove the saline in the balloon port and pull back gently until the catheter is free of the tip of the penis. Never remove an indwelling catheter without using a syringe to remove the saline from the balloon because it may damage the urinary sphincter. For a straight catheter, simply pull back gently to remove the catheter. Wash according to the home care instructions.

11. Remove your gloves and wash your hands, following standard precautions.

12. If the catheter is to remain in place, secure it to the patient's leg according to the home care instructions.

13. Document the procedure and assessment on the PCR.

To catheterize an adult female patient, follow these steps **Skill Drill 5**:

Skill Drill — 5

1. Help position the patient supine with the legs spread apart or side lying with the top knee flexed. Maintain privacy as much as possible.

2. Wash your hands and apply nonlatex gloves.

3. Open supplies including the urinary catheter and placement kit. Home care patients may reuse their catheters provided that they have been stored in a clean manner. Place necessary supplies onto a clean area within reach. If placing an indwelling catheter, use sterile technique throughout. Do not allow the catheter to be inserted to come into contact with anything that is not also sterile. If you are inserting an indwelling catheter, connect a syringe filled with saline to the balloon port. Also connect the indwelling catheter to the drainage system. There are no connecting ports for either a balloon or a drainage bag on a straight catheter.

4. Wash the perineal area with chlorhexidine solution, betadine solution, or another antiseptic depending on local protocols. First cleanse the outer area of the perineum, and then spread the labia minora and thoroughly wash

Skill Drill 4

Catheterizing an Adult Male Patient

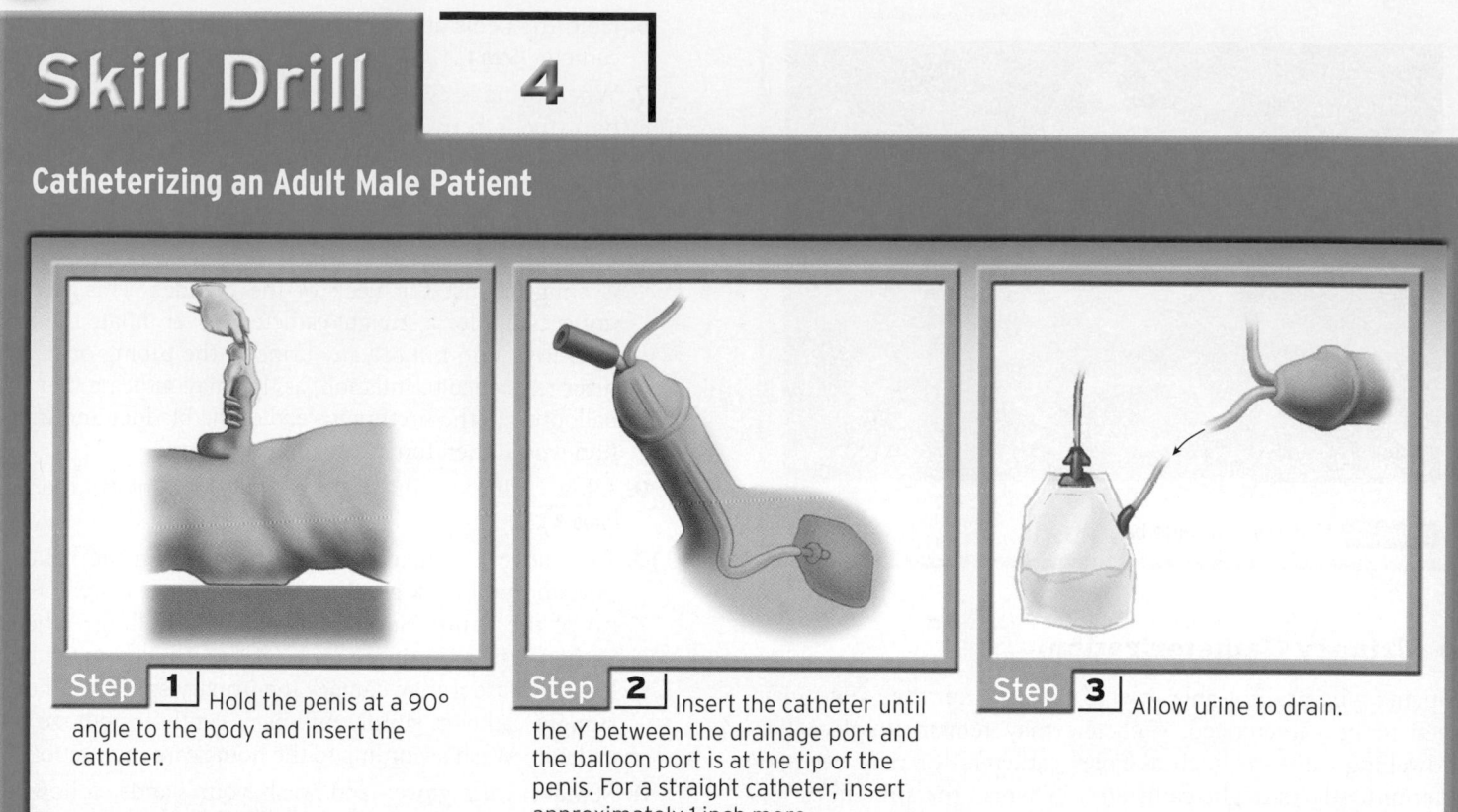

Step 1 Hold the penis at a 90° angle to the body and insert the catheter.

Step 2 Insert the catheter until the Y between the drainage port and the balloon port is at the tip of the penis. For a straight catheter, insert approximately 1 inch more.

Step 3 Allow urine to drain.

the mucosa surrounding the vagina and the urinary meatus. Dry with a clean towel.

5. Coat the end of the catheter with a water-soluble gel. An anesthetic gel is preferred for patients with sensation in the perineal area.

6. Locate the urinary meatus anterior to the vagina and insert the catheter **Step 1**.

7. When urine is evident in the tubing, insert the catheter another 1 to 3 inches **Step 2**.

8. Inflate the balloon and gently pull back on the catheter until you feel resistance, which indicates that the balloon is snug against the neck of the bladder. This step is unnecessary for a straight catheter.

9. Allow urine to drain. Note the amount and color **Step 3**.

10. To remove a catheter, remove the saline in the balloon port and pull back gently until the catheter is free of the tip of the meatus. Never remove an indwelling catheter without using a syringe to remove the saline from the balloon because it may damage the urinary sphincter. For a straight catheter, simply pull back gently to remove the catheter. If the catheter is to be reused, it should be cleaned.

11. Remove your gloves and wash your hands.

12. If the catheter is to remain in place, secure it to the patient's leg or abdomen according to the patient's needs.

13. Document the procedure and assessment on the PCR.

■ Dialysis

Patients undergo **dialysis** as a replacement for failed or failing kidneys. Kidney failure, also known as renal failure, may exist as a primary condition or occur as a consequence of another medical problem. Kidney failure is associated with cardiovascular disease, septic shock, liver failure, certain toxic chemicals or medications, diabetes, and many other acute or chronic conditions. As kidney function declines, fluids, excess electrolytes, and toxins accumulate within the body. If left untreated, these substances will cause death. Coma, cardiac dysrhythmia, and circulatory overload are late signs of kidney failure, requiring prompt intervention before death occurs.

Two types of dialysis are possible. **Hemodialysis** removes blood from the patient through a catheter or **fistula**. A fistula is a surgical connection between an artery and vein, usually in one of the patient's upper extremities **Figure 18**. Synthetic or animal-derived materials can also be used to create fistulas between a patient's artery and vein. Two needles are placed through the patient's skin into either side of the fistula. Blood exits the body

Skill Drill   5

Catheterizing an Adult Female Patient

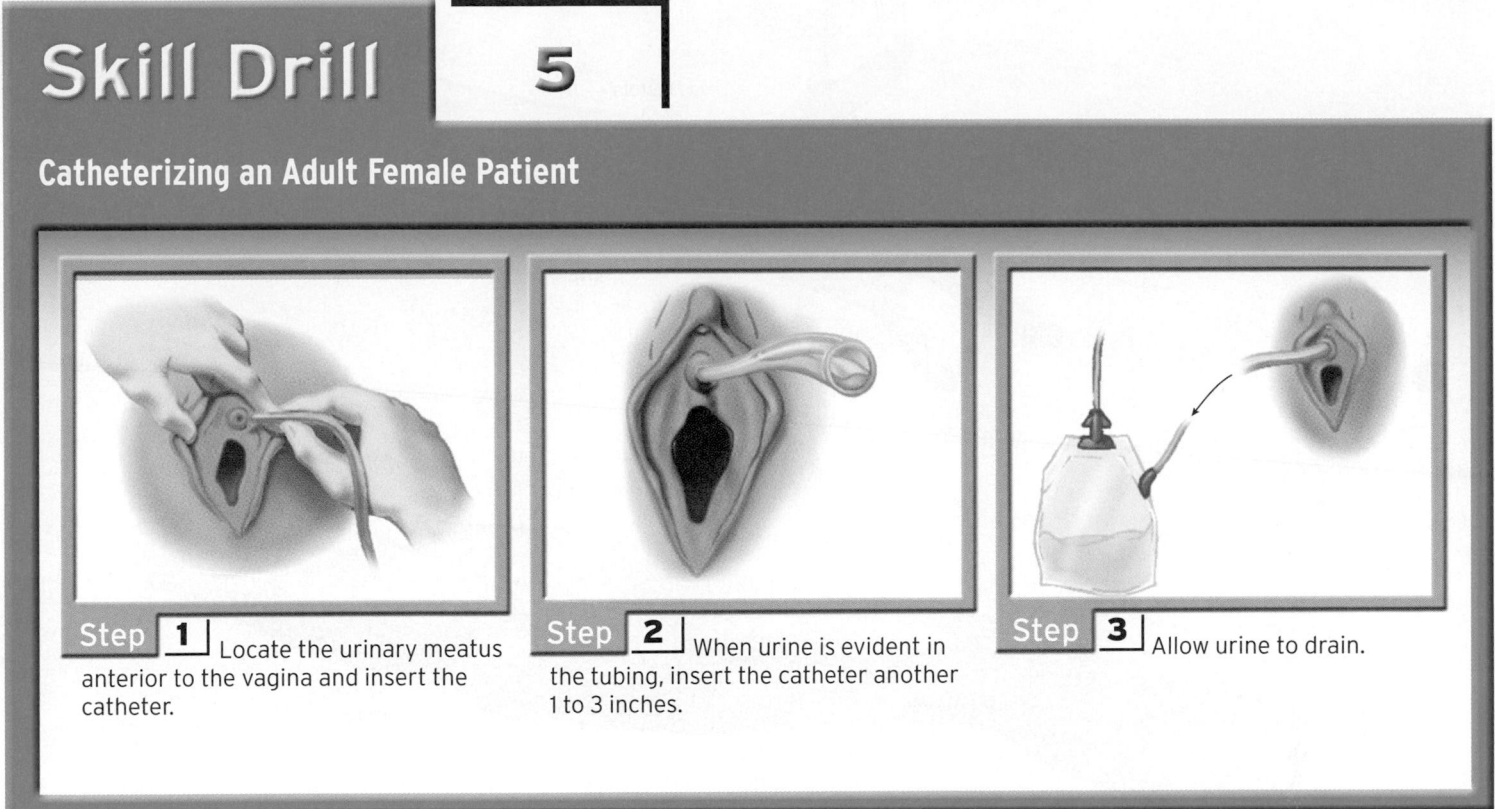

Step 1 Locate the urinary meatus anterior to the vagina and insert the catheter.

Step 2 When urine is evident in the tubing, insert the catheter another 1 to 3 inches.

Step 3 Allow urine to drain.

through one needle connected to tubing and returns to the body through the other. Blood cycles through a machine that returns blood to the patient with various toxins, electrolytes, and fluid removed.

Peritoneal dialysis involves instilling a special solution through a catheter into the patient's abdomen. The fluid draws toxins, electrolytes, and other fluids from the body, through the peritoneal membrane. These substances are then removed along with the original solution through the same catheter. Hemodialysis and peritoneal dialysis are performed in community-based centers as well as hospitals **Figure 19**. Peritoneal dialysis can be performed in a patient's home.

A wide variety of complications are possible during or following dialysis treatment. During dialysis, large volumes of fluid are moved in and out of the patient's body. Incorrect calculation during either method of dialysis can create massive abnormalities of fluids and electrolytes that cannot otherwise be compensated for. Both **hypovolemia** and fluid overload are possible during and after dialysis. Electrolyte abnormalities, including electrolyte depletion, may result from miscalculation. Infection at the site of the dialysis fistula for hemodialysis and an intra-abdominal infection for peritoneal dialysis can occur as well.

A severe, life-threatening hemorrhage can occur if the hemodialysis fistula is damaged or the catheter is improperly removed. Other problems with hemodialysis fistulas include **thrombosis** (blood clot) and **stenosis** (narrowing).

You need to use caution when you are treating patients who receive dialysis. Modest volumes of IV fluids may cause fluid overload, particularly in otherwise susceptible patients. IV fluids need to be monitored carefully and titrated judiciously to patient response. If too much IV fluid is given, it will be impossible to correct in the prehospital setting.

Patients with renal failure are prone to electrolyte abnormalities, particularly hyperkalemia, and an elevated blood potassium concentration. You need to avoid medications known to increase serum potassium levels such as succinylcholine (Anectine), digoxin, and beta-adrenergic (beta) blockers.

You must also use caution when a hemodialysis fistula is present. Dialysis fistulas are prone to both clots and infection. Avoid blood pressure measurements, blood draws, and IV access on the same arm as the dialysis fistula. Patients with impending dialysis may have already chosen which arm will be used for the fistula. This arm should also be avoided whenever possible. Both arterial and venous bleeding can occur from the fistula site, especially if improper care was taken during needle removal.

If you are called to respond to an emergency for a patient at a hemodialysis center, it is important to inquire whether the patient had received the dialysis treatment already. It is possible for a significant amount of the patient's blood to be in the dialysis machine during dialysis treatment. You and the dialysis center staff need to carefully coordinate when to remove the patient from the dialysis machine if dialysis is still in progress on your arrival.

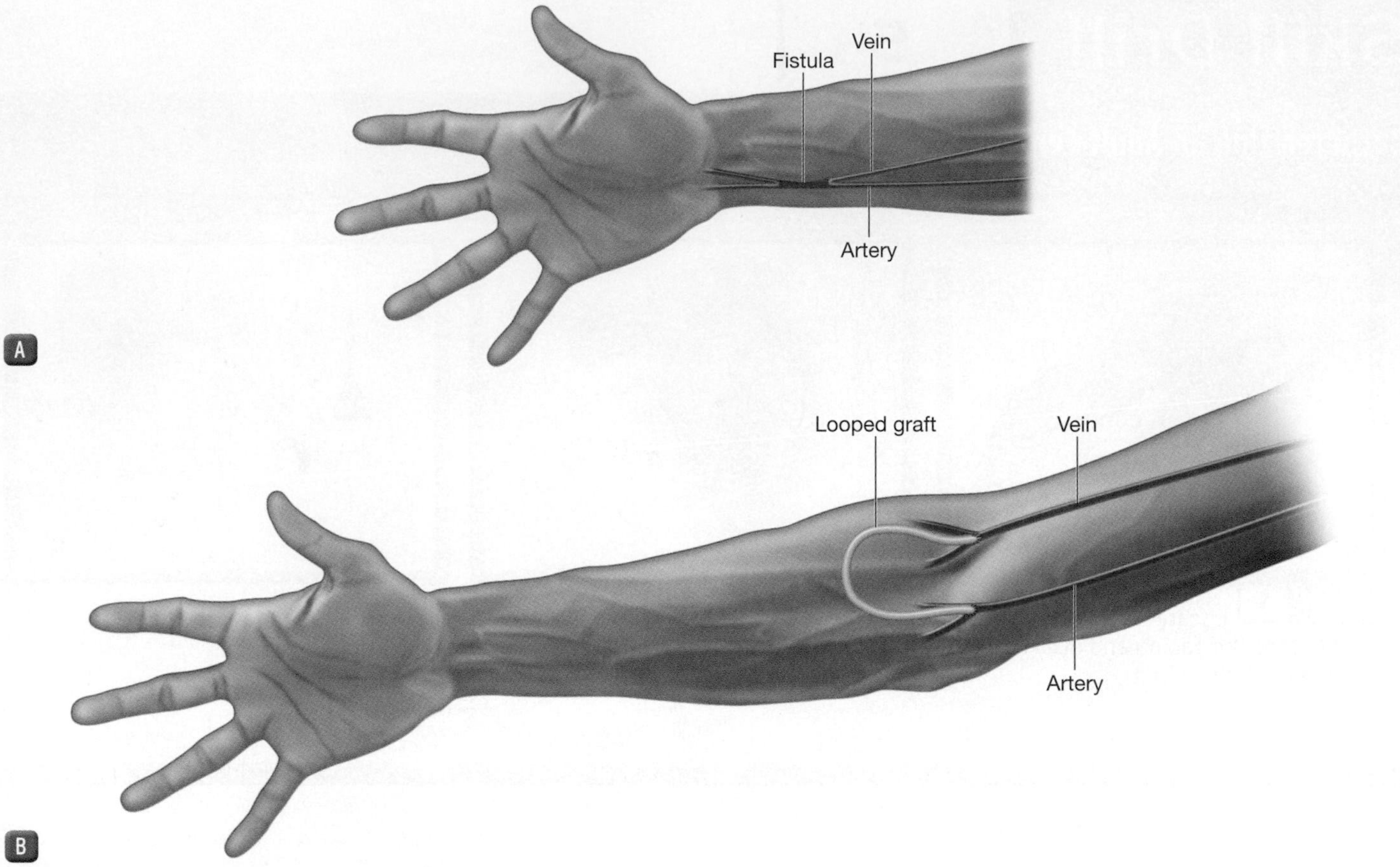

A

Fistula   Vein

Artery

B

Looped graft   Vein

Artery

Figure 18 **A.** With an arteriovenous (AV) fistula, a bulge is created beneath the skin by arterial pressure at the site where the artery and vein have been directly connected. **B.** An AV graft creates a raised area beneath the skin that looks like a large vessel.

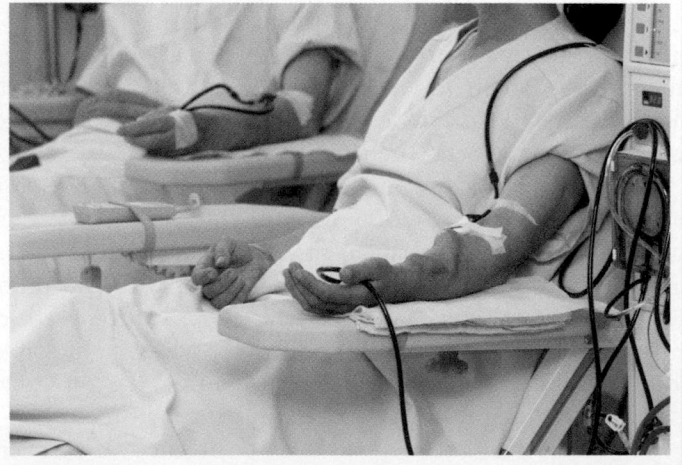

Figure 19 Patients may receive hemodialysis and peritoneal dialysis in community-based centers and hospitals; they may also receive peritoneal dialysis in their home.

Dialysis is both a lifesaving and life-sustaining therapy for patients in renal failure. Understanding dialysis will dramatically improve your ability to provide care to dialysis patients who become ill or injured.

Surgical Drains and Devices

Patients will be discharged to home or a long-term care facility soon after many surgical procedures. A variety of drains and devices are used following surgery to monitor and assist wound healing or closure **Figure 20** . Complications in the postoperative period can trigger requests for EMS assistance. Consequently, you potentially may have to provide care to patients with many different types of surgical drains and devices.

The list of possible surgical drains and devices that you will encounter is exhaustive. Wound drains prevent pockets of fluid from collecting at the surgical site while allowing health care providers to monitor volume, appearance, and composition of the fluid being drained. Other devices use mechanical forces to stabilize a particular surgical site and promote healing.

It is typically outside the paramedic scope of practice to manipulate many of these items. Improper manipulation or premature removal of a surgical drain or wound device can have significant complications for the patient including hemorrhage, infection, or the need for additional surgery.

You should contact online medical control in the event that additional guidance is needed. In most cases, any needed manipulation of a wound drain or other device will be done by an emergency department provider or other specialist.

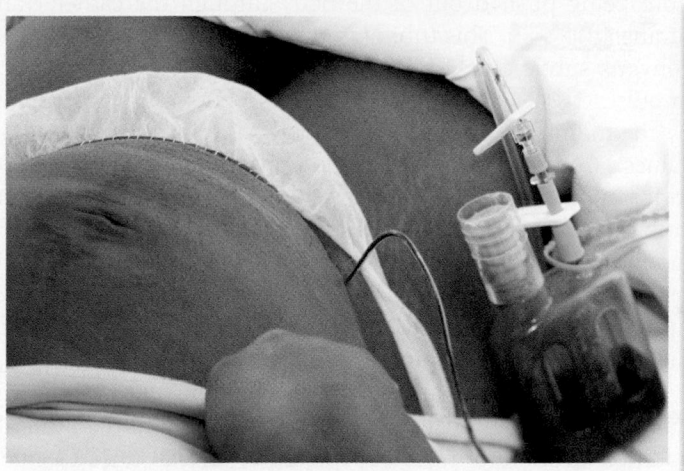

Figure 20 A surgical drain is used to monitor and assist wound healing and closure.

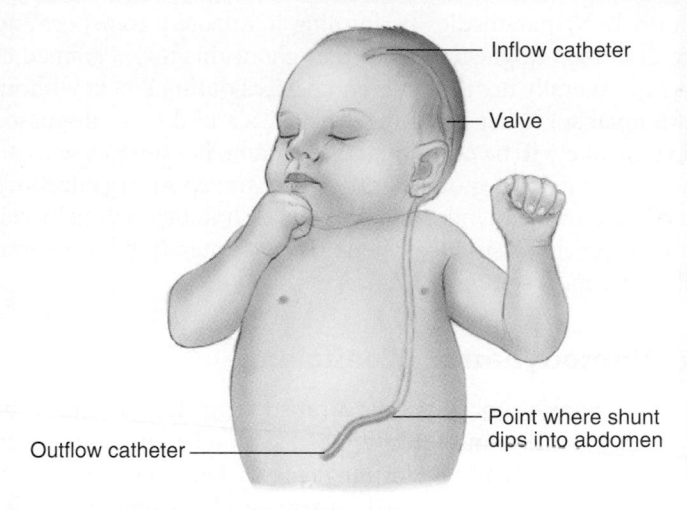

Inflow catheter

Valve

Point where shunt dips into abdomen

Outflow catheter

Figure 21 A CSF shunt, which drains excess CSF from the central nervous system, consists of the inflow (proximal) catheter, the valve, and the outflow (distal) catheter.

Orthotic devices, prosthetic limbs, and braces should also not be manipulated by paramedics. In many instances, these are fitted and adjusted for the needs of a particular patient. Improper adjustment may reduce the therapeutic benefit or lead to patient injury. Whenever possible, these devices should accompany the patient to the hospital, even if unrelated to the reason for EMS assistance.

Cerebrospinal Fluid Shunts

A condition called <u>hydrocephalus</u> can develop either before or after a person is born. Hydrocephalus is an excess volume of cerebrospinal fluid (CSF) around the brain. CSF is produced in the brain to protect, cushion, provide nourishment, and remove waste products from the brain and spinal cord. If the brain becomes injured, swelling of the brain can be offset by a reduction of CSF volume to maintain a lower intracranial pressure (ICP). Approximately 500 mL of CSF is produced daily by the choroid plexus of the brain. As CSF is being produced by the brain, it is constantly being reabsorbed by the bloodstream to maintain a balance within the central nervous system. The total volume of CSF is replaced almost four times each day. Excess production or decreased absorption of CSF causes hydrocephalus.

Excess CSF causes increased ICP. Increased ICP leads to signs and symptoms such as headaches, visual disturbances, unsteady gait, nausea and vomiting, seizures, altered mental status, and numerous other effects. Increased ICP will cause the relatively malleable skulls of fetuses, infants, and young children to enlarge, without generally distorting facial features.

Treatment of congenital hydrocephalus (occurring before birth) or acquired hydrocephalus (occurring after birth) involves surgical placement of a <u>cerebrospinal fluid shunt (CSF shunt)</u> to drain excess CSF from the central nervous system. The shunt consists of three parts: the inflow (proximal) catheter, the valve, and the outflow (distal) catheter **Figure 21**. The inflow catheter is typically placed into the ventricle of the brain of the patient. Occasionally, the inflow catheter is placed in CSF outside the

spinal cord. This catheter is connected to a tiny valve. The valve may have fixed opening pressure (pressure required to open the valve) and closing pressure (pressure at which the valve will close), or these may be adjustable. Newer valves can be adjusted by a physician using a magnet that is placed near the valve, outside the patient's body. The outflow catheter is most commonly placed into the patient's peritoneal cavity. This particular placement is known as a ventriculoperitoneal (VP) shunt. The outflow catheter can also be placed into the patient's right atrium or pulmonary cavity.

Patients often demonstrate substantial clinical improvement following CSF shunt placement. Improvement can be significant enough to eliminate the need for long-term care when the diagnosis of hydrocephalus is made in older adults and a CSF shunt is placed.

Patients and caregivers need to monitor closely for complications related to shunt malfunction. Many complications develop in the immediate postoperative period, often related to the surgery itself. Shunts will need periodic revisions as children grow or bodies change. Infection, shunt valve malfunction, and mechanical damage to either catheter will present with signs suggestive of increased ICP. You should suspect shunt malfunction in any patient with a CSF shunt who presents with a headache, visual disturbances, seizures, or altered mental status.

Medical Technology Used During Interfacility Transport

Paramedics perform both 9-1-1 emergency response and interfacility patient transport in many EMS systems and organizations. State EMS regulations and individual service medical directors determine which medications and procedures paramedics are permitted to use and under what circumstances. Medication infusion pumps, ventilators, and cardiac monitors are used routinely by paramedics performing interfacility transport and are discussed in greater detail throughout this text. Paramedics do not generally use the skills and devices outlined next without additional specialized training. The skills and devices discussed next are likely to be encountered as paramedics interact with air medical units and ground critical care transport organizations across the nation. Understanding this technology will help you provide greater assistance when it is encountered in the interfacility transport setting.

Hemodynamic Monitoring

Hemodynamic monitoring is a broad term that describes the movement and various forces applied to blood within the human body. You are actually performing cursory hemodynamic monitoring by assessing items such as patient blood pressure, pulse rate, pulse strength, urinary output over time, skin temperature, end-tidal CO_2, and mental status. Assessing these items provides you with valuable information regarding the effectiveness of perfusion to a patient's body organs, tissues, and cells.

Patients receive invasive hemodynamic monitoring when health care providers need to evaluate the effectiveness of specific components within the cardiovascular system or carefully guide fluid administration. Monitoring continues as medications are administered and procedures are performed to improve body function or the chances of survival following a critical illness, traumatic injury, or major surgery. Invasive monitoring includes values such as continuous arterial blood pressure, central venous pressure or right atrial pressure, pulmonary artery pressure, direct or indirect measurements of left atrial and left ventricular pressure, as well as systemic vascular resistance and pulmonary vascular resistance. Interpreting and manipulating these values allows you to optimize cardiovascular function in critically ill patients.

Hemodynamic monitoring technology is constantly evolving. The majority of current hemodynamic monitoring involves placement of different types of catheters into areas within the cardiovascular system, such as arteries, central veins, and various chambers of the heart Figure 22 . The catheter is connected to special tubing, typically filled with normal saline or heparinized solution (solution with heparin added to prevent clotting). The solution is placed on a pressure bag in order to prevent blood from being pushed out of the body through the catheter and tubing Figure 23 . This tubing is connected to a transducer that converts subtle changes in pressure of this fluid into electrical impulses Figure 24 . These electrical impulses are interpreted by the monitor and displayed as both waveforms and numeric values. Continuous interpretation of the values and waveforms allows providers to precisely titrate many inotropic and vasoactive medications to desired patient response. Invasive monitoring will identify impending heart failure, guide fluid resuscitation, demonstrate the effectiveness of compressions during CPR, help differentiate various shock states, and provide much potentially useful information in high-risk patients.

Arterial pressure monitoring is a component of hemodynamic monitoring that requires additional consideration. In addition to monitoring blood pressure, arterial lines (A-lines) are used as continuous access when critically ill patients require frequent blood tests or arterial blood gas sampling. Conditions such as sepsis, respiratory failure, diabetic ketoacidosis, or salicylate overdose require frequent testing of blood samples that may be impossible or impractical to obtain from repeated puncture of arteries or veins.

Paramedics may also encounter larger arterial sheaths that have been placed for a cardiac catheterization. These sheaths are placed into a femoral artery and provide a route to cardiac blood vessels. Arterial sheaths are occasionally left in place after a diagnostic cardiac catheterization if the patient needs to be transported to another hospital for further invasive cardiac care or cardiac surgery. Patients should remain supine with legs straight during placement of a femoral arterial sheath, and for a period of time after placement.

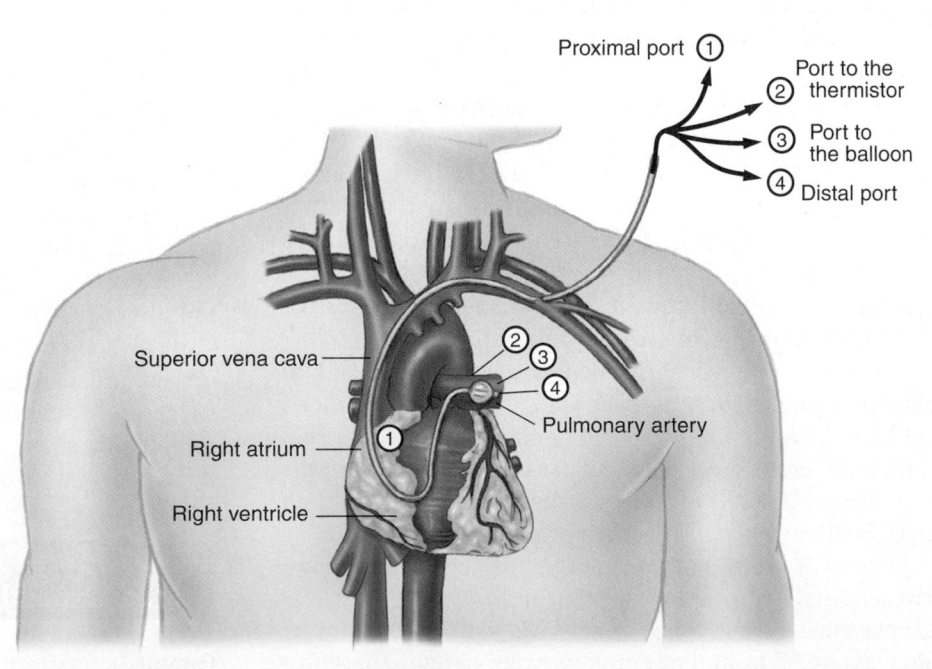

Proximal port ①
② Port to the thermistor
③ Port to the balloon
④ Distal port

Superior vena cava
Right atrium
Right ventricle
Pulmonary artery

Figure 22 An example of catheter placement for hemodynamic monitoring. This example shows pulmonary artery catheter placement.

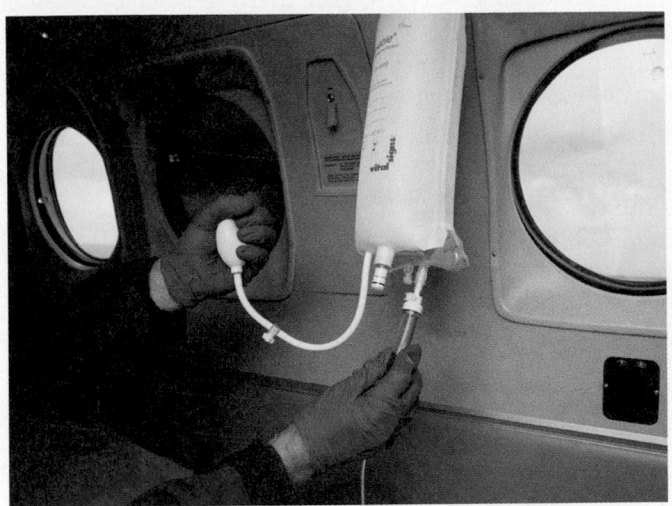

Figure 23 An inflated pressure bag used to increase fluid infusion rates.

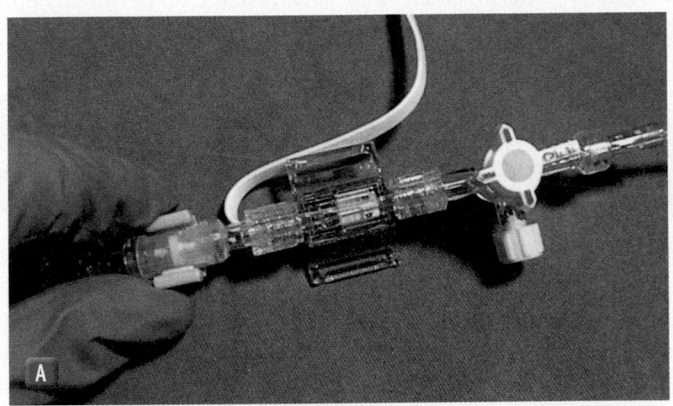

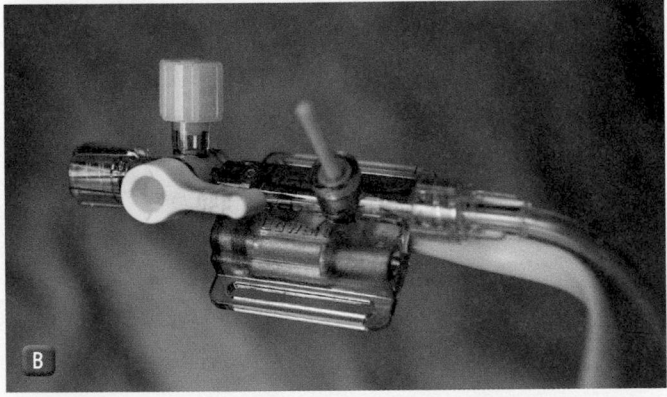

Figure 24 The two most common transducer flush system devices. **A.** Squeezable. **B.** Pull-style.

Bleeding associated with a displaced arterial catheter or arterial sheath can be immediately lifethreatening. Any time a catheter or sheath is in an artery, it must be continuously monitored by a trained health care provider. Patients have the potential to

quickly exsanguinate from unrecognized displacement of an arterial catheter. Large quantities of blood can become sequestered in a patient's groin area and stretcher linens before being recognized by transport personnel. You need to use extreme caution while moving or transporting a patient who has an arterial catheter or arterial sheath in place even if other trained health care personnel are present.

Intra-Aortic Balloon Pumps

Paramedics have the potential to assist with transport of patients being treated with an **intra-aortic balloon pump (IABP)**. IABPs are used to decrease cardiac workload and augment perfusion in patients with cardiogenic shock, structural abnormalities in the heart, or myocardial infarction, or following cardiac surgery. It is unlikely that a paramedic will be solely responsible for care of a patient on an IABP. It is quite conceivable, however, that paramedics will accompany a critical care transport team or other health care provider who is responsible for managing the IABP during interfacility transport of a patient.

IABPs consist of a relatively large machine, connecting tubing, monitor cables, and the balloon catheter itself **Figure 25**. A cylindrical balloon is inserted through the femoral artery and placed in the aorta, just outside the heart. Tubing connects the balloon catheter to the machine. Monitor leads from the

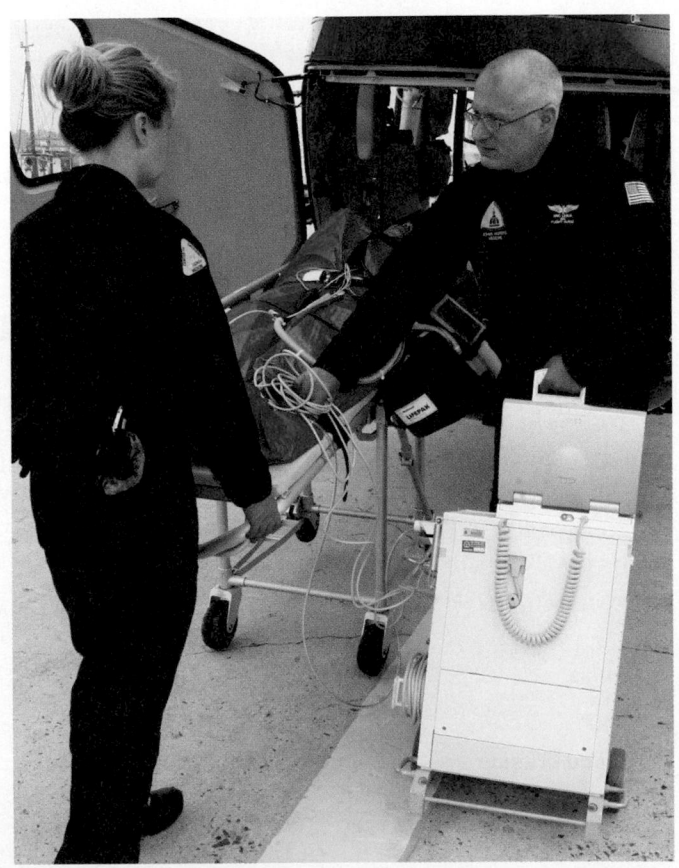

Figure 25 A patient being transported with an intra-aortic balloon pump.

machine are connected to the patient. Movement of both the patient and IABP machine requires careful planning and coordination among members of the transport team.

The balloon is inflated and actively deflated at precise times during the cardiac cycle. During diastole (relaxation of the heart), the balloon inflates, pushing blood forward into systemic circulation **Figure 26** . During systole (contraction of the heart), the balloon actively deflates, creating a brief vacuum, and reducing cardiac afterload. This process decreases myocardial oxygen demand, reduces cardiac workload, and improves systemic circulation.

The IABP is bulky and often difficult to move and secure in an ambulance. Additional straps need to be used to prevent the machine from injuring the patient or transport team in the

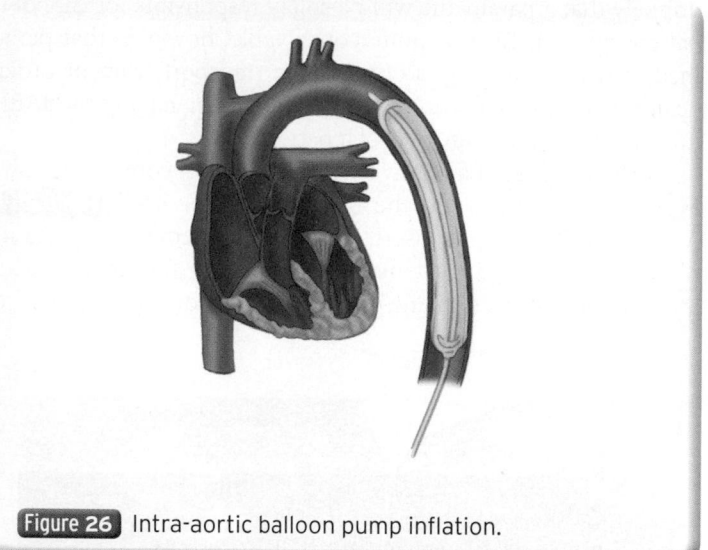

Figure 26 Intra-aortic balloon pump inflation.

event of an ambulance crash. Care needs to be taken when you are handling and securing the connecting tubing between the machine and balloon catheter. Accidental removal of the balloon catheter often creates a life-threatening emergency for the patient.

■ Intracranial Pressure Monitor

Patients with intracranial hemorrhage, severe head trauma, or having undergone neurosurgery may have an ICP monitor or drain placed. These devices allow health care providers to monitor ICP, evaluate the appearance of CSF, and allow drainage of CSF in order to maintain a lower ICP.

It is possible that you will assist other providers with interfacility transport of patients with these devices. Monitoring of ICP is similar to hemodynamic monitoring discussed previously, although newer technology is also in use. The transducer or drainage system is typically aligned at the same height as the patient's ear canal, which may take some creativity to accommodate in the back of an ambulance. Positioning of the drainage system is extremely important. Improper placement of an open drainage system can cause large volumes of CSF to quickly enter or leave the patient's central nervous system.

■ Care of Patients With Cognitive, Sensory, or Communication Impairment

The presence of a cognitive, sensory, or communication impairment can create unique challenges as you assess, treat, and provide transportation for a patient. Routine tasks become complicated, requiring creative approaches in order to provide

YOU are the Medic   PART 4

En route to the hospital you administer 86 mg of methylprednisolone (Solu-Medrol) IV and the second nebulizer. After the second breathing treatment Amanda states that it is slightly easier for her to breathe. Lung sounds after the second nebulizer treatment reveal increased air movement, expiratory wheezes, and rhonchi. While on your way to the hospital Amanda tells you that she feels this way each time she gets a lung infection and is worried that she will have to spend a long time in the hospital. You have a 12-minute transport time to the facility where Amanda typically receives her care.

Recording Time: 13 Minutes	
Respirations	26 breaths/min; labored with accessory muscle use; faint expiratory wheezes and rhonchi bilaterally
Pulse	118 beats/min, regular; strong radial pulses
Skin	Pink, warm, and dry
Blood pressure	116/70 mm Hg
Oxygen saturation (Spo$_2$)	93% at 12 L/min on nonrebreathing mask
Pupils	Equal and reactive to light

6. What changes in patient condition should you watch for during transport?

effective patient care. Patients and their caregivers are often valuable resources for paramedics providing care during EMS response or interfacility transportation. The special challenges discussed in this section, with the exceptions of autism and mental/emotional impairment, may appear early in life as a developmental disability or present later due to a medical condition or injury.

Developmental Disability

The United States Centers for Disease Control and Prevention (CDC) defines **developmental disability** as a diverse group of severe chronic conditions that are due to mental and/or physical impairments. These impairments appear prior to age 22 years and usually continue throughout the person's lifetime. Communication, movement, learning, behavior, the ability to care for one's self, prospects for employment, and a host of other important human attributes are adversely impacted. Profound vision or hearing impairment can disrupt other developmental progression, leading or contributing to a developmental disability. Certain conditions such as autism do not have a readily identifiable cause, although a variety of theories have been proposed. Known causes of other developmental disabilities are listed in Table 4.

Developmental Delay

Development delay is a broad term that describes an infant or child's failure to reach a particular developmental milestone by the expected time. Milestones include gross and fine motor skills such as crawling, walking, and hand-eye coordination along with cognitive skills (such as reaching, object permanence, or problem solving) and social skills (such as interaction and forming relationships with others). Language milestones include talking, listening, and comprehending. Signs of problems may be primarily in one developmental area such as language or social skills or there may be delays in multiple areas. Developmental delay is linked to many causes of developmental disabilities listed in Table 4. Down syndrome and autism are associated with potentially significant signs of developmental delay. Depending on the cause, developmental delays may persist into adulthood or resolve as a person's medical or social situation improves. Early intervention focused on children with developmental delays may allow these children to recover previously missed developmental milestones.

You may encounter children and adults with developmental delays that encompass the entire spectrum of possible severity. Cues from the patient and caregivers will help you determine how best to interact and communicate with a particular patient. Patients can regress to a lower developmental level following a stressful event, illness, or injury. You may find that experience and approaches used while treating younger children are useful when you are interacting with older children and adults with developmental delay. Additional time may be needed when you are assessing these patients, performing procedures, or preparing for transport.

Down Syndrome

Down syndrome is an inherited genetic disorder that is responsible for developmental delay, cognitive impairment, and a pattern of unusual physical features. Patients with Down syndrome can often be identified visually from certain telltale features of the person's head, face, and neck Figure 27. Features include a flattened face and nose, short neck, upward slanting eyes, and often a protruding tongue. Additionally, only a single crease is noted on the palms of the patient's hands.

Table 4	Known Causes of Development Disabilities
Genetic abnormality (for example, phenylketonuria, chromosomal disorder, or fragile X syndrome)
Hypoxia, malnutrition, or toxic exposure during fetal development (such as to tobacco, alcohol, or other drugs)
Maternal trauma, hemorrhage, or infection during fetal development
Premature birth, low birth weight
Malnutrition
Abuse or neglect; improper treatment of common childhood illnesses
Neurologic insult, injury, or infection
Severe metabolic abnormality
Toxic exposure (for example to lead, mercury, or another environmental toxin)
Inadequate stimulation during childhood
Near drowning
Hyperthermia
Trauma or hypoxia during delivery
Traumatic injuries

Original table by A. Bartkus, utilizing multiple sources.

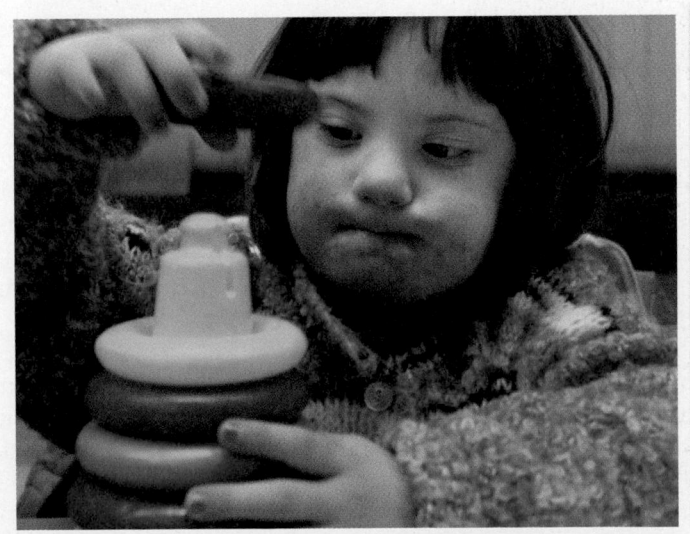

Figure 27 A child with Down syndrome.

Down syndrome is also known as trisomy 21. Normal human cells have 23 pairs of chromosomes that create the cell's genetic identity. In Down syndrome, an extra chromosome attaches to the 21st pair, thus becoming the third chromosome 21 or trisomy 21. The risk of an infant having Down syndrome is greater when a sibling or the mother has Down syndrome. The risk of Down syndrome also increases with older maternal age at the time of conception.

Chromosomal changes associated with Down syndrome may cause structural heart defects, seizures, numerous gastrointestinal problems, speech alterations, hearing loss, and many other abnormalities. Persons with Down syndrome also have a shorter life expectancy. Cognitive deficits with Down syndrome range from barely noticeable to profound impairment. Persons with Down syndrome, depending on their level of mental disability, may function relatively independently or require constant assistance with even basic tasks.

Mental Retardation

Mental retardation, sometimes known as intellectual disability, is a primarily cognitive disorder that appears during childhood and is accompanied by lack of "adaptive" behaviors. Adaptive behaviors include the ability to live and function independently or interact successfully with others. A variety of tests are available to support the diagnosis of mental retardation, but an intelligence quotient (IQ) below 70 is the defining characteristic.

Many causes of development delay listed in Table 4 will cause mental retardation. As with Down syndrome and autism, the clinical presentation and severity of symptoms will vary dramatically among people with this disorder.

Special Populations

Average: IQ = 70-130
Mild retardation: IQ = 52-69
Moderate retardation: IQ = 36-51
Severe retardation: IQ = 20-35
Profound retardation: IQ ≤ 19

Autism

Autism is a condition involving developmental delay that is being diagnosed with increased frequency in the United States. Increased rates of diagnosis may be due to better awareness and screening or an actual increase in the occurrence of autism in the population.

Patients with autism demonstrate a wide variety of symptoms that often relate to communication, social interaction, sensation of discomfort, the ability to purposefully shift attention, and the ability to play. A large number of people who are autistic will either be completely nonverbal throughout their lifetime or become nonverbal during periods of stress. Developmental regression in absence of another cause in young children should raise concerns for the possibility of autism. Cognitive function can vary significantly among people with autism. Some people

with autism may have impaired cognitive function, meeting the criteria for mental retardation discussed above. Other people with autism may have "savant" like abilities and demonstrate amazing skills with mathematics, puzzles, memory, or art.

When you are treating patients with autism, you should be extremely mindful of your actions when you are attempting to communicate and initiate physical contact. Commotion and excess stimuli may cause a patient with autism to have bizarre or aggressive behaviors. Any physical contact should be preceded by a careful explanation and go from distal to proximal on the patient. Any questions should be repeated to the patient in a variety of ways in order to determine whether there is a consistent response. Patients with autism may exhibit minimal reactions to significantly painful injuries or may experience great discomfort with minor physical contact or injuries.

You should be prepared for many possible challenges while providing care to patients with autism. Including the caregivers in assessment, treatment, and transport will often be extremely helpful. Additional information regarding EMS care of patients with autism is readily available on the Internet.

Mental/Emotional Impairment

Mental illness can occur in persons with mental or emotional disability just as it can arise in healthy people. (The care of mentally ill patients is discussed in depth in the chapter, *Psychiatric Emergencies.*) In the broader sense, a person's mental status can influence his or her physical well-being, and vice versa. Emotionally or mentally impaired patients may be difficult to assess due to the body's normal stress response, which may alter their respiratory rate, pulse rate, or perception of physical illness. Gathering a detailed history will be useful in the assessment and development of a treatment plan for these patients. Calmly ascertain the chief complaint and treat the patient accordingly, with care and understanding.

You may be particularly challenged when you encounter patients who demonstrate a conversion disorder, previously referred to as hysteria. Certain patients can present with focal neurologic abnormalities as a physical manifestation of an underlying mental illness. Blindness, paralysis, and impaired speech can occur as a response to stress in susceptible people. In this situation, the manifestations such as blindness or paralysis are not voluntary and the patient is not faking the sign or symptom. Diagnosis and treatment of conversion disorders require intervention from an experienced mental health provider and is beyond the scope of your training. When a conversion disorder is suspected, maintain a professional demeanor and continue to assess the patient for other potentially life-threatening causes of the sign or symptom.

Words of Wisdom

Use sirens judiciously, and when using them, protect your hearing... before it's too late.

Hearing Impairment

Over 30 million adults and children have some degree of hearing loss. Hearing loss inhibits communication, limits social interaction, interferes with infant development, and renders many safety and warning devices ineffective. Patients with profound hearing impairment can pose a considerable challenge to EMS providers.

Hearing impairment may be congenital (present since birth) or acquired. Genetic factors are believed to cause 50% of congenital hearing loss in children. The remaining 50% of congenital hearing loss is caused by such factors as maternal infection, Rh incompatibility, hypoxia, maternal diabetes, and pregnancy-induced hypertension.

The majority of acquired hearing loss in children and adults is a result of excessive exposure to loud noise. Other causes of acquired hearing loss include various infections including otitis media (middle ear infection), viral infections, tumors such as **acoustic neuroma**, ototoxicity of many kinds of medications, diseases such as **Meniere disease**, and degenerative processes associated with aging.

There are two types of hearing loss. Patients may have **conductive hearing loss**, which is an inability of sound to travel from the outer ear through to the inner ear. **Sensorineural hearing loss** is caused by problems with the uptake of sound through tiny hairs within the ear and subsequent conduction of nerve impulses. Patients may have hearing loss of either type or may have a combination of both conductive and sensorineural hearing loss (mixed hearing loss). It is also possible for patients to have normal hearing physiology but be unable to interpret sounds, particularly speech, due to **central auditory processing disorder (CAPD)**. CAPD is an auditory process deficit that can be characterized by difficulty interpreting speech when other background noises are present. Finally, **auditory neuropathy**, also known as auditory dyssynchrony, is a condition characterized by normal function of the structures of the ear without a corresponding stimulation of auditory centers of the brain. Auditory neuropathy is linked to prematurity, congenital anomalies, and several other neurologic conditions.

Patients with profound or total hearing loss, sometimes called **deafness**, may be able to communicate using sign language or written and printed words. Learning cursory sign language may prove extremely helpful for EMS providers who regularly provide care to large numbers of deaf patients **Figure 28**. The California Department of Social Services distributes a medical sign language reference card that is readily available for no charge on the Internet. Writing on simple notepads as well as many electronic devices will assist you in communicating with hearing-impaired patients who are able to read and write.

If patients have minimal or partial hearing loss, slow, deliberate, and sometimes repetitive speech will facilitate communication.

Hearing Aids

A hearing aid is essentially a device that makes sound louder. Hearing aids cannot restore hearing to normal, but they do improve hearing and listening ability. Several types of hearing aids are available **Figure 29**:

1. Behind-the-ear. All parts are contained in a plastic case that rests behind the ear.
2. Conventional body type. This older style is generally used by people with profound hearing loss.
3. In-the-canal and completely in-the-canal. These hearing aids are contained in a tiny case that fits partly or completely into the ear canal.
4. In-the-ear. All parts are contained in a shell that fits in the outer part of the ear.

Implantable hearing aids are also an option for patients with less profound hearing loss.

To insert a hearing aid, follow the natural shape of the ear. The device needs to fit snugly without forcing. If you hear a whistling sound, the hearing aid may not be in far enough to create a seal or the volume may be too loud. Try repositioning the hearing aid, or remove it and turn down the volume. If you cannot insert the hearing aid after two tries, put it in the box, take it with you, and document the transport and transfer of hearing aids to hospital personnel. Never try to clean hearing aids, and never get them wet.

If a patient's hearing aid is not working, try troubleshooting the problem. First, make sure the hearing aid is turned on **Figure 30**. Try a fresh battery, and check the tubing to make sure it is not twisted or bent. Check the switch to make sure it is set on M (microphone), not T (telephone). For a body aid, try a spare cord because the old one may be broken or shorted. Finally, check the ear mold to make sure it is not plugged with wax.

Visual Impairment

An estimated 2.5 million people in the United States are considered legally blind, with a corrected vision of worse than 20/200. When people who require glasses, contact lenses, or vision correction in order to function effectively with everyday tasks are included, the incidence of visual impairment is staggering.

Visual impairment can be caused by a variety of congenital and acquired conditions. Genetic factors may predispose people to develop vision loss later in life. Congenital causes include fetal exposure to cytomegalovirus, hypoxia during delivery, albinism, hydrocephalus, and retinopathy of prematurity. **Retinopathy** refers to any number of diseases of the retina of the eye that do

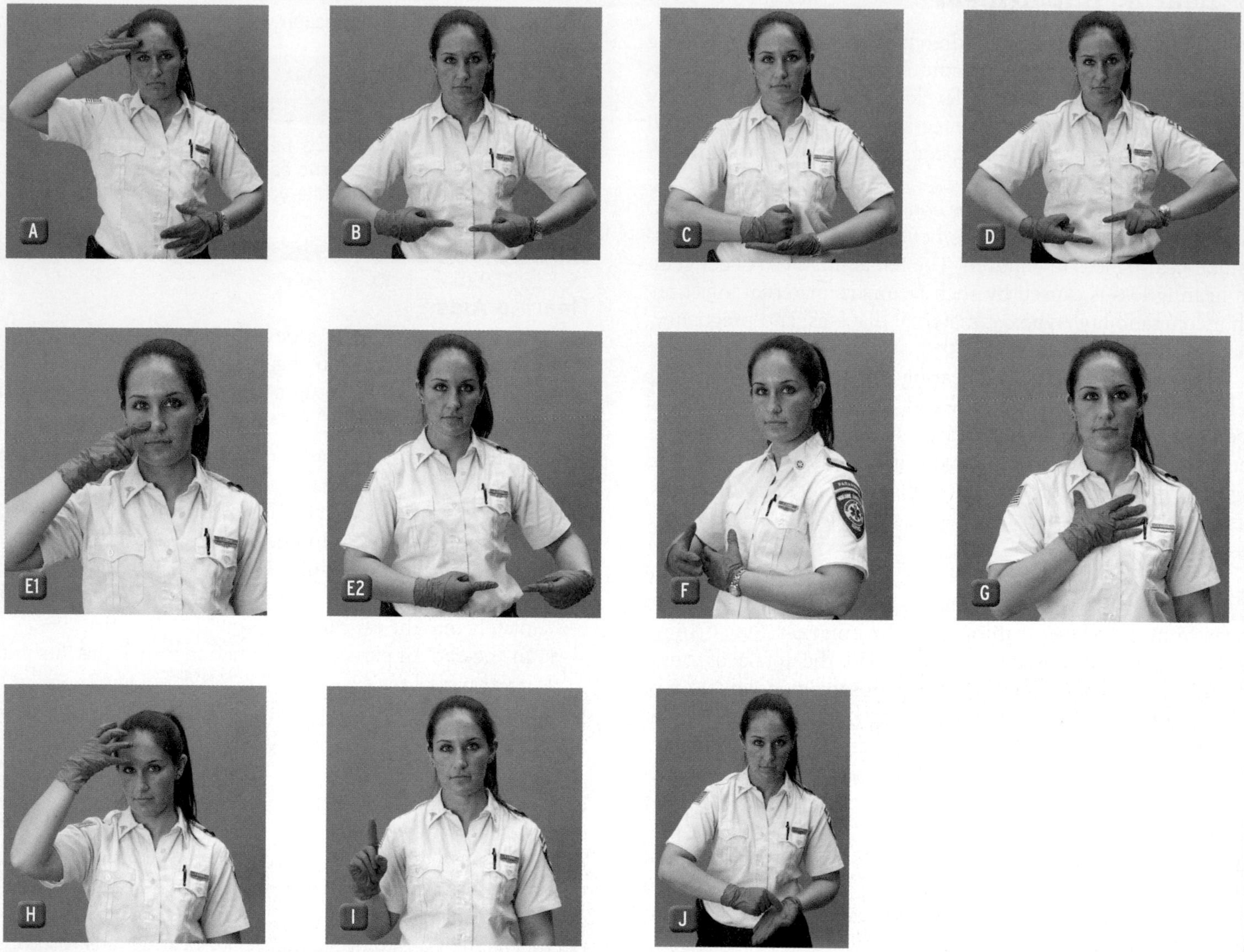

Figure 28 Consider learning the American Sign Language signs for common terms related to illness and injury. **A.** Sick. **B.** Hurt. **C.** Help. **D.** Ache/pain. **E.** Allergy. **F.** Breath. **G.** Chest. **H.** Dizziness. **I.** Where. **J.** Write.

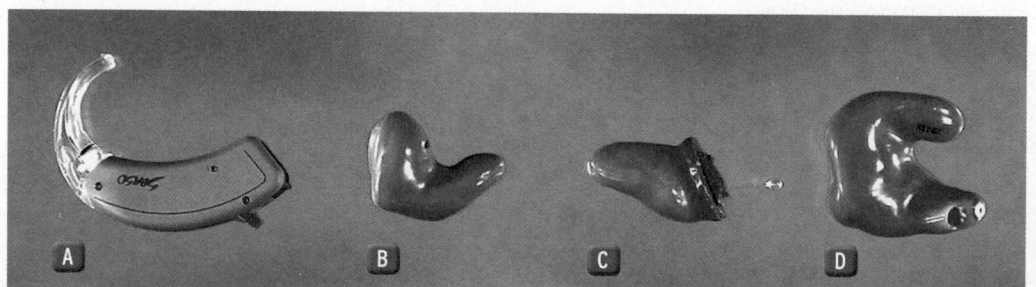

Figure 29 Different types of hearing aids. **A.** Behind-the-ear type. **B.** Conventional body type. **C.** In-the-canal type. **D.** In-the-ear type.

macular degeneration, **glaucoma** (increased pressure within the eye), **cataracts** (lens of the eye becomes opaque), uncontrolled hypertension, diabetic retinopathy, or degeneration of the eyeball, optic nerve, or nerve pathway (eg, with aging). Vitamin A deficiency is a significant cause of acquired visual impairment in many developing countries. Patients may have impaired vision due to **optic nerve hypoplasia**, a congenital condition characterized by failure of the optic nerve to completely develop. Over time, it is possible for optic nerve atrophy to occur following a cerebrovascular accident, brain tumor, certain toxic chemical exposure, trauma, and a variety of other causes. Optic nerve atrophy is permanent,

not involve inflammation. High levels of supplemental oxygen given to infants during the neonatal period have been linked to retinopathy of prematurity. Acquired causes of visual impairment include trauma, cerebrovascular accident, age-related

but prompt identification and treatment of the underlying cause may slow or stop further vision loss.

Visual impairment can present in several notable patterns. Table 5 outlines common patterns of visual impairment.

Hysterical blindness is an antiquated term for conversion disorder, a mental health condition. Blindness results as the body "converts" an extreme psychological stressor into a physical manifestation. Diagnosis and treatment of conversion disorders are often quite challenging.

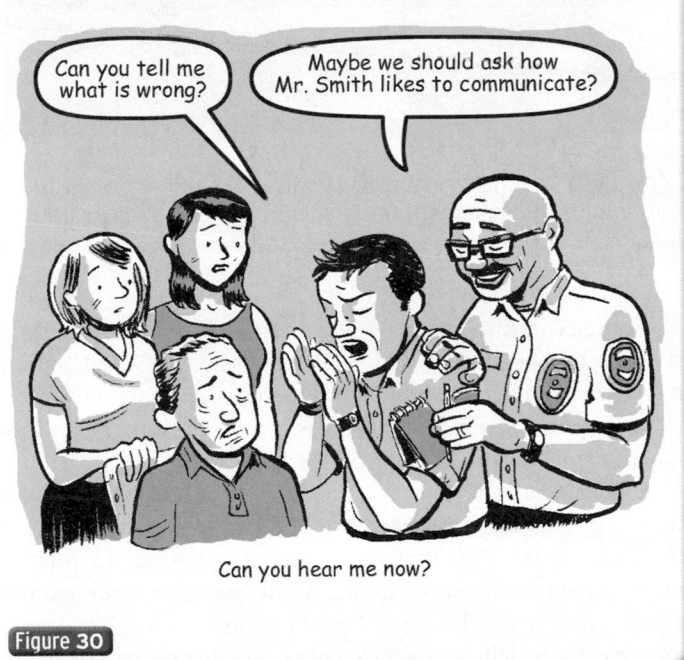

Figure 30

Table 5 Common Patterns of Visual Impairment

Type of Impairment	Characteristics
Amblyopia	Partial or complete vision loss in one eye
Blindness	Total visual impairment; patients may report the ability to see certain lights or shadows
Cortical visual impairment	Visual impairment caused by a brain abnormality
Hyperopia	Farsightedness; problem with light refraction that makes closer objects appear blurry
Myopia	Nearsightedness; problem with light refraction that makes distant object appear blurry
Presbyopia	Adult-onset farsightedness; problem with light refraction that makes closer objects blurry
Scotoma	Area missing from the visual field
Strabismus	Misaligned eyes

Acute angle-closure glaucoma (AACG) is a true ocular emergency. You should suspect AACG in patients who experience a sudden onset of unilateral eye or periorbital pain accompanied by visual changes. Prompt recognition and patient transport to an emergency department are imperative.

Other patients with profound visual impairment will benefit from explanation before any physical contact by EMS providers. You should warn your patient in advance if you are going to begin palpation of a body region or perform a procedure such as starting an IV line. A brief discussion with the patient prior to moving or transferring the patient will likely be greatly appreciated.

Speech Impairment

You may encounter patients exhibiting impaired speech. Changes in speech may be associated with neurologic injury, toxicologic exposure, anatomic abnormalities of the face or neck, and numerous other conditions. Speech impairment has the potential to adversely impact the information obtained during assessment and treatment of patients receiving EMS assistance.

Speech impairment may be divided into disorders impacting language, voice production, fluency, and articulation. Articulation disorders essentially involve forming particular words or sounds incorrectly. This may manifest as a lisp or a trouble with certain specific sounds. Voice disorders alter the pitch, volume, or tone of the patient's voice. Voices may appear muffled, raspy, or unusually high or low. Fluency disorders affect speech patterns. There may be unusual pauses or patterns to otherwise appropriate speech. Particular words or phrases may be prolonged, repeated, or avoided. Language disorders impair the manner that ideas, thoughts, and feelings are expressed or understood. A patient may cognitively understand what he or she is trying to say, but is unable to decide which words or phrases should be used to express the material. When difficulties with reading, spelling, or writing cause a person to fall behind expectations for a given age, the person has a **language-based learning disability**. Other types of language-based learning disabilities include problems with phonation. **Phonologic process disorders** impact a person's ability to produce sounds that combine into spoken words.

Autistic patients (discussed earlier) and others may present with a **semantic-pragmatic disorder** of speech. This condition is characterized by delayed language developmental milestones, with the person repeatedly using irrelevant phrases out of context, confusing word pairs such as the use of "I" and "you," and trouble following the conversations of others. A semantic-pragmatic disorder impacts both reception of communication and the person's ability to express himself or herself.

There are also two types of motor speech disorders that may adversely impact communication. **Dysarthria** is a failure of neurotransmission between the nervous system and muscles of the face and throat that causes impaired speech. Dysarthria is characterized by consistent repetition of the same impairment of speech. **Apraxia** is a neurologic impairment originating in the brain that inconsistently activates muscles needed to form particular sounds or words. The patient may understand what he or she is trying to say, but the pattern of muscle activation during attempts to form particular words becomes more or less random, resulting in the erratic production of sounds. The differentiation between apraxia and a phonologic process disorder is challenging and will likely require specialist consultation.

Impaired speech can be caused by many conditions other than intoxication. You may need to exercise patience and deliberation when you are communicating with patients who have speech impairment. Enlisting the help of family or caregivers familiar with the unusual speech can prove quite valuable, especially when specific information is needed from the patient.

Paralysis, Paraplegia, and Quadriplegia

Paralysis is simply defined as the inability to move. Muscles in affected areas of the body may become flaccid or fail to move because of continued spasm, known as **spastic paralysis**. Many chronic medical conditions discussed in this chapter can cause paralysis. Head trauma, cerebrovascular accident (CVA, stroke), spinal cord injury, malignancy, and other neuromuscular diseases can lead to long-term paralysis. Paralysis affecting the lower extremities but not upper extremities is known as **paraplegia**. If paralysis affects both the upper extremities and lower extremities, it is known as **quadriplegia**. In many instances, paralysis is accompanied by sensory deficits and loss of bowel or bladder control.

Patients with paralysis often experience serious complications. Paralysis of the respiratory muscles causes patients to be completely dependent on a mechanical ventilator or similar device. Interruption of assisted ventilation for even brief periods may have devastating consequences.

Pressure ulcers are a constant threat. Patients require frequent mechanical or caregiver assistance to change their position. Tissue perfusion to the coccyx region and over bony prominences becomes compromised when external pressure is applied to these areas for a long period of time. Approximately 60% of patients with quadriplegia have pressure ulcers. Infection related to pressure ulcers is a significant cause of mortality in these patients.

Patients who have paralysis related to spinal cord injury are at risk for a life-threatening condition known as autonomic dysreflexia. A stressor within the body, sometimes as simple as a full bladder, constipation, or pain, triggers a large release of catecholamines from the autonomic nervous system. This release causes vasodilation above the level of the spinal cord injury as well as massive arterial vasoconstriction. The patient's blood pressure can become dangerously high.

External devices such as halo rings and vests are used to stabilize structures of the spine following initial management of significant fractures or dislocations **Figure 31**. These devices require additional consideration and coordination while you are moving these patients. Halo rings and vests have substantial weight. It is necessary to support the halo ring and vest, without applying any force to this device during patient movement. In the event of cardiac arrest, there is typically an Allen/hex key attached to the anterior chest portion of the vest for removal only to perform external cardiac compressions. Paramedics and other prehospital providers should not attempt to reposition or adjust the halo ring or vest.

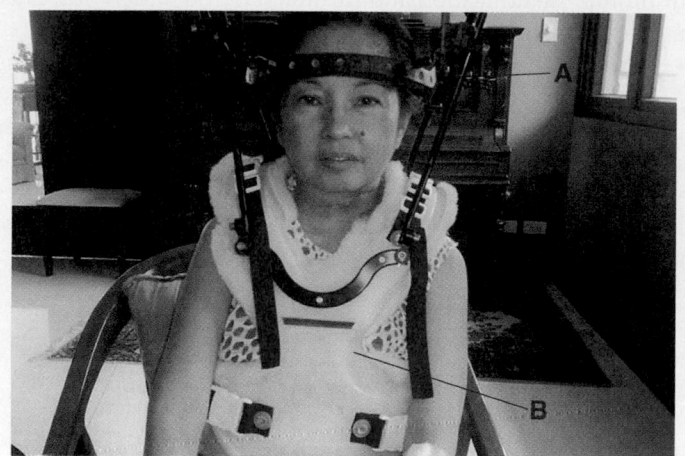

Figure 31 **A.** A halo ring. **B.** A vest used for spinal stabilization after initial management of significant fracture or dislocation.

Patients with paralysis are particularly susceptible to environmental extremes. It is often impossible for these patients to regulate perfusion to the skin. Fluctuations of the autonomic nervous system place patients at risk for both hypothermia and hyperthermia, particularly hyperthermia.

Paralysis does not always entail a loss of sensation. In some cases, the patient will have normal sensation or hyperesthesia (increased sensitivity) that may cause the patient to interpret touch as pain in the affected area. Conversely, for some patients, pressure that would be experienced by those with normal sensation may not be felt. Some male patients with a severe spinal cord injury will present with priapism, a prolonged penile erection, not at all related to sexual arousal. Depending on the pattern of sensation loss, the priapism may be associated with discomfort for the patient. You should maintain patient privacy and continue to provide interventions related to the patient's presenting complaint.

Scheduled urinary catheterization is required for many patients with paralysis. Urinary infection, urinary reflux, and autonomic dysreflexia are all possible if patients do not have regular bladder emptying.

Total lifting assistance is typically required for many patients with quadriplegia. These patients may or may not need to use a tracheostomy tube, indwelling urinary catheter, colostomy, or ventilator. You may need to request additional lifting assistance or specialty consultation regarding the ventilator or a similar device. Patients with significant paralysis have the potential to create serious challenges for EMS providers.

Trauma in Cognitively Impaired Patients

You are likely to encounter children or adults with a developmental disability at the scene or as a victim of a traumatic event. Many of the cognitive, sensory, and communication impairments discussed earlier will become particularly problematic when these patients experience a traumatic injury or become involved in a traumatic event such as a motor vehicle crash. Isolated sensory or communication impairments can cause additional anxiety, confusion, delays, and disruption of patient care or transport. Patients with severe cognitive impairments will have all of the above problems and may present with a variety of abnormal behavioral responses. You may need to significantly modify how communication, assessment, interventions, and patient transport are performed.

Cognitively impaired patients present a number of significant challenges for prehospital providers. These patients may have considerable difficulty communicating under normal circumstances, and when injury, stress, and the excitement of a traumatic event are added in, effective communication can become almost impossible. These patients may not be able to provide a thorough, accurate, or meaningful medical history. If the patient's caregiver is not available, you must rely on physical or behavioral cues when you are providing treatment to these patients. Environmental clues such as the type of business (group home), school (for example, school for the deaf), or lettering on the vehicle may provide you with hints regarding the nature of the disability. Altered or decreased pain sensation, concomitant neurologic disorders, and atypical presentation of physical signs and symptoms are characteristic of many people with profound cognitive impairment. Patients with autism may demonstrate unusual communication patterns or have an exaggerated reaction to physical contact by prehospital providers.

Consent for medical treatment may present some uncertainty. Adults with profound cognitive, sensory, or communication impairment may not have decision-making capacity to consent or refuse medical treatment. You may need to locate a valid surrogate decision-maker or initiate treatment under the doctrine of implied consent, particularly in emergency situations.

You will need to modify patient assessment techniques for patients with cognitive impairment. These patients may present with an education level at 6th grade or below. A second- or third-grade education level is not uncommon. Patients with cognitive impairment may have difficulty understanding or communicating the timing or relationship of particular events. The use of open-ended questions during patient assessment may offer clues regarding the patient's cognitive ability and decision-making capacity. Assess for understanding by having the patient paraphrase or repeat back information conveyed by you or your partner, especially in situations such as obtaining patient consent or refusal.

Caregivers can become valuable resources following a traumatic event with a cognitively impaired patient. Caregivers will be able to relay how that person normally communicates, his or her level of awareness and understanding, physical abilities such as motor skills or activity, as well as additional information such as sleep patterns and eating habits. Consider allowing the caregiver to remain with the patient during the physical exam or deferring measurement of the vital signs in patients who are outwardly demonstrating sufficient oxygenation, ventilation, and perfusion until the patient is calm and cooperative.

Interventions may require additional time, explanation, and holding assistance. The management of traumatic injuries with fluid resuscitation, airway and ventilation support, bleeding control, and immobilization are generally the same as for patients without cognitive impairment. You should expect many of these patients to have concomitant neurologic disorders

such as seizures, delirium, weakness, or muscle spasm. Psychiatric disorders, gastrointestinal abnormalities, and chronic or frequent infections are also common in this patient population. Assess for and treat preexisting injuries and remain alert for signs or clues of abuse and neglect.

Other Notable Chronic Medical Conditions

You should be aware of several notable medical conditions. These conditions may meet the criteria for developmental disability noted earlier, but are not primarily associated with sensory, cognitive, or communication impairment. The conditions discussed next are included to provide you with additional understanding of the impact of these chronic conditions when they are encountered in patients during an EMS response or interfacility transport.

Arthritis

Arthritis is an inflammation of joints between bones that can cause pain, stiffness, swelling, redness, and discomfort for patients. It may be caused by excessive use of a particular limb or joint, infection, autoimmune process, or at the site of a previous fracture. You may transport patients with arthritis who have other complications of autoimmune disease or have an entirely unrelated medical problem.

Osteoarthritis is the most common type of arthritis **Figure 32**. It is caused by cartilage loss or abnormal bone growth, usually in response to trauma or excess "wear and tear" on a joint over time (therefore, common in elderly patients). Treatment includes medications for analgesia and inflammation, topical creams, and injections directly into the affected joint and joint replacement in severe cases.

Rheumatoid arthritis (RA) is a systemic inflammatory disease that affects joints and other body systems. RA can be a mild and nonprogressive disease, or it can be a full-blown, fatal illness. In RA, significant bone erosion at the affected joints makes them more susceptible to fractures and dislocations.

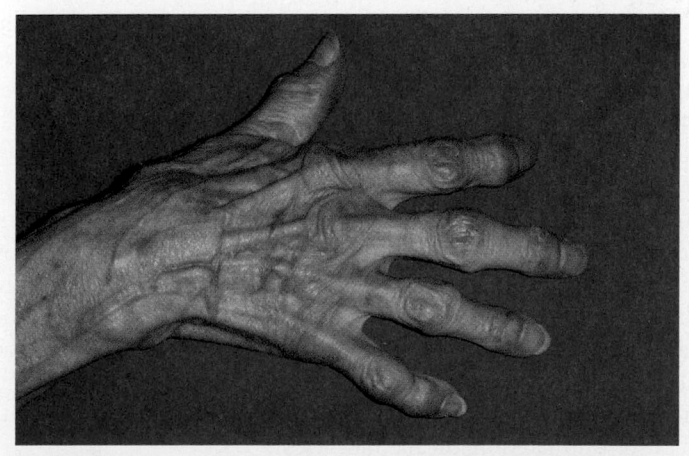

Figure 32 Osteoarthritis may cause substantial disfigurement.

You should remain alert when you are treating or transporting patients with arthritis associated with systemic lupus erythematosus (SLE), gout, or RA. In these patients, arthritis discomfort may be accompanied by other potential significant medical concerns. Symptoms associated with these diseases include chest pain, sensory changes or deficits, and skin changes. Patients with SLE can experience life-threatening cardiac, pulmonary, and neurologic events associated with this debilitating disease process. SLE is discussed in greater detail later in this chapter.

During EMS response or interfacility transport, you may administer analgesia medications and should attempt to maintain the patient's limb or joint in the most comfortable position possible. Assess the patient's current long-term medications to avoid problematic medication interactions. Many analgesic and sedative medications carried by paramedics have the potential to have adverse interactions with medications prescribed to these patients. Backboards and splints may require additional padding or support to best fit the patient and help avoid patient discomfort. Immobility of certain joints will interfere with physical examination of the patient. Problems with arm, wrist, or hand joints may make it difficult or impossible for you to obtain a blood pressure or initiate IV access. A hot, swollen joint or patient fever could indicate the presence of an infection within the joint that will require aggressive medical treatment.

Cancer

You are likely to become involved in the medical care or transportation of patients with active or successfully treated cancer. Cancer is a term applied to various conditions that result from excessive growth and division of abnormal cells within the body. This abnormal cell growth may linger for long periods of time with minimal clinical impact or progress rapidly, causing death in a relatively short period of time. Many body systems, tissues, and organs can be targeted and damaged by various types of cancer.

Cancer frequently targets organs and body systems such as the brain, breasts, skin, blood, stomach, liver, immune (lymphatic) system, and colon. Abnormal cells can multiply within a particular organ or body system, causing dysfunction of that particular organ or system. Cancer cells may also metastasize (spread) to another area of the body that is more susceptible to the effects of abnormal cell growth. In either scenario, critical illness or death may occur.

Signs, symptoms, clinical presentation, and treatment will largely depend on the present location of the cancer or the primary site of origin. Cancer conditions are typically treated by radiation therapy, chemotherapy medications, or some form of surgical removal. These treatment methods may be used alone or in combination, depending on the site or severity of the cancerous condition as well as specifics of a particular patient. Treatment for cancer may increase the susceptibility of patients to other unrelated medical conditions.

Chemotherapy medications are notorious for causing nausea and vomiting, anorexia, discomfort, and immune system compromise. When patients have a compromised immune system following chemotherapy, otherwise routine infections can become life-threatening emergencies. In many instances, patients will receive chemotherapy, analgesic medications, and blood product replacement through implanted ports and other long-term vascular access devices. These devices reduce patient discomfort and prevent irritation of smaller blood vessels while allowing reliable access for frequently administered medications. Long-term vascular access devices were discussed in greater detail previously in this chapter.

You may need to correct dehydration issues and administer pain or antiemetic medications for patients diagnosed or being treated for cancer. In addition to long-term vascular access devices, patients may also use transdermal patches for administration of analgesic or antiemetic medications. You should inquire about or inspect for transdermal medication patches prior to administering medications to these patients. These patients frequently receive hospice treatment (discussed earlier). You should inquire about the patient's wishes regarding resuscitation and obtain copies of advance directives or DNR paperwork when applicable.

Cerebral Palsy

Cerebral palsy (CP) is a potentially devastating, nonprogressive neurologic disorder that results from injury to brain tissue during brain development. Injury to the brain may occur during fetal development, labor and delivery, or during the child's first 2 years of life. CP may be caused by genetic defects that alter brain development, maternal infections during fetal development, fetal CVA (stroke), excessive fetal bilirubin (kernicterus) or hemolysis, hypoxia before or during birth, infant infection (eg, postpartum encephalitis, meningitis), or head trauma.

CP generally produces altered skeletal muscle function or contraction. Muscles are poorly controlled; they may be unusually contracted, flaccid, or paralyzed. Severity of this condition may range from almost unnoticeable, with children appearing and acting normal, to profoundly devastating with paralysis of the arms and legs, combined with severe mental retardation (discussed earlier). Children with mild symptoms may function well in regular school programs. More severely affected patients may present with an exhaustive list of chronic signs and symptoms, including seizure disorders, hearing loss, and a variety of neurologic disorders. It is possible for CP to primarily affect only certain body regions such as hemiplegia (one side of the body) or be more pronounced in either the arms or the legs (paraplegia) **Figure 33**. When CP affects all fours limbs, it is known as spastic tetraplegia. Movement disorders include tremors, unsteady gait (ataxia), and athetosis (involuntary writhing movement). Severe cases may present with seizures, loss of bladder control, inability to swallow, joint contractures, and impaired respiratory function. Often, severe manifestations of CP will require that the patient receive total assistance from caregivers.

Careful movement and positioning is essential during treatment and transport of the patient. These patients may have significant musculoskeletal changes that make patient assessment and safe movement extremely difficult. Seizures, infection, and

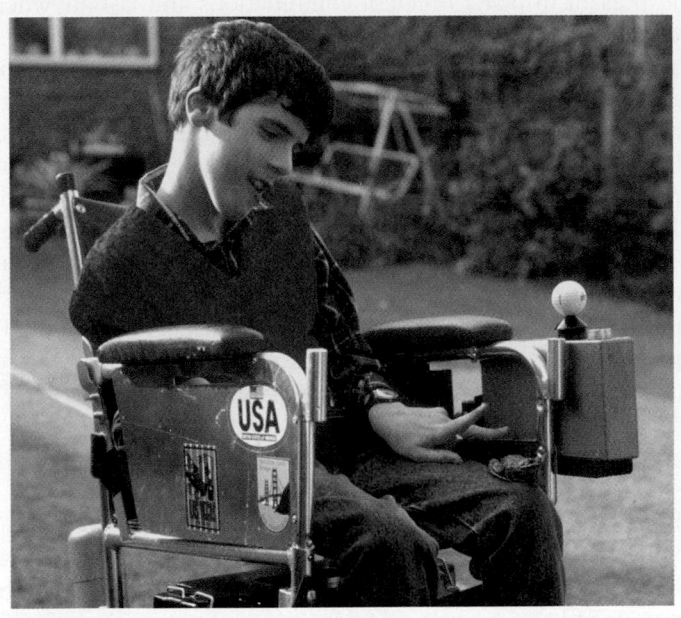

Figure 33 A young man with cerebral palsy.

respiratory distress, along with many other potential complications, may prompt requests for EMS assistance.

Cystic Fibrosis

Infants and young children may be diagnosed with **cystic fibrosis (CF)** (mucoviscidosis), a genetic disorder that is characterized by increased production of mucus in the lungs and digestive tract. CF is caused by a defective recessive gene, inherited from each parent, that makes it difficult for chloride to move through cells. This causes unusually high sodium loss (resulting in salty

skin). Mild cases can go undetected until after a patient reaches adulthood. Sweat glands, reproductive glands, and a variety of body systems may also become adversely affected. The increased mucus impairs respiration, disrupts digestion of food, and may become a life-threatening emergency in severe situations.

CF is suspected in newborn infants who present with meconium or odd-smelling or appearing stool (usually pale, greasy-looking, and foul-smelling). Gastrointestinal symptoms include nausea, anorexia, constipation, pancreatitis, and distended abdomen, as well as bowel obstruction or **ileus** (loss of gastrointestinal motility). CF impairs the release of pancreatic enzymes used to digest and absorb fats in the intestine. Patients with CF are prone to the development of venous thrombosis. Pulmonary manifestations include pneumonia, pneumothorax, cough, respiratory distress, and respiratory failure. Malnutrition and poor growth rate are not uncommon symptoms; in some cases a child with CF may fail to thrive. Other symptoms include infertility, chronic sinus congestion, and bone mineral loss.

Patients with CF receive frequent or continuous treatment with various antibiotics. These antibiotics may be administered intravenously through long-term vascular access devices (discussed earlier). Medical devices promoting lung function and removal of mucus may be used by patients with CF. Patients may be on intermittent or continuous home oxygen. A significant number of patients with CF await or receive lung transplants to prolong and improve the quality of life. It is possible that patients with CF will have a long, complex medical history and a vast array of clinical abnormalities requiring additional time for patient assessment. You may encounter patients with CF who may have minimal to profound respiratory or gastrointestinal compromise from this disorder. You should expect to administer oxygen, provide frequent deep suctioning, and assist ventilation for patients with CF. CF is usually diagnosed in infants and children, but 7% of cases, usually those people with

YOU *are the Medic*   **PART 5**

On arrival to the emergency department, you are met by an attending physician from the pediatric intensive care unit and a respiratory therapist. Amanda is diagnosed with pneumonia and is admitted to the pediatric intermediate care unit for continued treatment with bronchodilators, IV antibiotics, and chest physical therapy.

Recording Time: 25 Minutes	
Respirations	22 breaths/min; accessory muscle use noted
Pulse	110 beats/min, regular; weak peripheral pulses and strong central pulses
Skin	Pink, warm, and dry
Blood pressure	112/68 mm Hg
Oxygen saturation (Spo$_2$)	95% at 12 L/min on nonrebreathing mask
Pupils	Equal and reactive to light

7. Why is emotional support important when you are transporting a patient with cystic fibrosis?

mild or atypical symptoms, are diagnosed in adults. Diagnosis of CF requires specialized testing not available in the prehospital setting. You should alert receiving physicians if a strong suspicion for the possibility of CF exists.

Multiple Sclerosis

Multiple sclerosis (MS) is a severe, incurable degenerative disorder involving the central nervous system (brain and spinal cord). Immune cells within the body attack the myelin sheath of certain nerve fibers, ultimately destroying nerve fibers and preventing nerve transmission to other body tissues Figure 34. It is not entirely clear what causes MS, although some sources describe a connection between genetic predisposition, environmental factors, and possibly nutrition or exposure to a particular virus. This disease strikes women in their 20s to 40s two to three times more often than men. Approximately 350,000 Americans have MS, some with serious handicaps.

Patients typically present with problems related to muscle coordination, muscle tone, altered sensation, and gait disturbances. These patients report periods of varied improvement followed by relapse and progression of the disease. A vast array of signs and symptoms related to neurologic function are possible with MS. Patients may develop problems with the musculoskeletal system such as clumsiness and ataxia, constipation or bladder incontinence, fatigue, decreased sexual performance, extremities that feel heavy or weak, altered sensations (dizziness/vertigo), numbness or tingling in parts of the body, cognitive impairment, disruption of speech or swallowing, and visual impairment. Skin breakdown may result from immobility or poor positioning. Severe manifestations of the disease may render patients bedridden and incontinent. The patient's life span may be almost normal or markedly decreased depending on the presentation and the severity of the disease. Symptoms can present in many different combinations and last anywhere from several days to months, often interrupted by periods of absent or reduced symptoms. Life expectancy may be normal, but profound symptoms may cause significant disability or impairment depending on the severity of the disease process. MS is managed with medications, physical therapy, and counseling. There is no specific EMS treatment for MS. You should allow additional time for assessment due to cognitive or communication barriers. Because of the disease process, the patient may lack feeling, so the physical examination findings may be difficult to interpret. Other supportive measures include IV hydration, analgesic or muscle-relaxing medications, careful patient positioning, and assisted ventilation when indicated.

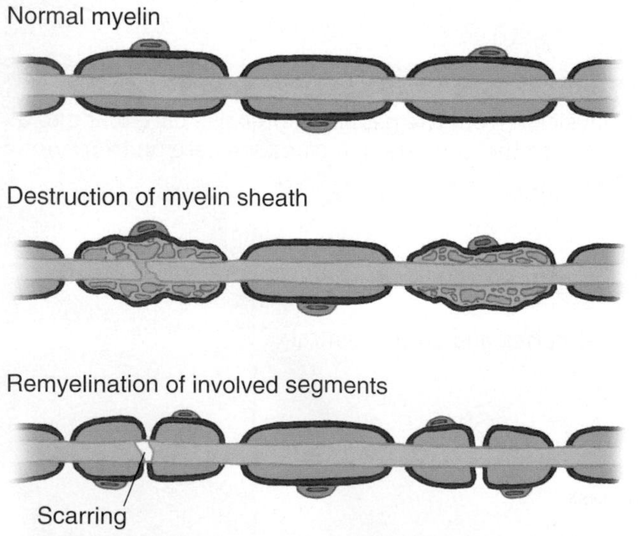

Muscular Dystrophy

Muscular dystrophy is a broad term that actually describes a category of incurable genetic diseases that cause a slow, progressive degeneration of the muscle fibers. In many cases, the destroyed fibers are replaced by fat or connective tissue. Specific diseases in this category can be diagnosed by certain genetic markers, age at the time of onset, rate at which the disease progresses, and gender of the patient in certain cases.

Children may present with obvious facial muscle changes, altered gait, delayed psychomotor developmental milestones, and changes in posture. Severe manifestations of certain specific diseases in this group include cardiomyopathy, cognitive impairment, and respiratory compromise. Muscular dystrophy may show obvious signs when an infant is born or have an onset as late as adulthood. Profound symptoms or death from muscular dystrophy may occur in children and teenagers in severe cases. Death typically occurs secondary to cardiac or respiratory dysfunction associated with the disease.

Duchenne muscular dystrophy (DMD), the most common type, is caused by a sex-linked, recessive gene that chiefly affects boys (1 of every 3,500 male births). This disorder is characterized by enlarged heart muscle tissue (dilated cardiomyopathy), heart dysrhythmias, scoliosis (abnormal curvature) of the spine, and gait disturbances. Children with DMD often require the use of a wheelchair by age 15.

EMS treatment is primarily limited to careful positioning, supportive treatment, and assisted ventilation in severe cases. Smaller or younger children with muscular dystrophy are typically relatively easy to examine or transport. Larger children or adults may require additional assistance during movement to or from an ambulance.

Myasthenia Gravis

Myasthenia gravis is a rare autoimmune disorder that suddenly or gradually impacts neuromuscular transmission, causing muscles to weaken and tire easily. Although it affects all ethnic groups and sexes, myasthenia gravis is most commonly found in women younger than 40 years (typically between 20 and 30 years) and men older than 60 years. This disease may remain localized to the eyelids and extraocular muscles in a manifestation known as ocular myasthenia gravis or become "generalized,"

Normal myelin

Destruction of myelin sheath

Remyelination of involved segments

Scarring

Figure 34 Progression of multiple sclerosis. **A.** Normal myelin. **B.** Destruction of myelin sheath. **C.** Remyelination of involved segments with scarring.

affecting respiratory muscles and a variety of skeletal muscles. Skeletal muscles of the face, jaw, neck, and upper extremities are most commonly affected. Patients often demonstrate difficulty speaking, chewing, or swallowing. Respiratory failure due to respiratory muscle fatigue is the most serious manifestation of myasthenia gravis, called a **myasthenic crisis**. A crisis may occur if the patient's respiratory muscles are damaged by infection, stress, side effects of medications, or even menstruation.

Signs and symptoms of this disease will fluctuate over time, either as the impact of the disease varies or in response to immune-based treatment or anticholinergic medication. Classic signs and symptoms include drooping eyelids; double vision; difficulty speaking, chewing, or swallowing; and muscle weakness in the extremities. You may be requested to transport patients with myasthenia gravis as complications of the disease develop or because patients request EMS assistance for unrelated needs. It is possible that symptoms will resolve completely with rest or during transient remission of the disease process. Treatment is generally supportive and based on patient presentation. Patients having a myasthenic crisis may require airway protection and assisted ventilation. No other specific treatment options are generally available in the prehospital setting.

Myelomeningocele (Spina Bifida)

Myelomeningocele, also known as spina bifida, is a birth defect caused by improper development of the fetal neural tube consisting of the brain and spinal cord.

During fetal development, a defect in the vertebral column creates an opening that exposes the spinal cord and meninges. There is also a corresponding defect in the overlying skin that exposes the spinal cord and meninges to the outside environment **Figure 35**. Spina bifida may be associated with hydrocephalus or occur as an isolated neurologic abnormality. Spinal cord involvement negatively impacts both bowel and urinary

elimination in almost all patients with spina bifida, similar to other patients with spinal cord injury. Scoliosis and other orthopaedic disorders frequently accompany spina bifida. Surgical treatment of spina bifida typically occurs within 1 to 2 days of the patient's birth although several specialized health care facilities are having significant success with repair of spina bifida while the fetus is still in the mother's uterus.

You may provide care to patients with spina bifida in one of two vastly different scenarios. It is possible that you may need to perform a prehospital delivery of a fetus with diagnosed or undiagnosed spina bifida. Spina bifida is typically diagnosed by routine prenatal ultrasound. If a patient has not received or followed up with prenatal care, it is conceivable that spina bifida could remain undiagnosed until after delivery. Successful vaginal delivery of a fetus with spina bifida is possible, particularly if hydrocephalus is not also present. Once the fetus is delivered, smaller spinal cord openings should be covered with a moist, sterile dressing. Larger openings should be covered with a sterile occlusive dressing to prevent neonatal hypothermia. The newborn should be placed in a prone or lateral position to keep pressure off of the spinal cord. Prompt transport to a hospital specializing in the care of critical newborns is required.

Modern medicine is able to keep patients with this disorder alive well into adulthood. You may also encounter infants, children, and adults with spina bifida who have already received surgical evaluation and correction of spina bifida. These patients may present with medical issues related to or completely unrelated to this disorder. These patients are likely to require careful positioning, related to the severity of vertebral column and orthopaedic abnormality.

Spina bifida may cause a wide range of clinical manifestations, ranging from minimal to severe. Most patients will present with some degree of bladder dysfunction, known as a neurogenic bladder, requiring frequent urinary catheterization. Scoliosis, an abnormal curvature of the spine, is also quite common, even after surgical correction of the initial abnormality. Patients may or may not have associated neurologic conditions such as a seizure disorder, hydrocephalus, CP, or mental retardation. Patients may also present with complete or partial paralysis of the legs as well as abnormalities of various bones or joints.

The severity of the spina bifida and presence of other neurologic abnormalities will determine the amount or type of interventions that you will need to provide. It is possible that spina bifida will not significantly impact patient care in certain situations. In more severe cases, you may require additional time or manpower to effectively assess or prepare these patients for transport.

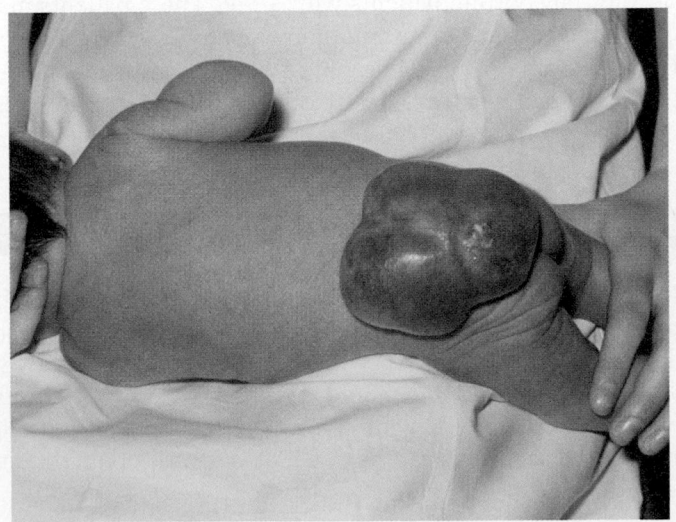

Figure 35 Spina bifida is characterized by exposure of part of the spinal cord.

Poliomyelitis/Postpolio Syndrome

Poliomyelitis (polio) is a devastating viral infection that has caused significant morbidity and mortality throughout the world. Since the 1950s, aggressive vaccination campaigns based on the Salk and Sabin vaccines have eradicated the polio virus in many countries, including the United States. Despite stopping the flow of new cases, over 500,000 people in the US live with sometimes-profound consequences of this problematic disease.

Humans are the only known hosts for the polio virus (poliovirus hominis). Polio initially presents similar to the common viral syndrome with headache, sore throat, fever, malaise, and vomiting. As the infection progresses, other somewhat generic symptoms present. Patients report back pain, diarrhea, leg pain, continued fever, and muscle discomfort or stiffness. Polio may or may not cause paralysis (paralytic and nonparalytic forms). In nonparalytic forms of polio, recovery is complete. In severe cases, muscle weakness evolves to paralysis of various muscles (most often the legs and lower trunk), muscle spasm, respiratory distress, drooling, difficulty swallowing, and other signs and symptoms. Any weakness or paralysis lasting longer than 12 months after the infection is a sign of permanent damage and disability. Complications include hypertension, respiratory failure, myocarditis, shock, loss of intestinal function, or death.

Those who survive an initial attack from the polio virus are still at risk for **postpolio syndrome**. This disorder is characterized by progressive or sudden worsening of muscle weakness, previously caused by the polio virus. Muscle atrophy also occurs. Patients are at renewed risk for developing respiratory insufficiency or respiratory failure, difficulty swallowing, or impaired speech. These adverse changes are frequently accompanied by significant pain or fatigue.

Polio may cause brief, mild symptoms lasting less than 72 hours, known as subclinical polio. Also, if polio did not initially involve the brain or spinal cord, a complete recovery occurs in over 90% of the patients. In either instance, the long-term prognosis is quite favorable.

The treatment for polio and postpolio syndrome remain primarily supportive. Patients with actual or impending respiratory failure require assisted ventilation and oxygenation. Movement and traditional EMS equipment are likely to cause patients significant discomfort. You should be prepared to assist patients with transfer or movement. Careful positioning and padding are essential. Patients with lower body paralysis may require assistance with urinary catheterization due to urinary retention.

Systemic Lupus Erythematosus

Systemic lupus erythematosus (lupus, SLE) is a chronic autoimmune disorder characterized by widespread inflammation of many body tissues. Antibodies in the body attack normal cells in the brain, kidneys, joints, digestive tract, and skin, although a variety of other organs and body systems may become affected.

Although the exact cause of SLE is unknown, it may be linked to a combination of genetic, environmental, and hormonal factors. SLE is more common in women than men and more common in Asian and African Americans than other groups.

Swelling and discomfort of joints are the most common manifestations of SLE. Patients may develop pleuritic-type chest discomfort, fevers, photosensitivity, swollen lymph nodes, and mouth sores. Severe manifestations include cardiac dysrhythmias, seizures, respiratory distress, and hemoptysis.

There is no specific prehospital treatment for SLE; care is supportive. You should monitor patients for potentially life-threatening conditions from a number of different body systems. IV hydration, analgesia medications, assisted ventilation, dysrhythmia management, and careful monitoring are interventions that you may need to perform during an EMS response or interfacility transport.

Traumatic Brain Injury

Traumatic brain injury (TBI) is a potentially devastating condition associated with many serious short- and long-term complications. You may encounter patients immediately after they experience the injury. Care of these patients in emergency situations is discussed in depth in the chapter, *Head and Spine Trauma*. Once the acute crisis has resolved, many of these patients continue to experience serious or life-altering long-term complications.

Patients may demonstrate a wide assortment of cognitive, emotional, behavioral, sensory, and communication disorders. Depending on the location and severity of the TBI, along with other associated injuries, these patients may also present with seizures, impaired movement, gastrointestinal dysfunction, urinary retention, paralysis, and almost any other conceivable problem.

You should be prepared to encounter a patient with a wide range of impairment or complications. The location or severity of the brain injury may cause you great difficulty during patient assessment and transport. In these situations, the caregiver's assistance is often essential as you interact with the patient or attempt to differentiate between new and preexisting signs and symptoms. Patients may not be cooperative or capable of providing a meaningful history or history of present illness. Communication and other common tasks may require additional time and attention while assessing, treating, and transporting patients with a TBI. These patients may not understand or voluntarily allow a physical examination or interventions such as initiating IV access. Patient restraint may be needed when the safety of the patient or prehospital providers is at risk.

Conclusion

The medical conditions, functional impairment, medical technology, and adverse situations discussed in this chapter create additional challenges for you when you are providing otherwise routine medical care. You should endeavor to become comfortable with these devices, conditions, and situations in order to provide optimal patient care during EMS response or interfacility transport.

YOU are the Medic   SUMMARY

1. **Using the pediatric assessment triangle as a guide, what is your general impression of the child?**

   By using the pediatric assessment triangle, you should be able to determine that Amanda is in respiratory distress and requires immediate attention. Her appearance and circulation are normal but her work of breathing is increased as evidenced by the tripod position and accessory muscle use. Careful attention to her respiratory status is required to prevent deterioration to respiratory failure.

2. **What information would you like to get from the mother?**

   The mother should be able to provide you with information regarding Amanda's past medical history and current illness. You should be asking the mother about childhood illnesses, medications, allergies, immunizations, events leading up to Amanda's present episode of respiratory distress, and if this episode varies from those in the past.

3. **What is cystic fibrosis?**

   Cystic fibrosis is a chronic genetic disease of the endocrine system that impairs the body's ability to move sodium through cells, resulting in the production of extremely thick, sticky mucus. Although anyone can be born with cystic fibrosis, it occurs predominantly in Caucasians of Northern European descent. Despite several medical advances over the past 10 to 20 years, many people who have cystic fibrosis do not survive beyond adolescence.

4. **Which body systems are most affected by cystic fibrosis?**

   Cystic fibrosis attacks several body systems, hitting the respiratory and digestive systems the hardest. The increased production of thick secretions sets up a perfect environment in the lungs to host bacteria and leaves the patient vulnerable to recurrent respiratory infections. Digestion is impaired by the mucus blocking the production of digestive enzymes inside the pancreas and blockage of the pancreas. Patients who have cystic fibrosis are usually smaller in height and weight because of their inability to properly absorb nutrients. Physical assessment findings common to patients with cystic fibrosis include tachypnea, productive cough, shortness of breath, and clubbing of the fingers.

5. **Your patient weighs 43 kg. How much methylprednisolone (Solu-Medrol) should you administer?**

   The pediatric dose of methylprednisolone (Solu-Medrol) is 1 to 2 mg/kg IV. The appropriate dose would be 43 to 86 mg IV.

6. **What changes in patient condition should you watch for during transport?**

   Patients with cystic fibrosis are chronically hypoxic, so a prolonged period of increased work of breathing can lead to further hypoxia and respiratory depression. Keep a watchful eye for dysrhythmias secondary to hypoxia and electrolyte imbalances.

7. **Why is emotional support important when you are transporting a patient with cystic fibrosis?**

   As mentioned above, many people who are diagnosed with cystic fibrosis do not live beyond their teenage years. Children such as Amanda who have been hospitalized on a regular basis develop close friends who form a support network for each other. Over time Amanda will watch her friends lose their fight against the disease, and she will eventually have to face her own mortality. It is important to be supportive and listen with an open mind and heart. Remember, sometimes the best treatment you can render is compassionate care.

YOU *are the Medic*   SUMMARY, *continued*

EMS Patient Care Report (PCR)

Date: 08-22-11	Incident No.: 07453	Nature of Call: Respiratory distress		Location: 2340 SW 20th Avenue	
Dispatched: 0912	En Route: 0913	At Scene: 0919	Transport: 0932	At Hospital: 0944	In Service: 0955

Patient Information

Age: 15 Sex: F Weight (in kg [lb]): 43 kg (95 lb)	Allergies: None known Medications: Albuterol, digestive enzymes, vitamins Past Medical History: Cystic fibrosis Chief Complaint: Respiratory distress

Vital Signs

Time: 0922	BP: 116/72	Pulse: 110	Respirations: 24	Spo$_2$: 92%
Time: 0926	BP: 118/74	Pulse: 115	Respirations: 24	Spo$_2$: 93%
Time: 0932	BP: 116/70	Pulse: 118	Respirations: 26	Spo$_2$: 93%
Time: 0944	BP: 112/68	Pulse: 110	Respirations: 22	Spo$_2$: 95%

EMS Treatment
(circle all that apply)

Oxygen @ _8 and 12_ L/min via (circle one): NC **(NRM)** Bag-mask device	Assisted Ventilation	Airway Adjunct	CPR
Defibrillation	**Bleeding Control**	**Bandaging**	**Splinting**	**(Other:)** Nebulizer: 2.5 mg Albuterol/3mLNS Nebulizer: 2.5 mg Albuterol/0.5mg Atrovent Solu-Medrol 86 mg IV Cardiac monitor

Narrative

Dispatched to the health department for a pt with respiratory distress. Upon arrival found 15-year-old girl sitting upright in a tripod position on an exam table. Faint expiratory wheezes audible. Pt's mother states the pt has been having an increase in respiratory distress for the past 2 days. Pt normally takes albuterol, but she has not had any for the past week due to the inability to pay for the medication. Mother denies any medical allergies. Pt is able to speak in short sentences. Pt awake, alert, and oriented to person, place, time, and event. PEARRL. No JVD or tracheal deviation noted. Accessory muscle use is noted. BBS equal with faint expiratory wheezes and rhonchi. Abdomen soft and nontender to palpation. PMS x 4. Pt placed on nebulizer with 2.5 mg albuterol/3 mL normal saline. Cardiac monitor shows sinus tachycardia at a rate of 110. IV started with 18-gauge left antecubital. 500-mL bag of normal saline hung running KVO. Pt reassessment after nebulizer treatment reveals no changes. Pt states she is still having trouble breathing. Medical control contacted for orders. Orders received for Solu-Medrol at 2 mg/kg and repeat nebulizer with 2.5 mg albuterol/0.5 mg Atrovent. 86 mg Solu-Medrol administered IV. Pt reassessment after second nebulizer reveals BBS with increased air movement, expiratory wheezing, and rhonchi. Pt states it is slightly easier for her to breathe. No further changes en route. Arrived at County Medical at 0944. Pt care turned over to Dr. Taylor. Available at 0955. **End of report**

Prep Kit

■ Ready for Review

- Paramedics will encounter patients with a variety of economic, psychological, and medical challenges.

- Patients with special challenges and their caregivers have likely become experts on a particular condition or impairment.

- Poverty and patients' lack of health insurance have a direct impact on EMS services nationwide. These patients may not receive preventive health services or may not purchase needed medications, thereby increasing the incidence and severity of disease, and making an emergency more likely.

- Homeless and low-income patients are prone to numerous chronic medical conditions.

- Federal laws require emergency departments to stabilize patients experiencing an emergency or active labor, regardless of the patient's ability to pay. Paramedics should become familiar with health care resources for low-income and homeless people.

- Abuse, neglect, and assault occur at all levels of society. Because maltreatment and assault are common reasons for calls to EMS, you must recognize the signs and symptoms of these problems.

- Child abuse includes any improper or excessive action that injures or otherwise harms a child or infant, including physical abuse, sexual abuse, neglect, and emotional abuse.

- Some benign physical findings may mimic child abuse. Toddlers are more prone to bruising and minor injuries as they develop psychomotor skills. Older children are prone to injuries from sports and recreational activities such as bicycling. Infants of Asian or African origin may have Mongolian spots on the buttocks or back. Other practices that may visually look like child abuse include coining and cupping.

- Your own safety is the number one priority when you are encountering an abusive situation. These situations can evoke powerful emotions; it is imperative that you remain calm and neutral while providing optimal clinical care. As always, treating life threats takes priority over collecting history.

- Careful, objective documentation of potential abuse or neglect is essential. Reporting of child abuse or neglect is mandatory in most states. Failure to report may lead to a variety of civil, criminal, or regulatory penalties.

- Terminal illnesses are those that cannot be cured. As health care providers, you and your team will sometimes be called on to assist a patient who is facing imminent death. With such a patient, always ask if there is an advance directive or DNR order.

- Obese (bariatric) patients may present significant clinical and logistical hurdles for EMS providers. For example, airway procedures and intravenous access are physically more difficult to perform. These patients may be too heavy for traditional EMS crews to package and transport safely and effectively. Careful planning and proper body mechanics are essential to avoid injury to emergency responders or the patient, and special equipment may be needed.

- Patients with communicable diseases deserve treatment with the same respect and dignity as any other patient.

- Many patients require physical support and care of chronic illnesses. This care that may take place in the home setting. Paramedics may need to troubleshoot these devices when they malfunction or incorporate this technology into traditional prehospital patient care.

- Like caregivers of patients with special challenges, family members who care for chronically ill patients are often the paramedic's best source of information and care guidelines.

- Medical technology likely to be encountered by EMS providers includes tracheostomy tubes, long-term ventilators, apnea monitors, long-term vascular devices, medical infusion pumps, insulin pumps, nasogastric or orogastric feeding tubes, colostomy, urostomy, dialysis, surgical drains/devices, and cerebrospinal fluid shunts.

- Patients with tracheostomy tubes may experience emergencies related to occlusion or accidental removal. In some patients, loss of a tracheostomy tube may become an immediate threat to life. Follow the DOPE acronym for troubleshooting tracheostomy tube problems (Dislodged/displaced/disconnected, Obstruction, Pneumothorax, Equipment).

- Patients may be on long-term ventilators at home for a variety of reasons, including spinal cord injury, neuromuscular disease, and lung injury. If you are called to an emergency for a patient who is on a long-term ventilator, ensure that the long-term ventilator is working effectively. It is possible to severely injure a patient by improperly adjusting his or her ventilator. If the ventilator appears to be adequate for the particular patient, it is typically best to leave the ventilator connected to the patient and unchanged.

- Long-term vascular access devices require guidance from medical control before removal, replacement, or flushing.

- Use extreme caution when you are treating patients who receive dialysis; IV fluid administration requires careful monitoring.

- Do not manipulate orthotic devices, prosthetic limbs, or braces; such equipment should always accompany the patient to the hospital.

- When you are assisting with interfacility transport, you may encounter any of the following: hemodynamic monitoring, intra-aortic balloon pumps, or intracranial pressure monitors.

- Use extreme caution when you are transporting a patient with an arterial sheath because any associated bleeding may be life threatening.

- Special challenges may include cognitive, sensory, or communication impairment in your patients.

- Developmental delay covers a spectrum of cognitive impairment. Early intervention may allow these children to recover previously missed developmental milestones. With these patients, it may be useful to use the same approaches used for working with young children.

- Autism is a developmental delay in which the patient displays verbal or nonverbal symptoms related to communication and the ability to purposefully shift attention. Autistic patients require a mindful approach to communication and physical contact. Limit external stimuli. These patients may have minimal reaction to pain or an exaggerated painful reaction to minor physical contact.

- Learning cursory sign language can help facilitate communication with hearing-impaired patients.

- Patients who are visually impaired may benefit from more detailed explanation of any physical contact or intervention before it occurs.

- Speech impairment can occur for a number of reasons and may be unrelated to cognitive impairment.

- Paramedics may encounter patients with spastic paralysis, paraplegia, or quadriplegia. Paralysis of respiratory muscles can make the patient dependent on a ventilator. The paralyzed patient is also prone to pressure ulcers. Paralyzed patients will likely require total lifting assistance.

- When caring for cognitively impaired patients who have experienced trauma, remember that these patients will not necessarily be able to give you a reliable medical history. You may need to locate a valid surrogate decision-maker. Interventions may require additional time, explanation, and holding assistance.

- Chronic conditions that EMS providers may encounter include arthritis, cancer, cerebral palsy, cystic fibrosis, multiple sclerosis, muscular dystrophy, myasthenia gravis, poliomyelitis, spina bifida, systemic lupus erythematosus, and traumatic brain injury. Become familiar with these conditions so that you can recognize them and manage emergencies in patients with these conditions.

■ Vital Vocabulary

abuse Any form of maltreatment that results in harm or loss. Maltreatment may be physical, sexual, psychological, or financial/material.

acoustic neuroma A slow-growing, benign tumor of the vestibular cochlear nerve that can lead to loss of hearing in the affected ear.

acute angle-closure glaucoma (AACG) Increased intraocular pressure that leads to ocular pain and decreased visual acuity; sudden onset is a medical emergency.

Adult Protective Services (APS) Organizations that investigate cases involving abuse and neglect and provide case management services in some cases.

apraxia A neurologic impairment in which the brain is intermittently unable to carry out the command for speech or other tasks.

arthritis Inflammation of the joints.

asynchrony Disturbance or lack of synchronization.

auditory neuropathy A condition characterized by normal function of the structures of the ear without a corresponding stimulation of auditory centers of the brain; also called auditory dyssynchrony.

autism A developmental disorder characterized by impairments of social interaction; may include severe behavioral problems, repetitive motor activities, and impairment in verbal and nonverbal skills.

bariatrics The medical specialty dedicated to prevention and treatment of obesity.

cancer Excessive growth and division of abnormal cells within the body that can occur in many body systems, tissues, and organs, and that can progress rapidly and cause death in a relatively short period of time.

cataract An eye condition caused by a clouding of the lens, leading to decreased vision.

central auditory processing disorder (CAPD) A disorder in which patients have difficulty interpreting speech and differentiating it from other sounds that are present.

cerebral palsy (CP) A developmental condition in which damage is done to the brain. It presents during infancy as a delay in walking or crawling, and can take on a spastic form in which muscles are in a nearly constant state of contraction.

cerebrospinal fluid shunt (CSF shunt) A tube placed in the body to relieve pressure by drawing excess cerebrospinal fluid away from the brain or spinal cord.

coining A cultural ritual intended to treat an illness by rubbing hot coins, often on the torso, which produces rounded and oblong red, patchy, flat skin lesions.

colostomy The surgical establishment of an opening between the colon and the surface of the body for the purpose of providing drainage of the bowel.

colostomy bag A plastic pouch or bag attached over a colostomy to collect stool.

comfort care Medical treatment aimed at symptom relief and providing comfort for the patient.

communicable disease An illness that can be transmitted from one person to another.

conductive hearing loss A type of hearing impairment due to problems with the middle ear bones' ability to conduct sounds from the outer ear to the inner ear.

contagious disease See communicable disease.

conversion disorder A psychological condition in which stress or mental conflict is converted into physical complaints.

cupping The cultural practice of placing warm cups on the skin to pull out illness from the body. The red, flat, rounded skin lesions are often more intensely red at the borders.

curative care Medical treatment aimed at curing an illness.

cystic fibrosis (CF) A genetic disorder of the endocrine system that makes it difficult for chloride to move through cells; primarily targets the respiratory and digestive systems.

deafness A complete or partial hearing loss.

developmental delay A broad term that describes an infant or child's failure to reach a particular developmental milestone by the expected time.

developmental disability Insufficient development of a portion of the brain, resulting in some level of dysfunction or impairment.

dialysis A medical process by which a patient's blood is cleansed of excess toxins by passing through a special machine.

Down syndrome A genetic chromosomal defect that can occur during fetal development and that results in mental retardation and certain physical characteristics, such as a round head with a flat occiput and slanted, wide-set eyes.

dysarthria A speech disorder caused by neuromuscular disturbance that causes speech to become slow and slurred.

emotional abuse A form of abuse that may be verbal (such as ridicule, threats, blaming, or humiliation), or nonverbal (caregiver ignores the victim or isolates the victim from others); causes a substantial change in the victim's behavior, emotional response, cognitive function, or may manifest as a variety of mental illnesses.

false lumen A term used to describe an area that a device was not intended to be inserted into—for example, when a tracheostomy tube is inserted into an area other than the trachea.

fenestrated Having perforations, holes, or openings.

fistula A surgical connection between an artery and a vein.

flange The part of a tracheostomy tube that is used to stabilize the tube to the patient's neck.

glaucoma An eye condition caused by increased intraocular pressure.

hemodialysis A form of dialysis in which blood is removed from the patient through a catheter or fistula, and then returns to the body through another needle, removing various toxins, electrolytes, and fluid in the process.

hemodynamic monitoring Monitoring and measurement of blood movement, volume, and pressure.

heparinized solution A saline solution mixed with heparin, an anticoagulant used to prevent blood clots from forming.

hospice A program and philosophy that attempt to help the patient maximize the quality of remaining life by providing social and emotional support, treating discomfort with pharmacologic and nonpharmacologic approaches, and helping patients and families cope with the prospect of impending death.

hydrocephalus A medical condition in which there is an abnormal buildup of cerebrospinal fluid in the skull; this can be acquired (occurring after birth) or congenital (developing before birth).

hypovolemia Low blood volume.

ileus Disruption or loss of normal gastrointestinal motility.

inner cannula The inner tube that is inserted into the outer cannula of a tracheostomy tube.

intra-aortic balloon pump A balloon that is inserted into the aorta and connected to a pump via a catheter; this therapy helps to increase the blood flow to the coronary arteries during diastole (inflation) and decrease afterload of blood from the left ventricle (deflation).

language-based learning disability A type of disability in which difficulties with reading, spelling, or writing cause a person to fall behind expectations for a given age.

mandatory reporter A category of professional required by some states to report suspicions of child maltreatment. Prehospital professionals may be included.

Meniere disease An inner ear disorder that causes vertigo, tinnitus, and hearing impairment.

mental retardation A primarily cognitive disorder that appears during childhood and is accompanied by lack of adaptive behaviors, such as the ability to live and function independently or interact successfully with others; the person generally has an intelligence quotient below 70; also known as intellectual disability.

Mongolian spots Lesions that resemble bruises, typically on the buttocks or back, that are present at birth on many infants of Asian or African origin.

multiple sclerosis (MS) An autoimmune condition in which the body attacks the myelin that insulates the brain and spinal cord, causing scarring.

muscular dystrophy A broad term that describes a category of incurable genetic diseases that cause a slow, progressive degeneration of the muscle fibers.

myasthenia gravis A condition in which the body generates antibodies against its own acetylcholine receptors, causing muscle weakness, often in the face.

myasthenic crisis A complication of myasthenia gravis in which weakened respiratory muscles lead to respiratory failure.

myelomeningocele A developmental anomaly in which a portion of the spinal cord or meninges protrudes outside the spinal column or even outside the body, usually in the area of the lumbar spine (the lower third of the spine); also called spina bifida.

neglect Refusal or failure on the part of the caregiver to provide life necessities, such as food, water, clothing, shelter, personal hygiene, medicine, comfort, and personal safety.

obese A term used when a person has a body mass index of greater than 30 kg per meters squared (kg/m^2).

obturator A solid plug at the end of a tracheostomy tube.

ocular myasthenia gravis An autoimmune disorder in which the extraocular muscles become weakened and are fatigued.

optic nerve hypoplasia A congenital condition characterized by failure of the optic nerve to completely develop, and possibly resulting in optic nerve atrophy over time.

osteoarthritis The degeneration of a joint surface caused by wear and tear that leads to pain and stiffness.

outer cannula The larger (outer) tube of a tracheostomy tube.

palliative care Medical care aimed at relief of pain and suffering in terminally ill patients.

paraplegia Paralysis of the lower extremities.

peritoneal dialysis A type of dialysis in which a special solution is instilled through a catheter into the patient's abdomen, and that draws toxins, electrolytes, and other fluids from the body through the peritoneal membrane.

phonologic process disorders A category of disorders that impact a person's ability to produce sounds that combine into spoken words.

physical abuse A form of abuse that involves an intentional act such as throwing, striking, hitting, kicking, burning, or biting a vulnerable person.

phytophotodermatitis A chemical reaction in which the skin becomes hypersensitive to sunlight.

poliomyelitis A viral infection that attacks and destroys motor axons. The disease can cause weakness, paralysis, and respiratory arrest. Because an effective vaccine has been developed, the incidence of the disease is now rare.

postpolio syndrome The death of nerve fibers as a late consequence of polio; the syndrome is characterized by swallowing difficulties, weakness, fatigue, and breathing problems.

quadriplegia Paralysis of the upper and lower extremities.

retinopathy Any eye disorder in which the retina becomes diseased, leading to partial or total vision loss.

rheumatoid arthritis (RA) An inflammatory disorder that affects the entire body and leads to degeneration and deformation of joints.

semantic-pragmatic disorder A condition characterized by delayed language developmental milestones, resulting in the person repeatedly using irrelevant phrases out of context, confusing word pairs, and having trouble following conversations.

sensorineural hearing loss A permanent lack of hearing caused by a lesion or damage of the inner ear.

sexual abuse A form of abuse that involves a vulnerable person being forced into unwanted sexual acts, or into involvement in sexual activities such as pornography.

sexual exploitation A form of abuse that involves forcing a vulnerable person to perform or be involved in sexual acts, or be involved in sexual activities such as pornography, in return for something they need or want, such as money, food, or shelter.

spastic paralysis A chronic form of paralysis in which the affected muscles experience continued spasm.

spastic tetraplegia A form of cerebral palsy in which all fours limbs are affected.

spina bifida A developmental anomaly in which a portion of the spinal cord or meninges protrudes outside the spinal column or even outside the body, usually in the area of the lumbar spine (the lower third of the spine); also called myelomeningocele.

stenosis Narrowing of a passageway in the body.

stoma A surgical opening, such as into the abdominal wall or trachea.

surrogate decision-maker A person legally authorized to make health care decisions on behalf of a patient who is incapable of making or communicating the decision on his or her own.

systemic lupus erythematosus A multisystem autoimmune disease.

terminal illness A sickness that a patient cannot be cured of; death is imminent.

thrombosis The formation of a blood clot in the circulatory system.

tracheostomy (trach) tube A plastic tube placed within the tracheostomy site (stoma).

transducer A device that converts energy or pressure into electrical signals.

traumatic brain injury (TBI) A traumatic insult to the brain capable of producing physical, intellectual, emotional, social, and vocational changes.

urostomy A surgically constructed opening for the urinary system.

Assessment in Action

While you are providing coverage in an unfamiliar zone, you and your partner are dispatched to a private residence for a child with difficulty breathing. On arrival you are met at the door by an anxious home health nurse who takes you to the living room where you observe a 5-year-old boy lying on a hospital bed receiving mechanical ventilation through a tracheostomy. He appears pale and anxious. You note that the child "bucks" the ventilator each time a breath is delivered, triggering an alarm. The home health nurse is able to provide limited information about the child because this is her first time caring for him. All she can tell you is the child has a history of muscular dystrophy and has required mechanical ventilation for the past 2 years.

1. What should be your initial action?
   A. Increase the rate on the ventilator until the child's work of breathing decreases.
   B. Administer a benzodiazepine to relax the child.
   C. Remove the child from the ventilator and attempt to ventilate with a bag-mask device.
   D. Start a nebulizer with albuterol and ipratropium.

2. Where is a tracheostomy placed?
   A. One inch below the vocal cords
   B. Below the cricoid ring
   C. At the level of the carina
   D. Above the fifth tracheal ring

3. How does a pediatric tracheostomy tube differ from an adult tracheostomy tube?
   A. Pediatric tubes are more flexible to accommodate for anatomic differences.
   B. A special adapter is needed for attaching a bag-mask device.
   C. All pediatric tubes have a cuff at the distal end that must be inflated after insertion.
   D. The pediatric tracheostomy tubes are one piece.

4. What should you do if you are unable to pass a suction catheter through the tracheostomy tube?
   A. Attempt to ventilate the patient with a bag-mask device.
   B. Perform an emergency cricothyrotomy.
   C. Use a larger catheter to force past the obstruction.
   D. Insert an endotracheal tube alongside the tracheostomy tube.

5. Which of the following is a complication associated with positive-pressure ventilation?
   A. Hypertension
   B. Decreased myocardial oxygen demand
   C. Hypotension
   D. Bronchospasm

6. Which of the following can cause the high-pressure alarm on the ventilator to trigger?
   A. Coughing as the ventilator delivers a breath
   B. Loose connections in the ventilator circuit
   C. Detachment of the circuit from the endotracheal tube
   D. Decreased respiratory rate

Additional Question

7. How can you overcome some of the difficulties you may experience while caring for a child who requires advanced technology in the home?

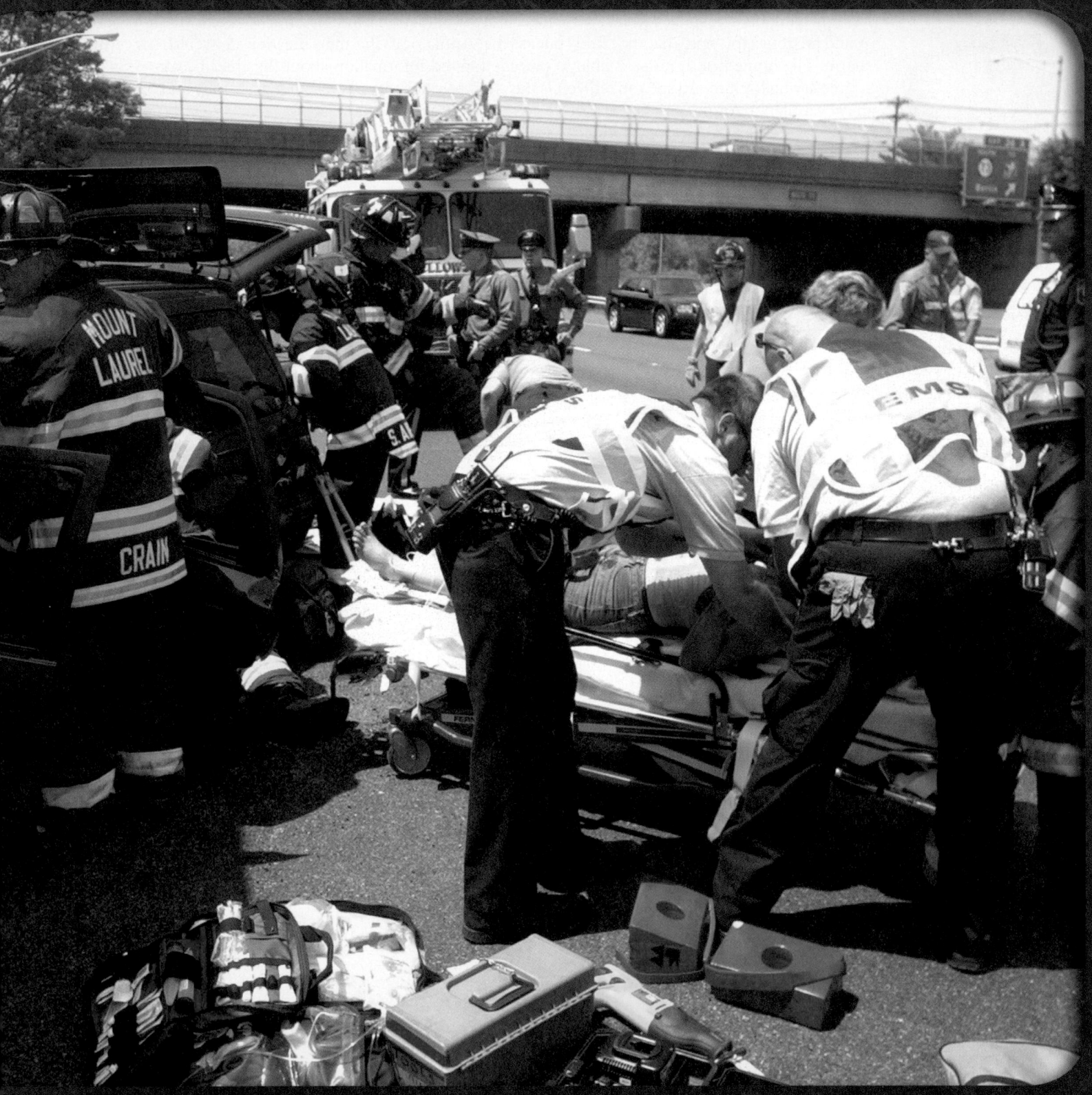

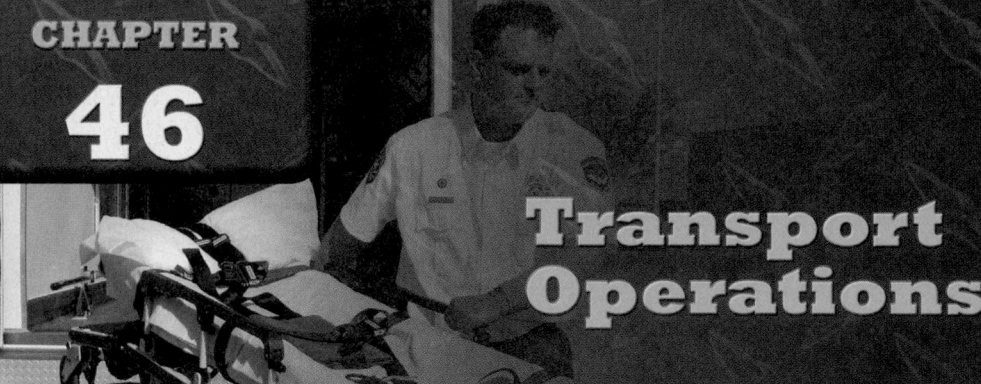

Transport Operations

National EMS Education Standard Competencies

EMS Operations

Knowledge of operational roles and responsibilities to ensure patient, public, and personnel safety.

Principles of Safely Operating a Ground Ambulance

- Risks and responsibilities of emergency response (pp 2173-2176)
- Risks and responsibilities of transport (pp 2178-2179)

Air Medical

- Safe air medical operations (pp 2188-2192)
- Criteria for utilizing air medical response (pp 2188-2189)
- Medical risks/needs/advantages (pp 2186-2192)

Medicine

Integrates assessment findings with principles of epidemiology and pathophysiology to formulate a field impression and implement a comprehensive treatment/disposition plan for a patient with a medical complaint.

Infectious Diseases

Awareness of
- A patient who may have an infectious disease (p 2179)
- How to decontaminate equipment after treating a patient (p 2179)

Assessment and management of
- A patient who may have an infectious disease (see chapter, *Infectious Diseases*)
- How to decontaminate the ambulance and equipment after treating a patient (p 2179)
- A patient who may be infected with a bloodborne pathogen (see chapter, *Infectious Diseases*)
  - Human immunodeficiency virus (HIV) (see chapter, *Infectious Diseases*)
  - Hepatitis B (see chapter, *Infectious Diseases*)
- Antibiotic-resistant infections (see chapter, *Infectious Diseases*)
- Current infectious diseases prevalent in the community (see chapter, *Infectious Diseases*)

Knowledge Objectives

1. Summarize the medical equipment, safety equipment, and operations equipment carried on an ambulance. (pp 2173-2174)
2. Discuss the importance of performing regular vehicle inspections, and list the specific parts of an ambulance that should be inspected daily. (pp 2173-2176)
3. Provide examples of some high-risk situations and hazards that may affect the safety of the ambulance and its passengers during both pretransport and transport. (pp 2178-2179)
4. Discuss specific considerations that are required for ensuring scene safety, including personal safety, patient safety, and traffic control. (p 2178)
5. Define the terms cleaning, disinfection, high-level disinfection, and sterilization, and explain how they differ. (p 2179)
6. Identify the dangers to consider when operating an ambulance in the emergency mode. (pp 2179-2186)
7. Discuss the guidelines for driving an ambulance safely and defensively, and identify key steps EMS personnel can take to improve safety while en route to the scene, the hospital, and the station. (pp 2180-2184)
8. Describe the elements that dictate the use of lights and siren to the scene and to the hospital and the factors required to perform a risk-benefit analysis regarding their use. (pp 2181; 2185)
9. Give examples of the specific, limited privileges that are provided to emergency vehicle drivers by most state laws and regulations. (pp 2185-2186)
10. Explain why using police escorts and crossing intersections pose additional risks to EMS personnel during transport, and discuss special considerations related to each. (pp 2185-2186)
11. Describe the capabilities, protocols, and methods for accessing air medical transport. (pp 2186-2192)
12. List the safety concerns when operating a landing zone for helicopter transport. (pp 2189-2192)
13. Describe key scene safety considerations when preparing for a helicopter medevac, including establishing a landing zone, securing loose objects, mitigating onsite hazards, and approaching the aircraft. (pp 2189-2192)

Skills Objectives

1. Demonstrate how to perform a daily inspection of an ambulance. (pp 2173-2176)
2. Demonstrate how to clean and disinfect the ambulance and equipment during the postrun phase. (p 2179)

Introduction

Today's ambulances are equipped with state-of-the-art technology, including defibrillators and monitors that can transmit information directly to the emergency department, blood and oxygen testing equipment, automatic ventilators, automated cardiopulmonary resuscitation (CPR) devices, global positioning systems (GPS), and computer-aided dispatch consoles. Even when all safety guidelines are being followed, the emphasis on rapid response places you and your crew members in great danger while driving to calls.

Driving an emergency vehicle is a tremendous responsibility. Not only do you have to be aware of the safety of your crew and passengers, but you are also responsible for the safe passage of other vehicles you encounter on the road. Activating the lights and sirens does not ensure that you will be heard or understood by other drivers. More importantly, the use of lights and sirens is usually only a request for the right of way.

This chapter discusses ambulance design and how to equip and maintain an ambulance. It also focuses on the techniques and judgment that you will need to learn to drive an ambulance or ambulance service vehicle, which includes parking considerations, emergency vehicle control and operation, the effects of weather on driving, and common hazards that are encountered in driving an ambulance. Finally, it describes how to work safely with air ambulances.

Emergency Vehicle Design

Current standards for ambulances are determined by the US General Services Administration. Design and manufacturing specifications are outlined in the **DOT KKK 1822** federal guidelines. These guidelines are reviewed and updated every 5 years based on recommendations from manufacturers and operators of the vehicles.

The original guidelines required that all ambulances be painted Omaha orange and white, allowing them to be easily recognized by other drivers. More recently, standards have been relaxed to allow for a variety of personalized paint schemes. The KKK Standards also established three major ambulance designs Figure 1 and Table 1 .

Improvements made to emergency vehicles over the years have not only made them safer for EMS personnel, but also more comfortable. One of the most significant developments in ambulance design has been the enlargement of the patient compartment. Improvements such as safety nets on the squad bench have made it easier to perform patient care activities with less risk of injury. The inclusion of padded cabinet corners has prevented paramedics from becoming injured while the vehicle is in motion. However, there is still room for improvement. In many ambulances, not everyone in the ambulance is restrained in a five-point harness and wearing a helmet.

Ambulance Equipment

In the patient compartment of an ambulance, every inch of space is dedicated to storing or securing the equipment it takes to do the job well. Much like a jigsaw puzzle, everything must fit tightly together to prevent injury, yet be easily accessible.

Many organizations have influenced the development of the supplies and equipment carried on today's units. The Occupational Safety and Health Administration (OSHA) makes recommendations regarding infection control practices to include all areas of personnel protective equipment, sharps containers, and disinfecting equipment. The American College of Surgeons (ACS) developed the first standardized list of equipment to be carried on an ambulance in 1970. The list is now published in a cooperative effort between the ACS, the American College of Emergency Physicians, and the National Association of EMS Physicians, and is continually updated as technologic advances are made in the field. In addition, the National Fire Protection Association (NFPA) has recently stepped into the arena of developing ambulance safety standards.

Checking the Ambulance

Getting ready to respond to a call is just as important as providing patient care. The crew is also responsible for ensuring that the unit is capable of responding safely and efficiently to calls.

At the beginning of each shift, crew members must check the ambulance to ensure the proper equipment is available and

YOU *are the Medic* **PART 1**

You and your partner are getting ready to order lunch at your favorite lunch spot when you are dispatched for a multi-vehicle crash on the interstate. It has been raining all day, so you are not surprised an accident has occurred. The interstate is nearby so you exit the parking lot and turn around to get to the closest on-ramp.

1. Explain the concept of "due regard."
2. What considerations should you make concerning your route to the interstate?

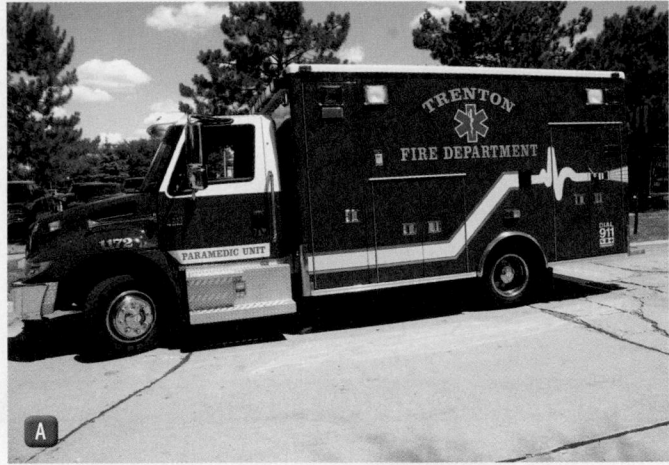

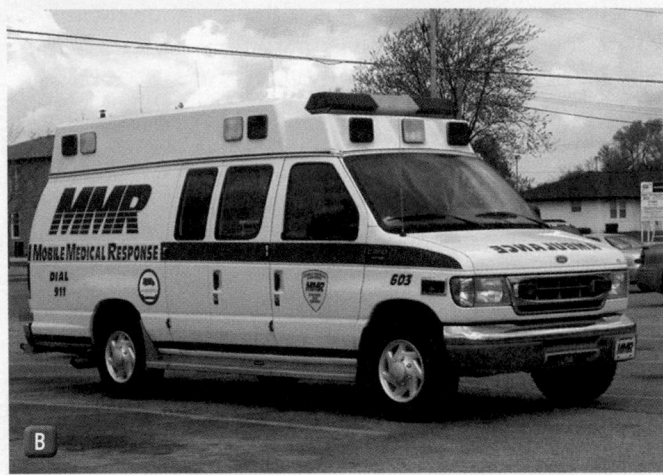

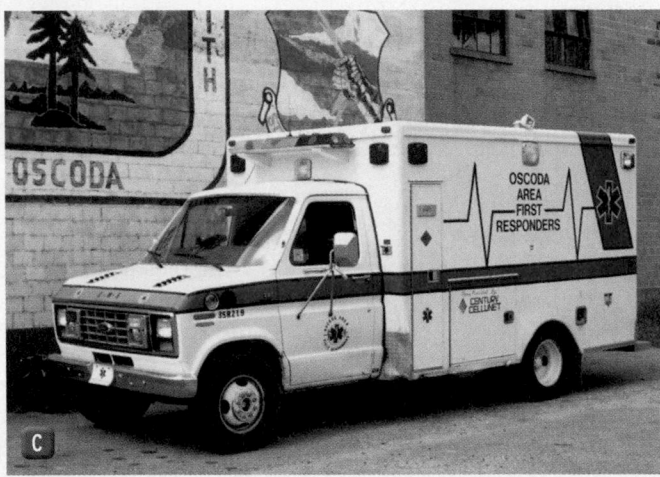

Figure 1 Basic ambulance designs. **A.** Type I (a heavy-duty type I is shown; a standard type I is shown in Figure 6). **B.** Type II. **C.** Type III.

Table 1	Basic Ambulance Designs
Type I ambulance	Conventional, truck-cab chassis with a modular ambulance body that can be transferred to a newer chassis as needed
Type II ambulance	Standard van, forward-control integral cab-body ambulance
Type III ambulance	Specialty van, forward-control integral cab-body ambulance
Heavy-duty ambulance	Extra heavy-duty vehicle

Documentation and Communication

Because the mechanical aspects of emergency work such as driving and moving patients have an impact on your safety and the safety of others, your service should have specific procedures for daily inspections. Following these procedures protects you physically, and documenting your compliance is an important legal protection. Procedures should call for dating and either signing or initialing the check sheets. Store these sheets where they can be found later if needed.

The ambulance inspection should include the following:

- Fuel levels
- Oil levels
- Transmission fluid levels
- Engine cooling system and fluid levels
- Batteries
- Brake fluid
- Engine belts
- Wheels and tires, including the spare, if there is one. Check inflation pressure and look for signs of unusual or uneven wear.
- All interior and exterior lights
- Windshield wipers and fluid
- Horn
- Siren
- Air conditioners and heaters
- Ventilating system
- Doors. Make sure they open, close, latch, and lock properly.
- Communication systems, vehicle and portable
- All windows and mirrors. Check for cleanliness and position.

All compartments in the ambulance should be checked regularly, both inside and out. Most ambulances carry stabilization and splinting equipment in the outside compartments for easy access when speed may be an important factor in patient care **Figure 2**. Medications and temperature-sensitive equipment are generally stored in the patient compartment area. It is important to maintain temperature control for certain medications; some ambulances have a medication refrigerator on board **Figure 3**.

in good working order. Each time supplies and equipment are used, they should be properly cleaned or replaced and returned to service for the next call. Medication expiration dates must be checked regularly to confirm that they have not expired. In addition, diagnostic equipment, such as defibrillators and pulse oximeters, must be tested or calibrated regularly.

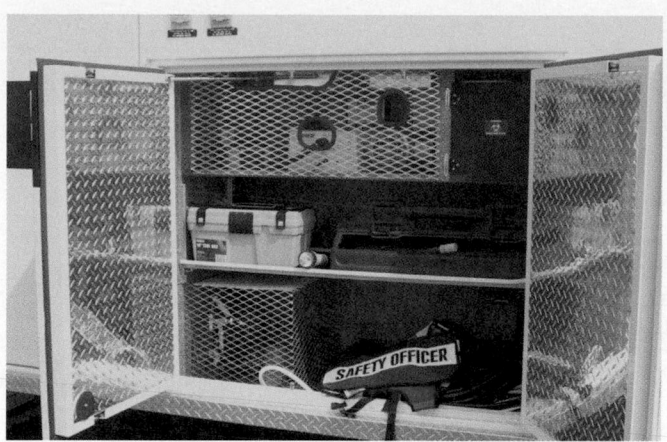

Figure 2 The ambulance should have a weatherproof compartment that can be reached from outside the patient compartment. It should hold equipment for safeguarding patients and crew, controlling traffic, and illuminating work areas.

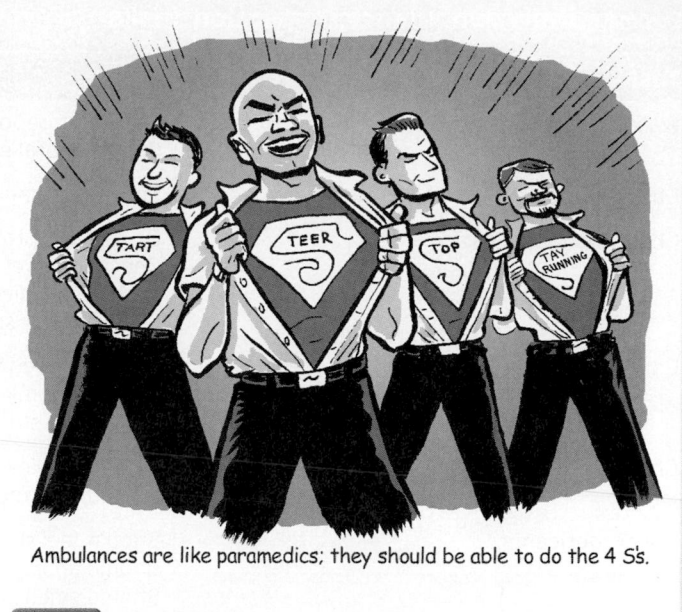

Ambulances are like paramedics; they should be able to do the 4 S's.

Figure 4

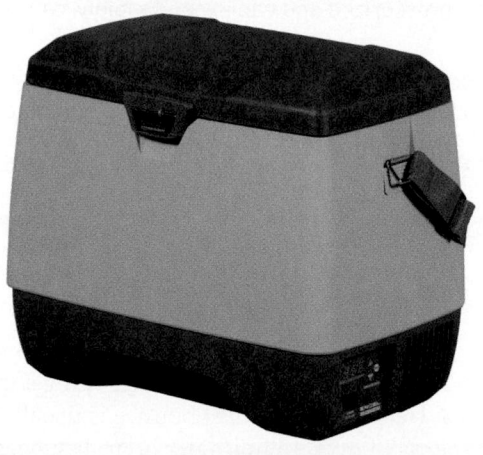

Figure 3 Some ambulances have a medication refrigerator on board. IV fluids may need to be chilled for post-cardiac arrest hypothermia therapy.

An ambulance needs to be able to do four things: start, steer, stop, and stay running **Figure 4**. Any threat to one of the "four S's" should prompt the operator to put the vehicle out of service immediately. A standard daily checklist is essential to ensure the ambulance is in good operating order. **Table 2** summarizes tasks that should be performed during the daily check of the ambulance.

It is also important for you to be cognizant of warning signs of impending problems. **Belt noise** is a chirping or squealing sound, synchronous with engine speed (not road speed). It is usually related to a load on one of the appliances operated by a drive belt—the power steering pump, the water pump, the vacuum pump (in a diesel), or the alternator. Belt noise is always significant and will eventually keep an ambulance from operating. It does not necessarily warrant taking a unit out of service immediately.

Brake fade is a sensation that an ambulance has lost its power brakes. Its most common causes are overheating of brake surfaces, loss of vacuum, loss of brake fluid, wet or greasy brake drums, or a failed master cylinder. Even a single instance of brake fade warrants taking your vehicle out of service immediately.

Generally, you should not hear, smell, or feel a vehicle's brakes, with occasional exceptions. Cold brakes may squeak intermittently in wet weather. Some kinds of brake pads are equipped with "telltale tabs"—small aluminum projections that are designed to rub on the disk surfaces and squeak, warning an operator when the pads are nearing the end of their useful life. Otherwise, a consistent squeaking or grinding sound warrants immediate attention by a mechanic.

Brake pull is a sensation that, when you depress the brake pedal, someone is trying to jerk the steering wheel to the left or right. It can indicate brake fluid or grease on a brake pad, or it can result from a serious mechanical malfunction. Remove the vehicle from service immediately.

Drift is a finding that when you let go of the steering wheel, the vehicle consistently wanders left or right. Any vehicle may normally drift slightly to the right, because most roads are built with a crown in the center (so water drains toward the gutters). A vehicle should not consistently drift to the left, however.

Steering pull is a persistent tug on the steering wheel that you can feel as the ambulance "drifts" to one side or the other. Its most common cause is uneven tire pressures (possibly a flat tire). Steering pull can also be caused by one or more misaligned wheels or another mechanical problem. It can cause loss of control in the event of a sudden stop. A vehicle's steering geometry is complex. To allow for its adjustment, the entire front suspension system is held together by clamps. Misalignment can occur when a vehicle hits a curb and dislodges one or more of these clamps. The result may be control problems as well as tire damage in short order.

Table 2 Daily Ambulance Inspection Tasks

Tasks	Tips
Walk around the ambulance.	Identify unreported body damage, major leaks, inoperative lighting, or damaged tires. Checking brake and back-up lights requires assistance of a second person.
Check fuel levels.	Some ambulances carry two fuel tanks; check both.
Check the motor oil.	Do this prior to starting the engine. Check for level and quality. Should be yellow or amber in a gasoline engine; gray or black in a diesel engine. Should never smell like fuel.
Check transmission fluid.	Often checked with motor running and the gear selector in "park." Should be pink or yellow. Should not smell like charcoal.
Check steering fluid.	Should be pink or yellow. Should not smell like charcoal.
Check lubricants.	Should feel slippery between the fingers. Should appear clean. Should smell like fresh oil.
Check brake fluid.	Should be clear or yellow when fresh; could be amber after a few years of service. Do not uncap brake fluid reservoir; fluid absorbs moisture from the atmosphere.
Check coolant.	May be either red or bright yellow-green. Do not uncap coolant reservoir; it is pressurized and can expand rapidly, causing burns.
Check the battery.	Should be clean. Top surfaces of battery should be dry. System voltage should be 12 to 12.5 volts at rest, 13.5 to 14.5 volts when engine is running. Should not be higher than 15. Should not smell like sewer gas; if so, take out of service immediately, leave hood closed, and do not start the engine.

A pulsating brake pedal—an up-and-down motion of the brake pedal during deceleration—is an abnormal condition, especially at low speeds. A pulsating brake pedal usually indicates warped brake rotors or drums, but can also suggest a bent wheel. This motion can be severe when the brakes are hot. This condition always warrants service.

Normally, little effort is required to steer an ambulance. Excessive effort to steer is therefore a serious finding and can be caused by inadequate steering fluid or a failed power steering pump or drive belt.

Steering play is a sensation of looseness or sloppiness in a vehicle's steering. This finding is important when accompanied by clunking or banging noises during steering, and it should never be noticeable in a new vehicle. This problem is typically caused by wear, but it can also result from underinflated tires. This situation warrants immediate inspection of the ambulance.

Tire squeal is a singing sound that occurs when you turn the vehicle, especially at parking speeds. Squealing is normal on smooth concrete, but not on asphalt. The most common cause is underinflated tires, but it can also result from misaligned wheels, especially in the presence of other signs. This situation warrants a mechanic's attention as soon as possible.

Wheel bounce is a vibration, synchronous with road speed, that you can feel in the steering wheel (suggesting a front wheel) or driver's seat (rear wheel). Wheel bounce is usually detectable at freeway speeds of over 45 miles per hour. It suggests a defective shock absorber, a bubble in a tire, or an improperly balanced wheel.

Wheel wobble is a common finding at low speeds when a vehicle has a bent wheel. You normally detect wobble in the steering wheel if it involves a front wheel, or in the driver's seat if it is in the rear wheel. Potholes are the most common cause.

■ Ambulance Staffing and Development

Ambulance staffing has been a major source of controversy over the past decade. Escalating costs for medical care, fuel, and the financial burden of operating an ambulance service have prompted the development of alternative strategies for managing EMS systems. For example, the development of "high-performance EMS systems" represents an effort to maximize personnel productivity and minimize response times. The key factors that are analyzed in an effective, cost-efficient service are summarized as follows.

- **Response times.** High-performance systems typically use a fractile response time standard in which a significant fraction (usually 90%) of all responses must be achieved in an established time—for example, 8 minutes or less in an urban area. These standards are based on the recommendations of the Commission on the Accreditation of Ambulances (CAAS).
- **Productivity.** The EMS provider measures how many patient transports per hour each ambulance accomplishes (known as "unit-hour utilization").
- **Unit costs.** Determined by the cost to respond to each call as well as the actual number of hours the units were actively operating, these costs include the paramedics' salaries plus the operational cost of vehicles and equipment (gas, routine maintenance, and repairs).
- **Taxpayer subsidies.** The local government may make a financial commitment to help lower user fees. Some services also offer annual subscription fees in return for free services during the year.

Ambulance and EMS Systems

In the United States, most first-response emergency medical service is delivered by fire department personnel who are cross-trained in EMS. Some emergency medical responders are trained in BLS; others have ALS training. These responders may be paid or volunteer, and they typically respond from fire stations located throughout the community. Many fire services also operate the ambulance service.

In other communities, the ambulance service is provided by a private, for-profit enterprise. In some areas, a public agency (not part of the fire department) delivers ambulance service; this system is known as the third service delivery model. Another type of model involves a public–private partnership.

Staffing of ambulances may be variable between and within EMS systems. Some systems have two or even three paramedics on each ambulance. Others staff ambulances with basic EMTs.

Some systems employ a tiered response system that attempts to assign ALS personnel only where they are needed.

System Status Management

System status management (SSM) is a concept that was developed by Jack Stout in 1983. The goals of SSM are to maximize efficiency and reduce response time. In SSM, historic data is compiled and used to determine ambulance service demands and it then takes into consideration fluctuations in demand to better organize service. For example, an increased demand for service may be noted during certain hours of the day or in certain geographic locations. These demands are termed **peak loads**. In an urban area, the demand for ambulance service may be higher during the daytime but lighter during the night. SSM attempts to arrange **strategic deployment** of ambulance resources in order to minimize response times. The strategic deployment of an ambulance to a location, known as **posting**, can take advantage of developments in satellite vehicle location and GPS technologies.

Another component of SSM is the capability to help organize peak demand staffing. Shift schedules are designed to provide a sufficient number of ambulances during peak load hours. For example, more ambulances might be staffed between noon and 6 PM than between midnight and 6 AM. One potentially negative aspect of SSM is the toll that it can take on personnel, who have less time to get out of the vehicle and relax in the ambulance station between calls.

Ambulance Stationing

The goals for establishing ambulance stations are to maximize efficiency and to minimize response times. In most urban and suburban areas, the distance factor may not be as important as the call volume. In a rural setting, both availability of first responders and distance may be equally important. Also,

YOU *are the Medic* **PART 2**

You arrive on scene and are directed to a vehicle where a woman is sitting in the driver's seat. There is minimal damage to the vehicle, which appears to have rear ended the vehicle in front of it. The patient states that she is fine but her knee hurts where it hit the bottom of the dashboard.

Recording Time: 1 Minute	
Appearance	Awake
Level of consciousness	Alert (oriented to person, place, and day)
Airway	Open
Breathing	Adequate
Circulation	Adequate

3. What equipment and supplies are typically taken from the ambulance to the patient's side?

4. What factors should be considered when you are operating an ambulance in inclement weather?

the district may have special facilities that create increased ambulance demand—long-term care facilities, for example. Other considerations in the design of ambulance stations include the need for maintenance of vehicles and equipment, storage, classrooms for training and meetings, and sleeping quarters for personnel who spend the night.

Mitigating Hazards Throughout the Call

En Route to the Scene

In many ways, the en route or response phase of the call is potentially very dangerous for you. Crashes between automobiles and emergency vehicles cause many serious injuries to EMS personnel. Techniques to make vehicle operation safer will be discussed later in this chapter. As you and your partner prepare to respond to the scene, make sure you fasten your seat belts and shoulder harnesses before you move the ambulance. At this point, you should inform dispatch that your unit is responding and confirm the nature and location of the call. This is also an excellent time to ask for any other available information about the location.

While en route, you and your team should prepare to assess and care for the patient. Review dispatch information about the nature of the call and the location of the patient. Assign specific initial duties and scene management tasks to each team member, and decide what type of equipment to take initially. Depending on your operation procedures, you may also decide which stretcher to bring to the patient.

Arrival at the Scene

On arrival at the incident, you will perform a scene size-up. After you complete your size-up, report to dispatch the nature of the incident if this is part of your local protocol. Also report any unexpected situations, such as the need for backup units, a heavy rescue unit, or a HazMat team. Do not enter the scene if there are any hazards to you. If there are dangerous hazards at the scene, the patient should be moved before you begin care. The patient may have to be moved by others if you are not appropriately equipped or trained. Immediately size up the scene by using the following guidelines:

- Look for safety hazards.
- Evaluate the need for additional units or other assistance.
- Determine the mechanism of injury in trauma patients or the nature of the illness in medical patients.
- Evaluate the need to stabilize the spine.
- Make sure that you follow standard precautions. The type of care that you expect to give will dictate what personal protective equipment you should wear.

If you are the first EMS provider at the scene of a multiple-casualty incident, quickly estimate the number of patients. Inform dispatch if additional units are needed at the scene. Multiple-casualty incidents involve complex organization of personnel under the incident command system (see the chapter, *Incident Management and Multiple-Casualty Incidents*).

In this system, individual EMS providers may be assigned roles to do such things as begin the triage process, assist in treating patients, and load patients for transportation to a hospital.

Traffic Control

After ensuring your own safety, your first responsibility at a crash scene is to care for the patients. Only when all the patients have been treated and the emergency situation is under control should you be concerned with restoring the flow of traffic. If the police do not arrive quickly at the scene, you might then need to take action.

The purpose of traffic control is to ensure an orderly traffic flow and to prevent another crash. Under ordinary circumstances, traffic control is difficult. A crash or disaster scene presents serious additional problems. Passing motorists often slow down and stare, paying little attention to the roadway in front of them. Some curiosity seekers may park down the road and return on foot, creating still other hazards. As soon as possible, place appropriate warning devices, such as reflectors, on both sides of the crash. Remember, the main objectives in directing traffic are to warn other drivers, to prevent additional crashes, and to keep vehicles moving in an orderly fashion so that care of injured patients is not interrupted.

Securing Equipment

It is important to make sure that all equipment (in the cab, rear, and compartments) is secured before placing a vehicle in motion. Driving rapidly through heavy traffic will cause things to shift in the rear compartment. Placing an item such as an open drug or equipment box on the squad bench for easy access may be convenient, but if a quick change in direction occurs, the contents will end up scattered all over the floor, or worse yet, broken. A piece of diagnostic equipment or a portable oxygen cylinder can become a lethal projectile if not secured correctly.

Safe Patient Transfer

Many patients have said that one of the most frightening parts of being suddenly ill or injured is the ambulance ride to the hospital. Already anxious, a patient may experience increased anxiety during a fast, bumpy ride with a siren blaring. Sometimes, such a ride is truly lifesaving. However, in most cases, excessive speed is unnecessary and dangerous. What is necessary is that the patient is safely transported to an appropriate medical care facility in the shortest practical time. This takes common sense and defensive driving techniques. Speed is no substitute for these qualities. In almost every case, you will provide lifesaving care right where you find the patient, before moving the patient to the ambulance. You may then begin less critical measures, such as bandaging and splinting. Next, you must package the patient for transport, securing him or her to a device such as a backboard, a scoop stretcher, or the wheeled ambulance stretcher. Then move to the ambulance, and properly lift the patient into the patient compartment.

No matter how careful the driver may be, a patient who is riding to the hospital while lying on his or her back on a stretcher can experience discomfort and possibly even danger. You need to secure the patient with at least three straps across the body. Use deceleration or stopping straps over the shoulders to prevent the patient from continuing to move forward in the event the ambulance suddenly slows or stops. Always follow your service's standard operating procedures on strapping the patient, and also the recommendations of the stretcher manufacturer.

Postrun Activities: Restocking, Cleaning, and Disinfection

As soon as you are back at the station, you should do the following:

- Clean and disinfect the ambulance and any equipment that was used, if you did not do so before leaving the hospital **Figure 5**.
- Restock any supplies you did not get at the hospital.

In order to maintain the ambulance so that it is safe and available on a moment's notice, you should perform routine inspections. Use a written checklist to document needed repairs or replacement of equipment and supplies.

It is also important to **decontaminate** the ambulance after the call. Terms related to decontamination include "cleaning," "disinfection," "high-level disinfection," and "sterilization." The definitions are as follows:

- **Cleaning**. The process of removing dirt, dust, blood, or other visible contaminants from a surface.
- **Disinfection**. The killing of pathogenic agents by directly applying a chemical made for that purpose to a surface.
- **High-level disinfection**. The killing of pathogenic agents by the use of potent means of disinfection.
- **Sterilization**. A process, such as the use of heat, that removes all microbial contamination.

You must ensure that the following steps are taken after each trip:

1. Strip used linens from the stretcher immediately after use, and place them in a plastic bag or in the designated receptacle in the emergency department.

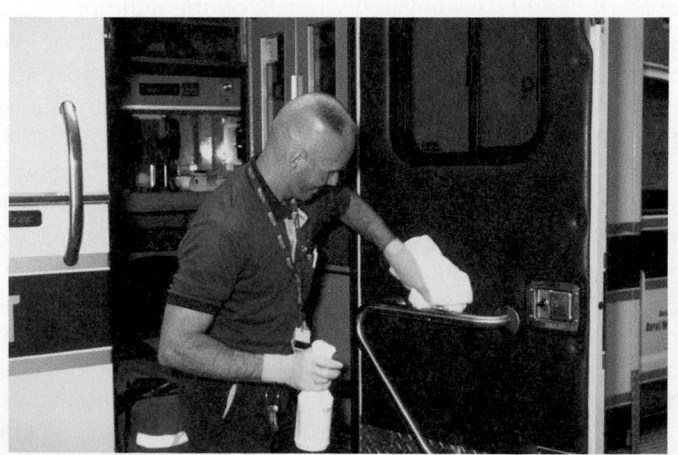

Figure 5 Be sure to clean and disinfect the ambulance and equipment at the station if you did not do so at the hospital.

2. In an appropriate receptacle, discard all disposable equipment used for care of the patient that meets your state's definition of medical waste. Most items will be considered general trash.
3. Wash all contaminated areas with soap and water. Scrub blood, vomitus, and other substances from the floors, walls, and ceilings with soap and water. For disinfection to be effective, cleaning must be done first. (You can use a 10% solution of bleach in water to clean the ambulance after any contamination.)
4. Disinfect all nondisposable equipment used in the care of the patient. For example, disassemble the bag-mask device and place the components in a liquid sterilization solution as recommended by the manufacturer.
5. Clean the stretcher with an EPA-registered germicidal/virucidal solution or bleach and water at 1:100 dilution.
6. If any spillage or other contamination occurred in the ambulance, clean it up with the same germicidal/virucidal or bleach/water solution.
7. Clean the outside of the ambulance as needed.
8. Replace or repair broken or damaged equipment without delay.
9. Replace any other equipment or supplies that were used.
10. Refuel the vehicle if the fuel tank is below required reserves. The oil level should be checked each time the vehicle is refueled.
11. Create a schedule for routine full cleaning for the vehicle.
12. Have a written policy/procedure for cleaning each piece of equipment. Refer to the manufacturer's recommendations as a guide.

Defensive Ambulance Driving Techniques

Every year there are more than 6,000 ambulances involved in crashes, some of them fatal. Between 1991 and 2001, the Centers for Disease Control and Prevention found that there were 300 fatal ambulance crashes with 275 pedestrians and motorists of other vehicles killed **Figure 6**, of the passengers onboard the ambulances, there were 82 fatalities, of which 27 were EMS personnel. These statistics do not include the thousands of injured pedestrians, motorists, ambulance passengers, and EMS personnel. Another troubling fact is that nearly half of ambulance operators involved in a crash had an earlier crash or moving violation in the 3 years prior to the incident.

Learning how to properly operate your vehicle is just as important as learning how to care for patients when you arrive on the scene. An ambulance that is involved in a crash delays patient care, at a minimum, and may take the lives of the EMS providers, or other motorists, or pedestrians at worst. The following section is provided to introduce you to safe driving techniques; however, you cannot become a proficient and safe ambulance driver without specialized training and practice. You are strongly encouraged to participate in an emergency driving program designed for the EMS-Vehicle Operator, such as those offered through your EMS organization, before attempting to

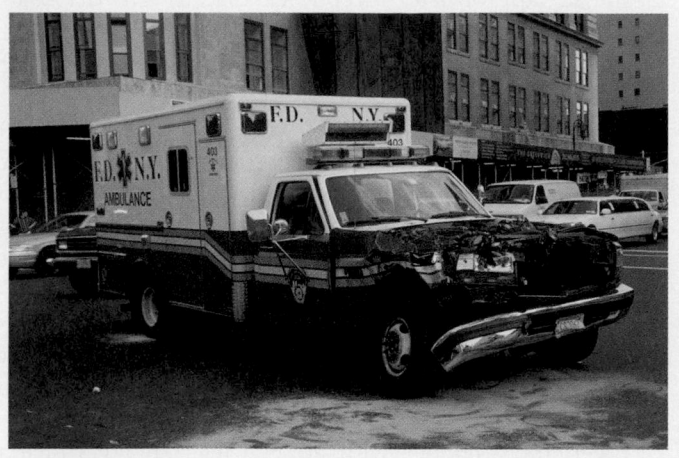

Figure 6 A wrecked ambulance (type 1 style).

operate an emergency vehicle. It is the responsibility of every ambulance service to ensure that personnel are not only safe drivers *before* they begin employment, but are given emergency vehicle operation courses *after* they are hired, and training in the service's policies, procedures, and state laws appropriate to operating an emergency vehicle.

Driver Characteristics

Not everyone who drives an automobile is qualified to drive an emergency vehicle. In some states, you must successfully complete an approved emergency vehicle operations course before you are allowed to drive the ambulance on emergency calls. In any state, diligence and caution are important characteristics, as are a positive attitude about your ability and tolerance of other drivers.

One basic requirement is physical fitness. Many crashes occur as a result of physical impairment of the driver. You should not be driving if you are taking medications that may cause drowsiness or slow your reaction times. These include cold remedies, analgesics, or tranquilizers. And, of course, you should never drive or provide medical care after drinking alcohol. Fatigue can also play a prominent role in accidents, so it is imperative to get as much rest as possible during down times. Driving alone may also be a factor on long transports.

Another requirement is emotional fitness. Emotions should not be taken lightly. A person's personality can change once he or she is behind a steering wheel. Emotional maturity and stability are closely related to the ability to operate under stress. In addition to knowing exactly what to do, you must be able to do it under difficult conditions.

Having the proper attitude is important for an ambulance driver. Never get behind the wheel of an emergency vehicle thinking that you can drive in any manner that pleases you. Great responsibility is placed on the driver of an ambulance.

In addition to training and experience, the good judgment and knowledge that you need to drive an ambulance require practice. Remember, even the best drivers can benefit from practice.

Safe Driving Practices

Route Planning and Navigation

When you are dispatched to an emergency, you must decide which route will be used to arrive at the scene safely. Make sure you have detailed street and area maps in the driver's compartment of the ambulance, along with directions to key locations, such as local hospitals. Even if you have access to and routinely rely on a GPS-enabled computer navigational system for directions, you should still have access to traditional maps in the event that the navigational system becomes disabled.

Become familiar with the roads and traffic patterns in your town or city so that you can plan alternative routes to common destinations. Avoid areas of heavy traffic if possible. Pay particular attention to ways around frequently opened bridges, congested traffic, or blocked railroad crossings. Often, switching to an alternative route will save more time than driving faster. School zones are especially dangerous at the beginning or ending of classes and should be avoided if possible. Be aware of construction zones in your area as well as railroad crossings. Also become familiar with special facilities and locations within your regional operating area, such as other medical facilities, airports, arenas and stadiums, and chemical or research facilities that might pose unusual problems (staging areas may be predefined for emergency operations).

Fatigue

Fatigue has many causes, such as stress, working the night shift, and lack of quality sleep in accordance with your body's circadian rhythms. As a result of these causes of fatigue, operating a large vehicle, such as an ambulance, creates a large risk. You must be able to recognize when you are fatigued. Do not be ashamed to admit it to yourself, your partner, or your supervisor. If you are feeling fatigued, you should be placed out of service for the remainder of the shift or until the fatigue has passed and you feel capable of operating the vehicle safely.

Distractions

With the availability of digital and electronic devices, there are many things that may distract the driver of an emergency vehicle from focusing on his or her driving. En route to a call it should not be the driver's responsibility to talk on the radio or operate the ambulance's audible devices. Personnel riding on the passenger side of the vehicle are not just there to read the road map and guide the driver to the destination. They serve as another set of eyes and ears to help arrive at a location safely.

GPS is a vital piece of equipment found on most vehicles today, but they can be a hazard if the driver is focused on its directions and not on the roadway. Do not totally rely on a device to lead you to every call, but use it as a supplement to your own territory knowledge base. Study your areas well before getting behind the wheel of an ambulance. Some ambulances come equipped with mobile data terminals. A driver should *never* attempt to type on the computer while driving the ambulance.

Driving is also not the time to be texting others or operating personal data devices. Many vehicle manufacturers are placing stereos or radios in the ambulance's cab. This is a nice feature when you are not committed to an ambulance call, but you should not listen to music when you are also listening to the service radio.

Eating or drinking in the ambulance may be convenient after a long transfer when personnel are being pressured to get back into service, but it is important for you to take the time to stop and recharge before jumping back into the emergency mode again. It may also be against OSHA guidelines. Driving alone while your partner is caring for a patient in the rear compartment is also a challenge, especially if it is in the middle of the night.

Use of Safety Restraints

Standard operating procedures should mandate that everyone in the ambulance use seat belts, not just the patient. Unless critical for patient care, all passengers including EMS personnel in the patient compartment should use the vehicle's restraint devices. For example, it is not acceptable or safe to allow parents to hold children in their laps even if both are on the ambulance stretcher. Children should not be transported on the stretcher unless properly restrained. It is not advisable to use adult seat belts for children. Most states now have policies in place that require that all pediatric patients be secured with age-appropriate restraints. Of course, when you are driving the ambulance you should always use a seat belt.

Speed

Do not allow the type of call to affect how you respond to it. When you hear that the call involves children or a severe trauma potential, you may have the urge to drive with less caution, feeling that speed is more important than safety. You may have the urge to speed up when you receive a call that involves another public safety worker. As a professional, you must not let the nature of the call affect your judgment—always drive with caution.

Siren Risk-Benefit Analysis

Despite improvements in the sophistication of 9-1-1 answering systems and in the accuracy of telephone triage protocols, most EMS ambulances use their lights and sirens most of the time when responding to calls. However, once a patient is loaded, a conscious decision should be made whether to use the ambulance warning devices en route to the patient destination or drive with the normal flow of traffic. Lights and sirens should never be used to transport a nonemergency patient. You should only drive in an emergency mode when the patient's condition warrants it. The paramedic riding in the rear compartment of the ambulance with the patient should be the person to make the decision to drive in an emergency mode to the patient destination. Great care must be taken in making that decision, and it should be guided by the stability of the patient and not by the surrounding traffic or closeness to the end of your shift.

Driver Anticipation

The one thing that is predictable about driving an ambulance in the emergency mode is that all other drivers are unpredictable. Do not expect them to pull to the right to allow your vehicle to pass on the left the way public safety vehicles are instructed to do. Expect other vehicles to pull to the left *or* right. Some drivers do not realize an ambulance is behind them because of loud music or inattentive behavior. Drivers may stop suddenly in front of you out of panic. You should always maintain a safe travel distance behind other vehicles.

If your ambulance is following too close behind, drivers may not know which lane is safe to move into because their vision is blocked by your unit. Also watch out for the aggressive actions of other drivers. Not everyone respects the passage of an emergency vehicle; some may refuse to grant the right of way. Do not respond aggressively in return, but wait until it is safe to pass before doing so.

A wise ambulance driver will not accelerate through all intersections, even if he or she has the right of way, but slow down or even stop in high traffic areas. It is important to make sure that all other drivers are aware of your presence. Make eye contact, especially with the lead vehicles and be ready to apply your brake until it appears that everyone is clear on your intentions. The ambulance driver should use the vehicle's turn signals the same way other drivers are expected to do. Never force a vehicle into oncoming traffic in an effort to get around; this creates a dangerous situation.

The Cushion of Safety

To operate an emergency vehicle safely, you must maintain a safe following distance from the vehicles in front of you and try to avoid being tailgated from behind. You must also leave enough space between your vehicle and the one in front when stopped at an intersection so that the ambulance can be safely manipulated around other vehicles when you are responding.

You also must ensure that the **blind spots** in your vehicle's mirrors do not prevent you from seeing vehicles or pedestrians on either side of the ambulance. Keeping a safe distance between your vehicle and the one in front of you, checking for tailgaters behind your ambulance, and keeping aware of vehicles potentially hiding in your mirror's blind spots are considered maintaining a **cushion of safety**. To ensure that you have enough reaction time and stopping distance from the vehicle in front of you, follow at a safe distance, allowing the motorist enough time to move over to the right. If the motorist does not move, you will need to allow for enough time to evade the vehicle. This entails driving about 4 or 5 seconds behind a vehicle traveling at an average speed.

When you are operating in emergency mode, tailgaters may follow your vehicle dangerously close in congested areas simply to use your ambulance to get through traffic. If the ambulance stops suddenly to avoid a crash, the tailgating vehicle could crash into the rear of the ambulance, possibly causing you to lose control and strike other vehicles or pedestrians. Always scan your rearview and side mirrors for cars that are following too closely.

If you are being tailgated, never speed up to create more distance. The tailgater may, in turn, increase his or her speed to continue to follow you through traffic. Slamming on your brakes to scare the other driver usually does not work either and may cause a crash. You can have your dispatcher contact the local police to let them know that someone is driving recklessly behind you.

Never, under any circumstance, get out of the ambulance to confront a driver. This will only delay your response to or transport of the patient and can lead to a dangerous situation.

Finally, there are three blind spots around the ambulance that you cannot see with the mirrors:

- The mirror itself creates a blind spot, obstructing the view ahead and preventing the driver from seeing objects such as a pedestrian or car. To eliminate this blind spot, you should lean forward in your seat so that the mirror does not obstruct the view, especially when making turns at intersections.
- The rear of the vehicle cannot be seen fully through the mirror and is therefore a blind spot. Because of the configuration of today's ambulances and the relative height of the vehicle, the rearview mirror generally gives the driver a view of the patient compartment, not the vehicle behind the ambulance. Because of this blind spot, many crashes occur when the ambulance is backing up.
- The side of the vehicle often cannot be seen through the driver and passenger mirrors at a certain angle. Entire cars may not be seen in the mirror, even though they are right next to the ambulance. To eliminate this problem, many EMS services place small rounded mirrors on the side mirrors to assist you in visualizing this blind spot. However, if these mirrors are not available, you need to lean forward or backward in the seat to help eliminate the blind spot. This is an especially important technique to use when changing lanes or making turns.

You should always scan your mirrors frequently for any new hazards. Remember that your mirrors can give you false information and may hide people or cars.

Vehicle Size and Distance Judgment

Vehicle length and width are critical factors when you are maneuvering, driving, and parking an emergency vehicle. They are especially important with types I and III vehicles, which are wider than they look from behind the steering wheel. To brake and pass effectively, you must know the width and length of your vehicle. Crashes often occur when the vehicle is backing up. Always use someone outside the ambulance as a ground guide when you are backing up, to avoid any accidents. Vehicle size and weight will greatly influence braking and stopping distances. Good peripheral vision and depth perception will help you to judge distances, but they are no substitute for intensive training, experience, and frequent evaluation of the vehicle.

Backing Up the Emergency Vehicle

Most EMS services have established a policy about emergency vehicle back up. Backing up a vehicle is the most common source of vehicle damage and may result in costly repairs. If possible, avoid situations in which the ambulance will have to be backed up. If it must be done, follow these rules:

- Use a **spotter** to guide you **Figure 7**.
- Agree with the spotter *before* you place the vehicle in reverse. You may be attempting to back to the left while your spotter is trying to direct you to the right.
- Keep your spotter in view at all times. If you lose sight of the spotter, stop until he or she is back in your line of sight.

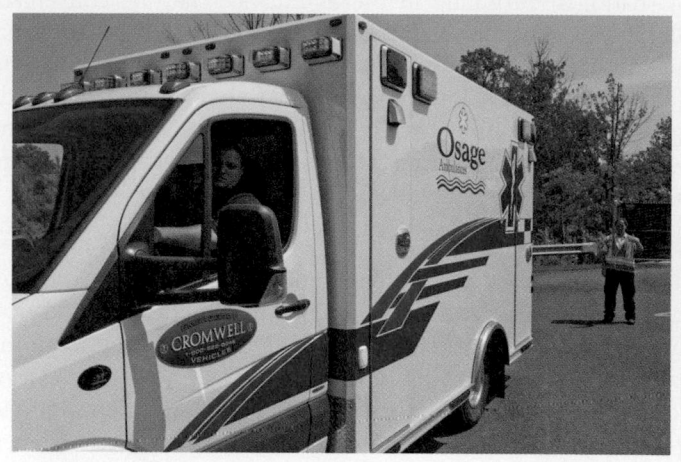

Figure 7 Always use a spotter when backing up the ambulance.

- Agree on hand signals with your spotter before moving. For example, some people have different ideas of which gesture means "Stop."
- Keep your window cracked or rolled down when in motion. This may allow you to hear people warning you of unseen dangers.
- Do a walk-around before getting behind the wheel and look up as well as down. Objects may not be visible once you start backing up.
- Use audible warning devices whenever the ambulance is in motion.
- Some vehicles have a back-up camera, which is helpful, but do not rely totally on the camera.

Parking at an Emergency Scene

When you are parking the ambulance, pick a position that will allow for efficient traffic control and flow around a crash scene. Do not park alongside the scene because you may block the movement of other emergency vehicles. Instead, park about 100 ft past the scene on the same side of the road. It is best to park uphill and/or upwind of the scene if smoke or hazardous materials are present. If you must park on the back side of a hill or curve, leave your warning lights or devices on. Do the same when you are parking at night. Always park so as to provide a cushion of space between your vehicle and operations at the scene. This can help prevent personnel from being struck if someone crashes into your vehicle on the scene. Maintain concern for others who are not involved in the incident. For example, if you are parking in an apartment complex, try not to block parked vehicles because the owners of those vehicles may need to leave while you are inside.

Stay away from any fires, explosive hazards, downed wires, or structures that might collapse. Be sure to set the parking brake. If your vehicle is blocking part of the roadway, leave the emergency warning lights on. If your vehicle has them, leave only the flashing yellow lights on. Other drivers tend to drive toward emergency vehicles with flashing red or red and white lights. Within these safety guidelines, you should try to park your ambulance as close to the scene as possible to facilitate emergency medical care. If necessary, you can temporarily block traffic to unload equipment and to load patients quickly and safely. If you must do this, try to do it quickly so that traffic is not blocked any longer than is absolutely necessary. Also, park in a location that will not hamper your departure from the scene.

When you are parking off the side of the road, you must be aware of the terrain **Figure 8**. In dry weather, the heat from underneath the vehicle could start a grass fire. In wet weather, the weight of the ambulance makes it susceptible to sinking into mud and getting stuck.

Parking on a roadway at night is especially dangerous **Figure 9**. Some drivers may have their attention distracted by the scene, and

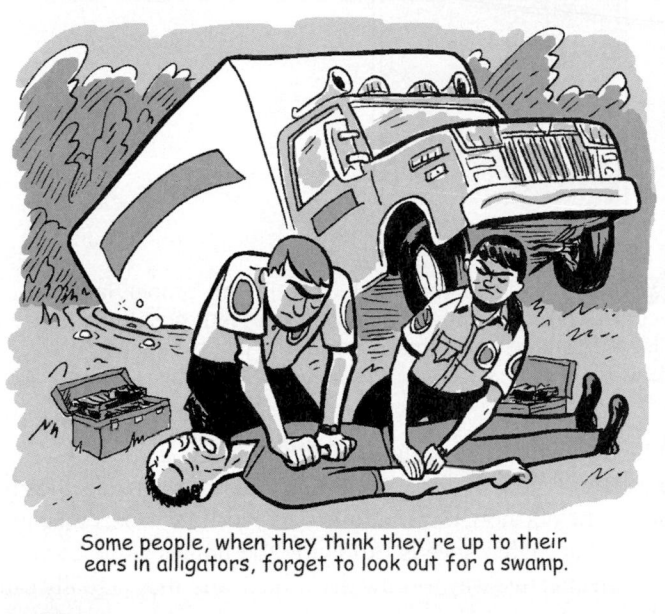

Some people, when they think they're up to their ears in alligators, forget to look out for a swamp.

Figure 8

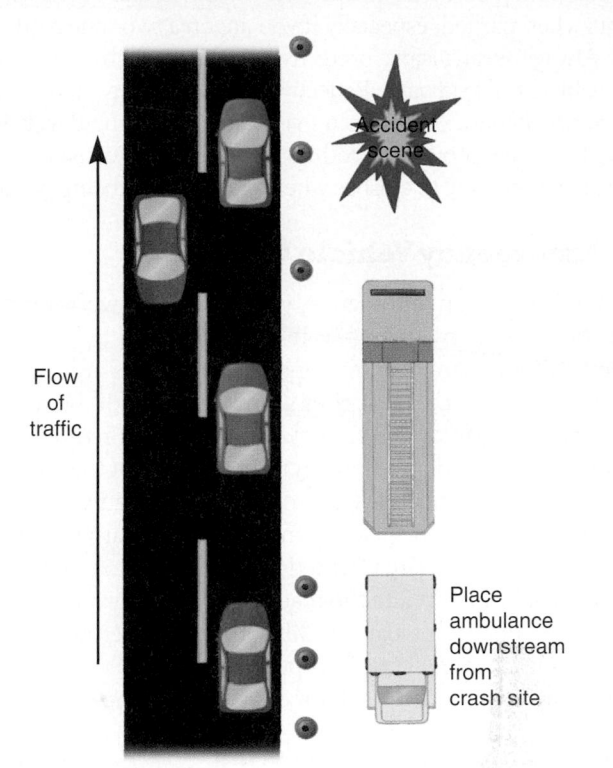

Figure 9 Position the vehicle to maximize your safety. Orange dots represent traffic cones separating flow of traffic from crash site.

YOU *are the Medic* **PART 3**

Your patient confirms that she was the driver of this vehicle. She is able to recall all events preceding the crash. Her primary and secondary assessments are unremarkable except for her right knee, which struck the base of the dash. You assess the knee and find it to be tender on palpation. There are good pulses in the lower leg and foot. The patient has limited range of motion. You place the patient in full spinal precautions and splint the knee per your protocol. You load the patient in your ambulance for transport.

Recording Time: 5 Minutes	
Respirations	14 breaths/min
Pulse	80 beats/min
Skin	Warm, dry, pink
Blood pressure	126/82 mm Hg
Oxygen saturation (Spo$_2$)	99% on room air
Pupils	Equal and reactive

5. Should lights and the siren be used while you are transporting this patient? Why or why not?

6. What actions should be taken before you depart the scene?

they may drift toward and collide with a parked emergency vehicle. Sometimes it may be safer to use your emergency flashers instead of all the overhead flashers. Likewise, to avoid blinding oncoming traffic, it may be better to turn off the emergency vehicle's headlights when parked, especially if you are on a two-lane road.

Always wear visible protective clothing when you get out of the vehicle on roadways. Reflective vests are lightweight and have the added benefit of increasing visibility during the day as well as at night. Heavy protective clothing should also be considered when you are responding to crashes where extrication is being performed.

■ Emergency Vehicle Control

As the driver of an ambulance, you have only two ways to control the vehicle: by changing its direction and by changing its speed. Either maneuver requires a continuous rolling contact between the surface of the tires and the surface of the road.

The tire's grip on the road may vary widely on different parts of the same road, depending on the condition of the surface, the age of the road, and the weather. Unpaved roadways may also present a challenge, especially in inclement weather. It also varies according to the tire's tread design and wear. As a driver, you must constantly evaluate the road surface: At a given speed, how much frictional force can the tires apply before the ambulance becomes unstable? This is especially important in cornering when additional centrifugal force is acting on the vehicle.

Road Positioning and Cornering

Road position refers to the position of the vehicle on the roadway relative to the inside or outside edge of the paved surface. To corner efficiently, you must know the vehicle's present position and its projected path. The aim is to take the corner at the speed that will put you in the proper road position as you exit the curve **Figure 10**. The apex of the turn through a curve is the point at which the vehicle is closest to the inside edge of the curve. If you reach the apex early in the curve, the vehicle will be forced toward the outside of the roadway as it exits the curve. If you reach the apex late in the curve, the vehicle will tend to stay on the inside of the roadway; this helps you to keep the vehicle in the proper lane and allows room for error if you enter the turn too fast.

■ Braking

Getting a feel for the proper brake pressure comes with experience and practice. Each vehicle has a different braking action. For example, the brakes on types I and III vehicles have a heavier feel than the brakes on a type II vehicle. Braking on a diesel-powered unit will be different from braking on an identically equipped gasoline-powered unit. Certain heavy vehicles use air brakes that have yet another feel. You should get to know each vehicle you drive, and be sure you understand its braking characteristics and the best downshifting techniques.

■ Controlled Braking

Controlled braking is the use of the brakes to control the vehicle. Brakes not only control the movement of the vehicle, causing it to slow or stop; they also help to control its direction. Braking

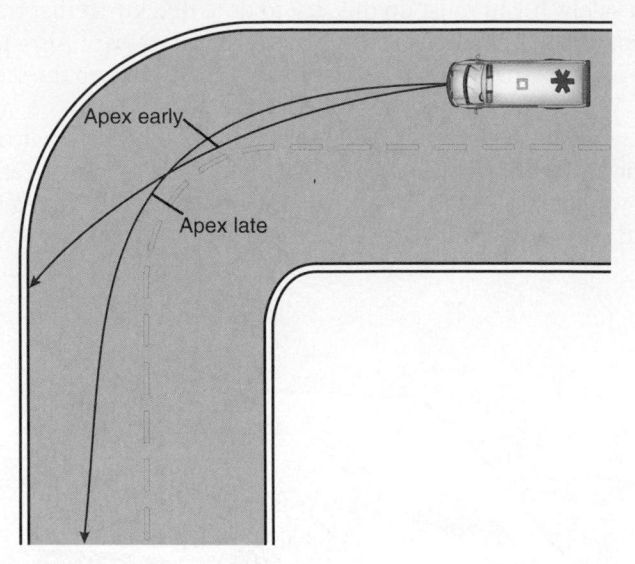

Figure 10 To keep the ambulance in the proper lane on a curve, you must know the vehicle's present position and projected path and take the corner at the correct speed.

while the vehicle is traveling in a straight line is the safest, most efficient method. Braking in a turn causes a loss of efficiency. You might not notice this at a low speed, but it becomes more apparent at higher speeds. Applying the brakes while cornering is not an effective way to slow the vehicle and may actually cause a skid or spin.

Words of Wisdom

Always brake in a straight line!

Weather and Road Conditions

Due to a higher center of gravity, most ambulances have the tendency to tip over if curves or turns are taken at too great of a speed. On rainy days there is an even greater danger for this to occur. Water can get trapped between the tires of vehicles with dual tires in the rear and cause the ambulance to start hydroplaning. You should use extreme caution and slow down in inclement weather to take the weight distributions of the vehicle into consideration. Remember that you will need more room to come to a complete stop when compared with driving a regular passenger vehicle. Also, remember that your line of sight is limited to what you can see in the side mirrors; make it a habit to use them frequently when you are driving both the ambulance and your own personal vehicle.

Hydroplaning On a wet road, at speeds of greater than 30 mph, the tire may be lifted off the road as water "piles up" under it; the vehicle feels as if it were floating. This is known as **hydroplaning**. At higher speeds on wet roadways, the front wheels may actually be riding on a sheet of water, robbing the driver of control of the vehicle. If hydroplaning occurs, you should gradually slow down without jamming on the brakes.

Water On the Roadway Wet brakes will slow the vehicle and pull it to one side or the other. If at all possible, avoid driving through large pools of standing water; often, you cannot tell how deep they are. If you must drive through standing water, make sure to slow down and turn on the windshield wipers. After driving out of the pool, lightly tap the brakes several times until they are dry. If the vehicle is equipped with anti-lock brakes, apply a steady, light pressure to dry the brakes. Finally, driving through moving water should be avoided at all times.

Decreased Visibility In areas where there is fog, smog, snow, or heavy rain, common sense tells you to slow down. At night, use only low headlight beams for maximum visibility without reflection. You should always use headlights during the day to increase your visibility to other drivers. Also, watch carefully for stopped or slow-moving vehicles.

Ice and Slippery Surfaces A light mist on an oily, dusty road can be just as slippery as a patch of ice. Good all-weather tires and an appropriate speed will reduce traction problems significantly. If you are in an area that often has snowy or icy conditions, consider using studded snow tires, if they are permitted by law. You should be especially careful on bridges and overpasses when temperatures are close to freezing. These road surfaces will freeze much faster than surrounding road surfaces because they lack the warming effect of the ground underneath.

■ Laws and Regulations

Regulations regarding vehicle operations vary from state to state and from city to city, but some things are the same everywhere. Drivers of emergency vehicles have certain limited privileges in every state. However, these privileges do not lessen their liability in a crash. In fact, in most cases, the driver is presumed to be guilty if a crash occurs while the ambulance is operating with warning lights and siren. Motor vehicle crashes are the single largest source of lawsuits against EMS personnel and services.

When you are on an emergency call, emergency vehicles typically are exempt from usual vehicle operations. If you are on an emergency call and are using your warning lights and siren, you may be allowed to do the following:

- Park or stand in an otherwise illegal location
- Proceed through a red traffic light or stop sign *after* stopping
- Drive faster than the posted speed limit
- Drive against the flow of traffic on a one-way street or make a turn that is normally illegal
- Travel left of center to make an otherwise illegal pass

Even if you are given specific exemptions to some traffic laws in an emergency, this privilege must be used sparingly.

Remember that these exemptions vary by state and local jurisdiction. Therefore, you should check your local statutes for regulations in your area.

Use of Warning Lights and Siren

Three basic principles govern the use of warning lights and siren on an ambulance:

1. The unit must be on a true emergency call to the best of your knowledge.
2. Both audible and visual warning devices must be used simultaneously.
3. The unit must be operated with due regard for the safety of all others, on and off the roadway.

The siren is probably the most overused piece of equipment on an ambulance. In general, the siren does not help you as you drive; nor does it really help other motorists. Motorists who are driving at the speed limit with the windows up, the radio on, and the air conditioner or heater set on high may not hear the siren until the ambulance is very close by. If the radio is particularly loud, they may not hear the siren at all.

If you do have to use the siren, be sure to warn the patient before you turn it on. Be especially mindful not to increase the speed of the ambulance just because the siren is in use. Always travel at a speed that will allow you to stop safely at all times, especially so that you are prepared for drivers who do not give you the right-of-way. Never assume that warning lights and sirens will allow you to drive through a congested area without stopping or slowing down. Slow down to ensure that all drivers are stopping as you approach an intersection, and then proceed with due caution.

Some ambulance headlights are equipped with a high-beam flasher unit. These are the most visible, effective warning devices for clearing traffic in front of the vehicle.

Right-of-way Privileges

A right-of-way privilege is just that: a privilege. State motor vehicle statutes or codes often grant an emergency vehicle, such as an ambulance, the right to disregard the rules of the road when responding to an emergency. However, in doing so, the operator of an emergency vehicle must not endanger people or property under any circumstances. Remember that use of lights and sirens does not give you the right-of-way; rather, it is asking for the right-of-way.

Right-of-way privileges for ambulances vary from state to state. Some states allow you to proceed through a red light or stop sign after you stop and make sure it is safe to proceed. Other states allow you to proceed through a controlled intersection "with **due regard**," using flashing lights and the siren. This means that you may proceed only if you consider the safety of all people who are using the highway. If you fail to use due regard, your service might be sued if a crash occurs. If you are found to be at fault, you may personally have to pay punitive damages or face both civil and criminal sanctions.

Get to know your local right-of-way privileges. Exercise them only when it is absolutely necessary for the patient's well-being. The use of lights and audible warning devices is a matter of state and local practice and protocol.

Use of Escorts

It is typically *not* a good idea to follow another emergency vehicle, such as a police car, through traffic as an escort. Many drivers will see only the first set of lights and sirens and assume that the way is clear once that vehicle has passed. If you are following another emergency vehicle, leave enough space between the vehicles so that other drivers (and you) have enough time to react and safely stop should someone pull in front of you unexpectedly.

Another potential danger occurs when family members follow closely behind you on the way to the hospital. Both the ambulance and other drivers may have difficulty seeing the vehicles that are following. If you need to stop suddenly, there may be no time to react and the vehicle could crash into the ambulance. Instruct family members before you leave the scene that they cannot drive closely behind you, and make sure they are aware of how to get to the hospital at a slower speed.

Sometimes family members will not heed your warning about following the ambulance to the hospital. If the patient's family members or another motorist begins to follow you when you are operating your ambulance using lights and siren, consider turning off your lights and siren and slowing down to normal speed, in an effort to prevent a collision.

Intersection Hazards

Intersection crashes are the most common and usually the most serious type of crash in which ambulances are involved. Always be alert and careful when you are approaching an intersection. If you are on an urgent call and cannot wait for traffic lights to change, you should still come to a momentary stop at the light; look around for other motorists and pedestrians before proceeding into the intersection.

Motorists who "time the traffic lights" present a serious hazard. You may arrive at an intersection while the light is green. At the same time, a motorist who is timing the lights on the cross street arrives at the intersection. The motorist has a red light but knows that it is about to turn green and is expecting to go through. The stage is now set for a serious crash.

Another common intersection hazard occurs when the driver of one emergency vehicle follows another emergency vehicle through an intersection without assessing the situation carefully. A motorist who has yielded the right-of-way to the first vehicle may proceed into the intersection without expecting a second vehicle. You should exercise extreme caution in these situations. To signal motorists that a second unit is approaching, use a siren tone that is different from that of the first vehicle.

Unpaved Roadways and Rural Settings

When you are required to drive the ambulance on an unpaved roadway, special care must be taken. Unpaved roads may be encountered when the patient's residence is far off the road, and may be inaccessible by ambulance. When you are responding on this type of roadway, you must operate the vehicle at a lower speed and maintain a firm grip on the steering wheel in an effort to maintain complete control of the ambulance at all times. Unpaved roadways often have uneven surfaces, as well as large potholes, and may be impassable in rain. Do not drive a heavy ambulance onto unpaved or grassy areas when the ground has been saturated with rain unless you are sure the unit will not get bogged down and stuck.

Rural EMS services usually have agreements with other agencies, such as the Forestry Service, to help them reach the remote locations. Watch out for animals entering the roadway, especially in the evenings when visibility is decreased. Large deer, moose, and even livestock can migrate onto the roadways, requiring the driver to be extra alert to avoid running into animals.

School Buses

An emergency vehicle is *never* allowed to pass a school bus that has stopped to load or unload children and is displaying its flashing red lights or extended "stop arm." If you approach a school bus that has its lights flashing, you should stop before reaching the bus and wait for the driver to make sure the children are safe, close the bus door, and turn off the warning lights. Only then may you carefully proceed past the stopped school bus.

School Zones

When you respond through a school zone with your emergency lights activated, it is important to remember that lights and sirens tend to attract children to the roadway and create a potential hazard. In many states, it is unlawful for an emergency vehicle to exceed the speed limit in school zones regardless of the condition of the patient.

Funeral Processions

There is also no exemption in most states when you are approaching a funeral procession while in the emergency mode. Some escorts will pull the procession over, but others may not. Out of respect, most emergency drivers will maintain the activation of the emergency lights, but turn off the audible devices and slowly pass the procession on the left, using due regard for other approaching drivers.

■ Air Medical Transports

Air medical transport—especially the use of helicopters—has done much to speed up the transfer of patients from the trauma scene to definitive care. This mode of transport presents certain risks, however, and it is only appropriate in certain circumstances. Several factors must be considered before calling for an **air ambulance**: Does the patient's condition warrant the risk of using air medical transport? Will use of the air ambulance truly save the patient time in getting to definitive care once all other factors are considered?

■ Rotor-Wing Versus Fixed-Wing Air Ambulances

Rotor-wing aircraft (helicopters) have become a standard of care for the transportation of critically injured patients from the scene to a regional trauma center **Figure 11**. Fixed-winged aircraft are used mainly for the transportation of patients over long distances. EMS personnel are frequently called to transport these patients from the airfield to definitive care facilities **Figure 12**.

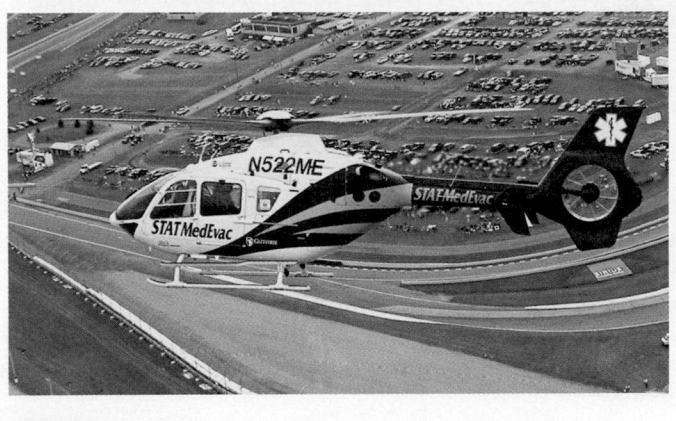

Figure 11 Rotor-wing air ambulance.

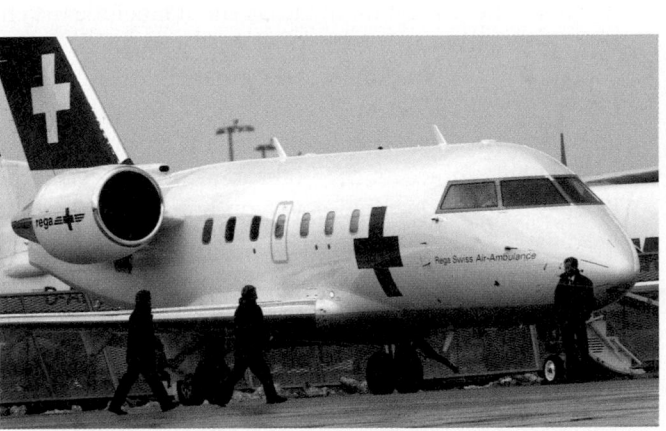

Figure 12 Fixed-winged aircraft.

Advantages of Using Air Ambulances

Air ambulances have an advantage over ground transport in that they reduce transport time if the transport distance is extreme and may help the patient receive definitive treatment within the golden hour. The decision to use rotor-winged transport (helicopter) should be made as early in the call as possible. If, after patient assessment, it is determined that the helicopter is not needed, it can always be returned to service. Some districts have "automatic send helicopter" procedures written into their protocols.

You should weigh all the factors that involve time when you are deciding whether the helicopter is appropriate. The machine must be started, personnel and gear loaded, and sometimes great distances covered. Once the helicopter is at the scene, time must be allotted to land the aircraft and transfer the patient to the air crew. Packaging the patient for air transport and loading the patient into the helicopter also require time. Especially in metropolitan areas, it can be difficult to justify use of the helicopter. Severe traffic congestion or prolonged extrication times may sometimes make the use of a helicopter appropriate in urban areas.

Use of an air ambulance may be warranted if the patient has a spinal injury and the terrain over which the patient must be carried is rough. Even though the patient is stabilized, ground transport in a vehicle that is bouncing on the road could further injure the patient. The paramedic on scene is the best judge of the patient's transportation needs. **Table 3** summarizes the advantages of using an air ambulance.

Disadvantages of Using Air Ambulances

Patients in cardiac arrest or those who appear to be in pre-cardiac arrest should be transported by ground. Treating a patient in cardiac arrest in the helicopter is difficult due to space limitations.

YOU *are the Medic* | PART 4 |

You are transporting your patient to the hospital and the rain has increased to a downpour. Your driver advises that she is slowing down due to weather conditions. You reassess your patient and find her to be resting comfortably with no change in condition.

Recording Time: 10 Minutes	
Respirations	14 breaths/min
Pulse	80 beats/min
Skin	Warm, pink, dry
Blood pressure	124/80 mm Hg
Oxygen saturation (Spo_2)	100% oxygen at 2 L/min via nasal cannula
Pupils	Equal and reactive

7. What should the emergency vehicle operator do if the patient's family is following the ambulance?

8. Are there any special privileges given to emergency vehicles when you are driving through a school zone?

Table 3 Advantages of Using an Air Ambulance
▪ Specialized skills or equipment is needed
▪ Rapid transport is possible
▪ Can provide access to remote areas
▪ Helicopter hospital helipads are available
▪ Availability of medical crew with advanced skills

Table 4 Disadvantages of Using an Air Ambulance
▪ Weather/environment
▪ Altitude limitations
▪ Airspeed limitations
▪ Aircraft cabin size
▪ Terrain
▪ Cost
▪ Patient's condition
▪ Restrictions on the number of caregivers
▪ Potential for crash

In addition, to ensure safety, air ambulances do not fly when there is poor visibility. The terrain also may make it difficult to land the helicopter safely. Uneven ground and loose objects such as rocks or debris should be taken into account before attempting to land the aircraft. Table 4 lists disadvantages of using the air ambulance.

Helicopter Medical Evacuation Operations

A medical evacuation is commonly known as a **medevac** and is generally performed exclusively by helicopters. Most rural and suburban EMS jurisdictions and many urban systems have the capability to perform helicopter medevacs or have a mutual aid agreement with another agency such as police or hospital-based medevac service to provide such service. You should become familiar with the medevac capabilities, protocols, and procedures of your particular EMS service because they vary from service to service.

Calling For a Medevac

Every agency has specific criteria for the type of patient who may receive medical evacuation and how and when to call for a medevac. These basic guidelines will help you to understand the process better.

- **Why call for a medevac?** The transport time to the hospital by ground ambulance is too long considering the patient's condition. Road, traffic, or environmental conditions limit or completely prohibit the use of a ground ambulance. The patient requires advanced care that you are unable to provide, such as administering pain medications or other specialized medications and inserting advanced airways. There are multiple patients who will overwhelm resources at the hospital reachable by ground transport.

- **Who receives a medevac?** Medical evacuations should be used for patients with time-dependent injuries or illnesses. They are widely used for patients suspected of having a stroke, heart attack, or serious spinal cord injury, such as injuries sustained in a motor vehicle crash or while diving into a pool or horseback riding. Serious conditions that may require the use of helicopter medevacs may be found in remote areas and involve scuba diving accidents, near-drownings, or skiing and wilderness accidents. Other patients who may warrant the use of medical evacuation are trauma patients and candidates for limb replantation (for amputations), a burn center, a hyperbaric chamber, or a venomous bite center. Because specific criteria differ between

services, you must be familiar with your local jurisdiction's criteria used to call for this lifesaving service.

- **Whom do you call?** Generally your dispatcher must be notified first. The request for medevac should include the chief complaint and the patient's weight, as many medevac helicopters have weight limits. (You should be aware the limitations of your local medevac service.) In some regions, after the medevac has been initiated, the ground EMS crew may be able to access the flight crew on a specially designated radio frequency for one-on-one communications. If available, it is important to keep this frequency clear of chatter and long, drawn-out communications. You may be asked to give a brief presentation or update on the patient's condition. In this case, you should gather your thoughts and speak clearly and concisely, avoiding information that is not immediately pertinent. Another important topic of communication between the ground and flight EMS crews will be where to land the helicopter.

Medevac Issues

While you are making the decision to request medevac, several important factors need to be taken into consideration. These factors are weather, the environment/terrain, altitude, airspeed limitations, cabin size, and cost. Typically, helicopters are unable to operate in severe weather such as thunderstorms, blizzards, and heavy rain. The environment may pose a risk as well. In mountainous or desert terrain, there may be too many hazards in the immediate vicinity to safely land the helicopter in the desired location.

As the elevation increases, the air thins, making it more difficult for pilots and patients to breathe. Because of this danger, helicopters have a maximum limit on flight elevations. Most helicopter services are limited to flying at 10,000 ft above sea level. This could create a problem if your patient is located at 13,500 ft above sea level. It is important to remember that medevac helicopters are not jets, and it takes time for them to arrive on the scene because of limitations in airspeed. Typically medevac helicopters fly between 130 and 150 mph.

Because of the helicopter cabin's confined space, helicopters are limited in the number of patients that can be safely transported and by the size of the patient whom they can safely transport. Although a helicopter may be able to safely lift off with a 500-lb patient, because of his or her size and girth, it may be impossible to safely fit and secure the patient into the cabin area.

Typical medevac flights cost in the range of $8,000 to $10,000, whereas the typical ambulance transport costs $400 to $1,000. The decision to request a medevac should not be based on the perceived ability of the patient to pay the bill, but rather on the medical necessity and flight conditions. However, the cost factor should be considered so as not to create any unnecessary financial hardship, while still providing the best care for the patient.

Establishing a Landing Zone

Although a helicopter can fly straight up and down, such movement is the most dangerous mode of operation. The safest and most effective way to land and take off is similar to that used by fixed-wing aircraft. Landing at a slight angle allows for safer operations. Takeoff combines a gradual lift and forward motion to travel up and out on a slight angle.

An important part of conducting a medevac is choosing the best location. Establishing a **landing zone** is the responsibility of the ground EMS crew. It involves more than simply looking for a clear space. You must be prepared to take action to make certain that the flight crew is able to land and take off safely. Actions to take and considerations to make when you are selecting and establishing a landing zone include the following:

- The area should be a hard or grassy level surface that measures 100 ft × 100 ft (recommended) and no less than 60 ft × 60 ft. If the site is not level, the flight crew must be notified of the steepness and direction of the slope.
- The area must be cleared of any loose debris that could become airborne and strike the helicopter or the patient and crew. This includes branches, trash bins, flares, accident tape, and medical equipment and supplies.
- You must survey the immediate area for any overhead or tall hazards such as power lines or telephone cables, antennas, and tall or leaning trees. The presence of these must be relayed immediately to the flight crew because an alternative landing site may be required. The flight crew may request that the hazard be marked or illuminated by weighted cones or by positioning an emergency vehicle with its lights turned on next to or under the potential hazard.
- To mark the landing site, use weighted cones or position emergency vehicles at the corners of the landing zone with headlights facing inward to form an X. This procedure is essential during night landings as well. Never use accident tape or people to mark the site. The use of flares is also not recommended, because not only can they become airborne, but they also have the potential to start a fire or cause an explosion.
- Make sure that all nonessential persons and vehicles are moved to a safe distance outside of the landing zone.
- If the wind is strong, radio the direction of the wind to the flight crew. They may request that you improvise some form of wind directional device to aid their approach. A bed sheet tightly secured to a tree or pole may be used to help the crew determine wind direction and strength. Never use tape.

Landing Zone Safety and Patient Transfer

You should be familiar with the capabilities, protocols, and methods for accessing helicopters in your area. Helicopter services provide training for EMS personnel in ground operations and safety. Interactions with flight personnel should be comprehensive. Patients should be packaged prior to arrival of the air ambulance and an extensive report given to the flight crew for transfer care. The following discussion is an introduction to safe operations, and is not intended to be substituted for the more extensive courses available locally.

Helicopter safety is nothing more than good common sense, along with a constant awareness of the need for personal safety. The types of helicopters that are used for medical operations vary, but the dangers are the same. If you are familiar with the way helicopters work and follow the pilot's instructions, you will minimize these dangers. You should be sure to do nothing near the helicopter and go only where the pilot or crew directs you. Keep the pilot in view at all times, and approach and depart the aircraft from the front, then move to the side as directed by the air crew.

The most important rule is to keep a safe distance from the aircraft whenever it is on the ground and "hot," which means when the tail rotor is spinning. Most of the time, the rotor blades will remain running because the flight crew does not generally expect to remain on the ground for a long time. This means that every EMS provider should stay outside the landing zone perimeter unless directed by the pilot or a member of the flight crew that they are to come to the aircraft. Usually, the flight crew will come to the crew carrying their own equipment and not require any assistance inside the landing zone. If you are asked to enter the landing zone, stay away from the tail rotor; the tips of its blades move so rapidly that they are invisible. Never approach the helicopter from the rear, even if it is not running. If you must move from one side of the helicopter to another, go around the front. Never duck under the body, the tail boom, or the rear section of the helicopter; the pilot cannot see you in these areas. The proper approach area is between the nine-o'clock and the three-o'clock positions as the pilot faces forward **Figure 13**.

Another area of concern is the height of the main rotor blade. On many aircraft, it is flexible and may dip as low as 4 ft off the ground **Figure 14**. When you approach the aircraft, walk in a crouched position. Wind gusts can alter the blade height without warning, so be sure to protect equipment as you carry it near the blades. Air turbulence created by the rotor blades can blow off hats and loose equipment. These, in turn, can become a danger to the aircraft and personnel in the area. Never carry anything above your head, and make sure that someone is always in charge of each piece of equipment when around the aircraft. Stretchers can easily roll into the tail rotors if no one is physically holding onto the cot after the patient is loaded into the helicopter.

When you are accompanying a flight crew member, you must follow directions exactly. Never try to open any aircraft door or move equipment unless a crew member tells you to. When you are told to approach the aircraft, use extreme caution and pay constant attention to hazards.

Keep the following guidelines in mind when you are operating at a landing zone:

- Pay close attention to direction by the flight crew when you are approaching the aircraft.
- Become familiar with helicopter hand signals used within your jurisdiction **Figure 15**.
- Do not approach the helicopter unless instructed and accompanied by flight crew.
- Make certain that all patient care equipment is properly secured to the stretcher and that the patient is fastened as well. This includes oxygen tanks, cervical collars, and head immobilizers. Any loose articles or belongings such as hats, coats, or bags that belong to the patient or crew should not be brought into the landing zone and will likely need to be transported to the hospital by ground.
- Be mindful that some helicopters may load patients from the side, whereas others have rear-loading doors. Regardless of where the patient is being loaded, always approach the aircraft from the front unless otherwise instructed by the flight crew. Always take the same path when you are exiting away from the helicopter, moving the patient headfirst.
- Smoking, open lights or flames, and flares are prohibited within 50 ft of the aircraft at all times.

Communicating With Other Agencies

When you are interacting with other agencies, there is always the possibility of communication issues. Medevacs are no exception. Whereas the typical EMS service has its specific and well-defined jurisdiction, medevacs respond to service requests throughout a large, multijurisdictional area. Because

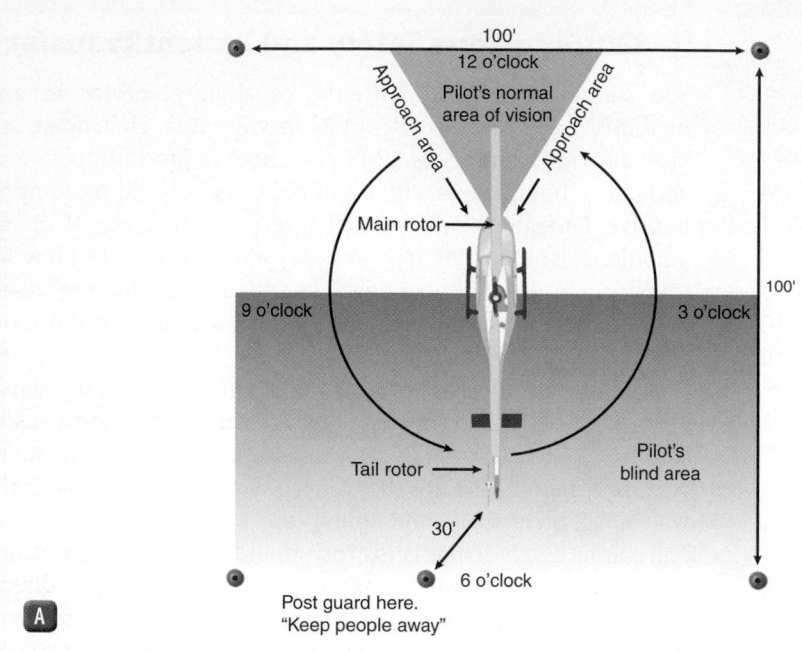

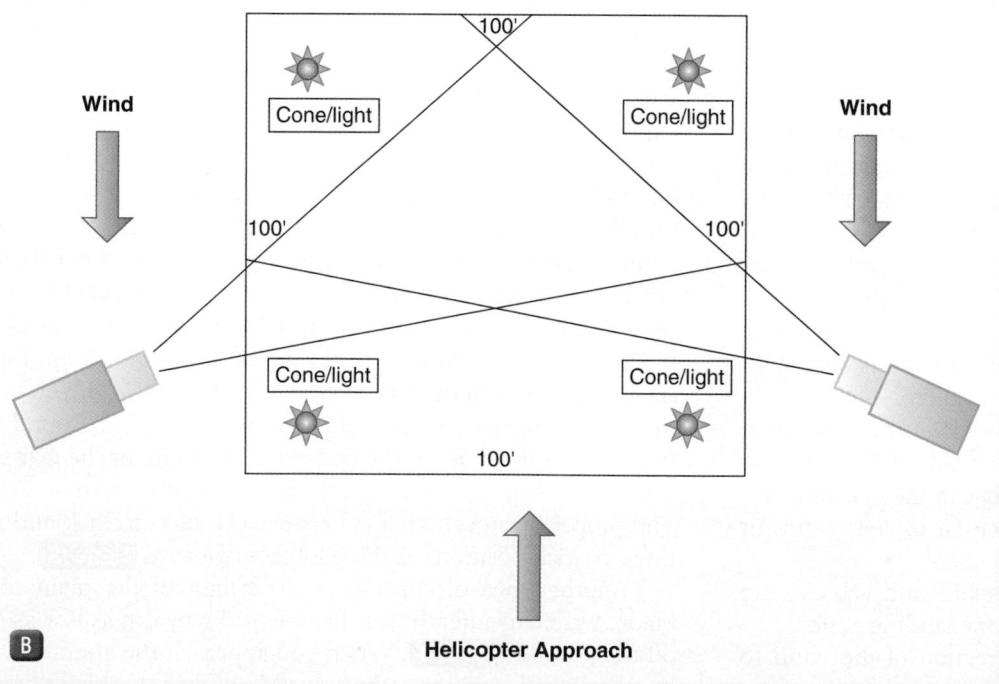

Figure 13 **A.** Approach a helicopter between the nine-o'clock and the three-o'clock positions as the pilot faces forward. **B.** Wind direction and helicopter approach are shown here. Nighttime operations can use ambulance headlights to light the area as shown.

of this large area with numerous jurisdictions, the medevac interacts with many services on a multitude of different radio frequencies.

To prevent any miscommunication, when the request is made for a medevac response, the request should include a ground contact radio channel (typically a preestablished mutual aid channel), as well as a call sign of the unit that the medevac should make contact with.

Special Considerations

Night Landings

Nighttime operations are considerably more hazardous than daytime operations because of the darkness. The pilot may fly over the area with the helicopter's lights on to spot obstacles and the shadows of overhead wires, which can be hard to see. Do not shine spotlights, flashlights, or any other lights in the air to help the pilot; they may temporarily blind the pilot. Instead, direct light beams toward the ground at the landing site. Even after the helicopter has landed, you should not aim lights anywhere near it. Of course, smoking, open lights or flames, and flares are prohibited within 50 ft of the aircraft at all times.

Landing on Uneven Ground

If the helicopter must land on a grade, extra caution is advised. The main rotor blade will be closer to the ground on the uphill side. In this situation, approach the aircraft from the downhill side only **Figure 16**. Do not move the patient to the helicopter

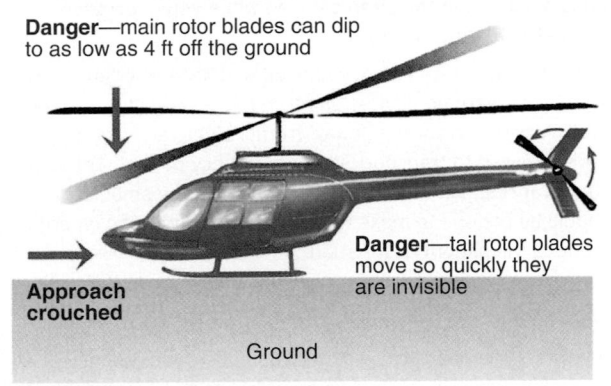

Figure 14 The main rotor blade of the helicopter is flexible and may dip as low as 4 ft off the ground.

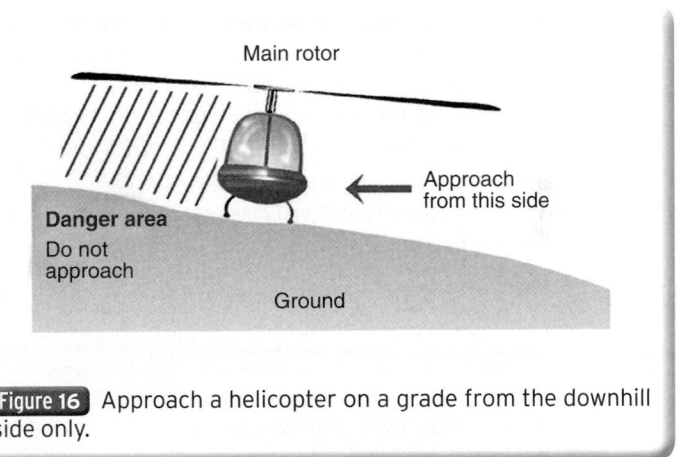

Figure 16 Approach a helicopter on a grade from the downhill side only.

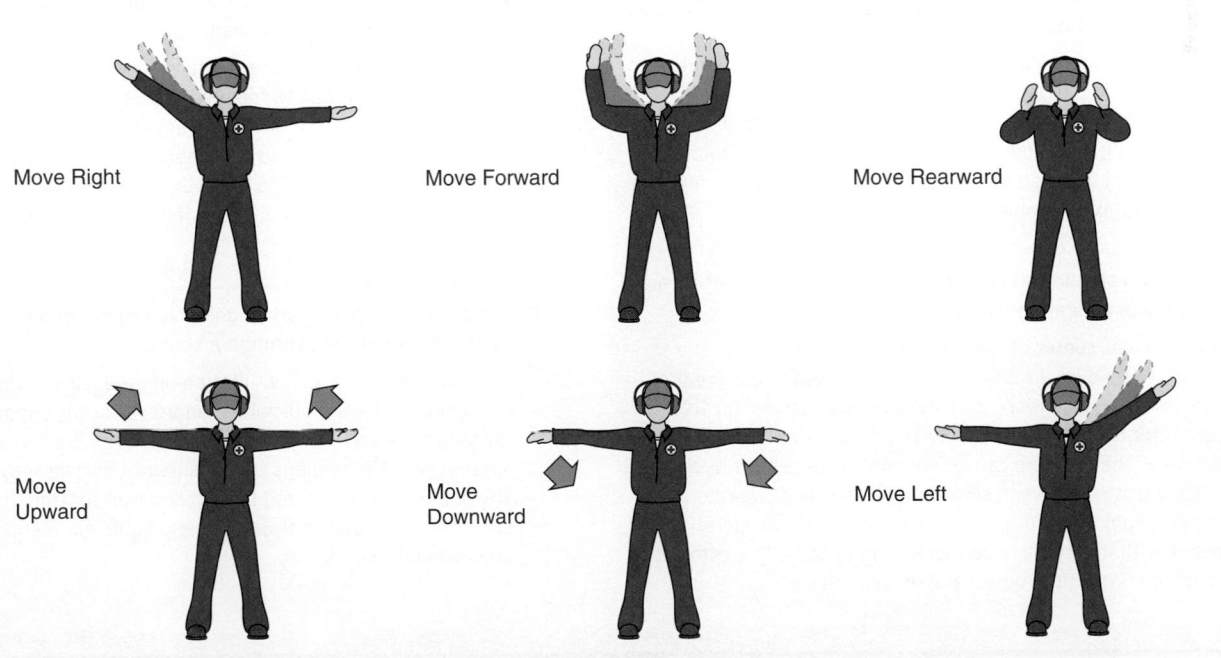

Figure 15 Some examples of helicopter hand signals. Be familiar with those used within your jurisdiction.

until the crew has signaled that they are ready to receive you. A flight crew member will direct and assist you in loading the patient.

Medevacs at Hazardous Materials Incidents

The flight crew must be notified immediately of the presence of hazardous materials at the scene. The aircraft generates tremendous wind and may easily spread any hazardous vapors present.

Always consult the flight crew and incident commander about the best approach and distance from the scene for a medevac. The landing zone should be established upwind and uphill from the hazardous materials scene. Any patients who have been exposed to a hazardous material must be properly decontaminated before they can be loaded into the aircraft. For proper procedures at hazardous materials incidents, refer to the chapter, *Incident Management and Multiple-Casualty Incidents*.

YOU *are the Medic*   SUMMARY

1. Explain the concept of "due regard."

Every state has laws regarding the use of lights and sirens when operating an emergency vehicle. The concept of due regard is an important part of those laws. Due regard means that you may use lights and sirens as a means to alert other drivers that you are in an emergency mode, but it does not exempt you from operating your vehicle with due regard for the safety of others.

2. What considerations should you make concerning your route to the interstate?

When you are dispatched to an emergency, you must decide which route will be used to arrive at the scene safely. Avoid areas of heavy traffic if possible. School zones are especially dangerous at the beginning or ending of classes and should be avoided if possible. Be aware of construction zones in your area as well as railroad crossings. Know the best routes in your district before you head out.

3. What equipment and supplies are typically taken from the ambulance to the patient's side?

Many provider agencies have a policy concerning what equipment is taken to the patient on every call. Usually this is an airway kit, oxygen assembly, and a response bag that contains a minimum of supplies and medications to stabilize a patient prior to transport. In the case of trauma patients, this will also include spinal precaution equipment.

4. What factors should be considered when you are operating an ambulance in inclement weather?

Due to a higher center of gravity, most ambulances have the tendency to tip over if curves or turns are taken at too great of a speed. On rainy days there is an even greater danger for this to occur. Water can get trapped between the tires of vehicles with dual tires in the rear and cause the ambulance to start hydroplaning. Use much caution and slow down in inclement weather to take the weight distributions of the vehicle into consideration. Remember that you will need more room to come to a complete stop, compared with a regular passenger vehicle.

5. Should lights and the siren be used while you are transporting this patient? Why or why not?

Once the patient is loaded, you need to decide whether to use the ambulance warning devices en route to the patient destination or drive with the normal flow of traffic. Lights and sirens should never be used to transport a nonemergency patient. The patient caregiver riding in the rear compartment of the ambulance should be the one to make the decision to drive in an emergency mode to the patient destination.

6. What actions should be taken before you depart the scene?

If your vehicle needs to be backed up, follow your agency's policy. At a minimum, walk around your vehicle to make sure cabinets are secured, and look at the scene behind your vehicle. If you are on a busy roadway such as an interstate, have a law enforcement officer help you by providing a break in the traffic flow so you can safely exit.

7. What should the emergency vehicle operator do if the patient's family is following the ambulance?

A potential danger occurs when family members follow closely behind you on the way to the hospital. Both the ambulance and other drivers may have difficulty seeing the vehicles that are following. If you need to stop suddenly, there may be no time to react and the vehicle could crash into the ambulance. Instruct family members before you leave the scene that they cannot drive closely behind you.

8. Are there any special privileges given to emergency vehicles when you are driving through a school zone?

In many states, it is unlawful for an emergency vehicle to exceed the speed limit in school zones regardless of the condition of the patient. Also, no specific exemption is allowed when you are approaching a school bus that has its warning devices activated. The ambulance is required to stop and wait for the driver of the school bus to drop the stop signs and lights on the bus before proceeding forward.

YOU are the Medic   SUMMARY, continued

EMS Patient Care Report (PCR)

Date: 02-02-11	Incident No.: 73542	Nature of Call: MVC		Location: 224 W/B I-80	
Dispatched: 1315	En Route: 1316	At Scene: 1321	Transport: 1328	At Hospital: 1342	In Service: 1400

Patient Information

Age: 25 Sex: F Weight (in kg [lb]): 50 kg (110 lb)	Allergies: No known drug allergies Medications: Pt denies Past Medical History: Pt denies Chief Complaint: Right knee pain

Vital Signs

Time: 1326	BP: 126/82	Pulse: 80	Respirations: 14	Spo$_2$: 99% on room air
Time: 1331	BP: 124/80	Pulse: 80	Respirations: 14	Spo$_2$: 100% oxygen at 2 L/min
Time:	BP:	Pulse:	Respirations:	Spo$_2$:

EMS Treatment
(circle all that apply)

Oxygen @ __2__ L/min via (circle one): (NC) NRM Bag-mask device	Assisted Ventilation	Airway Adjunct	CPR
Defibrillation	Bleeding Control	Bandaging	(Splinting) Knee splint	(Other) Spinal precautions

Narrative

Arrived to find 25-year-old-female driver of a midsize vehicle that rear ended a vehicle at low speed. The pt states she was wearing her seat belt. Pt denies any injury except for right knee pain. Pt believes her knee struck the lower dash on impact with the front vehicle. Air bags did not deploy. Primary and secondary assessments are within normal limits with the exception of the right knee. The pt has limited ROM but strong pulses in the lower leg and foot. Pt removed from vehicle using spinal precautions and knee splinted. Right leg assessed after splinting and no change noted. Pt transported to regional hospital without incident. Report to RN Sullivan upon arrival. **End of report**

Prep Kit

- Federal Regulation DOT KKK 1822 sets the standards for ambulance design and manufacturing specifications.
- Three body style types are identified:
  - Type I: Conventional, truck-cab chassis with a modular ambulance body that can be transferred to a new chassis as needed
  - Type II: Standard van, forward-control integral cab-body ambulance
  - Type III: Specialty van, forward-control integral cab-body ambulance
- Check the ambulance, including medical equipment and supplies, at the beginning of every shift to ensure that all equipment is available and in good working order.
- Preventive maintenance is just as important as operating skills. Looking for problems before the unit is in motion may prevent breakdowns while you are en route to calls.
- After the call, be sure to clean, disinfect, and restock. Perform a routine inspection to ensure that the ambulance is ready to respond to the next call.
- Learning how to properly operate your vehicle is just as important as learning how to care for patients when you arrive on the scene. The first rule of safe driving in an emergency vehicle is that speed does not save lives; good care does.

- Drivers must be qualified to drive the ambulance, must be physically and emotionally fit, and must have the proper attitude. The driver must know and follow safe driving practices, including wearing a seat belt, using an appropriate speed, using sirens appropriately, and maintaining a cushion of safety.
- All drivers and passengers should use appropriate safety restraints while a vehicle is in motion. Pediatric patients should be secured in devices designed for them.
- Make sure that all equipment is secured before leaving the scene.
- Lights and sirens should be used when you are responding to emergencies but used sparingly when transporting a patient to the hospital.
- Avoid backing up the vehicle if possible. If it is necessary, use a spotter to assist in the procedure. Make sure everyone is clear on where the unit is to be placed and that hand signals used are agreed upon.
- Use extreme caution when you are driving in heavy traffic areas or in rural areas where the roadways themselves may not be suitable for travel with a heavy ambulance. Watch out for other dangers such as animals running onto the roadway.
- Slow down in inclement weather, being aware that the ambulance requires greater travel time and distance to stop properly.

- Any specific exemption from traffic laws does not negate your responsibility to proceed with due regard to prevent ambulance crashes.
- Escorts should not be used due to the danger of motorists not seeing both the ambulance and the escort.
- Air ambulances are used to evacuate medical and trauma patients.
- A medical evacuation is commonly known as a medevac and is generally performed exclusively by helicopters.
- You must follow certain safety rules when you are working around landing zones and helicopters. Be sure that you are familiar with these rules before working any call involving air transport.

Vital Vocabulary

air ambulances Fixed-wing aircraft and helicopters that have been modified for medical care; used to evacuate and transport patients with life-threatening injuries to treatment facilities.

belt noise A chirping or squealing sound, synchronous with engine speed.

blind spots Areas of the road that are blocked from your sight by your own vehicle or mirrors.

brake fade A sensation that an ambulance has lost its power brakes.

brake pull A sensation that, when an operator depresses the brake pedal, the steering wheel is being pulled to the left or the right.

cleaning The process of removing dirt, dust, blood, or other visible contaminants from a surface.

cushion of safety Keeping a safe distance between your vehicle and other vehicles on any side of you.

decontaminate To remove or neutralize radiation, chemical, or other hazardous material from clothing, equipment, vehicles, and personnel.

disinfection The killing of pathogenic agents by direct application of chemicals.

DOT KKK 1822 Federal standards that regulate the design and manufacturing guidelines of emergency ambulances.

drift A finding that when the operator lets go of the steering wheel, a vehicle consistently wanders left or right.

due regard Driving with awareness and responsibility for other drivers on the roadways when you are operating an ambulance in the emergency mode, and making sure that other drivers are aware of your approach.

heavy-duty ambulance Extra heavy-duty vehicle.

high-level disinfection The killing of pathogenic agents by using potent means of disinfection.

hydroplaning A condition in which the tires of a vehicle may be lifted off the road surface as water "piles up" under them, making the vehicle feel as though it is floating.

landing zone Designated location for the landing of air ambulances.

medevac Medical evacuation of a patient by helicopter.

peak loads A time of day or day or week in which the call volume is at its highest.

posting The placement of an ambulance at a specific geographic location in order to cover larger areas of territory and reduce response times.

spotter A person who assists a driver in backing up an ambulance to compensate for blind spots at the back of the vehicle.

steering play A sensation of looseness or sloppiness in a vehicle's steering.

steering pull A drift that is persistent enough that an operator can feel a tug on the steering wheel.

sterilization A process, such as heating, that removes microbial contamination.

strategic deployment The staging of ambulances to strategic locations within a service area to allow for coverage of emergency calls.

Type I ambulance Conventional, truck-cab chassis with a modular ambulance body that can be transferred to a new chassis as needed.

Type II ambulance Standard van, forward-control integral cab-body ambulance.

Type III ambulance Specialty van, forward-control integral cab-body ambulance.

wheel bounce A vibration, synchronous with road speed that can be felt in the steering wheel.

wheel wobble A common finding at low speeds when a vehicle has a bent wheel.

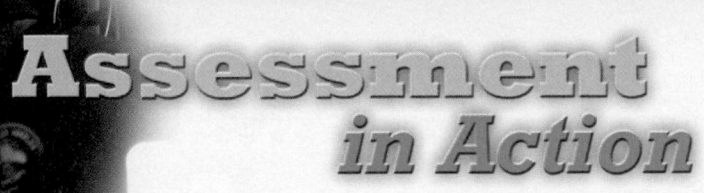
Assessment in Action

You are on scene with a critical trauma patient and are considering whether to transport the patient by ground or by air. You are 20 miles away from the closest trauma center, it is nighttime, and the weather is clear.

1. What is the most important factor in determining whether air transport is warranted?
   A. Weather conditions
   B. Will the difference in time make a difference in patient outcome
   C. Where the air transport vehicle will be starting from
   D. Can the air crew effectively care for the patient in small quarters

2. How does uneven terrain affect safety in a helicopter-landing zone?
   A. Inclines or depressions make it harder to judge rotor blade distance from the ground.
   B. Inclines or depressions make it harder to control the helicopter.
   C. Inclines or depressions make it harder to move the patient to the aircraft.
   D. Inclines or depressions in terrain do not affect a landing zone.

3. What is the recommended size of a standard helicopter landing zone?
   A. 25 ft × 25 ft
   B. 50 ft × 50 ft
   C. 100 ft × 100 ft
   D. 150 ft × 150 ft

4. What is the recommended method of marking a landing zone at night?
   A. Place a vehicle with emergency lights on at each corner of the zone.
   B. Place a single strobe light in the center of the zone.
   C. Place reflective tape at each corner of the zone.
   D. Place one strobe light at each corner of the zone.

5. When is it safe to approach a helicopter?
   A. When the patient care team exits the aircraft
   B. As soon as the helicopter lands
   C. When the rotor blades stop turning
   D. When the pilot signals you to approach

Additional Question

6. What are some standard objects that you have on scene that may interfere with a helicopter's operation?

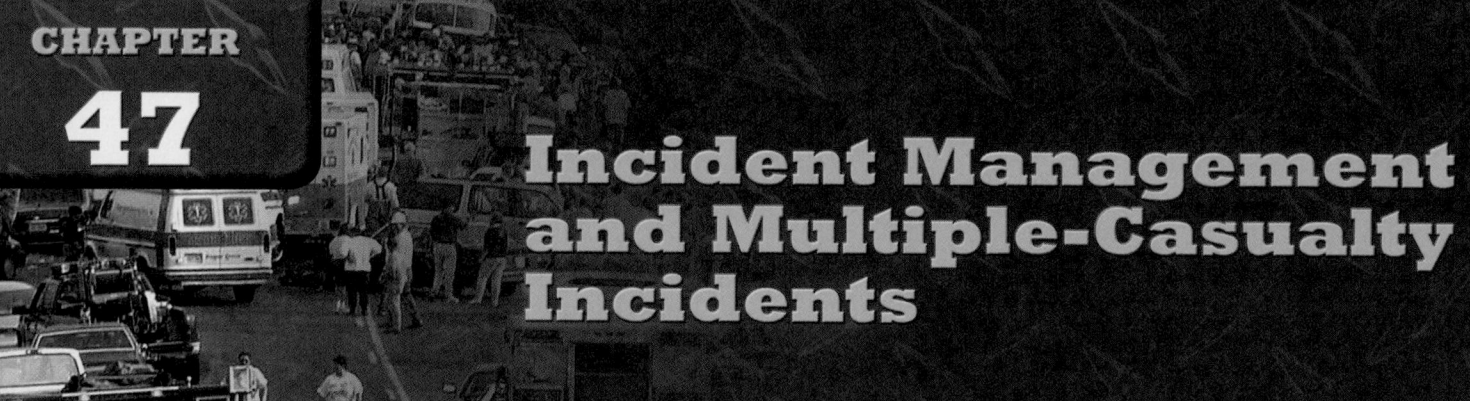

CHAPTER 47

Incident Management and Multiple-Casualty Incidents

National EMS Education Standard Competencies

EMS Operations

Knowledge of operational roles and responsibilities to ensure patient, public, and personnel safety.

Incident Management

Establish and work within the incident management system. (pp 2200-2207)

Multiple-Casualty Incidents

Triage principles (pp 2209-2213)

Resource management (pp 2207-2208)

Triage (pp 2209-2213)

- Performing (pp 2209-2213)
- Retriage (pp 2210-2212)
- Destination decisions (p 2213)
- Posttraumatic and cumulative stress (p 2213)

Knowledge Objectives

1. Explain the federal requirements for the minimum entry-level certifications of paramedics and other emergency personnel in incident command system training. (p 2199)
2. Describe the National Incident Management System (NIMS) and its major components. (pp 2199-2200)
3. Describe the purpose of the incident command system (ICS) and its organizational structure, and explain the role of EMS response within it. (pp 2200-2203)
4. Describe how the ICS assists the EMS in ensuring both personal safety and the safety of bystanders, health care professionals, and patients during an emergency. (pp 2203-2205)
5. Describe the role of the paramedic in establishing command under the ICS. (p 2204)
6. Explain the purpose of medical incident command within the incident management system, and describe its organizational structure within ICS. (pp 2205-2207)
7. Describe the specific conditions that would define a situation as a multiple-casualty incident (MCI) and give some examples. (pp 2207-2208)
8. Describe what occurs during primary and secondary triage, how the four triage categories are assigned to patients on the scene, and how destination decisions regarding triaged patients are made. (pp 2209-2213)
9. Describe how the START and JumpSTART triage methods are performed. (pp 2211-2212)
10. Explain the need for re-triaging of patients during multiple-casualty incidents. (pp 2210-2212)
11. Describe the purpose of critical incident stress management. (p 2213)

Skills Objectives

1. Demonstrate how to perform triage based on a fictitious scenario that involves a multiple-casualty incident. (pp 2199, 2201, 2204, 2210, 2214-2216)

Introduction

The most challenging situations you can be called to are disasters and multiple-casualty incidents (MCIs). These incidents can be overwhelming because you will find a large number of patients and a lack of specialized equipment and/or adequate help. When you respond to an event with a large number of patients, you must use a systematic approach to manage the incident most efficiently. By learning to use the principles of the incident command system (ICS), you will be able to do the greatest good for the greatest number. As a paramedic, you will typically be assigned to work within the EMS/medical branch or group under an ICS, but you may be asked to function in other areas (which will be discussed later in this chapter). To promote more efficient coordination of emergency incidents at the regional, state, and national levels, the National Incident Management System (NIMS) was developed. To reduce on-scene problems and to increase your efficiency, Homeland Security Presidential Directive (HSPD-5) specifies that students are required to complete entry-level certifications in FEMA IS-100 and IS-700 training and have a solid understanding of the basics of NIMS. These certifications can be prerequisites, co-requisites, or part of an entry-level course.

The NIMS

Although most incidents are handled at the local level, the president directed the Secretary of Homeland Security to implement the **National Incident Management System (NIMS)** in March 2004 **Table 1**. Major incidents require the involvement and coordination of multiple jurisdictions, functional agencies, and emergency response disciplines. The NIMS provides a consistent nationwide template to enable federal, state, and local governments, as well as private-sector and nongovernmental organizations, to work together effectively and efficiently. The NIMS is used to prepare for, prevent, respond to, and recover from domestic incidents, regardless of cause, size, or complexity, including acts of catastrophic terrorism and hazardous materials (HazMat) incidents.

Table 1 Development of the National Incident Management System

Year	Development
1973	First FIRESCOPE (FIrefighting RESources of California Organized for Potential Emergencies) technical team is established by the US Forestry and other major California fire departments
1982	Modifications are made to the FIRESCOPE management style, and the NIIMS (National Interagency Incident Management System) is developed
1987	NFPA (National Fire Protection Association) develops *NFPA 1561*–Standard on Fire Department Incident Management System
1990	National Fire Service Incident Management System (IMS) Consortium is created
2003	Homeland Security Presidential Directive (HSPD-5) mandates development of a national incident management system
2004	Homeland Security releases first NIMS training material

Two important underlying principles of the NIMS are flexibility and standardization. The organizational structure must be flexible enough to be rapidly adapted for use in any situation. The NIMS provides standardization in terminology, resource classification, personnel training, certification, and more. Another important feature of the NIMS is the concept of interoperability in which agencies of different types or from different jurisdictions can communicate with each other.

The ICS, which is the focus of this chapter, is one component of the NIMS. The major NIMS components are as follows:

- **Command and management.** The NIMS standardizes incident management for all hazards and across all levels of government. The NIMS standard incident command structures

YOU *are the Medic* PART 1

You have been dispatched to the scene of a motor vehicle crash involving a tour bus that hydroplaned during a recent thunderstorm. You are the first responding rescue/EMS unit to arrive on the scene. There are no identifiable hazards. The crash occurred on the interstate. The bus flipped on its side and is located on the northbound shoulder. Law enforcement personnel have determined that the scene is safe. From inside the ambulance, you see approximately 45 to 50 victims walking around or lying on the ground at the scene.

1. When does an event become a multiple-casualty incident (MCI)?
2. How can you prepare yourself for an MCI?
3. What is the goal of the incident command system?

are based on three key constructs: ICS, multiagency coordination systems, and public information systems.

- **Preparedness.** The NIMS establishes measures for all responders to incorporate into their systems in preparation to respond to all incidents at any time.
- **Resource management.** The NIMS sets up mechanisms to describe, inventory, track, and dispatch resources before, during, and after an incident. The NIMS also defines standard procedures to recover equipment used during the incident.
- **Communications and information management.** Effective communications, information management, and sharing are critical aspects of domestic incident management. The NIMS communications and information systems enable the essential functions needed to provide interoperability.
- **Supporting technologies.** The NIMS promotes national standards and interoperability for supporting technologies to successfully implement the NIMS and standard technologies for professions or incidents. It provides structure for the science and technology used in incident management.
- **Ongoing management and maintenance.** The US Department of Homeland Security will establish a multijurisdictional, multidisciplinary NIMS Integration Center. This center will provide strategic direction for and oversight of the NIMS, supporting routine maintenance and continuous improvement of the system in the long term.

The Incident Command System

It is important for you to be familiar with the terminology and concepts of the **incident command system (ICS)**. As you know, communication is the building block of good patient care. Common terminology and the use of "clear text" communications (plain English as opposed to 10-codes) help responders from multiple agencies work efficiently together.

Using the ICS gives you a modular organizational structure that is built on the size and complexity of the incident. The goal of the ICS is to make the best use of your resources to manage the environment around the incident and to treat patients during an emergency. Make certain to follow your local standard operating procedures for establishing the ICS. The ICS is designed to control duplication of effort and **freelancing**, in which individual units or different organizations make independent and often inefficient decisions about the next appropriate action.

One of the organizing principles of the ICS is limiting the **span of control** of any one person, keeping the supervisor/worker ratio at one supervisor for three to seven workers. A supervisor who finds that his or her effective span of control is exceeded—that is, has more than seven people reporting to him or her—needs to divide tasks and delegate supervision of some tasks to another person.

Organizational divisions may include sections, branches, divisions and groups, and resources **Figure 1**. In some regions, emergency operations centers may exist. The centers are usually operated by city, state, or federal governments. These centers will usually only be activated in a large catastrophic event that may go on for days, that has hundreds of patients, and that taxes the whole system.

The people who will participate in the many tasks in an MCI or a disaster should use the ICS. You should find out from your service if one exists, who is in charge, how it is activated, and what your expected role will be.

Incident Command System Roles and Responsibilities

There are many roles defined in the ICS. The general staff includes command, finance, logistics, operations, and planning roles. It is important for you to understand the specific duties of each and how they work in coordinating the response. **Command** functions include the public information officer (PIO), safety officer, and liaison officer.

Command

The **incident commander (IC)** is the person in charge of the overall incident. The IC will assess the incident, establish the strategic objectives and priorities, and develop a plan to manage the incident **Figure 2**. The number of command duties (public information, safety, and liaison) the IC takes on often varies by the size of the incident. Small incidents often mean the IC will do it all. In an incident of medium size or complexity, the IC may delegate some functions but retain others. For example, at a motor vehicle crash with multiple patients, the IC may designate a safety officer or assign a PIO but maintain responsibility for the other command functions. In a complex situation, the IC may appoint team members to all of the command roles.

Large MCIs, such as a hazardous materials incident, require a multiagency or multijurisdictional response and use of **unified command system**. In this case, plans are drawn up in advance by all cooperating agencies that assume a shared responsibility for decision making and cooperation. The response plan should designate the lead and support agencies in several kinds of

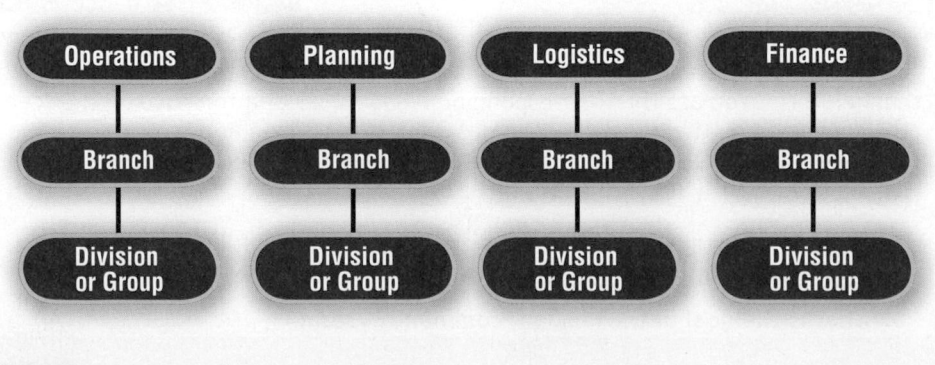

Figure 1 Organizational divisions may include sections, branches, divisions, and groups.

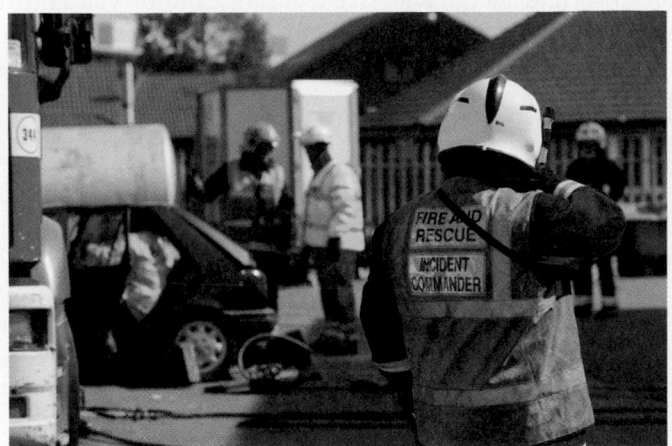

Figure 2 The person in command at an MCI oversees the incident and develops a plan for response.

MCIs. (The HazMat team will take the lead in a chemical leak, for example. However, the medical team might take the lead in a multivehicle car crash.) Agencies bordering each other should practice often with each other to ensure that a unified command system will function well and that communication among the people involved is well established before a real incident occurs.

A **single command system** is one in which one person is in charge, even if multiple agencies respond. It is generally used with incidents in which one agency has the majority of responsibility for incident management. Ideally, it is used for short-duration, limited incidents that require the services of a single agency.

Your IC should be on or near the scene in a clearly identified location, where he or she can easily communicate with all emergency responders operating at the scene. It is important that you know who the IC is, where the command post is located, and how to communicate with your supervisor. If the incident is large, you will be reporting to a supervisor working under the IC. (Remember the rule of span of control? The number of people who can be effectively supervised is between three and seven.) To make the IC easily identifiable, some type of garment can be worn, such as a brightly colored vest emblazoned with the word COMMAND. If the command post is set up in a vehicle, it should be well marked, and you should know its location. Make sure that your supervisor or the IC knows of any plans or operations before they are initiated.

This communication is particularly important if a **transfer of command** takes place. Because an MCI can be ever changing and ever increasing in scope, an IC may turn over command to someone with more experience in a critical area. This change, or transfer of command, must take place in an orderly manner and, if possible, face to face. In extreme situations, it could be done by phone, radio, or e-mail. Your agency should have standard operating procedures (SOPs) that govern the transfer of command. Make certain to follow those SOPs. When an incident draws to a close, there should be a **termination of command**. Your agency should have **demobilization** procedures to implement as the situation de-escalates or comes to an end.

Finance

The **finance** section chief is responsible for documenting all expenditures at an incident for reimbursement. A financial person is not usually needed at smaller incidents, but larger incidents demand keeping track of personnel hours and expenditures for materials and supplies and reporting at meetings of the general staff. Responding agencies and organizations may be eligible for some types of reimbursement after the incident, and an efficient finance section chief will help your agency to succeed in the reimbursement process. Finance personnel should be trained in the process of assessing expenditures with an eye to reimbursement long before an actual event.

YOU *are the Medic* | **PART 2** |

Once incident command has been established, you are assigned the role of triage supervisor. Patient 1 is an unresponsive man who has an obvious closed femur fracture.

Recording Time: 1 Minute	
Appearance	Pale, cool, moist skin
Level of consciousness	U (Unresponsive to verbal or painful stimuli)
Airway	Open
Breathing	Adequate
Circulation	Pulse rapid, weak, and regular

4. How should you triage this patient?

5. What are the four command functions within the incident command system?

6. How many people should be assigned to one supervisor?

The various functions within the finance section are the time unit, the procurement unit, the compensation/claims unit, and the cost unit. The time unit is responsible for ensuring the daily recording of personnel time and equipment use. The procurement unit deals with all matters concerning vendor contracts. The compensation and claims unit has two major purposes: dealing with claims as a result of the incident and injury compensation. Finally, the cost unit is responsible for collecting, analyzing, and reporting the costs related to an incident.

Logistics

The logistics section or section chief has responsibility for communications equipment, facilities, food and water, fuel, lighting, and medical equipment and supplies for patients and emergency responders. Local SOPs will list the medical equipment needed for the incident, depending on the type of incident. **Table 2** lists common MCI equipment and supplies. Logistics personnel are

Table 2	MCI Equipment and Supplies*
Airway control	PPE (gloves, face shield, HEPA or N95 mask)
	Oral airways, nasal airways
	Suction units (manual units)
	Rigid tip Yankauer and flexible suction catheters
	LMA, Combitube, ET tubes*
	Laryngoscope and blades*
	Tube check, tube restraint, tape, syringes, stylet*
	End-tidal CO_2 device
Breathing	Pocket mask and one-way valve
	Bag-mask device(s) (adult and child), spare masks
	Oxygen delivery devices (nonrebreathing mask, cannula, extension tubing)
	Oxygen tank, regulator
	Occlusive dressings
	Large-bore IV catheter for thoracic decompression*
Circulation	Dressings, bandages, tape
	Sphygmomanometer, stethoscope
	Burn dressings, burn sheets, sterile water for irrigation
	One-handed tourniquets
	1,000-mL bags of normal saline, IV start kits, catheters*
Disability	Rigid collars (one size fits all)
	Head beds, wide tape, backboard straps
	Flashlights, spare batteries
Exposure	Space blanket to cover patients
	Scissors
Logistic/ Command	Sector vests (triage, treatment, transport, staging, command, rescue)
	Pads of paper, pencils, pens, markers
	Triage tags or kits used by your regional system
	Assessment cards

Note: The items denoted by * could be packaged in an ALS kit.

trained to find food, shelter, and health care for you and the other responders at the scene of an MCI. In a large incident, it is often necessary for many people to handle logistics, even though only one person will report to the IC.

Operations

At a large incident, the operations section is responsible for managing the tactical operations job usually handled by the IC on routine EMS calls. In a complex incident, however, the IC must coordinate with other agencies and the media, engage in strategic planning, and ensure that logistics are functioning effectively. In these cases, the IC should appoint an operations section chief. The operations section chief will supervise the people working at the scene of the incident, who will be assigned to branches, divisions, and groups. Operations personnel often have experience in management within the fire department.

Planning

The planning section solves problems as they arise during the MCI. Planners obtain data about the problem, analyze the previous incident plan, and predict what or who is needed to make the new plan work. Planners need to work closely with the operations, finance, and, especially, logistics sections. Planners can and should call on technical experts to help with the planning process. Planners will also set out a course for demobilizing the response when needed.

Another function of the planning section is the development of an incident action plan, which is the central tool for planning during a response to a disaster emergency. The incident action plan is prepared by the planning section chief with input from the appropriate sections and units of the incident management team. It should be written at the outset of the response and revised continually throughout the response. In an initial response for an incident that is readily controlled, a written plan may not be necessary. Larger, more complex incidents will require an incident action plan to coordinate activities. The level of detail required in an incident action plan will vary according to the size and complexity of the response.

Command Staff

Three important positions that help the general staff (all staff described previously) and the IC are the safety officer, the PIO, and the liaison officer. The safety officer monitors the scene for conditions or operations that may present a hazard to responders and patients. The safety officer may need to work with environmental health and HazMat specialists. The importance of the safety officer cannot be underestimated—he or she has the authority to stop an emergency operation whenever a rescuer is in danger. A safety officer should remove hazards to paramedics and patients before the hazards cause injury.

The public information officer (PIO) provides the public and media with clear and understandable information. A wise PIO positions his or her headquarters well away from the incident command post and, most important, away from the incident, to minimize distractions. Also, the PIO must keep the media safe and from becoming part of the incident. The designated PIO may work in cooperation with PIOs from other agencies in a joint information center (JIC). In some circumstances, the PIO/JIC may be responsible for disseminating a message designed to help a situation, prevent panic, and provide evacuation directions.

The liaison officer (LNO) relays information and concerns among command, the general staff, and other agencies. If an agency is not represented in the command structure, questions and input should be given through the LNO.

Communications and Information Management

Communication has historically been the weak point at most major incidents. To minimize the effects of communications problems, it is recommended that communications be integrated. This means that all agencies involved should be able to communicate quickly and effortlessly via radios. Communications allow for accountability throughout the incident, as well as instant communication between recipients. As always, and more so during a large incident, it is important to maintain professionalism on all radio communications, remembering to communicate clearly, concisely, and using clear text (no codes).

Mobilization and Deployment

When an incident has been declared and the need for additional resources has been identified, a request is made for additional resources. Once a request is made, these resources are mobilized and deployed to a designated location or staging area. It is important to wait until the request is made, to minimize the potential for freelancing.

Check-in at the Incident

On arrival at an incident, you should check in with the finance section. Checking in accomplishes many different functions. It allows you to be assigned to a supervisor for job tasking and allows for personnel tracking throughout the incident. Checking in also ensures that costs, pay, and reimbursement can be calculated accurately.

Initial Incident Briefing

After the check-in process is complete, you should report to your supervisor for an initial briefing that will allow you to get information regarding the incident, as well as specific job functions and responsibilities.

Incident Record Keeping

Record keeping is important for financial reasons and for documentation purposes. If a large piece of equipment becomes inoperable, it may be possible for replacement costs to come from the incident. Record keeping also allows for tracking of time spent on the actual incident for reimbursement purposes.

Accountability

Because of the large number of responders at a large incident, accountability is important. Accountability means keeping your supervisor advised of your location, actions, and completed tasks. It also includes advising your supervisor of the tasks that you have been unable to complete and what tools you need to complete them.

Incident Demobilization

Once the incident has been stabilized and all of the hazards mitigated, the IC will determine which resources are needed or not needed and when to begin demobilization. This process allows for an expeditious return of resources to their parent organizations to be placed back in service.

EMS Response Within the Incident Command System

Preparedness

Preparedness involves the decisions made and basic planning done before an incident occurs. Every area can experience natural disasters, such as hurricanes, tornadoes, earthquakes, or wildfires. Therefore, preparedness in a given area would involve decisions and planning about the most likely natural disasters for the area, among other disasters.

Your EMS agency should have written disaster plans that you are regularly trained to carry out. A copy of the disaster plan should be kept in each EMS vehicle. EMS facilities should have disaster supplies for at least a 72-hour period of self-sufficiency. Your EMS service should have mutual aid agreements with surrounding organizations so that requests for help can be expedited in an emergency. All groups with mutual aid agreements should practice using the plans frequently. Practice with mock incidents involving 10 to 15 patients on a regular basis, rather than practicing a 100-patient incident every few years. Organizations should share a list of resources with each other so they will know early on what they can access. Also, your local EMS organizations should develop an assistance program for the families of EMS responders. If EMS responders have concerns about their families during a disaster, their effectiveness on the job could be diminished.

Of course, you should have a personal disaster plan for your family. Families need to be prepared and know what to expect should you be required to be a disaster responder. You should be up-to-date on immunizations for influenza, hepatitis A and B, and tetanus.

Scene Size-up

Remember that sizing up a scene starts with dispatch. If dispatch information indicates a possible unsafe scene, you should stay away from the scene or get only close enough to make an assessment without putting yourself in harm's way. When you arrive first on the scene of an MCI, you will perform a size-up and make some preliminary decisions. The size-up will be driven by three basic questions that responders must ask themselves:

- What do I have?
- What do I need to do?
- What resources do I need?

These questions have a symbiotic relationship. The answer from one helps answer the others, and each represents a piece to the puzzle. Work as team when you answer these questions because overlooking just one safety issue early on can start a chain of problems.

What Do I Have?

Start with scene safety. First, assess for hazards. Warn all other responders about hazardous materials, fuel spills, electrical hazards, or other safety concerns as soon as possible. Confirm the incident location. Establish whether the incident is open or closed. Estimate the number of casualties. Your immediate report to dispatch would be "Paramedic unit number one arriving on scene, multiple vehicles involved, full road blockage, no apparent hazards at this time. Paramedic unit number one is assuming command."

What Do I Need to Do?

You should keep the following priorities in mind:

- Safety
- Incident stabilization
- Preservation of property and the environment

You need to consider these priorities in the order they are given. Safety is paramount. Safety includes your life, your partner's life, and other rescuers' lives. Then, consider the safety of the patient and any bystanders. This will be difficult for anyone dedicated to saving lives, but it is important to put yourself and your partner first—you have the skills, and bystanders usually do not; the situation can be far worse if you do not put yourself first. Often, if a responder is injured, other responders will focus on "their own," removing available resources from the incident.

You may have to initially work to isolate or stabilize the incident before providing care to injured persons. This is another difficult concept for all emergency workers. Remember, you cannot help the injured if the scene is unstable. An unstable scene can lead to an injured paramedic.

What Do I Need?

Decide what resources are needed. You may need more EMS responders, ambulances, or other forms of transportation. If extrication is required, a rescue unit and fire department response may be needed. If there are hazardous materials issues, get a HazMat team immediately. Many large EMS systems deploy specialized MCI units or mobile emergency room vehicles that are able to treat dozens of patients on the scene **Figure 3**.

■ Establishing Command

Once you have performed a good scene size-up and answered the three basic questions, command should be established, notification to other responders should go out, and necessary resources should be requested. A command system ensures that resources are effectively and efficiently coordinated. Command must be established early, preferably by the first-arriving, most experienced public safety official. These officials may include police, fire, or EMS personnel.

■ Communications

Communications is often the key problem at an MCI or a disaster. The infrastructure can be damaged, or communications

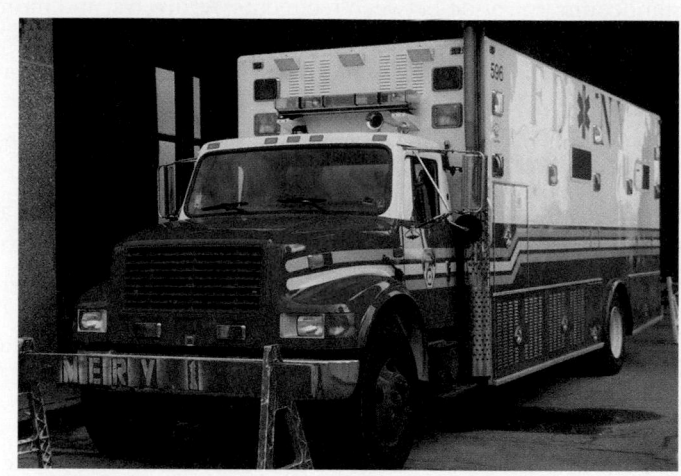

Figure 3 This mobile emergency room is staffed by EMTs, paramedics, and physicians who are able to provide advanced life support to multiple patients simultaneously on the scene of an MCI.

YOU are the Medic | PART 3

An elderly woman is walking toward you holding a cloth over a laceration on her forehead. You observe minimal venous bleeding.

Recording Time: 4 Minutes	
Appearance	Pink, warm, dry skin
Level of consciousness	Alert (oriented to person, place, and day)
Airway	Open
Breathing	Normal, adequate depth, nonlabored
Circulation	Radial pulse is normal, strong, and regular

7. How should you triage this patient?

8. What is the difference between primary and secondary triage?

Words of Wisdom

Participating in a simulated table-top MCI can help you better understand how command is established, how the scene is assessed, how scene objectives are determined, how an incident plan is created, how resources are requested, when ICS needs to expand, how communication is coordinated, and how EMS works with other agencies during a large emergency.

capabilities can be overwhelmed. If possible, use face-to-face communications to limit radio traffic. Some organizations responding to a disaster might not know how to use a radio. If you communicate via radio, do not use codes or signals. Most communications problems should be worked out before a disaster happens by designating channels strictly for command during a disaster. Whatever form of communications equipment is used, it is imperative that it is reliable, durable, and field-tested, and that there are backups in place if the primary communications system does not work. Some regions have mobile self-contained communications centers, whereas others use local radio groups such as HAM radio operators to assist with communications. Most important, your plan should include a "Plan B" in case of communications failure.

◾ Medical Incident Command

What has traditionally been referred to as **medical incident command** is also known as the medical (or EMS) branch of the ICS Figure 4. At incidents that have a significant medical factor, the IC should appoint someone as the medical branch director. This person will supervise the primary roles of the medical group—triage, treatment, and transport of the injured. The medical branch director should help ensure that EMS units responding to the scene are working within the ICS, each medical unit receives a clear assignment before beginning work at the scene, and personnel remain with their vehicle in the staging area until they are assigned their duties. Depending on the scale of the incident, EMS may be a branch or may fall under the logistics section as a unit.

◾ Triage Supervisor

The **triage supervisor** is ultimately in charge of counting and prioritizing patients. During large incidents, a number of triage personnel may be needed Figure 5. The primary duty of the triage unit is to ensure that every patient receives initial assessment of his or her condition. Paramedics doing triage will help move patients to the appropriate treatment sector. One of the most difficult parts of being a triage supervisor is that you must not begin treatment until all patients are triaged, or you will compromise your triage efforts.

◾ Treatment Supervisor

The **treatment supervisor** will locate and set up the treatment area with a tier for each priority of patient. Treatment supervisors ensure that secondary triage of patients is performed and that adequate patient care is given as resources allow. Treatment supervisors also have a responsibility to assist with moving patients to the transportation area. As treatment supervisors supervise the responders, they must communicate with the medical group leaders to request sufficient quantities of supplies, including bandages, burn supplies, airway and respiratory supplies, and patient packaging equipment.

◾ Transportation Supervisor

The **transportation supervisor** coordinates the transportation and distribution of patients to appropriate receiving hospitals. Transportation requires coordination with incident command to help ensure that enough personnel and ambulances are in staging

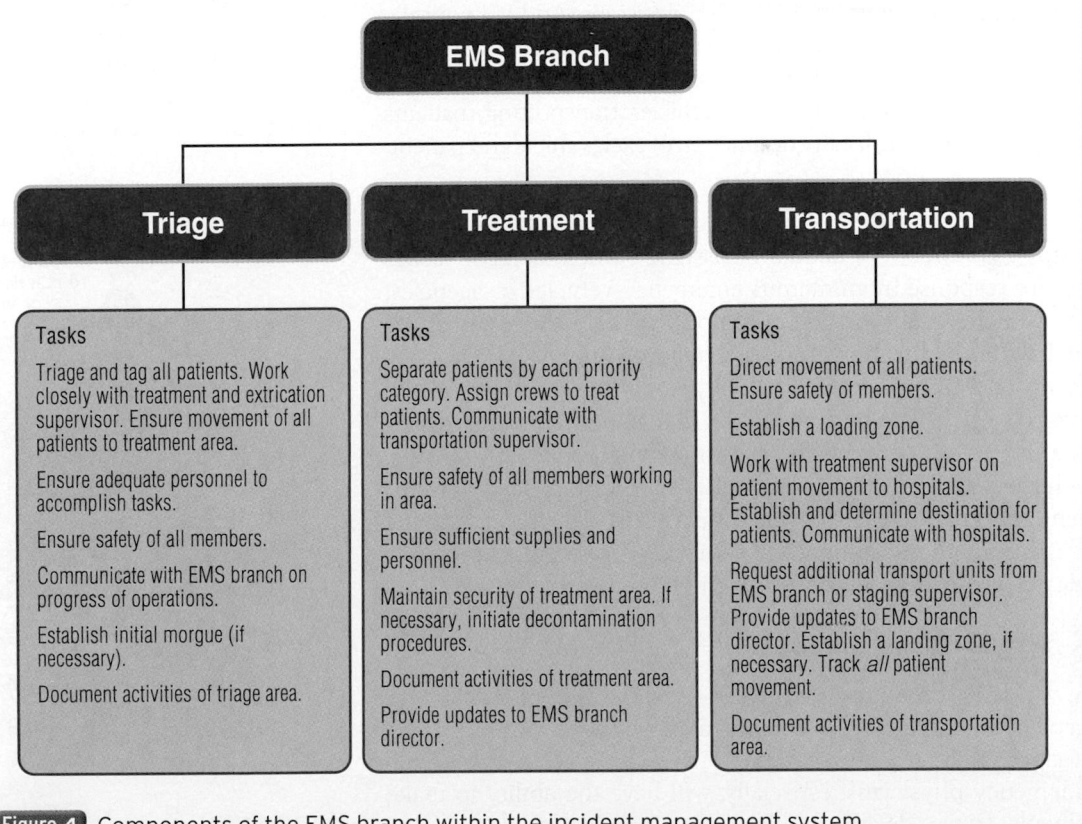

EMS Branch

Triage	Treatment	Transportation
Tasks	**Tasks**	**Tasks**
Triage and tag all patients. Work closely with treatment and extrication supervisor. Ensure movement of all patients to treatment area.	Separate patients by each priority category. Assign crews to treat patients. Communicate with transportation supervisor.	Direct movement of all patients. Ensure safety of members.
Ensure adequate personnel to accomplish tasks.	Ensure safety of all members working in area.	Establish a loading zone.
Ensure safety of all members.	Ensure sufficient supplies and personnel.	Work with treatment supervisor on patient movement to hospitals. Establish and determine destination for patients. Communicate with hospitals.
Communicate with EMS branch on progress of operations.	Maintain security of treatment area. If necessary, initiate decontamination procedures.	Request additional transport units from EMS branch or staging supervisor. Provide updates to EMS branch director. Establish a landing zone, if necessary. Track *all* patient movement.
Establish initial morgue (if necessary).	Document activities of treatment area.	
Document activities of triage area.	Provide updates to EMS branch director.	Document activities of transportation area.

Figure 4 Components of the EMS branch within the incident management system.

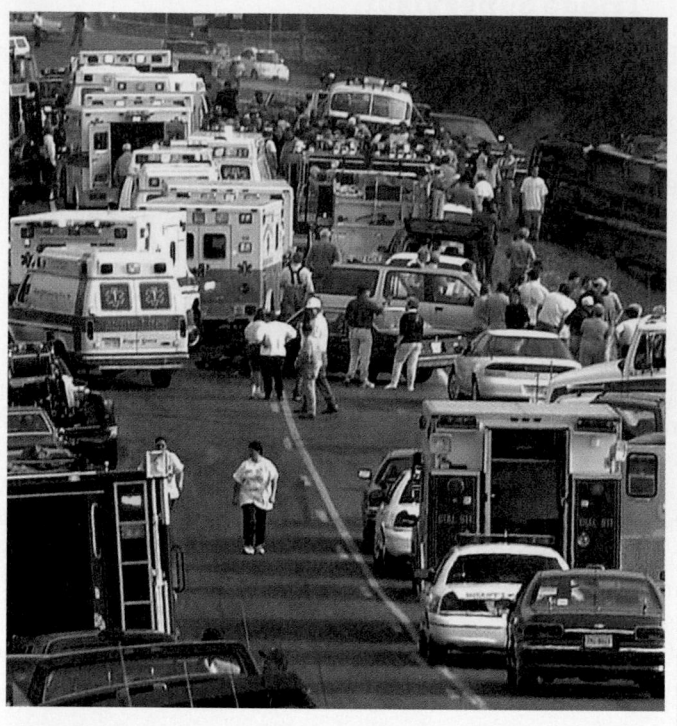

Figure 5 MCIs require triage.

or have been requested. A key role of the transportation supervisor is to communicate with the area hospitals to help determine where to transport the patients. Some regions may have planned for a designated hospital within a region to perform the coordination between hospitals on destination decisions. An MCI typically disrupts the everyday functioning of the region's trauma system, so good coordination is needed. The transportation supervisor documents and tracks the number of vehicles transporting, patients transported, and the facility destination of each vehicle and patient.

Staging Supervisor

A staging supervisor should be assigned when MCIs or scenes require response by numerous emergency vehicles or agencies. The vehicles cannot and should not drive into the scene of the MCI without direction from the staging supervisor. The staging area should be established away from the scene because the parked vehicles can be in the way. The staging supervisor locates an area to stage equipment and responders, tracks unit arrivals, and sends out vehicles as needed. This position plans for efficient access and exit from the disaster site and prevents traffic congestion among responding vehicles. The staging supervisor releases vehicles and supplies when ordered by command.

Physicians on Scene

In an MCI, some areas have plans in place for physicians on scene. Sometimes, even without a plan, the enormity of the situation may require that physicians be sent to the scene. Emergency physicians, especially, will have the ability to make difficult triage decisions. They also provide secondary triage decisions in the treatment sector, deciding which priority patients are to be transported first. Physicians can provide on-scene medical direction for paramedics, and they can provide care in the treatment sector as appropriate.

Rehabilitation Supervisor

In disasters or situations that will last for extended periods, a rehabilitation section for the responders should be established. The rehabilitation supervisor should establish an area that provides protection for responders from the elements and the situation. The rehabilitation area should be located away from exhaust fumes and crowds (especially members of the media) and out of view of the scene itself. Rehabilitation is where a responder's needs for rest, fluids, food, and protection from the elements are met **Figure 6**. The rehabilitation supervisor must also monitor responders for signs of stress. These signs may include fatigue, altered thinking patterns, and complete collapse. You should remember that all EMS personnel should be responsible to be aware of signs of stress. Your service might consider having a defusing or debriefing team in this area. Responders should be encouraged to take advantage of these services but should never be forced to participate.

Extrication and Special Rescue

Some disasters require search and rescue or extrication of patients **Figure 7**. An extrication supervisor or rescue supervisor may need to be appointed. These supervisors determine the type of equipment and resources needed for the situation. In some incidents, victims may need to be extricated or rescued before they can be triaged and treated. Because extrication and rescue are medically complex, the supervisors will usually function under the EMS branch of the ICS. The extrication and rescue supervisors identify the special equipment and personnel needed for the rescue. Extrication and rescue can be dangerous, so crew safety is of utmost importance.

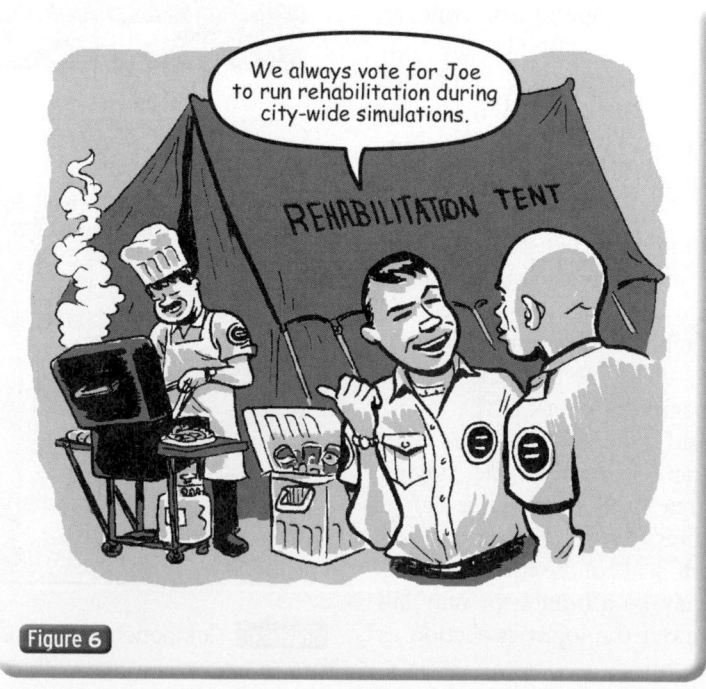

Figure 6

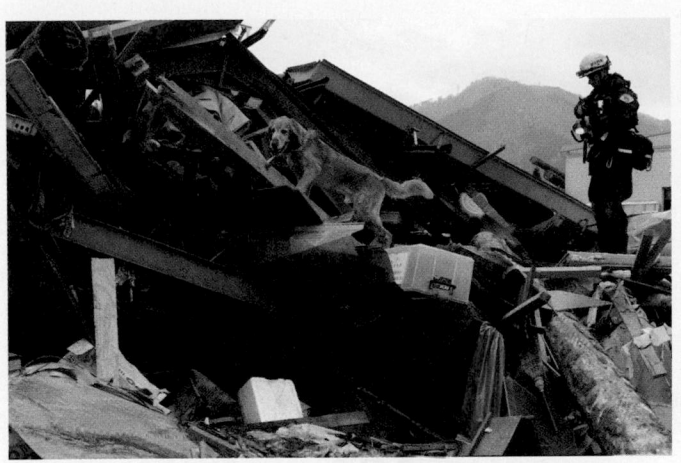

Figure 7 Some disasters will involve search and rescue or extrication.

Words of Wisdom

MCIs and disasters take a physical and emotional toll on emergency responders. Make certain that you are medically evaluated if you have been injured, come into contact with any hazardous substance, or inhale any dust, fumes, or smoke. Often, the health effects of such exposures do not manifest for years and are difficult to link to a particular event. Also, be aware of signs of stress in yourself and in your coworkers. Consider using the opportunity for stress debriefing after an incident.

Morgue Supervisor

In some disasters, there will be many dead patients. The **morgue supervisor** will work with area medical examiners, coroners, disaster mortuary assistance teams, and law enforcement agencies to coordinate removal of the bodies and even, possibly, body parts. The morgue supervisor should attempt to leave the dead victims in the location found, if possible, until a removal and storage plan can be determined. The location of victims may help in the identification of the dead victims in multiple-fatality situations, or there may be crime scene considerations. If it is determined that a morgue area is needed, the morgue supervisor should ensure that the morgue is out of view of the living patients and other responders because the psychological impact could worsen the situation, and that the morgue is secure from the public to prevent theft of any personal effects of the dead victims.

Multiple-Casualty Incidents

In this text, a **multiple-casualty incident (MCI)** refers to any call that involves three or more patients, any situation that places such a great demand on available equipment or personnel that

the system would require a **mutual aid response** (an agreement between neighboring EMS systems to respond to MCIs or disasters in each other's region when local resources are insufficient to handle the response), or any incident that has the potential to create one of the previously mentioned situations **Figure 8**. Bus or train crashes and earthquakes are obvious examples of MCIs. However, other causes of MCIs are far more common than such disasters and are usually much smaller in scope. **Figure 9** is a diagrammed example of a residential building fire confined to one apartment that may only produce one patient but that has the potential to generate dozens of patients from among the rescuers and residents. Loss of power to a hospital or nursing home with ventilator-dependent and nonambulatory victims is considered an MCI, although no one is injured.

Your response to MCIs will differ depending on the area of land covered by the incident, the location, and how spread out your patients are. You should be able to recognize an MCI as an open (uncontained) incident or a closed (contained) incident. An **open incident** has a number of casualties not yet located when you answer the initial call. Rescuers may have to search for patients and then triage or treat them in multiple locations. There also may be an ongoing situation that produces more patients while you are at the scene—for example, school shootings, tornadoes, a hazardous materials release, or rising floodwaters.

A **closed incident** is a situation that is not expected to produce more patients than initially present. The patients can be triaged and treated as they are removed. Although a closed incident is often easier to handle, a closed incident may suddenly become an open incident.

Communities may establish different standards for what constitutes an MCI or for when to implement the ICS, but experience with previous MCIs is helpful in making the determination as well. Agencies and jurisdictions that regularly use the

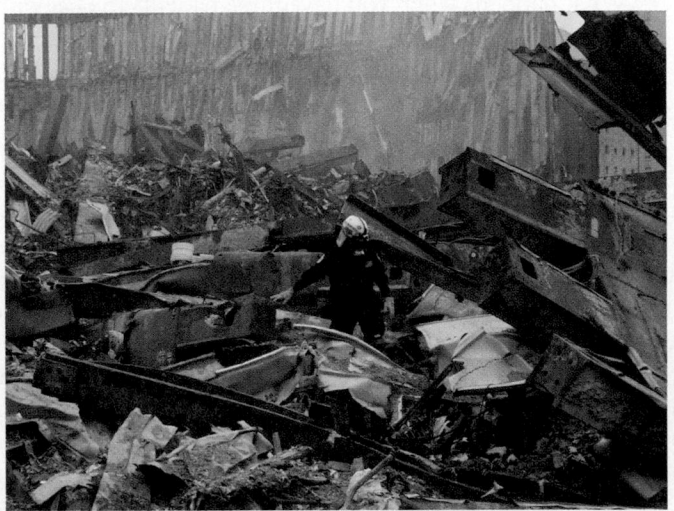

Figure 8 In large MCIs, such as the attack on September 11, 2001, mutual aid may be necessary from a large number of additional jurisdictions.

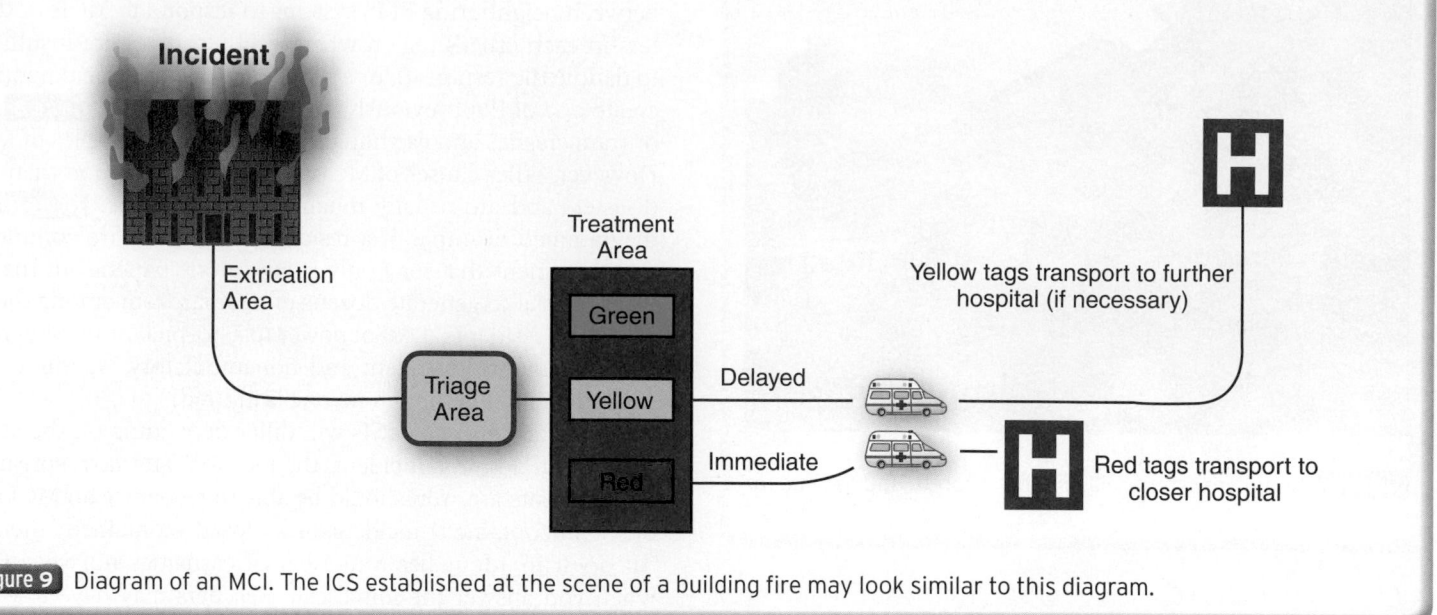

Figure 9 Diagram of an MCI. The ICS established at the scene of a building fire may look similar to this diagram.

ICS will gain valuable experience and will be better prepared to respond to an MCI or a disaster. You can make significant contributions to the safety of your community by participating in disaster planning drills, table-top MCI exercises, and other ICS training opportunities. By using the ICS and the NIMS and understanding the various roles and responsibilities of each position, the responders and/or IC can manage the incident in a smooth, organized manner.

All systems have different protocols for when to declare an MCI and initiate the ICS; however, as a paramedic, ask yourself the following questions when you are considering whether the call is an MCI:

- How many seriously injured or ill patients can you care for effectively and transport in your ambulance? One? Two?
- What happens when you have three patients to deal with?
- How long will it take for additional help to arrive?
- What do you do when a school bus crashes, resulting in eight critically injured patients, and you have only three ambulances available?

Obviously, you and your team cannot treat and transport all injured patients at the same time. At an MCI, you will often experience an increased demand for equipment and personnel. For example, you may realize that you are the only ambulance crew currently at the scene and there is a wait of 15 or more minutes before the next ambulance arrives. You should never leave the scene with patients who are loaded if there are still other patients present who are sick or wounded. This would leave patients at the scene without medical care and can be considered abandonment. If there are multiple patients and not enough resources to handle them without abandoning victims, you should declare an MCI (at least for the present time), request additional resources, and initiate the ICS and triage procedures (described later) **Figure 10** . Although this may cause some delay in initiating treatment to all patients, it will not adversely affect the patient care.

Always follow your local protocol. Many large EMS systems deploy specialized MCI units or mobile emergency room vehicles that are able to treat dozens of patients on the scene.

Words of Wisdom

The terminology used to describe an incident with multiple patients varies in different communities. Many communities use the term multiple-casualty incident to describe an emergency that involves more than one patient and the term mass-casualty incident to describe larger scale events, such as those with more than 20 patients. In this text, the term multiple-casualty incident is used to describe any call that involves three or more patients or a situation that overwhelms your available resources.

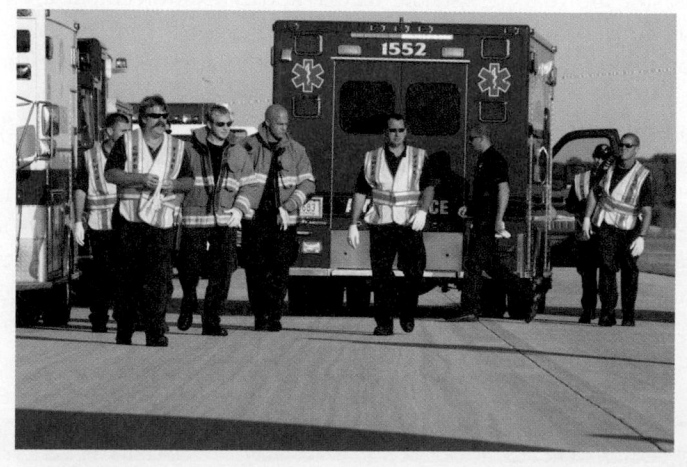

Figure 10 MCIs require additional ambulances and EMS providers from the immediate region.

■ Triage

Triage simply means "to sort" your patients based on the severity of their injuries Figure 11 . The goal of doing the greatest good for the greatest number means that the triage assessment is brief and the patient condition categories are basic. Primary triage is the initial triage done in the field, whereas secondary triage is done as patients are brought to the treatment area. During primary triage, patients are briefly assessed and then identified in some way, such as by attaching a triage tag. The main information needed on the tag is a unique number and a triage category. Rapid and accurate triage will help bring order to the chaos of the MCI scene. After the primary triage, the team leader should communicate the following information to the medical branch director:

- The total number of patients
- The number of patients in each of the triage categories
- Recommendations for extrication and movement of patients to the treatment area
- Resources needed to complete triage and begin movement of patients

When the initial triage has been completed, secondary triage, or retriage, can occur, allowing you to reassess all remaining patients and to upgrade or downgrade the triage category, as appropriate. Patient condition may change rapidly and with little warning; what may have appeared to be a delayed category initially could change to an immediate need, or even an expectant level, before transportation can be arranged. Frequent reevaluations of your triaged patients can help you identify these changes. Depending on your resources and available personnel, retriaging of patients should be performed as frequently as

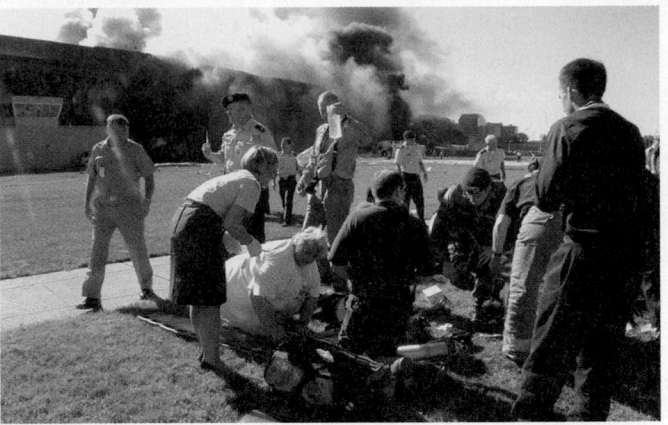

Figure 11 Triage is the process of sorting and prioritizing patients based on severity of conditions.

possible. In smaller MCI events, this step may not be necessary if enough resources have arrived on the scene at this point.

■ Triage Categories

There are four common triage categories. They can be remembered using the mnemonic IDME, which stands for Immediate (red), Delayed (yellow), Minimal (green; hold), and Expectant (black; likely to die or dead) Table 3 . This is the order of priority for treatment and transport of the patients at an MCI.

Immediate (red-tag) patients are your first priority. They will need immediate care and transport. They usually have problems with the ABCs, head trauma, or signs and symptoms of shock.

Table 3 Triage Priorities		
Triage Category	**Patient Description**	**Typical Injuries**
Red Tag: First Priority (immediate)	Patients who need immediate care and transport. Treat these patients first, and transport as soon as possible.	■ Airway and breathing difficulties ■ Uncontrolled or severe bleeding ■ Severe medical problems ■ Decreased mental status ■ Signs of shock (hypoperfusion) ■ Severe burns ■ Open chest or abdominal injuries
Yellow Tag: Second Priority (delayed)	Patients whose treatment and transport can be temporarily delayed.	■ Burns without airway problems ■ Major or multiple bone or joint injuries ■ Back injuries with or without spinal cord damage
Green Tag: Third Priority (walking wounded)	Patients who require minimal or no treatment and transportation can be delayed until last.	■ Minor fractures ■ Minor soft-tissue injuries
Black Tag: Fourth Priority (expectant; some areas call this Priority Zero)	Patients who are already dead or have little chance for survival. Treat salvageable patients before treating these patients.	■ Obvious death ■ Obviously nonsurvivable injury, such as major open brain trauma ■ Respiratory arrest (if limited resources) ■ Cardiac arrest

Delayed (yellow-tag) patients are the second priority and will need treatment and transport, but it can be delayed. Patients usually have multiple injuries to bones or joints, including back injuries with or without spinal cord injury.

Minimal (green-tag) patients are the third priority. Patients may require no field or only "minimal" treatment. In some parts of the world, this is the hold category. These patients are the "walking wounded" at the scene. If they have any apparent injuries, they are usually soft-tissue injuries such as contusions, abrasions, and lacerations.

The last priority is the expectant (black-tag) patients, who are dead or whose injuries are so severe that they have, at best, a minimal chance of survival. This category may include patients who are in cardiac arrest or who have an open head injury, for example. If you have limited resources, this category may also include patients in respiratory arrest. Patients in this category receive treatment and transport only after patients in the other three categories have received care.

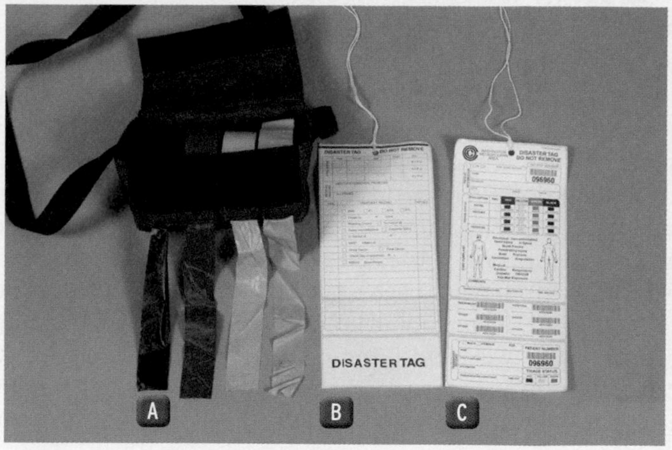

Figure 12 Triage tags (from left to right). **A.** Waterproof weapons of mass destruction tags. **B.** Back. **C.** Front.

Triage Tags

Whatever triage system is used, it is vital that a patient has a tag or some type of label. Tagging patients early assists in tracking them and can help keep an accurate record of their condition. Triage tags should be weatherproof and easily read **Figure 12**. The patient tags or tape should be color-coded and should clearly show the category of the patients. The combined use of symbols and colors to indicate the triage categories is important; in some cases rescuers are color blind.

The tags will become part of the patient's medical record. Most have a tear-off receipt with a number correlating with the number on the tag. When torn off by the transportation supervisor, it will assist him or her in tracking a patient. If the patient is unresponsive and cannot be identified at the scene, the tag will be an identifier for tracking purposes. Some areas use digital photography of patients to assist in later identification.

The photo is catalogued with the patient's tag number, and the patient's location is tracked with this. When family members are brought to crisis centers to help locate loved ones, the pictures may be of assistance. This technique has been used quite effectively in Europe and Israel with Polaroid and digital pictures. Another way of tracking and accounting for patients is to only issue 20 to 25 cards or tags at a time with a score card to mark how patients are triaged and their priority. When the responder returns for more tags, the scorecard will provide a patient count to help command and the staff develop a plan to respond and ensure that appropriate resources are available or summoned. Whatever labeling system is used, it is imperative for the transportation supervisor to be able to identify which patient went by which unit and to which destination, as well as the priority of the patient's condition.

YOU *are the Medic* | PART 4

A man reports not being able to feel or move his legs. He is currently pinned under debris.

Recording Time: 7 Minutes	
Appearance	Pale, warm, dry skin
Level of consciousness	Alert (oriented to person, place, and day)
Airway	Open
Breathing	Rapid and deep
Circulation	Radial pulses are slow and regular

9. How should you triage this patient?

10. What are the four common triage categories?

START Triage

START triage is one of the easiest methods of triage **Figure 13**. START stands for Simple Triage And Rapid Treatment. The staff members at Hoag Memorial Hospital, Newport Beach, CA, are responsible for developing this method of triage. It is easily mastered with practice and will give you the ability to rapidly categorize patients at an MCI. START triage uses a limited assessment of the patient's ability to walk, respiratory status, hemodynamic status, and neurologic status.

The first step of the START triage system is performed on arrival at the scene by calling out to the disaster site, "If you can hear my voice and are able to walk . . . " and then directing patients to an easily identifiable landmark. The injured persons in this group are the "walking wounded" and are considered minimal priority, or third-priority patients.

The second step in the START process is directed toward nonwalking patients. You move to the first nonambulatory patient and assess the respiratory status. If the patient is not breathing, you should open the airway by using a simple manual

Words of Wisdom

Another triage method is the Sort, Assess, Lifesaving interventions, and Treatment and/or Transport (SALT) triage system. This triage system begins by using a global sorting of patients. This first step identifies the patients who are able to understand verbal instructions and are therefore likely to have good perfusion. These patients are given a collection point to move to for further instructions. This is an attempt to decrease the number of patients leaving the scene and overwhelming local hospital resources before EMS can begin to move highest priority patients.

The SALT method differs from others in its lifesaving intervention steps, which include bleeding control, opening the airway, two rescue breaths for children, needle decompression for tension pneumothorax, and auto-injector antidotes. The START method uses respirations, pulse, and neurologic status to assign priority.

maneuver. A patient who still does not begin to breathe is triaged as expectant (black). If the patient begins to breathe, tag him or her as immediate (red) and place in the recovery position and move on to the next patient.

If the patient is breathing, a quick estimation of the respiratory rate should be made. A patient who is breathing faster than 30 breaths/min is triaged as an immediate priority (red). If the patient is breathing fewer than 30 breaths/min, move to the next step of the assessment.

The next step is to assess the hemodynamic status of the patient by checking for a radial pulse. An absent radial pulse implies the patient is hypotensive and should be triaged as an immediate priority. If the radial pulse is present, go to the next assessment.

The final assessment in START triage is to assess the patient's neurologic status, which simply means to assess the patient's ability to follow simple commands such as, "show me three fingers." This assessment establishes that the patient can understand

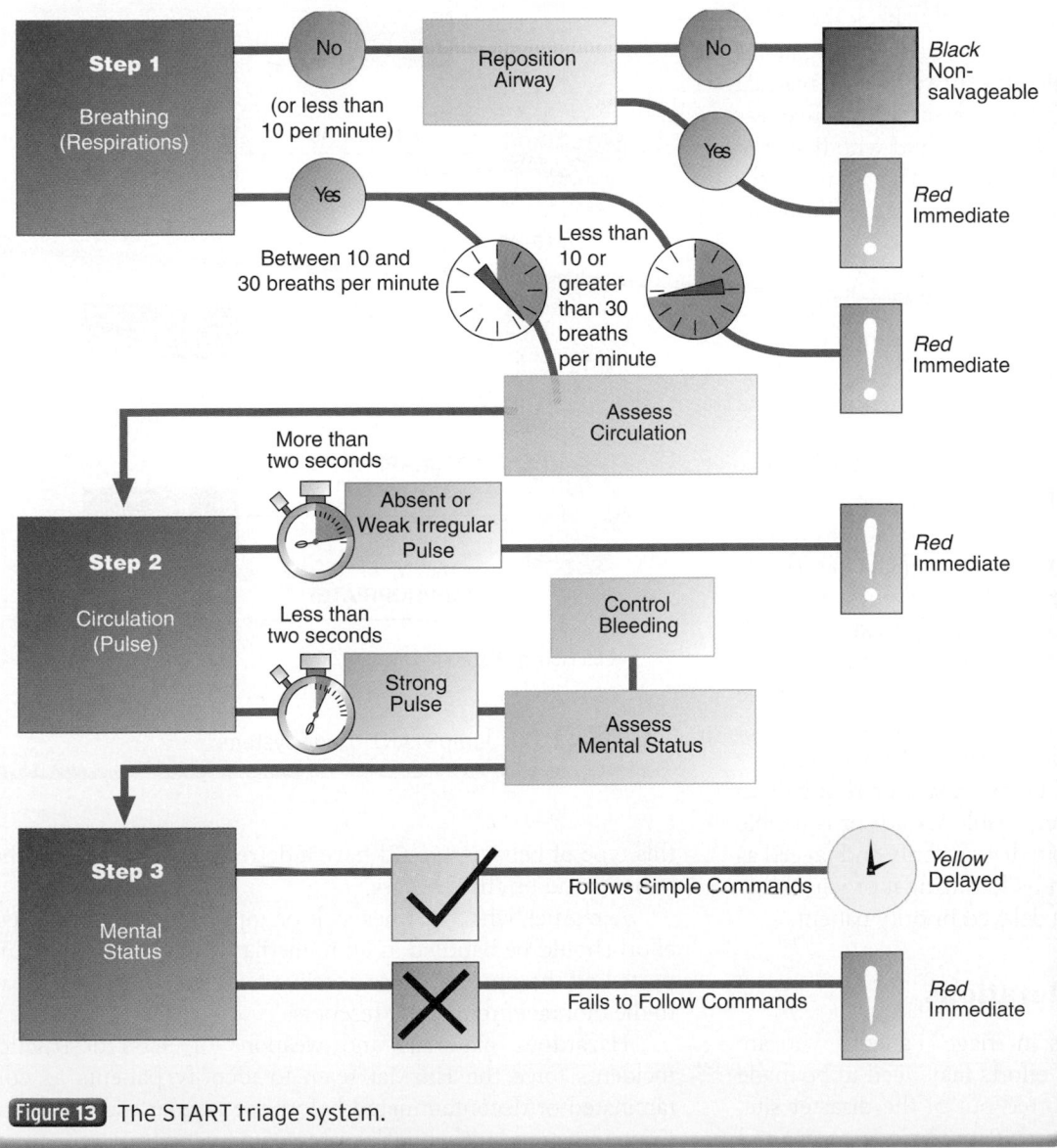

Figure 13 The START triage system.

and follow commands. A patient who is unresponsive or cannot follow simple commands is an immediate priority patient. A patient who complies with a simple command should be triaged in the delayed category.

JumpSTART Triage for Pediatric Patients

Lou Romig, MD, recognized that the START triage system does not take into account the physiologic and developmental differences of pediatric patients **Figure 14**. She developed the **JumpSTART triage** system for pediatric patients. JumpSTART is intended for use in children younger than 8 years or who appear to weigh less than 100 pounds. As in START, the JumpSTART system begins by identifying the walking wounded. Infants or children not developed enough to walk or follow commands (including children with special needs) should be taken as soon as possible to the treatment sector for immediate secondary triage. This action assists in getting children who cannot take care of their own basic needs into a caregiver's hands.

There are several differences within the respiratory status assessment compared with that in START. First, if you find that a pediatric patient is not breathing, immediately check the pulse. If there is no pulse, label the patient as expectant. If the patient is not breathing but has a pulse, open the airway with a manual maneuver. If the patient does not begin to breathe, give five rescue breaths and check respirations again. A child who does not begin to breathe should be labeled expectant. The primary reason for this difference is that the most common cause of cardiac arrest in children is respiratory arrest.

The next step of the JumpSTART process is to assess the approximate rate of respirations. A patient who is breathing fewer than 15 breaths/min or more than 45 breaths/min is tagged as immediate priority and you move on to the next patient. If the respirations are within the range of 15 to 45 breaths/min, the patient is assessed further.

The next assessment in JumpSTART triage is also the hemodynamic status of the patient. Just like in START, you are simply checking for a distal pulse. This does not need to be the brachial pulse; assess the pulse that you feel the most competent and comfortable checking. If there is an absence of a distal pulse, label the child as an immediate priority and move to the next patient. If the child has a distal pulse, move on to the next assessment.

The final assessment is for neurologic status. Because of the developmental differences in children, their responses will vary. For JumpSTART, a modified AVPU (Alert, Verbal, Pain, Unresponsive) score is used. A child who is unresponsive or responds to pain by posturing or with incomprehensible sounds or is unable to localize pain is considered an immediate priority and tagged as such. A child who responds to pain by localizing it or withdrawing from it or is alert is considered a delayed priority patient.

Triage Special Considerations

There are a few special situations in triage. Patients who are hysterical and disruptive to rescue efforts may need to be made an immediate priority and transported out of the disaster site, even if they are not seriously injured. Panic breeds panic, and

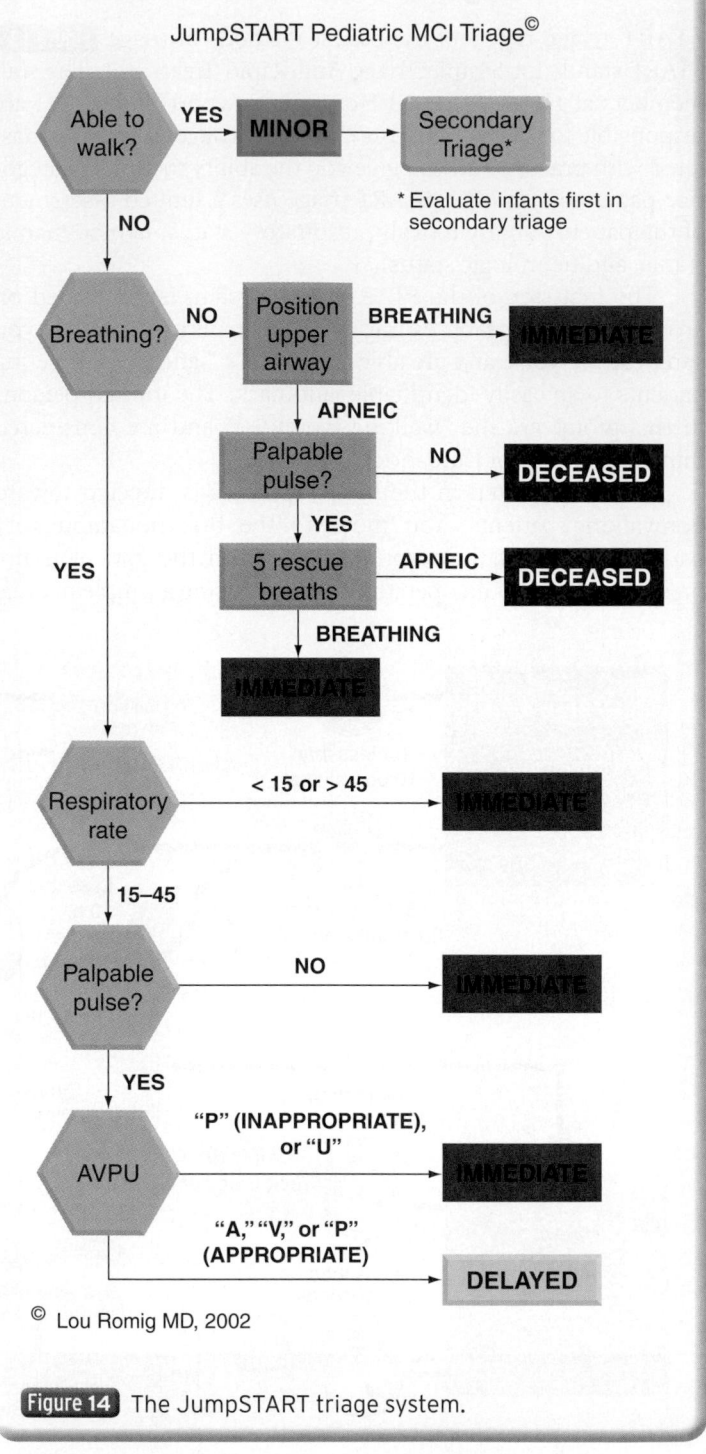

Figure 14 The JumpSTART triage system.

this type of behavior could have a detrimental impact on other patients and on the rescuers.

A rescuer who becomes sick or injured during the rescue effort should be handled as an immediate priority and be transported off the site as soon as possible to avoid a negative impact to the morale of remaining rescuers.

Hazardous materials and weapons of mass destruction incidents force the HazMat team to identify patients as contaminated or decontaminated before the regular triage process. Contamination by chemicals or biologic weapons in a treatment area, a hospital, or a trauma center could obstruct all systems and organizations coping with the MCI. Bear in mind that some incidents may require multiple triage areas or teams because the victims are located far apart.

Destination Decisions

Recall the 2011 American College of Surgeons Committee on Trauma (ACS-COT) field triage decision scheme shown in the chapter, *Trauma Systems and Mechanism of Injury*. The decision scheme outlines criteria for referral to a trauma center, including physiologic criteria, anatomic criteria, mechanism of injury criteria, and special considerations such as age or underlying health conditions. These guidelines help prehospital care providers recognize injured patients who are likely to benefit from transport to a trauma center, and are intended for individual patients. You may use this scheme in evaluating individual patients at large-scale incidents.

Another important consideration when you are choosing an appropriate facility for your patients will be the capabilities of local or even distant hospitals. Whereas some hospitals can handle dozens of patients with enough warning, others can be rapidly overwhelmed with only a few critical situations. In the event that a hospital is inundated with a large number of patients, most facilities have a **hospital surge capacity** plan in place to accommodate the overload. This may include rapidly deployed mobile units such as portable tents that can be put in place on site. In other cases, it may be necessary to transport some patients to specialty centers such as burn units or pediatric facilities that are more capable of handling the particular patient situation.

All patients triaged as immediate (red) or delayed (yellow) should preferably be transported by ambulance or air ambulance, if available. In extremely large situations, a bus may transport the walking wounded. If a bus is used for minimal priority patients, it is strongly suggested that they be transported to a hospital or clinic distant from the MCI or disaster site to avoid overwhelming the local area hospital resources. It is advisable when using a bus to plan for at least one EMT or paramedic to ride on the bus and to have an ambulance follow the bus. If a minimal patient's condition worsens, the patient could be moved to the ambulance and transported to a closer facility. The EMT or paramedic can stay with the patients triaged as needing minimal care until their arrival at the designated hospital. Any worsening of a patient's condition must be relayed to the receiving hospital as soon as possible in whatever manner the incident dictates.

Immediate priority patients should be transported two at a time until all are transported from the site. Then patients in the delayed category can be transported two or three at a time until all are at a hospital. Finally, the slightly injured are transported. Expectant patients who are still alive would receive treatment and transport at this time. Dead victims are handled or transported according to the SOP for the area.

It is important to remember that during an MCI, local hospitals may have their resources overwhelmed as well. Early notification to receiving facilities will allow for the hospitals to increase staffing and move patients within their facility as required. Typically EMS agencies will know a hospital's surge capacity, which will tell the agency how many patients of each category the hospital is able to safely handle and care for.

Critical Incident Stress Management

It is a misconception that emergency workers are immune from the psychological impacts of an MCI. Training and experience in the profession may allow some EMS providers to cope with horrific events they might be exposed to; however, there is no shame in using debriefing resources after an incident. Paramedics can be affected, sometimes permanently, by their roles at large-scale incidents. In the years since the 1995 bombing of the Alfred P. Murrah Federal Building in Oklahoma City, more focus has been given to the mental welfare of emergency workers in the performance of their duties.

The debriefing or defusing of emergency workers before, during, and after a major MCI should be considered as an included resource in your departmental disaster plan. At this point, this is considered somewhat controversial and will depend on your service director's and medical director's views of its usefulness. **Critical incident stress management (CISM)** should be considered for responders and should start within the rehabilitation sector. All responders are encouraged to participate, but stress management should not be imposed or forced. Forcing stress management can do more harm than good to the psychological well-being of rescuers.

Everyone should also have access to coping mechanisms after the incident, whether through a service's Employee Assistance Program (EAP), mental health professionals, or peer counselors trained in CISM debriefing. This assistance should be available without regard for a specific time frame. Some effects may not be seen until months after the incident and may present as drastic changes in daily routines, physical illnesses, mental illnesses, or even alienation from family members. The impact of the incident on all responders should be included as part of the post-incident evaluation.

After-Action Reviews

After any incident, an after-action review should be done. All agencies involved in the response should participate in the effort to improve future reactions to disasters. If something worked well in the plan, keep it. If something did not work at all, remove it or fix it.

No response is ever perfect, but it is up to all participants to keep perfecting their training, equipment, plans, and skills. Leaders in EMS suggest that all observations should be noted, in writing if possible, to allow future review. Discourage finger pointing, which is not problem solving. All MCIs are different; the way you react to each of them will be different, too. By keeping the basic goal of "doing the most good for the most patients" in the forefront, developing plans, using the ICS, and applying a systematic approach to triage, an MCI can be handled effectively. Practice plans often and they will become instinctive.

YOU *are the Medic* | SUMMARY

1. **When does an event become a multiple-casualty incident (MCI)?**

   An event becomes an MCI once the number of patients involved exceeds the resources available. This may vary in different areas based on location, the size of the department, and immediate resources. What may be easy for a large metropolitan department to handle may completely overwhelm a small rural system.

2. **How can you prepare yourself for an MCI?**

   A good place to start is your agency's policy and procedure manual. Familiarize yourself with the expectations for the roles you may be assigned. Then get involved! Participate in disaster planning drills, table-top MCI exercises, and other training opportunities. Consider becoming a member of a professional organization that focuses on disaster management. The educational and networking possibilities can provide you with valuable tools and information that you can share with your agency.

3. **What is the goal of the incident command system (ICS)?**

   The goal of the ICS is to make the best use of available resources to manage the environment around the incident and to treat patients in an emergency.

4. **How should you triage this patient?**

   The patient is unresponsive and presents with signs of shock and should be triaged red.

5. **What are the four command functions within the ICS?**

   The four command functions within the ICS are finance, logistics, operations, and planning.

6. **How many people should be assigned to one supervisor?**

   Effective supervision can be achieved when the supervisor/worker ratio is maintained at one supervisor for three to seven workers.

7. **How should you triage this patient?**

   This patient should be triaged green. She is walking, alert, and oriented to person, place, and time, has no immediate life threats, and displays no signs of shock.

8. **What is the difference between primary and secondary triage?**

   For the purpose of this chapter, primary triage is the initial triage performed at the scene. Secondary triage takes place later as the patient is brought to the treatment area. Other sources you read may refer to secondary triage as the assessment of a patient on arrival to the emergency department.

9. **How should you triage this patient?**

   This patient should be triaged yellow. Although the patient does not present with any immediate life threats, his complaint of not being able to feel or move his legs may indicate a spinal cord injury.

10. **What are the four common triage categories?**

    The four triage categories used most frequently are immediate (red), delayed (yellow), minimal or "walking wounded" (green), and expectant (black). Patients who are triaged red require immediate care and transport to correct life threats such as airway compromise, head injury, or shock. Patients who are triaged yellow will require care and transport; however, both can be delayed. Patients triaged green require minimal care or resources and therefore wait until the patients who are more critical are tended to. Patients who are dead or who are expected to die due to the severity of their injuries are categorized as black. An example of a patient who may be categorized black is a person in cardiac arrest.

YOU are the Medic · SUMMARY, continued

Patient No. 1

Triage Tag
No. 4862387

Move the Walking Wounded	MINIMAL
No respirations after head tilt	EXPECTANT
☐ Respirations–over 30 or less than 10	IMMEDIATE
☐ Perfusion–capillary refill over 2 seconds	IMMEDIATE
☒ Mental status–unable to follow simple commands	IMMEDIATE
Otherwise	DELAYED

MAJOR INJURIES: _Closed femur fracture_
HOSPITAL DESTINATION: _Mercy_
ORIENTED × 4   DISORIENTED ☐   UNRESPONSIVE ☒

TIME	PULSE	B/P	RESPIRATION
1136	Rapid, weak, and regular	N/A	Adequate
N/A	N/A	N/A	N/A

PERSONAL INFORMATION:
NAME: _Unknown_
MALE ☐   FEMALE   AGE: EST. 31   WEIGHT: EST. 175 lb
MEDICAL COMPLAINTS/HISTORY
Closed femur fracture

| EXPECTANT | No 4862387 |
| IMMEDIATE | No 4862387 |

Patient No. 2

Triage Tag
No. 4862388

Move the Walking Wounded	MINIMAL
No respirations after head tilt	EXPECTANT
☐ Respirations–over 30 or less than 10	IMMEDIATE
☐ Perfusion–capillary refill over 2 seconds	IMMEDIATE
☐ Mental status–unable to follow simple commands	IMMEDIATE
Otherwise	DELAYED

MAJOR INJURIES: _None_
HOSPITAL DESTINATION: _Concord North_
ORIENTED × 4   DISORIENTED ☐   UNRESPONSIVE ☐

TIME	PULSE	B/P	RESPIRATION
1139	Radial pulse is normal, strong, and regular	N/A	Normal, adequate depth, nonlabored
N/A	N/A	N/A	N/A

PERSONAL INFORMATION:
NAME: _Irva Mendez_
MALE ☐   FEMALE ☒   AGE: 88   WEIGHT: 125 lb
MEDICAL COMPLAINTS/HISTORY
Forehead laceration

EXPECTANT	No 4862388
IMMEDIATE	No 4862388
DELAYED	No 4862388
MINIMAL	No 4862388

YOU are the Medic   SUMMARY, continued

Patient No. 3

Triage Tag
No. 4862389

Move the Walking Wounded	MINIMAL
No respirations after head tilt	EXPECTANT
☐ Respirations—over 30 or less than 10	IMMEDIATE
☐ Perfusion—capillary refill over 2 seconds	IMMEDIATE
☐ Mental status—unable to follow simple commands	IMMEDIATE
(Otherwise)	DELAYED

MAJOR INJURIES: Leg injury
HOSPITAL DESTINATION: Mercy
(ORIENTED × 4)   DISORIENTED ☐   UNRESPONSIVE ☐

TIME	PULSE	B/P	RESPIRATION
1142	Radial pulses are slow and regular	N/A	Rapid and deep
N/A	N/A	N/A	N/A

PERSONAL INFORMATION:
NAME: Scott Melbourne
(MALE ☒)   FEMALE ☐   AGE: 52   WEIGHT: EST. 230 lb
MEDICAL COMPLAINTS/HISTORY
Leg pinned under debris

EXPECTANT   No 4862389

IMMEDIATE   No 4862389

DELAYED   No 4862389

Prep Kit

■ Ready for Review

- Major incidents require the involvement and coordination of multiple jurisdictions, functional agencies, and emergency response disciplines.
- The National Incident Management System (NIMS) provides a consistent nationwide template to enable federal, state, and local governments, as well as private-sector and nongovernmental organizations, to work together effectively and efficiently. The NIMS is used to prepare for, prevent, respond to, and recover from domestic incidents, regardless of cause, size, or complexity, including acts of catastrophic terrorism and hazardous materials (HazMat) incidents.
- The major NIMS components are command and management, preparedness, resource management, communications and information management, supporting technologies, and ongoing management and maintenance.
- The purpose of the incident command system (ICS) is to ensure responder and public safety, achieve incident management goals, and ensure the efficient use of resources.
- Using the ICS gives you a modular organizational structure that is built on the size and complexity of the incident.
- Preparedness involves the decisions made and basic planning done before an incident occurs.
- Your agency should have written disaster plans that you are regularly trained to carry out.
- General ICS staff roles include command, finance, logistics, operation, and planning.
- At incidents that have a significant medical factor, the incident commander should appoint someone as the medical branch director who will supervise triage, treatment, and transport of injured patients.
- A multiple-casualty incident refers to any call that involves three or more patients, any situation that places such a great demand on available equipment or personnel that the system would require a mutual aid response, or any incident that has a potential to create one of the previously mentioned situations.
- The goal of triage is to do the greatest good for the greatest number. This means that the triage assessment is brief and patient condition categories are basic.
- The four common triage categories are immediate (red), delayed (yellow), minimal (green), and expectant (black; likely to die or dead).
- It is vital to tag each patient during triage to help keep an accurate record of their condition. Triage tags become part of the patient's medical record.
- START triage (Simple Triage And Rapid Treatment) uses a limited assessment of the patient's ability to walk, respiratory status, hemodynamic status, and neurologic status to quickly and efficiently triage patients.
- JumpSTART triage modifies the START triage system to take into account the physiologic and developmental differences of pediatric patients. It is intended for use in children younger than 8 years or who appear to weigh less than 100 pounds.
- Consider critical incident management before, during, or after an event. It is normal to sometimes feel overwhelmed. Recognize the need for assistance in yourself as well as for others on the scene.

■ Vital Vocabulary

closed incident A contained incident in which patients are found in one focal location and the situation is not expected to produce more patients than initially present.

command In incident command, the position that oversees the incident, establishes the objectives and priorities, and from there develops a response plan.

critical incident stress management (CISM) A process that confronts responses to critical incidents and defuses them.

demobilization The process of directing responders to return to their facilities when work at a disaster or multiple-casualty incident has finished, at least for the particular responders.

extrication supervisor In incident command, the person appointed to determine the type of equipment and resources needed for a situation involving extrication or special rescue; also called the rescue supervisor.

finance In incident command, the position in an incident responsible for accounting of all expenditures.

freelancing When individual units or different organizations make independent and often inefficient decisions about the next appropriate action.

hospital surge capacity The capabilities of a receiving hospital to handle a large number of unexpected emergency patients, such as those seen in a multiple-casualty incident.

incident action plan An oral or written plan stating general objectives reflecting the overall strategy for managing an incident.

incident commander (IC) The overall leader of the incident command system to whom commanders or leaders of the incident command system divisions report.

incident command system (ICS) A system implemented to manage disasters and multiple-casualty incidents in which section chiefs, including finance, logistics, operations, and planning, report to the incident commander.

joint information center (JIC) An area designated by the incident commander, or a designee, in which public information officers from multiple agencies disseminate information about the incident.

JumpSTART triage A sorting system for pediatric patients younger than 8 years or weighing less than 100 pounds. There is a minor adaptation for infants because they cannot ambulate on their own.

liaison officer (LNO) In incident command, the person who relays information, concerns, and requests among responding agencies.

logistics In incident command, the position that helps procure and stockpile equipment and supplies during an incident.

medical incident command A branch of operations in a unified command system, whose three designated sector positions are triage, treatment, and transport.

morgue supervisor In incident command, the person who works with area medical examiners, coroners, and law enforcement agencies to coordinate the disposition of dead victims.

multiple-casualty incident (MCI) An emergency situation that can place great demand on the equipment or personnel of the EMS system or has the potential to overwhelm your available resources.

mutual aid response An agreement between neighboring EMS systems to respond to multiple-casualty incidents or disasters in each other's region when local resources are insufficient to handle the response.

National Incident Management System (NIMS) A Department of Homeland Security system designed to enable federal, state, and local governments and private-sector and nongovernmental organizations to effectively and efficiently prepare for, prevent, respond to, and recover from domestic incidents, regardless of cause, size, or complexity, including acts of catastrophic terrorism.

open incident An ongoing or uncontained incident in which rescuers will have to search for patients and then triage or treat them. The situation may produce more patients. Examples include school shootings, tornadoes, a hazardous materials release, and rising floodwaters.

operations In incident command, the position that carries out the orders of the commander to help resolve the incident.

planning In incident command, the position that ultimately produces a plan to resolve any incident.

primary triage A type of patient sorting used to rapidly categorize patients; the focus is on speed in locating all patients and determining an initial priority as their condition warrants.

public information officer (PIO) In incident command, the person who keeps the public informed and relates any information to the press.

rehabilitation supervisor In incident command, the person who establishes an area that provides protection for responders from the elements and the situation.

rescue supervisor In incident command, the person appointed to determine the type of equipment and resources needed for a situation involving extrication or special rescue; also called the extrication supervisor.

safety officer In incident command, the person who gives the "go ahead" to a plan or who may stop an operation when rescuer safety is an issue.

secondary triage A type of patient sorting used in the treatment sector that involves retriage of patients.

single command system A command system in which one person is in charge, generally used with small incidents that involve only one responding agency or one jurisdiction.

span of control In incident command, the subordinate positions under the commander's direction to which the workload is distributed; the supervisor/worker ratio.

staging supervisor In incident command, the person who locates an area to stage equipment and personnel and tracks unit arrival and deployment from the staging area.

START triage A patient sorting process that stands for simple triage and rapid treatment and uses a limited assessment of the patient's ability to walk, respiratory status, hemodynamic status, and neurologic status.

termination of command The end of the incident command structure when an incident draws to a close.

transfer of command In incident command, when an incident commander turns over command to someone with more experience in a critical area.

transportation supervisor In incident command, the person who coordinates transportation and distribution of patients to appropriate receiving hospitals.

treatment supervisor In incident command, the person responsible for locating, setting up, and supervising the treatment area.

triage To sort patients based on the severity of their conditions and prioritize them for care accordingly.

triage supervisor The person in charge of prioritizing patients, whose primary duty is to ensure that every patient receives initial triage.

unified command system A command system used in larger incidents in which there is a multiagency response or multiple jurisdictions are involved.

Assessment in Action

You are participating in an MCI exercise involving the county EMS agencies and local hospitals. The scenario is an early morning bomb blast at a chemical plant 5 miles from the university. You and your partner are assigned to the treatment sector and are waiting for patients to be brought to you. Initial reports indicate at least 75 people were in the vicinity of the explosion.

1. The National Incident Management System (NIMS) was developed to:
   A. determine allocation of federal resources during an MCI.
   B. provide a system for data collection following an MCI.
   C. promote more efficient coordination of an MCI.
   D. establish a method for triaging patients during an MCI.

2. Which type of command system is used during a large MCI that requires a multiagency or multijurisdictional response?
   A. Single command system
   B. Tiered command system
   C. Vertical command system
   D. Unified command system

3. In the incident command system, which section is responsible for procuring and stockpiling equipment and supplies during an MCI?
   A. Finance
   B. Logistics
   C. Planning
   D. Operations

4. Documentation and tracking of vehicles transporting, patients transported, and the facility destination is the responsibility of the:
   A. public information officer.
   B. planning officer.
   C. transportation supervisor.
   D. triage supervisor.

5. Which triage method uses a limited assessment of the patient's ability to walk, respiratory status, hemodynamic status, and neurologic status?
   A. JumpSTART
   B. START
   C. SALT
   D. SMART

6. The capabilities of a receiving hospital to handle a large number of unexpected emergency patients is known as:
   A. surge capacity.
   B. rapid expansion protocol.
   C. internal triage.
   D. hospital incident command.

7. Patient criteria used in the 2011 American College of Surgeons Committee on Trauma field triage decision scheme include:
   A. mechanism of injury.
   B. anatomy of the injury.
   C. physiologic status.
   D. all of the above.

8. What information should be communicated to the medical branch director following primary triage?
   A. Transportation assignment for each patient
   B. The number of patients in each of the triage categories
   C. Resources necessary to begin treating patients
   D. Contact information for next of kin

9. Which supervisor is responsible for releasing vehicles and resources when instructed by the incident commander?
   A. Planning officer
   B. Transportation supervisor
   C. Staging supervisor
   D. Resource supervisor

Additional Question

10. What are some of the ways you can be more involved in disaster management and planning?

Vehicle Extrication and Special Rescue

National EMS Education Standard Competencies

EMS Operations

Knowledge of operational roles and responsibilities to ensure patient, public, and personnel safety.

Vehicle Extrication

- Safe vehicle extrication (pp 2227-2237)
- Use of simple hand tools (p 2230)

••

Knowledge Objectives

1. Explain the three levels of training in technical rescue. (p 2222)
2. Discuss guidelines for assisting special rescue teams. (p 2222)
3. Discuss the steps of special rescue, including preparation, response, arrival and scene size-up, stabilization of the scene, access, disentanglement, removal, and transport of the patient. (pp 2223-2227)
4. Discuss specific hazards that may be encountered and identified during the arrival and scene size-up of a technical rescue incident. (p 2223)
5. Explain the importance of the incident management system during technical rescue incidents. (pp 2224-2225)
6. Discuss how to ensure safety at the scene of a rescue incident, including scene size-up and the selection of the proper personal protective equipment and additional necessary gear. (pp 2223-2227)
7. Provide examples of vehicle components that may be hazardous to responders and patients following a crash, and explain how to mitigate their dangers. (pp 2228-2230)

8. Discuss how to ensure situational safety at the site of a vehicle extrication, including controlling traffic flow, performing a 360° assessment, stabilizing the vehicle, dealing with unique hazards, and evaluating the need for additional resources. (pp 2229-2237)
9. Explain the simple methods used to access the patient during an incident that requires extrication. (pp 2232-2234)
10. Discuss disentanglement methods and considerations, including air bag safety, displacing the seat, removing the windshield, removing the roof, and displacing the dash. (pp 2234-2237)
11. Give examples of situations that would require special technical rescue teams and describe the paramedics' role in these situations. (pp 2238-2246)

Skills Objectives

1. Demonstrate how to stabilize a vehicle using wood cribbing. (pp 2230-2231)
2. Demonstrate how to gain access to the patient by opening the door. (p 2232)
3. Demonstrate how to gain access to the patient by breaking tempered glass using a spring-loaded center punch. (pp 2232-2234, Skill Drill 1)
4. Demonstrate how to gain access to the patient and provide initial medical care. (pp 2232-2234)
5. Describe how to remove or cut battery cables. (p 2235)
6. Demonstrate how to cut away the upholstery of the front seat in order to expose the metal frame and the areas of attachment. (p 2236)
7. Demonstrate how to stabilize a suspected spinal injury in the water. (pp 2242-2243, Skill Drill 2)

Introduction

Most EMS departments respond to a variety of special rescue situations **Figure 1**, including vehicle extrication, confined space, trench, water, and wilderness rescue. Often, the first emergency unit to arrive at a rescue incident is an ambulance with EMS providers. The initial actions taken by paramedics may determine the safety of both patients and paramedics. They may also determine how efficiently the rescue is completed.

"Rescue" means to deliver from danger or imprisonment. As an EMS provider, you must remove from peril or confinement every patient you encounter. Patients are found in every imaginable situation. Imagine you arrive at an extrication incident where a cement light pole has collapsed on the front end of a vehicle, trapping a person inside. Your assessment shows the patient is in stable condition; the treatment appears easy, but the rescue is difficult. You must extricate this patient.

This chapter discusses special rescue operation guidelines and procedures using vehicle extrication as a primary example. The chapter concludes with an overview of additional special rescue situations such as confined space, trench, water, and agricultural rescue. As a paramedic, you may not be responsible for special rescue and extrication. However, you need to be prepared for it and be aware of the associated hazards.

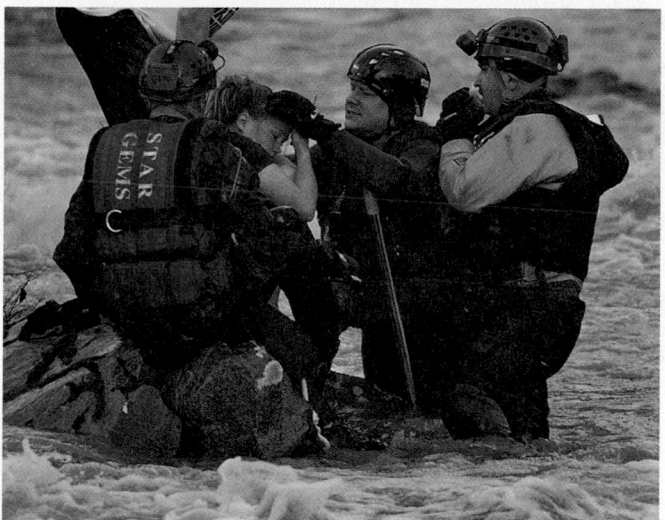

Figure 1 Most EMS departments respond to a variety of special rescue situations.

Words of Wisdom

One of the benefits of rescue awareness and operations education is that it helps you avoid rescue situations that you are not trained to handle.

YOU *are the Medic* PART 1

During the past 24 hours, approximately 10 inches of rain has fallen, saturating the ground and causing flooding to low-lying areas. It is midday and still raining when you and your partner are dispatched to a residential structure collapse located in a neighborhood affected by the flooding. Dispatch informs you that law enforcement personnel and the engine company have arrived at the scene and are reporting that a three-story brick house has collapsed and two people are trapped. Additional help including the technical response team are en route. On your arrival, incident command informs you that a 65-year-old woman is trapped from her lower chest down beneath concrete and other debris. She is screaming and crying for someone to find her grandson. A fire fighter provides initial information.

Recording Time: 1 Minute	
Appearance	65-year-old woman in obvious distress. Anxious and distraught.
Level of consciousness	Alert (oriented to person, place, and day)
Airway	Open
Breathing	Chest rise appears adequate
Circulation	Strong carotid pulse, slightly increased

1. What is a technical rescue incident?
2. Explain what the mnemonic "FAILURE" represents.

Awareness

All EMS providers must have some formalized education or training in rescue techniques. Most of the training and education EMS providers receive is aimed at the awareness level, enabling them to identify the hazards and secure the scene to prevent additional people from becoming patients.

Your function as a paramedic in rescue operations depends on the type of services you provide and the level of expertise your company has attained. Your primary concern is safety, and your primary role is to provide emergency medical care and prevent further injury to the patient. All providers must wear proper personal protective equipment (PPE) to allow them to access patients and safely administer treatment that will continue throughout the incident.

A **technical rescue incident (TRI)** is a complex rescue incident involving vehicle extrication, water/ice rescue, trench collapse, confined spaces, structural collapse, high-angle rescue, hazardous materials incidents, and wilderness search and rescue that requires specially trained personnel and special equipment. This chapter describes how to assist specially trained rescue personnel in carrying out the tasks, but it will not make you an expert in the skills that require specialized training.

Words of Wisdom

Just as in patient care, the first priority in rescue is "rescuer safety."

Training in technical rescue areas is conducted at three levels:

- **Awareness**. This training level is an introduction to the topic, with an emphasis on recognizing the hazards, securing the scene, and calling for appropriate assistance. There is no actual use of rescue skills at the awareness level.
- **Operations**. Geared toward working in the "warm zone" of an incident (the area directly around the hazard area), this kind of training will allow you to directly assist those conducting the rescue operation.
- **Technician**. At this level, you are directly involved in the rescue operation itself. Training includes the use of specialized equipment, care of patients during the rescue, and management of the incident and of all personnel at the scene.

Words of Wisdom

All rescue teams should have written safety procedures or SOPs that are familiar to every team member.

Guidelines for Rescue Operations

When you are assisting rescue team members, the following guidelines will prove useful:

- **Be safe:** Rescue situations have many hidden hazards, including combustible fuels, oxygen-deficient atmospheres, and strong water currents.
- **Follow orders:** The officers and the rescue teams you will work with on special rescue incidents have received extensive specialized training. They have been chosen for those duties because they have experience and skills in a particular area of rescue. It is critical to follow the orders of personnel who understand exactly what needs to be done to ensure everyone's safety and to mitigate the dangers involved in the rescue situation. Follow their orders exactly as given. If you do not understand what is expected of you, *ask*. Have the orders clarified so you will be able to complete your assigned task safely.
- **Work as a team:** Rescue efforts often require many people to complete a wide variety of tasks. Some personnel may be trained in specific tasks, such as vehicle extrication. However, they cannot do their jobs without the support and assistance of others. Rescue is a team effort, and you play an essential role on this team.
- **Think:** You must constantly assess and reassess the scene. If you think your assigned task may be unsafe, bring it to the attention of the incident commander (IC) or safety officer. Do not ignore what is happening around you because someone else is in charge. Observations that you should bring to the IC's attention include safety issues and broken equipment.
- **Follow the golden rule of public service:** When you are involved in carrying out a rescue effort, it is all too easy to concentrate on the technical aspects of the rescue and forget to focus on the patient, who needs your emotional support and encouragement. It is helpful to have a rescuer stay with the patient whenever possible, keeping the patient updated on which actions will be performed during the rescue process.

Words of Wisdom

F-A-I-L-U-R-E
The reasons for rescue failures can be referred to by the mnemonic "FAILURE":
F Failure to understand the environment, or underestimating it
A Additional medical problems not considered
I Inadequate rescue skills
L Lack of teamwork or experience
U Underestimating the logistics of the incident
R Rescue versus recovery mode not considered
E Equipment not mastered

Words of Wisdom

The paramedic's job at the scene of a crash is to take care of the patients.

Steps of Special Rescue

The role of the paramedic in special rescue operations is often vague and can change as a rescue operation progresses. Rescue and removal of patients involves several steps. You must access the patient and then quickly assess him or her for medical or trauma complications to determine which treatments should be started. Treatment in these situations is often difficult because of the circumstances surrounding the event. Once lifesaving treatment is initiated, the patient must be released or removed from **entrapment**, and medical care must continue throughout the incident. The most difficult process in any rescue is neither the rescue nor the treatment process, but rather the coordination and balance of both.

Although special rescue situations may take many different forms, all rescuers should perform the following steps to ensure the rescue is safe, effective, and efficient:

1. Preparation
2. Response
3. Arrival and scene size-up
4. Stabilization of the scene
5. Access
6. Disentanglement
7. Removal
8. Transport

Preparation

You can prepare for responses to emergency rescue incidents by training with fire departments and special rescue teams in your area. This educational process will prepare you to respond to a mutual aid call and teach you about the type of rescue equipment other departments have access to and the training levels of their personnel. Knowing the terminology used in the field will also make communicating with other rescuers easier and more effective. However, specialized training and certification is required before you are allowed to fully participate.

Prior to any technical rescue call, your department must consider the following issues:

- Does the department have the personnel and equipment needed to handle a TRI from start to finish?
- What equipment and which personnel will the department send on a TRI call?
- Do members of the department know the potential hazard areas in their response area? Have they visited those areas with local representatives?

Response

A dispatch protocol should be established for a TRI. If your department has its own **technical rescue team**, it will usually respond with a rescue squad, an ambulance, fire engine company, and fire chief. Otherwise, it will respond with a medic unit, engine company, and chief. In many EMS departments, the rescue squad will come from an outside agency. Often, it is necessary to notify utility companies during a TRI and seek their assistance. Many TRIs involve electricity, sewer pipes, or factors that may create the need for heavy equipment, to which utility companies have ready access.

Arrival and Scene Size-up

Beginning with the initial dispatch of the rescue call, you should be compiling facts and impressions about the call. Scene size-up begins with the information gained from the person reporting the incident and then from the bystanders at the scene on arrival. The information gathered when an emergency call is received is important to the success of the rescue operation. This information may include the location and nature of the incident, the condition and position of the patient, the number of patients trapped or injured, specific injuries, hazard information, and the name of the person calling and a number where the person can be reached. As you approach the scene of a TRI, however, you may not always know what kind of scene you are entering. Identify any life-threatening hazards, and take measures to avoid them or mitigate the hazards, if trained to do so. If additional resources are needed, they should be ordered by the IC. Determine whether the situation is a search, rescue, or recovery.

A rapid and accurate 360° scene size-up is needed to avoid placing rescuers in danger and to determine what additional resources may be needed. The scene size-up includes the *initial evaluation* of the following issues:

- Scope and magnitude of the incident
- Risk and benefit analysis
- Number of known and potential patients
- Hazards
- Access to the scene
- Environmental factors
- Available and necessary resources
- Establishment of a control perimeter

As a paramedic, you know that your own safety as well as the safety of your partner and the public is paramount. At a TRI, whereas you may be tempted to approach the patient or the accident area, it is critically important to slow down and properly *evaluate* the situation. *Consider* the potential general hazards and risks of utilities, environmental conditions, and hazards that are **immediately dangerous to life and health (IDLH)**. If hazards are identified, call for additional specialized resources at this time. Do *not* rush into the incident scene until an assessment of the situation is complete. EMS providers need to *stop and think about the dangers that may be present.* Do not make yourself part of the problem.

Stabilization of the Scene

Once resources are on the way, it is time to stabilize the incident. Look around you, and be sure you have identified and evaluated all hazards at the scene, observing the geographic area, noting the routes of access and exit, observing weather and wind conditions, and considering evacuation problems and transport distances. Remember, you may be the first to arrive on the scene. You may find yourself temporarily in command until an officer arrives.

The first arriving responder will immediately assume command and begin using the incident management system (IMS). The IMS is the foundation for mitigating a TRI. The IC will establish strategic objectives, coordinate and request additional resources, and unify command with other agencies that are involved.

Many TRIs will eventually become complex and require a large number of assisting units. Without the IMS in place, it will be difficult—if not impossible—to ensure the rescuers' safety. At any TRI, follow the IC's orders. Your ultimate goal is to protect the team and patients. No matter what type of rescue scene you enter, keep the following three guidelines in mind:

- Approach the scene cautiously.
- Position apparatus properly.
- Assist specialized team members as needed.

Emergency Vehicles

Determine where to locate your emergency vehicle, taking into account the safety of emergency workers, patients, and other motorists. Whenever possible, park emergency vehicles in a manner that will ensure safety and not disrupt traffic any more than necessary. Traffic flow is a hazard associated with any operation that takes place, especially if the operation is located on a highway. Do not hesitate to request that the road be closed if necessary. Provide a safe ambulance loading zone. Have staging areas away from the scene.

Use large emergency vehicles to provide a barrier against motorists who fail to heed emergency warning lights. Many departments place apparatus at an angle to the crash. This position ensures that the apparatus is pushed to the side in the event that it is struck from behind. You can also place traffic cones or fusees to direct motorists away from the crash site. Make sure there is no obvious fire hazard present.

You need to be visible. Use only essential warning lights because too many lights tend to distract or confuse other drivers. Turn off headlights and consider the use of amber lighting at the scene. Before exiting the ambulance at an emergency scene, be alert for any vehicles that might cause you injury. Do not assume that motorists will heed your warning lights, and let law enforcement personnel coordinate traffic control.

Control Zones

An outer perimeter needs to be established to keep the public and media out of the staging area, with a smaller perimeter maintained directly around the rescue area. The rescue area is the area that surrounds the incident site (eg, a motor vehicle crash). The size of the rescue area is proportional to the hazards that exist. The IC should coordinate with law enforcement personnel to help secure the scene. In addition, the fire department should implement a strict accountability system to control access to the rescue scene. As part of the scene stabilization effort, establish three controlled zones:

- **Hot zone**. This area is for entry teams and rescue teams only. This zone immediately surrounds the dangers of the site (eg, hazardous materials releases), and entry into this zone is restricted to essential properly equipped and prepared personnel.
- **Warm zone**. This area is for properly trained and equipped personnel only. The warm zone is where personnel and equipment decontamination and hot zone support take place.
- **Cold zone**. This area is for staging vehicles and equipment, and contains the command post. The public and the media should be kept clear of the cold zone at all times.

Police or fire line tape or barriers are often used to demarcate these controlled zones. Red tape is typically used for the hot zone, orange tape for the warm zone, and yellow tape for the cold zone. Of course, someone must ensure that the zones of the emergency scene are enforced. Scene control activities are sometimes assigned to law enforcement personnel.

Specific Hazards

During stabilization of the scene, atmospheric monitoring should be started to identify any IDLH environments for rescuers and patients. The U.S. Department of Transportation's (DOT) *Emergency Response Guidebook* (*ERG*) may be useful for rescuers who may potentially operate at a hazardous incident. The *ERG* is intended to help rescuers decide which preliminary actions to take. The guide provides information on approximately 4,000 chemicals that may be encountered at an incident scene.

Words of Wisdom

It is essential that a vehicle involved in a crash be stabilized with cribbing before gaining access to the patient. The fire department is usually responsible for stabilizing the vehicle. If the fire department is not on scene, depending on protocol, this may be a task that the paramedic can perform. This will be discussed in more detail later in the chapter.

Utility hazards require the assistance of trained personnel. For electrical hazards, such as downed lines, park at least one truck span away and do no park underneath damaged power lines **Figure 2**. Do not touch any wires, power lines, or other

Words of Wisdom

Treat all downed wires as if they are charged (live) until you receive specific clearance from the power company. Even if the lights are out along the street where the wires are down, never assume that the wires are dead. Be especially alert for downed wires after a storm that has blown down trees or tree limbs.

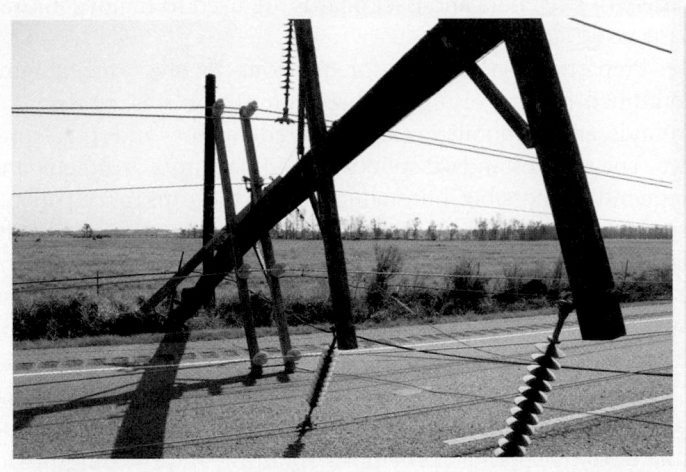

Figure 2 Downed electrical wires present a hazard for responding crews.

electrical sources until they have been de-energized by a power company representative. It is not just the wires that are hazardous; any metal that they touch is also energized. Metal fences or guardrails may become energized along their entire unbroken length. Be careful around running or standing water because water is an excellent conductor of electricity. The IC should ensure that the proper procedures are taken to shut off the utilities in the rescue area. Remember—utility hazards can be above or below ground, and the rescue situation will dictate which ones need to be addressed first.

Natural gas and liquefied petroleum gas are flammable. If a call involves leaking gas, call the gas company immediately. Follow your local protocol.

Protective Equipment

Most specialized teams carry unique items such as harnesses; smaller, lighter helmets; and jumpsuits that are easier to move in than turnout gear. When you are considering the use of protective head gear, you must use approved devices that meet certain standards and are appropriate for the rescue environment (eg, climbing helmets, fire fighter helmets). For example, your PPE should be bright to help ensure your visibility during daylight hours. Any PPE that is used at night needs to be equipped with reflective material to increase your visibility in the darkness. Footwear must be designed and certified for a specific rescue environment. The environment may require thermal protection (hot or cold), chemical protection, insole puncture barriers, and ankle support. Providers must also consider the use of American National Standards Institute (ANSI)-approved safety glasses or goggles, puncture- or cut-resistant gloves, flame- or flash-protective clothing that is highly visible, and appropriate footwear to support ankles and provide traction. Other useful items that are easily carried by paramedics include binoculars, chalk or spray paint for marking searched areas, a compass, first aid kits, a whistle, a handheld global positioning system, and cyalume-type light sticks. The IC and the technical rescue team

will help to determine what protective equipment you will need to wear while assisting at the rescue scene.

Accountability

Accountability should be practiced at all emergencies, no matter how small. The **accountability system** is an important process to ensure rescuers' safety. It tracks the personnel on the scene, including their identities, assignments, and locations. This system ensures that only rescuers who have been given specific assignments are operating within the area where the rescue is taking place. By using an accountability system and working within the IMS, an IC can track the resources at the scene, task out assignments, and ensure that every person at the scene operates safely.

Patient Contact

At any rescue scene, you must try to communicate with the patient. Technical rescue situations often last for hours, with the patient being left alone for long periods of time. If at all possible, you should attempt to communicate via a radio, cell phone, or yelling. Reassure the patient that everything is being done to ensure his or her safety.

If you succeed in making contact, it is important to stay in communication with the patient. Ideally, someone should be assigned to talk to the patient, while other personnel focus on making the rescue. Realize that the patient could be sick or injured and is probably frightened. If you are calm, your demeanor will in turn calm the patient:

- Make and keep eye contact with the patient.
- Tell the truth. Lying destroys trust and confidence. You may not always tell the patient everything, but if the patient asks a specific question, answer truthfully.
- Communicate at a level that the patient can understand.
- Be aware of your own body language.
- Always speak slowly, clearly, and distinctly. Do not use technical terminology.
- Address the patient properly. This will involve using the patient's surname, preceded by the proper qualifier (ie, Mr. or Ms.). Children and young adults should be addressed by their first names.
- If a patient is hard of hearing, speak clearly and directly at the person, so that he or she can read your lips.
- Allow time for the patient to answer or respond to your questions.
- Try to make the patient comfortable and relaxed whenever possible.

▇ Access

With the scene stabilized, now you must gain access to the patient. How is he or she trapped? Will accessing the patient require simple or complex tasks? For example, in a vehicle extrication incident, will the doors unlock and open to allow access, or will gaining access require the use of simple or specialized tools and equipment? **Simple access** may require hand tools such as a hammer, glass handsaw, Halligan, center punch, and come-along. **Complex access** may require special tools such as a hydraulic ram, spreader, or cutter. These tools require special training. Vehicle extrication courses can be taken separately, and topics covered include the use of pneumatic and hydraulic tools.

Remember that communication with patients during the rescue is essential to make sure they are not injured further by the rescue operation. Even if they are not injured, they need to be reassured that the team is working as quickly as possible to free them.

It is vitally important that the actions of EMS personnel be effectively coordinated into ongoing operations during rescue incidents. Their main functions are to treat patients and to stand by in case a rescue team member needs medical assistance. Throughout the course of the rescue operation, which may span many hours, EMS personnel must continually monitor and ensure the stability of all patients.

Gaining access to the patient will depend on the type of incident. For example, in an incident involving a motor vehicle, its location and position, the damage to the vehicle, and the position of the patient are important considerations. The means of gaining access to the patient must also take into account the nature and severity of the patient's injuries. The chosen means of access may change during the course of the rescue as the nature or severity of the patient's injuries becomes apparent.

■ Disentanglement

Emergency medical care should be initiated as soon as access to the patient is achieved. Some fire, EMS, and law enforcement departments have technical rescue paramedics; not only can these responders initiate IV lines and treat medical conditions, but they also know how to deal with the special equipment being used and the procedures taking place around them.

A team member should remain with the patient to direct the rescuers who are performing the disentanglement. For example, unless there is an immediate threat of fire, explosion, or other danger, you should perform a primary assessment and perform any critical interventions before disentanglement begins. This may include providing cervical spine immobilization, opening the airway, providing oxygen, ventilations, or controlling significant bleeding. Once life threats have been treated, disentanglement can begin.

Disentanglement involves freeing patients from what is trapping them. For example, in vehicle extrication, this would be the cutting of a vehicle (or machinery) away from trapped or injured patients, using rescue tools along with various methods to free the patient.

■ Removal

Once patients have been treated for life threats and disentangled from what was trapping them, efforts shift to removing the patients from the hazard area. In some instances, this may simply amount to having someone assist a patient out of the hazard area; in other situations, it may require removal with spinal immobilization in place due to possible injuries. A wide variety of stretchers and backboards are used to remove injured patients **Figure 3**.

Preparing the patient for removal involves maintaining continued control of all life-threatening problems, dressing all wounds, and immobilizing all suspected fractures and spinal injuries. The use of standard splints in confined areas is difficult and frequently impossible, but stabilization of the arms to the patient's trunk and of the legs to each other will often suffice until the patient is positioned on a backboard, with the backboard serving as the ultimate splint for the whole body. The short backboard, such as the Kendrick Extrication Device (KED) immobilization device, is typically used for stabilization of a sitting patient.

Sometimes a patient must be removed quickly (rapid extrication) because his or her general condition is deteriorating and time does not permit meticulous splinting and dressing procedures. Quick removal may also occur if hazards are present, such as spilled gas or other materials that could endanger the patient or rescue personnel. The only time the patient should be moved prior to completion of initial care, assessment, stabilization, and treatment is when the patient's or emergency responder's life is in immediate danger.

Packaging is preparing the patient for movement as a unit. It is often accomplished by means of a backboard or similar device. Backboards are essential for moving patients with potential or actual spine injuries.

Using a Basket Stretcher

Basket stretchers, often called stokes litters or stokes baskets, facilitate moving patients to a place of safety and can be used in a variety of situations. The manner in which a patient is packaged in a basket stretcher depends on his or her medical condition, the environment, and the manner in which the patient will be evacuated. Basket stretchers can be lifted by rope, carried by vehicles, or, most commonly, hand-carried by rescuers. In case of vertical evacuation, pack excess gear around the patient to prevent undue movement. While you are handling the patient, be sure to communicate and keep him or her apprised of the situation and your progress.

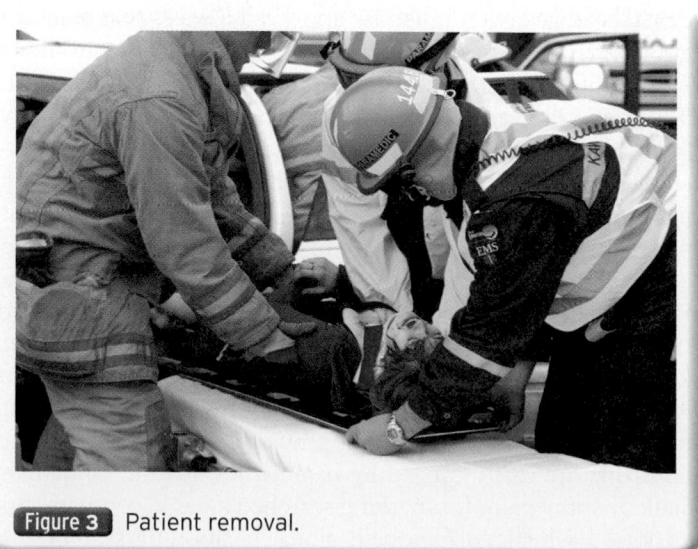

Figure 3 Patient removal.

The standard basket stretcher carry involves a team of six to eight rescuers distributed around the stretcher, three or four to a side. Normally, the person at the front of the left side is in charge and directs the activities of the others. This method has the advantages of being fast because little teamwork is required and it usually gives the patient a comfortable ride. Its disadvantages include the fact that this carrying method is tiring for the handlers because it puts constant strain on certain muscles, and ground vision is difficult, especially at night; a handler can easily trip over a rock and drop the stretcher.

More than one team will be needed if the stretcher must be carried over a distance farther than the team can cover in about 15 to 20 minutes. Team *leapfrogging* is a good method to use on long evacuations (one team takes the litter for a given distance whereas the other team goes ahead to rest and preplan the next stretch). At the pass-off point, the first team advances to the next point for rest and planning.

When footing is highly unstable, an obstacle prevents the team from progressing, or falling becomes a possible hazard, the caterpillar or lap pass is a useful option. When the stretcher reaches the obstacle, the team pauses while every extra person lines up on the route ahead of the difficult terrain or obstacles. The rescuers form two lines facing each other about the width of the stretcher apart and alternate (in other words, they are not all opposite each other). They usually sit down and try to make themselves as stable as possible. When everyone is set, rescuers pass the stretcher down between the two lines. As the stretcher passes a person, he or she gets up and carefully but quickly moves around the line in the direction of travel, and gets set to pass the stretcher again. Done correctly, this technique provides a stable and secure passage.

■ Transport

Once the patient has been removed from the hazard area, EMS will undertake transport to an appropriate medical facility. Depending on the severity of the patient's injuries and the distance to the medical facility, the type of transport will vary. For example, if a patient is critically injured or if the rescue is taking place some distance from the hospital, air transportation may be more appropriate than a ground ambulance.

Words of Wisdom

If you will be assisting a technical rescue team, training with the team is probably the most important step you can take so that you can work together effectively during a TRI. Training allows you to get a feel for how the team members operate; likewise, they can get an idea of which duties are within your level of expertise. The more knowledge you have, the more you will be able to do.

■ Vehicle Extrication

According to the National Highway Transportation Safety Administration (NHTSA), in 2009, an estimated 5,505,000 police-reported motor vehicle traffic crashes occurred. An aver-

YOU *are the Medic* | PART 2

Approximately 45 minutes after your arrival, the area by the patient has been declared safe for you and your partner to approach. Manual spinal immobilization has been maintained by one of the fire fighters. You ask him to continue to assist while you perform your primary assessment.

The patient tells you that it is difficult for her to "catch her breath" and repeatedly asks you where her grandson is. She states that she was playing with her 5-year-old grandson when the house began to shake. The next thing she knew she was lying in the mud trapped underneath the rubble. She is not sure whether she lost consciousness. The patient has a history of diabetes for which she takes metformin and insulin.

Recording Time: 5 Minutes	
Respirations	26 breaths/min, shallow
Pulse	Carotid pulse, 108 beats/min, regular and strong
Skin	Pale, cool, and diaphoretic
Blood pressure	Unable to obtain
Oxygen saturation (Spo₂)	Unable to obtain
Pupils	Equal and reactive to light

3. What are the three control zones that will be established while the scene is being stabilized?

4. Why is it important for the incident management system to be used during a technical rescue incident?

age of 93 people died each day in motor vehicle crashes in 2009. These statistics may have contributed to the inclusion of the vehicle extrication module in the National EMS Education Standards.

Vehicle Anatomy and Structural Components

To reduce confusion and mistakes at vehicle extrication scenes, it is important for you to use standardized terminology when referring to specific parts of vehicles. For example, the front of a vehicle normally travels down the road first. The hood is located on the front of the vehicle, and the rear of a vehicle is where the trunk is usually located.

The left side of a vehicle is on your left as you sit in the vehicle. In the United States and Canada, the driver's seat is on the left side of the vehicle. The right side of a vehicle is where the passenger's seat is located. Always refer to left and right as they relate to *the vehicle*—not as they refer to *your* left and right. It is also acceptable to refer to the left side of the vehicle as the driver side and the right side of the vehicle as the passenger side.

Roof posts (or pillars) are designed to add vertical support to the roof structure of a vehicle. The posts are generally labeled with an alphabetic type description (A-B-C). The A posts are located closest to the front of the vehicle; they form the sides of the windshield. In four-door vehicles, the B posts are located between the front and rear doors of a vehicle; in some vehicles, they do not reach all of the way to the roof. In four-door vehicles, the C posts are located behind the rear doors, if present **Figure 4**. D posts can be found on larger vehicles such as sport utility vehicles and vans that have windows behind the rear doors.

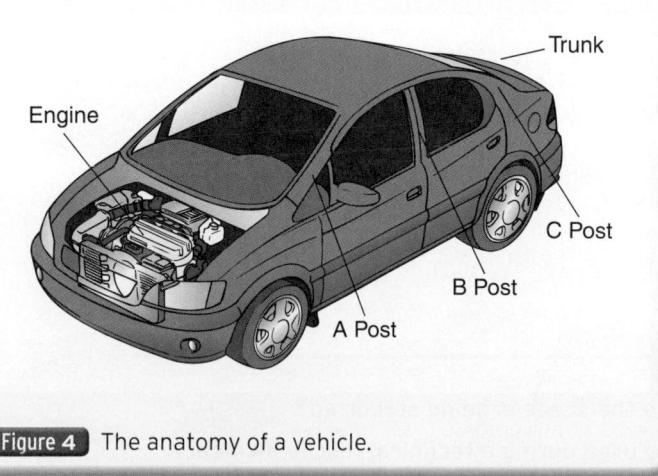

Figure 4 The anatomy of a vehicle.

The hood covers the engine compartment. The bulkhead divides the engine compartment from the passenger compartment. An insulating metal piece known as the firewall protects the passengers in the event of an engine fire. The passenger compartment includes the front and back seats. This part of a vehicle is sometimes called the occupant cage or occupant compartment.

There are two common types of vehicle frames: the *body-over-frame* construction and the unitized or *unibody* construction. These frames can be composed of steel (most common), aluminum, or carbon fiber/composite.

Body-over-frame construction uses two large beams tied together with cross member beams to fabricate the load-bearing frame of a vehicle. The engine, transmission, and body components are then attached to this basic platform frame. This type of frame is sometimes referred to as a ladder frame because of its similarity **Figure 5**. This type of frame construction is found primarily in trucks and sport utility vehicles; it is rarely found in smaller passenger cars. Body-over-frame construction provides a structurally sound base for stabilizing the vehicle and an anchor point for attaching cables or extrication tools. The potential for the body-over-frame design to be split in half with a severe crash is low, but you should be aware that the force distribution from the impact will be greater on the occupants.

Unibody construction, which is used for most modern cars, combines the vehicle body and the frame into a single component. The vehicle body is merged with the chassis, which consists of the braking, steering, and suspension system **Figure 6**. Unibody construction allows auto manufacturers to produce lighter weight vehicles. Unibody construction has the ability to absorb or redirect energy during a crash; it incorporates crumple zones into the front and sometimes the rear of the vehicle to redirect energy away from the passenger compartment. When an impact occurs, the crumple zones collapse, absorbing and diverting the force or energy of the crash and preventing intrusion into the cab of the vehicle. To fully understand this, you must understand the law of conservation of energy and particularly the mechanical energy system as it relates to the vehicle crash. Refer to the chapter, *Trauma Systems and Mechanism of Injury,* for more information. There is a negative

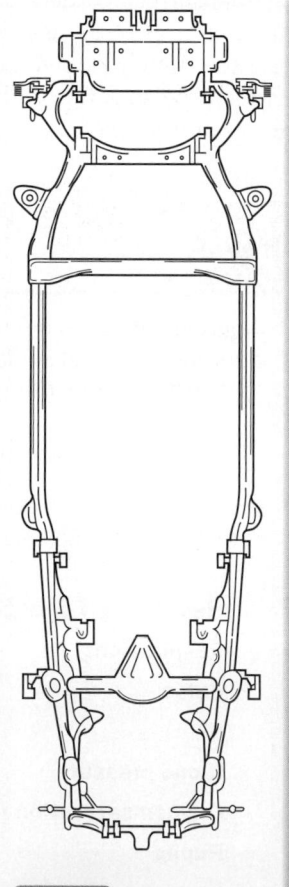

Figure 5 Body-over-frame construction has cross members that are similar to a ladder.

aspect of the unibody design. Because there is no frame structure, it is possible that the vehicle may split in half in a severe crash.

Alternative Powered Vehicles

Today, with advances in automotive technology, EMS responders should keep in mind that some vehicles on the road are alternative powered vehicles. <u>Alternative powered vehicles</u> may be powered by electricity and electricity/gasoline hybrids, or fuels such as propane, natural gas, methanol, or hydrogen. Caution should be used while working around alternative powered vehicles. Basic actions should be taken to secure the vehicle as soon as possible. This includes turning off the ignition key, setting the parking brake, and putting the vehicle in park. Trained rescue personnel may further secure the electrical system by disconnecting the battery.

Alternative powered vehicles are usually identified by markings on the vehicle **Figure 7** . You should not approach an alternative powered vehicle until properly trained and equipped rescuers can enter the scene. Toxic fumes and vapors from electric vehicle batteries can be carried in smoke or steam.

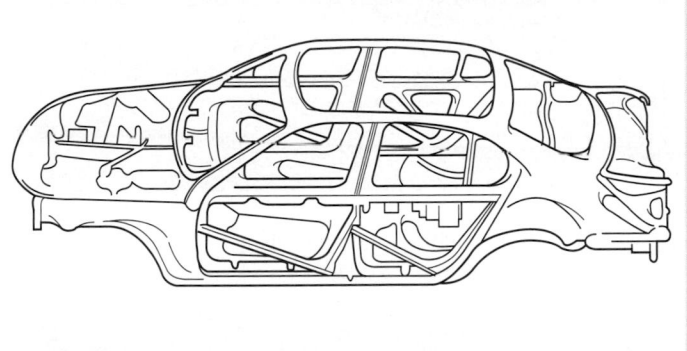

Figure 6 The unibody design.

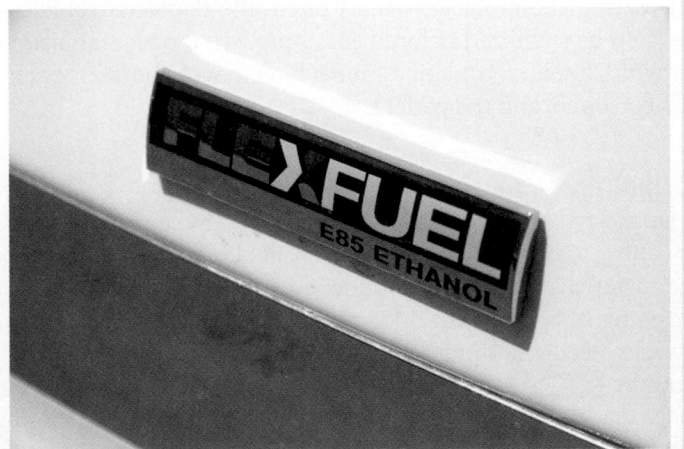

Figure 7 A flex fuel identification badge. Flex fuel vehicles are capable of running on gasoline alone or using an E85 blend of up to 85% ethanol and 15% gasoline for power.

In more than 40% of today's alternative powered vehicles, the batteries are not located in the engine compartment, but in other areas, such as the trunk or under the seats. Furthermore, there also may be more than one battery present. You must remain vigilant when you are presented with these alternative types of vehicles and their inherent dangers. For example, hybrid batteries have higher amperes than a traditional vehicle's battery, and these amperes can injure you.

Safety

A fire fueled by ethanol or methanol burns bright blue and can be difficult to see on a clear day.

Hazardous Materials

Vehicle extrication incidents could require specialized teams to manage hazardous materials, depending on the complexity of the incident. Before approaching a wreck, you should consider additional hazards from the vehicle or vehicles involved, such as fire hazards, electrical hazards, fuel sources, or fuel run-off, all of which are potential ignition sources. For example, an accident involving a tanker or semi-truck containing a known or unknown hazardous product would require hazardous materials personnel or a hazardous materials team to respond. In incidents involving hazardous materials, rescuers must follow a proper size-up and evaluation process. All too often in incidents involving hazardous materials, rescue personnel are unnecessarily exposed to dangerous agents because they rush into the incident site before they have gathered the necessary information pertaining to the material or agent. Although responders trained at the awareness level

Words of Wisdom

Tips for managing alternative powered vehicle hazards:

- Look for markings specific to alternative powered vehicles, and call early for assistance.
- Do not use flares to mark off the incident scene; use non-sparking markers such as cones.
- Stabilize the vehicle by turning off the ignition, setting the brakes, and using cribbing. Do not forget to turn off the valve to the fuel cylinder.
- A quiet hybrid is not necessarily turned off.
- Be aware of the potential for toxic vapors, gases, or fumes even if no fire is present. Also remember that during daylight hours it may be difficult to see flames from a fire fueled by methanol or ethanol.
- Avoid contact with any fluids leaking from the vehicle.
- Call for HazMat teams as soon as possible, and set up a safety zone around the perimeter to keep bystanders and rescue personnel safe.

perform only limited activities in such scenarios, they can certainly assist operations- and technician-level trained responders by looking through a set of binoculars and identifying placards, product labels, numbers, and other information. They can also assist in the response by preventing others from entering the incident site by sealing the site perimeter and referring to the DOT's *ERG* to identify the product, evacuation distances, the product's flammability and incompatibilities, and other pertinent data.

Hand Tools

A **hand tool** is any tool or equipment that operates from human power. Hand tools are the basis of all working tools. In some instances, hand tools may be more efficient than power tools. You should have a thorough working knowledge of the basic, simple hand tools used for any TRI.

Hand tools can be categorized as follows:

- Striking tools (eg, a hammer) **Figure 8**
- Leverage/prying/spreading tools (eg, a pry bar) **Figure 9**
- Cutting tools (eg, trauma shears, glass hand saw) **Figure 10**
- Lifting/pushing/pulling tools (eg, hooks, pike poles) **Figure 11**

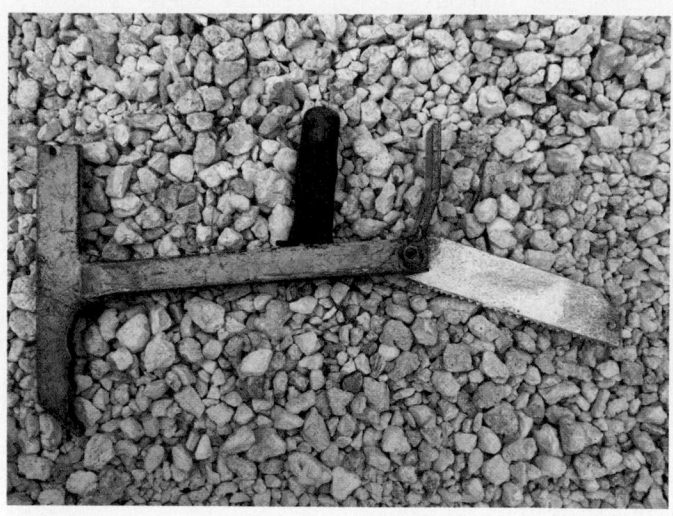

Figure 10 A cutting tool such as the Glass Master can be used to cut out a windshield.

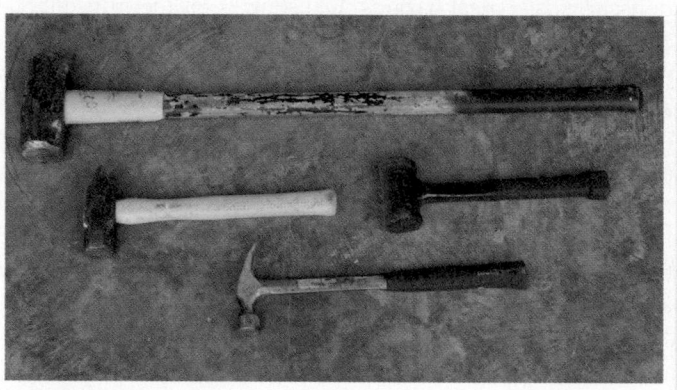

Figure 8 Striking tools.

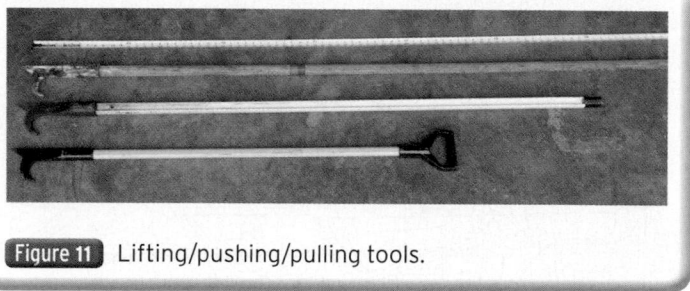

Figure 11 Lifting/pushing/pulling tools.

Vehicle Stabilization

Unstable objects pose a threat to both rescuers and victims of the crash. These objects—most often, the damaged vehicles—need to be stabilized before your approach. Proper stabilization provides a solid foundation from which to work, ensuring safety for personnel and the patient.

Cribbing

The most basic, physical tool used for vehicle stabilization is **cribbing**. Cribbing is commonly available as wood or composite materials, with some products being made of steel. Several cribbing designs are used for extrication incidents, such as step chocks, wedges, shims, and sections of timber cut at various lengths **Figure 12**. **Step chocks** are specialized cribbing assemblies made of wood or plastic/composite blocks in a step configuration. **Wedges** are objects used to snug loose cribbing under the load or to fill a void space. **Shims** are similar in design to a wedge, but their profile is much smaller.

Cribbing can be used regardless of the position of the vehicle **Figure 13**.

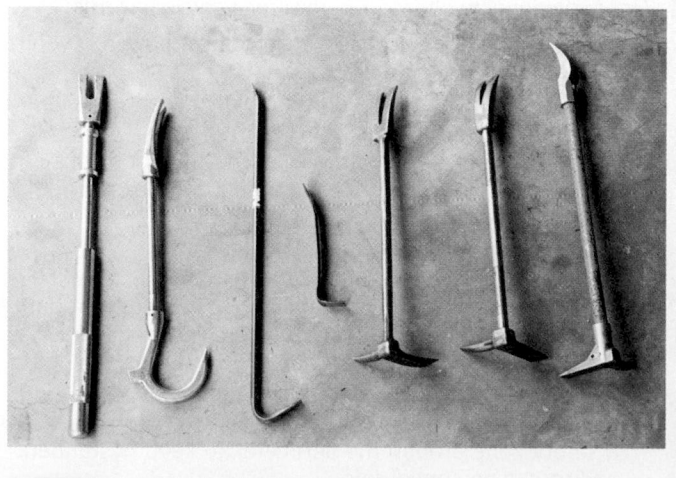

Figure 9 Leverage/prying/spreading tools.

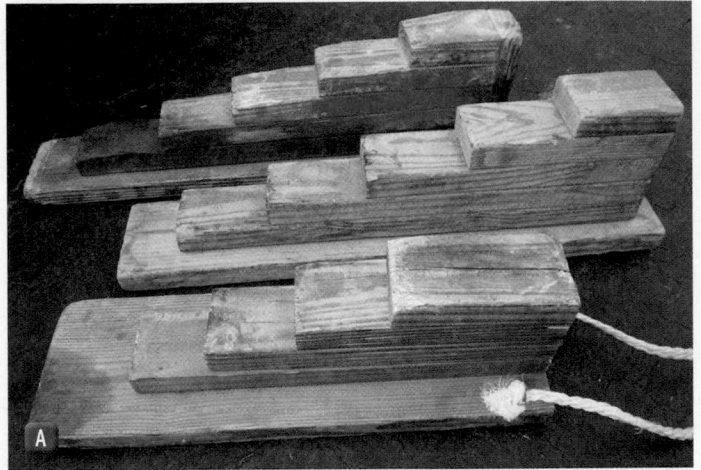

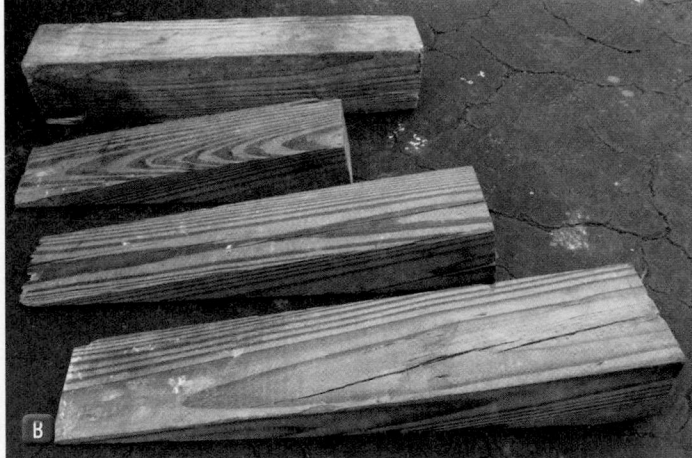

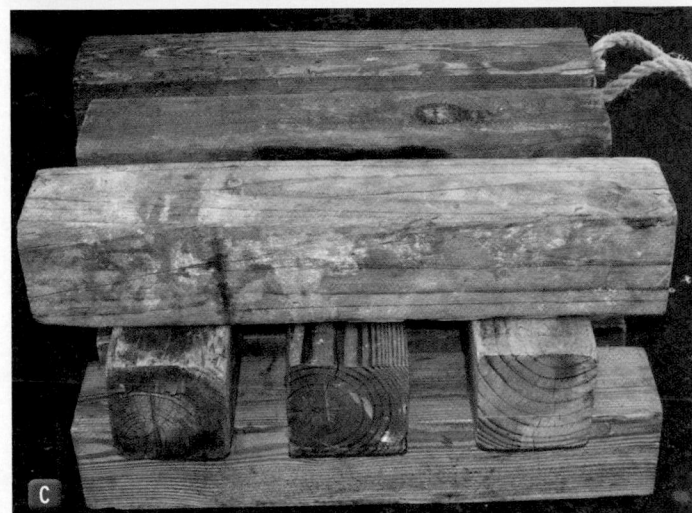

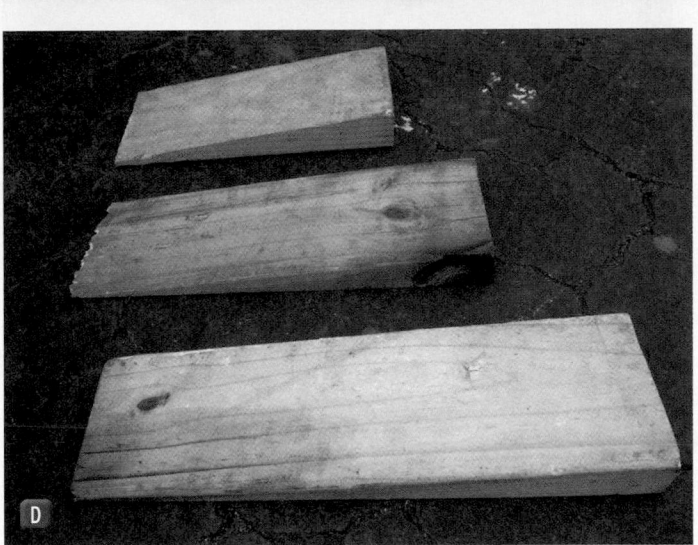

Figure 12 Wood cribbing designs. **A.** Step chocks. **B.** Wedges. **C.** Box crib. **D.** Shims.

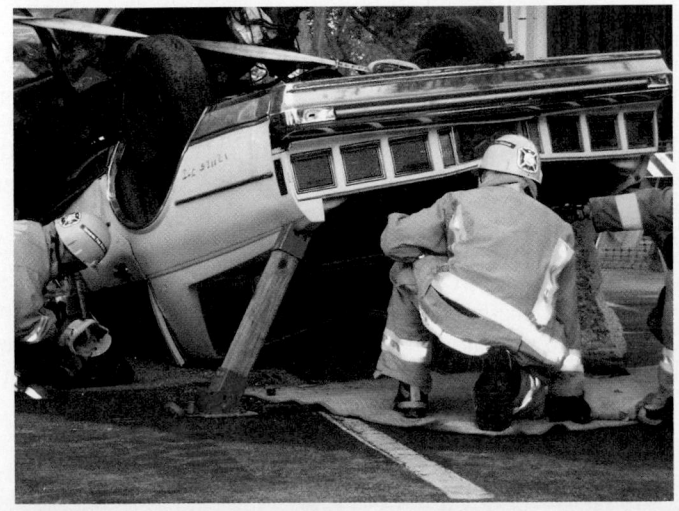

Figure 13 This vehicle is being stabilized on its roof using cribbing.

Words of Wisdom

Even vehicles that are positioned upright on all four wheels should be stabilized.

After cribbing has been placed, a vehicle may still move because of the give and motion generated by the suspension system. The five directional movements include horizontal movement, vertical movement, roll movement, pitch movement, and yaw movement **Figure 14**. These movements may occur as rescuers enter the vehicle and as the patients are extricated from the vehicle, and they can cause further injuries.

After the vehicle is completely stabilized, put the vehicle in park, set the parking brake, and turn the vehicle off.

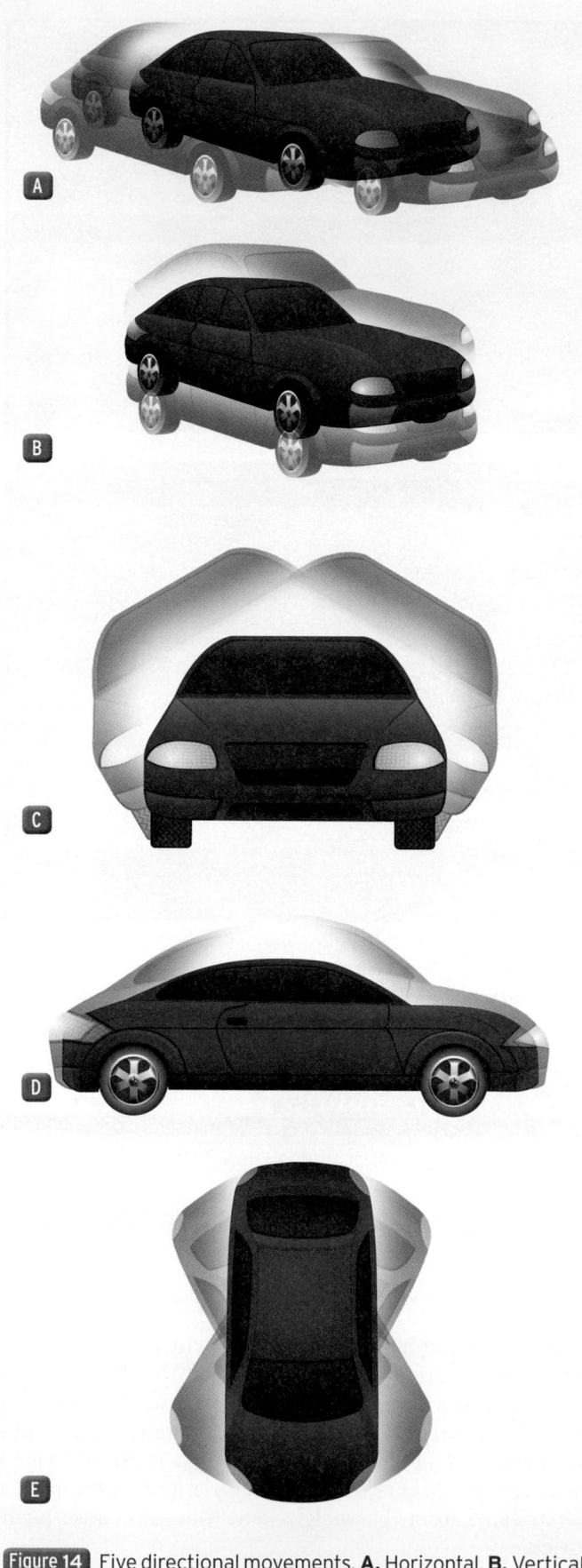

Figure 14 Five directional movements. **A.** Horizontal. **B.** Vertical. **C.** Roll. **D.** Pitch. **E.** Yaw.

■ Gaining Access to the Patient

This section discusses simple vehicle access techniques.

Words of Wisdom

An often-debated topic is whether the tires of the vehicle should be deflated after cribbing has been inserted. When the tires are deflated, a benefit is that the vehicle settles down onto the cribbing, creating a solid foundation to work from. A drawback of tire deflation is that the vehicle stability may shift. Some agencies do not advocate tire deflation because it may interfere with law enforcement's investigation by eliminating a means of measuring tire pressure. Always follow your local protocols.

Opening the Door

After stabilizing the vehicle, the simplest way to access a patient is to open a door. Try all of the doors first—even if they appear to be badly damaged. Make sure the locking mechanism is released. If the doors are locked, you might consider breaking a window using the techniques described in this chapter, and then attempt to manually release the locking mechanism to unlock the doors. It is a waste of time and energy to open a jammed door with heavy rescue equipment when another door can be opened without any special equipment.

Words of Wisdom

Energy-absorbing bumpers can explode when subjected to heat and can spring out when loaded.

Breaking Tempered Glass

If a patient's medical condition is serious enough to require immediate care and you cannot enter the vehicle through a door, consider breaking a window. Do not try to break and enter through the windshield because it is made of **laminated glass**, which is difficult to break. The side and rear windows are made of **tempered glass**, and will break easily into small pieces when hit Figure 15 . Sharp, pointed hand tools such as a spring-loaded center punch can be used to break the glass Figure 16 . Because these windows do not pose as great a safety threat, they can be your primary access route.

If you must break a window to unlock a door or gain access, try to break one that is far away from the patient. If the patient's

Words of Wisdom

The easiest way to enter an automobile is through a door. Try before you pry.

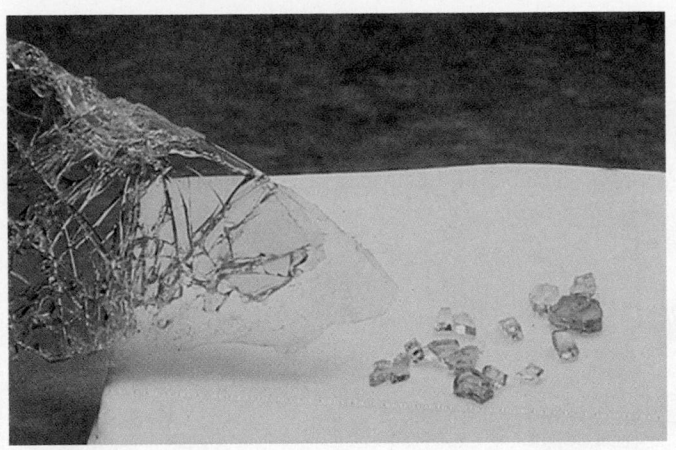

Figure 15 The two types of glass in vehicles: laminated glass (left) and tempered glass (right).

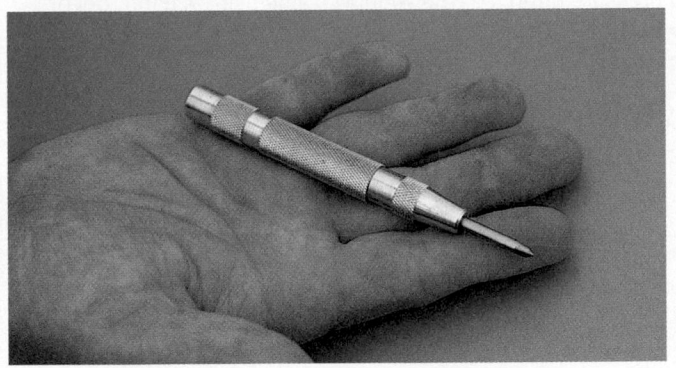

Figure 16 For tempered glass, a spring-loaded center punch is the most basic and common of all glass removal tools.

Words of Wisdom

Always warn trapped car passengers that you are going to break the glass!

condition warrants your immediate entry, however, do not hesitate to break the closest window. If access allows, place a blanket over the patient prior to breaking the glass.

During this step of the rescue, all rescuers should be in proper PPE, including dust mask, gloves, safety glasses, or

Words of Wisdom

Do not use a sledgehammer to crack a walnut. Use the right tool!

goggles. You should attempt to lower the windows as far as possible before breaking the glass. If you are using something other than a spring-loaded center punch, always aim for a low corner. The window frame will help prevent the tool (such as an axe or screwdriver) from entering the vehicle and striking the person inside. Other EMS personnel are given a verbal warning, "Breaking glass," unless a stop/freeze call is made. After breaking the window, use a hand tool to clean out the remaining glass in the window frame so it does not fall onto any passengers or injure any rescuers. Place the debris in a safe area to avoid injuries.

To break tempered glass using a spring-loaded center punch, follow the steps in Skill Drill 1:

Skill Drill 1

1. Don appropriate PPE.
2. Ensure the scene is safe and the vehicle is stable.
3. Ensure the patient is properly protected from flying glass particles. Warn personnel verbally, "Breaking glass!"
4. Using the window farthest from the patient, place the palm of your hand facedown against the lower corner of the window and frame, with your index finger and thumb facing upward.
5. Position and rest the body of the tool in the ridge section of the palm (V-section of your hand) between your index finger and thumb Step 1.
6. With the point of the center punch directly on the glass, apply forward pressure on the center punch until the spring is activated and the glass breaks Step 2.
7. Once the glass breaks, remove remaining glass segments around the window frame using a hand tool. Follow this procedure until all glass has been removed from the frame Step 3.

Once you have removed the pieces of glass from the frame, try to unlock the door again. Release the locking mechanism, and then use both the inside and outside door handles at the same time. This action may force a jammed locking mechanism, even in a door that appears to be badly damaged.

Breaking the rear window will sometimes provide an opening large enough to enable a rescuer to reach a patient if there is no other rapid means for gaining access. Using the simple techniques of opening a door or breaking the rear window will enable you to gain access to most patients in vehicle crashes, even those in upside-down vehicles.

If you cannot gain access to the vehicle by the methods already described, heavier extrication tools and trained personnel must be summoned to gain access to the patient.

Providing Initial Medical Care

Once entrance and access to the patient have been provided, you should begin to provide emergency medical care. This includes spinal immobilization and assessment and management of the ABCs. Being trapped in a damaged vehicle is a frightening

Skill Drill 1

Breaking Tempered Glass Using a Spring-Loaded Center Punch

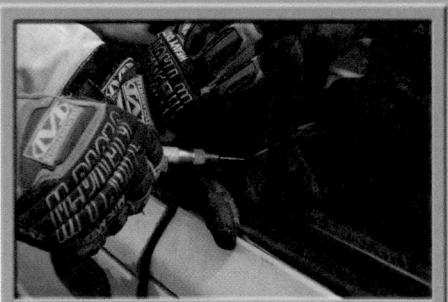

Step 1 Follow standard precautions using PPE. Assess the scene for hazards and stabilize the vehicle. Ensure that the patient is properly protected from flying glass particles. Warn all personnel and patients that you will be breaking the glass. Using the window farthest from the patient, place the palm of your hand facedown against the lower corner of the window and frame, with your index finger and thumb facing upward. Position and rest the body of the tool in the ridge section of the palm (V-section of your hand) between your index finger and thumb.

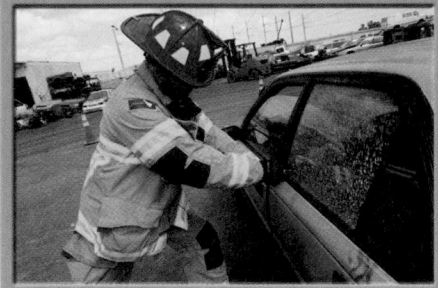

Step 2 With the point of the spring-loaded center punch directly on the glass, apply forward pressure until the spring is activated and the glass breaks.

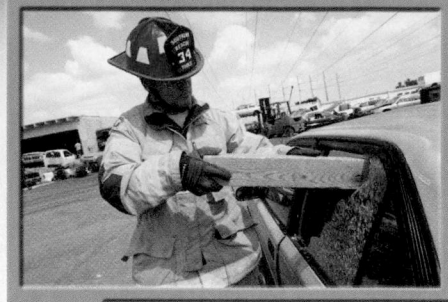

Step 3 Remove all loose tempered glass fragments from around the window frame using a hand tool or a piece of cribbing.

experience, so it is important that one caregiver remain with the patient and provide both emotional comfort and physical care. Patient care should occur simultaneously with extrication **Figure 17**. Although it may be necessary to delay some elements of these processes for a short period, it is important to work toward the goal of stabilizing the patient and removing him or her from the vehicle as quickly and safely as possible.

■ Disentangling the Patient

The next step in the vehicle extrication sequence is disentangling the patient, a measure that seeks to remove those parts of the vehicle that are trapping the patient. The goal here is to remove the sheet metal and plastic from around the patient—not to "cut the patient out of the vehicle."

Words of Wisdom

A good extrication is a safe extrication.

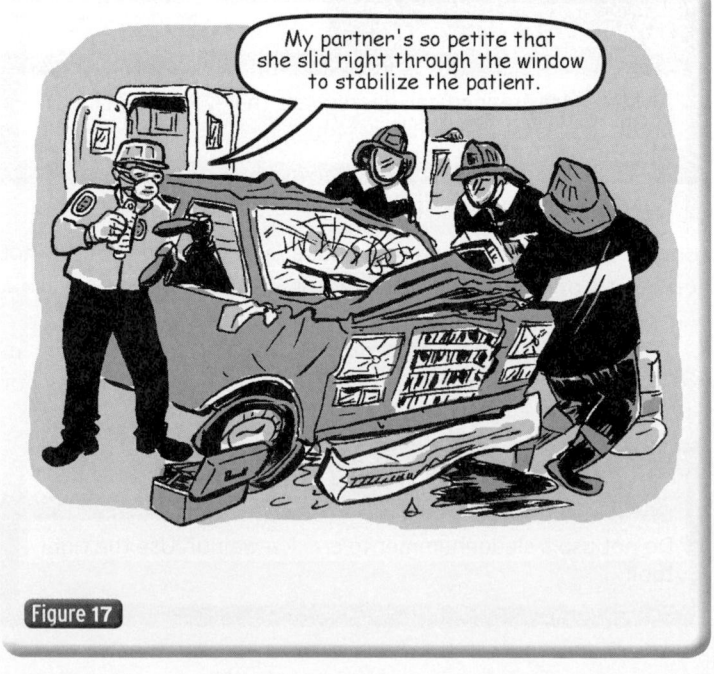

Figure 17

Before attempting disentanglement, study the situation. What is trapping the patient in the vehicle? Is the patient wearing a seat belt? Have all air bags been deployed? Only those disentanglement procedures that are necessary to remove the patient safely from the vehicle will be performed. The order in which these procedures are performed will be dictated by the specific conditions at the incident. Many times it will be necessary to perform one procedure before you can access the parts of the vehicle needed to perform another procedure. For example, the rescuer will need to find and disable undeployed air bags before removing the patient.

Before the patient is disentangled from the wrecked vehicle, the patient should be protected by covering him or her with a blanket or by using a backboard. Be sure that the patient understands what is being done—the sounds made by extrication procedures can be frightening for patients.

To learn all of the methods of disentangling a patient, you need to take an approved extrication course. The procedures presented below are the ones that are most commonly performed. Maintaining spinal alignment and immobilization is one of the main objectives of disentangling and actually removing a patient from the vehicle.

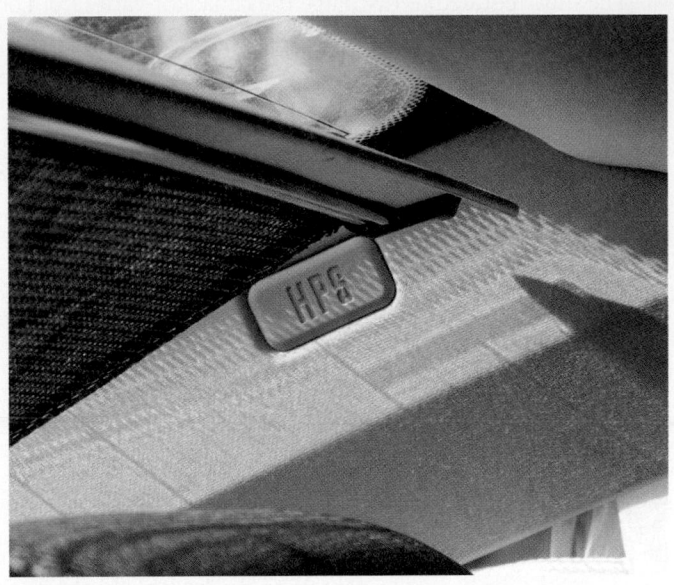

Figure 18 This air bag acronym stands for "head protection system."

Words of Wisdom

A seat belt pretensioning system is designed to automatically tighten or take up slack in a seat belt when a crash is detected. These systems can be activated in conjunction with the air bags or act independently.

Air Bag Safety

Before work can begin to remove the parts of the vehicle that are trapping the patient, a thorough inspection should be performed to identify and disable undeployed air bags. Undeployed air bags may deploy during extrication and cause harm to the patient and the rescuers. Air bag recognition and identification can be determined by the air bag badging or labeling system. These markings consist of acronyms that are generally located in proximity to the air bag inflator **Figure 18**. Never assume an air bag is dead just because power has been disconnected. A vehicle air bag system comes equipped with an energy capacitor that can store power for up to 30 minutes in some models. When you are working around air bags, your best defense is recognition and identification, disconnecting the power supply, and proper distancing.

Words of Wisdom

Vehicle extrication is a step-by-step technical process.

To disconnect power on a vehicle to disable an air bag system, remove the key from the ignition. Then, turn on an electrical component of the vehicle such as the emergency warning flashers to indicate whether the power is still connected. If the vehicle has electrical adjustable components such as electric seats or electric windows, you should adjust these components to provide better access before disabling power. To disable power, remove or cut the battery cables starting with the negative side **Figure 19**. Avoid the cables reconnecting with a terminal or the vehicle frame. Be aware that the main 12-volt DC battery may not be located in the traditional location under the engine compartment hood; it can also be found inside one of the wheel wells, under the rear/backseat, or in the trunk on some vehicles. Verify there is only one battery in the vehicle.

Remember the following when you are dealing with air bag systems:

- Steering wheels on most recently manufactured vehicles contain an air bag, which is a lifesaving safety feature for the occupants of the vehicle.
- If the air bag has deployed during the crash, it does not present a safety hazard for rescuers.
- If not deployed during the crash, an air bag presents a hazard for the passenger of the vehicle and for rescue personnel. It could potentially deploy if wires are cut or if it becomes activated during the rescue operation.
- If the air bag did not deploy, disconnect the battery and allow the air bag capacitor to discharge.

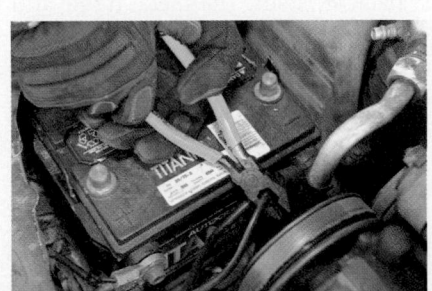

Figure 19 Remove or cut battery cables starting with the negative side.

The time required to discharge the capacitor varies from one model of air bag to another.

- Some newer-model vehicles have a switch mounted on or under the dash that allows drivers to disconnect or shut off the air bag.
- Do not place a hard object such as a backboard between the patient and an undeployed air bag.
- Do not attempt to cut a steering wheel if the air bag has not deployed.
- For your safety, never get in front of an undeployed air bag. You could sustain serious injuries if it is unexpectedly activated.
- Some vehicles contain side-mounted air bags or curtains that provide lateral protection for passengers. Check vehicles for the presence of these devices.

Displacing the Seat

In frontal and rear-end collisions, the vehicle may become compressed. As the front of the vehicle is pushed back, the space between the steering wheel and the seat becomes smaller. Displacing the seat can relieve pressure on the driver and give rescuers more space for removal.

If it is necessary to displace a seat backward, start with the simplest steps. Many times you can gain some room by moving the seat backward on its track, especially with short drivers who have the seat forward. To move a seat back, first be sure to provide spinal immobilization. With manually operated seats, you need to release the seat-adjusting lever and carefully slide the seat back as far as it will go. If the seat is electrically operated, check that the car has power, and engage the lever to electrically move the seat backward. With seats that have adjustable backs and adjustable heights, you can use these features to give the patient more room or lower the seat to help disentangle the patient.

If these methods are unsuccessful, perform a seat displacement.

Words of Wisdom

Remove the vehicle from the patient, not the patient from the vehicle.

In some cases, it may be helpful to remove the back of the seat. To do so, cut the upholstery away from the bottom of the seat back exposing the metal frame and the areas of attachment **Figure 20**. A reciprocating saw may be used to cut the supports for the seat back. If a technical rescuer is on scene, he or she may use an air chisel or a hydraulic cutter. Be certain that the patient is supported and protected during this procedure.

Removing the Windshield

A second technique that is often part of disentanglement is the removal of glass. Removing the rear window, side glass, or windshield improves communication between rescue personnel inside the vehicle and personnel outside the vehicle. Sometimes all you need to do is to roll a window down. Open windows provide a good route for passing medical care supplies to the

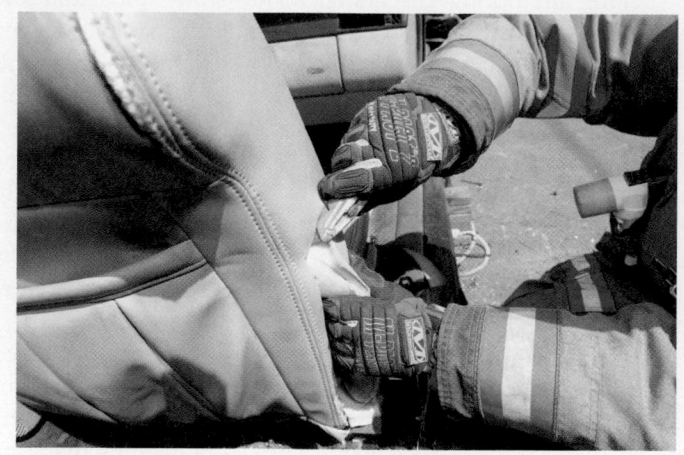

Figure 20 Cut away the upholstery of the front seat in order to expose the metal frame and the areas of attachment.

inside caregiver. When the roof of a vehicle must be removed, all of the glass must first be removed from the vehicle.

On most vehicles, the side windows and rear window are tempered glass that can be removed by striking the glass in a lower corner with a sharp object, such as a spring-loaded center punch. In contrast, windshields cannot be broken with a spring-loaded center punch. They consist of plastic laminated glass—a type of "sandwich," in which the two pieces of bread are thin sheets of specially constructed glass and the filling is a thin layer of a special flexible plastic. When laminated glass is struck by a sharp stone or by a spring-loaded center punch, a small mark is formed, but the structure of the glass remains intact. For this reason, the windshield must be removed in one large piece. The windshields of most passenger vehicles are glued in place with a strong, plastic-type adhesive.

Removing a windshield is an essential step before removing the roof of a vehicle. It will also provide added space when emergency medical care is being administered to an injured patient. The windshield of a damaged vehicle may be removed by a trained technical rescuer using a glass hand saw **Figure 21**.

Removing the Roof

Removing the roof of a vehicle allows equipment to be more easily passed in to the emergency medical provider. It also increases the amount of space available to perform medical care and increases the visibility and space for performing disentanglement. Both the provider and patient will benefit from the fresh air supply, too. The increased space helps to reduce the feeling of panic caused by the confined space of the wrecked vehicle. Removing the roof also provides a large exit route for the patient.

A key consideration in displacing the roof is to ensure the safety of rescuers and the patient inside the vehicle. In particular, as you cut the posts that support the roof, rescuers must support the roof to keep it from falling on the patient. The removal of a roof may be performed by a trained technical rescuer **Figure 22**.

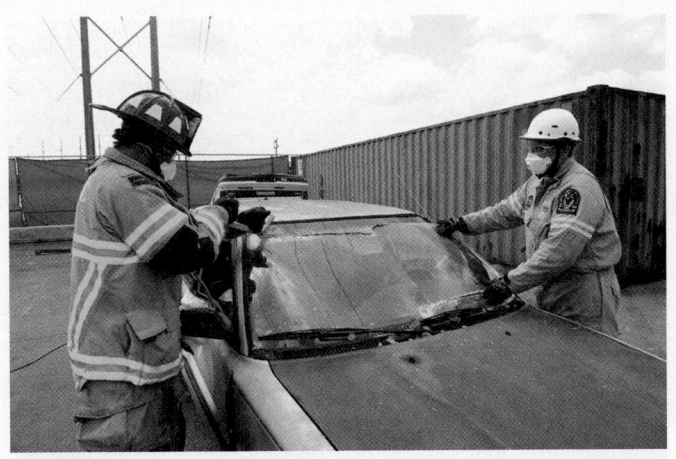

Figure 21 A technical rescuer removing the windshield with a glass handsaw.

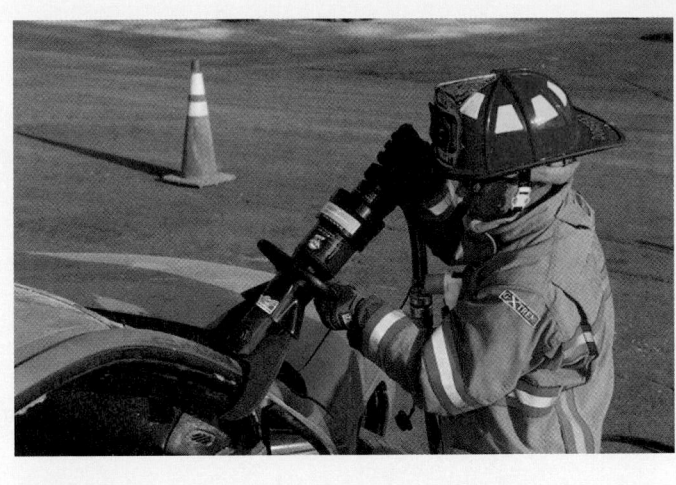

Figure 22 A technical rescuer removing the roof.

Displacing the Dash

During a frontal collision, the vehicle's dash may be pushed down or backward. When a patient is trapped by the dash, it must be moved using a technique called the dash roll technique. The objective of the dash roll technique is to lift the dash up and move it forward. The process involves pushing or rolling the entire front end of the vehicle, which encompasses the dashboard, steering wheel, and steering column, off of the entrapped occupant. The roof should be removed before this can be performed.

A dash roll technique requires a hydraulic cutter. A tool such as the hydraulic ram then pushes the dash forward, and cribbing maintains the opening made with these tools. A dash roll technique may be performed by a trained technical rescuer **Figure 23**.

YOU *are the Medic*   PART 3

The patient continues to be concerned and anxious about the safety of her grandson. You calmly reassure her that all efforts are being made to locate him and that you will let her know once he is found. You place the patient on a nonrebreathing mask at 15 L/min and try to coach her to take slow, deep breaths.

Twenty minutes later enough of the debris has been removed to allow for a full assessment. Assessment reveals tenderness to both sides of the rib cage with diminished breath sounds bilaterally and symmetric chest rise. The abdomen is soft and tender to palpation of the lower quadrants. You note bruising on the lower portion of the abdomen beneath the umbilicus. A 3-inch laceration to the left thigh with venous bleeding is found. At this time you ask your partner to dress the laceration while you obtain IV access with a 16-gauge catheter in the left antecubital space and initiate a normal saline drip using a 10-drop set running at 10 drops per minute. Your partner also performs a finger stick for a blood glucose level; the result is 183 mg/dL.

Recording Time: 30 Minutes	
Respirations	28 breaths/min, shallow
Pulse	Radial pulse, 126 beats/min, regular and strong
Skin	Pale, warm, diaphoretic
Blood pressure	104/62 mm Hg
Oxygen saturation (Spo$_2$)	96% on 15 L/min nonrebreathing mask
Pupils	Equal and reactive

5. Patients involved in situations requiring extrication frequently become anxious. What can you do to help calm the patient?

6. Why is the patient at risk for developing crush syndrome?

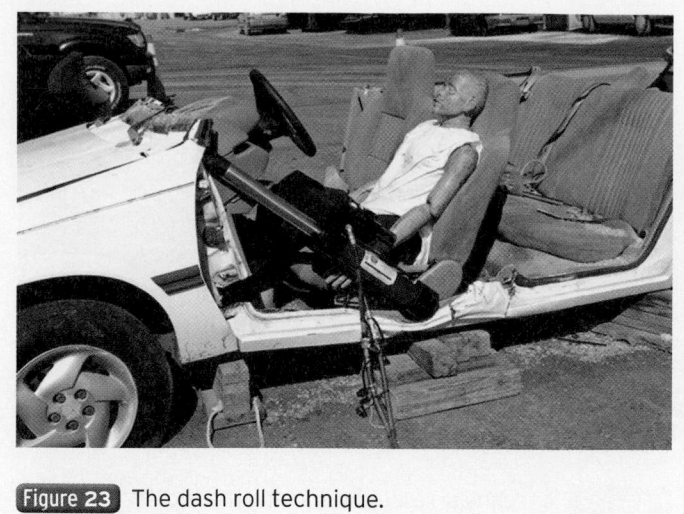

Figure 23 The dash roll technique.

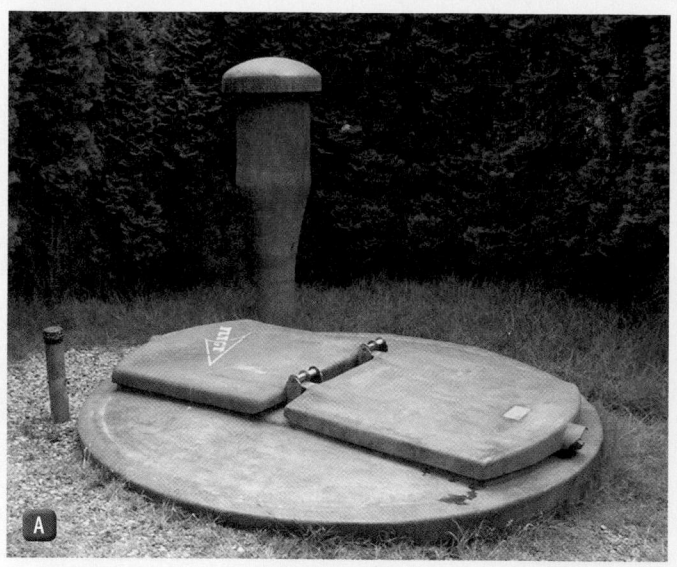

A

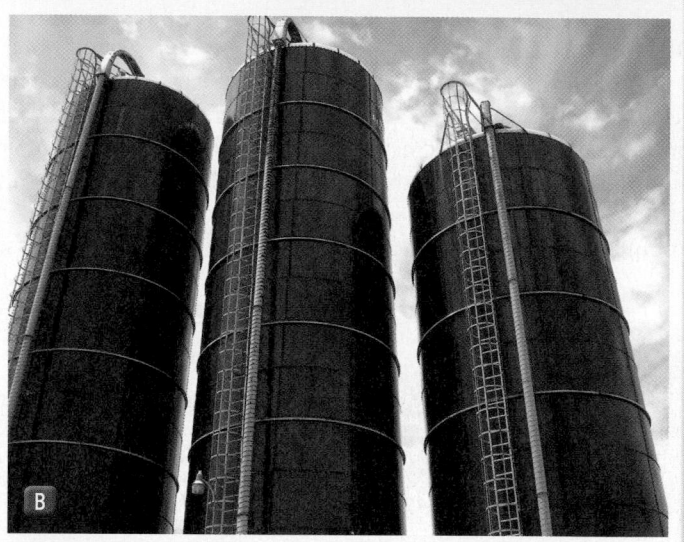

B

Figure 24 Confined spaces **A.** Below ground. **B.** Silo.

Additional Specialized Rescue Situations

Confined Spaces

A confined space is a location surrounded by a structure that is not designed for continuous occupancy. Confined spaces have limited openings for entrance and exit. Confined spaces can occur in farm, commercial, and industrial settings. Structures such as grain silos, industrial pits, tanks, and below-ground structures are all considered confined spaces. Automobile trunks are also considered confined spaces. Cisterns, well casings, and septic tanks are also confined spaces that are found in many residential settings Figure 24 .

Confined spaces present a special hazard because they may have limited ventilation to provide for air circulation and exchange, which can make them an oxygen-deficient atmosphere, or they may contain poisonous gases. Entering a confined space without testing the atmosphere for safety and without the proper breathing apparatus can result in death. Technical rescue teams will use air sampling monitors to check the atmosphere prior to making entry. Additionally, there is a risk of fire and explosion in confined spaces because inadequate ventilation may trap flammable mixtures. Grain silos and trenches can suddenly become "quicksand" and lead to engulfment. Machinery may often have confined spaces containing augers or screws that can be hazardous to rescue workers. All rescue personnel must consider the potential for stored electrical energy in any machinery and should never attempt any rescue without being properly trained.

Do not be overwhelmed by the urgency to start treating patients; scene safety must always be considered first. A confined-space call is sometimes dispatched as a heart attack or medical illness call, because the caller assumes the person who entered a confined space and became unresponsive experienced a heart attack or medical illness.

Words of Wisdom

Confined spaces such as manholes can be deceiving. They may look somewhat habitable but can contain minimal oxygen or deadly invisible toxins.

Oxygen Deficiency and Poisonous Gases

Hydrogen sulfide (H_2S) is a colorless, toxic, flammable gas that is released when bacteria break down organic matter in the absence of oxygen. It can be found in swamps, standing water, sewers, volcanic gases, natural gas, and in some wells. Hydrogen sulfide is heavier than air and has a pungent odor at first but deadens the sense of smell quickly.

Carbon monoxide (CO) is a colorless, odorless, tasteless gas that cannot be detected by your normal senses. Inhaling relatively small quantities of co gas can result in severe poisoning because it binds to red blood cells about 200 to 250 times more readily than oxygen. Therefore, a small quantity of co can "monopolize" the red blood cells and prevent them from transporting oxygen to all parts of the body. The signs and symptoms of co poisoning include headache, nausea, disorientation, and unconsciousness.

Carbon dioxide (CO_2) is a colorless gas associated with asphyxiation risks. It is actually the end product of a metabolism process in which sugar and fats combine with oxygen. Carbon dioxide is used to make dry ice and is found in fire extinguishers. It produces a sour taste in the mouth and a stinging sensation in the nose and mouth.

Methane (CH_4)—the principal component of natural gas—is not toxic but will cause burns if ignited. Flammable or explosive mixtures form at much lower concentrations than the concentrations at which asphyxiation risks arise. Methane is used as a fuel from natural gas fields but can also be generated from fermentation of organic matter (eg, manure, waste water, sludge, and municipal solid waste).

Ammonia (NH_3) is a toxic and corrosive chemical with a characteristic pungent odor. Because ammonia is lighter than air, it rises to the upper atmospheric level in confined spaces. It is typically found in rural areas and is used extensively for fertilizing agricultural crops.

Nitrogen dioxide (NO_2) is a reddish-brown gas that has a characteristic sharp, biting odor. It is most prominent in air pollution and is considered toxic by inhalation.

Safe Approach

As you approach a confined-space rescue scene, look for a bystander who might have witnessed the emergency. Information gathered prior to the technical rescue team's arrival will save valuable time during the actual rescue. Do not automatically assume that a person in a pit has simply experienced a heart attack; instead, assume that there is an IDLH atmosphere at any confined-space call. An IDLH atmosphere can immediately incapacitate anyone who enters the confined space without breathing protection. Toxic gases may be present, or oxygen levels may be insufficient to support life. Inevitably, it will take some time for qualified rescuers to arrive on the scene and prepare for a safe entry into the confined space. The victim of the original incident may have died before your arrival—do not become part of the problem and make an entry prior to atmospheric monitoring.

Assisting Other Rescuers

You and your partner can prevent a confined-space incident from becoming worse by recognizing it, securing the scene, and ensuring that no one enters the space until additional rescue resources arrive. As highly trained personnel arrive, you may provide help by giving these rescuers a situation report.

The first responding rescuers must share whatever information is discovered at the rescue scene with the arriving crew. Anything that may be important to the response should be noted by the first arriving unit. Observed conditions should be compared with reported conditions, and a determination should be made as to the relative change over the time period. Whether an incident appears to be stable or has changed significantly since the first report will affect the operation strategy for the rescue. A size-up should be quickly completed immediately on arrival, and this information should be relayed to the specialized rescue team members when they arrive at the scene. Other items of importance that should be included in a situation report are a description of any rescue attempts that have been made, exposures, hazards, extinguishment of fires, the facts and probabilities of the scene, the situation and resources of the fire company, the identity of any hazardous materials present, and a progress evaluation.

Confined-space rescues can be complex and can take a long time to complete. You may be asked to assist by bringing rescue equipment to the scene, maintaining a charged hose line, or providing crowd control. By understanding the hazards of confined spaces, you will be better prepared to assist a specialized team that is dealing with an emergency involving a confined space.

Trenches

Trench rescue may become necessary when earth is removed for placement of a utility line or for other construction and the sides of the excavation collapse, trapping a worker **Figure 25**. Entrapments may also occur when children play around a pile of sand or earth that collapses. Unfortunately, many entrapments occur because the required safety precautions were not taken.

Whenever a collapse occurs, you need to understand that the collapsed product is unstable and prone to further collapse. Earth and sand are heavy, and a person who is partly entrapped cannot simply be pulled out. Instead, the patient must be carefully dug out after **shoring** has stabilized the sides of the excavation.

Vibrations or additional weight on top of displaced earth will increase the probability of a **secondary collapse**. A secondary collapse occurs after the initial collapse; it can be caused by equipment vibrations, personnel standing at the edge of the trench, or water eroding away the soil. Safe removal of trapped persons requires a special rescue team that is trained and equipped to erect shoring that will protect the rescuers and the entrapped person from secondary collapse.

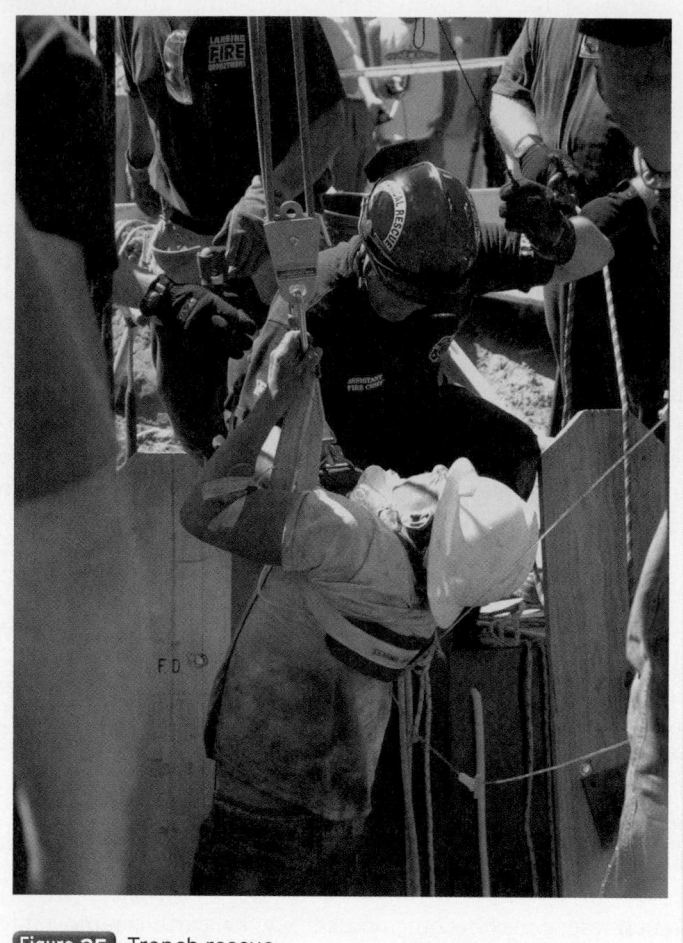

Figure 25 Trench rescue.

Safe Approach

Safety is of paramount importance when you are approaching a trench or excavation collapse. Walking close to the edge of a collapse can trigger a secondary collapse. Stay away from the edge of the site, and keep all workers and bystanders away. Vibrations from equipment and machinery can cause secondary collapses, so shut off all heavy equipment. Vibrations caused by nearby traffic can also cause collapse, so it may be necessary to stop or divert traffic.

Soil that has been removed from the excavation and placed in a pile is called the **spoil pile**. This material is unstable and may collapse if placed too close to the excavation. Avoid disturbing the spoil pile.

Make verbal contact with the trapped person if possible, but do *not* place yourself in danger while doing so. If you approach the trench, do so from the narrow end, where the soil will be more stable. However, it is best *not* to approach the trench unless absolutely necessary; EMS providers should stay out of a trench unless properly trained.

Provide reassurance by letting the trapped person know that a trained rescue team is on the way. By removing people from the edges of the excavation, shutting down machinery, and establishing contact with the patient, you start the rescue process.

You can also size up the scene, looking for evidence that would indicate where the trapped workers may be located. Hand tools and hard hats are one indicator of their presence. By questioning the workers, EMS providers may also determine where the patients were last seen.

▮ Water

Almost all EMS departments may potentially be called to perform a water rescue—whether from a small stream, a large river, a lake, the ocean, a reservoir, or a swimming pool. A static source such as a lake may have no current and is considered flat water or slow moving. In contrast, a whitewater stream or flooded river may have a swift current. During a flood, a dry wash in the desert can quickly become a site of raging water.

Rescuers may suddenly find themselves immersed in moving water during a water rescue, so they should be aware of self-rescue techniques. For example, for personnel who perform water rescues, the minimum PPE includes a **personal flotation device (PFD)**, thermal protection, a helmet appropriate for water rescue, a cutting device, a whistle, and contamination protection (if necessary). A PFD is essential. The most suitable PFD for rescue is known as type 3. Rescuers should use a properly sized PFD that is designed and certified for their specific mission. They must be familiar with the manufacturer's procedures for donning and removing their PFD. All straps should be tightened, with loose straps secured to prevent entanglement. Water rescue operations also require specialized foot protection such as wetsuit-type booties.

In addition, if rescue personnel are suddenly immersed in fast-moving water, they should adopt the **self-rescue position**. The first step is to roll into a faceup arched position with the lower back higher than the feet to avoid subsurface objects. Keep the feet together and facing in the direction of travel (feet first) with arms to the side. Use the hands for changing direction to avoid objects and for diversion to a safe area. Keep the head down, with the chin tucked in. This position protects the rescuer's head, face, and lower back from striking objects and provides a means for controlling direction.

Words of Wisdom

Do not attempt a water rescue unless you are specially trained. Pay close attention to the location where the patient was last seen going under the water.

Cold Water Rescue

Water temperature varies widely by season and by geographic area. Even on warm days, water temperatures can be low. Water causes heat loss 25 times greater than ambient air temperature. Indeed, any water temperature of less than 98.6°F (37°C) will cause hypothermia; patients who become hypothermic lose the ability to self-rescue. Maintaining body heat is critical because hypothermia becomes an immediate problem that progresses to unconsciousness and death. In extremely cold water

(35°F [1.7°C]), a submersion time of 15 to 20 minutes will cause the body to shut down and lead to death.

If you find yourself in cold water, make every effort to keep your face above water, protect your head, and assume the heat-escape-lessening position (HELP) **Figure 26** that helps keep heat in the core of your body. Immersion victims should minimize movement and assume the HELP position. In a group, victims should huddle together to share body warmth.

Words of Wisdom

Humans cannot maintain body heat in water that is less than 92°F. The colder the water, the faster the loss of heat. Compared with air, water causes a heat loss at a rate 25 times faster. Immersion for 15 to 20 minutes in 35°F water is likely to be fatal.

In water colder than 70°F (21°C), immersion victims may actually benefit from a phenomenon known as the <u>cold protective response</u>. Essentially, when a person is submerged in cold water, heat is conducted from the body to the water. The resulting hypothermia can protect vital organs from the lack of oxygen. In addition, exposure to cold water will occasionally activate certain primitive reflexes that may preserve body functions for prolonged periods. In one case, a 2½-year-old girl recovered after being submerged in cold water for at least 66 minutes. For this reason, you should continue to provide full resuscitative efforts for a victim of cold water submersion until the patient recovers or is pronounced dead by a physician (see the chapter, *Environmental Emergencies*, for a more detailed discussion of hypothermia).

Words of Wisdom

The HELP position can decrease body heat loss by 60% compared with treading water.

Whenever a person dives or jumps into cold water, the diving reflex (also known as the mammalian diving reflex)—the slowing of the heart rate caused by submersion in cold water—may cause immediate bradycardia. Although loss of consciousness may follow, the person may be able to survive for an extended time under water because of a lowering of the metabolic rate and decreased oxygen demand and consumption associated with hypothermia.

Words of Wisdom

Remember that hypothermic patients are dehydrated due to "cold diuresis" and should be removed from the water in a horizontal position to avoid orthostatic changes.

Other Water Rescue Situations

In North America, the most common swift water rescue scenario involves people who have attempted to drive vehicles through a pool of water created by a flooded stream. The vehicle stalls because of the depth of the water, leaving the vehicle occupants stranded in a rising stream with a swift current. If the water is high enough, the vehicle can be swept away. These incidents are especially dangerous for rescue personnel because it is difficult to determine the depth of the water around the vehicle.

In surface water rescues, rescuers must consider hazards such as the dangerous hydraulics created by moving water as well as "strainers" (objects in the water such as trees, branches, debris, or wire mesh that can pose a serious pinning risk for rescuers). Dams and hydroelectric sites are also treacherous for even the most skilled rescuers. It is important to remember that the height of a dam does not indicate the degree of hazard to rescuers. Intakes at the base of a dam can act like strainers. Low-head dams are often associated with recirculating currents (sometimes referred to as a "boil") **Figure 27** . These currents can trap victims and unwary rescuers alike, forcing them underwater, away from the dam, and back to the surface again, where

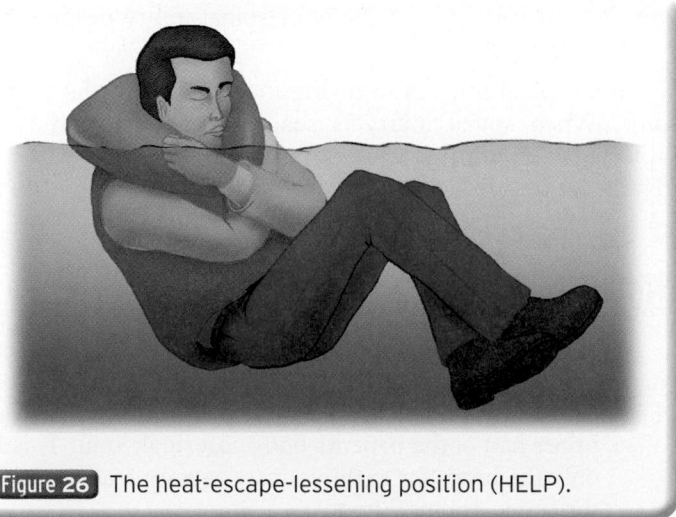

Figure 26 The heat-escape-lessening position (HELP).

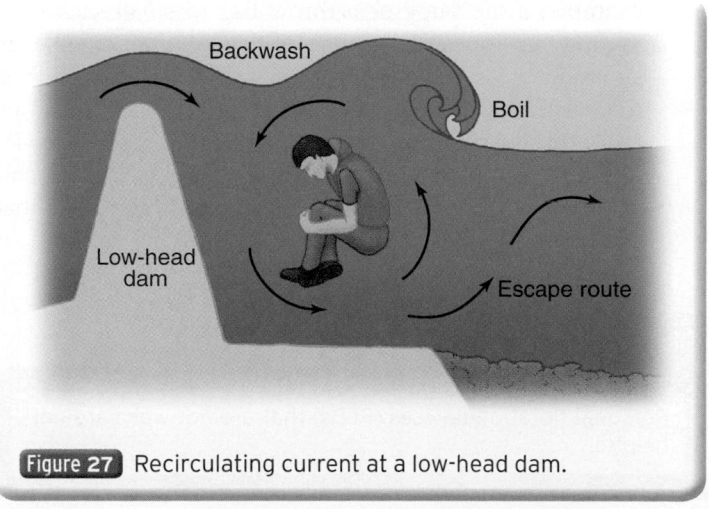

Figure 27 Recirculating current at a low-head dam.

the cycle repeats itself. For this reason, low-head dams are often referred to as "drowning machines." Never underestimate the power or intensity of moving water.

Safe Approach

When you are responding to water rescue incidents, your safety and the safety of other rescuers are your primary concerns. Your gear is not designed for water rescue activities. When you are working at a water rescue scene, you should use personal protective gear designed for water rescue. Whenever you are within 10 ft of the water, you should wear an approved PFD. Shoes that provide solid traction are preferable to boots.

Words of Wisdom

The hydraulics of moving water change with variables such as depth, velocity, and obstruction to flow.

If you are part of the first arriving ambulance's crew, and the endangered people are in a vehicle or holding on to a tree or other solid object, try to communicate with them. Let them know that more help is on the way.

Do not exceed your level of training. If you cannot swim, operating around or near water is not recommended. A person who is trained as a lifeguard for still water is not prepared to enter flowing water with a strong current, such as in a river, stream, or ocean. Make sure that bystanders do not try to rescue the patient and place themselves in a situation where they need to be rescued, too.

When you see a person struggling in the water, your first impulse may be to jump in to assist. However, that action may not result in a successful rescue and can endanger your life. The model most commonly used in water rescue is *reach-throw-row-go*:

- Attempt to *reach* out to the threatened person first, using any readily available object. If the person is close to shore, a branch, pole, oar, or paddle may be long enough.
- If you cannot reach the person, *throw* something—for example, a life buoy or a throw bag (a small sack containing two ropes and a piece of foam). In an emergency situation, a rescuer opens the bag, pulls out enough rope to grasp firmly (some rescuers prefer to wrap the rope around their backs), and then throws the bag to the victim. The victim should be instructed to grab the rope and not the bag, because the bag may contain more rope that can uncoil.

Words of Wisdom

Personal flotation devices (PFDs) that are not worn are not helpful!

- If you cannot reach the person by throwing something that floats, you may be able to *row* out to the drowning person if a small boat or canoe is available. Do so only if you know how to operate or propel the craft properly. Protect yourself by wearing an approved PFD.
- As a last resort, *go* into the water to save the victim. Enter the water only if you are a capable swimmer trained to the level of swift water rescue.

Many departments in colder regions have developed specialized equipment to assist in ice rescues. Throwing a rope or flotation device may be helpful initially. Ladders can be used to distribute the weight of the rescuer on ice-covered water. Specially designed hose lines have been used with end-caps and an air line to create a flotation buoy. Special rescue suits are available to prevent hypothermia and provide flotation for the rescuer. If your department is involved in ice rescues, you should receive training in these specialized procedures.

Recovery Situations

On occasion, you may be called to the scene of a drowning and find that the patient is not floating or visible in the water. An organized rescue effort in these circumstances calls for personnel who are experienced with recovery techniques and equipment, including snorkels, masks, and scuba gear. As a last resort, when standard procedures for recovery are unsuccessful, you may have to use a grappling hook or large hook to drag the bottom for the victim. Although the hook could seriously wound the patient, it may be the only effective way to bring him or her to the surface for resuscitative efforts.

■ Spinal Injuries in Submersion Incidents

Submersion incidents may be complicated by spinal fractures and spinal cord injuries. You must assume that spinal injury exists with the following conditions:

- The submersion has resulted from a diving mishap or fall.
- The patient is unconscious, and no information is available to rule out the possibility of a mechanism causing neck injury.
- The patient is conscious but reports weakness, paralysis, or numbness in the arms or legs.
- You suspect the possibility of spinal injury despite what witnesses say.

Most spinal injuries in diving incidents affect the cervical spine. When spinal injury is suspected, the neck must be protected from further injury. This means that you will have to stabilize the suspected injury while the patient is still in the water. Follow the steps in Skill Drill 2:

Skill Drill 2

1. Turn the patient supine. Two rescuers are usually required to turn the patient safely, although in some cases one rescuer will suffice. Always rotate the entire upper half of the patient's body as a single unit. Twisting only the head, for example, may aggravate any injury to the cervical spine (Step 1).

2. Open the airway and begin ventilation. Immediate ventilation is the primary treatment of all submersion patients as soon as the patient is faceup in the water. Use a pocket mask if it is available. Have the other rescuer support the head and trunk as a unit while you open the airway and begin artificial ventilation (Step 2).

3. Float a buoyant backboard under the patient as you continue ventilation (Step 3).

4. Secure the trunk and head to the backboard to eliminate motion of the cervical spine. Do not remove the patient from the water until this is done (Step 4).

5. Remove the patient from the water, on the backboard (Step 5).

6. Remove wet clothes and cover the patient with a blanket. Give supplemental oxygen if the patient is breathing adequately; give positive-pressure ventilation if apneic or breathing inadequately. Begin CPR (Step 6).

■ Rope Rescue

Rope rescue skills are the most versatile and widely used technical rescue skills. Sometimes a rope rescue is performed to remove a person from a position of peril.

Skill Drill 2

Stabilizing a Suspected Spinal Injury in the Water

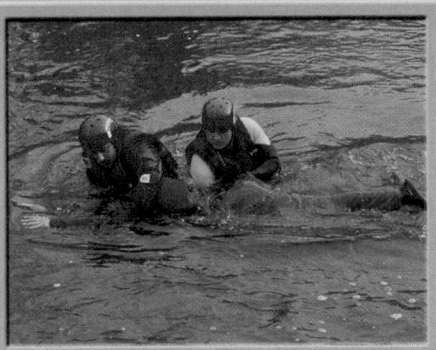

Step 1 Turn the patient supine by rotating the entire upper half of the patient's body as a single unit.

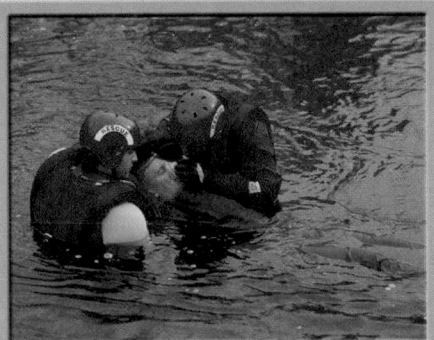

Step 2 As soon as the patient is turned, begin artificial ventilation using the mouth-to-mouth method or a pocket mask.

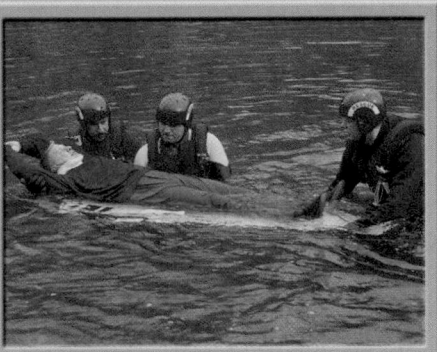

Step 3 Float a buoyant backboard under the patient as you continue ventilation.

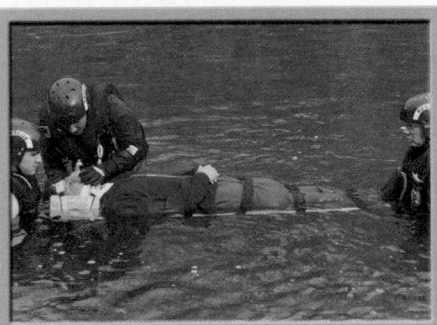

Step 4 Secure the trunk and head of the patient to the backboard to eliminate motion of the cervical spine.

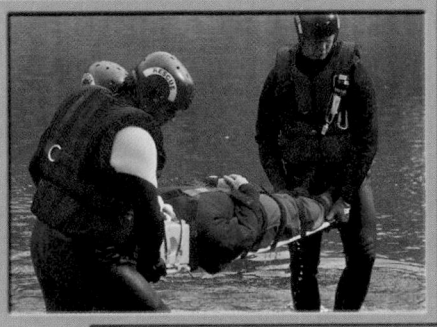

Step 5 Remove the patient from the water, on the backboard.

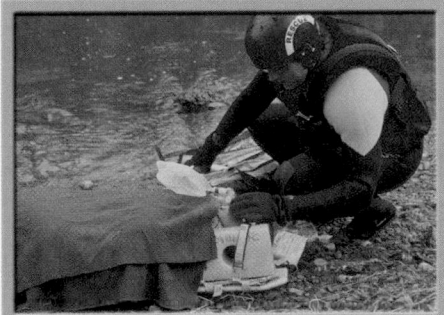

Step 6 Remove the patient's wet clothes and cover the patient with a blanket. Apply oxygen if breathing adequately; apply positive-pressure ventilation if apneic or breathing inadequately. Begin CPR if breathing and pulse are absent.

Types of Rope Rescue

Rope rescue incidents are divided into low-angle and high-angle operations. <u>Low-angle operations</u> are situations where the slope of the ground over which the rescuers are working is less than 45°. In these cases, rescuers depend on the ground for their primary support, and the rope system serves as a secondary means of support. An example of a low-angle system is a rope stretched from the top of an embankment and used for support by rescuers who are carrying a patient up an incline.

Low-angle operations are used when the scene requires ropes to be used only as assistance to pull or haul up a patient or rescuer. They are usually necessary when adequate footing is not present, in areas such as a dirt or rock embankment. In such an incident, a rope will be tied to the rescuer's harness and the rescuer will climb the embankment by himself or herself, using the rope to keep from falling. Low-angle operations also include lifelines placed during ice or water rescues.

> ### Words of Wisdom
>
> There should be a minimum of six rescuers on basket stretchers, and extra teams of six persons should be rotated when the patient needs to be carried a long distance.

Ropes can also be used to assist in raising or lowering a basket stretchers. This technique frees the rescuers from having to carry all of the weight over rough terrain. Rescuers at the top of the embankment can help to pull up or lower the basket using a rope system.

When rescue personnel are using any rope system to assist in rescue operations, a safety feature is to belay the rope. <u>Belay</u> in climbing is a technique of controlling the rope as it is fed out to the climbers to protect them in the event of a fall. A critical part of the climbing system, it can be accomplished with a self-belay or a secondary lifeline. One potential complication is that belays depend on the angle of operations; as a consequence, the entire load may be transferred to the belay line. This could prove dangerous depending on the load and the length of rope.

Another aspect of climbing or rescue situations is the act of descending. In some descents, the angle is so severe that a technique known as <u>rappelling</u> is performed. To rappel is to descend on a fixed rope. <u>Scrambling</u> is a method used to ascend rocky faces and ridges and can be considered a cross between hill climbing (where a person walks up a steep incline using both hands and feet) and rock climbing. These skills are technical rescue skills that require additional training beyond your paramedic course.

<u>High-angle operations</u> are situations where the slope of the ground is greater than 45°, and rescuers or patients are dependent on a life safety rope and not a fixed surface of support such as the ground. High-angle rescue techniques are used to raise or lower a person when other means of raising or lowering are not readily available. These rescues are extremely demanding and dangerous, and they should be attempted only by personnel who are thoroughly trained in proper procedures.

Safe Approach

If you respond to an incident that may require a rope rescue operation, consider both your safety and the safety of those around you. Rope rescues are among the most time-consuming calls that you will encounter. Extensive setup is necessary, and a considerable amount of equipment needs to be assembled prior to initiating any rescue. Protect your safety by remaining away from the area under the patient and away from any loose materials that might potentially fall. Work to control the scene, moving bystanders to an area where they will not be injured.

■ Wilderness Search and Rescue

Wilderness <u>search and rescue (SAR)</u> is an activity that is conducted by a limited number of departments. SAR missions consist of two parts: search (looking for a lost or overdue person) and rescue (removing a patient from a hostile environment).

Several types of situations may result in the initiation of SAR missions. Small children may wander off and be unable to find their way back to a known place. Older adults who have Alzheimer disease may fail to remember where they are going and become lost. People who are hiking, hunting, or participating in other wilderness activities may become lost because they lack the proper training or equipment. SAR missions may also be initiated if people are caught unaware by unexpected weather changes or if they become sick or injured.

Safe Approach

"Wilderness" can include many different environments, such as forests, mountains, deserts, natural parks, animal refuges, and rain forests. Depending on the terrain and environmental factors, the wilderness can be as little as a few minutes into the backcountry or a few feet off the roadway. Despite the short access time, the scene could require an extended evacuation and thus qualify as a wilderness incident. Terrain hazards include cliffs, steep slopes, caves, wells, mines, avalanches, rivers, streams, valleys, beaches, and rock slides.

When you participate in SAR missions, prepare for the weather conditions by bringing drinking water, food, suitable clothing, and the proper PPE for the mission. A handheld strobe light may help paramedics keep track of each other in a crowd or in rural or wilderness locations. When rescue personnel are working along highways, they can hook these lights onto their belts or attach them to their upper arms to provide additional visibility to oncoming vehicles. Strobe lights are lightweight, quite durable, and readily visible at night at a distance of approximately 1 mile.

Make sure that you do not exceed your physical limitations, and do not get in situations that are beyond your ability to handle in the wilderness. Call for a special wilderness rescue team, depending on the situation and your local protocols.

■ Lost Person Search and Rescue

When a person is lost in the outdoors and a search effort is initiated, an ambulance is usually summoned to the search base. Each search team will be organized to include a member who is EMS trained, carrying the essential equipment to provide simple immediate care. Your role is to stand by at the search base until the lost person or people have been found.

As soon as you arrive at the scene and have been briefed on the situation, you should isolate and prepare the equipment you will need to carry in to the patient's location so that no time is lost once the patient has been found or if a member of the search team becomes injured. The prepared carry-in equipment, including a backboard and other equipment you will need to immobilize the patient, should be left in the back of the ambulance so that it is protected from the weather. In addition, if the ambulance should need to be relocated, the equipment will not need to be reloaded or possibly be left behind. You will usually be given a portable radio that is tuned to the search frequency so that you can monitor the progress of the search and communicate with and be contacted by those in charge of the search operation.

Sometimes, you may be asked to stay with relatives of the lost person who are at the scene. Find out from relatives whether the lost person has any medical history that may need to be addressed, and pass this information on to those who are in charge of the search. Unless you have been instructed otherwise, only incident command should communicate any news or progress of the search to the family. For this reason, you must be sure that your radio is set at a discreet volume.

Safe Approach

Once the lost person has been found, you will be guided by search personnel to that location or a prearranged intersecting point where the patient will be carried to decrease the amount of time you need to reach the patient and begin treatment. You should be sure that the carry-in equipment is evenly distributed among personnel and that the pace is such that all personnel can easily stay together. Sometimes, the time and effort that are needed to reach and carry out the patient can be decreased by relocating the ambulance or, if available, by using a four-wheel drive or all-terrain vehicle. As with other technical rescues, although the ambulance crew will assume the responsibility for patient care once they are at the patient's side, a cooperative effort of both EMS and the search team is necessary to safely carry the patient to the base and waiting ambulance.

■ Structure Fires

In most areas, an ambulance is dispatched with the fire department apparatus to any structure fire, whether or not any injuries are reported. A fire in a house, apartment building, office, school, plant, warehouse, or other building is considered a structure fire. When you are responding to a major fire scene, you should determine whether, because of the fire, any special route will be necessary. Once you arrive at the scene, it is essential that the ambulance be parked far enough away from the fire to be safe from the fire itself or a collapsing building. You must also ensure that the ambulance will not block or hinder other arriving equipment or become blocked in by other equipment or hose lines. However, you must also make sure that the ambulance will be close enough to be visible and that patients can be brought to it easily. Finally, select a parking spot that will allow you unobstructed egress in the event you need to initiate

emergency transport of an injured patient. The fire officer who is the IC will determine this location. In some instances, EMS personnel will set up a rehabilitation sector for the fire crew.

Your next step is to determine whether there are any injured patients at the scene or whether you have been called to stand by. A number of ambulances may be dispatched to a major fire to ensure that one or more units will always remain immediately available at the scene if others leave to transport injured patients.

Safe Approach

As with other technical rescue situations, search and rescue in a burning building requires special training and equipment. Search and rescue is performed by teams of fire fighters wearing full turnout gear and self-contained breathing apparatus (SCBA), and carrying tools and fully charged hose lines. These teams will bring patients out of the burning building to the area where the ambulance is standing by. Therefore, unless otherwise ordered, you should always stay with the ambulance. You should remain present even after the fire is out, in the event a fire fighter becomes injured during salvage and overhaul. The ambulance should leave the scene only if you are transporting a patient or if the IC has released it.

■ Agricultural and Industrial Rescue

According to the National Agricultural Safety Database (NASD), 50% of farm fatalities involve tractors, and 14% are machine related. Tractors and machines have a great deal of power. Thus, in the agricultural or industrial setting, operators, workers, and family members are exposed to tremendous hazards. Rescue personnel should visit their local farms and industrial plants and learn as much as possible about the equipment that is used, how it operates, and how an operator can become entrapped in the equipment.

Typical machine hazards involve pinch points, wrap points, shear points, crush points, and pull-in points. These areas are typically protected with a shield or a guard; however, over time, guards may be removed or damaged and may not be replaced. To alleviate this problem, machines that are found in a factory are inspected routinely by the Occupational Safety and Health Association (OSHA) and other regulating agencies. However, the majority of farms in the United States are not covered under OSHA inspections or other mandates. This is an important consideration if you are in a farming community.

Safe Approach

A critical skill rescue personnel need to master is effective cribbing in order to stabilize a vehicle or equipment. During agricultural or industrial rescue, because of the uneven ground, large spaces, and heavy loads that will be supported, using the proper technique is essential for everyone's safety. Tractor rescue operations will use many cribbing blocks because of the large voids that need to be shored up and the need to provide a suitable platform for lifting processes.

Machinery is made of strong steel and cast material that will challenge most rescue tools that are designed for vehicle extrication. Farm machines can often be dismantled more easily than they can be cut apart if the right tools are available. Call for a special agricultural rescue team, depending on the situation and your local protocols.

Once rescuers are able to get close to the patient, they should observe the patient's entrapment carefully and determine how he or she is trapped. Rescue personnel need to ensure that parts of the machine on either side of the entrapped patient are secured to prevent any movement during disentanglement and extrication activities. This process is called isolating the injury site. This is the part of the machine that will receive the most focus. Once the injury site is isolated, study the machine to determine the alternative methods of disentangling the patient. At this point, the extent of the patient's injuries has not been determined. You should always have alternative plans of attack. One plan may be a slow and methodical approach while the other might be aggressive, such as if the patient's condition warrants a rapid disentanglement or extrication.

While rescue personnel are developing the plan(s) for disentanglement, EMS personnel must be assessing the patient and determining an index of suspicion based on the mechanism of injury and length of entrapment. A critical difference between an entrapment with farm machinery and entrapment with any other industrial machinery is the length of time for the entrapment. In a manufacturing setting, if an operator becomes entrapped in a machine, most likely a coworker is right there to shut off the power to that machine. Coworkers and maintenance people will then begin dismantling the machine and managing the stored energy before rescue personnel arrive. In many cases, they may actually have the patient extricated before rescue personnel arrive. Contrast that with a farmer who becomes entrapped out in a field while working alone. This patient may experience an extended delay between the time of injury and medical treatment because there is no witness to initiate the emergency response. Once the patient is assessed, discussion between the technical rescuers, EMS, and the IC needs to take place to decide which approach, whether methodical or aggressive, is needed.

■ Tactical Emergency Medical Support

EMS and law enforcement personnel frequently work together at the scene of violent crimes. A paramedic working in an urban environment may work closely with law enforcement personnel, almost on a daily basis. However, if the incident develops into a tactical situation, (eg, a high-risk warrant, hostage situation, or a barricaded suspect), law enforcement agencies may deploy use of specialized law enforcement tactical units or the special weapons and tactics (SWAT) team.

Nationally there is a trend to have a specially trained paramedic assigned to the tactical team. Many police departments have formed partnerships with EMS agencies to provide medical personnel. Once a paramedic becomes a member of the tactical team, he or she will undergo extensive training on tactical strategies and function as a member of the team. The tactical paramedic must also be proficient at providing medical care in extremely adverse situations. Advanced tactical EMS training courses that focus on teaching the student how to complete patient assessments in limited visibility, maintaining cover/concealment, and rapid patient extrication techniques are available. The tactical paramedic is trained to enter the hot zone with law enforcement personnel. They are equipped with the same PPE worn by the law enforcement officers. At a minimum, this would include body armor, ballistic helmet, and eye protection. The tactical paramedic must also have a compact medical kit that meets the needs of the incident, but does not dramatically encumber the medic's movements. Most of the medical equipment is designed to handle traumatic injuries, such as bleeding control, airway management, and fluid replacement. A complete set of ALS medical gear is usually cached in the warm zone.

The main duty of the tactical paramedic is to provide immediate medical care to people who may become injured during the incident. This may be a team member, a civilian, or the suspected criminal **Figure 28**. In most situations, the tactical paramedic will start providing medical care before the scene is declared safe for other personnel to enter.

When not responding to an emergency incident, the tactical paramedic will be responsible for maintaining medical records for each team member, conducting basic first aid training to team members, and providing suggestions for training evolutions.

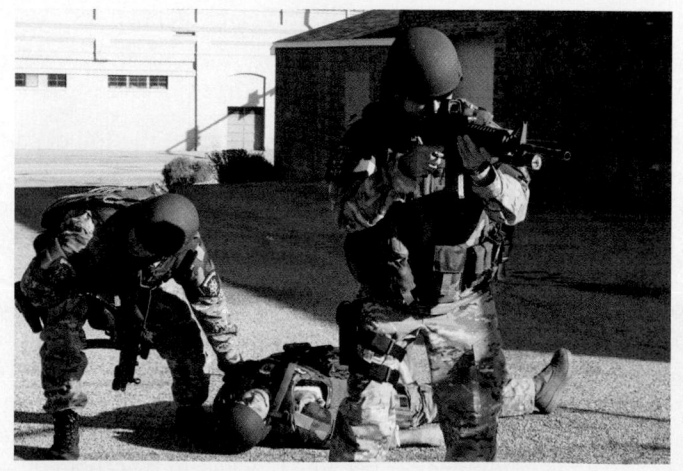

Figure 28 Tactical EMS providers move a downed officer; only the most basic medical care is provided in an unsecured area.

Words of Wisdom

Tips for responding to a tactical situation:

- Turn off lights and sirens as you approach the scene.
- Request direction from the incident commander when you arrive at the outer perimeter.
- An officer will guide you to the shielded, safe staging area selected for the ambulance and for patient care.
- When you are exiting the ambulance, stay low, and remain near the side of the vehicle unless you are directed to another place of safety.
- Do not turn on the vehicle's outside speakers. Turn down the volume of any radios that you are carrying.
- Do not look around the sides or over the top of any building or structure that may be serving to shield you.
- Stand by at the staging area to treat and package injured patients after the SWAT team or other law enforcement officers have evacuated them.
- When you are ready to transport a patient, ask a law enforcement officer to notify the incident commander. Leave only after the incident commander has verified that it is safe for the ambulance to move.
- When you are exiting the scene, follow the specific route indicated by the incident commander or law enforcement officer assigned to guide you. Proceed slowly for a good distance from the incident perimeter before using your emergency lights and siren.

◼ Patient Care

Many medical and trauma conditions can and will be assessed during the rescue process. In rescues that involve confined spaces, especially with cave-ins and trench rescues, EMS providers need to consider the potential for crush injuries—in particular, the possibility of crush syndrome. Crush syndrome may occur when large muscle groups are compressed for a prolonged period of time (usually 2 to 4 hours). When human tissue goes without an adequate supply of oxygen-enriched blood, tissue (cells) continues to metabolize (produce energy) without oxygen (anaerobic metabolism), producing lactic acid as a by-product. When entrapped or compressed areas of the body are eventually reperfused (the object causing compression is removed), these metabolic by-products are released into the circulation. Treatment with high-flow oxygen therapy or positive-pressure ventilations, along with administration of sodium bicarbonate, calcium chloride, and a fluid bolus, can help to reverse the effects of respiratory and metabolic acidosis. Electrocardiogram (ECG) abnormalities such as peaked T waves may be an early indicator of crush syndrome.

◼ Pain Management

Patients involved in many rescue situations will be experiencing pain from injuries received during the incident. Pain control should take the form of nonpharmacologic methods

YOU *are the Medic*   PART 4

The technical rescue personnel assist in packaging the patient using a vacuum splint and basket stretcher. As you are making your way back to the ambulance, the patient begins to report abdominal pain. A quick reassessment shows distention of the abdomen with pain on palpation to all quadrants. Her skin is now pale, cool, and diaphoretic and you are no longer able to feel a radial pulse. A carotid pulse is present and weak. Her respirations remain shallow and rapid. Breath sounds are present but diminished bilaterally. You increase the IV fluids to run wide open.

Ten minutes later you have secured the patient to the stretcher inside the ambulance and you reassess the patient. She is still reporting severe abdominal pain and is asking for something for the pain. As you are explaining that you are not able to give her any pain medication, one of the law enforcement officers opens the back door to the ambulance and lets the woman know that her grandson was found and has only scrapes and bruises. He will be brought to the same hospital by another rescue unit.

Recording Time: 45 Minutes	
Respirations	28 breath/min, shallow
Pulse	Carotid pulse, 136 beats/min, regular and weak
Skin	Pale, cool, and diaphoretic
Blood pressure	86/58 mm Hg
Oxygen saturation (Spo$_2$)	94% on 15 L/min nonrebreathing mask
Pupils	Equal and reactive

7. Why must pain medication be administered with caution, if at all, in the prehospital setting?

8. How should you manage your patient during transport?

such as splinting to minimize movement, gentle handling, or talking with patients to create a distraction during assessment and movement. EMS providers must also keep patients warm because a shivering patient will experience aggravated levels of pain with every movement.

Pharmacologic treatment in the prehospital setting remains controversial, and providers should consult with their medical directors on issues related to pain management. All medications are contraindicated in patients with a known hypersensitivity to the drug. Table 1 lists some of the medications that can be considered in the pain management of patients during rescue efforts. Because most analgesics have the potential to induce nausea and vomiting, all medications must be administered slowly and use of antiemetics should be considered.

Medical Supplies

Table 2 lists the basic medical supplies that you should carry in an off-road medical pack.

Patient Packaging

A number of special patient packaging tools are available to help you extricate patients out of their situation and up, down, or out to your ambulance. The basket stretcher or Stokes basket, for example, is a rigid framed structure that the patient is set into and then secured. It comes in two general types. The most common is the wire basket that consists of a rigid metal (aluminum, steel, or titanium) frame and ribs with a chicken-wire mesh attached to the frame. The other style is the plastic or fiberglass basket that consists of a steel or aluminum frame with a rigid plastic or fiberglass basket. Both types of baskets are available as one- or two-piece units that can be latched or joined together for easier packing into the rescue scene.

The wire basket is more suitable for water rescue and helicopter hoist situations because the wire mesh allows water or air to easily pass through it. Given that water weighs 8.37 pounds per gallon, this is a significant weight reduction. In the case of moving air (eg, a helicopter's rotor downwash) or moving water, such a basket allows the fluid or air to pass through it rather than spinning or dragging in response to the air or hydraulic forces being exerted on it.

Unfortunately, a wire basket catches every bit of debris and hooks on most any obstruction or obstacle. Thus for most other types of evacuations, a plastic or fiberglass basket is the superior choice because it more easily slides over the top of surfaces such as snow or debris, or down ladders.

Both types of baskets have a wheel device that can be attached to the bottom to facilitate movement over trails and low-level debris. Also, both devices have minimal (or no) belts or straps to secure the patient into the basket. Instead, a number of patient packaging systems may be used, including those featuring 5- to 6-mm cord or 1-inch tubular webbing. Each packaging system relies on the same basic principle: securing the patient's pelvis, which is the fulcrum of the body, into the basket. Separate securing techniques are then deployed to secure the patient's legs and/or chest, or to lash/lace the patient's entire body into the basket.

Table 1 Medications for Pain Management in Rescue Situations	
Medication	**Characteristics**
Morphine sulfate	Narcotic analgesic and central nervous system depressant often used in the treatment of myocardial infarction, kidney stones, and pulmonary edema. It is contraindicated in patients who are volume-depleted or experiencing severe hypotension.
Meperidine (Demerol)	Narcotic analgesic and central nervous system depressant primarily used for the treatment of moderate to severe pain. It is relatively contraindicated in patients with undiagnosed abdominal pain and head injuries.
Nitrous oxide (Nitronox, Entonox)	This central nervous system depressant with analgesic properties is used for musculoskeletal pain, fractures, and burns. It should not be used in patients who cannot follow verbal instructions, those with head injuries, COPD patients, and patients with thoracic injuries or possible pneumothorax. Use caution in environments of less than 21°F, which could make administration difficult to impossible.
Fentanyl citrate (Sublimaze)	Unrelated to morphine but with similar analgesic effects, it is considered 50 to 100 times more potent than morphine; however, its duration of action is much shorter. It can be used for rapid-sequence intubation and severe pain, but is contraindicated with severe hemorrhage, shock, or known hypersensitivity.
Butorphanol tartrate (Stadol)	This synthetic analgesic, with effects equal to a large dose of morphine, is indicated for the treatment of moderate to severe pain, but is contraindicated in patients with undiagnosed abdominal pain and head injuries.
Nalbuphine (Nubain)	Synthetic analgesic with the same effects as morphine. Nubain has the hemodynamic effects of morphine and is used in patients with moderate to severe pain. Like morphine, Nubain is contraindicated in patients with undiagnosed abdominal pain and head injuries.
Ketorolac (Toradol)	Classified as a nonsteroidal anti-inflammatory drug (NSAID), ketorolac has analgesic, anti-inflammatory, and antipyretic effects. It is considered in controlling moderate to severe pain. Its only true contraindication is in patients with a known hypersensitivity to the drug and patients with reported allergies to aspirin or NSAIDs.

Table 2 Supplies for an Off-Road Medical Pack

- Vinyl or latex gloves
- Face masks
- Hand sanitizer
- Mouth-to-mask resuscitation device
- 1 triangular bandage (cravat)
- Universal trauma dressings
- 4-inch × 4-inch and 5-inch × 9-inch sterile dressings
- Roller gauze bandage
- Gauze-adhesive strips
- Occlusive dressing for sealing chest wounds
- Adhesive tape
- Blankets
- Cold packs
- Alcohol pads
- One 12-mL or larger syringe for irrigation of wounds
- 2 glucose or energy gel packets
- Heat packs
- Abdominal dressing
- Survival blanket
- Scissors
- Irrigation fluid or wound cleansing soap
- Goggles
- SAM splint
- Butterfly bandages
- Cervical collars
- Blood pressure cuff
- Rapid immobilization straps
- Pocket flashlight
- Batteries

One difficulty that may arise is when you are packaging the patient with a fractured pelvis because these techniques will cause the patient an incredible amount of pain. Indeed, any sort of patient packaging that involves first anchoring the pelvis will result in a significant amount of patient "discomfort."

One highly effective solution to this problem is to secure the patient in a full-body vacuum mattress. Once the patient is adequately splinted and secured in this device, then the mattress is placed and secured inside the basket stretcher. Now the main attachment/focal point is the entire vacuum splint and not the patient's broken pelvis.

Another difficulty frequently encountered is the need to transport a spine-immobilized patient in a basket stretcher. Some devices have a leg divider portion for the lower extremities that prohibits use of a backboard. Also, most backboards are too wide and their rectangular shape will not readily fit inside a basket.

There are two solutions to this problem. The first is to place the patient in a Kendrick Extrication Device (KED) rather than a backboard and then secure the patient into the basket. The second is to hold the cervical spine, surround the patient with enough rescuers to lift/levitate the patient up while maintaining spinal immobilization, slide the basket underneath the patient, and then lower the patient back down into the basket. The patient may then be secured, with the basket serving as the spinal immobilization device.

Once the patient has been safely extricated or evacuated, you can reverse the process and lower/secure the patient to a backboard in preparation for transportation. This consideration is especially important in a multiple-patient rescue scenario, because most rescue services possess only one basket stretcher but have multiple backboards. Do not let the ambulance crew drive off with your basket stretcher unless you have a replacement for it. The loss of a specialized litter can put a rescue team out of service or necessitate having to improvise with alternative patient packaging.

When you are packaging a patient into a basket stretcher, you need to consider all of his or her needs. If you have placed the patient on supplemental oxygen, then the portable oxygen tank (preferably an aluminum one) must be secured in the stretcher as well. Likewise, the oxygen tubing to the mask or cannula must be secured because it might potentially catch on a piece of debris or inadvertently become entangled in the raising or lowering system. In addition, personnel must monitor the amount of oxygen in the cylinder. It could be hazardous to patient care if the oxygen supply runs out, especially when the patient is on a mask.

The same holds true for IV lines. You do not want to rely on a gravity-fed system if possible: The IV tubing may become hung up on something at best, or hung up on something and pulled out of your patient at worst. If the patient requires an IV line, use a pressure infuser and secure the IV line and tubing along with the patient prior to extrication and transportation.

Basket stretchers are poor insulators. Thus, when you are packaging the patient into the basket, you must also protect him or her from the elements. Keep the patient (and any IV lines) warm.

If you will be transporting a patient through or out of an area where falling debris such as rocks, ice, or building material is a factor, you should package your patient with head and eye protection. This may be as simple as placing a rock helmet and goggles or other protective glasses on the patient, or as comprehensive as using a shield to protect the patient's head and neck.

Some tight or confined spaces are so narrow that they cannot accommodate the passage of a basket stretcher. Your patient, however, may require spinal immobilization. In such a case, the solution is a KED or KED/SKED combination.

A KED is an excellent spinal immobilization device that captures the three planes of the spinal column (ie, the head, shoulders, and pelvis). This narrow-profile device was originally designed by an EMT for extrication of Formula One race car drivers. You apply the KED to the patient and then rig it for raising or lowering as you would an uninjured patient—namely, by using a seat harness and applying a chest harness around the patient and the KED. There are other devices similar to the KED that are rated as approved vertical lifting harnesses.

Another option is to place the patient in a KED and then secure both into a SKED device. A SKED litter is the classic example of a flexible, wrap-around litter. It is essentially a drag sheet made from heavy-duty polyethylene plastic that wraps around (cocoons) the patient with prerigged securing and attachment points. It is a great tool for sliding patients through narrow passageways and over rough surfaces.

Adaptability and improvisation are an essential part of EMS patient care practices. In rescue and extrication situations, the patient's needs, your resources, and the techniques used can change as the rescue process develops. Should you find yourself at a rescue situation without all the necessary equipment, you may have to use your ingenuity to improvise the tools needed to get the patient to safety. If necessary, you can always rely on the technique of splinting one body part to another, by attaching the upper extremities to the torso and the lower legs to each other. This is an effective means of splinting when no other devices are available.

YOU are the Medic | SUMMARY

1. What is a technical rescue incident?

A technical rescue incident is a challenging and complex rescue situation that will require the expertise of specially trained people and special equipment. Examples of technical rescue incidents include vehicle extrication, trench collapse, confined spaces, wilderness rescue, and water rescue.

2. Explain what the mnemonic "FAILURE" represents.

The mnemonic "FAILURE" can be used as a reminder of the reasons for rescue failures.

F- Failure to understand the environment, or underestimating it

A- Additional medical problems not considered

I- Inadequate rescue skills

L- Lack of teamwork or experience

U- Underestimating the logistics of the incident

R- Rescue versus recovery mode not considered

E- Equipment not mastered

3. What are the three control zones that will be established while the scene is being stabilized?

Control zones are necessary to ensure the safety of all parties involved. There are three areas or zones that need to be established. They are as follows:

- Hot zone—This area is for entry teams and rescue teams only. The hot zone immediately surrounds the dangers of the scene to protect personnel outside of the zone.

- Warm zone—Only properly trained and equipped personnel are permitted access to the warm zone. This is the site where personnel and equipment decontamination takes place. It is also the area used to support the hot zone.

- Cold zone—The purpose of the cold zone is to stage vehicles and equipment. The command post will be set up here.

4. Why is it important for the incident management system to be used during a technical rescue incident?

Technical rescue incidents often are complex and require the coordination of several resources. Using the incident management system will keep the scene organized and ensure the safety of those involved.

5. Patients involved in situations requiring extrication frequently become anxious. What can you do to help calm the patient?

The most important thing you can do is to maintain communication with your patient in a calm and collected manner.

Tips for successful communication include: (1) making and keeping eye contact with your patient; (2) tell the truth-your patient needs to hear honest answers and can often detect when they are being lied to; (3) communicate at a level the patient can understand and avoid the use of technical terms; (4) be aware of your own body language-you often reveal your feelings through nonverbal communication; (5) speak slowly, clearly, and distinctly so the patient can understand what you are saying; (6) use the patient's proper name-always address the patient using Mr. or Mrs. followed by their last name unless otherwise directed by the patient; (7) if the patient is hearing impaired, speak clearly and directly at the person so he or she can read your lips; (8) give the patient time to answer your questions; and (9) try to make the patient as comfortable and relaxed as the situation allows.

6. Why is the patient at risk for developing crush syndrome?

The patient was trapped under debris for a considerable amount of time. The areas of her body that were not able to receive oxygenated blood to feed the tissues switched to anaerobic metabolism for energy. As a result, lactic acids and other waste products formed and accumulated in the tissues. Once the pressure was released, the waste products were released into the bloodstream and carried throughout her body creating a potentially lethal situation.

7. Why must pain medication be administered with caution, if at all, in the prehospital setting?

The patient is demonstrating signs and symptoms of shock secondary to intra-abdominal bleeding. Although the patient is experiencing significant amounts of pain, the administration of pain medications may contribute to a further decrease in blood pressure and mask the source of the pain.

8. How should you manage your patient during transport?

As mentioned above, the patient is exhibiting signs and symptoms of shock. Your priority should be to support and maintain the ABCs. This may entail providing assisted ventilations, intubating, and administering medications to raise the blood pressure. Remember to also keep the patient warm. Multisystem trauma patients as well as patients in shock can lose significant amounts of body heat that can worsen their condition.

EMS Patient Care Report (PCR)

Date: 04-07-12	Incident No.: 11937	Nature of Call: Building collapse		Location: 40273 Poplar Drive	
Dispatched: 1232	En Route: 1234	At Scene: 1241	Transport: 1416	At Hospital: 1442	In Service: 1509

Patient Information

Age: 65	Allergies: None
Sex: F	Medications: Metformin, Insulin
Weight (in kg [lb]): 75 kg (165 lb)	Past Medical History: Diabetes
	Chief Complaint: Shortness of breath and abdominal pain

Vital Signs

Time	BP	Pulse	Respirations	Spo$_2$
Time: 1333	BP: N/A	Pulse: 108	Respirations: 26	Spo$_2$: N/A
Time: 1403	BP: 104/62	Pulse: 126	Respirations: 28	Spo$_2$: 96%
Time: 1414	BP: 86/58	Pulse: 136	Respirations: 28	Spo$_2$: 94%
Time: 1420	BP: 90/60	Pulse: 132	Respirations: 26	Spo$_2$: 96%
Time: 1427	BP: 94/60	Pulse: 130	Respirations: 26	Spo$_2$: 96%
Time: 1435	BP: 94/66	Pulse: 128	Respirations: 24	Spo$_2$: 96%
Time: 1442	BP: 96/58	Pulse: 131	Respirations: 24	Spo$_2$: 95%

EMS Treatment
(circle all that apply)

Oxygen @ __15__ L/min via (circle one): NC (NRM) Bag-mask device	Assisted Ventilation	Airway Adjunct	CPR
Defibrillation (Bleeding Control)	(Bandaging)	(Splinting)	Other

Narrative

Dispatched to residential building collapse with possible entrapment. En route informed that law enforcement and fire crew on-scene advising three-story brick house collapsed with reports of two people being trapped inside. Technical response team en route. Upon arrival incident commander advises our pt is a 65 year-old woman who is trapped from the lower portion of her chest down by concrete and other debris. Initial information provided by fire fighter Rodriguez: Pt is currently awake, alert, and oriented to person, place, time, and event. Airway is patent, and chest rise appears adequate. Carotid pulses are regular, strong, and elevated. The pt is complaining of difficulty breathing and is concerned about the location of her grandson. Initial pt contact was made at approximately 1330. Pt remains awake and alert and states "she can't catch her breath". Manual spinal immobilization held by fire fighter Rodriguez. Pt states that she was in her house playing with her grandson when the house began to shake. The next thing she recalls is being trapped beneath the rubble. Pt is unsure whether she lost consciousness. Pt states that she has a history of diabetes, takes metformin and insulin, and has no known drug allergies. Debris removed at approximately 1350 allowing for full assessment. Assessment reveals bilateral chest rise with tenderness to both sides of the ribcage. Breath sounds are diminished bilaterally. Abdomen is soft and tender to both lower quadrants. Bruising is noted to both lower quadrants beneath the umbilicus. A laceration approximately 3 inches in length was noted on the left thigh. Venous blood steadily coming from the wound. Bleeding controlled with direct pressure and bandage. Oxygen applied via nonrebreathing mask at 15 L/min. IV started in the left antecubital space with 16-gauge angiocath. Normal saline 1,000 mL hung with 10 gtt set and ran at 10 gtts per minute. Blood glucose is 183 mg/dL, which is normal pt. Pt had c-collar placed. No noted pain to the neck prior to collar. Back reveals no trauma or pain to palpation. The pt is packaged with a vacuum splint and basket stretcher. While the pt is being moved to the truck she begins to report severe abdominal pain. Reassessment reveals abdomen is distended and tender to palpation to all quadrants. Skin is pale, cool, and diaphoretic. Radial pulses are absent. Carotid pulses present and weak at a rate of 136 beats/min. IV opened to run wide open. Pt moved to stretcher and secured inside the ambulance. Pt still reports severe abdominal pain and requests pain medication. Explained to pt that she is unable to have any due to her condition. En route to Baptist Hospital at 1416. Head-to-toe assessment: Pupils equal and reactive. No noted trauma to the head or face. No fluids coming from the nose, mouth, or ears. No tracheal deviation or JVD noted. Bilateral breath sounds diminished bilaterally with pain upon palpation to the chest. Bruising now noted to the chest walls bilaterally. Abdomen distended and becoming rigid. Tender to palpation of all quadrants. Lower extremities have multiple abrasions. Bleeding from laceration on the left thigh has stopped. Upper extremities have multiple abrasions; no other trauma noted. PMS present in all four extremities. No further changes noted during transport. Arrived at Baptist trauma center at 1442. Report given and pt care turned over to RN Jenkins. **End of report**

Prep Kit

- "Rescue" means to deliver from danger or imprisonment.
- The most difficult process in any rescue is neither the rescue nor the treatment process, but rather the coordination and balance of both.
- A technical rescue incident (TRI) is a complex rescue incident involving vehicles, water, trench collapse, confined spaces, or wilderness search and rescue that requires specially trained personnel and special equipment.
- Technical rescue training occurs on three levels: awareness, operations, and technician. Most of the training and education EMS providers receive is aimed at the awareness level, enabling them to identify the hazards and secure the scene to prevent additional people from becoming patients.
- When you are assisting rescue team members, the following guidelines will prove useful:
  - Be safe.
  - Follow orders.
  - Work as a team.
  - Think.
  - Follow the golden rule of public service.
- Although special rescue situations may take many different forms, all rescuers should perform the following steps to perform these rescues in a safe, effective, and efficient manner:
  - Preparation
  - Response
  - Arrival and scene size-up
  - Stabilization of the scene
  - Access
  - Disentanglement
  - Removal
  - Transport
- At a technical rescue incident, it is critically important to slow down and properly evaluate the situation. Consider the potential general hazards and risks of utilities, confined spaces, and environmental conditions, as well as hazards that are immediately dangerous to life and health.
- The first arriving officer at a rescue scene should immediately assume command and start using the incident management system. This step is critically important because many technical rescue incidents will eventually become complex and require a large number of assisting units.
- Whenever possible, park emergency vehicles in a manner that will ensure safety and not disrupt traffic any more than necessary. Traffic flow is the largest single hazard associated with any operation that takes place on a highway.
- Accountability should be practiced at all emergencies, no matter how small.

- Basket stretchers facilitate moving patients to a place of safety and can be used in a variety of situations. The manner in which a patient is packaged in a basket stretcher depends on his or her medical condition, the environment, and the manner in which the patient will be evacuated.
- In 2009, an estimated 5,505,000 police-reported motor vehicle traffic crashes occurred. Vehicle extrication is therefore commonly necessary.
- Vehicles may be powered by electricity and electricity/gasoline hybrids, or fuels such as propane, natural gas, methanol, or hydrogen. There are many hazards associated with alternative powered vehicles.
- You should have a thorough working knowledge of the basic, simple hand tools. Hand tools can be categorized as striking tools, leverage/prying/spreading tools, cutting tools, and lifting/pushing/pulling tools.
- The most basic, physical tool used for vehicle stabilization is cribbing. Cribbing should be used regardless of the position of the vehicle.
- Simple vehicle extrication techniques include opening the door, breaking tempered glass, and providing initial medical care to the patients.
- During disentanglement, responders need to be mindful of undeployed air bags.
- Many vehicle extrication techniques require the use of specialized skills and training, as well as hydraulic or pneumatic tools.
- A confined space is a location surrounded by a structure that is not designed for continuous occupancy. Confined spaces have limited openings for entrance and exit.
- Confined spaces present a special hazard because they may have limited ventilation to provide for air circulation and exchange, which can make them an oxygen-deficient atmosphere, or they may contain poisonous gases.
- Trench rescues may become necessary when earth is removed for placement of a utility line or for other construction and the sides of the excavation collapse, trapping a worker.
- Because almost all EMS providers have the potential to be called to a water rescue situation, you should know how to properly don a personal flotation device as well as how to use the self-rescue position.
- Rope rescue incidents are divided into low-angle and high-angle operations.
  - Low-angle operations are situations where the slope of the ground over which the rescuers are working is less than 45°. Low-angle operations are used when the scene requires ropes to be used only as assistance to pull or haul up a patient or rescuer.

- High-angle operations are situations where the slope of the ground is greater than 45°, and rescuers or patients are dependent on a life safety rope and not a fixed surface of support such as the ground.

■ Wilderness search and rescue (SAR) missions consist of two parts: search (looking for a lost or overdue person) and rescue (removing a patient from a hostile environment).

■ During lost person search and rescue, your role is to stand by at the search base until the lost person or people have been found.

■ You should always stay with your ambulance during a structure fire. Search and rescue during a fire is performed by trained personnel.

■ If an incident develops into a tactical situation, law enforcement agencies may deploy use of specialized law enforcement tactical units or the SWAT team.

■ Pain control in rescue situations should take the form of nonpharmacologic methods, such as splinting to minimize movement, and gentle handling. Pharmacologic treatment in the prehospital setting remains controversial, and providers should consult with their medical directors on issues related to pain management.

■ A number of special patient packaging tools are available to help extricate patients out of their situation and up, down, or out to the ambulance. The basket stretcher is an example of a packaging tool.

■ Vital Vocabulary

accountability system A method of accounting for all personnel at an emergency incident and ensuring that only personnel with specific assignments are permitted to work within the various zones.

alternative powered vehicles A vehicle that uses fuels other than petroleum or a combination of petroleum and another fuel for power.

awareness The first level of rescue training provided to all responders, with an emphasis on recognizing the hazards, securing the scene, and calling for appropriate assistance. There is no actual use of rescue skills.

belay Technique of controlling the rope as it is fed out to climbers.

body-over-frame construction Vehicle design where the body of the vehicle is placed onto a frame skeleton and the frame acts as the foundation for the vehicle. The design consists of two large beams tied together by cross member beams.

cold protective response Phenomenon associated with cold water immersion in which reflexes in the body and a lowered metabolic rate help preserve basic body functions.

cold zone A safe area for those agencies involved in the operations; the incident commander (IC), command post, EMS providers, and other support functions necessary to control the incident should be located in the cold zone.

complex access Complicated entry that requires special tools and training and includes breaking windows or using other force.

confined space A space with limited or restricted access that is not meant for continuous occupancy, such as a manhole, well, or tank.

cribbing Short lengths of wood that are used to stabilize vehicles.

entrapment A condition in which a patient is trapped by debris, soil, or other material and is unable to extricate himself or herself.

hand tool Any tool or equipment operating from human power.

high-angle operations A rope rescue operation where the angle of the slope is greater than 45°; rescuers depend on life safety rope rather than a fixed support surface such as the ground.

hot zone The area immediately surrounding an incident site that is directly dangerous to life and health. All personnel working in the hot zone must wear complete and appropriate protective clothing and equipment. Entry requires approval by the IC or a designated sector officer. Complete backup, rescue, and decontamination teams must be in place at the perimeter before operations begin.

immediately dangerous to life and health (IDLH) An atmospheric concentration of any toxic, corrosive, or asphyxiant substance that poses an immediate threat to life or could cause irreversible or delayed adverse health effects. There are three general IDLH atmospheres: toxic, flammable, and oxygen-deficient.

laminated glass Type of window glazing that incorporates a sheeting material that stops the glass from breaking into shards.

low-angle operations A rope rescue operation on a mildly sloping surface (less than 45°) or flat land where rescuers are dependent on the ground for their primary support, and the rope system is a secondary means of support.

operations The technical rescue training level geared toward working in the warm zone of an incident. Training at this level allows responders to directly assist those conducting the rescue operation and to use certain rescue skills and procedures.

personal flotation device (PFD) Also commonly known as a life vest, a PFD allows the body to float in water.

rappelling To descend on a fixed rope.

scrambling A method used to ascend rocky faces and ridges and can be considered a cross between hill climbing and rock climbing.

search and rescue (SAR) The process of locating and removing a patient from the wilderness.

secondary collapse A collapse that occurs following the primary collapse. This can occur in trench, excavation, and structural collapses.

self-rescue position Position used in fast-moving water rescue situations. The rescuer rolls into a faceup arched position with the lower back higher than the feet to avoid objects below the surface. The feet should be together and facing in the direction of travel (feet first), with arms at the sides.

shims Objects that are smaller than wedges used to snug loose cribbing under a load or to fill void spaces.

shoring A method of supporting a trench wall or building components such as walls, floors, or ceilings using either hydraulic, pneumatic, or wood shoring systems. Shoring is used to prevent collapse.

simple access Access that is easily achieved with the use of simple hand tools or force.

special weapons and tactics (SWAT) team A specialized law enforcement tactical unit.

spoil pile The pile of dirt that has been removed from an excavation. The pile may be unstable and prone to collapse.

step chocks Specialized cribbing assemblies made out of wood or plastic in a step configuration.

tactical situation A high-risk situation where law enforcement agencies may deploy use of specialized law enforcement tactical units or the SWAT team.

technical rescue incident (TRI) A complex rescue incident involving vehicles or machinery, water or ice, rope techniques, a trench or excavation collapse, confined spaces, a structural collapse, wilderness search and rescue, or hazardous materials, and which requires specially trained personnel and special equipment.

technical rescue team A group of rescuers specially trained in the various disciplines of technical rescue.

technician The training level that provides a high level of competency in the various disciplines of technical or hazardous materials rescue for rescuers who will be directly involved in the rescue operation itself.

tempered glass A type of glass that is heat-treated so that it will break into small pieces.

unibody construction A vehicle design with no formal frame structure; the body and frame are one piece, which is considered to be the structural integrity of the vehicle.

warm zone The area located between the hot zone and the cold zone at an incident. Decontamination stations are located in the warm zone.

wedges Used to snug loose cribbing.

Assessment
in Action

It is 7 AM and the morning rush hour commute is getting under way. Visibility is down to a quarter mile due to a mix of dense fog and smoke from a forest fire. You and your partner are dispatched to the scene of a motor vehicle crash on a local back road where a SUV collided with a tractor trailer. The SUV struck the side of the tractor trailer and the entire engine compartment is wedged under the truck. The driver of the truck is out of the vehicle and claims he is uninjured. The driver of the SUV appears unconscious and is trapped in the vehicle.

1. Which of the following are potential scene hazards?
   A. Downed electrical lines
   B. Gasoline
   C. Air bags
   D. All of the above

2. What is the largest hazard associated with any operation that takes place on a highway?
   A. Visibility
   B. Traffic flow
   C. Access to the scene
   D. Bystanders and media

3. Vehicles can be stabilized with:
   A. steel-reinforced cables.
   B. stairs.
   C. air bags.
   D. cribbing.

4. What tool should be used to break tempered glass?
   A. Sledgehammer
   B. Spring-loaded center punch
   C. Axe
   D. Pike pole

5. If the air bag does not deploy at the time of impact, you should:
   A. disconnect the battery and allow the air bag capacitor to discharge.
   B. remove the steering wheel from the steering column.
   C. position a backboard between the patient and the air bag.
   D. attempt to manually discharge the air bag.

6. At what point during the rescue operation should initial medical care be rendered?
   A. Immediately on arrival at the scene
   B. After the patient has been disentangled from the vehicle
   C. Once the patient is in the ambulance
   D. Simultaneously with extrication

7. In order to be directly involved with the rescue operation itself, what level of training must you have completed?
   A. Master
   B. Technician
   C. Awareness
   D. Operations

Hazardous Materials

National EMS Education Standard Competencies

EMS Operations

Knowledge of operational roles and responsibilities to ensure patient, public, and personnel safety.

Hazardous Materials Awareness

Risks and responsibilities of operating in a cold zone at a hazardous material or other special incident. (pp 2268-2270)

....

Knowledge Objectives

1. Define the term hazardous material. (p 2257)
2. Describe the OSHA HAZWOPER regulation and recognize the entry-level training or experience requirements identified by the HAZWOPER regulation for a paramedic to respond to a hazardous materials incident. (pp 2257-2258)
3. Describe the hazard classification system used by the National Fire Protection Association (NFPA). (pp 2257-2258)
4. Explain the role of the paramedic during a hazardous materials incident both before and after the hazardous materials team arrives, including precautions required to ensure the safety of civilians and public service personnel. (pp 2258-2259)
5. Discuss the specific types of information and reference resources a paramedic can use to recognize a hazardous materials incident. (pp 2259-2262)

6. Describe some of the containers and vehicles used to transport hazardous materials on the roadway. (pp 2262, 2264-2268)
7. Explain how the three control zones are established at a hazardous materials incident, and discuss the characteristics of each zone, including the personnel who work within each one. (pp 2268-2269)
8. Describe the four levels of personal protective equipment (PPE) that may be required at a hazardous materials incident to protect personnel from injury by or contamination from a particular substance. (pp 2269, 2271-2272)
9. Describe how the route of the exposure, the dose and concentration of the hazard, and the length of time the hazard is in contact with the body affects the body. (pp 2272)
10. Provide examples of how understanding the chemical and physical properties of a substance may give you some valuable insight when it comes to providing care. (pp 2272-2275)
11. Describe decontamination techniques, including emergency decontamination, mass decontamination, and technical decontamination. (pp 2275-2279)
12. Describe patient care at a hazardous materials incident and explain special requirements for specific exposures. (pp 2277-2279)

Skills Objectives

1. Identify DOT labels, placards, and markings that are used to designate hazardous materials. (pp 2259-2262)
2. Demonstrate the ability to use a variety of reference materials to identify a hazardous material. (pp 2259-2262)

Introduction

One of the inevitable consequences of living in an industrialized world is the proliferation of hazardous materials. A <u>hazardous material</u>, as defined by the Department of Transportation (DOT), is any substance or material that is capable of posing an unreasonable risk to human health, safety, or the environment when transported in commerce, used incorrectly, or not properly contained or stored. The products of our civilization require the manufacture, transport, storage, use, and disposal of tens of thousands of potentially toxic substances. Thousands of hazardous materials releases occur each year, with the great majority of these being highway transportation incidents.

This chapter will take a broad look at some of the unique aspects you should consider when you are responding to hazardous materials incidents. The information provided here is not intended to be a comprehensive coverage of hazardous materials incident response procedures; certify you to any recognized level of hazardous materials response; or turn you into a hazardous materials expert. The material provided is intended to help you understand a hazardous materials incident, as well as help you understand the consequences of a person or persons who may become exposed to those substances, and understand where you fit into a hazardous materials incident. Operating at a hazardous materials scene presents many challenges that are not encountered during a normal EMS response. This includes the potential for you to be exposed to a toxic substance and turn into a victim like those patients already exposed, and the need for you to handle exposures properly and with confidence.

Regulations and Standards

The primary regulations for hazardous materials response are put forth by the US federal Occupational Safety and Health Administration (OSHA) and the US federal Environmental Protection Agency (EPA). The OSHA document containing the hazardous materials response competencies is commonly referred to as <u>**HAZWOPER (HAZardous Waste OPerations and Emergency Response)**</u>. The complete HAZWOPER regulation can be found in Title 29 of the Code of Federal Regulations (CFR), standard 1910.120 (q)(6)(i). The training levels found in the OSHA regulation are identified as awareness, operations, technician, specialist, and incident commander. According to OSHA, "first responders at the awareness level are individuals who are likely to witness or discover a hazardous substance release and who have been trained to initiate an emergency response sequence by notifying the proper authorities of the release. They would take no further action beyond notifying the authorities of the release." Based on the OSHA HAZWOPER regulation, first responders at the awareness level should have sufficient training or experience to objectively demonstrate competency in the following areas:

- An understanding of what hazardous substances are and the risks associated with them

YOU are the Medic   PART 1

You and your partner are en route to a chlorine leak at a water treatment plant. Initial reports state that approximately 20 people were in the immediate vicinity of the leak. The hazardous materials team is on scene setting up safety zones, and the incident management system has been established. On your arrival the Incident Commander assigns your unit to the treatment sector. When you arrive at the treatment sector, the sector leader provides you with the Material Safety Data Sheet (MSDS) for chlorine. Your patient, a middle-aged man, enters the treatment sector in respiratory distress.

Recording Time: 1 Minute	
Appearance	Anxious and restless
Level of consciousness	Alert (Oriented to person, place, and day)
Airway	Open
Breathing	Increased work of breathing with accessory muscle use and audible expiratory wheezes
Circulation	Strong radial pulse, slightly increased

1. What are some clues that might help you identify leaks or spills of hazardous materials?
2. How can the MSDS assist you with the treatment of your patient?

- An understanding of the potential outcomes of an incident
- The ability to recognize the presence of hazardous substances
- The ability to identify the hazardous substances, if possible
- An understanding of the role of the first responder awareness individual in the emergency response plan
- The ability to determine the need for additional resources and to notify the communication center

Consensus-based standards such as the National Fire Protection Association (NFPA) 472 standard, *Standard for Competence of Responders to Hazardous/Materials/Weapons of Mass Destruction Incidents* are also available to guide responders. Additionally, NFPA 473, *Standard for Competencies for EMS Personnel Responding to Hazardous Materials/Weapons of Mass Destruction Incidents* is a good resource to offer guidance to those EMS responders rendering medical care at hazardous materials incidents.

All EMS personnel should receive appropriate hazardous materials response training, based on the needs and requirements of the **authority having jurisdiction (AHJ)** and the local EMS agency. In many cases, the AHJ may decide that the awareness level of training may be appropriate. In other instances, the AHJ may choose to train EMS responders to a higher level of training, such as the operations or technician level. Refer to the chapter, *Vehicle Extrication and Special Rescue,* for a review of the three levels of training. Whatever the case, it is up to the AHJ to decide how much hazardous materials response training will be

required of EMS responders. The level of training will dictate when and where you might use your EMS skills.

Keep in mind that federal, state, and local regulations and standards govern the use, storage, and transportation of hazardous materials. These regulations and standards are designed to improve the public's ability to know and to help protect workers and emergency responders as they try to protect the public. You should become familiar with the laws of the state and locality in which you serve. In order to determine what level of hazardous materials training you may need, consult experts in the field from your local jurisdiction.

Paramedics and Hazardous Materials Incidents

Street smarts are not enough to identify potential hazardous materials scenes and determine how to safely operate if you are first on scene or called to provide medical support at a hazardous materials incident; you must also rely on training and reference sources. You should know how and when to access specific toxicologic information (reference sources, poison control center, medical control) and/or a hazardous materials team when the situation calls for it. You should understand how a hazardous materials scene is organized from a command and control perspective, including how you fit into the command structure and operational plan. You also need to be familiar with the different types of personal protective equipment (PPE) used at a hazardous materials scene, how the hazardous materials team or other responders will decontaminate patients, and how to assess and treat exposures. In addition, you may be called on to support hazardous materials teams through on-scene medical monitoring.

Hazardous materials incidents may include but are not limited to the following:

- A highway or rail incident in which a substance is leaking from a cargo tank or railroad tank car
- A leak, fire, or other emergency at an industrial plant, refinery, or other fixed facility where chemicals or explosives are produced, used, or stored
- A leak or rupture of an underground natural gas pipe
- Incidents in an agricultural setting in which insecticides may be in use or accidentally released
- Buildup of methane or other by-products of waste decomposition in sewers, sewage processing plants, or landfills
- An incident with criminal intent in which a suspected hazardous materials agent is intentionally released

Scene Size-up

When you first arrive at any scene and recognize the presence or potential presence of a hazardous material release, your most important job is to ensure your own safety. Unfortunately, identifying the hazard might not be possible, which could complicate your ability to rapidly understand the threat and initiate protective actions. In some cases, the presence of a hazardous materials agent can be recognized from warning signs such as victim/patient signs and symptoms, placards, labels, or other clues found at the scene. Placards or labels may be found:

- On buildings or in areas where hazardous materials are produced, used, or stored
- On trucks and rail cars that transport certain types/amounts of a hazardous material

- On drums or other storage vessels that contain a hazardous waste or hazardous material

Sometimes, transporters do not label containers or vessels appropriately, and the labeling of packages and transport vehicles can be misleading.

Always maintain a high index of suspicion as you perform your first assessment of the scene. Even the most mundane-looking scene could present significant dangers. Intentional ingestion of chemicals and illicit activities such as methamphetamine labs and potential terrorist activities may have no obvious warning signs. You could be well into the call before you have a firm grasp of what is really happening. In some cases, you may be able to identify leaks or spills by the following:

- A visible cloud or strange-looking smoke resulting from the escaping substance
- A leak or spill from a tank, container, truck, or railroad car with or without hazardous materials placards or labels
- An unusual, strong, noxious, acrid odor in the area

Some chemicals are odorized to indicate the presence of normally odorless gases (eg, propane and methane). However, there are a number of dangerous substances that are odorless and can only be detected by air monitoring instruments (carbon monoxide). To that end, never rely solely on your sense of smell to identify the presence of a hazardous material—if you smell it, you are exposed! Remember, a large number of people, including you, could be exposed before the presence of a hazardous materials incident is identified.

If you approach a scene where more than one person has collapsed or is unconscious or in respiratory distress, especially at a mass gathering event such as a political convention or sporting event, you should suspect the presence of a hazardous materials agent.

If you do not follow the proper safety measures when you are faced with a hazardous materials incident, you and many others could end up needlessly exposed or injured. The safety of you and your team, the other responders, and the public must be your most important concern. There will be times when your ambulance crew is the first set of responders to arrive at the scene. If, as you approach, any signs suggest that a hazardous materials incident has occurred, you should stop at a safe distance, upwind and uphill from the scene. After rapidly sizing up the scene, isolate the hazardous area to the best of your ability; deny entry to the affected area and call for additional resources. These resources may include law enforcement, fire, hazardous materials responders, or additional EMS responders. Once your safety is ensured, you may begin the process of identifying victims and beginning patient care if appropriate. There are, however, many factors that could impact your ability to provide care. More on this topic will be explored throughout the rest of the chapter. If you do not recognize the danger until you are too close, immediately leave the danger zone. Once you have reached a safe place, reassess the situation and provide as much information as possible when you are calling for additional resources. Examples of items to report include the following:

- Your exact location
- Atmospheric conditions if appropriate

- Size and shape of containers or cargo tankers
- The exact name of the substance if known
- The number of victims, including signs and symptoms if observed

- The type and number of additional resources requested
- Location of safe staging areas for incoming resources
- Location of incident command post

Do not reenter the scene or leave the area until you have been cleared by the hazardous material team, or you may contribute to the situation by spreading hazardous materials.

Identification of Hazardous Materials

Information is one of the most valuable commodities at a hazardous materials incident. This information can come to you in the form of your own observations; reports from bystanders; signs and symptoms of victims, and other sources including labels and placards, shipping papers, or material safety data sheets. In some cases, labels and placards will provide you with basic information about the materials involved in the release. Remember, take no risks, but when applicable, try to read the marking and placards required at hazardous materials storage sites and on vehicles.

The most recent edition of the DOT's *Emergency Response Guidebook* (*ERG*) should be carried on every emergency response vehicle **Figure 1**. The *ERG* is a guidebook for first responders during the initial phase of a dangerous goods/hazardous materials transportation incident. The *ERG* provides information

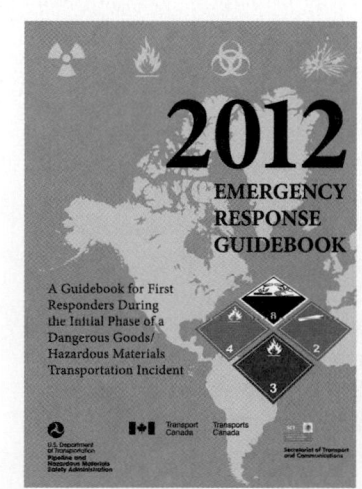

Figure 1 The *ERG* is a reference used as a base for your initial actions at a hazardous materials incident.

on specific properties and hazards of substances, what is shown on placards, and recommended isolation distances. The nine DOT chemical families recognized in the *ERG* are as follows:

- DOT Class 1: Explosives
- DOT Class 2: Gases
- DOT Class 3: Flammable combustible liquids
- DOT Class 4: Flammable solids; spontaneously combustible materials; and dangerous when wet materials/water-reactive substances
- DOT Class 5: Oxidizing substances and organic peroxides
- DOT Class 6: Toxic* substances and infectious substances
- DOT Class 7: Radioactive materials
- DOT Class 8: Corrosive substances
- DOT Class 9: Miscellaneous hazardous materials/products, substances, or organisms

*The word "poison" or "poisonous" is synonymous with the word "toxin."

You can download a free copy of the *ERG* by visiting the US DOT Pipeline and Hazardous Materials Safety Administration website.

Transportation Marking System

The US DOT marking system is an identification system characterized by labels, placards, and markings **Figure 2**. This marking system is used when materials are being transported from one location to another in the United States. The same marking system is also used in Canada by Transport Canada.

Placards are diamond-shaped indicators (at least 10.8 inches on each side) that are placed on all four sides of highway transport vehicles, railroad tank cars, and other forms of transportation carrying hazardous materials **Figure 3**. Placards identify the broad hazard class (flammable, poison, corrosive) to which the material inside belongs. The most

common placards show four-digit numbers that are part of the United Nations/North American coding system for identification of hazardous materials. This number identifies the specific material being transported and corresponds with information in the *ERG*. In addition to the numbers, different symbols are used to help identify different classes of hazardous materials.

Labels are smaller versions (at least 3.9 inches on each side) of placards; they are placed on the four sides of individual boxes

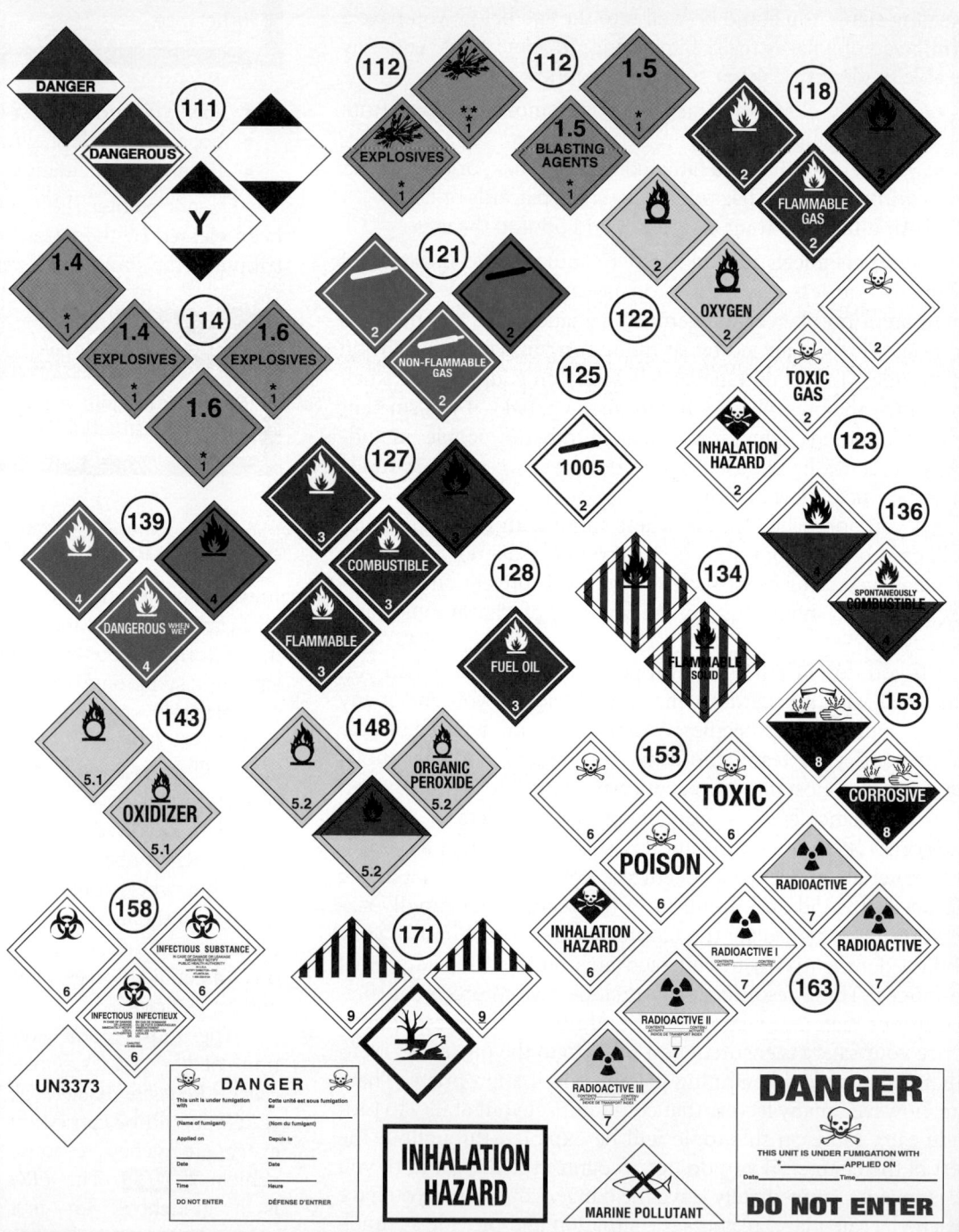

Figure 2 The DOT uses labels, placards, and markings (such as these found in the *Emergency Response Guidebook*) to give responders a general idea of the hazard inside a particular container or cargo tank.

and smaller packages being transported Figure 4 . A label on a box inside a delivery truck relates only to the potential hazard inside that particular package.

Placards, labels, and markings are intended to give responders a general idea of the hazard inside a particular container or cargo tank. However, the DOT system does not require that all chemical shipments be marked with placards or labels. In most cases the package or cargo tank must contain a certain amount of hazardous material before a placard is required. Conversely, some chemicals are so hazardous that shipping any amount requires placards or labels.

Other good sources of information for identifying hazardous materials in transport include the **bill of lading**, or freight bill, which should be carried by the truck driver in the cab, and the **waybill** or "consist" that is carried by the conductor of a train. Additionally, dispatchers may assist in collecting further information from organizations such as **CHEMTREC (Chemical Transportation Emergency Center)**, which

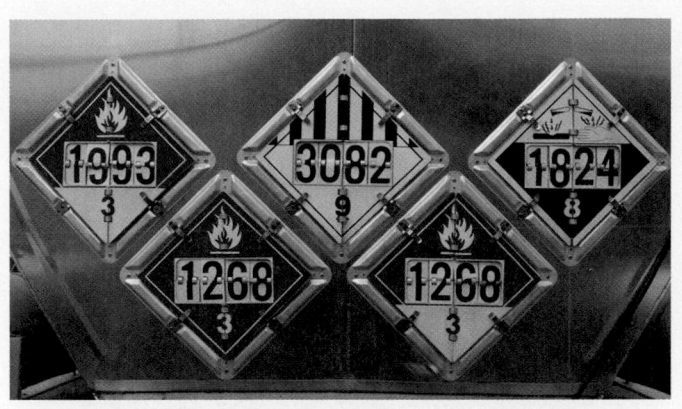

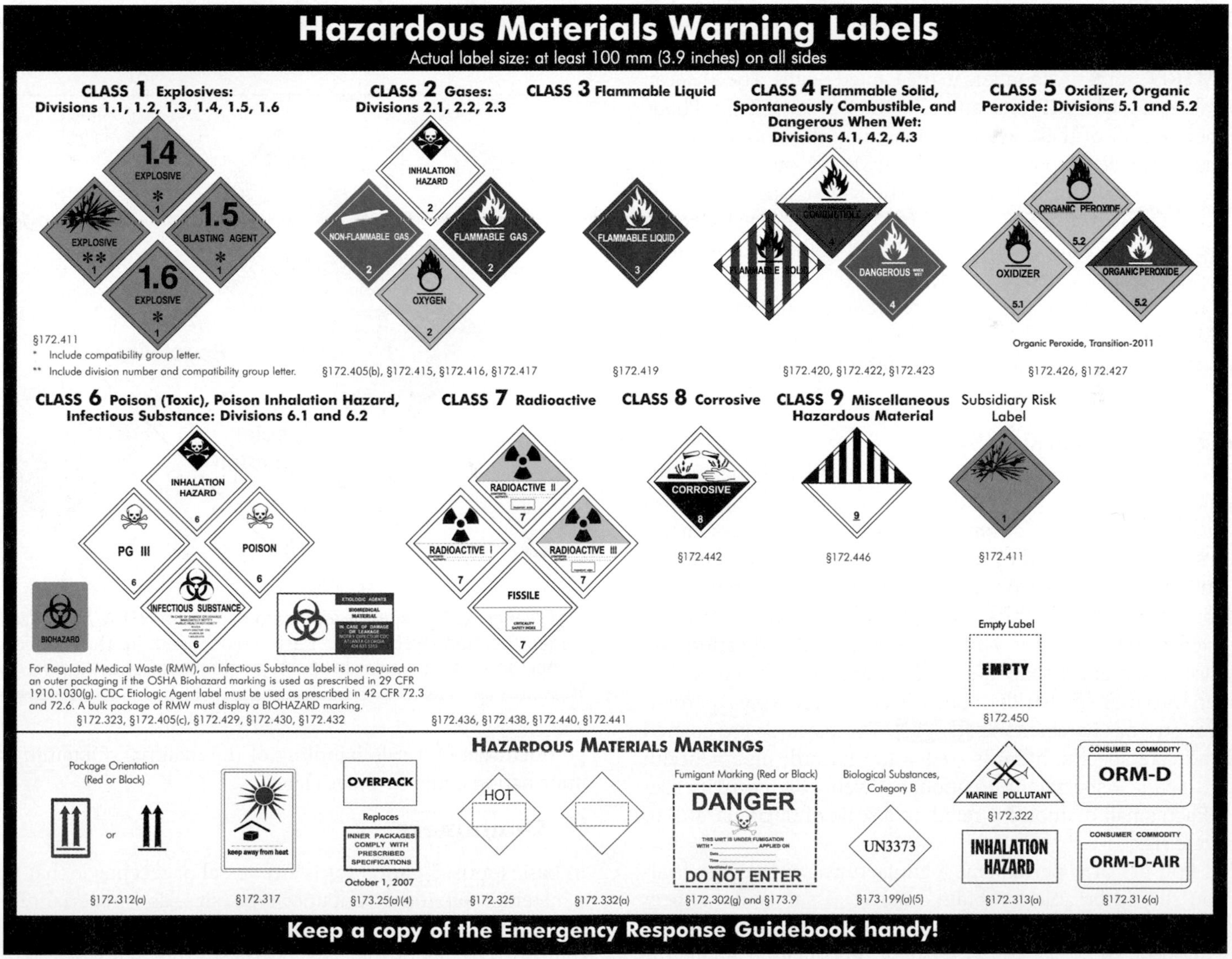

Figure 3 A placard is a large, diamond-shaped indicator that is placed on all sides of transport vehicles that carry hazardous materials. The numbers identify the specific material being transported.

Hazardous Materials Warning Labels
Actual label size: at least 100 mm (3.9 inches) on all sides

CLASS 1 Explosives:
Divisions 1.1, 1.2, 1.3, 1.4, 1.5, 1.6

CLASS 2 Gases:
Divisions 2.1, 2.2, 2.3

CLASS 3 Flammable Liquid

CLASS 4 Flammable Solid, Spontaneously Combustible, and Dangerous When Wet: Divisions 4.1, 4.2, 4.3

CLASS 5 Oxidizer, Organic Peroxide: Divisions 5.1 and 5.2

§172.411
* Include compatibility group letter.
** Include division number and compatibility group letter.

§172.405(b), §172.415, §172.416, §172.417

§172.419

§172.420, §172.422, §172.423

Organic Peroxide, Transition-2011

§172.426, §172.427

CLASS 6 Poison (Toxic), Poison Inhalation Hazard, Infectious Substance: Divisions 6.1 and 6.2

CLASS 7 Radioactive

CLASS 8 Corrosive

CLASS 9 Miscellaneous Hazardous Material

Subsidiary Risk Label

For Regulated Medical Waste (RMW), an Infectious Substance label is not required on an outer packaging if the OSHA Biohazard marking is used as prescribed in 29 CFR 1910.1030(g). CDC Etiologic Agent label must be used as prescribed in 42 CFR 72.3 and 72.6. A bulk package of RMW must display a BIOHAZARD marking.
§172.323, §172.405(c), §172.429, §172.430, §172.432

§172.436, §172.438, §172.440, §172.441

§172.442

§172.446

§172.411

Empty Label

EMPTY

§172.450

HAZARDOUS MATERIALS MARKINGS

Package Orientation (Red or Black)

§172.312(a)

§172.317

OVERPACK
Replaces
INNER PACKAGES COMPLY WITH PRESCRIBED SPECIFICATIONS
October 1, 2007
§173.25(a)(4)

HOT
§172.325

§172.332(a)

Fumigant Marking (Red or Black)
DANGER
THIS UNIT IS UNDER FUMIGATION WITH * APPLIED ON
Date
Time
DO NOT ENTER
§172.302(g) and §173.9

Biological Substances, Category B
UN3373
§173.199(a)(5)

MARINE POLLUTANT
§172.322
INHALATION HAZARD
§172.313(a)

CONSUMER COMMODITY
ORM-D
CONSUMER COMMODITY
ORM-D-AIR
§172.316(a)

Keep a copy of the Emergency Response Guidebook handy!

Figure 4 A label is a smaller version of the placard and is placed on boxes or smaller packages that contain hazardous materials.

operates a 24-hour telephone line (1-800-262-8200) and has an extensive database to assist emergency responders. CHEM-TREC has the ability to provide responders with technical chemical information via the telephone, fax, or other electronic media. Calls can be translated in over 180 languages. There is also a phone conferencing service that will put a responder in touch with thousands of shippers, subject matter experts, and chemical manufacturers. When you are calling CHEMTREC (a free service), be sure to have the following basic information ready:

- The name of the chemical(s) involved
- Name of the caller and callback telephone number
- Location of the actual incident or problem
- Shipper or manufacturer of chemical (if known)
- Container type
- Rail car or vehicle markings or numbers
- The shipping carrier's name
- Recipient of material
- Local conditions and exact description of the situation

The Canadian equivalent of CHEMTREC is known as CANUTEC (Canadian Transport Emergency Centre). This organization serves Canadian responders in much the same way CHEMTREC serves responders in the United States. The Mexican equivalent of CHEMTREC and CANUTEC is SETIQ. Phone numbers for all of these agencies, including the phone number for the National Response Center (NRC) and other important resources, can be found in the *ERG*. The NRC is operated by the US Coast Guard and serves as a central notification point, rather than a guidance center. Once the NRC is notified, it will alert appropriate state and federal agencies.

There are many legitimate reference sources available to EMS responders when it comes to hazardous materials response. It is up to you to be familiar with what is available within your AHJ.

Fixed-Facility Marking System

The NFPA has developed its own system for identifying hazardous materials. NFPA 704, *Standard System for the Identification of the Hazards of Materials for Emergency Response*, outlines a marking system characterized by a set of diamonds that are found on the outside of buildings, on doorways to chemical storage areas, and on fixed storage tanks. This marking system is designed for fixed-facility use. The NFPA 704 hazard identification system uses a diamond-shaped symbol of any size, which is itself broken into four smaller diamonds, each representing a particular property or characteristic **Figure 5**. The placards are colored and indicate specific hazards (red = fire hazard, blue = health hazard, white = special information, and yellow = reactivity hazard). Each small diamond is rated on a scale of 0 (no hazard) to 4 (severe risk).

If you are at a permanent manufacturing or storage facility, you should be able to obtain a **material safety data sheet (MSDS)** for in-depth information about the hazardous materials **Figure 6**. A MSDS provides basic information about the chemical makeup of a substance, the potential hazards it presents, appropriate first aid in the event of an exposure, and other

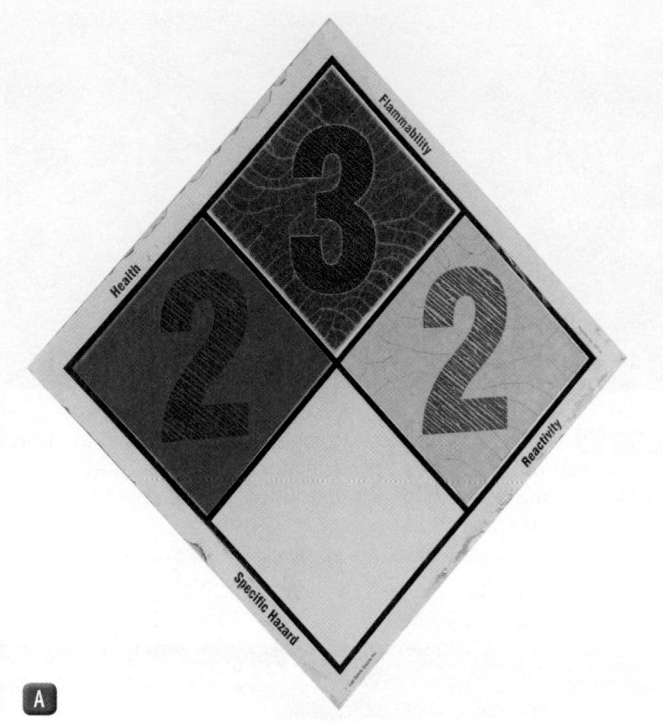

A

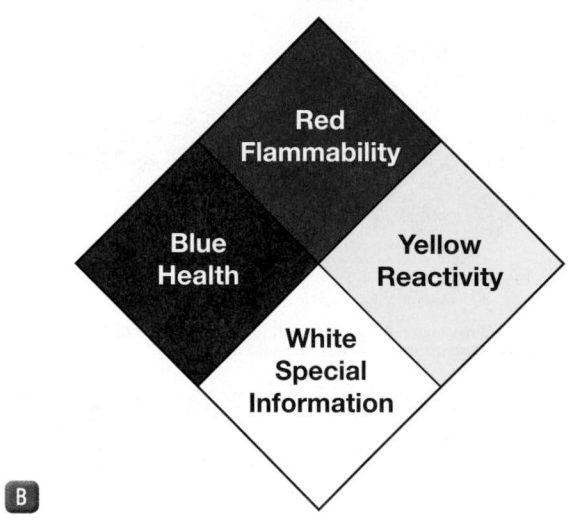

B

Figure 5 **A.** Example of a placard using the NFPA 704 hazard identification system. **B.** Each color used in the diamond represents a particular property or characteristic.

pertinent data for safe handling of the material. Obtaining this information could save lives later.

◼ Containers

In basic terms, a **container** is any vessel or receptacle that holds a material. Often the container type, size, and material of construction provide important clues about the nature of the substance inside. Nevertheless, you should not rely solely on the type of container when you are making a determination about hazardous materials.

MATERIAL SAFETY DATA SHEET

ANHYDROUS AMMONIA

TI

DISTRIBUTORS:

TANNER INDUSTRIES, INC.

DIVISIONS:

NATIONAL AMMONIA	NORTHEASTERN AMMONIA
HAMLER INDUSTRIES	BOWER AMMONIA & CHEMICAL

735 Davisville Road, Third Floor, Southampton, PA 18966; 215-322-1238

CORPORATE EMERGENCY TELEPHONE NUMBER: 800-643-6226 CHEMTREC: 800-424-9300

DESCRIPTION

CHEMICAL NAME: Ammonia, Anhydrous **CAS REGISTRY NO**: 7664-41-7
SYNONYMS: Ammonia **CHEMICAL FAMILY**: Inorganic Nitrogen Compound
FORMULA: NH_3 **MOL. WT**: 17.03 (NH_3) **COMPOSITION**: 99+% Ammonia

STATEMENT OF HEALTH HAZARD

HAZARD DESCRIPTION:
Ammonia is an irritant and corrosive to the skin, eyes, respiratory tract and mucous membranes. Exposure to liquid or rapidly expanding gases may cause severe chemical burns and frostbite to the eyes, lungs and skin. Skin and respiratory related diseases could be aggravated by exposure.

Not recognized by OSHA as a carcinogen.
Not listed in the National Toxicology Program.
Not listed as a carcinogen by the International Agency for Research on Cancer.

EXPOSURE LIMITS FOR AMMONIA: Vapor

OSHA	50 ppm,	35 mg / m^3 PEL	8 hour TWA
NIOSH	35 ppm,	27 mg / m^3 STEL 15 minutes	
	25 ppm,	18 mg / m^3 REL	10 hour TWA
	300 ppm,	IDLH	
ACGIH	25 ppm,	18 mg / m^3 TLV	8 hour TWA
	35 ppm,	27 mg / m^3 STEL 15 minutes	

TOXICITY: LD 50 (Oral / Rat) 350 mg / kg

PHYSICAL DATA

BOILING POINT: -28°F at 1 Atm.
PH: N/A
SPECIFIC GRAVITY OF GAS (air = 1): 0.596 at 32°F
SPECIFIC GRAVITY OF LIQUID (water = 1): 0.682 at 28°F (Compared to water at 39°F).
PERCENT VOLATILE: 100% at 212°F
APPEARANCE AND ODOR: Colorless liquid or gas with pungent odor.
CRITICAL TEMPERATURE: 271.4°F
GAS SPECIFIC VOLUME: 20.78 Ft^3/Lb at 32°F and 1 Atm.
VAPOR DENSITY: 0.0481 Lb/Ft^3 at 32°F
LIQUID DENSITY: 38.00 Lb/Ft^3 at 70°F
APPROXIMATE FREEZING POINT: -108°F
WEIGHT (per gallon): 5.15 pounds at 60°F
VAPOR PRESSURE: 114 psig at 70°F
SOLUBILITY IN WATER (per 100 pounds of water): 86.9 pounds at 32°F, 51 pounds at 68°F
SURFACE TENSION: 23.4 Dynes / cm at 52°F
CRITICAL PRESSURE: 111.5 atm

Revision: September 2005 Page 1 of 4 Prepared By: JRP

MATERIAL SAFETY DATA SHEET

EMERGENCY TREATMENT

EFFECTS OF OVEREXPOSURE:
Eye: Tearing, edema or blindness may occur.
Skin: Irritation, corrosive burns, blister formation may result. Contact with liquid may produce a caustic burn and frostbite.
Inhalation: Acute exposure may result in severe irritation of the respiratory tract, bronchospasm, pulmonary edema or respiratory arrest.
Ingestion: Lung irritation and pulmonary edema may occur. ***Extreme exposure may result in death from spasm, inflammation or edema. Brief inhalation exposure to 5,000 ppm may be fatal.***
EMERGENCY AID: Remove patient to uncontaminated area.
Eye: Flush with copious amounts of tepid water for a minimum of 20 minutes. Eyelids should be held apart and away from eyeball for thorough rinsing.
Skin: Flush with copious amounts of tepid water for a minimum of 20 minutes while removing contaminated clothing, jewelry and shoes. Do not rub or apply ointment on affected area. Clothing may initially freeze to skin. Thaw frozen clothing from skin before removing.
Inhalation: Remove to fresh air. If not breathing, administer artificial respiration. If trained to do so, administer supplemental oxygen, if required.
Ingestion: If conscious, give large amounts of water to drink. May drink orange juice, citrus juice or diluted vinegar (1:4) to counteract ammonia. If unconscious, do not give anything by mouth. **Do not induce vomiting!**

SEEK IMMEDIATE MEDICAL HELP FOR ALL EXPOSURES!

NOTE TO PHYSICIAN: **Respiratory injury may appear as a delayed phenomenon. Pulmonary edema may follow chemical bronchitis. Supportive treatment with necessary ventilation actions, including oxygen, may warrant consideration.**

FIRE AND EXPLOSION HAZARD DATA

FLASHPOINT: None.
FLAMMABLE LIMITS IN AIR: LEL/UEL 16% to 25%.(listed in the *NIOSH Pocket Guide to Chemical Hazards* 15% to 28%).
EXTINGUISHING MEDIA: Dry Chemical, CO_2, water spray or alcohol-resistant foam if gas flow cannot be stopped.
AUTO IGNITION TEMPERATURE: 1,204°F (If catalyzed) 1,570°F (If un-catalyzed).

SPECIAL FIRE-FIGHTING PROCEDURES:
Must wear protective clothing and a positive pressure SCBA. Stop source if possible. If a portable container (such as a cylinder or trailer) can be moved from the fire area without risk to the individual, do so to prevent the pressure relief valve of the trailer from discharging or the cylinder from rupturing. Fight fires using dry chemical, carbon dioxide, water spray or alcohol-resistant foam. Cool fire exposed containers with water spray. Stay upwind when containers are threatened. Use water spray to knock down vapor and dilute.

UNUSUAL FIRE AND EXPLOSION HAZARDS:
Outdoors, ammonia is not generally a fire hazard. Indoors, in confined areas, ammonia may be a fire hazard, especially if oil and other combustible materials are present. Combustion may form toxic nitrogen oxides.
If relief valves are inoperative, heat exposed storage containers may become explosion hazards due to over pressurization.

CHEMICAL REACTIVITY

STABILITY:
Stable at room temperature. Heating a closed container above room temperature causes vapor pressure to increase rapidly.
Anhydrous ammonia will react exothermically with acids and water. Will not polymerize.

CONDITIONS TO AVOID:
Anhydrous ammonia has potentially explosive reactions with strong oxidizers. Anhydrous ammonia forms explosive mixtures in air with hydrocarbons, chlorine, fluorine and silver nitrate. Anhydrous ammonia reacts to form explosive products, mixtures or compounds with mercury, gold, silver, iodine, bromine and silver oxide. Avoid anhydrous ammonia contact with chlorine, which forms a chloramine gas, which is a primary skin irritant and sensitizer. Avoid anhydrous ammonia contact with galvanized surfaces, copper, brass, bronze, aluminum alloys, mercury, gold and silver. A corrosive reaction will occur.

HAZARDOUS DECOMPOSITION PRODUCTS:
Anhydrous ammonia decomposes to hydrogen and nitrogen gases above 450°C (842°F). Decomposition temperatures may be lowered by contact with certain metals, such as iron, nickel and zinc and by catalytic surfaces such as porcelain and pumice.

Revision: September 2005 Page 2 of 4 Prepared By: JRP

MATERIAL SAFETY DATA SHEET

SPILL OR LEAK PROCEDURES

STEPS TO BE TAKEN:
Stop source of leak if possible, provided it can be done in a safe manner. Leave the area of a spill by moving laterally and upwind. Isolate the affected area. Non-responders should evacuate the area, or shelter in place. Only properly trained and equipped persons should respond to an ammonia release. Wear eye, hand and respiratory protection and protective clothing; see PROTECTIVE EQUIPMENT. Stay upwind and use water spray downwind of container to absorb the evolved gas. Contain spill and runoff from entering drains, sewers, and water systems by utilizing methods such as diking, containment, and absorption. CAUTION: ADDING WATER DIRECTLY TO LIQUID SPILLS WILL INCREASE VOLATILIZATION OF AMMONIA, THUS INCREASING THE POSSIBILITY OF EXPOSURE.

WASTE DISPOSAL:
Listed as hazardous substance under CWA (40 CFR 116.4, 40 CFR 117.3). Reportable Quantity 100 pounds. Classified as hazardous waste under RCRA (40CFR 261.22 Corrosive #D002). Comply with all regulations. Suitably diluted product may be disposed of on agricultural land as fertilizer. Keep spill from entering streams, lakes, or any water systems.

SPECIAL PROTECTION AND PROCEDURES

RESPIRATORY PROTECTION:
Respiratory protection approved by NIOSH/MSHA for ammonia must be used when applicable safety and health exposure limits are exceeded. For escape in emergencies, MSHA/NIOSH approved respiratory protection that consists of a full-face gas mask and canisters approved for ammonia is required. Refer to 29 CFR 1910.134 and ANSI: Z88.2 for requirements and selection. A positive pressure SCBA is required for entry into ammonia atmospheres at or above 300 ppm (IDLH).

EYE PROTECTION: Chemical splash goggles should be worn when handling anhydrous ammonia. A face shield can be worn over chemical splash goggles as additional protection. Do not wear contact lenses when handling anhydrous ammonia.

VENTILATION:
Local exhaust should be sufficient to keep ammonia vapor to 25 ppm or less.

PROTECTIVE EQUIPMENT:
At a minimum, splash proof, chemical safety goggles, ammonia resistant, gloves (such as rubber), and ammonia-impervious clothing should be worn to prevent contact during normal loading, unloading and transfer operations and handling small spills. Face shield and boots can be worn as additional protection.
Respiratory protection approved by NIOSH/MSHA for ammonia must be used when applicable safety and health exposure limits are exceeded. For a hazardous material release response, Level A and/or Level B ensemble including positive-pressure SCBA should be used. A positive pressure SCBA is required for entry into ammonia atmospheres at or above 300 ppm (IDLH). Refer to 29 CFR 1910.132 through 1910.138 for personal protective equipment requirements.

SPECIAL PRECAUTIONS

STORAGE AND HANDLING:
Only trained persons should handle anhydrous ammonia. Store in cool (26.7°C / 80°F) and well-ventilated areas, with containers tightly closed. OSHA 29 CFR 1910.111 prescribes handling and storage requirements for anhydrous ammonia as a hazardous material. Use only stainless steel, carbon steel or black iron for anhydrous ammonia containers or piping. Do not use plastic. Do not use any non-ferrous metals such as copper, brass, bronze, aluminum, tin, zinc or galvanized metals. Protect containers from physical damage. Keep away from ignition sources, especially in indoor spaces.

WORK-PLACE PROTECTIVE EQUIPMENT:
Protective equipment should be stored near, but outside of anhydrous ammonia area. Water for first aid, such as an eyewash station and safety shower, should be kept available in the immediate vicinity. See 29 CFR 1910.111 for workplace requirements.

DISPOSAL:
See WASTE DISPOSAL. Classified as RCRA Hazardous Waste due to corrosivity with designation D002, if disposed of in original form.

Revision: September 2005 Page 3 of 4 Prepared By: JRP

MATERIAL SAFETY DATA SHEET

LABELING AND SHIPPING

HAZARD CLASS: (US Domestic): 2.2 (Non-Flammable Gas) (International): 2.3 (Poison Gas) subsidiary 8 (Corrosive)

PROPER SHIPPING DESCRIPTION:
(US Domestic): Ammonia, Anhydrous, 2.2, UN1005, RQ, Inhalation Hazard
(International): Ammonia, Anhydrous, 2.3, (8), UN1005, RQ, Poison-Inhalation Hazard Zone "D"

PLACARD: **IDENTIFICATION NUMBER**: UN 1005
(US Domestic): Non-Flammable Gas
(International): Poison Gas, Corrosive (Subsidiary)

National Fire Protection Assoc. Hazardous Rating:

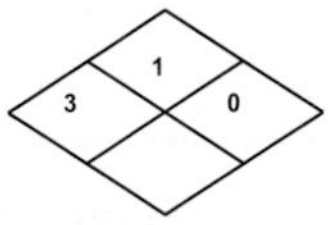

Hazardous Materials Identification System Labels:

ANHYDROUS AMMONIA	
HEALTH	3
FLAMMABILITY	1
REACTIVITY	0
PERSONAL PROTECTION	H

OTHER REGULATORY REQUIREMENTS

Under the Comprehensive Environmental Response, Compensation, and Liability Act of 1980 (CERCLA), Section 103, any environmental release of this chemical equal to or over the reportable quantity of 100 lbs. must be reported promptly to the National Response Center, Washington, D.C. (1-800-424-8802).

The material is subject to the reporting requirements of Section 304, Section 312 and Section 313, Title III of the Superfund Amendments and Reauthorization Act (SARA) of 1986 and 40 CFR 372. Emergency Planning & Community Right to Know Act, (EPCRA) extremely hazardous substance, 40 CFR 355, Title III, Section 302 – Ammonia, Threshold Planning Quantity (TPQ) 500 lbs.

EPA Hazard Categories - Immediate: Yes; Delayed: No; Fire: No; Sudden Release: Yes; Reactive: No.

Clean Air Act – Section 112(r): Material is listed under EPA's Risk Management Program (RMP), 40 CFR Part 68, at storage/process amounts greater than the Threshold Quantity (TQ) of 10,000 lbs.

DISCLAIMER

The information, data, and recommendations in this material safety data sheet relate only to the specific material designated herein and do not relate to use in combination with any other material or in any process. The information, data, and recommendations set forth herein are believed by us to be accurate. We make no warranties, either expressed or implied, with respect thereto and assume no liability in connection with any use of such information, data, and recommendations.

Revision: September 2005 Page 4 of 4 Prepared By: JRP

Figure 6 An example of a material safety data sheet (MSDS) for anhydrous ammonia.

Words of Wisdom

To ensure efficiency and safety when you are responding to a potential hazardous materials incident, you should learn the concepts and principles of the National Incident Management System (NIMS) and the Incident Command System (ICS) discussed in the chapter, *Incident Management and Multiple-Casualty Incidents*. Hazardous materials incident management may seem laborious, slow, or cumbersome to you, but the potentially extreme hazards and the need to protect rescuers, other health care personnel, and the public from harm mandate a cautious approach.

Red phosphorus from a drug laboratory, for example, might be found in an unmarked plastic container. In this case, there may be no legitimate markings to alert you to the possible contents. Gasoline or waste solvents may be stored in 55-gallon steel drums. Sulfuric acid, at 97% concentration, could be found in a polyethylene drum that might be colored black, red, white, or blue. In most cases, there is no correlation between the color of the drum and the possible contents. The same sulfuric acid might also be found in a 1-gallon amber glass container. Steel or polyethylene drums, bags, high-pressure gas cylinders, railroad tank cars, plastic buckets, above-ground and underground storage tanks, cargo tanks, and pipelines are all representative examples of how hazardous materials are packaged, stored, and shipped **Figure 7**.

Some recognizable chemical containers, such as 55-gallon drums and compressed gas cylinders, can be found in almost every type of manufacturing facility. Materials stored in a cardboard drum are usually in solid form. Stainless steel containers hold particularly dangerous chemicals, and cold liquids are kept in containers designed to maintain the appropriate temperature **Figure 8**.

One way to distinguish containers is to divide them into two categories based on their capacity: bulk and non-bulk storage containers.

Bulk Storage Vessels

Bulk storage containers include fixed tanks, highway cargo tanks, rail tank cars, totes, and intermodal tanks. In general, bulk storage containers are found in buildings that rely on and need to store large quantities of a particular chemical. Most manufacturing facilities have at least one type of bulk storage container. Often these bulk storage containers are surrounded by a supplementary containment system to help control an accidental release. <u>Secondary containment</u> is an engineered method to control spilled or released product if the main containment vessel fails. A 5,000-gallon vertical storage tank, for example, may be surrounded by a series of short walls that form a catch basin around the tank.

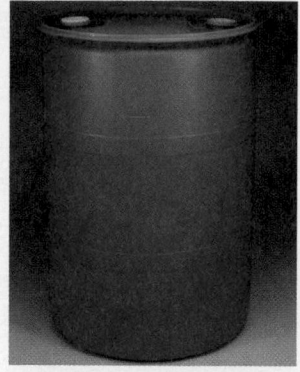

Figure 7 Drums may be constructed of many different types of materials, including cardboard, polyethylene, and stainless steel. The drum shown here is a polyethylene drum.

YOU are the Medic   PART 2

Your partner applies a nonrebreathing mask at 15 L/min while you begin your assessment. The patient is seated leaning forward in a tripod position. He has shallow, rapid respirations with intercostal and subcostal retractions. Audible expiratory wheezes are present. You place the patient on the cardiac monitor and observe a narrow complex tachycardia. A coworker is able to tell you that the patient was trapped in the room while the chlorine leak occurred for approximately 15 minutes. The patient has a past medical history of hypertension and asthma.

Recording Time: 5 Minutes	
Respirations	30 breaths/min; shallow
Pulse	Radial pulse, 127 beats/min; regular and strong
Skin	Pale, warm, and diaphoretic
Blood pressure	156/84 mm Hg
Oxygen saturation (Spo$_2$)	96% while receiving 15 L/min via nonrebreathing mask
Pupils	Equal and reactive to light

3. What should your initial treatment consist of?

4. Hazardous materials teams will establish safety zones at the scene. In which zone does patient triage and treatment take place?

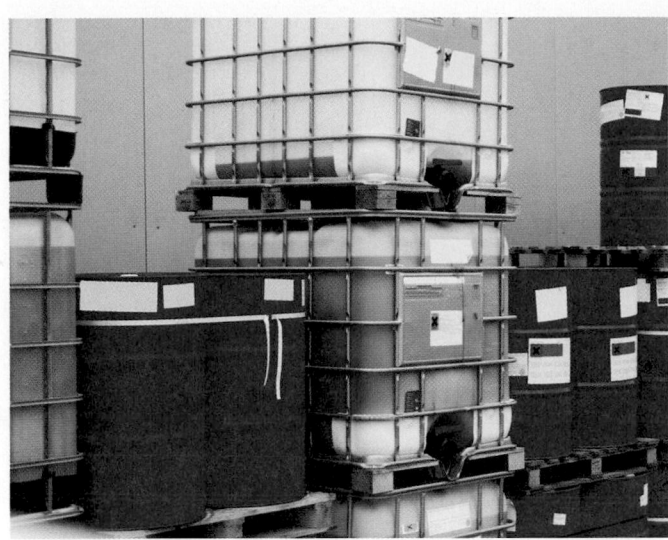

Figure 8 A series of chemical storage containers.

Words of Wisdom

When you consider locations for possible hazardous materials incidents, do not limit your thinking. You may be surprised by how many different kinds of containers you may find in your area.

Large-volume horizontal tanks are also common. When stored above ground, these tanks are referred to as aboveground storage tanks; if they are placed underground, they are known as underground storage tanks. These tanks can hold a few hundred gallons to several million gallons of product and are usually made of aluminum, steel, or plastic.

Another commonly encountered bulk storage vessel is the tote, also referred to as an intermediate bulk container. Totes have capacities ranging from 119 gallons to 703 gallons. These portable plastic tanks are surrounded by a stainless steel web that adds both structural stability and protection to the container. They can contain any type of chemical, including flammable liquids, corrosives, food-grade liquids, or oxidizers Figure 9 .

Shipping and storing totes can be hazardous. These containers often are stacked atop one another and moved with a forklift, such that a mishap with the loading or moving process can compromise the tote. Because totes have no secondary containment system, any leak has the potential to create a large puddle. In addition, the steel webbing around the tote makes it difficult to access and patch leaks.

Intermodal tanks are both shipping and storage vessels. They hold between 5,000 and 6,000 gallons of product and can be pressurized or nonpressurized. Intermodal tanks can also be used to ship and store gaseous substances that have been chilled until they liquefy, such as liquid nitrogen. In most cases, an intermodal tank is shipped to a facility, where it is stored and

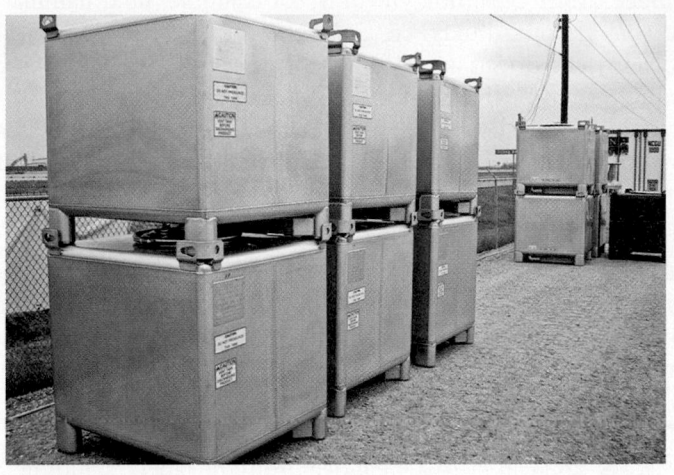

Figure 9 A tote is a commonly encountered bulk storage vessel.

used and then returned to the shipper for refilling. Intermodal tanks can be shipped by all methods of transportation—air, sea, and land Figure 10 .

Nonbulk Storage Vessels

Essentially, <u>nonbulk storage vessels</u> are all types of containers other than bulk containers. Nonbulk storage vessels can hold a few ounces to 119 gallons of product and include vessels such as drums, bags, compressed gas cylinders, cryogenic containers, and more. Nonbulk storage vessels hold commonly used commercial and industrial chemicals such as solvents, industrial cleaners, and compounds. This section describes the most commonly encountered types of nonbulk storage vessels.

Drums <u>Drums</u> are easily recognizable, barrel-like containers. They are used to store a wide variety of substances, including food-grade materials, corrosives, flammable liquids, and grease. Drums may be constructed of low-carbon steel, polyethylene, cardboard, stainless steel, nickel, or other materials. Generally, the nature of the chemical dictates the construction of the

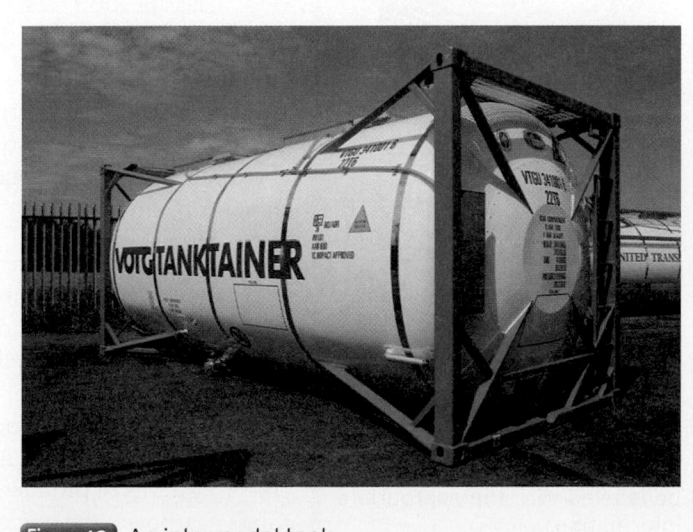

Figure 10 An intermodal tank.

storage drum. Steel utility drums, for example, hold flammable liquids, cleaning fluids, oil, and other noncorrosive chemicals. Polyethylene drums are used for corrosives such as acids, bases, oxidizers, and other materials that cannot be stored in steel containers. Cardboard drums hold solid materials such as soap flakes, sodium hydroxide pellets, and food-grade materials. Stainless steel or other heavy-duty drums generally hold materials too aggressive (ie, too reactive) for either plain steel or polyethylene.

Bags Bags are commonly used to store solids and powders such as cement powder, sand, pesticides, soda ash, and slaked lime. Storage bags may be constructed of plastic, paper, or plastic-lined paper. Bags come in different sizes and weights, depending on their contents.

Pesticide bags must be labeled with specific information **Figure 11**. You can learn a great deal from the label, including the following details:

- Name of the product
- Active ingredients
- Hazard statement
- The total amount of product in the container
- The manufacturer's name and address
- The EPA registration number, which provides proof that the product was registered with the EPA
- The EPA establishment number, which shows where the product was manufactured
- Signal words to indicate the relative toxicity of the material:
  - Danger—Poison: Highly toxic by all routes of entry
  - Danger: Severe eye damage or skin irritation
  - Warning: Moderately toxic
  - Caution: Minor toxicity and minor eye damage or skin irritation
- Practical first-aid treatment description
- Directions for use
- Agricultural use requirements
- Precautionary statements such as mixing directions or potential environmental hazards
- Storage and disposal information
- Classification statement on who may use the product

In addition, every pesticide label must carry the statement, "Keep out of reach of children."

Carboys Some corrosives and other types of chemicals are transported and stored in vessels called carboys **Figure 12**. A carboy is a glass, plastic, or steel container that holds 5 to 15 gallons of product. Glass carboys are often placed in a protective

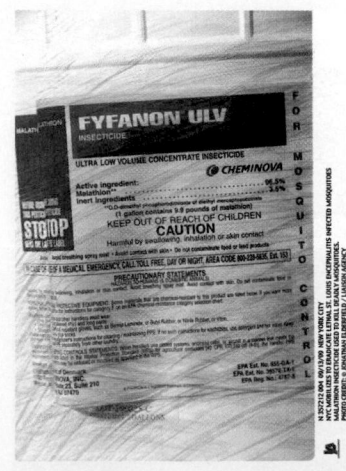

Figure 11 A pesticide bag must be labeled with the appropriate information.

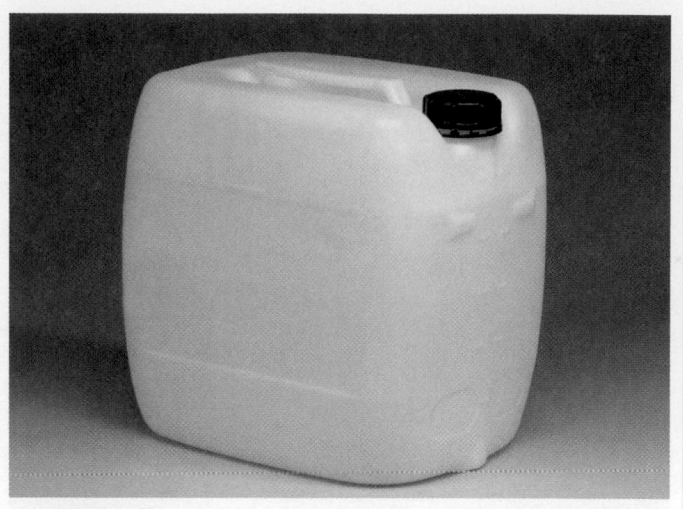

Figure 12 A carboy is used to transport and store corrosive chemicals.

wood, foam, fiberglass, or steel box to help prevent breakage. For example, nitric acid, sulfuric acid, and other strong acids are often transported and stored in thick glass carboys protected by a wooden or polystyrene (Styrofoam) crate to shield the glass container from damage during shipping.

Cylinders Several types of cylinders are used to hold liquids and gases. Uninsulated compressed gas cylinders are used to store substances such as nitrogen, argon, helium, and oxygen. They come in a range of sizes. As a paramedic, you are familiar with the shape of a cylinder; it holds the oxygen for your patients.

■ Roadway Transportation of Hazardous Materials

The most common method of hazardous material transport is over land, by roadway transportation vehicles. According to the CFR, 49 CFR 171.8(2), or local jurisdictional regulations (for example, Transport Canada), a cargo tank is bulk packaging that is permanently attached to or forms a part of a motor vehicle, or is not permanently attached to any motor vehicle, and that, because of its size, construction, or attachment to a motor vehicle, is loaded or unloaded without being removed from the motor vehicle. The US DOT does not view tube trailers (which consist of several individual cylinders banded together and affixed to a trailer) as cargo tanks.

One of the most common and reliable transportation vessels is the MC-306/DOT 406 flammable liquid tanker **Figure 13**. These tanks frequently carry liquid food-grade products, gasoline, or other flammable and combustible liquids. The oval-shaped tank is pulled by a diesel tractor and can carry between 6,000 gallons and 10,000 gallons of product. The MC-306/DOT 406 is nonpressurized (its working pressure is between 2.65 psi and 4 psi), usually made of aluminum or stainless steel, and offloaded through valves at the bottom of the tank. These cargo tanks have several safety features, including full rollover protection and remote emergency shut-off valves.

A vehicle that is similar to the MC-306/DOT 406 is the <u>MC-307/DOT 407 chemical hauler</u>. It has a round or horseshoe-shaped tank and is capable of holding 6,000 to 7,000 gallons of liquid Figure 14. The MC-307/DOT 407, which is also a tractor-drawn tank, is used to transport flammable liquids, mild corrosives, and poisons. This type of cargo tank may be insulated (horseshoe) or uninsulated (round) and may have a higher internal working pressure than the MC-306/DOT 406—in some cases up to 35 psi. Cargo tanks that transport corrosives may have a rubber lining to prevent corrosion of the tank structure.

The <u>MC-312/DOT 412 corrosive tanker</u> is commonly used to carry corrosives such as concentrated sulfuric acid, phosphoric acid, and sodium hydroxide Figure 15. This cargo tank has a smaller diameter than either the MC-306/DOT 406 or the MC-307/DOT 407 and is often identifiable by the presence of several heavy-duty reinforcing rings around the tank. The rings provide structural stability during transportation and in the event of a rollover. The inside of an MC-312/DOT 412 tanker operates at approximately 15 to 25 psi and holds approximately 6,000 gallons. These cargo tanks have substantial rollover protection to reduce the potential for damage to the top-mounted valves.

The <u>MC-331 pressure cargo tanker</u> carries materials such as ammonia, propane, Freon, and butane Figure 16. The liquid

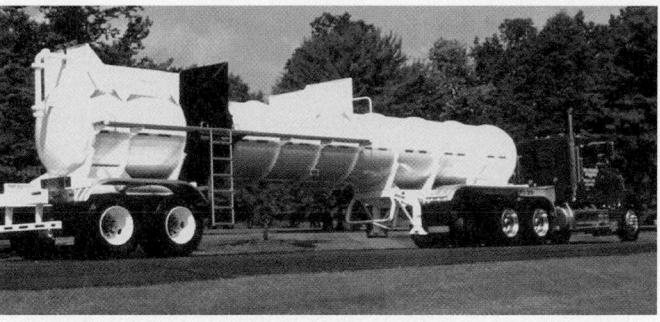

Figure 15 The MC-312/DOT 412 corrosive tanker is commonly used to carry corrosives such as concentrated sulfuric acid, phosphoric acid, and sodium hydroxide.

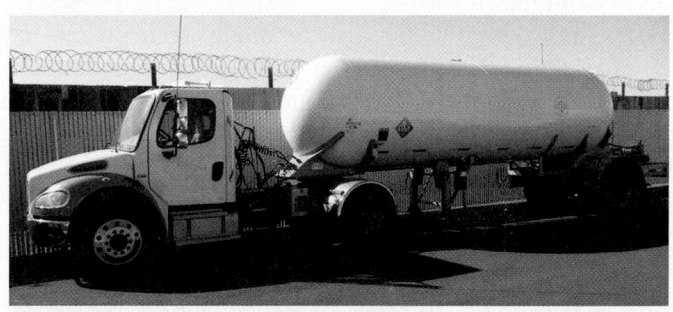

Figure 16 The MC-331 pressure cargo tanker carries materials such as ammonia, propane, Freon, and butane.

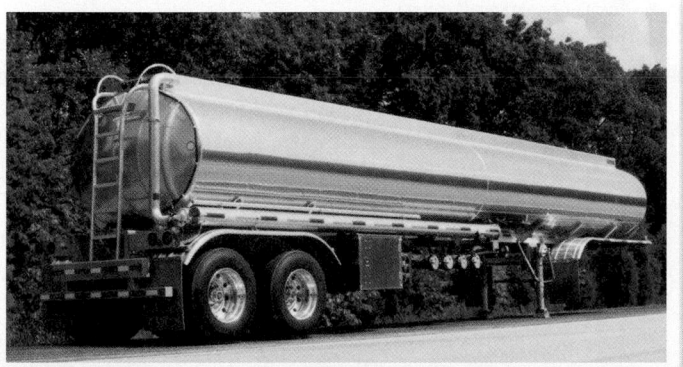

Figure 13 The MC-306/DOT 406 flammable liquid tanker typically hauls flammable and combustible liquid.

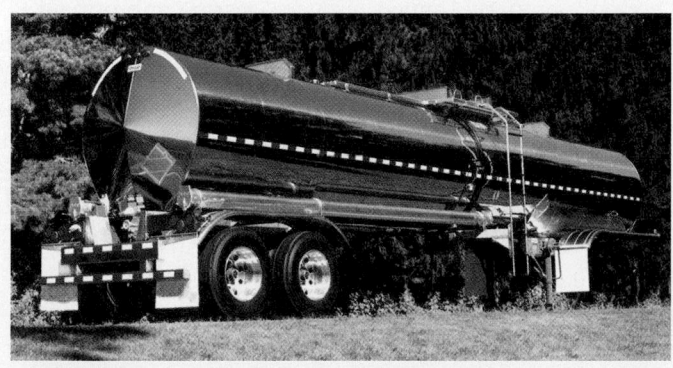

Figure 14 The MC-307/DOT 407 chemical hauler carries flammable liquids, mild corrosives, and poisons.

volume inside the tank varies, ranging from the 1,000-gallon delivery truck to the full-size 11,000-gallon cargo tank. The MC-331 cargo tank has rounded ends, typical of a pressurized vessel, and is commonly constructed of steel or stainless steel with a single tank compartment. The MC-331 operates at approximately 300 psi, with typical internal working pressures being in the vicinity of 250 psi. These cargo tanks are equipped with spring-loaded relief valves that traditionally operate at 110% of the designated maximum working pressure. A significant explosion hazard arises if a MC-331 cargo tank is impinged on by fire, however. Due to the nature of most materials carried in MC-331 tanks, a threat of explosion exists because of the inability of the relief valve to keep up with the rapidly building internal pressure. Responders must use great care when they are dealing with this type of transportation emergency.

The <u>MC-338 cryogenic tanker</u> is a low-pressure tanker that relies on tank insulation to maintain the low temperatures required for the cryogens it carries Figure 17. A boxlike structure containing the tank control valves is typically attached to the rear of the tanker. Special training is required to operate valves on this and any other tanker. An untrained person who attempts to operate the valves may disrupt the normal operation of the tank, thereby compromising its ability to keep the liquefied gas cold and creating a potential explosion hazard. Cryogenic tankers have a relief valve near the valve control box. From time to time, small puffs of white vapor will be vented from this valve. Responders should understand that this is a normal occurrence—the valve is working to maintain the proper internal pressure. In most cases, this vapor is not indicative of an emergency situation.

<u>Tube trailers</u> carry compressed gases such as hydrogen, oxygen, helium, and methane **Figure 18**. Essentially, they are high-volume transportation vehicles that are made up of several individual cylinders banded together and affixed to a trailer. The individual cylinders on the tube trailer are much like the smaller compressed gas cylinders discussed earlier in this chapter. These large-volume cylinders operate at working pressures of 3,000 to 5,000 psi. One trailer may carry several different gases in individual tubes. Typically, a valve control box is found toward the rear of the trailer, and each individual cylinder has its own relief valve. These trailers can frequently be seen at construction sites or at facilities that use large quantities of compressed gases.

<u>Dry bulk cargo tanks</u> are commonly seen on the road; they carry dry bulk goods such as powders, pellets, fertilizers, or grain **Figure 19**. These tanks are not pressurized, but may use pressure to offload the product. Dry bulk cargo tanks are generally V-shaped with rounded sides that funnel the contents to the bottom-mounted valves.

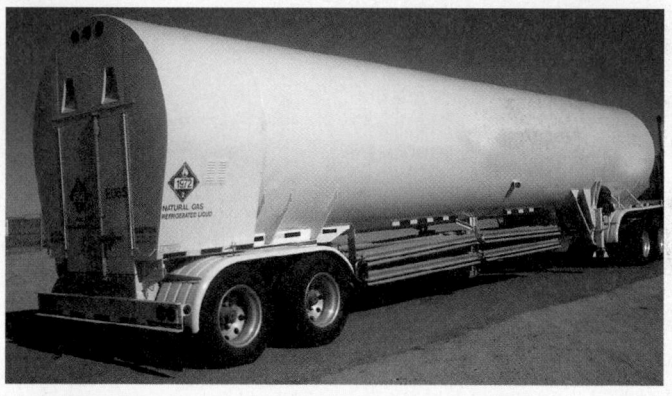

Figure 17 The MC-338 cryogenic tanker maintains the low temperatures required for the cryogens it carries.

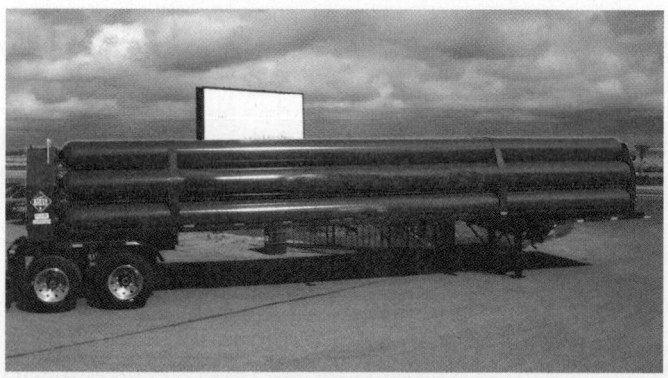

Figure 18 Tube trailers carry compressed gases such as hydrogen, oxygen, helium, and methane.

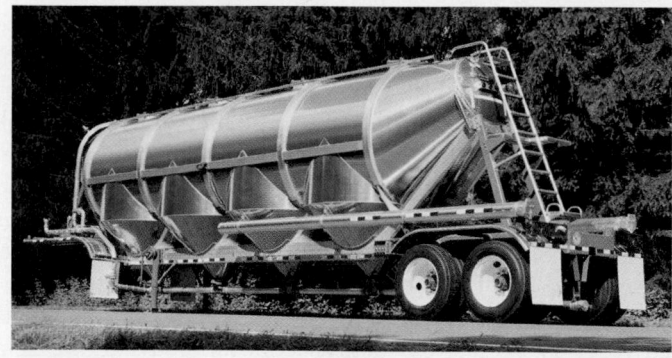

Figure 19 A dry bulk cargo tank carries dry goods such as powders, pellets, fertilizers, and grain.

Establishing Safety Zones

Until the hazardous materials technical team arrives to determine the hazard zone, you should be aware of the safety perimeters that are necessary for hazardous materials that are toxic (poisonous) and those that pose a danger of fire or explosion. If you are dispatched to a hazardous materials incident, you must take the following steps:

- Protect yourself first!
- Isolate the incident as much as possible to avoid the risk of further harm to other people—laypeople, EMS staff, fire fighters, and law enforcement responders. No one should risk his or her life or health at a hazardous materials incident. The *ERG*, which you should carry in your vehicle, can help determine initial isolation distances.
- Notify your dispatcher and any other EMS, fire, or law enforcement responders that a hazardous materials incident is in progress.
- Inform incoming responders of what you observe about wind direction, terrain features, and a safe response route.

As the hazardous materials incident progresses, hazardous materials specialists will establish the hot, warm, and cold zones. This is also discussed in the chapter, *Vehicle Extrication and Special Rescue.* The hot zone is the contamination zone where only properly trained rescuers wearing appropriate PPE are allowed. The warm zone surrounds the hot zone. Typically the decontamination corridor is located in the warm zone. This zone should only be entered by trained hazardous materials specialists wearing appropriate PPE. The cold zone provides a further buffer from the hazards present in the hot and warm zones. Paramedics normally perform triage and patient treatment in the cold zone **Figure 20**.

Initial Isolation and Protection Distance

There may be times when a decision must be made to shelter in place, evacuate, or rescue people in danger. In those instances, responders may need to consult printed and electronic reference sources for guidance on evacuation distances and other safety information. The most accessible resource for

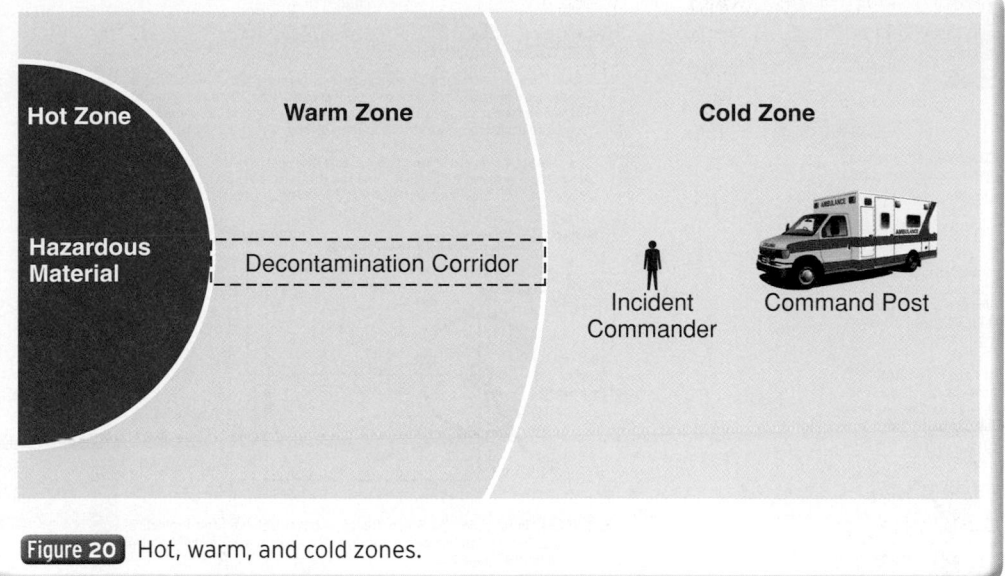

Hot Zone

Warm Zone

Cold Zone

Hazardous Material

Decontamination Corridor

Incident Commander

Command Post

Figure 20 Hot, warm, and cold zones.

evacuation distances is the green section of the *ERG* **Figure 21**. This reference book identifies and outlines predetermined evacuation distances and basic action plans for chemicals highlighted in the yellow or blue sections of the book, based on spill size estimates.

Hazardous materials teams also use air-monitoring equipment to help determine explosive limits, oxygen levels, and the concentration of hydrogen sulphide and carbon monoxide. They will also be able to determine the pH of spills and may have capability for specific agent testing using colorimetric devices.

There are also a number of computer programs such as Computer-Aided Management of Emergency Operations (**CAMEO**) to help predict downwind concentrations of hazardous materials based on the input of environmental factors into a computer model. When used properly, these computer programs can be a valuable source of information for predicting the size and direction of gas or vapor clouds. This type of program is typically used by hazardous materials responders, but may also be available to EMS personnel.

■ Personal Protective Equipment

You should be familiar with the PPE used at hazardous materials scenes even if you are not expected to use it. In most cases, the hazardous materials team or other trained responders will determine the appropriate PPE needed for a specific task or mission. Your job as an EMS provider is to recognize certain levels or combinations of PPE and understand the potential hazards encountered by the people inside the garments. It could be that the highest hazard is not posed by the released substance! EMS providers should consider the effects of heat and cold stress on the people inside the PPE in addition to the chemical threats posed by the hazardous materials agent. The astute EMS provider will evaluate the environmental conditions present at the scene, formulate a plan to deal with responders experiencing heat- or cold-related issues, determine the potential health risks that could be posed by

an exposure, and determine how that exposure should be treated along with the appropriate transport decision. A proactive EMS provider, operating at the scene of a hazardous materials incident already has a basic plan in place to treat civilians and responders alike.

Hazardous materials responders classify chemical protective clothing by Level A through Level D **Figure 22**. Most paramedic ambulances do not carry this equipment, but again, you should be familiar enough with it to understand what the wearer of the garment is experiencing.

A **level A ensemble** provides the greatest respiratory and skin protection from exposure to hazardous substances because it is "fully encapsulating." These garments fully cover the body and the self-contained breathing apparatus (SCBA) or other supplied air system worn by the responder. The suits are rigorously tested by manufacturers to determine resistance to many chemicals. Because they are considered to be "gastight," and completely cover the wearer, you may be asked to monitor or evaluate the technicians for heat stress. Additionally, you should familiarize yourself with the procedures for getting into and out of these types of garments in the event a responder has an in-suit emergency and you are called on to provide patient care.

A **level B ensemble** is called for when the responder needs a high level of respiratory protection, but the released substance does not pose a lethal threat via skin absorption. It is not fully encapsulating like level A, and it is worn with SCBA, or supplied air on the outside of the suit. Level B protection is oftentimes

<u>**HOW TO USE TABLE 1 - INITIAL ISOLATION AND**</u>
<u>**PROTECTIVE ACTION DISTANCES**</u>

(1) The responder should already have:

- Identified the material by its ID Number and Name; (if an ID Number cannot be found, use the Name of Material index in the blue-bordered pages to locate that number.)
- Found the three-digit guide for that material in order to consult the emergency actions recommended jointly with this table;
- **Noted the wind direction.**

(2) Look in Table 1 (the green-bordered pages) for the ID Number and Name of the Material involved in the incident. Some ID Numbers have more than one shipping name listed— look for the specific name of the material. (If the shipping name is not known and Table 1 lists more than one name for the same ID Number, use the entry with the largest protective action distances.)

(3) Determine if the incident involves a SMALL or LARGE spill and if DAY or NIGHT. Generally, a SMALL SPILL is one which involves a single, small package (e.g., a drum containing up to approximately 208 liters (55 US gallons)), a small cylinder, or a small leak from a large package. A LARGE SPILL is one which involves a spill from a large package, or multiple spills from many small packages. DAY is any time after sunrise and before sunset. NIGHT is any time between sunset and sunrise.

(4) Look up the INITIAL ISOLATION DISTANCE. Direct all persons to move, in a crosswind direction, away from the spill to the distance specified—in meters and feet.

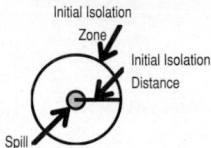

(5) Look up the initial PROTECTIVE ACTION DISTANCE shown in Table 1. For a given material, spill size, and whether day or night, Table 1 gives the downwind distance—in kilometers and miles— for which protective actions should be considered. For practical purposes, the Protective Action Zone (i.e., the area in which people are at risk of harmful exposure) is a square, whose length and width are the same as the downwind distance shown in Table 1.

(6) Initiate Protective Actions to the extent possible, beginning with those closest to the spill site and working away from the site in the downwind direction. When a water-reactive TIH producing material is spilled into a river or stream, the source of the toxic gas may move with the current or stretch from the spill point downstream for a substantial distance.

The shape of the area in which protective actions should be taken (the Protective Action Zone) is shown in this figure. The spill is located at the center of the small circle. The larger circle represents the INITIAL ISOLATION zone around the spill.

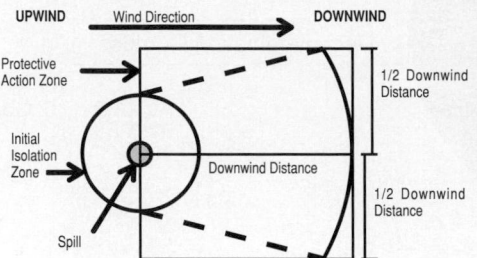

NOTE 1: See "Introduction To Green Tables – Initial Isolation And Protective Action Distances" under "Factors That May Change the Protective Action Distances" (page 285)

NOTE 2: See Table 2 – Water-Reactive Materials which Produce Toxic Gases for the list of gases produced when these materials are spilled in water.

Call the emergency response telephone number listed on the shipping paper or the appropriate response agency as soon as possible for additional information on the material, safety precautions and mitigation procedures.

TABLE 1 - INITIAL ISOLATION AND PROTECTIVE ACTION DISTANCES

ID No.		NAME OF MATERIAL	SMALL SPILLS (From a small package or small leak from a large package)						LARGE SPILLS (From a large package or from many small packages)					
			First ISOLATE in all Directions		Then PROTECT persons Downwind during-				First ISOLATE in all Directions		Then PROTECT persons Downwind during-			
					DAY		NIGHT				DAY		NIGHT	
			Meters	(Feet)	Kilometers	(Miles)	Kilometers	(Miles)	Meters	(Feet)	Kilometers	(Miles)	Kilometers	(Miles)
1051	117	Hydrocyanic acid, aqueous solutions, with more than 20% Hydrogen cyanide	60 m	(200 ft)	0.2 km	(0.1 mi)	0.6 km	(0.4 mi)	400 m	(1250 ft)	1.4 km	(0.9 mi)	3.8 km	(2.4 mi)
1051	117	Hydrogen cyanide, anhydrous, stabilized												
1051	117	Hydrogen cyanide, stabilized												
1052 *	125	Hydrogen fluoride, anhydrous	30 m	(100 ft)	0.1 km	(0.1 mi)	0.5 km	(0.3 mi)	300 m	(1000 ft)	1.5 km	(0.9 mi)	3.2 km	(2.0 mi)
1053	117	Hydrogen sulfide	30 m	(100 ft)	0.1 km	(0.1 mi)	0.4 km	(0.3 mi)	300 m	(1000 ft)	1.7 km	(1.0 mi)	5.6 km	(3.5 mi)
1053	117	Hydrogen sulphide												
1062	123	Methyl bromide	30 m	(100 ft)	0.1 km	(0.1 mi)	0.2 km	(0.2 mi)	100 m	(300 ft)	0.6 km	(0.4 mi)	1.9 km	(1.2 mi)
1064	117	Methyl mercaptan	30 m	(100 ft)	0.1 km	(0.1 mi)	0.3 km	(0.2 mi)	150 m	(500 ft)	1.0 km	(0.7 mi)	3.2 km	(2.0 mi)
1067	124	Dinitrogen tetroxide	30 m	(100 ft)	0.1 km	(0.1 mi)	0.4 km	(0.2 mi)	300 m	(1000 ft)	1.1 km	(0.7 mi)	2.7 km	(1.7 mi)
1067	124	Nitrogen dioxide												
1069	125	Nitrosyl chloride	30 m	(100 ft)	0.2 km	(0.2 mi)	1.1 km	(0.7 mi)	600 m	(2000 ft)	3.6 km	(2.3 mi)	9.5 km	(5.9 mi)
1071	119	Oil gas	60 m	(200 ft)	0.2 km	(0.1 mi)	0.2 km	(0.1 mi)	100 m	(300 ft)	0.4 km	(0.2 mi)	0.5 km	(0.3 mi)
1071	119	Oil gas, compressed												
1076	125	CG (when used as a weapon)	150 m	(500 ft)	0.8 km	(0.5 mi)	3.2 km	(2.0 mi)	1000 m	(3000 ft)	7.5 km	(4.7 mi)	11.0+ km	(7.0+ mi)
1076	125	Diphosgene	30 m	(100 ft)	0.2 km	(0.1 mi)	0.2 km	(0.1 mi)	30 m	(100 ft)	0.3 km	(0.2 mi)	0.5 km	0.3 mi)
1076	125	DP (when used as a weapon)	30 m	(100 ft)	0.2 km	(0.1 mi)	0.7 km	(0.4 mi)	200 m	(600 ft)	1.0 km	(0.7 mi)	2.4 km	(1.5 mi)
1076	125	Phosgene	100 m	(300 ft)	0.6 km	(0.4 mi)	2.7 km	(1.7 mi)	500 m	(1500 ft)	3.1 km	(1.9 mi)	10.8 km	(6.7 mi)
1079 *	125	Sulfur dioxide	100 m	(300 ft)	0.7 km	(0.4 mi)	2.8 km	(1.7 mi)	1000 m	(3000 ft)	5.6 km	(3.5 mi)	11.0+ km	(7.0+ mi)
1079 *	125	Sulphur dioxide												
1082	119P	Trifluorochloroethylene, stabilized	30 m	(100 ft)	0.1 km	(0.1 mi)	0.1 km	(0.1 mi)	60 m	(200 ft)	0.4 km	(0.2 mi)	0.9 km	(0.6 mi)
1092	131P	Acrolein, stabilized	150 m	(500 ft)	1.4 km	(0.9 mi)	4.0 km	(2.5 mi)	800 m	(2500 ft)	9.3 km	(5.8 mi)	11.0+ km	(7.0+ mi)
1098	131	Allyl alcohol	30 m	(100 ft)	0.1 km	(0.1 mi)	0.1 km	(0.1 mi)	60 m	(200 ft)	0.3 km	(0.2 mi)	0.5 km	(0.3 mi)

"+" means distance can be larger in certain atmospheric conditions   *** PLEASE ALSO CONSULT TABLE 3 FOR THIS MATERIAL**

Figure 21 Instructions and example pages from the Initial Isolation and Protective Action Distances table found in the *ERG*.

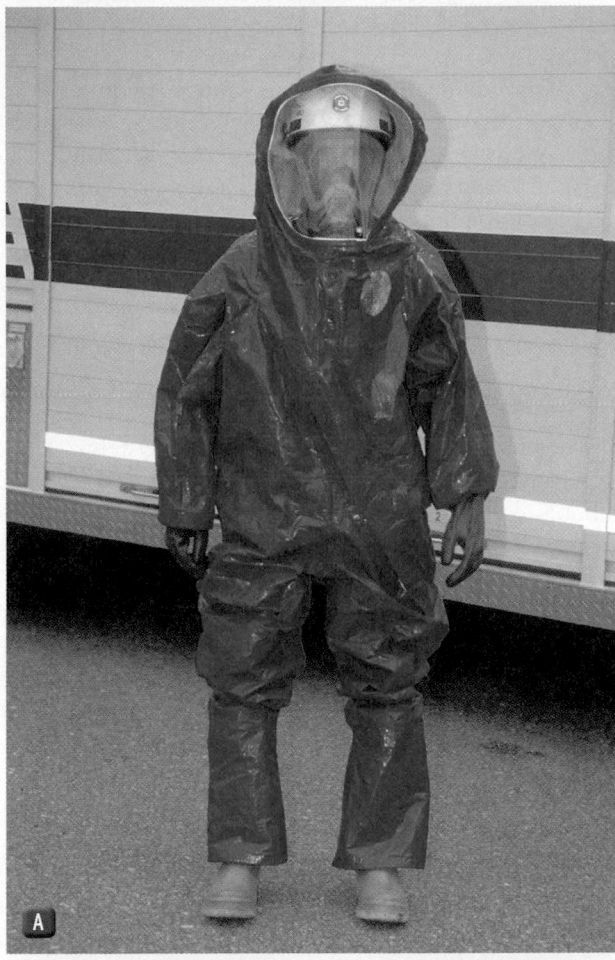

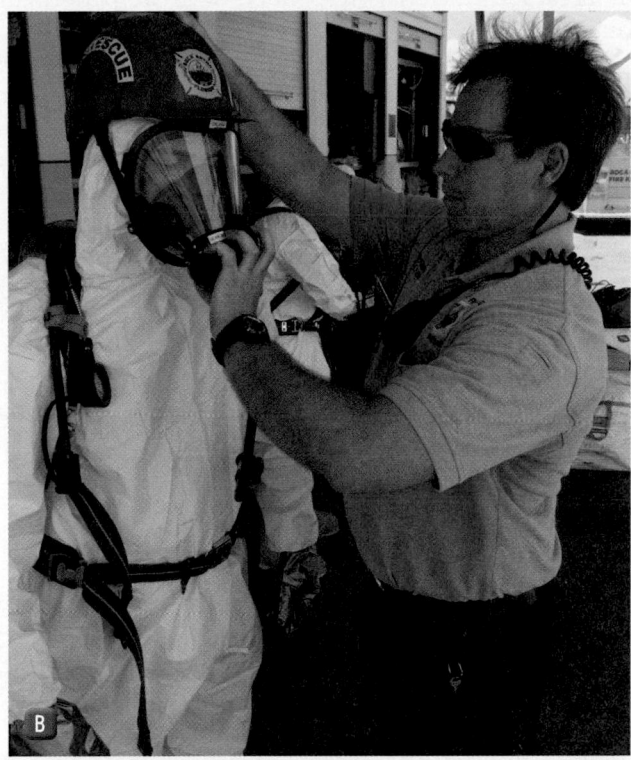

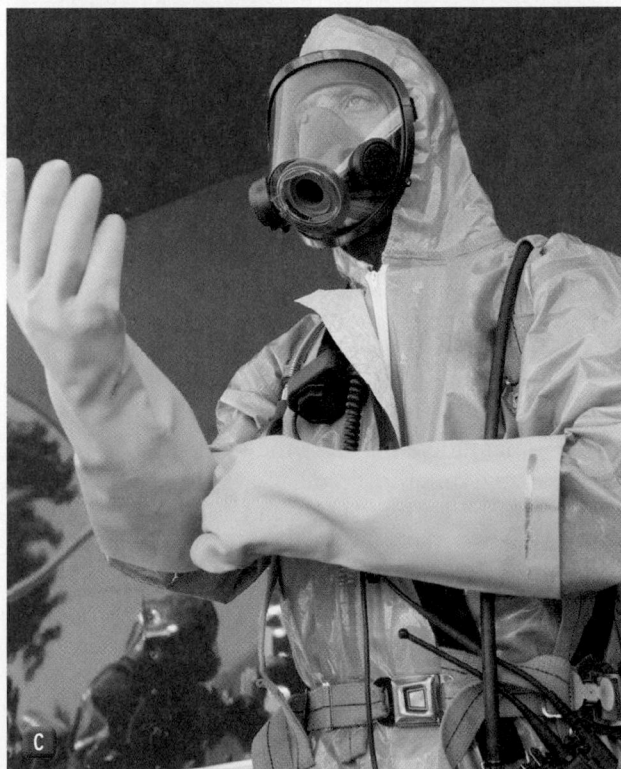

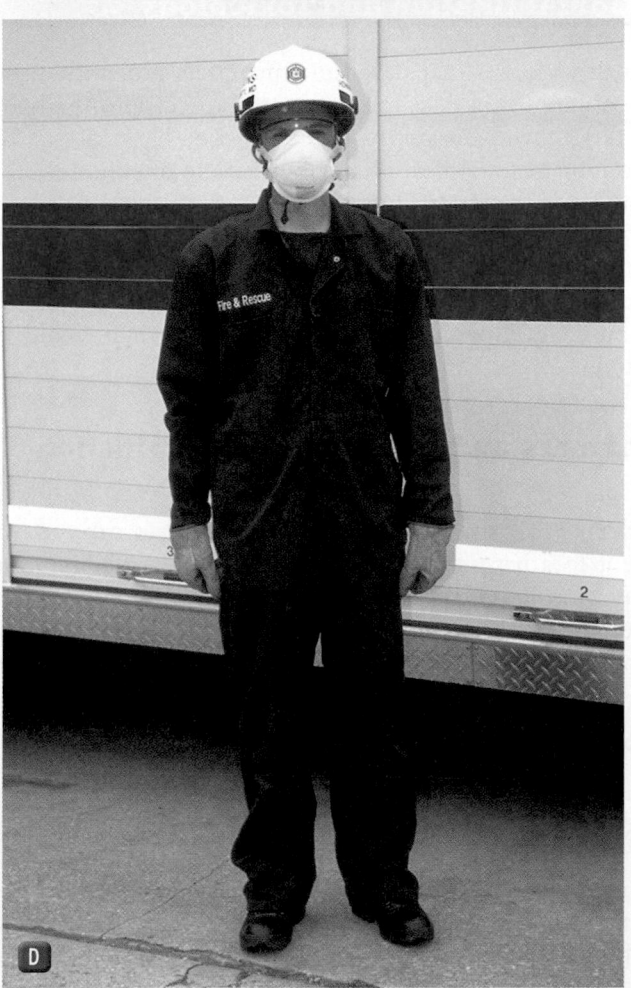

Figure 22 Four levels of protection. **A.** Level A protection. **B.** Level B protection. **C.** Level C protection. **D.** Level D protection.

worn by hazardous materials responders who are performing decontamination.

A level C ensemble is designed to protect against a known substance. The equipment provides minimal splash protection and is worn with an air-purifying respirator (APR) or powered air-purifying respirator (PAPR) that must have filters specifically chosen to provide protection against the known agent. Receivers of exposed patients in the emergency department (ED) and law enforcement officers providing perimeter protection at a scene would be good candidates for wearing level C protection.

A level D ensemble is typically not worn in hazardous materials incidents by anyone other than support personnel working in the cold zone. This level of protection is worn when there is little or no threat posed by the released substance, and the responder is wearing no respiratory protection other than perhaps a dust mask.

Words of Wisdom

If you are not dressed for the game, stay on the sidelines.

Contamination and Toxicology

The health hazards that hazardous materials present depend on the ability of the hazardous material to get into the body and interfere with the body's processes. The harm caused by a hazardous material is affected by the route of exposure, the dose and concentration, how long the toxin was in contact with the body, and whether it exhibits acute or delayed toxicity. If a patient has a chronic preexisting condition, like a respiratory ailment, then a minor chlorine spill in an enclosed warehouse could prove to be more dangerous than would be expected.

Primary and Secondary Contamination

There are two basic types of contamination, primary and secondary. Primary contamination is the direct exposure of a patient to a hazardous material. Secondary contamination takes place when a hazardous material is transferred to a person from another person or from contaminated objects (cross-contamination).

Routes of Exposure

The physical properties of hazardous materials and the physical surroundings at the hazardous materials incident can expose your patient in different ways. As described in the chapter, *Toxicology*, the four primary methods of entry are ingestion, inhalation, injection, and absorption. However, other factors will affect your treatment priorities, including air temperature, the concentration of the hazard, and the amount of time that a patient is exposed.

A local effect may be described as reddening of the skin, localized pain, or the formation of blisters. Some chemical substances may have a systemic effect on your patient. Carbon monoxide, for example, could be inhaled through the lungs without causing any damage to the airway, but ultimately render your patient unconscious, or in respiratory or cardiac arrest. These types of exposures are difficult to handle because the damage is occurring inside the body. Your job may entail identifying the exposure scenario and the substance involved, and providing supportive care during transport. In some patients, if it is within your scope of practice, you might be able to deliver an antidote to reverse the systemic effects of an exposure.

Some hazardous materials can have a significant adverse effect on the neurologic, renal, or hepatic systems. These toxic effects may be seen immediately in the field, or may be delayed for hours or even years later with the appearance of a form of cancer. When the reaction shows up hours or even days after your initial treatment, your careful documentation becomes invaluable to patients. Your records should include, among other elements required by the AHJ or your medical director, a description of the scene, anything the hazardous materials team told you about the substance, how your patient looked initially, the treatments rendered, and the positive or negative changes since initial contact.

Regardless of the route or type of exposure, the dose effect principle applies—the greater the length of time or the greater the concentration of the material, the greater the effect probably will be on the human body. For example, people who have a substance briefly splashed on their skin will be exposed to a much lower dose than if they were lying in a puddle of that same substance for 30 minutes. The cycle of poison action includes absorption into the body, delivery to target organs, and binding to the organs. The cycle continues with biotransformation and elimination of the toxin through the gastrointestinal, kidney, or respiratory systems. These concepts should be considered as decontamination decisions are made with the hazardous materials team.

Chemical Terms

When you are providing care and/or medical support at a hazardous materials incident, it is important to understand the terms and definitions used by the responders and how those terms and definitions relate to the released material. Additionally, understanding the chemical and physical properties of a substance may give you some valuable insight when it comes to providing care. For example, if your patient was rescued from a below-grade situation, and propane was released during the event, would you expect the vapors to collect in low-lying areas (where your patient might have been trapped) or rise up and away from the below-grade situation? Propane is heavier than air and does in fact collect in low-lying areas, so you might have an additional issue to deal with from a patient care perspective.

For the purpose of this chapter, the definition of <u>vapor pressure</u> will pertain to liquids held inside any type of closed container. When liquids are held in a closed 55-gallon drum or a 4-liter glass bottle, for example, some amount of pressure (in the headspace above the liquid) will develop inside. All liquids, even water, will develop a certain amount of pressure in the airspace between the top of the liquid and the container.

The key point to understanding vapor pressure is this: The vapors released from the surface of any liquid must be contained in order to exert pressure. What happens if the container is opened or spilled onto the ground to form a puddle? The liquid still has a vapor pressure, but it is no longer confined to a container. In this case, you can conclude that liquids with high vapor pressures will evaporate much more quickly than liquids with low vapor pressures. Vapor pressure directly correlates to the speed at which a material will evaporate once it is released from its container.

For example, motor oil has a low vapor pressure. When it is released, it will stay on the ground for a long time. Chemicals such as isopropyl alcohol or diethyl ether have the opposite reaction. When either of these materials is released and collects on the ground, it will evaporate rapidly. If the ambient air temperature or pavement temperature is elevated, the evaporation rate will increase. Wind speed, shade, humidity, and the surface area of the spill also influence how fast the chemical will evaporate.

<u>Vapor density</u> is another concept for figuring out where a gas or vapor might go once released from its container. Vapor density compares the hazardous material gas to air (air has a vapor density of 1). If the gas is heavier than air, the gas will sink into little valleys and ditches. Gases such as propane, butane, and carbon dioxide are heavier than air. But, if the vapor rises and dissipates as it travels with the wind, then the vapor density is less than that of the air. Gases like ammonia, acetylene, methane, and hydrogen are lighter than air. This is why you are taught to approach a scene from upwind and uphill!

Of course, the situation changes dramatically if a fire is involved. <u>Flash point</u> is an expression of the temperature at which a liquid fuel gives off sufficient vapors that, when an ignition source is present, will result in a flash fire. The flash fire involves only the vapor phase of the liquid and will go out once the vapor fuel is consumed.

For example, the flash point of gasoline is −45°F. When the temperature of gasoline reaches −45°F, either from an external source or from the surrounding environment, it gives off sufficient flammable vapors to support combustion. Diesel fuel, on the other hand, has a much higher flash point than gasoline, approximately 100°F to 160°F depending on the fuel grade. In either case, once the temperature of the liquid surpasses its flash point, the fuel will give off sufficient flammable vapors to support combustion. Because of this, responders should always be mindful of ignition sources at flammable/combustible liquid incidents. Low flash point liquids typically have high vapor pressures. Subsequently, low flash point liquids can be expected to produce a significant amount of flammable vapors at all but the lowest ambient temperatures.

<u>Ignition temperature</u> is the next important combustion landmark after flash point. When a liquid fuel is heated beyond its ignition temperature, it will ignite without an external ignition source. For example, think of a pan full of cooking oil being heated on the stove. For illustration purposes, assume

YOU are the Medic PART 3

While your partner prepares a nebulizer with 2.5 mg of albuterol and 0.5 mg of ipratropium (Atrovent), you establish an 18-g IV line in the patient's right antecubital space and draw up 125 mg of methylprednisolone (Solu-Medrol). During the breathing treatment, the patient begins to report increased difficulty breathing. Reassessment reveals diminished lung sounds with expiratory wheezing bilaterally and accessory muscle use. The patient appears to be fatigued.

Recording Time: 10 Minutes	
Respirations	28 breath/min; shallow
Pulse	Radial pulse, 134 beats/min; regular and strong
Skin	Pale, warm, and diaphoretic
Blood pressure	152/84 mm Hg
Oxygen saturation (Spo$_2$)	88% while receiving 8 L/min via nebulizer
Pupils	Equal and reactive to light

5. Explain the difference between primary and secondary contamination.

6. What are the four common types of decontamination methods used in the field?

that the ignition temperature of the oil is 300°F. What will happen if the burner is set on high, left unattended, and the oil is heated past 300°F? Once the temperature of the oil exceeds its ignition temperature, it will ignite; there is no need for an external ignition source. This is a common cause of stove fires.

Flammable range is another important term for you to understand. In broad terms, <u>flammable range</u> is an expression of a fuel/air mixture, defined by upper and lower limits, that reflects an amount of flammable vapor mixed with a given volume of air. Gasoline again can serve as the example. The flammable range for gasoline vapors is 1.4% to 7.6%. The two percentages, called the <u>lower flammable limit (LFL)</u> (1.4%) and the <u>upper flammable limit (UFL)</u> (7.6%), define the boundaries of a fuel/air mixture necessary for gasoline to burn properly. If a given gasoline/air mixture falls between the upper and lower flammable limits, and that mixture reaches an ignition source, there will be a flash fire.

Hazardous materials teams can, in many cases, cool down the heat or dissipate the concentration of vapors by pouring on streams of cool water. However, before any water is applied, the hazardous materials team will make critical decisions about whether or not the material may be <u>water reactive</u> or <u>water soluble</u>. If they are going to use water, they will also determine the hazardous material's <u>specific gravity</u>—whether or not the hazardous material will sink or float in water.

▮ Toxicology Terms

Chemistry experts and medical providers should communicate with each other using agreed-upon terms to describe the health hazards any incident might present. You will be a better provider and incident historian if you can master these terms.

The <u>threshold limit value (TLV)</u> is the maximum concentration of a toxin that someone can be exposed to for a 40-hour work week over a typical 30-year career. This value is established by the American Conference of Governmental Industrial Hygienists. The corresponding value, established by OSHA, is called the <u>permissible exposure limit (PEL)</u>. If you see both of these values listed in a reference source, you can assume the definitions are the same even if the values are different. OSHA is the law, but from an operational perspective, you should also pay attention to the more conservative of the two values if there is a conflict. The <u>threshold limit value/short-term exposure limit (TLV-STEL)</u> is the concentration that a person can be exposed to for a limited number of brief time periods (eg, four 15-minute exposures per day). The <u>threshold limit value/ceiling (TLV-C)</u> is the concentration that a person should never be exposed to. Keep in mind this value is established for workplace environments and, in many cases, hazardous materials responders will be operating in emergency environments that are many times greater than these values.

Lastly, the <u>threshold limit value/skin</u> indicates that direct or airborne contact with a material could result in possible and significant exposure from absorption through the skin, mucous membranes, and eyes.

Sometimes you will hear the experts refer to the lethal dose or lethal concentration value. The <u>lethal dose (LD)</u> of a material is a single dose that causes the death of a specified number of the group of test animals exposed by any route other than inhalation. The <u>lethal concentration (LC)</u> is defined as the concentration of the material in air that, on the basis of laboratory tests (inhalation route), is expected to kill a specified number of the group of test animals when administered over a specified period of time. You can use these values as rough guidelines in the field when you are gauging the amount of toxicity of a particular substance. From a toxicity standpoint, you should be more concerned with substances that can be harmful at low levels. The following information will give you an idea of how to gauge toxicity in the field if an LD or LC value is known.

Toxic, as defined by OSHA 29 CFR 1910.1200, is a chemical that falls in any of the following three categories:

- A chemical that has a LD_{50} of more than 50 milligrams per kilogram but not more than 500 milligrams per kilogram of body weight when administered orally to albino rats weighing between 200 and 300 grams each.
- A chemical that has a LD_{50} of more than 200 milligrams per kilogram but not more than 1,000 milligrams per kilogram of body weight when administered by continuous contact for 24 hours (or less if death occurs within 24 hours) with the bare skin of albino rabbits weighing between 2 and 3 kilograms each.
- A chemical that has a LC_{50} in air of more than 200 parts per million but not more than 2,000 parts per million by volume of gas or vapor, or more than 2 milligrams per liter but not more than 20 milligrams per liter of mist, fume, or dust, when administered by continuous inhalation for 1 hour (or less if death occurs within 1 hour) to albino rats weighing between 200 and 300 grams each.

Highly toxic, as defined by OSHA 29 CFR 1910.1200, is as follows:

- A chemical that has a LD_{50} of 50 milligrams or less per kilogram of body weight when administered orally to albino rats weighing between 200 and 300 grams each.
- A chemical that has a LD_{50} of 200 milligrams or less per kilogram of body weight when administered by continuous contact for 24 hours (or less if death occurs within 24 hours) with the bare skin of albino rabbits weighing between 2 and 3 kilograms each.
- A chemical that has a LC_{50} in air of 200 parts per million by volume or less of gas or vapor, or 2 milligrams per liter or less of mist, fume, or dust, when administered by continuous inhalation for 1 hour (or less if death occurs within 1 hour) to albino rats weighing between 200 and 300 grams each.

You might also hear the industrial hygienists or other hazardous materials responders use the term <u>immediately dangerous to life and health (IDLH)</u>, which means that the atmospheric concentration of any toxic, corrosive, or asphyxiant substance will pose an immediate threat to life, irreversible or delayed adverse effects, or serious interference for a team member's attempt to escape from the dangerous atmosphere. From a response perspective, this is the value you will be most concerned with and the value that is likely to be the cause of an exposure that requires some form of clinical intervention. Along with these toxicologic terms, when reference sources are available, you should also attempt to identify the expected signs and symptoms of exposure. This may help you make a differential diagnosis in the field or better correlate the patient's response to the exposure.

Decontamination and Treatment

Treating hazardous materials patients can be a difficult and emotionally challenging experience. Remember, your safety comes first. If you are first on the scene, you cannot immediately begin care until you fully understand the situation. Even if a patient is visible and in need of rescue, you must resist the temptation to enter the scene. Staying safe is a tough decision that requires discipline and emotional coolness. You must work as part of the team to prevent more casualties. When the substance presents an unacceptable risk to the responders, decontamination must be given the highest priority and you must wait until your patient(s) have been decontaminated. Then you can apply your knowledge and skills, in the cold or support zone, to treat the patient safely.

Words of Wisdom

Decontamination protects you and everyone else that provides care after you!

Decontamination

Decontamination methods will depend on the type of hazardous material involved; the stability of the scene; and the number, condition, and location of patients. In some cases, decontamination can be a form of treatment to reduce the dose of hazardous material in contact with the patient and decrease the risk of secondary contamination to others (including rescuers and ED personnel). Protection of the environment during decontamination is important and in most cases, plans should be made for containment of runoff. When lives are at stake, however, containing runoff is secondary.

There are four types of common decontamination methods you will see in the field—dilution, absorption, neutralization, and disposal. <u>Dilution</u> is the most common method and the easiest to perform in the field. Dilution typically relies on the use of copious amounts of water to flush the contaminant from the skin or eyes. This decreases the dose effect of the hazardous material on the patient. Sometimes a simple soap, such as tincture of green soap, is used in the decontamination process. Other decontamination agents are rarely used, although

vegetable or mineral oil is sometimes used if the contaminant is a water-reactive substance. Be cautious when you are using brushes; abrasion of a patient's skin increases the potential for hazardous material absorption. Pay special attention when your patient has been exposed to a solvent. Solvents are especially difficult to remove from the skin with water only; the patient may still have a solvent odor for quite some time after decontamination has been performed. Be aware of this during transport, or you may fall victim yourself to the off-gassing of solvents!

<u>Absorption</u> is accomplished with large pads that the hazardous materials team carries to soak up liquid and remove it from the patient. Towels can also be used in the same way. This is not the most effective way to remove contamination from the skin as a rule, but it is a method. <u>Neutralization</u> involves the use of a chemical to change the hazardous material into less harmful substances. Neutralization is almost never used when a person has been in contact with hazardous substances because of the dangers of uncontrolled exothermic reactions. When acids are used on bases, or vice versa, heat is generated as a by-product of the reaction. This could be detrimental to the patient and is an action that is almost always contraindicated. <u>Disposal</u> is not so much of a decontamination strategy as it is a result of the process. EMS responders should be mindful of removing as much of the patient's clothing as possible (in some cases this is all of it) in order to reduce the amount of contamination that contacts the body. Studies conducted by several branches of the US military have concluded that simply removing the clothing of a person exposed to chemicals can reduce the level of contamination by as much as 80%.

Emergency Decontamination in "Fast-Breaking" Situations

In some of the most difficult situations, you may be faced with the need to make an immediate decision about whether to treat patients despite the fact that they are contaminated. In this case, you may be responsible for deciding whether or not to proceed with rapid emergency decontamination. In all cases, you must ensure you have the appropriate protection to protect yourself against the threat and stay clear of the product. Do not make physical contact with it.

<u>Emergency decontamination</u> is the process of removing the bulk of contaminants off a person as quickly and completely as possible. Once you are properly protected, you should instruct the person to disrobe and remove as much of the hazardous materials from his or her body as possible; be prepared to provide assistance if necessary. If possible, give the person bags in which personal belongings and clothing can be placed. If the hazardous material is a powder, it should be brushed away first. If the hazardous material is water reactive, water should not be used for decontamination. Most often, however, water from whatever source is available (garden hose, fire hose, safety showers) is considered to be the universal decontamination solution. Again, when lives are at stake, controlling the runoff is secondary to getting the contaminant off the person. The goal is to get the victim clean enough to

allow you the opportunity to render care—this is the point at which the victim becomes a patient!

Mass Decontamination

In many cases, hose streams can be set up by the fire fighters to perform **mass decontamination**, or douse a large number of patients with copious amounts of water. Many agencies have commercial multiple-casualty decontamination systems as well. It is up to you to know what is used in your jurisdiction. In either case, the principle is the same—do the most good for the most people in the shortest amount of time possible.

An example of such a setup is the creation of an emergency decontamination corridor. A **decontamination corridor** is a controlled area within the warm zone where decontamination takes place. It is not a life safety action—it is the "normal course of business" decontamination that responders do as part of their mitigation efforts. A decontamination corridor may be formed by parking two fire engines parallel to each other and approximately 10 to 20 feet apart **Figure 23** . Nozzles can be attached to the side discharge ports of the engines and set to create a fine-particle fog-stream decontamination shower. Patients should disrobe on one end and enter the shower in single file. From a remote location, patients can be advised on how to decontaminate and directed to pay special attention to the areas of the body that are difficult to rinse such as the axilla, between fingers and toes, around the groin, the scalp, and between the buttocks. Soap and soft brushes should be made available. At the other end of the shower corridor, towels, blankets, and temporary garments should be available. It is at the *end* of this corridor that you would make initial contact with the patients and begin the triage process. Ideally, the runoff water from decontamination

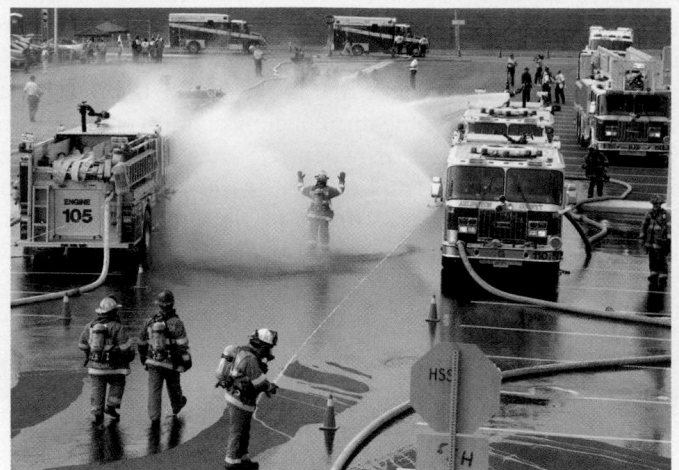

Figure 23   A decontamination corridor is located in the hot zone.

should be contained. At a minimum, the runoff should not be allowed to become a source of secondary contamination.

Technical Decontamination

Technical decontamination is the process used by the responders to clean PPE, tools, and equipment. It is a thorough cleaning process, often involving cleaning solutions and scrub brushes and a decontamination corridor. Keep in mind that the process and setup of technical decontamination may differ from jurisdiction to jurisdiction. There is not a single "right way" to do it, it is constructed more to accomplish the means, rendering the PPE, tools, and equipment free of contamination.

YOU are the Medic   PART 4

You request assistance to prepare the patient for transport. The patient is placed on continuous positive airway pressure (CPAP), 5 cm H_2O via mask and reassessed prior to being transferred to the ambulance stretcher. After 5 minutes of CPAP, the patient states that it is getting a little easier to breathe. You note a decreased work of breathing and anxiety. An additional nebulizer with 2.5 mg albuterol is attached to the CPAP mask and the patient is packaged for transport.

Recording Time: 17 Minutes	
Respirations	22 breaths/min; adequate depth and volume
Pulse	Radial pulse, 114 beats/min; regular and strong
Skin	Pale, warm, and dry
Blood pressure	146/80 mm Hg
Oxygen saturation (Spo$_2$)	94% while receiving 5 cm H_2O via CPAP
Pupils	Equal and reactive to light

7. Which areas of the body are difficult to clean and rinse when a patient is being decontaminated?

8. Depending on the type of exposure, the use of invasive procedures should be minimized if possible. Why is this important?

The following steps are intended to give you an idea of the technical decontamination process and to enhance your awareness of the dangers associated with hazardous materials and the constant need for proper decontamination techniques—it is not intended to make you proficient in accomplishing it yourself. You may receive additional training in hazardous materials response that will give you a better understanding of the task.

1. Responders exit the hot zone and approach the decontamination corridor.
2. Contaminated tools and equipment should be left behind at the hot zone end of the decontamination corridor.
3. Hazardous materials personnel are showered and washed using water, brushes, soap, or other appropriate decontamination agents to remove all surface contaminants. This is done with the assistance of other hazardous materials personnel (the decontamination team), who should wear not more than one step lower PPE than the entry team. Because technical decontamination is not aimed at life safety, it is done in a manner that will contain the runoff. Often this is accomplished inside a small wading pool or other disposable basin Figure 24 .
4. Paramedics should stay alert for signs of an ongoing primary or potential secondary contamination problem.
5. The team members move into an area of the decontamination corridor where they are helped out of their PPE by another member of the decontamination team. Contaminated protective clothing and equipment are placed into a bag or receptacle for later decontamination or disposal.
6. Respirators and/or SCBA masks and undergloves are removed last and placed in plastic bags or in other forms of containment.

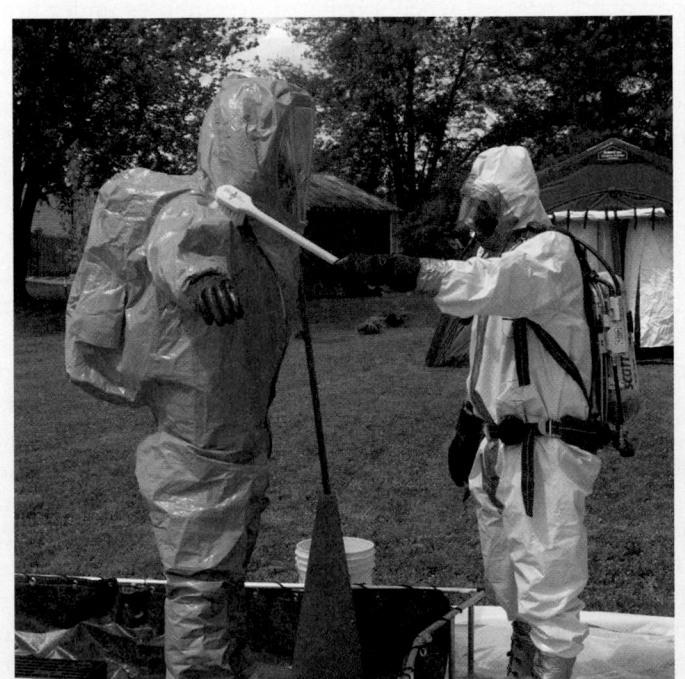

Figure 24 Technical decontamination is a thorough cleaning process to clean PPE, tools, and equipment.

7. Ideally, the responders should proceed to a location where they can take a personal shower to further reduce the potential for contamination. This is not always possible, but is the best course of action when possible.
8. Entry team personnel undergo medical evaluation.

Treatment of Patients Exposed to Hazardous Materials

In general, patients who are contaminated can be treated using the concepts learned in the chapters on burns and toxicology. Remember to apply the basics of patient care. However, there are some special considerations for hazardous materials patients. One of these is that invasive procedures should be minimized if possible. If you know from the hazardous materials team that your patient is contaminated, the process of endotracheal intubation may expose the patient to airway contamination. Placement of an IV or IO line may allow contamination to bypass the skin barrier. You will need to weigh the risks of invasive procedures against their benefits.

You should be familiar with references and how to access technical expertise when you are deciding how to treat patients from a hazardous materials incident. Some assistance may be obtained from the *ERG* and CHEMTREC. In addition, you may consult with poison control centers, the Agency for Toxic Substances and Disease Registry, and local medical control. The hazardous materials team may have comprehensive reference textbooks that can guide you in treatment decisions and also be of assistance to ED physicians. Never forget that you are the eyes and ears of the physician in the field. Share the knowledge you have gained from the hazardous materials team for your patient's sake.

The following categories of exposures are intended to serve as introductory information and should not be viewed as definitive treatment protocols or complete clinical interventions. They are intended to stimulate thinking and prompt you to learn more about the finer points of treating patients with chemical exposures.

Corrosives: Acids and Bases

Corrosives are chemicals that include both acids and bases. Some examples are toilet bowl cleaner, lye, and hydrochloric acid. Acids have a low pH (from 0 to 7), whereas bases have a high pH (7 to 14). Substances with both high and low pH can cause severe burns to the skin, eyes, and mucous membranes. Signs and symptoms include skin irritation, reddening or other discoloration, and blistering. Exposure of the mucous membranes to fumes can also cause burns, including severe life-threatening airway and lung burns.

Once the patient is decontaminated appropriately, treatment is generally supportive: ensure a patent airway, oxygenate the patient, treat for pain if indicated, and treat burns appropriately. Consider transport to a burn center if necessary. Patients showing signs of pulmonary edema secondary to an inhalation exposure may need to be treated for this with diuretics; however, you should always consult medical control to determine the proper course of action when you are treating patients with chemical exposures.

Solvents

Solvents may be liquids, solids, or gases. Common solvents include paint thinner and nail polish remover. <u>Solvents</u> are substances that are capable of dissolving other substances. Many solvents give off potent vapors that can be inhaled and can also be absorbed through the skin. Respiratory exposure in particular can cause immediate pulmonary symptoms such as pulmonary edema. Prolonged dermal exposure can cause symptoms as well, including cardiac dysrhythmias and seizures.

Solvent exposures may require extensive decontamination, almost to the point where it may be considered a form of treatment. Some solvents have additional hazards in that they can be metabolized into other toxic substances once absorbed by the body. Acetonitrile, for example, can be metabolized into a form of cyanide. It is important for you to research the substance the patient has been exposed to in order to understand what the substance is doing to the body and what the body may be doing to the substance. In general, solvent exposures require much of the same basic patient care as with any other exposure. Pay special attention to the potential for vomiting if a solvent has been ingested. This may complicate the patient's airway and be a cause for chemical pneumonitis.

Pesticides

Exposure to organophosphate and carbamate pesticides can produce severe signs and symptoms by interfering with the enzyme acetylcholinesterase, which promotes uptake of the neurotransmitter acetylcholine. In essence, these substances can cause runaway nervous system stimulation that produces a collection of signs known by the mnemonic <u>SLUDGEM</u> (Salivation, Lacrimation, Urination, Defecation, Gastrointestinal activity, Emesis, and Miosis). The mechanism of action of pesticides is similar to what you would find with most nerve agent exposures. It is recommended that you become more familiar with the mechanism of action of this unique group of chemical substances in order to fully understand the potential patient presentation. In addition to the SLUDGEM symptomology described, exposures can produce tachycardia or bradycardia, twitching muscles (unlike tonic-clonic seizures), and excessive pulmonary secretions. As always, you should protect yourself from secondary contamination, including that from emesis when the exposure has been gastrointestinal.

Treatment of pesticide poisoning includes aggressive decontamination, protection of the airway with intubation and frequent suctioning when necessary, high-flow oxygen, and the use of atropine to block the overstimulation of muscarinic receptors of the parasympathetic nervous system. Pralidoxime may also be recommended to restore the ability of the acetylcholinesterase to break down acetylcholine, which reverses the root cause of the exposure. This is a complicated set of chemical interactions and the full explanation is beyond the scope of this textbook. It is recommended that you fully educate yourself about the mechanism of action of organophosphates and carbamates and the recommended clinical interventions.

Chemical Asphyxiants

Any gas that displaces oxygen from the atmosphere is termed an <u>asphyxiant</u>. Colorless, odorless gases (eg, carbon monoxide and hydrogen sulfide) that are confined to an area may represent a deadly trap when would-be rescuers rush in to help a collapsed victim. Substances known as <u>chemical asphyxiants</u> interfere with the use of oxygen at the cellular level; <u>cyanide</u> is a common example of such an agent. Hydrogen cyanide is used in many industrial processes. The release of cyanide in Bhopal, India, was a major hazardous materials incident that caused thousands of fatalities. Cyanide poisoning can also occur during exposure to the by-products of combustion at structure fires, which is the most common exposure scenario for hydrogen cyanide.

Treatment of cyanide exposure (for non-smoke inhalation patients) begins with the use of amyl nitrite ampules that the patient should inhale for 15 seconds of every minute. This is followed by the IV administration of 300 mg of sodium nitrite, followed by 12.5 g of sodium thiosulfate. Follow the instructions found in the cyanide antidote kit for definitive treatment guidelines.

A treatment option for smoke inhalation cyanide poisoning is the antidote hydroxocobalamin, marketed in the United States and around the world as Cyanokit. This is an FDA-approved antidote for known or suspected smoke inhalation exposures. The drug is a precursor to vitamin B_{12} and is safe to use in the field to treat the cyanide component of a smoke exposure. Refer to the manufacturer's guidelines for use.

Another common exposure that results in a chemical asphyxiation is <u>carbon monoxide</u>. This gas ties up hemoglobin to the extent that oxygen in the blood becomes inaccessible to the cells. Treatment includes removal of the patient from the source and administration of 100% supplemental oxygen. Consider transport to an ED with hyperbaric oxygen capability.

Toxic Products of Combustion

<u>Toxic products of combustion</u> are the hazardous chemical compounds released when a material decomposes under heat. Remember that the process of combustion is a chemical reaction, and, like other reactions, will generate a given amount of by-products. You are well aware of the smoke produced by a structure fire, but have you really thought about what the smoke is made of or thought about the toxic gases that are liberated during a residential structure fire?

An easy way to think about it is to apply a long-standing phrase used in the world of chemistry: "garbage in, garbage out." This phrase reflects the idea that whatever objects are involved in the fire (eg, chairs, tables, and sofas) will break down in the heat and create a host of chemical by-products in the smoke. In short, the toxic gases and other chemical substances found in the smoke will be determined by what is burning. To that end, smoke is not "just smoke"—it is unique, to some degree, in each and every fire.

Burning wood may seem like simple combustion, but consider this: A burning piece of a common wood used in residential construction, Douglas fir, gives off more than 70 harmful chemical compounds. Other substances found in most fire smoke include soot, carbon monoxide, carbon dioxide, water vapor, formaldehyde, cyanide compounds, and many oxides of nitrogen. Each of these substances is unique in its chemical makeup and most are toxic to humans, even in small doses.

For example, carbon monoxide affects the ability of the human body to transport oxygen. The red blood cells cannot get oxygen to the cells and, subsequently, a person will die from tissue asphyxiation. Cyanide compounds also affect oxygen uptake in the body and are found to be a prevalent cause of civilian death in structure fires. Formaldehyde is found in many plastics and resins, and is one of the many components of smoke that causes eye and lung irritation. The oxides of nitrogen, including nitric oxide, nitrous oxide, and nitrogen dioxide are deep lung irritants that may cause a serious medical condition called pulmonary edema, or fluid buildup in the lungs.

Transportation Considerations

The ideal transportation scenario at a hazardous materials incident would be to have a team of paramedics who were not involved with decontamination or cold zone patient treatment standing by to transport patients to the ED. However, if the incident is a large one, the cold zone paramedics may need to both treat and transport patients.

You should remember that patients received after field decontamination should not be assumed to be completely decontaminated. Accordingly, you should take certain precautions to prepare yourself and your equipment for assuming care of the patient from the hazardous materials team and for getting the patient to the ED. First, you should wear appropriate PPE if indicated and be trained to wear the level required. The hazardous materials team may be able to supply some of the PPE if you do not have access to a splash-proof jumpsuit, for example. In addition, you should be given a complete report on what hazardous materials have been involved, what the patient's exposure has been, and what has been done to decontaminate and treat the patient. In no event should you transport a patient if decontamination has not been sufficient. An example of insufficient decontamination would be when hazardous material on the patient continues to produce toxic gases after a smoke exposure or perhaps a liquid splash exposure.

Before receiving and transporting a patient exposed to hazardous materials, you can do several things in preparation. One principle is to reduce the amount of supplies and equipment that the patient will come in contact with. You could remove the mattress from the stretcher because the patient will probably be carried on a backboard; removing the mattress will make later decontamination easier. In general, use as much disposable equipment as possible. Supplies and equipment inside the ambulance should be removed and set aside in a clean, safe place for later retrieval.

It is impractical and time-consuming to line the inside of the ambulance with plastic. Instead, plan to isolate the patient by wrapping him or her in a plastic barrier to reduce the potential for secondary contamination. A double-wrap procedure is preferable. In this procedure, the patient is first wrapped in a plastic blanket, preferably one that helps protect the patient from hypothermia. Then the patient is placed on a backboard and the backboard placed on the stretcher. You should know which EDs in your area have facilities for receiving patients with possible hazardous materials contamination. The ED should be given plenty of notice prior to the transport so that they can assemble the appropriately trained personnel and prepare

equipment. Often EDs will have a separate or dedicated treatment and decontamination room for these situations.

Medical Monitoring and Rehabilitation

You may be asked to assist with **medical monitoring** of the hazardous materials team. Wearing PPE often causes heat stress, and of course the toxins the team is working with can cause serious health effects. Factors that influence hazardous materials team members' health include level of physical fitness, activity, level of PPE, and environment factors such as temperature.

Medical monitoring should include documentation of the incident factors including the hazardous materials involved, their toxic effects, what PPE was worn, its resistance to permeability with the hazardous materials, and what type of decontamination was used. You should have a plan for treatment, transport, and potential availability of antidotes in the event that a hazardous materials team member needs medical assistance.

You might be asked to assess hazardous materials team members before they suit up for entry into the hot zone and then again after they come out. Your assessment should include a complete set of vital signs, as well as the ECG, temperature, and body weight. Team members should be encouraged to prehydrate with water or a sports drink. Working inside a level A suit is like being inside a sauna, with no way to lose heat through evaporation, conduction, convection, or radiation. A useful fact that can help you with your assessment is that some hazardous materials teams keep a file of their members' baseline medical status. Be sure to ask for this information.

Before being allowed to reenter the hot zone, the hazardous materials team should be evaluated by paramedics in the rehabilitation area (located in the cold zone) for hydration status, vital signs, and any potential symptoms of exposure to the toxic agent the incident involves Figure 25 . Team members

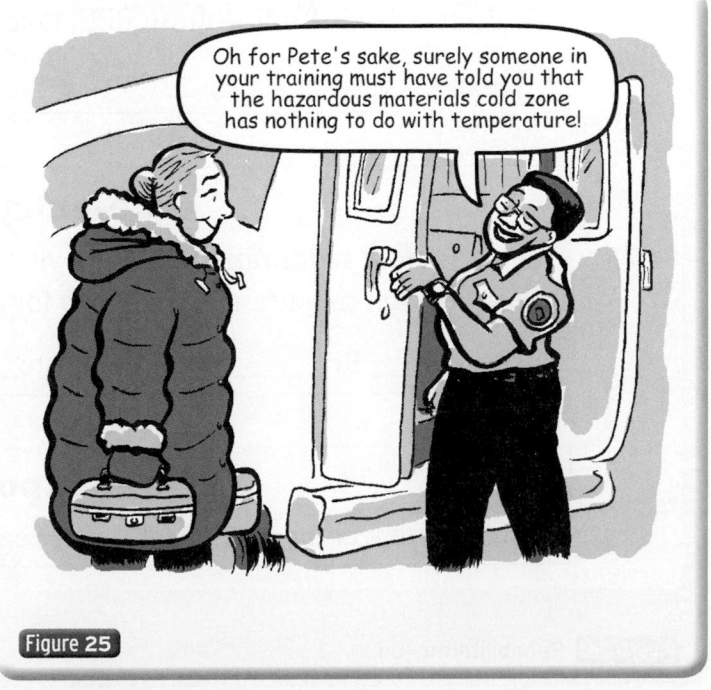

Oh for Pete's sake, surely someone in your training must have told you that the hazardous materials cold zone has nothing to do with temperature!

Figure 25

should remove their protective clothing and be given a chance to rest. Reassess vital signs and perform a neurologic assessment (eg, orientation to time, place, and events) as well as an assessment of fine motor skills. Team members with elevated temperatures should be monitored closely for possible heat stroke. The loss of body weight is a direct correlation to the loss of fluids and the risk of dehydration and hypovolemia. Members should be encouraged to rehydrate by drinking water or other appropriate fluids. If there are abnormalities in vital signs or if team members have signs or symptoms, they should not be allowed to return to work until their physical status returns to normal. An example of a hazardous materials team rehabilitation log that can assist you in the hazardous materials rehabilitation sector is shown in **Figure 26**.

HazMat Medical Monitoring Worksheet

Date:_____   Entry Person:_____

Incident #_____   Medical Monitor:_____

> **Important:** HazMat team members shall not be allowed to don PPE if any of the following conditions are present: systolic BP < 100 or > 160, diastolic BP > 100, pulse rate > 120, oral temperature > 99.8°F, Respirations > 24. Medical monitors must read and be familiar with the "Medical Monitoring Guidelines" before beginning medical evaluations.

Pre-entry Evaluation
Before donning PPE, take and record baseline vital signs.

Time_____ BP_____ Pulse Rate_____ Resp._____ Oral Temp._____°F

Post-entry Evaluation
Immediately after doffing PPE, take vital signs and assess for hyperthermia.

Time_____ BP_____ Pulse Rate_____ Resp._____ Oral Temp._____°F

Re-entry Evaluation
Before redonning PPE, take vital signs and reassess for hyperthermia.
Entry person must remain in rehab for a minimum of 30 minutes between entries.

Time_____ BP_____ Pulse Rate_____ Resp._____ Oral Temp._____°F

HazMat Exposure Suspected?
Immediately contact HazMat Team Leader and see "HazMat Exposure Protocols."

Figure 26 Rehabilitation log.

YOU *are the Medic*   SUMMARY

1. **What are some clues that might help you identify leaks or spills of hazardous materials?**

   Pay close attention to your surroundings—remember your safety comes first! DO NOT approach a substance if you do not know what it is and do not have proper protective equipment. From a safe distance you may observe a cloud or smoke coming from the area in question. You may see a leak or a spill coming from a tank, container, truck, or railway car with or without a hazardous material placard or label. Another word of caution, do not rely on your nose to identify the presence of a hazardous material. If you smell it, you are exposed!

2. **How can the MSDS assist you with the treatment of your patient?**

   The MSDS contains valuable information regarding all aspects of the chemical, from ingredients, physical data, and fire/explosion data to health hazard data. Reading the health hazard section will provide you with the signs and symptoms of exposure which then helps guide patient management.

3. **What should your initial treatment consist of?**

   Your patient presents in acute respiratory distress with bronchospasm. The MSDS tells you that chlorine is a respiratory irritant. On the basis of this information and the patient's presentation, initial treatment should include high-flow oxygen, IV access, and a nebulizer with bronchodilators.

4. **Hazardous materials teams will establish safety zones at the scene. In which zone does patient triage and treatment take place?**

   Treatment and triage will take place in the cold zone. The cold zone is established in a safe area with enough distance from the warm and hot zones to prevent harm to rescuers and patients.

5. **Explain the difference between primary and secondary contamination.**

   Primary contamination is the direct exposure of a patient to a hazardous material. Secondary contamination occurs when a hazardous material is transferred from one person to another or from contact with a contaminated object.

6. **What are the four common types of decontamination methods used in the field?**

   The four common types of decontamination methods used in the field are dilution, absorption, neutralization, and disposal. Dilution is the easiest method to perform, making it the most common type of decontamination in the field.

7. **Which areas of the body are difficult to clean and rinse when a patient is being decontaminated?**

   Several small areas on the body can be quite difficult to clean and rinse. These include the axilla, the area between the fingers and the toes, around the groin, the scalp, and between the buttocks. If you are assigned to assist with patient decontamination, make sure to pay close attention to these areas. Any remaining chemicals can be transferred to other rescuers and personnel via secondary contamination.

8. **Depending on the type of exposure, the use of invasive procedures should be minimized if possible. Why is this important?**

   Protecting the patient from further contamination is an important component of treatment. Any procedure such as endotracheal intubation or insertion of an IV line bypasses normal protective barriers of the body such as the skin and mucous membranes. This is not to say that these procedures should not be performed at all; just remember to weigh the risks against the benefits prior to doing so.

YOU *are the Medic*   **SUMMARY,** *continued*

EMS Patient Care Report (PCR)

Date: 01-15-12	Incident No.: 285972	Nature of Call: HazMat		Location: 674 Chestnut Drive	
Dispatched: 1417	En Route: 1418	At Scene: 1426	Transport: 1445	At Hospital: N/A	In Service: N/A

Patient Information

Age: 53 **Sex:** M **Weight (in kg [lb]):** 59 kg (130 lb)	**Allergies:** None **Medications:** Lisinopril, Albuterol **Past Medical History:** Asthma, hypertension **Chief Complaint:** Shortness of breath

Vital Signs

Time: 1431	BP: 156/84	Pulse: 127	Respirations: 30	Spo$_2$: 96%
Time: 1436	BP: 152/84	Pulse: 134	Respirations: 28	Spo$_2$: 88%
Time: 1443	BP: 146/80	Pulse: 114	Respirations: 22	Spo$_2$: 94%

EMS Treatment
(circle all that apply)

Oxygen @ __15__ L/min via (circle one): NC (NRM) Bag-mask device	Assisted Ventilation	(Airway Adjunct:) CPAP	CPR
Defibrillation	Bleeding Control	Bandaging	Splinting	(Other:) Nebulizer: 2.5 mg Albuterol, 0.5 mg Atrovent Solu-Medrol 125 mg IV Nebulizer: 2.5 mg Albuterol via CPAP

Narrative

Dispatched to water treatment plant for chlorine leak with multiple pts. Upon arrival unit assigned to treatment sector by Incident Command. Provided MSDS from treatment officer and assigned pt. Initial pt contact was made at 1500. Pt appeared in acute respiratory distress as evidenced by intercostal and subcostal retraction and audible expiratory wheezes. Pt was seated on tarp assuming tripod position with difficulty completing sentences. According to coworker, the pt was in the immediate area when the leak occurred and was trapped for approximately 15 minutes. Initial assessment reveals patent airway, rapid and shallow respirations, audible expiratory wheezes, and a regular, rapid radial pulse. Pt placed on NRB mask at 15 L/min. At 1426 a nebulizer with 2.5 mg albuterol and 0.5 mg ipratropium (Atrovent) was attached to mask and flow was decreased to 8 L/min. IV established with 18-gauge catheter in the right antecubital space. 125 mg methylprednisolone (Solu-Medrol) drawn up and administered IV. At approximately 1428 the pt stated he was having increased work of breathing. Reassessment revealed markedly diminished breath sounds with expiratory wheezing bilaterally. Accessory muscle use still present; however, the pt appeared fatigued. Pt placed on 5 cm H$_2$O CPAP via mask. After approximately 5 minutes after CPAP placed, the pt stated his work of breathing has become easier. Second nebulizer with 2.5 mg albuterol was attached to CPAP mask. Pt assessment prior to transport revealed: Pt awake and alert to person, place, time, and event. Pupils equal, round, and reactive to light. No JVD or tracheal deviation noted. Symmetric chest rise with bilateral expiratory wheezes. Accessory muscle use still noted though decreased from before. Abdomen soft and nontender on palpation. PMS present in all four extremities. Pt packaged for transport and care was turned over to medic O'Riley at 1445 for transport to Southport Regional Medical Center. **End of report**

Prep Kit

Ready for Review

- Thousands of hazardous materials incidents occur (and are reported) each year.
- Handling hazardous materials emergencies requires specialized training and equipment.
- You should never enter a hazardous materials scene without understanding the nature of the problem.
- According to OSHA, the levels of hazardous materials response training are: awareness, operations, technician, and specialist.
- The great majority of hazardous materials emergencies are transportation incidents, predominately occurring on roadways.
- When you are approaching an incident you should be alert for signs of hazardous materials. Signs of hazardous materials include vapor clouds, strange odors, spilled liquids, and multiple victims.
- Sources of information about hazardous materials include labels and placards, transport documents, material safety data sheets, and the DOT's *ERG*.
- Hazardous materials incident management follows NIMS and ICS principles.
- Hazardous material incidents have hot, warm, and cold zones.
- Without proper personal protective equipment and training, you should not enter the hot and warm zones.
- The four levels of hazardous materials PPE are level A, level B, level C, and level D.
- Primary hazardous materials contamination comes from direct contact with the toxin.
- Secondary contamination is spread by people (patients, the hazardous materials team, or EMS providers), clothing, or objects.
- Effects from hazardous materials exposure may be local on the body or systemic.
- Routes of exposure include inhalation, ingestion, absorption, and injection.
- Rescue and decontamination of victims is secondary to rescuer and public protection.
- Decontamination should be undertaken as a methodical process based on the nature of the contaminant.
- Treatment of hazardous materials victims is usually symptomatic and supportive of the ABCs. In some cases, antidotes are indicated and must be approved by the authority having jurisdiction.
- Invasive procedures should be carefully administered to avoid the risk of introducing contamination.
- Paramedics may be directed to support a hazardous materials operation with medical monitoring of the hazardous materials personnel.

Vital Vocabulary

absorption A type of decontamination that is done with large pads that the hazardous materials team use to soak up liquid and remove it from the patient.

asphyxiant Any gas that displaces oxygen from the atmosphere; can be deadly if exposure occurs in a confined space.

authority having jurisdiction (AHJ) An organization, office, or person responsible for enforcing the requirements of a code or standard, or for approving equipment, materials, an installation, or a procedure.

bill of lading A document carried by drivers of commercial vehicles that should provide specific information about what is carried on the vehicle.

CAMEO Computer-Aided Management of Emergency Operations; a tool to help predict downwind concentrations of hazardous materials based on the input of environmental factors into a computer model.

carbon monoxide A chemical asphyxiant that results in a cellular respiratory failure; this gas ties up hemoglobin to the extent that oxygen in the blood becomes inaccessible to the cells.

carboy A glass, plastic, or steel nonbulk storage container, ranging in volume from 5 to 15 gallons.

cargo tank Bulk packaging that is permanently attached to or forms a part of a motor vehicle, or is not permanently attached to any motor vehicle, and that, because of its size, construction, or attachment to a motor vehicle, is loaded or unloaded without being removed from the motor vehicle.

chemical asphyxiants Substances that interfere with the use of oxygen at the cellular level.

CHEMTREC (Chemical Transportation Emergency Center) A resource available to emergency responders via telephone on a 24-hour basis.

container Any vessel or receptacle that holds material, including storage vessels, pipelines, and packaging.

corrosives A class of chemicals with either high or low pH levels. Exposure can cause severe soft-tissue damage.

cyanide A chemical asphyxiant used in many industrial processes; exposure can occur from by-products of combustion at structure fires.

cylinders Portable, nonbulk, compressed gas containers used to hold liquids and gases. Uninsulated compressed gas cylinders are used to store substances such as nitrogen, argon, helium, and oxygen. They have a range of sizes and internal pressures.

decontamination corridor A controlled area within the warm zone where decontamination takes place.

dilution A type of decontamination method that uses copious amounts of water to flush the contaminant from the skin or eyes.

disposal A type of decontamination in which as much clothing and equipment as possible is disposed of to reduce the magnitude of the problem.

dose effect The principle that the longer a hazardous material is in contact with the body or the greater the concentration, the greater the effect will most likely be.

drums Barrel-like nonbulk storage vessels used to store a wide variety of substances, including food-grade materials, corrosives, flammable liquids, and grease. Drums may be constructed of low-carbon steel, polyethylene, cardboard, stainless steel, nickel, or other materials.

dry bulk cargo tanks Tanks designed to carry dry bulk goods such as powders, pellets, fertilizers, or grain. Such tanks are generally V-shaped with rounded sides that funnel toward the bottom.

emergency decontamination The process of removing the bulk of contaminants off of a victim without regard for containment. It is used in potentially life-threatening situations, without the formal establishment of a decontamination corridor.

evacuation The removal or relocation of people who may be affected by an approaching release of a hazardous material.

flammable range An expression of a fuel/air mixture, defined by upper and lower limits, that reflects an amount of flammable vapor mixed with a given volume of air.

flash point The minimum temperature at which a liquid or a solid releases sufficient vapor to form an ignitable mixture with air.

hazardous material Any substance that is toxic, poisonous, radio-active, flammable, or explosive and causes injury or death with exposure.

HAZWOPER (HAZardous Waste OPerations and Emergency Response) The federal OSHA regulation that governs hazardous materials waste site and response training. Specifics can be found in Title 29, standard number 1910.120. Subsection (q) is specific to emergency response.

ignition temperature The minimum temperature at which a fuel, when heated, will ignite in air and continue to burn. Also called the autoignition temperature.

immediately dangerous to life and health (IDLH) A phrase that means the atmospheric concentration of any toxic, corrosive, or asphyxiant substance will pose an immediate threat to life, irreversible or delayed adverse effects, or serious interference for a team member attempting to escape from the dangerous atmosphere; a respirator is mandatory.

intermodal tanks A bulk container that serves as both a shipping and a storage vessel. Such tanks hold between 5,000 and 6,000 gallons of product and can be pressurized or nonpressurized. Intermodal tanks may be shipped by all modes of transportation.

labels Signage at least 3.9 inches on each side that is often required on all four sides of individual packages and boxes that are being transported.

lethal concentration (LC) The concentration of a material in air that, on the basis of laboratory tests (inhalation route), is expected to kill a specified number of the group of test animals when administered over a specified period of time.

lethal dose (LD) A single dose that causes the death of a specified number of the group of test animals exposed by any route other than inhalation.

level A ensemble The highest level of protective suit worn by hazardous materials personnel. May also be referred to as fully encapsulating because the suit covers everything, including the breathing apparatus.

level B ensemble Personal protective equipment that is one step less protective than level A, but provides for a high level of respiratory protection.

level C ensemble A level of personal protective equipment that provides splash protection.

level D ensemble The level of protection that fire fighter turnout gear provides.

local effect An effect of a hazardous material on the body that is limited to the area of contact.

lower flammable limit (LFL) The minimum amount of gaseous fuel that must be present in the air for the air/fuel mixture to be flammable or explosive.

mass decontamination The physical process of reducing or removing surface contaminants from large numbers of victims in potentially life-threatening situations in the fastest time possible.

material safety data sheets (MSDS) Information documents that are supposed to be kept on site at workplaces for every potentially hazardous chemical at the workplace.

MC-306/DOT 406 flammable liquid tanker Such a vehicle typically carries between 6,000 gallons and 10,000 gallons of a product such as gasoline or other flammable and combustible materials. The tank is nonpressurized.

MC-307/DOT 407 chemical hauler A tanker with a rounded or horseshoe-shaped tank capable of holding 6,000 to 7,000 gallons of flammable liquid, mild corrosives, and poisons. The tank has a high internal working pressure.

MC-312/DOT 412 corrosive tanker A tanker that often carries aggressive (highly reactive) acids such as concentrated sulfuric and nitric acid. It is characterized by several heavy-duty reinforcing rings around the tank and holds approximately 6,000 gallons of product.

MC-331 pressure cargo tanker A tanker that carries materials such as ammonia, propane, Freon, and butane. This type of tank is commonly constructed of steel and has rounded ends and a single open compartment inside. The liquid volume inside the tank varies, ranging from the 1,000-gallon delivery truck to the full-size 11,000-gallon cargo tank.

MC-338 cryogenic tanker A low-pressure tanker designed to maintain the low temperature required by the cryogens it carries. A boxlike structure containing the tank control valves is typically attached to the rear of the tanker.

medical monitoring The process of assessing the health status of hazardous materials team members before and after entry to a hazardous materials incident site.

neutralization A type of decontamination that uses one chemical to change the hazardous material into two less harmful substances; rarely used by hazardous materials teams.

nonbulk storage vessels Any container other than bulk storage containers such as drums, bags, compressed gas cylinders, and cryogenic containers. Nonbulk storage vessels hold commonly used commercial and industrial chemicals such as solvents, cleaners, and compounds.

permissible exposure limit (PEL) The maximum concentration of a chemical that a person may be exposed to under OSHA regulations.

placards Signage at least 10.8 inches on each side that is often required to be on all four sides of transport vehicles identifying the hazardous contents of the vehicle.

primary contamination An exposure that occurs with direct contact with the hazardous material.

secondary containment An engineered method to control spilled or released product if the main containment vessel fails.

secondary contamination Exposure to a hazardous material by contact with a contaminated person or object.

shelter-in-place A method of safeguarding people located near or in a hazardous area by keeping them in a safe atmosphere, usually inside structures.

SLUDGEM A mnemonic that stands for salivation, lacrimation, urination, defecation, gastrointestinal activity, emesis, miosis, which are the signs and symptoms that can be produced by exposure to organophosphate and carbamate pesticides or other nerve-stimulating agents.

solvents Substances that are capable of dissolving other substances.

specific gravity The measure that indicates whether or not a hazardous material will sink or float in water.

systemic effect A physiologic effect on the entire body or one of the body's systems.

technical decontamination A multistep process of carefully scrubbing and washing contaminants off of a person or object, collecting runoff water, and collecting and properly handling all items.

threshold limit value (TLV) The concentration of a substance that is supposed to be safe for exposure no more than 8 hours per day and 40 hours per week.

threshold limit value/ceiling (TLV/C) The maximum concentration of hazardous material to which a worker should not be exposed, even for an instant.

threshold limit value/short-term exposure limit (TLV-STEL) The concentration of a substance that a worker can be exposed to for up to 15 minutes but no more than four times per day with at least 1 hour between each exposure.

threshold limit value/skin The concentration at which direct or airborne contact with a material could result in possible and significant exposure from absorption through the skin, mucous membranes, and eyes.

toxic products of combustion Hazardous chemical compounds that are released when a material decomposes under heat.

tube trailer A high-volume transportation device made up of several individual compressed gas cylinders banded together and affixed to a trailer. Tube trailers carry compressed gases such as hydrogen, oxygen, helium, and methane. One trailer may carry several different gases in individual tubes.

upper flammable limit (UFL) The maximum amount of gaseous fuel that can be present in the air if the air/fuel mixture is to be flammable or explosive.

vapor density The weight of an airborne concentration (vapor or gas) as compared with an equal volume of dry air.

vapor pressure For the purpose of this chapter, the pressure associated with liquids held inside any type of closed container.

water reactive A property that indicates that a material will undergo a chemical reaction (for example, explosion) when mixed with water.

water soluble A property that indicates that a material can be dissolved in water.

waybill A cargo document kept by the conductor of a train; also referred to as a consist.

Assessment
in Action

You are employed by a rural EMS system and are dispatched to the scene of an airplane crash with a possible hazardous materials exposure. A crop duster crashed into the terminal of the regional airport releasing an unknown chemical into the area. Prior to arrival, you are asked to stage 1 mile from the scene.

1. A hazardous material may enter the body through which of the following routes?
   A. Ingestion
   B. Inhalation
   C. Injection
   D. All of the above

2. Methods of decontamination include:
   A. evaporation.
   B. dilution.
   C. sterilization.
   D. autoclaving.

3. What type of protective clothing is worn only by personnel in the cold zone?
   A. Level D
   B. Level C
   C. Level B
   D. Level A

4. Organophosphates act on the body by inhibiting the breakdown of:
   A. epinephrine.
   B. acetylcholine.
   C. norepinephrine.
   D. serotonin.

5. The "S" in the mnemonic SLUDGEM stands for:
   A. stroke.
   B. seizures.
   C. salivation.
   D. shingles.

6. Which of the following drugs is administered to reduce the effects of organophosphate poisoning?
   A. Atropine
   B. Benadryl
   C. Dopamine
   D. Calcium chloride

7. Which chemical can produce signs and symptoms similar to those seen with organophosphates?
   A. Cyanide
   B. Hydrogen sulfide
   C. Ammonia
   D. Carbamates

Additional Question

8. What is a common method used to decontaminate patients during a multiple-casualty incident?

Terrorism

National EMS Education Standard Competencies

EMS Operations

Knowledge of operational roles and responsibilities to ensure patient, public, and personnel safety.

Mass-Casualty Incidents Due to Terrorism and Disaster

- Risks and responsibilities of operating on the scene of a natural or man-made disaster. (pp 2289-2311)

Knowledge Objectives

1. List key questions to consider when responding to a terrorist event. (pp 2289-2290)
2. Define international and domestic terrorism. (pp 2290-2291)
3. Define and specify types of terrorist groups. (pp 2291-2293)
4. List various examples of terrorist agendas. (pp 2291-2293)
5. Discuss the color-coded advisory system's replacement with the National Terrorism Advisory System (NTAS). (pp 2293-2294)
6. Discuss what actions paramedics should take during the course of their work to heighten their ability to respond to and survive a terrorist attack. (pp 2293-2297)
7. List various examples of potential terrorist targets. (pp 2293-2294)
8. Discuss factors to consider when responding to a potential weapon of mass destruction incident, including pre-incident indicators, the type of location, the type of call, the number of patients, and victims' statements. (pp 2293-2297)
9. Discuss key response actions to take at the scene of a terrorist event, including establishing scene safety, ensuring personal protection, notification procedures, requests for resources, and establishing or working within command. (pp 2294-2297)
10. Define secondary device, and discuss the importance of continually reassessing scene safety. (p 2297)
11. List the four main categories of weapons of mass destruction. (p 2297)
12. Discuss specific types of devices used by terrorists, including explosives, ammonium nitrate, and suicide bombers. (pp 2297-2298)
13. Define terms related to chemical agents, including persistency, volatility, contact hazard, and vapor hazard. (p 2298)

14. Describe specific vesicant agents. (pp 2298-2299)
15. Discuss signs, symptoms, and treatment for vesicant exposure. (pp 2298-2299)
16. Describe specific pulmonary agents. (pp 2299-2300)
17. Discuss signs, symptoms, and treatment for exposure to a pulmonary agent. (pp 2299-2300)
18. Describe specific nerve agents. (pp 2300-2302)
19. Discuss signs, symptoms, and treatment for exposure to a nerve agent. (pp 2300-2302)
20. Describe specific industrial chemicals and insecticides. (pp 2302-2303)
21. Discuss signs, symptoms, and treatment for exposure to a cyanide agent. (pp 2302-2303)
22. Define terms related to biologic agents, including dissemination, disease vector, communicability, and incubation. (p 2303)
23. Describe signs, symptoms, and treatment for smallpox. (pp 2304-2305)
24. Describe signs, symptoms, and treatment for viral hemorrhagic fevers. (pp 2304-2306)
25. Describe signs, symptoms, and treatment for inhalation and cutaneous anthrax. (p 2306)
26. Describe signs, symptoms, and treatment for plague. (pp 2306-2307)
27. Describe signs, symptoms, and treatment for exposure to botulinum toxin. (p 2307)
28. Describe signs, symptoms, and treatment for exposure to ricin. (pp 2307-2308)
29. Define syndromic surveillance, and discuss its importance during a potential terrorist event. (p 2308)
30. Define radiation, and describe the difference between alpha, beta, gamma, and neutron radiation. (pp 2309-2310)
31. Describe what a radiologic dispersal device, or dirty bomb, is and how it is used for terrorism. (p 2310)
32. List protective measures to take when responding to a radiologic event. (p 2311)
33. Discuss medical management of a patient who was potentially exposed to radiation. (p 2311)

Skills Objectives

1. Demonstrate how to use a nerve agent antidote kit. (p 2302)

Introduction

Over the last decade, the threat posed by international and domestic acts of terrorism has sharply increased. Several times a week a terror attack occurs someplace in the world. Preparing for response to an act of terror has become a reality for EMS workers in the United States and around the world. It is possible that you may respond to a terrorist event during the span of your career. International terrorists as well as domestic groups have increased their targeting of civilian populations with acts of terror. The question is not will terrorists strike again, but rather when and where they will strike. You must be mentally and physically prepared for the possibility of a terrorist event.

Your health and safety is a primary concern when you are called to respond to terrorist attacks. The threat that terrorism poses to the health and safety of paramedics was realized even before the September 11, 2001, attacks. The sarin attacks in Tokyo in 1996 sickened 135 of the 1,336 (approximately 10%) paramedics who rushed to the scene, because they lacked proper personal protective equipment (PPE). The attacks on September 11, 2001, brought emergency responder health and safety to the forefront because 450 emergency responders were killed on that day, representing over 15% of the total victims.

Many more paramedics and EMTs were injured, developed chronic disorders, or experienced depression and physiologic problems as a result of their response.

The chapter, *Disaster Response* discusses concerns related to disasters in general, but there are some issues specific to terrorist attacks that must be considered. Although it is difficult to anticipate and plan a response to many terrorist events, there are several key principles that apply to every response. This chapter describes how you can prepare to respond to these events by discussing types of terrorist events and patient management. You will also learn the signs, symptoms, and treatment of patients who have been exposed to chemical, biologic, radiologic, nuclear, and explosive (CBRNE) agents or injured by a suicide bomb and explosive attacks. Lastly, issues of responder health and safety at the scene of a terrorist attack will be discussed in detail. At the end of this chapter, you will be able to answer the following key questions:

- What are the most frequent sites for a terrorist attack?
- What are your initial actions when faced with a terrorist event?
- Who should you notify, and what should you tell them?
- What types of additional resources might you require?
- How do you ensure your own safety, your partner's safety, and the safety of victims?

YOU are the Medic   PART 1

You and your partner are dispatched to an unknown medical incident at the courthouse. The dispatcher informs you that the communications center is receiving multiple calls for persons having difficulty breathing within the courthouse where a high-profile murder trial was underway. Prior to arrival, you are asked to stage three blocks north of the courthouse until the scene is declared safe. The HazMat team is en route with an estimated time of arrival of 2 minutes. Incident command is being set up in a parking lot across the street from the courthouse.

Your unit is assigned to the treatment area. There are approximately 25 people outside of the courthouse with respiratory symptoms with an unknown number of patients inside. Initial reports indicate there was a strange odor throughout the second floor where the trial was being held. Decontamination areas are being established. Approximately 35 minutes into the call you receive your first patient.

Recording Time: 1 Minute	
Appearance	Man in his mid-20s, in respiratory distress. Patient appears confused.
Level of consciousness	Verbal (knows his name, but does not know where he is or how he got there)
Airway	Open
Breathing	Increased work of breathing with accessory muscle use and audible expiratory wheezes
Circulation	Strong radial pulse, decreased

1. What are some clues that might help you treat your patient?
2. Biologic agents can be modified in a laboratory to increase their impact on target populations. What are the primary types of biologic agents that you may encounter during a terrorist attack?

- How should you proceed to address the needs of the victims?
- What is the clinical presentation of a patient exposed to a weapon of mass destruction (WMD)?
- How are WMD patients to be assessed and treated?
- How do you avoid becoming contaminated or cross-contaminated with a WMD agent?
- How do you ensure your health after your response to the incident has concluded?

EMS providers are encouraged to seek additional training and participate in drills and exercises to hone the skills needed to respond safely to a terrorist event.

Terrorism

The US Department of Justice defines **terrorism** as a violent act dangerous to human life, in violation of the criminal laws of the United States or any state or subdivision thereof, to intimidate or coerce a government, the civilian population, or any segment thereof, in furtherance of political or social objectives. Mass destruction, assassinations, and kidnappings that are conducted with the aim to influence or affect a government are also defined as terrorism. Terrorists pose a threat to nations and cultures everywhere. Terrorism is commonly used as a form of **asymmetric warfare**, in which groups wage war against a population with unconventional weapons and covert tactics that are unequal—for example—when there are differences in military resources or capabilities, and are thus asymmetrical.

Terrorism is common around the world, with frequent attacks occurring across the Middle East, where terrorist groups frequently strike civilian populations in crowded outdoor markets, at sporting and religious events, and at weddings. In Colombia and oil-rich regions in Africa, political terrorist groups target oil resources (refineries, pipelines, and infrastructure) as a means to instill fear in multinational corporations and governments. Often, vulnerable innocent people are the victims of acts of political and economic terror. Terrorists often lack a sense of discrimination when selecting their targets, and have been known to intentionally attack children at schools and camps. In one such attack in 2004, over 30 heavily armed male and female terrorists and suicide bombers overran a school in Beslan, Russia, and held children as hostages over the course of 3 days. When the siege was over, 334 hostages were killed, many of them children, who were too weak after 3 days of starvation to escape the massacre **Figure 1**. In another attack in 2011 in Norway, a lone terrorist exploded a car bomb in Oslo and then targeted a summer camp, opening fire and killing 69 people.

International Terrorism

The US Federal Bureau of Investigation defines two types of terrorism: international terrorism and domestic terrorism. **International terrorism**, also known as cross-border terrorism, is defined as acts of terror committed by foreign agents. International terrorism can be further categorized into the following subgroups:

- **Non-state-supported terrorism**. Terrorism that is either indigenous or transnational, and that does not receive direction or support from a government.

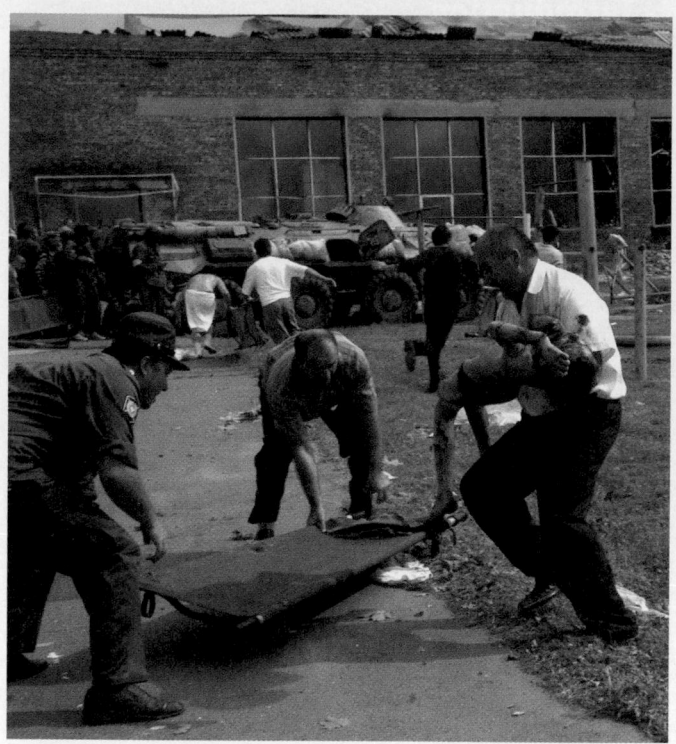

Figure 1 In 2004, a terrorist attack at a school in Beslan, Russia resulted in hundreds of deaths.

- **State-sponsored terrorism**. Terrorism that is funded or supported by a government; the government holds close ties with the terrorist group, but the terrorist group still acts independently.
- **State-directed terrorism**. Terrorism directed by a government; terrorists act as direct agents of the government.

The emergence of international terrorism has changed the lives of every American citizen and hundreds of millions more people around the globe. It has implications for paramedics who will respond to these events. Events such as the attack on New York's World Trade Center in 1993 and September 11, 2001 (9/11), have changed the way Americans live and travel **Figure 2** and **Figure 3**. In Mumbai, India international terrorists stormed two landmark hotels popular with Western tourists, in a coordinated attack that occurred at 11 sites (including a women and children's hospital and a train station) over the course of 3 days in November of 2008. These highly organized terror attacks killed over 160 people and injured more than 300.

Domestic Terrorism

Whereas terrorist attacks planned by foreigners have dominated the discussion and planning for emergency response, **domestic terrorism** is also a fact of life. Domestic terrorism is defined as when the perpetrators are citizens of the country that is being attacked. In the United States, domestic terrorists have planned attacks multiple times within the last several years post-9/11.

The Centennial Olympic Park bombing in Atlanta during the 1996 Summer Olympics injured over 100 people and killed 2 **Figure 4**. The destruction of the Alfred P. Murrah Federal

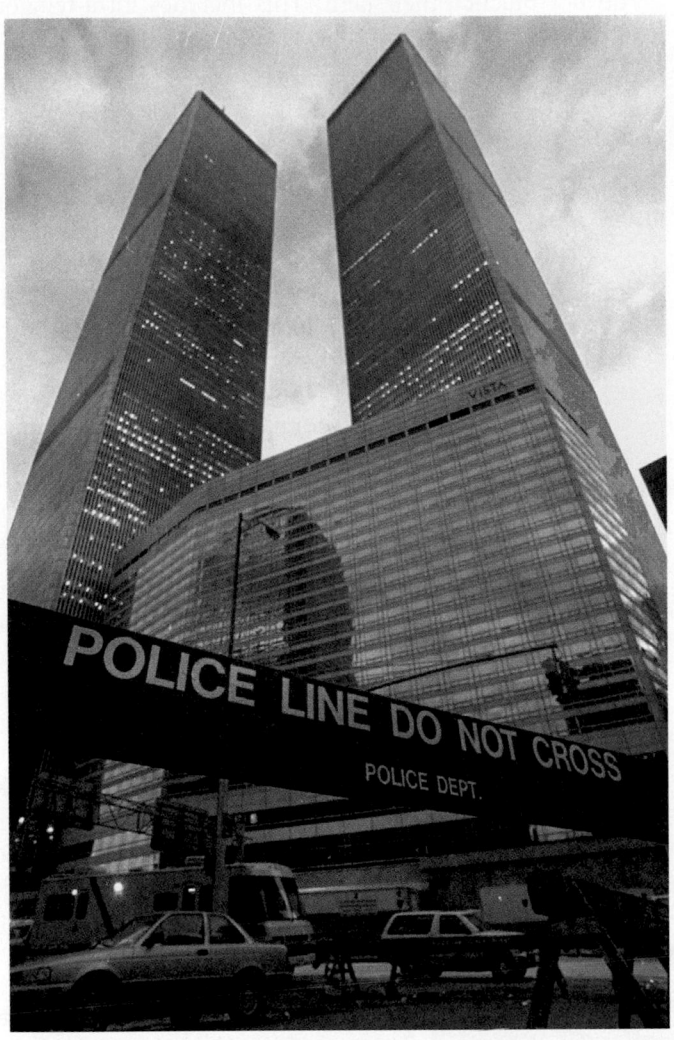

Figure 2 The terrorist attack on the World Trade Center in 1993.

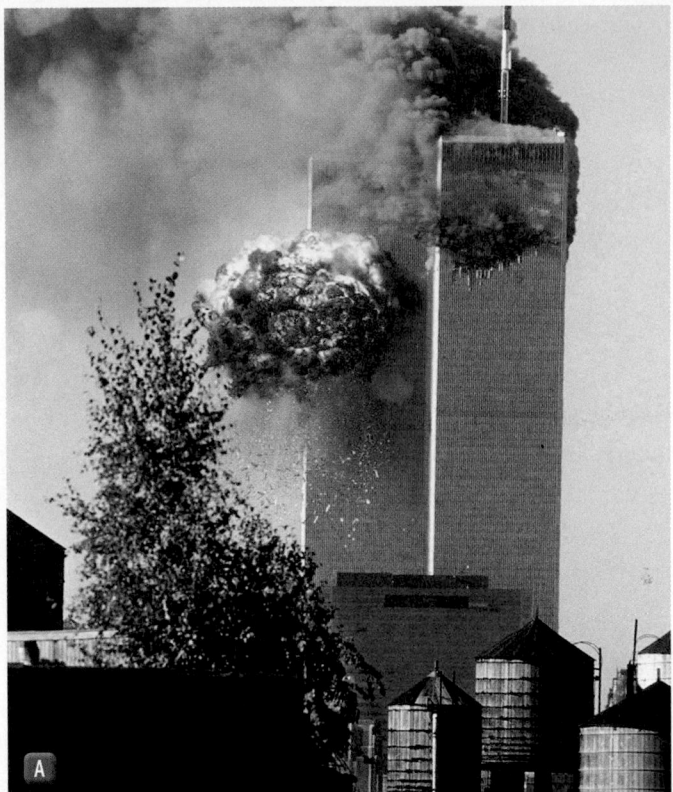

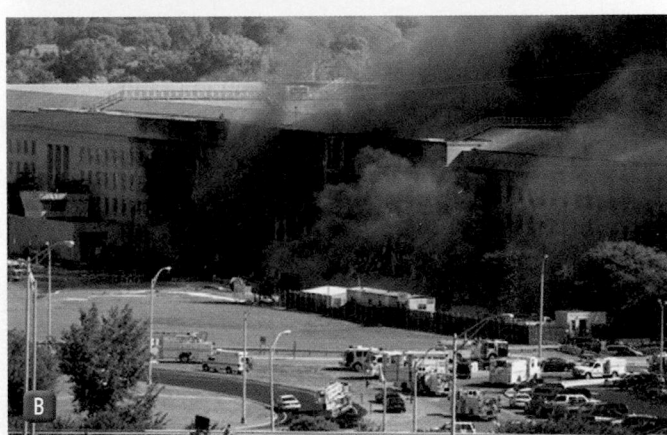

Figure 3 The September 11 attack on the World Trade Center accounted for the majority of the deaths caused by terrorists in 2001. **A.** The World Trade Center attack. **B.** The Pentagon attack.

Building in Oklahoma City in 1995 took the lives of 168 people, including 19 children **Figure 5**. These are early examples of domestic terrorist attacks. Post-9/11, there have been several domestic terrorist attacks in the United Kingdom, and a number of small-scale successful, failed, or thwarted plots in the US. Examples include the following events:

- The thwarted 2006 Sears Tower plot
- The thwarted 2006 Toledo, Ohio, terror plot
- 2007 Fort Dix, New Jersey, attack plot
- 2008 bombing of Armed Forces recruiting office in Times Square
- 2009 Fort Hood, Texas, shooting that killed 13 people and wounded 30 others
- 2009 Little Rock, Arkansas, Armed Forces recruiting office shooting that killed one recruiter and injured a second recruiter
- The thwarted 2009 New York subway and United Kingdom plots
- The failed 2010 Times Square car bombing
- 2010 Austin, Texas IRS office attack that killed one worker and the suicide attacker who flew his plane into the building

- The failed 2010 Portland, Oregon, car bomb plot
- 2011 mail bombings of two Maryland government buildings

These are just a few examples of domestic terror attacks and plots involving US citizens or legal residents.

Types of Terrorist Organizations

Terrorist organizations generally can be categorized as one or more of the following:

1. **Violent religious groups/doomsday cults.** These groups are especially dangerous because they often seek <u>apocalyptic violence</u> or mass murder as a means to their ends.

They see other religions or "nonbelievers" as worthy targets for death, and part of their apocalyptic doctrine is to eradicate or cleanse a region (or the entire earth) of those who

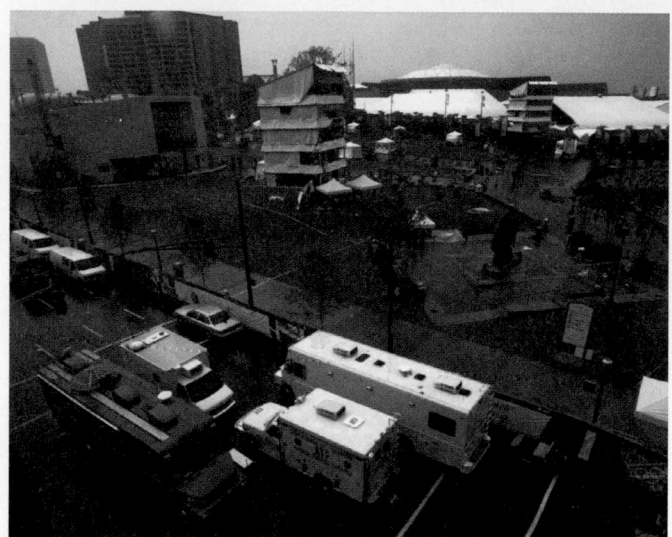

Figure 4 Domestic terrorists bombed the Centennial Olympic Park in Atlanta during the 1996 Summer Olympics.

do not practice their faith. This includes intra-religious terrorism, between two different sects of the same religion (such as Shiite vs. Sunni Muslims). These groups include terrorist organizations such as Aum Shinrikyo, who carried out sarin chemical attacks in Tokyo between 1994 and 1995.

2. **Extremist political/social groups.** These include violent separatist groups and those who seek political, economic, or social freedom. They may also seek to kill or evict foreigners, migrants, or those with different ethnic, racial, sociologic (poor or lower class), and/or cultural backgrounds from their region. They often use terror to influence economic or immigration politics and the drawing or redrawing of geopolitical borders to claim or reclaim land.

3. **Technology or "cyber" terrorists.** These groups attack a technologic infrastructure (power grid, Internet, intranet, telecommunications) using technology as a means to draw attention to their cause. Common methods used by these terrorists include "hacking" (gaining illegal access) into computer systems, and introducing corruptive computer programs such as viruses, worms, and "Trojan horses." These terrorists seek to extract valuable information stored in the computer systems, but may also seek to do harm to not just the computers but also the machines or processes that they control (security systems, mechanized work, electrical power). These attacks can be extremely difficult to detect early (if at all), and to shut down. Due to the level of sophistication of these types of attacks, these terrorists generally work in groups, take advantage of unsecured networks, and can even use an unsuspecting person's computer to launch an attack.

4. **Single-issue terrorist groups.** These include anti-abortion groups, animal rights groups, anarchists, racists, or even eco-terrorists who threaten or use violence as a means to advance their views or goals. These groups often represent the violent fringe or a splinter group of a legitimate non-violent group or movement that seeks to effect change through legal and socially acceptable means. However, if such non-violent methods are seen as ineffective, or time-consuming, or if there is a disagreement in methodology or philosophy

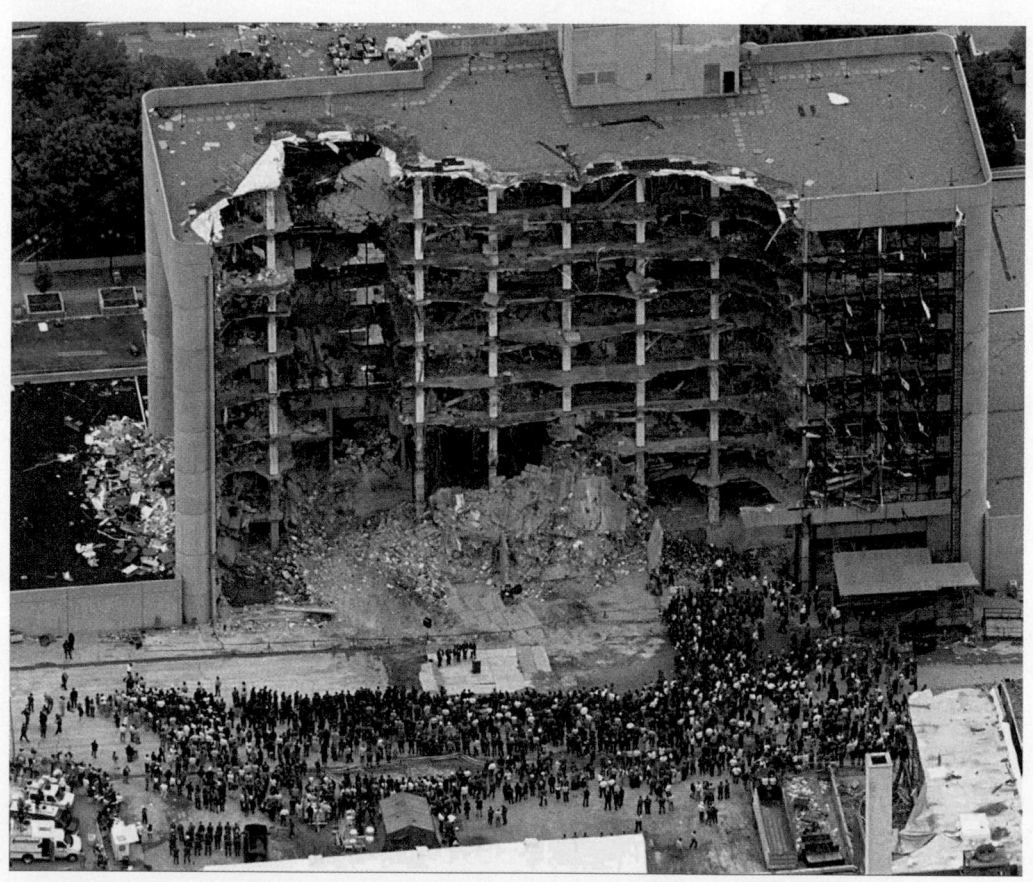

Figure 5 Domestic terrorists bombed the Alfred P. Murrah Federal Building in Oklahoma City in 1995.

between factions in the group, a smaller group may break off and look toward violence for a more immediate and effective response to their demands.

5. **Narcoterrorists.** Narcoterrorism is the use of terror to take control of a region, its politics, or government with the goal of manufacturing, distributing, and selling (trafficking) drugs without prosecution. They often target military, police, and anti-drug politicians or government officials (and their families), as well as innocent civilians in an effort to gain control over an entire region, usurping the power of the local authority. As a result of the revenue of the drugs that they manufacture and/or distribute, these groups are generally more heavily armed, organized, and funded than the local authorities. As such, they exert disproportionate and massive amounts of regional control. Other terrorist groups, such as extremist political or violent religious organizations, often use the drug trade to fund their terrorist activities. However, strictly speaking this would not classify as narcoterrorism, because they are not using terror for the furtherance of drug distribution.

Additional subcategories of terrorist groups include the following:

- **Hate groups.** Examples include the Ku Klux Klan, Skinheads, Neo-Nazis, Black Separatist, Neo-Confederates, and others targeting single issues such as homosexuality or affirmative action.
- **Patriot groups.** These frequently overlap with some of the hate groups.
- **Militia groups.** Minutemen, usually against central government, sometimes calling for secession of their states from the union.
- **Common-law groups.** Freeman; groups that distrust all government.
- **Cult groups.** Varied, many times religious-based doctrine.
- **Single-issue groups.** Fringe members of a group that is not a terrorist group, and who may commit terrorist acts, for example against animal laboratories.
- **Lone wolves.** Examples include people such as Ted Kaczynski (Unabomber) and Eric Rudolph (Olympic Park Bomber). These persons are extremely hard to detect and deter due to the lack of ties to an "umbrella" organization.

Terrorist groups may exhibit traits of several of these groups or even join forces with other groups that use different methods but strive for the same goals or wish to attack the same target. For example, a narcoterrorist group may join forces with technology terrorists or independently initiate a cyber attack on law enforcement's computer systems to eliminate records or gain information.

Al Qaeda is the most infamous international terrorist organization. Their influence and membership has spread across the Middle East over the last two decades, leading to multiple Al Qaeda offshoots or affiliated branches. The hallmark of these groups is violent, simultaneous, coordinated attacks. This is primarily meant to confuse, spread thin, and overwhelm emergency response to the incidents, but also to boast the level of sophistication and planning that they have put into committing the acts. These groups exhibit trends toward apocalyptic violence to affect a combination of political, geopolitical, and religious goals.

Terrorist organizations thrive in regions with weak or corrupt regional governments. This is an ideal environment for them to train terrorist recruits, store equipment, and plan and operate effectively. As such, many of these groups look to establish training camps and bases of operation in remote, austere locations where they can function with impunity, as well as protect themselves using **guerilla warfare** tactics.

Most terrorist attacks require precise coordination between multiple terrorists or "actors" working together. Recruiters identify willing actors and bring them into the organization, where they are trained, financed, and provided equipment and intelligence on their target(s), as well as transportation and often lodging. Twenty terrorists worked together to commit the worst act of terror in United States history on September 11, 2001, but there were dozens more people directly and indirectly involved in planning and helping to execute the attacks. Four terrorists worked together to carry out the London subway bombings on July 7, 2005, but many more were involved in their training, financing, and planning. However, in a few instances there has been a single "actor" terrorist who has struck with devastating results. Examples of terrorists who acted alone include those who carried out the Atlanta abortion clinic attacks, the 1996 Summer Olympics attack, and the Oklahoma City bombing.

Paramedic Response to Terrorism

Recognizing a Terrorist Event (Indicators)

Most acts of terror are **covert**, which means that the public safety community generally has no prior knowledge of the time, location, or nature of the attack. This element of surprise makes responding to an event more complex. You must constantly be aware of your surroundings and understand the possible risks for terrorism associated with certain locations, at certain times. It is therefore important that you know what locations or events in your jurisdiction would be considered high-value targets for terrorists. Examples of potential high-value targets for terrorists include the following:

- Military bases/installations and military recruiting centers
- Rail and metro transport systems
- Large bus depots
- Airports/seaports
- Chemical plants/chemical transfer stations or chemical transportation (pipelines, rail)
- Petrochemical (gasoline, natural gas, liquid natural gas) storage or transportation
- Dams and reservoirs
- Bio labs
- All large gathering spaces/places (stadiums, sporting arenas, parade routes)
- Government buildings (court houses, federal buildings, public safety headquarters)
- Hospitals (as secondary attack locations)

- Large religious venues (church, mosque, temple, synagogue)
- Large shopping centers and malls
- Large demonstrations or rallies
- Large financial centers (financial markets or exchanges)
- National symbols (monuments or memorials)

It is important to understand the **National Terrorism Advisory System (NTAS)**, which replaced the color-coded Homeland Security Advisory System that had been instituted in 2002 by the federal government through the Department of Homeland Security (DHS). NTAS alerts apply to threats to the United States and its territories. The NTAS alerts responders to the potential for an attack, and, as far as practicable, will give specifics of the current threat. If the information is available, the NTAS alert will provide specific details related to who will be potentially affected, such as the geographic area, transportation concerns, and the nature of the threat. It will also include steps that people or communities can take to protect themselves in response to the threat. The advisory will specify whether the threat is **elevated** (there is no specific information about the timing or location), or **imminent** (the threat is believed to be impending or expected to occur soon). The alert will be publically announced via posting at DHS.gov/alerts and releasing the alert to the news media. DHS will also distribute alerts via social media such as Facebook and Twitter. Updated NTAS alerts are issued if information related to the threat changes; updated alerts are distributed in the same manner as initial alerts. Alerts are automatically canceled on a designated expiration date.

The DHS has not issued specific recommendations for EMS personnel to follow in response to the alert system. Follow your local protocols, policies, and procedures. It is your responsibility to make sure you know the threat level at the start of your workday. Many EMS organizations are starting to display the NTAS system on boards where they can be seen by staff when they arrive for a shift. On the basis of the current information available, take appropriate actions and precautions while continuing to perform daily duties and responding to calls.

Understanding and being aware of the current threat is only the beginning of responding safely to calls. Once you are on duty, you must be able to make appropriate decisions regarding the potential for a terrorist event. In determining the potential for a terrorist attack, on every call you should observe the following:

- **Pre-incident indicators.** Has the NTAS posted a threat warning? Has there been a recent increase in violent political activism? Are you aware of any credible threats made against the location, gathering, or occasion?
- **Type of location.** Is the location a monument, infrastructure, government building, or a specific type of location such as a temple? Is there a large gathering such as a parade or political demonstration? Is there a special event taking place such as a college football game?
- **Type of call.** Is there a report of an explosion or suspicious device nearby? Does the call come into dispatch as someone having unexplained coughing and difficulty breathing? Are there reports of people fleeing the scene?
- **Number of patients.** Are there multiple patients with similar signs and symptoms? This is probably the single

most important clue that a terrorist attack or an incident involving a WMD has occurred.

- **Victims' statements.** This is probably the second best indication of a terrorist or WMD event. Are the patients fleeing the scene giving statements such as, "Everyone is passing out," "There was a loud explosion," or "There are a lot of people shaking on the ground." If so, something is occurring that you do not want to rush into, even if it is determined not to be a terrorist event.

Words of Wisdom

One of the easiest ways for you to distinguish between a nonterrorist multiple-casualty event and a terrorist event is that the intentional use of a WMD affects multiple persons. These casualties will generally exhibit the same signs and symptoms. It is highly unlikely for more than one person to experience a seizure at any given time. It is not uncommon to find multiple patients complaining of difficulty breathing at the scene of a fire. However, the same report in the subway at rush hour, when no smell of smoke has been reported, is certainly cause for suspicion. In these situations, you must use good judgment and resist the urge to "rush in and help," especially when there are multiple victims from an unknown cause.

▮ Response Actions

Once you suspect that a terrorist event has occurred or a WMD has been used, there are certain actions to take to ensure that you will be safe and be in the proper position to help the community:

- Ensure scene safety and personal safety
- Notify your dispatch and/or supervisor of the incident
- Request additional/specialized resources
- Establish command
- Initiate multiple-casualty incident procedures

Scene Safety

Ensure that the scene is safe. If you have any doubt that it may not be safe, do not enter. When you are dealing with a WMD scene, it is safe to assume that you will not be able to enter where the event has occurred—nor do you want to. The best location for staging is upwind and uphill from the incident. Wait for assistance from those who are trained in assessing and managing WMD scenes. Also remember the following:

- Failure to park your vehicle at a safe location can place you and your partner in danger **Figure 6** .
- If your vehicle is blocked in by other emergency vehicles or damaged by a secondary device (or event), you will be unable to provide patients with transportation, or escape yourself **Figure 7** .

Responder Safety (Personal Protection)

Emergency response by its nature is a dangerous profession; it is associated with exposure to a multitude of occupational hazards from ergonomics (lifting and carrying), to workplace violence, hazardous materials (HazMat), and vehicle crashes, to name just a few. Each day paramedics operate on the scene of hazardous and potentially life-threatening scenes, often without significant injuries or loss of life. However, when emergency workers respond to the scene of a major terrorist incident, research shows that responder health and safety suffer greatly. The uniqueness and uncertainty of terrorist and WMD incidents can cloud the decision-making process, and paramedics can develop tunnel vision—a situation in which a person does not see the overall picture, but focuses on only one aspect of it.

At large-scale events, you will arrive well before environmental health personnel or trained health and safety professionals arrive. For this reason, you need the following key resources when responding to potentially hazardous scenes:

- Awareness of measures to take for self-preservation
- A culture of safety within your organization
- Previous knowledge, fit-testing, experience, and comfort using multiple types and brands of PPE
- The proper PPE
- Self-enforcement of all protective measures

The best form of protection from a WMD agent is preventing yourself from coming into contact with the agent. The greatest threats facing you in a WMD attack are contamination and **cross-contamination**. Contamination with an agent occurs when you have direct contact with the WMD or are exposed to it. Cross-contamination occurs when you come into contact with a contaminated person who has not yet been decontaminated. Decontamination of patients is an important part of medical management of patients who have been exposed to or contaminated with a chemical, biologic, radiologic, or nuclear agent, or an explosive. Decontamination is covered in the chapter, *Hazardous Materials*. If EMS personnel have been appropriately

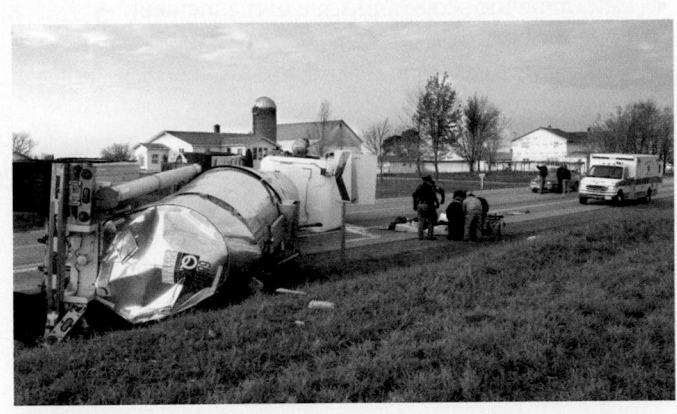

Figure 6 Park your vehicle at a safe location and distance.

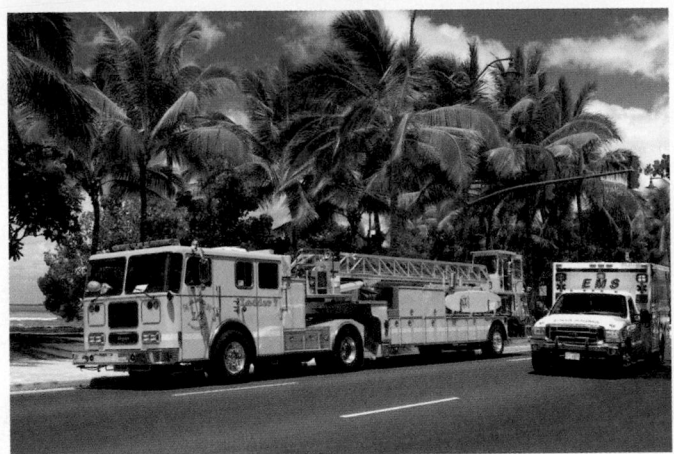

Figure 7 Make sure that your vehicle is not blocked in by other emergency vehicles.

YOU *are the Medic* | PART 2

Your partner quickly applies a nonrebreathing mask at 15 L/min while you begin your assessment. The patient is reporting chest pain and shortness of breath. You observe intercostal and supraclavicular retractions. Lung sounds are diminished but clear. The patient denies any past medical history or allergies to medications and is repeatedly asking you what happened.

Recording Time: 5 Minutes	
Respirations	28 breaths/min, shallow
Pulse	Radial pulse, 124 beats/min, regular and strong
Skin	Pink, warm, and dry
Blood pressure	172/86 mm Hg
Oxygen saturation (Spo$_2$)	96% on 15 L/min nonrebreathing mask
Pupils	Dilated, equal, and reactive to light

3. On the basis of the information you have, what do you think your patient was exposed to?

4. What should your initial treatment consist of?

trained in decontamination and have the appropriate PPE, they may be involved in decontamination per their protocols.

Notification Procedure/Resource Requests

When you suspect a terrorist or WMD event has taken place, notify the dispatcher, provided that communication is functioning properly. Vital information needs to be communicated effectively if you are to receive the appropriate assistance. Inform dispatch of the nature of the event, any additional resources that may be required, the estimated number of patients, and the upwind route of approach or optimal route of approach.

Words of Wisdom

IMPORTANT NOTE: In situations where there may be explosive agents present, paramedics are advised to restrict all radio and cell phone communications because they may trigger unexploded ordnance (weapons or other munitions or military equipment that may explode). Refer to your local or regional operations guidelines for response to suspicious packages or bomb threat procedures.

It is extremely important to establish a safe staging area where other units will converge. Be mindful of access and exit routes when you direct units to respond to a location. It is unwise to have units respond to the front entrance of a hotel or apartment building that has had an explosion, because perpetrators may plant secondary devices at entrances, expecting responders to enter there. Finally, trained responders in the proper protective equipment are the only persons equipped to handle the WMD incident. These specialized units, traditionally HazMat teams, must be requested as early as possible due to the time required to assemble and dispatch the team and their equipment. Many jurisdictions share HazMat teams, and the team may have to travel a long distance to reach the location of the event. It is always better to be safe than sorry; call the team early and the outcome of the call will be more favorable. Keep in mind that there may be more than one type of device or agent present.

Command

If the Incident Command System (ICS) is already in place, then you should immediately seek out the medical staging supervisor to receive your assignment.

The first arriving provider on the scene must begin to sort out the chaos and define his or her responsibilities under the ICS. As the first person on scene, the paramedic may need to establish "EMS or Medical Command" until additional personnel arrive. Depending on the circumstances, you and other paramedics may function as medical branch supervisors, triage supervisors, treatment supervisors, transportation or logistic supervisors, or staff. Generally, the most senior paramedic on the scene acts as the medical branch director until relieved by a supervisor or EMS physician. Initial tasks that the first arriving paramedic must perform are as follows:

- Report to incident command post (in unified command).
- Establish a medical branch under the operations section.

- Determine the scope and scale of the incident:
  - Type of incident
  - Hazards to responders and victims
  - Number of patients/deceased
  - Safe access, egress, and staging locations
  - Gather information on decontamination area(s), and hot, warm, and cold zones.
- Regularly gather and disseminate information to dispatch.
- Establish and assign a supervisor for the following areas:
  - Decontamination (if established)
  - Triage
  - Treatment
    - Minor/"walking wounded" (green tag)
    - Delayed (yellow tag)
    - Urgent (orange tag, used in some areas)
    - Immediate (red tag)
    - Deceased (black tag)
  - Transportation (departing units)
  - Staging (arriving personnel and units)
  - Rehabilitation (assessment and treatment for first responders only)
- Report all EMS activities to the operations section chief.

If the ICS is already in place, then you should immediately seek out the EMS staging supervisor to receive your assignment. The ICS and its components are discussed in further detail in the chapter, *Incident Management and Multiple-Casualty Incidents*.

Words of Wisdom

Secondary devices may include various types of electronic equipment such as cell phones or pagers that are detonated when "answered." They may also be set to a timer for when responders are anticipated to arrive. For these reasons, it is important that any uninjured person be directed from the scene to the triage area.

Paramedics should expect a heavy police presence at each EMS sector (treatment, triage, transportation). This is for several reasons:

1. To provide site security so that media and onlookers do not mingle with the wounded and interfere with their care.
2. To monitor all victims in the event the perpetrator or an accomplice (such as a look-out or secondary attacker) may be among the injured.
3. To canvas witnesses who may have valuable information.

Words of Wisdom

You are of no help to the public if you become a patient. More importantly, once you become a victim of the event, you place an additional burden on your fellow responders, who must treat you. Assess the scene and resist the urge to run in and help (do not develop tunnel vision). You may place your life and your partner in danger. Remember . . . do not become a victim.

Paramedics should fully comply with all law enforcement requests because they may be safety-related, or be intended to thwart additional planned attacks. Investigators may interview patients during triage or treatment, or ride along with them to the hospital to gather information on what they saw or know.

Secondary Device or Event (Reassessing Scene Safety)

Terrorists have been known to plant additional explosives that are set to explode after the initial bomb. This type of __secondary device__ is intended primarily to injure responders and to secure media coverage, because the media generally arrives on scene just after the initial response. Do not rely on others to secure your safety. It is every paramedic's responsibility to constantly assess and reassess the scene for safety. It is easy to overlook a suspicious package lying on the floor while you are treating casualties. Stay alert. Something as subtle as a change in the wind direction during a gas attack or an increase in the number of contaminated patients can place you in danger. Never become so involved with the tasks that you are performing that you do not look around and make sure that the scene remains safe.

Weapons of Mass Destruction

A __weapon of mass destruction (WMD)__ is anything used as a weapon designed to bring about mass death, casualties, and/or massive damage to property and infrastructure (bridges, tunnels, airports, and seaports). WMDs can be grouped into four major categories: explosive/incendiary devices, chemical, biologic, and radiologic/nuclear weapons and can include poison gas, grenades, rockets or missiles with a propellant charge or explosive, or a mine or similar device. To date, the preferred WMD for terrorists has been explosive devices. Terrorist groups have favored tactics that use truck or car bombs or pedestrian suicide bombers. Previous terrorist attempts to use either chemical or biologic weapons to their full capacity have been unsuccessful. Nonetheless, as a paramedic you should understand the destructive potential of these weapons, and be aware of the clinical symptomology that patients who have been exposed or infected with them may present with.

As discussed earlier, the motives and tactics of new-age terrorist groups have begun to change. As with doomsday cults, many terrorist groups participate in apocalyptic, indiscriminate killing. This doctrine of total carnage would make the use of WMDs highly desirable. WMDs are easy to obtain or create and are specifically geared toward killing large numbers of people. Had the proper techniques been used during the 1995 attack on the Tokyo subway, there may have been tens of thousands of casualties. With the fall of the former Soviet Union, the technology and expertise to produce WMDs may be available to terrorist groups with sufficient funding. Moreover, the technical recipes for making nuclear, biologic, and chemical (NBC) weapons and explosive devices can be found readily on the Internet; in fact, they have even been published on terrorist group websites.

The following sections describe the categories of WMDs that EMS personnel and their agencies should prepare to encounter in the field.

Explosives/Incendiary Weapons

Explosives are the most common weapon used by terrorists today **Figure 8**. Incendiary weapons involve agents and chemicals used to start fires. Incendiary agents, such as acetone, can be combined with chemicals to produce explosives capable of massive destruction. Ranging from suicide bombings on public buses to trucks loaded with explosives set to go off in underground parking garages of government buildings, these explosions can be destructive.

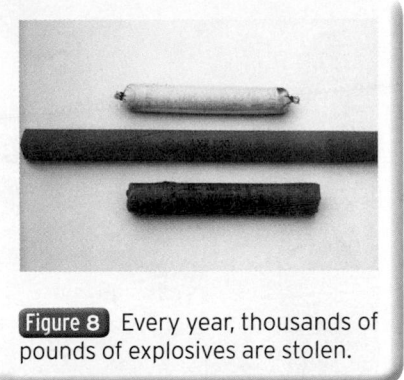

Figure 8 Every year, thousands of pounds of explosives are stolen.

Ammonium Nitrate or "Fertilizer" Bombs

__Ammonium nitrate__ is used commonly as an industrial-grade fertilizer that is not in itself dangerous to handle or transport. Yet in many regions, its sale and purchase requires a special license because when it is mixed with fuel such as diesel, and other easy to acquire components, it forms an extremely explosive compound. The attack on the Alfred P. Murrah Federal Building in Oklahoma City in 1995 (one of the deadliest terrorist attacks in the US) involved a homemade explosive device made from an ammonium nitrate and fuel oil mixture (ANFO). The perpetrators of that incident packed a van with 7,000 lb of ANFO to destroy the Alfred P. Murrah Federal Building and severely damage most buildings in the immediate vicinity. In 1993, Al Qaeda attacked the World Trade Center using an ANFO bomb, killing six people and wounding over 1,000.

Suicide Bombers (Human Bombs)

__Suicide bombers__ are by far the weapon of choice for modern-day terrorists. This concept merges the destructive power of military-grade explosives with the timing and accuracy of human guidance and triggering **Figure 9**. They are a low-cost, low-technology, and low-risk weapon. Weapons used by suicide bombers are easily concealed, carried, and delivered with accuracy to a selected target. Recruits for suicide bomb terrorism are readily available; they require little training and are generally deeply committed to killing others as well as themselves. In addition to men, women and children have acted as suicide bombers, making them even more difficult to prevent. Suicide bombers rely on the element of surprise and familiarity with the targeted area.

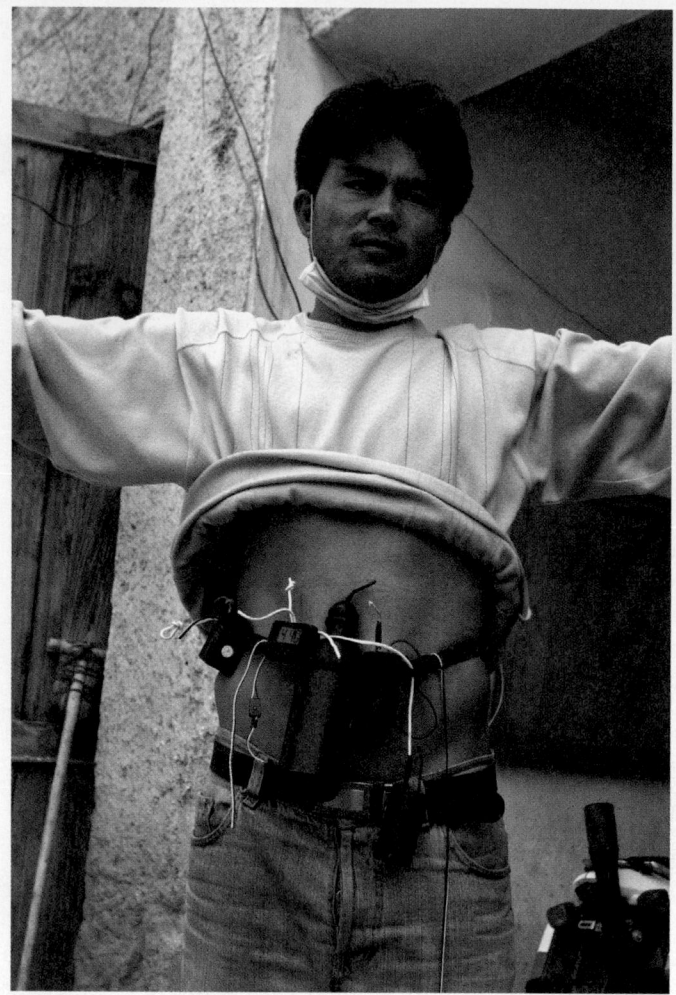

Figure 9 A suicide bomber merges the destructive power of explosives with human guidance and triggering.

In addition to their tactical advantages, suicide bombers' attacks are occasionally recorded by the terrorist organization as propaganda and to perpetuate fear in the population. Outside of the United States, media outlets exhibit little self-censorship and often broadcast graphic terrorist attacks and videos made by terrorists. This helps to spread the message of terror.

Words of Wisdom

REMEMBER: Two of the most common blast injuries are tympanic membrane rupture and barotraumas (damage to the structures of the inner ear). These types of injures make it difficult or impossible to communicate with patients who have been near a bomb blast because they may be disoriented from vertigo (as a result of inner ear damage) or have a greatly diminished or absent hearing. You will need to be aware of this when triaging and treating these patients because patients may not respond as expected to questions or the situation that they are in.

Chemical Agents

Chemical agents are man-made substances that can have devastating effects on living organisms. They can be produced in liquid, powder, or vapor form depending on the desired route of exposure and dissemination technique and are dispersed to kill or injure. First developed during World War I, these agents have been implicated in thousands of deaths since being introduced on the battlefield, and since then have been used to terrorize civilian populations. These agents can be categorized as follows:

- Vesicants or blister agents (eg, mustard gas and lewisite)
- Respiratory or choking agents (eg, phosgene or chlorine)
- Nerve agents (eg, sarin, soman, tabun, or V agent)
- Metabolic or blood agents (eg, hydrogen cyanide, cyanogen chloride)
- Irritating agents (eg, mace, chloropicrin, tear gas, capsicum/pepper spray, and dibenzoxazepine)

During the Cold War, many of these agents were perfected and stockpiled. Whereas the United States has long renounced the use of chemical weapons, many nations still develop and stockpile them. These agents are deadly and pose a threat if acquired by terrorists.

Chemical weapons have several classifications. The properties or characteristics of an agent can be described as liquid, gas, or solid material. **Persistency** and **volatility** are terms used to describe how long the agent will stay on a surface before it evaporates. Persistent or nonvolatile agents can remain on a surface for long periods of time, usually longer than 24 hours. Nonpersistent or volatile agents evaporate relatively fast when left on a surface in the optimal temperature range. An agent that is described as highly persistent (such as VX, a nerve agent) can remain in the environment for weeks to months, whereas an agent that is highly volatile (such as sarin, also a nerve agent) will turn from liquid to gas (evaporate) within minutes to seconds.

Route of exposure is a term used to describe how the agent most effectively enters the body. Chemical agents can have either a vapor or **contact hazard**. Agents with a **vapor hazard** enter the body through the respiratory tract in the form of vapors. Agents with a contact hazard (or skin hazard) give off little vapor or no vapors and enter the body through the skin.

Vesicants (Blister Agents)

The primary route of exposure of blister agents, or **vesicants**, is the skin (contact); however, if vesicants are left on the skin or clothing long enough, they produce vapors that can enter the respiratory tract. Vesicants cause burn-like blisters to form on the patient's skin as well as in the respiratory tract. The vesicant agents consist of sulfur mustard (H), lewisite (L), and phosgene oxime (CX) (the symbols H, L, and CX are military designations for these chemicals). The vesicants usually cause the most damage to damp or moist areas of the body, such as the armpits, groin, and respiratory tract. Signs of vesicant exposure on the skin include the following:

- Skin irritation, burning, and reddening
- Immediate intense skin pain (with L and CX)

- Formation of large blisters
- Gray discoloration of skin (a sign of permanent damage seen with L and CX)
- Swollen and closed or irritated eyes
- Permanent eye injury (including blindness)

If vapors were inhaled, the patient may experience the following:

- Hoarseness and stridor
- Severe cough
- Hemoptysis (coughing up of blood)
- Severe dyspnea

Sulfur mustard (agent H) is a brownish, yellowish oily substance that is generally considered persistent. When released, sulfur mustard has the distinct smell of garlic or mustard and is quickly absorbed into the skin and/or mucous membranes. As the agent is absorbed into the skin, it begins an irreversible process of damage to the cells. Absorption through the skin or mucous membranes usually occurs within seconds, and damage to the underlying cells takes place within 1 to 2 minutes.

Sulfur mustard is considered a **mutagen**, which means that it mutates, damages, and changes the structures of cells. Eventually, cellular death will occur. On the surface, the patient will generally not produce any signs or symptoms until 4 to 6 hours after exposure (depending on concentration and amount of exposure) Figure 10 .

The patient will experience a progressive reddening of the affected area, which will gradually develop into large blisters. These blisters are similar in shape and appearance to those associated with thermal second-degree burns. The fluid within the blisters does not contain any of the agent; however, the skin covering the area is considered to be contaminated until decontamination by trained personnel has been performed.

Sulfur mustard also attacks vulnerable cells within the bone marrow and depletes the body's ability to reproduce white blood cells. As with burns, the primary complication associated with vesicant blisters is secondary infection. If the patient does survive the initial direct injury from the agent, the depletion of the white blood cells leaves the patient with a decreased resistance

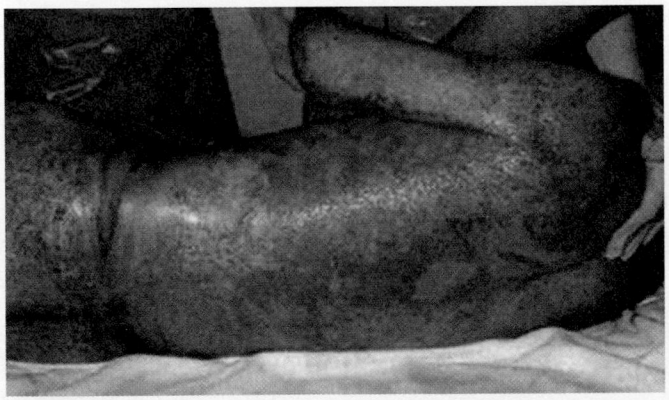

Figure 10 Skin damage resulting from exposure to sulfur mustard (agent H).

to infections. Although sulfur mustard is regarded as persistent, it does release enough vapors when dispersed to be inhaled. This creates upper and lower airway compromise. The result is damage and swelling of the airways. The airway compromise makes the patient's condition far more serious.

Lewisite (L) and **phosgene oxime (CX)** produce blister wounds similar to sulfur mustard. They are highly volatile and have a rapid onset of symptoms, as opposed to the delayed onset seen with sulfur mustard. These agents produce immediate intense pain and discomfort when contact is made. The patient may have a grayish discoloration at the contaminated site. While tissue damage also occurs with exposure to these agents, they do not cause the secondary cellular injury that is associated with sulfur mustard.

Vesicant Agent Treatment

There are no antidotes for sulfur mustard or CX exposure. BAL (British Anti-Lewisite) is the antidote for agent L; however, it is not carried by civilian EMS. You must ensure that the patient has been decontaminated (usually by soap and copious amounts of water) before ABCs are initiated. The patient may require prompt airway support if any agent has been inhaled, but this should not occur until after decontamination. Initiate transport and gain IV access as soon as possible. Generally, burn centers are best equipped to handle the wounds and subsequent infections produced by vesicants. Follow your local protocols when you are deciding what facility to transport the patient to.

■ Pulmonary Agents (Choking Agents)

The pulmonary agents are gases that cause immediate harm to persons exposed to them. The primary route of exposure for these agents is through the respiratory tract, which makes them an inhalation or vapor hazard. Once inside the lungs, they damage the lung tissue and fluid leaks into the lungs. Pulmonary edema develops in the patient, resulting in difficulty breathing due to the inability for air exchange. These agents produce respiratory-related symptoms such as dyspnea, tachypnea, and pulmonary edema. This class of chemical agents consists of **chlorine (CL)** and **phosgene**.

CL was the first chemical agent ever used in warfare. It has a distinct odor of bleach and creates a green haze when released as a gas. Initially it produces upper airway irritation and a choking sensation. The patient may later experience the following signs and symptoms:

- Shortness of breath
- Chest tightness
- Hoarseness and stridor due to upper airway constriction
- Gasping and coughing

With serious exposures, patients may experience pulmonary edema, complete airway constriction, and death. The fumes from a mixture of household bleach (CL) and ammonia create an acid gas that produces similar effects. Each year, such mixtures overcome hundreds of people when they try to mix household cleaners.

Phosgene should not be confused with phosgene oxime, a blistering agent, or vesicant. Not only has phosgene been produced for chemical warfare, but it is a product of combustion such as might be produced in a fire at a textile factory or house, or from metalwork or burning Freon (a liquid chemical used in refrigeration). Therefore, you may encounter a patient who was exposed to this gas during the course of a normal call or at a fire scene. Phosgene is a potent agent that has a delayed onset of symptoms, usually hours. Unlike CL, when phosgene enters the body, it generally does not produce severe irritation that might possibly cause the patient to leave the area or hold his or her breath. In fact, the odor produced by the chemical is similar to that of freshly mown grass or hay. The result is that much more of the gas is allowed to enter the body unnoticed. The initial symptoms of a mild exposure may include the following signs and symptoms:

- Nausea
- Chest tightness
- Severe cough
- Dyspnea on exertion

The patient with a severe exposure may present with dyspnea at rest and excessive pulmonary edema (the patient will actually expel large amounts of fluid from their lungs). The pulmonary edema that is seen with a severe exposure produces such large amounts of fluid from the lungs that the patient may actually become hypovolemic and subsequently hypotensive.

Pulmonary Agent Treatment

The best initial treatment for any pulmonary agent is to remove the patient from the contaminated atmosphere. This should be done by trained personnel in the proper PPE. Aggressive management of the ABCs should be initiated, paying particular attention to oxygenation, ventilation, and suctioning if required. Do not allow the patient to be active because this will worsen the condition much faster. There are no antidotes to counteract the pulmonary agents. Performing the ABCs, gaining IV access, allowing the patient to rest in a position of comfort with the head elevated, and initiating rapid transport are the primary goals for care provided in the prehospital setting. Pharmacotherapy of this patient may include the standard treatment for bronchospasm, pulmonary edema, potential corticosteroid use (per local medical direction), and positive-pressure ventilation with supplementary oxygen.

◼ Nerve Agents

The **nerve agents** are among the most deadly chemicals developed. Designed to kill large numbers of people with small quantities, nerve agents can cause cardiac arrest within seconds to minutes of exposure. Nerve agents, discovered while in search of a superior pesticide, are a class of chemical called **organophosphates**, which are found in household bug sprays, agricultural pesticides, and some industrial chemicals, at far lower strengths than in nerve agents.

There are almost 900 different pesticides available for use in the United States. Approximately 37 of these belong to a class of insecticides known as organophosphates. The chemicals in this class kill insects by disrupting their brains and nervous systems. Unfortunately, these chemicals or nerve agents (at greater strengths) also can harm the brains and nervous systems of animals and humans. These chemicals block the essential enzyme in the nervous system called cholinesterase from working, causing the body's organs to become overstimulated and burn out.

G agents came from the early nerve agents, the G series, which were developed by German scientists (hence the G) in the period after WWI and into WWII. There are three G series agents, which are all designed with the same basic chemical structure with slight variations to produce different properties. The two variations of these agents are lethality and volatility.

YOU are the Medic PART 3

While you are performing your primary assessment, the sector leader informs you that the HazMat team located an empty gas cylinder by the air intake of the air conditioning system and has confirmed the presence of cyanide. A few people from inside the courthouse described the odor as "almond-like." You obtain IV access in the right antecubital space with an 18-gauge angiocath and hang a bag of normal saline running it to keep the vein open. Before you can prepare any medications, the patient becomes unresponsive and hypotensive.

Recording Time: 10 Minutes	
Respirations	18 breaths/min, shallow
Pulse	Radial pulse, 116 beats/min, regular and weak
Skin	Pink, warm, dry
Blood pressure	92/56 mm Hg
Oxygen saturation (Spo$_2$)	96% on 15 L/min nonrebreathing mask
Pupils	Dilated, equal, and slow to react

5. Will the smell of almonds always be present with a cyanide exposure?

The following G agents are listed from high volatility to low volatility:

- **Sarin (GB)**. Highly volatile colorless and odorless liquid. Turns from liquid to gas within seconds to minutes at room temperature. Highly lethal, with an LD_{50} of 1,700 mg/70 kg (about 1 drop, depending on the purity). The **LD_{50}** is the amount that will kill 50% of people who are exposed to this level. GB is primarily a vapor hazard, with the respiratory tract as the main route of entry. This agent is especially dangerous in enclosed environments such as office buildings, shopping malls, or subway cars. When this agent comes into contact with skin, it is quickly absorbed and evaporates. When GB is on clothing, it has the effect of **off-gassing**, which means that the vapors are continuously released over a period of time (like perfume). This renders the patient as well as the patient's clothing contaminated.
- **Soman (GD)**. Twice as persistent as GB and five times as lethal. It has a fruity odor as a result of the type of alcohol used in the agent and generally has no color. GD is both a contact and inhalation hazard that can enter the body through skin absorption and through the respiratory tract. A unique additive in GD causes it to bind to the cells so that it attacks faster than any other agent. This irreversible binding is called aging, which makes it more difficult to treat patients who have been exposed.
- **Tabun (GA)**. Approximately half as lethal as GB and 36 times more persistent; under the proper conditions, it will remain for several days. It also has a fruity smell and an appearance similar to GB. The components used to manufacture GA are easy to acquire and the agent is easy to manufacture, which make it unique. GA is both a contact and inhalation hazard that can enter the body through skin absorption as well as through the respiratory tract.
- **V agent (VX)**. Clear oily agent that has no odor and looks like baby oil. VX was developed by the British after WWII and has similar chemical properties to the G series agents. The difference is that VX is over 100 times more lethal than GB and is extremely persistent **Figure 11**. In fact, VX is so persistent that given the proper conditions it will remain relatively unchanged for weeks to months. These properties make VX primarily a contact hazard because it lets off little vapor. It is easily absorbed into the skin, and the oily residue that remains on the skin's surface is extremely difficult to decontaminate.

Nerve agents all produce similar symptoms but have varying routes of entry. Nerve

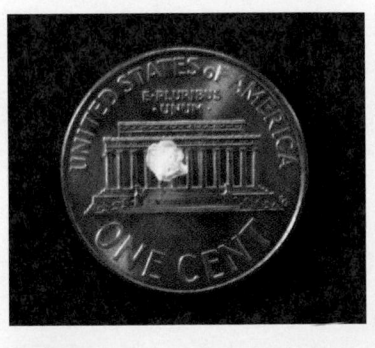

Figure 11 VX is the most toxic chemical ever produced. The dot on the penny demonstrates the amount needed to achieve the lethal dose.

agents differ slightly in lethal concentration or dose and also differ in their volatility. Some agents are designed to become a gas quickly (nonpersistent or highly volatile), whereas others remain liquid for a period of time (persistent or nonvolatile). These agents have been used successfully in warfare and to date represent the only type of chemical agent that has been used successfully in a terrorist act. Once the agent has entered the body through skin contact or through the respiratory system, the patient will begin to exhibit a pattern of predictable symptoms. Like all chemical agents, the severity of the symptoms will depend on the route of exposure and the amount of agent to which the patient was exposed. The resulting symptoms are described using the military mnemonic SLUDGEM and the medical mnemonic DUMBELS. These two mnemonics are used to describe the symptoms of nerve agent exposure and are shown in **Table 1**. The medical mnemonic is more useful to you because it lists the more dangerous symptoms associated with exposure to nerve agents.

There are only a handful of medical conditions that are associated with the bilateral pinpoint constricted pupils (**miosis**) seen with nerve agent exposure. Conditions such as a suspected stroke, basilar skull fracture, direct light to both eyes, and an opiate drug overdose all can cause bilateral constricted pupils. You should therefore assess the patient for all of the SLUDGEM/DUMBELS signs and symptoms to determine whether the patient has been exposed to a nerve agent.

Miosis is the most common symptom of nerve agent exposure and can remain for days to weeks. This symptom, along with

Table 1	Symptoms of Persons Exposed to Nerve Agents
Military Mnemonic: SLUDGEM	
S	Salivation
L	Lacrimation
U	Urination
D	Defecation
G	GI distress
E	Emesis
M	Miosis
Medical Mnemonic: DUMBELS	
D	Defecation
U	Urination
M	Miosis
B	Bradycardia, Bronchorrhea
E	Emesis
L	Lacrimation
S	Salivation

the others listed in Table 1, will help you recognize exposure to a nerve agent early. The seizures that are associated with nerve agent exposure are unlike those found in patients with a history of seizure. The patient will continue to seize until death or until treatment is given with a nerve agent antidote (DuoDote or MARK 1).

Nerve Agent Treatment

Fatalities from severe exposure occur as a result of respiratory complications, which lead to respiratory arrest. Once the patient has been decontaminated, you should be prepared to treat these patients aggressively, if they are to be saved. You can greatly increase the patient's chances of survival simply by providing airway and ventilatory support. As with all emergencies, managing the ABCs is the best and most important treatment that you can provide. Often patients exposed to these agents will begin seizing and will not stop. These patients will require administration of nerve agent antidote kits in addition to support of the ABCs.

Fortunately, there is an antidote for nerve agent exposure. The DuoDote Antidote Kit contains a single injection of both atropine (2 mg) and 2-PAM chloride (pralidoxime chloride) (600 mg). You may also have access to a MARK 1 kit, also known as Nerve Agent Antidote Kits (NAAK), but these kits are no longer made. The MARK 1 kit contains the same medications that are in the DuoDote Antidote Kit (atropine and 2-PAM chloride), but they are administered with two separate auto-injectors. In some regions, paramedics may carry DuoDote or MARK 1 kit on the unit and will be called on to administer it. These medications are delivered using the same technique as the EpiPen auto-injector; however, multiple doses may need to be administered. Also, a benzodiazepine may need to be administered due to the concurrent seizure activity.

Atropine is used to block the nerve agent's overstimulation of the body. However, because the nerve agent may remain in the body for long periods of time, 2-PAM chloride is used to eliminate the agent from the body. The 2-PAM antidote is effective at relieving the respiratory muscle paralysis and twitching caused by the nerve agent. Many of the symptoms described in the DUMBELS mnemonic will be reversed with the use of atropine; however, many doses may need to be administered to see these results. If your service carries a NAAK, please refer to your medical director and local protocols for dose and usage information.

Table 2 has been provided for quick reference and comparison of the nerve agents.

Industrial Chemicals/Insecticides

As previously mentioned, the basic chemical ingredient in nerve agents is organophosphate. This is a common chemical that is used in lesser concentrations for insecticides. Whereas industrial chemicals do not possess sufficient lethality to be effective WMDs, they are easy to acquire, inexpensive, and would have similar effects as the nerve agents. Crop-duster planes could be used to disseminate these chemicals. You should be cautious when you are responding to calls where insecticide equipment is stored and used, such as a farm or supply store that sells these products. The symptoms and medical management of patients poisoned by organophosphate insecticide are identical to those of the nerve agents.

Metabolic Agents (Cyanides)

Hydrogen cyanide (AC) and cyanogen chloride (CK) are both agents that affect the body's ability to use oxygen. Cyanide is a colorless gas that has an odor similar to almonds. The effects of the cyanides begin on the cellular level and are rapidly seen at the organ system level. Beside the nerve agents, metabolic agents are the only chemical weapons known to kill within seconds to minutes. Unlike nerve agents, however, these deadly gases

Table 2 Nerve Agents

Name	Code Name	Odor	Special Features	Onset of Symptoms	Volatility	Route of Exposure
Tabun	GA	Fruity	Easy to manufacture	Immediate	Low	Both contact and vapor hazard
Sarin	GB	None (if pure) or strong	Will off-gas while on victim's clothing	Immediate	High	Primarily respiratory vapor hazard; extremely lethal if skin contact is made
Soman	GD	Fruity	Ages rapidly, making it difficult to treat	Immediate	Moderate	Contact with skin; minimal vapor hazard
V agent	VX	None	Most lethal chemical agent; difficult to decontaminate	Immediate	Very low	Contact with skin; no vapor hazard (unless aerosolized)

are commonly found in many industrial settings. Cyanides are produced in massive quantities throughout the United States every year for industrial uses such as gold and silver mining, photography, lethal injections, and plastics processing. They are often present in fires associated with textile or plastic factories. In fact, cyanide is naturally found in the pits of many fruits in low doses. There is little difference in the symptoms found between AC and CK. In low doses, these chemicals are associated with dizziness, light-headedness, headache, and vomiting. Higher doses will produce symptoms that include the following:

- Shortness of breath and gasping respirations
- Tachypnea
- Flushed skin color
- Tachycardia
- Altered mental status
- Seizures
- Coma
- Apnea
- Cardiac arrest

Words of Wisdom

Always make sure your patients have been thoroughly decontaminated by trained personnel before you come into contact with them. Chemical agents are primarily a vapor hazard, and all of the patient's clothing must be removed to prevent off-gassing. Finally, never perform mouth-to-mouth or mouth-to-mask ventilation on a victim of a chemical agent. Many of the vapors may linger in the patient's airway, and cross-contamination may occur.

The symptoms associated with the inhalation of a large amount of cyanide will all appear within several minutes. Death is likely unless the patient is treated promptly.

Cyanide Agent Treatment Cyanide binds with the body's cells, preventing oxygen from being used. Several medications act as antidotes, but many services do not carry them. Once trained personnel wearing the proper PPE have removed the patient from the source of exposure, even if there is no liquid contamination, all of the patient's clothes must be removed to prevent off-gassing in the ambulance. Trained and protected personnel must decontaminate any patients who may have been exposed to liquid contamination before you can initiate treatment. Then you should support the patient's ABCs and gain IV access. Mild effects of cyanide exposure will generally resolve by simply removing the victim from the source of contamination and administering supplementary oxygen. Severe exposure, however, will require aggressive oxygenation and perhaps ventilation with supplementary oxygen. Always use a bag-mask device or oxygen-powered ventilator device to ventilate a patient exposed to a metabolic agent. The agent can easily be passed on from the patient to you through mouth-to-mouth or mouth-to-mask ventilations. If no antidote is available, initiate transport immediately.

Table 3 summarizes the chemical agents. The odors of the particular chemicals are provided for informational purposes only. The sense of smell is a poor tool to use to determine whether there is a chemical agent present. Many persons are unable to smell the agents, and the odor could be derived from another source. This information is useful to you if you receive reports from victims claiming to smell bleach or garlic, for example. You should never enter a potentially hazardous area and "smell" to determine whether a chemical agent is present.

■ Biologic Agents

Biologic agents are organisms that cause disease or death. They are generally found in nature; for terrorist use, however, they are cultivated, synthesized, and mutated in a laboratory. The **weaponization** of biologic agents is performed to artificially maximize the target population's exposure to the germ, thereby exposing the greatest number of people and achieving the desired result.

The primary types of biologic agents that you may come into contact with during a biologic event include the following:

- Viruses
- Bacteria
- Neurotoxins

Biologic agents pose many difficult issues when used as a WMD. Biologic agents can be almost completely undetectable. Also, most of the diseases caused by these agents will be similar to other minor illnesses commonly seen by paramedics.

Biologic agents may be spread in various ways. **Dissemination** is the means by which a terrorist will spread the agent—for example, poisoning the water supply or aerosolizing the agent into the air or ventilation system of a building. A **disease vector** is an animal that spreads disease, once infected, to another animal. For example, the plague can be spread by infected rats, smallpox by infected persons, and West Nile virus by infected mosquitoes. How easily the disease is able to spread from one human to another human is called **communicability**. Some diseases, such as those caused by human immunodeficiency virus (HIV), are difficult to spread by routine contact. Therefore, communicability is considered low. In other instances when communicability is high, such as with smallpox, the person is considered **contagious**. Typically, your standard precautions are enough to prevent contamination from contagious biologic organisms.

Incubation describes the period of time between the person becoming exposed to the agent and when symptoms begin. The incubation period is especially important for you to understand. Although your patient may not exhibit signs or symptoms, he or she may be contagious.

You need to be aware of when you should suspect the use of biologic agents. If the agent is in the form of a powder, such as in the October 2001 incidents involving anthrax powder mailed in letters, the call must be handled by HazMat specialists. Patients who have come into direct contact with the agent need to be decontaminated before any EMS contact or treatment is initiated.

Table 3 Chemical Agents

Class	Military Designations	Odor	Lethality	Onset of Symptoms	Volatility	Primary Route of Exposure
Vesicants	Mustard (H) Lewisite (L) Phosgene oxime (CX)	Garlic (H) Geranium (L)	Causes large blisters to form on victims; may severely damage upper airway if vapors are inhaled; severe intense pain and grayish skin discoloration (L, CX)	Delayed (H) Immediate (L, CX)	Very low (H, L) Moderate (CX)	Primarily contact; with some vapor hazard
Pulmonary agents	Chlorine (CL) Phosgene (CG)	Bleach (CL) Cut grass (CG)	Causes irritation; choking (CL); severe pulmonary edema (CG)	Immediate (CL) Delayed (CG)	Very high	Vapor hazard
Nerve agents	Tabun (GA) Sarin (GB) Soman (GD) V agent (VX)	Fruity or none	Most lethal chemical agents can kill within minutes; effects are reversible with antidotes	Immediate	Moderate (GA, GD) Very high (GB) Low (VX)	Vapor hazard (GB) Both vapor and contact hazard (GA, GD) Contact hazard (VX)
Cyanide agents	Hydrogen cyanide (AC) Cyanogen chloride (CK)	Almonds (AC) Irritating (CK)	Highly lethal chemical gases; can kill within minutes; effects are reversible with antidotes	Immediate	Very high	Vapor hazard

Viruses

Viruses are germs that require a living host to multiply and survive. A virus is a simple organism and cannot thrive outside of a host (living body). Once in the body, the virus will invade healthy cells and replicate itself to spread through the host. As the virus spreads, so does the disease that it carries. Viruses survive by moving from one host to another by using its transport system—vectors.

Viral agents that may be used during a biologic terrorist release pose an extraordinary problem for health care providers, especially those in EMS. Although some viral agents do have vaccines, there is no treatment for a viral infection other than antivirals for some agents. Because of this characteristic, the following viruses have been used as terrorist agents.

Smallpox

Smallpox is a highly contagious disease. All forms of standard precautions must be used to prevent cross-contamination to health care providers. Simply by wearing examination gloves, a HEPA-filtered respirator, and eye protection, you will greatly reduce your risk of contamination. The last natural case of smallpox in the world was seen in 1977. Before the rash and blisters show, the illness will start with a high fever and body aches and headaches. The patient's temperature is usually in the range of 101°F to 104°F.

An easy, quick way to differentiate the smallpox rash from other skin disorders is to observe the size, shape, and location of the lesions. In smallpox, all the lesions are identical in their development. In other skin disorders, the lesions will be in various stages of healing and development. Smallpox blisters also begin on the face and extremities and eventually move toward the chest and abdomen. The disease is in its most contagious phase when the blisters begin to form **Figure 12**. Unprotected contact with these blisters will promote transmission of the disease. There is a vaccine to prevent smallpox; however, it has been linked to medical complications and in rare cases, death **Table 4**. Vaccination against the disease is part of a national strategy to respond to a terrorist threat. Because the vaccine does have some risk, only first responders have been offered the vaccine. Should an outbreak occur, the vaccine would be offered to people at risk.

Viral Hemorrhagic Fevers

Viral hemorrhagic fevers (VHFs) consist of a group of diseases that include the Ebola, Rift Valley, and yellow fever viruses,

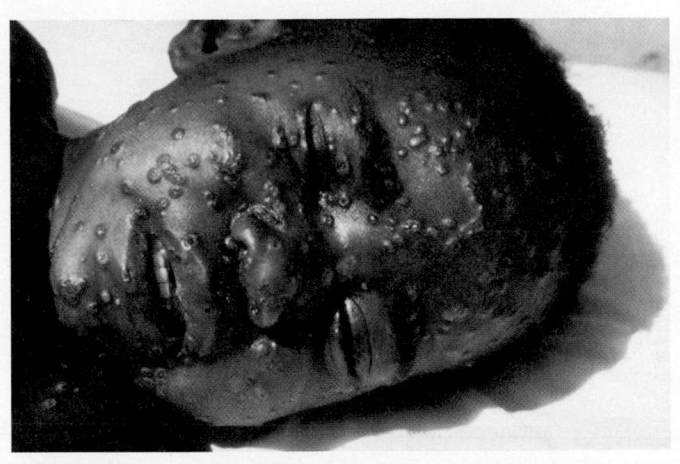

Figure 12 In smallpox, all the lesions are identical in their development. In other skin disorders, the lesions will be in various stages of healing and development.

among others. This group of viruses causes the blood in the body to seep out from the tissues and blood vessels **Figure 13**. Initially, the patient will have flu-like symptoms, progressing to more serious symptoms such as internal and external hemorrhaging. Outbreaks are not uncommon in Africa and South America. Outbreaks in the United States, however, are extremely rare. All standard precautions must be taken when you are treating these illnesses. Mortality rates can range from 5% to 90%, depending on the strain of virus, the patient's age and health condition, and the availability of a modern health care system **Table 5**.

■ Bacteria

Unlike viruses, **bacteria** do not require a host to multiply and live. Bacteria are much more complex and larger than viruses and can grow up to 100 times larger than the largest virus. Bacteria contain all the cellular structures of a normal cell and are completely self-sufficient. Most importantly, bacterial infections can be fought with antibiotics.

Table 4   **Characteristics of Smallpox**

Dissemination	Aerosolized for warfare or terrorist uses
Communicability	High from infected persons or items (such as blankets used by infected patients). Person-to-person transmission is possible.
Route of entry	Through inhalation of coughed droplets or direct skin contact with blisters.
Signs and symptoms	Severe fever, malaise, body aches, headaches, small blisters on the skin, bleeding of the skin and mucous membranes. Incubation period is 10 to 12 days and the duration of the illness is approximately 4 weeks.
Medical management	Standard precautions. There is no specific treatment for smallpox victims. Patients should be provided with supportive care (ABCs).

YOU *are the Medic*   PART 4

Your partner provides positive-pressure ventilation with a bag-mask device attached to 100% oxygen while you increase the flow of the IV line and prepare for intubation. The patient's airway is secured with a 7.5-mm ETT. Tube placement is confirmed with waveform capnography and the patient is manually ventilated by your partner. Per your protocols, you mix 5 g of hydroxocobalamin into a 250-mL bag of normal saline and set it to run over 15 minutes. After the hydroxocobalamin infusion is finished, you help prepare the patient for transport.

Recording Time: 15 Minutes	
Respirations	12 breaths/min, adequate depth and volume, manual ventilation
Pulse	Radial pulse, 114 beats/min, regular and weak
Skin	Pink, warm, and dry
Blood pressure	96/60 mm Hg
Oxygen saturation (Spo$_2$)	96% on 100% oxygen via bag-mask
Pupils	Dilated, equal, and slow to respond

6. **What is the treatment of choice for a patient with cyanide toxicity?**

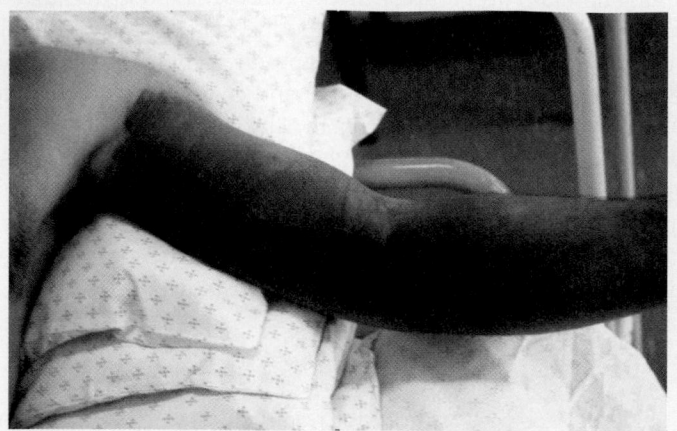

Figure 13 Viral hemorrhagic fevers cause the blood vessels and tissues to seep blood. The end result is ecchymosis, hemoptysis, and blood in the patient's stool. Notice the severe discoloration in this patient with Crimean Congo hemorrhagic fever, indicating internal bleeding.

Table 5	Characteristics of Viral Hemorrhagic Fevers
Dissemination	Direct contact with an infected person's body fluids. It can also be aerosolized for use in an attack.
Communicability	Moderate from person to person or from contaminated items.
Route of entry	Direct contact with an infected person's body fluids.
Signs and symptoms	Sudden onset of fever, weakness, muscle pain, headache, and sore throat. All of these symptoms are followed by vomiting and as the virus runs its course, internal and external bleeding.
Medical management	Standard precautions. There is no specific treatment for viral hemorrhagic fever. Patients should be provided supportive care (ABCs) and treatment for shock and hypotension, if present.

Most bacterial infections will generally begin with flu-like symptoms, which make it quite difficult to identify whether the cause is a biologic attack or a natural epidemic. Biologic agents have been developed and used for centuries during times of war.

Inhalation and Cutaneous Anthrax (*Bacillus anthracis*)

__Anthrax__ is a deadly bacterium that lies dormant in a spore (protective shell). When exposed to the optimal temperature and moisture, the germ will be released from the spore. The routes of entry for anthrax are inhalation, cutaneous, or gastro-intestinal (from consuming food that contain spores) **Figure 14**.

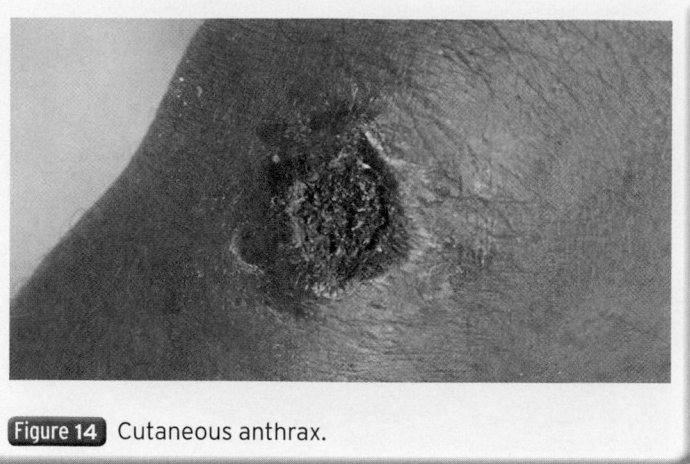

Figure 14 Cutaneous anthrax.

The inhalational form or pulmonary anthrax is the most deadly and often presents as a severe cold. Pulmonary anthrax infections are associated with a 90% death rate if untreated. Antibiotics can be used to treat anthrax successfully. There is also a vaccine to prevent anthrax infections **Table 6**.

Plague–Bubonic/Pneumonic

Of all the infectious diseases known to humans, none has killed as many as the plague. The 14th century plague that ravaged Asia, the Middle East, and finally Europe (the Black Death) killed an estimated 33 to 42 million people. Later on, in the early 19th century, almost 20 million people in India and China perished due to the plague. The plague's natural vectors are infected rodents and fleas. When a person is either bitten by an infected flea or comes into contact with an infected rodent (or the waste of the rodent), that person can contract bubonic plague.

__Bubonic plague__ infects the __lymphatic system__ (a passive circulatory system in the body that bathes the tissues in lymph and works with the immune system). When this occurs, the

Table 6	Characteristics of Anthrax	
Dissemination	Aerosol
Communicability	Only in the cutaneous form (rare)
Route of entry	Through inhalation of spore or skin contact with spore or direct contact with skin wound (cutaneous)
Signs and symptoms	Flu-like symptoms, fever, respiratory distress with tachycardia, shock, pulmonary edema and respiratory failure after 3 to 5 days of flu-like symptoms
Medical management	Pulmonary/inhalation: Standard precautions, supplemental oxygen, ventilatory support for pulmonary edema or respiratory failure, and transport. Cutaneous: Standard precautions, apply dry sterile dressing to prevent accidental contact with wound and fluids.

patient's <u>lymph nodes</u> (area of the lymphatic system where infection-fighting cells are housed) become infected and grow. The glands of the nodes will grow large (up to the size of a tennis ball) and round, forming <u>buboes</u> Figure 15 . If left untreated, the infection may spread through the body, leading to sepsis and possibly death. This form of plague is not contagious and is not likely to be seen in a bioterrorist incident.

Pneumonic plague is a lung infection, also known as plague pneumonia, which results from inhalation of plague bacteria. This form of the disease is contagious and has a much higher death rate than the bubonic form. This form of plague therefore would be easier to disseminate (aerosolized), has a higher mortality rate and is contagious Table 7 .

Neurotoxins

<u>Neurotoxins</u> are the most deadly substances known to humans. The strongest neurotoxin is 15,000 times more lethal than VX and 100,000 times more lethal than GB. These toxins are produced from plants, marine animals, molds, and bacteria. The route of entry for these toxins is through ingestion, inhalation from aerosols, or injection. Unlike viruses and bacteria, neurotoxins are not contagious and have a faster onset of symptoms. Although these biologic toxins have immense destructive potential, they have not been used successfully as a WMD.

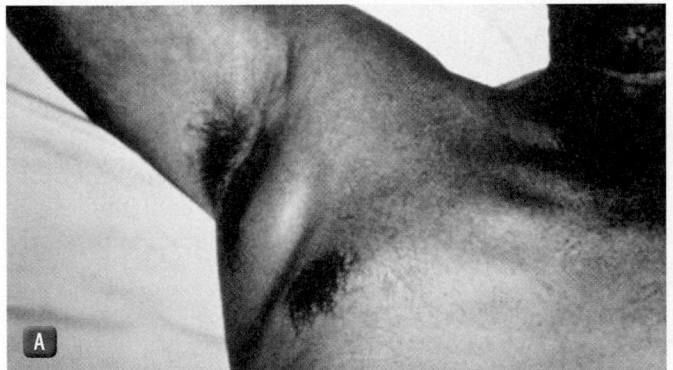

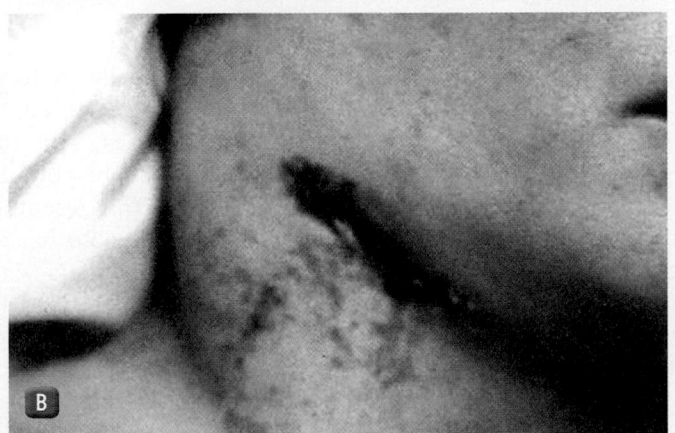

Figure 15 **A.** Plague buboe at lymph node under arm. **B.** Plague buboe at lymph node on neck.

Table 7 Characteristics of Plague

Dissemination	Aerosol
Communicability	Bubonic: Low, only from contact with fluid in buboe Pneumonic: High, from person to person
Route of entry	Ingestion, inhalation, or cutaneous
Signs and symptoms	Fever, headache, muscle pain and tenderness, pneumonia, shortness of breath, extreme lymph node pain and enlargement (bubonic)
Medical management	Standard precautions, ABCs, provide supplemental oxygen, and transport

Botulinum Toxin

The most potent neurotoxin is <u>botulinum</u>, which is produced by bacteria. When introduced into the body, this neurotoxin affects the nervous system's ability to function. Voluntary muscle control will diminish as the toxin spreads. Eventually the toxin will cause muscle paralysis that begins at the head and face and travels downward throughout the body. The patient's accessory muscles and diaphragm will become paralyzed, and the patient will go into respiratory arrest Table 8 .

Ricin

While not as deadly as botulinum, <u>ricin</u> is still five times more lethal than VX. This toxin is derived from mash that is left from the castor bean Figure 16 . When introduced into the body, ricin causes pulmonary edema and respiratory and circulatory failure, leading to death Table 9 .

The clinical picture depends on the route of exposure. The toxin is quite stable and extremely toxic by many routes of

Table 8 Characteristics of Botulinum Toxin

Dissemination	Aerosol or food supply sabotage or injection
Communicability	None
Route of entry	Ingestion or gastrointestinal
Signs and symptoms	Dry mouth, intestinal obstruction, urinary retention, constipation, nausea and vomiting, abnormal pupil dilation, blurred vision, double vision, drooping eyelids, difficulty swallowing, difficulty speaking, and respiratory failure due to paralysis
Medical management	ABCs, provide supplemental oxygen, and transport. Ventilatory support may be needed due to paralysis of the respiratory muscles. A vaccine is available.

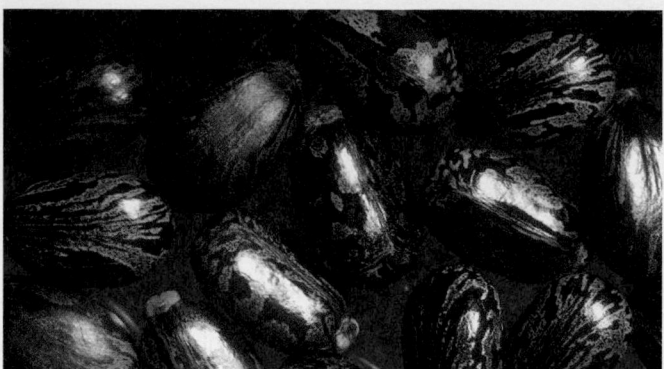

Figure 16 These seemingly harmless castor beans contain the key ingredient for ricin, one of the most potent toxins known to humans.

Table 9   **Characteristics of Ricin**

Dissemination	Aerosol or contamination of a food or water supply by sabotage
Communicability	None
Route of entry	Inhalation, ingestion, injection
Signs and symptoms	Inhaled: Cough, difficulty breathing, chest tightness, nausea, muscle aches, pulmonary edema, and hypoxia Ingested: Nausea and vomiting, internal bleeding, and death Injection: No signs except swelling at the injection site and death
Medical management	ABCs. No treatment or vaccine exists.

exposure, including inhalation. Perhaps 1 to 3 mg of ricin can kill an adult, and the ingestion of one seed can probably kill a child.

Although all parts of the castor bean are actually poisonous, it is the seeds that are the most toxic. Castor bean ingestion causes a rapid onset of nausea, vomiting, abdominal cramps, and severe diarrhea, followed by vascular collapse. Death usually occurs on the third day in the absence of appropriate medical intervention.

Ricin is least toxic by the oral route. This is probably a result of poor absorption in the gastrointestinal tract, some digestion in the gut, and, possibly, some expulsion of the agent as caused by the rapid onset of vomiting. Ingestion causes local hemorrhage and necrosis of the liver, spleen, kidneys, and gastrointestinal tract. Signs and symptoms appear 4 to 8 hours after exposure.

Signs and symptoms of ricin ingestion are as follows:

- Fever
- Chills
- Headache

- Muscle aches
- Nausea
- Vomiting
- Diarrhea
- Severe abdominal cramping
- Dehydration
- Gastrointestinal bleeding
- Necrosis of liver, spleen, kidneys, and gastrointestinal tract

Inhalation of ricin causes nonspecific weakness, cough, fever, hypothermia, and hypotension. Symptoms occur about 4 to 8 hours after inhalation, depending on the inhaled dose. The onset of profuse sweating some hours later signifies the termination of the symptoms.

Signs and symptoms of ricin inhalation are as follows:

- Fever
- Chills
- Nausea
- Local irritation of eyes, nose, and throat
- Profuse sweating
- Headache
- Muscle aches
- Nonproductive cough
- Chest pain
- Dyspnea
- Pulmonary edema
- Severe lung inflammation
- Cyanosis
- Convulsions
- Respiratory failure

Treatment is supportive and includes both respiratory support and cardiovascular support as needed. Early intubation, ventilation, and positive end-expiratory pressure, combined with treatment of pulmonary edema, are appropriate. IV fluids and electrolyte replacement are useful for treating the dehydration caused by profound vomiting and diarrhea. **Table 10** summarizes the biologic agents.

Other Paramedic Roles During a Biologic Event

Syndromic Surveillance

Syndromic surveillance is the monitoring, usually by local or state health departments, of patients presenting to emergency departments and alternative care facilities, and the recording of EMS call volume and the use of over-the-counter medications. Patients with signs and symptoms that resemble influenza are particularly important. Local and state health departments monitor for an unusual influx of patients with these symptoms in hopes of discovering an outbreak early. The EMS role in syndromic surveillance is a small one, yet valuable in the overall tracking of a biologic terrorist event or infectious disease outbreak. Quality assurance and dispatch operations need to be aware of an unusual number of calls from patients with "unexplainable flu" coming from a particular region or community.

Table 10 Biologic Agents

Disease	Transmission Person to Person	Incubation Period	Duration of Illness	Lethality (approximate case fatality rates)
Smallpox	High	7 to 17 d (average 12 d)	4 wk	High to moderate
Viral hemorrhagic fevers	Moderate	4 to 21 d	Death between 7 to 16 d	High to moderate, depending on type of fever
Inhalation anthrax	No	1 to 6 d	3 to 5 d (usually fatal if untreated)	High
Pneumonic plague	High	2 to 3 d	1 to 6 d (usually fatal)	High unless treated within 12 to 24 h
Botulinum	No	1 to 5 d	Death in 24 to 72 h; lasts months if patient does not die	High without respiratory support
Ricin	No	18 to 24 h	Days; death within 10 to 12 d for ingestion	High

Points of Distribution

<u>Points of distribution (PODs)</u> (Strategic National Stockpile) are strategically placed facilities that have been preestablished for the mass distribution of antibiotics, antidotes, vaccinations, and other medications and supplies. These medications may be delivered in large containers known as "push packs" by the Centers for Disease Control and Prevention Figure 17 . These containers have a targeted delivery time of within 12 hours anywhere in the country and contain antibiotics, chemical antidotes, antitoxins, life-support medications, IV administration, airway maintenance supplies, and medical/surgical items. In some regions, local and state municipalities have started to stockpile their own supplies to reduce the time delay.

Paramedics may be called on to assist in the delivery of the medications to the public (depending on local emergency management planning). The paramedic's role may include triage, treatment of seriously ill patients, and patient transport to the hospital. Most plans for PODs include at least one ambulance on standby for the transport of seriously ill patients.

■ Radiologic/Nuclear Devices

There have been only two publicly known incidents involving the use of a nuclear device. During WWII, Hiroshima and Nagasaki were devastated when they were targeted with nuclear bombs. It has been estimated that a death toll of 214,000 people occurred due to the two bombs and their associated effects. The awesome destructive power demonstrated by the attack ended WWII and has since served as a deterrent to nuclear war.

There are also nations that hold close ties with terrorist groups (state-sponsored terrorism) and have obtained some degree of nuclear capability. It is also possible for a terrorist to secure radioactive materials or waste to perpetrate an act of terror. Such materials are far easier for the determined terrorist to acquire and require less expertise to use. The difficulties in

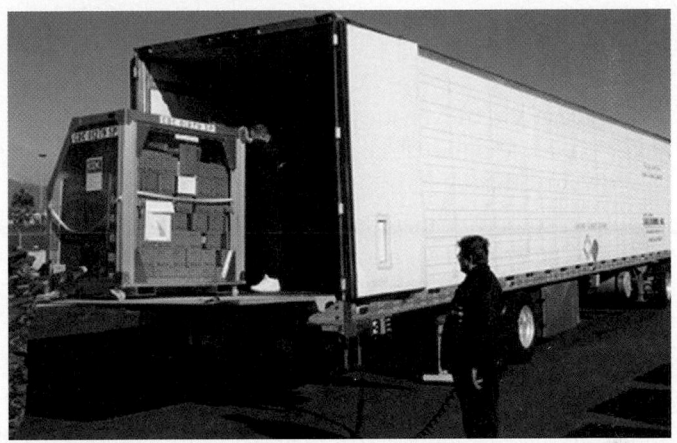

Figure 17 The Centers for Disease Control and Prevention Strategic National Stockpile can deliver one of many push packs to any location in the country within 12 hours of an emergency.

developing a nuclear weapon are well documented. Radioactive materials, however, such as those in radiologic dispersal devices (RDDs, discussed later), can cause widespread panic and civil disturbances.

■ Radiation

<u>Ionizing radiation</u> is energy that is emitted in the form of rays, or particles. This energy can be found in <u>**radioactive material**</u>, such as rocks and metals. Radioactive material is any material that emits radiation. This material is unstable, and it attempts to stabilize itself by changing its structure in a natural process called <u>**decay**</u>. As the substance decays, it gives off radiation until it stabilizes. The process of radioactive decay can take from as little as minutes to billions of years; meanwhile, the substance remains radioactive.

The energy that is emitted from a strong radiologic source is either <u>alpha</u>, <u>beta</u>, <u>gamma (x-rays)</u>, or <u>neutron radiation</u> Figure 18 . Alpha is the least harmful penetrating type of radiation and cannot travel fast or through most objects. In fact, a sheet of paper or the body's skin easily stops it. Beta radiation is slightly more penetrating than alpha and requires a layer of clothing to stop it. Gamma or x-rays are far faster and stronger than alpha and beta rays. These rays easily penetrate through the human body and require either several inches of lead or concrete to prevent penetration. Neutron energy is the fastest moving and most powerful form of radiation. Neutrons easily penetrate through lead and require several feet of concrete to stop them.

Sources of Radiologic Material

There are thousands of radioactive materials found on the earth. These materials are generally used for purposes that benefit humankind, such as medicine, killing germs in food (irradiating), and construction work. Once radiologic material has been used for its purpose, the material remaining is called radiologic waste. Radiologic waste remains radioactive but has no more usefulness. These materials can be found at the following locations:

- Hospitals
- Colleges and universities
- Chemical and industrial sites
- Power plants

Not all radioactive material is tightly guarded, and the waste is often not guarded. This makes use of radioactive material and substances appealing to terrorists.

Radiologic Dispersal Devices

A <u>radiologic dispersal device (RDD)</u> is any container that is designed to disperse radioactive material. This would generally

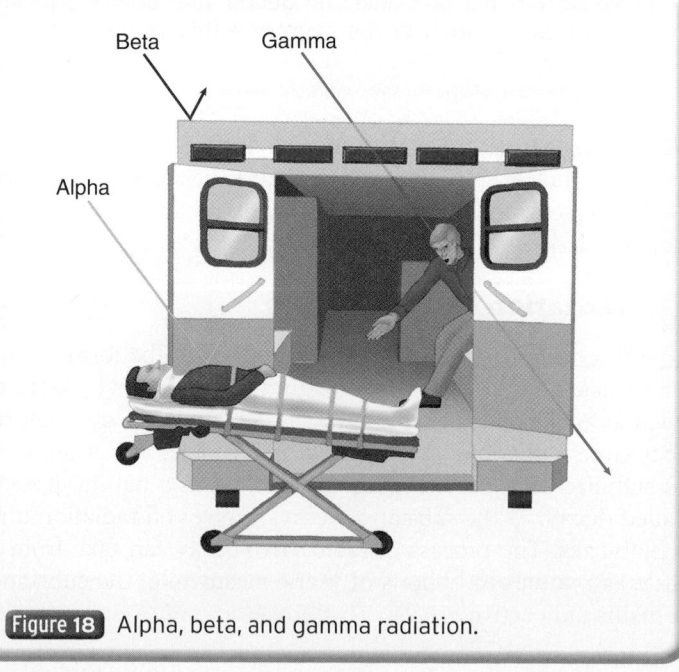

Figure 18 Alpha, beta, and gamma radiation.

require the use of a bomb, hence the nickname <u>dirty bomb</u>. A dirty bomb carries the potential to injure victims with not only the radioactive material but also the explosive material used to deliver it. Just the thought of an RDD creates fear in a population, and so the ultimate goal of the terrorist—fear—is accomplished. In reality, however, the destructive capability of a dirty bomb is limited to the explosives that are attached to it. Therefore, if the explosive is sufficient to kill 10 persons without radioactive material, it will also kill 10 persons with the radioactive material added. There may be long-term injuries and illness associated with the use of an RDD, yet not much more than the bomb by itself would create. In short, the dirty bomb is an ineffective WMD in terms of physical damage, but can be psychologically potent in terms of the fear it can create.

Nuclear Energy

Nuclear energy is artificially released by altering (splitting) radioactive atoms. The result is an immense amount of energy that usually takes the form of heat. Nuclear material is used in medicine, weapons, naval vessels, and power plants. Nuclear material gives off all forms of radiation including neutrons (the most deadly type). Like radioactive material, when nuclear material is no longer useful it becomes waste that is still radioactive.

Nuclear Weapons

The destructive energy of a nuclear explosion is unlike any other weapon in the world. That is why nuclear weapons are kept only in secure facilities throughout the world. There are nations that have ties to terrorists and that have actively attempted to build nuclear weapons. However, the ability of these nations to deliver a nuclear weapon, such as a missile or bomb, is, as of yet, incomplete. There is also the deterrent of complete mutual annihilation. Therefore, the likelihood of a nuclear attack is extremely remote.

Unfortunately, due to the collapse of the former Soviet Union, the whereabouts of many small nuclear devices is unknown. These small suitcase-sized nuclear weapons are called <u>special atomic demolition munitions (SADMs)</u>. SADM, or "suitcase nuke," was designed to destroy individual targets, such as important buildings, bridges, tunnels, or large ships. The estimate is that perhaps as many as 80 are missing as of 1998. No other information or updates on the whereabouts of these devices have been made public.

How Radiation Affects the Body

The effects of radiation exposure will vary depending on the amount of radiation that a person receives and the route of entry. There are three levels of radiation exposure:

- **Radioactive exposure.** Exposure to radioactive material occurred, but the body is not necessarily contaminated.
- **External contamination.** The skin was contaminated with radioactive material, but the inside of the body is not necessarily contaminated yet.
- **Internal contamination.** The inside of the body is contaminated.

Radiation can be introduced into the body by all routes of entry as well as through the body (irradiation). The patient can inhale radioactive dust from nuclear fallout or from a dirty bomb, or have radioactive liquid absorbed into the body through the skin. Once in the body, the radiation source will irradiate the person from within rather than from an external source (such as x-ray equipment). Some common signs of acute radiation sickness are nausea, vomiting, and diarrhea. Additional injuries will occur with a nuclear blast such as thermal and blast trauma, trauma from flying objects, and eye injuries.

Words of Wisdom

The inverse square law is derived from physics and describes how radiation travels from its source. If you double your distance from a radiologic source, you will decrease the amount of radiation that you are exposed to by a factor of four. For example: if the radiation dose at 2 feet from the source is 20R, at 4 feet it will decrease to 5R, and at 6 feet away it will be 1.25R. Therefore, the farther away you get from a radioactive source the better, but moving even a small distance away greatly reduces your exposure. Remember that your best allies are time, distance, and shielding.

Medical Management

Being exposed to a radiation source does not make a patient contaminated or radioactive. However, when patients have a radioactive source on their body (such as debris from a dirty bomb), they are contaminated and must be initially cared for by a HazMat responder. Once the patient is decontaminated and there is no threat to you, you may begin treatment with the ABCs and treat the patient for any burns or trauma.

Protective Measures

There are no suits or protective gear designed to completely shield you from radiation. Those people who work in high-risk areas do wear some protection (lead-lined suits); however, this equipment is not available to the paramedic. The best ways to protect yourself from the effects of radiation are to use time and distance, and shield yourself in Level C protection from the source (protection levels are discussed in the chapter, *Hazardous Materials*).

- **Time.** Radiation has a cumulative effect on the body. The less time that you are exposed to the source, the less the effects will be. If you realize that the patient is near a radiation source, leave the area immediately.
- **Distance.** Radiation is limited as to how far it can travel. Depending on the type of radiation, often moving only a few feet is enough to remove you from immediate danger (inverse square law). You should take this into account when you are responding to a nuclear or radiologic incident and make certain that responders are stationed far enough from the incident.
- **Shielding.** As discussed earlier, the path of all radiation can be stopped by a specific object. It will be impossible for you to recognize the type of radiation being emitted, or even from which direction it is coming. Therefore, you should always assume that you are dealing with the strongest form of radiation and use concrete shielding (such as buildings or walls) between yourself and the incident. The importance of shielding cannot be overemphasized. In one atomic test, a car was parked on the side of a house, opposite the direction of the oncoming blast. The house was completely destroyed, yet the car that was directly next to it sustained almost no damage.

YOU are the Medic | SUMMARY

1. What are some clues that might help you treat your patient?

Pay close attention to the information being provided, not only from those in command but from the general impression of your patient. You know that the toxic substance was released into the air and that its effects are rapid in onset and target multiple body systems. The patient presents in acute respiratory distress, with an altered mental status and a slow pulse rate.

2. Biologic agents can be modified in a laboratory to increase their impact on target populations. What are the primary types of biologic agents that you may encounter during a terrorist attack?

The primary types of biologic agents that you may come into contact with during a terrorist attack include viruses, bacteria, and toxins.

3. On the basis of the information you have, what do you think your patient was exposed to?

The information that you have so far can be indicative of several agents that enter the body through inhalation and have immediate physiologic effects. Potential substances that can present with symptoms similar to those of your patient include phosgene, chlorine, Freon, and cyanide.

4. What should your initial treatment consist of?

As with any patient, initial treatment should focus on identifying and correcting any problems related to airway, breathing, and circulation. The patient's primary presenting problem is respiratory distress, so oxygen therapy is an appropriate place to start. Because you do not have any information regarding the toxin, specific treatment aimed at reversing its effects cannot be provided.

5. Will the smell of almonds always be present with a cyanide exposure?

This is one of those times when the nose does not always know. Not everyone is able to detect the bitter almond smell associated with the presence of cyanide. Treat the patient based on signs and symptoms until the identity of the substance is known.

6. What is the treatment of choice for a patient with cyanide toxicity?

Several medications act as antidotes, but many services do not carry them. Your response cannot begin until trained personnel wearing the proper PPE remove the patient from the source of exposure, remove the patient's clothes, and decontaminate any patients who may have been exposed to liquid contamination.

Once those measures have occurred, support the patient's ABCs, including administering supplementary oxygen, and gain IV access. Severe exposure will require aggressive oxygenation and perhaps ventilation with supplementary oxygen. Always use a bag-mask device or oxygen-powered ventilator device to ventilate a patient exposed to a metabolic agent. The agent can easily be passed on from the patient to you through mouth-to-mouth or mouth-to-mask ventilations. If no antidote is available, initiate transport immediately.

YOU *are the Medic* | **SUMMARY,** *continued*

Triage Tag
No. 35572009

Move the Walking Wounded	MINIMAL
No respirations after head tilt	EXPECTANT
☐ Respirations—over 30 or less than 10	IMMEDIATE
☐ Perfusion—capillary refill over 2 seconds	IMMEDIATE
☐ Mental status—unable to follow simple commands	IMMEDIATE
Otherwise	DELAYED

MAJOR INJURIES: None

HOSPITAL DESTINATION: Southport

ORIENTED × 4   DISORIENTED ☐   UNRESPONSIVE ☐

TIME	PULSE	B/P	RESPIRATION
1050	124 beats/min, strong	172/86 mm Hg	28 breaths/min, shallow, labored
1055	116 beats/min, weak	92/56 mm Hg	18 breaths/min, shallow
1100	114 beats/min, weak	96/60 mm Hg	12 breaths/min, manual ventilation

PERSONAL INFORMATION:

NAME: Brett Murphey

MALE ☐   FEMALE ☐   AGE: EST. 22   WEIGHT: EST. 83 KG (165 lb)

MEDICAL COMPLAINTS/HISTORY

Respiratory distress; chemical exposure

EXPECTANT	No 35572009

IMMEDIATE	No 35572009

Prep Kit

- As a result of the increase in terrorist activity, it is possible that you could be called to respond to a terrorist event. You must be mentally and physically prepared for this possibility.
- The use of weapons of mass destruction (WMDs) further complicates the management of the terrorist incident. Be aware of your surroundings at all times. The best form of protection from a WMD agent is to avoid contact with the agent.
- Terrorism is a violent act that is dangerous to human life, in violation of the criminal laws of the United States, to intimidate or coerce a government, the civilian population, or any segment thereof, in furtherance of political or social objectives.
- Terrorists are either international or domestic, and can be categorized as violent religious groups/doomsday cults, extremist political/social groups, technology or cyber terrorists, single-issue terrorist groups, and narcoterrorists.
- The National Terrorism Advisory System (NTAS) replaced the color-coded Homeland Security Advisory System. The NTAS alerts responders to the potential for an attack, provides specifics of the threat if practical, and advises on measures to take for protection. The threat level can be elevated or imminent.
- On the basis of the current threat level, take appropriate actions and precautions. Be aware of established policies that your organization may have regarding the current threat level.
- Indicators that may give you clues as to whether the emergency is the result of an attack include the type of location, type of call, number of patients, patients' statements, and preincident indicators.
- If you suspect that a terrorist or WMD event has occurred, ensure that the scene is safe. If you have any doubt that it may not be safe, do not enter. Wait for assistance.
- Notification of the dispatcher is essential. Inform dispatch of the nature of the event, any additional resources that may be required, the estimated number of patients, and the upwind route of approach or optimal route of approach.
- Establish a staging area, where other units will converge. Be mindful of access and exit routes.
- Terrorists may set secondary devices to explode after the initial bomb to injure responders and secure media coverage. Constantly assess and reassess the scene for safety.
- A weapon of mass destruction is any weapon or agent designed to bring about mass death, casualties, and/or massive damage to property and infrastructure (bridges, tunnels, airports, and seaports). These can be nuclear, chemical, biologic, and explosive weapons.
- Explosives are the most common weapon used by terrorists. Incendiary weapons involve agents and chemicals used to start fires. Ammonium nitrate bombs and suicide bombers are two weapons commonly used by terrorists.
- Chemical agents include vesicants or blister agents, respiratory or choking agents, nerve agents, metabolic or blood agents, and irritating agents. When a patient has been exposed to one of these, decontamination is a necessary first step. Do not approach the patient until hazardous materials responders have declared that the patient is decontaminated. Treatment will usually include airway management, IV access, and rapid transport.
- Patients exposed to a nerve agent can be treated with an antidote. This is delivered as an auto-injector. Multiple doses may be needed. Follow your local protocols.
- Biologic agents include viruses such as smallpox and those that cause viral hemorrhagic fevers, bacteria such as those that cause anthrax and plague, and neurotoxins such as botulinum toxin and ricin.
- Standard precautions are extremely important when you are treating patients who were potentially exposed to a biologic agent.
- Nuclear or radiologic weapons can create a massive amount of destruction. Radioactive material may be used in a radiologic dispersal device, or dirty bomb, but the majority of the damage from such a bomb is caused by the explosives, not from the radioactive material.
- As with exposure to chemical agents, patients who were potentially exposed to radioactive material must be decontaminated before you have any contact. Time, distance, and shielding are the best ways to protect yourself from radiation exposure.

■ Vital Vocabulary

alpha Type of energy that is emitted from a strong radiologic source; it is the least harmful penetrating type of radiation and cannot travel fast or through most objects.

ammonium nitrate A commonly used industrial-grade fertilizer that is not in itself dangerous to handle or transport, but when mixed with fuel and other components, forms an extremely explosive compound.

anthrax A deadly bacteria (*Bacillus anthracis*) that lies dormant in a spore (protective shell); the germ is released from the spore when exposed to the optimal temperature and moisture. The route of entry is inhalation, cutaneous, or gastrointestinal (from consuming food that contains spores).

apocalyptic violence A type of violence sought by some terrorists, such as violent religious groups and doomsday cults, in which they wish to bring about the end of the world.

asymmetric warfare A type of warfare in which groups wage war with unconventional weapons and covert tactics that are unequal—for example, when there are differences in military resources or capabilities.

bacteria Microorganisms that reproduce by binary fission. These single-cell creatures reproduce rapidly. Some can form spores (encysted variants) when environmental conditions are harsh.

beta Type of energy that is emitted from a strong radiologic source; is slightly more penetrating than alpha, and requires a layer of clothing to stop it.

botulinum A very potent neurotoxin produced by bacteria; when introduced into the body, this neurotoxin affects the nervous system's ability to function and causes muscle paralysis.

buboes Enlarged lymph nodes (up to the size of tennis balls) that are characteristic of people infected with the bubonic plague.

bubonic plague An epidemic that spread throughout Europe in the Middle Ages, causing over 25 million deaths, also called the Black Death; transmitted by infected fleas and characterized by acute malaise, fever, and the formation of tender, enlarged, inflamed lymph nodes that appear as lesions, called buboes.

chlorine (CL) The first chemical agent ever used in warfare. It has a distinct odor of bleach, and creates a green haze when released as a gas. Initially it produces upper airway irritation and a choking sensation.

communicability The ease with which a disease spreads from one human to another human.

contact hazard A hazardous agent that gives off little or no vapors; the skin is the primary route for this type of chemical to enter the body; also called a skin hazard.

contagious An adjective used to describe the ability of a person infected with a highly communicable disease to pass that disease to another person.

covert Act in which the public safety community generally has no prior knowledge of the time, location, or nature of the attack.

cross-contamination Occurs when a person is contaminated by an agent as a result of coming into contact with another contaminated person.

cyanide Agent that affects the body's ability to use oxygen. It is a colorless gas that has an odor similar to almonds. The effects begin on the cellular level and are very rapidly seen at the organ system level.

decay A natural process in which a material that is unstable attempts to stabilize itself by changing its structure.

dirty bomb Name given to a bomb that is used as a radiologic dispersal device (RDD).

disease vector An animal that, once infected, spreads a disease to another animal.

dissemination The means with which a terrorist will spread a disease—for example, by poisoning the water supply or aerosolizing the agent into the air or ventilation system of a building.

domestic terrorism Terrorism that is carried out by native citizens against their own country.

DuoDote A nerve agent antidote kit that contains a single injection of both atropine (2 mg) and 2-PAM chloride (pralidoxime chloride) (600 mg).

elevated A threat level in which a terrorist event is suspected, but there is no specific information about its timing or location.

G agents Early nerve agents that were developed by German scientists in the period after WWI and into WWII. There are three such agents: sarin, soman, and tabun.

gamma (x-rays) Type of energy that is emitted from a strong radiologic source that is far faster and stronger than alpha and beta rays. These rays easily penetrate through the human body and require either several inches of lead or concrete to prevent penetration.

guerilla warfare A form of warfare in which a small group that is not part of the official military engages in combat that uses the element of surprise, such as raids and ambushes; sometimes used by terrorists to protect their training camps and bases of operation.

imminent A threat level in which a terrorist event is known to be impending or will occur very soon.

incubation Describes the period of time from a person being exposed to a disease to the time when symptoms begin.

international terrorism Terrorism that is carried out by those not of the host's country; also known as cross-border terrorism.

ionizing radiation Energy that is emitted in the form of rays, or particles.

LD_{50} The amount of an agent or substance that will kill 50% of people who are exposed to this level.

lewisite (L) A blistering agent that has a rapid onset of symptoms and produces immediate intense pain and discomfort on contact.

lymphatic system A passive circulatory system that transports a plasma-like liquid called lymph, a thin fluid that bathes the tissues of the body.

lymph nodes Area of the lymphatic system where infection-fighting cells are housed.

MARK 1 A nerve agent antidote kit containing two auto-injector medications, atropine and 2-PAM chloride (pralidoxime chloride); also known as a nerve agent antidote kit (NAAK).

miosis Bilateral pinpoint constricted pupils.

mutagen A substance that mutates, damages, and changes the structures of DNA in the body's cells.

National Terrorism Advisory System (NTAS) The US system for informing citizens of a potential terrorist threat; replaced the color-coded Homeland Security Advisory System.

nerve agents A class of chemicals called organophosphates; they function by blocking an essential enzyme in the nervous system, which causes the body's organs to become overstimulated and burn out.

neurotoxins Biologic agents that are the most deadly substances known to humans; they include botulinum toxin and ricin.

neutron radiation Type of energy that is emitted from a strong radiologic source; the fastest moving and most powerful form of radiation; the particles easily penetrate through lead, and require several feet of concrete to stop them.

non-state-supported terrorism Terrorism that is either indigenous or transnational, and that do not receive direction or support from a government.

off-gassing The emitting of an agent after exposure—for example, from a person's clothes that have been exposed to the agent.

organophosphates A class of chemical found in many insecticides used in agriculture and in the home; nerve agents fall into this class of chemicals.

persistency Term used to describe how long a chemical agent will stay on a surface before it evaporates.

phosgene A pulmonary agent that is a product of combustion, such as might be produced in a fire at a textile factory or house, or from metalwork or burning Freon; a very potent agent that has a delayed onset of symptoms, usually hours.

<u>phosgene oxime (CX)</u> A blistering agent that has a rapid onset of symptoms and produces immediate intense pain and discomfort on contact.

<u>pneumonic plague</u> A lung infection, also known as plague pneumonia, that is the result of inhalation of plague bacteria.

<u>points of distribution (PODs)</u> Strategically placed facilities that have been preestablished for the mass distribution of antibiotics, antidotes, and vaccinations, along with other medications and supplies.

<u>radioactive material</u> Any material that emits radiation.

<u>radiologic dispersal device (RDD)</u> Any container that is designed to disperse radioactive material.

<u>ricin</u> Neurotoxin derived from mash that is left from pressing oil from a castor bean; causes pulmonary edema and respiratory and circulatory failure, leading to death.

<u>route of exposure</u> Manner by which a toxic substance enters the body.

<u>sarin (GB)</u> A nerve agent that is one of the G agents; a highly volatile colorless and odorless liquid that turns from liquid to gas within seconds to minutes at room temperature.

<u>secondary device</u> Additional explosives used by terrorists, which are set to explode after the initial bomb.

<u>smallpox</u> A highly contagious disease; it is most contagious when blisters begin to form.

<u>soman (GD)</u> A nerve agent that is one of the G agents; twice as persistent as sarin and five times as lethal; it has a fruity odor as a result of the type of alcohol used in the agent, and is both a contact and inhalation hazard that can enter the body through skin absorption and through the respiratory tract.

<u>special atomic demolition munitions (SADMs)</u> Small suitcase-sized nuclear weapons that were designed to destroy individual targets, such as important buildings, bridges, tunnels, or large ships.

<u>state-directed terrorism</u> Terrorism directed by a government; the terrorists act as direct agents of the government.

<u>state-sponsored terrorism</u> Terrorism that is funded or supported by nations that hold close ties with terrorist groups, but the terrorist group still acts independently.

<u>suicide bombers</u> People who are terrorists who wear or carry a weapon, such as an explosive, and trigger its detonation, killing themselves in the process to achieve terrorism.

<u>sulfur mustard (H)</u> A vesicant; it is a brownish-yellowish oily substance that is generally considered very persistent; has the distinct smell of garlic or mustard and, when released, it is quickly absorbed into the skin and/or mucous membranes and begins an irreversible process of damaging the cells.

<u>syndromic surveillance</u> The monitoring, usually by local or state health departments, of patients presenting to emergency departments and alternative care facilities, the recording of EMS call volume, and the use of over-the-counter medications.

<u>tabun (GA)</u> A nerve agent that is one of the G agents; is 36 times more persistent than sarin and approximately half as lethal; has a fruity smell and is unique because the components used to manufacture the agent are easy to acquire and the agent is easy to manufacture.

<u>terrorism</u> A violent act dangerous to human life, in violation of the criminal laws of the United States or any segment to intimidate or coerce a government, the civilian population, or any segment thereof, in furtherance of political or social objectives.

<u>V agent (VX)</u> One of the G agents; it is a clear, oily agent that has no odor and looks like baby oil; over 100 times more lethal than sarin and is extremely persistent.

<u>vapor hazard</u> An agent that enters the body through the respiratory tract.

<u>vesicants</u> Blister agents; the primary route of entry is through the skin.

<u>viral hemorrhagic fevers (VHFs)</u> A group of diseases that include the Ebola, Rift Valley, and yellow fever viruses, among others. This group of viruses causes the blood in the body to seep out from the tissues and blood vessels.

<u>viruses</u> Germs that require a living host to multiply and survive.

<u>volatility</u> Term used to describe how long a chemical agent will stay on a surface before it evaporates.

<u>weapon of mass destruction (WMD)</u> Any agent designed to bring about mass death, casualties, and/or massive damage to property and infrastructure (bridges, tunnels, airports, and seaports).

<u>weaponization</u> The creation of a weapon from a biologic agent generally found in nature and that causes disease; the agent is cultivated, synthesized, and/or mutated to maximize the target population's exposure to the germ.

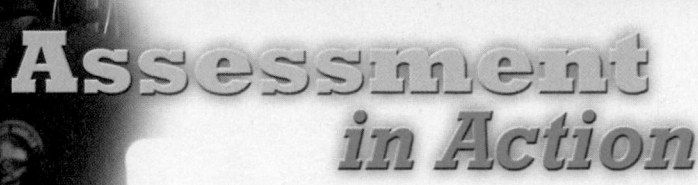
Your city will be hosting the Super Bowl next year. As part of the preparation, the local hospitals are hosting a continuing education seminar on the emergency treatment of patients during an act of terrorism.

1. Which type of radiation cannot travel fast or through most objects?
   A. Delta
   B. Gamma
   C. Alpha
   D. Beta

2. _____ affects the nervous system's ability to function and causes muscle paralysis.
   A. Tabun
   B. Botulinum
   C. Ricin
   D. Sarin

3. Ebola is an example of a:
   A. plague.
   B. neurotoxin.
   C. mutagen.
   D. viral hemorrhagic fever.

4. What was the first chemical agent ever used in warfare?
   A. Chlorine
   B. Phosgene
   C. Mustard gas
   D. Cyanide

5. The routes of entry for anthrax include:
   A. inhalation.
   B. cutaneous.
   C. gastrointestinal.
   D. All of the above

6. The most deadly substances known to humans are:
   A. pulmonary agents.
   B. neurotoxins.
   C. organophosphates.
   D. vesicants.

7. Some toxins can be derived from certain plants and flowers. Which of the following toxins is made from the castor bean?

A. Sarin
B. Ricin
C. Mustard gas
D. Phosgene

8. An example of a disease that infects the lymphatic system is:
   A. botulism.
   B. Rift Valley fever.
   C. bubonic plague.
   D. anthrax.

9. Potential sources of radiologic waste include:
   A. hospitals.
   B. universities.
   C. power plants.
   D. All of the above

10. Strategically placed facilities that have been preestablished for the mass distribution of antibiotics, antidotes, vaccinations, and other medications and supplies are called:
    A. strategic warehouses.
    B. points of distribution.
    C. rapid deployment units.
    D. central response centers.

Additional Question

11. What are some of the challenges that will be faced if medical resources become scarce?

Disaster Response

National EMS Education Standard Competencies

EMS Operations

Knowledge of operational roles and responsibilities to ensure patient, public, and personnel safety.

Mass-Casualty Incidents Due to Terrorism and Disaster

- Risks and responsibilities of operating on the scene of a natural or man-made disaster. (pp 2326-2339)

Knowledge Objectives

1. Define disaster, including the types of critical infrastructure that can be affected by a disaster. (p 2319)
2. Explain what is meant by an all-hazards approach to disaster planning. (p 2319)
3. List items to consider when preplanning for a disaster of any sort. (pp 2320-2322)
4. Discuss preplanning questions to consider related to general items, such as geography, the infrastructure, and the population. (pp 2320, 2321)
5. Discuss preplanning considerations related to available EMS resources, such as mutual aid, fire, police, and hospitals. (pp 2320-2321)
6. Discuss other resources that should be considered when preplanning for a disaster event, such as nongovernmental organizations, disaster relief agencies, and local businesses. (p 2321)
7. Discuss other preplanning considerations for disaster planning, including communications, supplies, training, transportation, and media and legal concerns. (pp 2320, 2321, 2322)
8. List items to consider when responding to a disaster emergency. (pp 2322-2325)
9. Describe early measures to take when responding to a disaster, including early preparation when a warning is received, inventory of supplies, mobilization of personnel, and command setup. (pp 2322-2323)
10. Discuss other general considerations for responding to a disaster, including personnel physical and mental needs, resupplying, surveillance, and media. (pp 2323, 2324, 2325)
11. List items to consider after responding to a disaster. (pp 2325-2326)
12. Discuss actions to take after responding to a disaster, including the after-action report, retraining, and reimbursement. (p 2326)
13. Discuss concerns related to specific natural disasters, including natural fires, snow and ice storms, tornadoes, hurricanes, tsunamis, earthquakes, landslides, cave-ins, volcanic eruptions, flooding, sandstorms, prolonged cold weather, drought, heat wave, meteors, and pandemics. (pp 2326-2334)
14. Discuss concerns related to specific man-made disasters, including structural fires, construction failures, power failures, riots and stampedes, strikes, snipers and hostage situations, explosions, and technology disruptions. (pp 2334-2339)

Skills Objectives

There are no skills objectives for this chapter.

Introduction

The EMS system responds to small, medium, and large emergencies every day, every hour, everywhere. A main function of EMS is responding to disasters. A **disaster** is any calamitous event that causes or has the potential to cause injury or death, destruction, and distress. A disaster can be man-made or natural. Disasters overwhelm EMS and community resources because critical infrastructure has been damaged or destroyed **Figure 1**. **Critical infrastructure** includes the electrical power grid, communication systems, fuel for vehicles, water, sewage removal, food, hospitals, and transportation systems. In smaller, rural services, anything that overwhelms the capabilities of EMS and community resources may also be classified as a disaster. Two critical patients with only one ambulance crew responsible for their care can surely become a disaster if not handled properly. **Disaster management** requires planners to take a broad look at preparedness, planning, training, response, and after-action review.

This chapter will cover the general rules that should apply to all EMS responses to disasters, such as planning, and will also cover specific man-made and natural emergencies. The chapters, *Incident Management and Multiple-Casualty Incidents*, *Hazardous Materials*, and *Terrorism* address those specific emergencies; therefore they are not discussed here. Refer to those chapters for specific information on those particular incidents.

Disaster Response Planning

Federal, state, and local governments have plans in place to manage disasters. Large and small companies also have plans, as do military, educational, and similar institutions. EMS agencies are, or should be, no different. Plans should be suited to the geography, population, and potential risks specific to the area. The best way to plan for a disaster is to think, "What could happen here?" and "What plans do we have in place for this possibility?"

The key for any EMS response unit or provider when responding to a disaster is planning. The act of conducting comprehensive preplanning for all types of disasters is called an

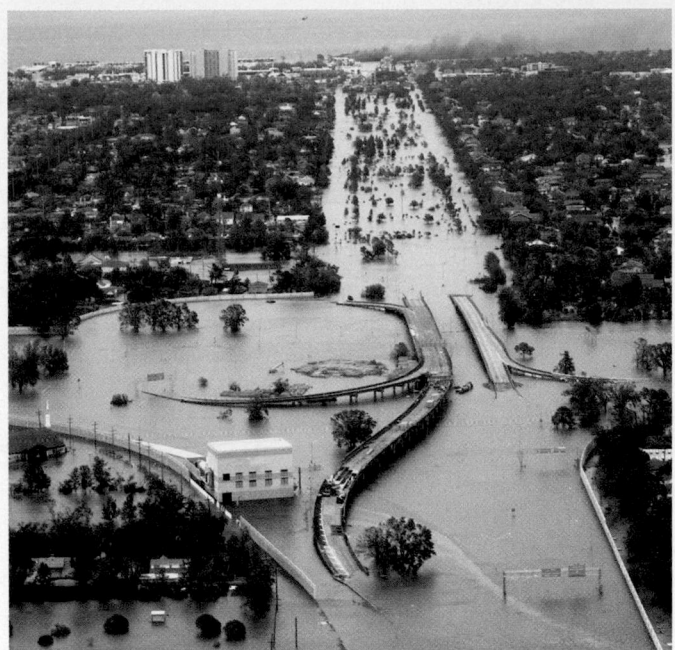

Figure 1 Disasters can overwhelm EMS resources and can damage critical infrastructure.

all-hazards approach. Before addressing specifics particular to the disaster, general considerations that apply to any disaster must be addressed, such as the number of personnel needed, equipment required, and which hospital(s) to transport patients to.

Phases of a Disaster Response Plan

Disaster response by EMS is improving and changing as threats and knowledge of them evolve. The key to any disaster response is planning. The key to planning is thinking, meeting, and brainstorming. A good motto to remember is that if it's bad and it's out there—it will happen. With the right plans and mindset, EMS will be ready. The three phases of any plan of response are before the event (preplanning), during the event, and after the event.

YOU *are the Medic*   PART 1

You and your partner have been working in the aftermath of a major storm that caused a large amount of damage in your response area. You have been on duty for the past 24 hours with no end in sight and have seen many patients who were injured because of the storm. Currently, you and your partner are assigned to a large-scale incident at an apartment complex that collapsed during the storm.

1. What is the definition of a disaster?
2. What does the term all-hazards approach mean in disaster planning?

Before the Event

Preplanning is the process in which EMS agencies prepare for a potential event. EMS agencies evaluate emergency incident factors that responders may or may not have control over to develop logical steps to effectively deal with potential incidents. When it comes to preplanning, certain issues are relevant to all involved. Table 1 lists some of the main items to consider when preplanning for a disaster. Depending on a responder's position within an EMS organization, certain questions will come to mind during the preplanning process. This section does not address every issue, but it should give you an idea of what to consider before an event occurs. Management considerations for specific disasters are discussed in the latter half of this chapter.

While no disaster is predictable, some events are more likely to occur than others. For example, an EMS agency in the Northeast may preplan for a snowstorm, whereas an agency in the Midwest may develop a response plan in the event of a tornado. However, natural disasters such as the tornado that tore through Springfield, Massachusetts, in 2011, and the earthquake centered in Virginia in the same year have proven that unlikely events do occur. General disaster preplanning with an all-hazards approach will put your agency in the best position to handle any disaster that may befall your area.

Geography of Response Area Your area may be prone to a particular type of natural disaster (eg, flood, earthquake, tornado). During the preplanning process, hazards and life threats associated with a particular type of natural disaster can be identified. Advance knowledge of factors that can affect response, including obstacles (eg, flooded roads) as well as terrain features (eg, hills, rivers) that can hinder access for equipment and entry into a facility, helps to prepare responders for a more successful response. You should consider how particular factors such as snow, ice, or smoke may impact your response Figure 2. For example, in the event of flooding, you should be familiar with secondary routes identified by your agency to avoid obstacles such as downed bridges and blocked roads. Remember, as a paramedic, especially in times of disaster, you could easily become the lead EMS worker. Knowledge of your response area and its hazards are key to preparation.

Population Is the population spread out, densely packed, or, as in most communities, mixed? Is the daytime population the same as the night-time population? For example, many cities have as much as six times more people present during business hours than at night because businesses and shops are open primarily during daytime hours. There may be language differences or cultural aspects to consider during preplanning. Your area may include different types of facilities (eg, retirement community, handicapped facilities, prisons) that may be of special concern to EMS agencies because they present numerous hazards, evacuation issues, and the condition of the people residing within these facilities may vary greatly. Special equipment (eg, special medications, special moving devices) and training may be needed to care for these populations in the event of a disaster.

EMS Resources Preplanning allows for the designation, acquisition, and movement of items needed to respond effectively and efficiently to an incident. Resources may include additional staff or personnel, specialized staff (eg, critical transport personnel), medical supplies, and equipment to handle tasks. Your agency must be able to cover its area of responsibility even if resources are dispatched to other communities to assist in a disaster response. Some important resources are mutual aid agreements, supplies on hand, transportation assets, and maps.

Table 1 Disaster Response Preplanning Considerations
Geography of response area
Population (urban, rural, mixed, special needs)
EMS resources (mutual aid, medical supplies, transportation, maps)
Access to business assets
Nongovernmental organizations and disaster relief agencies
Fire and police response
Training standards
Infrastructure
Internal communication
Hospitals
Media
Liaison to next higher level
Immunizations of personnel
Sheltering (of personnel, patients)
Animal control

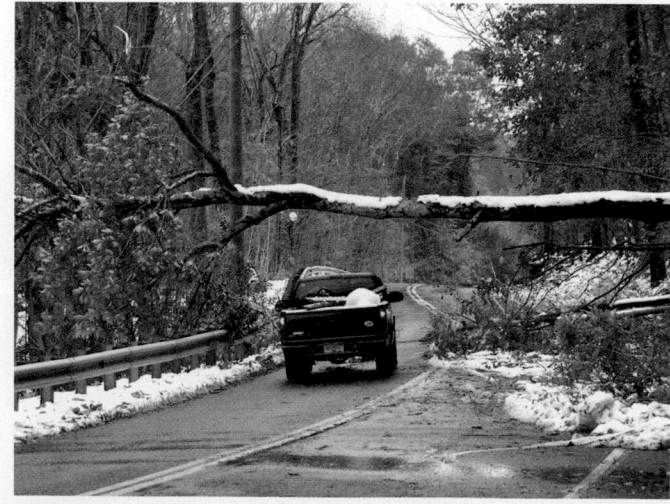

Figure 2 Considering the geography of your response area can help you to anticipate potential obstacles that could occur in a disaster.

Mutual aid agreements (MAAs), sometimes called automatic fill-in/send-up policies, formally define the relationships between two or more agencies or municipalities and the support that those organizations will provide to each other when requested. EMS is normally accustomed to MAAs that allow EMS agencies and fire departments in neighboring jurisdictions to cover emergency calls.

Your agency may have a "disaster stash" (supplies on hand just for emergencies). It is important to keep your agency's inventory up to date. The inventory list should be a living document whose quantities and items can be changed based on the threat. Who in your agency is responsible for predicting inventory needs (eg, extra supply of gloves and air purifying respirators for a predicted pandemic)? Who is the person responsible for ordering these? Many agencies have a designated supply officer or an inventory stored electronically with minimum stock lows and highs for disaster items.

Your agency may have access to special transportation equipment that can be used for a particular type of disaster situation. For example, if you are in a flood-prone zone, your agency may have access to boats or other water vehicles. It is important that drivers are trained and familiar with specialized vehicles and how to operate them in difficult conditions.

Emergency vehicles may be equipped with GPS; however, in the event of satellite loss, you may need to use laptop or paper maps. These maps should be updated to include information such as road closures and flood paths and the means to secure them. EMS personnel must be able to read maps, use compasses, and use protractors.

Access to Business Assets Businesses in your area may be able to help your agency in a disaster (eg, a local lumber company may be able to supply wood for additional makeshift backboards). Your agency can determine what expertise is available to you from the private sector in your response area (eg, mechanics, electricians) and may have written agreements with local businesses that include information regarding how to contact business personnel after hours if a disaster occurs.

Nongovernmental Organizations and Disaster Relief Agencies Nongovernmental organizations and disaster relief agencies such as the Salvation Army or Red Cross may also have the capability to provide support during a disaster. Your agency will determine the best method for contacting these organizations. You may be required to attend training programs offered by such organizations or your agency may invite them to your planning sessions.

Fire and Police Response Your agency's disaster response plan will outline fire and police response during an event **Figure 3** . Plans should include a rehabilitation area for fire fighters, paramedics, and other personnel. It is important to have drills on a **unified command system** within the **incident command system (ICS)** to ensure that you understand how your agency will work within a unified command structure during a disaster. Unified command allows representatives from multiple jurisdictions and agencies to share command authority and responsibility, thereby working together as a joint incident command team. Before a disaster strikes, it is important to have an

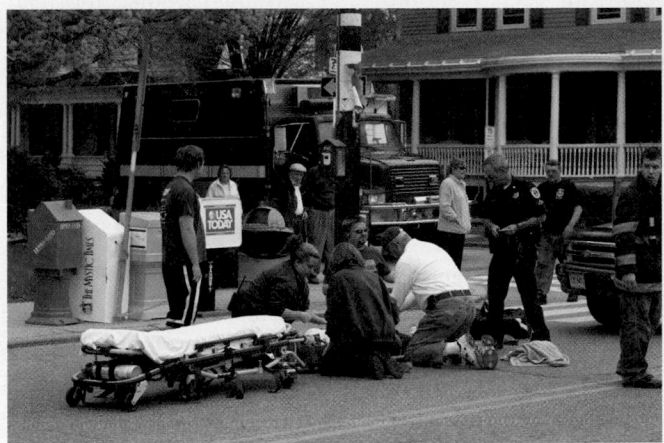

Figure 3 Emergency plans must be coordinated with those of local fire and police departments, as you will likely all be working together at a disaster scene.

understanding of how your agency will work within a unified command structure.

Training Standards One of the benefits of preplanning is that it permits organizations to conduct training on tasks they may be required to perform at a later time. Training is usually done in phases that follow a set process, progressing from individual tasks, to intermediate tasks, to crew training, to agency training, and then to interagency training. Your agency will frequently train and update EMS providers on procedures to follow during a disaster, including personal protective equipment (PPE) protocols, safety procedures, and operation of new and specialized equipment.

Infrastructure It is important to be familiar with your agency's communication backup plan to be prepared when telephone landlines are down, when cell phones are overwhelmed, and when power grids fail. The backup plan will also include information about other backup procedures such as how vehicles will be refueled when there are natural gas interruptions or no fuel deliveries.

Internal Communication Your agency's plan will include a way to maintain communication with all its members (those at base camp, those off base camp, and those working with other agencies such as the fire or police departments) as well as backup methods of communication to stay in touch with all involved parties. Vehicles may be equipped to communicate with each other or specific radio frequencies and cell phones may be reserved for such use.

Hospitals You must be familiar with the level of care available in your area. Local hospitals may have limitations on the number of patients they can accept during a disaster. Your agency might participate with local hospitals during disaster drills, and there may be an agreement in place between your agency and local hospitals to provide personnel to your agency or vice versa.

Media Your agency should have a trained public information officer or a person trained to use the media to your agency's advantage. This person should be familiar with the Health Insurance Portability and Accountability Act (HIPAA), which protects personal health information? Also, it is helpful to designate someone as a backup public information officer, in case the public information officer is out of town or unable to reach the command post, for example, due to road disruptions.

Liaison to the Next Higher Level It is important for members of your agency to know when and how to contact the next higher level of authority. Your agency and dispatch system should have a list of contacts at the state and federal levels, and those contacts should be verified on a regular basis. Redundancy is built into the plan to ensure that all necessary parties remain informed as an incident evolves. Has the system been tested at least semiannually? It should be clear what steps should be taken to ensure that higher levels of authority know who you are, where you are, and what you are going to do.

Immunizations of Personnel Your agency requires that its members' immunization records are on file and up to date. A paramedic is responsible for keeping his or her medical records up to date, based on the instruction of the agency's medical director, and under the protection of HIPAA. The designated infection control officer or your service's medical director should be aware of the health status of all employees. They should be on top of making sure timely titers have been drawn. It is important to familiarize yourself with your agency's plan for inoculations pursuant to a specific emergency. For example, personnel will receive immunization against cholera or typhus during emergencies where they could contract these diseases.

Sheltering Your agency's disaster plan will include procedures for sheltering members of the community as well as on-duty and off-duty personnel **Figure 4**. In addition, your agency may have an adult supervision plan for children of personnel or patients who cannot be cared for due to duty or incapacitation. Methods

of supplying food, water, and bath facilities for personnel and patients will be outlined in the plan as well.

Animal Control If your agency plans to assist in evacuations, your plan should address animals such as pets that must be left behind. If you are in a rural area, precautions must be in place to manage carcasses. If there are any zoos, wildlife refuges, or veterinarian facilities in your area, it is important for your agency to plan for concerns related to these facilities. For example, your agency may identify a need for access to rabies prophylaxis for patients and personnel.

Special Populations

What is your agency's policy regarding pets? When involved in an evacuation, many patients will not leave without their pets, or at least some confirmation of the pet's security. Will pets be allowed at a makeshift field hospital? Now is the time to get these procedures written into your disaster plans.

During the Event

Once a disaster strikes, it is best to stick to the plan if possible, but remember that changing conditions and oversights in preplanning may require modifying the initial plan. Plans are not written in stone; they are guidelines to help EMS provide care in the safest and most efficient manner **Table 2**.

Table 2   Considerations During a Disaster
Inventory
Mobilization of personnel
Command setup or response
Unification of command
Personal protective and safety equipment
Equipment resupply
Triage and classification
Patient tracking
Assignment of personnel
Personnel physical needs
Personnel mental needs
Hospital updates
Providing and accepting relief
Surveillance
Media
Legal issues
Unit leadership reinforcement

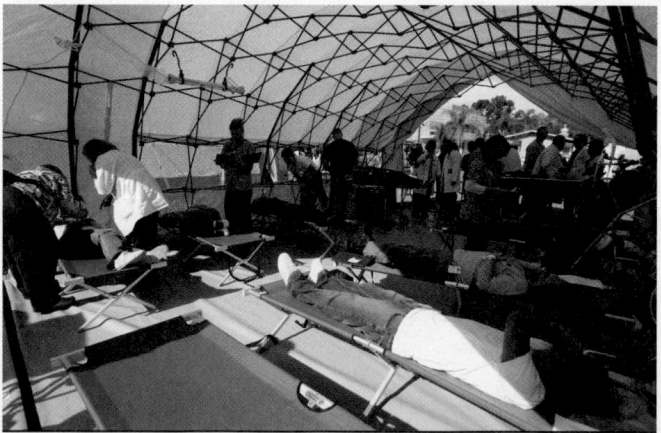

Figure 4 Emergency plans must include plans for sheltering patients as well as EMS personnel.

You may have advance warning of the upcoming event, such as a tornado or ice storm. If you do, the advance notice may be long or it may be incredibly brief. You must use this time to your advantage to "fine tune" your plan to the specific disaster predicted. Make sure you stay updated on the latest information.

Inventory During the alert or preparation period, take immediate inventory of supplies on hand. For a snowstorm, put a couple of shovels in the ambulance as well as some rock salt. For a cold-weather emergency, pack some extra blankets. Try to anticipate what you will need; determine how much space is available on the ambulances, at the stations, and at supply dumps; and prepare for the worst, mentally and physically. Then take a deep breath, take an inventory of yourself and your crew, and remember the emergency rule: "You can only do what you can do safely."

Mobilization of Personnel Another important step is to gather the crew and activate the notification system. Personnel must be briefed and notified of changes to the plans as soon as possible and as often as needed. Agencies will assign jobs as needed, making sure that everyone realizes that assignments can change based on the circumstances as they unfold. The agency will also start an IS-211 form to track personnel, noting who reported, when and where they were assigned, and any additional comments. It is essential to have a constant and continual inventory of where people are and what they are doing. Finally, each paramedic must have the necessary credentials on his or her person.

Command Setup or Response As a paramedic, you will either be setting up a command or reporting to a command. In either case, command must be visible (the incident commander and the location of incident command must be easily identifiable; for example, the incident commander should wear a command vest and helmet, and the command post as well as specific areas such as triage and treatment should be marked with panels or flags) and all responding personnel must be assimilated into the ICS properly.

Unification of Command Command unity is essential to optimize operations effectiveness, and reduce the problems and potential for miscommunication at responses to incidents. Fire, police, EMS, and other agencies should all be represented in the command structure with a lead agency directing the efforts. The lead agency can change many times depending on the course of events during an emergency. Cooperation is essential; egos must be "checked at the door." In major disasters, a state or federal government entity usually leads the command structure.

Personal Protective and Safety Equipment PPE and safety gear can wear out during a crisis. Personnel safety is always a primary concern during an emergency. PPE must be replaced immediately; measures must be in place to replace gear as needed. This is a command and personal responsibility. Personnel must not take shortcuts or neglect to wear the gear assigned to them for their protection.

Equipment Resupply Like PPE, equipment gets worn out, broken, or expended during the crisis. Resupply of disposables and recharging of battery-operated equipment are just a couple examples of gear that must be resupplied during the event. The command structure should have plans in place or formulated for equipment resupply. Keep in mind that new incoming personnel might not use exactly the same equipment as the assisted agency, so plans for either similar equipment or on-the-spot training should be enacted.

YOU *are the Medic* | PART 2

You arrive at the staging area and check in. You are immediately assigned to transport one priority yellow patient to a local receiving hospital. You report to the transportation supervisor and she directs you to the yellow tarp. You take a report on a 24-year-old woman from the paramedic caring for the patients in the yellow area.

Recording Time: 1 Minute	
Appearance	Awake
Level of consciousness	Alert (oriented to person, place, and day)
Airway	Open
Breathing	Adequate
Circulation	Adequate

3. What is pre-event planning, and how can an event be predicted in advance?

4. Why are preplanned mutual aid agreements essential to your operation?

Triage and Classification Patient classification may be disaster-dependent in some cases. For example, in a pandemic situation, patients who need ventilators would receive much more intense care than would patients who need palliative care or basic support. Triage and classification will be a constant and ongoing process, depending not only on patient needs, but also on availability, safety, and sustainability of EMS providers **Figure 5**. As discussed in the chapter, *Incident Management and Multiple-Casualty Incidents*, methods of triage include START triage and SALT triage.

Patient Tracking During the event, you must make a record for every patient you see or assist. This is typically done with a triage tag. If you are involved in transporting patients, you must complete a patient care report for the patients you transported. The transportation supervisor must maintain a log of all patients and the hospitals to which they are transported. Some areas use innovative methods for tracking patients, such as using barcoded tags. Information you may collect includes patient names, their injury categories, which units transported, and where the patient was transported. This information should be listed, updated, and given to the incident commander. The incident commander can disclose this information to the proper authorities. This information is not a violation of HIPAA.

Assignment of Personnel Assessment of new resource personnel must be done before they begin working, preferably in the staging areas, especially when receiving aid from other communities. The choice of appropriate personnel for patient care will depend on several factors, such as the level of training of EMS workers, the duration of event, and the amount of stress related to the event.

Personnel Physical Needs Patients and personnel need to eat, drink, and use bathroom facilities **Figure 6**. In long-lasting emergencies, personnel will require sleep areas and a way to communicate with their loved ones. It is imperative that the plan address methods of supplying the basic and fundamental needs of patients and EMS providers during a disaster.

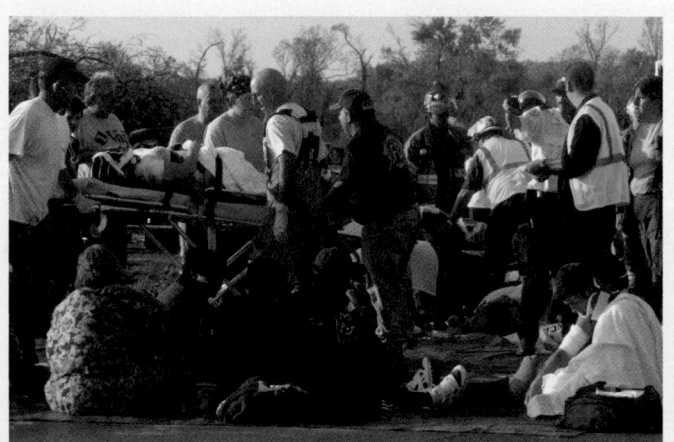

Figure 5 Patient triage is a constant, ongoing process that will occur throughout the disaster.

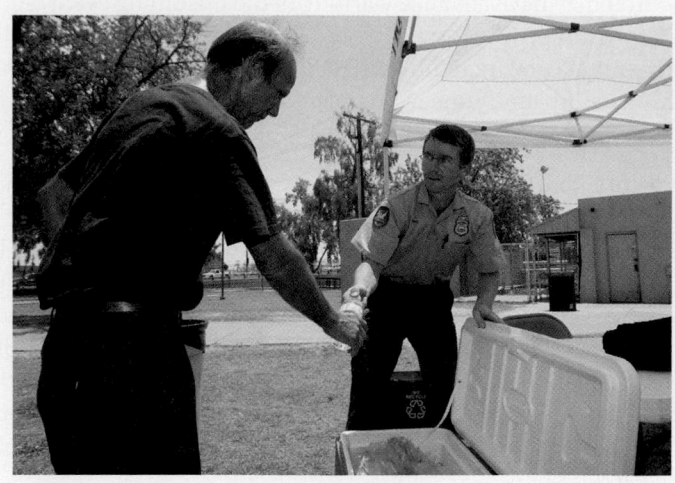

Figure 6 Plan for food, drink, and bathroom facilities to be supplied for patients and personnel working at disasters.

Personnel Mental Needs Disaster response is hard work! People become stressed, tired, aggravated, and burned-out. Use a "buddy system" approach to monitor these problems. In a long-lasting event, agencies should provide some downtime and an area where the EMS workers can "unwind." EMS providers should be encouraged to talk about their experiences. Remember that light humor and a constant supply of information are often helpful. Be alert for mental issues and incident fatigue in yourself and among your coworkers.

Hospital Updates It is important to maintain communication with your destination hospitals. You need to know whether they can take more patients, and if so, what kind. These hospitals may be able to resupply your equipment and supplies. Do they need some of your agency's personnel or could your agency use some of theirs? You must keep the hospitals updated on field conditions so that they can readjust their priorities, if necessary. Your help may be needed to set up an off-site hospital.

Providing and Accepting Relief If your agency is providing relief, it must ensure that it has enough coverage in its home area of responsibility. If a crew is sent to another area, it may need to be self-sustaining for 48 to 72 hours. Before you go, make sure your equipment is compatible. For example, your radios will need to be able to work on the same frequencies as other radios at the scene. Your ECG monitors may require adaptors to be used in another setting, and ECG leads need to be able to be switched from one machine to another, because the crew that transports the patient may be different than the crew that treated the patient. A phone call to the asset-requesting agency is a good way to double-check this information. If your agency is accepting relief, the rules for providing relief apply in reverse. Also, the credentials of the incoming personnel must be checked, and the agency accepting relief must ensure that these personnel have the proper PPE.

Surveillance Depending on the incident, your observations and field updates could make all the difference in the progression of an event. In a terrorism event, as discussed in the chapter, *Terrorism*, suspicious people or packages should be reported. In a flooding environment, EMS providers can assist with disease monitoring by reporting on evolving trends in their patients such as diarrhea, vomiting, and rashes not normally encountered. Each agency should keep its personnel attuned to exactly what they should be on the lookout for.

Media Your agency will need to determine if there is a need for it to supply a public information officer Figure 7 . Members of your agency may be trained to respond to questions from the press and measures in place to control rumors. It might be necessary to set up a press area and to direct questioners to this area. Your agency should use the press to its advantage; for example, inform the public to stay indoors or to provide self-care in non-emergent cases or until help can be sent to them. Consider a press briefing location and provide prompt briefing so all the facts that you are allowed to release about the incident can be communicated through the media.

Legal Issues Proper documentation during a crisis is essential; it is the best way to describe any events or issues that arise during an event. Most legal issues will be resolved long after the event, but eyewitness testimony and patient care issues are almost always helped by clear, concise write-ups. During a disaster, all patients who are transported should have a patient care report written, in addition to the triage tag.

Unit Leadership Reinforcement During the crisis, if possible, it is best if a commander or supervisor performs occasional field checks to stay aware of conditions, complaints, and concerns. A strong, concerned unit commander can do a lot to bolster morale by listening to the field pulse. Many issues can be resolved with the early intervention of a concerned supervisor.

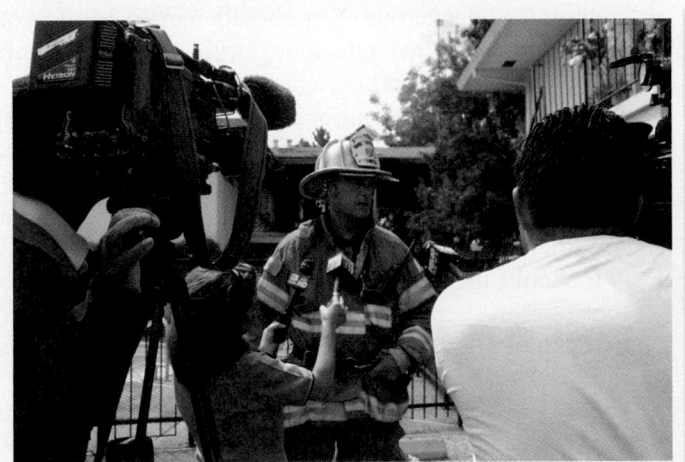

Figure 7 The public information officer or another responder must be trained in how to speak appropriately with the media regarding emergencies.

After the Event

There are specific measures to take after the event has occurred. These are listed in Table 3 . The time period after the event can be very useful: personnel can recover, supplies can be restocked, reimbursement can occur, and training needs can be identified.

Accountability Your agency must account for every worker and patient that was involved in an event. Duty rosters must be completed for each EMS provider to include, date(s) and times worked, duties, and any additional comments. A patient care report or triage tag is required for every patient seen, transported, or assisted.

Resupply and Repair All equipment used during the event must be replaced. All equipment that was not used must be checked to see if it was weathered or contaminated during the response. Finally, repair equipment that needs it, and service the vehicles that were used during the event.

Inventory After resupply and repair, a complete inventory of all physical assets should be done. This may be the time to reconsider equipment carried based on lessons learned during the crisis. The complete inventory will probably help in determining the reimbursement.

Stress Reaction Review Posttraumatic stress disorder is a real occurrence. Your agency may consider using critical incident stress management teams, especially for long-term events or those with a high mortality rate. As you work with colleagues, note subtle or dramatic changes in behavior in yourself and your coworkers, such as changes in mood or appetite. Any concerns should be immediately reported to your supervisor for further professional evaluation, in line with your agency's employee assistance program (EAP) or critical incident stress debriefing (CISD) program plans. Open communication should be encouraged, and your agency should provide a receptive environment for those exposed to tragedy.

Physical Examination of Personnel All injured personnel should be examined by a physician. This examination is useful for future workers' compensation claims in the event of

Table 3 Considerations After the Event
Accountability
Resupply and repair
Inventory
Stress reaction review
Physical examination of personnel
Brainstorm
After-action report
Finance and reimbursement
Acknowledgment

claimed disability. Physicians' comments should be maintained with the protected personnel records. The EMS provider should be notified of test results as soon as they are received. Also, counseling services should be made available, if requested or required.

Brainstorm Your agency should solicit input from its staff when evaluating the agency's response to a disaster. This process has a twofold benefit. The first is that EMS providers have a chance to share their observations and requests, making them stakeholders in the event. The second is that this feedback provides input for the after-action review.

After-action Report The <u>after-action report (AAR)</u> is your official internal report of the entire event. It should contain a chronological and accurate description of the facts of the incident. On the basis of this report, an agency can review the incident in its entirety. The after-action report and all accumulated anecdotal evidence can be used to provide a basis for retraining in specific areas. On the basis of the after-action report, EMS crews may become aware of areas of deficiency or skills that need to be refreshed. A plan for reinforcement of skills and knowledge should be prepared based on this data.

Finance and Reimbursement In large incidents, monies spent on equipment, personnel, and losses may be covered by government organizations or insurance. This is one of the reasons why a "declaration of a disaster" is important and may open up the door to state or federal disaster relief funds and low-interest loans. The key to reimbursement is accurate and specific documentation. It is also possible that some monies may be owed; again, itemization is the key.

Acknowledgment New paramedics may not be accustomed to being in a supervisory role, but may be the most senior person in the crew once working as a paramedic. Good performance should be praised so that EMS providers feel good about their service. Learn to praise often, immediately, and honestly. Awards dinners and plaques are justified in this selfless profession and do wonders to increase morale and retention of trained personnel.

Up until this point, we have discussed concerns that apply to every emergency response. The next sections will discuss specific disaster responses.

Natural Disasters

There are two types of disasters: natural and man-made. Some disasters are a combination of both types. For example, riots and looting may occur after a hurricane. Table 4 lists some examples of natural disasters.

As discussed previously, there are certain general actions to take before, during, and after every event. However, concerns related to specific disasters, must be considered, as well. These concerns should be addressed during the preplanning phase along with the general concerns that must be addressed for every event.

Table 4 Examples of Natural Disasters
Forest and brush fires
Snow and ice storms
Tornadoes
Hurricanes
Tsunamis
Earthquakes
Landslides, avalanches, mudslides
Cave-ins
Volcanoes
Flooding
Sandstorms and dust storms
Prolonged cold weather
Drought
Heat wave
Meteors and space debris
Pandemics

Forest and Brush Fires

Fires can be either natural or man-made. The response to forest and brush fires should be considered differently than the response to structural fires Figure 8. The following considerations apply to forest, brush, and lightning strike fires; some of these considerations apply to structural fires as well (discussed later).

- As a paramedic, remember that you are not there to fight fire. You will be directed to a safe staging or treatment area.
- Lightning is dangerous. You should remain inside your vehicle or in another safe spot during strikes. Minimize your chances for becoming a target for lightning.
- Try to predict which kind of injuries you will be treating. Fire fighters will most likely need care for smoke inhalation, exhaustion, and burns. Civilians will need care for exposure, physical and mental trauma, burns, exhaustion, and smoke inhalation.
- PPE should include proper gear in addition to infection control gear, such as bunker gear, air-purifying respirator (APR) masks, and heavy-duty gloves. Make sure you have extinguishers and protective blankets on board.
- Follow the directions of fire command and stay in touch at all times with the command post. Be prepared to move away immediately and have a couple of preplanned routes to safety.
- Firefighting is taxing; expect cardiac events, even in fire fighters who appear young and healthy.

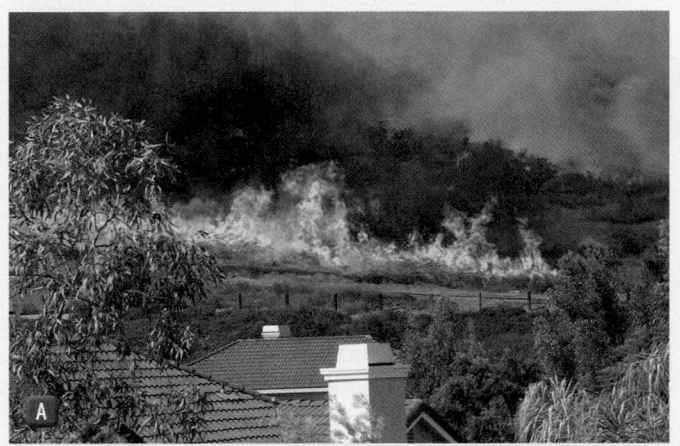

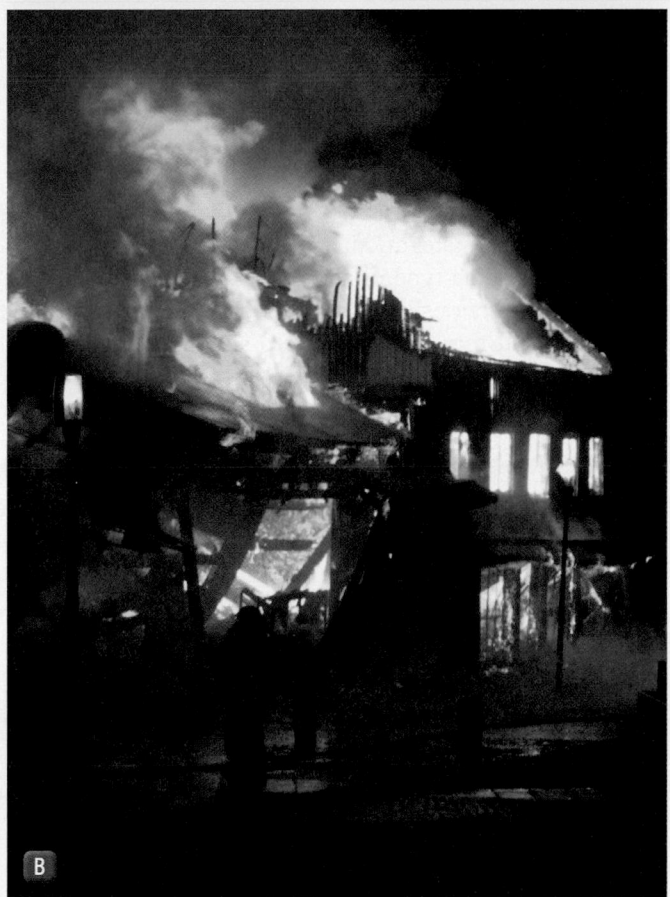

Figure 8 **A.** Most natural-occurring fires are forest or brush fires. **B.** Most man-made fires are structural.

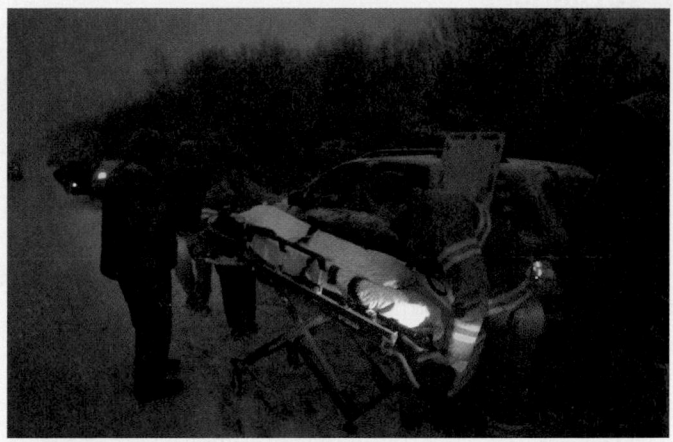

Figure 9 Working in a snow or ice storm requires proper gear and presents challenges when driving.

Snow and Ice Storms

The northern regions of the United States experience snow and ice storms regularly; however, these storms can occur anywhere in the country **Figure 9**. Personnel who do not have experience working in these conditions may have to adapt in a short period. It is important to make sure that your agency's vehicles are "snow ready." This includes using snow tires, possibly studded, or equipped with drop-down or freestanding chains. Also, be sure to check the vehicle's antifreeze and coolant levels. Cold weather motor oil should be used in vehicles.

Slow down! It is important that drivers of emergency vehicles understand the braking differences and the traction problems when driving in inclement conditions. It is tough to train for driving in snow and ice in areas that do not get much, but there are training programs available. Consider sending a team to a colder climate for hands-on practice. Remember that you may have four-wheel drive vehicles, but you do not have four-wheel brakes; four-wheel drive will not help once your vehicle is in a skid. Put a couple of snow shovels in the back of the ambulance just in case you need to dig a path through the snow. Kitty litter, calcium chloride crystals, and rock salt should also be on board to provide traction. If you are heading out to unplowed/unsalted streets, coordinate with your local municipal or state department of transportation to get you there safely. Many times municipal public works will take your transportation requests seriously. They may be able to reprioritize their tasks based on your needs.

Some important points to remember when working in snow and ice storms include the following:

- Clothing should be weather ready. Prepare for the conditions. You will need warm coats, pants, gloves, boots, hats, and lip balm.
- Your agency may have ancillary equipment such as snowmobiles, snow blowers, and plows. EMS providers should receive training on the equipment they may need to use during snow or ice storms.
- Take your time. Stretchers do not roll well in snow. You might not be able to park close to the scene; therefore, you may have to carry the patient(s) further. Plastic basket stretchers (Stokes litters) will be helpful. Make sure your crew has enough people.
- Look at the roof before entering a structure. EMS and fire personnel have been killed by snow and ice slides.
- If your company is on a standby status, prepare portable warm-up shelters or access to coffee, water, and hot chocolate.

Tornadoes

Tornadoes can and do occur anywhere in the country. Most commonly, they occur in the Midwest and South. The warnings may be timely or there may be none. Before the event, if possible, disperse and forward supplies in tornado-proof shelters to avoid destruction of these supplies if they are in the tornado's path. Whenever possible, store vehicles in storm-proof shelters until the storm has passed. During the tornado and until it is declared safe, keep your crews in tornado-proof shelters, preferably underground. After the tornado passes through, be ready to stage in a **directed area** to await instructions. A directed area is an area considered by engineering expertise to be a safe place to stage until directed otherwise.

It is likely that radio communication and cell phones will not be reliable, especially in the early stages of the tornado. Be prepared to act independently based on your storm protocols. Make use of amateur **radio operators** and communication experts who can "patch" through a temporary communication setup.

Important points to remember when working in tornadoes include the following:

- After a tornado hits, landmarks may be gone; use lights to direct displaced people toward emergency services. You might be collecting uninjured patients and bringing them to collection points. In the case of many casualties, casualty collection points can be set up to pick up lightly treated, stable patients by buses and trucks.
- Remember, helicopters and air assets probably will not be available. Air currents, **thermals** (changes in temperature and wind speed in the air), and rain make flying dangerous or impossible. Calling for medevac will not be an option during the initial aftermath.

- EMS should be represented both in the **emergency operations center (EOC)** and in the unified command center. This means having a physical presence as well as communications capability with those in the field.
- Situational awareness is essential. Again, landmarks may be gone and GPS may be knocked out. Members should be able to read a map and determine their location at all times.
- Tornadoes come with bad weather. Be prepared for foul weather and severe winds.
- As in many big disasters, dignitaries may visit the site of the incident for various reasons. This will present issues such as crowd control and EMS protection for the visitors.
- Consider leaving landmarks in the field in place of street signs that have been blown over. These landmarks can include spray-painted directions on curbs and flags planted on street corners.
- You may need to help set up field hospitals and first aid stations at **casualty collection points**.

Hurricanes

Hurricanes (ie, cyclones), can occur anywhere, but tend to happen in the southern states and in coastal regions. Usually, but not always, there is some type of warning. These warnings should always be taken seriously. Hurricanes come in five categories, ranging from category 1 (winds 74 to 95 mph; minimal damage expected) up to a category 5 (winds greater than 155 mph; severe damage expected). It is a good idea to plan on at least one level higher than the worst prediction.

Hurricane Katrina and the response, or lack of response, to it has become the new standard for the EMS world in terms of lessons learned. EMS and hospital communities did truly

YOU *are the Medic* | **PART 3**

Your patient fell from a second floor window when she tried to escape from her collapsed apartment. She is responsive and able to speak with you. She has obvious fractures of the left lower leg and right ankle that have been splinted. There is an intravenous lock in place. You move the patient to your stretcher and then to your unit. The transportation supervisor reports that you will transport your patient to Regional Hospital.

Recording Time: 5 Minutes	
Respirations	18 breaths/min
Pulse	96 beats/min
Skin	Cool, dry, pink
Blood pressure	140/86 mm Hg
Oxygen saturation (Spo_2)	98% prior to oxygen administration
Pupils	Equal and react to light

5. How does the transportation supervisor know which hospital you should transport to?

6. What additional patient assessment should you accomplish en route to the hospital?

heroic things during the hurricane, but that does not prevent criticism.

One lesson learned during and after Hurricane Katrina was that people's frustration can lead to feelings of fear or abandonment, which in turn can lead them to resort to violence to secure medical resources. If the situation is possibly dangerous to EMS worker (and personal) safety, do not go out without a security presence. If the situation is serious enough, the National Guard, Coast Guard, or State Police, may be available to assist.

Safety is first, always. You cannot help if you are injured or stranded. You will only add to the current problem if your response is not well thought out. If you are told to "hunker down," do it. Most EMS work will come after the storm. Is your staging site hurricane proof? You may be able to use the time before the storm hits to fill sandbags and restock equipment. In addition to PPE, make sure you have wet weather gear, personal flotation devices, and access to boats and other specialized equipment.

After the storm has passed, make sure to stay updated on post-storm failures such as levees that are overcome as well as bridges and roads that are flooded **Figure 10**. Your agency must have a means to communicate these changing developments with field personnel.

If you do not know the depth of the water, do not drive through it. You might want to consider high-axle vehicles such as ambulances as opposed to "fly car" sedans (for example, if you are meeting a BLS crew at a scene), that may sit too low for water driving.

Tsunamis

Tsunamis (also called tidal waves) are large waves with major destructive power. Tsunamis can travel thousands of miles, and can hit the shore at speeds of 250 to 600 mph, or more.

In 2011, the tsunami disaster in Japan showed the world the destructive power of a tidal wave and its potential for local annihilation **Figure 11**. Tsunamis and storm surges have the potential to occur in coastal areas of the United States and in Hawaii, Puerto Rico, and the US Virgin Islands. Unlike hurricanes, these events cannot always be predicted with the same amount of accuracy. There can be very little time, if any, for advance preparation. Also, mental health issues, in both workers and civilians, are common in these events.

Remember that your personal safety is essential. If you know a tsunami is coming, get out of the way. Move inland and get uphill. Your work will begin after the event. It is safe to assume that nothing that the water hits will survive. Bring all of your vehicles uphill and inland, and bring as many supplies as you can with you. If items need to be secured, plans should be made for tie-down stakes or for the use of tents or safes to secure supplies and drugs.

Tsunamis can come in a series. Even if subsequent events are less severe, your first-line defenses have probably been overwhelmed. If subsequent events are even more intense, you may need to move farther inland and onto higher elevation. Buildings will have a hard time sustaining that kind of an impact, which may be successive in nature.

Some important points relating to EMS response to tsunamis include the following:

- Pay strict attention to the warning systems in place and comply with instructions. Monitor systems at all times and have a backup receiving system in place. There should be someone, preferably in the EOC or command post, keeping up with current changes.

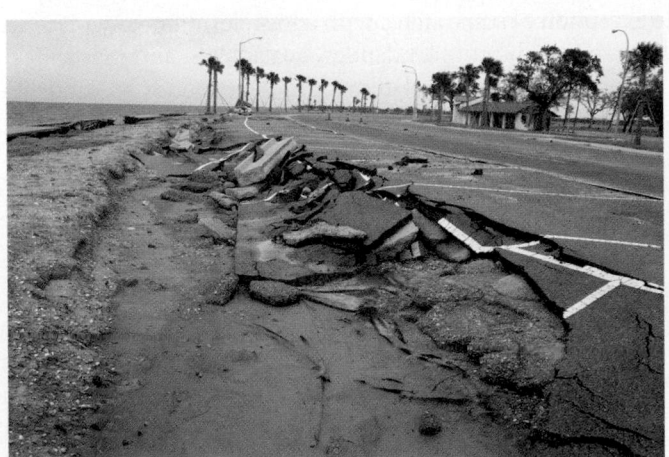

Figure 10 It is important to stay updated on post-storm failures such as levees that are overcome and bridges and roads that are awash.

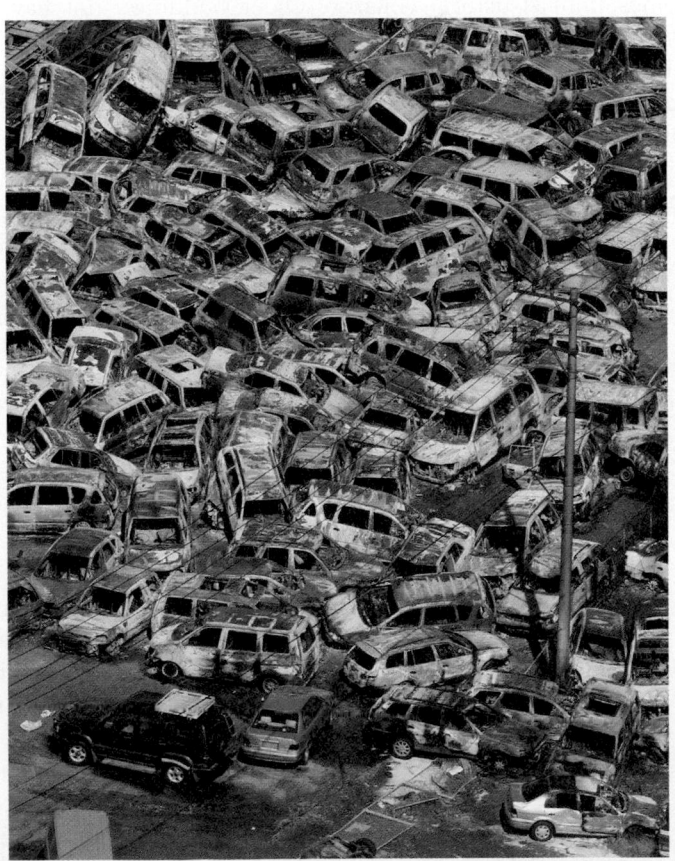

Figure 11 Tsunamis can cause local annihilation.

- It may seem like your initial patients would be drowning victims, but those who drowned will likely already be dead by the time EMS can reach them. Instead, you should primarily prepare for trauma patients who have been struck by or entangled in debris. Exposure will also become problematic, especially as time goes on.
- Your agency should plan to set up a temporary morgue site to accommodate patients who are beyond EMS help.

Remember that you cannot respond until the tsunami has done its damage. Until the danger has passed, resources and personnel must be kept safe. Patient care and cleanup begin once the safety of EMS personnel can be ensured. Your response will depend on what kind of access you will have once the tsunami has passed.

Earthquakes

On August 23, 2011, a magnitude 5.8 earthquake struck Mineral, Virginia, affecting major population centers in the entire northeastern United States. This was a rare occurrence and despite the minimal damage and very few injuries that resulted, it demonstrates that no region of the country is safe from earthquake damage. As in other disasters, there may be little or no warning. Earthquakes, depending on their size, duration, and strength can cause thousands of deaths and billions of dollars of damage within minutes. Aftershocks will occur regularly after the initial earthquake and can be substantial. In some cases, they can last for days.

The biggest immediate danger resulting from an earthquake comes from structural collapse. Older buildings, not having been subject to newer building codes, are the most problematic. Also, severed gas and electrical power lines as well as fuel tanks spilling their fumes and contents contribute to fires during and after the event.

Important points related to EMS response to earthquakes include the following:

- If you have advance warning, or if you are in an area along an earthquake fault line, your building and vehicle contents should be secured. Straps, springs, and bungee cords can be used to secure contents. Look at your buildings and imagine something shaking them violently from the outside, then think about what you could do to secure items so that they do not fall or become damaged.
- During and after an earthquake, roads will likely be damaged or cut off. Stay in touch with your local EOC and keep up with conditions in your response area.
- A phenomenon known as **dust suffocation** can occur during the quake. This is caused by particles of dust and debris loosened and released into the air. These produce both a toxic and hypoxic atmosphere. Breathing will be difficult, and face masks, at the very least, should be worn during the recovery efforts.
- If you are responding to patients at the scene of a building collapse, leave the rescue to the trained rescue personnel. If a patient is outside the building and easy to reach, make sure your footing is good and that the patient platform is stable.

When in doubt, do not go out! Your weight and that of your crew could make the bearing structure untenable.

- Rescuers will need ongoing rehabilitation. It is easy for personnel in these situations to develop tunnel vision and not recognize situations dangerous to them, such as fatigue, dehydration, and posttraumatic stress disorder.
- If possible, have extra food and water on board. This is not just for you and your crew, but also for civilians, patients, and other rescuers. It will take time for authorities to get food and water delivery services up and running.
- Call your local hospitals and find out if they are able to receive patients. Find out whether the hospitals sustained damage. They may need you to set up a field hospital or assist a **forward surgical team** (a team, usually staffed with physicians, nurses, and EMS providers, that performs minor surgical procedures and debridements in the field, taking some of the load from the hospital facility).
- When you are out in the field, take note of hazards such as unstable buildings and severed gas lines. Make a list and report these to the EOC as soon as possible. This will, at the least, make others aware of the danger and help to get repairs scheduled.

Finally, if your local hospitals, schools, businesses, government offices, or fire departments participate in regular earthquake drills, try to become a part of them.

Landslides, Avalanches, and Mudslides

There are many reasons for landslides, avalanches, and mudslides based on natural occurrences throughout the country. These include severe winter storms, heavy rainfall, wildfires and past wildfires, flash flooding, major and minor earthquakes, hurricanes and typhoons, and intentional landslides performed to clear massive vegetation for urbanization. This happens because the surface tension in the earth and bedrock changes drastically—for example due to winter storms. Southern California experiences earthquakes almost every year. Many western ski resorts have daily avalanche patrols and experience these numerous times throughout the winter season. With the possible exception of some states with a low elevation, any place with a hill can be subject to landslides, avalanches, and mudslides.

Important points related to EMS response to landslides, avalanches, and mudslides include the following:

- Cliffs, high hills, and anything in the gravity path of a landslide, avalanche, or mudslide would obviously be in the danger area. If time permits, consider moving out of the target area and stage at a safer location.
- When a landslide occurs, it can cause such a buildup of soil and vegetation that it can block a stream or river, causing a lake to be formed. You may need to consider putting water rescue procedures in place.
- Underground piping, conduit for electrical lines, and telephone lines can be damaged. Plan for alternate water delivery and waste systems; generators and cell phones may need to be employed, as well.

- EMS may be initially deployed to assist in evacuation efforts.
- Mudslides or mudflows are similar to a river of concrete. Do not venture into these, or into the path of gravity, on foot or in vehicles. Indeed, you may treat many people who were trapped in cars that were swept away by the mud.
- The intense heat of brushfires seals the soil surface, making mudslides, avalanches, and landslides move even faster over terrain. Consider the history of the area when preplanning. Past landslide events predict what could happen again; review past incident reports as a normal part of preplanning.
- Equipment that may be planned for in advance should include backhoes and earth movers.

Cave-ins

Cave-ins occur naturally for the same reasons that landslides, mudslides, and avalanches occur. However, in cave-ins, the bedrock is not as important a consideration as is the actual soil composition. Cave-ins can be caused by rapid freezing and thawing, heavy rain, or excess vibration such as that associated with earthquakes and tremors **Figure 12A**.

Considerations for EMS response during a cave-in include the following:

- If a cave-in occurs in your response area, check with your local utility company to make sure power lines are not severed or unstable **Figure 12B**. Remember, underground mining can cause overhead lines to fail.
- Be watchful for loose rock in the collapse area. In cave-ins, EMS personnel are under the command of trench rescue responders. They will identify safe zones based on shoring and sloping techniques.
- In a cave-in there will almost always be accumulation of water. Expect that patients will have been trapped in water, and be prepared to treat the patient(s) for hypothermia. Pumping out accumulated water can cause further damage in the area of collapse; therefore, keep an eye on the run-off if the pump is still in service at the scene. If you are pumping out water, make sure the water that is being pumped is not degrading the area you are working on.
- There are three ways to secure the area of excavation: sloping, benching, and shoring **Figure 12C**. Unless you are qualified in these techniques, do not enter an area of collapse or potential collapse.
- The atmosphere in cave-ins is generally toxic. You can assume that any patient brought out of a cave-in has been in an oxygen-deficient atmosphere.
- If the patient care area is located in the collapse area, continuous monitoring of the lower explosive limit, carbon monoxide (CO), hydrogen sulfide gas, and oxygen levels is essential.
- Cave-ins can release sewer and chemical gases. After atmosphere security, consider positive-pressure ventilation in the patient care area.

Volcanic Eruptions

It may surprise you to learn that the United States follows only Japan and Indonesia in having the highest number of volcanic eruptions in the world. Ten percent of the world's eruptions take place in the United States, and they occur primarily

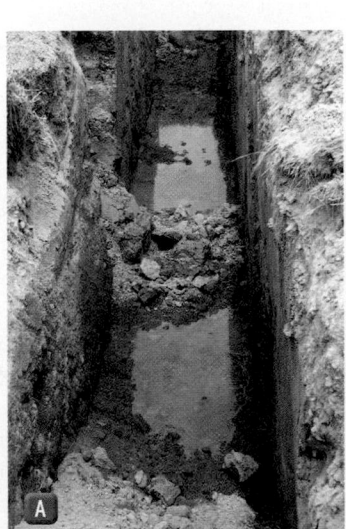
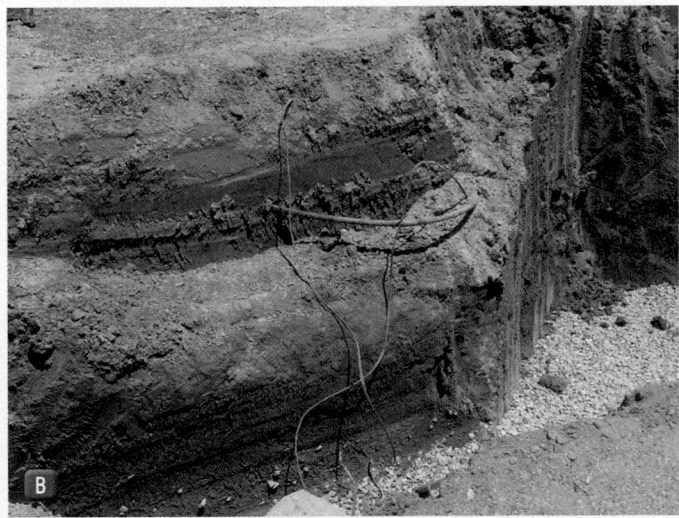
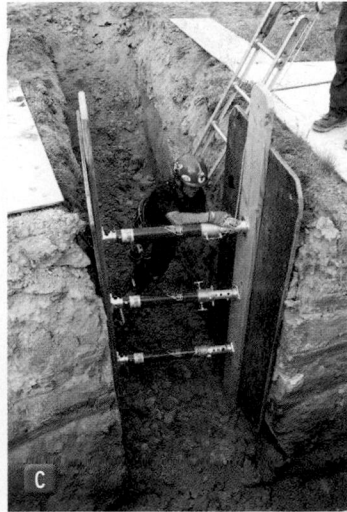

Figure 12 Cave-ins are associated with many dangers and require specially-trained rescue personnel. Do not enter a cave-in scene until directed to do so by the incident commander. **A.** The presence of water can make a cave-in more likely. **B.** Electrical wires must be secured before entering the area. **C.** Walls must be secured with specialty techniques such as sloping, benching, and shoring. This photo shows a top shore being installed.

in Alaska, Hawaii, and the Pacific Northwest **Figure 13**. The primary emergencies come from **pyroclastic explosions**, which are the explosions that occur in the bubbling magma. These are associated with release of hot ash and gas emissions. Lava flow is rarely a problem as its course is slow and predictable.

Since volcanic eruptions usually occur at a height, rescue workers may be affected by secondary problems, including melting ice and snow and the resultant water flows. Landslides may also occur with mudflows.

During preplanning, identify buildings that are "volcano proof" (ie, made of fire retardant construction materials), including your squad buildings. Are there warning systems in place? EMS crews should be trained to respond based on the projected timeline.

Consider the following when responding to a volcanic eruption:

- If a population is located close to an eruption and the warning is late or nonexistent, panic may spread. Evacuation will become the prime concern.
- Expected injuries include burns, respiratory problems, and crush trauma injuries. Respiratory problems will be continuous and serious. Acid rain and acid-based debris will also contribute to respiratory, eye, and skin problems.
- **Ashfall** is the residue left behind from the eruption. This can cause inhalation issues. Masks should be issued to everyone (crews and patients) in downrange positions. Ingestion also becomes a problem because ash gets into the food and water supply chains. Packaged food and water must be provided. The weight of ashfall can cause roofs to collapse. Try to shovel the ash to keep your agency's roofs clear, and clean the ash from windshields to make driving less difficult. Drive carefully because ash can make roads slippery.
- Try to make the public aware of the importance of wearing respiratory protection, even after the initial danger is resolved.

■ Flooding

Although the flooding associated with Hurricane Katrina in 2005 was well publicized, severe flooding happens annually all over the United States. For example, flooding from Hurricane Irene covered the Northeast in 2011 and was devastating in terms of the economy, lives lost, and number of people injured. Never underestimate the power of a rising river.

Most preparations for flooding occur during preplanning. Typically, the regions that will be affected can be predicted; therefore, during the preplanning process, agencies should identify the amount of time needed to execute response plans. Long-term consequences of flooding cannot be judged as easily.

Issues to watch for during EMS response to flooding are **overtopping** (reservoirs overflowing their borders); slow degradation of levees and banks; and debris flow, which contains large debris such as logs or cars and has a greater impact force

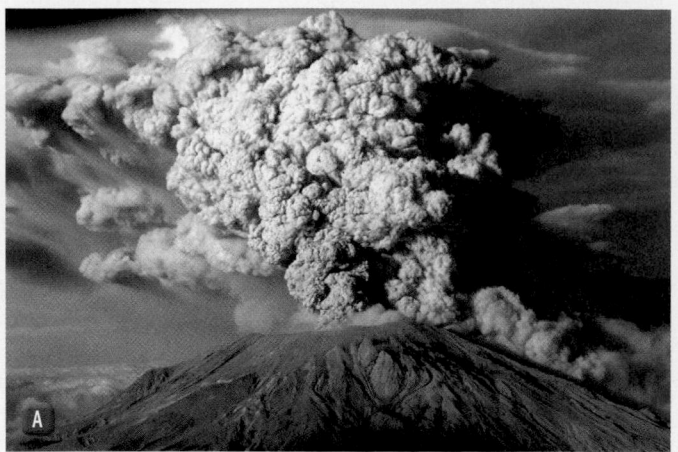

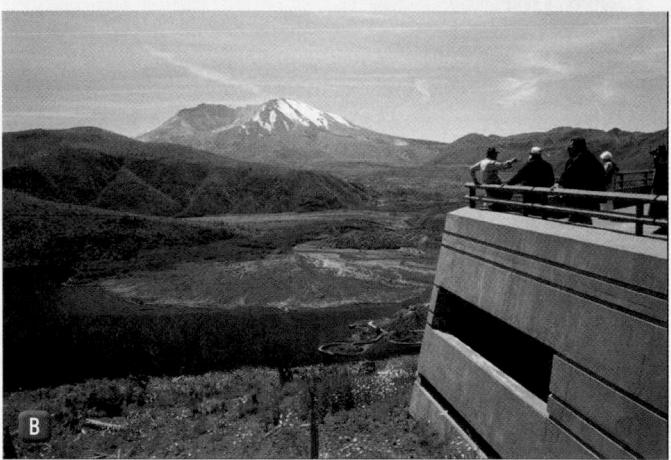

Figure 13 In 1980, Mount St Helens in Washington state experienced the most devastating volcanic eruption recorded in US history. **A.** The explosion. **B.** Regrowth of the area almost 30 years after the eruption.

than water that does not contain such debris. Also watch for sudden catastrophic degradation of levees, which tend to cause a "chain reaction" destructive effect. As one section of sandbags fails, the flow washes away the remaining bags.

Additional considerations for flood response include the following:

- Wear proper wet weather gear, and use personal flotation devices as well as **tag lines** (safety ropes tied around rescuers so they can be pulled to safety) when necessary.
- Driving through water can be challenging. Make sure you use only high-axle vehicles, such as ambulances, fire trucks, fire engines, and SUVs, not cars. Moving water as low as 2 inches can easily move a car.
- Walking in moving water that is over 6 inches deep will likely result in a fall, and you may be swept away. Make sure that you and your team members are connected with tag lines or at least link arms when walking through moving water.

Damage can be surveyed after the flood and when the water starts to recede. This is also when the contaminants and residue left behind by the floods can cause serious health problems. Cleanup is essential and should start as soon as practical.

Sandstorms and Dust Storms

Sandstorms and dust storms are common in arid and semiarid regions of the country, especially after a prolonged period of drought. For the EMS provider, most of the problems associated with these storms are directly related to the abrasive and visual effects of the storm. Considerations for responding to a sandstorm or dust storm include the following:

- During a sandstorm sensory input becomes difficult. You may lose your orientation and should consider shelter-in-place until the storm subsides.
- Eye protection should be worn. It should cover the entire eye area because sand will come in from the side of standard EMS goggles.
- Do not rub your eyes, nose, or skin during a storm. Sand is an abrasive (like sandpaper) and can cause permanent injury, specifically to the eyes.
- Respiratory protection should be worn. Properly fitted APRs and N-95 masks will seal out more of the fine particles of sand than will a standard surgical mask.
- Lip balm as well as some kind of a cloth barrier over your whole head is a good idea during the storm.
- Driving is a challenge, even during a minor event. If you employ your windshield washer fluid, you will create a muddy windshield. Be prepared to stop and manually clean the windshield if you cannot see (ensure that you have windshield cleaner and a squeegee in your vehicle). Before heading out, you may wish to consider applying one of the chemical spray-on appliques available that will make the windshield more slippery, which can prevent sand from accumulating as quickly.
- Objects may be hidden by the blowing sand. Keep low and be aware.

Prolonged Cold Weather

Prolonged cold weather is relative; EMS workers in some regions of the country such as the northern states are used to working in cold conditions and have relatively little trouble adapting. What is cold to a person from Georgia compared with a Minnesota native might be dramatically different. In areas that do not regularly get a lot of cold weather, especially for a long period of time, EMS response can become challenging.

People who are exposed to cold weather for long periods of time, even though sheltered, can develop a condition called cold stress. This is similar to seasonal affective disorder (SAD) and can take a serious psychological toll on EMS crews. EMS providers and management should monitor each other for changes in personality and work habits. The cold weather itself is taxing to EMS providers.

If maintenance or repair issues can wait until warmer weather, let them. If repairs must be done, try to make them during the warmest part of the day. Things like washing the vehicles may not be necessary, unless there are decontamination problems. Try to limit physical demands, if possible. For example, it is not a good idea to shovel snow or chop ice for hours and then have to respond to an EMS call.

Additional considerations for working in prolonged cold weather include the following:

- Dress loosely and in layers. Avoid tight clothing that can restrict blood flow. Have dry, clean replacement clothes with you, especially boots and socks. Hats and good gloves are important, as well.
- If you have to do standbys, try to switch crews frequently. If possible, have warm-up tents or sheds set up on a long scene. Hot liquids should be placed on the vehicles or delivered to field crews.
- Keep an eye on older EMS providers—for example, those older than 55 years. They may not handle the cold as well as younger workers. Also watch crew members who may have minor medical issues or may be pregnant.

Drought

Drought is caused by a lack of water available to the public and is primarily based on a lack of precipitation over a length of time. Drought causes a myriad of problems for the medical community. Heat injuries are more common during droughts. Dust storms and wildfires are more common during droughts, with their concurrent problems. Snakes migrate more often during drought, increasing the risk of snake bite injuries. Finally, both water quality and quantity are significantly reduced. Infections increase, as does the possibility of surface contamination, because the remaining standing pools are highly concentrated with more bacteria and sediment from human waste.

Your agency may have to secure its working water supply. Civil unrest could spread if townspeople think EMS crews have water. EMS could require protection and security from police.

Heat Wave

EMS personnel are very cognizant of the three main types of heat injury in patients: heat cramps, heat exhaustion, and heatstroke. They are less familiar with working in these conditions every day. In Chicago, Illinois, in 1995, a heat wave occurred in which 495 people died of heat-related causes and 23 of 42 hospitals were placed on diversion or bypass status. In 2003, a European heat wave killed thousands. The following are some of the problems and potential solutions to issues that occur during a heat wave:

- Vigilance is the key. If possible, work in pairs, monitoring each other for heat-related problems.
- Water must be consumed at all times. Small, constant sips of water throughout the day are best. You may also consider some electrolyte fluid replacement in addition to the water.
- Small, more frequent meals are better than large ones. Eat foods that are heavy in fluids, such as vegetables, fruits, and salads.

- Set up "water trains." As you empty your water bottles, have them refilled. Your agency must ensure that it has a good, clean source of water. Use of <u>water buffalo trailers</u> (500-gallon water containers on trailers), <u>lister bags</u> (100-liter canvas bags that can be hung from trees), and portable water backpacks is advisable.
- If you have air conditioning in your buildings or vehicles, use it!
- Wet towels placed on the head or on the body can help reduce body temperature.
- Try to break up work schedules during the hottest part of the day. Take frequent rest breaks, in a cool, shady place, if possible. Schedule manual labor for evening or morning shifts if possible.

Meteors and Space Debris

Meteors, asteroids, space debris, and <u>space junk</u> are not just the stuff of science fiction novels. Meteors regularly hit the earth, though mostly in desert areas. As meteors and asteroids approach earth's atmosphere, they become micrometeoroids and, for the most part, burn up. Space debris (natural materials, such as micrometeoroids) or space junk (man-made items), also burn up when entering the atmosphere. Space junk can be any man-made material, whereas meteors are generally stones with a high content of iron.

Most space debris and large meteors coming from space can be detected. The problem is ascertaining just where they will land and how great the impact will be.

Other things can fall from the sky, such as spent bullets and waste products from aircraft. There is really no way to be prepared for them all. Keep an open mind when a patient has a history of sudden sharp pain with local bruising.

Pandemics

An <u>epidemic</u> is illness that affects a disproportionately large geographic area and number of people. A <u>pandemic</u> is an extensive epidemic. The H1N1 influenza outbreak of 2009 is a good example of a pandemic. Not all pandemics are influenza. The bubonic plague of the 16th century and various diseases such as SARS and AIDS were also considered pandemics.

The most important consideration during these situations will always be personal protection from the disease. Gloves and goggles may not be enough. You may need N-95 or APR-type respiratory protection as well as gowns. Handwashing and sanitizing is the best first line of defense. In addition, prophylaxis, such as vaccination should be administered free of charge to all health care workers in the crew (EMS providers as well as other health care workers, and their families, if possible). If vaccination is not available, after-care medicine should be provided.

The best method of detecting disease in workers is direct observation and reports from crew members. If someone appears to be sick, that person should be pulled from duty. Sick EMS providers should be sent home or to the hospital.

The <u>6-feet rule</u> should be applied. A person can transmit a sneeze or cough from a distance of 6 feet. Try to stay out of this area. Even though you should be wearing a mask, the patient may not be. Staying more than 6 feet away becomes particularly challenging in the back of an ambulance, if not impossible. In those cases, maintain as much distance as possible.

Realize that in a pandemic situation, the full work force will not be present. They will be sick or caring for sick loved ones. Your agency's <u>continuity of operations plan (COOP)</u> should be in effect.

The public should be instructed via 9-1-1 dispatch, your public information officer, EOC, or phone or radio on how to care for sick people in place. In conjunction with your medical director, your agency should set specific guidelines for which emergencies you will respond to, and which calls will have to wait until more serious cases have been handled.

Your agency may have to set up field hospitals or care stations. Your agency may be called on to become a <u>point of distribution (POD)</u> for medicine or vaccination with minimal additional training provided. A POD is a temporary supply and inoculation or medicine distribution area.

Man-Made Disasters

Many types of disasters are caused by humans. Several examples are listed in Table 5. The next section discusses these, with the exception of weapons of mass destruction and hazardous materials incidents, which are discussed in the chapters, *Terrorism* and *Hazardous Materials*, respectively. Remember that as with natural disasters, general actions must be taken before, during, and after every event.

Structural Fires

Wildland fires are horrendous, but structural fires, whether intentional or accidental, have a much higher death and injury rate Figure 14. Structural fires are different from forest and brush fires in that structural fires occur in populated areas and

Table 5 Examples of Man-Made Disasters

Structural fires
Construction failures and building collapse
Power failures or disruptions
Riots, civil disturbances, and stampedes
Strikes and labor disputes
Sniper, shooter, and hostage situations
Explosions (intentional and unintentional)
IT (cyber) disruptions
Incidents involving weapons of mass destruction
Hazardous materials incidents

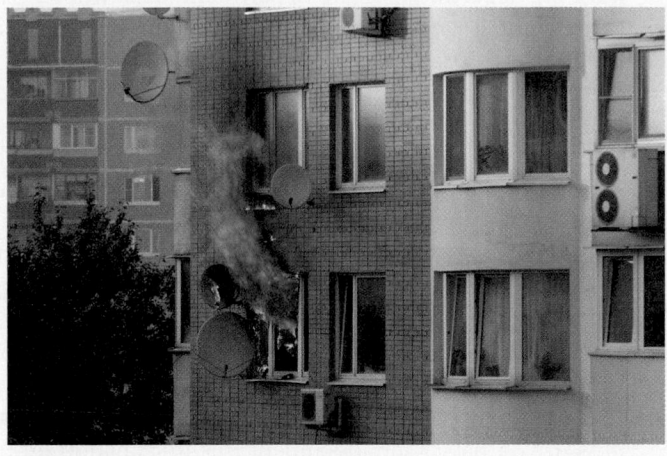

Figure 14 Structural fires have a much higher death and injury rate than wildland fires.

involve products of combustion that can be explosive, toxic, fast-spreading, and very unpredictable. Structural fires have the added hazard that if they were set by an arsonist, he or she may be strategically planning to entrap fire fighters.

Remember to let the fire fighter fight the fire. EMS crews probably do not have the proper bunker gear, training, or expertise to contain the conflagration or to rescue people from a burning building. Personnel must be staged properly at a safe, visible distance from the scene where vehicles or equipment will not interfere with firefighting operations or apparatus placement. Your agency must ensure that it has someone in the unified command who will have face-to-face contact with command as the event materializes.

Additional key points for EMS response to structural fires include the following:

- Watch for falling or collapsing items. Roofs can collapse, and people, ice, or severed power lines can fall rapidly from above.
- Prepare to treat burns and respiratory problems. Injuries to fire fighters will include exhaustion, heat injuries, cold injuries, CO poisoning, and trauma.
- Stay upwind. Smoke from artificial resins carries many toxins and carcinogens. You cannot always see the products of complete and incomplete combustion (CO and cyanide). At a minimum, wear a surgical mask; APRs provide even more protection.
- Be prepared to evacuate your position quickly. Fires double in size every minute if unchecked. Plan a few routes away from the scene, just in case.
- Be ready for cardiac events. These are the number one killer of fire fighters at the scene of fires. CO and cyanide poisoning can cause ECG abnormalities such as T-wave aberrancies.

Construction Failures and Building Collapse

In July 1981, a recently completed walkway collapsed in the Hyatt Regency Hotel in Kansas City, Missouri, killing 114 people and seriously injuring 216. EMS learned many lessons from this disaster, especially in the triage role. New and old constructions fail all the time, everywhere. EMS crews and agencies must be ready to handle all eventualities to the best of their abilities.

As part of preplanning, check out the new construction in your area. A building or other large structure is most dangerous

YOU *are the Medic* | PART 4

You assess the patient's legs for pulses, motor function, and sensation, and all appear unchanged. The patient's vital signs remain stable. The intravenous lock is accessible and flushes easily. You begin administering oxygen to the patient via nasal cannula. Your partner reports that there is a large stretch of damaged roadway between your current location and the hospital.

Recording Time: 10 Minutes	
Respirations	18 breaths/min
Pulse	96 beats/min
Skin	Warm, pink, dry
Blood pressure	140/84 mm Hg
Oxygen saturation (Spo$_2$)	100% with oxygen administration
Pupils	Equal and react to light

7. What actions should be taken after a disaster to ensure your wellbeing?

8. What is the purpose of the after-action report?

while under construction. Review the site and preplan access and egress routes. Note conditions, dirt roads, and placement of equipment such as cranes. Update these plans frequently. Your agency can take pictures to share with its crews. Your agency can also talk to the construction foreman to determine what could go wrong.

While considering EMS care at these sites, consider what special PPE you might need such as helmets, steel toe safety boots, eye protection, knee pads, and heavy-duty work gloves **Figure 15**.

Considerations when responding to construction failures and building collapses include the following:

- If there is a lock out/tag out information sheet on site, review it. This sheet contains information regarding the number of people and conditions in the danger zone. In addition, all fixed buildings are required to have a current Material Safety Data Sheet on file at the site and the local building department or fire department. This will tell you the quantities and types of materials your patients may have been exposed to.
- During response, particularly response to a large collapse, crews may be called on to do a perimeter search for patients. This includes only the farthest reaches of the perimeter where patients could have wandered off or been directed, not the collapse area. Once you find these victims, get them to a safe area, and start both the accountability and triage processes. Use your sector tags and flags to prevent confusion.
- When victims are brought to you, try to elicit from them information such as the position in which the patient was found, initial patient complaints, and level of consciousness. If you have time, document this information on the patient care report or triage tag and include the names of rescuers who brought the patient to you.
- You may need to supply backboards, straps, and Stokes baskets to the rescuers. Make sure they know how to use the equipment and, if possible, rig it in advance to make it easier for rescuers to use.
- At big events, be wary of locating a triage or treatment center in an area with a bowstring- or truss-type roofing configuration. These are notorious for weakening when under stress or fire.

Power Failures or Disruptions

Power failures and electrical disruptions are, at best, annoying. In the EMS world, they can be truly life threatening. These are common problems that happen frequently in all parts of the country, and these failures and disruptions last for various lengths of time. EMS must be prepared.

If your squad building has electric locks on its doors or equipment rooms, your agency should consider getting a manual override device. Remember that agency refrigerators and heaters will not be working. If fluids and medications are stored in there, your agency should have an alternate source for heating or cooling (eg, in its vehicles).

Backup generators must be checked on a regular basis. They should be turned on and run for at least half an hour each month. Fuel must be topped off and there should be an ample supply of fuel stored in a flame-proof container. Remember that these devices need oil too. The operating manuals should be kept near the device.

Make sure to have battery-powered backup devices. For example, if you have an electric suction device, make sure it has a battery- or oxygen-powered backup. Manual suctions are crude, but they do work. Make sure you and your colleagues are trained to use them.

Have an ample supply of batteries (all types) available. When the failure occurs, particularly if it lasts a long time, you will not be able to purchase them anywhere at any price. Crew members may bring their own flashlights, cell phones, and headlamps, which may take batteries that you do not normally use. Stock up on the common types necessary to power these devices.

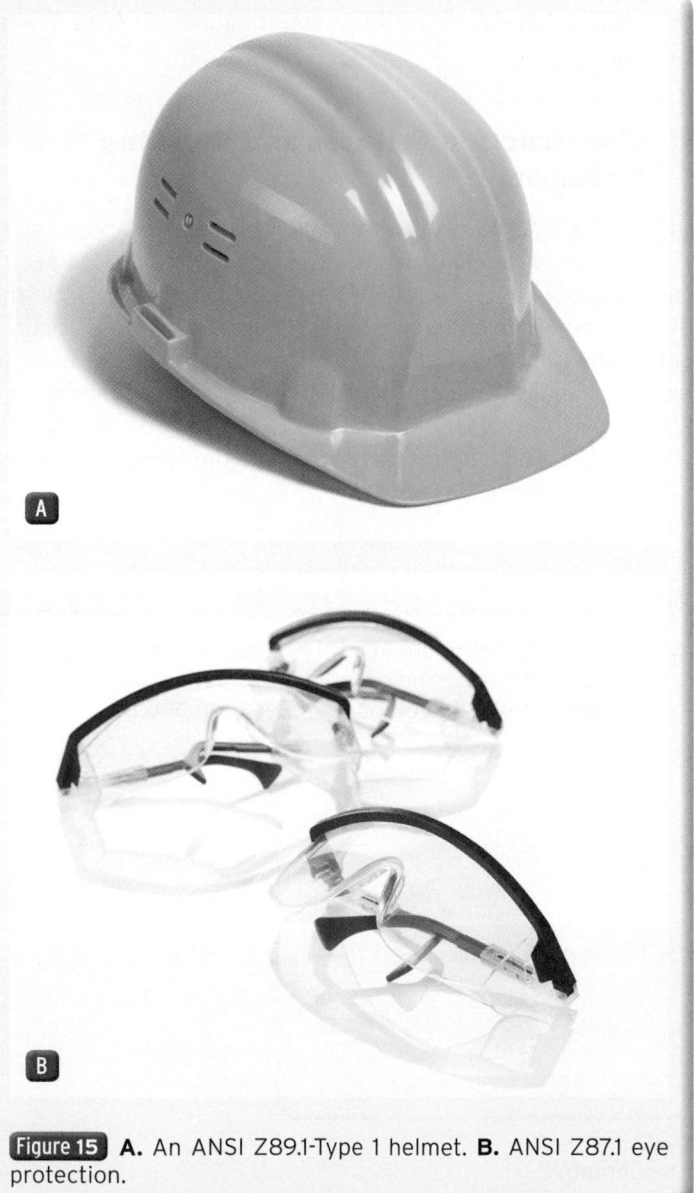

Figure 15 **A.** An ANSI Z89.1-Type 1 helmet. **B.** ANSI Z87.1 eye protection.

Make a list of all patients who use electrically powered life-saving devices, such as ventilators, at home. Your crew may need to manually supply ventilations to such patients. Ahead of time, find out whether you have a home dialysis patient in your area; he or she may need your assistance in the event of a power failure.

Computers will be down, so you will not be able to download electronic patient care reports, at least for a while. Make sure you have written versions of the patient care report or triage tags to use as a substitute. Because cell phones and GPS may be out of service, be ready to use radios and paper maps; they work just as well, with a little patience.

Riots, Civil Disturbances, and Stampedes

EMTs and paramedics are accustomed to being exposed to dangers such as violent patients, cars speeding past on the freeway, family hysteria, and verbal and physical abuse; it comes with the job. Multiply those dangers by hundreds or even thousands—that is the scenario in riots, civil disturbances, and stampedes. In these events, many people will be in panic mode. Even peaceful protests such as the Occupy movements of 2011 and 2012 can quickly degenerate into violent confrontations, as did the protests in Oakland, California in 2011 **Figure 16**. Always plan for and expect the worst.

Before and during the response, get as much information as possible from dispatch, police, or command about the scene you are entering. It is crucial to stay updated and maintain communication with these organizations. These events can change quickly. You do not want to get into a situation that you cannot get out of.

Considerations during an EMS response to riots, civil disturbances, and stampedes include the following:

- Once a safe route is transmitted to you, do not report to or set up a staging area until you are sure the scene is safe or that you will have physical police presence. Ascertain the location of the command post and establish communications with it. Frequent updates are the key to safety.
- Determine what is happening right now and what could potentially happen. For example, if tear gas or pepper spray has been used, you will need to protect yourselves from the gas and you will need lots of water to treat a large number of patients. If rocks or other missiles have been thrown, you should be ready to treat these traumas. Do not drive over broken glass, and if the crowd is still there, consider using a ground guide to walk in front of the slow moving vehicle for safety. Is there smoke from protestors burning tires and bonfires? Make sure you have respiratory protection and watch out for limited visibility concerns.
- Your situational awareness is paramount. The chaotic scene may not be familiar to you. Use the buddy system; do not split up. Make sure you always have a 360° view of the scene. GPS could be necessary if you need assistance. Most handheld GPS devices can identify

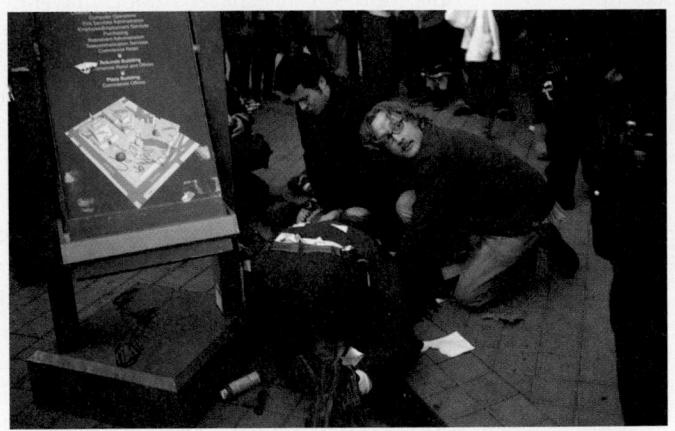

Figure 16 Protests can quickly degenerate into violent confrontations, as did this Occupy protest in Oakland, California in 2011.

your location to within 10 meters. You must have a radio—make sure that it is turned on! Do not make the mistake of thinking your radio is very quiet, only to discover that you failed to turn it on. Headsets become a real advantage especially when there is a lot of noise or yelling, and are also helpful because you need two hands for patient care.

- Police escort is crucial during riots, civil disturbances, and stampedes. If police escort is unavailable, keep command notified of your location and your movements.
- Consider wearing body armor, a helmet, and an APR, and carry more than one flashlight.
- Anything you see at the scene could later be used in criminal or civil court. Document everything as thoroughly as you can, or have a running commentary taped while you are out in the field. Do not count on your memory to serve you well during a chaotic situation; you have enough to think about.

Strikes and Labor Disputes

Strikes and labor disputes are another everyday occurrence in the United States. These disputes can involve large groups of people nationwide and may last a long time. Others may be

Controversies

Some people in EMS think that EMTs and paramedics should be armed. They argue that EMS providers will be better able to protect themselves, and will be able to assist the police with firepower. The counterargument is that weapons training would involve adding even more hours to an already daunting curriculum. And if the provider is busy engaging a target, who is taking care of the patient?

small and may last only hours; the general public may never hear of them. Even though most strikes and labor disputes involve disagreements, they are generally peaceful. However, even in peaceful disputes, people on both sides of the picket line can get sick or injured, which presents EMS with some of the following tactical and ethical considerations:

- Should EMS providers cross the picket line? Many EMS providers are members of a union or may sympathize with the strikers. Crossing the picket line to help a patient does not mean that you are taking sides. Remember that you do not know whether you are responding for a striker, management, or an uninvolved civilian. You are there to care for the patient. Ask yourself the following question, "What is in the best interest of the patient?" and follow that answer. However, this does not mean that you should sacrifice your safety in any way. Secure police escort and get away from a violent situation immediately. You cannot help anyone if you are hurt. However, remember that failure to cross a picket line to care for an ill or injured patient simply because you support the cause of the strikers constitutes abandonment, gross negligence, and represents grounds for suit and grounds for disciplinary action relative to your license or certification.
- If the patient is ambulatory, he or she might be safely brought to you.
- Television coverage of an event, especially a volatile one, can act as a deterrent to verbal or physical attacks on EMS providers in front of a large audience. This may be a false security, but should give you something to think about. You may be able to use this to your advantage.
- Again, document and record all your findings, particularly if participants on either side of the labor action appeared to have delayed EMS response or patient care.

■ Sniper, Shooter, and Hostage Situations

In all shooter and sniper scenarios, EMS should be staged out of gun range (the kill zone). You need to be out of the line of fire. In an indirect fire situation such as mortar or a rocket, you need to be out of the effective range. If gunshot victims are still exposed, do not go to help them. Trained people will either get them under cover or eliminate the threat. If you can see or hear about their wounds, you can tell a police officer or SWAT member how to stop bleeding by applying a tourniquet or how to open an airway.

In a hostage situation, the perpetrators may want EMS to examine or treat a hostage or a fellow perpetrator. Entering such a situation is very dangerous; perpetrators are usually mentally unstable.

The press and news media will probably be located near you in a safe area. Do not say anything to the press about the incident. Refer them to the public information officer at the scene. Be careful if they are lurking, listening to updates on your radio. You are responsible for communications security on your end. They may praise and compliment you in an effort to win your trust to get you to say something "off the record." This will come back to haunt you and could jeopardize the scenario.

Try to anticipate the type of injuries that you may need to treat. Are perpetrators going to use tear gas? Prepare to treat respiratory problems. Obviously, gunshot wounds and other violent trauma must be expected. If it is a long standoff, do not lose your sense of urgency regarding security. The situation can be just as dangerous, maybe more so, as the event goes on. Stay hydrated, fed and, if possible, rested.

■ Explosions

Explosions can be intentional or unintentional. The end result is the same: predictable injuries. Explosions were covered in the chapter, *Trauma Systems and Mechanism of Injury*, but here are a few additional considerations:

- Secondary and tertiary explosives may have been placed. The first bomb may have been set to draw in responders. Improvised explosive devices (IEDs) and vehicle-borne improvised explosive devices (VBIEDs) have been used in new waves of explosive attacks. These devices can be concealed in cars, trash containers, or anywhere near the safe zone. Keep your eyes open and stay alert. The Internet has made bomb making a "do-it-yourself" project for many people.
- When you begin treating patients, carefully record anything a seriously injured patient has to say. This patient may not recover, and the information could prove valuable to the investigators.
- Ear injuries are common. Remember to speak loudly and face the patient.
- Air particles are probably contaminated. Wear your APR during patient care.
- Your agency may consider setting up a field hospital at the scene because local hospitals may be overwhelmed. Physicians, physician's assistants, nurse practitioners, EMS providers, and security personnel from your multiple-casualty incident plan can staff this facility.

■ IT (Cyber) Disruptions

Internet technology has helped EMS in many ways. In the field, you can transmit ECGs and can send real-time, visual patient presentations to hospitals thousands of miles away. However, there is a downside: hackers can penetrate EMS security to steal patient information. Worse yet, hackers may be able to electronically access secure places. EMS agencies must remain vigilant and use the latest security patches and systems.

Test your systems relentlessly. Every agency likely has a person who is computer savvy. Your agency may consider seeking this person's help in testing your agency's system to identify its weak points. Drilling and practicing cyber security is just as important as patient care.

Use of your computer system should be limited to your agency. Limit access to those fields necessary; for example, a person who does basic life support does not need computer access to see what controlled substances are in stock. Password protect systems, and change passwords frequently. Appoint a cyber security officer.

Finally, should you recognize a cyber threat, immediately report it to your supervisor and stop using the threatened browser or program.

YOU are the Medic   SUMMARY

1. What is the definition of a disaster?

A disaster is any calamitous event that causes or has the potential to cause injury or death, destruction, and distress. A disaster can be natural or man-made. Disasters overwhelm EMS and community resources.

2. What does the term all-hazards approach mean in disaster planning?

The act of conducting comprehensive preplanning for a disaster is called an all-hazards approach. Before addressing specifics particular to the disaster that has occurred, general considerations that apply to any disaster must be addressed, such as the number of personnel and equipment needed and which hospital(s) to transport to.

3. What is pre-event planning, and how can an event be predicted in advance?

Pre-event planning is the stage in which EMS providers prepare for any potential event. Table 1 lists main items to consider when preplanning for a disaster. While no disaster is predictable, some events are more likely to occur than others. For example, it is a good idea to prepare for a snowstorm in the Northeast and a tornado in the Midwest. However, the tornado that tore through Springfield, Massachusetts in 2011, and the earthquake centered in Virginia in the same year have proven that unlikely events do occur. General disaster preplanning with an all-hazards approach will put your agency in the best position to handle any disaster that may befall your area.

4. Why are preplanned mutual aid agreements essential to your operation?

Mutual aid agreements, sometimes called automatic fill-in/send-up policies, describe how your agency will access help from other areas when needed. It is important to identify the person who will request additional resources and the person who has the authority to grant permission to release resources. All parties listed in the plan should be aware of this plan. All providers must train frequently on the plan. Preplanning mutual aid agreements is essential to ensure that your agency has needed backup resources to provide patient care during a disaster.

5. How does the transportation supervisor know which hospital you should transport to?

This determination must be made in advance of a disaster; a preplanning assessment of your area hospitals is essential!

Preplanning includes knowing the level of care available in your area, the limitations on patient numbers at your local hospitals, which personnel local hospitals can supply to your agency, and vice versa. It is important that your agency participate with local hospitals in disaster drills.

6. What additional patient assessment should you accomplish en route to the hospital?

Because the patient's legs were splinted prior to patient contact, you must continually reassess pulses, motor function, and sensation en route to the hospital. You should also check the patency of the intravenous lock. Your regular 5-minute serial assessments should continue as normal.

7. What actions should be taken after the event to ensure your well-being?

You should be assessed physically as well as emotionally. Posttraumatic stress disorder is a real occurrence. Critical incident stress management teams should be considered, especially for long-term events or those with a high mortality rate. Be alert for behavioral changes in yourself and your coworkers. Open communication should be encouraged, and your agency should provide a receptive environment for those exposed to tragedy. All personnel should be checked by a physician. This will help with future workers' compensation claims in the event of a claimed disability. Physician's comments should be maintained with the protected personnel records. Notifications of disease or injury should be made the EMS provider as soon as they are received. Also, counseling services should be made available, if requested or required.

8. What is the purpose of the after-action report?

The AAR is your official internal report of the entire event. It should contain the facts of the incident reflected in a chronologic, accurate manner. Based on this report, an agency can review the entire incident in its totality. The AAR and all anecdotal evidence can be accumulated to provide a basis for additional training in areas that need scrutiny. Also, based on the incident, EMS crews may notice areas of deficiency or skills that need to be refreshed. An outline for reinforcement of skills and knowledge should be prepared based on this data.

YOU *are the Medic*   **SUMMARY,** *continued*

EMS Patient Care Report (PCR)

Date: 11-06-11	Incident No.: 2456	Nature of Call: Leg fractures		Location: Dawn Apartment Complex	
Dispatched: N/A	En Route: N/A	At Scene: 2041	Transport: 2046	At Hospital: 2105	In Service: 2130

Patient Information

Age: 24 Sex: F Weight (in kg [lb]): 59 kg (130 lb)	Allergies: Denies Medications: Denies Past Medical History: Denies Chief Complaint: Bilateral leg fractures

Vital Signs

Time: 2046	BP: 140/86	Pulse: 96	Respirations: 18	Spo$_2$: 98%
Time: 2051	BP: 140/84	Pulse: 96	Respirations: 18	Spo$_2$: 100%

EMS Treatment
(circle all that apply)

Oxygen @ __4__ L/min via (circle one): (NC) NRM Bag-mask device	Assisted Ventilation	Airway Adjunct	CPR
Defibrillation	**Bleeding Control**	**Bandaging**	**Splinting**	**Other**

Narrative

Arrived from the Dawn Apartment staging area to the Priority Yellow treatment area for this pt. Pt is a 24-year-old woman who fell from a second-story window when the apartment building partially collapsed. Pt was triaged, moved, splinted, bandaged, and an IV lock was started prior to our pt contact. Pt report from the yellow sector treatment supervisor states the pt has an obvious fx of left tib/fib and a fx of her right ankle. All PMS assessments are reported acceptable. Pt moved to our stretcher for transport to Regional Hospital as directed by the transportation supervisor. Reassessment shows no change in pt condition. Due to rough road conditions, pain control was discussed with the pt who consented to analgesia. Pt denies any medical hx or allergy to medications. 2 mg MS IVP administered at 2050 hrs. Pt remained comfortable and stable throughout the remainder of the transport. Report to charge nurse Mary on arrival at Regional Hospital. **End of report**

Prep Kit

▪ Ready for Review

- A disaster is any calamitous event that causes or has the potential to cause injury or death, destruction, and distress.
- Disaster management requires planners to take a broad look at preparedness, planning, training, response, and after-action report.
- EMS agencies must have comprehensive plans in place to address all potential disasters. The act of conducting comprehensive preplanning that will address any disaster situation is called an all-hazards approach.
- The three phases of any plan of response are before the event (preplanning), during the event, and after the event.
- Preplanning is a crucial stage in disaster management. Preplanning should take into account general, predictable factors, such as the local geography, makeup of the population, EMS resources and supplies on hand, infrastructure, places to shelter, and potential assets that can be used.
- During a disaster, it is best to stick to the preplanned measures, if possible. Items to consider during the event include warnings, inventory, mobilization of personnel, personnel needs, command structure, equipment, hospital capabilities, surveillance, and media concerns, among others.
- Specific measures to take after a disaster event include ensuring accountability, resupply, repair, stress reaction review, retraining, reimbursement, the after-action report, and acknowledging EMS providers.
- A disaster can be man-made or natural. Natural disasters include forest and brush fires; earthquakes; landslides; cave-ins; tsunamis; flooding; sandstorms; weather events such as tornadoes, hurricanes, snowstorms, cold weather, heat waves, and droughts; and pandemics.
- Examples of man-made disasters include structural fires, construction failures, building collapses, power failures, riots, civil disturbances, strikes, sniper and hostage situations, explosions, IT disruptions, and hazardous materials incidents.
- Natural and man-made disasters should be handled with the all-hazards measures identified during preplanning, with additional measures used as needed based on the nature of the specific event.

▪ Vital Vocabulary

6-feet rule A guideline to follow regarding the distance to place between oneself and a person who sneezes or coughs, to avoid exposure to germs.

after-action report (AAR) The official internal report of the entire event, such as a disaster, which should contain the facts of the incident reflected in a chronologic, accurate manner.

all-hazards approach The act of conducting comprehensive preplanning that will apply to any disaster.

ashfall The residue left behind from a volcanic eruption.

casualty collection points Areas where slightly injured or noninjured displaced persons can be gathered together and transported by bus or truck for further treatment.

cold stress A psychological condition that can develop in people who are exposed to cold weather for long periods of time, even if sheltered.

continuity of operations plan (COOP) The detailed plan describing the functioning of the agency in situations that disrupt normal operations.

critical infrastructure The external foundation in communities made up of structures and services critical in the day-to-day living activities of humans: energy sources, fuel, water, sewage removal, food, hospitals, and transportation systems.

directed area An area away from the command post or emergency operations center, considered by engineering expertise to be a safe place to stage until directed otherwise.

disaster A widespread event that disrupt community resources and functions, in turn threatening public safety, lives, and property.

disaster management A planned, coordinated response to a disaster that involves cooperation of multiple responders and agencies and enables effective triage and provision of care according to triage decisions.

dust suffocation A phenomenon that can occur during an earthquake, in which particles of dust and debris are loosened and released into the air, producing a toxic and hypoxic atmosphere.

emergency operations center (EOC) A central command and control facility, found at all government levels, responsible for strategic overview; tactical decisions are left to incident commanders.

epidemic Sickness that is larger than expected, area-wise and population-wise.

forward surgical team A team, usually staffed with physicians, nurses, and EMS providers, that performs minor surgical procedures and débridements in the field, taking some of the load from the hospital facility.

incident command system (ICS) A system implemented to manage disasters and multiple-casualty incidents in which section chiefs, including finance, logistics, operations, and planning, report to the incident commander.

lister bags Heavy canvas bags that can be hung from trees containing water in amounts from 40 to 100 gallons.

mutual aid agreements (MAAs) Documents that preplan how you will access help from other areas when needed.

overtopping A situation in which a reservoir overflows its borders.

pandemic An extensive epidemic.

point of distribution (POD) An area where medications or supplies can be administered on a temporary basis.

pyroclastic explosions Blasts from flowing or standing lava that can have a wide dispersal circumference, spewing ash and magma.

radio operators Amateur radio operators who have a formal emergency communications set of SOPs. Most are licensed by the FCC.

seasonal affective disorder (SAD) Depression that can affect persons in long periods of bad weather, usually winter.

shelter-in-place Securing one's position in the state found during an emergency; sometimes as simple as shutting the windows, going to the cellar, or turning off the heating and air conditioning systems.

space junk Debris from satellites and other man-made objects that reenter the earth's atmosphere.

tag lines Rope or cord tied to a person who is entering a dangerous environment. Used for quick retrieval, usually in conjunction with a harness.

thermals Differing temperatures and swirling patterns of moving air with changes in wind speed.

unified command system A command system used in larger incidents in which there is a multiagency response or multiple jurisdictions are involved.

water buffalo trailers Portable trailers that contain from 500 to 3,000 gallons of water.

Assessment in Action

You and your coworkers have received a notice that a major storm is expected in your response area in 24 hours and that a state of emergency is being issued. Your department has informed you to prepare to report to work with supplies for 72 hours. As you are packing for the deployment, you review your agency's policy, procedures, and definitions.

1. Any calamitous event that causes or has the potential to cause injury, death, destruction, and distress is called a(n):
   A. event.
   B. disaster.
   C. MCI.
   D. terrorism.

2. All of the following are items to consider during preplanning, and should have been addressed in preplanning for an event such as this storm, except:
   A. geography.
   B. sheltering of personnel.
   C. specific personnel assignments.
   D. immunizations.

3. Your supervisor indicates that fire, police, and EMS will be operating together to form a command during this response. This is called:
   A. unified command.
   B. command structure.
   C. incident command.
   D. joint powers command.

4. You see your supervisor filling out an ICS-211 form. What is this form used for?
   A. Ordering supplies
   B. Tracking personnel
   C. Tracking patients
   D. Changing command

5. Two days later, when your agency's response to this storm is complete, your supervisor meets with you and your crew to discuss the official report of the entire event. This report is called an:
   A. incident command system report.
   B. end-of-shift report.
   C. after-event report.
   D. after-action report.

6. The two types of disasters are:
   A. natural and man-made.
   B. biologic and chemical.
   C. terrorism and natural.
   D. natural and nuclear.

7. Examples of natural disasters include all of the following, except:
   A. tornadoes.
   B. ice storms.
   C. civil disturbance.
   D. pandemic.

Additional Question

8. Discuss five considerations to take while you are working during a disaster.

Crime Scene Awareness

National EMS Education Standard Competencies

EMS Operations

Knowledge of operational roles and responsibilities to ensure patient, public, and personnel safety.

Knowledge Objectives

1. Understand the significance of potential violence that can occur on an EMS call, including specific settings in which violence is more likely to occur. (pp 2345-2347)

2. Discuss practical measures that can be taken to reduce the likelihood of a paramedic becoming a victim on the scene, including uniform style and body armor. (p 2346)

3. Describe factors to assess during scene size-up that can help determine whether the scene is safe, including specific indicators of violence. (pp 2346-2347)

4. Discuss the role of standard operating procedures at a potentially violent incident. (p 2347)

5. Describe how to park and position your emergency vehicle when responding to a call involving another motor vehicle. (pp 2347-2348)

6. Describe the safest way to approach a passenger-style motor vehicle. (pp 2348-2349)

7. Describe the safest way to approach a van. (pp 2348-2349)

8. Describe how to retreat from danger. (pp 2349-2350)

9. Describe how to approach a residence safely. (p 2350)

10. Discuss types of exits, including primary exit and secondary exit. (p 2350)

11. List items that can potentially be used as a weapon. (p 2350)

12. Discuss techniques to use when responding to a call involving potential domestic violence. (p 2351)

13. Discuss concerns related to clandestine drug laboratories. (p 2351)

14. Discuss concerns related to gang territories and measures that the paramedic can take to work safely in these areas. (pp 2351-2353)

15. Discuss procedures the paramedic should follow at mass shootings and at scenes involving active shooters or snipers. (pp 2353, 2355)

16. Define cover and concealment, and provide examples of each. (p 2355)

17. Describe measures the paramedic can take to increase his or her safety in a hostage situation. (pp 2355-2356)

18. Discuss the role self-defense can play in the practice of paramedicine. (pp 2358-2359)

19. Discuss measures the paramedic can take to preserve evidence at a crime scene, while still providing optimal patient care. (pp 2359-2361)

Skills Objectives

There are no skills objectives for this chapter.

Introduction

FACT: EMS can be a dangerous and potentially fatal profession. Thousands of times each year, paramedics face potentially violent situations. With any call, you may find yourself in the middle of a physical altercation when you are responding to a sick or injured patient **Figure 1**. You may encounter a call where there are violent or attack animals being raised, or a methamphetamine lab or other drug-producing process is housed at the location. From reading the many cautions in this textbook about potentially violent and dangerous scenes, remember that paramedics have been severely injured or killed in violent incidents while attempting to reach and treat sick and injured people. During 2009, the Bureau of Labor Statistics estimated that 200 EMS workers were reported to have sustained injuries from assaults alone. Many experts agree that even these figures are underreported, and that many assaults that do not result in serious injury or lost time are not reported. Whereas reporting on occupational illness and injuries specific to EMS personnel is a relatively recent event and research is scant, most studies suggest that EMS work is on par with other hazardous occupations including firefighting and law enforcement. Between 1992 and 1997, there were 10 homicide-related on-duty EMS fatalities, with 7 EMS personnel victims of a gunshot. More recently, a 2008 Bureau of Labor Statistics report listed EMS workers as third in the nation in occupations with high rates of injuries, surpassing construction workers, roofers, and welders. As the research suggests, assault can be attributed to these numbers.

As an educated and effective health care provider, you need to know how to avoid violence when possible and how to protect yourself when violence erupts. Because all emergency services agencies respond to potentially life-threatening situations daily, you should actively seek out and encourage your organization to offer self-protection courses that are geared specifically toward EMS providers. Sound survival skills training will help you identify and avoid potentially dangerous situations. Once you recognize a violent situation, your goal is to retreat to a safe location and await the assistance of law enforcement personnel. *Your main mission is to return home safely at the end of each shift. Remember: Not only can you not help anyone if you become a victim, but you become a burden to other responders who must now take care of you in addition to the original patient(s).*

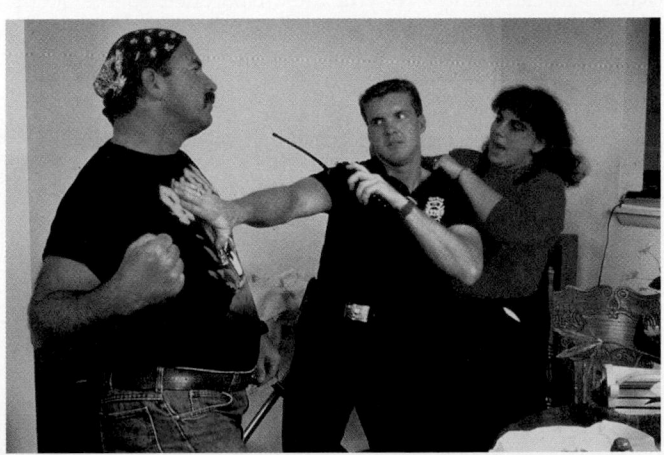

Figure 1 The most routine call can quickly turn violent.

Awareness

You may be surprised to hear how serious and widespread attacks against emergency responders have become. Violence is not only an urban event; a call in a rural area can be just as deadly as a call in a large city. In many rural areas, paramedics may arrive at the scene of an emergency long before law enforcement personnel. You should never be complacent about the possibility of encountering violence. Violence comes in many forms, ranging from obvious to subtle. Problems can occur at every social and economic level and in every size of community. The paramedic who has a healthy sense of self-preservation will be the paramedic who is more likely to go home to his or her family safely at the end of the shift.

Before you begin patient care, you need to perform a scene size-up with an eye toward your safety, which includes looking for indicators of potential violence and escape routes. If you feel the scene is not safe, contact law enforcement personnel, retreat

YOU *are the Medic*   PART 1

You and your partner are dispatched to a single-family residence in an upscale gated community for an unknown type of incident. As you are responding, the dispatcher informs you that the call was made by a neighbor who heard a woman screaming for help in the house next door. The dispatcher also states that attempts are being made to get more information from the caller, and a request has been made for additional law enforcement personnel.

1. On the basis of the limited amount of information available, do you have any concern for entering this scene?
2. What factors should you take into consideration because the residence is in an upscale, gated community?

to your ambulance, and wait for them to secure the scene. Remember: If you rush into a scene and are injured by violence, you become a burden to your partner and fellow EMS responders, not a trained care provider.

Paramedics Mistaken for Law Enforcement Personnel

Many patients and bystanders mistake paramedics for police officers. In many jurisdictions EMS personnel wear similar color uniforms, utility belts, and even badges as their police counterparts. Aggressive behavior intended for the police may be unintentionally directed at you. Your options for defending yourself may be severely limited. To counteract this, many agencies have adopted a more casual uniform for paramedics, such as golf shirts with only the department's logo printed on the shirt. If possible, advocate that your service adopt uniforms that differ from local law enforcement, and are clearly marked "EMS", "Paramedic", or "Medic" **Figure 2**.

Body Armor

Most police officers routinely wear soft body armor, and some EMS agencies offer this protective garment as an option, especially for those providers working in neighborhoods with high rates of drugs and violent crimes. Remember that there is no such thing as a "bulletproof vest." Body armor is not bulletproof; there are six levels of protection. Body armor does not shield your neck or head, so whatever your level of protection, you will still be vulnerable to injury. Consult with your department and local law enforcement officials to decide if you need protection and at what level. Remember that using sound survival skills to avoid dangerous situations gives you more protection than body armor.

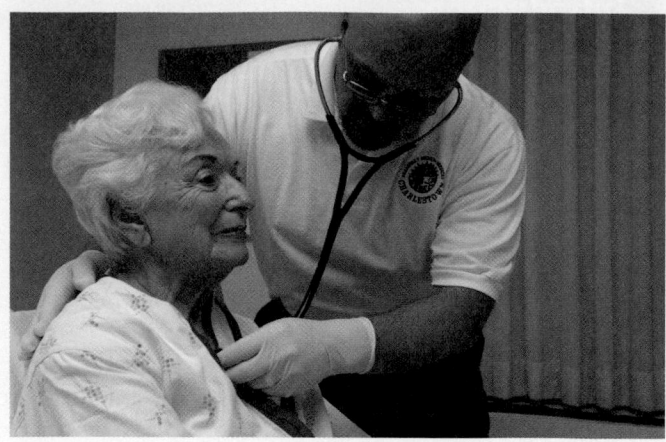

Figure 2 Many EMS agencies have provided a less formal uniform for their members that is not only more comfortable, but decreases the likelihood that staff will be confused with law enforcement personnel.

Indicators of Violence

Violence can often be predicted, as most experienced EMS providers already know. If you are dispatched to the scene of a shooting, stabbing, or attempted suicide, the potential for violence can be obvious. You should always expect aggressive behavior when you arrive at the scene of an injured person. The patient may be upset for having been a victim of violence. Family members can also be agitated, pacing the room with fists clenched and using profane language because they perceive that it took you too long to reach the scene, or because they feel you are moving too slowly in your treatment of their loved one. Once you have determined that the scene is safe and

YOU *are the Medic* | PART 2 |

You arrive at the main gate of the community and the guard informs you that one of their security officers is on the way to the residence in a golf cart. When you clear the gatehouse, your dispatcher tells you the caller now reports the screams have stopped and all appears quiet. The caller stated that someone from the house has driven away in a car. The caller believes the home is now empty. You continue to the residence and find an empty golf cart parked in front of the home.

Recording Time: 1 Minute	
Appearance	Unknown
Level of consciousness	Unknown
Airway	Unknown
Breathing	Unknown
Circulation	Unknown

3. Is the scene safe to enter?

4. Should you enter the scene prior to the arrival of law enforcement personnel?

you begin to render care, be aware of the potential for someone to burst through the door in rage as you are treating their relative or loved one who has been the victim of domestic violence. The potential for such behavior to escalate to physically violent behavior should not be discounted. You must quickly identify potentially dangerous situations and act to remove yourself, your team, and, if possible the patient, to a safe place. Even after your initial scene size-up, you must continuously evaluate scenes for the potential for secondary violence. You must not become so completely involved with patient care that you fail to see the possibility of physical harm to the patient or other EMS providers. Experts call this <u>tunnel vision</u>.

> ### Words of Wisdom
>
> You need to realize that scene safety is a dynamic process because scenes that involve crimes or violence are dynamic. Just because the scene is safe when you first enter, does not mean it will continue to remain safe.

Standard Operating Procedures

Some agencies or regions have developed standard operating procedures (SOPs) for dealing with potentially violent incidents. Specific procedures for response to methamphetamine labs, civil disturbances, and hostage or barricade incidents provide paramedics with specific steps to be taken at such scenes. In many parts of the country, paramedics have advanced protocols that allow them to sedate patients who are emotionally disturbed and pose a threat to themselves and others. If your agency has an SOP manual, take time to review the contents so that you will be familiar with directions on handling specific situations. Remember that SOPs and protocols cannot possibly cover all of the circumstances that you may find yourself in. Always use them as the basis for your approach to the scene or patient care, but be prepared to abandon them if they interfere with the preservation of your or your partner's life.

Highway and Rural Road Incidents

Highway incidents account for the bulk of serious injuries to EMS personnel, accounting for an estimated 67 EMS deaths out of 114 deaths of EMTs and paramedics in a 6-year span from 1992 to 1997. Law enforcement dashboard cameras mounted in vehicles have provided the public a rare view of the dangers routinely faced by law enforcement officers when approaching vehicles on the side of the road. You face similar dangers whenever you walk to the door of a motor vehicle. Calls to a "man slumped over the steering wheel" or an "unresponsive person in a vehicle" can be disastrous for an unsuspecting paramedic. In 2010, two law enforcement officers were exposed to hazardous materials when responding to a vehicle in which a chemical suicide had occurred; one officer had to be treated for the exposure. In 2011, a paramedic in Bellmore, New York, was shot by the driver of a car that was involved in a crash. The driver, who was

heavily armed and determined to commit murder, was only stopped when he was killed by police during a shootout. Not only must you be mindful of the obvious hazards posed by fast-moving vehicles and curious drivers gawking at the incident, but you must also still be aware of potentially violent patients. The motor vehicle crash that you respond to may not be just a routine incident, but rather could be the culmination of a number of circumstances such as armed robbery, drug use, stolen vehicles, or perpetrators fleeing the scene of a violent crime.

Approach and Vehicle Positioning

For your maximum safety when you are arriving at incidents with a single vehicle in which the potential for danger is high, and you are the first vehicle to respond, your vehicle should be positioned a minimum of 21 ft behind the stopped vehicle at a 10° angle to the driver's side facing the shoulder **Figure 3** . The front wheels should be turned all the way to the left. In this position, the wheels and the motor block will provide limited protection in the event of gunfire. If you are not the first vehicle to arrive at the scene, ask the incident commander (IC) where he or she would like you to park your vehicle or try to park downstream of the incident, and let the police use one of their cruisers or properly placed flares behind the car that was in the crash.

Your agency may have specific policies regarding the use of light after dark. For example, you may use your vehicle's high beams and spotlights to illuminate the interior and exterior of the patient's vehicle. Bright light will also conceal you as you approach the vehicle; however, some agencies prohibit the use of high beams so as not to blind passing traffic. Do not walk between the spotlight and the vehicle because you will provide a silhouette in the patient's rearview mirror and alert any responsive occupants to your position.

Do not approach a vehicle if you have an uneasy feeling about it. In most every case, law enforcement will be the first to respond to the scene. You must always wait for them to declare

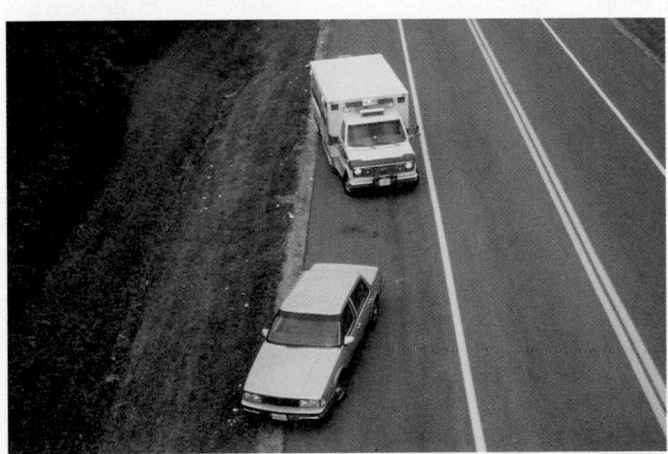

Figure 3 When you are the first vehicle to respond, position the unit a minimum of 21 ft behind the stopped vehicle at a 10° angle to the left if you are the only emergency vehicle on the scene. Then call for law enforcement and set some flares if they will be delayed.

the scene safe before you approach. If law enforcement is not present and there is any potential that the scene is not safe, request them and remain in your vehicle until they declare the scene to be safe.

If you do approach a vehicle, before leaving yours, consider notifying the dispatcher of the situation, your location, and the license number and state of the motor vehicle. You may also consider documenting this information. If something happens to you and your partner, a record of the motor vehicle will exist. This information will allow your agency to react quickly. Follow your department's policy.

Approaching the Motor Vehicle

A systematic approach to a motor vehicle with people inside is not usually needed in cases of personal injury collisions at a busy intersection, collisions where the motor vehicle is found torn wide open, or situations with bystanders already around the motor vehicle. Here are some procedures that you can use.

When there are two or more paramedics in the unit, the person riding in the right front seat, the IC of the emergency vehicle, makes the approach. All other members of the emergency response team remain with the ambulance or medical unit in the event there is a problem.

Proceed to the rear passenger-side trunk area **Figure 4**. Look out for people hiding in the trunk of a motor vehicle, and check the trunk lid to ensure that it is properly closed. Use only a light touch on the trunk seam to detect motion or an unsecured trunk lid. If the trunk is open, retreat to your vehicle. Using a belly-in movement, proceed to the "C" post on the passenger side of the motor vehicle **Figure 5**. Moving belly-in toward the motor vehicle creates as small an image as possible for the occupants of the motor vehicle to see.

Stop at the left C post and look in the rear and side windows **Figure 6**. Notice the number of people in the vehicle. Pay particular attention to the location of their hands. Any attempt to stab, strike, or shoot will be accomplished using the hands. Try to see if there are items lying on the seat or

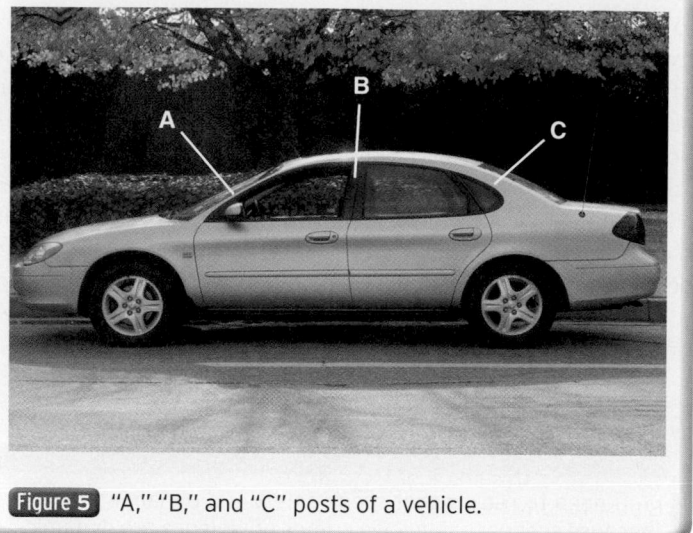

Figure 5 "A," "B," and "C" posts of a vehicle.

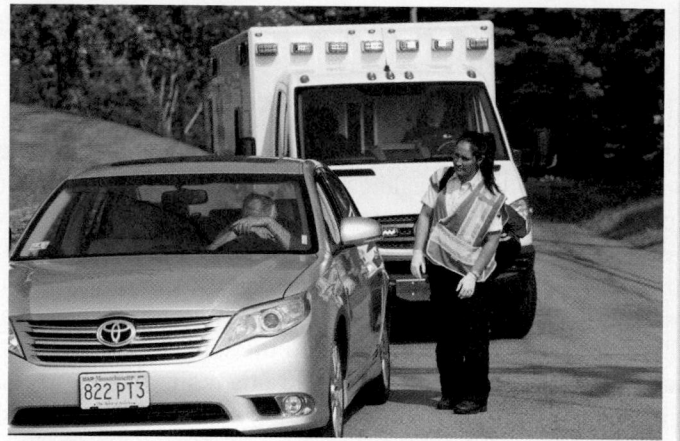

Figure 6 Stop at the right C post and look in the rear and side windows.

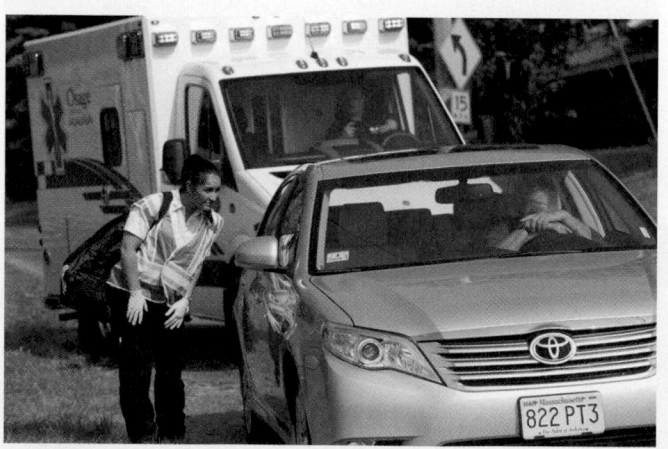

Figure 4 The IC moves from the right front of the unit directly to the right rear-trunk area of the vehicle.

on the floor. Look for weapons. These might include the obvious guns or knives, but may also include baseball bats, beer bottles, or pieces of pipe. If you see a deadly weapon, a gun, or a knife, retreat to a safe location, and call for law enforcement assistance. Wait for law enforcement. Officers are trained to retrieve and secure weapons; you are not. *Never* attempt to unload a weapon. And although you cannot retreat every time you see a bat or pipe, your awareness that the object is within reach of the people in the car gives you time to react if that object becomes a weapon.

If the back seat is occupied, do not pass the C post. If you pass the C post, the back-seat passengers will be behind you. You will have to divide your attention between the front and rear seats.

If there are no passengers in the back seat, move forward to the B post with the same belly-in movement **Figure 7**. As with the C post, the B post will conceal you from the passengers of the vehicle. Examine the front-seat area. Where are the occupants' hands? What are the occupants doing? Are any weapons visible? When you are ready to let the driver know that

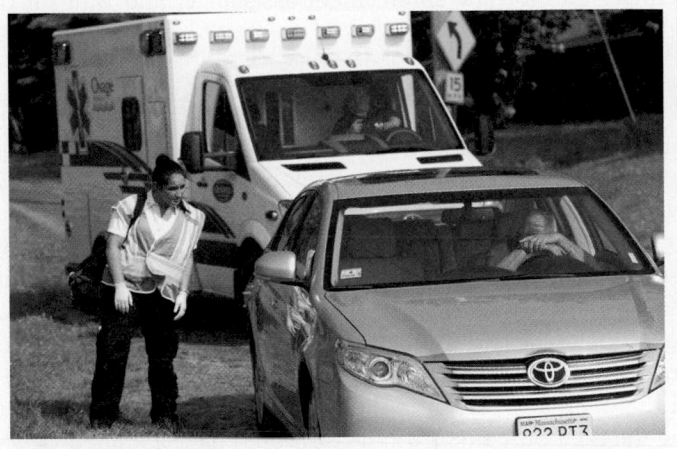

Figure 7 At this stage of the approach, do not move past the B post for any reason.

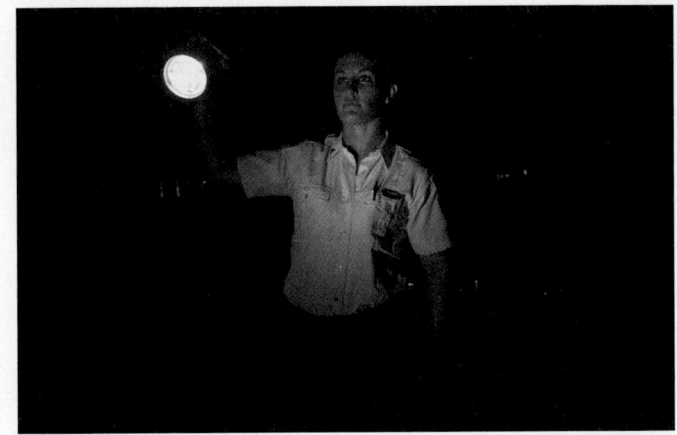

Figure 8 Because a light makes a good target, hold a flashlight away from your body when illuminating an area.

Words of Wisdom

Weapon locations:

- Glove box
- On top of the sun visor
- Arm rest
- Under either side of the seat
- In the center console
- In side-door pockets
- Next to driver's right thigh

you are there, do so without moving past the B post into the driver's door area. Law enforcement personnel refer to this area as the kill zone. Tap lightly on the window of the vehicle to get the driver's attention and announce yourself: "Paramedic. Do you need help?"

After the IC declares that the incident scene is safe and determines that the occupants of the motor vehicle need medical or other assistance, you should follow the SOPs for your department.

Keep your flashlight off until you need it. Hold the light at arms-length and away from your body before you turn it on **Figure 8**. Illuminate the scene for only a few seconds during each use.

Take special precautions when you approach vans. Vans can carry many types of cargo, and your inability to see that cargo is a danger. A van can carry a large number of people or a large quantity of weapons.

A safe approach to a van is modified from the approach made to the passenger side of a standard motor vehicle. When you exit the unit with the jump kit, move 10 to 15 ft away from the passenger side of the van. If you are belly-in to the van, an occupant may suddenly open the side door and grab you. Instead, remain clear of the side door of the van throughout the approach **Figure 9**. From this distance, walk parallel to

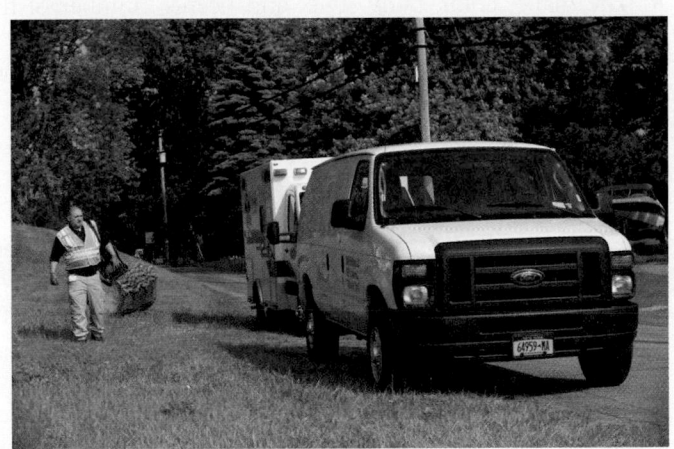

Figure 9 Until you are 45° forward of the A post, maintain 10 to 15 ft between yourself and the passenger side of the van.

the van until you are approximately 45° forward of the A post. This position gives you the greatest visibility inside of the van but keeps you at a safe distance until you can determine that the situation is secure **Figure 10**.

Retreating From Danger

You will be in situations in which unsafe circumstances dictate your retreat to a safe area. The safest means of retreat is to back away and call for law enforcement assistance. If your partner is injured while approaching a motor vehicle, the best way to ensure help will arrive quickly is to back away and call for assistance yourself. Back away from the danger zone, remain in your vehicle, and provide the dispatcher with all the needed information. This would include:

- The number of aggressors involved
- The number and type of injuries
- The number and type of weapons involved

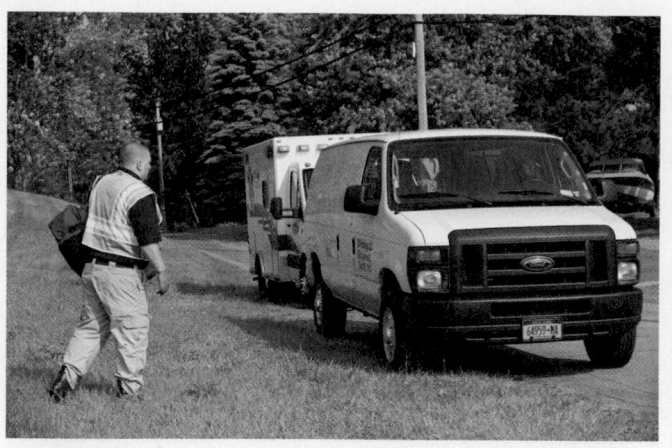

Figure 10 Position yourself 45° forward of the A post before making contact with the occupants of a van.

- The make, color, body style, and license number of the vehicle involved
- The direction of travel if the vehicle leaves the scene before the law enforcement personnel arrive

In addition, make certain to document in detail why you had to leave the scene.

Residential Incidents

Warning Signs

Emergency response personnel are frequently called to residential areas to assist someone injured in an assault, domestic dispute, shooting, or stabbing. These calls require an obvious level of caution. But many routine calls have the potential for violent outcomes. An attempted suicide may turn into a homicide, with you as the victim. Your response to an "injured person" may be a planned intentional attack by a person who remains on the scene as you arrive.

Your standard procedure for responding to any call involving violence should be to allow law enforcement personnel to both arrive and secure the scene before your entry because securing a scene demands more than the simple presence of a law enforcement officer. You must ensure that the scene is safe before going in to provide patient care, and continually reevaluate the situation while providing patient care.

Approaching a Residence

Information provided to dispatchers may be limited, and a complete picture of the circumstances at the scene may not be available to paramedics. Keep in mind that all calls have a potential for violence. When you are arriving at a residence, listen for loud, threatening voices. Glance through available windows for signs of a struggle. In addition, look for visible weapons. By obtaining such information, you can make a decision about the relative safety of the scene. Any time you perceive danger, abort the approach and back away to your vehicle. Call for law enforcement assistance, and wait for the officers to arrive.

Entering a Residence

Law enforcement officers consider entry doors to residences extremely dangerous. Many law enforcement officers have been shot and killed while standing in front of a door after knocking to gain entry. Most bullets pass easily through all but the heaviest doors. Use an alternative path while approaching, rather than using the path to the front door. Once at the front door, you should stand to the doorknob side of the door when you are preparing to knock **Figure 11**. If you stand on the hinged side of the door, any person in the room can observe you by opening the door only slightly, and you would have a limited view of conditions inside the room. Knock on the door and announce: "Paramedics," "Fire department," or "Rescue squad." In doing so, you will not be mistaken for a law enforcement officer. Ask whoever answers the door to lead you to the patient. If you do this, you will not only get to the patient quickly, but the person who leads you acts as a shield for you and gives you a few extra moments to react if the situation deteriorates.

When you are entering any type of structure, you should pick a **primary exit** and a **secondary exit**. Your primary exit is usually the door that was used to enter the building. A secondary exit might be a rear door or, in an emergency, a window. Whenever you are in a building, try to keep at least one means of escape accessible at all times.

As you arrive at the patient's location, scan the room for weapons. If there is a gun or knife, back your way out of the residence and call for law enforcement assistance. Many people keep loaded firearms in the house for personal protection. A nightstand, a dresser drawer, and a table next to a comfortable chair are popular locations to conceal these weapons. Be aware that objects like ashtrays, scissors, bottles, fireplace pokers, and knitting needles can be used as weapons. Move any potential weapon out of the patient's reach.

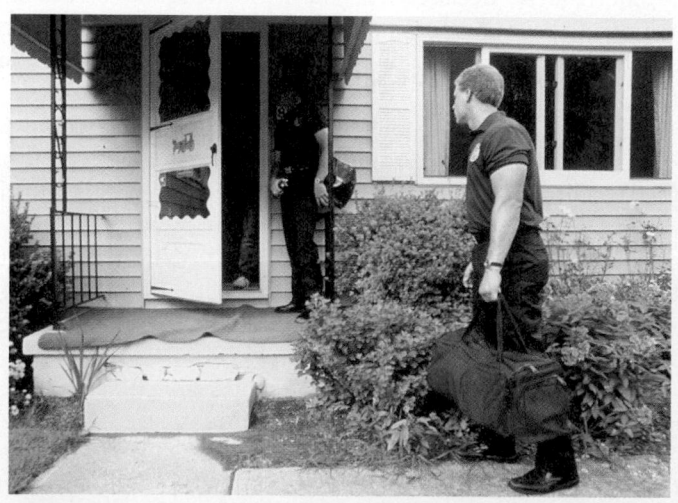

Figure 11 Stand on the doorknob side of the entrance when announcing your arrival.

Domestic Violence

Domestic disturbances are among the most dangerous situations faced by law enforcement officers and paramedics. As a paramedic, you must be aware of the dangers involved and handle these incidents with extreme caution.

If a violent or physical dispute is in progress when you arrive at a residence, wait for law enforcement assistance before you enter. Tempers may flare while you are treating a patient. Using good communication skills in conjunction with eye contact and appropriate body language can help defuse the situation. Your voice is the most effective tool you can use to keep out of trouble in a dispute. Knowing what words to use or not to use in a situation is only part of your goal. You must also be aware of the tone, pacing, pitch, and rhythm of your voice. Talk to people with the same respect that you expect from them, regardless of your personal opinion of them. A good paramedic is always respectful because it puts patients at ease and can suppress the anger of a violent person who is not the patient. That person may turn on you, and the situation can quickly deteriorate to a dangerous level if you do not use respectful language, body posture, and tone.

You may also use a technique known as **contact and cover**, which will be described in greater depth later in the chapter. One aspect of the technique involves one paramedic making contact with the patient to provide care. The second paramedic obtains patient information, and more important, gauges the level of tension and warns his or her partner at the first sign of trouble.

Your most important mandate is to conduct yourself as a professional when you are providing patient care. Your duty is to act in a professional manner, no matter how unpleasant or difficult the situation.

Most paramedics are not trained as marriage counselors, psychologists, psychiatrists, or clergy. Crisis intervention is not part of your job and should be left to the professionals. You may be required by law to report certain conditions such as domestic violence or child abuse to local authorities. Be sure to check your state's statutes and your community's laws to learn your mandatory reporting duties.

Violence on the Streets

The increase in gang activity and the prevalence of clandestine drug laboratories pose unique challenges to paramedics. Multiple-casualty shootings, resulting from what law enforcement characterizes as an active shooter, have struck fear in many communities. In addition, you may be responding to an assault or robbery scene before law enforcement personnel arrive.

Clandestine Drug Laboratories

Clandestine drug laboratories are a growing problem. The most popular substance manufactured in clandestine labs is methamphetamine, known on the street as meth, speed, and crank. With a small investment of a few hundred dollars, a drug producer, or "cooker," can begin producing methamphetamine Figure 12.

Everything associated with a clandestine lab is hazardous! Because of the highly flammable properties of some chemicals

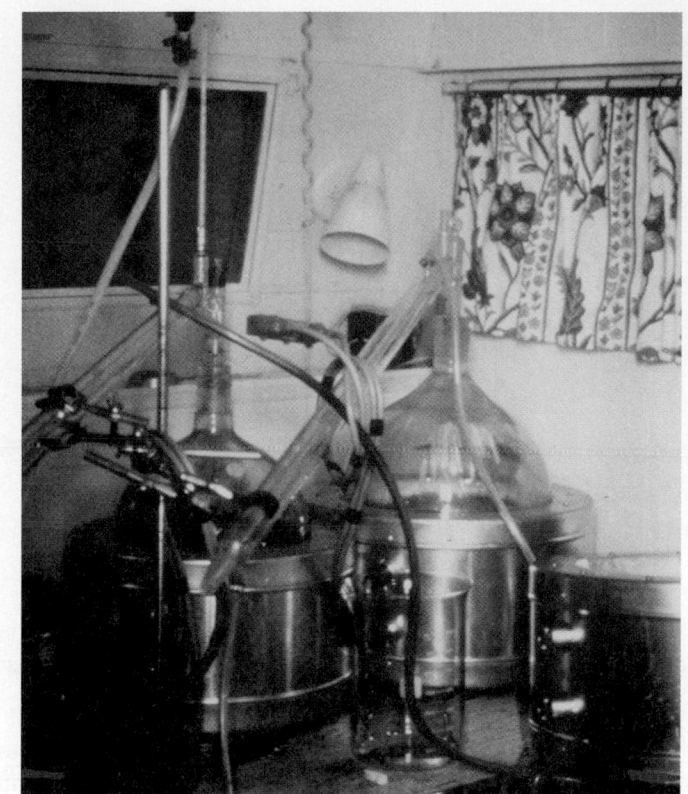

Figure 12 Some methamphetamine labs may resemble a high school chemistry laboratory. Do not touch anything!

associated with cooking methamphetamine and the toxic nature of others, extreme caution must be exercised when a lab is found. Although some methamphetamine "cooking" operations may look like a typical high school chemistry laboratory, others are much harder to recognize. Large quantities of over-the-counter cold remedies containing ephedrine or pseudoephedrine, gallon containers of camping fuel, and sulfuric acid in the form of lye may be the only signs of methamphetamine production. Almost every chemical involved is a hazardous material Figure 13.

In addition to the chemical hazards found at clandestine labs, some cookers use booby traps to safeguard their operations. These may include fragmentation and incendiary devices, animal traps, and impaling stakes.

Once a clandestine laboratory is identified, it is your job to remain clear of the area until the scene is secured by trained law enforcement personnel and hazardous materials specialists. If possible, take any patients with you if you can do so without exposing yourself and your team to additional danger. Remember that patients should always be decontaminated by specially trained hazardous materials personnel before you approach them and before they enter the ambulance.

Gangs

Gangs pose an increasing threat in communities across the nation. What was once a problem only in major cities is now a problem in smaller suburban and rural communities. According

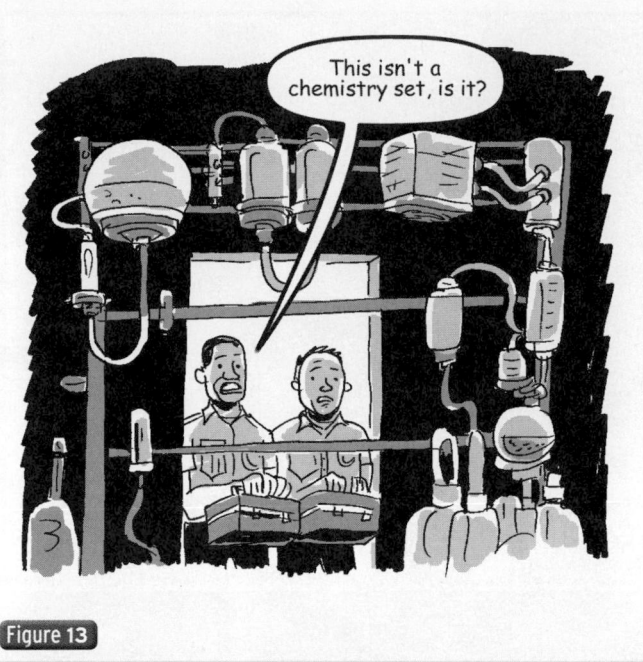

Figure 13

extend their influence, recruit new members, and promote drug trafficking into virgin territories. The FBI estimates that almost every community across the nation either has some level of gang activity or is affected by gang activity. Today's gangs operate at a low level such as retail or street-level drug sales, all the way up to major drug trafficking, rivaling the activity of international drug cartels.

Words of Wisdom

Youths usually join gangs for the following reasons:
- Identity
- Respect
- Recognition
- Love
- Belonging
- Money
- Fear

to a 2009 FBI report, there are approximately 20,000 violent street gangs, motorcycle gangs, and prison gangs with more than 1 million members operating in the United States. Gang activity has migrated from the cities into suburban and rural areas, in part to evade law enforcement and other gangs, as well as to

Gangs predominantly survive through the drug trade. In 2008, gangs accounted for roughly 50% of the drug activity in powder and crack cocaine, heroin, marijuana, and illicit pharmaceutical drug distribution. Whereas they thrive on the drug trade, they also earn money through robbery, extortion, human smuggling and human trafficking, gun-running, prostitution rings, insurance and bank fraud, and identity theft. There are

YOU *are the Medic*   PART 3

As you park in front of the residence, the community security guard comes out of the front door to meet you. He states a woman has been assaulted by her husband who has left the scene. He says she looks "bad." Two sheriff's deputies arrive on the scene and take a report from the security guard. The deputies tell you a vehicle drove through the closed security gate and officers are looking for it.

Once law enforcement personnel have returned from assessing the scene and have indicated that it is safe to enter, you and your partner gather your equipment and enter the residence. You find a 30-year-old woman lying on a tile floor with a copious amount of blood around her torso. You notice a knife on the floor next to the patient's left shoulder. The patient tells you that her husband stabbed her.

Recording Time: 10 Minutes	
Respirations	36 breaths/min, shallow
Pulse	116 beats/min
Skin	Cool, moist, and pale
Blood pressure	90/60 mm Hg
Oxygen saturation (Spo$_2$)	93% prior to high-flow O$_2$ administration
Pupils	Equal and slow to react to light

5. What is your first priority for this patient?

6. Do you feel this scene is now secure?

three different types of gangs: street gangs, prison gangs, and motorcycle gangs. All operate differently with rules on sex, age, race, religion, and national origin, but all have similar codes with regard to committing violence. They recruit children as young as age 12 years from schools, and are a growing cause of school violence and drug proliferation. In some states such as California, Illinois, and New Mexico, the FBI estimates that gang members outnumber law enforcement personnel by a ratio of as much as 6 to 1, and account for up to 80% of the crime in some areas. While many people are familiar with the "gang signs" Figure 14 , most gang communication is far more sophisticated, using multiple prepaid cell phones that are easily discarded, text messaging, email, and even satellite communications in more remote areas. Like many of us, gang members use Internet social networks such as Myspace and Facebook, and even employ voiceover phone (VoIP; Internet phone) and Skype. Gang membership is so pervasive that, according to the FBI, over 19 different gangs have representation in the US Armed Forces, with the intent on receiving military weapons and tactics training to pass on to other members, as well as to spread their influence.

Knowing this, you should contact your local law enforcement to ask about and be aware of known gang territories. Many gangs have literally carved out sections of the map where they operate, and that no other gangs may enter Figure 15 . When you are entering these areas, you must always be mindful of the threat of gang violence, and of what types of activities the local gangs are involved in. Often local law enforcement has a "gang unit" that keeps its finger on the pulse of gang activity and shares information with fire and EMS for your protection, as well as providing assistance. You should encourage your service or agency to work with local law enforcement to share information such as new gangs that may be entering the area and looking to make a name for themselves, "turf wars"

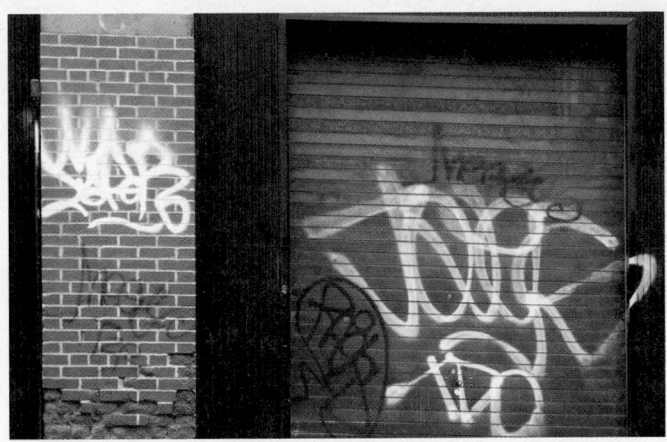

Figure 15 Many gangs use graffiti to mark off their territories. It is imperative that paramedics be aware of when they are entering a gang's area.

that are ongoing or may start, and illegal activities that are on the rise. You and your agency need to concern yourselves with these issues because when you are responding to an incident in a gang's territory, it is best to have as much knowledge as possible. Remember: the last thing a rival gang wants to see is the paramedics coming to rescue the person that they just shot or stabbed. In all potentially violent situations, the paramedic's best and often only defense is <u>situational awareness</u>. That means knowing your surroundings, the players, the climate of violence or strife, and synthesizing that information quickly so that you can make rapid, effective decisions even while under stress.

■ Mass Shootings, Active Shooters, and Snipers

The last decade has been especially violent with regard to mass shootings Table 1 . You, as the paramedic, are an integral part of emergency operations at these scenes. Paramedics must prepare, plan, and train for these complex and difficult violent incidents. Mass shootings unfortunately are on the rise, and show no signs of tapering off. Those persons bent on murder wish to "go out with a bang," as many of their notes and video-taped confessions left for after their death describe. Mass shootings garner a tremendous amount of media coverage, and, as such, afford those persons an opportunity to be infamous. Many of the mass shootings that have occurred over the last decade have been protracted events, associated with long standoffs and hostage-taking, and often culminating in the death of the perpetrator. As such, you may find yourself on the scene with an <u>active shooter</u>—a gunman who has begun to fire on people and is still at large. These scenes are especially tense because persons who appear to be released hostages could in fact be the perpetrators or their accomplices.

Paramedics must take direction from law enforcement personnel on the scene and may even be instructed as to *whom* to treat and *when* a victim can be treated (but never *how* to treat). This is not your normal triage situation because law enforcement has absolute control of the scene, and they may dictate that you initiate or withhold treatment not based on medical necessity,

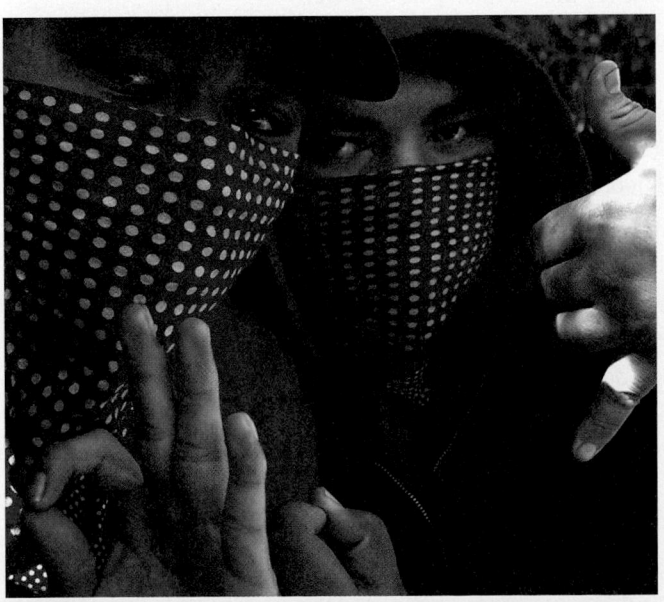

Figure 14 This form of hand communication is still used today, although gangs employ more sophisticated means of communicating such as the Internet and satellite phones.

Table 1 A Decade of Mass Shootings (2001–2011)

Year	Month	Incident
2001	March	A 15-year-old boy killed two fellow students and wounded 13 others at Santana High School in Santee, California.
2002	October	A series of sniper shootings crippled the Washington, DC, area for weeks, leaving 10 people dead.
2003	August	In Chicago, a laid-off worker shot and killed six of his former workmates.
2004	November	A hunter killed six other hunters and wounded two others after an argument in Birchwood, Wisconsin.
2005	March	A man opened fire on members of his own church during a service in Brookfield, Wisconsin, killing seven people before killing himself.
	March	A 16-year-old student killed nine people, including five fellow students, a teacher, and a security guard at Red Lake High School in Red Lake, Minnesota. Seven students were wounded. He also killed his grandfather, his grandfather's friend, and himself at home.
2006	October	A truck driver killed five schoolgirls and seriously wounded six others in an Amish school in Nickel Mines, Pennsylvania, before killing himself.
2007	April	A student shot and killed 32 people and wounded 15 others at Virginia Tech in Blacksburg, Virginia, before shooting himself, making it the deadliest mass shooting in the United States after 2000.
	December	A 19-year-old man killed nine people and injured five others in a shopping center in Omaha, Nebraska, before killing himself.
	December	A woman and her boyfriend shot dead six members of her family on Christmas Eve in Carnation, Washington.
2008	February	A shooter tied up and shot six women at a suburban clothing store in Chicago, leaving five dead and one injured.
	February	A former student opened fire in a lecture hall at Northern Illinois University in DeKalb, Illinois, killing five students and wounding 16 others.
	September	A mentally ill man shot eight people in Alger, Washington, leaving six of them dead.
	December	A man dressed in a Santa Claus suit opened fire at a family Christmas party in Covina, California, and then set the house on fire and killed himself. Nine people died.
2009	March	A laid-off worker opened fire while driving a car through several towns in Alabama, killing 10 people including his mother and four other relatives before taking his own life.
	March	A heavily armed man shot and killed eight people at a rehabilitation center for the elderly and sick in North Carolina.
	March	A man shot six people dead including his two children and three other relatives before killing himself in an affluent neighborhood in Santa Clara, California.
	April	A heavily armed gunman shot dead 13 people at an immigration center in Binghamton, New York.
	November	A US army psychologist opened fire at a military base in Fort Hood, Texas, leaving 13 dead and 42 others wounded. This was classified as an act of terrorism.
2010	February	A University of Alabama Huntsville biology professor opened fire on colleagues during a department faculty meeting. Three faculty members were killed; another three were injured.
	March	A gang-related drive-by shooting by two adults and one juvenile in Washington, DC, resulted in 10 people being shot, four of whom died.
	July	A 17-year-old boy shot and injured nine people, between the ages of 10 and 19, at Indiana Black Expo's Summer Celebration in Indianapolis.
2011	January	A lone gunman opened fire at a political gathering outside a grocery in Tuscon, Arizona, killing six people including a 9-year-old girl and wounding 12 more. A US congresswoman, Gabrielle Giffords, was severely injured with a gunshot wound to the head, and was one of the survivors.

but rather on public safety. You should carefully document any requests or demands to deviate from your local protocols, which includes being instructed to withhold treatment, or being prevented from treating a patient who clearly requires emergency medical care. Whereas law enforcement personnel are charged with public safety, and they discharge that duty to the fullest of their extent, you may encounter situations where you feel that your medical ethics are being compromised. However, the time to dispute the ethics of what is being asked of you is not while there is an active shooter at large. Refer any serious matters to your on-scene supervisor, or if one is not on scene yet, contact your dispatcher only if time permits. Otherwise, it is a crime scene, and you MUST follow the directives of law enforcement personnel until the scene has been secured.

As with any other shooting or stabbing incident, responding paramedic units should remain in the staging area until the scene is secured by law enforcement personnel. Staging, treatment, and triage areas may need to be one half to 1 mile away from the actual scene. Line-of-sight and, thus, line-of-fire from windows must be avoided when you are establishing these sites. Although parking lots or playing fields at schools may seem to be ideal locations for staging, they could allow an assailant a wide field of fire, causing a chaotic situation to deteriorate even further **Figure 16**.

Paramedics who unknowingly respond to a mass or active shooting scene need to know how to use <u>cover</u> and <u>concealment</u>. You need to know the difference between objects that provide cover and those that offer concealment only. Cover objects, such as trees, utility poles, mail collection boxes, dumpsters, curbs, vehicles, and depressions in the ground are usually impenetrable to bullets. Tall grass, shrubbery, and dark shadows

are areas of concealment. When cover is not readily available, use concealment to provide some protection while you assess your position. Your job at that point is to find cover until either the scene is secure, or until you can retreat to a position of safety. Remember: people are going to need your help; do not do anything that could get you or your partner injured.

Paramedics should consider having a training session with local police on how to assess the police officer who has been shot, to address specific topics such as the removal of full-body armor and the officer's duty belt. The protocol for who removes the officer's weapons, and how, should be established before a potential incident.

Many services are using <u>tactical paramedics</u> in mass shootings and other scenes where there is actual violence or the potential for violence. In most jurisdictions, their primary function is to care for law enforcement teams making tactical entry into violent situations; however, these specially trained paramedics can also provide care for barricaded patients, patients being held hostage, and other special operations in which a paramedic without special training might not be able to work. Tactical paramedics are a critical link in providing medical care in hostile situations, including mass shootings. Training in this newly emerging subspecialty is widely available from reputable training centers **Figure 17**.

Hostage Situations

EMS personnel sometimes arrive on a scene before it is secure. Once again, hostage situations are under the jurisdiction of law enforcement until the scene is secure. Have you considered what you would do if you met an armed adversary? Because no hard and fast rules apply, you should take additional training about handling armed people in the field. The possibility of being taken hostage is extremely remote, but it exists. If you are taken hostage, remember that most hostage incidents in the United States last between 4½ and 5 hours. Your behavior can greatly enhance your chances of surviving the ordeal.

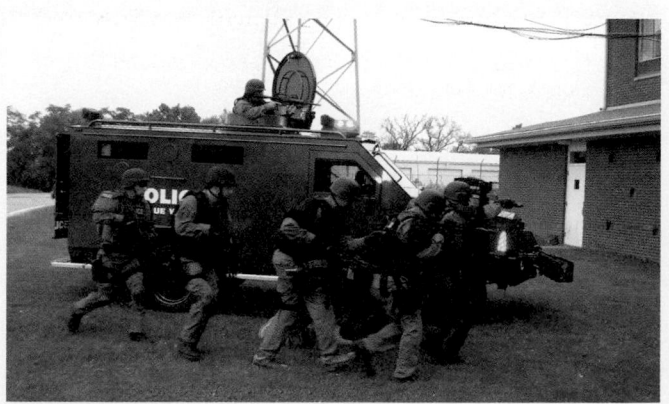

Figure 16 At a shooting or stabbing incident, a SWAT team may be employed. Remain in your safe staging area and follow all instructions from law enforcement.

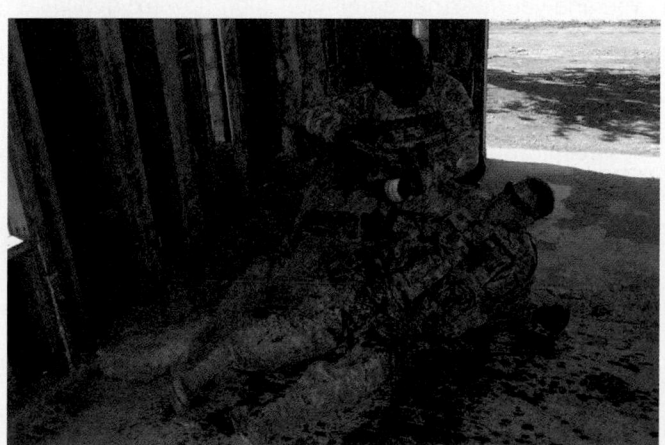

Figure 17 Many systems have specially trained tactical paramedics who can render care in violent and dangerous situations.

Hostages are usually held as a form of human collateral to ensure compliance with a promise. If you are taken hostage, you can increase your chances of survival if you can anticipate the feelings and actions of the hostage taker and the negotiators.

The psychological results of being held hostage are of greater concern than physical problems. Even if you are physically unharmed, you may experience strong psychological reactions during the incident. A person who has been held hostage can develop posttraumatic stress disorder (PTSD). It is often wise to seek professional counseling after your release, even if you do not think you need it, to prevent long-term problems later. Knowing what to expect if you are held hostage can help you keep your psychological equilibrium during the situation and help you deal with the psychological stress that often accompanies your release.

If you are taken hostage, manage yourself and your personal environment. Do not do anything that will attract unwanted attention, and do not stare at your captors. If the hostage takers believe you are in their way or you irritate them, they may kill you. Remember that any one of your captors can walk in and kill you at any time. Your only chance for survival is to maintain your role as a bargaining chip.

Because you are wearing a uniform, other hostages may look to you for guidance and strength. Your captors may consider this image of authority as a threat. Anything that draws attention to you increases the possibility of violence. Make every effort to be inconspicuous. Develop a nonthreatening image by removing the badge, collar pins, and patches from your uniform, or turn your uniform shirt inside out so these items are not visible. Ask to treat the wounded, if possible, even for minor injuries. This will serve to help you gauge the intentions of your captors, as well as make you seem less threatening. It will also keep your mind sharp, by performing tasks that you are used to doing as opposed to sitting around like the other captives, and hopefully offer the other captives some comfort. You may also consider offering to treat the injuries of any captors. This may seem ethically inconceivable, but not only is it consistent with your code of ethics and training (paramedics do not discriminate nor withhold treatment, regardless of the circumstances), but it may also help your captors perceive you as less of a threat, and make you more valuable.

■ Contact and Cover

In any violent situation, you must never assume that you will not be harmed because you are clearly identified as a paramedic. Always assume that the person with a gun will shoot anyone in sight. If you see law enforcement personnel seeking cover, you must not remain in the immediate vicinity.

Remember the difference between objects that provide cover and those that offer concealment only. You should make your body conform to the shape of the object as much as possible **Figure 18**.

People shooting from a higher position than you (such as in an upper floor window or on a roof) can usually see the upper part of your torso or head over the top of your cover, especially if you are using a wall or motor vehicle as cover **Figure 19**. If this occurs, use the engine block and wheel area of a motor vehicle as cover. Avoid the area near the fuel tank, and do not use the area between the wheels as cover **Figure 20**. Even though the aggressor cannot see you if you are between the wheels, a skilled

YOU are the Medic | PART 4

The law enforcement officers note the knife on the floor and you report that the patient was stabbed in the left lateral chest. You and your partner administer high-flow oxygen via a nonrebreathing mask, seal the chest wound, start two large-bore IV lines of NaCl, and transport the patient to the trauma center.

Recording Time: 15 Minutes	
Respirations	30 breaths/min, shallow
Pulse	114 beats/min
Skin	Cool, pale, moist
Blood pressure	94/66 mm Hg
Oxygen saturation (Spo$_2$)	97% with high-flow O$_2$ administration
Pupils	Equal and slow to react to light

7. Should you take the knife with you to the trauma center?

8. Should you report the circumstances of this event to the hospital in your radio report or when you arrive at the facility?

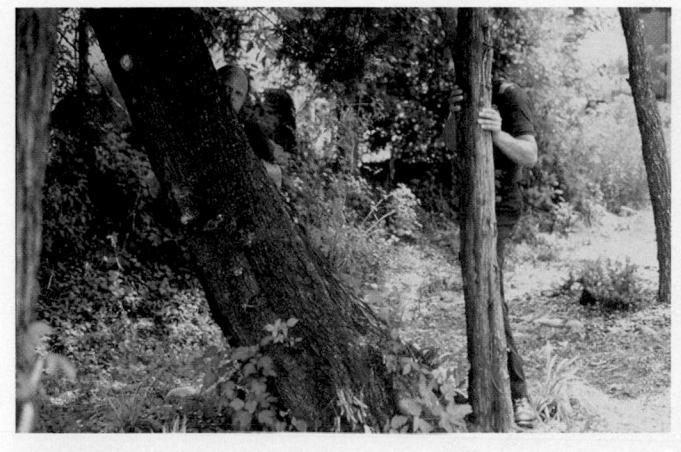

Figure 18 Choose a tree that is large enough to conceal all of your body.

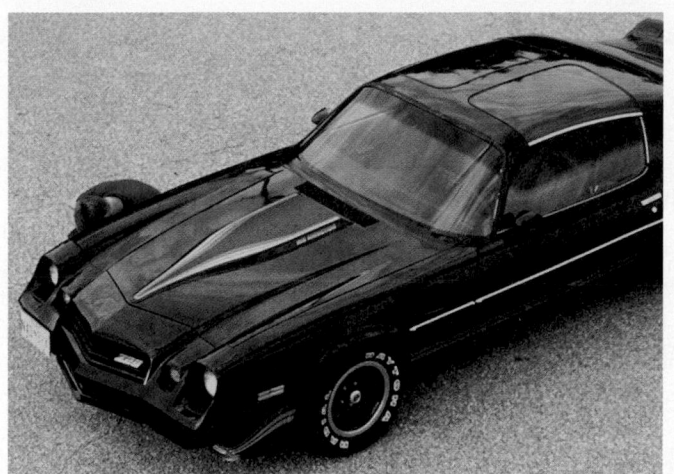

Figure 19 A sniper who is shooting from a higher position than you can see part of your body from above your position of cover.

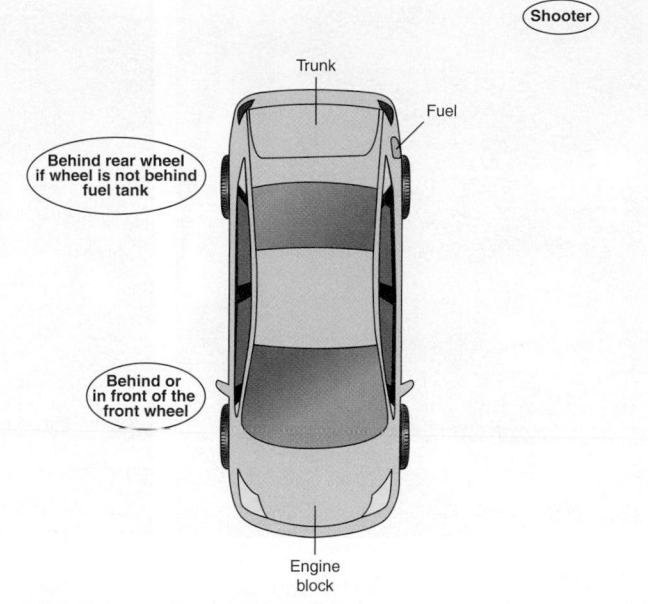

Figure 20 The engine block and the wheel area of a motor vehicle can be used as cover when shooting is occurring from overhead, but avoid the area near the fuel tank and the area between the wheels.

shooter can hit you by ricocheting bullets off the pavement in front of you.

Select a fire hydrant as cover only if you cannot immediately find larger objects. You will soon become uncomfortable trying to match your body to the small hydrant. There is a real possibility in such a situation that you could be shot in the arm, knee, or shoulder. However, your central body mass vital organs will be protected. If this is the only cover available, it is better than remaining in the open.

If you are not outdoors, items inside a structure and the structure itself can provide cover or concealment, depending on their construction. Furniture and appliances, such as a solid oak desk or a refrigerator, can be used for cover because they can stop a bullet. If you position yourself behind a sofa or a stuffed chair, you have concealed yourself but you are not protected by cover.

Using Walls as Cover

You cannot assume that a wall will provide safe cover—many provide only concealment. For your safety and survival, you must determine whether the type of wall you have chosen gives you cover or concealment only. For example, brick and concrete block walls are much safer than cinder block walls. The porous nature of cinder blocks will not absorb the bullet's energy and stop it. However, most interior walls are constructed with wood or aluminum studs and covered with drywall or siding. They may conceal you but they are not good cover because they are not impenetrable. If your only protection is behind a frame wall, try to stand near the door or window frames. These areas are usually constructed with extra framing materials and contain more wood than other areas of the wall.

Evasive Tactics

Change locations only if the new location is better cover, farther from the hostile atmosphere, and can be reached without revealing yourself to the attacker. Do not change your position of cover just for the sake of changing. Before changing locations, quickly look out from your cover several times **Figure 21**. Look from a different height and angle each time. Use this "quick-peek" technique to evaluate the advisability of changing locations. Always return to cover as quickly as possible.

If you decide that you would be safer in another location, do not run directly away from the assailant's position; run in a zigzag pattern. You have less chance of being hit if your movement takes you across the assailant's field of view.

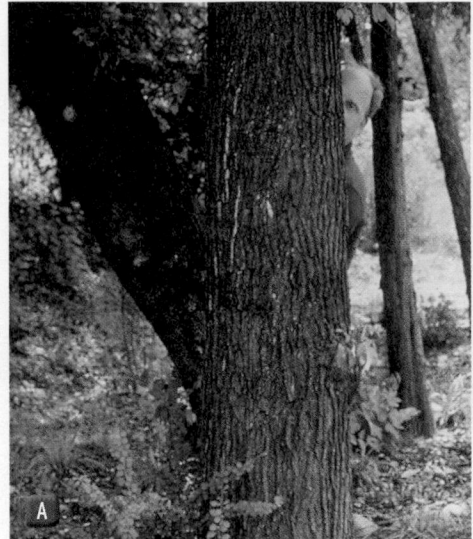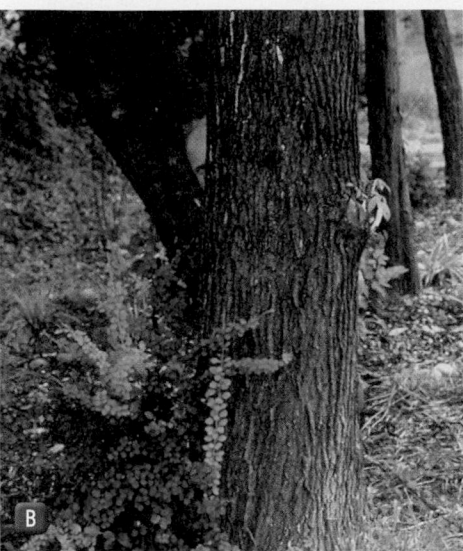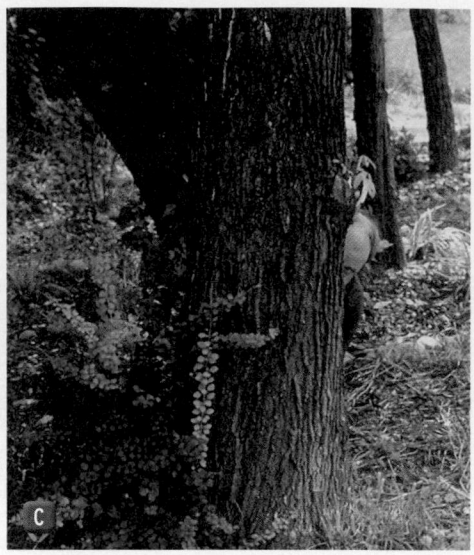

Figure 21 If you must analyze your position, look from a different height and angle each time. **A.** Look from one side. **B.** Look from the other side. **C.** Look from a different height.

Concealment Techniques

Tall grass, shrubbery, and dark shadows are considered areas of concealment. When cover is not readily available, use concealment to provide some protection while you assess your position and seek cover.

Areas of concealment are more common after dark than during daylight hours. If you are involved in a violent situation at night, move into the darkness or shadows and stand still. The assailant cannot see you and may not shoot. If the assailant fires shots at random, chances are you will not be hit.

In rural areas, tall grass or a cornfield can conceal you whether it is day or night. Remain motionless so that the foliage does not move. After you finish analyzing the situation, move toward cover.

Self-Defense

Recognizing the potential for violence when you arrive on the scene gives you time to request support and protection from law enforcement officers. With their protection, you should be able to treat your patient safely after the scene is secure. However, you must also consider what to do if the violence is ongoing or breaks out while you are providing care. If you know some effective defensive moves, you may be able to resolve the situation without getting hurt yourself. Self-defense must be physically practiced to be learned effectively; consider taking a self-defense course to learn techniques that can help you on the job.

If someone prevents you from reaching your patient, identify yourself. Instruct the person to move away. Inform the person that your patient may die if you are not allowed to provide assistance (although be mindful that this may actually be his or her intent). If the person blocking your way moves, you have attained your goal, but you should radio your dispatcher and request that law enforcement personnel respond just in case the person becomes uncooperative again. If the person does not

move, take a side step and repeat the verbal challenge. Inform the person, "If you do not get out of the way, then we will summon the police." This threat may make the person move, but not always in the direction you wanted.

You can control an unexpected attack. Always make sure that your exit path is not blocked, and that you can easily retreat the way you came. Use household objects to try to obstruct the assailant's path toward you as you retreat. Stretchers and equipment are also excellent obstructions, but you should be ready to leave them behind if you need to make a swift escape.

Self-Defense in Armed Encounters

Distraction techniques are useful in breaking the chain of events (turn, locate, focus, and fire) in a shooting incident and in preventing attacks with knives or other sharp objects. Again, the purpose of the distraction is to increase your chances of survival by giving you time to escape. The distraction does not have to be elaborate.

When you see something is coming at you, your initial instinct is to blink or flinch. Consider what happens when you are driving during a heavy rain and a passing vehicle throws water on your car's windshield. Even though you know the water is not going to hit you, you still blink or flinch when the water strikes the windshield. This is the reaction you want to provoke.

Throwing whatever you have handy, such as your patient care report pad, or even your pen or pen light at the person provides the same distraction as the water hitting the windshield. It interrupts the chain of events long enough to permit you to get out of the line of fire and run to safety.

If the patient takes aggressive action during your initial interview, one technique is to throw a light object directly at the aggressor's nose. Use only a lightweight object such as the ones previously mentioned. A hard or heavy object such as an aluminum report book, metal clipboard, laptop computer, or portable radio may cause needless (and permanent) injuries and later result in legal issues. A soft or light object will not cause undue harm.

After you throw the object, do not wait for a reaction. As soon as it is out of your hand, turn toward your vehicle, get out of the possible line of fire, and run to safety.

Put as much distance as possible between you and the aggressor. If possible, run to your vehicle 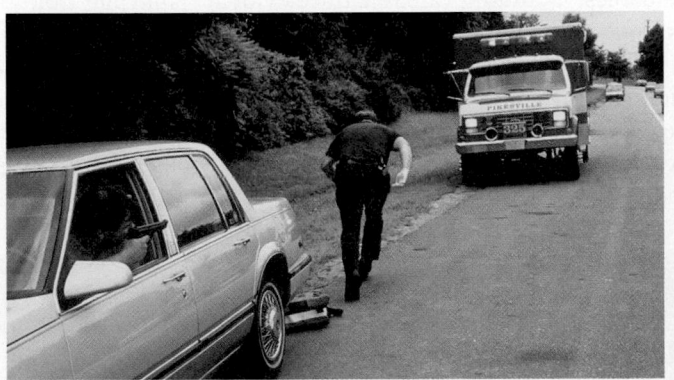 Figure 22 . You can call for help or drive to a safer location. If you are cut off from the ambulance, evaluate the surrounding area for the best possible cover and concealment.

Use physical force as a defensive technique, not an aggressive motion. Properly executed defensive motions can be as effective as physical strikes and are easier to defend if you face civil liability charges.

The amount of defensive force needed to protect yourself varies with each incident. If you believe that your life is in imminent danger, any action that gets you out of the situation is a reasonable level of force.

Words of Wisdom

Undoubtedly, you will encounter situations where things unpredictably get out of hand. Having a heightened sense of awareness, knowing your escapes routes, and being able to effectively use cover, concealment, and evasive techniques may be the difference between you getting hurt, and being able to get away without injury.

■ Crime Scenes

As a paramedic, you will respond to assist the victims of violent crime. Your first responsibility is your own safety, then your partner's safety, then the patient's safety, and then bystander safety. However, you also have a responsibility to the community at large. By assisting law enforcement personnel to maintain the integrity of the crime scene, you increase the probability that a suspect will be captured and convicted.

Figure 22 While the aggressor flinches and attempts to refocus, run toward the unit.

■ Preserving Evidence

Generally, there are two types of evidence: testimonial and real or physical. <u>Testimonial evidence</u> is the oral documentation by a witness of the facts. Real or <u>physical evidence</u> ties a suspect or a victim to a crime and includes body materials, objects, and impressions. You should be acutely concerned with not disturbing, damaging, or potentially altering physical evidence at the scene. Small blood stains on the wall or floor unperceivable to the untrained eye can yield critical forensic information that can be used to apprehend the perpetrator **Figure 23** . Unnecessary

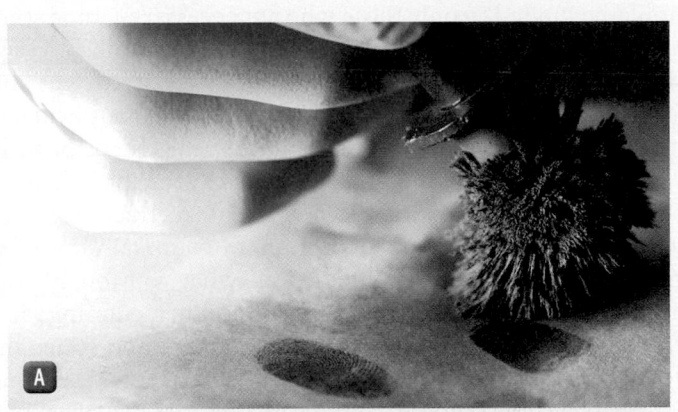

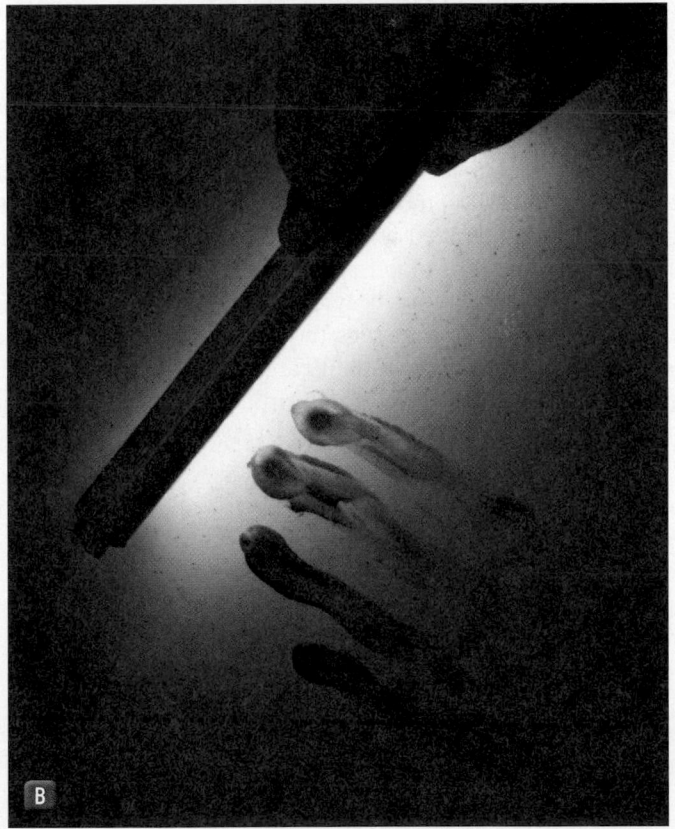

Figure 23 Fingerprints can be left on the scene in a variety of mediums. **A.** Some fingerprint marks can be dusted with a powder that adheres to residue on the print. **B.** Ultraviolet light can be used in other cases; this example shows a bloody fingerprint smear.

cutting or removal of clothes can potentially destroy or dislodge fibers, hair, or other evidence deposited by the perpetrator **Figure 24**.

Law enforcement personnel should collect evidence. If you must remove a piece of evidence (for example, clothing) in order to treat the patient, place each piece of evidence into a brown paper bag. If the item is saturated, then place the paper bag into a plastic bag for biohazard control.

Follow law enforcement direction when you are asked to park in a specific area or to avoid a certain location. Officers may be attempting to safeguard tire imprints, bullet casings, or blood. The number of EMS personnel entering the scene should be limited to only those who are necessary. Crime scene investigators commonly wear full-body Tyvex suits **Figure 25**. This is because every time they enter a crime scene, not only do they deposit evidence (in the form of DNA), but evidence can collect on their clothes and damage the evidence or make it less useful. You should also keep these principles in mind whenever you enter a crime scene. Every interaction with a space or surface entails the deposition of your DNA onto that area. Limit your time and interaction (what you touch) with the crime scene and ALWAYS wear gloves when entering. First responders are typically the first to enter a crime scene and view it in its most pristine condition. Once you enter the scene, regardless of how careful you are to preserve evidence, that scene is inexorably altered. This is often why paramedics are called to speak with investigators and prosecutors and appear at trials and pretrial hearings (ie, grand jury). These people will want to know exactly what you saw, what you touched, what you smelled, what you heard (radio, TV, fan, alarm clock), and what you did while you were there. You must not clean up the scene, alter items, or move bodies unless doing so is essential to establish the need for resuscitation. Be mindful of bullet casings, weapons, blood spatter, and puddles. Whenever possible, walk around such evidence **Figure 26**. Do not pick up expended cartridge casings to determine the caliber; that is irrelevant to rendering patient care. Do not use telephones, flush toilets, or turn on water in a sink. In each case, valuable

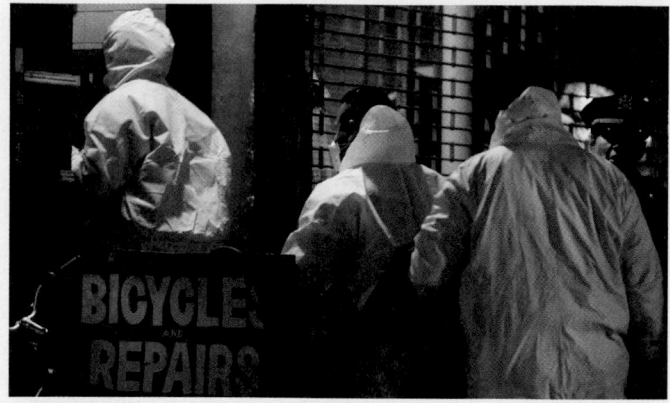

Figure 25 This joint NYC CSI team is comprised of various agencies, whose members use suits that prevent them from depositing their own false evidence on the scene, and also prevents them from collecting any on their body.

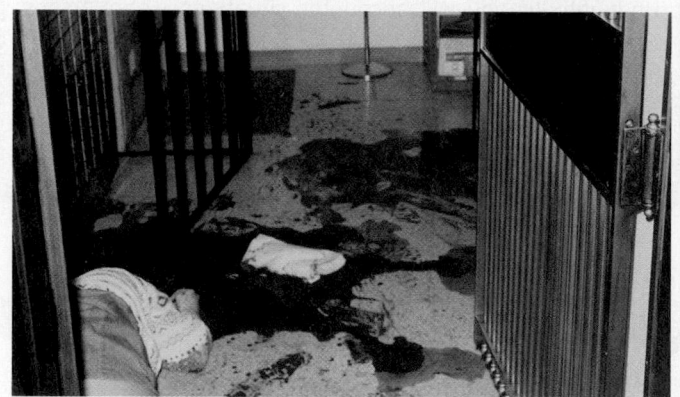

Figure 26 Do not disturb bullet casings, and avoid stepping in blood spatter and puddles.

evidence can be lost. When you remove clothes to expose a wound, do not cut through bullet holes, knife cuts, or tears. Once the clothes are removed, do not shake them because valuables, including valuable trace evidence, may fall from the pockets to the floor.

Because it is highly likely that you may be called to provide testimonial evidence in court regarding what you saw or heard at the scene of a crime, it is imperative that the incident be properly documented. Often, much time will elapse between the actual call and when you are asked to provide additional

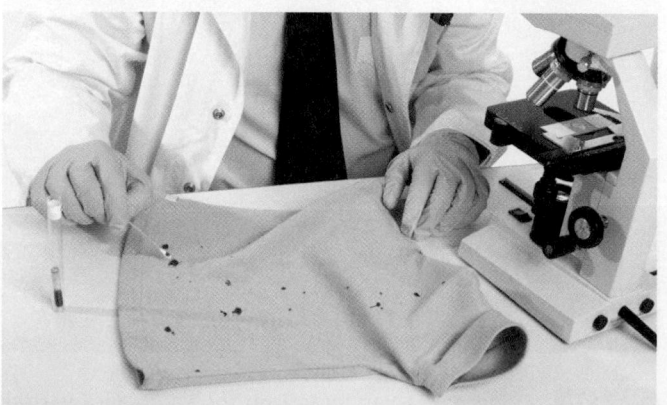

Figure 24 Hair, fibers, or body fluid containing DNA (blood, sweat, semen) can be found and analyzed in articles of clothing months to years after the transfer has occurred.

Documentation and Communication

Remember to document as much as you can at the crime scene. Your documentation may become evidence in a court case. If you are called to testify, your documentation will help you remember the specifics of the call.

Documentation and Communication

Your report should answer the following questions:

What did you see?
- Overturned or damaged furniture
- Weapons
- Position of victim and other persons at the scene

What did you hear?
- Arguing or screams
- Weapons being chambered or talk of the use of a weapon
- Incriminating statements by persons on the scene
- Television/radio left on
- Alarm clock or timer
- Phone left off the hook

What did you smell?
- Gunpowder or smoke
- Rotten food or garbage
- Putrefaction (decomposition)

What were you told?
- By police or fire personnel
- Bystanders or neighbors
- Family members or caregivers

What was done with evidence or personal effects taken from the victim?
- Clothing
- Weapons (Law enforcement personnel should secure weapons whenever possible)
- Medications
- Identification/wallet or purse

What did you alter or disturb?
- Where you went (and where you did not go)
- What you had to move in order to get to or assess the patient
- What you looked in (refrigerator, medicine cabinet, or drawer)?
- For what purpose you moved, altered, or disturbed something?
- Document your use of gloves and any other PPE that you wore that would prevent the spread of your DNA throughout the crime scene.

As always, PRINT LEGIBLY!

information or testimony about it. Sometimes years may have passed. Therefore, it is imperative whenever you encounter a crime scene that you clearly (legibly) and properly document what you find. This document may be read by dozens of people (and potentially a jury), and the quality of your report will speak volumes to your level of professionalism and credibility. More practically, the better your documentation is of the scene, the more likely that you will recall what you witnessed years later when all you have is your patient care report to refresh your memory.

The following are the elements of proper documentation: document what you saw; what you heard; what you were told; what you smelled (if there were any odors); what you moved, altered, or disturbed; and the chain of custody of any items that were presented to you, or that you found on the patient or decedent. Documentation should include a description of the scene. How many patients or decedents? Was the victim supine or prone? Where was the weapon? Were any characteristics of the scene noteworthy? Do not draw conclusions or overstate facts. Any statements made by the patient during transfer to a medical facility should be documented.

YOU *are the Medic* | SUMMARY

1. On the basis of the limited amount of information available, do you have any concern for entering this scene?

You should have concern for your safety and your crew's safety any time there is limited information for a call that may indicate violence. It is not usual for screams to come from a residence that are loud enough for a neighbor to be concerned. Listen to your instincts and if something does not sound safe or indicates a potential for violence, request assistance from law enforcement personnel.

2. What factors should you take into consideration because the residence is in an upscale, gated community?

The fact that the call is to an upscale, gated community does not add anything extra to take into consideration. Unfortunately, violence knows no economic or social boundaries. It is extremely important that you remember that the most important consideration on any call is your safety and that of your crew. You can do nothing for your patient if you are injured.

3. Is the scene safe to enter?

The scene may be safe to enter, but at this point you do not have enough information to make that decision. Security guards who work in gated communities are typically unarmed and are not sworn law enforcement officers. The empty golf cart in front of the residence indicates nothing in relation to your safety. You do not know where the security guard is, or why he or she did not meet you in front of the residence. At this point, you do not know if a potential perpetrator is still on the scene.

4. Should you enter the scene prior to the arrival of law enforcement personnel?

Your standard procedure for responding to any call involving violence should be to allow law enforcement personnel to arrive and secure the scene before your entry. Securing a scene demands more than the simple presence of a law enforcement officer at the scene. Responding paramedics must ensure that the scene is safe before going in to provide patient care.

5. What is your first priority for this patient?

A stab wound to the left lateral chest can injure many critical structures including the heart, great vessels, and lungs. Your first priority for the patient is to maintain her airway and administer high-flow oxygen. Assess the wound and seal it to maintain the atmospheric pressure necessary for respiration. Because this is a violent crime and the patient is responsive, your calm demeanor is essential to demonstrate to the patient that things are under control.

6. Do you feel this scene is now secure?

Not yet. No one has accounted for the person and vehicle that left the scene. Your crew and the patient are currently in a vulnerable position; you are performing patient care and are not ready for transport.

7. Should you take the knife with you to the trauma center?

No. The knife is considered evidence. Every effort should be made to not disturb weapons or other items that may have been used in the assault. The exception is if any of these items must be moved to continue patient care. If you move an item, inform law enforcement of the original location and where you moved it.

8. Should you report the circumstances of this event to the hospital in your radio report or when you arrive at the facility?

You must report to the hospital that you are transporting a patient who has been stabbed. This is necessary for internal notifications and to prepare for your arrival. The actual circumstances of the stabbing can wait until your arrival. Full details should be documented in your patient care report as well. Finally, law enforcement will typically send an officer to the hospital to obtain information.

YOU *are the Medic*   **SUMMARY**, *continued*

EMS Patient Care Report (PCR)

Date: 12-10-11	**Incident No.:** 5544	**Nature of Call:** Unknown		**Location:** 1 Shady Glen Manor	
Dispatched: 2041	**En Route:** 2041	**At Scene:** 2045	**Transport:** 2105	**At Hospital:** 2115	**In Service:** 2140

Patient Information

Age: 30
Sex: F
Weight (in kg [lb]): 79.5 kg (175 lb)

Allergies: Denies
Medications: Denies
Past Medical History: Denies
Chief Complaint: Difficulty breathing

Vital Signs

Time: 2055	**BP:** 90/60	**Pulse:** 116	**Respirations:** 36	**Spo$_2$:** 93%
Time: 2100	**BP:** 94/66	**Pulse:** 114	**Respirations:** 30	**Spo$_2$:** 97%
Time:	**BP:**	**Pulse:**	**Respirations:**	**Spo$_2$:**

EMS Treatment
(circle all that apply)

Oxygen @ __15__ L/min via (circle one): NC (NRM) Bag-mask device	**Assisted Ventilation**	**Airway Adjunct**	**CPR**
Defibrillation	(Bleeding Control)	(Bandaging)	**Splinting**	(Other:) IV, NaCL

Narrative

Arrived to find law enforcement securing scene. After 10 minutes, scene declared safe. Entered to find this 30-year-old female lying supine on a tile floor with a 1-inch penetrating wound to her left lateral chest approx. 2 inches below the mid axilla. A large amount of blood is noted on the floor. Pt is responsive and states her husband stabbed her, and then left the house. O$_2$ 15 L/min via NRM applied, chest wound dressed with an Asherman Seal. Lung sounds diminished on left in all fields, WNL on right all fields. IV NS started in left A/C with 14-ga titrating fluid to BP. Pt moved to unit for transport to University Hospital Trauma Center. No changes to the pt's condition en route. Report to Dr. Emory upon arrival and pt delivered to Trauma Room 1.
End of report

Prep Kit

■ Ready for Review

- EMS can be a dangerous profession. Always remember that your mission, beyond providing optimal patient care, is to return safely at the end of each shift. An injured paramedic cannot care for patients.

- No community, socioeconomic group, race, or religion is immune to violence. The use of sound survival skills will reduce the potential for you to fall victim to an act of violence while on an emergency call.

- Before performing patient care, perform a scene size-up for indicators of potential violence and escape routes. If you feel a scene is not safe, retreat to your ambulance and wait for law enforcement personnel to secure the scene.

- Obvious indicators of violence include calls for shootings, stabbings, or attempted suicides; body language such as clenched fists; and use of profane language or yelling.

- Also be aware of the possibility that secondary violence can occur during a call, even if indicators of violence were not present at the outset.

- Your agency will have standard operating procedures for dealing with potentially violent incidents. Become familiar with these and be sure to follow them.

- When you are responding to a vehicle on a road, park your vehicle a minimum of 21 ft behind the stopped vehicle, at a 10° angle to the driver's side facing the shoulder. Turn your front wheels all the way to the left; this provides limited protection in the event of gunfire.

- When you are approaching a vehicle such as a standard automobile, use your vehicle's high beams, but do not walk in the spotlight. Approach the vehicle with your abdomen facing the vehicle, checking the trunk and the inside of the vehicle before reaching the B post. If the back seat is occupied, do not proceed past the C post.

- When you are approaching a van, remain clear of the side door of the van throughout your approach. Walk parallel to the van until you are approximately 45° forward of the A post.

- When a dangerous situation develops, retreat from the scene and alert your dispatcher of the situation, including details such as the number of aggressors involved.

- When you are approaching a residence, stand to the side of the door. Do not stand on the hinged side; this will provide a view of you as the person inside opens the door.

- When you are entering a structure, always identify a primary exit as well as a secondary exit, should the primary exit become inaccessible.

- Clandestine drug laboratories are extremely hazardous. Once such a site is identified, remain clear of it until trained law enforcement and hazardous materials specialists have secured it.

- Gang activity can present hazards to EMS crews. Work with local law enforcement so you are aware of areas gangs may be affiliated with.

- In situations that involve an active shooter or sniper, follow law enforcement's direction, even if it means a patient cannot receive care immediately.

- You may need to use cover and concealment if a scene becomes dangerous. Cover includes objects or areas that are difficult or impossible for bullets to penetrate. Concealment includes objects or areas where it is difficult or impossible for you to be seen, but that could still be penetrated by bullets.

- Consider taking a self-defense course to help increase your ability to survive should dangerous situations develop.

- When you are working at a crime scene, make every attempt not to disturb, damage, or potentially alter the scene or physical evidence. Properly and thoroughly document these scenes and the actions you performed.

■ Vital Vocabulary

active shooter A gunman who has begun to fire on people and is still at large.

clandestine drug laboratories Locations where illegal drugs such as methamphetamine, lysergic acid diethylamide (LSD), ecstasy, and phencyclidine hydrochloride (PCP) are manufactured.

concealment Protection from being seen.

contact and cover Technique that involves one paramedic making contact with the patient to provide care, while the second paramedic obtains patient information, gauges the level of tension, and warns his or her partner at the first sign of trouble.

cover Obstacles that are difficult or impossible for bullets to penetrate.

physical evidence The evidence that ties a suspect or victim to a crime. It may include body materials, objects, and impressions.

primary exit The main means of escape should violence erupt. This is usually the door you used to enter the building.

secondary exit Any other means of egress, including windows and rear doors.

situational awareness Knowing your surroundings, the people and groups in your environment, and the climate of violence or strife.

tactical paramedics Specially trained medics who provide care for SWAT team members conducting operations, barricaded patients, patients being held hostage, and other special operations.

testimonial evidence The oral documentation by a witness of the facts of a criminal act.

tunnel vision Dangerous situation when a paramedic becomes so completely involved with patient care that he or she fails to see the possibility of physical harm to the patient or other care providers.

Assessment in Action

You are dispatched to a subdivision for a victim of a fight. The dispatcher tells you there were reports of four to five people fighting in the street. Two of them got into a vehicle that crashed into a pole across the street from the address you are given. The other people went into the home. As you arrive, you look at the front of the vehicle and see moderate damage in front of the driver's side A post. Inside the vehicle are two occupants who are actively yelling at each other. You look at the residence and find the front door is standing open. There are two large windows and you see no one inside. Law enforcement personnel are arriving on scene right behind you.

1. Being so completely involved with patient care that you fail to see anything else is called:
   A. concentration.
   B. tunnel vision.
   C. exclusionary.
   D. concealment.

2. When you are approaching the vehicle, which post on a standard passenger vehicle should you approach first?
   A. A
   B. B
   C. C
   D. D

3. When you enter this residence, the door you enter through is called the:
   A. primary exit.
   B. secondary exit.
   C. front exit.
   D. back exit.

4. An example of a secondary exit includes all of the following except:
   A. a back door.
   B. the door you entered.
   C. a window.
   D. a fire escape.

5. When you are assessing the patients in the vehicle, what is the most effective tool you can use to keep you out of trouble in a dispute?
   A. Your vehicle
   B. Your partner
   C. Your radio
   D. Your voice

6. What is the name of the technique in which one crew member is in a position to warn other crew members of increasing tension or a threat of violence?
   A. Contact and cover
   B. Contact and assess
   C. Concealment and cover
   D. Cover and call

7. In the event that you are in the open and someone in the vehicle has a firearm, you can use objects such as trees, utility poles, dumpsters, vehicles, and depressions in the ground, which are examples of:
   A. concealment.
   B. contact.
   C. cover.
   D. shadows.

Additional Question

8. What is the difference between testimonial evidence and physical evidence?

Glossary

6 Ps of musculoskeletal assessment Pain, Paralysis, Parasthesias, Pulselessness, Pallor, and Pressure.

6-feet rule A guideline to follow regarding the distance to place between oneself and a person who sneezes or coughs, to avoid exposure to germs.

abduction Movement *away* from the midline of the body.

abortion Expulsion of the fetus, from any cause, before the 20th week of gestation.

abrasion An injury in which a portion of the body is denuded of the epidermis by scraping or rubbing.

abruptio placenta A premature separation of the placenta from the wall of the uterus.

absence seizures The type of seizures characterized by a brief lapse of attention in which the patient may stare and not respond; formerly known as petit mal seizures.

absorption A type of decontamination that is done with large pads that the hazardous materials team use to soak up liquid and remove it from the patient.

abuse Any form of maltreatment that results in harm or loss. Maltreatment may be physical, sexual, psychological, or financial/material.

acceleration (a) The rate of change in velocity; speeding up.

accountability system A method of accounting for all personnel at an emergency incident and ensuring that only personnel with specific assignments are permitted to work within the various zones.

acetabulum The cup-shaped cavity in which the rounded head of the femur rotates.

acoustic neuroma A slow-growing, benign tumor of the vestibular cochlear nerve that can lead to loss of hearing in the affected ear.

acrocyanosis Cyanosis of the extremities due to a decrease in the amount of oxygen delivered to the extremities; the hands and feet turn blue because of narrowing (constriction) of small arterioles (tiny arteries) toward the end of the arms and legs.

acromion Lateral extension of the scapula that forms the highest point of the shoulder.

active shooter A gunman who has begun to fire on people and is still at large.

acute angle-closure glaucoma (AACG) Increased intraocular pressure that leads to ocular pain and decreased visual acuity; sudden onset is a medical emergency.

acute lung injury A condition in which lung tissue is damaged, characterized by hypoxemia, low lung volume, and pulmonary edema.

acute mountain sickness (AMS) An altitude illness characterized by headache plus at least one of the following: fatigue or weakness, gastrointestinal symptoms (nausea, vomiting or anorexia), dizziness or light-headedness, or difficulty sleeping.

acute radiation syndrome The clinical course that usually begins within hours of exposure to a radiation source. Symptoms include nausea, vomiting, diarrhea, fatigue, fever, and headache. The long-term symptoms are dose-related and are hematopoietic and gastrointestinal.

adduction Movement *toward* the midline of the body.

adipose tissue Fat tissue.

Adult Protective Services (APS) Organizations that investigate cases involving abuse and neglect and provide case management services in some cases.

aerobic metabolism Metabolism that can proceed only in the presence of oxygen.

after-action report (AAR) The official internal report of the entire event, such as a disaster, which should contain the facts of the incident reflected in a chronologic, accurate manner.

afterdrop Continued fall in core temperature after a victim of hypothermia has been removed from a cold environment, due at least in part to the return of cold blood from the body surface to the body core.

afterload The pressure in the aorta against which the left ventricle must pump blood; increasing this can decrease cardiac output.

air ambulances Fixed-wing aircraft and helicopters that have been modified for medical care; used to evacuate and transport patients with life-threatening injuries to treatment facilities.

all-hazards approach The act of conducting comprehensive preplanning that will apply to any disaster.

alpha Type of energy that is emitted from a strong radiologic source; it is the least harmful penetrating type of radiation and cannot travel fast or through most objects.

alternative powered vehicles A vehicle that uses fuels other than petroleum or a combination of petroleum and another fuel for power.

altitude illnesses Conditions caused by the effects from hypobaric (low atmospheric pressure) hypoxia on the central nervous system and pulmonary systems as a result of unacclimatized people ascending to altitude; range from acute mountain sickness (AMS) to high-altitude cerebral edema (HACE) and high-altitude pulmonary edema (HAPE).

alveolar ridges   The ridges between the teeth that are covered with thickened connective tissue and epithelium.

alveoli   Small pits or cavities, such as the sockets for the teeth.

Alzheimer disease   A progressive organic condition in which neurons die, causing dementia.

ammonium nitrate   A commonly used industrial-grade fertilizer that is not in itself dangerous to handle or transport, but when mixed with fuel and other components, forms an extremely explosive compound.

amniotic fluid   A clear, slightly yellowish liquid that surrounds the fetus during pregnancy; contained in the amniotic sac.

amniotic fluid embolism   An extremely rare, life-threatening condition that occurs when amniotic fluid and fetal cells enter the pregnant woman's pulmonary and circulatory system through the placenta via the umbilical veins, causing an exaggerated allergic response from the woman's body.

amniotic sac   The fluid-filled, baglike membrane in which the fetus develops.

amputation   An injury in which part of the body is completely severed.

anaerobic metabolism   Metabolism that takes place in the absence of oxygen.

anaphylactic shock   A severe hypersensitivity reaction that involves bronchoconstriction and cardiovascular collapse.

anchoring bias   Occurs when an initial reference point distorts your estimates.

angioedema   Recurrent large areas of subcutaneous edema of sudden onset, usually disappearing within 24 hours, which is seen mainly in young women, frequently as a result of allergy to food or drugs.

angle of impact   The angle at which an object hits another; this characterizes the force vectors involved and has a bearing on patterns of energy dissipation.

angle of Louis   Prominence on the sternum that lies opposite the second intercostal space.

angulation   The presence of an abnormal angle or bend in an extremity.

anisocoria   A condition in which the pupils are not of equal size.

anterior chamber   The anterior area of the globe between the lens and the cornea that is filled with aqueous humor.

anterior cord syndrome   A condition that occurs with flexion injuries or fractures, resulting in the displacement of bony fragments into the anterior portion of the spinal cord; findings include paralysis below the level of the insult and loss of pain, temperature, and touch sensation.

anterior tibial artery   The artery that travels through the anterior muscles of the leg and continues to the foot as the dorsalis pedis.

anterograde (posttraumatic) amnesia   Loss of memory relating to events that occurred after the injury.

anthrax   A deadly bacteria (*Bacillus anthracis*) that lies dormant in a spore (protective shell); the germ is released from the spore when exposed to the optimal temperature and moisture. The route of entry is inhalation, cutaneous, or gastrointestinal (from consuming food that contains spores).

aortic sclerosis   A condition in which the aortic valve thickens due to fibrosis and calcification, obstructing blood flow from the left ventricle.

aortic stenosis   A condition in which the aortic valve does not open fully, decreasing blood flow from the heart.

Apgar score   Scale used to assess the status of a newborn 1 and 5 minutes after birth (range, 0 to 10); assigns a number value to each of five areas of assessment.

apnea   Respiratory pause greater than or equal to 20 seconds.

apocalyptic violence   A type of violence sought by some terrorists, such as violent religious groups and doomsday cults, in which they wish to bring about the end of the world.

apparent life-threatening event (ALTE)   An unexpected sudden episode of color change, tone change, or apnea that requires mouth-to-mouth resuscitation or vigorous stimulation.

appendicular skeleton   The part of the skeleton comprising the upper and lower extremities.

apraxia   A neurologic impairment in which the brain is intermittently unable to carry out the command for speech or other tasks.

aqueous humor   The clear, watery fluid in the anterior chamber of the globe.

arachnoid   The middle membrane of the three meninges that enclose the brain and spinal cord.

arterial air embolism   Air bubbles in the arterial blood vessels.

arterial gas embolism (AGE)   The resultant gaseous emboli from the forcing of gas into the vasculature from barotrauma.

arteriosclerosis   A pathologic condition in which the arterial walls become thickened and inelastic.

arthritis   Inflammation of the joints.

articulations   The locations where two or more bones meet; joints.

ashfall   The residue left behind from a volcanic eruption.

asphyxia   Condition of severely deficient supply of oxygen to the body leading to end organ damage.

asphyxiant Any gas that displaces oxygen from the atmosphere; can be deadly if exposure occurs in a confined space.

asymmetric warfare A type of warfare in which groups wage war with unconventional weapons and covert tactics that are unequal—for example, when there are differences in military resources or capabilities.

asynchronous In CPR, when two rescuers perform ventilations and compressions individually and not timed or waiting for the other rescuer to pause.

asynchrony Disturbance or lack of synchronization.

ataxia Inability to coordinate the muscles properly; often used to describe a staggering gait.

atelectasis Alveolar collapse that prevents use of that portion of the lungs for ventilation and oxygenation.

atherosclerosis A disorder in which cholesterol and calcium build up inside the walls of the blood vessels, forming plaque, which eventually leads to partial or complete blockage of blood flow.

atmosphere absolute (ATA) A measurement of ambient pressure; the weight of air at sea level, equivalent in pressure to 33 feet of seawater (fsw).

atrial septal defect (ASD) A hole in the atrial septal wall that allows oxygenated and deoxygenated blood to mix; patients with this hole have a higher incidence of stroke.

atrophy Wasting away of a tissue.

auditory neuropathy A condition characterized by normal function of the structures of the ear without a corresponding stimulation of auditory centers of the brain; also called auditory dyssynchrony.

auditory ossicles The bones that function in hearing and are located deep within cavities of the temporal bone.

auricle The large outside portion of the ear through which sound waves enter the ear; also called the pinna.

authority having jurisdiction (AHJ) An organization, office, or person responsible for enforcing the requirements of a code or standard, or for approving equipment, materials, an installation, or a procedure.

autism A developmental disorder characterized by impairments of social interaction; may include severe behavioral problems, repetitive motor activities, and impairment in verbal and nonverbal skills.

automated external defibrillator (AED) A "smart" defibrillator that can analyze the patient's ECG rhythm and determine whether a defibrillating shock is needed.

autonomic dysreflexia A potentially life-threatening late complication of spinal cord injury in which a massive, uninhibited, uncompensated cardiovascular response occurs due to stimulation of the sympathetic nervous system below the level of injury; also known as autonomic hyperreflexia.

autoregulation An increase in mean arterial pressure to compensate for decreased cerebral perfusion pressure; compensatory response of the body to shunt blood to the brain; manifests clinically as hypertension.

avascular necrosis Tissue death resulting from the loss of blood supply.

avulsing A tearing away or forcible separation.

avulsion An injury that leaves a piece of skin or other tissue partially or completely torn away from the body.

avulsion fracture A fracture that occurs when a piece of bone is torn free at the site of attachment of a tendon or ligament.

awareness The first level of rescue training provided to all responders, with an emphasis on recognizing the hazards, securing the scene, and calling for appropriate assistance. There is no actual use of rescue skills.

axial skeleton The part of the skeleton comprising the skull, spinal column, and rib cage.

axilla The armpit.

axillary artery The artery that runs through the axilla, connecting the subclavian artery to the brachial artery.

axon Long, slender extension of a neuron (nerve cell) that conducts electrical impulses away from the neuronal soma.

Babinski reflex When the toe(s) moves upward in response to stimulation to the sole of the foot. Under normal circumstances, the toe(s) moves downward.

bacteria Microorganisms that reproduce by binary fission. These single-cell creatures reproduce rapidly. Some can form spores (encysted variants) when environmental conditions are harsh.

bacterial tracheitis An invasive exudative bacterial infection of the soft tissues of the trachea.

bacterial vaginosis An overgrowth of bacteria in the vagina, characterized by itching, burning, or pain, and possibly a "fishy" smelling discharge.

bandage Material used to secure a dressing in place.

bariatrics The medical specialty dedicated to prevention and treatment of obesity.

barometric energy The energy that results from sudden changes in pressure as may occur in a diving accident or sudden decompression in an airplane.

baroreceptors Receptors in the blood vessels, kidneys, brain, and heart that respond to changes in pressure in the heart or main arteries to help maintain homeostasis.

barotrauma Injury resulting from pressure disequilibrium across body surfaces.

basal ganglia Structures located deep within the cerebrum, diencephalon, and midbrain that have an important role in coordination of motor movements and posture.

basal metabolic rate (BMR) The heat energy produced at rest from normal body metabolic reactions, determined mostly by the liver and skeletal muscles.

basilar skull fractures Usually occur following diffuse impact to the head (such as falls, motor vehicle crashes); generally result from extension of a linear fracture to the base of the skull and can be difficult to diagnose with a radiograph (x-ray).

Battle sign Bruising over the mastoid bone behind the ear commonly seen following a basilar skull fracture; also called retroauricular ecchymosis.

belay Technique of controlling the rope as it is fed out to climbers.

belt noise A chirping or squealing sound, synchronous with engine speed.

bereavement Sadness from loss; grieving.

beta Type of energy that is emitted from a strong radiologic source; is slightly more penetrating than alpha, and requires a layer of clothing to stop it.

bill of lading A document carried by drivers of commercial vehicles that should provide specific information about what is carried on the vehicle.

biomechanics The study of the physiology and mechanics of a living organism using the tools of mechanical engineering.

Biot respirations Characterized by an irregular rate, pattern, and volume of breathing with intermittent periods of apnea; also called ataxic respirations.

blast front The leading edge of the shock wave.

blastocyst The term for an oocyte once it has been fertilized and multiplies into cells.

blind spots Areas of the road that are blocked from your sight by your own vehicle or mirrors.

blood The fluid tissue that is pumped by the heart through the arteries, veins, and capillaries and consists of plasma and formed elements or cells, such as red blood cells, white blood cells, and platelets.

bloody show A plug of mucus, sometimes mixed with blood, that is expelled from the dilating cervix and discharged from the vagina.

blow-by technique A method of delivering oxygen by holding a face mask or similar device near an infant's or a child's face; used when a nonrebreathing mask is not tolerated.

blowout fracture A fracture to the floor of the orbit usually caused by a blow to the eye.

blunt trauma An impact on the body by objects that cause injury without penetrating soft tissues or internal organs and cavities.

body-over-frame construction Vehicle design where the body of the vehicle is placed onto a frame skeleton and the frame acts as the foundation for the vehicle. The design consists of two large beams tied together by cross member beams.

botulinum A very potent neurotoxin produced by bacteria; when introduced into the body, this neurotoxin affects the nervous system's ability to function and causes muscle paralysis.

bowing fracture An incomplete fracture typically occurring in children in which the bone becomes bent as the result of a compressive force.

boxer's fracture A fracture of the head of the fifth metacarpal that usually results from striking an object with a clenched fist.

Boyle's law At a constant temperature, the volume of a gas is inversely proportional to its pressure (if you double the pressure on a gas, you halve its volume); written as PV = K, where P = pressure, V = volume, and K = a constant.

brachial artery The artery that runs through the arm and branches into the radial and ulnar arteries.

bradycardia A pulse rate of less than 100 beats/min in the newborn.

brain Part of the central nervous system located within the cranium; contains billions of neurons that serve a variety of vital functions.

brainstem The midbrain, pons, and medulla, collectively.

brake fade A sensation that an ambulance has lost its power brakes.

brake pull A sensation that, when an operator depresses the brake pedal, the steering wheel is being pulled to the left or the right.

breath-hold diving Also called free diving, this type of diving does not require any equipment, except sometimes a snorkel.

breech presentation A delivery in which the buttocks come out first.

brisance The shattering effect of a shock wave and its ability to cause disruption of tissues and structures.

bronchiolitis A condition seen in children younger than 2 years, characterized by dyspnea and wheezing.

bronchopulmonary dysplasia A spectrum of lung conditions found in premature neonates who require long periods of high-concentration oxygen and ventilator support, ranging from mild reactive airways to debilitating chronic lung disease.

Brown-Séquard syndrome A condition associated with penetrating trauma with hemisection of the spinal cord and complete damage to all spinal tracts on the involved side.

buboes Enlarged lymph nodes (up to the size of tennis balls) that are characteristic of people infected with the bubonic plague.

bubonic plague An epidemic that spread throughout Europe in the Middle Ages, causing over 25 million deaths, also called the Black Death; transmitted by infected fleas and characterized by acute malaise, fever, and the formation of tender, enlarged, inflamed lymph nodes that appear as lesions, called buboes.

buckle fracture A common incomplete fracture in children in which the cortex of the bone fractures from an excessive compression force; also called a torus fracture.

buddy splinting Securing an injured digit to an adjacent uninjured one to allow the intact digit to act as a splint.

burn shock The shock or hypoperfusion caused by a burn injury and the tremendous loss of fluids; capillaries leak, resulting in intravascular fluid volume oozing out of the circulation and into the interstitial spaces, and cells take in increased amounts of salt and water.

bursa A fluid-filled sac located adjacent to joints that reduces the amount of friction between moving structures.

bursitis Inflammation of a bursa.

calcaneus The heel bone; the largest of the tarsal bones.

CAMEO Computer-Aided Management of Emergency Operations; a tool to help predict downwind concentrations of hazardous materials based on the input of environmental factors into a computer model.

cancellous bone Trabecular or spongy bone.

cancer Excessive growth and division of abnormal cells within the body that can occur in many body systems, tissues, and organs, and that can progress rapidly and cause death in a relatively short period of time.

candidiasis A vaginal infection that is not technically a sexually transmitted infection, and which can occur in a pregnant or nonpregnant female, but which is more common in pregnancy; also called thrush or a yeast infection.

capacitance vessels The smallest venules.

carbon monoxide A chemical asphyxiant that results in a cellular respiratory failure; this gas ties up hemoglobin to the extent that oxygen in the blood becomes inaccessible to the cells.

carboy A glass, plastic, or steel nonbulk storage container, ranging in volume from 5 to 15 gallons.

cardiac output (CO) The volume of blood pumped by the heart per minute. Calculated by multiplying the stroke volume by the heart rate per minute.

cardiac tamponade A condition in which the atria and right ventricle are collapsed by a collection of blood or other fluid within the pericardial sac, resulting in a diminished cardiac output.

cardiogenic shock A condition caused by loss of 40% or more of the functioning myocardium; the heart is no longer able to circulate sufficient blood to maintain adequate oxygen delivery.

cardiovascular collapse Failure of the heart and blood vessels; shock.

cargo tank Bulk packaging that is permanently attached to or forms a part of a motor vehicle, or is not permanently attached to any motor vehicle, and that, because of its size, construction, or attachment to a motor vehicle, is loaded or unloaded without being removed from the motor vehicle.

carpal tunnel syndrome Compression of the median nerve at the wrist where it passes through the carpal canal, causing numbness and tingling in the hand, and possibly pain.

carpals The eight small bones of the wrist.

cartilage Tough, elastic substance that covers opposable surfaces of moveable joints and forms part of the skeleton.

cartilaginous joints Joints that are spanned completely by cartilage and allow for minimal motion.

casualty collection points Areas where slightly injured or noninjured displaced persons can be gathered together and transported by bus or truck for further treatment.

cataract A clouding of the lens of the eye or its surrounding transparent membrane; normally a result of aging; leads to decreased vision.

cauda equina The location where the spinal cord separates, composed of nerve roots.

cauda equina syndrome A neurologic condition caused by compression of the bundle of nerve roots located at the end of the spinal cord.

cavitation Cavity formation; shock waves that push tissues in front of and lateral to the projectile and may not necessarily increase the wound size or cause permanent injury but can result in cavitation.

cellulitis An acute inflammation in the skin caused by a bacterial infection.

central auditory processing disorder (CAPD) A disorder in which patients have difficulty interpreting speech and differentiating it from other sounds that are present.

central cord syndrome A condition resulting from hyperextension injuries to the cervical area that cause damage with hemorrhage or edema to the central cervical segments; findings include greater loss of function in the upper extremities with variable sensory loss of pain and temperature.

central cyanosis Bluish coloration of the skin due to the presence of deoxygenated hemoglobin in blood vessels near the skin surface.

central nervous system (CNS) The system containing the brain and spinal cord.

central neurogenic hyperventilation Deep, rapid respirations; similar to Kussmaul, but without an acetone breath odor; commonly seen following brainstem injury.

central shock A condition that consists of cardiogenic shock and obstructive shock (Weil-Shubin classification).

central venous catheter A catheter inserted into the vena cava to permit intermittent or continuous monitoring of central venous pressure and to facilitate obtaining blood samples for chemical analysis.

central vision The visualization of objects directly in front of you.

cephalopelvic disproportion A situation in which the head of the fetus is larger than the woman's pelvis; in most cases, cesarean section is required for such a delivery.

cerebellum The region of the brain essential in coordinating muscle movements in the body; also called the athlete's brain.

cerebral concussion Occurs when the brain is jarred around in the skull; a mild diffuse brain injury that does not result in structural damage or permanent neurologic impairment.

cerebral contusion A focal brain injury in which brain tissue is bruised and damaged in a defined area.

cerebral cortex The largest portion of the cerebrum; regulates voluntary skeletal movement and one's level of awareness—a part of consciousness.

cerebral edema Cerebral water; causes or contributes to swelling of the brain.

cerebral palsy (CP) A developmental condition in which damage is done to the brain. It presents during infancy as a delay in walking or crawling, and can take on a spastic form in which muscles are in a nearly constant state of contraction.

cerebral perfusion pressure (CPP) The pressure of blood flow through the brain; the difference between the mean arterial pressure (MAP) and intracranial pressure (ICP).

cerebrospinal fluid (CSF) Fluid produced in the ventricles of the brain that flows in the subarachnoid space and bathes the meninges.

cerebrospinal fluid shunt (CSF shunt) A tube placed in the body to relieve pressure by drawing excess cerebrospinal fluid away from the brain or spinal cord.

cerebrum The largest portion of the brain; responsible for higher functions, such as reasoning; divided into right and left hemispheres, or halves.

cervical canal The interior of the cervix.

cervix The narrowest portion of the uterus that opens into the vagina.

chemical asphyxiants Substances that interfere with the use of oxygen at the cellular level.

chemical energy The energy released as a result of a chemical reaction.

chemoreceptors Sense organs that monitor the levels of oxygen and carbon dioxide and the pH of cerebrospinal fluid and blood and provide feedback to the respiratory centers to modify the rate and depth of breathing based on the body's needs at any given time.

chemotactic factors The factors that cause cells to migrate into an area.

CHEMTREC (Chemical Transportation Emergency Center) A resource available to emergency responders via telephone on a 24-hour basis.

Cheyne-Stokes respirations The respirations that are fast and then become slow, with intervening periods of apnea; commonly seen following brainstem injury.

chilblains Itchy reddish and purple swollen lesions that occur primarily on the extremities, due to longer exposure to temperatures just above freezing or sudden rewarming after exposure to cold.

child abuse Any improper or excessive action that injures or otherwise harms a child or infant; it includes physical abuse, sexual abuse, neglect, and emotional abuse.

child protective services (CPS) An agency that is the community legal organization responsible for protection, rehabilitation, and prevention of child maltreatment and neglect; it has the legal authority to temporarily remove children from homes if there is reason to believe they are at risk for injury or neglect and to secure foster placement.

chlamydia A sexually transmitted disease (STD) caused by the bacterium *Chlamydia trachomatis*; has the highest incidence in sexually transmitted diseases; signs and symptoms include inflammation of the urethra, epididymis, cervix, and fallopian tubes, and discharge from the urethra.

chlorine (CL) The first chemical agent ever used in warfare. It has a distinct odor of bleach, and creates a green haze when released as a gas. Initially it produces upper airway irritation and a choking sensation.

choanal atresia A narrowing or blockage of the nasal airway by membranous or bony tissue; a congenital condition, meaning it is present at birth.

cholestasis A disease of the liver that occurs only during pregnancy, in which hormones affect the gallbladder by slowing down or blocking the normal bile flow from the liver; the most common symptom is profuse, painful itching, particularly of the hands and feet.

choroid plexus Specialized cells within the hollow areas in the ventricles of the brain that produce cerebrospinal fluid.

chronic hypertension A blood pressure that is equal to or greater than 140/90 mm Hg, which exists prior to pregnancy, occurs before the 20th week of pregnancy, or continues to persist postpartum.

chronotropic effect The rate of contraction of the heart.

circumferential burns Burns on the neck or chest that may compress the airway or on an extremity that might act like a tourniquet.

clandestine drug laboratories Locations where illegal drugs such as methamphetamine, lysergic acid diethylamide (LSD), ecstasy, and phencyclidine hydrochloride (PCP) are manufactured.

classic heatstroke Also called passive heatstroke, this is a serious heat illness that usually occurs during heat waves and is most likely to strike very old, very young, or bedridden people.

clavicle An S-shaped bone, also called the collarbone, that articulates medially with the sternum and laterally with the shoulder.

cleaning The process of removing dirt, dust, blood, or other visible contaminants from a surface.

cleft lip An abnormal defect or fissure in the upper lip that failed to close during development. It is often associated with cleft palate.

cleft palate A fissure or hole in the palate (roof of the mouth) that forms a communicating pathway between the mouth and nasal cavities.

closed abdominal injury An injury in which there is soft-tissue damage inside the body, but the skin remains intact.

closed fracture A fracture in which the skin is not broken.

closed incident A contained incident in which patients are found in one focal location and the situation is not expected to produce more patients than initially present.

closed wound An injury in which damage occurs beneath the skin or mucous membrane but the surface remains intact.

coarctation of the aorta (CoA) Pinching or narrowing of the aorta that obstructs blood flow from the heart to the systemic circulation.

cochlea The shell-shaped structure within the inner ear that contains the organ of Corti.

cochlear duct A canal within the cochlea that receives vibrations from the ossicles.

code team leader The code team member who has the responsibility for managing the rescuers or team members during a cardiac arrest, as well as choreographing the effort of the group.

code team member A member of the resuscitation team trying to revive the patient.

coining A cultural ritual intended to treat an illness by rubbing hot coins, often on the torso, which produces rounded and oblong red, patchy, flat skin lesions.

cold diuresis Secretion of large amounts of urine in response to cold exposure and the consequent shunting of blood volume to the body core.

cold protective response Phenomenon associated with cold water immersion in which reflexes in the body and a lowered metabolic rate help preserve basic body functions.

cold stress A psychological condition that can develop in people who are exposed to cold weather for long periods of time, even if sheltered.

cold zone A safe area for those agencies involved in the operations; the incident commander (IC), command post, EMS providers, and other support functions necessary to control the incident should be located in the cold zone.

collagen A protein that gives tensile strength to the connective tissues of the body.

colostomy The surgical establishment of an opening between the colon and the surface of the body for the purpose of providing drainage of the bowel.

colostomy bag A plastic pouch or bag attached over a colostomy to collect stool.

comedo A noninflammatory acne lesion.

comfort care Medical treatment aimed at symptom relief and providing comfort for the patient.

command In incident command, the position that oversees the incident, establishes the objectives and priorities, and from there develops a response plan.

comminuted fracture A fracture in which the bone is broken into three or more pieces.

commotio cordis An event in which an often fatal cardiac dysrhythmia is produced by a sudden blow to the thoracic cavity.

communicability The ease with which a disease spreads from one human to another human.

communicable disease An illness that can be transmitted from one person to another.

compartment syndrome A condition that develops when edema and swelling result in increased pressure within soft tissues, causing circulation to be compromised, possibly resulting in tissue necrosis.

compensated shock (classes I and II) The early stage of shock, in which the body can still compensate for blood loss. The systolic blood pressure and brain perfusion are maintained.

complete abortion Expulsion of all products of conception from the uterus.

complete fracture A fracture in which the bone is broken into two or more completely separate pieces.

complete spinal cord injury Total disruption of all tracts of the spinal cord, with all cord-mediated functions below the level of transection lost permanently.

complex access Complicated entry that requires special tools and training and includes breaking windows or using other force.

complex febrile seizures An unusual form of seizure that occurs in association with a rapid increase in body temperature.

complex partial seizures Seizures characterized by alteration of consciousness with or without complex focal motor activity.

compound fracture An open fracture; a fracture beneath an open wound.

concealment Protection from being seen.

conduction Transfer of heat to a solid object or a liquid by direct contact.

conductive hearing loss A type of hearing impairment due to problems with the middle ear bones' ability to conduct sounds from the outer ear to the inner ear.

confined space A space with limited or restricted access that is not meant for continuous occupancy, such as a manhole, well, or tank.

confirmation bias Occurs with the tendency to gather and rely on information that confirms your existing views and to avoid or downplay information that does not conform to your preexisiting hypothesis or field differential.

congenital adrenal hyperplasia (CAH) Inadequate production of cortisol and aldosterone by the adrenal gland.

congenital heart disease (CHD) The most common birth defect; associated with hypoxia in the newborn period requiring intervention during the first months of life; often lead to cyanosis.

conjunctiva A thin, transparent membrane that covers the sclera and internal surfaces of the eyelids.

conjunctivitis An inflammation of the conjunctivae that usually is caused by bacteria, viruses, allergies, or foreign bodies; should be considered highly contagious if infectious in orgin; also called pink eye.

Consensus formula A formula that recommends giving 4 mL of normal saline for each kilogram of body weight, multiplied by the percentage of body surface area burned; sometimes used to calculate fluid needs during lengthy transport times; formerly called the Parkland formula.

contact and cover Technique that involves one paramedic making contact with the patient to provide care, while the second paramedic obtains patient information, gauges the level of tension, and warns his or her partner at the first sign of trouble.

contact burn A burn produced by touching a hot object.

contact hazard A hazardous agent that gives off little or no vapors; the skin is the primary route for this type of chemical to enter the body; also called a skin hazard.

contagious An adjective used to describe the ability of a person infected with a highly communicable disease to pass that disease to another person.

contagious disease See communicable disease.

container Any vessel or receptacle that holds material, including storage vessels, pipelines, and packaging.

continuity of operations plan (COOP) The detailed plan describing the functioning of the agency in situations that disrupt normal operations.

contusion A bruise; an injury that causes bleeding beneath the skin but does not break the skin.

convection Mechanism by which body heat is picked up and carried away by moving air currents.

conversion disorder A psychological condition in which stress or mental conflict is converted into physical complaints.

core body temperature (CBT) The temperature in the part of the body comprising the heart, lungs, brain, and abdominal viscera.

cornea The transparent anterior portion of the eye that overlies the iris and pupil.

coronal suture The point where the parietal bones join with the frontal bone.

corpus luteum The remains of a follicle after an oocyte has been released, and which secretes progesterone.

corrosives A class of chemicals with either high or low pH levels. Exposure can cause severe soft-tissue damage.

coup-contrecoup injury Dual impacting of the brain into the skull; coup injury occurs at the point of impact; contrecoup injury occurs on the opposite side of impact, as the brain rebounds.

cover Obstacles that are difficult or impossible for bullets to penetrate.

covert Act in which the public safety community generally has no prior knowledge of the time, location, or nature of the attack.

cranial vault The bones that encase and protect the brain, including the parietal, temporal, frontal, occipital, sphenoid, and ethmoid bones; also called the cranium or skull.

craniofacial disjunction A Le Fort III fracture involves a fracture of all of the midfacial bones, thus separating the entire midface from the cranium.

crepitus A grating sensation made when two pieces of broken bone rub together or subcutaneous emphysema is palpated.

cribbing Short lengths of wood that are used to stabilize vehicles.

cribriform plate A horizontal bone perforated with numerous foramina for the passage of the olfactory nerve filaments from the nasal cavity.

crista galli A prominent bony ridge in the center of the anterior fossa and the point of attachment of the meninges.

critical incident stress management (CISM) A process that confronts responses to critical incidents and defuses them.

critical infrastructure The external foundation in communities made up of structures and services critical in the day-to-day living activities of humans: energy sources, fuel, water, sewage removal, food, hospitals, and transportation systems.

critical minimum threshold Minimum cerebral perfusion pressure required to adequately perfuse the brain; 60 mm Hg in the adult.

critical patients Patients in either pre-morbid conditions, with major trauma, or in the peri-arrest period.

cross-contamination Occurs when a person is contaminated by an agent as a result of coming into contact with another contaminated person.

croup A common disease of childhood due to upper airway obstruction and characterized by stridor, hoarseness, and a barking cough.

crown The part of the tooth that is external to the gum.

crowning The appearance of the newborn's body part (usually the head) at the vaginal opening at the beginning of labor.

crush injury An injury in which the body or part of the body is crushed, preventing tissue function and, possibly, resulting in permanent tissue damage.

crush syndrome A condition that arises after a body part that has been compressed for a significant period is released, leading to the entry of potassium and other metabolic toxins into the systemic circulation.

cubital tunnel syndrome Compression of the ulnar nerve at the tunnel along the outer edge of the elbow, causing numbness, tingling, and possible partial loss of function of the little finger and medial aspect of the ring finger.

cupping The cultural practice of placing warm cups on the skin to pull out illness from the body. The red, flat, rounded skin lesions are often more intensely red at the borders.

curative care Medical treatment aimed at curing an illness.

Cushing triad Hypertension (with a widening pulse pressure), bradycardia, and irregular respirations; classic trio of findings associated with increased intracranial pressure.

cushion of safety Keeping a safe distance between your vehicle and other vehicles on any side of you.

cusps Points at the top of a tooth.

cutaneous Pertaining to the skin.

cyanide A colorless gas that has an odor similar to almonds, and which is a chemical asphyxiant used in many industrial processes; exposure can occur from by-products of combustion at structure fires.

cylinders Portable, nonbulk, compressed gas containers used to hold liquids and gases. Uninsulated compressed gas cylinders are used to store substances such as nitrogen, argon, helium, and oxygen. They have a range of sizes and internal pressures.

cystic fibrosis (CF) A genetic disorder of the endocrine system that makes it difficult for chloride to move through cells; primarily targets the respiratory and digestive systems.

cytomegalovirus (CMV) A herpesvirus that can produce the symptoms of prolonged high fever, chills, headache, malaise, extreme fatigue, and an enlarged spleen.

Dalton's law Each gas in a mixture exerts the same partial pressure that it would exert if it were alone in the same volume, and the total pressure of a mixture of gases is the sum of the partial pressures of all the gases in a mixture.

deafness A complete or partial hearing loss.

decay A natural process in which a material that is unstable attempts to stabilize itself by changing its structure.

deceleration A negative acceleration—that is, slowing down.

decerebrate (extensor) posturing Abnormal posture characterized by extension of the arms and legs; indicates pressure on the brainstem.

decompensated shock (class III) The late stage of shock, when blood pressure is falling.

decompression illness (DCI) A term for decompression sickness (DCS) and air gas embolism (AGE).

decompression sickness (DCS) A broad range of signs and symptoms caused by nitrogen bubbles in blood and tissues coming out of solution on ascent.

decontaminate To remove or neutralize radiation, chemical, or other hazardous material from clothing, equipment, vehicles, and personnel.

decontamination corridor A controlled area within the warm zone where decontamination takes place.

decorticate (flexor) posturing Abnormal posture characterized by flexion of the arms and extension of the legs; indicates pressure on the brainstem.

deep fascia A dense layer of fibrous tissue below the subcutaneous tissue; composed of tough bands of tissue that ensheath muscles and other internal structures.

deep frostbite A type of frostbite in which the affected part looks white, yellow-white, or mottled blue-white and is hard, cold, and without sensation.

deep vein thrombosis (DVT) The formation of a blood clot within the larger veins of an extremity, typically following a period of prolonged stabilization.

defibrillation The use of an unsynchronized direct current electric shock to terminate ventricular fibrillation or ventricular tachycardia.

degloving A traumatic injury that results in the soft tissue of a part of the body being drawn downward like a glove being removed.

degranulate To release granules into the surrounding tissue.

delirium An acute confusional state characterized by global impairment of thinking, perception, judgment, and memory.

dementia A chronic deterioration of mental functions.

demobilization The process of directing responders to return to their facilities when work at a disaster or multiple-casualty incident has finished, at least for the particular responders.

dentin The principal mass of the tooth that is made up of a material that is much more dense and stronger than bone.

depressed skull fractures Result from high-energy direct trauma to a small surface area of the head with a blunt object (such as a baseball bat to the head); commonly result in bony fragments being driven into the brain, causing injury.

depression fracture A fracture in which the broken region of the bone is pushed deeper into the body than the remaining intact bone.

dermatomes Areas of the body innervated by sensor components of spinal nerves.

dermis The inner layer of skin containing hair follicle roots, glands, blood vessels, and nerves.

desquamation The continuous shedding of the dead cells on the surface of the skin.

devascularization The loss of blood to a part of the body.

developmental delay A broad term that describes an infant or child's failure to reach a particular developmental milestone by the expected time.

developmental disability Insufficient development of a portion of the brain, resulting in some level of dysfunction or impairment.

dialysis A medical process by which a patient's blood is cleansed of excess toxins by passing through a special machine.

diaphragm Large skeletal muscle that plays a major role in breathing and separates the chest cavity from the abdominal cavity.

diaphragmatic hernia Passage of loops of bowel with or without other abdominal organs, through a developmental defect in the diaphragm muscle; occurs as the bowel from the abdomen "herniates" upward through the diaphragm into the chest (thoracic) cavity.

diaphysis The shaft of a long bone.

diastasis An increase in the distance between the two sides of a joint.

diencephalon The part of the brain between the brainstem and the cerebrum that includes the thalamus, subthalamus, and hypothalamus.

differential field diagnosis The short list of the potential causes of the patient's presenting condition.

diffuse axonal injury (DAI) Diffuse brain injury that is caused by stretching, shearing, or tearing of nerve fibers with subsequent axonal damage.

diffuse brain injury Any injury that affects the entire brain.

diffusion A process in which molecules move from an area of higher concentration to an area of lower concentration.

digital arteries The arteries that supply blood to the fingers and toes.

dilated cardiomyopathy (DCM) A condition in which the heart becomes weakened and enlarged, making it less efficient and causing a negative impact to the pulmonary, hepatic, and other systems.

dilution A type of decontamination method that uses copious amounts of water to flush the contaminant from the skin or eyes.

diplopia Double vision.

directed area An area away from the command post or emergency operations center, considered by engineering expertise to be a safe place to stage until directed otherwise.

dirty bomb Name given to a bomb that is used as a radiologic dispersal device (RDD).

disaster A widespread event that disrupt community resources and functions, in turn threatening public safety, lives, and property.

disaster management A planned, coordinated response to a disaster that involves cooperation of multiple responders and agencies and enables effective triage and provision of care according to triage decisions.

disease vector An animal that, once infected, spreads a disease to another animal.

disinfection The killing of pathogenic agents by direct application of chemicals.

dislocation The displacement of a bone from its normal position within a joint.

displaced fracture A break in which the ends of the fractured bone move out of their normal positions.

disposal A type of decontamination in which as much clothing and equipment as possible is disposed of to reduce the magnitude of the problem.

dissemination The means with which a terrorist will spread a disease—for example, by poisoning the water supply or aerosolizing the agent into the air or ventilation system of a building.

distraction injury An injury that results from a force that tries to increase the length of a body part or separate one body part from another.

distributive shock A condition that occurs when there is widespread dilation of the resistance vessels, the capacitance vessels, or both.

domestic terrorism Terrorism that is carried out by native citizens against their own country.

dorsal Referring to the back or posterior side of the body or an organ.

dorsiflex To bend the foot or hand backward.

dose effect The principle that the longer a hazardous material is in contact with the body or the greater the concentration, the greater the effect will most likely be.

DOT KKK 1822 Federal standards that regulate the design and manufacturing guidelines of emergency ambulances.

Down syndrome A genetic chromosomal defect that can occur during fetal development and that results in mental retardation and certain physical characteristics, such as a round head with a flat occiput and slanted, wide-set eyes.

dressing Material used to directly cover a wound.

drift A finding that when the operator lets go of the steering wheel, a vehicle consistently wanders left or right.

dromotropic effect The effect on the velocity of conduction.

drowning The process of experiencing respiratory impairment from submersion or immersion in liquid.

drums Barrel-like nonbulk storage vessels used to store a wide variety of substances, including food-grade materials, corrosives, flammable liquids, and grease. Drums may be constructed of low-carbon steel, polyethylene, cardboard, stainless steel, nickel, or other materials.

dry bulk cargo tanks Tanks designed to carry dry bulk goods such as powders, pellets, fertilizers, or grain. Such tanks are generally V-shaped with rounded sides that funnel toward the bottom.

due regard Driving with awareness and responsibility for other drivers on the roadways when you are operating an ambulance in the emergency mode, and making sure that other drivers are aware of your approach.

duodenum The first part of the small intestine.

DuoDote A nerve agent antidote kit that contains a single injection of both atropine (2 mg) and 2-PAM chloride (pralidoxime chloride) (600 mg).

dura mater The outermost layer of the three meninges that enclose the brain and spinal cord; it is the toughest meningeal layer.

dust suffocation A phenomenon that can occur during an earthquake, in which particles of dust and debris are loosened and released into the air, producing a toxic and hypoxic atmosphere.

dysarthria A speech disorder caused by neuromuscular disturbance that causes speech to become slow and slurred.

dysconjugate gaze Paralysis of gaze or lack of coordination between the movements of the two eyes.

dysphagia Difficulty swallowing.

ecchymosis Extravasation of blood under the skin to produce a "black-and-blue" mark.

eclampsia Seizures that result from severe hypertension in a pregnant woman.

ectopic pregnancy An egg that attaches outside the uterus, typically in a fallopian tube.

effacement Thinning and shortening of the cervix; this is a normal process that occurs as the uterus contracts.

ejection fraction (EF) The percentage of blood that leaves the heart each time it contracts.

elastin A protein that gives the skin its elasticity.

elective abortion Intentional expulsion of the fetus.

electrical energy The energy delivered in the form of high voltage.

elevated A threat level in which a terrorist event is suspected, but there is no specific information about its timing or location.

embryo The fetus in the earliest stages after fertilization.

emergency decontamination The process of removing the bulk of contaminants off of a victim without regard for containment. It is used in potentially life-threatening situations, without the formal establishment of a decontamination corridor.

emergency operations center (EOC) A central command and control facility, found at all government levels, responsible for strategic overview; tactical decisions are left to incident commanders.

emotional abuse A form of abuse that may be verbal (such as ridicule, threats, blaming, or humiliation), or nonverbal (caregiver ignores the victim or isolates the victim from others); causes a substantial change in the victim's behavior, emotional response, cognitive function, or may manifest as a variety of mental illnesses.

endometrium The innermost layer of tissue in the uterus.

endosteum The inner lining of a hollow bone.

entrapment A condition in which a patient is trapped by debris, soil, or other material and is unable to extricate himself or herself.

entry wound The point at which a penetrating object enters the body.

envenomation The injecting of venom via a bite or sting.

environmental emergencies Medical conditions caused or exacerbated by the weather, terrain, or unique atmospheric conditions such as high altitude or underwater.

epidemic Sickness that is larger than expected, area-wise and population-wise.

epidermis The outermost layer of the skin.

epidural hematoma An accumulation of blood between the skull and dura.

epiglottitis Inflammation of the epiglottis.

epiphysis The end region of a long bone extending between the metaphysis and the articulate (joint) surface.

episiotomy An incision in the perineal skin made to prevent tearing during childbirth.

epistaxis Nosebleed.

epithelialization The formation of fresh epithelial tissue to heal a wound.

Erb palsy Lack of movement at the shoulder due to nerve injury resulting from the stretching of the cervical nerve roots (C5 and C6 most commonly) during delivery of the newborn's head during birth. The effect is usually transient, but can be permanent.

erythema Reddening of the skin.

erythrocytes Red blood cells.

escharotomy A surgical cut through the eschar or leathery covering of a burn injury to allow for swelling and minimize the potential for development of compartment syndrome in a circumferentially burned limb or the thorax.

evacuation The removal or relocation of people who may be affected by an approaching release of a hazardous material.

evaporation The conversion of a liquid to a gas.

evisceration Displacement of an organ outside the body.

exercise-associated hyponatremia A condition due to prolonged exertion in hot environments coupled with excessive hypotonic fluid intake that leads to nausea, vomiting, and, in severe cases, mental status changes and seizures (also known as exertional hyponatremia).

exertional heatstroke A serious type of heatstroke usually affecting young and fit people exercising in hot and humid conditions.

exit wound The point at which a penetrating object leaves the body, which may or may not be in a straight line from the entry wound.

exophthalmos Protrusion of the eyes from the normal position within the socket.

external auditory canal The area in which sound waves are received from the auricle (pinna) before they travel to the eardrum; also called the ear canal.

external ear One of three anatomic parts of the ear; it contains the pinna, the ear canal, and the external portion of the tympanic membrane.

extrication supervisor In incident command, the person appointed to determine the type of equipment and resources needed for a situation involving extrication or special rescue; also called the rescue supervisor.

facet joint The joint on which each vertebra articulates with adjacent vertebrae.

facial nerve The seventh cranial nerve; supplies motor activity to all muscles of facial expression and anterior two thirds of the tongue; and also relates to the sense of taste and cutaneous sensation to the external ear, tongue, and palate.

fallopian tubes The vehicles of transportation of the ova from the ovaries to the uterus; also called oviducts.

false lumen A term used to describe an area that a device was not intended to be inserted into—for example, when a tracheostomy tube is inserted into an area other than the trachea.

fascia A strong, fibrous membrane that covers, supports, and separates muscles.

fasciitis Inflammation of the fascia.

fasciotomy A surgical procedure that cuts away fascia to relieve pressure.

fatigue fractures   Fractures that result from multiple compressive loads.

feet of seawater (fsw)   An indirect measure of pressure under water, equal to one atmosphere absolute (ATA).

femoral artery   The main artery supplying the thigh and leg.

femoral shaft fractures   A break in the diaphysis of the femur.

femur   The proximal bone of the leg that extends from the pelvis to the knee.

fenestrated   Having perforations, holes, or openings.

fetal macrosomia   A situation in which a fetus is large, usually defined as weighing more than 4,500 grams or almost 9 pounds; also known as "large for gestational age."

fetal transition   The process through which the fluid in the fetal lungs is replaced with air, the ductus arteriosus constricts, and the newborn begins adequate oxygenation of its own blood.

fetus   The developing, unborn infant inside the uterus.

fibrous joints   The joints that contain dense fibrous tissue and allow for no motion.

fibula   The smaller of the two bones of the lower leg.

Fick principle   A principle that states the movement and use of oxygen in the body is dependent on an adequate concentration of inspired oxygen, appropriate movement of oxygen across the alveolar-capillary membrane into the arterial bloodstream, adequate number of red blood cells to carry the oxygen, proper tissue perfusion, and efficient offloading of oxygen at the tissue level.

finance   In incident command, the position in an incident responsible for accounting of all expenditures.

first stage of labor   The stage of labor that begins with the onset of regular labor pains, crampy abdominal pains, during which the uterus contracts and the cervix effaces.

fistula   A surgical connection between an artery and a vein.

flail chest   An injury that involves two or more adjacent ribs fractured in two or more places, allowing the segment between the fractures to move independently of the rest of the thoracic cage.

flame burn   A thermal burn caused by flames touching the skin.

flammable range   An expression of a fuel/air mixture, defined by upper and lower limits, that reflects an amount of flammable vapor mixed with a given volume of air.

flange   The part of a tracheostomy tube that is used to stabilize the tube to the patient's neck.

flash burn   An electrothermal injury caused by arcing of electric current.

flash point   The minimum temperature at which a liquid or a solid releases sufficient vapor to form an ignitable mixture with air.

flat bones   Bones that are thin and broad, such as the scapula.

flexion injury   A type of injury that results from forward movement of the head, typically as the result of rapid deceleration, such as in a car crash, or with a direct blow to the occiput.

flexor tenosynovitis of the hand   A closed-space infection of the hand.

focal brain injury   A specific, grossly observable brain injury.

follicle-stimulating hormone (FSH)   A hormone produced by the anterior pituitary gland that is important in the menstrual cycle.

fontanelles   The soft spots in the skull of a newborn and infant where the sutures of the skull have not yet grown together.

foramen magnum   The large opening at the base of the skull through which the spinal cord exits the brain.

foramen ovale   An opening in the septum of the heart that closes after birth.

foramina   Small natural openings, perforations, or orifices, such as in the bones of the cranial vault; plural of foramen.

forward surgical team   A team, usually staffed with physicians, nurses, and EMS providers, that performs minor surgical procedures and débridements in the field, taking some of the load from the hospital facility.

fracture   A break or rupture in the bone.

free-flow oxygen   Oxygen administered via oxygen tube and a cupped hand on patient's face.

freelancing   When individual units or different organizations make independent and often inefficient decisions about the next appropriate action.

frontal lobe   The portion of the brain that is important in voluntary motor actions and personality traits.

frostbite   Localized damage to tissues resulting from prolonged exposure to extreme cold.

frostnip   Early frostbite, characterized by numbness and pallor without significant tissue damage.

full-thickness burn   A burn that extends through the epidermis and dermis into the subcutaneous tissues beneath; previously called a third-degree burn.

fundus   The dome-shaped top of the uterus.

G agents   Early nerve agents that were developed by German scientists in the period after WWI and into WWII. There are three such agents: sarin, soman, and tabun.

galea aponeurotica Tough, tendinous layer of the scalp.

gamma (x-rays) Type of energy that is emitted from a strong radiologic source that is far faster and stronger than alpha and beta rays. These rays easily penetrate through the human body and require either several inches of lead or concrete to prevent penetration.

gangrene An infection commonly caused by *Clostridium perfringens*. The result is tissue destruction and gas production that may lead to death.

gastrostomy tube (G-tube) A tube that is surgically placed directly into the patient's stomach through the skin in order to provide nutrition or medications.

generalized seizure Seizure activity that is bilateral, synchronous, and nonmigratory; indicate involvement of both cerebral hemispheres.

geriatrics The assessment and treatment of disease in someone 65 years or older.

gestation Period of time from conception to birth. For humans, the full period is normally 9 months (or 40 weeks).

gestational period The time that it takes for the fetus to develop in utero, normally 38 weeks.

Glasgow Coma Scale (GCS) A widely accepted method of assessing level of consciousness that is based on three independent measurements: eye opening, verbal response, and motor response.

glaucoma A disease of the eye caused by an increase in intraocular pressure; when severe enough, this may damage the optic nerve and potentially cause permanent loss of vision.

glenoid fossa Socket in the scapula in which the head of the humerus rotates.

globe The eyeball.

glomerular filtration The first step in the formation of urine; calculated to determine renal function.

glossopharyngeal nerve Ninth cranial nerve; supplies motor fibers to the pharyngeal muscle, providing taste sensation to the posterior portion of the tongue, and carrying parasympathetic fibers to the parotid gland.

gonorrhea A sexually transmitted disease (STD) that results in infection caused by the gonococcal bacteria, *Neisseria gonorrhoeae*; signs and symptoms include pus-containing discharge from the urethra and painful urination in men and signs and symptoms of an acute abdomen in women.

gout A painful disorder characterized by the crystallization of uric acid within a joint.

granulocytes Cells that contain granules.

gravid The total number of times pregnant, including the current pregnancy.

gravidity A term used to refer to the number of times a woman has been pregnant, regardless of the outcome.

gravity (g) The acceleration of a body by the attraction of the earth's gravitational force, normally 32.2 ft/sec^2.

greenstick fracture A type of fracture occurring most frequently in children in which there is incomplete breakage of the bone.

ground substance Material between cells.

grunting A short, low-pitched sound at the end of exhalation, present in children with moderate to severe hypoxia; reflects poor gas exchange because of fluid in the lower airways and air sacs.

guerilla warfare A form of warfare in which a small group that is not part of the official military engages in combat that uses the element of surprise, such as raids and ambushes; sometimes used by terrorists to protect their training camps and bases of operation.

habitual abortion Three or more consecutive pregnancies that end in miscarriage.

hand tool Any tool or equipment operating from human power.

hard palate The bony anterior part of the palate that forms the roof of the mouth.

hazardous material Any substance that is toxic, poisonous, radioactive, flammable, or explosive and causes injury or death with exposure.

HAZWOPER (HAZardous Waste OPerations and Emergency Response) The federal OSHA regulation that governs hazardous materials waste site and response training. Specifics can be found in Title 29, standard number 1910.120. Subsection (q) is specific to emergency response.

head injury A traumatic insult to the head that may result in injury to soft tissue, bony structures, or the brain.

heat cramps Acute and involuntary muscle pains, usually in the lower extremities, the abdomen, or both, that occur because of profuse sweating and subsequent sodium losses in sweat.

heat exhaustion A clinical syndrome characterized by volume depletion and heat stress that is thought to be a milder form of heat illness and on a continuum leading to heatstroke.

heat illness The increase in core body temperature due to inadequate thermolysis.

heat syncope An orthostatic or near-syncopal episode that typically occurs in nonacclimated people who may be under heat stress.

heatstroke The least common and most deadly heat illness, caused by a severe disturbance in thermoregulation, usually characterized by a core temperature of more than 104°F (40°C) and altered mental status.

heavy-duty ambulance Extra heavy-duty vehicle.

hematemesis Vomited blood.

hematochezia Passage of stools containing bright red blood.

hematocrit A blood test that measures the portion of red blood cells in whole blood.

hematoma A mass of blood in the soft tissues beneath the skin; indicates bleeding into soft tissues and may be the result of a minor or a severe injury.

hematopoiesis The generation of blood cells.

hematuria Blood in the urine.

hemodialysis A form of dialysis in which blood is removed from the patient through a catheter or fistula, and then returns to the body through another needle, removing various toxins, electrolytes, and fluid in the process.

hemodynamic monitoring Monitoring and measurement of blood movement, volume, and pressure.

hemoglobin The oxygen-carrying pigment in red blood cells.

hemoperitoneum The presence of extravasated blood in the peritoneal cavity.

hemophilia A bleeding disorder that is primarily hereditary, in which clotting does not occur or occurs insufficiently.

hemopneumothorax A collection of blood and air in the pleural cavity.

hemoptysis Coughing up blood.

hemorrhage Bleeding.

hemorrhagic shock Volume lost as blood.

hemostasis Stopping hemorrhage.

hemothorax The collection of blood within the normally closed pleural space.

Henry's law The amount of gas dissolved in a liquid is directly proportional to the partial pressure of the gas above the liquid.

heparinized solution A saline solution mixed with heparin, an anticoagulant used to prevent blood clots from forming.

herniation Process in which tissue is forced out of its normal position, such as when the brain is forced from the cranial vault, either through the foramen magnum or over the tentorium.

herpes An infection of the genitals, buttocks, or anal area caused by herpes simplex virus, type 1 or type 2.

herpes zoster Shingles; a contagious condition caused by the reactivation of the varicella virus on nerve roots.

high-altitude cerebral edema (HACE) An altitude illness in which there is a change in mental status and/or ataxia in a person with acute mountain sickness or the presence of mental status changes and ataxia in a person without acute mountain sickness.

high-altitude pulmonary edema (HAPE) An altitude illness characterized by at least two of the following: dyspnea at rest, cough, weakness or decreased exercise performance, or chest tightness or congestion. Also, at least two of the following signs: central cyanosis, audible rales or wheezing in at least one lung field, tachypnea, or tachycardia.

high-angle operations A rope rescue operation where the angle of the slope is greater than 45°; rescuers depend on life safety rope rather than a fixed support surface such as the ground.

high-level disinfection The killing of pathogenic agents by using potent means of disinfection.

high-pressure injection injuries Types of injuries that occurs when a foreign material is forcefully injected into soft tissue.

homeostasis A tendency to constancy or stability in the body's internal environment; body processes that balance the supply and demand of the body's needs.

hospice A program and philosophy that attempt to help the patient maximize the quality of remaining life by providing social and emotional support, treating discomfort with pharmacologic and nonpharmacologic approaches, and helping patients and families cope with the prospect of impending death.

hospital surge capacity The capabilities of a receiving hospital to handle a large number of unexpected emergency patients, such as those seen in a multiple-casualty incident.

hot zone The area immediately surrounding an incident site that is directly dangerous to life and health. All personnel working in the hot zone must wear complete and appropriate protective clothing and equipment. Entry requires approval by the IC or a designated sector officer. Complete backup, rescue, and decontamination teams must be in place at the perimeter before operations begin.

human immunodeficiency virus (HIV) An infection that causes acquired immune deficiency syndrome or AIDS.

human papilloma virus (HPV) The most common sexually transmitted disease that can cause genital warts and some types of cancer.

humerus The bone of the upper arm.

hydramnios A condition in which there is too much amniotic fluid; also known as polyhydramnios.

hydrocephalus A medical condition in which there is an abnormal buildup of cerebrospinal fluid in the ventricles of the brain; this can be acquired (occurring after birth) or congenital (developing before birth).

hydroplaning   A condition in which the tires of a vehicle may be lifted off the road surface as water "piles up" under them, making the vehicle feel as though it is floating.

hyoid bone   A bone at the base of the tongue that supports the tongue and its muscles.

hyperemesis gravidarum   A condition of persistent nausea and vomiting during pregnancy.

hyperesthesia   Hyperacute pain to touch.

hyperextension   Extension of a limb or other body part beyond its usual range of motion.

hyperkalemia   An increased level of potassium in the blood.

hyperphosphatemia   An increased level of phosphate in the blood.

hyperpyrexia   A high body temperature.

hyperthermia   Unusually elevated body temperature.

hypertrophic cardiomyopathy (HCM)   A condition in which the heart muscle is unusually thick, which means that the heart has to pump harder to get blood to leave.

hypertrophic scar   An abnormal scar with excess collagen that does not extend over the wound margins.

hypertrophy   An increase in size.

hyperuricemia   High levels of uric acid in the blood.

hyphema   Bleeding into the anterior chamber of the eye; results from direct ocular trauma.

hypoglossal nerve   Twelfth cranial nerve; provides motor function to the muscles of the tongue and throat.

hypoglycemia   A deficiency of glucose in the blood caused by too much insulin or too little glucose; in the newborn it is a level of less than 40 mg/dL, and in older neonates it is a level of less than 60 mg/dL.

hypoperfusion   A condition that occurs when the level of tissue perfusion decreases below that needed to maintain normal cellular functions; also called shock.

hypopituitarism   A condition in which the pituitary gland does not produce normal amounts of some or all of its hormones, can be congenital; secondary to tumors, infection, strokes, or develop after trauma or radiation therapy.

hypoplastic left heart syndrome (HLHS)   Underdevelopment of the aorta, aortic valve, left ventricle, and mitral valve; this defect involves the entire left side of the heart.

hypothalamus   The most inferior portion of the diencephalon; responsible for control of many body functions, including heart rate, digestion, sexual development, temperature regulation, emotion, hunger, thirst, and regulation of the sleep cycle.

hypothermia   A condition in which the core body temperature is significantly below normal (less than 35°C [95°F]).

hypotonia   Low or poor muscle tone (floppy).

hypovolemia   Low blood volume.

hypovolemic shock   A condition that occurs when the circulating blood volume is inadequate to deliver adequate oxygen and nutrients to the body.

hypoxic ischemic encephalopathy   Damage to cells in the central nervous system (the brain and spinal cord) from inadequate oxygen.

ignition temperature   The minimum temperature at which a fuel, when heated, will ignite in air and continue to burn. Also called the autoignition temperature.

ileus   Disruption or loss of normal gastrointestinal motility.

ilium   The broad, uppermost bone of the pelvis.

immediately dangerous to life and health (IDLH)   An atmospheric concentration of any toxic, corrosive, or asphyxiant substance that poses an immediate threat to life or could cause irreversible or delayed adverse health effects. There are three general IDLH atmospheres: toxic, flammable, and oxygen-deficient; a respirator is mandatory.

imminent   A threat level in which a terrorist event is known to be impending or will occur very soon.

imminent abortion   A spontaneous abortion that cannot be prevented.

impacted fracture   A broken bone in which the end of one bone becomes wedged into another bone, as could be the case in a fall from a significant height.

implosion   A bursting inward.

inborn errors of metabolism (IEM)   A group of congenital conditions that cause either accumulation of toxins or disorders of energy metabolism in the neonate. These conditions are characterized by an infant's failure to thrive and by vague signs such as poor feeding.

incident action plan   An oral or written plan stating general objectives reflecting the overall strategy for managing an incident.

incident command system (ICS)   A system implemented to manage disasters and multiple-casualty incidents in which section chiefs, including finance, logistics, operations, and planning, report to the incident commander.

incident commander (IC)   The overall leader of the incident command system to whom commanders or leaders of the incident command system divisions report.

incision   A wound usually made deliberately, as in surgery; a clean cut, as opposed to a laceration.

incomplete abortion   Expulsion of the fetus that results in some products of conception remaining in the uterus.

incomplete fracture   A fracture in which the bone does not fully break.

incomplete spinal cord injury   Spinal cord injury in which there is some degree of cord-mediated function; initial dysfunction may be temporary and there may be potential for recovery.

incubation   Describes the period of time from a person being exposed to a disease to the time when symptoms begin.

index of suspicion   Anticipating the possibility of specific types of injury.

indirect injury   An injury that results from a force that is applied to one region of the body but leads to an injury in another area.

infantile hypertrophic pyloric stenosis (IHPS)   Marked hypertrophy and hyperplasia of the two (circular and longitudinal) muscular layers of the pylorus, resulting in the pylorus becoming thick and obstructing the end of the stomach.

inner cannula   The inner tube that is inserted into the outer cannula of a tracheostomy tube.

inner ear   One of three anatomic parts of the ear; it consists of the cochlea and semicircular canals.

inotropic effect   Affecting the contractility of muscle tissue, especially cardiac muscle.

integument   The skin.

intercostal retractions   Skin sucking in between the ribs, seen when a patient creates increased negative intrathoracic pressure to breathe.

intercostal space   The space between two ribs, named according to the number of the rib above it, that contains the intercostal muscles and neurovascular bundle.

intermodal tanks   A bulk container that serves as both a shipping and a storage vessel. Such tanks hold between 5,000 and 6,000 gallons of product and can be pressurized or nonpressurized. Intermodal tanks may be shipped by all modes of transportation.

international terrorism   Terrorism that is carried out by those not of the host's country; also known as cross-border terrorism.

intertrochanteric fractures   Fractures that occur in the region between the lesser and greater trochanters.

intestinal atresia   A congenital condition in which part of the bowel does not develop.

intestinal stenosis   A congenital condition in which part of the bowel is narrow.

intra-aortic balloon pump   A balloon that is inserted into the aorta and connected to a pump via a catheter; this therapy helps to increase the blood flow to the coronary arteries during diastole (inflation) and decrease afterload of blood from the left ventricle (deflation).

intracerebral hematoma   Bleeding within the brain tissue (parenchyma) itself; also referred to as an intraparenchymal hematoma.

intracranial pressure (ICP)   The pressure within the cranial vault; normally 0 to 15 mm Hg in adults.

intussusception   An event where one part of the intestine folds into another part of the intestines leading to a blockage.

ionizing radiation   Energy that is emitted in the form of rays, or particles.

iris   The colored portion of the eye.

irregular bones   Bones with unique shapes that allow them to perform a specific function and that do not fit into the other categories based on shape.

irreversible shock (class IV)   The final stage of shock, prior to death.

ischium   The lowermost dorsal bone of the pelvis.

joint   The point at which two or more bones articulate, or come together.

joint capsule   A saclike envelope that encloses the cavity of a synovial joint.

joint information center (JIC)   An area designated by the incident commander, or a designee, in which public information officers from multiple agencies disseminate information about the incident.

Joule's law   A description of the relationship between heat production, current, and resistance.

jugular vein distention (JVD)   A prominence of the jugular veins due to increased volume or increased pressure within the central venous system or the thoracic cavity.

JumpSTART triage   A sorting system for pediatric patients younger than 8 years or weighing less than 100 pounds. There is a minor adaptation for infants because they cannot ambulate on their own.

Kehr sign   Left shoulder pain that may indicate a ruptured spleen.

keloid scar   An abnormal scar commonly found in people with darkly pigmented skin. It extends over the wound margins.

kinetic energy (KE)   The energy associated with bodies in motion, expressed mathematically as half the mass times the square of the velocity.

kinetics   The study of the relationship among speed, mass, vector direction, and physical injury.

Klumpke paralysis   An injury of childbirth affecting the spinal nerves C7, C8, and T1 of the brachial plexus. It can be contrasted to Erb palsy, which affects C5 and C6.

labels Signage at least 3.9 inches on each side that is often required on all four sides of individual packages and boxes that are being transported.

labor The mechanism by which the fetus and the placenta are expelled from the uterus.

laceration A wound made by tearing or cutting tissues.

lacrimal apparatus The structures in which tears are secreted and drained from the eye.

lactic acid A metabolic end product of the breakdown of glucose that accumulates when metabolism proceeds in the absence of oxygen.

lambdoid suture The point where the occipital bones attach to the parietal bones.

lamina Arise from the posterior pedicles and fuse to form the posterior spinous processes.

laminated glass Type of window glazing that incorporates a sheeting material that stops the glass from breaking into shards.

landing zone Designated location for the landing of air ambulances.

language-based learning disability A type of disability in which difficulties with reading, spelling, or writing cause a person to fall behind expectations for a given age.

laryngospasm Severe constriction of the larynx in response to allergy, noxious stimuli, or illness.

lateral compression A force that is directed from the side toward the midline of the body.

law of conservation of energy The principle that energy can be neither created nor destroyed; it can only change form.

LD50 The amount of an agent or substance that will kill 50% of people who are exposed to this level.

Le Fort fractures Maxillary fractures that are classified into three categories based on their anatomic location.

lens A transparent body within the globe that focuses light rays.

lethal concentration (LC) The concentration of a material in air that, on the basis of laboratory tests (inhalation route), is expected to kill a specified number of the group of test animals when administered over a specified period of time.

lethal dose (LD) A single dose that causes the death of a specified number of the group of test animals exposed by any route other than inhalation.

leukocytes White blood cells.

level A ensemble The highest level of protective suit worn by hazardous materials personnel. May also be referred to as fully encapsulating because the suit covers everything, including the breathing apparatus.

level B ensemble Personal protective equipment that is one step less protective than level A, but provides for a high level of respiratory protection.

level C ensemble A level of personal protective equipment that provides splash protection.

level D ensemble The level of protection that fire fighter turnout gear provides.

lewisite (L) A blistering agent that has a rapid onset of symptoms and produces immediate intense pain and discomfort on contact.

liaison officer (LNO) In incident command, the person who relays information, concerns, and requests among responding agencies.

ligaments Tough bands of tissue that connect bone to bone around a joint or support internal organs within the body.

lightening In pregnancy, a feeling of relief of pressure in the upper abdomen; a premonitory sign of labor.

limbic system Structures within the cerebrum and diencephalon that influence emotions, motivation, mood, and sensations of pain and pleasure.

linear fracture A fracture that runs parallel to the long axis of a bone.

linear skull fractures Account for 80% of skull fractures; also referred to as nondisplaced skull fractures; commonly occur in the temporal-parietal region of the skull; not associated with deformities to the skull.

lister bags Heavy canvas bags that can be hung from trees containing water in amounts from 40 to 100 gallons.

local effect An effect of a hazardous material on the body that is limited to the area of contact.

lochia The vaginal discharge of blood and mucus that occurs following delivery of a newborn; usually lasts several days and then gradually decreases over the weeks following delivery.

logistics In incident command, the position that helps procure and stockpile equipment and supplies during an incident.

long bones Bones that are longer than they are wide.

low-angle operations A rope rescue operation on a mildly sloping surface (less than 45°) or flat land where rescuers are dependent on the ground for their primary support, and the rope system is a secondary means of support.

lower flammable limit (LFL) The minimum amount of gaseous fuel that must be present in the air for the air/fuel mixture to be flammable or explosive.

loxoscelism A potentially fatal condition resulting from a brown recluse spider bite that begins with a painful, inflamed vesicle that may progress to a gangrenous sloughing of the skin.

Lund and Browder chart A detailed version of the rule of nines chart that takes into consideration the changes in body surface area brought on by growth.

luteinizing hormone (LH) A hormone released by the anterior pituitary gland that stimulates the process of ovulation.

luxation A complete dislocation.

lymph nodes Area of the lymphatic system where infection-fighting cells are housed.

lymphangitis Inflammation of a lymph channel.

lymphatic system A passive circulatory system that transports a plasma-like liquid called lymph, a thin fluid that bathes the tissues of the body.

lymphocytes White blood cells that function to remove invading pathogens.

macroglossia Large tongue size.

macrophages Cells that are responsible for protecting the body against infection.

malignant hyperthermia A condition that can result from common anesthesia medications (notably succinylcholine) and present with hyperthermia, muscular rigidity, altered mental status, and a hyperdynamic state.

malleolus The large, rounded, bony protuberance on either side of the ankle joint.

mallet finger An avulsion fracture of the extensor tendon of the distal phalynx caused by jamming a finger into an object.

malocclusion Misalignment of the teeth.

malrotation A congenital anomaly of rotation of the midgut, the small bowel is found predominantly on the right side of the abdomen. Results in increased incidence of intestinal volvulus.

malrotation with volvulus A condition that occurs when there is a twisting of the bowel around its mesenteric attachment to the abdominal wall.

mandatory reporter A category of professional required by some states to report suspicions of child maltreatment. Prehospital professionals may be included.

mandible The movable lower jaw bone.

mandibular nerve A sensory and motor nerve that supplies the muscles of chewing and skin of the lower lip, chin, temporal region, and part of the external ear.

manual defibrillation A mode available on automated external defibrillators, allowing the paramedic to interpret the cardiac rhythm and determine whether defibrillation is indicated (rather than the monitor making the determination).

manubrium The superior segment of the sternum; its lower border defines the angle of Louis.

march fractures *See* fatigue fractures.

MARK 1 A nerve agent antidote kit containing two auto-injector medications, atropine and 2-PAM chloride (pralidoxime chloride); also known as a nerve agent antidote kit (NAAK).

mass decontamination The physical process of reducing or removing surface contaminants from large numbers of victims in potentially life-threatening situations in the fastest time possible.

mastication The process of chewing with the teeth.

mastoid process A cone-shaped section of bone at the base of the temporal bone.

material safety data sheets (MSDS) Information documents that are supposed to be kept on site at workplaces for every potentially hazardous chemical at the workplace.

maxillary nerve A sensory nerve; supplies the skin on the posterior part of the side of the nose, lower eyelid, cheek, and upper lip.

MC-306/DOT 406 flammable liquid tanker Such a vehicle typically carries between 6,000 gallons and 10,000 gallons of a product such as gasoline or other flammable and combustible materials. The tank is nonpressurized.

MC-307/DOT 407 chemical hauler A tanker with a rounded or horseshoe-shaped tank capable of holding 6,000 to 7,000 gallons of flammable liquid, mild corrosives, and poisons. The tank has a high internal working pressure.

MC-312/DOT 412 corrosive tanker A tanker that often carries aggressive (highly reactive) acids such as concentrated sulfuric and nitric acid. It is characterized by several heavy-duty reinforcing rings around the tank and holds approximately 6,000 gallons of product.

MC-331 pressure cargo tanker A tanker that carries materials such as ammonia, propane, Freon, and butane. This type of tank is commonly constructed of steel and has rounded ends and a single open compartment inside. The liquid volume inside the tank varies, ranging from the 1,000-gallon delivery truck to the full-size 11,000-gallon cargo tank.

MC-338 cryogenic tanker A low-pressure tanker designed to maintain the low temperature required by the cryogens it carries. A boxlike structure containing the tank control valves is typically attached to the rear of the tanker.

mean arterial pressure (MAP) The average (or mean) pressure against the arterial wall during a cardiac cycle; the blood pressure required to sustain organ perfusion; roughly 60 mm Hg in the average person.

mechanical energy   The energy that results from motion (kinetic energy) or that is stored in an object (potential energy).

mechanism of injury (MOI)   The way in which traumatic injuries occur; the forces that act on the body to cause damage.

Meckel diverticulum   One of the most common congenital malformations of the small intestines, which presents with painless rectal bleeding.

meconium   A dark greenish black material that, when appearing in the amniotic fluid, indicates fetal distress; can be aspirated into the fetus' lungs during delivery; the fetus's first bowel movement.

medevac   Medical evacuation of a patient by helicopter.

mediastinitis   Inflammation of the mediastinum, often a result of the gastric contents leaking into the thoracic cavity after esophageal perforation.

mediastinum   Space within the chest that contains the heart, major blood vessels, vagus nerve, trachea, and esophagus; located between the two lungs.

medical incident command   A branch of operations in a unified command system, whose three designated sector positions are triage, treatment, and transport.

medical monitoring   The process of assessing the health status of hazardous materials team members before and after entry to a hazardous materials incident site.

medulla   Continuous inferiorly with the spinal cord; serves as a conduction pathway for ascending and descending nerve tracts; coordinates heart rate, blood vessel diameter, breathing, swallowing, vomiting, coughing, and sneezing.

medullary canal   The hollow center portion of a long bone.

melanin   The pigment that gives skin its color.

melena   Passage of dark, tarry stools.

Meniere disease   An inner ear disorder in which endolymphatic rupture creates increased pressure in the cochlear duct, which then leads to damage to the organ of Corti and the semicircular canal; symptoms include severe vertigo, tinnitus, and sensorineuronal hearing loss.

meninges   A set of three tough membranes, the dura mater, arachnoid, and pia mater, that encloses the entire brain and spinal cord.

meningitis   Inflammation of the meningeal coverings of the brain and spinal cord; usually caused by a virus or bacterium; the viral type is less severe than the bacterial; the bacterial type can result in brain damage, hearing loss, learning disability, or death.

mental retardation   A primarily cognitive disorder that appears during childhood and is accompanied by lack of adaptive behaviors, such as the ability to live and function independently or interact successfully with others; the person generally has an intelligence quotient below 70; also known as intellectual disability.

mesentery   A membranous double fold of tissue in the abdomen that attaches various organs to the body wall.

metacarpals   The five bones that form the palm and back of the hand.

metaphysis   The region of the long bone between the epiphysis and diaphysis.

metatarsals   The five long bones extending from the tarsus to the phalanges of the foot.

middle ear   One of three anatomic parts of the ear; it consists of the inner portion of the tympanic membrane and the ossicles.

miosis   Bilateral pinpoint constricted pupils.

missed abortion   A situation in which a fetus has died during the first 20 weeks of gestation, but has remained in utero.

missile fragmentation   A primary mechanism of tissue disruption from certain rifles in which pieces of the projectile break apart, allowing the pieces to create their own separate paths through tissues.

Mongolian spots   Lesions that resemble bruises, typically on the buttocks or back, that are present at birth on many infants of Asian or African origin.

morgue supervisor   In incident command, the person who works with area medical examiners, coroners, and law enforcement agencies to coordinate the disposition of dead victims.

mottling   A condition of abnormal skin circulation, caused by vasoconstriction or inadequate perfusoin.

mucopolysaccharide gel   One of the complex materials found, along with the collagen fibers and elastin fibers, in the dermis of the skin.

multifocal seizure   Seizure activity that involves more than one site, is asynchronous, and is usually migratory.

multiple sclerosis (MS)   An autoimmune condition in which the body attacks the myelin that insulates the brain and spinal cord, causing scarring.

multiple-casualty incident (MCI)   An emergency situation that can place great demand on the equipment or personnel of the EMS system or has the potential to overwhelm your available resources.

multiple-organ dysfunction syndrome (MODS)   A progressive condition usually characterized by combined failure of several organs, such as the lungs, liver, and kidneys, along with some clotting mechanisms, which occurs after severe illness or injury.

multisystem trauma   Trauma caused by generalized mechanisms which affect numerous body systems.

muscle fatigue The condition that arises when a muscle depletes its supply of energy.

muscular dystrophy A broad term that describes a category of incurable genetic diseases that cause a slow, progressive degeneration of the muscle fibers.

mutagen A substance that mutates, damages, and changes the structures of DNA in the body's cells.

mutual aid agreements (MAAs) Documents that preplan how you will access help from other areas when needed.

mutual aid response An agreement between neighboring EMS systems to respond to multiple-casualty incidents or disasters in each other's region when local resources are insufficient to handle the response.

myalgia Muscle pain.

myasthenia gravis A condition in which the body generates antibodies against its own acetylcholine receptors, causing muscle weakness, often in the face.

myasthenic crisis A complication of myasthenia gravis in which weakened respiratory muscles lead to respiratory failure.

myelomeningocele A developmental anomaly in which a portion of the spinal cord or meninges protrudes outside the spinal column or even outside the body, usually in the area of the lumbar spine (the lower third of the spine); also called spina bifida.

myocardial contractility The ability of the heart to contract.

myocardial contusion Blunt force injury to the heart that results in capillary damage, interstitial bleeding, and cellular damage in the area.

myocardial rupture An acute traumatic perforation of the ventricles, atria, intraventricular septum, intra-atrial septum, chordae, papillary muscles, or valves.

myocarditis Inflammation of the myocardium.

myoglobin A protein found in muscle that is released into the circulation after a crush injury or other muscle damage and whose presence in the circulation may produce kidney damage.

myometrium The middle layer of tissue in the uterus.

myositis Inflammation of the muscle, usually caused by infection.

myotomes Regions of the body innervated by the motor components of spinal nerves.

nasal cavity The chamber inside the nose that lies between the floor of the cranium and the roof of the mouth.

nasal flaring Intermittent outward movements of the nostrils with each inspiration; indicates an increase in the work needed to breathe.

nasal septum The separation between the right and left nostrils.

nasolacrimal duct The passage through which tears drain from the lacrimal sacs into the nasal cavity.

National Incident Management System (NIMS) A Department of Homeland Security system designed to enable federal, state, and local governments and private-sector and nongovernmental organizations to effectively and efficiently prepare for, prevent, respond to, and recover from domestic incidents, regardless of cause, size, or complexity, including acts of catastrophic terrorism.

National Terrorism Advisory System (NTAS) The US system for informing citizens of a potential terrorist threat; replaced the color-coded Homeland Security Advisory System.

necrotizing fasciitis Death of tissue from bacterial infection, caused by more than one infecting organism—most commonly, *Staphylococcus aureus* and hemolytic streptococci; this condition has a high mortality rate.

needle decompression Also referred to as a needle thoracentesis, this procedure introduces a needle or angiocath into the pleural space in an attempt to relieve a tension pneumothorax.

negative wave pulse The phase of an explosion in which pressure from the blast is less than atmospheric pressure.

neglect Refusal or failure on the part of the caregiver to provide life necessities, such as food, water, clothing, shelter, personal hygiene, medicine, comfort, and personal safety.

neonate Infant during the first month after birth.

neovascularization Development of new blood vessels to aid in healing injured soft tissue.

nerve agents A class of chemicals called organophosphates; they function by blocking an essential enzyme in the nervous system, which causes the body's organs to become overstimulated and burn out.

nerve root injury Injury to a nerve at the level of the spinal cord.

neurogenic shock Shock caused by paralysis of the nerves that control the size of the blood vessels, leading to widespread dilation and pooling of blood in the peripheral vessels to the extent that adequate perfusion cannot be maintained; seen in patients with spinal cord injuries.

neuroleptic malignant syndrome (NMS) A condition caused by antipsychotic and even common antiemetic medications that presents with hyperthermia, muscular rigidity, altered mental status, and a hyperdynamic state.

neuronal soma The body of a neuron (nerve cell).

neurotoxins   Biologic agents that are the most deadly substances known to humans; they include botulinum toxin and ricin.

neurovascular bundle   A closely placed grouping of an artery, vein, and nerve that lies beneath the inferior edge of a rib.

neurovascular compromise   The loss of the nerve supply, blood supply, or both to a region of the body, typically distal to a site of injury; characterized by alterations in sensation, including numbness and tingling, or by a loss or decrease of motor function; vascular compromise is indicated by weak or absent pulses, poor skin color, and cool skin.

neutralization   A type of decontamination that uses one chemical to change the hazardous material into two less harmful substances; rarely used by hazardous materials teams.

neutron radiation   Type of energy that is emitted from a strong radiologic source; the fastest moving and most powerful form of radiation; the particles easily penetrate through lead, and require several feet of concrete to stop them.

newborn   Infant within the first few hours after birth.

Newton's first law of motion   The principle that a body at rest will remain at rest unless acted on by an outside force.

Newton's second law of motion   The principle that the force that an object can exert is the product of its mass times its acceleration.

nitrogen narcosis   A state resembling alcohol intoxication produced by nitrogen gas dissolved in the blood at high ambient pressure; also called rapture of the deep.

nonbulk storage vessels   Any container other than bulk storage containers such as drums, bags, compressed gas cylinders, and cryogenic containers. Nonbulk storage vessels hold commonly used commercial and industrial chemicals such as solvents, cleaners, and compounds.

nondisplaced fracture   A break in which the bone remains aligned in its normal position.

non-hemorrhagic shock   Shock that occurs as a result of fluid loss contained within the body, such as in dehydration, burn injury, crush injury, and anaphylaxis.

non-state-supported terrorism   Terrorism that is either indigenous or transnational, and that do not receive direction or support from a government.

nuchal cord   A situation in which the umbilical cord is wrapped around the fetus's neck; cord compression may occur during labor, causing the fetal heart rate to slow and resulting in fetal distress.

nuchal rigidity   A stiff or painful neck; commonly associated with meningitis.

nursemaid's elbow   The subluxation of the radial head that often results from pulling on an outstretched arm.

obese   A term used when a person has a body mass index of greater than 30 kg per meters squared (kg/m^2).

oblique fracture   A fracture that travels diagonally from one side of the bone to the other.

obstructive shock   Shock that occurs when there is a block to blood flow in the heart or great vessels, causing an insufficient blood supply to the body's tissues.

obtunded   A condition when the patient is dulled to pain and sensation.

obturator   A solid plug at the end of a tracheostomy tube.

occipital condyles   Articular surfaces on the occipital bone in which the skull articulates with the atlas on the vertebral column.

occipital lobe   The portion of the brain that is responsible for the processing of visual information.

ocular myasthenia gravis   An autoimmune disorder in which the extraocular muscles become weakened and are fatigued.

oculomotor nerve   Third cranial nerve; innervates the muscles that cause motion of the eyeballs and upper eyelid.

odynophagia   Painful swallowing.

off-gassing   The emitting of an agent after exposure—for example, from a person's clothes that have been exposed to the agent.

Ohm's law   The formula that describes the relationship between voltage and resistance. Current (I) = Voltage (V) divided by Resistance (R).

old-age dependency ratio   A formula used to determine the number of older people in a society as compared with the number of potential workers who are theoretically capable of providing resources to sustain the whole population. It is the number of older people (65 years and older) for every 100 adults (potential caregivers) between the ages of 18 and 64 years.

olecranon   The proximal bony projection of the *ulna* at the elbow; the part of the ulna that constitutes the "funny bone."

olfactory nerves   Nerves that participate in the transmission of scent impulses.

oligohydramnios   Decreased volume of amniotic fluid during a pregnancy; a risk factor associated with abnormalities of the urinary tract, postmaturity (birth after a prolonged pregnancy), and intrauterine growth retardation.

oocyte   An egg produced from the female ovary.

open abdominal injury   An injury in which there is a break in the surface of the skin or mucous membrane, exposing deeper tissue to potential contamination.

open fracture   Any break in a bone in which the overlying skin has been damaged.

open incident   An ongoing or uncontained incident in which rescuers will have to search for patients and then triage or treat them. The situation may produce more patients. Examples include school shootings, tornadoes, a hazardous materials release, and rising floodwaters.

open pneumothorax   The result of a defect in the chest wall that allows air to enter the thoracic space.

open wound   An injury in which there is a break in the surface of the skin or the mucous membrane, exposing deeper tissue to potential contamination.

open-book pelvic fracture   A life-threatening fracture of the pelvis caused by a force that displaces one or both sides of the pelvis laterally and posteriorly.

operations   In incident command, the technical rescue training level geared toward working in the warm zone of an incident. Training at this level allows responders to directly assist those conducting the rescue operation and to use certain rescue skills and procedures.

ophthalmic nerve   A sensory nerve that supplies the skin of the forehead, the upper eyelid, and conjunctiva.

optic nerve   Either of the second cranial nerves that enter the eyeball posteriorly, through the optic foramen.

optic nerve hypoplasia   A congenital condition characterized by failure of the optic nerve to completely develop, and possibly resulting in optic nerve atrophy over time.

orbits   Bony cavities in the frontal part of the skull that enclose and protect the eyes.

organ of Corti   A structure located in the cochlea that contains hairs that are stimulated by vibrations to form nerve impulses that travel to the brain and are perceived as sound.

organophosphates   A class of chemical found in many insecticides used in agriculture and in the home; nerve agents fall into this class of chemicals.

orthostatic hypotension   A drop in systolic blood pressure when moving a patient from a recumbent position to a sitting position, or a sitting to a standing position.

ossicles   The three small bones in the middle ear that transmit vibrations to the cochlear duct at the oval window.

ossification center   Areas where cartilage is transformed through calcification into a new area of bone.

osteoarthritis (OA)   The degeneration of a joint surface caused by wear and tear that lead to pain and stiffness.

osteoporosis   A condition characterized by decreased bone density and increased susceptibility to fractures.

outer cannula   The larger (outer) tube of a tracheostomy tube.

oval window   An oval opening between the middle ear and the vestibule.

overriding   The overlap of a bone that occurs from the muscle spasm that follows a fracture, leading to a decrease in the length of the bone.

overtopping   A situation in which a reservoir overflows its borders.

ovulation   A process in which an ovum is released from a follicle.

ovum   A mature oocyte.

palatine bone   An irregularly shaped bone found in the posterior part of the nasal cavity.

palliative care   Medical care aimed at relief of pain and suffering in terminally ill patients.

pandemic   An extensive epidemic.

panhypopituitarism   The inadequate production or absence of the pituitary hormones, including adrenocorticotropic hormone (ACTH), cortisol, thyroxine, luteinizing hormone (LH), follicle-stimulating hormone (FSH), estrogen, testosterone, growth hormone, and antidiuretic hormone (ADH).

para   The number of live births.

paranasal sinuses   The sinuses, or hollowed sections of bone in the front of the head, that are lined with mucous membrane and drain into the nasal cavity.

paraplegia   Paralysis of the lower extremities.

parasympathetic nervous system   Subdivision of the autonomic nervous system; involved in control of involuntary, vegetative functions, mediated largely by the vagus nerve through the chemical acetylcholine.

paresthesias   Abnormal sensations such as burning, numbness, or tingling.

parietal lobe   The portion of the brain that is the site for reception and evaluation of most sensory information, except smell, hearing, and vision.

parity   Number of live births a woman has had.

Parkinson disease   A neurologic condition in which the portion of the brain responsible for production of dopamine has been damaged or overused, resulting in tremors.

paronychia   Infection of the area around the fingernail bed.

partial pressure   The amount of the total pressure contributed by various gases in solution.

partial seizures   Seizures that involve only one part of the brain

partial-thickness burn   A burn that involves the epidermis and part of the dermis, characterized by pain and blistering; previously called a second-degree burn.

patella   The kneecap.

patent ductus arteriosus (PDA) A situation in which the ductus arteriosus, which assists in fetal circulation, does not transition as it should after birth to become the ligamentum arteriosum; the result is that the connection between the pulmonary artery and the aorta remains, allowing some oxygenated blood to move back into the heart rather than all of it moving out of the aorta and into the systemic circulation.

pathogenic gastroesophageal reflux (GER) A condition in which stomach acid rises into the esophagus on a regular or frequent basis, potentially causing irritation and damage; a common cause of vomiting.

pathologic fracture A fracture that occurs in an area of abnormally weakened bone.

pathway expansion The tissue displacement that occurs as a result of low-displacement shock waves that travel at the speed of sound in tissue.

peak loads A time of day or day or week in which the call volume is at its highest.

pectoral girdle The shoulder girdle.

Pediatric Assessment Triangle (PAT) An assessment tool that allows rapid formation of a general impression of the type and level of illness or injury in an infant or child without touching him or her; consists of assessing appearance, work of breathing, and circulation to the skin.

pedicle A narrow strip of tissue by which an avulsed piece of tissue remains connected to the body; also, thick lateral bony struts that connect the vertebral body with the spinous and transverse processes and make up the lateral and posterior portions of the spinal foramen.

pelvic girdle The large bone that arises in the area of the last nine vertebrae and sweeps around to form a complete ring.

penetrating trauma Injury caused by objects that pierce the surface of the body, such as knives and bullets, and damage internal tissues and organs.

perfusion The delivery of oxygen and nutrients to the cells, organs, and tissues of the body.

peri-arrest period The period either just before or just after cardiac arrest when the patient is critical and care must be taken to prevent progression or regression into cardiac arrest.

pericardial sac The potential space between the layers of the pericardium.

pericardiocentesis A procedure in which a needle or angiocath is introduced into the pericardial sac to relieve cardiac tamponade.

pericardium Double-layered sac containing the heart and the origins of the superior vena cava, the inferior vena cava, and the pulmonary artery.

perimetrium The outer protective layer of tissue in the uterus.

periorbital ecchymosis Bruising under or around the orbits that is commonly seen following a basilar skull fracture; also called raccoon eyes.

periosteum The fibrous tissue that covers bone.

peripheral nerve injury Injury to a nerve anywhere in the body that is outside of the spinal cord.

peripheral shock A condition that consists of hypovolemic shock and distributive shock (Weil-Shubin classification).

peripheral vision Visualization of lateral objects while looking forward.

peritoneal dialysis A type of dialysis in which a special solution is instilled through a catheter into the patient's abdomen, and that draws toxins, electrolytes, and other fluids from the body through the peritoneal membrane.

peritoneal space The area in the abdomen encased in the peritoneum, and which consists of an upper and lower part. The upper portion contains the diaphragm, liver, spleen, stomach, gallbladder, and transverse colon. The lower portion contains the small bowel, sigmoid colon, parts of the descending and ascending colon, and, in women, the internal reproductive organs.

peritoneum A membrane in the abdomen encasing the liver, spleen, diaphragm, stomach, and transverse colon.

peritonitis Inflammation of the peritoneum that results from either blood or hollow organ contents spilling into the abdominal cavity.

periumbilical Pertaining to the area around the umbilicus.

permanent cavity The path of crushed tissue produced by a missile traversing part of the body.

permissible exposure limit (PEL) The maximum concentration of a chemical that a person may be exposed to under OSHA regulations.

persistency Term used to describe how long a chemical agent will stay on a surface before it evaporates.

persistent pulmonary hypertension Delayed transition from fetal to neonatal circulation.

personal flotation device (PFD) Also commonly known as a life vest, a PFD allows the body to float in water.

pertussis An acute infectious disease characterized by catarrhal stage, followed by a paroxysmal cough that ends in a whooping inspiration; also called whooping cough.

petechial Characterized by small purplish, nonblanching spots on the skin.

phalanges The bones of the fingers or toes.

phonologic process disorders A category of disorders that impact a person's ability to produce sounds that combine into spoken words.

phosgene A pulmonary agent that is a product of combustion, such as might be produced in a fire at a textile factory or house, or from metalwork or burning Freon; a very potent agent that has a delayed onset of symptoms, usually hours.

phosgene oxime (CX) A blistering agent that has a rapid onset of symptoms and produces immediate intense pain and discomfort on contact.

physical abuse A form of abuse that involves an intentional act such as throwing, striking, hitting, kicking, burning, or biting a vulnerable person.

physical evidence The evidence that ties a suspect or victim to a crime. It may include body materials, objects, and impressions.

physis The growth plate in long bones.

phytophotodermatitis A chemical reaction in which the skin becomes hypersensitive to sunlight.

pia mater The innermost and thinnest of the three meninges that enclose the brain and spinal cord; rests directly on the brain and spinal cord.

Pierre Robin sequence A condition present at birth marked by a small lower jaw (micrognathia). The tongue tends to fall back and downward (glossoptosis), and there is a cleft soft palate.

pinna The large outside portion of the ear through which sound waves enter the ear; also called the auricle.

placards Signage at least 10.8 inches on each side that is often required to be on all four sides of transport vehicles identifying the hazardous contents of the vehicle.

placenta The tissue attached to the uterine wall that nourishes the fetus through the umbilical cord.

placenta previa A condition in which the placenta develops over and covers the cervix.

planning In incident command, the position that ultimately produces a plan to resolve any incident.

plantar Referring to the sole of the foot.

plantar flexion Bending of the foot toward the ground.

plasma The fluid portion of the blood from which the cells have been removed.

platelets Small cells in the blood that are essential for clot formation.

pleura Membrane lining the outer surface of the lungs (visceral pleura), the inner surface of the chest wall, and the thoracic surface of the diaphragm (parietal pleura).

plexus A cluster of nerve roots that permits peripheral nerve roots to rejoin and function as a group.

pneumonia An inflammation of the lungs caused by bacterial, viral, or fungal infections or infections with other microorganisms.

pneumonic plague A lung infection, also known as plague pneumonia, that is the result of inhalation of plague bacteria.

pneumothorax The collection of air within the normally closed pleural space.

point of distribution (PODs) Strategically placed facilities that have been preestablished for the mass distribution of antibiotics, antidotes, and vaccinations, along with other medications and supplies.

point tenderness The tenderness that is sharply localized at the site of the injury, found by gently palpating along the bone with the tip of one finger.

poliomyelitis A viral infection that attacks and destroys motor axons. The disease can cause weakness, paralysis, and respiratory arrest. Because an effective vaccine has been developed, the incidence of the disease is now rare.

polycythemia Abnormally high red blood cell count.

polyhydramnios An excessive amount of amniotic fluid. May cause preterm labor.

polyneuropathy A type of disorder in which multiple nerves become dysfunctional.

polypharmacy The use of multiple medications.

pons Lies below the midbrain and above the medulla and contains numerous important nerve fibers, including those for sleep, respiration, and the medullary respiratory center.

popliteal artery The artery in the area or space behind the knee joint.

positive wave pulse The phase of the explosion in which there is a pressure front with a pressure higher than atmospheric pressure.

positive-pressure ventilation (PPV) Method for assisting ventilation (bag-mask or intubated) with high-flow air or supplemental oxygen.

posterior chamber The posterior area of the globe between the lens and the iris.

posterior cord syndrome A condition associated with extension injuries with isolated injury to the dorsal column; presents as decreased sensation to light touch, proprioception, and vibration while leaving most other motor and sensory functions intact.

posterior spinous process Formed by the fusion of the posterior lamina, this is an attachment site for muscles and ligaments.

posterior tibial artery The artery that travels through the calf muscles to the plantar aspect of the foot.

posting The placement of an ambulance at a specific geographic location in order to cover larger areas of territory and reduce response times.

postpartum The period of time after a woman has given birth.

postpolio syndrome The death of nerve fibers as a late consequence of polio; the syndrome is characterized by swallowing difficulties, weakness, fatigue, and breathing problems.

post-term Any pregnancy that lasts more than 42 weeks.

potential energy The amount of energy stored in an object, the product of mass, gravity, and height, that is converted into kinetic energy and results in injury, such as from a fall.

preeclampsia A condition of late pregnancy that involves gradual onset of hypertension, headache, visual changes, and swelling of the hands and feet; also called pregnancy-induced hypertension or toxemia of pregnancy.

pregnancy-induced hypertension High blood pressure that develops after the 20th week of pregnancy, in women with previously normal blood pressures, and resolves spontaneously in the postpartum period.

preload The initial stretching of the cardiac muscles prior to contraction as the volume of blood builds up.

premature Underdeveloped; the condition of an infant born too soon. Refers to infants delivered before 37 weeks from the first day of the last menstrual period.

premorbid condition A condition preceding the onset of disease.

prenatal The state of the pregnant woman before birth.

presbycusis Progressive hearing loss, particularly in the high frequencies, along with lessened ability to discriminate between a particular sound and background noise.

pressure ulcers Ulcers that occur when pressure is applied to body tissue, resulting in a lack of perfusion and ultimately necrosis.

preterm Used to describe an infant delivered at less than 37 completed weeks.

primary apnea Apnea caused by oxygen deprivation; usually corrected with stimulation, such as drying or slapping the newborn's feet. Primary apnea is typically preceded by an initial period of rapid breathing.

primary brain injury An injury to the brain and its associated structures that is a direct result of impact to the head.

primary contamination An exposure that occurs with direct contact with the hazardous material.

primary exit The main means of escape should violence erupt. This is usually the door you used to enter the building.

primary spinal cord injury Injury to the spinal cord that is a direct result of trauma—for example, transection of the spinal cord from penetrating trauma or displacement of ligaments and bone fragments, resulting in compression of the spinal cord.

primary triage A type of patient sorting used to rapidly categorize patients; the focus is on speed in locating all patients and determining an initial priority as their condition warrants.

primigravida First pregnancy.

progesterone A hormone that influences the second phase of the menstrual cycle, when the oocyte is either fertilized or dies.

prolapsed cord When the umbilical cord presents itself outside of the uterus while the fetus is still inside; an obstetric emergency during pregnancy or labor that acutely endangers the life of the fetus; can happen when the amniotic sac breaks and with the gush of amniotic fluid the cord comes along.

pronation The act of turning the palm of the hand backward or downward, performed by internal rotation of the forearm.

proprioception The ability to perceive the position and movement of one's body or limbs.

psychogenic shock A sudden reaction of the nervous system that produces a temporary, generalized vascular dilation, resulting in syncope (vasovagal syncope).

pubic symphysis The midline articulation of the pubic bones.

pubis One of two bones that form the anterior portion of the pelvic ring.

public information officer (PIO) In incident command, the person who keeps the public informed and relates any information to the press.

pulmonary blast injuries Pulmonary trauma resulting from short-range exposure to the detonation of high explosives.

pulmonary contusion Injury to the lung parenchyma that results in capillary hemorrhage into the tissue.

pulmonary embolism Obstruction of a pulmonary artery or arteries by solid, liquid, or gaseous material swept through the right side of the heart into the lungs.

pulmonary hypertension Elevated blood pressure in the pulmonary arteries from constriction; causes problems with the blood flow in the lungs, and makes the heart work harder.

pulmonary overpressurization syndrome (POPS) Also called "burst lung," this diving emergency can occur during rapid ascent and can cause pneumothorax, mediastinal and subcutaneous emphysema, alveolar hemorrhage, and the lethal arterial gas embolism (AGE).

pulmonary stenosis Narrowing of the pulmonary valve.

pulp Specialized connective tissue within the cavity of a tooth.

pulse pressure The difference between the systolic and diastolic pressures.

pulsus paradoxus A drop in the systolic blood pressure of 10 mm Hg more than during inspiration; commonly seen in patients with cardiac tamponade or severe asthma.

puncture wound A stab injury from a pointed object, such as a nail or a knife.

pupil The circular opening in the center of the eye through which light passes to the lens.

purpuric Pertaining to bruising of the skin.

pyloric stenosis Hypertrophy (enlargement) of the pyloric sphincter of the stomach; ultimately leads to intestinal obstruction, often in infants.

pylorus A circumferential muscle at the end of the stomach that acts as a valve between the stomach and duodenum.

pyroclastic explosions Blasts from flowing or standing lava that can have a wide dispersal circumference, spewing ash and magma.

quadriplegia Paralysis of the upper and lower extremities.

rabid Describes an animal that is infected with rabies.

raccoon eyes Bruising under or around the orbits that is commonly seen following a basilar skull fracture; also called periorbital ecchymosis.

radial artery The artery pertaining to the wrist.

radiation Emission of heat from an object into surrounding, colder air.

radio operators Amateur radio operators who have a formal emergency communications set of SOPs. Most are licensed by the FCC.

radioactive material Any material that emits radiation.

radiologic dispersal device (RDD) Any container that is designed to disperse radioactive material.

radius The bone on the thumb side of the forearm.

range of motion (ROM) The arc of movement of an extremity at a joint in a particular direction.

rappelling To descend on a fixed rope.

recruitment The process of signaling additional muscle fibers to contract to create a more forceful contraction.

rehabilitation supervisor In incident command, the person who establishes an area that provides protection for responders from the elements and the situation.

rescue supervisor In incident command, the person appointed to determine the type of equipment and resources needed for a situation involving extrication or special rescue; also called the extrication supervisor.

resistance vessels The smallest arterioles.

respiratory arrest The absence of respirations with detectable cardiac activity.

respiratory distress A clinical state characterized by increased respiratory rate, effort, and work of breathing.

respiratory failure A clinical state of inadequate oxygenation, ventilation, or both.

respiratory syncytial virus (RSV) A virus that affects the upper and lower respiratory tracts, but disease, namely pneumonia and bronchiolitis, is more prevalent in the lower respiratory tract.

reticular activating system (RAS) Located in the upper brainstem; responsible for maintenance of consciousness, specifically one's level of arousal.

retina A delicate 10-layered structure of nervous tissue located in the rear of the interior of the globe that receives light and generates nerve signals that are transmitted to the brain through the optic nerve.

retinal detachment Separation of the inner layers of the retina from the underlying choroid, the vascular membrane that nourishes the retina.

retinopathy Any eye disorder in which the retina becomes diseased, leading to partial or total vision loss.

retinopathy of prematurity A disease of the eye that affects prematurely born infants, thought to be caused by disorganized growth of retinal blood vessels resulting in scarring and retinal detachment; can lead to blindness in serious cases.

retractions Skin pulling between and around the ribs and clavicles during inhalation; a sign of respiratory distress.

retrograde amnesia Loss of memory relating to events that occurred before the injury.

retroperitoneal space The area in the abdomen containing the aorta, vena cava, pancreas, kidneys, ureters, and portions of the duodenum and large intestine.

return of spontaneous circulation (ROSC) The return of spontaneous heart beat and blood pressure during the resuscitation of a patient in cardiac arrest.

Revised Trauma Score (RTS) A scoring system used for patients with head trauma.

Rh factor A protein found on the red blood cells of most people; when a woman without this protein is impregnated by a man with this protein, the woman's body can create antibodies against the protein and attack future pregnancies.

rhabdomyolysis The destruction of muscle tissue leading to a release of potassium and myoglobin.

rheumatoid arthritis (RA) An inflammatory disorder that affects the entire body and leads to degeneration and deformation of joints.

ricin Neurotoxin derived from mash that is left from pressing oil from a castor bean; causes pulmonary edema and respiratory and circulatory failure, leading to death.

rotation-flexion injury A type of injury typically resulting from high acceleration forces; can result in a stable unilateral facet dislocation in the cervical spine.

round bones The small bones that are found adjacent to joints that assist with motion.

route of exposure Manner by which a toxic substance enters the body.

rubella A viral disease similar to measles, best known by the distinctive red rash on the skin; not nearly as infectious or severe as measles.

rule of nines A system that assigns percentages to sections of the body, allowing calculation of the amount of skin surface involved in the burn area.

rule of palms A system that estimates total body surface area burned by comparing the affected area with the size of the patient's palm, which is roughly equal to 1% of the patient's total body surface area; also called rule of ones.

sacroiliac joints The points of attachment of the *ilium* to the sacrum.

safety officer In incident command, the person who gives the "go ahead" to a plan or who may stop an operation when rescuer safety is an issue.

sagittal suture The point of the skull where the parietal bones join.

sarin (GB) A nerve agent that is one of the G agents; a highly volatile colorless and odorless liquid that turns from liquid to gas within seconds to minutes at room temperature.

saturation diving A type of diving in which the diver remains at depth for prolonged periods.

scald burn A burn produced by hot liquids.

scaphoid The wrist bone that is found just beyond that most distal portion of the radius.

scapula A large, flat, triangular bone along the posterior thorax that articulates with the clavicle and humerus; the shoulder blade.

scar revision A surgical procedure to improve the appearance of a scar, reestablish function, or correct disfigurement from soft-tissue damage, surgical incision, or lesion.

sclera The white part of the eye.

scrambling A method used to ascend rocky faces and ridges and can be considered a cross between hill climbing and rock climbing.

search and rescue (SAR) The process of locating and removing a patient from the wilderness.

seasonal affective disorder (SAD) Depression that can affect persons in long periods of bad weather, usually winter.

sebaceous gland A gland located in the dermis that secretes sebum.

sebum An oily substance secreted by the sebaceous glands.

second stage of labor The stage of labor in which the newborn's head enters the birth canal, during which contractions become more intense and more frequent.

secondary apnea When asphyxia continues after primary apnea, infant responds with a period of gasping respirations, falling pulse rate, and falling blood pressure. Positive-pressure ventilation is indicated to reverse secondary apnea.

secondary brain injury The "after effects" of the primary injury; includes abnormal processes such as cerebral edema, increased intracranial pressure, cerebral ischemia and hypoxia, and infection; onset is often delayed following the primary brain injury.

secondary collapse A collapse that occurs following the primary collapse. This can occur in trench, excavation, and structural collapses.

secondary containment An engineered method to control spilled or released product if the main containment vessel fails.

secondary contamination Exposure to a hazardous material by contact with a contaminated person or object.

secondary device Additional explosives used by terrorists, which are set to explode after the initial bomb.

secondary exit Any other means of egress, including windows and rear doors.

secondary spinal cord injury Injury to the spinal cord, thought to be the result of multiple factors that result in a progression of inflammatory responses from primary spinal cord injury.

secondary triage A type of patient sorting used in the treatment sector that involves retriage of patients.

segmental fracture A bone that is broken in more than one place.

seizure A paroxysmal alteration in neurologic function—ie, behavioral and/or autonomic function.

self-contained underwater breathing apparatus The expansion of the acronym (SCUBA) for specialized underwater breathing equipment.

self-rescue position Position used in fast-moving water rescue situations. The rescuer rolls into a faceup arched position with the lower back higher than the feet to avoid objects below the surface. The feet should be together and facing in the direction of travel (feet first), with arms at the sides.

semantic-pragmatic disorder A condition characterized by delayed language developmental milestones, resulting in the person repeatedly using irrelevant phrases out of context, confusing word pairs, and having trouble following conversations.

sensitization Developing sensitivity to a substance that initially caused no allergic reaction.

sensorineural hearing loss A permanent lack of hearing caused by a lesion or damage of the inner ear.

sepsis A pathologic state, usually in a febrile patient, resulting from the presence of invading microorganisms or their poisonous products in the bloodstream.

septic abortion A life-threatening emergency in which the uterus becomes infected following any type of abortion.

septic arthritis Inflammation of a joint based on a bacterial or fungal infection.

septic shock Shock caused by severe infection, usually a bacterial infection.

sexual abuse A form of abuse that involves a vulnerable person being forced into unwanted sexual acts, or into involvement in sexual activities such as pornography.

sexual exploitation A form of abuse that involves forcing a vulnerable person to perform or be involved in sexual acts, or be involved in sexual activities such as pornography, in return for something they need or want, such as money, food, or shelter.

shallow water blackout A diving emergency that occurs when a person hyperventilates just before submerging underwater and loses consciousness before resurfacing due to hypoxemia and cerebral vasoconstriction.

shearing An applied force or pressure exerted against the surface and layers of the skin as tissues slide in opposite but parallel planes.

shelter-in-place A method of safeguarding people located near or in a hazardous area by keeping them in a safe atmosphere, usually inside structures.

shims Objects that are smaller than wedges used to snug loose cribbing under a load or to fill void spaces.

shock An abnormal state associated with inadequate oxygen and nutrient delivery to the metabolic apparatus of the cell; also called hypoperfusion.

shoring A method of supporting a trench wall or building components such as walls, floors, or ceilings using either hydraulic, pneumatic, or wood shoring systems. Shoring is used to prevent collapse.

short bones The bones that are nearly as wide as they are long.

shoulder dystocia A complication of delivery in which there is difficulty delivering the shoulders of a newborn; the shoulder cannot get past the woman's symphysis pubis.

sickle cell disease (SCD) A disease that causes red blood cells to be misshapen, resulting in a poor oxygen-carrying capability and potentially resulting in lodging of the red blood cells in blood vessels or the spleen.

silver fork deformity The dorsal deformity of the forearm that results from a Colles fracture.

simple access Access that is easily achieved with the use of simple hand tools or force.

simple febrile seizures A brief, self-limited, generalized seizure in a previously healthy child between ages 6 months and 6 years that is associated with the onset of or sudden increase in fever.

simple partial seizures Focal seizures that involve a motor or sensory abnormality in a patient who remains conscious.

single command system A command system in which one person is in charge, generally used with small incidents that involve only one responding agency or one jurisdiction.

situational awareness Knowing your surroundings, the people and groups in your environment, and the climate of violence or strife.

skeletal muscle Muscle that is attached to bones and usually crosses at least one joint; striated or voluntary muscle.

skull The structure at the top of the axial skeleton that houses the brain and consists of 28 bones that comprise the auditory ossicles, the cranium, and the face.

slipped capital femoral epiphysis (SCFE) A dislocation of the epiphyseal end of the femur, usually found in children and adolescents.

SLUDGEM A mnemonic that stands for salivation, lacrimation, urination, defecation, gastrointestinal activity, emesis, miosis, which are the signs and symptoms that can be produced by exposure to organophosphate and carbamate pesticides or other nerve-stimulating agents.

small for gestational age An infant whose size and weight are considerably less than the average for infants of the same age.

smallpox A highly contagious disease; it is most contagious when blisters begin to form.

SMART An acronym used to describe a prehospital program's objectives: Specific, Measurable, Attainable and Achievable, Realistic and Relevant, and Timely.

sniffing position An upright position in which the patient's head and chin are thrust slightly forward to keep the airway open; appears to be sniffing.

snuffbox The region at the base of the thumb where the scaphoid may be palpated.

solvents Substances that are capable of dissolving other substances.

soman (GD) A nerve agent that is one of the G agents; twice as persistent as sarin and five times as lethal; it has a fruity odor as a result of the type of alcohol used in the agent, and is both a contact and inhalation hazard that can enter the body through skin absorption and through the respiratory tract.

somatic motor neurons The nerve fibers that transmit impulses to a muscle.

somatic pain Localized pain, usually felt deeply, which represents irritation or injury to tissue, causing activation of peripheral nerve tracts.

space junk Debris from satellites and other man-made objects that reenter the earth's atmosphere.

spalling Delaminating or breaking off into chips and pieces.

span of control In incident command, the subordinate positions under the commander's direction to which the workload is distributed; the supervisor/worker ratio.

spastic paralysis A chronic form of paralysis in which the affected muscles experience continued spasm.

spastic tetraplegia A form of cerebral palsy in which all fours limbs are affected.

special atomic demolition munitions (SADMs) Small suitcase-sized nuclear weapons that were designed to destroy individual targets, such as important buildings, bridges, tunnels, or large ships.

special weapons and tactics (SWAT) team A specialized law enforcement tactical unit.

specific gravity The measure that indicates whether or not a hazardous material will sink or float in water.

sphincters Circular muscular walls of capillaries that constrict and dilate, acting as a gate to increase or decrease blood flow.

spina bifida A developmental anomaly in which a portion of the spinal cord or meninges protrudes outside the spinal column or even outside the body, usually in the area of the lumbar spine (the lower third of the spine); also called myelomeningocele.

spinal clearance The act of declaring that a spinal injury is not present.

spinal cord The part of the central nervous system that extends downward from the brain through the foramen magnum and is protected by the spine.

spinal shock The temporary local neurologic condition that occurs immediately after spinal trauma; swelling and edema of the spinal cord begin immediately after injury, with severe pain and potential paralysis.

spinal stenosis Narrowing of the spinal canal, causing back pain that worsens with standing or walking.

spiral fracture A break in a bone that appears like a spring on a radiograph.

spoil pile The pile of dirt that has been removed from an excavation. The pile may be unstable and prone to collapse.

spondylosis Degenerative condition resulting in decreased mobility of vertebral joints and compression of neural elements.

spontaneous abortion Expulsion of the fetus that occurs naturally; also called miscarriage.

spotter A person who assists a driver in backing up an ambulance to compensate for blind spots at the back of the vehicle.

sprain An injury including a stretch or a tear, to the ligaments of a joint that commonly leads to pain and swelling.

staging supervisor In incident command, the person who locates an area to stage equipment and personnel and tracks unit arrival and deployment from the staging area.

START triage A patient sorting process that stands for simple triage and rapid treatment and uses a limited assessment of the patient's ability to walk, respiratory status, hemodynamic status, and neurologic status.

state-directed terrorism Terrorism directed by a government; the terrorists act as direct agents of the government.

state-sponsored terrorism Terrorism that is funded or supported by nations that hold close ties with terrorist groups, but the terrorist group still acts independently.

status epilepticus A condition in which seizures recur every few minutes, or in which seizure activity lasts more than 30 minutes.

steam burn A burn that has been caused by direct exposure to hot steam exhaust, as from a broken pipe.

steering play A sensation of looseness or sloppiness in a vehicle's steering.

steering pull A drift that is persistent enough that an operator can feel a tug on the steering wheel.

stenosis Narrowing of a passageway in the body.

step chocks Specialized cribbing assemblies made out of wood or plastic in a step configuration.

sterilization A process, such as heating, that removes microbial contamination.

sternum   Also known as the breastbone, this bony structure along the midline of the thorax provides a point of anterior attachment for the thoracic cage.

stoma   A surgical opening, such as into the abdominal wall or trachea; in the context of the airway, the resultant orifice of a tracheostomy that connects the trachea to the outside air; located in the midline of the anterior part of the neck.

straddle fracture   A fracture of the pelvis that results from landing on the perineal region.

strain   Stretching or tearing of a muscle by excessive stretching or overuse.

strategic deployment   The staging of ambulances to strategic locations within a service area to allow for coverage of emergency calls.

stress fracture   A fracture that results from exaggerated stress on the bone caused by unusually rapid muscle development.

striated muscle   Skeletal muscle that is under voluntary control.

stroke volume (SV)   The amount of blood that the left ventricle ejects into the aorta per contraction.

subarachnoid hemorrhage   Bleeding into the subarachnoid space, where the cerebrospinal fluid circulates.

subarachnoid space   The space located between the pia mater and the arachnoid.

subclavian artery   The artery that travels from the aorta to each upper extremity.

subconjunctival hematoma   The collection of blood within the sclera of the eye, presenting as a bright red patch of blood over the sclera but not involving the cornea.

subcutaneous   Beneath the skin.

subcutaneous emphysema   A physical finding of air within the subcutaneous tissue.

subcutaneous layer   Beneath the skin.

subdural hematoma   An accumulation of blood beneath the dura but outside the brain.

subgaleal hemorrhage   Bleeding between the periosteum of the skull and the galea aponeurosis.

subglottic space   The narrowest part of the pediatric airway.

subluxation   A partial or incomplete dislocation.

subthalamus   The part of the diencephalon that is involved in controlling motor functions.

sudden infant death syndrome (SIDS)   The abrupt and unexplained death of an apparently healthy child younger than 1 year.

suicide bombers   People who are terrorists who wear or carry a weapon, such as an explosive, and trigger its detonation, killing themselves in the process to achieve terrorism.

sulfur mustard (H)   A vesicant; it is a brownish-yellowish oily substance that is generally considered very persistent; has the distinct smell of garlic or mustard and, when released, it is quickly absorbed into the skin and/or mucous membranes and begins an irreversible process of damaging the cells.

superficial burn   A burn involving only the epidermis, producing very red, painful skin; previously called a first-degree burn.

superficial frostbite   A type of frostbite characterized by altered sensation (numbness, tingling, or burning) and white, waxy skin that is firm to palpation, but the underlying tissues remain soft.

supination   To turn the forearm laterally so that the palm faces forward (if standing) or upward (if lying supine).

supine hypotensive syndrome   Low blood pressure resulting from compression of the inferior vena cava by the weight of the pregnant uterus when the woman is supine.

supracondylar fractures   Fractures of the distal humerus that occur just proximal to the elbow.

supragaleal hematoma   Bleeding between the subgaleal area of the skull and the galea aponeurosis.

supraglottic   Located above the glottic opening, as in the upper airway structures.

suprasternal notch   The indentation formed by the superior border of the manubrium and the clavicles, often used as a landmark for procedures such as subclavian vein access.

surface-tended diving   A type of diving in which air is piped to the diver through a tube from the surface.

surfactant   A substance formed in the lungs that helps keep the small air sacs or alveoli from collapsing and sticking together; a low level in a premature infant contributes to respiratory distress syndrome.

surrogate decision-maker   A person legally authorized to make health care decisions on behalf of a patient who is incapable of making or communicating the decision on his or her own.

sympathetic eye movement   The movement of both eyes in unison.

sympathetic nervous system   Subdivision of the autonomic nervous system that governs the body's fight-or-flight reactions by inducing smooth muscle contraction or relaxation of the blood vessels and bronchioles.

synchronized cardioversion   The use of synchronized direct current (DC) electric shock to convert tachydysrhythmias (such as atrial fibrillation) to normal sinus rhythm.

syndromic surveillance   The monitoring, usually by local or state health departments, of patients presenting to emergency departments and alternative care facilities, the recording of EMS call volume, and the use of over-the-counter medications.

synovial joints Joints that permit movement of the component bones.

synovial membrane The lining of a joint that secretes synovial fluid into the joint space.

syphilis A sexually transmitted disease caused by the bacterium *Treponema pallidum*, which manifests in three stages—primary, secondary, and late—and is transmitted through direct contact with open sores; characterized by an ulcerative lesion or chancre of the skin or mucous membrane at the site of infection, commonly in the genital region.

systemic effect A physiologic effect on the entire body or one of the body's systems.

systemic lupus erythematosus A multisystem autoimmune disease.

systemic vascular resistance (SVR) The resistance to blood flow within all of the blood vessels except the pulmonary vessels.

tabun (GA) A nerve agent that is one of the G agents; is 36 times more persistent than sarin and approximately half as lethal; has a fruity smell and is unique because the components used to manufacture the agent are easy to acquire and the agent is easy to manufacture.

tactical paramedics Specially trained medics who provide care for SWAT team members conducting operations, barricaded patients, patients being held hostage, and other special operations.

tactical situation A high-risk situation where law enforcement agencies may deploy use of specialized law enforcement tactical units or the SWAT team.

tag lines Rope or cord tied to a person who is entering a dangerous environment. Used for quick retrieval, usually in conjunction with a harness.

talus The bone of the foot that articulates with the tibia.

tarsals The ankle bones.

technical decontamination A multistep process of carefully scrubbing and washing contaminants off of a person or object, collecting runoff water, and collecting and properly handling all items.

technical rescue incident (TRI) A complex rescue incident involving vehicles or machinery, water or ice, rope techniques, a trench or excavation collapse, confined spaces, a structural collapse, wilderness search and rescue, or hazardous materials, and which requires specially trained personnel and special equipment.

technical rescue team A group of rescuers specially trained in the various disciplines of technical rescue.

technician The training level that provides a high level of competency in the various disciplines of technical or hazardous materials rescue for rescuers who will be directly involved in the rescue operation itself.

tempered glass A type of glass that is heat-treated so that it will break into small pieces.

temporal lobe The portion of the brain that has an important role in hearing and memory.

temporomandibular joint (TMJ) The joint between the temporal bone and the posterior condyle that allows for movements of the mandible.

tendinitis Inflammation of a tendon that most commonly results from overuse.

tendons The fibrous portions of muscle that attach to bone.

tension lines The pattern of tautness of the skin, which is arranged over body structures and affects how well wounds heal.

tension pneumothorax A life-threatening collection of air within the pleural space; the volume and pressure have both collapsed the involved lung and caused a shift of the mediastinal structures to the opposite side.

tenting A condition in which the skin slowly retracts after being pinched and pulled away slightly from the body; a sign of dehydration.

tentorium A structure that separates the cerebral hemispheres from the cerebellum and brainstem.

term Used to describe a newborn delivered at 38 to 42 weeks of gestation.

terminal illness A sickness that a patient cannot be cured of; death is imminent.

termination of command The end of the incident command structure when an incident draws to a close.

terrorism A violent act dangerous to human life, in violation of the criminal laws of the United States or any segment to intimidate or coerce a government, the civilian population, or any segment thereof, in furtherance of political or social objectives.

testimonial evidence The oral documentation by a witness of the facts of a criminal act.

tetralogy of Fallot (ToF) A cardiac anomaly that consists of four defects: a ventricular septal defect, pulmonary stenosis, right ventricular hypertrophy, and an overriding aorta.

thalamus The part of the diencephalon that processes most sensory input and influences mood and general body movements, especially those associated with fear or rage.

thermal burn An injury caused by radiation or direct contact with a heat source on the skin.

thermals Differing temperatures and swirling patterns of moving air with changes in wind speed.

thermogenesis The production of heat in the body.

thermolysis The liberation of heat from the body.

thermoregulation The process by which the body maintains temperature through a combination of heat gain by metabolic processes and muscular movement and heat loss through respiration, evaporation, conduction, convection, and perspiration.

third stage of labor The stage of labor in which the placenta is expelled.

Thompson test Squeezing of the calf muscle to evaluate for plantar flexion of the foot to determine whether the Achilles tendon is intact.

thoracic inlet The superior aspect of the thoracic cavity, this ring-like opening is created by the first vertebral vertebra, the first rib, the clavicles, and the manubrium.

thorax The part of the body between the neck and the diaphragm, encased by the ribs.

threatened abortion Expulsion of the fetus that is attempting to take place but has not occurred yet; usually occurs in the first trimester.

threshold limit value (TLV) The concentration of a substance that is supposed to be safe for exposure no more than 8 hours per day and 40 hours per week.

threshold limit value/ceiling (TLV/C) The maximum concentration of hazardous material to which a worker should not be exposed, even for an instant.

threshold limit value/short-term exposure limit (TLV-STEL) The concentration of a substance that a worker can be exposed to for up to 15 minutes but no more than four times per day with at least 1 hour between each exposure.

threshold limit value/skin The concentration at which direct or airborne contact with a material could result in possible and significant exposure from absorption through the skin, mucous membranes, and eyes.

thrombocytopenia A reduction in the number of platelets in the blood.

thromboembolic disease The condition in which a patient has a deep vein thrombosis or pulmonary embolism.

thrombosis The formation of a blood clot in the circulatory system.

tibia The shinbone.

tonic-clonic seizures Seizures that feature rhythmic back-and-forth motion of an extremity and body stiffness.

torus fracture *See* buckle fracture.

total anomalous pulmonary venous return (TAPVR) A rare congenital defect in which the four pulmonary veins do not connect to the left atrium; instead, the pulmonary veins connect to the right atrium, resulting in diminished oxygen and an increased load on the right ventricle.

toxic products of combustion Hazardous chemical compounds that are released when a material decomposes under heat.

toxoplasmosis An infection caused by a parasite that pregnant women may get from handling or eating contaminated food or exposure from handling cat litter; the fetus can become infected.

tracheal transection Traumatic separation of the trachea from the larynx.

tracheostomy (trach) tube A plastic tube placed within the tracheostomy site (stoma).

transducer A device that converts energy or pressure into electrical signals.

transfer of command In incident command, when an incident commander turns over command to someone with more experience in a critical area.

transportation supervisor In incident command, the person who coordinates transportation and distribution of patients to appropriate receiving hospitals.

transposition of the great arteries (TGA) A defect in which the great vessels are reversed; the aorta is connected to the right ventricle, and the pulmonary artery is connected to the left ventricle.

transverse fracture A fracture that runs in a straight line from one edge of the bone to the other and that is perpendicular to each edge.

transverse presentation A delivery in which the fetus lies crosswise in the uterus; one hand may protrude through the vagina.

transverse spinous process The junction of each pedicle and lamina on each side of a vertebra; these project laterally and posteriorly and form points of attachment for muscles and ligaments.

trauma Acute physiologic and structural change that occurs in a victim as a result of the rapid dissipation of energy delivered by an external force.

trauma score A score that relates to the likelihood of patient survival with the exception of a severe head injury. It is calculated on a scale from 1 to 16, with 16 being the best possible score. It takes into account the Glasgow Coma Scale score, respiratory rate, respiratory expansion, systolic blood pressure, and capillary refill.

traumatic aortic disruption Dissection or rupture of the aorta.

traumatic asphyxia A pattern of injuries seen after a severe force is applied to the thorax, forcing blood from the great vessels and back into the head and neck.

traumatic brain injury (TBI) A traumatic insult to the brain capable of producing physical, intellectual, emotional, social, and vocational changes.

treatment supervisor In incident command, the person responsible for locating, setting up, and supervising the treatment area.

trench foot A process similar to frostbite but caused by prolonged exposure to cool, wet conditions.

triage To sort patients based on the severity of their conditions and prioritize them for care accordingly.

triage supervisor The person in charge of prioritizing patients, whose primary duty is to ensure that every patient receives initial triage.

trichomoniasis A parasitic infection caused by a single-cell parasite that is transmitted through sexual contact, with the vagina being the most common site of infection; infected person may be asymptomatic or may experience frothy, yellow-green vaginal discharge with a strong odor, irritation, and itching of the female genital area, discomfort during intercourse, dysuria, and lower abdominal pain.

tricuspid atresia The absence of a tricuspid valve, which normally separates the right atrium and the right ventricle.

trigeminal nerve Fifth cranial nerve; supplies sensation to the scalp, forehead, face, and lower jaw and innervates the muscles of mastication, the throat, and the inner ear.

tripoding An abnormal position to keep the airway open; involves leaning forward onto two arms stretched forward.

trismus Clenching of the teeth owing to spasm of the jaw muscles.

truncus arteriosus A condition in which the pulmonary artery and the aorta are combined into one.

tube trailer A high-volume transportation device made up of several individual compressed gas cylinders banded together and affixed to a trailer. Tube trailers carry compressed gases such as hydrogen, oxygen, helium, and methane. One trailer may carry several different gases in individual tubes.

tunnel vision Dangerous situation when a paramedic becomes so completely involved with patient care that he or she fails to see the possibility of physical harm to the patient or other care providers.

twisting injuries Injuries that commonly occur during athletic activities in which an extremity rotates around a planted foot or hand.

tympanic membrane The eardrum; a thin, semitransparent membrane in the middle ear that transmits sound vibrations to the internal ear by means of the auditory ossicles.

Type I ambulance Conventional, truck-cab chassis with a modular ambulance body that can be transferred to a new chassis as needed.

Type II ambulance Standard van, forward-control integral cab-body ambulance.

Type III ambulance Specialty van, forward-control integral cab-body ambulance.

ulna The larger bone of the forearm, on the side opposite the thumb.

ulnar artery The artery of the forearm that travels along its medial aspect.

umbilical cord The conduit connecting the pregnant woman to the fetus via the placenta; contains two arteries and one vein.

umbilical vein The blood vessel in the umbilical cord used to administer emergency medications.

unibody construction A vehicle design with no formal frame structure; the body and frame are one piece, which is considered to be the structural integrity of the vehicle.

unified command system A command system used in larger incidents in which there is a multiagency response or multiple jurisdictions are involved.

upper flammable limit (UFL) The maximum amount of gaseous fuel that can be present in the air if the air/fuel mixture is to be flammable or explosive.

urostomy A surgically constructed opening for the urinary system.

uterine cavity The interior of the body of the uterus.

uterine inversion A potentially fatal complication of childbirth in which the placenta fails to detach properly and results in the uterus turning inside out.

uterus A muscular inverted pear-shaped organ that lies situated between the urinary bladder and the rectum.

V agent (VX) One of the G agents; it is a clear, oily agent that has no odor and looks like baby oil; over 100 times more lethal than sarin and is extremely persistent.

vagina A tubular organ lined with mucous membranes, that is the lower portion of the birth canal.

vapor density The weight of an airborne concentration (vapor or gas) as compared with an equal volume of dry air.

vapor hazard An agent that enters the body through the respiratory tract.

vapor pressure For the purpose of this chapter, the pressure associated with liquids held inside any type of closed container.

vasoconstriction   Narrowing of the diameter of the blood vessels.

velocity (V)   The distance an object travels per unit time.

ventilation-perfusion mismatch   A pathologic state in which there is an imperfect match between the areas of the lung being ventilated and the areas being perfused.

ventricles   Specialized hollow areas in the brain.

ventricular septal defect (VSD)   A hole in the septum separating the ventricles, allowing blood from the left ventricle to flow into the right ventricle.

ventricular shunt   A surgically inserted tube draining cerebrospinal fluid from the cerebral ventricles into a body cavity, often the peritoneal cavity or the right atrium.

vertebral body   Anterior weight-bearing structure in the spine made of cancellous bone and surrounded by a layer of hard, compact bone that provides support and stability.

vertical compression   A type of injury typically resulting from a direct blow to the crown of the skull or rapid deceleration from a fall through the feet, legs, and pelvis, possibly causing a burst fracture or disk herniation.

vertical shear   The type of pelvic fracture that occurs when a massive force displaces the pelvis superiorly.

vesicants   Blister agents; the primary route of entry is through the skin.

viral hemorrhagic fevers (VHFs)   A group of diseases that include the Ebola, Rift Valley, and yellow fever viruses, among others. This group of viruses causes the blood in the body to seep out from the tissues and blood vessels.

viruses   Germs that require a living host to multiply and survive.

visceral pain   Crampy, aching pain deep within the body, the source of which is usually difficult to pinpoint; common with genitourinary problems.

visual cortex   The area in the brain where signals from the optic nerve are converted into visual images.

vitreous humor   A jellylike substance found in the posterior compartment of the eye between the lens and the retina.

volar   Pertaining to the palm or sole; referring to the flexor surfaces of the forearm, wrist, or hand.

volatility   Term used to describe how long a chemical agent will stay on a surface before it evaporates.

Volkmann contracture   Contraction of the fingers and, sometimes, the wrist, with loss of muscular power with death and resultant contracture of the forearm musculature, that sets in rapidly after severe injury around the elbow joint; associated with compartment syndrome.

voluntary muscle   Muscle that can be controlled by a person.

von Willebrand disease   The most common heritable disorder of coagulation. Its presentation can mimic hemophilia A.

Waddell triad   A pattern of automobile-pedestrian injuries in children and people of short stature in which (1) the bumper hits pelvis and femur, (2) the chest and abdomen hit the grille or low hood, and (3) the head strikes the ground.

warm zone   The area located between the hot zone and the cold zone at an incident. Decontamination stations are located in the warm zone.

water buffalo trailers   Portable trailers that contain from 500 to 3,000 gallons of water.

water reactive   A property that indicates that a material will undergo a chemical reaction (for example, explosion) when mixed with water.

water soluble   A property that indicates that a material can be dissolved in water.

waybill   A cargo document kept by the conductor of a train; also referred to as a consist.

weapon of mass destruction (WMD)   Any agent designed to bring about mass death, casualties, and/or massive damage to property and infrastructure (bridges, tunnels, airports, and seaports).

weaponization   The creation of a weapon from a biologic agent generally found in nature and that causes disease; the agent is cultivated, synthesized, and/or mutated to maximize the target population's exposure to the germ.

wedges   Used to snug loose cribbing.

wheel bounce   A vibration, synchronous with road speed that can be felt in the steering wheel.

wheel wobble   A common finding at low speeds when a vehicle has a bent wheel.

whiplash   An injury to the cervical vertebrae or their supporting ligaments and muscles, usually resulting from hyperextension as a result of the head moving abruptly forward or backward; can be difficult to differentiate from injuries that involve cervical bony structures and the spine.

wind chill factor   The factor that takes into account the temperature and wind velocity in calculating the effect of a given ambient temperature on living organisms.

xiphoid process   An inferior segment of the sternum often used as a landmark for cardiopulmonary resuscitation.

zone of coagulation   The reddened area surrounding the leathery and sometimes charred tissue that has sustained a full-thickness burn.

zone of hyperemia In a thermal burn, the area that is least affected by the burn injury. This is an area of increased blood flow where the body is attempting to repair injured but otherwise viable tissue.

zone of stasis The peripheral area surrounding the zone of coagulation that has decreased blood flow and inflammation.

This area can undergo necrosis within 24 to 48 hours after the injury, particularly if perfusion is compromised due to burn shock.

zygomatic arch The bone that extends along the front of the skull below the orbit.

Index

Figures and tables are indicated with *f* and *t* following the page numbers.

Butorphanol tartrate (Stadol), 2248t
Bystander CPR, reluctance issues in, 1855

C

C posts of vehicles, 2228, 2228f, 2348, 2348f
C1 (atlas), 1649, 1649f
C2 (axis), 1649, 1649f
Calcaneus, 1757, 1757f
  fractures, 1789
Calcium chloride, 1944
Calcium gluconate, 1839
Callus, 1765
CAMEO (Computer-Aided Management of Emergency Operations), 2269
Cancellous bone, 1767t
Cancer, 1684–1685, 1793, 2054–2056, 2158
Candidiasis, 1933–1934
CANUTEC (Canadian Transport Emergency Centre), 2262
Cao gio, 2127. See also Coining
Capacitance vessels, 1907
Capillaries, 1522, 1892–1893
Capillary refill, 1910, 2018
Caput succedaneum, 1990
Car seat displacement, vehicle extrication and, 2236, 2236f
Carbon dioxide (CO₂), 2239
Carbon monoxide (CO), 1910, 2238–2239, 2278
Carbon monoxide intoxication, 1580–1581, 1582f
Carboys, for hazardous materials, 2266, 2266f
Cardiac arrest and cardiac arrest management
  advanced cardiac life support, 1866, 1868, 1868f
  electrical contact with body and, 1596
  electrical injuries and, 1597
  "H" and "T" questions of, 1869t, 1885t
  improving response to, 1851–1854, 1852–1853f
  labor and, 1926
  lightning and, 1598
  maternal, 1954
  possible causes and treatment of, 1869t
Cardiac contusions, 2009.
  See also Myocardial contusion
Cardiac cycle, 1520–1521
Cardiac dysrhythmias, 1931
Cardiac muscle, 1761f
Cardiac output (CO), 1520, 1698, 1886, 1926, 1952
Cardiac tamponade
  chest trauma and, 1701t, 1713–1714, 1713f
  in critical patients, 1906–1907
  needle aspiration in, 1715f
  in pediatric patients, 2009
  physical findings of tension pneumothorax vs., 1714t
  possible causes and treatment of, 1869t

shock and, 1525t, 1900
Cardiogenic shock
  characteristics, 1899t, 1904, 1905t, 1906
  in pediatric patients, 2040
  as pump failure, 1525t
  volume expanders and, 1903
Cardiomyopathy, 2044
Cardiopulmonary arrest, pediatric, 2035, 2043
Cardiopulmonary resuscitation (CPR).
  See also Resuscitation
  for adults, 1854–1855, 1855f, 1857f
  for commotio cordis, 1716
  defibrillation and, 1862, 1865
  early, Chain of Survival and, 1851–1852, 1852f
  high-quality, 1856
  for infants and children, 1856–1860, 1858t, 1859–1861f
    with foreign body airway obstruction, 2021–2022
  for newborns, 1975–1977, 1976f
  starting and stopping, 1872–1873
  2010 guidelines, 1853–1854, 1853f, 1866–1867t, 2022
  two or more rescuers, 1856
Cardiovascular collapse, 1894
Cardiovascular system
  aging and changes in, 2082–2083, 2082f
  bleeding emergencies and, 1530
  geriatric emergencies, 2093–2095, 2093f
  in infants and children, 2008–2009, 2008t
  lightning and, 1598
  pediatric emergencies, 2040–2044, 2045t
  perfusion and, 1887–1888, 1887f
  as perfusion triangle, 1889, 1890f
Cardioversion, 1861
  synchronized, 2042
Caregiver substance abuse, 2124–2125
Cargo tanks, 2266
Carpal navicular fractures, 1783
Carpal tunnel syndrome, 1794–1795
Carpals, 1756
Cartilage, 1757, 1759
Cartilaginous joints, 1758, 1761f
Castor beans, 2308, 2308f
Casualty collection points, 2328
Cataract surgery, anisocoria and, 1626
Cataracts, 2083, 2154
Catheters, hemodynamic monitoring, 2148, 2148f
Cauda equina, 1650
Cauda equina syndrome, 1672, 1793
Cave-ins, 2331, 2331f
Cavitation, 1498, 1499
CBRNE (chemical, biologic, radiologic, nuclear, and explosive) agents, 2289
Cecum, 1731
Cellular respiration, 1518
Cellulitis, 2107, 2107f
Centennial Olympic Park bombing, Atlanta (1996), 2290, 2292f
Centers for Disease Control and Prevention (CDC)

on ambulance crashes, 2179
on death due to trauma, 1483, 1734
on developmental disabilities, 2151
on diabetes and aging, 2085
on drownings, 1821
on field triage decisions, 1507
on hypothermia-related deaths, 1805
on nursing homes, 2080
points of distribution and, 2309, 2309f
on shock and unintentional death, 1525
on thoracic trauma, 1695
Central auditory processing disorder (CAPD), 2153
Central cord syndrome, 1672
Central cyanosis, 1969
Central nervous system (CNS), 1644, 1894.
  See also Head and spine trauma
Central neurogenic hyperventilation, 1659t
Central shock, 1904
Central venous catheters, 2069–2070
Central vision, 1611
Centruroides (bark scorpion) stings, 1839, 1839f
Cephalhematoma, 1990
Cephalic presentation, in childbirth, 1948
Cephalopelvic disproportion, 1948, 1990
Cerebellum, 1647, 1647f
Cerebral concussion, 1665–1666
Cerebral contusions, 1666
Cerebral cortex, 1645
Cerebral edema, 1664
Cerebral herniation, 1654, 1654t, 1665
Cerebral palsy (CP), 2158–2159, 2159f
Cerebral perfusion pressure (CPP), 1664–1665
Cerebrospinal fluid (CSF)
  hemorrhaging from nose, ears, and mouth and, 1531
  leakage
    head injuries and, 1669
    nasotracheal intubation and, 1620
  meninges and, 1648, 1648f
Cerebrospinal fluid shunts, 2147, 2147f
Cerebrovascular disease, 2109t
Cerebrum, 1645, 1647f
Certec bag, 1832
Cervical canal, 1923
Cervical collars, for pediatric patients, 1676
Cervical nerve roots, 1650, 1652f
Cervical plexus, 1650, 1652f
Cervical spine (vertebrae), 1646f, 1648, 1649, 1649f
Cervical spine injuries, 1620, 1632, 2065–2066, 2065–2067f
Cervix, 1923, 1939
Chain of Survival, 1851–1852, 1852f
Chemical, biologic, radiologic, nuclear, and explosive (CBRNE) agents, 2289
Chemical agents as terrorist weapons, 2298, 2304t
  industrial chemicals/insecticides, 2302–2303
  nerve agents, 2300–2302, 2301f, 2301t, 2302t
  pulmonary agents, 2299–2300
  vesicants, 2298–2299, 2299f

Infantile hypertrophic pyloric stenosis (IHPS), 1987

Infants and neonates. *See also* Delivering babies; Neonatal care; Pediatric emergencies; Pediatric patients
  asthma and, 2025
  burns to, 1586*t*
  CPR for, 1858*t*, 1859–1860, 1860–1861*f*, 1866–1867*t*
  defibrillation paddle sizes for, 1864*t*, 1865
  face and neck trauma in, 1613
  growth and development, 2005, 2005*t*
  heat illness and, 1809
  long backboard spinal immobilization for, 1656
  normal skull of, 1645*f*
  removing foreign body obstruction in, 2021–2022, 2021*f*

Infection
  in newborns, core temperature and, 1988, 1989
  wound healing and, 1550, 1558

Infectious diseases
  bacterial tracheitis, 2023
  Haemophilus influenzae, type B, 2023
  heatstroke and, 1813
  pregnancy and, 1933–1935

Inferior nasal concha, 1609

Inferior vena cava, 1520, 1521*f*

Inflammation, 1549

Inflatable splints, 1777–1778, 1777*f*

Information management, ICS, 2203. *See also* Communications

Infraorbital hypoesthesia, 1619

Infrared rays and eye injury, 1625

Infrastructure. *See also* Communications
  disaster response planning and, 2321

Inhalation anthrax, 2309*t*

Inhalation burns, 1580, 1590, 1593, 1593*t*

Inner cannula, 2133, 2133*f*

Inner ear, 1612, 1613*f*

Inotropic effects, 1891*t*

Insect bites, 1834–1835

Insecticides, 2302–2303, 2304*t*

Inspiration, 1696*f*

Insulin pumps, 2140

Integument, 1545–1546, 1575. *See also* Skin

Integumentary (skin) system
  in geriatric patients, 2085–2086, 2107, 2107*f*
  in pediatric patients, 2010
    circulation to, 2013–2014, 2014*f*, 2014*t*

Intellectual disability, 2152

Intercostal retractions, 1971

Intercostal space, 1696

Intermediate bulk containers (totes), 2265, 2265*f*

Intermodal tanks, 2265, 2265*f*

Internal communication, 2321. *See also* EMS communications

Internal contamination, by radiation, 2310–2311

Internal hemorrhage, 1524, 1527, 1536*f*

International terrorism, 2290, 2291*f*. *See also* Terrorism

Internet technology disruptions, 2338–2339

Intersection hazards, for ambulances, 2186

Intertrochanteric fractures, 1786–1787

Intervertebral disks, 1650, 1650*f*, 1683
  degenerative disease of, 1685
  herniated, 1650, 1650*f*, 1685

Intestinal atresia in newborns, 1987

Intestinal stenosis in newborns, 1987

Intestines, 1730*f*, 1731, 1743

Intra-abdominal injury, in newborns, 1990

Intra-aortic balloon pump (IABP), 2149–2150, 2150*f*

Intracerebral hematoma, 1668, 1668*f*

Intracranial hemorrhage, 1666–1668, 1667–1668*f*, 1984*t*

Intracranial pressure (ICP). *See also* Head and spine trauma
  assessment, 1659, 1659*t*
  exacerbating, 1655
  monitors, 2150
  primary assessment, 1653
  pupillary sensitivity to, 1658–1659, 1659*f*
  traumatic brain injury and, 1664–1665

Intraosseous (IO) infusion, 2038–2039, 2039*f*

Intraosseous needle, 2038*f*

Intrauterine fetal death, 1947

Intravenous (IV) therapy
  basket stretchers and, 2249
  for hypovolemic shock, 1910
    in pediatric patients, 2037–2039*f*
  neurogenic shock and, 1908
  in newborns, 1977, 1977–1978*f*
  shock and, 1900, 1901–1902, 1903*f*

Intubation
  burns and, 1587–1588
  nasotracheal, head trauma and, 1620
  neonatal care and, 1966*t*
  for newborns, 1972, 1974–1975, 1974*f*
  spine injuries and, 1653–1654

Intuition, 1883

Intussusception, 1987, 2050

Inventory
  after disaster response, 2325
  during disaster response, 2323

Inverse square law, 1600, 2311

Ionizing radiation, 2309

Ipratropium bromide (Atrovent), 2024

Iris, 1611, 1612*f*

Irregular bones, 1757

Irreversible shock (class IV), 1526, 1526*t*, 1896–1897

Irrigating the eye, 1627, 1627*f*

IS-211 forms, personnel tracking with, 2323

Ischium, 1756

J

J wave, 1818*f*

Jaundice, neonatal, 1988, 2049–2050

Jaw-thrust maneuver, 2026, 2026*f*

Jejunostomy (J) tubes, 2140

Jitteriness, seizures in newborns vs., 1984*t*

Joint capsule, 1758

Joint information center (JIC), ICS, 2202–2203

Joints, 1754, 1757, 1760–1761*f*, 1776, 1793–1794

Joule's law, 1595

Jugular foramen, 1646*f*

Jugular veins, 1631–1632

Jugular vein distention (JVD), 1700–1701, 1700*f*, 1709

JumpSTART triage for pediatric patients, 2212, 2212*f*

K

Kallikrein-kinin system, 1894

KED/SKED device, 2249

Kehr sign, 1745

Keloid scars, 1550

Kendrick Extrication Device (KED), 2249

Ketorolac (Toradol), 2248*t*

Kidney failure, pregnancy and, 1931

Kidneys. *See also* Renal system
  assessment of injuries to, 1745
  injuries to, 1743, 1744, 1744*f*
  labor and, 1940
  multiple-organ dysfunction syndrome and, 1894
  perfusion and, 1523
  pregnancy and, 1925

Kinetic energy (KE), 1484, 1485

Kinetics, 1484, 1485–1486

King LT airway, 1865

KKK Standards, on emergency vehicle design, 2173

Klumpke paralysis, 1990

Knee injuries, 1560, 1788, 1791–1792, 1792

Kneeling births, 1940, 1941*f*

Kyphosis, 1678, 2108

L

Labels, hazardous materials, 2260–2261, 2261*f*

Labetalol (Normodyne, Trandate), 1932

Labor
  cardiac arrest and, 1926
  complications, 1945–1946
  false vs. true, 1929*t*
  history taking, 1928–1929
  precipitous, 1946
  premature, birth complications and, 1964*t*
  prolonged, birth injuries and, 1990
  prolonged, postpartum hemorrhage and, 1951
  stages of, 1939, 1939*t*

Labor disputes, 2337–2338

Lacerations, 1560, 1561*f*, 1951
  ear, 1629, 1629*f*
  eye, 1621–1622, 1622*f*, 1625–1626
  facial, 1618
  fractures and, 1769
  scalp, 1669–1670, 1669*f*

Lacrimal apparatus, 1611–1612, 1612*f*

Lacrimal bones, 1609, 1610*f*

Lactate monitors, 1898, 1899*f*

Lactated Ringer's (LR) solution, 1903, 1978

Lactic acid, 1761

Lacunae, 1924

Photo Credits

Section Opener 7 © Keith Muratori/ShutterStock, Inc.

Chapter 29

Opener Courtesy of Rhonda Beck; **29-1** ©Shout Pictures/Custom Medical Stock Photo; **29-2** © jcpjr/ShutterStock, Inc.; **29-4** © Terry Dickson, Florida Times-Union/AP Photos; **29-5** © Jack Dagley Photography/ShutterStock, Inc.; **29-6** Courtesy of Captain David Jackson, Saginaw Township Fire Department; **29-10** © Alexander Gordeyev/ShutterStock, Inc.; **29-11** © Dennis Wetherhold, Jr.; **29-12** © iStockphoto/Thinkstock; **29-14** © Michael Ledray/ShutterStock, Inc.; **29-19A** © Chuck Stewart, MD; **29-19B** © Willoughby/Custom Medical Stock Photo; **29-21** Adapted from Centers for Disease Control and Prevention, Morbidity and Mortality Weekly Report (MMWR), January 13, 2012; **29-22** Courtesy of Mark Woolcock

Chapter 30

30-8 © Sam Medical Products®; **30-10** Courtesy of Medtrade Products Ltd., UK

Chapter 31

Opener © Mark C. Ide; **31-3** Courtesy of Rhonda Beck; **31-4** © Mark C. Ide; **31-5** Courtesy of Matthew J. Belan, MD; **31-8** © E. M. Singletary, MD. Used with permission; **31-11A** Courtesy of Rhonda Beck; **31-13** © Custom Medical Stock Photo; **31-15** © E. M. Singletary, MD. Used with permission; **31-16A** Courtesy of Moose Jaw Police Service; **31-16B** © Chuck Stewart, MD

Chapter 32

Opener © Siphiwe Sibeko/Reuters/Landov; **32-1** © Dale A. Stock/ShutterStock, Inc.; **32-2** © Dr. P. Marazzi/Photo Researchers, Inc.; **32-6** © J. Yakwichuk/Custom Medical Stock Photo; **32-7** Courtesy of Health Resources and Services Administration (HRSA), Maternal and Child Health Bureau (MCHB), Emergency Medical Services for Children (EMSC) Program; **32-8** © Kevin Frayer/AP Photos; **32-9A** © Amy Walters/ShutterStock, Inc.; **32-9B** © E. M. Singletary, M.D. Used with permission; **32-13** Adapted from Lund, C. C., and Browder, N. C. Surg. Gynecol. Obstet. 1944. 79: 352–358; **32-14** Courtesy of Water-Jel® Technologies; **32-18** Courtesy of MorTan, Inc.; **32-19A–32-20** © Chuck Stewart, MD; **32-21** © 2007 British Association of Plastic, Reconstructive and Aesthetic Surgeons

Chapter 33

Opener © E. M. Singletary, M.D. Used with permission; **33-15** Courtesy of Rhonda Beck; **33-17** © Eddie M. Sperling; **33-20** Courtesy of John T. Halgren, MD, University of Nebraska Medical Center; **33-32** © E. M. Singletary, MD. Used with permission

Chapter 34

Opener © Mark C. Ide; **34-17** © Kristin Smith/ShutterStock, Inc.; **34-20** Courtesy of Thomas E.M.S.; **34-40** © Mark C. Ide

Chapter 35

Opener Courtesy of ED, Royal North Shore Hospital/NSW Institute of Trauma & Injury; **35-1** © PhotoStock-Israel/Alamy Images; **35-5** Courtesy of Rhonda Beck; **35-20** © SIU Bio Med Comm./Custom Medical Stock Photo; **35-21** © Chuck Stewart, MD

Chapter 36

Opener © Mark C. Ide; **36-11** © Dr. P. Marazzi/Photo Researchers, Inc.; **36-13** © Custom Medical Stock Photo

Chapter 37

Opener © Mark C. Ide; **37-9** Courtesy of Tim Arnett/University College London; **37-19** Courtesy of Rhonda Beck; **37-20** © Chuck Stewart, MD; **37-21** © iStockphoto/Thinkstock; **37-22** Courtesy of Andrew N. Pollak, MD, FAAOS; **37-33B** Courtesy of Andrew N. Pollak, MD, FAAOS; **37-34** EMS facility courtesy of St. Charles County Ambulance District, Missouri, © Ray Kemp/911 Imaging; **37-36A–37-36B** Courtesy of Andrew N. Pollak, MD, FAAOS; **37-37** Courtesy of Anand M. Murthi, MD

Chapter 38

Opener Courtesy of BM1 Kevin Erwin/U.S. Coast Guard; **38-1** © Martin Pisek/ShutterStock, Inc.; **38-2** © Earl Neikirk/AP Photos; **38-5** © Peter Bernik/ShutterStock, Inc.; **38-7A** Courtesy of Neil Malcom Winkelmann; **38-9** Courtesy of Dr. Jack Poland/CDC; **38-10** © Andy Barrand, The Herald Republican/AP Photos; **38-11** © Jim Cole/AP Photos; **38-12** From 12-Lead ECG: The Art of Interpretation, courtesy of Tomas B. Garcia, MD; **38-13** Adapted from American Heart Association; **38-14** Courtesy of Cincinnati Sub-Zero Products, Inc.; **38-17** Courtesy of Perry Baromedical Corporation; **38-18** Courtesy of Mass Communication Specialist 2nd Class Rebecca J. Moat/U.S. Navy; **38-19** © Alan Heartfield/ShutterStock, Inc.; **38-20** © 2007 British Association of Plastic, Reconstructive and Aesthetic Surgeons; **38-21** © Stuart Elflett/ShutterStock, Inc.; **38-23A** © Photos.com; **38-23B** Courtesy of Ray Rauch/U.S. Fish & Wildlife Service; **38-23C** © SuperStock/Alamy Images; **38-23D** Courtesy of Luther C. Goldman/U.S. Fish & Wildlife Service; **38-25** © Crystal Kirk/ShutterStock, Inc.; **38-26** Courtesy of Kenneth Cramer, Monmouth College; **38-27A** Courtesy of Department of Entomology, University of Nebraska; **38-27B** Courtesy of Department of Entomology, University of Nebraska; **38-28** © Visual&Written SL/Alamy Images; **38-29** © Joao Estevao A. Freitas (jefras)/ShutterStock, Inc.

Section Opener 8 © Mark C. Ide

Chapter 39

Opener © Imageshop/Alamy Images; **39-5B** Courtesy of Defibtech, LLC; **39-9** Courtesy of Advanced Circulatory Systems, Inc.; **39-10** Courtesy of ZOLL; **39-11** Courtesy of Michigan Instruments, Inc.; **39-12** Courtesy of Physio-Control, Inc.; **39-13** ©Mark Pagani Photography/ShutterStock, Inc.

Chapter 40

Opener © Mark C. Ide; **40-1** © Mark C. Ide; **40-9** Courtesy of EKF Diagnostics www.ekfdiagnostics.com; **40-10** © SPL/Photo Researchers, Inc.

Chapter 41

41-1A © Claude Cortier/Photo Researchers, Inc.; **41-1B** © Nestle/Petit Format/Photo Researchers, Inc.; **41-18** © Hattie Young/Photo Researchers, Inc.

Chapter 42

Opener © JHP Public Safety/Alamy Images; **42-7** Courtesy of Marianne Gausche-Hill, MD, FACEP, FAAP; **42-9** Used with permission of the American Academy of Pediatrics, Textbook of Neonatal Resuscitation, 6th Edition. © American Academy of Pediatrics; **42-15** Courtesy of CDC; **42-T04** Adapted from: American Academy of Pediatrics Neonatal Resuscitation Program

Chapter 43

Opener © CORBIS/age fotostock; **43-2** Used with permission of the American Academy of Pediatrics, Pediatric Education for Prehospital Professionals, © American Academy of Pediatrics, 2000; **43-3** © Joyce Marrero/ShutterStock, Inc.; **43-4–43-5** Courtesy of Health Resources and Services Administration (HRSA), Maternal and Child Health Bureau (MCHB), Emergency Medical Services for Children (EMSC) Program; **43-7** Courtesy of Health Resources and Services Administration (HRSA), Maternal and Child Health Bureau (MCHB), Emergency Medical Services for Children (EMSC) Program; **43-9** From Hockenberry MJ, Wilson D, Wikelstein ML: Wong's Essentials of Pediatric Nursing, 8th ed, St. Louis, 2009, p. 1259. Used with permission. © Mosby; **43-19** Courtesy of Ronald Dieckmann, MD; **43-20** Courtesy of Moose Jaw Police Service; **43-21** Courtesy of Ronald Dieckmann, MD; **43-22** © Dr. P. Marazzi/Photo Researchers, Inc.; **43-23** Used with permission of the American Academy of Pediatrics, Pediatric Education for Prehospital Professionals, © American Academy of Pediatrics, 2000; **43-25** © Mark C. Ide; **43-27** Courtesy of Cindy Bissell; **43-SD4-8** Courtesy of James P. Thomas, M.D. www.voicedoctor.net

Chapter 44

Opener © Glen E. Ellman; **44-2** © Photodisc; **44-4** © Maxx-Studio/ShutterStock, Inc.; **44-12** © Dr. P. Marazzi/Science Photo Library; **44-16** © Photofusion Picture Library/Alamy Images

Chapter 45

Opener © Richard Levine/Alamy Images; **45-3A–45-5B** Courtesy of Ronald Dieckmann, MD; **45-6** © Dr. P. Marazzi/Photo Researchers, Inc.; **45-7** Used with permission of the American Academy of Pediatrics, Pediatric Education for Prehospital Professionals, © American Academy of Pediatrics, 2000; **45-8** © Cora Reed/ShutterStock, Inc.; **45-9** © Mark C. Ide; **45-10** Portex® Blue Line® Ultra Tracheostomy courtesy of Smiths Medical; **45-12** © ResMed 2012. Used with permission;